learning system

To access your Student Resources, visit:

http://evolve.elsevier.com/Copstead

Evolve® Student Learning Resources for *Pathophysiology* offer the following features:

- **Case Studies**

  Patient case studies that initiate the critical thinking process will assist you in the application of pathophysiologic concepts in clinical situations.

- **Disease Profiles**

  An outlined, at-a-glance review provides you with a quick study of clinically significant conditions.

- **Key Questions**

  Provides the answers to the Key Questions included in each chapter opener in the book in an effort to reinforce key concepts and allow self-study.

- **Key Points Review**

  The Key Points boxes are provided here for quick review of the main points from each chapter.

- **WebLinks**

  This useful resource links you to hundreds of websites carefully chosen to supplement the content of your textbook. The Weblinks are regularly updated, with new ones added as they develop.

ELSEVIER

PATHOPHYSIOLOGY

Fourth Edition

PATHOPHYSIOLOGY

Lee-Ellen C. Copstead, PhD, RN
Associate Professor
College of Nursing and Health Sciences
University of Wisconsin – Eau Claire
Eau Claire, Wisconsin

Jacquelyn L. Banasik, PhD, ARNP
Associate Professor
Intercollegiate College of Nursing
Washington State University
Spokane, Washington

11830 Westline Industrial Drive
St. Louis, Missouri 63146

PATHOPHYSIOLOGY, FOURTH EDITION

1-4160-5543-6 / 978-1-4160-5543-3

Notice

Pathophysiology is an ever-changing field. Standard safety precautions must be followed, but as new research and clinical experience broaden our knowledge, changes in treatment and drug therapy may become necessary or appropriate. Readers are advised to check the most current product information provided by the manufacturer of each drug to be administered to verify the recommended dose, the method and duration of administration, and contraindications. It is the responsibility of the licensed prescriber, relying on experience and knowledge of the patient, to determine dosages and the best treatment for each individual patient. Neither the publisher nor the author assumes any liability for any injury and/or damage to persons or property arising from this publication.

The Publisher

International Standard Book Number   1-4160-5543-6 / 978-1-4160-5543-3

Library of Congress Cataloging in Publication Data

Copstead, Lee Ellen.
  Pathophysiology/Lee-Ellen C. Copstead, Jacquelyn (Jackie) L. Banasik.— 4th ed.
    p. ; cm.
  Includes bibliographical references and index.
  ISBN-13: 978-1-4160-5543-3 (hardcover: alk. paper)
  ISBN-10: 1-4160-5543-6 (hardcover: alk. paper) 1. Physiology, Pathological. I.
Banasik, Jacquelyn L. II. Title.
  [DNLM: 1. Disease. 2. Pathology. QZ 140 C785p 2010]
  RB113. P45 2010
  616. 07—dc22

                                            2008048295

Executive Editor: Darlene Como
Acquisitions Editor: Sandra E. Clark
Developmental Editor: Charlene R.M. Ketchum
Editorial Assistant: Brooke Bagwill
Publishing Services Manager: Jeff Patterson
Project Manager: Jeanne Genz
Designer: Margaret Reid

Printed in Canada

Last digit is the print number: 9 8 7 6 5 4 3 2 1

To:

The memory of my father for his guiding wisdom and common sense;

The memory of my mother for her creativity, sense of humor, and compassion;

The memory of my husband for his unbending devotion to his family;
and with much love and admiration,
My now teenaged daughter, Amelia Charlotte Kirkhorn,
who reminds me daily that there is always more to learn.

LECK

To:

The memory of my mother
Lueria Ella Petersen

JLB

Contributors

Carol L. Danning, MD
Physician, Rheumatology
Gundersen Lutheran Medical Center
La Crosse, Wisconsin

Lorrie J. Dawson, PhD, ARNP-BC
Assistant Professor
College of Nursing
Washington State University
Vancouver, Washington

E. Ruth Diestelmeier, MSN, RN
Clinical Instructor
College of Nursing and Health Sciences
University of Wisconsin—Eau Claire
Eau Claire, Wisconsin

Michael R. Diestelmeier, MD, FAAD
Dermatologist
Luther Midelfort Mayo Health System
Eau Claire, Wisconsin

Roberta J. Emerson, PhD, RN, CCRN Emeritus
Associate Professor
Intercollegiate College of Nursing
Washington State University
Spokane, Washington

Linda Felver, PhD, RN
Associate Professor
School of Nursing
Oregon Health & Science University
Portland, Oregon

Patricia Garber, PhDc, RN, MS, MSN, CNTP
Associate Professor Emerita
College of Nursing and Health Sciences
University of Wisconsin—Eau Claire
Eau Claire, Wisconsin

Dan Guerra, PhD, MS, BS
Adjunct Professor
Department of Veterinary and Comparative Anatomy,
    Pharmacology and Physiology
Washington State University
Pullman, Washington

Rosemary Jadack, PhD, RN
Professor
College of Nursing and Health Sciences
University of Wisconsin—Eau Claire
Eau Claire, Wisconsin

Marie L. Kotter, PhD, CLS
Professor and Department Chair
Health Sciences
Weber State University
Ogden, Utah

Naomi Lungstrom, MN, ARNP, FNP, CCRN Emerita
Clinical Assistant Professor/Faculty
Intercollegiate College of Nursing
Washington State University
Spokane, Washington

Joni D. Nelsen-Marsh, MN, RN, ARNP
Family Nurse Practitioner
South Hill Family Medicine
Spokane, Washington

Nirav Patel, MD, FACS
Trauma Director
Gundersen Lutheran Medical Center
La Crosse, Wisconsin

Faith Young Peterson, BS, MS, MPA, FNP
Family Nurse Practitioner and Clinic Manager
Terry Reilly Health Services, Marsing Clinic
Marsing, Idaho

Jeffrey S. Sartin, MD
Internal Medicine and Infectious Disease Physician
Gundersen Lutheran Medical Center
La Crosse, Wisconsin

Lorna Schumann, PhD, ACNP-BC, NP-C, ACNS-BC, CCRN, ARNP, FAANP
Associate Professor
Intercollegiate College of Nursing
Washington State University
Spokane, Washington

Sheila Smith, PhD, APRN, BC
Professor
Assistant Dean, College of Nursing and Health Sciences
University of Wisconsin—Eau Claire
Eau Claire, Wisconsin

Angela Starkweather, PhD, ACNP, CCRN, CNRN
Assistant Professor
College of Nursing
Washington State University
Spokane, Washington

Susan G. Trevithick, RN, MS, CNA
Associate Clinical Professor
University of Utah College of Nursing
Salt Lake City, Utah
Associate Chief Nursing Service for Critical Care
VA Salt Lake City Healthcare System
Salt Lake City, Utah

Marvin J. Van Every, MD
Urologist
Gundersen Clinic
La Crosse, Wisconsin

Reviewers

Jennifer J. Donwerth, MSN, RN, ANP-BC, GNP-BC
Faculty, Department of Nursing
Tarleton State University
Stephenville, Texas

Roberta J. Emerson, PhD, RN, CCRN Emeritus
Associate Professor
Intercollegiate College of Nursing
Washington State University
Spokane, Washington

Kathleen Murphy-Ende, RN, PhD, AOCNP
Nurse Practitioner
University of Wisconsin Hospital and Clinics
American Family Children's Hospital
University of Wisconsin School of Nursing
Madison, Wisconsin

Jeffrey S. Sartin, MD
Internal Medicine and Infectious Disease Physician
Gundersen Lutheran Medical Center
La Crosse, Wisconsin

Jo A. Voss, PhD, RN, CNS
Associate Professor
College of Nursing
South Dakota State University
Rapid City, South Dakota

Diane Young, PhD, CNE, RN
Professor
Allen College
Waterloo, Iowa

Preface

The scientific basis of pathophysiology is rapidly expanding and becoming increasingly well understood at the genetic and cellular levels. Accelerated progress in human genetics has virtually transformed our understanding of the living world. To be clinically relevant and useful to health care students and professionals, a text must be able to synthesize a vast amount of knowledge about a multitude of individual structures, functions, and dysfunctions into overarching concepts that can be applied to individual diseases. In the fourth edition of *Pathophysiology*, attention has been given to the development of practical, student-centered learning aids that support learning and mastery of content. Discussions of relevant biochemistry, genetics, and cell physiology are used to help students understand concepts at a deeper level. This fourth edition has been updated extensively with sensitivity to the unique needs of today's students to better prepare them as practitioners in an ever-changing health care environment.

ORGANIZATION

Pathophysiology is a comprehensive text and reference that uses a systems approach to content, beginning with a thorough treatment of normal physiology, followed by pathophysiology and application of concepts to specific disorders. The text is organized into 15 units, each of which includes a particular system or group of interrelated body systems and the pertinent pathophysiology concepts and disorders.

Unit I (**Chapters 1 and 2**) sets the stage for understanding major elements of the pathophysiologic processes in individuals and population groups. The purpose of these chapters is to give students an appreciation for the complex nature of disease and illness, including sociocultural influences and the significant contributions of stress, adaptation, and coping. The unifying concepts of pathophysiologic processes—etiology, pathogenesis, clinical manifestations, and implications for treatment of disease—are explained.

Unit II (**Chapters 3 to 7**) addresses cellular mechanisms. Chapter 3 describes normal cells to give students an insight into how cells function, with an emphasis on cellular signaling and communication. Chapter 4 discusses cellular pathology and the processes of injury, apoptosis, aging, and death.

Chapters 5 and 6 describe gene structure and function, development, and genetic and congenital disorders. Chapter 7 describes the cellular biology of tumor growth, focusing on the roles of proto-oncogenes and tumor suppressor genes. Revisions reflect new knowledge about apoptosis, genetics, and cancer biology.

Unit III (**Chapters 8 to 12**) addresses key cellular defense mechanisms and the basic processes of infectious disease, inflammation, immunity, autoimmune disease, hypersensitivity, hematologic malignancies, and HIV-AIDS. Unit III was revised to reflect new knowledge about immune mechanisms and therapy for HIV disease.

Unit IV (**Chapters 13 to 16**) includes content pertaining to the transport of oxygen in the circulation, hemostasis, vascular regulation of flow, blood pressure regulation, and the pathologies relevant to these functions. The content on blood pressure was extensively revised.

Unit V (**Chapters 17 to 20**) includes concepts related to cardiac physiology and pathophysiology. Content has been updated to reflect new knowledge in the areas of acute coronary syndrome, heart failure, and shock.

Unit VI (**Chapters 21 to 23**) provides a thorough description of pulmonary anatomy and physiology including concepts of ventilation, perfusion, and gas exchange. The content on asthma has been updated.

Unit VII (**Chapters 24 and 25**) describes concepts basic to understanding the alterations in fluid, electrolyte, and acid-base homeostasis that accompany many disease processes.

Unit VIII (**Chapters 26 to 29**) provides a thorough description of renal anatomy and physiology, abnormalities of renal function, bladder dysfunction, and strategies for interpreting common laboratory values in the context of kidney or bladder diseases. The chapters on renal disorders and chronic kidney disease have been extensively revised.

Unit IX (**Chapters 30 to 34**) includes extensive information on male and female genital anatomy and reproductive physiology as well as common disorders. Chapter 34 provides thorough coverage of common sexually transmitted infections.

Unit X (**Chapters 35 to 38**) provides a review of normal gastrointestinal anatomy, physiology, and disorders, with separate chapters dedicated to pancreatic and biliary dysfunction and liver disease.

Unit XI (**Chapters 39 to 42**) addresses alterations in endocrine control, metabolism, and nutrition. The chapter on normal endocrine physiology has been extensively rewritten to include a detailed discussion of hormone synthesis, activity, and regulation. A separate chapter is dedicated to the growing problem of diabetes mellitus.

Unit XII (**Chapters 43 to 47**) includes a review of neurologic anatomy and physiology, acute and chronic neuronal disorders, disorders of special senses, and pain. Content has been updated to reflect new information on Alzheimer disease and Parkinson disease.

Unit XIII (**Chapters 48 and 49**) covers current concepts in the pathophysiology of psychobiology including anxiety, mood, thought, and personality disorders.

Unit XIV (**Chapters 50 to 52**) includes alterations in musculoskeletal support and movement, with separate chapters dedicated to normal bone and muscle anatomy and physiology, disorders of bone and muscle, and rheumatic disorders.

Unit XV (**Chapters 53 and 54**) includes alterations affecting the largest system of the body—the integumentary system. Chapter 53 includes normal integumentary structure and function and a survey of common skin disorders. Chapter 54 covers burn injury, emphasizing the multiple stresses that are encountered in patients with these complex injuries.

FEATURES

An understanding of normal structure and function of the body is necessary for any detailed understanding of its abnormalities and pathophysiology. The first chapter in most units includes a fully illustrated *review of normal physiology*. Changes in structure and function as a result of normal development and aging are also addressed where appropriate. Changes due to aging are highlighted in *Geriatric Considerations* boxes.

Each unit opens with a short essay that engages students by encouraging them to relate the material to frontiers of research and new developments in the field. Each chapter opens with *Key Questions*, which are designed to develop a strong pathophysiology knowledge base and to serve as the foundation for critical thinking. These Key Questions integrate the essential information in each chapter, emphasizing *concepts* rather than small details. *Chapter Outlines* are also included at the beginning of each chapter to help the reader locate specific content. Within every chapter, *Key Points* are identified at the end of every major discussion and are presented in short bulleted lists. These recurring summaries help readers to focus on the main points.

Nearly 1000 illustrations elucidate both normal physiology and pathophysiologic changes. The entire book is in *full color*, with color used generously in the illustrations to better explain pathophysiologic concepts.

To help students master the new vocabulary of pathophysiology, key terms appear in boldface within each chapter, and these terms are defined in a comprehensive *Glossary*, which appears at the end of the text. Throughout this text, the nonpossessive forms of eponyms (e.g., Down syndrome) are used consistently when referring to the person for whom a disease is named. Clinical and laboratory values are provided in the *Appendix*.

ANCILLARIES

CD Companion

This **CD-ROM**, which comes with every new copy of the book, contains a variety of useful tools for additional study, review, and exploration, including *Review Questions and Answers* for every chapter (500 questions in all); the *Glossary* from the book, which is enhanced on the CD with audio pronunciations for selected terms; and *Animations*, to help readers visualize pathophysiologic processes.

Student Learning Resources on Evolve

The student section of the book's website hosted on Evolve offers *Case Study Worksheets, Disease Profiles,* answers to *Key Questions* and *Key Points Review* and *WebLinks* to hundreds of carefully chosen Internet sites pertaining to pathophysiology. Visit the Evolve website at **http://evolve.elsevier.com/Copstead/**.

Study Guide

Pathophysiology can be a daunting subject for students because of the large volume of factual material to be learned. The student **Study Guide** is designed to help students focus on important pathophysiologic concepts. Questions to check recall of normal anatomy and physiology are included for each system. A number of activities that help the student focus on similarities and differences between often confused pathologic processes are included. More than 1500 *Self-assessment test questions* with answers are included to help students check their understanding and build confidence for examinations. *Case studies* with rationales for correct and incorrect answers are used to help students begin to apply pathophysiologic concepts to clinical situations.

Instructor Learning Resources on Evolve

The **Instructor's Course Resources on Evolve** provides a number of instructional aids for instructors who require the text for their students. The materials include a *Test Bank* presented in both Word and ExamView with approximately 1200 test items, a *PowerPoint lecture guide* with more than 550 slides to facilitate classroom presentations, answers to the *Case Studies* in the Student Learning Resources, an *Image Collection* of more than 600 color images from the text, and 2 to 3 questions for audience response systems (*iClicker*) for each chapter.

Acknowledgments

Many creative and unique efforts grace the pages of this work. It is exceedingly difficult to know how to best recognize every one. Writing this text has been possible only because of the tremendous dedication of authors, artists, reviewers, and editors. Our sincere gratitude goes to all who helped with this and previous editions. In particular, grateful appreciation is extended to all of the contributing authors—recognized experts—who gave exhaustively of their time to write chapters and create illustrations. Special thanks to Linda Felver for her outstanding contributions to the online companion course. We are also indebted to the many thoughtful experts who gave of their time to read and critique manuscripts and help ensure excellence in chapter content throughout the text.

No project of this magnitude could be accomplished without wonderfully supportive colleagues and students who provided a source of continual motivation and encouragement. We are most keenly aware of the inspiration provided by the faculty, staff, and students of Washington State University Intercollegiate College of Nursing and the University of Wisconsin-Eau Claire College of Nursing and Health Sciences. Grateful recognition is made to the staff at Elsevier. In particular, developmental editor, Charlene Ketchum, deserves our heartfelt thanks for helping with the content, illustrations, and the many details to keep our project on track. Jeanne Genz, our project manager, paid excellent attention to the copyediting, proofreading, and page layout. Margaret Reid's elegant and colorful design helped give the book its polished format, and Jeannie Robertson contributed extensively to the art program of the third edition, which was used as a template for the present edition. In addition, Sandra Clark believed in the book and oversaw the revision from beginning to end.

We would like to recognize those who provided a foundation for the revised text through their contributions to the first edition: Mary Sanguinetti-Baird, Linda Belsky-Lohr, Tim Brown, Karen Carlson, Leslie Evans, Jo Annalee Irving, Debby Kaaland, Rick Madison, Maryann Pranulis, Edith Randall, Bridget Recker, Cleo Richard, Gary Smith, Pam Springer, Martha Snider, Patti Stec, Julie Symes, Lorie Wild, and Debra Winston-Heath. We also would like to thank those who contributed to the second and third editions of the book: Arnold A. Asp, Katherina P. Choka, Cynthia F. Corbett, Mark Puhlman, Barbara Bartz, Arnold Norman Cohen, Karen Groth, Christine M. Henshaw, Carolyn Hoover, Marianne Genge Jagmin, Linda Denise Oakley, Anne Roe Mealey, David Mikkelsen, Billie Marie Severtsen, and Jacqueline Siegel.

To the late Dr. Michael J. Kirkhorn, we give acknowledgment and thanks for writing the first, second, and third edition's provocative and thoughtful essays that begin each unit.

Contents

PART 3
Alterations in Immune and Inflammatory Response

UNIT III
Defense

PART 5
Alterations in Fluid Balance, Excretion, and Reproduction

PART 6
Alterations in Metabolism and Nutrition

UNIT X
Gastrointestinal Function

PART 1

Alterations in Homeostasis

Frontiers of Research

The Complex Nature of Disease

Sheila K. Smith • Lee-Ellen C. Copstead • Michael J. Kirkhorn

Over the past 50 years, our understanding of health and disease has become increasingly complex. Concepts of health are now explored from philosophical, experiential, spiritual, and political perspectives, in addition to the physiologic perspectives central to medicine and the biological sciences. We speak of the health of individuals, families, work environments, organizations, populations, and nations. In all these perspectives, health brings connotations of balance, effective functioning, well-being, dynamic interaction with the environment, and the capacity for growth, reorganization, and change. Margaret Newman, noted nurse theorist, described health not as a state but as a process, as the informational capacity of a system to interact with its environment. From this point of view, disease processes or limited functional capacity are not the absence of health but simply the specific manifestations of health patterning for that specific individual.

In many ways these varied and complex understandings of concepts of health represent the use of health as a metaphor. Health represents wholeness, harmony, renewal, and change. From the perspective of physiology, health indicates correct, effective, and dynamic functioning of the complex physical and chemical systems of life.

Disease, on the other hand, indicates the limitations of these processes over time. In the world of cell physiology, infinitesimally small alterations can result in the eventual expression of large deficits: incorrect copying of genetic material, broken protein strands, oxidatively altered chemical bonds, the misinterpretation of cellular communication, failure to recognize incorrectly incorporated cellular components-all can lead to additive effects and the eventual expression of disease. When a DNA error is not repaired, the cell passes on its defective gene to new cells, which may lead to many biochemical events over time that cause normal tissues to become diseased. When lipid molecules cause injury to vascular walls, complex inflammatory cascades lead to eventual arterial occlusion and major organ system disease. In our attempts to put health and disease into a simple framework, the terms normal or abnormal can be easily misapplied, because determining norms in health and disease often involves the assessment of individuals who vary greatly in their susceptibilities and in their abilities to withstand, cope, and even thrive while they are living through what is considered a diseased state.

Pathophysiology is concerned with the science of disease-all the complex processes, mechanisms, theoretical models, underlying causes, risk factors, progressions, variations, consequences, and approaches to care. Today we know more about the processes of disease than ever before. Our models are more detailed and sophisticated. Advances especially in the areas of genetic research and cellular communication are some of the most dramatic. We are vastly increasing our information about age, racial/ethnic and gender differences, and other factors that allow us to see disease not as an "evil visitor" but as an inherent factor in the spectrum of possibilities presented to each human being at

Cell nuclei. (From Gartner LP, Hiatt JL: Color textbook of histology, *ed 2, Philadelphia, 2001, Saunders, p 52.)*

Pathophysiologic Processes

birth. We also know more about the effects of outside factors, such as environmental pollution or exposure to toxins, which may turn susceptibility or inherited weakness into actual disease. Lifestyle health practices, such as tobacco smoking, diet, physical activity, and alcohol use, also are increasingly implicated in the development of chronic disease. High levels of stress have now been clearly linked to the release of excess catecholamines and stimulation of the sympathetic nervous system. Over time, these adaptive responses can contribute maladaptively to cardiovascular disease, kidney disease, metabolic abnormalities, and, possibly, autoimmune disorders.

Looking into the future, environmental, public health, and epidemiologic research will become increasingly important in advancing knowledge of disease. We have become a global community. Within a few short generations, populations once widely isolated from one another are now in frequent daily contact, sharing food and water resources, and making families with one another. With increased human mobility communicable disease transmission patterns are changing. This includes alterations in the antigenicity of organisms that shift from animal to human hosts, as previously undeveloped ecosystems become home to human communities. Practices as simple and widespread as heating food in the microwave raises questions about the long-term safety of microwave exposure and ingesting molecules from plastics. Modern agricultural practices raise questions about antibiotic, growth hormone, and pesticide exposures through our food sources. These questions now join some of the more traditional environmental health concerns of air and water pollution in redefining human health threats of the 21st century. Epidemiologists also remind us, however, to keep a clear sense of balance when we think about disease. Some diseases are highly publicized, often for good reason and with beneficial effects, but public health epidemiologists notice that a community may suffer as much or more when its citizens encounter an epidemic of a mundane illness, such as influenza.

Our understanding of the nature of disease and therefore of health is proceeding with unusual speed and confidence. Researchers expect that in the near future, genetic research could produce a number of cures, as well as new kinds of diagnosis, immunization, prevention, anticipation of disease, and preemptive therapy. Genetic research into the nature of disease promises to locate the origin of many diseases and thus allows us to either prevent or correct them with therapies unavailable to past generations. Disease is being tracked to its most secret refuge-where it is naturally coded in the body. Current research also promises prevention of life-threatening diseases, including diseases that seem to arise without warning and kill prematurely. In breast cancer, for example, research into T-cell vaccines and T-cell therapy indicates that the cancer patient's own immune system can be strengthened to fight the cancer and possibly develop protection against relapse.

Hippocrates would have been impressed.

chapter

1

Introduction to Pathophysiology

Lee-Ellen C. Copstead • Jacquelyn L. Banasik

MEDIA RESOURCES

Additional Material for Study, Review, and Further Exploration

 CD Companion ▪ Review Questions and Answers ▪ Glossary (with audio pronunciations for selected terms) ▪ Disease Profiles ▪ Animations

evolve **Website** at http://evolve.elsevier.com/Copstead/
▪ Case Studies ▪ Disease Profiles ▪ WebLinks ▪ Key Points Review

KEY QUESTIONS

▪ What is pathophysiology?
▪ How are etiology and pathogenesis used to predict clinical manifestations and response to therapy?
▪ How are normal and abnormal physiologic parameters defined?

▪ What general factors affect the expression of disease in a particular person?
▪ What kinds of information about disease can be gained through understanding concepts of epidemiology?

CHAPTER OUTLINE

Pathophysiology derives from the intersection of two older, related disciplines: pathology (from *pathos*, suffering) and physiology (from *physis*, nature). Pathology is the study and diagnosis of *disease* through examination of *organs, tissues, cells* and *bodily fluids*. Physiology is the study of the mechanical, physical, and biochemical functions of living organisms. Together as *pathophysiology,* the term refers to the study of abnormalities in physiologic functioning of living beings.

Pathophysiology seeks to reveal physiologic responses of an organism to disruptions in its internal or external environment. Because humans exhibit considerable diversity, healthy structure and function are not precisely the same in any two individuals. However, discovering the common and expected responses to abnormalities in physiologic functioning is useful, and it allows a general prediction of clinical progression, identification of possible causes, and selection of interventions that are most likely to be helpful. Thus, pathophysiology is studied in terms of common or "classic" presentations of disorders.

Historically, descriptions of diseases were based on observations of those individuals who came to medical attention because they exhibited abnormal signs or complained of symptoms. Over time, cases with similar presentations were noted and treatments that had been successful before were used again. In some cases, similarities among individuals pointed to possible common causes. With the advent of more sophisticated measurements of physiologic and biochemical function, such as blood pressure, blood chemistries, x-ray imaging, and DNA analysis, the wide variability in the expression of diseases and disorders in the population became apparent, as did the opportunity to discover diseases at earlier stages, before they were clinically obvious. Screening programs that evaluated large segments of the population revealed the complexity and diversity of disease expression, even in persons with the same genetic defect. Thus, while the study of pathophysiology is necessarily a study of the usual and expected responses of the body to a given disruption, individuals often vary significantly from a classic presentation, making the diagnostic process complex and challenging.

Advances in genomic and epigenomic characterization, innovative technologies, and revolutionary approaches to the analysis of genetic variation and function have made studies and treatments possible that were not even imaginable just a few years ago. As a result, definitions of the living world have been virtually transformed and permeate every branch of biological science. Benefits of this new biology include a deeper understanding of evolution, greater insights into immune mechanisms, and nearly every advance against cancer and acquired immunodeficiency syndrome (AIDS).

Genetic manipulation also raises sensitive and complex ethical and moral questions that did not exist half a century ago. Scientists are able to experiment with what genes do and how they do it—dramatically altering medical practice—especially the management of inhrited diseases. New capabilities have led to experimental treatments such as gene therapy–molecular surgery powerful enough to cure and alter the next generation. The study of pathophysiology takes on even greater significance as genetic research reveals fresh insights and hopeful new treatments for human diseases.

Pathophysiology examines disturbances of normal mechanical, physical, and biochemical functions, either caused by a disease or resulting from a disease or abnormal syndrome or condition. For example, from the field of infectious disease would be the study of a toxin released by a bacterium, and what that toxin does to the body to cause harm-one possible result being sepsis. Another example is the study of the chemical changes that take place in body tissue as the result of inflammation.

While individual study of specific diseases undertaken in medical pathology textbooks helps students identify subtle differences between similar diseases, the study of pathophysiology is dynamic and conceptual, seeking to explain processes and relationships common to a number of pathologies. For example, the pathophysiology of inflammation, hypotension, fluid volume deficit, hypoxia, and ischemia is important to the understanding of a large number of different pathologies, but each separate process is not necessarily a specific disease.

Pathophysiology includes four interrelated topics: etiology, pathogenesis, clinical manifestations, and treatment implications—the framework used throughout this textbook. Specific diseases will be used as illustrative examples of conditions in which particular pathophysiologic processes may occur.

FRAMEWORK FOR PATHOPHYSIOLOGY

Etiology

Etiology, in its most general definition, is the study of the causes or reasons for phenomena.[1] A description of etiologic process includes the identification of those causal factors that, acting in concert, provoke a particular disease or injury. When the cause is unknown, a condition is said to be *idiopathic.* If the cause is the result of an unintended or unwanted medical treatment, the resulting condition is said to be *iatrogenic.* Most disorders are multifactorial, having several different etiologic factors that contribute to their development. For example, coronary heart disease is a result of the interaction of genetic predisposition, diet, exposure to cigarette smoke, elevated blood pressure, and perhaps numerous other lifestyle and hormone factors acting in concert. None of these individual factors can be said to cause the disease. When the link between an etiologic factor and development of a disease is less than certain, but the probability is increased when the factor is present, it is termed a *risk factor.* The identification of risk factors is important for disease prevention and is the focus of the epidemiology section at the end of this chapter.

Some diseases are closely linked with etiologic factors, such that they are said to be the causative agents in the disease. For example, microbial pathogens are considered to be causative agents for infectious diseases; human immunodeficiency virus causes HIV disease, influenza viruses cause the flu, and *Mycobacterium tuberculosis* causes pulmonary tuberculosis.

Etiologic Classification of Diseases

Congenital (inborn) diseases or birth defects
Degenerative diseases
Iatrogenic diseases
Idiopathic diseases
Immunologic diseases
Infectious diseases
Inherited diseases
Metabolic diseases
Neoplastic diseases
Nutritional deficiency diseases
Physical agent-induced diseases
Psychogenic diseases

These diseases do not occur unless the pathogen is present in the body; however this does not mean that the infection will have the same consequences in each case, because many host factors affect the clinical course. Even when the link between disease and etiologic agent is strong, only a portion of the population exposed to the factor may develop the disease. For example, in persons who consume large quantities of alcohol and develop liver cirrhosis, it is the alcohol consumption that is considered to be the cause, yet only a portion of persons who drink heavily will develop cirrhosis.[2] Thus sorting out the probable etiologies for diseases is a long, difficult research process and, not surprisingly, the exact causes of most disorders remain incompletely understood. Several classification schemes have been proposed to categorize diseases according to etiology. Box 1-1 summarizes an example of an etiologic classification system. No classification system is truly comprehensive and some diseases fall into multiple categories. Some diseases may receive different designations in the future, as further research reveals new data.

Pathogenesis

Pathogenesis refers to the development or evolution of a disease, from the initial stimulus to the ultimate expression of the manifestations of the disease.[3] The sequence of physiologic events that occurs in response to an etiologic agent is a dynamic interplay of changes in cell, tissue, organ, and systemic function. As the ways in which intricate intercellular communication networks control physiologic function are discovered, pathogenesis is being increasingly understood on the cellular level. One of the best examples of this communication network is the immune system and its interactions with essentially every other cell in the body. A disruption in the delicate system of checks and balances between immune tolerance of normal cells and immune surveillance for abnormal cells and foreign antigens is at the root of a large number of degenerative and inflammatory diseases.

Pathologic disruptions in cellular behavior lead, in turn, to changes in organ and system function that may be detected by clinical or laboratory examination. Most pathophysiology texts take a systems approach to presenting information. This approach builds on the way in which students learn anatomy and physiology and has its roots in medical specialization. Usually the clinical examination of a patient is also conceptualized by a systems approach. Although the division into systems is useful for breaking up the content into conceptual pieces, it is important to remember that the organism functions as an integrated whole and the intercellular communication networks are not confined within single systems. In summary, pathogenesis is a description of how etiologic factors are thought to alter physiologic function and lead to the development of clinical manifestations that are observed in a particular disorder or disease.

Clinical Manifestations

Manifestations of disease that are observed are termed *signs of disease*. Such objective data may be gathered by clinical examination or by biochemical analysis, diagnostic imaging, and other laboratory tests. The subjective feelings of an abnormality in the body are termed *symptoms*. By definition, symptoms are subjective and can only be reported by the affected individual to an observer. For example, the feeling of nausea is a symptom, whereas vomiting is objectively observed and is a sign. Some signs and symptoms, such as fever and headache, are nonspecific and, while indicating that something is amiss, they do not indicate a specific cause. In this case further examination and, often, laboratory tests, are needed to narrow down the possible causes of the signs and symptoms. Many diseases and disorders are characterized by a particular constellation of signs and symptoms, the knowledge of which is essential for accurate detection and diagnosis. When the etiology of a particular set of signs and symptoms has not yet been determined, the disorder may be termed a *syndrome*. For example, AIDS was originally detected as a set of signs and symptoms related to a deficiency of helper T cells of unknown cause, now known to be a late stage of HIV infection.[4]

The clinical manifestations of some diseases may change significantly over time, resulting in a completely different clinical presentation at different stages. Knowledge of the possible stages of a disease is helpful in making an appropriate diagnosis and anticipating the clinical course.

Stages and Clinical Course

Early in the development of a disease, the etiologic agent or agents may provoke a number of changes in biological processes that can be detected by laboratory analysis, although no recognition of these changes by the patient has occurred. The interval between exposure of a tissue to an injurious agent and the first appearance of signs and symptoms may be called a latent period or, in the case of infectious diseases, an incubation period. The prodromal period, or prodrome, refers to the appearance of the first signs and symptoms indicating the onset of a disease. Prodromal symptoms often are nonspecific, such as headache, malaise, anorexia, and nausea. During the stage of manifest illness, or the acute phase, the disease reaches its full intensity, and signs and symptoms attain their greatest severity. Sometimes during the course of a disease, the signs and symptoms may become mild or even disappear for a time. This interval may be called a silent period or latent period. For example, in the total-body irradiation syndrome, a latent period may occur between the prodrome and the stage of manifest illness. Another example is syphilis, which may have two latent periods: one occurring between the primary and secondary clinical stages and another occurring between the secondary and tertiary stages.[5]

A number of diseases have a subclinical stage, during which the patient functions normally, although the disease processes are well established. It is important to understand that the structure and function of many organs provide a large reserve or safety margin, so that functional impairment may become evident only when organ damage has become advanced. For example, chronic renal disease can completely destroy one kidney and partly destroy the other before any symptoms related to a decrease in renal function are perceived.[6]

The clinical course of a disease is often classified as acute or chronic. An acute condition has relatively severe manifestations but runs a short course measured in hours, days, or a few weeks. A chronic condition lasts for months to years. Sometimes chronic disease processes begin with an acute phase and become prolonged when the body's defenses are insufficient to overcome the causative agent or stressor. In other cases, chronic conditions develop insidiously and never have an acute phase.

Some diseases (e.g., some types of autoimmune diseases) follow a course of alternating exacerbations and remissions. An exacerbation is a relatively sudden increase in the severity of a disease or any of its signs and symptoms. A remission is an abatement or decline in severity of the signs and symptoms of a disease. If a remission is permanent (sometimes defined as longer that 5 years), the person is said to be cured.

Convalescence is the stage of recovery after a disease, injury, or surgical operation. Occasionally a disease produces a subsequent pathologic condition called a sequela (plural: sequelae). For example, the sequela of an inflammatory process might be scarring. The sequelae of acute rheumatic inflammation of the heart might be scarring and deformation of cardiac valves. In contrast, a complication of a disease is a new or separate process that may arise secondarily because of some change produced by the original problem. For example, bacterial pneumonia may be a complication of viral infection of the respiratory tract.

Treatment Implications

An understanding of the etiology, pathogenesis, and clinical consequences of a particular disorder may suggest, or "imply," that certain treatments could be helpful. For example, understanding that a person with septic shock has excessive dilation of blood vessels which contributes to hypotension implies that fluid administration would likely be helpful. In contrast, most patients with cardiogenic shock have fluid overload, and hypotension in this case is unlikely to improve with fluid administration. Care must be taken not to rely on theoretical

implications when evidence-based treatment recommendations are available. When subjected to evaluation by rigorous randomized clinical trials, many treatments that seem as though they should help based on pathophysiology fail to pass the test of application.

The treatment implications discussed in pathophysiology texts usually are general statements rather than specific prescriptions. For example, the pathophysiology of heart failure is characterized by fluid overload, which implies that diuretic therapy would be useful; however, the exact selection of a drug and the dosing schedule would depend on a number of factors particular to the individual patient. Specific treatment recommendations are beyond the scope of a pathophysiology text and can be found in pharmacology and clinical practice texts.

KEY POINTS

- Pathophysiology includes four interrelated topics: etiology, pathogenesis, clinical manifestations, and treatment implications.
- Etiology refers to study of the proposed cause or causes of a particular disease process. Etiology is a complex notion because most diseases are multifactorial, resulting from interplay between genetic constitution and environmental influences.
- Pathogenesis refers to the proposed mechanisms whereby an etiologic stimulus leads to typically observed clinical manifestations. Pathogenesis describes the direct effects of the initiating event, as well as the usual physiologic responses and compensatory mechanisms.
- Clinical manifestations describe the signs and symptoms that typically accompany a particular pathophysiologic process. Manifestations may vary depending on the stage of the disorder, individual variation, and acuity or chronicity.
- An understanding of the etiology, pathogenesis, and clinical consequences of a particular disorder may imply that certain treatments could be helpful.

CONCEPTS OF NORMALITY IN HEALTH AND DISEASE

The ability to measure numerous structural, physiologic, biochemical, and genetic parameters in an individual allows the evaluation of information that is helpful in the diagnosis and monitoring of clinical diseases. Many of these same measures are commonly used to screen for disease or to evaluate the risks of a disease occurring in the future. To determine whether a certain finding is indicative of disease or "abnormal," it must be compared with what is "normal." The obviousness of this statement belies the difficulty in determining what is normal and the degree of deviation from normal that would be considered abnormal. Many clinical parameters are evaluated by direct observation by the examiner. Skin color, warmth, quality of pulses, briskness of pupil reactions to light, mental acuity, muscle strength, joint mobility, heart sounds, lung sounds, bowel sounds, balance, psychological affect, and level of consciousness are but a few examples of assessments that are subjectively interpreted based on the examiner's observations. Deciding whether a clinical finding is normal, a normal variation, or an abnormality indicative of a disorder is essential. Reliability of data obtained from observation is dependent upon the examiner's skill and experience. Often the clinical examination is not sufficient to determine definitively the underlying pathophysiologic processes, and diagnostic testing is undertaken to provide more information.

Statistical Normality

Some of the variables that are measured to diagnose disease are relatively easy to declare as normal or abnormal because they occur in only two states. For example, a bone is either broken or not broken on x-ray examination. But most diagnostic variables occur in the population according to a "bell curve" or normal distribution.[7] This means that a large enough sample taken from the population should give a good estimate of the range of values in the population. Statistics are often used to determine the standard deviation of the variable in question, and then a normal range is suggested as the mean +/- 2 standard deviations. This means that 95% of the values in the population are expected to fall in the normal range and 5% will be either higher or lower (Figure 1-1). The "population" chosen to serve as the normal reference population must be carefully selected to represent the individual to be tested for disease, because many variables are influenced by age and gender.

For example, bone density can be measured in the population by radiologic imaging and then a mean and standard deviation can be calculated. Women typically have lower bone density than men, and older women have lower bone density than younger women. If an elderly woman's bone density is compared to women of her own age group, it may fall within the normal range, but when compared to a group of younger women, it is more than 2 standard deviations below the mean.

Which is the right comparison group to use to determine if she has osteoporosis? There is controversy on this point because, in this situation, it is difficult to determine the difference between disease and the effects of normal aging.

Often, when assessing a person's health status, a change in some value or factor is more significant than the actual value of the factor. A blood pressure of 90/70 mm Hg may not be significant if that is the usual value. However, if a person usually has a blood pressure of 120/80 mm Hg, a reading of 90/70 mm Hg could indicate a significant change. Individuals are typically evaluated more than once—generally two or three times—to establish deviation from their usual value.

Reliability, Validity, and Predictive Value

The accurate determination of whether a specific condition is present or absent depends on the quality and adequacy of the data collected, as well as the skill of interpretation. Decisions about the data needed are based on the initial clinical presentation and a working knowledge of pathophysiology, which guide hypothesis generation about probable etiologies. During the clinical examination, data are analyzed and a number of likely explanations for the clinical presentation may emerge. These possible explanations are "probabilities" based on knowledge and past experience with similar cases. The purpose of further data collection, particularly laboratory and diagnostic testing, is to refine the initial probability estimates and identify the most likely diagnosis. The success of this approach depends on the selection of appropriate tests based on the pretest probabilities, as well as on the validity, reliability, and predictive value of the tests.

Validity, or accuracy, is the degree to which a measurement reflects the true value of the thing it is intended to measure. For example, a pulse oximeter is designed to measure arterial oxygen saturation, and the closeness of the reading to a direct measurement of oxygen saturation in an arterial blood sample reflects its accuracy. Reliability, or precision, is the ability of a test to give the same result in repeated measurements.

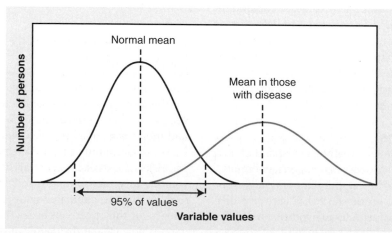

FIGURE 1-1 Representative example of a normal bell curve for a physiologic variable. Many physiologic variables are normally distributed within the population, so the mean +/- 2 standard deviations include 95% of the normal values in the sample. Approximately 2.5% of values will be above the normal range and 2.5% will be below it. There may be overlap between the values in a normal sample and those in the population with a disease, making interpretation difficult in some cases.

An instrument or laboratory test can be reliable, yet inaccurate. Repeated measurements with the pulse oximeter could give the same result each time, but if those values are significantly different from the "gold standard" of an arterial blood sample, the oximeter data would have poor validity.

Some measurements vary according to the reagents and laboratory methods used. For example, prothrombin time (PT) is sensitive to the reagent used. In one method of determining PT, the reagent-a substance composed of thromboplastin and calcium-is added to decalcified plasma to create a reaction resulting in clot formation. The PT is then determined by measuring the length of time it takes for clotting to occur after this reagent is added and compared to the normative average. Portions of the same blood sample sent to several different laboratories could return significantly different PT results. In fact this is such a problem that laboratories now use a correction procedure to normalize the PT values across labs. The corrected PT value is reported as the International Normalized Ratio (INR), which has higher reliability than the PT.[8]

The predictive value of a test is the extent to which the test can differentiate between the presence or absence of a condition in an individual. The positive predictive value is an estimate of the probability that disease is present if the test is positive. The negative predictive value is an estimate of the probability that disease is absent if the test is negative. The predictive value of a test depends in part upon the sensitivity and specificity of the test and in part upon the probability of the disease being present before the test is obtained. Most tests are not perfectly specific and sensitive so the results must be interpreted probabilistically in view of the diagnostic hypotheses being tested.

Sensitivity and specificity are measures of how well a given test can discriminate between persons with and without a given condition. Sensitivity is the probability that the test will be positive when applied to a person with the condition. For example, if a kit for testing a throat swab for the presence of streptococcal infection has a sensitivity of 80%, then 20% of a group of people with streptococcal throat infection would erroneously test negative for the condition (false negative rate). Another example is the blood test for HIV antibodies, which has a sensitivity of 99% and would fail to detect the condition in only 1% of a group of individuals who had HIV antibodies in their blood. Specificity is the probability that a test will be negative when applied to a person who does not have a given condition. If the streptococcal throat swab kit has a specificity of 95%, then 5% of those tested who do not actually have the condition would erroneously test positive (false positive rate). The importance of evaluating the accuracy and precision of data is paramount as inappropriate diagnoses and clinical management could occur if decisions are predicated on invalid or unreliable data.

The positive predictive value of a test is improved when sensitivity and specificity are high and the test is applied to individuals who have a high probability of having the condition being tested. If the likelihood of a condition in the population being tested is low, say a 2% prevalence rate, then a positive result in a test with 99% specificity and 99% sensitivity would only have a 67% positive predictive value.[9] This means that testing low-likelihood or low-risk individuals would produce a high percentage of false positive results (33% in the example above). Therefore decisions about who to test for a given condition based on the probability of the condition being present is as important as the sensitivity and specificity of the test. A good working knowledge of pathophysiology is necessary to generate the hypotheses that guide collection of appropriate data and facilitate the diagnostic process.

Individual Factors

Variations in physiologic processes may be a result of factors other than disease or illness. Age, gender, genetic and ethnic background, geographic area, and time of day may influence various physiologic parameters.[10] Care must be taken to interpret "abnormal" findings in the light of these possible confounding factors. In addition, the potential for spurious findings always exists. Thus, trends and changes in a particular individual are more reliable than single observations. Single measurements, observations, or laboratory results that seem to indicate abnormality must always be judged in the context of the entire health picture of the individual. One slightly elevated blood glucose level does not mean clinical diabetes, a single high blood pressure reading does not denote hypertension, and a temporary feeling of hopelessness does not indicate clinical depression.

Cultural Considerations

Each culture defines health and illness in a manner that reflects its experience. Cultural factors determine which signs, symptoms, or behaviors are perceived as abnormal. An infant from an impoverished culture with endemic chronic diarrhea and a degree of malnutrition would be viewed as abnormal in a progressive culture, such as a well-baby clinic in Sweden. Given cultural variations that affect definitions of normal and abnormal, the resulting pattern of behaviors or clinical manifestations affects what the culture labels as illness.[11]

Age Differences

Many biological factors vary with age, and the normal value for a person at one age may be abnormal at another. Physiologic changes, such as hair color, skin turgor (tension), and organ size, vary with age. In general, most organs shrink; exceptions are the male prostate and the heart, which enlarge with age.[12] Special sensory changes, such as severely diminished nearsight, high-tone hearing loss, and loss of taste discriminations for sweet and salty, are normal in an elderly adult and abnormal in a middle-aged adult or child. There are fewer sweat glands and less thirst perception in an elderly person than in a young adult or child. Elderly persons have diminished temperature sensations and can therefore sustain burn injuries—from a heating pad or bath water—because they do not perceive heat with the same intensity as do middle-aged adults. A resting heart rate of 120 beats per minute is normal for an infant but not for an adult.

Gender Differences

Some laboratory values, such as levels of sex and growth hormones, show gender differences. The complete blood cell count shows differences by gender in hematocrit, hemoglobin, and red blood cell (RBC) count.[13] For example, the normal range of hemoglobin concentration for adult women is lower than that for adult men. For adult women, the normal range is 12 to 16 g/100 ml of blood; for adult men the normal range is 13 to 18 g/100 ml of blood.[13] There are also gender differences in the erythrocyte sedimentation rate (ESR). Normally, in males, the ESR is less than 13 mm/hr; it is slightly higher in females.[13] There are differences by gender in creatinine values. For females, the normal serum creatinine level is 0.4 to 1.3 mg/dl; for males, the normal range is 0.6 to 1.5 mg/dl.[13] Research into gender differences also suggests that, on average, males snore more, have longer vocal cords, have better daylight vision, have higher metabolic rates, and are more likely to be left-handed than females.[14] Research suggests, too, that females and males have different communication styles and respond differently to similar conditions.

Situational Differences

In some cases, a deviation from the usual value may occur as an adaptive mechanism, and whether the deviation is considered abnormal depends on the situation. For example,

the RBC count increases when a person moves to a high altitude.[15] The increase is a normal adaptive response to the decreased availability of oxygen at a high altitude and is termed *acclimatization*. A similar increase in the RBC count at sea level would be abnormal.

Time Variations

Some factors vary according to the time of day; that is, they exhibit a circadian rhythm or diurnal variation. In interpreting the result of a particular test, it may be necessary to know the time at which the value was determined. For example, body temperature and plasma concentrations of certain hormones (such as growth hormone and cortisol) exhibit diurnal variation. Reflecting fluctuation in plasma levels, the peak rate in urinary excretion for a particular steroid (17-ketosteroid) occurs between 8 AM and 10 AM for persons who customarily get up early in the morning and is about two to three times greater than the lowest rate in the same people, which occurs between midnight and 2 AM, usually during sleep.[16] The urinary excretion of ions (e.g., potassium) also exhibits diurnal variation. Figure 1-2 illustrates circadian rhythms of several physiologic variables for persons living on a standard day-active schedule.

FIGURE 1-2 Circadian rhythms of several physiologic variables in a human subject depict the effect of light and dark. In an experiment with lights on (*open bars* at top) for 16 hours and off (*black bars* at top) for 8 hours, temperature, plasma growth hormone, plasma cortisol, and urinary potassium levels exhibit diurnal variation. (Redrawn from Vander AJ et al: *Human physiology,* ed 7, New York, 1998, McGraw-Hill.)

KEY POINTS

- Determining whether clinical findings are normal, abnormal, or normal variation is an essential but often difficult process in evaluating for the presence or absence of disease.
- Normal ranges for laboratory tests are typically defined as the mean +/– 2 standard deviations; thus, 5% of the normal population may fall outside the normal range despite the absence of disease. Laboratory tests must be evaluated in concert with clinical information.
- The predictive value of a clinical test is the extent to which it can differentiate between presence and absence of disease in an individual. Tests with high sensitivity and specificity generally have better predictive value.
- Variations in physiologic processes may be a result of factors other than disease or illness. Age, gender, genetic and ethnic background, geographic area, and time of day may influence various physiologic parameters.
- Trends and changes in a particular individual are more reliable than single observations.

CONCEPTS OF EPIDEMIOLOGY

Differences among *individuals* are, of course, very important in determining the diseases to which they are susceptible and their reactions to the diseases once contracted. But epidemiology, or the study of *patterns of disease* involving aggregates of people (Figure 1-3), provides yet another important dimension. Information may be gained by examining the occurrence, incidence, prevalence, transmission, and distribution of diseases in large groups of people or populations.

FIGURE 1-3 The aggregate focus in disease: crowds at a public market in Russia. (Photographed by LE Copstead.)

A disease that is native to a local region is called an *endemic disease*. If the disease spreads to many individuals at the same time, the situation is called an *epidemic*. Pandemics are epidemics that affect large geographic regions, perhaps spreading worldwide. Because of the speed and availability of human travel around the world, pandemics are more common than they once were. Almost every flu season, a new strain of influenza virus quickly spreads from one continent to another.

Factors Affecting Patterns of Disease

Principal factors affecting patterns of disease in human populations include the following: (1) age (i.e., time in the life cycle), (2) ethnic group, (3) gender, (4) socioeconomic factors and lifestyle considerations, and (5) geographic location.

Age

In one sense, life is entirely different during the 9 months of gestation. The structures and functions of tissues are different: they are primarily dedicated to differentiation, development, and growth. Certainly the environment is different; the individual is protected from the light of day, provided with predigested food (even preoxygenated blood), suspended in a fluid buffer, and maintained at incubator temperature. This is fortunate because the developing embryo or fetus has relatively few homeostatic mechanisms to protect it from environmental change. (The factors that produce disease in utero are discussed in Chapter 6.) Diseases that arise during the postuterine period of life and affect the neonate include immaturity, respiratory failure, birth injuries, congenital malformations, nutritional problems, metabolic errors, and infections. These conditions are discussed in separate chapters.

Accidents, including poisoning, take their toll in childhood. Infections in children reflect their increased susceptibility to agents of disease. Consideration of other childhood diseases is addressed in each chapter, as appropriate. The study of childhood processes and of changes that occur in this period of life is the domain of pediatrics; specific diseases that occur during maturity (ages 15 to 60) are the primary emphasis of this text.

The changes in function that occur during the early years of life are termed *developmental processes*. Those that occur during maturity and postmaturity (age 60 and beyond) are called *aging processes*. The study of aging processes and other changes that occur during this period of life is called *gerontology*. The effects of aging on selected body systems are so important physiologically that they receive separate consideration throughout the text. The immune, cardiac, respiratory, musculoskeletal, neurologic, special sensory, endocrine, gastrointestinal, and integumentary systems are all affected by the process of aging.

Ethnic Group

It is difficult to differentiate sharply between the effects of ethnicity on patterns of disease and the socioeconomic factors, religious practices, customs, and geographic considerations with which ethnicity is inseparably bound. For example, carcinoma of the penis is virtually unknown among Jews and Muslims who practice circumcision at an early age (avoiding the carcinogenic stimulus that comes from accumulation of smegma about the glans penis).

However, comparisons reveal significant differences in occurrence of certain disease states in ethnic groups that seem to be more closely related to genetic predisposition than to environmental factors. For example, sickle cell anemia has a much higher rate of occurrence in African populations, whereas pernicious anemia occurs more frequently among Scandinavians and is rare among black populations worldwide.

The study of racial and ethnic group variation in disease states is the domain of medical anthropology. Volumes have been written about disease-specific differences that relate to racial or ethnic group differences. In clinical practice, recognition of diversity in disease risk by racial or ethnic group is useful in disease diagnosis, prevention, and management. Ethnic group-specific differences, where important, are presented in individual chapters.

Gender

Particular diseases of the genital system obviously show important differences between the sexes; men do not have endometriosis nor do women have hyperplasia of the prostate, and carcinoma of the breast is more common in women than in men. Pyelonephritis is more common in young women than in men of comparable age (before they develop prostatic hyperplasia) because the external urethral orifice of women is more readily contaminated, and bacteria can more easily travel up a short urethra than a long one. Less obviously related to the reproductive system, the onset of severe atherosclerosis in women is delayed some 20 years or so over that in men, presumably because of the protective action of estrogenic hormone.

There are also gender-specific factors that defy explanation.[17] For example, systemic lupus erythematosus is much more common in women.[18] Toxic goiter and hypothyroidism are also more common in women.[19] Rheumatoid arthritis is more common in women, but osteoarthritis affects men and women with equal frequency.[20] Thromboangiitis obliterans (a chronic, recurring, inflammatory peripheral vascular disease) occurs more commonly in men.[21] Gender differences in predisposition to cancer and other diseases are presented throughout the text.

Socioeconomic Factors and Lifestyle Considerations

The environment and the political climate of countries determine how people live and the health problems that are likely to ensue. The importance of poverty, malnutrition, overcrowding, and exposure to adverse environmental conditions, such as extremes of temperature, is obvious. Volumes have been written about the effects of socioeconomic status on disease. Sociologists study the influence of these factors. Social class influences education and the type of occupation a person is likely to have.

Disease is related to occupational exposure to such agents as coal dust, noise, or extreme stress.[22] Lifestyle considerations are closely related to socioeconomic factors. People living in the United States, for example, consume too much food, alcohol, and tobacco and do not exercise enough. Childhood obesity is a problem in the United States. Arteriosclerosis; cancer; diseases of the kidney, liver, and lungs; and accidents cause most deaths in the United States. By contrast, people living in developing nations suffer and frequently die from undernutrition and infectious diseases.

However, infectious disease is not limited to developing countries.[23] The Centers for Disease Control and Prevention (CDC) estimates that 2 million people annually acquire infections while hospitalized and 90,000 people die of those infections. More than 70% of hospital-acquired infections have become resistant to at least one of the drugs commonly used to manage them, largely due to the overprescribing of antibiotics.[24] *Staphylococcus,* the leading cause of hospital infections,

FIGURE 1-4 Risk factors for schistosomiasis include the widespread use of irrigation ditches that harbor the intermediate snail host.

is now resistant to 95% of first-choice antibiotics and 30% of second-choice antibiotics. Poor hygiene is considered the leading source for infections acquired during hospitalizations. Sadly, efforts to get medical workers to improve safety through means as simple as more frequent and thorough hand washing have met with only modest success.

The incidence of many parasitic diseases is closely tied to socioeconomic factors and lifestyle considerations. Worm infections, for example, are related to the use of human feces as fertilizer. In some areas, such as Africa and tropical America, the frequency of schistosomiasis (a parasitic infestation by blood flukes) is tied directly to the widespread use of irrigation ditches that harbor the intermediate snail host.[25] The fact that children play in the ditches or that clothes are washed there gives adequate opportunity for human infection (Figure 1-4).

Trichinosis, a disease caused by the ingestion of *Trichinella spiralis,* comes almost entirely from eating inadequately cooked, infected pork. People who are fond of raw meat and inadequately cooked sausage are at highest risk.

Education is often very effective in changing lifestyle patterns that contribute to disease. In Tokyo, for example, mass public education about minimizing the use of sodium-a common ingredient in most traditional Japanese cooking-has been effective in changing current dietary practices, thus affecting the control of hypertension.

Examples of educational efforts directed at lifestyle modification in the United States are numerous.[26-28] Antidrug, antismoking, and pro-fitness messages fill the media and are prevalent on the Internet. Choosing healthy alternatives over unhealthy ones is made easier through positive peer pressure and support groups.

Geographic Location

Patterns of disease vary greatly by geographic location. Certainly there is considerable overlap with ethnicity, socioeconomic factors, and lifestyle choices, but physical environment also is an important aspect. Obviously, frostbite in Antarctica and dehydration in the Sahara are examples of disorders that are more prevalent in specific geographic settings. But important patterns of disease occur within individual

Distribution of *falciparum* malaria

FIGURE 1-5 Geographic distribution of malaria. (From Thibodeau GA, Patton KT: *Anatomy and physiology,* ed 6, St. Louis, 2007, Mosby, p 1206.)

countries. For example, the incidence and kind of malnutrition vary tremendously by geographic region.

Many diseases have a geographic pattern for reasons that are clear. For example, malaria, an acute and sometimes chronic infectious disease resulting from the presence of protozoan parasites within red blood cells, is transmitted to humans by the bite of an infected female *Anopheles* mosquito. The *Anopheles* mosquito can live only in certain regions of the world (Figure 1-5).[29]

Fungal diseases are both more common and more serious in hot, humid regions. But some infectious diseases are highly limited geographically for reasons that are not well understood. For example, bartonellosis, which is also called Carrión disease, is found only in Peru, Ecuador, Chile, and Colombia.[30] This disease resembles malaria superficially in that the minute rickettsia-like organisms invade erythrocytes and destroy them. Humans are infected by the bite of the sand fly. Although conditions in other parts of the world should be favorable for this disease, it remains limited geographically.

Taking a world view, there is widespread recognition of the importance of geographic factors in influencing human disease.[31] The World Health Organization (WHO) and the National Institutes of Health (NIH) have been deeply concerned with geographic problems in disease. Consult WHO and NIH home pages on the World Wide Web for additional information. (Web locations are provided on the Evolve site.)

Levels of Prevention

Prevention of ill health is too narrow to be the goal of health care. What is needed instead is some notion of positive health or physical "wholeness" that extends beyond the absence of ill health. WHO defines health as complete physical, mental, and social well-being, and not merely the absence of disease or infirmity.[31] For some individuals, health implies the ability to

do what they regard as worthwhile and to conduct their lives as they want. Aging and ill health are not synonymous, and many elders enjoy excellent health, even in the face of chronic disease (Figure 1-6).

Epidemiologists suggest that treatment implications fall into categories called *levels of prevention.* There are three levels of prevention: primary, secondary, and tertiary. Primary prevention is prevention of disease by altering susceptibility or reducing exposure for susceptible individuals. Secondary prevention (applicable in early disease, i.e., preclinical and clinical stages) is the early detection, screening, and management of the disease. Tertiary prevention (appropriate in the stage of advanced disease or disability) includes rehabilitative and supportive care and attempts to alleviate disability and restore effective functioning.[32]

Primary Prevention

Prolongation of life has resulted largely from decreased mortality from infectious disease. Primary prevention in terms of improved nutrition, economy, housing, and sanitation for those living in developed countries is also responsible for increased longevity. Certain childhood diseases—measles, poliomyelitis, pertussis (whooping cough), and neonatal tetanus—are decreasing, owing to a rapid increase in coverage by immunization programs. More than 120 million children younger than age 5 in India were immunized against poliomyelitis in a single day in 1996.[33] Globally, coverage of children immunized against six major childhood diseases increased from 5% in 1974 to 80% in 1995.[33] In 1985, Rotary International launched the PolioPlus program to protect children worldwide from the cruel and fatal consequences of polio. In 1988, the World Health Assembly challenged the world to eradicate polio. Since that time, Rotary's efforts and those of partner agencies, including the WHO, the United Nations Children's Fund, the CDC, and governments around the world, have achieved a 99% reduction in the number of polio cases worldwide.[33]

Cardiovascular diseases in developed countries (except those in Eastern Europe) are on the wane, thanks to the spread of health education and promotion. Infant and child mortality rates and the overall death rate are continuing to decrease globally.

High school education programs about abstinence from sex and ways to say no to drugs, alcohol, and tobacco are other examples of primary prevention making a difference in the lives of people. Primary prevention also includes adherence to safety precautions, such as wearing seat belts, observing the posted speed limit on highways, and taking precautions in the use of chemicals and machinery. Violent crimes involving dangerous weapons must be stopped to achieve primary prevention of the traumatic or fatal injuries they cause.

Environmental pollutants poison the organs. Some experts fear an epidemic of cancer due to carcinogenic chemicals blighting the environment.[34] Public health measures to ensure clean food, air, and water prevent many diseases, including cancer. As air, water, and soil quality is improved, the risk of exposure to harmful carcinogens is minimized.

FIGURE 1-6 Healthy aging: elders exercising in an aerobics class **(A)** and painting **(B)** illustrate the concept that aging and disease are not synonymous. The artist, a healthy woman in her mid-70s, is also a breast cancer survivor. (Photographed by Therese A. Capal, Rockville, Md.)

Secondary Prevention

Yearly physical examinations and routine screening are examples of secondary prevention that lead to the early diagnosis of disease and, in some cases, cures. The routine use of Papanicolaou (Pap) smears has led to a decline in the incidence of invasive cancer of the uterine cervix. Also, more women are examining their own breasts monthly for cancer; thus, earlier diagnoses are achieved.

Prenatal diagnosis of certain genetic diseases is possible. New diagnostic laboratory techniques provide definitive information for the genetic counseling of parents. This information can aid in predicting chances of involvement or noninvolvement of offspring for a given genetic disorder (e.g., Down syndrome). One technique, *amniocentesis,* consists of removing a small amount of fluid from the amniotic sac that surrounds the fetus and analyzing the cells and chemicals in the fluid. Blood samples can also be obtained from the fetus by amniocentesis; the amniotic fluid and fetal blood are then studied for defects in enzymes, to determine gender, and to measure substances associated with defects in the spinal cord and brain.

Tertiary Prevention

Once a disease becomes established, treatment—within the context of traditional Western medicine—generally falls into one of the following two major categories: medical (including such measures as physical therapy, pharmacotherapy, psychotherapy, radiation therapy, chemotherapy, immunotherapy, and experimental gene therapy) and surgical. Numerous other subspecialties of medicine and surgery also have evolved to focus on a given organ or technique. In a clinical setting, a large array of professional caregivers provides rehabilitative and supportive tertiary prevention to the diseased individual.

Every professional brings the perspective of his or her discipline to the caregiving situation. Each makes clinical judgments about the patient's needs and problems and decides which goals and intervention strategies are most beneficial.

KEY POINTS

- Epidemiology is the study of patterns of disease in human populations.
- Age, ethnicity, gender, lifestyle, socioeconomic status, and geographic location are epidemiologic variables that influence the occurrence and transmission of disease.
- Understanding the epidemiologic aspects of a disease is essential for effective prevention and treatment.

SUMMARY

Most people recognize what it is to be healthy and would define disease or illness as a change from or absence of that state. Under closer scrutiny, the concept of health is difficult to describe in simple, succinct terms. Correspondingly, the concepts of disease and illness also are complex. Environment, genetic constitution, socioeconomic status, lifestyle, and previous physical health all affect the timing and ultimate expression of disease in individuals.

Because humans exhibit considerable diversity, healthy structure and function are not precisely the same in any two individuals. By discovering common and expected patterns of responses to abnormalities, general prediction of etiology, pathogenesis, clinical manifestations, and targeted levels of prevention and intervention become possible.

REFERENCES

1. *Stedman's medical dictionary,* ed 28, Philadelphia, 2005, Lippincott Williams & Wilkins.
2. Cargiulo T: Understanding the health impact of alcohol dependence, *Am J Health Syst Pharm* 64(5 Suppl 3):S5-11, 2007.
3. MedicineNet.com. Available at http://www.medterms.com/script/main/art.asp?articlekey=6385. Accessed 3/26/08.
4. Office of AIDS Research, National Institutes of Health. Available at http://www.oar.nih.gov/about/research/etiology/oaretio.htm. Accessed 3/26/08.
5. Pickering LK: Syphilis. In *Red book,* Elk Grove Village, IL, 2006, American Academy of Pediatrics, pp 631-644.
6. Vassalotti JA, Stevens LA, Levey AS: Testing for chronic kidney disease: a position statement from the National Kidney Foundation, *Am J Kidney Dis* 50(2):169-180, 2007.
7. *How to define and determine reference intervals in the clinical laboratory: approved guideline-second edition.* Wayne, PA, 2000, Clinical and Laboratory Standards Institute. NCCLS document C28-A2.
8. Lindahl TL, et al: INR calibration of Owren-type prothrombin time based on the relationship between PT% and INR utilizing normal plasma samples, *Thromb Haemost* 91(6):1223-1231, 2004.
9. Smith J, Winkler R, Fryback D: The first positive: computing positive predictive value at the extremes, *Ann Intern Med* 132:804-809, 2000.
10. Bocklandt S, Vilain E: Sex differences in brain and behavior: hormones versus genes, *Adv Genet* 59:245-266, 2007.
11. Gerber A, Hentzelt F, Lauterbach KW: Can evidence-based medicine implicitly rely on current concepts of disease or does it have to develop its own definition? *J Med Ethics* 33(7):394-399, 2007.
12. Linton AD, Lach HW: *Matteson & McConnell's gerontological nursing: concepts and practice,* ed 3, Philadelphia, 2006, Saunders.
13. Wu AHB: *Tietz clinical guide to laboratory tests,* ed 4, Philadelphia, 2006, Saunders.
14. Blair ML: Sex-based differences in physiology: what should we teach in the medical curriculum? *Adv Physiol Educ* 31(1):23-25, 2007.
15. Hopfl G, Ogunshola O, Gassmann M: Hypoxia and high altitude. The molecular response, *Adv Exp Med Biol* 543:89-115, 2003.
16. Buckley TM, Schatzberg AF: On the interactions of the hypothalamic-pituitary-adrenal (HPA) axis and sleep: normal HPA axis activity and circadian rhythm, exemplary sleep disorders, *J Clin Endocrinol Metab* 90(5):3106-3114, 2005.
17. Wizemann TM, Pardue M-L, editors: *Exploring the biological contributions to human health: does sex matter?* Washington, DC, April 25, 2001, Institute of Medicine Board of Health Sciences Policy.
18. Walsh SJ, Rau LM: Autoimmune diseases: a leading cause of death among young and middle-aged women in the United States, *Am J Public Health* 90(9):1463-1466, 2000.
19. Surks MI, et al: Subclinical thyroid disease: scientific review and guidelines for diagnosis and management, *JAMA* 291:228-238, 2004.
20. Klippel JH: *Primer on the rheumatic diseases,* ed 12, Atlanta, 2001, Arthritis Foundation, pp 86-93, 184-190, 2001.
21. Puechal X, Fiessinger JN: Thromboangiitis obliterans or Buerger's disease: challenges for the rheumatologist, *Rheumatology (Oxford)* 46:192-199, 2007.
22. Division of Cancer Epidemiology & Genetics: Cancer, organic solvents and other industrial chemicals. National Cancer Institute US National Institutes of Health. Available at http://www.cancer.gov. Accessed 3/26/08.
23. Trends in tuberculosis incidence-United States, 2006, *JAMA* 297:1765-1767, 2007.
24. Sartin J, et al: Medical management issues surrounding community-acquired pneumonia in adults, *Gundersen Lutheran Med Found J* 1(2):6-9, 2003.
25. World Health Organization: Tropical diseases research. Available at http://www.who.int/en/. Accessed 3/26/08.
26. Daynard RA: Lessons from tobacco control for the obesity control movement, *J Public Health Policy* 24(3-4):274-290, 2003.
27. Wadden TA, et al: Randomized trial of lifestyle modification and pharmacotherapy for obesity, *N Engl J Med* 353(20):2111-2120, 2005.
28. McCabe BW, et al: Practice of health-promoting behaviors by nursing home residents, *West J Nurs Res,* 27(12):1000-1016, 2005.
29. World Health Organization: World malaria situation. Available at http://www.who.int/en/. Accessed 3/26/08.
30. O'Neill J: Environmental values through thick and thin, *Conservation and Society* 3:479-500, 2005.
31. World Health Organization. Available at http://www.who.int/en/. Accessed 3/26/08.
32. Jekel JF: *Epidemiology, biostatistics, and preventive medicine,* Philadelphia, 2001, Saunders.
33. Rotary.org: Facts about polio. Available at http://www.rotary.org. Accessed 4/10/08.
34. Laden F, et al: Reduction in fine particulate air pollution and mortality: extended follow-up of the Harvard Six Cities study, *Am J Respir Crit Care Med* 173:667-672, 2006.

Homeostasis and Adaptive Responses to Stressors

Roberta J. Emerson

MEDIA RESOURCES

Additional Material for Study, Review, and Further Exploration

CD Companion ■ Review Questions and Answers ■ Glossary (with audio pronunciations for selected terms) ■ Disease Profiles ■ Animations

evolve **Website** at http://evolve.elsevier.com/Copstead/
■ Case Studies ■ Disease Profiles ■ WebLinks ■ Key Points Review

KEY QUESTIONS

- What is the relationship between homeostasis and allostasis?
- How do the sympathetic nervous system and neuroendocrine system respond to stress?
- What are the key features of Selye's General Adaptation Syndrome?

- What factors affect the stress response?
- How does allostatic overload contribute to the development of disease?

CHAPTER OUTLINE

Survival of the human species is dependent on its ability to respond to changes in the environment. Changes in the external environment, such as moving outside from a warm house on a cold winter day, demand physiologic adjustments in the body's internal environment beyond the simple addition of layers of clothing to the outside of the body. Variations in the internal environment, such as a fever caused by infection, also necessitate physiologic responses to bring the body's temperature back into the normal range. The human organism maintains a variety of highly complex interactions with both the internal and external environments. These interactions facilitate ongoing compensatory changes designed to support the organism physically and psychologically. This process is necessary, allowing the perpetuation of both the individual and the species. However, researchers have found that the body's efforts to adapt to profound or extraordinarily demanding environmental changes may be associated with many physical and psychological health problems. This chapter explores the historical and current perspectives of homeostasis and stress responses, and their relationship to illness.

HOMEOSTASIS AND ALLOSTASIS

Homeostasis

The word *homeostasis* is derived from the Greek, *homeo* or same, and *stasis* or stable, and means remaining stable by remaining the same.[1] The concept of homeostasis has historically contributed greatly to the fields of physiology, psychology, and pathophysiology. Homeostasis is conceptualized as a state of being in which all systems are in balance at a particular ideal "set-point." Bodily changes formerly seen as conflicting are understood as adaptive or compensatory to the maintenance of homeostasis within the body as a whole. It is well accepted that homeostasis describes a tendency to stabilize an organism's functional systems, despite changes both internally and externally. Deviations from homeostasis resulting from these changes require complex systems to support its reestablishment. There has been a great deal of discussion in the literature over the past several decades criticizing the inadequacy of the definition of homeostasis to encompass the entire process of maintaining a stable state in complex organisms. But the fact remains that homeostatic concepts are an essential starting point for an exploration of stress, adaptation, and disease.

The origins of the concept that is known today as homeostasis reach back thousands of years to the Greeks.[2] Terms and concepts such as *balance, harmony, equilibrium,* and *steady-state* as a fundamental attribute of life were introduced by them. They recognized that when menacing energies were present, other energies were activated to counteract them.[2] The Greek philosopher Heraclitus (540-480 BC) was the first to suggest that a static, unchanged state was not the natural condition, and the capacity to undergo constant change was intrinsic to all things.[2,3] Shortly afterward, the philosopher Empedocles (495-435 BC) proposed the corollary that all matter consisted of elements and qualities that were in dynamic opposition or alliance to one another, and that balance or harmony was a necessary condition for the survival of living organisms. Following those hypotheses, Hippocrates (460-375 BC) equated health to the harmonious balance of the elements, and illness and disease to the systematic disharmony of these elements.[2,3] The terms *dyscrasia* and *idiosyncrasy* are derived from hippocratic concepts of health and disease and are defined, respectively, as the defective and peculiar mixing of the elements.[3] Hippocrates also suggested that the disturbing forces that produced disharmony (disease) and counterbalancing (adaptive) forces were both derived from natural rather than supernatural sources.[2,3] He introduced the idea that nature is the healer of disease.[2,3] Epicurus (341-270 BC) believed the quality of life was enhanced by coping with emotional

incidences and the "impermeability" of mind, which he called *ataraxia*.[2] Hippocrates' beliefs were later echoed by Roman references to counterbalancing forces as *vis medicatrix naturae,* or the healing powers of nature.[2,3] During the European Renaissance, Thomas Sydenham expanded the hippocratic concept of disease as a system of disharmony brought about by disturbing forces by adding that an individual's adaptive response could itself be capable of producing pathologic changes.[3] These concepts were supported well into the seventeenth century.[2]

Nearly 150 years ago, Claude Bernard published his seminal work, declaring that the maintenance of the internal environment, the *milieu intérieur,* surrounding the body's cells, was essential for the life of the organism.[4] In 1929, Walter B. Cannon published his first extrapolation from Bernard's 1865 work; he named his theory "homeostasis."[2,4-6] Homeostasis, according to Cannon, was a process of synchronized adjustments in the internal environment resulting in the maintenance of specific physiologic variables within defined parameters.[2,4,6-7] These variables were quite precise—blood pressure, temperature, pH—with clearly identified "normal" ranges or steady-states. Threats to homeostasis, Cannon affirmed, could originate from the external environment (e.g., temperature extremes, traumatic injury) or the internal environment (e.g., pain, infection), and could be physical or psychological, as in emotional distress.[4]

Maintenance of this internal physical and psychological balance, homeostasis, demands an internal network of communication, with sensors capable of identifying deviations from the acceptable ranges and effectors to return those deviations back within acceptable limits.[4] Cannon identified these negative feedback systems and emphasized that, regardless of the nature of the danger to the maintenance of homeostasis, the response he mapped within the body would be the same.[4]

Allostasis

Typically, the homeostatic response was seen as a mechanistic, predictable series of orchestrated internal activities. As knowledge has expanded, efforts to apply homeostatic concepts in a broader fashion have seemed forced and inadequate. The simplistic view has been challenged, even by Cannon himself, and over the decades by many others.[8-10] The innate complexity of biological organisms requires hierarchies of response mechanisms; changes occur but in some cases, set points are readjusted and desired changes in one body system may be detrimental to another, yet ultimately support the survival of the organism as a whole.[5,8] For instance, in shock, when the continuation of the life of the organism is at risk, blood flow to essential organs (brain and heart) is maintained by reducing perfusion to the kidneys, skin, and the gastrointestinal tract.

In 1988, Sterling and Eyer coined a new term, **allostasis,** in recognition of the complexity and variable levels of activity necessary to reestablish or maintain homeostasis.[4,5] Like homeostasis, *allostasis* is a derivation from Greek.[1] *Allo* means variable, and added to stasis (same), accentuates the role of allostatic systems in maintaining the organism's

---

BOX 2-1

Examples of Homeostatic Systems

Baroreceptor response to acute changes in blood pressure

Vasopressin/antidiuretic hormone release from the posterior pituitary in response to changes in serum osmolality

Hypothalamic-mediated responses to changes in body core temperature

Central chemoreceptor responses to changes in $PaCO_2$

Parathyroid gland response to changes in serum calcium level

---

stability through the capacity for change.[1] Allostasis is a process that supports homeostasis; the organism's overall stability is accomplished through change.[7] Homeostasis, from this perspective, is seen as a steady-state as originally conceived of by the Greeks. There are some homeostatic systems designed to support the life of the organism in the most basic sense, as shown in Box 2-1. Allostasis then refers to a superordinate set of systems that support homeostasis in light of environmental and life changes.[7,11] Allostasis comes into play in the complexity of social interactions, changes in the weather, reproduction, even the hibernation patterns of bears and migration of birds. Although the concept is occasionally challenged,[12] it has garnered broad support in the past decade in both the physical and behavioral sciences. It seems especially applicable to subsequent discussions of adaptation and disease.

KEY POINTS

- Contemporary concepts of homeostasis have a long history, reaching back to the ancient Greeks.
- Homeostasis is a state of equilibrium, of balance within the organism.
- Homeostatic responses refer to systems whose purpose is specifically to normalize selected physiologic variables.
- Allostasis is the overall process of adaptive change necessary to maintain survival and well-being.

STRESS AS A CONCEPT

Stress is something of an ambiguous term today. It is most often interpreted as a physical, chemical, or emotional factor resulting in tension in the body or the mind ("He's experiencing a lot of stress"). But it can also mean the actual state that the tension produces ("I feel stressed"). These disparate definitions have not changed the fact that stress is one of the concepts most frequently addressed in the biomedical literature.[2] It is a natural outgrowth of the concept of homeostasis but is even more applicable to the dynamic concept of allostasis.

Although Cannon wrote extensively about homeostasis, he never defined stress and he used the term itself infrequently.[5] From his writings, it has been deduced that he saw stress as one harmful feature of the environment. But his attention

was broadly on his concept of homeostasis as a collection of steady-states that was the ideal outcome of synchronized body functions.[5] Nearly simultaneous with the work of Cannon, a new voice was heard. It took Hans Selye (1907-1982) to popularize the concept of stress.[4] Selye used the word *stress* in a rather sloppy and, according to many, inopportune fashion that continues to dominate the literature today.[2] He intended the word to be an extrapolation from physics, and in his initial publication in 1956 he referred to a *strain reaction* resulting in *stress*.[4,5] It was this strain reaction phenomenon that he had intended to focus on, but the resulting acceptance of stress as the pivotal concept forced him to create the word *stressor* for the causation and *stress* as the resulting response. Selye's definition of stress was a condition that evoked a shared set of responses to any demand that was placed on it.[5] To this point, the roles of specific stress effectors that had been identified and the mechanisms involved in achieving stability were not integrated; it was Selye who accomplished this.[2] Today, **stress** is seen as a direct consciously or indirect unconsciously sensed threat to stability of the organism.[4,7] Stress has a degree of specificity, depending to a certain extent on the stressor itself, and one's perceptions of its significance and ability to successfully adapt.[4,13]

Selye was experimenting with hormonal preparations in rats when he serendipitously uncovered a biological basis for stress.[4,14,15] He was expecting to find different changes in rats injected with different hormonal preparations but, to his amazement, the same three changes occurred each time. In every animal tested, the cortex of the adrenal gland enlarged, lymphatic organs (thymus, spleen, and lymph nodes) shrank, and in the stomach and duodenum, bleeding ulcers developed. When Selye experimented with noxious stimuli, the same three changes occurred. To Selye, the changes seemed to occur simultaneously and did not appear to be related to any particular kind of injury.[4] Any kind of harmful physical stimuli he used produced the same observed physiologic changes. Selye termed the harmful stimuli **stressors** and concluded that the changes observed represented a nonspecific response to any noxious stimulus, a general "stress response."[4] Because so many different agents caused the same changes, Selye called this process a **general adaptation syndrome (GAS)** with three components: an *alarm reaction*, a *stage of resistance*, and a *stage of exhaustion*. According to Selye's theory, when confronted by an injurious stimulus, individuals move through the first two stages repeatedly and consequently become adapted or habituated to the stressors they encounter during day-to-day life.[7,14,15] This nonspecific response to stress is now seen as a part of allostasis.

Selye's work in the 1920s concentrated on stimuli of a physical nature.[11] Beginning in the 1970s, researchers began to realize that perception of these stimuli was important to individuals' responses to stress, and that responses could be physiologic, as Selye described, as well as behavioral in nature. When stress is generated by extreme psychological or environmental demands, balance is disrupted, and allostatic reactions are initiated to endeavor to restore balance.[11] The discussion that follows presents the GAS as a reflection of the responses to these diverse stimuli and incorporates much of the knowledge acquired since the 1920s.

The General Adaptation Syndrome and Allostasis

Components of the GAS can be subdivided into three unique, largely physiologic stages (Table 2-1). Examining the stages separately is the best way to understand the entire GAS. The specific chemicals involved are among those seen today as integral to the broader view of allostatic responses to stress in the maintenance of homeostasis. All will be discussed later in the chapter.

Alarm Stage

The alarm stage has been called the **fight-or-flight response,** derived from Cannon's work, because it provides a surge of energy and physical alterations to either run from or confront danger (Figure 2-1). This stage begins when the hypothalamus, as it monitors the internal and external environment, senses a need to activate the GAS in response to a stimulus, a stressor placing the balance of homeostasis at risk. The stressor might be physical or emotional, positive or negative—an argument with a friend, an upper respiratory tract infection, running a marathon, or winning the lottery. The hypothalamus then mediates the activation of the sympathetic nervous system,

which in turn stimulates the adrenal medulla. Increased catecholamines enable the body to rapidly take action and the sympathetic nervous system coordinates multiple responses designed to fight or flee. The hypothalamus, through the secretion of corticotropic-releasing hormone (CRH), also stimulates the anterior pituitary gland to secrete adrenocorticotropic hormone (ACTH). ACTH then causes the adrenal cortex to release substantial amounts of the glucocorticoids, specifically cortisol, eliciting its diverse responses. This cascade of effects is termed the *hypothalamic-pituitary-adrenal* (HPA) axis. Once the pituitary gland is activated, the alarm stage cannot be turned off or deactivated; it must run its course, progressing to the stage of resistance. This coordinated systemic response to stress is illustrated in Figure 2-2.

The **allostatic state** is essentially the activity of these and other mediators integrating the various responses to evoke changes that return the organism to homeostasis. The allostatic state includes, but is not limited to, this specific stress response. Mediators of allostasis include these same hormones and neurotransmitters of the HPA axis and the autonomic nervous system,[16] and others presented later in this chapter.

Resistance

If the alarm stage were to persist, the body would soon suffer undue wear and tear and become subject to permanent damage.[14,15] Selye's resistance stage supports the allostatic return

TABLE 2-1

Stages of the General Adaptation Syndrome

Alarm	Resistance	Exhaustion
Increased secretion of glucocorticoids and responses	Normalization of glucocorticoid secretion	Increased glucocorticoid secretion followed by significant reduction
Increased sympathetic nervous system activity	Normalization of sympathetic nervous system activity	Triad of stress findings (hypertrophied adrenal glands, atrophied thymus and lymph nodes, bleeding ulcerations in stomach and duodenum)
Increased secretion of epinephrine from the adrenal medulla	Normalization of epinephrine secretion from adrenal medulla	
Fight-or-flight manifestations	Resolution of fight-or-flight manifestations	Loss of resistance to stressor; possible death of organism
Reduced resistance to stressors	Increased resistance (adaptation) to stressor	

FIGURE 2-1 Steps of Selye's Alarm Stage of the General Adaptation Syndrome. (Redrawn from McKenry L et al: *Mosby's pharmacology in nursing,* ed 22, St. Louis, 2006, Mosby.)

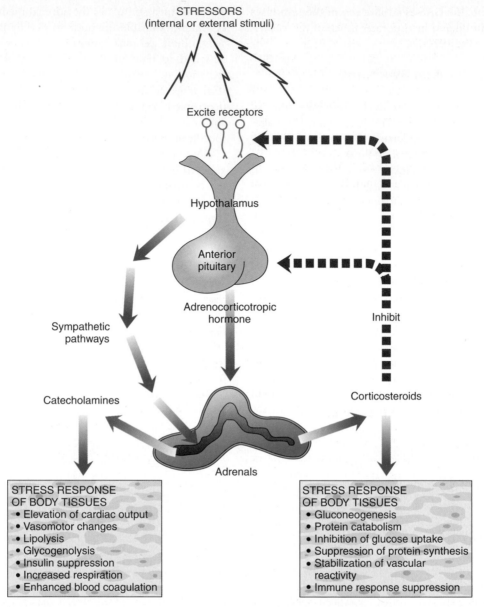

STRESSORS
(internal or external stimuli)

Excite receptors

Hypothalamus

Anterior
pituitary

Sympathetic
pathways

Adrenocorticotropic
hormone

Inhibit

Catecholamines

Corticosteroids

Adrenals

STRESS RESPONSE
OF BODY TISSUES
• Elevation of cardiac output
• Vasomotor changes
• Lipolysis
• Glycogenolysis
• Insulin suppression
• Increased respiration
• Enhanced blood coagulation

STRESS RESPONSE
OF BODY TISSUES
• Gluconeogenesis
• Protein catabolism
• Inhibition of glucose uptake
• Suppression of protein synthesis
• Stabilization of vascular
  reactivity
• Immune response suppression

FIGURE 2-2 Neuroendocrine interactions in response to a stressor. Receptors are excited by stressful stimuli and relay the information to the hypothalamus. The hypothalamus signals the adrenal cortex (by way of the pituitary) and the sympathetic pathways (by way of the autonomic nervous system). The stress response is then mediated by the catecholamines, epinephrine and norepinephrine, and by the glucocorticoids, predominantly cortisol.

to a state of homeostasis. As the body moves into the stage of resistance, the sympathetic nervous system and adrenal medulla and cortex are functioning at full force. If the stressor is adequately addressed and resolved, the organism returns to its steady-state; all of the mechanisms activated by the alarm stage return to their baseline level of functioning. This process described by Selye is clearly a part of the more recently described process of allostasis.

Exhaustion

Exhaustion occurs when the body is no longer able to bring about a return to homeostasis.[14,15] Selye postulated that when energy resources are completely depleted, death occurs because the organism is no longer able to adapt. He speculated

that individuals have both superficial and deep adaptive energy. Superficial adaptive energy can be replaced from deeper adaptive energy stores. However, when these deep adaptive energy stores are depleted, no other resource exists to facilitate recovery. It is with this stage that Selye's findings of a pathologic triad (hypertrophy of adrenal glands, atrophy of lymphoid tissues, and bleeding gastrointestinal ulcers) were associated.[14]

Stress is frequently psychosocial or psychological rather than physical in origin,[11] and the GAS theory fails to recognize this. Efforts to apply Selye's GAS theory to include psychosocial stress-related illness had significant limitations. The concept of allostasis addresses this gap. Conceptually, allostasis includes the stress response as the mechanism through which physiologic stability is maintained.[7] Adaptation efforts and pathologies evolving when these efforts fail are also compatible with the conceptualization of allostasis. Allostasis provides the link between the routine experiences of life and the more capricious disruptions, physical and psychological, that may arise across the life span.[7] The collective effect of an allostatic state on the organism is termed **allostatic load.**[5,7,10-11,16-19] When the mechanisms that facilitate the adjustments to life's demands are chronically over- or underactivated, the resulting bodily wear and tear is termed *allostatic load.*[10] Allostatic load is basically composed of the typical demands that are part of day-to-day life. However, with chronic, unremitting, or excessive demands, allostatic load can become an overload. This **allostatic overload** reflects the "cost" to the body's organs and tissues for an allostatic response that is excessive or ineffectively regulated.[16] It is essentially a reenvisioning of the effect of wear and tear on the body, both acutely and chronically, and is a more useful definition than homeostasis in discussions of pathophysiology.

Stressors and Risk Factors

Stressors are agents or conditions that are capable of producing stress and endangering homeostasis, initiating allostasis in order to return to a stable state. Every day the human organism encounters stressors. These may be external to the individual (e.g., air pollution, a motor vehicle accident) or internal (e.g., low blood glucose level or a threat to self-esteem). Common general stressors are physical (e.g., extreme hot or cold air temperature), chemical (e.g., auto exhaust), biological (e.g., bacteria and viruses), social (e.g., overcrowding and relationships), cultural (e.g., behavioral norms), or psychological (e.g., feelings of hopelessness). Stressors of an emotional or mental origin may be actually present or anticipated, and may lie in a neurochemical imbalance in the brain or the recollection of prior traumatic events. Less commonly noted but extremely powerful stressors are psychosocial experiences over which a person may have little or no personal control. Racial stressors[20,21] and socioeconomic stressors[22,23] can produce many of the manifestations of stress described in this chapter.

Stressors vary in their scope, intensity, and duration. A stressor of less intensity can still have a significant impact if it persists for some time. A glass of water held at arm's length poses little stress initially, but as minutes turn into hours the stress on the body escalates. Even events associated with happiness may serve as stressors—holidays, childbirth, and vacations. Stressors of all types challenge human adaptation.

The identification of specific stressors in isolation provides little insight into today's complex global society. Over the past several decades, research has explored innumerable factors that can indirectly increase or decrease the impact of stressors. It is now generally well accepted that inherent personal characteristics allow for a great deal of variation in the way humans respond to stressors.[24-27] The activation of the sympathetic nervous system response occurs with a wide variety of physical, mental, and psychosocial activities, whereas the HPA axis seems to respond more notably to psychosocial stressors when the individual's sense of self is involved.[26] Personality characteristics have been found to be associated with variations in cortisol release in the stress response.[25] Indeed, the effect of personality on the stress response differs with the situational context, that is, the characteristics of the stressor and the attributes of the available social support.[24]

Beginning in the early 1970s, researchers started to examine gender differences related to stress and recent research has continued to expand what is known about these differences between men and women.[17,26,28-30] For example, one study in the 1980s examined the differences in performance and stress responses of men and women under controlled laboratory conditions.[30] When subjected to a stressful task, there was a 50% to 100% increase in epinephrine release in men, whereas there was little if any increase noted in women, who were also found to perform as well or better than their male counterparts. Women did have an elevation in epinephrine release in a more real-life stress situation, an academic examination, but these elevations remained well below those of men.[30] Although some researchers consider these differences to be related to gender-associated roles and psychological factors as opposed to biological ones,[17] more recent researchers attribute these variances to the effect of the sex hormones on the stress response.[26,28] Variations in HPA axis function are noticeable during adolescence, when sex hormone secretion is significantly elevated in both males and females.[28] A prolonged HPA activation in response to stress in childhood has been documented in both genders when compared with that of adults. This physiologic finding has been suggested to impact the vulnerability of brain development in adolescents exposed to high levels of stress during this period.[28] Adult women during the period between menarche and menopause have lower stress responses than men of the same age.[26] It has been hypothesized that this is a physiologic evolutionary effort to protect the fetus from the effects of exposure to elevated levels of cortisol especially. Post-menopause, the responses of both the sympathetic nervous system and the HPA axis appear to increase.[26] The effects of gender are often inseparable from those of age, in human as well as animal models.[29,31] Clearly, stressors can affect the same person in different ways at different times over the course of a lifetime.

Risk factors are not of themselves stressors, but rather conditions or situations that increase the likelihood of encountering or experiencing a stressor. Eating while driving is a risk factor for having a motor vehicle accident; running in the dark is a risk factor for falling; inadequate immunization is a risk factor for certain illnesses or injuries. Risk factors include genetic predispositions as well as early life experiences.[16,18] By being aware of risk factors, it is possible to decrease the probability of exposure to certain stressors and their inevitable threat to homeostasis.

NEUROHORMONAL MEDIATORS OF STRESS AND ADAPTATION

Numerous hormones and signaling molecules are involved in the day-to-day maintenance of homeostasis through allostatic processes. These mediators are briefly described here, and their roles in allostasis, adaptation, and disease are discussed in later parts of this chapter. A key idea to the understanding of homeostasis is that once the allostatic load has been resolved, levels of these chemicals should return to their baselines. However, in cases of allostatic overload, pathologies of a physiologic, psychological, or behavioral nature may result.

Catecholamines: Norepinephrine and Epinephrine

Canon identified that the body's response to threats resulted in the activation of the adrenal medulla and sympathetic nervous system.[4] He deemed this "sympathico-adrenal system" ultimately responsible for what he termed the "*fight or flight*" reaction, whose purpose is the maintenance of the physical and psychological integrity of the organism.[5] He likewise underscored that dissimilar threats to homeostasis would elicit the same effect by activating the sympathoadrenal response. The catecholamine neurotransmitters play an integral role in allostasis.[16]

Release of catecholamine is initiated through the activation of the hypothalamus gland, a collection of nerve centers gathered together near the third ventricle near the base of the brain (see Chapter 39). It receives informational input from the body's internal environment, and the external environment as well. In response to these stressors, the hypothalamus prompts the release of **norepinephrine** from the sympathetic branch of the autonomic nervous system and epinephrine from the adrenal medulla. Norepinephrine is released by sympathetic neurons directly into the synaptic clefts near the effector organs and tissues. Preganglionic fibers from the sympathetic nervous system neurons synapse at the adrenal medulla, stimulating the release of epinephrine and, to a lesser extent, norepinephrine. Adrenal catecholamines are released into the bloodstream, and travel to effector organs and tissues (endocrine). These circulating catecholamines have essentially the same effects as sympathetic nerve stimulation and are often seen as an extension of the sympathetic nervous system. The responses on the part of the sympathetic nervous system and the adrenal medulla may differ according to the stimulus.[5] During situations such as exposure to temperature extremes, precipitous decreases in blood pressure, and slight exercise, the sympathetic nervous system response dominates. However, emotional distress or acute hypoglycemia cause the greatest response from the adrenal medulla.[5]

The effects of catecholamines are profound. They affect cardiovascular function; control fluid volume by activating the renin-angiotensin-aldosterone mechanism; have a role in inflammation and immunity; impact metabolism; and in the central nervous system, they are associated with attentiveness, arousal, and memory formation.[16] Norepinephrine is the primary constrictor of smooth muscle in all blood vessels. It therefore regulates blood flow through tissues and its distribution through the organs, as well as, importantly, maintenance of blood pressure. It also reduces gastric secretion and innervates the iris and ciliary muscles of the eyes, increasing night and far vision. Epinephrine enhances myocardial contractility, increases heart rate and venous return to the heart, thus increasing cardiac output and blood pressure. Epinephrine also has the metabolic effects of increasing glycogenolysis and the release of glucose from the liver. In the brain, the increased blood flow and availability of glucose lead to increases in mental attention and alertness. The effects of these catecholamines are summarized briefly in Table 2-2. For more detail, see Chapter 43.

Adrenocortical Steroids: Cortisol and Aldosterone

Among the most versatile hormones in the human body, glucocorticoids have regulatory roles in the cardiovascular system and fluid volume, and contribute to metabolism, immunity, and inflammatory responses, brain function, and even reproduction (Table 2-3).[16] Glucocorticoids are lipid-soluble hormones, allowing them to pass through cell membranes to bind with receptors in the cytosol or nucleus and initiate changes in cellular activities. Practically every body tissue has intracellular glucocorticoid receptors.[16] As opposed to the catecholamines, the onset of their effects is slower, but the duration is longer. Cushing is credited with identifying the role of the adrenocortical hormones in the maintenance of homeostasis, and particularly the effects of the glucocorticoid hormone, cortisol, and the results of its prolonged secretion at high levels.[2]

TABLE 2-2	
Brief Summary of Effects of Catecholamines on Tissues and Organs of the Body	
Tissue/Organ	**Catecholamine Effect**
Heart	Increases rate
	Increases speed of impulse conduction
	Increases contractility
Vascular smooth muscle	
Skin, mesenteric bed, kidneys	Constricts to reduce perfusion
Skeletal muscle, lungs, heart	Dilates to increase perfusion
Peripheral vasculature	Constricts to increase blood pressure
Gastrointestinal tract	Decreases peristalsis
	Contracts sphincters
Eyes	Contracts radial muscle to dilate iris
	Relaxes ciliary muscle for far vision
Liver	Glycogenolysis and gluconeogenesis for increased energy
Central nervous system	Promotes arousal, attention, and vigilance

TABLE 2-3	
Major Effects of Glucocorticoids in the Stress Response	
Metabolism	Catabolism of muscle, fat, lymphoid tissue, skin and bone
	Liver gluconeogenesis
	Opposes insulin in transport of glucose into cells
	Increased appetite
Fluid balance	Sodium and water retention
Inflammation and infection	Suppressed inflammatory response
	Increased neutrophil release
	Decreased new antibody release
	Decreased T lymphocyte production and function
	Decreased production of eosinophils, basophils, and monocytes
Support catecholamines	Increased epinephrine synthesis
	Enhanced vasoconstriction

The **glucocorticoids** are so named because of their significant role in glucose metabolism. The primary glucocorticoid, **cortisol,** is secreted by the adrenal cortex in response to ACTH from the anterior pituitary. Release of ACTH is itself affected by another releasing hormone, CRH from the hypothalamus.

The actions of the HPA axis may synergize or antagonize the effects of the catecholamines.[16] Catecholamines facilitate the release of ACTH, therefore helping to maintain the function of the HPA axis and release of cortisol. Glucocorticoids promote adrenal medulla synthesis of epinephrine through the control of the major enzyme, phenylethanolamine N methyl transferase (PNMT). Glucocorticoids also support the actions of the catecholamines in the maintenance of normal blood pressure and, therefore, cardiac output. In skeletal muscle, catecholamines antagonize the catabolic glucocorticoid effects by impeding the breakdown of somatic protein.[16] Together, the catecholamines and glucocorticoids facilitate the brain's development of memory, which is especially important when hazardous circumstances have occurred.[7]

The metabolic effects of cortisol are significant. Cortisol affects protein metabolism. It has an *anabolic* effect leading to increased rates of protein synthesis in the liver. However, it has a *catabolic* effect in muscle, lymphoid, and adipose tissues, and on skin and bone. This protein breakdown produces increased circulating amino acids. The resulting pooling of amino acids from catabolized proteins ensures their availability for the liver. Cortisol then stimulates gluconeogenesis in the liver and a six- to tenfold increase in the rate of amino acid conversion to ketoacids and glucose.

Gluconeogenesis ensures an adequate supply of glucose for body tissues in general, but nerve cells have priority. Cortisol may act to preserve available glucose for nerve cell use by limiting the uptake and oxidation of glucose by other cells in the body. Cortisol also promotes appetite and food-seeking behaviors.[16]

Glucocorticoids are known for their significant role in the control of the immune response. They suppress the acute-phase response to infection and inflammation, helping to curtail the possible effects of overactivity.[16] This is accomplished by inhibiting production of immune cytokines (signaling molecules), and in some cases by directly inhibiting the proliferation and activation of specific immune system cells.[16] At the same time, when the acute stress of tissue injury or infection occurs, the resulting release of glucocorticoids and catecholamines assists the movement of the necessary immune cells to that location.[7,16]

Aldosterone is the primary **mineralocorticoid** secreted by the adrenal cortex. Stimulation of the sympathetic nervous system activates the renin-angiotensin system, and the release of aldosterone is the final chemical outcome. The specific stressor of volume depletion also activates the release of renin, initiating this sequence of hormones. The primary effect of this steroid hormone, once bound to receptors in the kidneys' distal tubules and collecting ducts, is reabsorption of sodium and an increase in the excretion of potassium. Through osmotic force, water tends to follow sodium; therefore, enhanced reabsorption of sodium leads to increased extracellular fluid volume and increased blood pressure. Endogenous glucocorticoids have a small amount of mineralocorticoid effect, but the greatest effect on circulating volume is through aldosterone. Additionally, angiotensin II, whose formation stimulates aldosterone release, is a potent vasoconstrictor. This chemical mediator provides support for the catecholamine-induced increase in blood pressure.[16]

Endorphins and Enkephalins and Immune Cytokines

Stress naturally activates the inhibition of pain, through release of small peptides called endorphins and enkephalins.[32] **Endorphins** and enkephalins are endogenous opioids first discovered in 1975 that are produced within the central nervous system and released in response to stressors, by certain foods (most notably chocolate), laughter, massage, and acupuncture.[33] The term *endorphin* comes from *endogenous* and *morphine*. Like the opiate drug morphine, endorphins raise the pain threshold and produce sedation and euphoria. Some immune cells (T lymphocytes, granulocytes, and monocytes) also produce several types of endorphins that are released in response to stressors, CRH, antiinflammatory cytokines, and catecholamines.[32] Opioid receptors also have been identified on immune cells, and when activated, modulate both cell proliferation and function. Activated immune cells (mast cells, neutrophils, macrophages, and T lymphocytes) also release proinflammatory cytokines that add to pain.[32,34,35] Pain is a classic manifestation of the inflammatory response (Chapter 9). Thus the central and peripheral nervous systems and the immune system maintain a "pain-related" communication that serves as part of the allostatic mechanism to bring the system back toward homeostasis.[32]

Another example of the interaction between stress, the nervous system, and the immune system is interleukin-1, one of the cytokines secreted by macrophages, which is capable of impacting the production of CRH by the hypothalamus. Leukocytes are also capable of producing some of the hormones, such as ACTH, that are involved in the signaling system.[36,37] Some researchers propose that stressors of relatively short duration (less than 2 hours) could augment facets of immune function.[36] Most notable of these is the emigration of immune cells from the lymphoid tissues to the skin and peripheral components of the vascular system.[36] Numerous studies over the years have shown that severe and persistent psychological stress can down-regulate, or suppress, immune functioning through innumerable and complex mechanisms.[36,37] Immune system suppression brought about by severe or persistent stress represents a direct link between stress and illness. Expanded understanding of the interrelationships between the nervous, endocrine, and immune systems holds great promise in the identification of new therapeutic interventions.[36,37]

Sex Hormones: Estrogen, Testosterone, and Dehydroepiandrosterone

As noted previously, women during the period between menarche and menopause have a different stress response than men of the same age, and this may be attributable to influences of sex hormones on allostasis. Cortisol exerts inhibiting effects on the female reproductive system by suppressing release of luteinizing hormone, estradiol, and progesterone. Excessive stress appears, in general, to inhibit female reproduction. However, sexual stimulation may cause the gonadal axis to be resistant to suppression by the HPA axis. Estradiol down-regulates glucocorticoid receptor binding in the brain and alters regulatory feedback control. Androgens, such as testosterone and dehydroepiandrosterone (DHEA), may also inhibit the effects of glucocorticoids.[16] Androgens oppose the catabolic effects of glucocorticoids on bone and the impact of glucocorticoids on lymphoid tissues, inflammatory cytokines, and leukocytes. DHEA interacts with numerous neurotransmitters in the brain, counteracting the depressive tendencies often noted with glucocorticoids.[16] Numerous stressful stimuli, such as illness, surgery, heavy physical exercise, heart failure, and stressful academic programs result in a significant reduction in circulating testosterone levels. In combination with another hormone, vasopressin, testosterone enhances blood pressure and heart rate reactivity and enhances the "fight or flight" response. Estrogen, in combination with the hormone oxytocin, described below, is thought to produce a calming effect during times of stress, resulting in the notion that women may have a "tend and befriend" response, rather than a "fight or flight" response in some situations.

Growth Hormone, Prolactin, and Oxytocin

Growth hormone (somatotropin) is released from the anterior pituitary gland and affects protein, lipid, and carbohydrate metabolism. It has anabolic effects, increasing protein synthesis and fat mobilization while decreasing the rate of carbohydrate utilization by the body.[16] Growth hormone is normally secreted in a cyclic basal pattern according to developmental proscriptions. Serum levels of growth hormone also increase following a variety of intensely stressful physical or psychological stimuli, such as strenuous exercise or extreme fear.[10,16] Growth hormone appears to enhance immune function.

Prolactin is similar in structure to growth hormone and is also secreted from the anterior pituitary in response to stress, sexual activity, and suckling. Numerous tissues have receptors for prolactin in addition to the breast, including kidney, liver, and adrenal glands. Lymphocytes also have prolactin receptors, suggesting a role for prolactin in immune regulation. A significant increase in growth hormone or prolactin tends to require more intense stimuli than the stress that increases catecholamines and glucocorticoids.

Oxytocin is produced during childbirth, lactation, and orgasm (in both genders) and has been associated with promoting bonding and social attachment. Oxytocin is thought to moderate the stress response and have a calming effect, with reductions in HPA activation and reduced perceived anxiety.

Through interactions of the primary stress hormones, catecholamines, and glucocorticoids, as well as numerous other mediating influences, the allostatic process needed to sustain the human organism is achieved. In some cases, these stress-related hormones have similar and synergistic effects and in others they work in opposition. This state of counterbalancing helps to control allostasis, ideally moving back toward homeostasis.

KEY POINTS

- The foundations of modern views of allostatic maintenance of homeostasis in the face of stress are primarily derived from an understanding of negative feedback, as well as the roles of the sympathetic nervous system and the glucocorticoid, cortisol.

- The primary role of the sympathetic nervous system is appraisal of a stressful stimulus and release of norepinephrine. Norepinephrine released from sympathetic nerve endings increases heart rate and contractility, constricts blood vessels, enhances blood flow to skeletal muscle, reduces gastrointestinal motility and secretion, and dilates the pupils.

- Stress simultaneously stimulates sympathetic activation of the adrenal medulla to release epinephrine. Epinephrine's actions are similar to those of norepinephrine and are particularly important for increasing cardiac performance and the release of glucose from the liver.

- Cortisol, from the adrenal cortex, has widespread effects on numerous tissues that are both synergetic and antagonistic with catecholamines, and has an antiinflammatory role.

- Aldosterone promotes volume expansion and increases blood pressure.

- Confronted by painful stressors, release of endorphins in the central nervous system (CNS) increases, leading to decreased perception of pain, sedation, and euphoria. Immune cells in the periphery also contribute to pain modulation.

- Understanding of the role of the immune system in the response to stressors is rapidly expanding. Immune cells respond to the hormones released by the HPA axis and sympathetic nervous system. They also release cytokines that in turn affect the functioning of these systems.

- Sex hormones and differential release of growth hormone, prolactin, and oxytocin produce mediating effects on the stress response that may differ between genders.

ADAPTATION, COPING, AND ILLNESS

Although much has been learned about the dynamic biological systems and human environment interactions involved, stress is personal in that individual stress responses change with time and circumstances. Indeed, the effects of stress on each individual are impacted by genetics and culture, prior susceptibilities, preexisting health status, allostatic state, and individual abilities to manage stress.[2] Clearly, the maintenance of homeostasis requires the human organism to routinely initiate allostatic responses to the stressors of day-to-day life, as well as the less frequent severe assaults on the integrity of the body and the mind, responsible for allostatic load. The roles of the sympathetic nervous system and the HPA axis have been defined and supportive chemical mediators described. Systemically, allostasis may be seen as beginning with some degree of the alarm stage/fight-or-flight activation, and ideally moving to an effective resolution through adaptation, ultimately culminating in a return to homeostasis. The effects of this process are seen in allostatic load and the occasional allostatic overload. The prolonged effects of allostatic overload—the long-term wear-and-tear costs of adaptation efforts—provide a conceptual foundation for examining the long-term consequences of stress to health.[5] What Selye called "diseases of adaptation" are the outcome of allostatic overload exacerbating pathophysiologic change.[38]

Adaptation and Coping

Adaptation, seen from the perspective of allostasis rather than simply Selye's stage of the GAS, broadly refers to the biopsychosocial process of change in response to new or altered circumstances, internal and external in origin.[10,39] Encountering favorable or unfavorable stressors requires multiple levels of biological, personal, and social change or adaptation. *Maladaptation,* a less frequently used term, refers to ineffective, inadequate, or inappropriate change in response to new or altered circumstances. **Coping** is another term used and is most often seen as a behavioral adaptive response to a stressor. Coping mechanisms are typically culturally based, and so vary with the individual within the parameters of what is acceptable to the given culture. The coping behavior is usually dictated by the specific stressor; thus, it commonly varies with the circumstances, but individuals typically embrace a specific repertoire of behaviors. These behavioral adaptations allow an individual or a group to withstand successfully the stressful experience or the stress response generated by the experience. A coping strategy can be considered effective or functional if it helps resolve either the situation or the feelings. In some cases, such as exercise, the coping method can promote health.[10] A coping strategy is considered ineffective or dysfunctional if it does not achieve the desired goal. Coping that achieves unintended goals is considered dysfunctional. Being complex organisms, adaptation may result in the adoption of less than desirable coping behaviors, such as excessive eating or alcohol consumption, smoking or other types of substance abuse.[7] Unfortunately, these dysfunctional coping behaviors can ultimately be damaging to overall health.[10] Smoking and overeating contribute to atherosclerosis, the underlying pathophysiology of coronary artery disease and a risk factor for hypertension. Excess weight accumulated through overeating is a contributing factor for type 2 diabetes mellitus. Although coping is customarily interpreted as behavioral adaptation only, the terms *coping* and *adapting* often are used interchangeably.

Perception and expectations of the stressor can affect its interpretation, and therefore the behavior evoked by it. Perceptions can be related to uncertainty about the meaning of the stressor. Consider the stressor of undue noise. The "bang" of a car backfiring could also be the sound of a gun being fired. Depending upon the environment and circumstances, one or the other etiology would be more expected, dictating different adaptive responses. The term *distress* describes the experience of perceiving an inability to cope with a stressor.[5] This distress further activates the HPA axis, escalating levels of circulating mediators, and may exacerbate existing allostatic load and preexisting pathophysiologic conditions.[5] For instance, the person with asthma who is experiencing an episode of acute shortness of breath is likely to become even more so on finding an inhaler is not readily available.

Adaptation to a particular stressor can come about in several ways. Loud noise is a known stressor. Yet people who live close to busy airports often reach a point at which they barely notice the noise of airplanes flying over their homes. They become *habituated* to the stressor (loud noise). One important way to habituate to a stressor is to manipulate or "train" the hypothalamus to react less forcefully to a perceived threat or stressor. Repeatedly ignoring a specific stressor prevents the inappropriate triggering of the GAS. The result is a more acceptable level of stress response. Techniques that accomplish this **desensitization** change the predominant brain waves of the individual from beta to alpha waves, which are slower and more normal. Biofeedback, visualization, and meditation are examples of therapies that use this principle. Practicing these techniques for 20 to 30 minutes daily can enhance the ability to alter how a stressor is perceived and modulate the stress response. These techniques have documented efficacy in modulating immune function.[36] Desensitization methods have been found to be beneficial for common stress-related conditions, such as migraine headache, chronic back pain, and hypertension.

Allostatic Overload and Illness

When adaptation mechanisms are inadequate or the total amount of allostatic load is excessive, overwhelming allostasis capacities, the result is allostatic overload. There are several ways in which allostatic load can accumulate in an individual: (1) the response may diminish due to repetitive exposure to a specific stimulus; (2) the response may fail to terminate once the stimulus is removed; (3) the response may decrease over time when the stress is ongoing for a lengthy period; (4) there may be insufficient quantities of the chemicals required to maintain the response.[11,16,39,40] Homeostasis, the steady-state that previously existed, cannot be attained. Instead, allostatic overload occurs and the resulting maladaptation can be reflected in a range of pathophysiologic states that cut across the traditional boundaries of health care, from psychiatric and endocrine disorders to inflammatory disease.

Hair loss, emotional tension, mouth sores, asthma, heart palpitations, neuromuscular movement disorders (tics), tension headaches, muscle contraction backache, digestive disorders, and irritable bladder are just a few of the common disorders that can be caused by or worsened by stress. Skin outbreaks such as acne, reproductive disorders such as menstrual irregularity in women, and male impotence also have been linked with the effects of allostatic overload. Box 2-2 summarizes some of the physiologic and psychological effects of excessive stress. Figure 2-3 depicts the multiple body organs

---

BOX 2-2

Physical and Behavioral Indicators of High Stress

Physical Indicators
Elevated blood pressure
Increased muscle tension
Elevated pulse
Increased respiration
Sweaty palms
Cold extremities (hands and feet)
Fatigue
Tension headache
Upset stomach: nausea, vomiting, diarrhea
Change in appetite
Change in weight
Increased blood catecholamine level
Hyperglycemia
Restlessness
Insomnia

Behavioral and Emotional Indicators
Anxiety (nonspecific fears)
Depression
Increased use of mind-altering substances (e.g., alcohol, chemical substances)
Change in eating, sleeping, or activity pattern
Mental exhaustion
Feelings of inadequacy; loss of self-esteem
Increased irritability
Loss of motivation
Decreased productivity
Inability to make good judgments
Inability to concentrate
Increased absenteeism and illness
Increased proneness to accidents

---

and systems in which the effects of insufficient or overactive stress responses may be seen.

There is a clear physiologic basis for the role of the chemical mediators of stress and illness. Cortisol being released from the adrenal cortex supports resistance but may also be accountable for pathologic changes.[4,39,40] The same can be said of the catecholamines and the other chemical mediators. Because these blood-borne chemicals have such broad effects systemically, the impact of excessive or inadequate amounts is understandably wide reaching. In some cases, the relationships have been well substantiated by research; in others, they are hypothesized based upon knowledge of the effects of these chemicals.

The relationship between excessive catecholamine levels and what have been called "stress-related" illnesses historically has been most often associated with cardiovascular pathologies such as hypertension, stroke, and myocardial infarction.[10,17] Abdominal fat cells are well supplied with cortisol receptors.[17] Excessive secretion of cortisol results in the collection of fat in this area. When this fat is released into the bloodstream, the resulting increase in circulating free fatty acids plays a role in cardiovascular risk.[17] Repeated or prolonged elevation of the blood pressure, especially in combination with the metabolic effects of elevated cortisol levels, promotes the development of

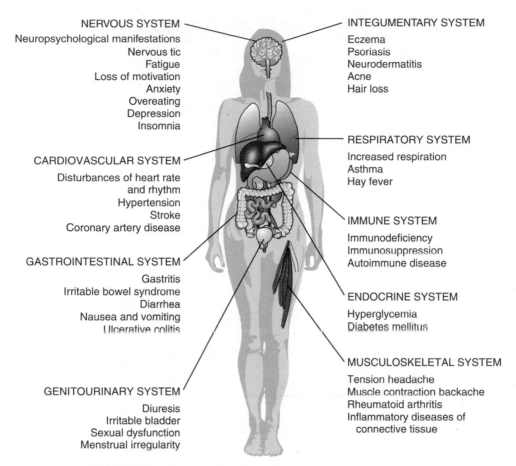

NERVOUS SYSTEM

Neuropsychological manifestations
Nervous tic
Fatigue
Loss of motivation
Anxiety
Overeating
Depression
Insomnia

CARDIOVASCULAR SYSTEM

Disturbances of heart rate
and rhythm
Hypertension
Stroke
Coronary artery disease

GASTROINTESTINAL SYSTEM

Gastritis
Irritable bowel syndrome
Diarrhea
Nausea and vomiting
Ulcerative colitis

GENITOURINARY SYSTEM

Diuresis
Irritable bladder
Sexual dysfunction
Menstrual irregularity

INTEGUMENTARY SYSTEM

Eczema
Psoriasis
Neurodermatitis
Acne
Hair loss

RESPIRATORY SYSTEM

Increased respiration
Asthma
Hay fever

IMMUNE SYSTEM

Immunodeficiency
Immunosuppression
Autoimmune disease

ENDOCRINE SYSTEM

Hyperglycemia
Diabetes mellitus

MUSCULOSKELETAL SYSTEM

Tension headache
Muscle contraction backache
Rheumatoid arthritis
Inflammatory diseases of
connective tissue

FIGURE 2-3 Effects of allostatic overload on body organs and systems.

atherosclerosis and, ultimately, the development of the many cardiovascular pathologies.[38] Catecholamines not only contribute to the development of atherosclerosis, they increase platelet activity resulting in clot formation and serum lipid levels, significant factors in the pathogenesis of myocardial infarction.[17,19] Cardiac hypertrophy is one outcome of prolonged hypertension and compensation following myocardial infarction.[4] Chronically elevated sympathetic nervous system activity accelerates this process, which ultimately results in heart failure.[4]

The field of psychoneuroimmunology has provided substantive evidence of the role of the stress hormones in the brain. In the central nervous system, specifically the brain, the mediators of adaptation facilitate learning, memory, neuroendocrine and autonomic regulation.[10,19] This heightened memory allows the individual to be more aware of the potential stressor in the future.[38] Chronic over- or underactivity results in atrophy and death of some nerve cells, impairing memory,[10,38] whereas others have been found to proliferate, resulting in an increase in fear.[38] Enhanced cognitive function supports allostasis, whereas allostatic overload results in impaired cognitive function.[17] Stress hormones have been found to be elevated in major depressive illness.[19] In addition, other effects of long-term cortisol dysregulation, including demineralization of bone and increased abdominal fat deposits, are

noted. The normal pattern of cortisol secretion is impaired, elevated androgen levels have been found in women, and increased levels of growth hormone are all documented in major depressive illness.[19] Studies have found levels of cortisol and certain cytokines from immune cells to be elevated in depressed patients with fibromyalgia[41] and multiple sclerosis.[42] Depression is common with chronic disease, and the elevated cortisol levels associated with allostatic overload may be a significant finding in association with depression and the progression of some of the diseases.

Allostatic mediators activate and maintain energy reserves, whereas obesity, diabetes, and atherosclerosis are associated with their chronic activation.[10,17,38,40] The food-seeking behavior initiated by cortisol is beneficial in the short term, but when cortisol levels are increased by chronic stress of either a physiologic or psychological origin, this adaptation gone awry results in obesity. Obesity is a risk factor for decreased effectiveness of glucose transport into the cells (insulin resistance), the pathophysiologic basis for type 2 diabetes.[38] Elevated cortisol levels also directly increase insulin resistance.[4,17]

In acute stress, activation of the immune system allows for the coordinated defense of the body from damage.[10,38] Chronic activation of these same mediators produces immunosuppression and increases the risk of infection[10,7,36,38] and has been implicated in the development of autoimmune diseases.[10] Such overaction also prolongs existing infections.[36] Research supports the hypothesis that physical and emotional stress and dysfunctional coping mechanisms impair both antibody and T cell-mediated responses to viruses and antiviral and antibacterial vaccines. Stressors of more than 1 month's duration have been found to be the greatest predictors of the development of colds. Cumulated evidence, in both human and animal models, supports the role that stress-induced dysregulation of the cellular and humoral arms of the immune system increases risk of infectious disease. Stress has been found by numerous studies to accelerate the progression of HIV infection. Immune dysregulation can also include the excessive production of cytokines that have actions supporting the inflammatory response. Both physical and psychological stressors have been found to accomplish this, sensitizing the overall inflammatory response so that subsequent activations are markedly increased. This is important because many diseases are associated with inflammation: cancer, acute coronary syndrome resulting in myocardial infarction, chronic inflammatory bowel disease, and asthma, to name but a few. Wound healing is impaired by multiple mediators of stress in excessive amounts.[36,37]

KEY POINTS

- Adaptation, or allostasis, is a network of biopsychosocial processes of responding to a stressor with the goal of reestablishing homeostasis. Coping mechanisms are usually seen as behavioral adaptations to stress but are often used interchangeably with adaptation.
- The effect of adaptation on the body and mind is the allostatic load. It reflects the cumulative cost of adaptation.
- A number of disorders are thought to be related to excessive stress or inappropriate stress responses—allostatic overload. These are a result of the dysregulation of the mechanisms and mediators involved in the stress response.

SUMMARY

Homeostasis is the state of balance of the body's biopsychosocial systems. Stressors evoke a stress response and initiate adaptive efforts, an allostatic process, designed to return to this steady-state. The response to stressors is affected by a wide variety of factors. Recently there has been an exponential increase in knowledge regarding the complex interactions of the HPA axis, the sympathetic nervous system, and their chemical mediators of the stress response.

Excessive or prolonged stress and over- or underactivity of these chemical mediators produce disproportionate responses in the body, a condition of allostatic overload known as stress-induced illness. As humans strive to adapt to the constant changes of modern life, the study of stress and stress-related disease has become vital to public health and contributes to the development of increasingly sophisticated models of health and illness.

REFERENCES

1. McEwen B, Lasley EN: All stressed out? Here's what to do about it, *Consumers' Res* 1:10-13, 29, 2003.
2. Moal ML: Historical approach and evolution of the stress concept: a personal account, *Psychoneuroendocrinology* 32:S3-S9, 2007.
3. Clendening L: *Sourcebook of medical history,* New York, 1942, Dover Publications.
4. Goldstein DS, Kopin IJ: Evolution of concepts of stress, *Stress* 10:109-120, 2007.
5. Goldstein DS, McEwen B: Allostasis, homeostasis, and the nature of stress, *Stress* 5:55-58, 2002.
6. Buchman TG: The community of the self, *Nature* 420:246-251, 2002.
7. McEwen BS, Wingfield JC: The concept of allostasis in biology and biomedicine, *Horm Behav* 43:2-15, 2003.
8. Carpenter RHS: Homeostasis: a plea for a unified approach, *Adv Physiol Educ* 28:S180-S187, 2004.
9. Powers WT: *Behaviour: The control of perception,* London, 1973, Wildwood House.
10. McEwen BS: Stress, adaptation, and disease: allostasis and allostatic load, *Ann NY Acad Sci* 840:33-44, 1998.
11. Stewart JA: The detrimental effects of allostasis: allostatic load as a measure of cumulative stress, *J Physiol Anthropol* 25:133-145, 2006.
12. Day TA: Defining stress as a prelude to mapping its neurocircuitry: no help from allostasis, *Prog Neuropsychopharmacol Biol Psychiatry* 29:1195-1200, 2005.
13. Goldstein DS: *The autonomic nervous system in health and disease,* New York, 2001, Marcel Decker, Inc.
14. Selye H: The general adaptation syndrome and the diseases of adaptation, *J Clin Endocrinol* 6:117-230, 1946.
15. Selye H: *The stress of life,* ed 2, New York, 1976, McGraw-Hill.
16. McEwen B: Interacting mediators of allostasis and allostatic load: towards an understanding of resilience in aging, *Metabolism* 52:10-16, 2003.
17. Lundberg U: Stress hormones in health and illness: the roles of work and gender, *Psychoneuroendocrinology* 30:1017-1021, 2005.
18. McEwen B: Early life influences on life-long patterns of behavior and health, *Ment Retard Dev Disabil Res Rev* 9:149-154, 2003.
19. McEwen B: Mood disorders and allostatic load, *Biol Psychiatry* 54:200-207, 2003.
20. Khaylis A, Waelde LC, Bruce EJ: The role of ethnic identity in the relationship of race-related stress to PTSD symptoms among young adults, *J Trauma Dissociation* 8:91-105, 2007.
21. Choi H, Meininger JC, Roberts RE: Ethnic differences in adolescents' mental distress, social stress, and resources, *Adolescence* 41:263-283, 2006.
22. Dowd JB, Goldman N: Do biomarkers of stress mediate the relation between socioeconomic status and health? *J Epidemiol Community Health* 60:633-639, 2006.
23. Suchday S, Krantz DS, Gottdiener JS: Relationship of socioeconomic markers to daily life ischemia and blood pressure reactivity in coronary artery disease patients, *Ann Behav Med* 30:74-84, 2005.
24. DeLongis A, Holtzman S: Coping in context: the role of stress, social support, and personality in coping, *J Pers* 73:1633-1656, 2005.
25. Oswald LM et al: Relationship between cortisol responses to stress and personality, *Neuropsychopharmacology* 31:1583-1591, 2006.
26. Kajantie E, Phillips DI: The effects of sex and hormonal status on the physiological response to acute psychosocial stress, *Psychoneuroendocrinology* 31:151-178, 2005.
27. Glei DA et al: Do chronic stressors lead to physiological dysregulation? Testing the theory of allostatic load, *Psychosom Med* 69:769-776, 2007.
28. McCormick CM, Mathews IZ: HPA function in adolescence: role of sex hormones in its regulation and the enduring consequences of exposure to stressors, *Pharmacol Biochem Behav* 86:220-233, 2007.

29. Luine VN et al: Chronic stress and neural function: accounting for sex and age, *J Neuroendocrinol* 19:743-751, 2007.

30. Frankenhaeuser M: The sympathetic-adrenal and the pituitary-adrenal resonse to challenge: comparison between the sexes. In Dembroski TM, Smidt TH, Blumchen G, editors: *Biobehavioral bases of coronary heart disease,* New York, 1983, Karger, pp 91-105.

31. Neupert SD, Almeida DM, Charles ST: Age differences in reactivity to daily stressors: the role of personal control, *J Gerontol B Psychol Sci Soc Sci* 62:P216-225, 2007.

32. Machelska H: Targeting of opioids-producing leukocytes for pain control, *Neuropeptides* 41:355-363, 2007.

33. Davidson MW: The endorphin collection, Florida State University. Available at http://micro.magnet.fsu.edu/micro/gallery/endorphin/endorphins.html

34. Zhang J, Huang Y: The immune system: a new look at pain, *Chin Med J* 119:930-938, 2006.

35. Thacker MA et al: Pathophysiology of peripheral neuropathic pain: immune cells and molecules, *Anesth Analg* 105:838-847, 2007.

36. Glaser R, Kiecolt-Glaser JK: Stress-induced immune dysfunction: implications for health, *Nat Rev Immunol* 5:243-251, 2005.

37. Godbout JP, Glaser R: Stress-induced immune dysregulation: implications for wound healing, infectious diseases and cancer, *J Neuroimmune Pharmacol* 1:421-427, 2006.

38. McEwen BS: Stressed or stressed out: What is the difference? *J Psychiatry Neurosci* 30:316-318, 2005.

39. Schulkin J: *Rethinking homeostasis: allostatic regulation in physiology and pathophysiology,* Cambridge, Mass, 2003, MIT Press.

40. Schulkin J: *Allostasis, homeostasis and the costs of physiological adaptation,* New York, 2004, Cambridge Press.

41. Van Houdenhove B, Luyten P: Stress, depression and fibromyalgia, *Acta Neurol Belg* 106:149-156, 2006.

42. Pucak ML, Carroll KA, Kerr DA, Kaplin AL: Neuropsychiatric manifestations of depression in multiple sclerosis: neuroinflammatory, neuroendocrine, and neurotrophic mechanisms in the pathogenesis of immune-mediated depression, *Dialogues Clin Neurosci* 9:125-139, 2007.

PART 2

Alterations in Cellular Function, Genetics, and Development

Frontiers of Research

Genes and Genetic Disorders

Sheila K. Smith

Genes are the reproductive material that carry information for making proteins. Genes direct the activities of cells, regulate organ system functions, and influence visible and invisible inherited traits of individuals and families. Genomics is the study of human genes, including study of interactions between genes, the environment, and human health and disease. In 2003, the Human Genome Project was completed. This was a 13-year effort to map the approximately 25,000 genes that comprise human DNA. Completion of this project was a milestone in molecular biology and genetics. Much of the information from the Human Genome Project is now being used in the development of new medical theory, treatment approaches, and disease prevention.

2007 has been established as the year in which the science of genomics became available to individuals for personal use, with direct-to-consumer genetic risk testing now available for a range of diseases. For about $350,000 it is now possible to obtain one's full genome sequence; for about $1,000 one can order an assay indicating personal risk for approximately 1 million genetic variations.

By studying the entire genome of large numbers of persons with specific diseases, specific genetic variations have been identified that increase the risk for developing Alzheimer disease, Crohn disease, type 1 and type 2 diabetes, bipolar disorder, rheumatoid arthritis, and coronary artery disease. Rearrangements of large chunks of DNA—replications, deletions,

Chromosome painting with a library of chromosome 22-specific DNA probes. The presence of three fluorescent chromosomes indicates that the patient has trisomy 22. (From Kumar V et al: Robbins and Cotran pathologic basis of disease, ed 7, Philadelphia, 2005, Saunders, p 173. Courtesy Dr. Charleen M. Moore, The University of Texas Health Science Center at San Antonio, Tex.)

Cellular Function

reorganizations—have been found to be involved in certain disease susceptibilities and human genetic variations. These large structural differences have been particularly identified within the immune system.

Important advances in stem cell research have occurred as well. Stem cell research has been a highly controversial area of genetic research, relying upon the use of human embryonic stem cell lines. Stem cells are unique in that they are pluripotent, meaning they can differentiate into any type of specialized tissue. They also have the capacity to reproduce indefinitely in their undifferentiated state. Because of this, stem cells have been invaluable in the treatment of diseases such as lymphomas and leukemias, in which the diseased individual's own lymphocyte or white blood cell production has become severely deregulated or destroyed. By exposing human skin cells to specific genes, stem cell researchers were able to develop cells that act like stem cells. This development may provide an approach to conducting stem cell research without the difficult ethical questions that arise from the use of human embryo cell lines or from therapeutic cloning. It also may allow a way to develop stem cells that are genetically matched to the individual, an enormous advantage due to the dangers of tissue rejection with stem cell transplantation.

Cell Structure and Function

Jacquelyn L. Banasik

MEDIA RESOURCES

Additional Material for Study, Review, and Further Exploration

CD Companion ■ Review Questions and Answers
■ Glossary (with audio pronunciations for selected terms)
■ Disease Profiles ■ Animations

evolve **Website** at http://evolve.elsevier.com/Copstead/
■ Case Studies ■ Disease Profiles ■ WebLinks ■ Key Points Review

Online Course (Module 1)

KEY QUESTIONS

■ What are the major cellular structures and their functions?
■ How do cells acquire and use energy?
■ How are substances transported across the cell membrane?
■ Why is it that some cells can produce action potentials and others cannot?

■ How do cells in a multicellular organism communicate with one another?
■ What are the normal mechanisms of cellular growth control?

CHAPTER OUTLINE

basic principle of biology states that the cell is the fundamental unit of life. As more diseases are understood on the cellular and molecular levels, it appears that the cell is also the fundamental unit of disease. A knowledge explosion is currently occurring in the fields of cell and molecular biology, leading to a better understanding of human physiology and the cellular aspects of disease. Detailed knowledge of cellular dysfunction has led to the development of more specific and appropriate prevention and treatment modalities for many disease processes. Thus, an understanding of cellular mechanisms is essential for health care providers and fundamental to the discussions of pathophysiologic processes presented throughout the remainder of this text.

Cells are complex, membrane-bound units packed with a multitude of chemicals and macromolecules. They are able to replicate and thus form new cells and organisms. The very first cells on earth probably arose from the spontaneous association of organic (carbon-containing) and inorganic molecules about 3.5 billion years ago.[1] Over billions of years, the self-replicating molecules now known as deoxyribonucleic acid (DNA) and ribonucleic acid (RNA) are believed to have evolved by chance association and natural selection. Evolution

of the cell membrane created a closed compartment that provided a selective advantage for the cell and accomplished the first separation of life (inside) from nonlife (outside). In this protected environment, the early cells continued to evolve and develop. Today, a number of different cell types exist, but many of the basic biochemical mechanisms of these cell types are remarkably similar. Scientists believe that all modern cells, from bacteria to human neurons, evolved from common primordial cells.[2] It is therefore possible to unlock many of the secrets of human cellular physiology by studying easily grown and rapidly proliferating cells, such as yeasts and bacteria.

Much of our knowledge of cell physiology has derived from study of the class of cells known as **prokaryotic,** which includes bacteria and archaea. Prokaryotic cells are smaller and simpler than **eukaryotic** cells, having no defined nucleus or cytoplasmic organelles. Fungi, plants, and animals belong to the eukaryotic class of cells, which possess a membrane-bound nucleus and a host of cytoplasmic organelles (Figure 3-1). In this chapter, the essentials of eukaryotic cell structure, physiology, metabolism, and communication are reviewed.

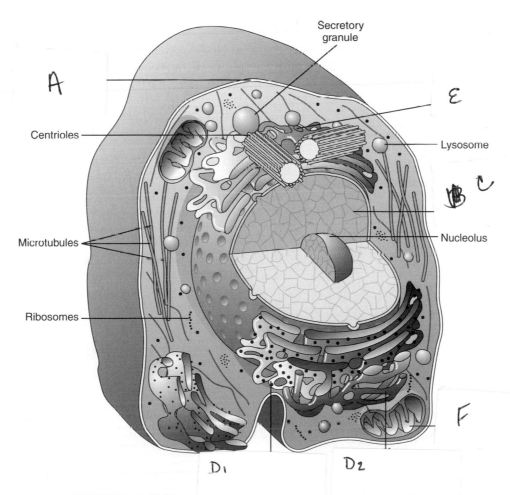

FIGURE 3-1 Structure o   wing intracellular organelles.

PLASMA MEMBRANE
Membrane Structure

All cells are enclosed by a barrier composed primarily of lipid and protein called the **plasma membrane** (plasmalemma). This cell membrane is a highly selective filter that shields internal cell contents from the external environment. The plasma membrane performs a variety of functions, including transport of nutrients and waste products, generation of membrane potentials, and cell recognition, communication, and growth regulation. The cell membrane is a sensor of signals and enables the cell to respond and adapt to changes in its environment.

According to the fluid mosaic model first described in the 1960s by Singer and Nicolson,[3] the plasma membrane is a dynamic assembly of lipid and protein molecules. Most of the lipids and proteins move about rapidly in the fluid structure of the membrane. As shown in Figure 3-2, the lipid molecules are arranged in a double layer, or **lipid bilayer,** which is highly impermeable to most water-soluble molecules, including ions, glucose, and proteins. A variety of proteins embedded or "dissolved" in the lipid bilayer perform most of the membrane's functions. Some membrane proteins are involved in the transport of specific molecules into and out of the cell; others function as enzymes or respond to external signals; and some serve as structural links that connect the plasma membrane to adjacent cells. The lipid structure of the plasma membrane is similar to the membrane that surrounds the cell's organelles (nucleus, mitochondria, endoplasmic reticulum, Golgi apparatus, lysosomes).

Lipid Bilayer

The bilayer structure of all biological membranes is related to the special properties of lipid molecules that cause them to spontaneously assemble into bilayers. The three major types of membrane lipids are cholesterol, phospholipids, and glycolipids. All three have a molecular structure that is **amphipathic;** that is, they have a hydrophilic (water-loving) charged or polar end and a hydrophobic (water-fearing) nonpolar end.[1] This amphipathic nature causes the lipids to form bilayers in aqueous solution. A typical phospholipid molecule is shown in Figure 3-3. The hydrophobic nonpolar tails tend to associate with other hydrophobic nonpolar-tail groups to avoid association with polar water molecules. The hydrophilic polar head groups preferentially interact with the surrounding aqueous environment. A bilayer, with tails sandwiched in the middle, allows both portions of the lipid molecules to be chemically "satisfied." In addition, the lipid bilayers tend to close on themselves, forming sealed, spherical compartments (Figure 3-4). If the membrane is punctured or torn, it will spontaneously reseal itself to eliminate contact of the hydrophobic tails with water.

For the most part, individual lipid and protein molecules can diffuse freely and rapidly within the plane of the bilayer, but flip from one side to the other infrequently.[4] The degree of membrane fluidity depends on the lipid composition. Saturated lipids have straight tails that can pack together and tend to stiffen the membrane, whereas lipids with bent, unsaturated hydrocarbon tails tend to increase fluidity. About 50% of the lipid in eukaryotic cell membranes is cholesterol, which serves to decrease membrane permeability and prevent leakage of small water-soluble molecules. In addition to affecting fluidity by the degree of saturation of tail groups, the phospholipids that inhabit the membrane also differ in the size, shape, and charge of the polar head groups. Figure 3-5 shows the structures of the four most prevalent membrane phospholipids: phosphatidylethanolamine, phosphatidylserine, phosphatidylcholine, and sphingomyelin. Some membrane-bound proteins require specific phospholipid head groups to function properly. Some lipids—sphingolipids and cholesterol in particular—may bind together transiently to form rafts in the sea of moving lipids. These rafts may surround and help organize membrane proteins into functional units. For example, a membrane receptor and its intracellular target proteins may associate together in a raft to facilitate transfer of information across the membrane.[4]

Glycolipids contain one or more sugar molecules at the polar head region. Interestingly, glycolipids and glycoproteins are found only in the outer half of the lipid bilayer, with the sugar groups exposed at the cell surface (Figure 3-6). The functional significance of membrane glycolipids remains largely a mystery, although they are thought to be involved in cell recognition and cell-to-cell interactions.[5]

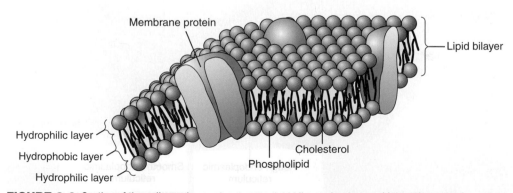

FIGURE 3-2 Section of the cell membrane showing the lipid bilayer structure and integral membrane proteins.

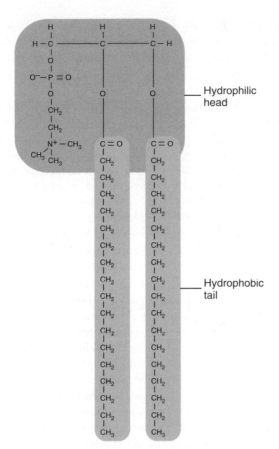

FIGURE 3-3 Schematic drawing of a typical membrane phospholipid molecule showing the amphipathic nature of the structure.

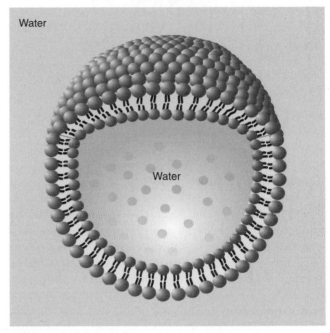

FIGURE 3-4 The amphipathic nature of membrane lipids results in bilayer structures that tend to form spheres.

Phosphatidylethanolamine   Phosphatidylserine   Phosphatidylcholine   Sphingomyelin

FIGURE 3-5 Chemical structures of the four most common membrane phospholipids.

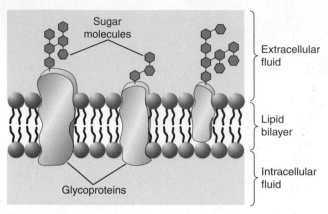

FIGURE 3-6 Portion of the cell membrane showing orientation of membrane glycoproteins toward the outer surface of the cell.

Membrane Proteins

Approximately 50% of the mass of a typical cell membrane is composed of protein. The specific types of membrane proteins vary according to cell type and environmental conditions. Some membrane proteins, called *transmembrane proteins,* extend across the membrane bilayer and are in contact with both the extracellular and intracellular fluids. Transmembrane proteins serve a variety of functions, including transport of charged and polar molecules into and out of cells and transduction of extracellular signals into intracellular messages. Other peripheral membrane proteins are less tightly anchored to the membrane. The common structural orientations of membrane proteins are shown in Figure 3-7. The amino acid structure of membrane proteins determines the way they are arranged in the membrane. Nonpolar amino acids tend to inhabit the hydrophobic middle of the membrane, whereas charged and polar amino acids stick out into the aqueous fluid or associate with polar lipid head groups. The three-dimensional structure of many membrane proteins is complex, with numerous twists and turns through the lipid bilayer.

The type of membrane proteins in a particular cell depends on the cell's primary functions. For example, a kidney tubule cell has a large proportion of transmembrane proteins, which are needed to perform the kidney's function of electrolyte and nutrient reabsorption. In contrast, the human red blood cell (RBC) contains mainly peripheral proteins attached to the inner surface of the membrane.[6] One of these proteins, spectrin, has a long, thin, flexible rodlike shape that forms a supportive meshwork or **cytoskeleton** for the cell. It is this cytoskeleton that enables the RBC to withstand the membrane stress of being forced through small capillaries.

Although proteins and lipids are generally free to move within the plane of the cell membrane, many cells are able to confine certain proteins to specific areas. Using the example of the kidney tubule cell again, it is important for the cell to keep transport proteins on its luminal side to reabsorb filtered molecules (Figure 3-8). This segregation of particular proteins is thought to be accomplished primarily by intercellular connections called **tight junctions,** which connect neighboring

cells and function like a fence to confine proteins to an area of membrane. Membrane proteins also can be immobilized by tethering them to cytoskeleton or extracellular matrix structures.

ORGANIZATION OF CELLULAR COMPARTMENTS

Cytoskeleton

Eukaryotic cells have a variety of internal compartments, or **organelles,** that are membrane bound and carry out distinct cellular functions. The cell's organelles are not free to float around haphazardly in the cytoplasmic soup; rather, they are elaborately organized by a protein network called the *cytoskeleton* (Figure 3-9).[7] The cytoskeleton maintains the cell's shape, allows cell movement, and directs the trafficking of substances within the cell. Three principal types of protein filaments make up the cytoskeleton: actin filaments, microtubules, and intermediate filaments.

All three types of filaments are made up of small proteins that can assemble (polymerize) into filaments of varying length. The filament structures are dynamic and can be rapidly disassembled and reassembled according to the changing needs of the cell.[7] Actin filaments, also known as microfilaments, play a pivotal role in cell movement. As one might expect, muscle cells are packed with actin filaments, which allows the cell to perform its primary function of contraction. However, nonmuscle cells also possess actin filaments that are important for complex movements of the cell membrane, such as cell crawling and phagocytosis. Such movements of the cell membrane are mediated by dense networks of actin filaments that cluster just beneath the plasma membrane and interact with specific proteins embedded in it. Actin and some of the other cytoskeletal proteins make specific contacts with and through the plasma membrane and are involved in information transfer from the extracellular environment to signaling cascades within the cell.

Organization of the cytoplasm and its organelles is achieved primarily by microtubules. In animal cells, microtubules originate at the cell center, or **centrosome,** near the nucleus and radiate out toward the cell perimeter in fine lacelike threads. Microtubules guide the orderly transport of organelles in the cytoplasm as well as the equal distribution of chromosomes during cell division. Intermediate filaments, so named because

FIGURE 3-7 Structural orientation of some proteins in the cell membrane. **A,** Membrane-associated protein with noncovalent attachment to plasma lipids. **B,** Membrane protein with noncovalent attachment to another membrane protein. **C,** Transmembrane protein extending through the lipid bilayer. **D,** Covalently attached peripheral membrane protein.

FIGURE 3-8 Transport proteins may be confined to a particular portion of the cell membrane by tight junctions. Segregation of transport proteins is important for the absorptive functions of the kidney epithelial cells. *N,* Nucleus.

FIGURE 3-9 Schematic of the cytoskeleton of a resting platelet showing actin proteins. (From Hoffman R et al: *Hematology: Basic principles and practice,* ed 4, Philadelphia, 2005, Churchill Livingstone, p 1877.)

their size is between that of microtubules and actin filaments, are strong, ropelike, fibrous proteins. Their primary function seems to be mechanical support of the cell. A variety of intermediate filaments that differ from tissue to tissue have been identified. In addition to the three main groups of cytoskeletal filaments described above, a large number of accessory proteins are essential for cytoskeletal function. For example, the accessory protein, myosin, is needed to bind with actin to achieve motor functions. Different accessory proteins are present in different cell types.

Nucleus

The largest cytoplasmic organelle is the **nucleus,** which contains the genetic information for the cell in the form of **DNA.** The human genome contains approximately 25,000 genes that code for proteins, representing less than 2% of the total DNA structure composed of more than 6 billion base pairs.[8] The nuclear contents are enclosed and protected by the nuclear envelope, which consists of two concentric membranes. The inner membrane forms an unbroken sphere around the DNA and contains protein-binding sites that help to organize

FIGURE 3-10 A, Structure of the double-membrane envelope that surrounds the cell nucleus. **B,** Detail of a nuclear pore.

the chromosomes inside. The outer nuclear membrane is continuous with the endoplasmic reticulum (ER) (see below) and closely resembles it in structure and function (Figure 3-10). The nucleus contains many proteins that help mediate its functions of genetic control and inheritance. These proteins, including histones, polymerases, and regulatory proteins, are manufactured in the cytosol and transported to the nucleus through holes in the membrane called *nuclear pores*. The nuclear pores are selective as to which molecules are allowed access to the nuclear compartment, and in this way they protect the genetic material from enzymes and other molecules in the cytoplasm. The nuclear pores also mediate the export of products such as RNA and ribosomes that are synthesized in the nucleus but function in the cytosol. Ribosomes are manufactured in a specialized portion of the nucleus called the *nucleolus*. Nuclear pores are complexes of proteins that span across both the inner and outer nuclear membrane, creating a pathway between the cytoplasm and the nuclear lamina (see Figure 3-10).

A major function of the nucleus is to protect and preserve genetic information so that it can be replicated exactly and passed on during cell division. However, the nucleus is continuously functioning even when the cell is not actively dividing. The nuclear DNA controls the production of cellular enzymes, membrane receptors, structural proteins, and other proteins that define the cell's type and behavior. (The structure and function of DNA are discussed in Chapter 5.)

During mitosis, the complex structure of the nuclear membrane and its pore-forming proteins breaks up into small bits that diffuse through the cell cytoplasm. After cell division is complete, bits of nuclear membrane surround and gather up the chromosomes and then fuse together to form a new nuclear membrane. Nuclear proteins and pore structures are then recruited back to their normal nuclear locations.[9]

Endoplasmic Reticulum

The ER is a membrane network that extends throughout the cytoplasm and is present in all eukaryotic cells (Figure 3-11). The ER is thought to have a single continuous membrane that separates the lumen of the ER from the cytosol—it could be likened to a "gastrointestinal tract" in the cell. The ER plays a central role in the synthesis of membrane components, including proteins and lipids, for the plasma membrane and cellular organelles, as well as in the synthesis of products to be secreted from the cell. The ER is divided into rough and smooth types based on its appearance under the electron microscope. The **rough ER** is coated with ribosomes along its outer surface. **Ribosomes** are complexes of protein and RNA that are formed in the nucleus and transported to the cytoplasm. Their primary function is the synthesis of proteins (see Chapter 5). Depending on the destination of the protein to be created, ribosomes may float free in the cytosol or may bind to the ER membrane. Proteins synthesized by free-floating ribosomes are released within the cytosol of the cell. Proteins to be transported into the ER have a special sequence of amino acids that directs the ribosome responsible for its synthesis to the ER membrane. Special proteins called signal recognition particles (SRP) bind to the leading sequence of the protein and then bind to a receptor on the ER membrane. As the ribosome adds

In addition to synthetic functions, the ER also sequesters large amounts of calcium ions by pumping them from the cytoplasm. In response to specific signals, the ER releases calcium ions as part of important second-messenger cascades. Muscle cells have extensive smooth ER (sarcoplasmic reticulum) dedicated to the sequestration of calcium. When the cell is stimulated, the sarcoplasmic reticulum releases the calcium ions needed to accomplish muscle contraction.

Golgi Apparatus

The **Golgi apparatus** or Golgi complex is composed of a stack of smooth membrane-bound compartments resembling a stack of hollow plates (see Figure 3-11). These compartments or *cisternae* are organized in a series of at least three processing compartments. The first compartment (*cis* face) lies next to the ER and receives newly synthesized proteins and lipids by way of ER transport vesicles. These transport vesicles bud off from the ER membrane and diffuse to the Golgi, where they bind and become part of the Golgi apparatus membrane. The proteins and lipids then move through the middle compartment (medial) to the final compartment (*trans* face), where they depart for their final destination. As the lipid and protein molecules pass through the sequence of Golgi compartments, they are modified by enzymes that attach or rearrange sugar molecules. After specific arrangement of these sugars has occurred, the lipids and proteins are packaged into Golgi transport vesicles (secretory vesicles). The particular configuration of sugar molecules on the lipid or protein is thought to serve as an "address label," directing them to the correct destination within the cell. Golgi vesicles transport their contents primarily to the plasma membrane and to lysosomes.

Lysosomes and Peroxisomes

Transport of Golgi vesicles to the membrane-bound bags of digestive enzymes known as **lysosomes** has been well described and provides a model for Golgi sorting and transport to other destinations. Lysosomes are filled with more than 40 different acid hydrolases, which are capable of digesting organic molecules, including proteins, nucleotides, fats, and sugars.[12] Lysosomes obtain the materials they digest from three main pathways.[12] The first is the pathway used to digest products taken up by endocytosis. In this pathway, endocytotic vesicles bud off from the plasma membrane to fuse with endosomes. Endosomes mature into lysosomes as the Golgi delivers lysosomal enzymes to them; the pH inside the lysosome acidifies, and active digestion occurs. The second pathway is autophagy, whereby damaged and obsolete parts of the cell itself are destroyed. Unwanted cellular structures are enclosed by a membrane from the ER, which then fuses with the lysosome, leading to autodigestion of the cellular components. Autophagy also may occur during cell starvation or disuse, leading to a process called **atrophy,** in which the cell becomes smaller and more energy efficient. The third pathway providing materials to the lysosomes is present only in specialized phagocytic cells. White blood cells (WBCs), for example, are capable of ingesting large particles, which then form a **phagosome** capable of

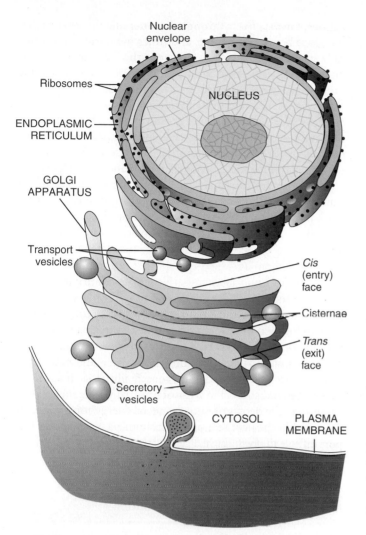

FIGURE 3-11 Schematic drawing of the endoplasmic reticulum and its relationship to the Golgi apparatus and nuclear envelope.

amino acids to the growing protein chain, it is pushed into the lumen of the ER through a pore in the ER membrane called a *translocon*.[10] After processing in the ER and Golgi apparatus, the protein is eventually transported to the appropriate organelle or secreted at the cell surface. Free-floating and rough ER ribosomes are identical and interchangeable; their location depends on the amino acid structure of the protein they are producing at the time.[11]

Regions of ER that lack ribosomes are called **smooth** ER. The smooth ER is involved in lipid metabolism. Most cells have very little smooth ER, but cells specializing in the production of steroid hormones or lipoproteins may have significant amounts of smooth ER. For example, the hepatocyte (liver cell) has abundant smooth ER-containing enzymes (P450) responsible for the manufacture of lipoproteins as well as the detoxification of harmful lipid-soluble compounds, such as alcohol. The cellular smooth ER can double in surface area within a few days if large quantities of drugs or toxins enter the circulation. Cells in the adrenal cortex and gonads that produce steroid hormones also have abundant smooth ER.

fusing with a lysosome. The final products of lysosomal digestion are simple molecules, such as amino acids, fatty acids, and sugars, which can be used by the cell or secreted as cellular waste at the cell surface.

Discovery of the mechanism for sorting and transport of lysosomal enzymes was aided by studying patients suffering from the lysosomal storage diseases.[13] Patients with I-cell (inclusion cell) disease, for example, accumulate large amounts of debris in lysosomes, which appear as spots or "inclusions" in the cells. These lysosomes lack nearly all of the hydrolases normally present and thus are unable to perform lysosomal digestion. However, all the hydrolases missing from the lysosomes can be found in the patient's bloodstream. The abnormality results from "mis-sorting" by the Golgi apparatus, which erroneously packages the enzymes for extracellular secretion rather than sending them to the lysosomes. Studies of this rare genetic disease resulted in the discovery that all lysosomal enzymes have a common marker, mannose-6-phosphate, which normally targets the enzymes to the lysosomes. Persons with I-cell disease lack the enzyme responsible for attaching this marker.

Peroxisomes (microbodies), like lysosomes, are membrane-bound bags of enzymes that perform degradative functions. They are particularly important in liver and kidney cells, where they detoxify various substances, such as alcohol. In contrast to lysosomes, which contain hydrolase enzymes, peroxisomes contain oxidative enzymes. These enzymes use molecular oxygen to break down organic substances by an oxidative reaction that produces hydrogen peroxide. The hydrogen peroxide is then used by another enzyme (catalase) to break down other organic molecules, including formaldehyde and alcohol. Catalase also prevents accumulation of excess hydrogen peroxide in the cell by converting it to water and oxygen. Peroxisomes also oxidize fatty acids (β oxidation) to produce acetyl coenzyme A (acetyl CoA) that is used in cellular metabolism. Unlike lysosomes, which acquire their enzymes from Golgi vesicles, peroxisomes import enzymes directly from the cytoplasm.

Mitochondria

The **mitochondria** have been aptly called the "powerhouses of the cell" because they convert energy to forms that can be used to drive cellular reactions. A distinct feature of mitochondria is the large amount of membrane they contain. Each mitochondrion is bound by two specialized membranes. The inner membrane forms an enclosed space, called the *matrix,* which contains a concentrated mix of mitochondrial enzymes. The highly convoluted structure of the inner membrane with its numerous folds, called cristae (Figure 3-12), provides a large surface area for the important membrane-bound enzymes of the respiratory chain. These enzymes are essential to the process of oxidative phosphorylation, which generates most of the cell's **adenosine triphosphate (ATP).** The outer membrane contains numerous porin transport proteins forming large aqueous channels that make the membrane porous like a sieve. Fairly large molecules, including proteins up to 5000

daltons, can pass freely through the outer membrane such that the space between the outer and inner membranes is chemically similar to the cytosol. However, the inner membrane is quite impermeable even to small molecules and ions. Specific protein transporters are required to shuttle the necessary molecules across the inner mitochondrial membrane.

Mitochondria are believed to have originated as bacteria that were engulfed by larger cells but that still retain some of their own DNA. Mitochondrial DNA codes for 22 transfer RNA molecules, 2 ribosomal RNAs, and 13 proteins.[14-16] During evolution the majority of mitochondrial genes were transferred to locations within the nuclear genome. Thus only a few of the mitochondrial enzymes are produced from DNA located in the mitochondria; the majority are transcribed from nuclear DNA. Nuclear genes are translated into protein in the cytoplasm and then transported to the mitochondria, whereas mitochondrial gene-derived proteins are made within the mitochondria. There are several rare disorders associated with mitochondrial gene defects (see Chapter 6). The number and location of mitochondria differ according to cell type and function. Cells with high energy needs, such as cardiac or skeletal muscle, have many mitochondria. These mitochondria may pack between adjacent muscle fibrils, such that ATP is delivered directly to the areas of unusually high energy consumption. The details of mitochondrial energy conversion are discussed in the next section. Mitochondria also have an important role in programmed cell death, called *apoptosis,* which is discussed in Chapter 4.

KEY POINTS

- The cytoskeleton is made up of actin, microtubules, and intermediate filaments. These proteins regulate cell shape, movement, and the trafficking of intracellular molecules.
- The nucleus contains the genomic DNA. These nuclear genes code for the synthesis of proteins. There are about 25,000 protein-coding genes in the human genome.
- The endoplasmic reticulum and the Golgi apparatus function together to synthesize proteins and lipids for transport to lysosomes or to the plasma membrane.
- Lysosomes and peroxisomes are membrane-bound bags of digestive enzymes that degrade intracellular debris.
- Mitochondria contain enzymes necessary for oxidative phosphorylation to produce ATP. Mitochondria have their own small number of genes that code for some of the mitochondrial proteins.

CELLULAR METABOLISM

All living cells must continually perform essential cellular functions such as movement, ion transport, and synthesis of macromolecules. Many of these cellular activities are energetically unfavorable (i.e., they are unlikely to occur

FIGURE 3-12 Electron micrograph **(A)** and schematic drawing **(B)** of the mitochondrial structure. The highly convoluted inner membrane provides a large surface area for membrane-bound metabolic enzymes. (**A,** From Alberts B et al, editors: *Molecular biology of the cell,* ed 5, New York, 2008, Garland Science, p 28. Micrograph courtesy of Daniel S. Friend © DS Friend, All rights reserved. Used under license from The American Society for Cell Biology. Available at http://cellimages.ascb.org)

spontaneously). Unfavorable reactions can be driven by linking them to an energy source such as ATP, which is a molecule that contains high-energy phosphate bonds. In normal cells where the ATP concentration is high, approximately 11 to 13 kcal of energy per mole of ATP is liberated when one of the phosphate bonds is hydrolyzed (broken with the aid of water) in a chemical reaction.[15] Enzymes throughout the cell are able to capture the energy released from ATP hydrolysis and use it to break or make other chemical bonds. In this way, ATP serves as the "energy currency" of the cell. A specific amount of ATP is "spent" to "buy" a specific amount of work. Most cells contain only a small amount of ATP, sufficient to maintain cellular activities for just a few minutes. Because ATP cannot cross the plasma membrane, each cell must continuously synthesize its own ATP to meet its energy needs; ATP cannot be "borrowed" from other cells or "banked" in any significant quantity within a cell. ATP is synthesized primarily from the breakdown of glycogen and fat.

An average adult has enough glycogen stores (primarily in liver and muscle) to supply about 1 day's needs, but enough fat to last for a month or more. After a meal, the excess glucose entering the cells is used to replenish glycogen stores or to synthesize fats for later use. Fat is stored primarily in adipose tissue and is released into the bloodstream for other cells to use when needed. When cellular glucose levels fall, glycogen and fats are broken down to provide glucose and fatty acyl molecules, which are ultimately metabolized to provide ATP. During starvation, body proteins can also be used for energy production by a process called *gluconeogenesis.*

Cellular metabolism is the biochemical process whereby foodstuffs are used to provide cellular energy and biomolecules. Cellular metabolism includes two separate and opposite phases: anabolism and catabolism. **Anabolism** refers to *energy-using* metabolic processes or pathways that result in the synthesis of complex molecules such as fats. **Catabolism** refers to the *energy-releasing* breakdown of nutrient sources such as glucose to provide ATP to the cell. Both of these processes require a long, complex series of enzymatic steps. The catabolic processes of cellular energy production are briefly discussed below. (See Chapter 42 for a detailed discussion of metabolism.)

Glycolysis

The catabolic process of energy production begins with the intestinal digestion of foodstuffs into small molecules: proteins into amino acids, polysaccharides into simple sugars, and fats into fatty acids and glycerol. The second stage of catabolism occurs in the cytosol of the cell, where sugar molecules are further degraded by **glycolysis** into pyruvate (three-carbon atoms). Glycolysis involves 10 enzymatic steps to break the six-carbon glucose molecule into a pair of three-carbon pyruvate molecules (Figure 3-13).[15] Glycolysis requires the use of two ATP molecules in the early stages but produces four ATP molecules in the later steps, for a net gain of two ATP molecules per glucose molecule. The production of ATP through glycolysis is relatively inefficient, and the pyruvate

end products still contain substantial chemical energy that can be released by further catabolism in stage 3. However, glycolysis is an important provider of ATP under *anaerobic* conditions because oxygen is not required. Thus, ATP production by glycolysis becomes important during conditions of reduced cellular oxygenation, which may accompany respiratory and cardiovascular disorders. The pyruvate that accumulates during prolonged anaerobic conditions is converted to lactate and excreted from the cell into the bloodstream. Lactic acidosis is a dangerous condition that may result from excessive lactate production owing to severe or prolonged lack of oxygen (see Chapter 20). In addition to the two molecules of ATP and pyruvate, each glucose molecule produces two reduced nicotinamide adenine dinucleotide (NADH) molecules, which contain high-energy electrons that are transferred to the electron transport chain in the mitochondria. Cells that do not contain mitochondria, such as RBCs, must rely totally on glycolysis for ATP production.

Citric Acid Cycle

For most cells, glycolysis is only a prelude to the third stage of catabolism, which takes place in the mitochondria and results in the complete oxidation of glucose to its final end products, CO_2 and H_2O. The third stage begins with the citric acid cycle (also called the Krebs cycle or the tricarboxylic acid cycle) and ends with the production of ATP by oxidative phosphorylation.[15] The purpose of the citric acid cycle is to break, by oxidation, the C-C and C-H bonds of the compounds produced in the second stage of catabolism. Pyruvate and fatty acids enter the mitochondrial matrix, where they are converted to acetyl CoA (Figure 3-14). The pyruvate dehydrogenase complex cleaves pyruvate to form one CO_2, one NADH, and one acetyl CoA molecule. Fatty acids are cleaved by a process called β oxidation to form one NADH and one reduced flavin adenine dinucleotide (FADH$_2$, another type of electron carrier). No CO_2 is produced by β oxidation of fatty acids. Patients who have difficulty excreting CO_2 because of respiratory disease are sometimes given a high-fat, low-carbohydrate diet to take advantage of the lower CO_2 production that accompanies fat metabolism.

In the first reaction of the citric acid cycle, the two-carbon acetyl group is transferred from coenzyme A to a four-carbon oxaloacetate molecule. This results in the formation of the six-carbon molecule citrate, for which the cycle is named. In a series of enzymatic oxidations, carbon atoms are cleaved off in the form of CO_2 (Figure 3-15); this CO_2 is free to diffuse from the cell and be excreted by the lungs as a waste product. Two carbon atoms are removed to form two CO_2 molecules for each complete turn of the cycle. The extra oxygen molecules needed to create CO_2 are provided by the surrounding H_2O; therefore, the citric acid cycle does not require molecular oxygen from respiration. However, the cycle will shut down in the absence of oxygen because the carrier molecules, NADH and FADH$_2$, cannot unload their electrons onto the electron transport chain (which does require oxygen) and thus are unavailable to accept electrons from the citric acid cycle.

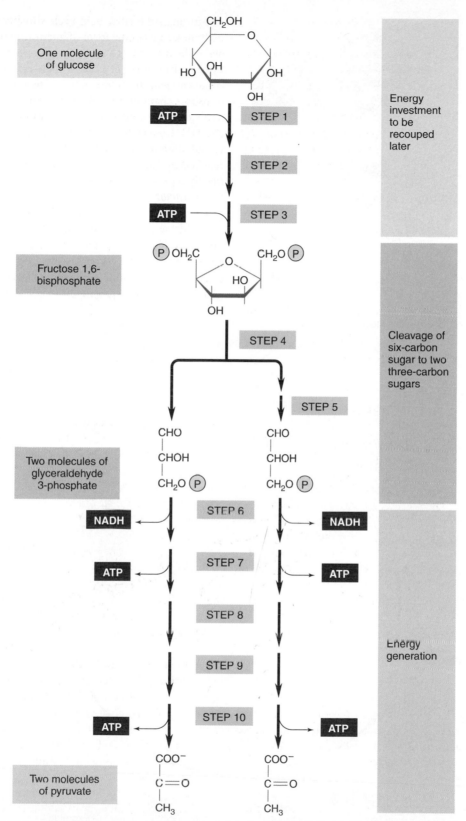

FIGURE 3-13 Glycolysis involves 10 enzymatic steps to break glucose into two three-carbon pyruvate molecules. A net gain of two ATP molecules is achieved. (From Alberts B et al, editors: *Molecular biology of the cell*, ed 5, New York, 2008, Garland Science, p 89.)

Although the citric acid cycle directly produces only one ATP molecule (in the form of guanosine triphosphate [GTP]) per cycle, it captures a great deal of energy in the form of activated hydride ions (H^-). These high-energy ions combine with larger carrier molecules, which transport them to the electron transport chain in the mitochondrial membrane. Two important carrier molecules are nicotinamide adenine dinucleotide (NAD^+), which becomes NADH when reduced by H^-, and flavin adenine nucleotide (FAD), which becomes $FADH_2$ when reduced by H^-. The energy carried by these molecules is ultimately used to produce ATP through a process called *oxidative phosphorylation*.

Oxidative Phosphorylation

Oxidative phosphorylation follows the processes of glycolysis and the citric acid cycle and results in the formation of ATP by the reaction adenosine diphosphate (ADP) + inorganic phosphate (P_i) → ATP. The energy to drive this unfavorable reaction is provided by the high-energy hydride ions (H^-) derived

FIGURE 3-14 Space-filling model of acetyl CoA.

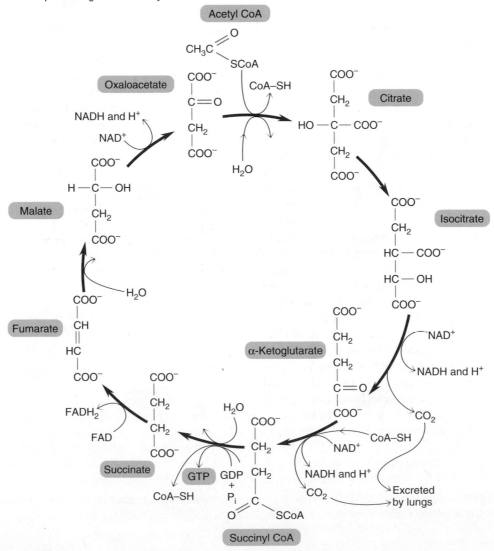

FIGURE 3-15 Chemical structures of the compounds of the citric acid cycle (Krebs cycle). In a series of enzymatic reactions, carbon atoms are cleaved to form CO_2 and high-energy hydride ions, which are carried by FAD and NAD.

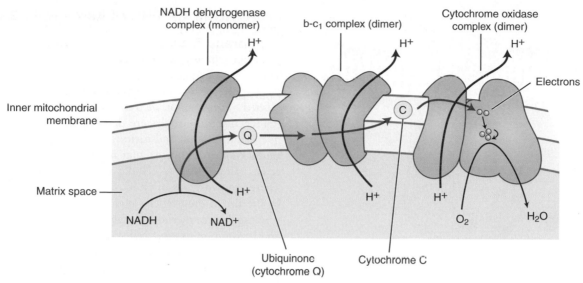

FIGURE 3-16 A representation of the electron transport chain located in the inner mitochondrial membrane. High-energy electrons are passed along the chain until they combine with oxygen to form water. The energy released at each electron transfer is used to pump H+ across the membrane

from the citric acid cycle. This energy is not used to form ATP directly; a series of energy transfers is required.[15] In eukaryotic cells, this series of energy transfers occurs along the **electron transport chain** on the inner mitochondrial membrane. The transport chain consists of three major enzyme complexes and two mobile electron carriers that shuttle electrons between the protein complexes (Figure 3-16). The hydrogen molecules and their associated electrons are transported to the electron transport chain by the carrier molecules NADH or $FADH_2$. Each NADH carries two electrons and donates them readily to the first enzyme in the respiratory chain complex. The path of electron flow is NADH → NADH dehydrogenase complex → ubiquinone → b-c_1 complex → cytochrome c → cytochrome oxidase complex. As the electrons pass from one complex to the next they transfer energy, which is used to pump hydrogen ions (H+) out of the mitochondrial matrix. Each transfer of one electron provides enough energy to pump one or two protons across the membrane. At the very end of the transport chain, low-energy electrons are finally transferred to O_2 to form H_2O. Oxidative phosphorylation is called *aerobic* because of this oxygen-requiring step. The last enzyme in the chain, cytochrome oxidase, collects four electrons and then transfers all four at once to a molecule of O_2 to create two water molecules. If electrons are not transferred to oxygen in the correct ratio, then oxygen free radicals may be produced and damage the cell. Free radical generation is discussed in Chapter 4.

Thus far, little ATP synthesis has been accomplished. However, the enzymes of the transport chain have harnessed energy from the transported electrons in the form of a proton (H+) gradient. Finally, the proton gradient is used to power the synthesis of ATP. A special enzyme in the inner mitochondrial membrane (ATP synthase) allows protons to flow back into the mitochondria down their electrochemical gradient. The energy of the proton flow is used to drive ATP synthesis

(Figure 3-17). A total of about 30 ATP molecules is formed from the complete oxidation of glucose into CO_2 and H_2O. Two of these are from glycolysis, two from the citric acid cycle (in the form of GTP), and the remainder from oxidative phosphorylation.[15] The ATP formed within the mitochondria is transported to the cytosol by protein transporters in the mitochondrial membrane. The ATP is then available to drive a variety of energy-requiring reactions within the cell.

KEY POINTS

- Energy-requiring reactions within cells are driven by coupling to ATP hydrolysis.
- ATP is not stored and must be continuously synthesized by each cell to meet the cell's energy needs.
- Glycolysis is an anaerobic process that produces two ATP molecules, two NADH molecules, and two pyruvate molecules per glucose molecule. Pyruvate enters the mitochondria and is converted to acetyl CoA with release of a CO_2 molecule. Pyruvate can also be converted to lactate when oxygen supply is insufficient for oxidative processes.
- The citric acid cycle in the mitochondrial matrix oxidizes the acetyl groups supplied by acetyl CoA to form large quantities of H- (hydride ions), which are carried to the respiratory chain by NADH and $FADH_2$.
- The respiratory chain enzymes capture the energy from electron transfer and use it to produce an H+ (proton) gradient. Molecular oxygen is required at this stage (aerobic) to accept the electrons from the last enzyme in the transport chain.
- ATP is produced by ATP synthase, a protein in the mitochondrial membrane. ATP synthase produces ATP by capturing the energy of the proton gradient and using it to form a bond between ADP and P_i. In total, about 30 ATP molecules are produced per glucose molecule.

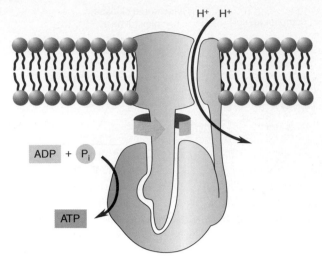

FIGURE 3-17 The inner mitochondrial ATP synthetase captures the potential energy of the H⁺ gradient in a manner similar to a turbine. The proton gradient drives the synthesis of ATP from adenosine diphosphate *(ADP)* and inorganic phosphate *(Pᵢ).*

FUNCTIONS OF THE PLASMA MEMBRANE

Membrane Transport of Macromolecules

Endocytosis and Exocytosis

The transport of large molecules, such as proteins and polysaccharides, across the plasma membrane cannot be accomplished by the membrane transport proteins discussed earlier. Rather, macromolecules are ingested and secreted by the sequential formation and fusion of membrane-bound vesicles. **Endocytosis** refers to cellular ingestion of extracellular molecules. The process of cellular secretion is called **exocytosis.** There are two types of endocytosis, which are differentiated by the size of the particles ingested. **Pinocytosis,** or "cellular drinking," is the method of ingesting fluids and small particles and is common to most cell types. **Phagocytosis,** or "cellular eating," involves the ingestion of large particles, such as microorganisms, and is practiced mainly by specialized phagocytic WBCs. Endocytosis begins at the cell surface by the formation of an indentation or "pit" in the plasma membrane, which is coated with special proteins, including clathrin *(coated pit).* The indentation invaginates and then pinches off a portion of the membrane to become a **vesicle** (Figure 3-18). Each vesicle

0.1 μm

FIGURE 3-18 A, A representation of the steps of endocytosis. An invagination of the membrane occurs and pinches off to form a vesicle. Exocytosis progresses in essentially the reverse. **B,** Electron micrograph showing the steps of endocytosis. **(B,** From Perry M, Gilbert A: Yolk transport in the ovarian follicle of the hen *[Gallus domesticus]:* lipoprotein-like particles at the periphery of the oocyte in the rapid growth phase, *J Cell Sci* 39:257-272, 1979.)

thus formed is internalized, sheds its coat, and fuses with an endosome. The contents of these endocytic vesicles generally end up in lysosomes, where they are degraded.

Endocytosis of certain macromolecules is regulated by specific receptors on the cell surface. These receptors bind the molecules (ligands) to be ingested and then cluster together in coated pits. The receptor-ligand complexes are internalized by the invagination process described above. The vesicles generally fuse with endosomes where the ligand is removed from the receptor for processing by the cell. The receptor may be degraded in the lysosome or may be recycled to the cell surface to be used again. Receptor-mediated endocytosis allows the cell to be selective about the molecules ingested and to regulate the amount taken into the cell. The cell can produce greater numbers of cell surface receptors to ingest more ligand.

An example of receptor-mediated endocytosis is cellular uptake of cholesterol. The process of cholesterol uptake by cells is shown in Figure 3-19. Most cholesterol in the blood is transported by protein carriers called low-density lipoproteins (LDLs). The cell can regulate the number of LDL receptors on its cell surface to increase or decrease the uptake of cholesterol. Once the LDL binds to its receptor, this complex is rapidly internalized in a coated pit. The coated vesicle thus formed sheds its coat and fuses with an endosome. In the endosome, the LDL receptor is retrieved and recycled to the cell surface to be used again. The LDL is transported to lysosomes

and degraded to release free cholesterol, which the cell uses for synthesis of biomolecules, such as steroid hormones.

Dangerously high blood cholesterol levels occur in some individuals who lack functional LDL receptors. These individuals inherit defective genes for making LDL receptor proteins (familial hyperlipidemia) and are incapable of taking up adequate amounts of LDL. Accumulation of LDL in the blood predisposes these individuals to development of atherosclerosis and heart disease (see Chapter 18).

Exocytosis is essentially the reverse of endocytosis. Substances to be secreted from the cell are packaged in membrane-bound vesicles and travel to the inner surface of the plasma membrane. There the vesicle membrane fuses with the plasma membrane and the contents of the vesicle arrive at the cell surface. Some secreted molecules may remain embedded in the cell membrane, others may be incorporated into the extracellular matrix, and still others may enter the extracellular fluids and travel to distant sites. Many substances synthesized by the cell, including new membrane components, are constantly being packaged and secreted. This continuously operative and unregulated pathway is termed *constitutive*. In some specialized cells, selected proteins or small molecules are packaged in secretory vesicles, which remain in the cell until the cell is triggered to release them. These special secretory vesicles are typically regulated by stimulation of cell surface receptors. For example, the mast cell, a special type of WBC,

FIGURE 3-19 Steps in the process of re   ...ocytosis of cholesterol. Cholesterol is carried in the blood by LDL. The uptake of LDL with its associated cholesterol is mediated by a specific LDL-receptor protein on the cell surface. Once internalized, the cholesterol is removed from the LDL-receptor complex and used by the cell. The LDL receptors are sent back to the cell surface to bind more LDL.

releases large amounts of histamine when its cell surface receptors are activated (Chapter 9).

Membrane Transport of Small Molecules

All cells must internalize essential nutrients, excrete wastes, and regulate intracellular ion concentrations. However, the lipid bilayer is extremely impermeable to most polar and charged molecules. Transport of small water-soluble molecules is achieved by specialized transmembrane proteins called *transporter proteins*.[17] Most membrane transporters are highly specific—a different transporter protein is required for each type of molecule to be transported. Only lipid-soluble molecules can permeate the lipid bilayer directly by simple diffusion.

Membrane transport proteins are of three basic kinds: ATP-driven pumps, carriers, and channel proteins. Channel proteins are the simplest of the three, forming a water-filled pore through the lipid bilayer. These pores are able to open and close to allow ions to pass through the membrane. The particular structure of the protein channel ensures that only ions of a certain size and charge can move through. Pumps and carrier proteins, however, bind to the solute to be transported and move it through the membrane by undergoing a structural, or conformational, change. Pumps and carriers have a transport maximum that is much lower than that of channels because they must bind to the molecules to be transported and then move them through the membrane. Pumps and carriers, which transport ions and nonelectrolyte molecules (e.g., glucose and amino acids) are also highly specific for the substances they transport.

Lipid-soluble particles can cross the lipid bilayer directly by simple diffusion through the hydrophobic lipid portion of the membrane. Diffusion of ions occurs passively owing to an **electrochemical gradient.** The electrochemical gradient exists because of differences in intracellular and extracellular charge and/or concentration of chemicals. Passive transport is governed by laws of physics. (See Chapter 24 for a discussion of electrolyte chemistry.) Polar or charged molecules must cross the membrane via protein channels or carriers. Transport through membrane proteins may be a passive or an active process. Passive transport through membrane proteins is called *facilitated diffusion*. Channel proteins and carrier proteins allow particles to move down their electrochemical or concentration gradients passively by facilitated diffusion. Some carriers use the movement of one ion flowing down its concentration gradient (usually Na+ moving into the cell) to move another substance uphill against its gradient.[17] This process is called *secondary active transport* because ATP is not used directly; however, ATP is necessary to run the pumps that maintain the sodium gradient. The lipid bilayer is quite impermeable to water because of its polar structure. Water moves across the plasma membrane through channels called *aquaporins.* Nearly all cells have aquaporins present in their cell membranes at all times, with the exception of a few specialized cells in the kidney tubules. Net movement of water across a membrane (osmosis) occurs in response to differences in osmotic pressure on either side of the membrane and is a passive process.

Active Transport Pumps

Active transport is the process whereby protein transport pumps move solutes across the membrane against an electrochemical or concentration gradient. Primary active transport requires metabolic energy, which is supplied by ATP hydrolysis. There are three families of ATP-driven pumps: the F-type ATPases that move H+; the P-type ATPases that pump ions across membranes; and the ATP-binding cassette (ABC) transporters that transport a wide range of solutes. The ATP synthase located on the inner mitochondrial membrane is an example of an F-type pump; however, in that location it runs backward, allowing H+ to run down its electrochemical gradient and using the energy to form a bond between ADP and P_i (see Figure 3-17). As a general principle, pumps, carriers, and channels can transport either direction depending on the concentration of substrate on either side of the membrane.

Sodium-Potassium Ion Pump. The sodium-potassium (Na^+-K^+) pump is a P-type ATPase present in the plasma membranes of virtually all animal cells. It serves to maintain low sodium and high potassium concentrations in the cell.[18] The Na^+-K^+ transporter must pump ions against a steep electrochemical gradient. Almost one third of the energy of a typical cell is consumed by the Na^+-K^+ pump. ATP hydrolysis provides the energy to drive the Na^+-K^+ transporter. The Na^+-K^+ pump behaves as an enzyme in its ability to split ATP to form ADP and P_i, leading to the protein being termed *Na^+-K^+ ATPase.*

Transport of sodium and potassium ions through the Na^+-K^+ carrier protein is *coupled;* that is, the transfer of one ion must be accompanied by the simultaneous transport of the other ion. The transporter moves three sodium ions *out* of the cell for every two potassium ions moved *into* the cell (Figure 3-20). The Na^+-K^+ pump is important in maintaining cell volume. It controls the solute concentration inside the cell, which in turn affects the osmotic forces across the membrane. If Na^+ is allowed to accumulate within the cell, the cell will swell and could burst. The role of the Na^+-K^+ pump can be demonstrated by treating cells with digitalis, a drug that inhibits Na^+-K^+ ATPase. Cells thus treated will indeed swell and often burst. The Na^+-K^+ pump is responsible for maintaining a steep concentration gradient for Na^+ across the plasma membrane. This gradient can be harnessed to transport small molecules across the membrane in a process called secondary active transport. Carriers that use ATP directly are engaging in primary active transport.

Membrane Calcium Transporters. Numerous important cellular processes, such as cell contraction and growth initiation, are dependent on the intracellular calcium concentration. Intracellular calcium concentration is normally very low and tightly regulated. Two important calcium pumps present in the plasma membrane and, in the endoplasmic reticulum (sarcoplasmic reticulum of muscle cells), function to remove calcium from the cell cytoplasm.[19] These transporters use ATP

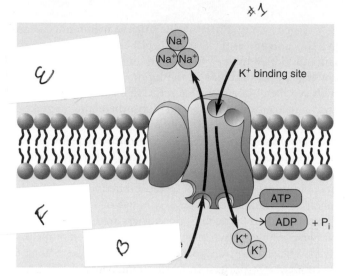

FIGURE 3-20 Schematic drawing of the sodium-potassium transport protein, which uses ATP to pump Na^+ out of the cell and K^+ into the cell against steep electrochemical gradients. This transporter is responsible for maintaining a low intracellular concentration of Na^+ and a large Na^+ gradient across the membrane. The energy of this Na^+ gradient can be harvested by other transporters to actively transport substances.

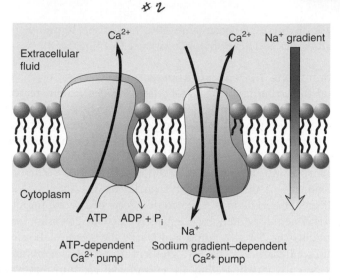

FIGURE 3-21 Two transporters of calcium ions are present in some cell membranes. One uses ATP as the energy source to pump calcium against a gradient (primary active transport). The other captures the potential energy of the sodium gradient to pump calcium out of the cell (secondary active transport).

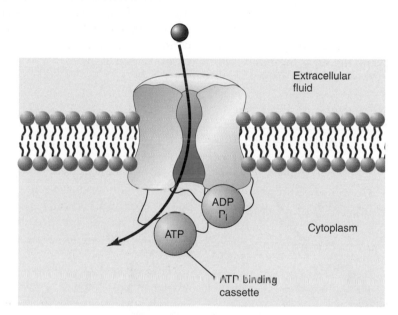

FIGURE 3-22 The ABC transporters are the largest known family of membrane transport proteins. They are characterized by an ATP-binding domain that causes a substrate pocket to be exposed first on one side of the membrane and then on the other as ATP is bound and hydrolyzed to ADP and P_i.

as the energy source, much as the Na^+-K^+ transporter does (Figure 3-21).

If calcium levels in the cytoplasm become dangerously elevated, calcium pumps in the mitochondrial membrane swing into action. Calcium ions are actively pumped into the mitochondria using the energy of the proton (H^+) gradient. This is the same proton gradient that the mitochondria uses to synthesize ATP, and ATP production falls when the mitochondria are called on to sequester Ca^{2+}. A high intracellular calcium level is even more dangerous to the cell than a reduction in ATP production.

ABC Transporters. Another important class of ATP-driven transporters is the ABC transporter family. These transporters all have a common ATP-binding domain, called the *ATP binding cassette* (ABC), which hydrolyzes ATP to provide energy for the transport process (Figure 3-22). This family of membrane transporters is the largest of all, but the members of the family and their functions are just beginning to be described. A clinically important member of this family is a chloride channel in the plasma membrane of epithelial cells. A defect in this transporter is responsible for cystic fibrosis, a common genetic disorder that affects the lungs and pancreas (see Chapter 22). Bacteria use ABC transporters to pump out antibiotics and develop drug resistance (see Chapter 8).

Membrane Transport Carriers

Na⁺-Driven Carriers. In animal cells, the Na^+ gradient created by the Na^+-K^+ pump is used to power a variety of transporters by secondary active transport. An important Ca^{2+} transporter located in the plasma membrane of cardiac muscle cells uses the electrochemical gradient of Na^+ to power the transport of Ca^{2+} out of the cell (see Figure 3-21). The dependence of this calcium transporter on the sodium gradient helps explain the inotropic effects of the commonly prescribed drug digitalis. Digitalis is a cardiac glycoside that inhibits the Na^+-K^+ pump and allows the accumulation of intracellular Na^+. The Na^+ gradient across the membrane is thus decreased, leading to less efficient calcium removal by the Na^+-dependent Ca^{2+} pump. A more forceful cardiac muscle contraction results from the increased intracellular Ca^{2+}. Another example of a transporter that uses secondary active transport is the Na^+-H^+ exchange carrier, which uses the Na^+ gradient to pump out excess hydrogen ions to help maintain intracellular pH balance. The Na^+ gradient also can be used to bring substances into the cell. For example, glucose and amino acid transport into epithelial cells is coupled to Na^+ entry. As Na^+ moves through the transporter, down its electrochemical gradient, the sugar or amino acid is "dragged" along. Entry of the nutrient will not occur unless Na^+ also enters the cell. The epithelial cells that line the gut and kidney tubules have large numbers of these nutrient transporters present in the luminal (apical) surfaces of their cell membranes. In this way, large amounts of glucose and amino acids can be effectively absorbed. The reuptake of numerous types of neurotransmitters from synapses also occurs by way of Na^+-driven carrier proteins. The movement of Na^+ through carriers located in the presynaptic neuron drags the neurotransmitter from the synapse back into the nerve terminal, where it can be repackaged for reuse or metabolized by cellular enzymes.

Passive Transport Carriers. Some carriers are not linked to the Na^+ gradient and move substances across the membrane passively. The glucose transporters in many cell types belong to this class of transporters. In β cells of the pancreas, for example, the glucose transporters (Glut-2) are always present in the plasma membrane and let glucose into the cell according to its concentration in the extracellular fluid. In this way the pancreas detects blood glucose levels and releases an appropriate amount of insulin. In insulin-sensitive cells, such as muscle, liver, and adipose cells, the glucose carriers are sequestered inside the cell until insulin binds to its receptor at the cell surface. Receptor activation causes the glucose carriers (Glut-4) to move to the cell surface, where they allow passive influx of glucose (Figure 3-23).

FIGURE 3-23 In response to insulin binding to its receptor on the cell surface, carrier proteins that transport glucose *(Glut-4)* are moved to the cell surface where they passively transport glucose into the cell (facilitated diffusion).

Membrane Channel Proteins

In contrast to carrier proteins, which bind molecules and move them across the membrane by a conformational transformation, channel proteins form water-filled pores in the membrane. Nearly all channel proteins are involved in transport of ions and may be referred to as ion channels. Ions can flow through the appropriate channel at very high rates (100 million ions/sec); this is much faster than carrier-mediated transport.[17,20] However, channels are not linked to an energy source, so ions must flow passively down an electrochemical gradient. The channel proteins in the plasma membranes of animal cells are highly selective, permitting only a particular ion or class of ions to pass. Humans have about 400 genes that encode channel proteins.[21] Ion channels are particularly important in allowing the cell to respond rapidly to a variety of external stimuli. Most channels are not continuously open, but they open and close according to membrane signals. Ion channels may be stimulated to open or close in three principal ways: (1) *voltage-gated* channels respond to a change in membrane potential; (2) *mechanically gated* channels respond to mechanical deformation; and (3) *ligand-gated* channels respond to the binding of a signaling molecule (a hormone or neurotransmitter) to a receptor on the cell surface (Figure 3-24). In addition, some channels open without apparent stimulation and are referred to as *leak* channels. Ion channels are responsible for the development of membrane potentials and are of vital importance in nerve and muscle function, as discussed in the next section.

KEY POINTS

- Large, lipid-insoluble molecules are transported across the plasma membrane by endocytosis and exocytosis.
- Small, lipid-insoluble molecules are transported across the plasma membrane by three kinds of membrane proteins: ATP-driven pumps, carriers, and channels.

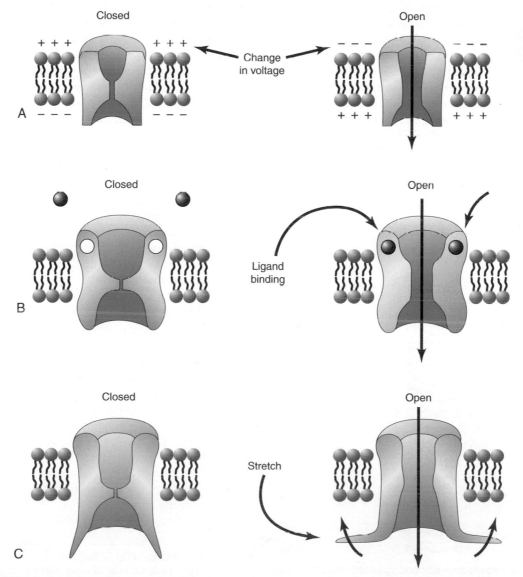

FIGURE 3-24 Gating of ion channels. **A,** Voltage-gated channel. **B,** Ligand-gated channel. **C,** Mechanically gated channel.

- Pumps use the energy of ATP to move solutes against a gradient. Examples of ATP-driven active transport include proton pumps, Na^+-K^+ pumps, Ca^{2+} pumps, ABC transporters.
- Carriers may be passive or use the Na^+ gradient for secondary active transport. Neurotransmitter reuptake carriers and those that transport glucose and amino acids across the gut and renal tubules are examples of Na^+ driven carriers. Passive carriers include those that allow glucose entry into insulin-sensitive cells.
- Channels are always passive and allow ions to move down their electrochemical gradients when open. Channels open and close in response to specific signals, such as voltage changes, ligand binding, and mechanical pressure.

Cellular Membrane Potentials

Animal cells typically have a difference in the electrical charge across the plasma membrane. There is a slight excess of negative ions along the inner aspect of the membrane and extra positive ions along the outer membrane. This separation of charges creates a membrane potential that can be measured as a voltage. Positive and negative ions separated by the plasma membrane have a strong attraction to one another that can be used by the cell to perform work, such as the transmission of nerve impulses. A relatively large membrane potential is created by the separation of a very small number of ions along the membrane (Figure 3-25).

FIGURE 3-25 A relatively large membrane potential results from the separation of a very small number of ions across the plasma membrane.

Resting Membrane Potential

When there is no net ion movement across the plasma membrane, the electrical charge present inside the cell is called the *resting membrane potential* (RMP). The major determinant of the resting membrane potential is the difference[17,22] in potassium ion concentration across the membrane. The concentration of potassium inside the cell is much greater (about 30 times greater) than the extracellular potassium concentration. At rest, the membrane is permeable to K^+, but not to other positively charged cations, including Na^+ and Ca^{2+}. Potassium ions remain inside the cell because of the attraction of fixed intracellular anions (negatively charged organic molecules such as proteins that cannot diffuse out of the cell). Because the cell membrane is impermeable to Na^+ and Ca^{2+}, only K^+ is available to balance these negative intracellular ions. Thus, two opposing forces are acting on the potassium ion. The negative cell interior attracts K^+ into the cell, whereas the huge K^+ concentration gradient favors movement of K^+ out of the cell. When the cell is at rest and not transmitting impulses, these forces are balanced and although the membrane is permeable to K^+, there is no net movement. The voltage required to exactly balance a given potassium concentration gradient can be calculated mathematically.*

The measured membrane potential is very close to that predicted mathematically and varies directly with changes in extracellular K^+ ion concentration.

For example, a typical nerve cell has a normal resting potential of about -85 mV. If the extracellular K^+ level is increased, fewer K^+ ions will leave the cell, owing to the reduced concentration gradient. These extra positive intracellular ions will neutralize more of the negative cellular anions, and the cell will *hypopolarize,* or become less negative. Conversely, if extracellular K^+ levels fall, more K^+ will exit the cell, owing to a greater concentration gradient. Fewer intracellular anions will be neutralized, and the cell interior will become more negative, or *hyperpolarized* (Figure 3-26). Changes in RMP can have profound effects on the ease of action potential generation in cardiac and nerve cells.

The RMP is described by the potassium equilibrium potential because the cell is relatively impermeable to other ions at rest. Under certain conditions, the membrane may become highly permeable to an ion other than potassium. The membrane potential will reflect the equilibrium potential of the most permeant ions.

Long-term maintenance of the potassium concentration gradient across the cell membrane is accomplished primarily by the Na^+-K^+ pump. The Na^+-K^+ pump also contributes to the negative RMP in that it extrudes *three* Na^+ for every *two* K^+ brought into the cell. However, this pump can be inhibited for minutes to hours in some tissues with little immediate effect on the resting membrane potential.

---

*The numerical value of the resting potential *(M)* can be calculated from the ratio of extracellular to intracellular K^+ using the Nernst equation: M (in millivolts) = 61 log ($K^+_{outside} \div K^+_{inside}$)

FIGURE 3-26 The effects of changes in extracellular K+ on the resting membrane potential. A high level of serum K+ results in a hypopolarization of the membrane. A low serum K+ level results in membrane hyperpolarization. With high serum K+ levels, the resting membrane potential is closer to threshold, making it easier to achieve an action potential. A low serum K+ level moves the resting membrane potential away from threshold, making it more difficult to achieve an action potential.

Action Potential

Nearly all animal cells have negative resting membrane potentials, which may vary from -20 to -200 mV, depending on the cell type and organism. The cell membranes of some specialized cell types, mainly nerve and muscle, are capable of rapid changes in their membrane potentials. These cells are electrically "excitable" and can generate and propagate action potentials. In classic experiments, action potentials were determined to be rapid, self-propagating electrical excitations of the membrane that are mediated by ion channels that open and close in response to changes in voltage across the membrane (voltage-gated ion channels).[23-27] An action potential is triggered by membrane depolarization.

In nerve and muscle cells, the usual trigger for depolarization is binding of a neurotransmitter to cell surface receptors. Transmitter binding causes channels or pores in the membrane to open, allowing ions (primarily Na+) to enter the cell. This influx of positive ions results in a shift in the membrane potential to a less negative value, resulting in depolarization. *Threshold* is reached when a patch of the membrane becomes sufficiently depolarized (approximately -65 mV in animal neurons) to activate voltage-gated sodium channels in the membrane. At threshold, these channels open rapidly and transiently to allow the influx of Na+ ions. A self-propagating process follows whereby Na+ influx in one patch of membrane causes membrane depolarization of the next patch and opens more voltage-gated Na+ channels, allowing more Na+ to enter the cell. This process repeats over and over again as the action potential proceeds along the length of the cell (Figure 3-27). In this way, action potentials can transmit information rapidly over relatively long distances.

A typical neuronal action potential is shown in Figure 3-28. The various changes in membrane potential during the time course of the action potential are attributable to the flow of ions through membrane ion channels. The steep upstroke of the action potential corresponds to Na+ influx through "fast" sodium channels, as described above. *Fast channels* are so termed because they open and close rapidly, with the entire process lasting less than a millisecond. This phase of rapid depolarization is terminated when the fast Na+ channels suddenly close and the repolarization phase begins. Fast Na+ channels are interesting in that they can assume at least three conformations (three-dimensional forms).[28] In addition to the open and closed conformations, the fast Na+ channel has a refractory form during which the channel will not open again in response to another depolarizing stimulus (Figure 3-29). This refractory period limits the rate at which action potentials can be generated.

Two major factors contribute to cellular repolarization: sodium conductance (inflow) is stopped by closing Na+ channels, as described previously, and K+ conductance (outflow) through voltage-gated K+ channels increases. These K+ channels respond to depolarization of the membrane in the same manner as fast Na+ channels, but they take much longer to open and close. When K+ channels open, K+ flows out of the cell, owing to the concentration gradient and the loss of intracellular negativity that accompanies Na+ influx. The loss of positive intracellular potassium ions helps to quickly return the membrane potential to its negative RMP value.

Action potentials in muscle cells are more complex than the neuronal ones just described. Recall that muscle contraction depends on the presence of intracellular calcium ions. Because Ca2+ carries a charge, its entry into the cell is reflected

FIGURE 3-27 The action potential *(AP)* in excitable cells is propagated along the membrane by the sequential opening of voltage-gated sodium channels in adjacent sections of membrane. **A,** An action potential is initiated by the opening of sodium channels in a section of membrane. **B,** The action potential is regenerated in adjacent sections of membrane as more sodium channels open. The initial segment repolarizes as sodium channels close and potassium ions move out of the cell.

in the membrane potential. In skeletal muscle, most of the free cytosolic calcium ions come from intracellular stores (sarcoplasmic reticulum) that are released when the cell is depolarized. In cardiac muscle cells, Ca^{2+} entry through voltage-gated channels in the plasma membrane is also important. Calcium conductance into the cell tends to prolong the action potential, resulting in a plateau phase (Figure 3-30). This is of functional importance in cardiac tissue, as it allows time for muscular contraction before another impulse is conducted and prevents the potentially disastrous condition of cardiac muscle tetany. (For a more thorough discussion of cardiac electrophysiology, see Chapter 17.)

KEY POINTS

- The negative value of the RMP is determined by the ratio of intracellular to extracellular K^+ ion concentration. Changes in serum K^+ can have profound effects on the RMP.
- Cells with voltage-gated ion channels are excitable and can produce and conduct action potentials. An action potential results from the opening of "fast" Na^+ channels, which allows Na^+ to rush into the cell.
- Repolarization is caused by closure of Na^+ channels and efflux of K^+ from the cell. In cardiac muscle, repolarization is prolonged owing to Ca^{2+} influx through "slow" Ca^{2+} channels.

INTERCELLULAR COMMUNICATION AND GROWTH

Cell Signaling Strategies

Cells in multicellular organisms need to communicate with one another and respond to changes in the cellular environment. Coordination of growth, cell division, and the functions of various tissues and organ systems is accomplished by three principal means of communication: (1) Through gap junctions that directly connect the cytoplasm of adjoining cells; (2) By direct cell-to-cell contact of plasma membranes or the extracellular molecules associated with the cell (extracellular matrix); and (3) By secretion of chemical mediators (ligands) that influence cells some distance away (Figure 3-31).[29]

Gap junctions are found in large numbers in most tissues. They are connecting channels between adjacent cells that allow the passage of small molecules from one cell to the next. These junctions are formed by special transmembrane proteins that associate to form pores of about 1.5 nm in width. Small molecules, such as inorganic ions, sugars, amino acids, nucleotides, and vitamins, may pass through the pores, whereas macromolecules (proteins, polysaccharides, and nucleic acids) are too large to pass through. Gap junctions are particularly important in tissues in which synchronized functions are required, such as cardiac muscle contraction and intestinal peristaltic movements. Gap junctions appear to be important in embryogenesis as well. Cellular differentiation

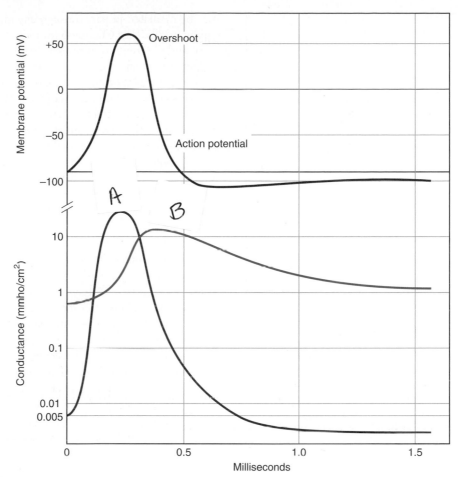

FIGURE 3-28 A typical neuronal action potential showing changes in membrane potential and the associated ion conductances. Note: mmho is a measure of conductance (amperes per volt), also called millisiemens (mS). The steep upstroke of the action potential is attributed to the sudden influx of Na$^+$ through voltage-gated "fast" sodium ion channels. Voltage-gated K$^+$ channels open more slowly and stay open longer to allow K$^+$ efflux from the cell, which aids in repolarization.

FIGURE 3-29 The three possible states of the voltage-gated sodium channel. In the open state, Na$^+$ is allowed to pass. In the refractory state, the channel is blocked by the inactivation gate and will not open in response to a depolarizing stimulus. In the closed state, the channel will open in response to a membrane depolarization.

FIGURE 3-30 A typical cardiac muscle cell action potential showing the ion fluxes associated with each phase. Note that the repolarization phase is prolonged in comparison to the nerve action potential in Figure 3-28. This occurs because Ca^{2+} influx offsets the repolarizing effect of K^+ efflux and a plateau in the membrane potential is seen. When the Ca^{2+} channels close, the membrane quickly repolarizes.

may be mediated in part through chemical signaling through gap junctions. (See Chapter 5 for a discussion of the development and differentiation of tissue types.)

Direct contact of cell membrane receptors with signaling molecules present on the surface of other cells or extracellular matrix is an important means of local communication among cells in tissues. Contact-dependent signaling is particularly important for the development of the immune response. Such cell-to-cell contact during fetal development is thought to allow the cells of the immune system to discriminate between foreign and self tissues and to develop self tolerance. If cell-to-cell contact does not occur during fetal life, the immune cells may later attack the body's own cells, leading to the development of autoimmune diseases. (See Chapter 10 for a discussion of autoimmunity.) There are four major families of cell adhesion molecules (CAMs): immunoglobulin-cell adhesion molecules (Ig-CAMs); cadherins; integrins; and selectins. These cell adhesion proteins make contacts between cells and with the extracellular matrix and provide signals that maintain cell survival and differentiated cell types (Figure 3-32).

The best understood form of cell communication is signaling through secreted molecules or *ligands*. Three strategies of intercellular chemical signaling have been described, relating to the distances over which they operate (Figure 3-33). *Synaptic* signaling is confined to the cells of the nervous system and occurs at specialized junctions between the nerve cell and its target cell. The neuron secretes a chemical

REMOTE SIGNALING BY SECRETED MOLECULES

DIRECT SIGNALING BY PLASMA MEMBRANE–BOUND MOLECULES OR EXTRACELLULAR MATRIX

DIRECT SIGNALING VIA GAP JUNCTIONS

FIGURE 3-31 Methods used for intercellular communication.

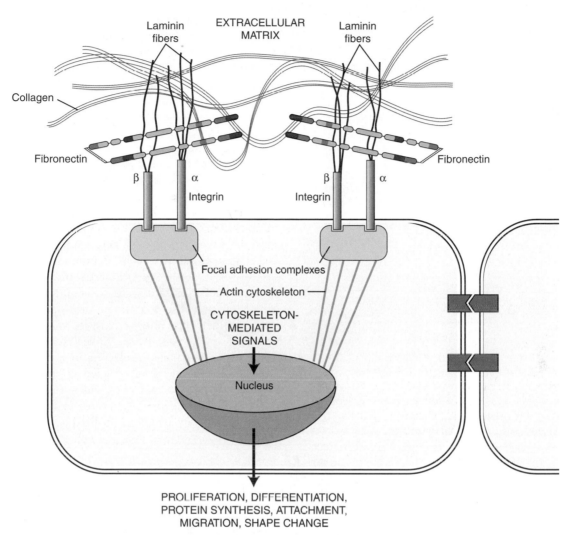

FIGURE 3-32 Cell adhesion proteins interact with the extracellular matrix (integrins) and with neighboring cells to maintain cell survival and differentiation. (Redrawn from Kumar V et al, editors: *Robbins basic pathology,* ed 8, Philadelphia, 2007, Saunders, p 69.)

neurotransmitter into the space between the nerve and target cell; the neurotransmitter then diffuses across and binds receptors on the postsynaptic cell. Synaptic signaling occurs over very small distances (50 nm) and involves only one or a few postsynaptic target cells. In *paracrine* signaling, chemicals are secreted into a localized area and are rapidly destroyed, so that only cells in the immediate area are affected. Growth factors (GFs), for example, act locally to promote wound healing without affecting the growth of the entire organism. *Endocrine* signaling is accomplished by specialized endocrine cells that secrete hormones that travel via the bloodstream to target cells widely distributed throughout the body. Endocrine signaling is slow in comparison to nervous signaling, because it relies on diffusion and blood flow to target tissues.

Autocrine signaling occurs when cells are able to respond to signaling molecules that they secrete. Autocrine communication provides a feedback signal to the secreting cell and is commonly linked to pathways that regulate ligand secretion rates. Abnormal autocrine stimulation is thought to be a mechanism in some forms of cancer (see Chapter 7).

Target cells respond to ligand signaling through specific protein *receptors.* Cells can respond to a particular ligand only if they possess the appropriate receptor. For example, all cells of the body are exposed to thyroid-stimulating hormone (TSH) as it circulates in the blood, but only thyroid cells respond because they alone possess TSH receptors. However, cells that possess the same receptor may respond very differently to a particular ligand. For example, binding of acetylcholine to its receptor on a glandular cell may induce secretion, whereas binding to the same receptor on a cardiac muscle cell causes a decrease in contractile force. The cellular response to signaling molecules is regulated both by the array of receptors the cell carries and by the internal machinery to which the receptors are linked.

Cell Surface Receptor-Mediated Responses

Most hormones, local chemical mediators, and neurotransmitters are water-soluble molecules that are unable to pass through the lipid bilayer of the cell. These ligands exert their effects through binding with a receptor on the surface of the target cell, which then changes or transduces the external

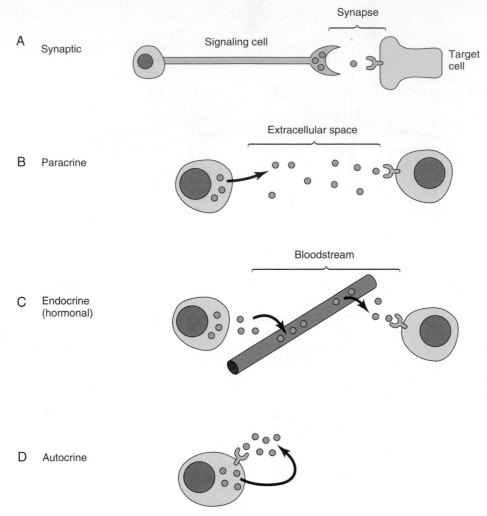

FIGURE 3-33 Signaling by secreted ligands can occur over variable distances. **A,** Synaptic signaling over a very small distance between neuron and target cell. **B,** Paracrine signaling through the extracellular fluid between cells in a tissue. **C,** Long-range signaling from endocrine cells through the bloodstream to distant targets. **D,** Localized autocrine signaling in which the secreting cell is also the target cell.

signal into an intracellular message. There are at least three major classes of cell surface receptor proteins: ion channel–linked, enzyme-linked, and G-protein-linked (Figure 3-34).[29]

Ion channel-linked receptors bind neurotransmitters, causing specific ion channels in the membrane to open or close. This type of signaling is prevalent in the nervous system, where rapid synaptic signaling between neurons is required. *Enzyme-linked* receptors catalyze enzyme reactions when they are activated by appropriate ligands. Nearly all enzyme-linked receptors function as *protein kinases;* that is, they mediate the transfer of phosphate groups from ATP (or GTP) to proteins (phosphorylate), and thus affect the activity of those proteins. The insulin receptor and most GF receptors are protein kinase receptors that phosphorylate and activate intracellular enzyme cascades. A large number of signaling ligands bind to *G-protein-linked receptors.* More than half of known drugs have their effects through G-protein-linked cascades.

G-protein-linked receptors act indirectly through a membrane-bound trimeric G-protein that binds and hydrolyzes GTP. The activated G-protein then activates target enzymes

or ion channels within the membrane. The target enzymes of G-protein receptors produce second messengers that trigger specific intracellular cascades and alter cell function (Figure 3-35). The alpha subunit of G-proteins has intrinsic enzyme activity that degrades GTP into GDP and P_i after a time. When GTP is bound, the G-protein is in the right conformation to activate its downstream targets, but when GTP is hydrolyzed to GDP and P_i, the G-protein resumes its inactive conformation and activity of the signaling cascade turns off.

There are three principal G-protein-linked signaling systems that, when activated, alter the intracellular concentration of one or more second messengers (Figure 3-36). Numerous G-protein-linked receptors activate trimeric G-proteins whose α subunit stimulates adenylyl cyclase to produce the second messenger cyclic adenosine monophosphate (cAMP). These G-proteins are called G_s. An increase in cAMP is linked to different signaling cascades in different cell types. For example, cAMP causes glycogen breakdown in liver cells, increased force of contraction in cardiac cells, and increased secretion by glandular cells. Various cell types respond differently to

FIGURE 3-34 There are three major types of cell surface receptor proteins. **A,** Ion channel-linked receptors are also called ligand-gated channels. When the ligand binds, they open to allow specific ions through the membrane. **B,** Enzyme-linked receptors become activated kinases when a ligand binds to them. Kinases phosphorylate target proteins and change their activity. **C,** G-protein-linked receptors have seven membrane-spanning segments with a ligand binding pocket on the outside and a G-protein-activating portion on the inside. G-protein-linked receptors activate G-proteins, which in turn activate enzymes that produce second messengers.

The metabolic process of introducing a phosphate group into an organic molecule.

FIGURE 3-35 Schematic of the proposed role of guanosine triphosphate *(GTP)*-binding proteins in the transduction of extracellular signaling messages. When the ligand binds the receptor, an intracellular domain is changed into an active configuration that can interact with inactive trimeric G proteins. The receptor induces the G protein to release its bound GDP and P$_i$ in exchange for a GTP molecule. When GTP binds to the α subunit of the G protein, it is activated and diffuses away from the $\gamma\beta$ subunits to find its target enzyme. The α GTP stimulates its target enzyme to produce a second messenger, which in turn activates a signaling cascade within the cell. After a time, the α subunit hydrolyzes its GTP to GDP and P$_i$ and becomes inactive. The α subunit is now in the correct conformation to reassociate with the $\gamma\beta$ subunits and await another signal from the receptor.

G_s Pathway

G_q Pathway

G_i Pathway

FIGURE 3-36 Ligand binding to membrane receptors leads to activation of G-proteins, which in turn regulate membrane-bound enzymes (adenylyl cyclase *[AC]* and phospholipase C). These enzymes catalyze the formation of second messengers (cyclic adenosine monophosphate *[cAMP]*, inositol 1,4,5-triphosphate *[IP₃]*, diacylglycerol *[DAG]*). Second messengers then activate enzyme cascades within the cell or affect intracellular Ca^{2+} concentration. **A,** The G_s pathway increases the production of cAMP. **B,** The G_q pathway increases the production of IP₃ and DAG, and releases intracellular Ca^{2+}. **C,** The G_i pathway is inhibitory to the production of cAMP. In some cases the γβ unit also has functional activity and may regulate ion channels. *PKC,* Protein kinase C; *ER,* endoplasmic reticulum.

the same second messenger because of differences in enzymes and other proteins in the cell.

Another important G-protein-linked cascade is mediated by G-proteins called G_q whose α subunit stimulates the enzyme phospholipase C. Phospholipase C cleaves a membrane phospholipid ($PI[4,5]P_2$) to form two second messengers, inositol 1,4,5-trisphosphate (IP_3) and diacylglycerol (DAG) (see Figure 3-36). The IP_3 travels to the endoplasmic reticulum, where it stimulates the release of Ca^{2+} into the cytoplasm. The Ca^{2+} then triggers a change in cell function. DAG remains bound to the inner surface of the plasma membrane and can trigger several different intracellular cascades. Two important targets are the protein kinase C pathway and the eicosanoid pathway. Protein kinase C is a key enzyme in the growth response. The eicosanoid pathway results in the production of several arachidonic acid derivatives, including prostaglandins. These products are often secreted by the cell as signaling molecules to other nearby cells. Prostaglandins are important mediators of inflammation and platelet function.

The third trimeric G-protein type is called G_i because it is inhibitory to the production of cAMP. G-protein-linked receptors such as the acetylcholine receptor in the heart activate G_i whose α subunit then inhibits adenylyl cyclase (see Figure 3-36). In this case, the $\gamma\beta$ subunit of G_i is also activated and opens membrane potassium channels in the heart, which tend to slow the heart rate.

In addition to the four second messengers already mentioned (cAMP, IP_3, DAG, and Ca^{2+}) there is a fifth called *cyclic guanosine monophosphate* (cGMP), which is produced by the enzyme guanylyl cyclase (Figure 3-37). The primary activator of guanylyl cyclase is a small lipid-soluble gas molecule called *nitric oxide*. Nitric oxide is an important signaling molecule with widespread targets. It functions as a neurotransmitter in the brain and is an important smooth muscle relaxant in the vascular system. cGMP is also produced by a special class of enzyme-linked receptors (see Figure 3-37).

To be effective at communicating signals, all the receptor systems must be quickly turned off so that they can be responsive to the next incoming signal. A variety of strategies are used to quench the signaling cascades (Figure 3-38). For example, phosphodiesterases are enzymes that convert the cyclic nucleotides cAMP and cGMP to their inactive forms, AMP and GMP, and help to remove these second messengers soon after they are formed. Some drugs, such as caffeine and sildenafil citrate (Viagra), are phosphodiesterase inhibitors that slow the normal breakdown of cyclic nucleotides and prolong their activity. Many of the intracellular signaling cascades rely on kinases that phosphorylate their target proteins so as to change their activity. The action of kinases is countered by numerous phosphatase enzymes that quickly cleave the phosphates back off the target proteins and inhibit their activity.

The cell also can regulate the activity and number of receptors on the cell surface.[29] Generally a cell decreases the number or activity of receptors when it is exposed to excessive concentrations of signaling molecules (see Figure 3-38). Receptors can be internalized in the cell where they are inactive but are available for later use, or they can be sent to lysosomes for degradation. Destruction of receptors in lysosomes is called *down-regulation*. (The production of extra receptors is called *up-regulation*.) Receptors that remain in the membrane also can be inhibited by phosphorylation, which blocks them from interacting with their intracellular targets. Receptors that can bind ligand but do not produce a response are said to be uncoupled. The proteins that phosphorylate G-protein receptors are called G-protein-receptor kinases (GRKs). The mechanisms that "turn off" signaling cascades are vitally important to maintaining a responsive communication system.

Intracellular Receptor-Mediated Responses

A small number of hormones are lipid soluble and can pass directly through the cell membrane to interact with receptors *inside* the cell. These receptors are located in the cell cytosol

FIGURE 3-37 Cyclic GMP *(cGMP)* is an important second messenger. **A,** It can be synthesized by enzyme-linked receptors that are activated by water-soluble ligands. **B,** Nitric oxide is an important signaling molecule that is lipid soluble and can diffuse across the cell membrane. Nitric oxide binds to and stimulates the enzyme guanylyl cyclase to produce cGMP.

FIGURE 3-38 A variety of mechanisms exist to inhibit receptor-mediated signaling cascades. **A,** Phosphorylation of the receptor by receptor kinases such as G-protein receptor kinase *(GRK)* uncouples the enzyme from its intracellular cascade. **B,** Receptor internalization temporarily reduces the number of receptors displayed at the cell surface. **C,** Receptor degradation results in a long-term reduction in receptors (down-regulation). **D,** The cyclic nucleotide second messengers can be degraded by phosphodiesterase enzymes to stop the intracellular cascade. **E,** Phosphatase enzymes counteract the phosphorylating activities of kinases and inhibit the intracellular cascade.

(e.g., cortisol) or may be associated with the cell nucleus (e.g., thyroid). Intracellular receptors are specific for a particular ligand, just as surface receptors are. Binding of the ligand causes the receptor to become activated. The activated cytosolic receptor then travels to the nucleus, where it binds with specific genes and regulates their activity (Figure 3-39). Because lipid-soluble ligands enter the cell directly, no second messengers are needed. Steroid hormones such as cortisol usually bind to receptors in the cytosol, whereas the thyroid receptor is already bound to DNA in the absence of its ligand. When thyroid hormone finds its nuclear receptor, the complex dissociates and removes an inhibitory influence on gene transcription. Cellular responses to these gene regulatory receptor complexes are slow in comparison to the cell surface receptor responses and generally last longer.

Regulation of Cellular Growth and Proliferation

In multicellular organisms such as humans, the growth and proliferation of cells and tissues must be strictly controlled to maintain a balance between cell birth rate and cell death rate. The system must be capable of rapidly increasing proliferation of a particular tissue to replace cells lost to injury

and normal wear and tear while simultaneously inhibiting unwanted growth or proliferation of other cells. Special intercellular communication systems function to regulate the replication of individual cells in the body. Two important strategies of cell cycle control have been described. First, a variety of protein mitogens and growth factors are required in specific combinations for growth and proliferation of particular cell types. Second, cells respond to spatial signals from the extracellular matrix and neighboring cells that indicate how much room is available. When conditions favor cell proliferation, the cell proceeds through the stages of the cell cycle (Figure 3-40). Dormant cells remain in G_1 phase indefinitely. Cycling cells proceed through G_1, S phase (synthesis), G_2, M phase (mitosis), and cell division. S phase is characterized by duplication of DNA and synthesis of intracellular components in preparation for cell division. M phase, or mitosis, proceeds through six stages, beginning with prophase, in which the chromosomes condense and become visible, and ending with cytokinesis, when cell division is accomplished. The chromosomes of body cells are duplicated and distributed equally to the cell's progeny when it divides by mitosis, such that each daughter cell receives an identical full

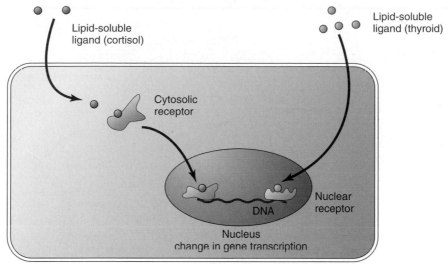

FIGURE 3-39 Lipid-soluble ligands, such as steroid hormones, thyroid hormones, and gases, can diffuse across the cell membrane and interact with receptors located within the cell cytoplasm or nucleus. When the ligand binds to its intracellular receptor, it forms a functional gene regulatory protein that affects the rate of transcription of its target genes. The response of the cell to intracellular ligands is generally slow and long lasting.

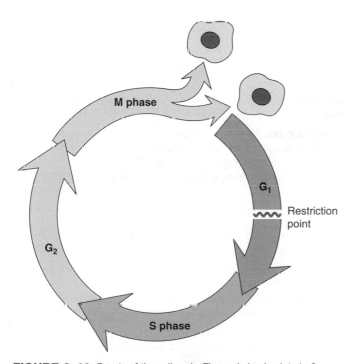

FIGURE 3-40 Events of the cell cycle. The cycle begins late in G_1 when the cell passes a restriction point. The cell then proceeds systematically through the S phase (synthesis), G_2, and M phase (mitosis).

set of 46 chromosomes. The stages of mitotic cell division are explained in Figure 3-41. Mitosis is responsible for the proliferation of body cells in which little genetic variation is needed or desired. A more elaborate cell division process, meiosis, occurs in the germ cells (egg and sperm), where significant chromosomal rearrangements occur (see Chapter 6).

The **cell cycle** has been the subject of intense study in recent years because of its importance in cancer biology. Cancer cells continue to grow and divide unchecked, despite the lack of

appropriate signals to stimulate them. A clearer understanding of the roles of numerous genes in regulating the cell cycle is beginning to emerge. Of particular interest are the events that prod the cell from its dormant state and cause it to begin the cycle. A simplified picture of a major component of this complex process is shown in Figure 3-42. The Rb protein (or pRb) is of central importance in preventing a cell from proceeding through the cell cycle.[30] The Rb protein functions to bind up gene regulatory factors called *E2F* so that they are unable to bind to DNA promoter regions and begin the processes of cell replication. The Rb protein can be induced to let go of the E2F transcription factors when appropriate mitogen signals arrive at the cell surface. These proliferation-promoting signals at the cell surface are transmitted to the Rb protein by way of cyclin-dependent signaling pathways within the cell. Proteins called *cyclins* accumulate in the cell and then bind to and activate cyclin-dependent kinases (cdk). The cdk then phosphorylates the Rb protein, changing its affinity for E2F so that it lets go. The E2F then translocates to specific regions of DNA where it promotes gene transcription, allowing cell replication to begin.

To respond to a mitogen or GF, a cell must have the corresponding receptor on its cell surface. Many cells in the body synthesize and secrete mitogens and GFs, which then influence the proliferation of other cell types in a paracrine or endocrine fashion. Platelet-derived growth factor (PDGF) was one of the first mitogens to be discovered. It is secreted by platelets when they form blood clots in response to an injury. PDGF stimulates fibroblasts and smooth muscle cells in the damaged area to divide and replace cells lost to the injury. Numerous mitogens have been identified, and most cells require an appropriate combination of mitogen signals before they can enter the cell cycle.[31] There are many signaling steps in the pathway from mitogen receptor to DNA activation. Some growth factors promote an increase in cell size, whereas mitogens

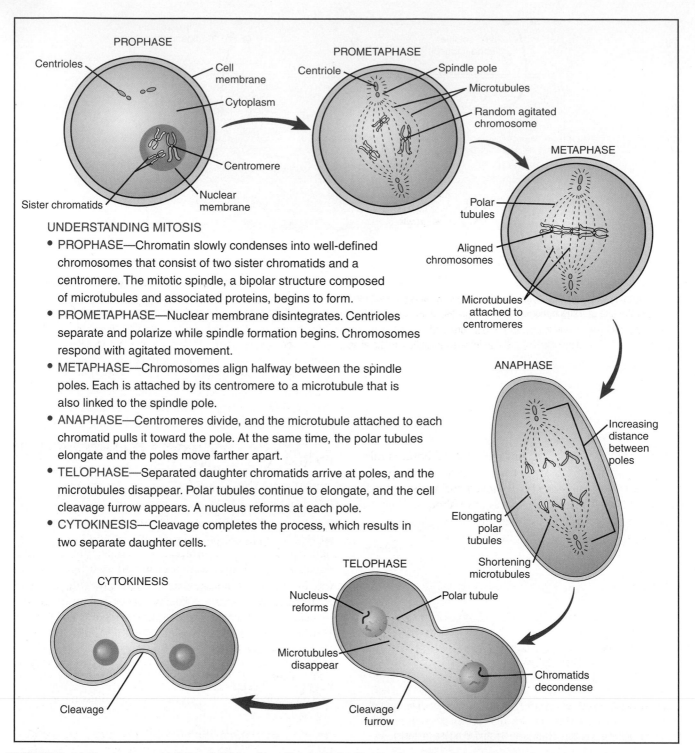

UNDERSTANDING MITOSIS

- PROPHASE—Chromatin slowly condenses into well-defined chromosomes that consist of two sister chromatids and a centromere. The mitotic spindle, a bipolar structure composed of microtubules and associated proteins, begins to form.
- PROMETAPHASE—Nuclear membrane disintegrates. Centrioles separate and polarize while spindle formation begins. Chromosomes respond with agitated movement.
- METAPHASE—Chromosomes align halfway between the spindle poles. Each is attached by its centromere to a microtubule that is also linked to the spindle pole.
- ANAPHASE—Centromeres divide, and the microtubule attached to each chromatid pulls it toward the pole. At the same time, the polar tubules elongate and the poles move farther apart.
- TELOPHASE—Separated daughter chromatids arrive at poles, and the microtubules disappear. Polar tubules continue to elongate, and the cell cleavage furrow appears. A nucleus reforms at each pole.
- CYTOKINESIS—Cleavage completes the process, which results in two separate daughter cells.

FIGURE 3-41 The six stages of mitotic cell division. (From Nichols FH, Zwelling E, editors: *Maternal-newborn nursing: theory and practice,* Philadelphia, 1997, Saunders, p 307.)

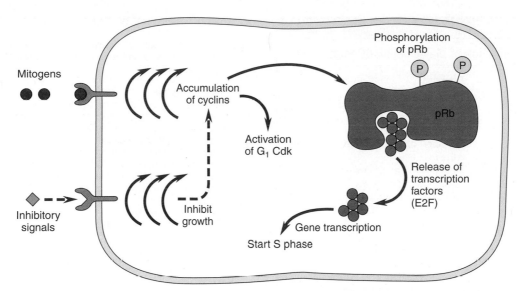

FIGURE 3-42 The mechanism of initiation of cellular replication requires appropriate stimulation by extracellular growth factors that bind their complementary receptors on the cell surface. Activation of the receptor stimulates signaling pathways within the cell that increase cyclin proteins. The cyclins bind to cyclin-dependent kinases *(Cdk)* to form active enzyme complexes. The active cyclin-Cdk enzymes phosphorylate Rb protein *(pRb)*, inducing it to let go of E2F transcription factors that initiate replication. In the absence of appropriate growth factor signals, the Rb protein functions to inhibit unwanted cell proliferation.

stimulate cell division, and many appear to do both. Similar signaling pathways are used to trigger cell death (apoptosis) when cells have to be reduced or removed during tissue development and remodeling. The processes of abnormal cellular proliferation and cancer are further detailed in Chapter 7. The process of apoptosis is described in Chapter 4.

KEY POINTS

- Intercellular communication is accomplished by three principal means: (1) Gap junctions, which directly connect the cytoplasm of adjoining cells; (2) Direct cell-to-cell surface contact; and (3) Secretion of chemical mediators (ligands). Most ligands are water-soluble molecules that interact with receptors on the cell surface. These receptors are of three general types: ion channel linked, enzyme linked, and G-protein linked.
- Binding of a ligand to a G-protein receptor usually results in the production of second messengers (cAMP, IP_3, DAG, Ca^{2+}) within the target cell that initiate a change in cell function.
- Somatic cells divide by a process called *mitosis* in which daughter cells each receive an identical and complete set of 46 chromosomes.
- Cell replication normally requires specific extracellular mitogens that activate signaling systems within the cell. Cyclin proteins and cyclin-dependent kinases alter the function of RB protein, causing it to release transcription factors that begin the process of cell replication.

SUMMARY

Detailed knowledge of cell physiology is essential to understanding disease processes. Cells are complex, membrane-bound units that perform a variety of functions necessary to the maintenance of life. The major cell components and their functions are summarized in Table 3-1. The cell membrane is an important cellular structure that protects the cell interior and mediates information transfer to and from the extracellular environment. Proteins embedded in the membrane lipid bilayer perform most of the membrane functions, including transduction of extracellular messages, membrane transport, electrical excitation, and cell-to-cell communication.

Human cells have several important intracellular organelles. These include the cytoskeleton, which organizes the intracellular compartment; the nucleus, which holds the cell's genetic material and directs the day-to-day activities of the cell; the endoplasmic reticulum and the Golgi apparatus, which produce, package, and transport proteins and lipids to the plasma membrane and lysosomes; the lysosomes and peroxisomes, which perform the task of intracellular digestion of organic waste; and the mitochondria, which produce cellular energy in the form of ATP. The energy released by ATP hydrolysis is used by the cell to drive the many energetically unfavorable reactions needed to maintain cellular functions. Multicellular organisms have developed complex communication systems to control cell behavior, such as growth and differentiation into specialized cell types. Disruption of these cellular processes is at the root of pathophysiologic processes and disease.

TABLE 3-1

Structure and Function of Major Cellular Components

Cellular Structure	Functions
Plasma membrane	Protective barrier separates life from nonlife
	Extracellular message transduction
	Transport of materials into and out of the cell
	Maintenance and transmission of membrane potentials
	Cell-to-cell recognition, interaction
Cytoskeleton	Maintenance of cell shape
	Cell movement
	Trafficking within the cell
Nucleus	Protection of genetic material
	Regulation of cell type and function through control of protein synthesis
Endoplasmic reticulum	Protein and lipid synthesis
	Lipid metabolism and detoxification
Golgi apparatus	Protein and lipid modification and sorting
	Transport of proteins and lipids to appropriate destinations
Lysosomes	Hydrolytic breakdown of organic waste
Peroxisomes	Oxidative breakdown of organic waste
Mitochondria	Cellular energy production (ATP)

ATP, Adenosine triphosphate.

REFERENCES

1. Alberts B et al: Cells and genomes. In Alberts B et al, editors: *Molecular biology of the cell,* ed 5, New York, 2008, Garland Science, pp 1-44.
2. Lahava N, Nira S, Elitzurb A: The emergence of life on Earth, *Progr Biophys Mol Biol* 75:75-120, 2001.
3. Singer SJ, Nicolson GL: The fluid mosaic model of the structure of cell membranes, *Science* 175:720-731, 1972.
4. Alberts B et al: Membrane structure. In Alberts B et al, editors: *Molecular biology of the cell,* ed 5, New York, 2008, Garland Science, pp 617-650.
5. Hakomori S: Structure, organization, and function of glycosphingolipids in membrane, *Curr Opin Hematol* 10(1):16-24, 2003.
6. Bennett V, Baines A: Spectrin and ankyrin-based pathways: metazoan inventions for integrating cells into tissues, *Physiol Rev* 81:1353-1392, 2001.
7. Alberts B et al: The cytoskeleton. In Alberts B et al, editors: *Molecular biology of the cell,* ed 5, New York, 2008, Garland Science, pp 965-1062.
8. Pollard T, Earnshaw W: *Cell biology,* ed 2, Philadelphia, 2008, Saunders, p 191.
9. Lenart P, Ellenberg J: Nuclear envelope dynamics in oocytes: from germinal vesicle breakdown to mitosis, *Curr Opin Cell Biol* 15(1):88-95, 2003.
10. Pollard T, Earnshaw W: *Cell biology,* ed 2, Philadelphia, 2008, Saunders, p 348.
11. Johnson AE et al: Structure, function, and regulation of free and membrane-bound ribosomes: the view from their substrates and products, *Cold Spring Harb Symp Quant Biol* 66:531-541, 2001.
12. Alberts B et al: Intracellular vesicular traffic. In Alberts B et al, editors: *Molecular biology of the cell,* ed 5, New York, 2008, Garland Science, pp 779-784.
13. Cheng SH, Smith AE: Gene therapy progress and prospects: gene therapy of lysosomal storage disorders, *Gene Ther* 10(16):1275-1281, 2003.
14. Chinnery PF, Schon EA: Mitochondria, *J Neurol Neurosurg Psychiatry* 74(9):1188-1199, 2003.
15. Alberts B et al: Energy conversion: mitochondria and chloroplasts. In Alberts B et al, editors: *Molecular biology of the cell,* ed 5, New York, 2008, Garland Science, pp 813-878.
16. Pollard T, Earnshaw W: *Cell biology,* ed 2, Philadelphia, 2008, Saunders, p 332.
17. Alberts B et al: Membrane transport of small molecules and the electrical properties of membranes. In Alberts B et al, editors: *Molecular biology of the cell,* ed 5, New York, 2008, Garland Science, pp 651-694.
18. Clausen T: The sodium pump keeps us going, *Ann N Y Acad Sci* 986:595-602, 2003.
19. Martonosi AN, Pikula S: The network of calcium regulation in muscle, *Acta Biochim Pol* 50(1):1-30, 2003.
20. Karpen JW, Ruiz M: Ion channels: does each subunit do something on its own?, *Trends Biochem Sci* 27(8):402-409, 2002.
21. Pollard T, Earnshaw W: *Cell biology,* ed 2, Philadelphia, 2008, Saunders. p 149.
22. Lamas JA, Reboreda A, Codesido V: Ionic basis of the resting membrane potential in cultured rat sympathetic neurons, *Neuroreport* 13(5):585-591, 2002.
23. Hodgkin AL: *The conduction of the nervous impulse,* Liverpool, England, 1971, Liverpool University Press.
24. Baker PF, Hodgkin AL, Shaw T: The effects of changes in internal ionic concentrations of the electrical properties of perfused giant axons, *J Physiol* 164:355-374, 1962.
25. Hodgkin AL, Huxley AF: Currents carried by sodium and potassium ions through the membrane of the giant axon of *Loligo, J Physiol* 116:449-472, 1952.
26. Hodgkin AL, Huxley AF, Katz B: Measurement of current-voltage relations in the membrane of the giant axon of *Loligo, J Physiol* 116:424-448, 1952.
27. Hodgkin AL, Katz B: The effect of sodium ions on the electrical activity of the giant axon of the squid, *J Physiol* 108:37-77, 1949.
28. Bezanilla F: Voltage sensor movements, *J Gen Physiol* 120(4):465-473, 2002.
29. Alberts B et al: Mechanisms of cell communication. In Alberts B et al, editors: *Molecular biology of the cell,* ed 5, New York, 2008, Garland Science, pp 879-964.
30. Stiegler P, Giordano A: The family of retinoblastoma proteins, *Crit Rev Eukaryot Gene Expr* 11(1-3):59-76, 2001.
31. Alberts B et al: The cell cycle. In Alberts B et al, editors: *Molecular biology of the cell,* ed 5, New York, 2008, Garland Science, pp 1101-1114.

Cell Injury, Aging, and Death

Jacquelyn L. Banasik

MEDIA RESOURCES

Additional Material for Study, Review, and Further Exploration

CD Companion ▪ Review Questions and Answers
▪ Glossary (with audio pronunciations for selected terms)
▪ Disease Profiles ▪ Animations

ℯvolve **Website** at http://evolve.elsevier.com/Copstead/
▪ Case Studies ▪ Disease Profiles ▪ WebLinks ▪ Key Points Review

 Online Course (Module 1)

KEY QUESTIONS

▪ What are the usual cellular responses to reversible injury?
▪ How are reversible and irreversible cellular injuries differentiated?
▪ How do necrosis and apoptosis differ?

▪ To what kind of injuries are cells susceptible?
▪ What are the usual physiologic changes of aging and how are these differentiated from disease?

CHAPTER OUTLINE

D isease and injury are increasingly being understood as cellular and genetic phenomena. Although pathophysiologic processes are often presented in terms of systemic effects and manifestations, ultimately it is the *cells* that make up the systems that are affected. Even complex multisystem disorders such as cancer ultimately are the result of alterations in cell function. As the mysterious mechanisms of diseases are understood on the cellular and molecular levels, more specific methods of diagnosis, treatment, and prevention can be developed. This chapter presents the general characteristics of cellular injury, adaptation, aging, and death that underlie the discussions of systemic pathophysiologic processes presented in later chapters of this text.

Cells are confronted by many challenges to their integrity and survival and have efficient mechanisms for coping with an altered cellular environment. Cells respond to environmental changes or injury in three general ways: (1) If the change is mild or short lived, the cell may withstand the assault and completely return to normal. This is called a *reversible cell injury*. (2) The cell may adapt to a persistent but sublethal injury by changing its structure or function. Generally, adaptation also is reversible. (3) Cell death may occur if the injury is too severe or prolonged. Cell death is irreversible and may occur by two different processes termed *necrosis* and *apoptosis*. Necrosis is cell death caused by external injury, whereas apoptosis is triggered by intracellular signaling cascades that result in cell suicide. Necrosis is considered to be a pathologic process associated with significant tissue damage, whereas apoptosis may be a normal physiologic process in some instances and pathologic in others.

REVERSIBLE CELL INJURY

Regardless of the cause, reversible injuries and the early stages of irreversible injuries often result in cellular swelling and the accumulation of excess substances within the cell. These changes reflect the cell's inability to perform normal metabolic functions owing to insufficient cellular energy in the form of adenosine triphosphate (ATP) or dysfunction of associated metabolic enzymes. Once the acute stress or injury has been removed, by definition of a reversible injury, the cell returns to its preinjury state.

Hydropic Swelling

Cellular swelling due to accumulation of water, or hydropic swelling, is the first manifestation of most forms of reversible cell injury.[1] Hydropic swelling results from malfunction of the sodium-potassium (Na^+-K^+) pumps that normally maintain ionic equilibrium of the cell. Failure of the Na^+-K^+

pump results in accumulation of sodium ions within the cell, creating an osmotic gradient for water entry. Because Na^+-K^+ pump function is dependent on cellular ATP, any injury that results in insufficient energy production also will result in hydropic swelling (Figure 4-1).[1] Hydropic swelling is characterized by a large, pale cytoplasm, dilated endoplasmic reticulum, and swollen mitochondria. With severe hydropic swelling, the endoplasmic reticulum may rupture and form large water-filled vacuoles. Generalized swelling in the cells of a particular organ will cause the organ to increase in size and weight. Organ enlargement is indicated by the suffix *-megaly* (e.g., *splenomegaly* denotes an enlarged spleen, *hepatomegaly* denotes an enlarged liver).

Intracellular Accumulations

Excess accumulations of substances in cells may result in cellular injury because the substances are toxic or provoke an immune response, or merely because they occupy space needed for cellular functions. In some cases, accumulations do not in themselves appear to be injurious but rather are indicators of cell injury. Intracellular accumulations may be categorized as (1) excessive amounts of normal intracellular substances such as fat, (2) accumulation of abnormal substances produced by the cell because of faulty metabolism or synthesis, and (3) accumulation of pigments and particles that the cell is unable to degrade (Figure 4-2).

Normal intracellular substances that tend to accumulate in injured cells include lipids, carbohydrates, glycogen, and proteins. Faulty metabolism of these substances within the cell results in excessive intracellular storage. In some cases, the enzymes required for breaking down a particular substance are absent or abnormal as a result of a genetic defect. In other cases, altered metabolism may be due to excessive intake, toxins, or other disease processes.

A common site of intracellular lipid accumulation is the liver, where many fats are normally stored, metabolized, and

FIGURE 4-1 Cellular swelling in kidney tubule epithelial cells. **A,** Normal kidney tubule with cuboidal cells; **B,** early ischemic changes showing surface blebs and swelling of cells. (From Kumar V et al: *Robbins basic pathology,* ed 8, Philadelphia, 2007, Saunders, p 8. Photograph courtesy Drs. Neal Pinckard and M.A. Venkatachalam, University of Texas Health Sciences Center, San Antonio.)

FIGURE 4-3 Fatty liver showing large intracellular vacuoles of lipid. (From Kumar V et al: *Robbins basic pathology*, ed 8, Philadelphia, 2007, Saunders, p 24. Photograph courtesy Dr. James Crawford, Department of Pathology, University of Florida School of Medicine, Gainesville, Florida.)

FIGURE 4-2 General mechanisms of intracellular accumulation: (1) abnormal metabolism as in fatty change in the liver, (2) mutations causing alterations in protein folding and transport so that defective proteins accumulate, (3) deficiency of critical enzyme responsible for lysosomal degradation, and (4) an inability to degrade phagocytosed particles such as coal dust. (From Kumar V et al: *Robbins basic pathology*, ed 8, Philadelphia, 2007, Saunders, p 23.)

synthesized. Fatty liver is often associated with excessive intake of alcohol.[2] Mechanisms whereby alcohol causes fatty liver remain unclear, but it is thought to result from direct toxic effects as well as the preferential metabolism of alcohol instead of lipid (see Chapter 38 for a discussion of fatty liver). Lipids

may also contribute to atherosclerotic diseases and accumulate in blood vessels, kidney, heart, and other organs. Fat-filled cells tend to compress cellular components to one side and cause the tissue to appear yellowish and greasy (Figure 4-3). In several genetic disorders, the enzymes needed to metabolize lipids are impaired; these include Tay-Sachs disease and Gaucher disease, in which lipids accumulate in neurologic tissue.

Glycosaminoglycans (mucopolysaccharides) are large carbohydrate complexes that normally make up the extracellular matrix of connective tissues. Connective tissue cells secrete most of the glycosaminoglycan into the extracellular space, but a small portion remains inside the cell and is normally degraded by lysosomal enzymes. The *mucopolysaccharidoses* are a group of genetic diseases in which the enzymatic degradation of these molecules is impaired and they collect within the cell. Mental retardation and connective tissue disorders are common findings.

Like other disorders of accumulation, *excessive glycogen storage* can be the result of inborn errors of metabolism, but a common cause is diabetes mellitus.[1] Diabetes mellitus is associated with impaired cellular uptake of glucose, which results in high serum and urine glucose levels. Cells of the renal tubules reabsorb the excess filtered glucose and store it intracellularly as glycogen. The renal tubule cells also are a common site for abnormal accumulations of proteins. Normally, very little protein escapes the bloodstream into the urine. However, with certain disorders, renal glomerular capillaries become leaky and allow proteins to filter through. Renal tubule cells recapture some of the escaped proteins through endocytosis, resulting in abnormal accumulation.

Cellular stress may lead to accumulation and aggregation of denatured proteins. The abnormally folded intracellular proteins may cause serious cell dysfunction and death if they

REPAIR OF PROTEIN DAMAGE

Chaperone

STRESS
(UV, heat, free radical injury, etc.)

Protein

Nonfunctional proteins
and aggregates

CELL DEATH

Ubiquitin

Proteasome

Degraded peptide
fragments

FIGURE 4-4 Roles of chaperone proteins in protein refolding and ubiquitin in protein degradation after stress-induced protein damage. (From Kumar V et al: *Robbins basic pathology,* ed 7, Philadelphia, 2003, Saunders, p 17.)

are allowed to persist in the cell. A family of stress proteins (also called chaperone or heat-shock proteins) is responsible for binding and refolding aberrant proteins back into their correct three-dimensional form (Figure 4-4). If the chaperones are unsuccessful in correcting the defect, the abnormal proteins form complexes with another protein called *ubiquitin*. Ubiquitin targets the abnormal proteins to enter a proteosome complex, where they are digested into fragments that are less injurious to cells (see Figure 4-4).

In some cases, the accumulated substances are not metabolized by normal intracellular enzymes. In diabetes, for instance, high serum glucose levels result in excessive glucose uptake by neuronal cells because they do not require insulin for glucose uptake. Neurons possess an enzyme (aldose reductase) that converts the glucose to sorbitol.[3] The sorbitol is not metabolized by normal glycolytic enzymes and thus accumulates in the cell, where some of it is converted to fructose. Excessive activation of the aldose reductase pathway may cause oxidative stress that damages neurons, or sorbitol may alter intracellular osmolality and interfere with nerve impulse conduction in the person with diabetes. (Diabetes mellitus is discussed in Chapter 41.)

Finally, a variety of pigments and inorganic particles may be present in cells. Some pigment accumulations are normal, such as the accumulation of melanin in tanned skin, whereas others signify pathophysiologic processes. Pigments may be produced by the body (endogenous) or may be introduced from outside sources (exogenous). In addition to melanin, the iron-containing substances hemosiderin and bilirubin are endogenous pigments that, when present in excessive amounts, indicate disease processes. Hemosiderin and bilirubin are derived from hemoglobin. Excessive amounts may indicate abnormal breakdown of hemoglobin-containing red blood cells (RBCs), prolonged iron administration, and hepatobiliary disorders. Inorganic particles that may accumulate include calcium, tar, and mineral dusts such as coal, silica, iron, lead, and silver. Mineral dusts generally are inhaled and accumulate in lung tissue (Figure 4-5). Inhaled dusts cause chronic inflammatory reactions in the lung, which generally result in destruction of pulmonary alveoli and capillaries and the formation of scar

FIGURE 4-5 Accumulations of silicon dust in tissues of the lung. (From Kumar V et al: *Robbins basic pathology,* ed 8, Philadelphia, 2007, Saunders, p 498. Photograph courtesy Dr. John Goldeski, Brigham and Women's Hospital, Boston.)

tissue. Over many years, the lung may become stiff and difficult to expand because of extensive scarring (see Chapter 23).

Deposits of calcium salts occur in conditions of altered calcium intake, excretion, or metabolism. Impaired renal excretion of phosphate may result in the formation of calcium phosphate salts that are deposited in the tissues of the eye, heart, and blood vessels. Calcification of the heart valves may cause obstruction to blood flow through the heart or interfere with valve closing. Calcification of blood vessels may result in narrowing of vessels and insufficient blood flow to distal tissues. Dead and dying tissues often become calcified (filled with calcium salts) and appear as dense areas on x-ray films. For example, lung damage resulting from tuberculosis often is apparent as calcified areas, called *tubercles.*

With the exception of inorganic particles, the intracellular accumulations generally are reversible if the causative factors are removed.

CELLULAR ADAPTATION

The cellular response to persistent, sublethal stress reflects the cell's efforts to adapt. Cellular stress may be due to an increased functional demand or a reversible cellular injury. Although the term **adaptation** implies a change for the better, in some instances an adaptive change may not be beneficial. The common adaptive responses are atrophy (decreased cell size), hypertrophy (increased cell size), hyperplasia (increased cell number), metaplasia (conversion of one cell type to another), and dysplasia (disorderly growth) (Figure 4-6). Each of these changes is potentially reversible when the cellular stress is relieved.

Atrophy

Atrophy occurs when cells shrink and reduce their differentiated functions in response to a variety of normal and injurious factors. The general causes of atrophy may be summarized as (1) disuse, (2) denervation, (3) ischemia, (4) nutrient starvation, (5) interruption of endocrine signals, (6) persistent cell injury, and (7) aging. Apparently, atrophy represents an effort by the cell to minimize its energy and nutrient consumption by decreasing intracellular organelles and other structures.

A common form of atrophy is the result of a reduction in functional demand, sometimes called **disuse atrophy.** For example, immobilization by bed rest or casting of an extremity results in shrinkage of skeletal muscle cells. On resumption of activity, the tissue resumes its normal size. Denervation of skeletal muscle results in a similar decrease in muscle size caused by loss of nervous stimulation. Inadequate blood supply to a tissue is known as **ischemia.** If the blood supply is totally interrupted, the cells will die, but chronic sublethal ischemia usually results in cell atrophy. The heart, brain, kidneys, and lower leg are common sites of ischemia. Atrophic changes in the lower leg due to ischemia include thin skin, muscle wasting, and loss of hair. Atrophy also is a consequence of chronic nutrient starvation, whether the result of poor intake, absorption, or distribution to the tissues. Many glandular tissues throughout the body depend on growth-stimulating (trophic) signals to maintain size and function. For example, the adrenal cortex, thyroid, and gonads are maintained by trophic hormones from the pituitary gland and will atrophy in their absence. Atrophy that results from persistent cell injury is most commonly related to chronic inflammation and infection.

The biochemical pathways that result in cellular atrophy are imperfectly known; however, two pathways for protein degradation have been implicated. The first is the previously mentioned ubiquitin-proteosome system, which degrades targeted proteins into small fragments (see Figure 4-4). The second involves the lysosomes that may fuse with intracellular structures leading to hydrolytic degradation of the components. Certain substances apparently are resistant to degradation and remain in the lysosomal vesicles of atrophied cells. For example, lipofuscin is an age-related pigment that accumulates in residual vesicles in atrophied cells, giving them a yellow-brown appearance.

Hypertrophy

Hypertrophy is an increase in cell mass accompanied by an augmented functional capacity. Cells hypertrophy in response to increased physiologic or pathophysiologic demands. Cellular enlargement results primarily from a net increase in cellular protein content.[4] Like the other adaptive responses, hypertrophy subsides when the increased demand is removed; however, the cell may not entirely return to normal because of persistent changes in connective tissue structures. Organ enlargement may be a result of both an increase in cell size (hypertrophy) and an increase in cell number (hyperplasia). For example, an increase in skeletal muscle mass and strength in response to repeated exercise is primarily the result of hypertrophy of individual muscle cells, although some increase in cell number is also possible because muscle stem cells (satellite cells) are able to divide. Physiologic hypertrophy occurs in

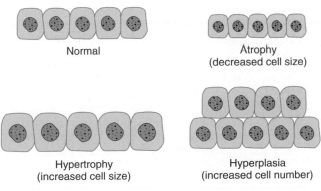

Normal

Atrophy
(decreased cell size)

Hypertrophy
(increased cell size)

Hyperplasia
(increased cell number)

Metaplasia
(conversion of one cell
type to another)

Dysplasia
(disorderly growth)

FIGURE 4-6 The adaptive cellular responses of atrophy, hypertrophy, hyperplasia, metaplasia, and dysplasia.

response to a variety of trophic hormones in sex organs—the breast and uterus, for example. Certain pathophysiologic conditions may place undue stress on some tissues, causing them to hypertrophy. Liver enlargement in response to bodily toxins and cardiac muscle enlargement in response to high blood pressure (Figure 4-7) represent hyperplastic and hypertrophic adaptations to pathologic conditions. Hypertrophic adaptation is particularly important for cells, such as differentiated muscle cells, that are unable to undergo mitotic division.

Hyperplasia

Cells that are capable of mitotic division generally increase their functional capacity by increasing the number of cells (**hyperplasia**) as well as by hypertrophy. Hyperplasia usually results from increased physiologic demands or hormonal stimulation. Persistent cell injury also may lead to hyperplasia. Examples of demand-induced hyperplasia include an increase in RBC number in response to high altitude and liver enlargement in response to drug detoxification. Trophic hormones induce hyperplasia in their target tissues. Estrogen, for example, leads to an increase in the number of endometrial and uterine stromal cells. Dysregulation of hormones or growth

factors can result in pathologic hyperplasia, such as that which occurs in thyroid or prostate enlargement.

Chronic irritation of epithelial cells often results in hyperplasia. Calluses and corns, for example, result from chronic frictional injury to the skin. The epithelium of the bladder commonly becomes hyperplastic in response to the chronic inflammation of cystitis.

Metaplasia

Metaplasia is the replacement of one differentiated cell type with another. This most often occurs as an adaptation to persistent injury, with the replacement cell type better able to tolerate the injurious stimulation.[1] Metaplasia is fully reversible when the injurious stimulus is removed. Metaplasia often involves the replacement of glandular epithelium with squamous epithelium. Chronic irritation of the bronchial mucosa by cigarette smoke, for example, leads to the conversion of ciliated columnar epithelium to stratified squamous epithelium. Metaplastic cells generally remain well differentiated and of the same tissue type, although cancerous transformations can occur. Some cancers of the lung, cervix, stomach, and bladder appear to derive from areas of metaplastic epithelium.

Dysplasia

Dysplasia refers to the disorganized appearance of cells because of abnormal variations in size, shape, and arrangement. Dysplasia occurs most frequently in hyperplastic squamous epithelium, but it may also be seen in the mucosa of the intestine. Dysplasia probably represents an adaptive effort gone astray. Dysplastic cells have significant potential to transform into cancerous cells and are usually regarded as *pre*neoplastic lesions. (See Chapter 7 for a discussion of cancer.) Dysplasia that is severe and involves the entire thickness of the epithelium is called *carcinoma in situ*. Mild forms of dysplasia may be reversible if the inciting cause is removed.

FIGURE 4-7 A, Hypertrophy of cardiac muscle in the left ventricular chamber. **B,** Compare with the thickness of the normal left ventricle. This is an example of cellular adaptation to an increased cardiac workload. (From Kumar V et al: *Robbins basic pathology,* ed 8, Philadelphia, 2007, Saunders, p 2.)

KEY POINTS

- Adaptive cellular responses indicate cellular stress caused by altered functional demand or chronic sublethal injury.
- Hypertrophy and hyperplasia generally result from increased functional demand. Atrophy results from decreased functional demand or chronic ischemia. Metaplasia and dysplasia result from persistent injury.

IRREVERSIBLE CELL INJURY

Pathologic cellular death occurs when an injury is too severe or prolonged to allow cellular adaptation or repair. Two different processes may contribute to cell death in response to injury: necrosis and apoptosis. Necrosis usually occurs as a consequence of ischemia or toxic injury and is characterized by cell rupture, spilling of contents into the extracellular fluid, and inflammation. Apoptosis (from a Greek word meaning falling off, as in leaves from a tree) occurs in response to injury that does not directly kill the cell but triggers intracellular cascades that activate a cellular suicide response. Apoptotic cells generally do not rupture and are ingested by neighboring cells with minimal disruption of the tissue and without inflammation. Apoptosis is not always a pathologic process and occurs as a necessity of development and tissue remodeling.

Necrosis

Necrotic cells demonstrate typical morphologic changes, including a shrunken (pyknotic) nucleus that is subsequently degraded (karyolysis), a swollen cell volume, dispersed ribosomes, and disrupted plasma and organelle membranes (Figure 4-8). The disruption of the permeability barrier of the plasma membrane appears to be a critical event in the death of the cell.[5]

Localized injury or death of tissue is generally reflected in the entire system as the body attempts to clear away dead cells and works to compensate for loss of tissue function. Several manifestations indicate that the system is responding to cellular injury and death. A general inflammatory response is often present, with general malaise, fever, increased heart rate, increased white blood cell (WBC) count, and loss of appetite. With the death of necrotic cells, intracellular contents are released and often find their way into the bloodstream. The presence of specific cellular enzymes in the blood is used as an indicator of the location and extent of cellular death. For example, an elevated serum amylase level indicates pancreatic damage, and an elevated creatine kinase (MB isoenzyme) or cardiac troponin level indicates myocardial damage. The location of pain due to tissue destruction may also aid in the diagnosis of cellular death.

Four different types of tissue necrosis have been described: coagulative, liquefactive, fat, and caseous (Figure 4-9). They differ primarily in the type of tissue affected. *Coagulative* necrosis is the most common. Manifestations of coagulative necrosis are the same, regardless of the cause of cell death. In general, the steps leading to coagulative necrosis may be summarized as follows: (1) ischemic cellular injury, leading to (2) loss of the plasma membrane's ability to maintain electrochemical gradients, which results in (3) influx of calcium ions and mitochondrial dysfunction, and (4) degradation of plasma membranes and nuclear structures (Figure 4-10). The area of coagulative necrosis is composed of denatured proteins and is relatively solid. The coagulated area is then slowly dissolved by proteolytic enzymes and the general tissue architecture is preserved for a relatively long time (weeks). This is in contrast to liquefactive necrosis.

When the dissolution of dead cells occurs very quickly, a liquefied area of lysosomal enzymes and dissolved tissue may result and form an abscess or cyst. This type of necrosis, called *liquefactive necrosis,* may be seen in the brain, which is rich in degradative enzymes and contains little supportive connective tissue. Liquefaction may also result from a bacterial infection that triggers a localized collection of WBCs. The phagocytic

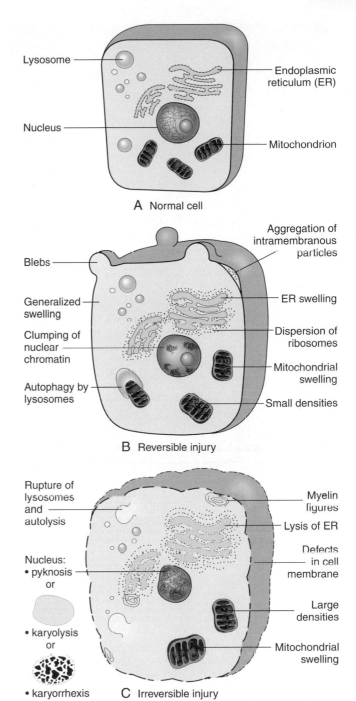

FIGURE 4-8 Cellular features of a normal cell **(A)** compared with a reversibly injured cell **(B)** and a necrotic cell **(C)**. (From Kumar V et al: *Robbins basic pathology,* ed 7, Philadelphia, 2003, Saunders, p 22.)

WBCs contain potent degradative enzymes that may completely digest dead cells, resulting in liquid debris.

Fat necrosis refers to death of adipose tissue and usually results from trauma or pancreatitis. The process begins with the release of activated digestive enzymes from the pancreas or injured tissue. The enzymes attack the cell membranes of fat cells, causing release of their stores of triglycerides. Pancreatic lipase can then hydrolyze the triglycerides to free fatty acids,

FIGURE 4-9 The four primary types of tissue necrosis. **A,** Coagulative; **B,** liquefactive; **C,** fat; **D,** caseous. (**A** from Crowley L: *Introduction to human disease,* ed 4, Boston, 1996, Jones and Bartlett Publishers, p 302, Sudbury, MA. www.jbpub.com; reprinted with permission. **B-D** from Kumar V et al: *Robbins basic pathology,* ed 8, Philadelphia, 2007, Saunders, p 11.)

which precipitate as calcium soaps (saponification). Fat necrosis appears as a chalky white area of tissue.

Caseous necrosis is characteristic of lung tissue damaged by tuberculosis. The areas of dead lung tissue are white, soft, and fragile, resembling clumpy cheese. Dead cells are walled off from the rest of the lung tissue by inflammatory WBCs. In the center, the dead cells lose their cellular structure but are not totally degraded. Necrotic debris may persist indefinitely.

Gangrene is a term used to describe cellular death involving a large area of tissue. Gangrene usually results from interruption of the major blood supply to a particular body part, such as the toes, leg, or bowel. Depending on the appearance and subsequent infection of the necrotic tissue, it is described as dry gangrene, wet gangrene, or gas gangrene. *Dry* gangrene is a form of coagulative necrosis characterized by blackened, dry, wrinkled tissue that is separated from adjacent healthy tissue by an obvious line of demarcation (see Figure 4-9, *A*). It generally occurs only on the extremities. Liquefactive necrosis may result in *wet* gangrene, which is typically found in internal organs, appears cold and black, and may be foul smelling owing to the invasion of bacteria. Rapid spread of tissue damage and the release of toxins into the bloodstream make wet gangrene a life-threatening problem. *Gas* gangrene is characterized by the formation of bubbles of gas in damaged muscle tissue. Gas gangrene is the result of infection of necrotic tissue by anaerobic bacteria of the genus *Clostridium*. These bacteria produce toxins and degradative enzymes that allow the infection to spread rapidly through the necrotic tissue. Gas gangrene may be fatal if not managed rapidly and aggressively.

FIGURE 4-10 Cellular injury as a consequence of intracellular calcium overload. (From Kumar V et al: *Robbins basic pathology*, ed 8, Philadelphia, 2007, Saunders, p 15.)

Apoptosis

The number of cells in tissues is tightly regulated by controlling the rate of cell division and the rate of cell death. If cells are no longer needed, they activate a cellular death pathway resulting in cell suicide. In contrast to necrosis, which is messy and results in inflammation and collateral tissue damage, apoptosis is tidy and does not elicit inflammation. Apoptosis is not a rare event; large numbers of cells are continually undergoing cell suicide as tissues remodel. During fetal development, for example, more than half of the nerve cells that form undergo apoptosis. It is estimated that more than 95% of the T lymphocytes that are generated in the bone marrow are induced to undergo apoptosis after reaching the thymus. These are normal physiologic processes that regulate normal system function. Apoptosis also has been implicated in pathologic cell death and disease. For example, it has been estimated that the area of tissue death following a myocardial infarction (heart attack) is about 20% necrotic and 80% apoptotic.[6] It is difficult to measure the degree of apoptotic cell death because neighboring cells rapidly ingest their apoptotic neighbors and few are ever present in the tissue.[7] Death of cancer cells in response to radiation or chemotherapy is believed to be primarily caused by apoptotic mechanisms. When the rate of apoptosis is greater than the rate of cell replacement, tissue or organ function may be impaired. Apoptosis is now recognized as a primary factor in diseases such as heart failure (Chapter 19) and dementia (Chapter 45). The mechanisms regulating apoptosis are complex, and only major concepts are included here.

There are two types of environmental or extrinsic signals that may induce apoptosis. First, apoptosis may be triggered by withdrawal of "survival" signals that normally suppress the apoptotic pathways.[7] Normal cells require a variety of signals from neighboring cells and from the extracellular matrix in order to stay alive (Figure 4-11). If these contacts or signals are removed, the cell suicide cascade is activated. Cancer cells are notorious for their ability to survive despite the lack of appropriate survival signals from their environment (see Chapter 7). A second mechanism of triggering apoptosis involves extracellular signals, such as the *Fas* ligand, that bind to the cell and trigger the death cascade though activation of "death receptors" (Figure 4-12).

FIGURE 4-11 Each cell displays a set of receptors that enable it to respond to extracellular signals that control growth, differentiation, and survival. **A,** Extracellular signals are provided by the neighboring cells, secreted signaling molecules, and the extracellular matrix. **B,** Withdrawal of these survival signals induces the cell to initiate apoptosis.

FIGURE 4-12 Induction of apoptosis by *Fas* ligand. **A,** Target cell binds to *Fas* ligand on a signaling cell. **B,** Active *Fas* receptors organize and activate caspases. **C,** The caspases degrade the nucleus and trigger cell death.

Apoptosis can also be triggered by intrinsic pathways. Cells have ways to monitor their condition and usefulness internally. When excessive, irreparable damage occurs to the cell's DNA or other vital structures, growth and division stalls for a while to permit repair. If the damage is too great, the cell will trigger its own death. Mitochondrial damage with leakage of cytochrome c into the cytoplasm is a critical activator of the intrinsic apoptotic pathway. This pathway is governed in part by a protein called p53. The amount of p53 in a cell is normally quite low but increases in response to cellular DNA damage. If high levels of p53 are sustained, apoptosis will occur.[8] Thus p53 is important in preventing the proliferation of cells with damaged DNA. A large number of cancers (50%) are associated with a mutation in the *P53* gene, which allows cancer cells to escape this monitoring system.[8]

Regardless of the initiating event, apoptosis involves numerous intracellular signals and enzymes (Figure 4-13). A family of enzymes called caspases is the main component of the proteolytic cascade that degrades key intracellular structures leading to cell death. The caspases are proenzymes that are activated in a cascade. Activation of a few *initiator* caspases at the beginning of the cascade results in a rapid domino effect of caspase activation. Some caspases cleave key proteins, such as the nuclear lamina, to destroy the nuclear envelope, whereas others activate still more enzymes that chop up the DNA. All of this destruction is contained within an intact plasma membrane, and the cell remnants are then assimilated by its neighbors. Neighboring cells are prompted to ingest apoptotic cells because a phospholipid that is normally located only on the cytoplasmic side of a healthy cell (phosphatidylserine) flips to the outside of the lipid bilayer. This membrane lipid signals

neighbors and tissue macrophages to bind and assimilate the cell components and suppresses the inflammatory response that normally accompanies phagocytosis.[7]

KEY POINTS

- Necrosis occurs when the injury is too severe or prolonged to allow adaptation and is usually a consequence of disrupted blood supply.
- Local and systemic indicators of cell death include pain, elevated serum enzyme levels, inflammation (fever, elevated WBC count, malaise), and loss of function.
- Different tissues exhibit necrosis of different types: heart (coagulative), brain (liquefactive), lung (caseous), and pancreas (fat).
- Gangrene refers to a large area of necrosis that may be described as dry, wet, or gas gangrene. Gas gangrene and wet gangrene may be rapidly fatal.
- Apoptosis is cell death resulting from activation of intracellular signaling cascades that cause cell suicide. Apoptosis is tidy and not usually associated with systemic manifestations of inflammation.

ETIOLOGY OF CELLULAR INJURY

Cellular injury and death result from a variety of cellular assaults, including lack of oxygen and nutrients, infection and immune responses, chemicals, and physical and mechanical factors. The extent of cell injury and death depends in part on the duration and severity of the assault and in part on the prior condition of the cells. Well-nourished and somewhat

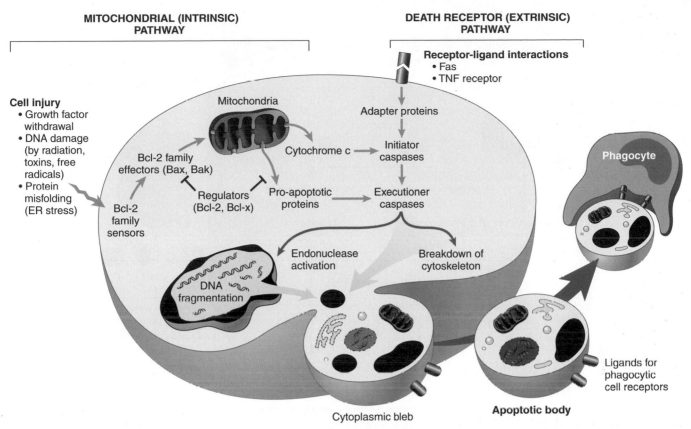

FIGURE 4-13 Schematic of the events of apoptosis. Numerous triggers can initiate apoptosis through intrinsic cell-injury pathways (mitochondrial), such as withdrawal of survival factors, various cell injuries, and protein overload or misfolding; or through extrinsic (death receptors), such as binding to *Fas* or tumor necrosis factor receptors. A number of intracellular regulatory proteins may inhibit or promote the activation of caspases, which, when activated begin the process of cellular degradation and apoptotic cell fragmentation. Fragments are internalized by phagocytic cells. (From Kumar V et al: *Robbins basic pathology,* ed 8, Philadelphia, 2007, Saunders, p 21.)

adapted cells may withstand the injury better than cells that are poorly nourished or unadapted. Common causes of cellular injury include hypoxic injury, nutritional injury, infectious and immunologic injury, chemical injury, and physical and mechanical injury.

Ischemia and Hypoxic Injury

Living cells must receive a continuous supply of oxygen to produce ATP to power energy-requiring functions. Lack of oxygen (**hypoxia**) results in power failure within the cell. Tissue hypoxia is most often caused by *ischemia,* or the interruption of blood flow to an area, but it may also result from heart failure, lung disease, and RBC disorders. Ischemia is the most common cause of cell injury in clinical medicine and injures cells faster than hypoxia alone. Faster injury occurs because ischemia not only disrupts the oxygen supply, it also allows metabolic wastes to accumulate and deprives the cell of nutrients for glycolysis. The cellular events that follow oxygen deprivation are shown in Figure 4-14. Decreased oxygen delivery to the mitochondria causes ATP production in the cell to stall and ATP-dependent pumps, including the Na+-K+ and Ca2+ pumps, to fail. Sodium accumulation within the cell creates an osmotic gradient favoring water entry, resulting in hydropic swelling. Excess intracellular calcium collects in the mitochondria, further interfering

with mitochondrial function. A small amount of ATP is produced by anaerobic glycolytic pathways, which break down cellular stores of glycogen. The pyruvate end products of glycolysis accumulate and are converted to lactate, causing cellular acidification. Lactate can escape into the bloodstream, resulting in **lactic acidosis,** which can be detected by laboratory tests. Cellular proteins and enzymes become progressively more dysfunctional as the pH falls. Up to a point, ischemic injury is reversible, but when the plasma, mitochondrial, and lysosomal membranes are critically damaged, cell death ensues.[1]

Cell death resulting from ischemia may be slow to develop, generally taking many minutes to hours. In fact, most cellular damage occurs after the blood supply to the tissues has been restored—a so-called *reperfusion injury.* Ischemia-reperfusion is a complex phenomenon, but three critical components have been identified: (1) calcium overload, (2) formation of reactive oxygen molecules (free radicals), and (3) subsequent inflammation.

Restoration of blood flow to ischemic cells bathes them in a fluid high in calcium ions at a time when their ATP stores are depleted and they are unable to control ion flux across the cell membrane. Accumulation of calcium ions in the cytoplasm can trigger apoptosis or activate enzymes that degrade lipids in the membrane (lipid peroxidation).

ISCHEMIA

MEMBRANE DAMAGE

FIGURE 4-14 Mechanisms of ischemia-induced cell injury. Cellular damage often occurs through the formation of reactive oxygen radicals. (From Kumar V et al: *Robbins basic pathology,* ed 7, Philadelphia, 2003, Saunders, p 23.)

The ischemic episode also primes cells for abnormal generation of reactive oxygen molecules, such as superoxide (O_2^-), peroxide (H_2O_2), and hydroxyl radicals (OH^-).[9] These reactive oxygen molecules are free radicals that have an unpaired electron in an outer orbital. They steal hydrogen atoms and form abnormal molecular bonds. Molecules that react with free radicals are in turn converted to free radicals, continuing the destructive cascade. Reactive oxygen species damage cell membranes, denature proteins, and disrupt cell chromosomes. Oxygen free radicals also have been linked to initiation of the inflammatory cascade (see Figure 4-14).

Ischemia primes cells for the generation of oxygen radicals by allowing the buildup of ATP precursors, such as adenosine diphosphate (ADP) and pyruvate, during the period of hypoxia. When oxygen supply is reestablished, there is a disorganized burst of high-energy electrons that partially reduce oxygen and form oxygen radicals. The ischemia-reperfusion event frequently is followed by a generalized inflammatory state,[10] which may lead to ongoing cellular and organ damage for days and weeks following the initial event. WBCs recruited to the area stick and release enzymes and other chemicals that further damage the cells in the area. (Mechanisms and causes of ischemic tissue injury are described further in Chapter 20.)

Nutritional Injury

Adequate amounts of fats, carbohydrates, proteins, vitamins, and minerals are essential for normal cellular function. Most of these essential nutrients must be obtained from external sources because the cell is unable to manufacture them. The cell is unable to synthesize many of the 20 amino acids needed to form the proteins of the body. Likewise, most vitamins and minerals must be obtained from exogenous sources. Cell injury results from deficiencies as well as excesses of essential nutrients.

Certain cell types are more susceptible to injury from particular nutritional imbalances. Iron deficiency, for example, primarily affects RBCs, whereas vitamin D deficiency affects bones. All cell types must receive glucose for energy, and fatty acid and amino acid building blocks to synthesize and repair cellular components. Nutritional deficiencies result from poor intake, altered absorption, impaired distribution by the circulatory system, or inefficient cellular uptake. Common causes of malnutrition include (1) poverty, (2) chronic alcoholism, (3) acute and chronic illness, (4) self-imposed dietary restrictions, and (5) malabsorption syndromes.[11] Vitamin deficiencies are common even in industrialized countries because of pervasive use of processed foods. Some examples of vitamin deficiency disorders are shown in Table 4-1. Deficiencies of minerals, especially iron, also are common (Table 4-2).

Nutritional excesses primarily result from excessive intake, although deficient cellular uptake by one cell type may contribute to excess nutrient delivery to other cell types. For example, in the condition of diabetes mellitus, some cell types have deficient receptors for insulin-dependent glucose uptake, which causes excessive amounts of glucose to remain in the bloodstream. As a result, cells that do not require insulin to

TABLE 4-1

Vitamins: Major Functions and Deficiency Syndromes

Vitamin	Functions	Deficiency Syndromes
Fat Soluble		
Vitamin A	A component of visual pigment	Night blindness, xerophthalmia, blindness
	Maintenance of specialized epithelia	Squamous metaplasia
	Maintenance of resistance to infection	Vulnerability to infection, particularly measles
Vitamin D	Facilitates intestinal absorption of calcium and phosphorus and mineralization of bone	Rickets in children Osteomalacia in adults
Vitamin E	Major antioxidant; scavenges free radicals	Spinocerebellar degeneration
Vitamin K	Cofactor in hepatic carboxylation of procoagulants—factors II (prothrombin), VII, IX, and X; and protein C and protein S	Bleeding diathesis
Water-Soluble		
Vitamin B$_1$	As pyrophosphate, is coenzyme in decarboxylation reactions	Dry and wet beriberi, Wernicke syndrome, ? Korsakoff syndrome
Vitamin B$_2$ (riboflavin)	Converted to coenzymes flavin mononucleotide and flavin adenine dinucleotide, cofactors for many enzymes in intermediary metabolism	Ariboflavinosis, cheilosis, stomatitis, glossitis, dermatitis, corneal vascularization
Niacin	Incorporated into nicotinamide adenine dinucleotide (NAD) and NAD phosphate, involved in a variety of redox reactions	Pellagra – "three Ds": dementia, dermatitis, diarrhea
Vitamin B$_6$ (pyridoxine)	Derivatives serve as coenzymes in many intermediary reactions	Cheilosis, glossitis, dermatitis, peripheral neuropathy
Vitamin B$_{12}$	Required for normal folate metabolism and DNA synthesis Maintenance of myelinization of spinal cord tracts	Combined system disease (megaloblastic pernicious anemia and degeneration of posterolateral spinal cord tracts)
Vitamin C	Serves in many oxidation-reduction (redox) reactions and hydroxylation of collagen	Scurvy
Folate	Essential for transfer and use of 1-carbon units in DNA synthesis	Megaloblastic anemia, neural tube defects
Pantothenic acid	Incorporated in coenzyme A	No nonexperimental syndrome recognized
Biotin	Cofactor in carboxylation reactions	No clearly defined clinical syndrome

From Kumar V et al: *Robbins basic pathology,* ed 8, Philadelphia, 2007, Saunders, p 314.
NAD, Nicotinamide adenine dinucleotide.

take in glucose, such as neurons, may have abnormally high intracellular glucose levels. An excess of caloric intake above metabolic use produces overweight and obesity syndromes. Excess body fat can be estimated by measuring the ratio of body weight (in kilograms) to height (in meters squared) to derive the body mass index (BMI). A BMI greater than 27 kg/m^2 imparts a health risk and a BMI greater than 30 kg/m^2 is considered to be obesity.[12] Numerous health problems are associated with excess body fat, including heart and blood vessel disease, musculoskeletal strain, diabetes, hypertension, and gallbladder disease.

Infectious and Immunologic Injury

Bacteria and viruses are common infectious agents that may injure cells in a variety of ways. The virulence of a particular biological agent depends on its ability to gain access to the cell and its success in altering cellular functions. (See Chapter 8 for a detailed discussion of infectious processes.) Some of the injurious effects are directly due to the biological agent, but added injury may be done indirectly by triggering the body's immune response.

Most bacteria do not gain entry into the cell and so accomplish their injurious effects from the outside. (Notable exceptions include *Mycobacterium tuberculosis, Shigella, Legionella, Salmonella,* and *Chlamydia.*) Some bacteria produce and secrete powerful destructive enzymes that digest cellular membranes and connective tissues. For example, collagenase and lecithinase are produced by *Clostridium perfringens.* Other bacteria produce **exotoxins,** which interfere with specific cellular functions when released from the bacterium. *Clostridium botulinum* and *Clostridium tetani,* for example, produce life-threatening toxins that disrupt normal neuromuscular transmission. Cholera and diphtheria are well-known examples of exotoxin-related diseases. Exotoxins are primarily proteins and are generally susceptible to destruction by extremes of heat. Certain gram-negative bacteria (e.g., *Escherichia coli, Klebsiella pneumoniae*) contain another type of toxin, **endotoxin,** in their cell wall. On lysis of the bacteria, the endotoxin is released, causing fever, malaise, and even circulatory shock.[13]

The indirect cellular injury due to the bacteria-evoked immune response may be more damaging than the direct effects of the infectious agent. White blood cells secrete many

TABLE 4-2

Selected Trace Elements and Deficiency Syndromes

Element	Function	Basis of Deficiency	Clinical Features
Zinc	Component of enzymes, principally oxidases	Inadequate supplementation in artificial diets Interference with absorption by other dietary constituents Inborn error of metabolism	Rash around eyes, mouth, nose, and anus called acrodermatitis enteropathica Anorexia and diarrhea Growth retardation in children Depressed mental function Depressed wound healing and immune response Impaired night vision Infertility
Iron	Essential component of hemoglobin as well as a number of iron-containing metalloenzymes	Inadequate diet Chronic blood loss	Hypochromic microcytic anemia
Iodine	Component of thyroid hormone	Inadequate supply in food and water	Goiter and hypothyroidism
Copper	Component of cytochrome c oxidase, dopamine β-hydroxylase, tyrosinase, lysyl oxidase, and unknown enzyme involved in cross-linking collagen	Inadequate supplementation in artificial diet Interference with absorption	Muscle weakness Neurologic defects Abnormal collagen cross-linking
Fluoride	Mechanism unknown	Inadequate supply in soil and water Inadequate supplementation	Dental caries
Selenium	Component of glutathione peroxidase Antioxidant with vitamin E	Inadequate amounts in soil and water	Myopathy Cardiomyopathy (Keshan disease)

From Kumar V et al: *Robbins basic pathology,* ed 8, Philadelphia, 2007, Saunders, p 315.

enzymes and chemicals meant to destroy the invading organism, including histamines, kinins, complement, proteases, lymphokines, and prostaglandins. Normal body cells may be exposed to these injurious chemicals because they are too close to the site of immunologic battle. Immune cells are particularly adept at producing free radicals, which can attack host cell membranes and induce significant cell injury.

Viruses are small bits of genetic material that are able to gain entry into the cell. They may be thought of as intracellular parasites that use the host cell's metabolic and synthetic machinery to survive and replicate. Viral infections tend to follow two distinct pathways. In some cases the virus remains in the cell for a considerable time without inflicting lethal injury. In other cases the virus causes rapid lysis and destruction of the host cell. The mechanisms that determine which course the virus will take are poorly understood.

The polio virus is an example of a virus that is directly cytopathic: it can kill the host cell directly without immune system participation.[14] The polio virus is made up of RNA, which the cell recognizes as any other messenger RNA molecule and translates into viral proteins. Some of the virally coded proteins insert into the plasma membrane of the cell, forming pores or channels that allow ions to diffuse across. The cell dies as the vital ion gradients are dissipated.

Other viruses remain in the cell for long periods, unobtrusively making and releasing viral copies of themselves without causing lethal cell injury. The virally infected cells may not escape death, however, because they express cell surface proteins that are foreign to the host's immune system. The hepatitis B virus is an example of such an indirectly cytopathic virus that causes immune-mediated cell death. The hepatitis B virus consists of double-stranded DNA that gets incorporated into the host cell's nucleus, where it can be transcribed by the normal DNA polymerases. The mRNA transcripts of the viral genes are transported to the cytoplasm and translated into structural proteins and enzymes, which are used to make more copies of the virus. Such virally infected cells may remain functional virus factories until they are destroyed by the host's immune system.

Chemical Injury

Toxic chemicals or poisons are plentiful in the environment (Tables 4-3 and 4-4). Some toxic chemicals cause cellular injury directly, whereas others become injurious only when metabolized into reactive chemicals by the body. Carbon tetrachloride (CCl_4) is an example of the latter.[15] Carbon tetrachloride, a formerly used dry-cleaning agent, is converted to a highly toxic **free radical,** $CCl_3^{\cdot}$, by liver cells. The free radical is very reactive, forming abnormal chemical bonds in the cell and ultimately destroying the cellular membranes of liver cells, causing liver failure. In high doses, acetaminophen, a commonly used analgesic, may have similar toxic effects on the liver.

TABLE 4-3

Health Effects of Outdoor Air Pollutants

Pollutant	Populations at Risk	Effects
Ozone	Healthy adults and children Athletes, outdoor workers Asthmatics	Decreased lung function Increased airway reactivity Lung inflammation Decreased exercise capacity Increased hospitalizations
Nitrogen dioxide	Healthy adults Asthmatics Children	Increased airway reactivity Decreased lung function Increased respiratory infections
Sulfur dioxide	Healthy adults Patients with chronic lung disease Asthmatics	Increased respiratory symptoms Increased mortality Increased hospitalization Decreased lung function
Acid aerosols	Healthy adults Children Asthmatics	Altered mucociliary clearance Increased respiratory infections Decreased lung function Increased hospitalizations
Particulates	Children Patients with chronic lung or heart disease Asthmatics	Increased respiratory infections Decreased lung function Excess mortality Increased attacks

See Chapters 22 and 23 for a discussion of respiratory disorders.
From Kumar V et al: *Robbins basic pathology,* ed 8, Philadelphia, 2007, Saunders, p 282.

TABLE 4-4

Health Effects of Indoor Air Pollutants

Pollutant	Population at Risk	Effects
Carbon monoxide	Adults and children	Acute poisoning
Nitrogen dioxide	Children	Increased respiratory infections
Wood smoke	Children	Increased respiratory infections
Formaldehyde	Adults and children	Eye and nose irritation, asthma
Radon	Adults and children	Lung cancer
Asbestos fibers	Maintenance and abatement workers	Lung cancer; mesothelioma
Manufactured mineral fibers	Maintenance and construction workers	Skin and airway irritation
Bioaerosols	Adults and children	Allergic rhinitis, asthma

From Kumar V et al: *Robbins basic pathology,* ed 7, Philadelphia, 2003, Saunders, p 267.

Many toxins are inherently reactive and do not require metabolic activation to exert their effects. Common examples are heavy metals (e.g., lead and mercury), toxic gases, corrosives, and antimetabolites. Some toxins have an affinity for a particular cell type or tissue, whereas others exert widespread systemic effects. For example, carbon monoxide binds tightly and selectively to hemoglobin, preventing the red cell from carrying sufficient oxygen. Lead poisoning, however, has widespread effects, including effects on nervous tissue, blood cells, and the kidney. Extremely acidic or basic chemicals are directly corrosive to cellular structures. Certain chemicals interfere with normal metabolic processes of the cell. Some of these antimetabolites have been put to use in the form of cytotoxic agents for the management of cancer.

Physical and Mechanical Injury

Injurious physical and mechanical factors include extremes of temperature, abrupt changes of atmospheric pressure, mechanical deformation, electricity, and ionizing radiation.[11]

Extremes of cold result in the hypothermic injury known as frostbite. Before actual cellular freezing, severe vasoconstriction and increased blood viscosity may result in ischemic injury. With continued exposure to cold, a rebound vasodilatory response may occur, leading to intense swelling and peripheral nerve damage. The cytoplasmic solution may freeze, resulting in the formation of intracellular ice crystals and rupture of cellular components. Frostbite generally affects the extremities, ears, and nose, and is often complicated by gangrenous necrosis.

Extremes of heat result in hyperthermic injury or burns. High temperatures cause microvascular coagulation and may speed up metabolic processes in the cell. Burns result from direct tissue destruction by high temperatures and are classified according to the degree of tissue destruction. Burns are discussed in Chapter 54.

Abrupt changes in atmospheric pressure may result from high-altitude flying, deep sea diving, and explosions. Pressure changes may interfere with gas exchange in the lungs, cause the formation of gas emboli in the bloodstream, collapse the thorax, and rupture internal organs. A well-known example of pressure injury is the condition of "the bends," which afflicts deep-sea divers who surface too quickly. The rapid decrease in water pressure results in the formation of bubbles of nitrogen gas in the blood, which may obstruct the circulation and cause ischemic injury.

Destruction of cells and tissues resulting from mechanical deformation ranges from mild abrasion to severe lacerating trauma. Cell death may result from direct trauma to cell membranes, resulting blood loss, or obstruction of blood flow and hypoxia. Nonpenetrating trauma generally results from physical impact with a blunt object such as a fist, a car steering wheel, or the pavement. Surgery is a common cause of tissue trauma. Other causes of penetrating trauma are bite, knife and gun wounds. Trauma-induced inflammatory swelling may further compromise injured tissues.

Electrical injury may occur when the cells of the body act as conductors of electricity. The electrical current damages tissues in two ways: (1) by disrupting neural and cardiac impulses, and (2) by hyperthermic destruction of tissues. Resistance to the flow of electrons results in heat production, which damages the tissues. The current tends to follow the path of least resistance—through neurons and body fluids—causing violent muscle contractions, thermal injury, and coagulation in blood vessels. In general, greater injury is suffered with high-voltage alternating current applied to a low-resistance area (wet skin).

There are many forms of electromagnetic radiation, ranging from low-energy radio waves to high-energy γ rays or photons (Figure 4-15). Radiation is capable of injuring cells directly by breakage of chemical bonds and indirectly by generating free radicals.[11] Cellular DNA is particularly susceptible to damage from radiation exposure.[16] A direct hit of the radiant energy on the DNA molecule may result in breakage of the chemical bonds holding the linear DNA together. This type of direct bond breakage generally results from the high-energy forms of radiation, such as x and γ rays. The molecular bonds of DNA also may be indirectly disrupted by ionizing radiation. *Ionization* refers to the ability of the radiant energy to split water molecules by knocking off orbital electrons (**radiolysis**). Radiolysis creates activated free radicals that steal electrons from other molecules and disrupt chemical bonds. Many forms of radiation are capable of ionization, but the medium-energy α and β particles that result from decay of atomic nuclei are especially destructive. Low-energy electromagnetic radiation, such as that from microwaves, ultrasound, computers, and infrared light, cannot break chemical bonds, but it can cause rotation and vibration of atoms and molecules.[17] The rotational and vibrational energy is then converted to heat. It is probable that the resulting localized hyperthermia may result in cellular injury. Early studies reported a higher incidence of certain cancers in persons occupationally exposed to radio-frequency microwave electromagnetic radiation, but further analysis failed to confirm these findings.[11]

At the cellular level, radiation has two primary effects: (1) genetic damage and (2) acute cell destruction (Figure 4-16). The vulnerability of a tissue to radiation-induced genetic damage depends on its rate of proliferation. Genetic damage to the DNA of a long-lived, nonproliferating cell may be of little consequence, whereas tissues with rapid cellular division have less opportunity to repair damaged DNA before passing it on to the next generation of cells. (Genetic mutation is discussed in Chapter 6.) Hematopoietic, mucosal, gonadal, and fetal cells are particularly susceptible to genetic radiation damage.

Radiation-induced cell death is attributed primarily to the radiolysis of water, with resulting free radical damage to the plasma membrane. Whole-body exposure to sufficiently high levels of radiation (300 rad) results in acute radiation sickness with hematopoietic failure, destruction of the epithelial

FIGURE 4-15 Types of electromagnetic radiation.

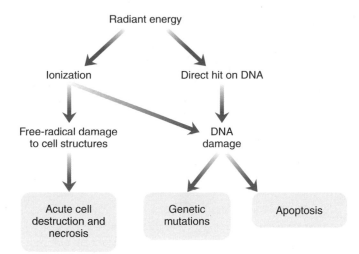

FIGURE 4-16 The mechanism of radiation-induced genetic and cell injury.

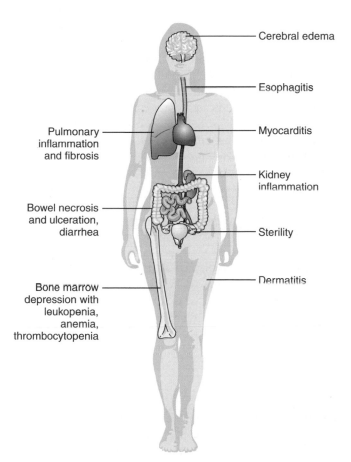

FIGURE 4-17 Signs and symptoms of acute radiation sickness.

layer of the gastrointestinal tract, and neurologic dysfunction. The high levels of irradiation that cause acute radiation sickness are associated with events such as nuclear accidents and bombings. Radiation exposure from diagnostic x-rays, cosmic rays, and natural radiant chemicals in the earth are far below the level that would result in acute radiation sickness. The signs and symptoms of acute radiation sickness are shown in

Figure 4-17. The fact that radiation induces cell death in proliferating cells is used to advantage in the management of some forms of cancer. Radiation therapy may be used when a cancerous growth is confined to a particular area. Injury associated with radiation therapy is generally localized to the irradiated area. Small arteries and arterioles in the area may be damaged, leading to blood clotting and fibrous deposits that compromise tissue perfusion. Most irradiated cells are thought to die through the process of apoptosis rather than from direct killing effects of radiation.[18] Radiation induces cell damage that triggers the apoptotic pathway in cells that cannot efficiently repair the damage. Cells most susceptible to apoptotic death are those that tend to have high rates of division.

KEY POINTS

- Hypoxia is an important cause of cell injury that usually results from poor oxygenation of the blood (hypoxemia) or inadequate delivery of blood to the cells (ischemia).
- Reperfusion injury to cells may occur when circulation is restored, owing to the production of partially reduced oxygen molecules that damage cell membranes and trigger immune-mediated injury.
- Nutritional injury is a common cause of dysfunction and disease. Malnutrition is rampant in many poor countries, whereas industrialized nations are facing an epidemic of obesity-related disorders, including heart disease and diabetes.
- Cellular damage due to infection and immunologic responses is common. Some bacteria and viruses damage cells directly, whereas others stimulate the host's immune system to destroy the host's cells.
- Chemical, physical, and mechanical factors cause cell injury in various ways. Chemicals may interfere with normal metabolic processes in the cell. Injury resulting from physical factors, such as burns and frostbite, causes direct destruction of tissues. Radiation-induced cell death is primarily a result of radiolysis of water, with resulting free radical damage to the cell membrane.

CELLULAR AGING

The inevitable process of aging and death has been the subject of interest and investigation for centuries. Despite scientific study and the search for the fountain of youth, a satisfactory explanation for the process of cellular aging and methods for halting the aging process have not been revealed. The maximal human life span has remained constant at about 90 to 110 years, despite significant progress in the management of diseases.[19] It seems apparent that aging is distinct from disease, and that the life span is limited by the aging process itself rather than by the ravages of disease. Although the elderly are certainly more vulnerable to diseases, the aging process and disease processes are generally viewed as different phenomena. In practice, the distinction between aging and disease may be difficult to make. For example, the aging skeleton normally loses some bone mass, but too much bone loss results in osteoporosis—a disease process. Likewise, a loss of blood vessel elasticity is generally viewed as a normal aging change, but at what point does too much arterial stiffness become abnormal? This confusion results from the continued inability to identify the irreversible and universal processes of cellular aging as separate from the potentially reversible effects of disease.

Cellular Basis of Aging

Cellular aging is the cumulative result of a progressive decline in proliferative and reparative capacity of cells coupled with exposure to environmental factors that cause accumulation of cellular and molecular damage. Several mechanisms are thought to be responsible for cellular aging. These include DNA damage, reduced proliferative capacity of stem cells, and accumulation of metabolic damage.

Damage to cellular DNA is a common phenomenon resulting from various factors, including ultraviolet radiation, oxidative stress from normal metabolism, and errors in DNA replication. A host of DNA repair mechanisms is present in normal cells to prevent accumulation of DNA damage. With aging these repair systems appear to become less able to keep up with DNA damage, and cell replication may be inhibited or apoptosis initiated. Support for this idea comes from the premature aging syndromes that are associated with defective DNA repair mechanisms.

The *programmed senescence theory* holds that aging is the result of an intrinsic genetic program. Support for the theory of a genetically programmed life span comes primarily from studies of cells in culture. In classic experiments by Hayflick, fibroblastic cells in culture were shown to undergo a finite number of cell divisions.[20] Fibroblasts taken from older individuals underwent fewer cell divisions than those from younger individuals. Given an adequate environment, the information encoded in the cellular genome is thought to dictate the number of possible cell replications, after which damaged or lost cells are no longer replaced. It has been postulated that cells undergo a finite number of replications because the chromosomes shorten a bit with each cell division until some critical point is reached (Figure 4-18), at which time the cell becomes dormant or dies. The end caps of the chromosomes, called **telomeres,** are the sections that shorten with each cell division.[21] Certain cells (germ cells, such as egg and sperm) are able to replenish their telomeres, which gives them potential immortality. The enzyme that rebuilds the telomeres has been named *telomerase.* Stem cells, which are capable of mitosis, also express telomerase, but at low levels. Progressive loss of telomerase gene expression with aging may contribute to reduced proliferative capacity. Interestingly, a number of cancer cell types have been found to produce telomerase, whereas most normal cells do not (Chapter 7).

Aging may also be a result of accumulated metabolic cell damage over time. The *free radical theory* was prompted

FIGURE 4-18 The end caps of the chromosomes are called *telomeres.* In most body cells, the telomeres progressively shorten with each cell replication until a critical point is reached, at which time the cell becomes dormant or dies.

in part by the observation that larger animals, which have slower metabolic rates, generally have longer life spans.[1] Metabolic rate, in turn, determines the production of activated oxygen free radicals. Aging is thought to result from the cumulative and progressive damage to cell structures, particularly the cell membrane, by these oxygen radicals. Protection from metabolic damage is provided by a number of antioxidant mechanisms. Over time these protective mechanisms may become less efficient, allowing metabolic damage to accumulate in cells. Accumulated damage may eventually trigger apoptotic mechanisms leading to tissue degeneration.

Physiologic Changes of Aging

All the body systems show age-related changes that can be generally described as a decrease in functional reserve or inability to adapt to environmental demands. An overview of the tissue and systemic changes of aging is presented in Table 4-5. The details of age-related changes in the various body systems are described in later chapters of this book.

KEY POINTS

- Aging is theoretically distinct from disease. The maximal life span is limited by the aging process itself rather than by the ravages of disease.
- Aging is thought to be the result of accumulated DNA damage, decreased proliferative capacity of stem cells, and accumulation of metabolic damage. Cells may age more quickly when DNA repair mechanisms are faulty and when metabolic damage is excessive because of reduced antioxidant activity.
- Age-related changes in body systems can generally be described as a decrease in functional reserve and a reduced ability to adapt to environmental demands.

TABLE 4-5	

Overview of the Physiologic Changes of Aging

System	Physiologic Changes
Cardiovascular	↓ Vessel elasticity caused by calcification of connective tissue (↑ pulmonary vascular resistance) ↓ Number of heart muscle fibers with ↑ size of individual fibers (hypertrophy) ↓ Filling capacity ↓ Stroke volume ↓ Sensitivity of baroreceptors Degeneration of vein valves
Respiratory	↓ Chest wall compliance resulting from calcification of costal cartilage ↓ Alveolar ventilation ↓ Respiratory muscle strength Air trapping and ↓ ventilation due to degeneration of lung tissue (↓ elasticity)
Renal/urinary	↓ Glomerular filtration rate due to nephron degeneration (↓ one third to one half by age 70) ↓ Ability to concentrate urine ↓ Ability to regulate H^+
Gastrointestinal	↓ Muscular contraction ↓ Esophageal emptying ↓ Bowel motility ↓ Production of HCl, enzymes, and intrinsic factor ↓ Hepatic enzyme production and metabolic capacity Thinning of stomach mucosa
Neurologic/sensory	Nerve cells degenerate and atrophy ↓ Of 25%-45% of neurons ↓ Neurotransmitters ↓ Rate of conduction of nerve impulses Loss of taste buds Loss of auditory hair cells and sclerosis of eardrum
Musculoskeletal	↓ Muscle mass Bone demineralization Joint degeneration, erosion, and calcification
Immune	↓ Inflammatory response ↓ In T cell function owing to involution of thymus gland
Integumentary	↓ Subcutaneous fat ↓ Elastin Atrophy of sweat glands Atrophy of epidermal arterioles causing altered temperature regulation

SOMATIC DEATH

Death of the entire organism is called *somatic death*. In contrast to localized cell death, no immunologic or inflammatory response occurs in somatic death. The general features of somatic death include the absence of respiration and heartbeat. However, this definition of death is insufficient because, in some cases, breathing and cardiac activity may be restored by resuscitative efforts. Within several minutes of cardiopulmonary arrest, the characteristics of irreversible somatic death become apparent. Body temperature falls, the skin becomes pale, and blood and body fluids collect in dependent areas. Within 6 hours, the accumulation of calcium and the depletion of ATP result in perpetual actin-myosin cross-bridge formation in muscle cells. The presence of stiffened muscles throughout the body after death is called *rigor mortis*. Rigor mortis gives way to limpness or flaccidity as the tissues of the body begin to deteriorate. Tissue deterioration or putrefaction becomes apparent 24 to 48 hours after death.[22] Putrefaction is associated with the widespread release of lytic enzymes in tissues throughout the body, a process called *postmortem autolysis*.

The determination of "brain death" has become necessary because of the technological ability to keep the heart and lungs working through artificial means, even though the brain is no longer functional. Criteria for determining brain death as proof of somatic death may vary by geographic area but generally include unresponsiveness, flaccidity, absence of brain stem reflexes (e.g., swallowing, gagging, pupil and eye movements), absence of respiratory effort when the subject is removed from the mechanical ventilator, absence of electrical brain waves, and lack of cerebral blood flow.

KEY POINTS

- Somatic death is characterized by the absence of respirations and heartbeat. Definitions of brain death have been established to describe death in instances in which heartbeat and respiration are maintained mechanically.
- After death, body temperature falls, blood and body fluids collect in dependent areas, and rigor mortis ensues. Within 24 to 48 hours the tissues begin to deteriorate and rigor mortis gives way to flaccidity.

SUMMARY

Cells and tissues face many challenges to survival, including injury from lack of oxygen and nutrients, infection and immune responses, chemicals, and physical and mechanical factors. Cells respond to environmental changes or injury in three general ways: (1) If the change is mild or short lived, the cell may withstand the assault and return to its preinjury status. (2) The cell may adapt to a persistent but sublethal injury by changing its structure or function. (3) Cell death by apoptosis or necrosis may occur if the injury is too severe or prolonged. Characteristics of reversible cell injury include hydropic swelling and the accumulation of abnormal substances. Cell necrosis is characterized by irreversible loss of function, release of cellular enzymes into the bloodstream, and an inflammatory response. The disruption of the permeability barrier of the plasma membrane appears to be a critical event in necrotic cellular death. Apoptosis is characterized by a tidy, noninflammatory autodigestion of the cell.

Aging is a normal physiologic process characterized by a progressive decline in functional capacity and adaptive ability. The biological basis of aging remains largely a mystery, but several theories have been proposed to explain certain aspects of the process. At present, most sources differentiate between the biological alterations of aging and the alterations consequent to disease processes. In practice, however, the distinction may be difficult to make.

REFERENCES

1. Kumar V, Abbas A, Fausto N, Mitchell R: Cell injury, cell death, and adaptations. In Kumar V, Abbas A, Fausto N, Mitchell R, editors: *Robbins basic pathology,* ed 8, Philadelphia, 2007, Saunders, pp 1-30.
2. Kumar V, Abbas A, Fausto N, Mitchell R: The liver, gallbladder, and biliary tract. In Kumar V, Abbas A, Fausto N, Mitchell R, editors: *Robbins basic pathology*, ed 8, Philadelphia, 2007, Saunders, pp 631-674.
3. Kumar V, Abbas A, Fausto N, Mitchell R: The endocrine system. In Kumar V, Abbas A, Fausto N, Mitchell R, editors: *Robbins basic pathology*, ed 8, Philadelphia, 2007, Saunders, pp 780-781.
4. Yarasheski KE: Exercise, aging, and muscle protein metabolism, *J Gerontol A Biol Sci Med Sci* 58(10):M918-M922, 2003.
5. Han SI, Kim TH, Kim YS: Role of apoptotic and necrotic cell death under physiologic conditions, *BMB reports* 41(1):1-10, 2008.
6. Nadal-Ginard B et al: Myocyte death, growth, and regeneration in cardiac hypertrophy and failure, *Circ Res* 92:139-150, 2003.
7. Alberts B et al: Apoptosis. In Alberts B et al, editors: *Molecular biology of the cell*, ed 5, New York, 2008, Garland Science, pp 1115-1129.
8. Alberts B et al: Mechanisms of cell communication. In Alberts B et al, editors: *Molecular biology of the cell*, ed 5, New York, 2008, Garland Science, pp 879-964.
9. Wong CH, Crack PJ: Modulation of neuro-inflammation and vascular response by oxidative stress following cerebral ischemia-reperfusion injury, *Curr Med Chem* 15(1):1-14, 2008.
10. Chan RK et al: Ischaemia-reperfusion is an event triggered by immune complexes and complement, *Br J Surg* 90(12):1470-1478, 2003.
11. Kumar V, Abbas A, Fausto N, Mitchell R: Environmental and nutritional diseases. In Kumar V, Abbas A, Fausto N, Mitchell R, editors: *Robbins basic pathology*, ed 8, Philadelphia, 2007, Saunders, pp 279-318.
12. *Clinical guidelines on the identification, evaluation, and treatment of overweight and obesity in adults*, NIH Publication No. 98-4083, National Institutes of Health, 1998.
13. van der Poll T, Opal SM: Host-pathogen interactions in sepsis. *Lancet Infect Dis* 8(1):32-43, 2008.
14. Kumar V, Abbas A, Fausto N, Mitchell R: General pathology of infectious diseases. In Kumar V, Abbas A, Fausto N, Mitchell R, editors: *Robbins basic pathology*, ed 8, Philadelphia, 2007, Saunders, pp 319-338.
15. Weber LW, Boll M, Stampfl A: Hepatotoxicity and mechanism of action of haloalkanes: carbon tetrachloride as a toxicological model, *Crit Rev Toxicol* 33(2):105-136, 2003.
16. Huang L, Snyder AR, Morgan WF: Radiation-induced genomic instability and its implications for radiation carcinogenesis, *Oncogene* 22(37):5848-5854, 2003.
17. Osepchuk JM, Petersen RC: Historical review of RF exposure standards and the International Committee on Electromagnetic Safety (ICES), *Bioelectromagnetics* 24(suppl 6):S7-S16, 2003.
18. Rupnow BA, Knox SJ: The role of radiation-induced apoptosis as a determinant of tumor responses to radiation therapy, *Apoptosis* 4(2):115-143, 1999.
19. Troen BR: The biology of aging, *Mt Sinai J Med* 70(1):3-22, 2003.
20. Hayflick L: The biology of human aging, *Adv Pathobiol* 7(2): 80-99, 1980.
21. Jiang H, Ju Z, Rudolph KL: Telomere shortening and ageing, *Z Gerontol Geriatr* 40(5):314-324, 2007.
22. Shennan T: *Postmortems and morbid anatomy,* ed 3, Baltimore, 1935, William Wood.

Molecular Genetics and Tissue Differentiation

Jacquelyn L. Banasik

MEDIA RESOURCES

Additional Material for Study, Review, and Further Exploration

CD Companion ■ Review Questions and Answers
- Glossary (with audio pronunciations for selected terms)
- Disease Profiles ■ Animations

ⓔvolve **Website** at http://evolve.elsevier.com/Copstead/
- Case Studies ■ Disease Profiles ■ WebLinks ■ Key Points Review

Online Course (Module 2)

KEY QUESTIONS

- How is genetic information stored in the cell and transmitted to progeny during replication?
- How does the simple four-base structure of DNA serve as a template for synthesis of proteins that may contain 20 varieties of amino acids?
- What roles do genes play in determining cell structure and function?

- How is gene expression regulated?
- By what mechanisms can the cells of an organism, which all contain identical genes, become differentiated into divergent cell types?
- What are the general structures and functions of the four main tissue types: epithelial, connective, muscle, and nerve?

CHAPTER OUTLINE

The ability of scientists to study and manipulate genes has evolved at an incredible pace, including the complete sequencing of all 6.4 billion nucleotides in an entire human genome. A better understanding of the role that genetics plays in cellular function and disease has spurred efforts to develop therapies to correct genetic abnormalities. The science of genetics developed from the premise that invisible, information-containing elements called **genes** exist in cells and are passed on to daughter cells when a cell divides. The nature of these elements was at first difficult to imagine: what kind of molecule could direct the day-to-day activities of the organism and be capable of nearly limitless replication? The answer to this question was discovered in the late 1940s and was almost unbelievable in its simplicity. It is now common knowledge that genetic information is stored in long chains of stable molecules called **deoxyribonucleic acid (DNA).** The human genome contains approximately 25,000 genes encoded by only four different molecules. These molecules are the deoxyribonucleotides containing the bases *adenine* (A), *cytosine* (C), *guanine* (G), and *thymine* (T). Genes are composed of varying sequences of these four bases, which are linked together by sugar-phosphate bonds. By serving as the templates for the production of body proteins, genes ultimately affect all aspects of an organism's structure and function. With the completed sequencing of an entire human genome in 2004 and development of methods to rapidly survey the DNA sequences of a particular person, genetics is an increasingly important consideration in the etiology, pathogenesis, and pharmacologic treatment of a variety of diseases. Knowledge of the basic principles of genetics and gene regulation is therefore prerequisite not only to understanding conventional genetic diseases, but nearly every pathophysiologic process. This chapter examines the biochemistry of genes (molecular genetics), regulation of gene expression, and the processes of tissue differentiation. Principles of genetic inheritance precede the discussion of genetic diseases in Chapter 6.

MOLECULAR GENETICS

Structure of DNA

In humans, DNA encodes genetic information in 46 long double-stranded chains of nucleotides called chromosomes.[1] The **nucleotides** consist of a 5-carbon sugar (deoxyribose),

a phosphate group, and one of the four nucleotide bases (Figure 5-1). The nucleotide bases are divided into two types based on their chemical structure. The pyrimidines, cytosine and thymine, have single-ring structures. The purines, guanine and adenine, have double-ring structures (Figure 5-2). DNA polymers are formed by the chemical linkage of these nucleotides. The sugar-phosphate linkages, also called *phosphodiester bonds,* join the phosphate group on one sugar (attached to the 5-carbon) to the 3-carbon of the next sugar (see Figure 5-1). The four kinds of bases (A, C, G, T) are attached to the repeating sugar-phosphate chain. The bases of one strand of DNA form weak bonds with the bases of another strand of DNA. These noncovalent hydrogen bonds are specific and complementary (Figure 5-3). The bases G and C always bond together and the bases A and T always bond together. Nucleotides that are able to bond together in this complementary way are called *base pairs.*

In the early 1950s, Watson and Crick proposed that the structure of DNA was a double helix.[2] In this model, DNA can be envisioned as a twisted ladder, with the sugar-phosphate bonds as the sides of the ladder and the bases forming the rungs (see Figure 5-3). There is one complete turn of the helix every 10 base pairs. The two strands of DNA must be complementary to form the double helix; that is, the bases of one strand must pair exactly with their complementary bases on the other strand. The helix is wound around proteins called histones to form *nucleosomes* (Figure 5-4). DNA coupled

FIGURE 5-1 A nucleotide consists of a sugar (deoxyribose), a phosphate group, and one of the four nucleotide bases. Nucleotides are joined by repeating sugar-phosphate bonds to form long chains, called *polymers. A,* Adenine; *C,* Cytosine; *G,* Guanine; *T,* Thymine.

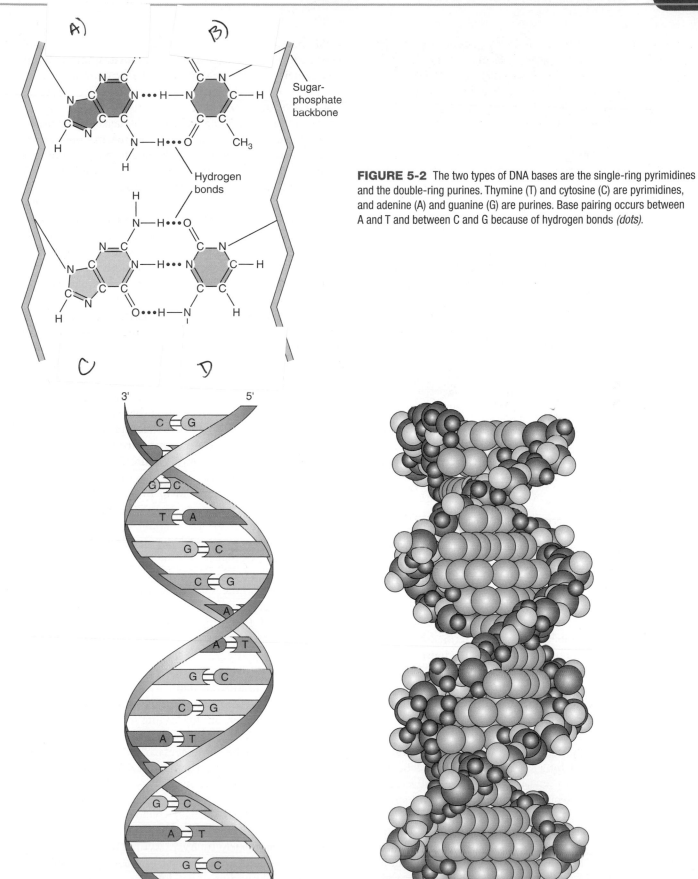

FIGURE 5-2 The two types of DNA bases are the single-ring pyrimidines and the double-ring purines. Thymine (T) and cytosine (C) are pyrimidines, and adenine (A) and guanine (G) are purines. Base pairing occurs between A and T and between C and G because of hydrogen bonds *(dots)*.

FIGURE 5-3 A schematic and space-filling model of the DNA double helix as proposed by Watson and Crick. The pairing of bases is specific and complementary: Cytosine *(C)* always pairs with guanine *(G)*, and adenine *(A)* always pairs with thymine *(T)*.

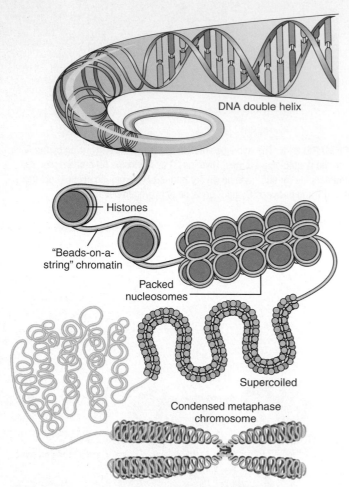

DNA double helix

Histones

"Beads-on-a-string" chromatin

Packed nucleosomes

Supercoiled

Condensed metaphase chromosome

FIGURE 5-4 DNA is packaged by wrapping around protein complexes called histones to form beadlike structures called *nucleosomes*. During cell division, the coiled DNA becomes very condensed into chromosomes that are visible under the light microscope. During interphase and when genes are being transcribed, the DNA is more loosely packaged and not visible.

to histones and other nuclear proteins is termed *chromatin*. When a cell is not dividing, the chromatin is loosely packed within the nucleus and not visible under the light microscope. During cell division, the chromatin becomes tightly condensed into the 46 chromosomes that become visible during mitosis.

The discovery of the double-helix model was profound because it immediately suggested how information transfer could be accomplished by such simple molecules. Because each DNA strand carries a nucleotide sequence that is exactly complementary to the sequence of its partner, both strands can be used as templates to create an exact copy of the original DNA double helix. When a cell divides to form two daughter cells, each daughter cell must receive a complete copy of the parent cell's DNA. The process of DNA replication requires separation of the DNA double helix by breaking the hydrogen bonds between the base pairs. Specific replication enzymes then direct the attachment of the correct (complementary) nucleotides to each of the single-stranded DNA templates.

In this way, two identical copies of the original DNA double helix are formed and passed on to the two daughter cells during cell division.

DNA Replication

Although the underlying principle of gene replication is simple, the cellular machinery required to carry out the replication process is complex, involving a host of enzymes and proteins.[3] These "replication machines" can duplicate DNA at a rate of 1000 nucleotides per second and complete the duplication of the entire genome in about 8 hours.[4] The DNA double helix must first separate so that new nucleotides can be paired with the old DNA template strands. The DNA double helix is normally very stable: the base pairs are locked in place so tightly that they can withstand temperatures approaching the boiling point. In addition, DNA is wrapped around histones and bound by a host of DNA binding proteins through which the replication machinery must navigate. DNA replication is started by special proteins (initiator protein) that pry the DNA strands apart at specific places along the chromatin, called *replication origins.* Then special enzymes (DNA helicases) are needed to rapidly unwind and separate the DNA strands, whereas helix-destabilizing proteins (also called single-stranded DNA-binding proteins) bind to the exposed DNA strands to keep them apart until replication can be accomplished (Figure 5-5). As the DNA is unwound in the replication fork, it becomes overly twisted downstream, so another set of enzymes, topoisomerases, cuts nicks in the DNA and allows it to unwind to prevent tangling. Ligases repair the nicks.

Once a portion of the DNA double helix has been separated, an enzyme complex, DNA polymerase, binds the single strands of DNA and begins the process of forming a new complementary strand of DNA. The polymerases match the appropriate base to the template base and catalyze the formation of the sugar-phosphate bonds that form the backbone of the DNA strand. Replication proceeds along the DNA strand in one direction only: from the 3′ end toward the 5′ end.[4] The ends of the DNA strands are labeled 3′ and 5′ according to the exposed carbon atom at that end. Because two complementary DNA strands are antiparallel, DNA replication is asymmetrical; one strand, the leading strand, is replicated as a continuous polymer, but the lagging strand must be synthesized in short sections in a "backstitching" process (see Figure 5-5). The backstitched fragments of DNA, called Okazaki fragments, are then sealed together by DNA ligase to form the unbroken DNA strand. DNA polymerase is unable to replicate DNA located at the very ends of the chromosomes (the telomeres), so another special enzyme complex, telomerase, is needed for this. The telomeres are fairly short, being composed of approximately 1000 repeats of a GGGTTA sequence. When the telomeres are replicated, one side of the double helix (3′ end) is always longer and loops around and tucks back in. This prevents nuclear enzymes from mistaking the ends of the chromosomes as broken DNA ends and trying to attach them to each other. In many somatic cell types, telomerase is

FIGURE 5-5 Summary of the major proteins of the DNA replication fork. Helicase unwinds the DNA double helix, whereas helix-destabilizing proteins keep the strands from reuniting. Okazaki fragments are formed in a "backstitching" direction and then sealed together with DNA ligase.

not present in sufficient levels and the cell's chromosomes get a bit shorter with each cell division. Chromosomal shortening has been proposed as a mechanism of "counting" the number of replications and may be important in cellular aging and prevention of cancer (see Chapter 7). DNA replication is said to be semiconservative because each of the two resulting DNA double helices contains one newly synthesized strand and one original (conserved) strand (Figure 5-6).

The DNA polymerase also has the ability to proofread the newly synthesized strands for errors in base pairing. If an error is detected, the enzyme will back up, remove the incorrect nucleotide, and replace it with the correct one. The fidelity of copying during DNA replication is such that only about one error is made for every 10^9 base-pair replications.[5] The self-correcting function of the DNA polymerases is extremely important because errors in replication will be passed on to the next generation of cells.

Genetic Code

How do an organism's genes influence its structural and functional characteristics? A central theory in biology holds that a gene directs the synthesis of a protein. It is the presence (or absence) and relative activity of various structural proteins and enzymes that produce the characteristics of the cell. This definition of genes as protein-coding elements is not entirely

correct because many genes code for ribonucleic acid (RNA) molecules as their final functional products and some genes may code for more than one protein product through alternate splicing of the RNA messages. Protein synthesis still holds a predominant place in understanding how genes direct cell structure and function. One of the surprising outcomes of the human genome projects was how little of the DNA in chromosomes contains coding segments (less than 2%) and how few genes there are (25,000). Prior to the genome project, it was estimated that the human genome contained 100,000 genes.

Proteins are composed of one or more chains of amino acids (polypeptides) that fold into complex three-dimensional structures. Cells contain 20 different types of amino acids that join together in a specific sequence to form a particular protein (Table 5-1). Each type of protein has a unique sequence of amino acids that dictates its structure and activity.

If genes are to direct the synthesis of proteins, the information contained in just four kinds of DNA nucleotide bases must code for 20 different amino acids. This so-called genetic code was deciphered in the early 1960s.[6,7] It was determined that a series of three nucleotides (triplet) was needed to code for each of the 20 amino acids. Because there are four different bases, there are 4^3, or 64 different possible triplet combinations. This is far more than needed to code for the 20 known amino acids. Three of the nucleotide triplets or **codons** do not

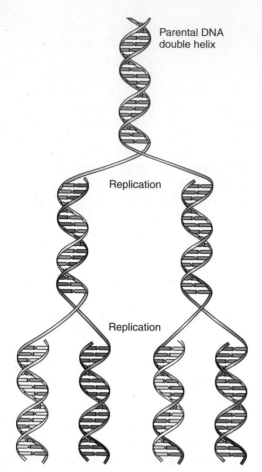

FIGURE 5-6 DNA replication is semiconservative. Each of the new DNA double helices contains one newly synthesized strand and one original strand.

TABLE 5-1

RNA Codons for the Different Amino Acids and for Start and Stop

Amino Acids	RNA Codons					
Alanine	GCU	GCC	GCA	GCG		
Arginine	CGU	CGC	CGA	CGG	AGA	AGG
Asparagine	AAU	AAC				
Aspartic acid	GAU	GAC				
Cysteine	UGU	UGC				
Glutamic acid	GAA	GAG				
Glutamine	CAA	CAG				
Glycine	GGU	GGC	GGA	GGG		
Histidine	CAU	CAC				
Isoleucine	AUU	AUC	AUA			
Leucine	CUU	CUC	CUA	CUG	UUA	UUG
Lysine	AAA	AAG				
Methionine	AUG					
Phenylalanine	UUU	UUC				
Proline	CCU	CCC	CCA	CCG		
Serine	UCU	UCC	UCA	UCG	AGC	AGU
Threonine	ACU	ACC	ACA	ACG		
Tryptophan	UGG					
Tyrosine	UAU	UAC				
Valine	GUU	GUC	GUA	GUG		
Start (CI)	AUG					
Stop (CT)	UAA	UAG	UGA			

CI, Chain initiation; *CT,* chain termination.

code for amino acids and are called *stop codons* because they signal the end of a protein code. The remaining 61 codons code for one of the 20 amino acids (see Table 5-1). Obviously, some of the amino acids are specified by more than one codon. For example, the amino acid arginine is determined by six different codons. The code has been highly conserved during evolution and is essentially the same in organisms as diverse as humans and bacteria.

Several intermediate molecules are involved in the process of DNA-directed protein synthesis, including the complex protein-synthesizing machinery of the ribosomes and several types of **RNA.** With few exceptions, the flow of information transfer is from DNA to RNA to protein. RNA is structurally similar to DNA, except that the sugar molecule is ribose rather than deoxyribose, and one of the four bases is different in that uracil replaces thymine. Because of the biochemical similarity of uracil and thymine, both can form base pairs with adenine. In addition, RNA forms stable single-stranded molecules, whereas DNA strands anneal together, forming a double-stranded molecule.

Several functionally different types of RNA are involved in protein synthesis and cell function. Some transcription units code for functional RNA molecules that have direct activities in cells and do not code for protein. Ribosomal RNA (rRNA) is found associated with the ribosome (see Chapter 3) in the cell cytoplasm. Messenger RNA (mRNA) is synthesized from the DNA template in a process termed **transcription** and carries the protein code to the cytoplasm, where the proteins are manufactured. The amino acids that will be joined together to form proteins are carried in the cytoplasm by a third type of RNA, transfer RNA (tRNA), which interacts with mRNA and the ribosome in a process termed **translation.** Several other forms of RNA are active in the nucleus, performing mRNA splicing, ribosome assembly, and quality control of RNA messages before they are sent out to the cytoplasm. Some RNA molecules have enzymatic activity independent of proteins. The role of many types of RNA in cellular function is still incompletely understood. A list of the principal types of RNA is shown in Box 5-1.

Transcription

Transcription is the process whereby mRNA is synthesized from a single-stranded DNA template. The process is similar in some respects to DNA replication. Double-stranded DNA must be separated in the region of the gene to be copied, and specific enzyme complexes (DNA-dependent RNA polymerases) orchestrate the production of the mRNA polymer. Only one of the DNA strands contains the desired gene sequence and serves as the template for the synthesis of mRNA. This strand is called the *sense strand*. The other strand is termed the *nonsense* or *antisense strand* and is not transcribed into an RNA message.

Some genes are continuously active in certain cells, whereas others are carefully regulated in response to cellular needs and environmental signals. Special sequences of DNA near a desired gene may enhance or inhibit its rate of transcription. In general, a gene is transcribed when the RNA polymerase-enzyme complex binds to a promoter region just upstream of the gene's start point. This binding event requires the

BOX 5-1

Types of RNA Produced in Cells

mRNA—messenger RNA; codes for proteins
rRNA—ribosomal RNA; within ribosomes, catalyzes protein synthesis
tRNA—transfer RNA; adaptors between mRNA and amino acids in protein synthesis
snRNA—small nuclear RNA; splicing of pre-mRNA in the nucleus
snoRNA—small nucleolar RNA; processing of rRNA in the nucleolus
scaRNA—small cajal RNA; modifies snoRNA and snRNA
miRNA—micro RNA; regulates gene expression by blocking mRNA translation
siRNA—small interfering RNA; turns off gene expression through alteration in chromatin

cooperative function of numerous DNA-binding proteins. Most gene regulation is accomplished through control of polymerase binding and is discussed later in this chapter. Once bound at the promoter, the RNA polymerase directs the separation of the DNA double helix and catalyzes the synthesis of the RNA message by matching the appropriate RNA bases to the DNA template (Figure 5-7). The RNA message is directly complementary to the DNA sequence, except that uracil replaces thymine.

In higher organisms, the DNA template for a particular protein is littered with stretches of bases that must be removed from the original RNA transcript (pre-mRNA) before it can be translated into a protein. These unwanted areas, called **introns,** are removed in the nucleus by a complex splicing process, resulting in an mRNA sequence that contains only the wanted segments, called **exons.** Introns range from 10 to 100,000 nucleotides in length.[8] On average a gene contains about 27,000 nucleotides, but only about 1300 remain in the final mRNA transcript; thus, a single gene may contain dozens of introns that must be precisely removed. The function of introns remains largely a mystery, although they are believed to be important in the evolution of new genetic information and in gene regulation. Many of these intron sequences are conserved across species, which implies an important function. The removal of introns and splicing of the RNA transcript is mediated by a group of small RNA molecules located in specialized areas of the nucleus called the *spliceosomes.* The *snRNAs,* or small nuclear RNAs, cause the introns to loop out like a lariat, bringing the adjacent exons close together, followed by cutting and splicing. Another group of RNA-protein complex molecules called *small nuclear ribonucleoproteins* (snRNP) attach to

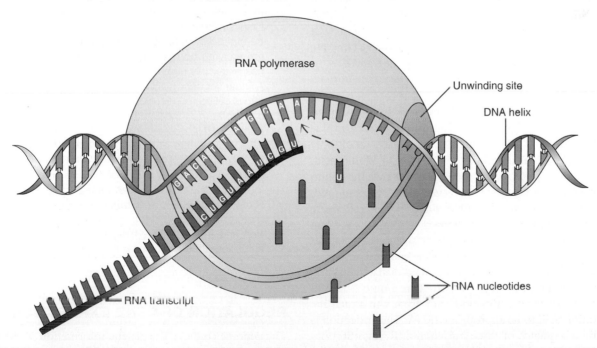

FIGURE 5-7 A moving RNA polymerase complex unwinds the DNA helix ahead of it while rewinding the DNA behind. One strand of the DNA serves as the template for the formation of mRNA.

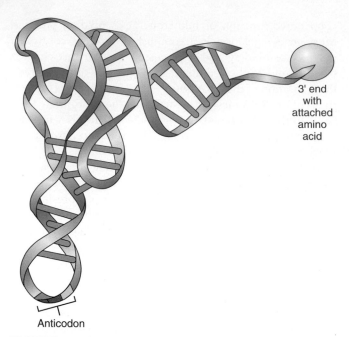

3' end
with
attached
amino
acid

Anticodon

FIGURE 5-8 Schematic drawing of a transfer RNA (tRNA) molecule. Each tRNA binds a specific amino acid, which corresponds with the three-base sequence at the anti-codon end.

the pre-mRNA and prevent its escape through the nuclear envelope until all the necessary splicing has been accomplished.[9] Most pre-mRNA transcripts can be spliced in different ways to increase the number of different protein forms produced by a single gene.[8]

The processed mRNA is finally transported to the cell cytoplasm through pores in the nuclear membrane that contain complexes that inspect the mRNA for certain structural characteristics that distinguish it from RNA debris. The mRNA then directs the synthesis of a protein in cooperation with tRNA and the ribosomes. Each mRNA may serve as a template for thousands of copies of protein before it is degraded.

Translation

Translation is the process whereby messenger RNA is used to direct the synthesis of a protein. The mRNA is read in linear fashion from one end to the other, with each set of three nucleotides serving as a codon for a particular amino acid. The codons in the mRNA do not directly recognize the amino acids. Intermediary molecules or "translators" are required. These intermediaries are the tRNA molecules. A schematic drawing of a tRNA molecule is shown in Figure 5-8, illustrating its L-shaped, three-dimensional structure. A codon reading area (anticodon) is located at one end and an amino acid attachment at the other. A group of specialized enzymes that have a binding pocket for a particular amino acid and a reading pocket for the anticodon are needed to attach the correct amino acid to its appropriate tRNA. The anticodon is formed by a sequence of three nucleotides. Recognition between the mRNA codon and the tRNA anticodon is accomplished by the same kind of complementary base pairing as

was described for DNA. The complex machinery of the ribosome is needed to line up the tRNA on the mRNA and to catalyze the peptide bonds that hold the amino acids together. **Ribosomes** are large complexes of protein and RNA. Each ribosome is composed of two subunits that are first assembled in a special part of the nucleus called the *nucleolus* and then transported through the nuclear pores to the cytoplasm. The smaller subunit binds the mRNA and the tRNA, whereas the larger subunit catalyzes the formation of peptide bonds between the incoming amino acids. The ribosome must first find the appropriate starting place on the mRNA to set the correct reading frame for the codon triplets. Then the ribosome moves along the mRNA, translating the nucleotide sequence into an amino acid sequence, one codon at a time (Figure 5-9).[10] The newly synthesized protein chain is released from the ribosome when a "stop codon" signaling the end of the message is reached. The new protein is typically bound by "chaperone" proteins that help it fold into its final three-dimensional shape.

REGULATION OF GENE EXPRESSION

The genome contains the genetic information of the cell and ultimately determines its form and function. All the various cells in a multicellular organism contain the same genome,

FIGURE 5-9 Synthesis of a protein by the ribosomes attached to a mRNA molecule. Ribosomes attach near the start codon and catalyze the formation of the peptide chain. The mRNA strand is read in groups of three nucleotides (codons) until the stop codon is reached and the peptide is released. Several ribosomes may translate a single mRNA into multiple copies of the protein.

and differences in cell type are thought to be to the result of differences in DNA *expression*. To maintain the cell's phenotype, some genes must be actively transcribed, whereas others remain quiescent. In addition, the cell must be able to change the expression of certain genes to respond and adapt to changes in the cellular environment. At any one time, a cell expresses 30% to 60% of its approximately 25,000 genes.[11] There is evidence that gene expression can be regulated at each of the steps in the pathway from DNA to RNA to protein synthesis. The proteins made by a cell can be controlled in the following ways: (1) regulating the rate and timing of gene transcription; (2) controlling how the mRNA is spliced; (3) selecting which mRNAs are transported to the cytoplasm; (4) selecting which mRNAs are translated by ribosomes; (5) selectively destroying certain mRNAs in the cytoplasm; or (6) selectively controlling the activity of the proteins after they have been produced.[11]

For a majority of genes, the most important regulators of expression are the transcriptional controls. Cells contain DNA-binding proteins that are able to enhance or inhibit gene expression. These gene regulatory proteins recognize and bind only particular DNA sequences and thus are specific to the genes they regulate.[12] The genome contains about 2000 different genes that code for gene-regulatory proteins, each of which works in combination with others to control numerous genes. The ability to regulate gene expression allows the cell to alter its structure and function in response to signals from its environment.

Transcriptional Controls

The gene regulatory proteins described in the preceding paragraphs are thought to control gene transcription by binding near the promoter sequence of DNA, where the RNA polymerase must attach to initiate transcription of the gene.[13]

Binding of the regulatory proteins may either enhance or inhibit RNA polymerase binding and subsequent transcription of the gene. This is sometimes referred to as "turning on" or "turning off" a gene. The DNA-binding proteins are able to recognize their specific binding sites because of small variations in structure of the external surface of the DNA double helix and do not require separation of the strands to bind. These regulatory DNA-binding proteins can be categorized as positive controls that turn on or activate transcription (*activators*) or negative controls that inhibit transcription (*repressors*).

In humans, the strategies for gene regulation are complex. Gene regulatory proteins often bind DNA segments far from the gene being regulated, and binding of several gene regulatory proteins in combination is often necessary. A critical step in initiating gene transcription in human cells is the assembly of general transcription factors at the promoter region.[14] General transcription factors are a group of DNA-binding proteins necessary for RNA polymerase activity, and initiation of transcription does not occur without them. Regulatory gene activator proteins help to collect the transcription factors at the promoter of the correct gene by first recognizing and binding to a specific DNA sequence and then coordinating the assembly of the transcription factors (Figure 5-10).

Inhibition of transcription is achieved by gene repressor proteins, which also recognize and bind specific DNA sequences but inhibit the assembly of transcription factors at the site. Some repressor proteins may work simply by binding to and physically blocking the promoter region, but most appear to exert their effects through more complex mechanisms, such as compacting the DNA to make it difficult to pry open, interfering with activator proteins, and binding up or

FIGURE 5-10 Gene activator proteins coordinate the assembly of general transcription factors at the promoter region of the gene to be transcribed. RNA polymerase is unable to bind and begin transcription until the requisite transcription factors are in place.

inhibiting transcription factors. Inappropriate transcription of genes in a particular cell may have dire consequences for the cell or for the organism as a whole and is therefore a carefully regulated process. The presence, position, and activity of gene regulatory proteins may be regulated by various signaling cascades within the cell. Many of these signaling cascades are triggered by changes in the cell's environment, which then alter gene transcription. This process is very complex, with numerous signaling pathways often converging on a particular gene regulatory system.

KEY POINTS

- All the cells in an individual have essentially the same DNA; however, cells differ greatly in structure and function. This occurs because genes are selectively expressed in particular cells.
- Gene expression can be regulated at any step in the pathway from DNA to RNA to protein synthesis. The most important regulators are transcriptional controls.
- A critical step for initiation of gene transcription is the assembly of general transcription factors at the promoter region of the gene.
- The actions of general transcription factors and RNA polymerase are controlled by a large number of regulatory proteins that specifically bind to DNA. The presence of certain DNA-binding proteins at specific sites can activate or repress the transcription of a particular gene in response to signals in the cell's environment.

DIFFERENTIATION OF TISSUES

Cell Diversification and Cell Memory

The cells of a multicellular organism tend to specialize to perform particular functions in coordination with other cells and tissues of the body. Cells not only must become different

during development, they must also remain different in the adult, after the original cues for cell diversification have disappeared. The differences among cell types are ultimately the result of the differentiating influences experienced in the embryo. Differences are maintained because the cells retain the effects of those past influences and pass the memory on to their descendants. When a skin cell divides to replace lost skin cells, the daughter cells are also skin cells; when a liver cell divides, its daughter cells are liver cells; and so on. The behavior of cells of higher organisms is governed by their genome and their present environment, as well as by their developmental history.

There is substantial evidence that the differences in tissue structure and function in a particular organism are not due to deletions or additions to the genome.[15] All the cells of an organism contain essentially the same genes. Many genes are expressed in nearly all cell types (e.g., the so-called *housekeeping genes* that code for RNA and proteins essential for cell viability). It is the expression of a relatively few tissue-specific genes that results in differences among cell types.[11] The exact mechanisms leading to the stable expression of tissue-specific genes in particular cell types are partly unknown; however, differences in DNA packaging and the combination of gene regulatory proteins passed on during cell division are thought to be important. The DNA in human cells is extensively packaged, so that 40 inches of linear DNA can be compacted to fit into the cell nucleus. However different regions of chromosomes can be more or less condensed[1] (see Figure 5-4).

Some regions of DNA, called **heterochromatin,** are so condensed that they are not open to transcription. It is thought that the pattern of packaging as well as the DNA-binding proteins that regulate it are transmitted to progeny when a cell divides such that the pattern of gene expression is maintained as the cell's developmental memory. An example of this mechanism is the inactivation of one of the X chromosomes in females.[16] In mammals, all female cells contain two X chromosomes

(XX), whereas male cells contain an X and a Y chromosome (XY). One of the X chromosomes in females is permanently inactivated early in development by condensed packaging. This apparently occurs to prevent a double dose of the X gene products. Which of the two X chromosomes is inactivated in a particular cell is a random event. However, the same X chromosome will be inactive in all of the cell's progeny. Segments of other chromosomes are also highly condensed into heterochromatin, which varies in different cell types. The processes that initiate variations in DNA packaging are not well understood; however, the pattern of inactivated genes in a particular cell type is "remembered" in subsequent generations of cells and may explain, in part, how differentiated tissues remain differentiated in the adult.

Mechanisms of Development

Embryonic development is associated with selective gene expression that controls four essential processes to enable a single cell to develop into a complex organism: (1) cell proliferation, (2) cell specialization, (3) cell-to-cell interactions, and (4) cell movement and migration.[17] Each time a cell divides it must retain memory of the developmental events that have preceded the division so that it can progress along a developmental pathway toward becoming a differentiated tissue. Cells have a genetic memory: the genes a cell expresses and the way it behaves depend on the cell's past as well as its present environment. There is no overall controlling center; each cell must make its own developmental decisions.

There are two major classes of proteins that are particularly important for multicellular development: (1) transmembrane proteins in the cell surface that participate in cell adhesion and communication; and (2) DNA-binding proteins that regulate gene transcription. Differences between cells in an embryo are a necessary prelude to development of a multicellular organism and arise in various ways. Very early in embryonic development, cells begin to divide asymmetrically so that daughter cells are not identical—those on the outside of the group of cells receive different environmental cues than those on the inside, which are surrounded by other cells. These simple differences in cell-to-cell adhesion may alter the transcription of a set of genes. The altered genetic expression will then be passed on to daughter cells in the next cell division, making them diverge further from the original cell. Subsequently the cell will respond differently to environmental influences, which further alter the cell's structure and function. Thus cells become committed to a developmental pathway over the course of many cell divisions that pass on the history of previous exposures through sequential changes in gene expression.

Continued interactions with nearby cells, chemical gradients, and extracellular matrix components provide clues to guide the cell to its appropriate form and location in the developing organism. Chemicals that control the patterning of fields of nearby tissue are termed **morphogens.** For example, cells in the head region may specialize to secrete a "position signal" for other cells. The morphogen is progressively degraded as it diffuses through the neighboring tissue, such that it has higher concentration close to the source. A particular cell will have information regarding its proximity to the head region based on the surrounding concentration of the chemical. Morphogens are thought to be effective only over small distances. Thus the gross distinctions, between head and tail, for example, must be made very early in the embryo, and morphogens can provide only a general pattern for future development. Successive levels of detail can be filled in later by other positional signals.

The organization of molecules surrounding the cell surface also provides positional information. The extracellular matrix is composed of a large meshwork of molecules that is produced locally by cells in the area. Some common components include the proteins collagen and elastin, long polysaccharide chains called *glycosaminoglycans,* and a variety of peptides, growth factors, and hormones. The extracellular matrix is highly organized, with components binding to each other and to the cell membrane in specific ways. The extracellular matrix is thought to be important in cell development through its ability to screen or modulate the transport of molecules, such as growth factors, to the cell membrane and through direct contacts with the cell membrane that bring about changes in cell structure and function.[18]

The extracellular matrix surrounding the cells in different locations may provide positional information to cells that must migrate to their final destination.[18] In vertebrates, connective tissue cells appear to provide much of this positional information. As the migratory cell travels through the connective tissue, it may continually "test" the surroundings, searching for cues to guide it. Migratory cells with specific cell surface receptors may interact differentially with the extracellular matrix in different areas. In this way the migratory cell can be guided along particular paths and induced to settle in particular areas. Once the migratory cell has settled, local extracellular matrix molecules may further affect the cell's growth rate, differentiation, and likelihood of survival.

Interactions between the extracellular matrix and nearby cells are mediated primarily by binding proteins called **integrins.**[19] Integrins are transmembrane proteins that tie the cell's cytoskeleton to particular matrix structures. They enable the cytoskeleton and extracellular matrix to communicate across the plasma membrane in specific ways. In addition to inducing cells to bind in a particular location, integrins have been shown to activate intracellular signaling pathways, which may influence cell behavior in numerous ways (e.g., cell shape, polarity, metabolism, development, and differentiation).

The steps leading to the development of differentiated tissues in a multicellular organism are such that, once differentiated, a cell type generally does not revert to earlier forms. Some tissues are said to be terminally differentiated and have limited capacity to change form or replicate. Other tissues maintain less-differentiated stem cells that are able to develop into a variety of cell types, depending on environmental cues.

TABLE 5-2

Major Categories and Location of Body Tissues

Tissue Type	Locations
Epithelium	
Simple squamous	Lining of blood vessels, pulmonary alveoli, Bowman capsule
Simple cuboidal	Thyroid, sweat, and salivary glands; kidney tubules
Simple columnar	Lining of intestine, glandular ducts
Pseudostratified (mixed cell shapes)	Male urethra, respiratory passages
Stratified squamous	Skin, mucous membranes
Stratified columnar	Epiglottis, anus, parts of pharynx
Stratified transitional (layers of different cell shapes)	Bladder
Connective Tissue	
Loose	Widespread locations, dermis of skin, adipose, tissue organs
Dense/supportive	Cartilage, bone, tendons, joints, fascia surrounding muscles
Hematopoietic	Bone marrow, lymph tissue, plasma
Muscle	
Skeletal	Voluntary muscles of body
Cardiac	Heart (myocardium)
Smooth	Intestine, blood vessels, bladder, uterus, airways
Myoepithelial	Mammary, sweat, and salivary glands
Nervous	
Neurons	Central and peripheral nerves
Neuroglia	Primarily central nervous system

Differentiated Tissues

The more than 200 different cell types in the adult human are generally classified into four major tissue categories: epithelium, connective tissue, muscle, and nerve.[20] The tissue types with some of their subtypes are summarized in Table 5-2. Most of the organ systems of the body are combinations of these four tissue types mixed together in a highly organized and cooperative manner.

Epithelial Tissue

Epithelial cells cover the majority of the external surfaces of the body and line the glands, blood vessels, and internal surfaces. Epithelial cells adopt a variety of shapes and functions, depending on their locations. For example, the *stratified* epithelium that makes up the epidermis of the skin is several layers thick and is primarily protective in function. New epithelial skin cells are formed from stem cells in the deepest part of the epidermis, where it contacts the basal lamina. As cells mature, they move outward toward the surface until they become keratinized and finally flake away (Figure 5-11). Keratin is a tough protective protein that is present in large quantities in the outer skin layers of flattened, dead epithelial cells. The epidermis in humans is completely replaced about once per month, but turnover can occur more rapidly after injury to the skin.[20]

In addition to stratified epithelium, the epithelium may be characterized as simple or pseudostratified according to the number and arrangement of cell layers (Figure 5-12). *Simple* epithelium consists of a single layer of cells, all of which contact the basement membrane. Simple epithelium is found in

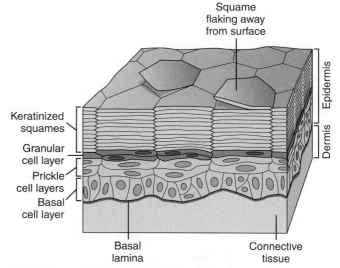

FIGURE 5-11 Organization of epidermal skin layers, showing the flattened keratinized outer layer. Epithelial cells are continually produced by stem cells at the basal lamina and then migrate to the surface.

the lining of blood vessels and body cavities, in many glands, and in the alveoli of the lungs. The simple epithelium that lines the blood vessels is called *endothelium*. Simple epithelium also forms the kidney tubules and lines the intestine, where absorption is its primary function. *Stratified* epithelium consists of two or more layers of epithelial cells and is found in mucous membranes, such as the mouth, and in the skin, as mentioned previously. Epithelium that appears to be more than one layer thick because of a mixture of cell shapes but

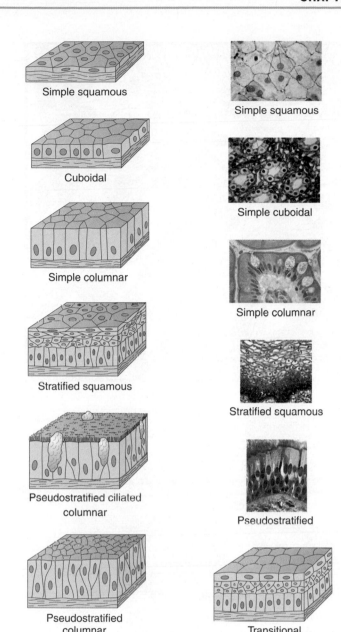

FIGURE 5-12 Various epithelial tissue shapes and layering.

Simple squamous

Cuboidal

Simple columnar

Stratified squamous

Pseudostratified ciliated columnar

Pseudostratified columnar

Simple squamous

Simple cuboidal

Simple columnar

Stratified squamous

Pseudostratified

Transitional

is actually a single layer is called *pseudostratified* epithelium. The linings of the respiratory tract and some glands contain pseudostratified epithelium.

Epithelial cells may also be classified according to cell shape. The three basic cell shapes are squamous, cuboidal, and columnar. Squamous cells are thin in comparison to their surface area and have a flattened appearance. Cuboidal cells are approximately equal in width and height, similar to a cube. Columnar cells are a bit taller than they are wide, resembling a rectangular column. Several classifications of epithelial tissue are given in Table 5-2, using both shape and layering as criteria.

Connective Tissue

Connective tissue is the most abundant and diverse tissue in the body, including cell types as different as bone cells, fat cells, and blood cells.[20] Connective tissue commonly functions as a scaffold on which other cells cluster to form organs, but it does much more than hold tissues together. Connective tissue cells often form an elaborate extracellular matrix, which is thought to be important in the maintenance of cell differentiation (Figure 5-13). Connective tissue cells play an important part in the support and repair of nearly every tissue and organ in the body. Three major classifications of connective tissue are commonly identified: loose connective tissue, dense or supportive tissue, and hematopoietic tissue.

Loose connective tissue appears unstructured, with a fair amount of space between fibers of the extracellular matrix. The matrix contains a number of cell types and an elaborate meshwork of protein and other molecules (Figure 5-14). The primary protein constituents are collagen, elastin, and reticular fibers. Collagen is composed of tough, nonelastic bundles of protein fibers that are secreted by fibroblasts. It gives structural strength to skin, tendons, ligaments, and other tissues. The ability of a structure to withstand deforming and stretching forces is due, in large part, to elastin, which can return to its original length after being stretched, like a rubber band. Elastin is important to the function of structures such as the aorta, which must expand to accept the blood ejected from the heart during systole and bounce back to its original shape during diastole. Reticular fibers are short branching fibers that provide networks for the attachment of connective tissue to other cell types, such as epithelial cell attachments in glands, hematopoietic cells in bone marrow, and the parenchymal cells (functional cells) in organs. Cell types associated with loose connective tissue include the fibroblasts, mast cells, and adipocytes (fat cells).

Dense or supportive connective tissue is rich in collagen, which gives strength to structures such as cartilage, tendon, bone, and ligaments. The collagen fibers are more organized and densely packed than in loose connective tissue. Cartilage cells, or chondrocytes, may be found in the trachea, joints, nose, ears, vertebral disks, organs, and the young skeleton. Once formed, the collagenous extracellular matrix structures require little maintenance and do not receive a blood supply. Bone is a very dense form of connective tissue composed of a mixture of tough collagen fibers and solid calcium phosphate crystals in approximately equal proportions. Throughout the bone's hard extracellular matrix are channels and cavities occupied by living cells (osteocytes) (Figure 5-15). These cells incessantly model and remodel their bony environment, responding to environmental signals. These osteocytes are of two kinds: the cells that erode old bone are called *osteoclasts,* whereas the cells that form new bone are called *osteoblasts.* Osteoblasts detect when a bone is subjected to a greater load stress and adapt by strengthening the bone mass. Conversely, when the load is removed, as during bed rest, the osteoclasts busily digest the bone away, often resulting in some of the common complications of immobility. Osteoclasts, like macrophages, are derived from monocytes that are produced in the bone marrow. The monocytes travel via the bloodstream and collect at sites of bone resorption, where they fuse together to become osteoclasts.[21] Osteocyte activity is essential for

FIGURE 5-13 A schematic drawing of loose connective tissue. (From Thibodeau G and Patton K: *Anatomy & physiology,* ed 6, St. Louis, 2007, Mosby, p 147. Courtesy Ed Reschke.)

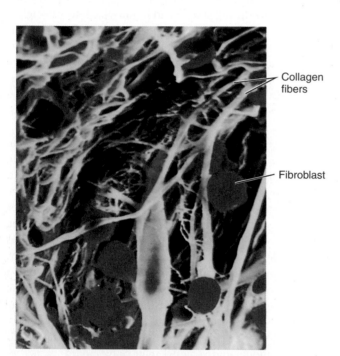

Collagen fibers

Fibroblast

Loose connective tissue

FIGURE 5-14 Scanning electron micrograph of fibroblasts in loose connective tissue of a rat cornea. The matrix is composed primarily of collagen fibers (magnification ×440). (From Solomon EP: *Introduction to human anatomy and physiology,* ed 3, Philadelphia, 2009, Saunders, p 36.)

Lacunae

Haversian canal

Matrix

Bone

FIGURE 5-15 Photomicrograph of a section of compact bone showing circular networks formed by the action of osteoclasts and osteoblasts as they remodel the bone. The osteocytes occupy the lacunae and canals. (From Solomon EP: *Introduction to human anatomy and physiology,* ed 3, Philadelphia, 2009, Saunders, p 36.)

bone growth and the repair of bone injuries. (See Chapter 50 for a detailed description of the musculoskeletal system.)

The blood-forming organs of the body are formed by a specialized type of connective tissue called *hematopoietic* tissue. The blood cells include the red cell, or **erythrocyte,** which is specialized for the transport of oxygen; the platelet, or **thrombocyte,** which is important in blood coagulation; and a host of white cells, or **leukocytes,** which mediate immune function. Blood-forming tissue is located in the bone marrow, spleen, and lymphatic tissue. Hematopoietic cells are necessarily nomadic, traveling to distant areas of the body, sometimes settling in a particular organ, sometimes moving continuously (Figure 5-16). Blood cells have a short life span in comparison to other cells and must continually be replenished. This is accomplished by the hematopoietic stem cells. Stem cells reside primarily in the bone marrow and are multipotent; they may differentiate into any of the blood cell types. This results in a system that can respond quickly to the changing needs of the body.

5 µm

FIGURE 5-16 Scanning electron micrograph of red and white blood cells in the lumen of a blood vessel. Red cells are smooth and concave, whereas white cells are rough and rounded. (From Alberts B et al, editors: *Molecular biology of the cell*, ed 5, New York, 2008, Garland Science, p 1451. Courtesy Ray Moss.)

Muscle Tissue

The term *muscle* refers to tissues that are specialized for contraction. Muscle cells, or myocytes, are usually long and thin and packed with the proteins actin and myosin, which make up the contractile apparatus. In mammals, there are four main categories of muscle cells: skeletal, cardiac, smooth, and myoepithelial (Figure 5-17).[20] Contraction in all four types depends on intracellular calcium and occurs because of interactions between actin and myosin filaments. Actin and myosin filaments differ among cell types with regard to amino acid sequence, arrangement within the cell, and the mechanisms that control contraction. The mechanism of muscle contraction has been called *the sliding filament hypothesis* or *cross-bridge theory*. These terms describe the interactions of the actin and myosin filaments as they form bonds and pull past each other, causing the muscle cell to shorten. Contraction is initiated by an increase in intracellular free calcium and requires energy in the form of adenosine triphosphate (ATP). A detailed description of actin-myosin cross-bridging and the role of calcium, troponin, and tropomyosin can be found in Chapter 17.

Skeletal muscle is responsible for nearly all voluntary movements. Skeletal muscle cells fuse together to form long multinucleated fibers that can be huge, up to 0.5 m in length. Once fused and differentiated into mature skeletal muscle cells, they cannot enter the cell cycle and divide to produce new cells. Skeletal muscle stem cells (satellite cells) are retained in the muscle tissue and can proliferate in response to muscle damage. The actin and myosin proteins in skeletal muscle are aligned in orderly arrays, giving the tissue a striped appearance under the microscope, which in turn has led to the term

striated muscle. Skeletal muscle contracts in response to stimulation from the motor neurons of the nervous system. As in other types of muscle, stimulation results in an increase in free calcium within the cell. In skeletal muscle, the calcium comes from internal storage sites in the sarcoplasmic reticulum. Contraction is initiated when the calcium binds troponin, a regulatory protein attached to the actin filament. Because of the high energy requirements of contracting skeletal muscle, the cells are packed with energy-producing mitochondria.

Like skeletal muscle, *cardiac muscle* also has a striated appearance due to the systematic organization of its actin and myosin filaments. Cardiac muscle cells are linked by special structures, called *intercalated disks*, that cause the tissue to behave as a **syncytium:** all the cells contract synchronously. Cardiac muscle contracts in response to autonomic innervation and blood-borne chemicals, but it also has the special property of automaticity. *Automaticity* refers to the inherent ability of the cell to initiate an action potential without outside stimulation. The contractile mechanisms of cardiac muscle are similar to those of skeletal muscle, requiring free calcium to interact with troponin, resulting in the formation of actin-myosin cross-bridges. In cardiac muscle, some of the free calcium comes from the sarcoplasmic reticulum, but diffusion into the cell through channels in the cell membrane is also necessary. These membrane calcium channels represent an important difference from skeletal muscle, as they can be manipulated by drugs (calcium channel blockers) without disrupting skeletal muscle control. (Cardiac muscle is discussed in Chapter 17.)

Smooth muscle comprises a diverse group of tissues located in organs throughout the body. Smooth muscle generally is

FIGURE 5-17 The four classes of muscle cells. **A,** Skeletal muscle. **B,** Heart (cardiac) muscle. **C,** Smooth muscle (bladder). **D,** Myoepithelial cells in a mammary gland. (**A** and **C,** From Alberts B et al, editors: *Molecular biology of the cell*, ed 5, New York, 2008, Garland Science, p 1451. **A,** Courtesy Junzo Deskati. **B,** From Fujiwara T: Cardiac muscle. In Canal ED, editor: *Handbook of microscopic anatomy*, Berlin, 1986, Springer-Verlag. **C,** Courtesy Satoshi Nakasiro. **D,** From Nagato T et al: A scanning electron microscope study of myoepithelial cells in exocrine glands, *Cell Tissue Res* 209:1-10, 1980.)

not under voluntary control and therefore is called *involuntary muscle*. Some types of smooth muscle are able to contract intrinsically, and most are influenced by the autonomic nervous system. Smooth muscle is found in blood vessels and in the walls of hollow organs, such as those of the gastrointestinal tract, uterus, and large airways.

The structure of smooth muscle differs considerably from that of skeletal and cardiac muscle, and therefore some classification schemes consider it to be a member of the connective tissue family.[20] The actin and myosin filaments are less organized in smooth muscle, and the muscle does not have striations. Smooth muscle contraction tends to be slower and can be maintained indefinitely. This is critical to the function of blood vessels, which must maintain a degree of contraction or vascular tone to maintain the blood pressure. Smooth muscle differs in the way actin-myosin cross-bridges are formed and in the calcium-binding regulatory proteins. When calmodulin, the calcium-binding protein in smooth muscle, binds calcium, it activates the enzyme, myosin light chain kinase (MLCK), which phosphorylates myosin and stimulates the rate of cross-bridge formation. Smooth muscle contraction is highly dependent on the diffusion of extracellular calcium into the cell through calcium channels in the plasma membrane (sarcolemma). Thus, like cardiac muscle, smooth

muscle can also be affected by drugs that alter the calcium channel's ability to conduct calcium. For example, calcium channel-blocking drugs are used to cause the smooth muscle in arterial blood vessels to relax as a treatment for high blood pressure.

Myoepithelial cells represent the fourth class of muscle cells. They are located in the ducts of some glands (e.g., mammary, sweat, and salivary). Unlike all other types of muscle, myoepithelial cells lie in the epithelium and are derived from embryonic ectoderm, whereas skeletal, cardiac, and smooth muscle are derived from embryonic mesoderm. Myoepithelial cells contract in response to specific stimuli (e.g., oxytocin in the mammary gland) and serve to expel the contents from the gland.

Nervous Tissue

Nervous tissue is widely distributed throughout the body, providing a rapid communication network between the central nervous system and various body parts. Nerve cells are specialized to generate and transmit electrical impulses very rapidly. Like muscle, nerves are excitable; they respond to stimulation by altering their electrical potentials. This excitability is caused by the presence of voltage-sensitive ion channels located in the plasma membrane of the nerve cell. Movement

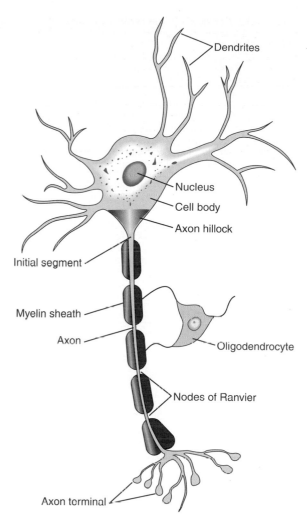

FIGURE 5-18 Diagram of a typical neuron showing the cell body, axon, and dendrites. Neurons have many shapes and sizes.

Labels in figure:
- Dendrites
- Nucleus
- Cell body
- Axon hillock
- Initial segment
- Myelin sheath
- Axon
- Oligodendrocyte
- Nodes of Ranvier
- Axon terminal

In addition to neurons, nervous tissue contains a variety of supportive cells, termed **neuroglia** ("nerve glue"), that nourish, protect, insulate, and clean up debris in the central nervous system. These include the astrocytes, oligodendroglia, ependymal cells, and microglia. (See Chapter 43 for a detailed description of nervous system anatomy and physiology.)

KEY POINTS

- The structure and function of cells are influenced by the genome and environment as well as by developmental history.
- Embryonic development is associated with selective gene expression that controls four essential processes to enable a single cell to develop into a complex organism: (1) cell proliferation; (2) cell specialization; (3) cell-to-cell interactions; and (4) cell movement and migration.
- Differentiated cell types have different capacities to divide. Some tissues, such as nerve and cardiac muscle, are terminally differentiated and have limited ability to divide. Other cell types, such as skin and bone marrow, maintain more stem cells, which have great capacity to proliferate.
- Different cell types in the adult human are classified into four major categories: epithelium (e.g., skin, glands, endothelium), connective tissue (e.g., bone, cartilage, fat, blood), muscle (e.g., skeletal, cardiac, smooth), and nervous tissue (e.g., neuronal, glial).

SUMMARY

The development, differentiation, and day-to-day activities of a cell are directed by its genes. Genes are sequences of nucleotides that provide the template for the production of RNA or cellular proteins. In large part, the kinds and amounts of cellular proteins determine cell structure and function. All the cells of the body possess essentially the same DNA, but through complex processes of differentiation they become specialized to perform particular functions. It is believed that different sets of genes are active in different cell types. The four major classes of differentiated tissues are epithelial, connective, muscle, and nerve. These four tissues interdependently form the functioning systems of the body.

of ions through these channels results in the production and propagation of action potentials along the length of the neuron. Neurons communicate their action potentials to other nerve and muscle cells through synapses. At the synapse, the presynaptic neuron releases a chemical neurotransmitter into the space between itself and the next neuron (synaptic cleft), where it diffuses across and interacts with receptors on the postsynaptic neuron.

A typical neuron is composed of three parts: a cell body, an axon, and one or more dendrites (Figure 5-18). The cell body contains the nucleus and other cytoplasmic organelles. The axon is generally long (as long as 1 m) and may be encased in a myelin sheath. The axons usually conduct impulses away from the cell body, whereas the dendritic processes usually receive information and conduct impulses toward the cell body. Neurons are classified on the basis of the number of projections extending from the cell body. Neurons are terminally differentiated and incapable of replicating. However, some neural stem cells are located in certain areas of the brain and may replicate to form either neurons or glial cells in response to specific signals (see Chapter 43).

REFERENCES

1. Alberts B et al: DNA chromosomes, and genomes. In Alberts B et al, editors: *Molecular biology of the cell*, ed 5, New York, 2008, Garland Science, pp 195-262.
2. Watson JD, Crick FHC: Molecular structure of nucleic acids: a structure for deoxyribose nucleic acid, *Nature* 171:737-738, 1953.
3. Hubscher U, Seo YS: Replication of the lagging strand: a concert of at least 23 polypeptides, *Mol Cell* 12(2):149-157, 2001.

4. Alberts B et al: DNA replication, repair and recombination. In Alberts B et al, editors: *Molecular biology of the cell*, ed 5, New York, 2008, Garland Science, pp 263-328.

5. Kunkel TA, Bebenek K: DNA replication fidelity, *Annu Rev Biochem* 69:497-529, 2000.

6. Crick FHC: The genetic code: III, *Sci Am* 215(4):55-62, 1966.

7. Frisch L, editor: The genetic code. In *Cold Spring Harbor symposia on quantitative biology*, Cold Spring Harbor, NY, 1966, Cold Spring Harbor Laboratory.

8. Alberts B et al: How cells read the genome: from DNA to protein. In Alberts B et al, editors: *Molecular biology of the cell*, ed 5, New York, 2008, Garland Science, pp 329-410.

9. Gravely BR: Sorting out the complexity of SR functions, *RNA* 6(9):1197-1211, 2000.

10. Frank J: The ribosome: a macromolecular machine par excellence, *Chem Biol* 7:R133-R141, 2000.

11. Alberts B et al: Control of gene expression. In Alberts B et al, editors: *Molecular biology of the cell*, ed 5, New York, 2008, Garland Science, pp 411-499.

12. Emerson BM: Specificity of gene regulation, *Cell* 109(3):267-270, 2003.

13. Hochheimer A, Tjian R: Diversified transcription initiation complexes expand promoter selectivity and tissue-specific gene expression, *Genes Dev* 17(11):1309-1320, 2003.

14. Thomas MC, Chiang CM: The general transcription machinery and general transcription factors, *Critical Rev Biochem Mol Biol* 41:105-178, 2006.

15. Gurdon JB: The developmental capacity of nuclei taken from intestinal epithelium cells of feeding tadpoles, *J Embryol Exp Morphol* 10:622-640, 1962.

16. Georgel PT: Role of chromatin/epigenetic modifications on DNA accessibility, *Drug News Perspect* 20(9):549-556, 2007.

17. Alberts B et al: Development of multicellular organisms. In Alberts B et al, editors: *Molecular biology of the cell*, ed 5, New York, 2008, Garland Science, pp 1305-1416.

18. Lock JG, Wehrle-Haller B: Cell-matrix adhesion complexes: master control machinery of cell migration, *Sem Cancer Biol* 18(1):65-67, 2008.

19. Bokel C, Brown NH: Integrins in development: moving on, responding to, and sticking to the extracellular matrix, *Dev Cell* 3:311-321, 2002.

20. Alberts B et al: Specialized tissues, stem cells, and tissue renewal. In Alberts B et al, editors: *Molecular biology of the cell*, ed 5, New York, 2008, Garland Science, pp 1417-1484.

21. Teitelbaum SL: Osteoclasts: what do they do and how do they do it? *Am J Pathol* 170(2):427-435, 2007.

Genetic and Developmental Disorders

Jacquelyn L. Banasik

MEDIA RESOURCES

Additional Material for Study, Review, and Further Exploration

CD Companion ■ Review Questions and Answers
■ Glossary (with audio pronunciations for selected terms) ■ Disease Profiles ■ Animations

ⓔvolve **Website** at http://evolve.elsevier.com/Copstead/
■ Case Studies ■ Disease Profiles ■ WebLinks ■ Key Points Review

Online Course (Module 2)

KEY QUESTIONS

■ How are genes transmitted from parent to offspring?
■ How is pedigree analysis used to determine if a trait is inherited as autosomal dominant, autosomal recessive, or X-linked?
■ How might abnormal meiosis lead to alterations in chromosome number or structure?

■ What are the inheritance patterns and general clinical features of some common genetic disorders?
■ What is the role of the environment in development of congenital disorders?
■ What methods of genetic testing are available?

CHAPTER OUTLINE

Geneticists and parents alike have marveled at the development of a recognizable human baby, with eyes and ears, toes and fingers, from its simple beginning as a single cell containing one set of genes. Considering the enormous list of potentially disastrous genetic and environmental influences, the birth of a healthy normal child does indeed seem like a miracle. Although the risk of bearing a child with mental or physical defects is small for most parents, it is real and is often a source of worry during the prenatal period. It has been estimated that most people harbor one or two defective genes that are recessive and therefore of little consequence until they are transmitted to offspring.[1] In addition, there are many known and unknown environmental hazards to which the parent and fetus may be exposed. Disorders that are present at birth are called *congenital* and are generally grouped according to genetic or environmental causes. Some congenital disorders are associated with structural defects that are due to errors in fetal development and are called **congenital malformations.** Malformations are frequently associated with genetic causes; however, environmental influences (teratogens) also may adversely affect the developing fetus. It is estimated that about 3% of newborns have a major malformation of cosmetic or functional significance.[2,3] Approximately one half of all birth malformations are associated with genetic factors.[3,4] The incidence of chromosomal abnormalities in neonates is approximately 1 in 200, and the incidence of single gene disorders is approximately 1 in 100.[3] Not all inherited genetic disorders are apparent at birth and therefore are not considered congenital. Some single-gene defects and many polygenic disorders do not become apparent until later in childhood or adulthood. In this chapter, the general principles of inheritance; genetic and environmental causes of congenital disorders; and the principles of diagnosis, counseling, and gene therapy are described.

PRINCIPLES OF INHERITANCE

"Whom does the baby look like?" is frequently asked of new parents. It is common knowledge that traits tend to run in families, but Gregor Mendel, a nineteenth-century monk turned geneticist, was the first to notice that traits were transmitted in a predictable way from parent to offspring.[5] Height, weight, skin color, eye color, and hair color are some of the physical traits that characterize an individual. **Phenotype** refers to the physical and biochemical attributes of an individual that are outwardly apparent. These traits are a result of the expression of the individual's unique genetic makeup, or **genotype.** In humans, these genes are organized into 46 different chromosome units that become visible under the microscope only during cell division (see Chapter 5).

During meiosis, chromosomes look like Xs of varying sizes and shapes. The X-shaped chromosome is really made up of two identical linear chromosome units, called **chromatids,** which separate during meiosis. The point at the middle of the X at which the two sister chromatids are joined together

FIGURE 6-1 Scanning electron micrograph of a chromosome showing the two sister chromatids attached at the centromere. Sister chromatids separate during meiosis with one chromatid being distributed to each daughter cell. (From Pollard T et al: *Cell biology,* ed 2, Philadelphia, 2007, Saunders, p 224.)

is the **centromere** (Figure 6-1). Human chromosomes are **diploid;** they occur as pairs. One member of the pair comes from the mother, and one member comes from the father. Under the microscope the members of a pair appear to be identical (**homologous**), although they are different in DNA sequence. Chromosomes are characterized on the basis of total size, length of the arms of the X, and their characteristic banding patterns when exposed to certain stains (karyotype) (Figure 6-2).

Of the 23 pairs of chromosomes, 22 are homologous and are called **autosomes.** The remaining pair, the **sex** chromosomes, differs in males and females. Females receive an X chromosome from each parent (homologous), whereas males receive an X chromosome from their mothers and a Y chromosome from their fathers (hemizygous). Thus, the genotype is a result of the union of 23 maternal and 23 paternal chromosomes at conception. Sexual reproduction allows the mixing of genomes from two different individuals to produce offspring that differ genetically from one another and from their parents. This source of genetic variability is advantageous to the species because it allows for adaptation and evolution in a changing environment.

For two germ cells (egg and sperm) to combine to form a cell with the normal complement of 46 chromosomes (23 pairs), each germ cell must contribute only half of the total. **Meiosis** refers to this special form of cell division, which results in germ cells that are **haploid;** they have half of the normal number of chromosomes. In contrast to mitosis (see Chapter 3), meiosis involves two divisions of the chromosomal DNA. A comparison of meiotic and mitotic cell division is shown in Figure 6-3.

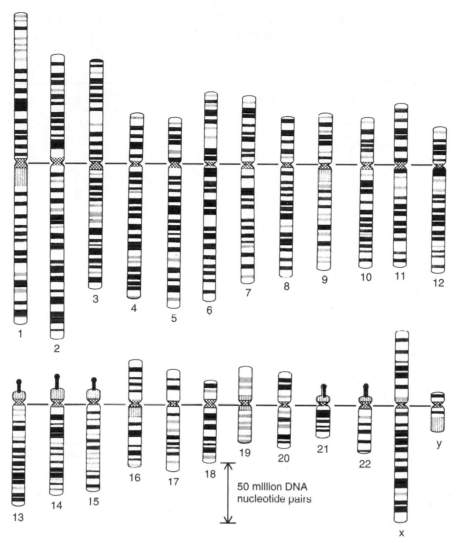

FIGURE 6-2 A standard map of the banding pattern of each of the 23 chromosomes of the human. Somatic cells contain two copies of each chromosome. The centromere region is marked by the line. (From Alberts B et al, editors: *Molecular biology of the cell,* ed 5, New York, 2008, Garland Science, p 203.)

During the first phase of meiosis, duplicated sister chromatids come in close contact with their homologous pairs. Portions of the homologous chromosomes are exchanged in a process called *crossing over* (Figure 6-4). This results in a mixing of the maternal and paternal genes of the cell to form a new combination of genes within the chromosomes. Genetic recombination is very precise, such that genes are exchanged intact and not interrupted in the middle. On average, each homologous pair of chromosomes has two or three crossover events occurring during the first meiotic division.[6] The first cellular division of meiosis results in two cells, each with 46 chromosomes. These two cells undergo a second division in which the sister chromatids are pulled apart (similar to normal mitosis), resulting in four cells, each having only 23 chromosomes. Each of the germ cells has a different combination of genes that, when passed on through sexual reproduction, will form a new, genetically unique individual.

The genes that code for a particular trait, such as eye color, are located at a particular position (locus) on the chromosome and come in several forms, or alleles. In the case of eye color, there are two common alleles, blue and brown. A person actually has two alleles for each gene, one received from each parent. If both alleles for a trait are identical, the individual is homozygous for that trait. If two different alleles are present, the individual is heterozygous for the trait. Using the eye color example again, if an individual receives a blue eye color allele from each parent, he or she is homozygous for eye color. If a blue eye color allele is received from one parent and a brown eye color allele is received from the other parent, the individual is heterozygous for that trait.

Some traits, like eye color, involve only one gene locus and are called single-gene traits. (Variations in shade may be determined by other genes.) The transmission of single-gene traits from parent to offspring follows predictable patterns that can be demonstrated using the Punnett square (Figure 6-5). In the Punnett square, the alleles for a gene are represented by capital and lowercase letters. The capital letter represents the **dominant** allele, and the lowercase letter is the **recessive** allele.

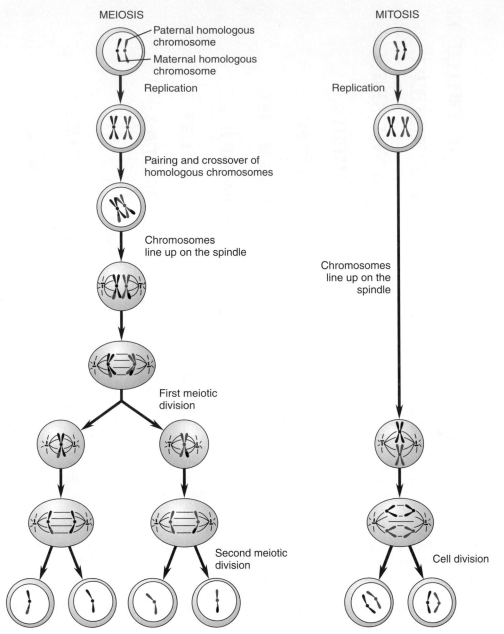

FIGURE 6-3 A comparison of meiosis and normal mitotic cell division, showing only one homologous chromosome pair. In meiosis, the homologous chromosomes form a pair and exchange sections of DNA in a process called *crossing over*. Two nuclear divisions are required in meiosis to form the haploid germ cells.

As the term implies, the trait of the dominant allele is apparent and will mask the recessive allele. A recessive trait is apparent only if *both* alleles for the trait are recessive (homozygous). Dominant genes often code for functional enzymes or structural proteins, and recessive genes code for nonfunctional ones. The Punnett square is based on the Mendelian principle that all genes are independent and will be inherited in a random manner. Thus, if both parents are heterozygous for a dominant trait (Aa), the offspring will have a 25% probability of being AA, a 50% probability of being Aa, and a 25% probability of being aa. Persons having the AA and Aa genotypes will *express* the trait in a similar manner. The trait will be absent in the aa genotype. Many genetic diseases are carried

in the recessive allele and are manifested only by the homozygous (aa) genotype (e.g. cystic fibrosis, phenylketonuria). Persons who are heterozygous for the disease (Aa) are said to be **carriers** because they are able to pass the defective recessive gene to their offspring even though they do not exhibit the trait.

Some alleles are not clearly dominant or recessive and result in a blending or *codominant* expression of the trait. Blood type, for example, has three distinct alleles: A, B, and O. The A and B alleles may both be expressed together, resulting in the AB blood type. Other traits result from the interaction of several gene loci and are called **polygenic** or multifactorial. Polygenic traits are heritable, but predicting their occurrence is more

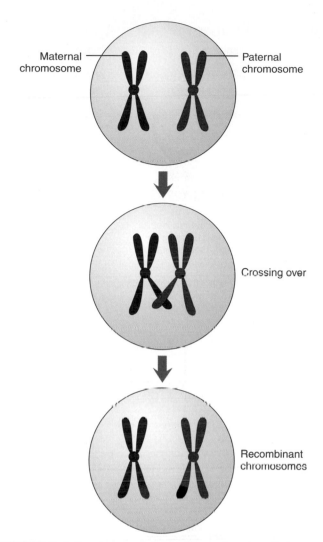

FIGURE 6-4 Crossing over during meiotic prophase I results in a reassortment of genes between homologous chromosomes.

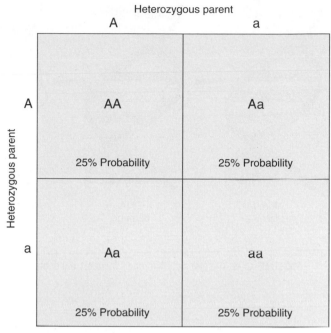

FIGURE 6-5 A Punnett square shows the distribution of parental genes to their offspring. This example shows the mating of two heterozygous individuals. *A*, Dominant genes; *a*, recessive genes.

difficult. Polygenic traits are often affected by environmental factors. As examples, height, weight, and blood pressure are polygenic traits; however, dietary intake certainly influences the ultimate expression of these genes.

DNA Mutation and Repair

The term **mutation** refers to a permanent change in DNA structure. Genetic mutation is a rare event despite the daily exposure of cells to numerous mutagenic influences. Radiation, chemicals, viruses, and even some products of normal cellular metabolism are all potential **mutagens.** In a typical cell, more than 5000 adenine and guanine DNA bases are lost and more than 100 cytosine bases are damaged each day owing to thermal disruption.[7] Many other types of DNA damage also occur, but only a few of these changes result in permanent alterations (mutations). The stability of the genes, and thus the low mutation rate, depends on efficient DNA repair mechanisms.

There are a variety of cellular DNA repair mechanisms. Most require the presence of a normal complementary DNA template to correctly repair the damaged strand of DNA. Single-stranded breaks or loss of bases from only one DNA strand are readily repaired. Double-stranded breaks, involving both strands of complementary DNA, may result in permanent loss of genetic information at the break point where the broken strands are reunited. Different types of DNA damage are detected and repaired by different enzyme systems. The steps in one type of DNA repair are shown in Figure 6-6.

Genetic mutations are generally of two types: a point mutation, which involves a single base pair substitution, or a frameshift mutation, which often changes the genetic code dramatically. A sequence of three DNA bases (codon) is required to code for each amino acid. A point mutation in the gene may cause the affected codon to signify an abnormal amino acid. The inclusion of the abnormal amino acid in the sequence of the protein may or may not be of clinical significance. Sickle cell anemia and α_1-antiprotease deficiency are examples of point mutation disorders in which a single amino acid substitution causes significant dysfunction. A frameshift mutation is due to the addition or removal of one or more bases, which changes the "reading frame" of the DNA sequence. The DNA sequence is normally "read" in groups of three bases, with no spaces between. All of the codon triplets will be changed in the DNA region downstream from the mutation, resulting in a protein with a greatly altered amino acid sequence (Figure 6-7). Numerous genetic disorders are due to mutations in the DNA that codes for a particular protein. These are termed *single-gene* or *Mendelian* disorders. Mutations may also alter chromosome structure through loss, gain, or translocation of chromosome segments. These processes are discussed later in the chapter.

| Normal DNA | DNA damage | Removal of damaged base pair (step 1) | DNA polymerase inserts new base pair using good strand as a template (step 2) | DNA ligase repairs nick (step 3) |

FIGURE 6-6 The steps of DNA repair. In step 1 the damaged section is removed; in steps 2 and 3 the original DNA sequence is restored.

FIGURE 6-7 Schematic illustration of mutations that alter the messenger RNA sequence and the resulting protein amino acid sequence. **A,** Point mutation alters one amino acid. **B,** Frameshift mutation alters all downstream amino acids.

KEY POINTS

- Human DNA is organized into 46 chromosomes (23 pairs). Paired chromosomes look similar under the microscope but differ in DNA sequence. One member of each pair is inherited from the mother, and the other from the father.
- Twenty-two pairs of chromosomes are autosomes. The remaining pair, the sex chromosomes, confers maleness (XY) or femaleness (XX).
- During meiotic cell division, the chromosomes are distributed to daughter cells. Meiosis results in four daughter cells, each having one-half the normal number of chromosomes (23).

- Genes that code for a particular trait come in several forms or alleles. Genotype refers to the particular set of alleles an individual receives. Phenotype refers to an individual's observable attributes. People with different genotypes may have similar phenotypes.
- Some traits involve only one gene locus and are called *single-gene traits.* The transmission of these traits from parent to offspring follows predictable patterns. The expression of single-gene traits is determined by whether the gene is dominant or recessive. Dominant genes usually code for functional enzymes; recessive genes do not. Traits resulting from the interaction of several genes are polygenic and do not follow predictable patterns of inheritance.

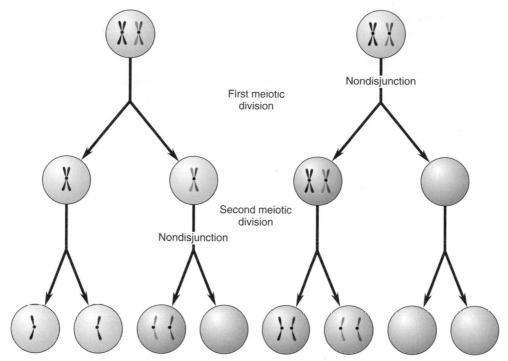

FIGURE 6-8 Mechanism of nondisjunction leading to aneuploidy. For simplicity, only one pair of chromosomes is shown.

Genetic Disorders

Genetic disorders may be apparent at birth or may not be clinically evident until much later in life. The great majority of genetic disorders are inherited from the affected individual's parents. However, 15% to 20% represent new mutations that arise during fetal development.[4] The genetic disorders encountered clinically are only a small percentage of those that occur, representing the less extreme aberrations that permit live birth. It has been estimated that about 50% of spontaneous first-trimester abortions have demonstrable chromosomal abnormalities, and many more may have hidden genetic defects.[4]

Disorders that are genetic in origin traditionally have been divided into three groups: (1) chromosomal aberrations, (2) Mendelian single-gene disorders, and (3) multifactorial or polygenic disorders. A fourth group encompasses a number of single-gene defects that do not follow the classic Mendelian patterns of inheritance. This group includes triplet-repeat mutations, mitochondrial gene mutations, and mutations influenced by genomic imprinting. General principles of transmission and selected examples are included for each of the four groups.

CHROMOSOMAL ABNORMALITIES

Chromosomal defects are generally due to an abnormal number of chromosomes or alterations in the structure of one or more chromosomes. These defects usually result from errors in the separation or crossing over of chromosomes during meiosis or mitosis. Approximately 1 in 200 newborn infants has some form of chromosomal abnormality.[3,4]

Aberrant Number of Chromosomes

The union of sperm and egg results in a fertilized egg (zygote) with the full complement of 46 chromosomes: 22 pairs of autosomes and 2 sex chromosomes (euploid). **Aneuploidy** refers to an abnormal number of chromosomes—in humans, either more or less than 46. The usual causes of aneuploidy are nondisjunction and anaphase lag.[8] **Nondisjunction** means that the paired homologous chromosomes fail to separate normally during either the first or second meiotic division (Figure 6-8). The resulting germ cells then have an abnormal number of chromosomes: one will have 22 chromosomes and one will have 24. When the chromosomes from the abnormal germ cell are combined with a normal germ cell containing 23 chromosomes, the fertilized cell will either be deficient by one chromosome (45) or have an extra chromosome (47). In anaphase lag, one chromosome lags behind and is therefore left out of the newly formed cell nucleus. This results in one daughter cell with the normal number of chromosomes and one with a deficiency of one chromosome, a condition called **monosomy. Polysomy** refers to the condition of having too many chromosomes.

The causes of abnormalities in chromosome number are poorly understood. Radiation, viruses, and chemicals have been implicated because they can interfere with mitosis and meiosis in experimental animals. Their role in causing aneuploidy in humans is unproved. Two conditions are known to increase the risk of abnormalities in chromosome number in humans: advanced maternal age and abnormalities in parental chromosome structure.[9] There is no precise explanation for the higher risk of nondisjunction with these conditions.

In general, monosomy involving the autosomes is not compatible with life. Autosomal polysomy may result in a viable fetus. The extra autosomal chromosomes are nearly always associated with severe disability (e.g., trisomy 21—Down syndrome). Disorders involving extra or missing sex chromosomes are more common and less debilitating.

Abnormal Chromosome Structure

Alterations in chromosome structure are usually due to breakage and loss or rearrangement of pieces of the chromosomes during meiosis or mitosis. During meiosis, the homologous chromosomes normally pair up and exchange genetic alleles in a process called *crossing over*. Normal crossing over involves precise gene exchange between homologues only, with no net gain or loss of DNA. When the normal process of crossing over goes awry, portions of chromosomes may be lost, attached upside down, or attached to the wrong chromosome. Mitosis also presents opportunities for chromosomal breakage and rearrangement. The severity of the chromosomal rearrangement ranges from insignificant to lethal, depending on the number and importance of the gene loci involved. Gene locations can be described by their location on the long arm (q arm) or the short arm (p arm) of the chromatid. For example, the gene locus 2p13 is located on the short arm of chromosome 2 at region 1, band 3 (Figure 6-9). The common types of chromosomal rearrangements are translocations, inversions, deletions, and duplications (Figure 6-10).

Chromosomal *translocations* result from the exchange of pieces of DNA between nonhomologous chromosomes. If no genetic material is lost, as in a reciprocal translocation, the individual may have no symptoms of the disorder. However, an individual with a reciprocal translocation is at increased risk of producing abnormal gametes. The exchange of a long chromatid arm for a short one results in the formation of one very large chromosome and one very small chromosome (see Figure 6-10). This is called a Robertsonian translocation and is responsible for a rare hereditary form of Down syndrome, discussed later in the chapter. Isochromosomes occur when the sister chromatids separate incorrectly at the centromere such that the two identical short arms remain together, as do the two long arms.

Inversion refers to the removal and upside-down reinsertion of a section of chromosome (see Figure 6-10). Like balanced translocations, inversions involve no net loss or gain of genetic material and are often without consequence to the individual. Difficulties result, however, when homologous chromosomes attempt to pair up during meiosis. The chromosome with an inverted section may not pair up properly, resulting in duplications or loss of genes at the time of crossing over. Thus, the offspring of an individual harboring an inversion may be affected.

Loss of chromosomal material is called *deletion*. Deletions result from a break in the arm of a single chromosome, resulting in a fragment of DNA with no centromere. The piece is then lost at the next cell division. Chromosomal deletions have been associated with some forms of cancer, including

FIGURE 6-9 Metaphase chromosome showing location of centromere and long and short arms of the chromatids. Gene loci are described by the chromosome number, location on short *(p)* or long *(q)* arm, region, and band.

retinoblastoma (see Chapter 7). Deletions at both ends of a chromatid may cause the free ends to attach to one another, forming a ring chromosome.

In contrast to a deletion, where genes are lost, *duplication* results in extra copies of a portion of DNA. The consequences of duplications are generally less severe than those from loss of genetic material.

Examples of Autosomal Chromosome Disorders

Trisomy 21 (Down Syndrome). Trisomy 21 is a chromosomal disorder in which individuals have an extra 21st chromosome. It is the most common of the chromosomal disorders and a leading cause of mental retardation, occurring in about 1 in 700 live births.[10] A lower incidence of about 1 in 1000 live births has been reported in many countries because of a trend toward prenatal diagnosis and termination of pregnancies.[10] The syndrome, first described by Langdon Down in 1866,[11] includes mental retardation, protruding tongue, low-set ears, epicanthal folds, poor muscle tone, and short stature (Figure 6-11). Children with Down syndrome often are afflicted with congenital heart deformities, such as atrial septal defect, and an increased susceptibility to respiratory infections and leukemia. A majority of fetuses known to have trisomy 21 are either stillborn or aborted.[10]

A rare form of Down syndrome (occurring in about 4% of cases) is due to a chromosomal translocation of the long arm of chromosome 21 to another chromosome. It is believed that inheritance occurs by passing of the chromosome from parent to offspring. In contrast, the cause of trisomy

FIGURE 6-10 Types of chromosomal rearrangement. (Adapted from Kumar V et al: *Robbins basic pathology,* ed 8, Philadelphia, 2007, Saunders, p 243.)

FIGURE 6-11 Typical clinical manifestations of trisomy 21 (Down syndrome).

TABLE 6-1

Frequency of Trisomy 21 (Down Syndrome) in Relation to Maternal Age

Age of Mother at Birth (year)	Frequency of Trisomy 21 at Birth
20	1/1470
25	1/1333
30	1/935
35	1/353
37	1/200
39	1/112
41	1/68
43	1/46
45	1/36
50	1/26

Data from Morris JK, et al: Comparison of models of maternal age-specific risk for Down syndrome live births, *Prenat Diagn* 23:252-258, 2003.

FIGURE 6-12 Typical clinical manifestations of Klinefelter syndrome. (From Moore KL, Persuad TVN: *The developing human: clinically oriented embryology,* ed 8, Philadelphia, 2007, Saunders, p 466.)

21 is not well understood, although it is clearly associated with advanced maternal age.[12] Table 6-1 demonstrates a rise in the incidence of Down syndrome from maternal age 20 to 50 years. The reason for increased susceptibility of the ovum to nondisjunction with age remains unknown. In 95% of cases, the extra chromosome 21 is thought to be of maternal origin.[4]

Trisomy 18 (Edwards Syndrome) and Trisomy 13 (Patau Syndrome). Trisomy of chromosomes 18 or 13 is much less common than trisomy 21 and more severe. Mental retardation is quite severe, and average life expectancy is only a few weeks beyond birth. Trisomies involving chromosomes 8, 9, and 22 also have been described but are extremely rare.

Cri du Chat Syndrome. Deletion of the short arm of chromosome 5 results in a syndrome characterized by severe mental retardation, round face, and congenital heart anomalies. The syndrome was so named because of the characteristic cry of the affected infant, which resembles a cat crying. Some children afflicted with this syndrome survive to adulthood, and they generally thrive better than those with the trisomies.

Examples of Sex Chromosome Disorders

Klinefelter Syndrome. The incidence of Klinefelter syndrome is about 1 in 500 to 1 in 1000 live births, making it one of the most common genetic diseases of the sex chromosomes.[13] Individuals with Klinefelter syndrome usually have an extra X chromosome (an XXY genotype). However, individuals with more than one extra X (XXXY and XXXXY) have also been described. The presence of the Y chromosome determines the sex of these individuals to be male; however, the extra X chromosomes result in abnormal sexual development and feminization. The condition is rarely diagnosed prior to puberty, when lack of secondary sex characteristics becomes apparent. Associated symptoms reflect a lack of testosterone and include testicular atrophy and infertility, tall stature with long arms and legs, feminine hair distribution, gynecomastia (breast enlargement), high-pitched voice, and impaired intelligence (Figure 6-12).[14] Testosterone therapy can achieve a dramatic reduction in the feminine characteristics associated with Klinefelter syndrome.

Turner Syndrome. Also known as monosomy X, Turner syndrome is associated with the presence of only one normal X chromosome and no Y chromosome. The absence of the Y chromosome results in a female phenotype; however, the ovaries fail to develop, and affected individuals are sterile. In some cases of Turner syndrome, the second X chromosome is not entirely missing but is structurally abnormal. In the great majority of cases, the missing or damaged X chromosome is of paternal origin and may be related to advanced age of the father. Only about 3% of infants with monosomy X survive to birth, and there is a high postnatal mortality rate as well. The incidence is about 1 in 3000 female births.[15] Principal characteristics of Turner syndrome include short stature, webbing of the neck, fibrous ovaries, sterility, amenorrhea, a wide chest, and congenital heart defects (Figure 6-13).

Multiple X Females and Double Y Males. A relatively common disorder of the sex chromosomes is the presence of an extra copy of the X chromosome in females (XXX) or of the Y chromosome in males (XYY). Most individuals appear normal; however, females may experience menstrual abnormalities, and males will generally be taller than average.

FIGURE 6-13 Typical clinical manifestations of Turner syndrome. (From Connor JM, Ferguson-Smith MA: *Essential medical genetics,* ed 5, London, 1997, Blackwell Scientific, p 123.)

A tendency toward mental retardation has been noted in females with more than four X chromosomes.

MENDELIAN SINGLE-GENE DISORDERS

In contrast to the chromosomal disorders described above, Mendelian disorders result from alterations or mutations of single genes. The affected genes may code for abnormal enzymes, structural proteins, or regulatory proteins. An individual has two variants or alleles of each gene (one allele from each parent). A recessive gene is expressed only when the individual is homozygous for the gene, that is, the individual has two identical copies. Dominant genes require only one allele in order to be expressed. Mendelian disorders are generally classified according to the *location* of the defective gene (autosomal or sex chromosome) and

the *mode of transmission* (dominant or recessive). The great majority of Mendelian disorders are familial (mutant genes inherited from the parents), but 10% to 15% represent new mutations. In many cases, the particular gene responsible for a Mendelian disease has not been identified. A detailed **pedigree** may be used to trace the transmission of the disease through the history of a family. The pedigree chart (Figure 6-14), showing family relationships and which members have been affected by the disease, is a useful tool in determining the pattern of inheritance as recessive, dominant, or sex linked. Mendelian genetics is based on the principle that single genes are randomly and independently transmitted to offspring such that there is a 50:50 chance of receiving one or the other of a parent's alleles for a particular gene. It is important to note that there are many exceptions to these rules, but they generally are useful in predicting transmission patterns for a number of single-gene disorders. Prevalence rates for several single-gene disorders are shown in Table 6-2. The number of known single-gene traits and disorders is nearly 17,000.[3] A comprehensive database of the chromosomal location and sequence of these single-gene traits and disorders, called *Online Mendelian Inheritance in Man,* can be accessed at http://www.ncbi.nlm.nih.gov/omim.

Autosomal Dominant Disorders

Autosomal dominant disorders are due to a mutation of a dominant gene located on one of the autosomes. Autosomal dominant disorders follow predictable patterns of inheritance (Figure 6-15), which may be summarized as follows:

- Males and females are equally affected.
- Affected individuals usually have an affected parent.
- Unaffected individuals do not transmit the disease.
- Offspring of an affected individual (with normal mate) have a 1 in 2 chance of inheriting the disease.
- The rare mating of two individuals, each carrying one copy of the defective gene (heterozygous), results in a 3 in 4 chance of producing an affected offspring.

The list of known autosomal dominant disorders is long. Many are described in later chapters as they relate to system pathophysiology. A partial list is presented in Table 6-3. In general, autosomal dominant disorders involve key structural proteins or regulatory proteins, such as membrane receptors. Marfan syndrome and Huntington disease are commonly cited examples of autosomal dominant disorders and are briefly described here.

Marfan Syndrome. Marfan syndrome is a disorder of the connective tissues of the body. Individuals with Marfan syndrome are typically tall and slender with long, thin arms and legs (Figure 6-16). Because of the long, thin fingers, this syndrome has also been called *arachnodactyly* ("spider fingers"). It is commonly suggested that President Abraham Lincoln may have had this disorder. Although skeletal and joint deformities are problematic, the cardiovascular lesions are the most life threatening. The medial layer of blood vessels, particularly the aorta, tends to be weak and susceptible to dilation and rupture. Dysfunction of the heart valves may occur from poor

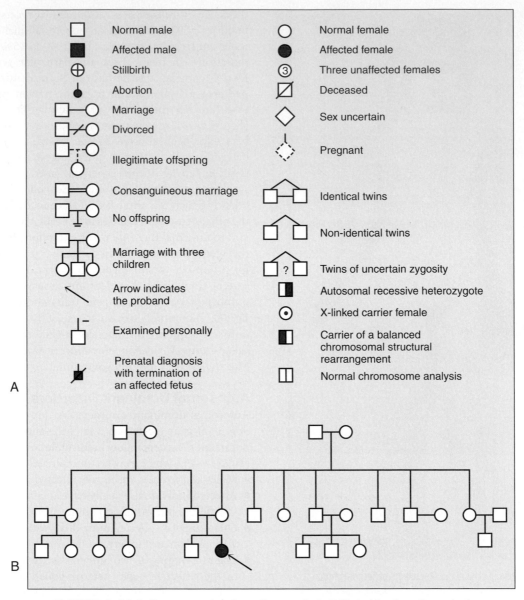

FIGURE 6-14 A, Common symbols for pedigree analysis. **B,** Typical family pedigree chart.

connective tissue support. Marfan syndrome has been traced to mutations in the fibrillin 1 gene on chromosome 15.[16] Fibrillin 1 is a glycoprotein secreted by fibroblasts into the extracellular matrix. It provides important scaffolding for deposition of other matrix proteins such as elastin. Marfan-type fibrillin 1 appears to be more susceptible to proteolytic degradation than normal fibrillin, leading to the weakened connective tissues typical of the disease.

Huntington Disease. Huntington disease is an autosomal dominant disease that primarily affects neurologic function. The symptoms of mental deterioration and involuntary movements of the arms and legs do not appear until approximately age 40 years. The disease was formerly called Huntington chorea (from the Greek *khoreia,* "dance") because of the uncontrolled movements of the limbs. The delayed onset

of symptoms means that the disease may be transmitted to offspring before the parent is aware that he or she harbors the defective gene. The prevalence rate is about 1 in 10,000 persons.

The gene abnormality in Huntington disease has been localized to chromosome 4, where an abnormally large number of triplet repeats (CAG) has been noted.[17,18] Triplet repeats of more than 39 are reliably associated with development of the disease, and the greater the number of triplet repeats, the earlier the onset of symptoms.[18] The Huntington disease protein (huntingtin) has a long segment of glutamine amino acids that are coded for by the CAG triplet repeat. The protein forms aggregates in brain tissue, which are thought to contribute to the pathogenesis of neurodegeneration.[19] Clinical manifestations and pathophysiology of Huntington disease are discussed in Chapter 45.

TABLE 6-2

Prevalence of Selected Single-Gene Disorders Among Liveborn Infants

Disorder	Estimated Prevalence
Autosomal Dominant	
Familial hypercholesterolemia	1 in 500
Polycystic kidney disease	1 in 1250
Huntington disease	1 in 2500
Hereditary spherocytosis	1 in 5000
Marfan syndrome	1 in 20,000
Autosomal Recessive	
Sickle cell anemia	1 in 625 (U.S. blacks)
Cystic fibrosis	1 in 2000 (Caucasians)
Tay-Sachs disease	1 in 3000 (U.S. Jews)
Phenylketonuria	1 in 12,000
Mucopolysaccharidoses (all types)	1 in 50,000
Galatosemia	1 in 57,000
X-Linked	
Duchenne muscular dystrophy	1 in 7000
Hemophilia	1 in 10,000

From Kumar V et al: *Robbins basic pathology,* ed 8, Philadelphia, 2007, Saunders, p 228.

TABLE 6-3

Autosomal Dominant Disorders

System	Disorder
Nervous	Huntington disease
	Neurofibromatosis
	Myotonic dystrophy
	Tuberous sclerosis
Urinary	Polycystic kidney disease
Gastrointestinal	Familial polyposis coli
Hematopoietic	Hereditary spherocytosis
	Von Willebrand disease
Skeletal	Marfan syndrome
	Ehlers-Danlos syndrome (some variants)
	Osteogenesis imperfecta
	Achondroplasia
Metabolic	Familial hypercholesterolemia
	Acute intermittent porphyria

From Kumar V et al: *Robbins basic pathology,* ed 8, Philadelphia, 2007, Saunders, p 228.

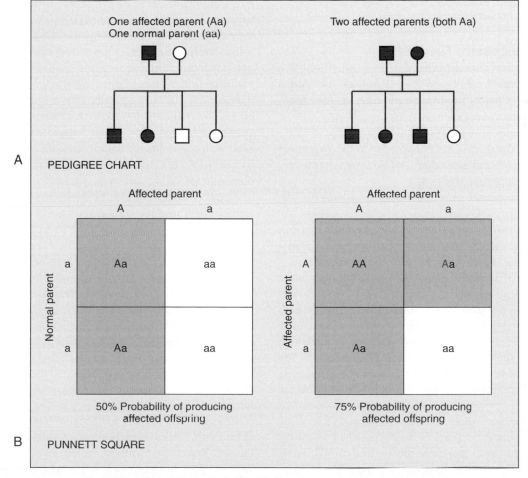

FIGURE 6-15 Typical pattern of inheritance of an autosomal dominant trait (e.g., Marfan syndrome). **A,** Pedigree chart. **B,** Punnett square.

FIGURE 6-16 Typical clinical manifestations of Marfan syndrome. Skeletal deformities such as pectus excavatum and abnormal curvature of the thoracic spine are common findings. (From Connor JM, Ferguson-Smith MA: *Essential medical genetics,* ed 5, London, 1997, Blackwell Scientific, p 142.)

Autosomal Recessive Disorders

Autosomal recessive disorders are due to a mutation of a recessive gene located on one of the autosomes. Autosomal recessive disorders follow predictable patterns of inheritance (Figure 6-17), which may be summarized as follows:

- Males and females are equally affected.
- In most cases, the disease is not apparent in the parents or relatives of the affected individual, but both parents are carriers of the mutant recessive gene.
- Unaffected individuals may transmit the disease to offspring.
- The mating of two carriers (heterozygous) results in a 1 in 4 chance of producing an affected offspring and a 2 in 4 chance of producing an offspring who carries the disease.

It is believed that nearly everyone carries one or more mutant recessive genes. Related individuals are more likely to carry the *same* recessive genes. Because recessive diseases are only expressed when both alleles for a particular gene are mutant (homozygous), they are often associated with **consanguinity**—the mating of related individuals.[1] The closer the biological relationship, the greater the proportion of shared genes and the greater the risk of producing affected offspring.

Recessive disorders often involve abnormal enzymatic functions. The gene for a particular enzyme may be absent or present in a mutant, and therefore nonfunctional, form. The enzyme deficiency usually is not apparent in heterozygotes carrying one normal gene and one mutant gene because the normal gene produces enough of the necessary enzyme. In the homozygous state, neither gene for the enzyme is functional, resulting in an enzyme deficiency. A partial list of the large number of autosomal recessive disorders that have been identified is given in Table 6-4. Many of these diseases involve inability to metabolize nutrients (inborn errors of metabolism) or to synthesize cellular components because of enzyme deficiencies. Albinism, phenylketonuria, and cystic fibrosis are described here as representative examples. Other disorders are described in the discussions of system pathophysiology in later chapters.

Albinism. Albinism refers to a lack of pigmentation of the hair, skin, and eyes. There are at least six different forms of oculocutaneous albinism, all of which are transmitted as autosomal recessive disorders. Some forms of albinism are associated with organ defects. The defect in one form of albinism has been traced to lack of the enzyme tyrosinase, which catalyzes the formation of dopa from tyrosine. Dopa is a precursor of the pigment melanin. Individuals with albinism are at risk for sunburn and skin cancer, and generally exhibit impaired vision and photosensitivity.[20]

Phenylketonuria. Phenylketonuria (PKU) results from an inability to metabolize the amino acid phenylalanine due to lack of the enzyme phenylalanine hydroxylase. It is one of several enzyme deficiencies that are often referred to as *inborn errors of metabolism.* The symptoms of the disorder are due to the buildup of dietary phenylalanine in the body, which primarily affects the nervous system. Children with PKU tend to be overly irritable and tremorous and have slowly developing mental retardation. Excess phenylalanine is excreted in the urine in the form of phenylketones; hence the name phenylketonuria. Infants typically have a musty odor because of excess phenylalanine by-products in the sweat and urine. The enzyme deficiency can be detected soon after birth and managed with a low-phenylalanine diet. Because treatment must be instituted very early to prevent mental retardation, routine screening for PKU is performed at birth.

Cystic Fibrosis. Cystic fibrosis is one of the most common single-gene disorders, with about 5% of Caucasian Americans harboring the defective gene.[4] The incidence of cystic fibrosis is approximately 1 in 3200 live births.[3] The clinical abnormalities associated with cystic fibrosis have been traced to a defect in a membrane transporter for chloride ions in epithelial cells. The alteration in chloride transport is associated with production of abnormally thick secretions in glandular tissues. The lung bronchioles and pancreatic ducts are primarily affected, often resulting in progressive destruction of these organs (see Chapter 22).

The cystic fibrosis gene was isolated in 1989 and mapped to chromosome 7. A number of different mutations of this gene have been identified, all of which cause a defect in chloride transport across the cell membrane, however the severity of chloride channel dysfunction varies widely with different mutations. The most common mutation, accounting for about 70% of cystic fibrosis cases, is due to a deletion of three nucleotides that normally code for a phenylalanine at position

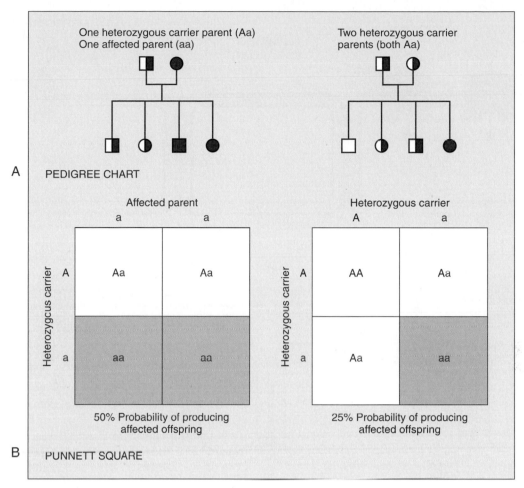

FIGURE 6-17 Typical pattern of inheritance of an autosomal recessive trait (e.g., cystic fibrosis, sickle cell anemia). **A,** Pedigree chart. **B,** Punnett square.

TABLE 6-4	
Autosomal Recessive Disorders	
System	**Disorder**
Metabolic	Cystic fibrosis
	Phenylketonuria
	Galactosemia
	Homocystinuria
	Lysosomal storage disease
	α_1-Antitrypsin deficiency
	Wilson disease
	Hemochromatosis
	Glycogen storage diseases
Hematopoietic	Sickle cell anemia
	Thalassemias
Endocrine	Congenital adrenal hyperplasia
Skeletal	Ehlers-Danlos syndrome (some variants)
	Alkaptonuria
Nervous atrophies	Neurogenic muscular
	Friedreich ataxia
	Spinal muscular atrophy

From Kumar V et al: *Robbins basic pathology,* ed 8, Philadelphia, 2007, Saunders, p 229.

508.[21] The absence of this single amino acid apparently causes the protein to fold abnormally, preventing its release from the endoplasmic reticulum, where it is eventually degraded. A schematic of the normal chloride transporter (called *cystic fibrosis transmembrane conductance regulator protein,* CFTR) is shown in Figure 6-18. This transporter belongs to the family of ABC transporters that bind and hydrolyze ATP (see Chapter 3).

The discovery and characterization of the cystic fibrosis gene and CFTR protein have made it possible to envision effective gene therapy for this disorder. Clinical trials have been published, however efficiency for delivering genes to target cells has been low.[22] Reliable genetic screening for the common forms of cystic fibrosis is readily available, making prevention and early management possible.

Sex-Linked (X-Linked) Disorders

Sex-linked disorders are due to a mutation of the sex chromosomes. Disorders linked to the Y chromosome are extremely rare, and for that reason the terms *sex-linked* and *X-linked* are often used interchangeably. Nearly all X-linked disorders are recessive. Females express the X-linked disease only in the rare

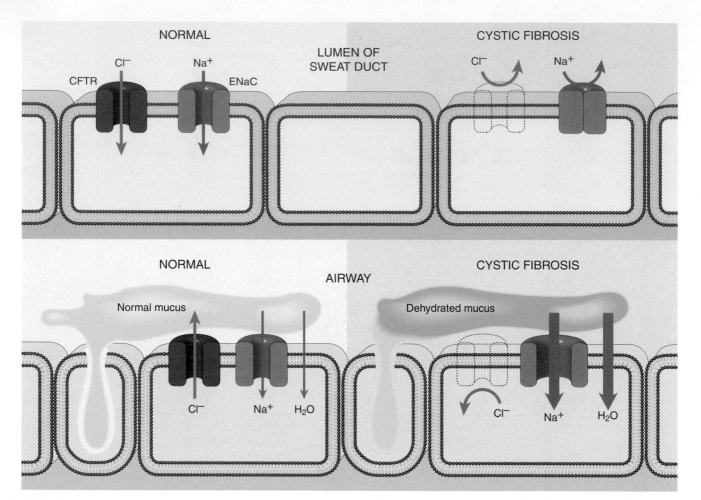

FIGURE 6-18 Schematic illustration of the cystic fibrosis transmembrane conductance regulator *(CFTR)* located in an epithelial cell. CFTR is a transmembrane protein that transports chloride from the cytoplasm into the lumen of the bronchiole. Mutations in the CFTR transporter gene are believed to cause the thick secretions typical of cystic fibrosis. (From Kumar V et al: *Robbins basic pathology,* ed 8, Philadelphia, 2007, Saunders, p 265.)

instance in which both X chromosomes carry the defective gene. Males, however, do not have the safety margin of two X chromosomes and express the disease if their one and only X chromosome is abnormal. X-linked disorders follow predictable patterns of inheritance (Figure 6-19), which are dependent on the sex of the offspring, and may be summarized as follows:

- Affected individuals are almost always male.
- Affected fathers transmit the defective gene to none of their sons but to all of their daughters.
- Unaffected males do not carry the defective gene.
- A carrier female has a 1 in 2 chance of producing an affected son and a 1 in 2 chance of producing a carrier daughter.
- Females are affected only in the rare homozygous state that may occur from the mating of an affected or carrier mother and an affected father.

Several X-linked recessive disorders have been identified, as presented in Table 6-5. A well-known example of an X-linked disease is hemophilia A.

Hemophilia A. Hemophilia A is a bleeding disorder associated with a deficiency of factor VIII, a protein necessary for blood clotting. Individuals afflicted with hemophilia A bleed easily and profusely from seemingly minor injuries (see Chapter 14). The transmission of hemophilia A in the European royal families constitutes one of the best-known pedigrees available (Figure 6-20). Queen Victoria of England was the first known carrier of the disease. A number of her male descendants were affected by it.

NONMENDELIAN SINGLE-GENE DISORDERS

Transmission of certain single-gene disorders does not follow the classic Mendelian principles of random and independent assortment. Three such categories have been described: (1) disorders caused by long triplet repeat mutations, such as fragile X syndrome; (2) disorders due to mitochondrial DNA mutations; and (3) disorders associated with genomic imprinting.

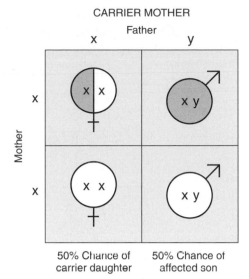

FIGURE 6-19 Typical inheritance pattern for X-linked disorders. The risk of disease varies according to the gender of the offspring.

TABLE 6-5	
X-Linked Recessive Disorders	
System	**Disorder**
Musculoskeletal	Duchenne muscular dystrophy
Blood	Hemophilias A and B
	Chronic granulomatous disease
	Glucose-6-phosphate dehydrogenase deficiency
Immune	Agammaglobulinemia X-linked severe combined immunodeficiency (SCID)
	Wiskott-Aldrich syndrome
Metabolic	Diabetes insipidus
	Lesch-Nyhan syndrome
Nervous	Fragile X syndrome

From Kumar V et al: *Robbins basic pathology*, ed 8, Philadelphia, 2007, Saunders, p 230.

Triplet Repeat Mutations

Fragile X syndrome is a prototypical example of disorders characterized by long repeating sequences of three nucleotides, called *triplet repeat mutations*. Fragile X syndrome is the most common cause of familial mental retardation, exhibiting a prevalence rate of about 1 in 4000.[23] A typical constriction on the long arm of the X chromosome can be detected on cytogenic studies. The area is composed of long repeating triplets of the sequence CGG. Normal individuals have an average of 29 CGG triplet repeats at this gene locus. Persons with fragile X syndrome have significantly more: 200 to 4000 triplet repeats. Persons who have an intermediate number of repeats (52 to 200) are said to have a *pre*mutation and are at significant risk for producing affected offspring, although they themselves are unaffected.[3]

The premutation is unstable and predisposed to amplification during oogenesis, but not spermatogenesis. As the premutation is passed on through the female lineage, the number of triplet repeats tends to increase as does the risk of mental retardation in the offspring. As might be guessed, the transmission patterns of this disorder are quite unusual. Males with fragile X syndrome tend to be more severely affected, apparently because the presence of a second X chromosome in females moderates the clinical symptoms. The protein normally produced by the fragile X gene *(FMR1)* is a ribosome-associated protein.[23] It is found in the dendrite area of neurons and may be involved in regulating synthesis of neuronal proteins.

Mitochondrial Gene Mutations

Nearly all cellular genes are located in the cell nucleus; however, several mitochondrial genes are passed on to daughter cells within the mitochondria when a cell divides. Essentially all mitochondria are contributed to a zygote by the egg, and therefore mitochondrial genes are of maternal origin because sperm contain few if any mitochondria.[4] Mothers transmit mitochondrial DNA to both sons and daughters, but only daughters transmit the mitochondrial genes to their offspring. Mitochondrial DNA codes for enzymes involved in oxidative phosphorylation reactions, and mutations tend to cause dysfunction in tissues with high utilization of ATP such as nerve, muscle, kidney, and liver. Mitochondrial gene disorders exhibit tricky inheritance patterns and are very rare.

Genomic Imprinting

The concept of genomic imprinting challenges the long-held belief that the parental origin of a gene does not matter to the cells that inherit them. Genomic imprinting is a process whereby maternal and paternal chromosomes are marked

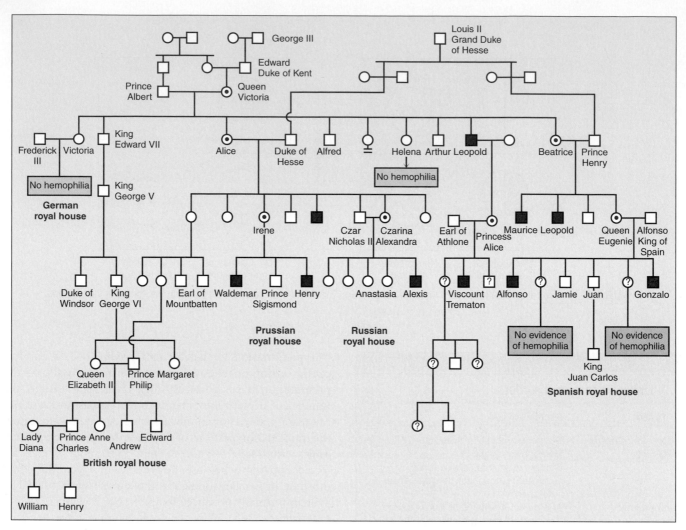

FIGURE 6-20 Pedigree chart for the transmission of the X-linked disease hemophilia A in the royal families of Europe.

differentially within the cell (by methylation of DNA for example). Genomic imprinting can be illustrated by considering two very different syndromes, which at first glance appeared to be a result of the same chromosomal defect. Prader-Willi syndrome and Angelman syndrome both result from a deletion at the same location on chromosome 15.[4] Prader-Willi syndrome is characterized by mental retardation, short stature, obesity, poor muscle tone, and hypogonadism. Patients with Angelman syndrome are also mentally retarded, but they have ataxia and tend to laugh inappropriately. The fact that two different syndromes resulted from the same mutation was puzzling until it was discovered that the Prader-Willi mutation is always on the paternally derived chromosome 15, whereas the Angelman syndrome mutation is always on the maternally derived chromosome 15. Two genes are normally present in the region, the "Angelman gene" is normally active on a maternal chromosome and silent (imprinted) on the paternal chromosome, whereas the "Prader-Willi" gene is normally active on only the paternal chromosome and silent on the maternal chromosome.

Thus normal cells have only one functional copy of each gene. The disorders arise when there is a deletion mutation of chromosome 15. A different syndrome arises if the area on a maternal chromosome is deleted compared to the paternal one (Figure 6-21). These findings imply that the cell is not blind to the parental origin of chromosomes and that homologous chromosomes may be marked and function differently within the cell.

MULTIFACTORIAL (POLYGENIC) DISORDERS

Differences in traits between identical twins indicated to early researchers that environmental influence has a role in gene expression. Many traits, such as blood pressure, have a "bell curve" distribution in the population and are known to be influenced by environmental factors such as dietary intake. These traits and disorders are called *multifactorial* or *polygenic*. Multifactorial traits do not follow clear-cut modes of inheritance but do tend to "run in families." Characteristics that are

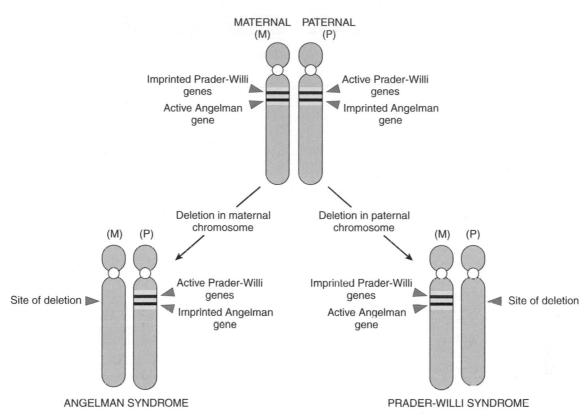

MATERNAL   PATERNAL
(M)   (P)

Imprinted Prader-Willi genes

Active Angelman gene

Active Prader-Willi genes

Imprinted Angelman gene

Deletion in maternal chromosome

Deletion in paternal chromosome

(M)   (P)

Site of deletion

Active Prader-Willi genes

Imprinted Angelman gene

(M)   (P)

Imprinted Prader-Willi genes

Active Angelman gene

Site of deletion

ANGELMAN SYNDROME

PRADER-WILLI SYNDROME

FIGURE 6-21 Angelman and Prader-Willi syndromes are examples of genetic imprinting, where the location of a mutation on the maternal or paternal homologous chromosome produces a different outcome. (From Kumar V et al: *Robbins basic pathology,* ed 8, Philadelphia, 2007, Saunders, p 251.)

governed by multifactorial inheritance tend to have a range of expression in the population and are thought to be produced by the interaction of several genes, each contributing a small additive effect. For example, height, weight, and intelligence are multifactorial. Most multifactorial disorders also present a range of severity, although a few disorders are either present or absent. In the latter case, it may be that a certain threshold number of defective genes must be inherited before the disease is expressed.[4]

It is extremely difficult to predict the risk of occurrence of multifactorial disorders based on family history. The risk of recurrence of a typical multifactorial disorder is in the range of 2% to 7%.[4] Thus, the parents of one affected child have a 2% to 7% chance of bearing a second affected child. The risk rises to about 9% after the birth of a second affected child. The number of genes contributing to the disorder, the degree to which the disease is expressed, and environmental influences (most of which may be undetermined) all affect the true risk of recurrence.

In contrast to single-gene and chromosomal abnormalities, which are rare, multifactorial disorders are very common. High blood pressure, cancer, diabetes mellitus, cleft lip, and several forms of congenital heart defects are governed by multifactorial inheritance. This list is destined to grow as knowledge of the role of genetic mechanisms in cellular function and disease expands.

KEY POINTS

- Genetic disorders are of three general types: chromosomal aberrations, single-gene disorders, and polygenic disorders.
- Chromosome disorders result from an abnormality in number or structure. The presence of only one chromosome of a homologous pair is termed *monosomy* (e.g., Turner syndrome), and the presence of an excessive number of chromosomes is called *polysomy* (e.g., Down syndrome). Abnormal rearrangement of portions of the chromosomes (translocation, inversion, deletion, duplication) can result in loss or unusual expression of genes.
- Single-gene disorders result from mutations that alter the nucleotide sequence of one particular gene. Mendelian disorders are transmitted predictably and include autosomal dominant (e.g., Huntington disease), autosomal recessive (e.g., cystic fibrosis), and sex-linked (e.g., hemophilia) disorders.
- Some single-gene disorders have unusual transmission patterns, which violate Mendel's laws. These include triplet repeat mutations, mitochondrial DNA mutations, and genomic imprinting disorders.
- Multifactorial disorders are very common and result from the interaction of multiple genes. Disorders such as high blood pressure, cancer, and diabetes are polygenic.

ENVIRONMENTALLY INDUCED CONGENITAL DISORDERS

Adverse influences during intrauterine life are a significant cause of errors in fetal development that result in congenital malformations. The study of developmental anomalies is called *teratology* (from the Greek *teras,* or "monster"). Most malformations are associated with genetic causes; however, numerous environmental influences that may adversely affect the developing fetus, such as chemicals, radiation, and viral infections, have been identified (Table 6-6). Factors that cause congenital malformation are called **teratogens.** Many substances are thought to have teratogenic potential, based on experiments in animals, but few are proved in humans. Exposure to a known teratogen may, but need not, result in a congenital malformation. Susceptibility to a teratogen depends on the amount of exposure, the developmental stage of the fetus when exposed, the prior condition of the mother, and the genetic predisposition of the fetus.[4]

Periods of Fetal Vulnerability

The timing of the exposure to a teratogen greatly influences fetal susceptibility and the resulting type of malformation. The intrauterine development of humans can be divided into two stages: (1) the embryonic period, which

TABLE 6-6

Causes of Congenital Malformations in Humans

Cause	Malformed Live Births (%)
Genetic	
Chromosomal aberrations	10-15
Mendelian inheritance	2-10
Environmental	
Maternal/placental infections (e.g., rubella, toxoplasmosis, syphilis, cytomegalovirus infection, human immunodeficiency virus infection)	2-3
Maternal disease states (e.g., diabetes, phenylketonuria, endocrinopathies)	6-8
Drugs and chemicals (e.g., alcohol, folic acid antagonists, phenytoin, thalidomide, warfarin 13-cis-Retinoic acid)	~1
Irradiation	~1
Multifactorial	20-25
Unknown	40-60

Adapted from Stevenson RE et al, editors: *Human malformations and related anomalies,* New York, 1993, Oxford University Press, p 115. In Kumar V et al: *Robbins basic pathology,* ed 8, Philadelphia, 2007, Saunders, p 255.

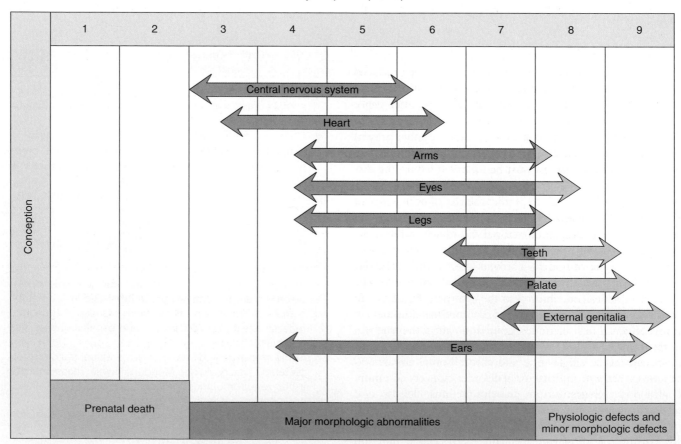

FIGURE 6-22 The vulnerable periods of fetal organ development.

extends from conception to 9 weeks of development, is followed by (2) the fetal period, which continues until birth. Prior to the third week of gestation, exposure to a teratogen generally either damages so few cells that the embryo develops normally, or damages so many cells that the embryo cannot survive and spontaneous abortion occurs. Between the third and ninth week of gestation the embryo is very vulnerable to teratogenesis, with the fourth and fifth weeks being the time of peak susceptibility.[4] Organ development (organogenesis) occurs during this period and is very sensitive to injury, regardless of the cause. Each organ has a critical period during which it is most vulnerable to malformation (Figure 6-22). Unfortunately, an embryo may be exposed to teratogens during the vulnerable period because the mother does not yet realize she is pregnant. The fetal period, from 3 to 9 months, is primarily concerned with further growth and maturation of the organs, and susceptibility to errors of morphogenesis is significantly less. Fetal insults occurring after the third month are more likely to result in growth retardation or injury to normally formed organs.

Teratogenic Agents

The teratogenic potential of many agents is unknown. Several chemicals, some infections, and large doses of radiation are definitely associated with a higher risk of congenital disorders. In general, teratogens cause errors in morphogenesis by interfering with cell proliferation, migration, or differentiation. The specific mechanisms of action of most teratogens are unknown.

Chemicals and Drugs

The list of proven teratogenic chemicals and drugs includes thalidomide, alcohol, anticonvulsants, warfarin, folate antagonists, androgenic hormones, angiotensin-converting enzyme inhibitors, and organic mercury. Almost no drugs or chemicals are considered to be totally safe, and the current trend is to discourage pregnant women from using *any* drugs or chemicals. A classification system for determining relative risk of medications in pregnancy has been developed (Table 6-7). Two agents, thalidomide and alcohol, illustrate the teratogenic potential of chemicals.

In the 1960s, a jump in the incidence of congenital limb deformities was traced to maternal use of thalidomide, a tranquilizer, between the 28th and 50th day of pregnancy.[2] Exposure during the vulnerable period was associated with a very high risk (50% to 80%) of fetal malformation. Typically, the arms were short and flipperlike, although deformities ranged from mild abnormalities of the digits to complete absence of the limbs. Damage to other structures, particularly the ears and heart, also occurred. Thalidomide is one of the most potent teratogens known.

The chronic ingestion of large amounts of alcohol is known to cause a group of congenital anomalies referred to as *fetal alcohol syndrome* (FAS). It is estimated that between 0.5 and 2.0 of every 1000 newborns suffer from alcohol-induced anomalies.[24] The incidence in the United States is greater than

TABLE 6-7

Pregnancy Categories for Medication Administration

CATEGORY	INTERPRETATION
A	Adequate, well-controlled studies in pregnant women have not shown an increased risk of fetal abnormalities to the fetus in any trimester of pregnancy.
B	Animal studies have revealed no evidence of harm to the fetus, however, there are no adequate and well-controlled studies in pregnant women. **OR** Animal studies have shown an adverse effect, but adequate and well-controlled studies in pregnant women have failed to demonstrate a risk to the fetus in any trimester.
C	Animal studies have shown an adverse effect, and there are no adequate and well-controlled studies in pregnant women. **OR** No animal studies have been conducted, and there are no adequate and well-controlled studies in pregnant women.
D	Adequate well-controlled or observational studies in pregnant women have demonstrated a risk to the fetus. However, the benefits of therapy may outweigh the potential risk. For example, the drug may be acceptable if needed in a life-threatening situation or serious disease for which safer drugs cannot be used or are ineffective.
X	Adequate well-controlled or observational studies in animals or pregnant women have demonstrated positive evidence of fetal abnormalities or risks. The use of the product is contraindicated in women who are or may become pregnant.

in Europe and is highly associated with low socioeconomic status. Affected infants suffer from growth retardation, neurologic disorders, malformations of the head and face, and atrial septal heart defects. Data are insufficient to determine what, if any, level of alcohol intake during pregnancy is safe. It is clear that factors other than the absolute amount of alcohol intake during pregnancy are important in determining risk of FAS. Low socioeconomic status may be a permissive factor, allowing the teratogenic effects of alcohol to affect the fetus to a greater extent.[25] The mechanisms of alcohol teratogenesis include maternal-fetal hypoxia and excessive free radical production. Alcohol causes acute and transient collapse of the umbilical cord, which could damage the fetus by interrupting its oxygen supply. Complete abstinence from alcohol during pregnancy is generally recommended.

Infectious Agents

A number of perinatal infections have been implicated in the development of congenital malformations.[2] Certain viral infections appear to carry the greatest threat, although

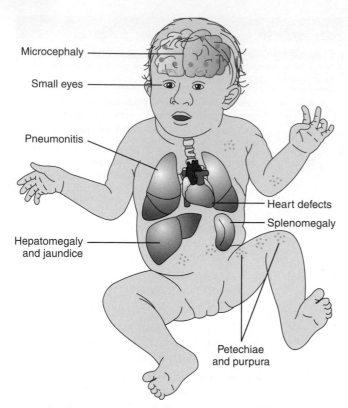

Microcephaly

Small eyes

Pneumonitis

Hepatomegaly
and jaundice

Heart defects

Splenomegaly

Petechiae
and purpura

FIGURE 6-23 Major clinical findings in the TORCH (toxoplasmosis, others, rubella, cytomegalovirus, herpes) complex of infective congenital disorders.

protozoa and bacteria have also been implicated. As with other teratogens, the gestational age of the fetus at the time of infection is critically important. Perhaps the best known viral teratogen is rubella. The risk period for rubella infection begins just prior to conception and extends to 20 weeks gestation, after which the virus rarely crosses the placenta. Rubella-induced defects vary but typically include cataracts, deafness, and heart defects. Several other organisms cause a similar constellation of congenital defects, so the acronym **TORCH** was developed to alert clinicians to the potential teratogenicity of these infections. TORCH stands for toxoplasmosis, others, rubella, cytomegalovirus, herpes.[4] The major features of the TORCH complex are shown in Figure 6-23. The category of "others" includes several less frequently seen causes: hepatitis B, coxsackievirus B, mumps, poliovirus, and others. All microorganisms of the TORCH complex are able to cross the placenta and infect the fetus.

Toxoplasmosis is a protozoal infection that can be contracted from ingestion of raw or undercooked meat and from contact with cat feces. Cytomegalovirus and herpes simplex virus are generally transmitted to the fetus by chronic carrier mothers. Cytomegalovirus and herpes simplex virus often colonize the genital area of the mother. Infants who escape infection in utero may still acquire the virus as they pass through the birth canal (see Chapter 34).

Radiation

In addition to being mutagenic, radiation is also teratogenic. The teratogenic potential of radiation became apparent from the increased incidence of congenital malformations in children born to women who underwent irradiation of the cervix for cancer and in the children of atomic bomb victims in World War II. It is not known if lower levels of radiation, such as those used in diagnostic x-rays, are teratogenic. It is generally recommended that pregnant women avoid diagnostic x-rays or use appropriate lead shielding.

Other Disorders of Infancy

An infant may be afflicted with a variety of problems at birth that do not fall into the category of genetic or developmental malformations. These problems generally arise later in uterine life and often involve mechanical factors or problems with the health of the mother and placenta. For example, babies with low birth weight or immaturity at birth may have difficulty breathing and taking in adequate nutrition. Interruption of the placental oxygen supply due to maternal hemorrhage, sedation, or blood incompatibility may result in fetal brain injury. A difficult labor and delivery may result in a variety of injuries during the birth process. The details of these disorders of infancy and childhood may be found in specialized texts.

KEY POINTS

- Environmental factors that adversely affect the developing fetus are called teratogens. Exposure to teratogens is particularly dangerous during the third to ninth weeks of gestation.
- Known teratogens include chemicals and drugs, infections, and radiation. The teratogenic potential of many chemicals and drugs is unknown, so pregnant women are usually advised to avoid all drugs if possible.
- Of the infectious agents, viruses are the most teratogenic, particularly organisms of the TORCH variety (toxoplasmosis, others, rubella, cytomegalovirus, herpesvirus).

DIAGNOSIS, COUNSELING, AND GENE THERAPY

In recent years, the ability to diagnose and manage genetic and developmental disorders has improved dramatically. Although pedigree analysis continues to be an important method for identifying at-risk individuals, for a number of disorders it is now possible to determine if parents carry defective genes or if a particular fetus is afflicted. Currently, the ability to detect genetic mutations far exceeds the ability to offer definitive genetic treatment, giving rise to many ethical concerns. Unfortunately, many individuals at risk for transmitting recessive genetic diseases are not identified until the birth of an afflicted child. Genetic counseling and prenatal assessment then become extremely important in assisting the family in regard to future pregnancies.

Prenatal Diagnosis and Counseling

A number of conditions are associated with a higher risk of congenital anomalies and are indications for instituting counseling and prenatal diagnostic examination. These conditions include (1) maternal age of 35 years or greater; (2) having borne a child with a chromosomal disorder (such as trisomy 21); (3) having a known family history of X-linked disorders; (4) having a family history of inborn errors of metabolism; (5) the occurrence of neural tube anomalies in a previous pregnancy; and (6) being a known carrier of a recessive genetic disorder. As diagnostic methods become more cost effective, general screening for other risk factors may be undertaken. Samples for prenatal testing of the fetus are usually obtained by amniocentesis, chorionic villus biopsy, or umbilical cord blood. Postnatal genetic analysis is usually done on peripheral blood samples of lymphocytes.

Ultrasound and amniocentesis are mainstays of prenatal diagnostic examination. **Ultrasound** is a noninvasive procedure that uses sound waves to produce a reflected image of the fetus. It is commonly used to determine gestational age, fetal position, and placental location. Ultrasound is also useful in detecting visible congenital anomalies such as spina bifida (neural tube defect); heart defects; and malformations of the face, head, body, and limbs.

Amniocentesis may be performed to determine genetic and developmental disorders not detectable by ultrasound. During amniocentesis, a needle is inserted through the abdomen or vagina and into the uterus. A sample of amniotic fluid containing skin cells shed by the fetus is removed for analysis. The amniotic fluid can be analyzed for abnormal levels of certain substances secreted by the fetus, such as α-fetoprotein, which may indicate neural tube defects. The live skin cells can be cultured and subjected to biochemical and chromosomal analysis. Only certain genetic and developmental disorders can be reliably detected by these procedures, and they may not provide the needed information until relatively late in the pregnancy. Amniocentesis cannot generally be performed prior to the 16th week of gestation. **Chorionic villus sampling** involves the removal of a bit of tissue directly from the chorion (the outer membrane of the fetal sac). It can be performed at 8 weeks gestation. Cells obtained from the fetus can be used to obtain small amounts of DNA that can then be amplified into a larger quantity by a process called polymerase chain reaction (PCR). This DNA can then be analyzed by a variety of methods to determine the genetic sequence, presence or absence of particular genes, or mutations. A genome can be scanned for particular genes by exposing the processed DNA to microchips that are coated with thousands of genetic sequence probes in specific locations. Complementary base pairing between the probes fixed on the microchip and the DNA being tested is used to detect the presence of particular gene sequences.

Embryoscopy allows direct visualization of the embryo as early as the first trimester of pregnancy. The scope is inserted through the cervix and into the uterus. Embryoscopy can be used to identify developmental progress and to diagnose structural anomalies. An exciting application of this technique is the potential to directly manage genetic disorders with targeted gene or stem cell therapy. The early diagnosis of congenital disorders allows a greater number of treatment options. Some disorders can be managed in utero; others may require early delivery, immediate surgery, or cesarean section to minimize fetal trauma. Early warning of fetal difficulties allows parents time to prepare emotionally for the birth of the child. In some instances, termination of the pregnancy may be the treatment of choice.

Genetic Analysis and Therapy

An exciting outcome of the human genome project is the potential for gene therapy—the treatment of genetic disease by replacing the defective gene with a normal, healthy one. This idea once sounded like science fiction, but clinical trials are under way to manage a number of genetic disorders.[76] The first federally approved gene therapy procedure was performed in 1990 to treat a child who suffered from a rare condition called *severe combined immunodeficiency* (SCID) by introducing a functional gene for the enzyme adenosine deaminase. In the past, children who suffered from SCID had severely compromised immune systems and generally died from overwhelming infections unless their environment was strictly controlled. Use of gene therapy has been successful in improving immune function and allowing these children to live in the outside world.

Gene therapy has the potential for alleviating human suffering by curing genetic diseases, but it is accompanied by a number of moral and ethical dilemmas. Tampering with the human gene pool could have serious implications for human evolution. There is also the potential for using the technology to create "new and improved" human beings or human clones.

Recombinant DNA Technology

Over the past 30 years, DNA has gone from being the hardest cellular molecule to study to being the easiest. The great advances in molecular genetics during this time are due to the development of recombinant DNA technologies. It is now possible to select a specific region of DNA, produce unlimited copies of it, determine its nucleotide sequence, use it to make unlimited quantities of a desired protein, or alter its DNA sequence at will (genetic engineering) and reinsert it into a living cell. These tools provide the means to uncover the nucleotide sequence of the entire human genome, to create DNA probes to explore an individual's genetic makeup for specific mutations, to mass produce therapeutic proteins and vaccines, and to cure genetic disorders by replacing mutant cellular genes with normally functioning ones.

Recombinant DNA technology comprises a number of techniques, the most important of which are briefly described here.

- The long, difficult-to-handle DNA strands are more easily studied if cut into smaller pieces. This is accomplished by restriction enzymes that cleave DNA at specific sites. The resulting pieces then can be separated by electrophoresis

FIGURE 6-24 Fluorescence in situ hybridization assay showing an interphase nucleus from a male patient with suspected trisomy 18. Three different fluorescent probes have been used: The red probe hybridized to the Y chromosome, the green probe hybridized to the X chromosome, and the blue probe hybridized to the centromere of chromosome 18. Three copies of chromosome 18 are identified, confirming the diagnosis. (From Kumar V et al: *Robbins basic pathology,* ed 8, Philadelphia, 2007, Saunders, p. 274. Photograph courtesy Dr. Nancy R. Schneider and Jeff Doolittle, University of Texas Southwestern Medical Center, Dallas.)

according to their size. A section of DNA can be collected and efficiently sequenced by automated means.

- Nucleic acid hybridization techniques take advantage of the natural tendency for DNA and RNA to find and bind to a complementary nucleotide sequence. A labeled piece of DNA or RNA can therefore be used to search for or "probe" for its complementary sequence among the many millions of sequences in a cell or cell extract. For example, in a fluorescence in situ hybridization assay, a probe for a specific site on a chromosome is attached to a fluorescent label and incubated with a cell. The fluorescence then identifies the location and number of copies of the particular chromosome sequence (Figure 6-24). Without the hybridization technique, finding a desired gene among the 10^9 base pairs in the human genome could take many years of intense effort, like finding the proverbial needle in a haystack. Hybridization is also the method behind the "gene chip assay" technology. As an outcome of the human genome project, the DNA sequence for the thousands of human genes and common mutations have been identified. Specific DNA sequence probes for these genes can be synthesized and attached to a fixed position on a plate (microchip). The DNA of interest can then be exposed to the chip, and the probes will preferentially bind to DNA segments having complementary bases. The position of the probe and the degree of DNA binding can then be analyzed by computer to produce a specific genetic analysis of gene mutations.

- DNA cloning is the technique used to produce many identical copies of a DNA sequence containing a gene of interest. The availability of large quantities of a purified gene sequence makes study and gene manipulation possible. A number of different techniques can be used to clone DNA. The polymerase chain reaction (PCR) technique is very efficient if the DNA sequence is already partially known. Basically, the DNA sequence of interest is mixed with special DNA polymerases that use the DNA sequence as a template to produce double-stranded DNA. Each DNA thus produced can in turn act as a template for production of another DNA. Large quantities can be produced very rapidly by PCR. The DNA can also be cloned by inserting it into bacteria by use of a viral or plasmid vector. Bacteria that take up the desired gene are identified by hybridization with a labeled probe. The desired bacteria then are allowed to proliferate, making a copy of the DNA sequence along with their own genome with each cell division.

- Genetic engineering refers to a process whereby a gene of interest is altered from its original form. The changed (mutant) genes can be reintroduced into a cell to disclose the effect on cell function and thus elucidate the normal function of the original gene and its protein product. Genetic engineering has been applied to plants to increase their value as food crops. Genetically engineered cells can be turned into protein factories to produce hormones, such as insulin, in large quantity.

Gene therapy relies heavily on these techniques to facilitate identification of genetic mutations, study of gene function, and development of methods to repair or replace mutant genes. Many more applications of recombinant DNA technology will become apparent as research on the genetic basis of human function and disease proceeds.

KEY POINTS

- Risk factors that indicate the need for prenatal diagnostic examination and counseling include advanced maternal age (older than 35 years), a family history of recessive or sex-linked disorders, and the previous birth of a child with chromosomal or neural tube defects.
- Ultrasound, amniocentesis, and chorionic villus sampling are the mainstays of prenatal assessment for genetic disorders.
- DNA sequences that are complementary to a gene of interest can be synthesized and used to probe the genome to determine if and where the gene is present. These hybridization techniques make screening for genetic disorders relatively fast and simple.
- Gene therapy is the treatment of genetic disease by replacing defective genes with normal genes. Gene therapy is possible because of the advances attained in recombinant DNA technology over the past 30 years.

SUMMARY

Genetic and developmental disorders are responsible for a number of congenital malformations. Congenital disorders are caused by genetic and environmental factors that disrupt normal fetal development. Genetic disorders are classified as (1) chromosomal alterations, including structural and numeric abnormalities; (2) Mendelian disorders, including autosomal dominant autosomal recessive, and X-linked disorders; (3) non-Mendelian single-gene disorders, including triplet repeats, mitochondrial gene defects, and genetic imprinting disorders; and (4) polygenic disorders. Known environmental teratogens include radiation, infectious organisms, and various chemicals and drugs. The embryo is particularly susceptible to teratogens during the period of organogenesis, which extends from the third to the ninth week of gestation. Pedigree analysis, ultrasound, amniocentesis, and chorionic villus biopsy may provide helpful information regarding genetic risk and the prenatal condition of at-risk infants. DNA sequencing of normal and mutant genes has made it possible to efficiently screen for genetic disorders and develop gene therapies for a variety of genetic diseases.

REFERENCES

1. Modell B, Darr A: Science and society: genetic counselling and customary consanguineous marriage, *Nat Rev Genet* 3(3): 225-229, 2002.
2. Kalter H: Teratology in the 20th century: environmental causes of congenital malformations in humans and how they were established, *Neurotoxicol Teratol* 25(2):131-282, 2003.
3. Turnpenny P, Ellard S: *Emersy's elements of medical genetics,* ed 13, Philadelphia 2007, Churchill-Livingstone.
4. Kumar V, Maitra A: Genetic and pediatric diseases. In Kumar V, Cotran RS, Robbins ST, editors: *Robbins basic pathology,* ed 8, Philadelphia, 2007, Saunders, pp 225-278.
5. Bateson W: *Mendel's principles of heredity*, London, 1902, Cambridge University Press.
6. Alberts B et al: Sexual reproduction: meiosis, germ cells and fertilization. In Alberts B et al, editors: *Molecular biology of the cell*, ed 5, New York, 2008, Garland Science, pp 1269-1304.
7. Alberts B et al: DNA replication, repair, and recombination. In Alberts B et al, editors: *Molecular biology of the cell*, ed 5, New York, 2008, Garland Science, pp 263-328.
8. Pellestor F, Tal H: The occurrence of aneuploidy in human: lessons from the cytogenetic studies of human oocytes, *Eur J Med Genet* 49(2):103-116, 2006.
9. Sherman SL et al: Risk factors for nondisjunction of trisomy 21, *Cytogenet Genome Res* 111(3-4):273-280, 2005.
10. Roizen NJ, Patterson D: Down's syndrome, *Lancet* 361(9365): 1281-1289, 2003.
11. Down JHL: Observations on an ethnic classification of idiots, *Clin Lect Rep London Hosp* 3:259-262, 1866.
12. Morris JK et al: Comparison of models of maternal age-specific risk for Down syndrome live births, *Prenat Diagn* 23(3):252-258, 2003.
13. Morris JK et al: Is the prevalence of Klinefelter syndrome increasing? *Eur J Hum Genet* 16(2):163-170, 2008.
14. Bojesen A, Claus HG: Klinefelter syndrome in clinical practice, *Nat Clin Pract Urol* 4(4):192-204, 2007.
15. De Vigan C et al: EUROSCAN Working Group: contribution of ultrasonographic examination to the prenatal detection of chromosomal abnormalities in 19 centres across Europe, *Ann Genet* 44(4):209-217, 2001.
16. Faivre L et al: Effect of mutation type and location on clinical outcome in 1,013 probands with Marfan syndrome or related phenotypes and FBN1 mutations: an international study, *Am J Hum Genet* 81(3):454-466, 2007.
17. The Huntington's Disease Collaborative Research Group: A novel gene containing a trinucleotide repeat that is expanded and unstable on Huntington's disease chromosomes, *Cell* 72:971, 1993.
18. Stack EC, Ferrante RJ: Huntington's disease: progress and potential in the field, *Expert Opin Investig Drugs* 16(12): 1933-1953, 2007.
19. Bates G: Huntingtin aggregation and toxicity in Huntington's disease, *Lancet* 361(9369):1642-1644, 2003.
20. Okulicz JF et al: Oculocutaneous albinism, *J Eur Acad Dermatol Venereol* 17(3):251-256, 2003.
21. Bobadilla JL et al: Cystic fibrosis: a worldwide analysis of CFTR mutations—correlation with incidence data and application to screening, *Hum Mutat* 19(6):575-606, 2002.
22. Flotte TR: Viral vector-mediated and cell-based therapies for treatment of cystic fibrosis, *Mol Ther* 15(2):229-241, 2007.
23. Pfeiffer BE, Huber KM: Fragile X mental retardation protein induces synapse loss through acute postsynaptic translational regulation, *J Neurosci* 27(12):3120-3130, 2007.
24. Green RF, Stoler JM: Alcohol dehydrogenase 1B genotype and fetal alcohol syndrome: a HuGE minireview, *Am J Obstet Gynecol* 197(1):12-25, 2007.
25. Abel EL, Hannigan JH: Maternal risk factors in fetal alcohol syndrome: provocative and permissive influences, *Neurotoxicol Teratol* 17(4):445-462, 1995.
26. Cotrim AP, Baum BJ: Gene therapy: some history, applications, problems, and prospects, *Toxicol Pathol* 36(1):97-103, 2008.

chapter 7

Neoplasia

Jacquelyn L. Banasik

MEDIA RESOURCES

Additional Material for Study, Review, and Further Exploration

CD Companion ■ Review Questions and Answers
■ Glossary (with audio pronunciations for selected terms) ■ Disease Profiles ■ Animations

evolve **Website** at http://evolve.elsevier.com/Copstead/
■ Case Studies ■ Disease Profiles ■ WebLinks ■ Key Points Review

 Online Course (Module 3)

KEY QUESTIONS

■ How do neoplastic cells differ from normal cells?
■ In what ways do benign and malignant tumors differ?
■ How might overexpression of proto-oncogenes lead to abnormal cellular proliferation?
■ How might underexpression of tumor suppressor genes lead to abnormal cellular proliferation?
■ What properties are gained during tumor progression that contribute to malignant behavior and metastasis?

■ How are tumor grading and staging used to guide the selection of cancer therapies?
■ How might lifestyle and carcinogen exposure contribute to cancer risk?
■ What treatment options are available for benign and malignant tumors?

CHAPTER OUTLINE

Neoplasia means "new growth." In common use, the term implies an *abnormality* of cellular growth and may be used interchangeably with the term *tumor*. It is no surprise that the discovery of a tumor in an individual can evoke feelings of disbelief, anger, and dread. Characterization of the tumor cells is of critical importance to determine whether the tumor is benign or malignant. The term *cancer* is applied only to malignant neoplasms. The diagnosis of a **benign** growth is received with great relief inasmuch as the tumor is generally easily cured. The diagnosis of a **malignant** cancer, on the other hand, may herald months of intensive and often uncomfortable treatment with uncertain outcomes. Cancer remains the second leading cause of death in the United States for both men and women.

It is increasingly clear that cancer is associated with *altered expression of cellular genes* that normally regulate cell proliferation and differentiation. A unified theory of cancer causation has emerged, and new methods for cancer therapy continue to be developed. Cancer is a complex, multifaceted disorder with each individual cancer having some unique properties. A better understanding of the molecular characteristics of individual cancers is encouraging the development of specific therapies that target each cancer's weaknesses.

BENIGN VERSUS MALIGNANT GROWTH

Characteristics of Benign and Malignant Tumors

The terms *benign* and *malignant* refer to the overall consequences of a tumor to the host. Generally, malignant tumors have the potential to kill the host if left untreated, whereas benign tumors do not. This difference is not strict because some benign tumors may be located in critical areas. For example, a benign tumor may be life threatening if it causes pressure on the brain or blocks an airway or blood vessel. Histologic examination of a tumor is the primary mode for determining its benign or malignant nature. Certain tumor

characteristics have historically been shown to indicate malignant potential. Important considerations include localization of the tumor and the degree of tumor cell differentiation.

Benign tumors do not invade adjacent tissue or spread to distant sites. Many benign tumors are encapsulated by connective tissue, which is an indication of strictly local growth. Any evidence that tumor cells have penetrated local tissues (invasiveness), lymphatics, or blood vessels suggests a malignant nature with potential to spread to distant sites (metastasize).

As a general rule, benign cells more closely resemble their tissue type of origin (e.g., skin, liver) than do malignant cells. The degree of tissue-specific differentiation has traditionally been used to predict malignant potential. A lack of differentiated features in a cancer cell is called **anaplasia,** and a greater degree of anaplasia is correlated with a more aggressively malignant tumor.[1] Anaplasia is indicated by variation in cell size and shape within the tumor, enlarged nuclei, abnormal mitoses, and bizarre-looking giant cells (Figure 7-1). Regardless of histologic appearance, invasion of local tissue or evidence of **metastasis** to distant sites confirms the diagnosis of malignancy.

Other differences between benign and malignant tumors have been noted (Table 7-1). Benign tumors generally grow more slowly, have little vascularity, rarely have necrotic areas, and often retain functions similar to those of the tissue of origin. Conversely, malignant tumors often grow rapidly and may initiate vessel growth in the tumor. They frequently have necrotic areas and are dysfunctional.

Tumor Terminology

General rules for the naming of tumors have been developed to indicate the tissue of origin and the benign or malignant nature of the tumor. The suffix *-oma* is used to indicate a benign tumor, whereas *carcinoma* and *sarcoma* are used to indicate malignant tumors. Carcinoma refers to malignant tumors of epithelial origin and sarcoma to malignant tumors

FIGURE 7-1 A, Normal Papanicolaou smear from the uterine cervix showing large, flat epithelial cells with small nuclei. **B,** Typical histologic appearance of anaplastic tumor cells showing variation in cell size and shape, with large, hyperchromic nuclei. (From Kumar V et al: *Robbins basic pathology,* ed 8, Philadelphia, 2007, Saunders, p 220. Courtesy Dr. Richard M. DeMay, Department of Pathology, University of Chicago.)

TABLE 7-1

General Characteristics of Benign and Malignant Tumors

Characteristic	Benign	Malignant
Histology	Typical of tissue of origin Few mitoses	Anaplastic, with abnormal cell size and shape Many mitoses
Growth rate	Slow	Rapid
Localization/metastasis	Strictly local, often encapsulated/no metastasis	Infiltrative/frequent metastases
Tumor necrosis	Rare	Common
Recurrence after treatment	Rare	Common
Prognosis	Good	Poor if untreated

of mesenchymal (nerve, bone, muscle) origin. Thus a benign tumor of glandular tissue would be called an adenoma, but a malignant tumor of the same tissue would be called an adeno-carcinoma (Table 7-2). Some notable exceptions to the rules are lymphomas, hepatomas, and melanomas, which are all highly malignant despite their *-oma* suffix. Leukemia refers to a malignant growth of white blood cells. The great majority of human cancers (90%) are carcinomas from malignant trans-formation of epithelial cells.[2]

The Malignant Phenotype

Cells growing in normal tissue have predictable relation-ships with neighboring cells. In a particular tissue, the rate of cell proliferation is precisely matched to the rate of cell death. Normal cells require constant reassurance in the form of survival signals from their environment that their con-tinued existence is desirable, and they proliferate only when space is available and appropriate mitogen-stimulating signals are present. Normal cells also respond to signals instructing them to actively destroy themselves in a process called *apop-tosis* (see Chapter 4). Cancer cells, however, do not obey the rules; they have escaped the normal mechanisms of growth control. A number of antisocial properties develop in malig-nant cells that allow them to proliferate at the expense of other cells and tissues of the body. These abnormal behaviors can be summarized as follows:

- Cancer cells proliferate despite lack of growth-initiating sig-nals from the environment.
- Cancer cells escape signals to die and achieve a kind of immortality in that they are capable of unlimited replication.
- Cancer cells lose their differentiated features and contribute poorly or not at all to the function of their tissue.
- Cancer cells are genetically unstable and evolve by accu-mulating new mutations at a much faster rate than normal cells.
- Cancer cells invade their local tissue and overrun their neighbors.
- Perhaps worst of all, cancer cells gain the ability to migrate from their site of origin to colonize distant sites where they do not belong.

Most cancers are thought to arise from stem cells that are present in tissues. Tissue stem cells are capable of unlimited proliferation, entering the cell cycle to produce two daughter cells, one of whom retains the original stem cell properties and the other becomes a more differentiated cell, but still capable of proliferation. Normally, the partially differenti-ated cells can undergo only a limited number of cell divisions before they permanently leave the cell cycle and become senescent.[2] Either a stem cell or a partially differentiated cell has the potential to acquire the genetic mutations necessary to become malignant.

KEY POINTS

- Malignant tumors have the potential to kill the host, whereas benign tumors generally do not. The primary difference between malignant and benign tumors is the propensity of malignant tumors to invade adjacent tis-sue and spread to distant sites (metastasize).
- The suffix *-oma* is used to indicate a benign tumor (e.g., fibroma). *Carcinoma* and *sarcoma* are used to indicate malignancy (e.g., fibrosarcoma). Exceptions include melanomas, lymphomas, hepatomas, and leukemia, all of which are malignant.
- Malignant cells exhibit antisocial properties that al-low them to ignore growth-controlling signals from the environment. Cancer cells proliferate excessively, become immortal, invade locally, and may travel to dis-tant sites where they establish new colonies.

EPIDEMIOLOGY AND CANCER RISK FACTORS

Cancer accounts for approximately 25% of all deaths, which makes it the second leading cause of death in the United States. Most cancer deaths (77%) occur in persons older than 55 years. The American Cancer Society estimates that men have almost a 1 in 2 lifetime risk of developing cancer,

TABLE 7-2

Nomenclature for Neoplastic Diseases

Cell or Tissue of Origin	Benign	Malignant
Tumors of Epithelial Origin		
Squamous cells	Squamous cell papilloma	Squamous cell carcinoma
Basal cells	—	Basal cell carcinoma
Glandular or ductal epithelium	Adenoma	Adenocarcinoma
	Cystadenoma	Cystadenocarcinoma
Transitional cells	Transitional cell papilloma	Transitional cell carcinoma
Bile duct	Bile duct adenoma	Bile duct carcinoma (cholangiocarcinoma)
Liver cells	Hepatocellular adenoma	Hepatocellular carcinoma
Melanocytes	Nevus	Malignant melanoma
Renal epithelium	Renal tubular adenoma	Renal cell carcinoma
Skin adnexal glands		
Sweat glands	Sweat gland adenoma	Sweat gland carcinoma
Sebaceous glands	Sebaceous gland adenoma	Sebaceous gland carcinoma
Germs cells (testis and ovary)	—	Seminoma (dysgerminoma), embryonal carcinoma, yolk sac carcinoma
Tumors of Mesenchymal Origin		
Hematopoietic/lymphoid tissue	—	Leukemia, lymphoma, Hodgkin disease, multiple myeloma
Neural and retinal tissue		
Nerve sheath	Neurilemmoma, neurofibroma	Malignant peripheral nerve sheath tumor
Nerve cells	Ganglioneuroma	Neuroblastoma
Retinal cells (cones)	—	Retinoblastoma
Connective tissue		
Fibrous tissue	Fibromatosis (desmoid)	Fibrosarcoma
Fat	Lipoma	Liposarcoma
Bone	Osteoma	Osteogenic sarcoma
Cartilage	Chondroma	Chondrosarcoma
Muscle		
Smooth muscle	Leiomyoma	Leiomyosarcoma
Striated muscle	Rhabdomyoma	Rhabdomyosarcoma
Endothelial and related tissues		
Blood vessels	Hemangioma	Angiosarcoma
		Kaposi sarcoma
Lymph vessels	Lymphangioma	Lymphangiosarcoma
Synovium	—	Synovial sarcoma
Mesothelium	—	Malignant mesothelioma
Meninges	Meningioma	Malignant meningioma

From Murphy GP, Lawrence W, Lenhard RE, editors: *American Cancer Society textbook of clinical oncology*, Atlanta, 1995, American Cancer Society, p 77. Reproduced by permission of the American Cancer Society.

and women have slightly higher than a 1 in 3 risk. The 5-year relative survival rate for all cancers combined is about 66%.[3] The 5-year survival rate doesn't distinguish between those who were cured and those who have relapsed or are still in treatment. Fortunately, the current view of cancer causation predicts that most cancer is preventable. Indeed, one third of cancer-related deaths may be attributed to lifestyle factors. Lifestyle factors of particular importance are tobacco use, nutrition, and obesity. Sun exposure is a significant risk factor for skin cancer (Chapter 53), and sexual exposure to certain strains of human papillomavirus predisposes to cervical cancer (Chapter 34). The high incidence and relative ease of screening for breast, cervical, colorectal, and prostate cancers has prompted the development of guidelines for early detection of these cancers. The current recommendations for

early detection of cancer in average-risk, asymptomatic persons are shown in Table 7-3. Statistics regarding some of the major forms of cancer are shown in Figure 7-2. Further discussions of particular cancers can be found in chapters relating to corresponding body systems.

Tobacco Use

The impact of tobacco use on cancer-related death can be most vividly seen by looking at cancer death rates in the United States from 1930 to 2004 (Figure 7-3). Whereas all other cancer-related death rates declined or remained relatively stable, the death rate from lung cancer increased dramatically. The increase is attributable almost entirely to smoking. Lung cancer remains the leading cause of cancer death in both men and women, accounting for 30% of all cancer deaths. Lung

TABLE 7-3

Screening Guidelines for the Early Detection of Cancer in Asymptomatic People

Site	Recommendation
Breast	Yearly mammograms are recommended starting at age 40. The age at which screening should be stopped should be individualized by considering the potential risks and benefits of screening in the context of overall health and status and longevity. Clinical breast exam should be part of a periodic health exam, about every 3 years for women in their 20s and 30s, and every year for women 40 and older. Women should know how their breasts normally feel and report any breast change promptly to their health care providers. Breast self-exam is an option for women starting in their 20s. Women at increased risk (e.g. family history, genetic tendency, past breast cancer) should talk with their doctors about the benefits and limitations of starting mammography screening earlier, having additional tests (i.e., breast ultrasound and MRI), or having more frequent exams.
Colon and rectum	Beginning at age 50, men and women should begin screening with 1 of the examination schedules below: ■ A fecal occult blood test (FOBT) every year or fecal immunochemical test (FIT) every year ■ A flexible sigmoidoscopy (FSIG) every 5 years ■ Annual FOBT or FIT and flexible sigmoidoscopy every 5 years* ■ A double-contrast barium enema every 5 years ■ A colonoscopy every 10 years *Combined testing is preferred over either annual FOBT or FIT, or FSIG every 5 years alone. People who are at moderate or high risk for colorectal cancer should talk with a doctor about a different testing schedule.
Prostate	The PSA test and the digital rectal examination should be offered annually, beginning at age 50, to men who have life expectancy of at least 10 years. Men at high risk (African-American men and men with a strong family history of 1 or more first-degree relatives diagnosed with prostate cancer at an early age) should begin testing at age 45. For both men at average risk and high risk, information should be provided about what is known and what is uncertain about the benefits and limitations of early detection and treatment of prostate cancer so that they can make an informed decision about testing.
Uterus	*Cervix:* Screening should begin approximately 3 years after a woman begins having vaginal intercourse, but no later than 21 years of age. Screening should be done every year with regular Pap tests or every 2 years using liquid-based test. At or after age 30, women who have had 3 normal test results in a row may get screened every 2 to 3 years. Alternatively, cervical cancer screening with HPV DNA testing and conventional or liquid-based cytology could be performed every 3 years. However, doctors may suggest a woman get screened more often if she has certain risk factors, such as HIV infection or a weak immune system. Women 70 years and older who have had 3 or more consecutive normal Pap tests in the last 10 years may choose to stop cervical screening. Screening after total hysterectomy (with removal of the cervix) is not necessary unless the surgery was done as a treatment for cervical cancer. *Endometrium:* The American Cancer Society recommends that at the time of menopause all women should be informed about the risks and symptoms of endometrial cancer, and strongly encouraged to report any unexpected bleeding or spotting to their physicians. Annual screening for endometrial cancer with endometrial biopsy beginning at age 35 should be offered to women with or at risk for hereditary nonpolyposis colon cancer (HNPCC).
Cancer-related checkup	For individuals undergoing periodic health examinations, a cancer-related checkup should include health counseling and, depending on a person's age, might include examinations for cancers of the thyroid, oral cavity, skin, lymph nodes, testes, and ovaries, as well as for some nonmalignant diseases.

From American Cancer Society. *Cancer Facts and Figures 2008.* Atlanta: American Cancer Society, Inc.

American Cancer Society guidelines for early cancer detection are assessed annually in order to identify whether there is new scientific evidence sufficient to warrant a reevaluation of current recommendations. If evidence is sufficiently compelling to consider a change or clarification in a current guideline or the development of a new guideline, a formal procedure is initiated. Guidelines are formally evaluated every 5 years regardless of whether new evidence suggests a change in the existing recommendations. There are nine steps in this procedure, and these "guidelines for guideline development" were formally established to provide a specific methodology for science and expert judgment to form the underpinnings of specific statements and recommendations from the Society. These procedures constitute a deliberate process to ensure that all Society recommendations have the same methodological and evidence-based process at their core. This process also employs a system for rating strength and consistency of evidence that is similar to that employed by the Agency for Health Care Research and Quality (AHCRQ) and the U.S. Preventive Services Task Force (USPSTF).

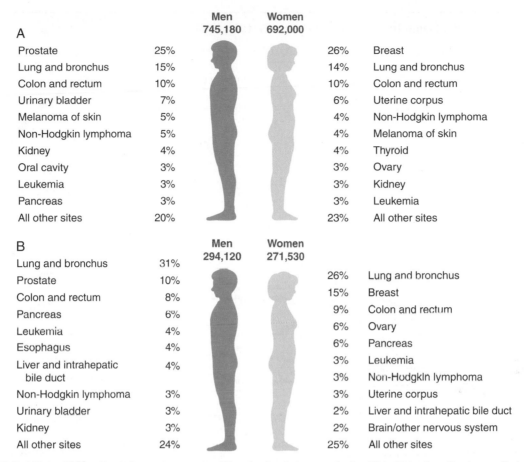

FIGURE 7-2 United States 2008 estimated new cancer cases **(A)** and estimated cancer deaths **(B)** in 10 leading sites by sex. Excludes basal and squamous cell skin cancers and in situ carcinomas except urinary bladder. (Data from American Cancer Society: *Cancer facts and figures—2008*, Atlanta, 2008, The Society.)

cancer has one of the worst survival rates of all cancers—only 15%. In addition to lung cancer, tobacco use has been linked with cancer of the pancreas, bladder, kidney, mouth, esophagus, and cervix (Figure 7-4). Smoking prevalence among adults in the United States declined from 42% in 1965 to 21% in 2004 and has remained stable at 21%, with rates being approximately 5% lower in women than in men. An estimated 45 million U.S. adults currently smoke cigarettes. Approximately 23% of high school students reported being cigarette smokers in 2005. In 2006, only 8% of college graduates were current smokers, compared to 21% in 1983.[3]

Carcinogens can be grouped into two major types: those that cause genetic damage (initiators) and those that promote growth of the tumor (promoters). Tobacco smoke contains hundreds of compounds, many of which have known genotoxicity (e.g., polycyclic aromatic hydrocarbons, nicotine derivatives) and probably serve as initiators. Tobacco smoke also contains promoters, which spur the mutant cells to proliferate. Second-hand smoke contains more than 4000 chemicals, of which over 5% are known or suspected to cause cancer.[3] The American Cancer Society estimates that about 3000 nonsmoking adults die from lung cancer each year as a result of exposure to second-hand smoke.[3]

Nutrition

The results of studies on the relationship between cancer and certain nutrients remain confusing and contradictory. The general opinion is that diet is associated with cancer risk, but there is little agreement as to what that association might be. A lack of fruits and vegetables in the diet may be a significant contributor to cancer risk, but the mechanisms are unclear. Dietary factors believed to be related to cancer risk include fat, fiber, alcohol, and antioxidants. It is not yet clear how single nutrients, nutrient combinations, overnutrition, or body fat distribution affect the risk of developing cancer, and more research is needed.[4]

Fat

Several epidemiologic studies done in the 1970s and early 1980s suggested a relationship between high-fat diets and the development of breast, colon, and prostate cancer. In some studies, however, higher fat intake was found to be protective against some cancers. A pooled analysis of seven large studies found no link between fat intake and the risk of breast cancer.[5] The results of one large, randomized clinical trial investigating the effect of a low-fat diet on the occurrence of invasive breast cancer found no difference between the control and low-fat groups after 8 years of follow up in postmenopausal

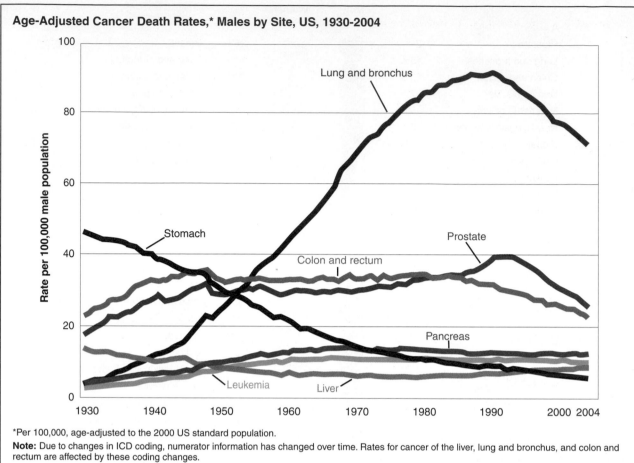

Age-Adjusted Cancer Death Rates,* Males by Site, US, 1930-2004

*Per 100,000, age-adjusted to the 2000 US standard population.

Note: Due to changes in ICD coding, numerator information has changed over time. Rates for cancer of the liver, lung and bronchus, and colon and rectum are affected by these coding changes.

Source: US Mortality Data 1960 to 2004, US Mortality Volumes 1930 to 1959, National Center for Health Statistics, Centers for Disease Control and Prevention, 2006.

American Cancer Society, Surveillance Research, 2008

A

FIGURE 7-3 U.S. age-adjusted cancer death rates for selected sites in men **(A)** and women **(B)** from 1930 to 2004. (Redrawn from American Cancer Society: *Cancer facts and figures—2008*, Atlanta, 2008, The Society.)

women.[6] Fat or calorie intake and high production of insulin may affect breast cancer outcomes depending on tumor cell type and hormone responsiveness. Further research on the specific type of fat intake and other cofactors is needed to clarify the fat-cancer relationship. Several studies in animals have shown that regardless of fat intake, tumor growth may be inhibited by caloric restriction. Some investigators have proposed a link between high insulin production and breast cancer. The American Cancer Society suggests that controlling body fat through calorie restriction and increased activity may help reduce the risk of cancer.

Fiber

Fiber is a general term for nondigestable dietary substances that remain in the intestinal lumen, increase fecal bulk, and improve bowel regularity. Fiber includes a diversity of compounds such as cellulose, bran, and pectin. An association between fiber intake and colorectal cancer proposed in the early 1970s was based on a study comparing the incidence of certain ailments in Americans and Africans.[7] A number of correlational and comparison studies done since that time have yielded conflicting results, and large randomized trials failed to show a benefit.[8] Part of the difficulty may be linked to the way that different studies define dietary fiber. Because fiber is associated with beneficial effects on digestion and elimination, fiber intake in the range of 10 to 13 g per 1000 calories consumed is generally recommended.

Alcohol

Alcohol intake has been linked to a number of cancers, including breast, esophageal, laryngeal, and liver cancer. Alcohol may exert its cancer-promoting effects through impairment of the liver's ability to metabolize harmful substances and endogenous hormones. Moderate alcohol intake has been shown to increase estrogen levels, which may account for its promoting effects on breast cancer.[9] As a carbohydrate-dense substance, alcohol may contribute to cancer risk through its effects on insulin secretion. Insulin is a general growth factor for a number of tissues. Limiting alcohol intake may provide a modest reduction in cancer risk.

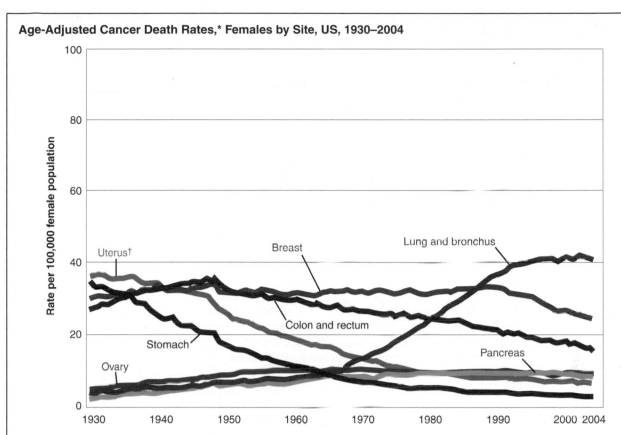

Age-Adjusted Cancer Death Rates,* Females by Site, US, 1930–2004

*Per 100,000, age-adjusted to the 2000 US standard population. †Uterus cancer death rates are for uterine cervix and uterine corpus combined.

Note: Due to changes in ICD coding, numerator information has changed over time. Rates for cancer of the lung and bronchus, colon and rectum, and ovary are affected by these coding changes.

Source: US Mortality Data 1960 to 2004, US Mortality Volumes 1930 to 1959, National Center for Health Statistics, Centers for Disease Control and Prevention, 2006.

American Cancer Society, Surveillance Research, 2008

B

FIGURE 7-3 cont'd.

Antioxidants

Until recently, the emphasis of cancer prevention has been on the identification and avoidance of cancer-causing agents. However, increasing interest has been shown in finding substances with cancer-protective properties. The fact that DNA damage is an important step in cancer initiation, coupled with the knowledge that oxygen free radicals can impart this damage, led to the idea that antioxidants may have protective effects for cancer.

Vitamin A and the antioxidant trio of vitamin E, beta carotene, and vitamin C have been most widely studied. The use of antioxidants to prevent cancer sounds like a good idea; however, several large-scale studies have failed to reveal a benefit and some have found that the risk of cancer may be increased. For example, two studies using beta carotene supplementation in smokers and asbestos-exposed individuals found a higher incidence of lung cancer in the group receiving the antioxidants.[10,11] A meta-analysis of twelve trials, 9 of high methodological quality, including a total subject population of 104,196 reported that antioxidant supplementation did not significantly reduce total cancer incidence or mortality or any site-specific cancer incidence.[12] Beta carotene supplementation was associated with an increase in the incidence of cancer among smokers. Selenium supplementation was associated with reduced cancer incidence in men, but not in women. Vitamin E supplementation had no apparent effect on overall cancer incidence or cancer mortality. Further research is needed before the role of antioxidant supplementation can be defined. At present, it may be prudent to consume a diet high in natural fruit and vegetable sources of antioxidants.

KEY POINTS

- The risk of developing cancer increases with age. It is estimated that men have almost a 1 in 2 lifetime chance of developing cancer, whereas women have a little more than a 1 in 3 chance.
- The development of many cancers is related to lifestyle, particularly tobacco use and nutrition. Smoking cessation is considered important in reducing cancer risk. Guidelines regarding nutrition are less clear. Limiting excessive fat, carbohydrate, and alcohol intake while increasing dietary fiber, fruit, and vegetables may be of benefit.

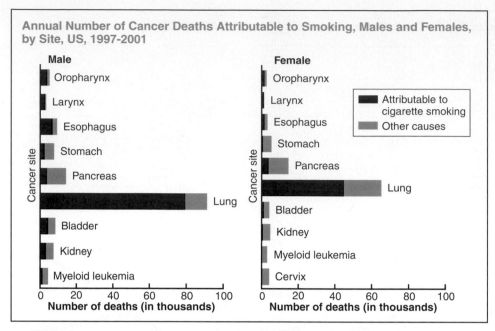

FIGURE 7-4 Annual cancer deaths attributable to smoking in males and females in the U.S. (Centers for Disease Control and Prevention, Annual smoking-attributable mortality, years of potential life lost, and productivity losses—United States, 1997-2001. *MMWR Morb Mortal Wkly Rep* 54(25): 625-628, 2005.)

GENETIC MECHANISMS OF CANCER

Despite much progress in our understanding of how mechanisms of growth control and cellular differentiation may go awry, there is still no simple answer to the question, "What causes cancer?" It is increasingly evident, however, that cancer is primarily a disorder of gene expression. Early support for a genetic basis of cancer came from the observation that cancer often resulted from agents known to damage deoxyribonucleic acid (DNA). In the 1970s a number of potential cancer-causing agents (**carcinogens**) were identified by demonstrating their mutagenic potential.[13] The suggestion that mutant genes were the basis for cancer launched intense research to identify the cancer-causing gene or genes.

Cancer-critical genes are grouped into two broad classes, according to whether over-activity of the gene contributes to cancer (gain-of-function mutations) or whether too little gene activity is the problem (loss-of-function mutations). Both categories of genes result in similar effects in enhancing cell proliferation and survival.[2] Genes in the first category are called **proto-oncogenes,** which normally code for components of the cellular growth-activating pathways. A proto-oncogene in its mutant, overactive or over-expressed form is called an *oncogene.* Genes in the second category of cancer-related genes are called **tumor suppressor genes,** which normally inhibit cell proliferation. Cancers may arise when tumor suppressor gene function is lost or abnormally inhibited. To achieve malignant transformation, a cell must generally suffer mutations in a combination of these growth regulatory genes. A cell thus transformed passes on these mutations to its progeny when it divides and forms a clone of abnormally proliferating cells. Numerous studies have begun to unravel the details of how proto-oncogenes and tumor suppressor genes may dysfunction and contribute to the malignant phenotype. In addition to the genes that regulate the cell cycle, a third category of genes that monitor and maintain the genome contributes indirectly to the development of cancer. This class includes the DNA-repair genes and the genes that regulate apoptosis (see Chapter 4).

Proto-Oncogenes

Proto-oncogenes were the first of the tumor-associated genes to be discovered, and hundreds have been described to date.[2] As often happens in the study of genes, a gene associated with a disease process is identified long before its normal cellular function is elucidated. Thus genes associated with cancer are traditionally named for the cancer in which they were first discovered (in mutant form) rather than their normal cellular function. Many of the first cancer-associated genes, called **oncogenes,** were initially identified in viruses and still retain the name reflecting their viral discovery. The term *proto-oncogene* was created to label the normal cellular gene that can be transformed into an oncogene by activating (gain-of-function) mutations. A representative list of known proto-oncogenes is shown in Table 7-4.

The majority of proto-oncogenes described to date code for components of cell-signaling systems that promote cell proliferation.[2] These components can be lumped into four broad categories: (1) growth factors, (2) receptors, (3) cytoplasmic signaling molecules, and (4) nuclear transcription factors (Figure 7-5). Excessive activity in any of these components may release the cell from environmental feedback and allow it to proliferate abnormally.

TABLE 7-4

Examples of Gain-of-Function Proto-Oncogenes and Their Mechanisms of Action

Factor	Type of Cancer
Mitogens and Growth Factors	
PDGF	Glioma (brain)
FGF	Melanoma
EGF	Breast
TGF-α	Breast, numerous others
Cell Membrane Receptors	
ERBB1 (EGF receptor)	Breast, brain
HER-2 (ERBB2)	Breast, ovarian
RET	Thyroid
Cytoplasmic Signaling Molecules	
RAS	Lung, ovarian, colon, pancreatic
ABL	Leukemia
Transcription Factors	
C-MYC	Leukemia, breast, lung
N-MYC	Neuroblastoma
L-MYC	Lung
MYB	Various
JUN	Various
FOS	Various
REL	Various

EGF, epidermal growth factor; *FGF*, fibroblast growth factor; *PDGF*, platelet-derived growth factor; *TGF*, transforming growth factor.

Growth Factors (Mitogens)

The first proto-oncogenes to be discovered coded for growth factors. A great deal of intercellular communication is accomplished through the cell-to-cell transmission of growth factors. Growth factors are small peptides that are manufactured by cells and secreted into the extracellular space. They diffuse to nearby cells and interact with receptors on the target cell surface. Binding of growth factors to cell surface receptors activates signaling cascades within the cell that enhance proliferation. As a general principle, cells do not independently produce growth factors sufficient to stimulate their own proliferation. The proliferation signals must be produced by the cell's environment. The cell's environment also conveys growth-inhibiting signals. Overproduction of stimulatory growth factors by a mutant proto-oncogene can shift the balance of signals and produce excessive self-stimulated growth (**autocrine signaling**). Examples of tumor-secreted growth factors include platelet-derived growth factor, transforming growth factor-α, and epidermal growth factor. Certain cancer types typically secrete particular growth factors. For example, platelet-derived growth factor is commonly oversecreted in glial cell cancers (brain tumors) and connective tissue cancers (sarcomas).

Growth Factor Receptors

Peptide growth factors (mitogens) cannot penetrate the cell membrane directly, so their presence at the cell surface must be transmitted intracellularly by cell surface receptors. Receptors

FIGURE 7-5 Possible effects of proto-oncogene activation on growth signaling pathways. **A,** Production of growth factors (mitogens). **B,** Production of growth factor receptors. **C,** Intracellular pathway disturbances. **D,** Activation of transcription factors for growth.

are transmembrane proteins with the mitogen-binding area on the outside of the cell and an enzyme-activating area on the inside of the cell. These receptors are extremely specific; they will bind with only one particular mitogen. Binding activates a series of reactions within the cell that eventually leads to cell proliferation.

A mutational event may allow the expression of receptors that should not be present at all or allow excessive amounts of normally present receptors, or it may produce receptors with abnormally high affinity. All of these changes result in excessive responsiveness to the mitogens normally present in the cell's environment. Some mutant receptors may even be active in the absence of growth factors and spur the cell to divide despite the absence of environmental signals to do so. An important example of a receptor abnormality is the over-expression of human epidermal growth factor receptor type 2 (HER2) receptors in about 25% of breast cancers. The overactive receptors stimulate proliferation of tumor cells even when there is little or no epidermal growth factor bound to them.

Cytoplasmic Signaling Pathways

A third way in which oncogenes may facilitate proliferation is by the manufacture of excessive or abnormal components of the intracellular signaling pathways. These pathways involve numerous enzymes and chemicals that normally function to transmit signals from activated receptors at the cell surface to the cell nucleus. A mutant proto-oncogene that codes for excessive or abnormal cytoplasmic signaling components could cause activation of the pathway even though no signal was received at the cell surface. The best understood example of this mechanism is mutations of the *ras* gene family. Proteins encoded by *ras* genes are monomeric G proteins that transmit signals from receptors at the cell surface into the interior of the cell. The *ras* protein is active when it has guanosine triphosphate (GTP) bound to it, but it quickly hydrolyzes the GTP, thus automatically turning itself off after a brief period of activity. A mutation in the *ras* gene can code for a protein that is unable to hydrolyze GTP, so it remains persistently active and stimulates cell proliferation inappropriately. Mutations of the *ras* genes occur in about 30% of all human cancers, including leukemias and lung, ovarian, colon, and pancreatic cancer.

Transcription Factors

The entire proliferation pathway, including the growth factor (mitogen), the receptor, and the intracellular cascade, ultimately affects transcription of a set of genes in the nucleus that spur the cell to enter S phase. A number of proto-oncogenes have been identified that code for transcription factors in the nucleus. Transcription factors are proteins that must be assembled at the promoter area to begin gene transcription (see Chapters 3 and 5). Transcription factors are normally sequestered and prevented from indiscriminate activity until appropriate signals cause their release. Mutations in transcription factor genes may cause overproduction of transcription factors or interfere with the normal mechanisms for keeping them in check. *Myc*, *jun*, and *fos* are examples of proto-oncogenes that code for

nuclear transcription factors. Abnormalities of the *myc* genes are found in numerous cancers, including lung and breast cancer, leukemia, and neuroblastoma.

From Proto-Oncogene to Oncogene

Proto-oncogenes become activated oncogenes when mutations alter their activity so that proliferation-promoting signals are generated inappropriately. At least four general ways in which proto-oncogenes can be activated are known (Figure 7-6): (1) Oncogenes may be introduced into the host cell by a retrovirus; (2) a proto-oncogene within the cell may suffer a mutagenic event that changes its structure and function; (3) a DNA sequence that normally regulates proto-oncogene expression may be damaged or lost and allow the proto-oncogene to become abnormally active; and (4) an error in chromosome replication may cause extra copies of the proto-oncogene to be included in the genome (amplification).

In the early 1960s it was discovered that certain viruses were associated with cancer in various animal models. Researchers speculated that a virus could introduce a mutant, cancer-causing gene (oncogene) into the host's cells. Indeed, malignant cells containing the cancer-causing viruses were shown to have incorporated a small number of viral genes into their cellular DNA.[14] The presence of these oncogenes was required to maintain the malignant state of the cell.

Only a few types of human cancers are thought to be associated with viruses. The clearest associations involve viruses called *retroviruses*. At least three retroviruses are thought to be causative factors in some human cancers: Human immunodeficiency virus is associated with Kaposi sarcoma, Epstein-Barr virus with Burkitt lymphoma, and human T-lymphocyte virus type I with adult T-cell leukemia-lymphoma.

Retroviruses are composed of RNA and possess a unique enzyme, reverse transcriptase, which directs the synthesis of a DNA copy of the viral RNA. The DNA copy can then be incorporated into the cellular DNA and become part of the host's genome. The degree of viral oncogene expression depends on where the oncogene is inserted in the host DNA. Insertion near a promoter sequence may result in continuous transcription of the oncogene. Viral oncogenes are not subject to normal DNA transcription controls and are thus not responsive to growth-suppressing signals. Where did the viral oncogenes originate? Apparently, the tendency of retroviruses to slip in and out of host genomes allows them to pick up some of the host's genes, namely, the growth-promoting proto-oncogenes.

Proto-oncogene expression is tightly regulated in a normal cell. A number of different mutations can affect proto-oncogene expression and activity. A point mutation in the coding region of the proto-oncogene can alter the structure of its protein product and make it hyperactive. An example of this mechanism is the abnormal *ras* protein described earlier. Even though the protein is made in normal quantity, its activity is enhanced. Other mutations may lead to overproduction of a protein with normal structure. Gene amplification and chromosomal rearrangement during mitosis may release the proto-oncogene from its normal regulation and allow excessive transcription (Figure 7-7).

FIGURE 7-6 Mechanisms of proto-oncogene activation. **A,** Retroviral insertion. **B,** Proto-oncogene mutation. **C,** Regulatory sequence mutation. **D,** Proto-oncogene amplification. *RT,* Reverse transcriptase.

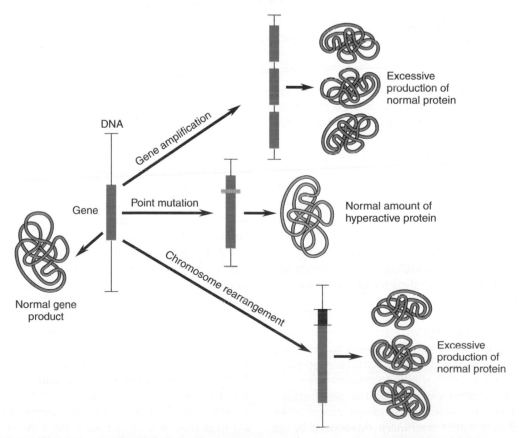

FIGURE 7-7 Overactivity of proto-oncogenes may be due to normal production of an abnormal protein (mutation in coding sequence) or excessive production of a normal protein (gene amplification or chromosome rearrangement).

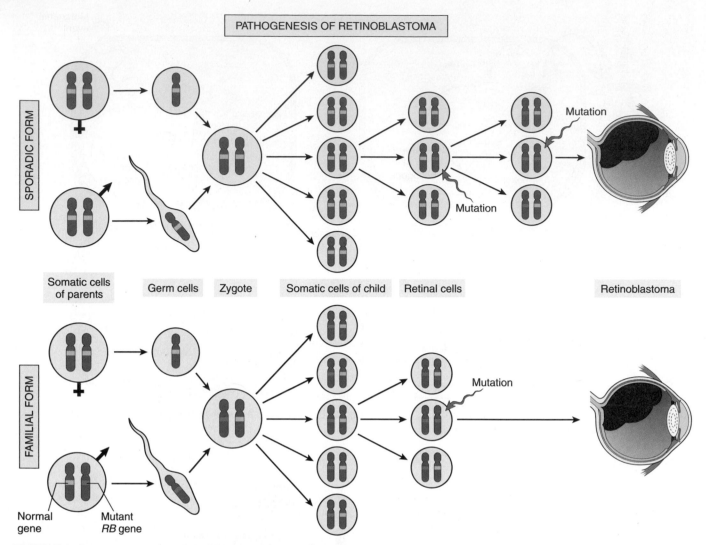

PATHOGENESIS OF RETINOBLASTOMA

SPORADIC FORM

FAMILIAL FORM

Somatic cells of parents | Germ cells | Zygote | Somatic cells of child | Retinal cells | Retinoblastoma

Mutation

Normal gene | Mutant *RB* gene

FIGURE 7-8 Both DNA copies (alleles) of the *Rb* tumor suppression gene must be dysfunctional for retinoblastoma to occur. Inheriting a defective *Rb* gene predisposes an individual to the development of cancer because only a single mutational event is required to inactivate *pRb* function. (From Kumar V et al: *Robbins Basic pathology,* ed 8, Philadelphia, 2007, Saunders, p 193.)

In summary, mutational events in the cell's genome may cause overexpression of normal proto-oncogene products or production of altered and hyperactive proteins. Most known oncogenes act by releasing the cell from its dependence on growth and survival signals in its environment. This effect usually is accomplished by gain-of-function abnormalities in the proliferation pathways that involve growth factors (mitogens), receptors, cytoplasmic signaling molecules, or nuclear transcription factors.

Tumor Suppressor Genes

To become malignant, cells must devise ways to evade the normal inhibitory mechanisms that keep the brakes applied to cell division. It is not enough to simply overstimulate growth-promoting signals. Critical elements of the proliferation-inhibiting pathways are defective in most cancers. The components of the inhibitory machinery are specified by the so-called *tumor suppressor genes.* Tumor suppressor genes

are difficult to study because they contribute to cancer only when they are not there. The first tumor suppressor gene to be discovered was the *Rb* gene, so named because of its role in retinoblastoma, a cancer of the eye.[15] A familial form of retinoblastoma is associated with the transmission of a genetic defect; a portion of chromosome 13 is missing, which is where the *Rb* gene is normally located. An absent *Rb* gene predisposes an individual to cancer, but cancer will not develop unless the other copy of the *Rb* gene (from the other parent) is also damaged (Figure 7-8).

Since the initial discovery of the *Rb* tumor suppressor gene, researchers have compiled an impressive list of other genes that appear to function as inhibitors of cellular proliferation (Table 7-5). As with the *Rb* gene, both copies of the tumor suppressor genes usually are inactivated when cancer develops. A person who inherits a defective copy of a tumor suppressor gene from one parent has a much higher risk of cancer than one who inherits two healthy copies. Knowledge about

TABLE 7-5

Examples of Tumor Suppressor Genes

Gene	Chromosome Location	Cancer
Rb	13q14	Retinoblastoma, sarcoma
P53	17p13	Li-Fraumeni syndrome, 50% of all tumors
DCC	18q21	Colorectal carcinoma
APC	5q21	Colorectal, stomach, pancreatic
BRCA1	17q21	Breast, ovarian
BRCA2	13q12	Breast, ovarian, prostate
WT1	11p13	Wilms tumor
WT2	11p15	Rhabdomyosarcoma
NF1	17q11	Neurofibromatosis type 1, astrocytoma
NF2	22q12	Neurofibromatosis type 2, meningioma
VHL	3p25	Renal cell carcinoma
MEN1	11q23	Multiple endocrine neoplasia
MTS1	9p21	Melanoma, leukemia, sarcomas, several carcinomas

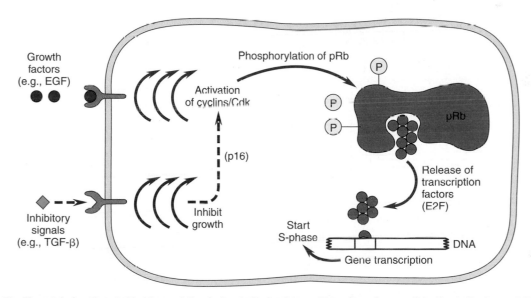

FIGURE 7-9 The Rb protein functions to bind transcription factors in the nucleus and keep them from participating in the transcription of cell cycle–related genes. pRb is induced to release its hold on the E2F transcription factors when it is sufficiently phosphorylated by cyclin-dependent kinases *(Cdk)*. Cyclin-dependent kinases are activated by cyclin proteins that accumulate when growth factors bind to receptors and stimulate growth pathways. Other signals, such as transforming growth factor-β *(TGF-β)*, inhibit the activity of cyclin/Cdk through activation of inhibitory proteins such as p16. A loss of pRb function removes the "major brake" on cell division. *P,* Phosphate group; *EGF,* epidermal growth factor.

the sequence of many of these genes provides the opportunity to screen individuals with familial cancers to determine whether they carry a defective gene. Detection of defective tumor suppressor genes is easier than figuring out their normal cellular functions, but steady progress is being made.

Why do tumor suppressor genes stop functioning? As with proto-oncogene activation, genetic mutations are the usual culprits. Chromosome deletions, point mutations, or chromosome loss through nondisjunction may knock out tumor suppressor gene function. Tumor suppressor gene function may also be lost through an "epigenetic" process that "silences" the gene. Epigenetic influences do not change the DNA sequence (no mutation is required), but change the packaging

of DNA and chemically modify it (e.g. methylation) so that the gene is inactivated. This inactivation can be passed on to daughter cells during mitosis.

The *Rb* Gene

The *Rb* gene codes for a large protein in the cell nucleus (pRb) that has been labeled the "master brake" of the cell cycle (see Chapter 3). It blocks cell division by binding transcription factors (primarily E2F) and thereby inhibiting them from transcribing the genes that initiate the cell cycle (Figure 7-9). The Rb protein can be induced to release the transcription factors when it is sufficiently phosphorylated. Proliferation-promoting signals in the cell increase cyclin-dependent kinase

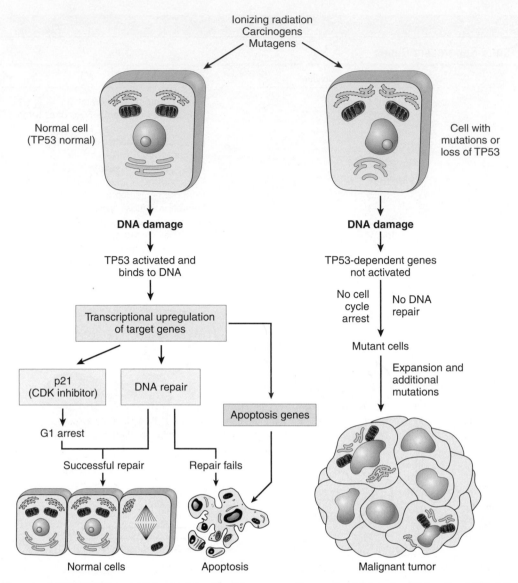

FIGURE 7-10 The role of *P53* (TP53) in maintaining the integrity of the genome. Damage to DNA in cells with functional *P53* stalls the cell cycle so that DNA can be repaired. If repair fails, then the cell undergoes apoptosis to prevent the proliferation of DNA-damaged cells. If the *P53* is not functional, genetically unstable cells may be allowed to survive and proliferate. (Redrawn from Kumar V et al: *Robbins basic pathology,* ed 8, Philadelphia, 2007, Saunders, p 196.)

(cdk) enzymes and promote pRb phosphorylation, whereas growth-inhibiting signals prevent phosphorylation. Thus an inactivating mutation of the *Rb* genes removes one of the major restraints on cell division. Defective pRb is common to a number of different cancers.

The *P53* Gene

The most common tumor suppressor gene defect identified in cancer cells involves *P53,* so named because of the protein's molecular mass of 53 kd (also called TP53). More than half of all types of human tumors lack functional *P53.* The p53 protein, like pRb, inhibits cell cycling. Unlike pRb, however, normally very little p53 is found in cells, and it accumulates only after cellular, particularly DNA, damage. P53 binds to damaged DNA and stalls cell division, presumably

to allow time for DNA repair before DNA replication in S phase (Figure 7-10). In the face of excessive damage (or other distress signals), p53 may direct the cell to initiate apoptosis. A defect in p53 function disrupts this important quality control system, allowing genetically damaged and unstable cells to survive and continue to replicate (see Figure 7-10). Genetically unstable cells have a propensity to accumulate more cancer-promoting mutations as they proliferate. The *P53* gene is important for therapeutic reasons as well. Chemotherapy- and radiation-induced cell death is mediated in large part by p53. These agents usually do not kill cancer cells directly; rather, they cause enough cellular damage in the target cell to trigger p53-mediated cell suicide. Cancer cells that lack functional p53 may therefore be resistant to some radiation and chemotherapeutic protocols.

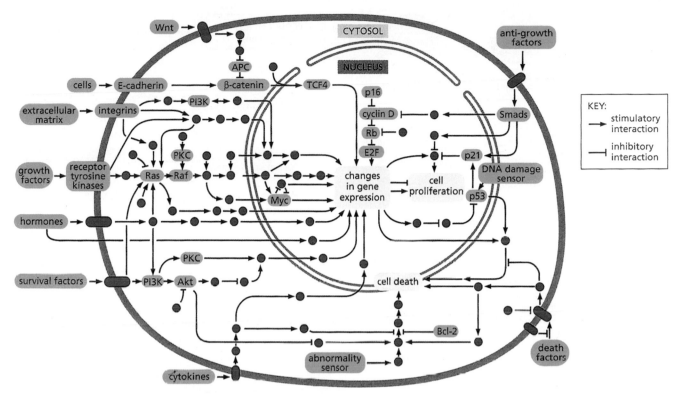

FIGURE 7-11 Diagram of the major signaling pathways relevant to human cancer. Overactivity of proto-oncogenes and underactivity of tumor suppressor genes result in enhanced cell proliferation and inhibition of appropriate cell death. More than 100 proto-oncogene products and numerous tumor suppressor gene products have been identified. (From Alberts B et al, editors: *Molecular biology of the cell,* ed 5, New York, 2008, Garland Science, p 1243.)

BRCA1 and BRCA2

Many tumor suppressor genes have been identified through studies of inherited predisposition to certain types of cancer. The breast cancer genes *BRCA1* and *BRCA2* are important examples. Women with a family history of breast cancer and an inherited defect in the *BRCA1* gene have about an 85% risk of developing breast cancer and a 40% to 60% risk of ovarian cancer.[16] The age of onset of inherited breast cancer is earlier than the onset of noninherited (sporadic) forms, and the prevalence of bilateral breast cancer is higher. Inherited forms of breast cancer account for only about 5% to 10% of all cases of breast cancer, but study of the genes involved is providing important insights into breast cancer biology in general.

Defects in numerous other tumor suppressor genes have been identified in certain types of cancers (see Table 7-5), including *APC* and *DCC* in colorectal cancer, *NF1* and *NF2* in neurofibromatosis, and *VHL* in renal cell cancers. The functions of tumor suppressor genes are varied, but most appear to inhibit proliferation or induce apoptosis in defective cells.

Figure 7-11 summarizes the major known cellular signaling pathways that are relevant to the development of cancer. The functions of oncogenes and tumor suppressor genes are shown to interact to determine cell proliferation, cell survival, and cell death. In general, any cellular alteration that promotes proliferation or inhibits cell death can contribute to an increased risk of tumor development.

KEY POINTS

- Cancer is thought to develop when proto-oncogenes become inappropriately activated in a cell or when tumor suppressor genes become inactivated. This change in gene function is usually due to mutations in the cell's DNA.
- Mutant proto-oncogenes disrupt the intercellular communication pathway that normally regulates cell proliferation. This disruption may occur through abnormal production of growth factors, receptors, cytoplasmic signaling molecules, or nuclear transcription factors.
- Both copies of a tumor suppressor gene usually must be inactivated to eliminate its function. Tumor suppressor genes inhibit cellular proliferation in various ways. The Rb protein serves as a "master brake" on cell proliferation by inhibiting transcription factors. P53 inhibits cell cycling when the cell is damaged to allow time for DNA repair. P53 is also important in initiating apoptosis of damaged or unwanted cells.

MULTISTEP NATURE OF CARCINOGENESIS

From the preceding discussion, it might seem that simply activating an oncogene in a normal cell or knocking out a tumor suppressor gene would be sufficient to transform it into

FIGURE 7-12 Synergy between oncogenes may be necessary to initiate malignant growth. **A,** The *ras* gene only. **B,** The *myc* gene only. **C,** Synergy between *ras* and *myc* genes.

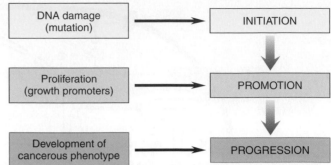

FIGURE 7-13 Theoretical steps in the development of cancer include initiation, promotion, and progression.

a malignant cell. Such has not proved to be the case. Growth regulation of mammalian cells appears to be organized in such a manner that a single aberrant gene is unable to induce conversion to full malignancy. Different genes work in distinct ways and may affect only a subset of the changes necessary to achieve full malignancy. For example, introduction of the *ras* oncogene into normal cells in culture causes them to show anchorage independence, but they are unable to form tumors when inoculated into an animal. Anchorage independence is a typical feature of most transformed cells and means that they are capable of proliferating even if they are not attached to a matrix. Normal cells will not divide and will initiate apoptosis if they do not have a space on the matrix on which to anchor themselves. Similarly, the *myc* oncogene allows cells to grow indefinitely in culture, but these immortal cells are still unable to induce tumor formation. However, when both the *ras* and *myc* oncogenes are introduced into normal cells, they become fully malignant (Figure 7-12).[17]

These culture experiments support the clinical observation that carcinogenesis is a multistep phenomenon.[2] The steps of carcinogenesis have been labeled *initiation, promotion,* and *progression* (Figure 7-13).

Initiation

Initiating events are thought to be the genetic mutations that inappropriately activate proto-oncogenes and inactivate tumor suppressor genes. However, the genetic mutations are not evident until the mutant cell proliferates. *Proliferation* is a requirement for cancer development, and nonproliferating cells cannot cause cancer. This explains why terminally differentiated tissues that have few or no stem cells, such as

cardiac and neurons, rarely become cancerous. It has been suggested that several mutations may be necessary to achieve full malignancy.[18] The development of colorectal cancer is a well-documented example of these sequential changes (Figure 7-14). Each individual cancer is likely to have its own unique combination of mutations that eventually lead to malignant behavior.

A number of etiologic agents are thought to be important initiators of cancer. The term *carcinogen* is applied to agents and substances capable of inducing cancer. Some carcinogens are complete carcinogens in that they are capable of the initiation of genetic damage as well as the promotion of cellular proliferation, whereas many others are only partial carcinogens. Partial carcinogens are often promoters that stimulate growth but are incapable of causing genetic mutations sufficient to initiate cancer by themselves. Examples of known carcinogens are ultraviolet and ionizing radiation, certain viruses, asbestos, and numerous chemicals. Most known chemical carcinogens are encountered through repeated occupational exposure (Table 7-6).

Promotion

Promotion is the stage during which the mutant cell proliferates. The transition from initiation to promotion may involve the activation of another oncogene or the inactivation of a tumor suppressor gene that has kept proliferation in check. Nonmutating factors may also be important in promoting cellular proliferation. For example, nutritional factors and infection may provide a stimulus for cellular proliferation. As previously described, proliferation is regulated by numerous hormonal growth factors. It is not surprising, then, that hormones may act as promoters of certain types of cancer.

The relationship between estrogen hormones and breast, ovarian, and uterine cancer is an important example. Epidemiologic studies indicate that the greater the number of menstrual cycles experienced, the higher the risk of these types of cancer developing. Women with early menarche, late first pregnancy, lack of breast-feeding, and late menopause have a greater risk of developing breast, uterine, and ovarian cancer. This enhanced susceptibility is thought to occur in part because of the greater lifetime estrogen exposure. Estrogen

FIGURE 7-14 The development of colorectal cancer illustrates the concept of multistep carcinogenesis. Derangement of several genes is likely to occur in most types of cancer. (Redrawn from Alberts B et al, editors: *Molecular biology of the cell,* ed 5, New York, 2008, Garland Science, p 1255.)

TABLE 7-6

Carcinogenicity to Humans for Selected Substances from the IARC Monograph Database

Chemical Family	Category*	Chemical Family	Category^
PAHs		**Metals (as compounds)**	
TCDD (dioxin)	1	Nickel	1
2,3,7,8-tetrachlorodibenzo-*p*-dioxin benzo[a]pyrene	2A	Chromium	1
		Cadmium	1
Benzo[a]anthracene	2A	Arsenic	1
PCBs (polychlorinated biphenyls)	2A	Beryllium	1
Benzo[b]fluoranthene	2B	Cobalt	2B
AAs		**Fibers**	
4-Aminobiphenyl	1	Silica (asbestos)	1
Benzidine	1	Wood dust	1
IQ (2-amino-3-methlimidazo[4,5-*f*]quinoline)	2A	Ceramic fibers	2B
MeIQ (2-amino-3,4-dimethylimidazo [4,4-*f*]quinoline)	2B	Glasswool	2B
		Acrylic fibers	3
PhIP (2-amino-1-methy-6-phenylimidazo [4,5-*b*]pyridine)	2B	**Others**	
4-Nitropyrene	2B	Vinyl chloride	1
		Tobacco smoke	1
Alkylating Agents		Tobacco products	1
Sulfur mustard	1	Cyclophosphamide	1
DMS, DES, ENU	2A	Sulfur mustard	1
EDB (ethylene dibromide)	2A	Nitrogen mustard	1
NNK (4-[*N*-nitrosomethylamino]- 1-[3-pyridyl]-1-butanone)	2B	Formaldehyde	2A
		Cisplatin	2A
Many nitrosamines	2B	Methylene chloride	2B
DMN (*N*-nitrosodimethylamine)	2A	Hydrazine	2B
		Hydrogen peroxide	3
Mycotoxins		Ethylene	3
Aflatoxins (naturally occurring)	1		
Aflatoxin M1	2B		
Sterigmatocystin	2B		

From Loechler E, Henry B, Seo K: Cellular responses to chemical carcinogens. In Coleman W, Tsongalis G, editors: *The molecular basis of human cancer,* Totowa, NJ, 2002, Humana Press, p 204.

*Categorization by group based on the following criteria of evaluation for agents as stated in the Preamble to the IARC Monographs. Group 1, The agent is carcinogenic to humans. This category is used when there is sufficient evidence of carcinogenicity in humans. Group 2, This category includes agents for which, at one extreme, the degree of evidence of carcinogenicity in humans is almost sufficient, as well as those for which, at the other extreme, there are no human data but for which there is evidence of carcinogenicity in experimental animals. Agents are assigned to either group 2A (probably carcinogenic to humans) or group 2B (possibly carcinogenic to humans). Group 3, The agent is not classifiable as to its carcinogenicity to humans. This category is used most commonly for agents, mixtures, and exposure circumstances for which the evidence of carcinogenicity is inadequate in humans and inadequate or limited in experimental animals. Group 4, The agent (mixture) is probably not carcinogenic to humans.

is a trophic hormone for these tissues and may therefore be viewed as having promoter effects. Treatment protocols using antiestrogen agents (tamoxifen) indicate that breast cancer risk may be reduced by blocking the effects of estrogen.[19,20] However, estrogen is not considered to be carcinogenic and does not cause genetic mutations.

A similar relationship has been identified for prostate cancer and testosterone hormones. In males, testosterone is secreted primarily from the testes under the influence of pituitary gonadotropins. Testosterone is a growth factor for the prostate gland and can act as a promoter of tumor formation in this tissue. This relationship is supported by the fact that therapeutic blocking of testosterone activity in persons with prostate cancer can help shrink the tumor.

Progression

Progression is the stage during which the mutant, proliferating cells begin to exhibit malignant behavior. The mutations suffered during initiation are not sufficient to cause all the biochemical changes necessary for malignant behavior. The proliferating cells are genetically unstable and undergo chance mutations that give them a growth advantage. Clones of mutant cells exhibit a wide variation in phenotype. *Phenotype* refers to the cell's traits, such as morphology, metabolism, and biochemical makeup. Cells whose phenotype gives them a growth advantage proliferate more readily. With each cycle of proliferation, an opportunity for chance variation arises. In the end, highly evolved tumor cells are generated that differ significantly from their normal ancestors. These cells have developed characteristics such as laminin receptors, lytic enzymes, and anchorage independence that enable them to behave malignantly.[21]

Cancer cells often have numerous abnormalities of chromosome structure, and the karyotype can be quite bizarre with bits and pieces of chromosomes attached in the wrong places and extra or missing chromosomes. An example of the chromosomes obtained from an ovarian cancer cell is shown in Figure 7-15. The color stains are specific for a particular chromosome, and each chromosome pair should be one color. Note the numerous multicolored chromosomes indicating multiple translocations of chromosome pieces.

To become malignant, cancer cells must also overcome the normal limits on the number of cell replications allowed before a cell stops dividing and enters senescence or dies. In the early 1970s it was discovered that normal somatic cells replicate only a finite number of times in culture: Fetal cells may replicate 80 or so times, whereas cells from older individuals divide only 20 or 30 times.[22] A mechanism whereby cells can track their history of cell division, as well as the way in which cancer cells may overcome it, has been proposed.[23] Each time a cell divides, it must replicate its DNA, but DNA polymerase is unable to copy the DNA strands all the way to the very tips of the chromosomes (called *telomeres*). The telomere thus shortens a bit with each cell division until some critical length is reached and cell division stops (see Chapter 4). Unicellular organisms and germ cells produce an enzyme called *telomerase* that promotes synthesis of the telomere ends and permits these cell types to replicate indefinitely. Most cancer cells begin to synthesize telomerase as they acquire the malignant phenotype, thus rescuing themselves from critical telomere shortening and gaining a mechanism for achieving immortality. In addition, the majority of cancers are deficient in p53 activity, which allows them to escape apoptosis despite gross derangements in DNA structure.

The fact that conversion from a normal cell type to a malignant cell type requires multiple steps implies many opportunities to intervene in the process. Prevention of the initiating mutation may be difficult inasmuch as carcinogens

FIGURE 7-15 Fluorescent images from human ovarian cancer (CH1) cells. A representative karyotype of CH1 cell line shows the balanced *t*(15;20) chromosomes (arrows). The size of one of the chromosome 2 (arrowhead) is slightly bigger than normal, which contains a duplication. (From Xueying Mao et al: Subtle genomic alterations and genomic instability revealed in diploid cancer cell lines, *Cancer Letters,* 267[1]: 49-54, August 2008.)

are ubiquitous; however, therapies to prevent promotion and progression could render the initial mutation harmless. As the biochemical processes governing promotion and progression become clearer, strategies for blocking these stages continue to be developed.

METASTASIS

Metastasis is the process whereby cancer cells escape their tissue of origin and initiate new colonies of cancer in distant sites. For tumor cells to gain access to the blood or lymphatic circulation, they must first escape the basement membrane of the tissue of origin, move through the extracellular space, and penetrate the basement membrane of the vessel. This process is thought to involve loss of cell-to-cell adhesion and binding to matrix components such as laminin via specific laminin receptors on the tumor cell, followed by release of enzymes such as proteases and collagenases that digest the basement membrane.[24] The cancer cell then squeezes through the rift by ameboid movement. The process is repeated at the vessel basement membrane to access the blood or lymphatic vessel. When the cell reaches the tissue to be colonized, it must again traverse the basement membranes by using similar mechanisms (Figure 7-16). Once in a new tissue setting, the cancer cell colony must acquire nutrients and a blood supply and cope with an environment that may differ considerably from its origin. In general, less differentiated cancer cells are better able to adapt to foreign tissues and survive.

FIGURE 7-16 The mechanisms of tumor invasion allow tumor cells to escape the site of origin, penetrate the basement membrane, and travel to distant sites. **A,** Tumor cells decrease cell-to-cell attachments via cadherins that allow detachment and migration toward the basement membrane. **B,** Enzymes that break down proteins are released into the area to form a rift. **C,** The tumor cell migrates away from the site of origin using laminin and fibronectin receptors to pull through the tissue. **D,** Finally the cell moves through a rift in the matrix. (From Kumar V et al: *Robbins basic pathology,* ed 8, Philadelphia, 2008, Saunders, p 202.)

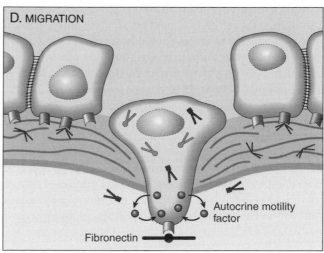

Patterns of Spread

The survival of tumor cells in the circulation is not guaranteed. They may be detected by immune cells and destroyed, or they may undergo apoptosis unless they quickly find a matrix on which to stick. Fewer than 1 in 10,000 of the cancer cells that enter the circulation survive to form a new tumor at a distant site.[24] Some tumor cell types appear to prefer specific target organs. Sometimes the pattern of metastasis is related to the circulatory flow. For example, metastatic tumors from the colon often seed the liver because they travel within the portal vein. The localization of most metastatic tumors is not so easily explained by blood flow patterns, and some tumor cells appear to "home" to specific targets. This homing tendency is poorly understood but may involve chemotactic signals from the organ to which the tumor cells respond. Cell surface receptors of the integrin and cell adhesion molecule families, which mediate cell-to-matrix and cell-to-cell adhesion, are likely to influence the choice of tissues that cancer cells invade. Spread via lymphatics is somewhat more predictable than spread by blood flow. Generally, the lymph nodes that immediately drain the tissue of cancer origin are colonized first, and then the tumor cells tend to spread contiguously from node to node. Hodgkin disease, a lymphoma, is particularly noted for its orderly spread via the lymphatics.

Because tumor cells exhibit various degrees of differentiation or resemblance to the parent tissue of origin, it may be difficult to determine the metastatic cancer's tissue of origin. **Tumor markers** are substances associated with tumor cells that may be helpful in identifying their tissue type. Identification of the tissue of origin has important implications for prognosis and selection of treatment. Tumor markers rely on the retention of at least some characteristics of the parent tissue type. Some tumor markers are released into the circulation, whereas others must be identified through biopsy of the metastatic tissue. Enzymes and other proteins that are specific to a particular cell type are commonly used as tumor markers. For example, production of thyroglobulin protein is specific for thyroid tumor cells. Melanoma cells express the antigens HMB-45 and S-100, which is helpful in identification as melanocytes. Unfortunately, most tumor markers are not very specific for cancer since the normal cells in the tissue of origin also produce them. Tumor markers are most useful as indicators for further diagnostic evaluation and to track the tumor activity. An increasing blood concentration of a specific tumor marker may indicate progression and proliferation of the cancer cells (increased tumor burden). See Table 7-7 for other examples of antigen, hormone, isoenzyme, and immunoglobulin markers used to identify tumor cell types.

Angiogenesis

Tumors cannot enlarge more than about 2 mm in diameter unless they grow blood vessels into the tumor mass to provide oxygen and nutrients. Angiogenesis is the process of forming new blood vessels. Most tumors do not induce angiogenesis until late in the stage of cancer development and so remain small and nonvascularized for years. The triggers that spur

TABLE 7-7

Selected Markers Useful for Tumor Identification

Marker	Commonly Associated Tumor
Antigens	
Carcinoembryonic antigen (CEA)	Adenocarcinoma of colon, pancreas, breast, ovary, lung, stomach
Desmin	Myogenic (muscle) sarcoma
CA 125	Ovarian, uterus, cervix, pancreas, others
CA 19-9	GI, pancreatic carcinoma; melanoma
CA 15-3	Breast cancer
CA 27-29	Breast cancer
HMB-45	Melanoma
S-100 protein	Melanoma
α-Fetoprotein	Hepatic carcinoma, gonadal tumors
Prostate-specific antigen (PSA)	Prostate cancer
Hormones	
Human chorionic gonadotropin	Gonadal tumors
Calcitonin	Medullary thyroid cancer
Thyroglobulin	Thyroid carcinoma
Isoenzymes	
Prostatic acid phosphatase	Prostate adenocarcinoma, leukemia, non-Hodgkin lymphoma
Neuron-specific enolase	Small cell carcinoma of lung, neuroblastoma
Immunoglobulins	
Monoclonal Ig	Multiple myeloma

Data from National Cancer Institute, National Institutes of Health, website: http://www.nci.nih.gov.

the cancer to begin angiogenesis are not completely understood. Tumor cells may begin to produce angiogenic factors such as vascular endothelial growth factor (VEGF) in response to hypoxia or other signals. VEGF stimulates proliferation of vascular endothelial cells, which then migrate to the tumor and orchestrate blood vessel development. Metastatic tumors must also initiate angiogenesis in their new locations or they will not survive. Therefore inhibition of angiogenesis is an important therapeutic goal to limit tumor growth and metastasis and continues to be an area of active research.

Grading and Staging of Tumors

Grading and staging of tumors are done to predict the clinical behavior of a malignant tumor and to guide therapy. **Grading** refers to the histologic characterization of tumor cells and is basically a determination of the degree of anaplasia. Most grading systems classify tumors into three or four classes of increasing degrees of malignancy. A greater degree of anaplasia indicates a greater malignant potential. The correlation between the grade of the tumor and its biological behavior is not perfect. Some low-grade tumors have proved to be quite malignant.

The choice of treatment modality is usually influenced more by the stage of the tumor than by its histologic grade. **Staging** describes the location and pattern of spread of a tumor within the host. Factors such as tumor size, extent of local growth, lymph node and organ involvement, and presence of distant metastases are considered. Several staging systems exist; however, the international TNM (*tumor*, *node*, *metastasis*) system is used extensively as a general framework for staging tumors.[25] Particular staging criteria vary with tumors in different organ systems. Examples of staging criteria for breast and colon cancer are shown in Tables 7-8 and 7-9.

In the past, tumor staging was based primarily on results of radiography and exploratory surgery. The availability of computed tomography (CT), magnetic resonance imaging (MRI), positron emission tomography (PET), as well as other highly sophisticated imaging techniques, has revolutionized cancer detection.[26] These imaging modalities allow noninvasive exploration of the tissues of the entire body. The computer-generated images can then be scrutinized for any signs of abnormality that might signal the presence of hidden tumors. CT and MRI rely primarily on detection of differences in tissue density and are therefore not totally specific for tumors. They can, however, guide the selection of sites for exploration and biopsy and potentially reduce unnecessary surgery. Positron emission tomography is a promising staging technology because it facilitates cancer detection based on molecular and biochemical processes within the tumor tissues (Figure 7-17). PET may be used in certain clinical situations in which CT has known limitations, such as differentiation of benign from malignant lymph nodes or other lesions, differentiation of residual tumor from scar tissue, or detection of unsuspected distant metastases.[26]

Antibodies can also be used to track down cancer cells in the body. Antibodies can be raised against specific antigens present on the surface of tumor cells. The antibodies are also bound to a tracer (e.g., a radioactive isotope such as iodine 125), which can be detected by imaging. As methods for identifying tumor antigens and raising specific antibodies have improved, this technology provides the potential for finding very small numbers of tumor cells hidden in the body.

The results of the staging procedure will determine which of the mainstays of cancer treatment—surgery, radiation therapy, or chemotherapy—may be used, singly or in combination, to destroy the cancer cells. Localized tumors may be managed with surgery and radiation therapy, whereas evidence of metastasis generally necessitates the addition of chemotherapy.

KEY POINTS

- Malignant cells produce specialized enzymes and receptors to enable them to escape their tissue of origin and metastasize.
- The spread of tumors generally occurs by way of the bloodstream or lymphatics. Tumor cells often lodge in the capillary beds of the organs that drain them, such as liver and lung. Some tumors appear to "home" to certain tissues.
- Grading and staging are done to predict tumor behavior and guide therapy. Grading is the histologic characterization of tumor cells, whereas staging describes the location and pattern of tumor spread within the host.
- The TNM staging system is used to describe the tumor size, lymph nodes affected, and degree of metastasis.

EFFECTS OF CANCER ON THE BODY

The effects of cancer on the host vary widely, depending on the location of the tumor and the extent of metastasis. Early-stage cancer may be asymptomatic. As the tumor increases in size and spreads through the body, a number of symptoms typically become apparent, including pain, cachexia, immune suppression, and infection. Once treatment has begun, patients may also suffer hair loss and sloughing of mucosal membranes. The American Cancer Society has published the seven warning signs of cancer as a way of encouraging the public to seek early evaluation of potential cancers (Box 7-1). The presentation of cancer in children differs from that in adults, and special warning signs have been identified for the pediatric population (Box 7-2).

Pain is a common and feared complication of the disease process. Pain may be due to invasion of metastatic cells into organs or bone and subsequent activation of pain and pressure receptors in these tissues. Tissue destruction and inflammation may contribute to cancer pain. Cancer treatment may contribute to overall pain because of procedures requiring biopsy and intravenous drug administration. Pain can usually be controlled through the use of analgesics. The use of patient-controlled analgesia has been effective in reducing patient fears of inadequate therapy for pain (see Chapter 47).

Cachexia refers to an overall weight loss and generalized weakness (Figure 7-18). Many factors contribute to cancer cachexia, including loss of appetite (anorexia) and increased metabolic rate. Anorexia accompanies many disease processes and may result from toxins released by the cancer cells or immune cells. Cancer patients may have aversions to specific foods and may feel full after only a few bites. Nausea and vomiting are common complications of cancer therapy and contribute to decreased nutrient intake. Despite the minimal nutrient intake, body metabolism remains high. Production of tumor necrosis factor (TNF) and other immune cytokines is thought to be important in producing the hypermetabolic state. Nutrients are mobilized from fat and protein stores in the body and consumed by the hypermetabolic cells (see Chapter 42). Some patients may require nutritional supplementation by enteral or parenteral routes.

Individuals with cancer often demonstrate deficits in immune system competence. Cancer cells secrete substances that suppress the immune system. Individuals with cancer may have reduced populations of T and B cells and may respond poorly to injected antigens. The mechanisms by which cancer

TABLE 7-8

TNM Staging Criteria for Breast Cancer

Primary Tumor (T)

TX	Primary tumor cannot be assessed
T0	No evidence of primary tumor
Tis	Carcinoma in situ, intraductal carcinoma, lobular carcinoma in situ, or Paget disease of the nipple with no tumor
T1	Tumor 2 cm or less in greatest dimension
T1mic	Microinvasion 0.1 cm or less in greatest dimension
T1a	Tumor 0.5 cm or less in greatest dimension
T1b	Tumor more than 0.5 cm but not more than 1 cm in greatest dimension
T1c	Tumor more than 1 cm but not more than 2 cm in greatest dimension
T2	Tumor more than 2 cm but not more than 5 cm in greatest dimension
T3	Tumor more than 5 cm in greatest dimension
T4	Tumor of any size with direct extension to chest wall or skin
T4a	Extension to chest wall, not including pectoralis muscle
T4b	Edema (including peau d'orange) or ulceration of skin of the breast or satellite nodules confined to the same breast
T4c	Both T4a and T4b
T4d	Inflammatory carcinoma

Lymph Node (N)

NX	Regional lymph nodes cannot be assessed (e.g., previously removed)
N0	No regional lymph node metastasis
N1	Metastasis to movable ipsilateral axillary lymph node(s)
N2	Metastasis to ipsilateral axillary lymph node(s) fixed to one another or to other structures
N2a	Metastasis in ipsilateral axillary lymph nodes fixed to one another (matted) or to other structures
N2b	Metastasis only in clinically apparent* ipsilateral internal mammary nodes and in the *absence* of clinically evident axillary lymph node metastasis
N3	Metastasis in ipsilateral infraclavicular lymph node(s) with or without axillary lymph node involvement, or in clinically apparent* ipsilateral internal mammary lymph node(s) and in the *presence* of clinically evident axillary lymph node metastasis; or metastasis in ipsilateral supraclavicular lymph node(s) with or without axillary or internal mammary lymph node involvement
N3a	Metastasis in ipsilateral infraclavicular lymph node(s)
N3b	Metastasis in ipsilateral internal mammary lymph node(s) and axillary lymph node(s)
N3c	Metastasis in ipsilateral supraclavicular lymph node(s)

Distant Metastasis (M)

MX	Presence of distance metastasis cannot be assessed
M0	No distant metastasis
M1	Distant metastasis

Stage Grouping

Stage 0	Tis	N0	M0
Stage I	T1	N0	M0
Stage IIA	T0	N1	M0
	T1	N1	M0
	T2	N0	M0
Stage IIB	T2	N1	M0
	T3	N0	M0
Stage IIIA	T0	N2	M0
	T1	N2	M0
	T2	N2	M0
	T3	N1	M0
	T3	N2	M0
Stage IIIB	T4	Any N	M0
Stage IIIC	Any T	N3	M0
Stage IV	Any T	Any N	M1

Adapted from Greene F: *AJCC cancer staging handbook,* ed 6, New York, 2002, Springer-Verlag, pp 263-266.

Clinically apparent is defined as detected by imaging studies (excluding lymphoscintigraphy) or by clinical examination or grossly visible pathologically.

TABLE 7-9

TNM Staging Criteria for Colon Cancer

Primary Tumor (T)

TX	Primary tumor cannot be assessed
T0	No evidence of primary tumor
Tis	Carcinoma in situ: intraepithelial or invasion of lamina propria
T1	Tumor invades submucosa
T2	Tumor invades muscularis propria
T3	Tumor invades through the muscularis propria into the subserosa, or into nonperitonealized pericolic or perirectal tissues
T4	Tumor directly invades other organs or structures, and/or perforates visceral peritoneum

Regional Lymph Nodes (N)

NX	Regional lymph nodes cannot be assessed
N0	No regional lymph node metastasis
N1	Metastasis in 1-3 regional lymph nodes
N2	Metastasis in 4 or more regional lymph nodes

Distant Metastasis (M)

MX	Distant metastasis cannot be assessed
M0	No distant metastasis
M1	Distant metastasis

Stage Grouping

Stage 0	Tis	N0	M0
Stage I	T1	N0	M0
	T2	N0	M0
Stage IIA	T3	N0	M0
Stage IIB	T4	N0	M0
Stage IIIA	T1-T2	N1	M0
Stage IIIB	T3-T4	N1	M0
Stage IIIC	Any T	N2	M0
Stage IV	Any T	Any N	M1

Adapted from Greene F: *AJCC cancer staging handbook,* ed 6, New York, 2002, Springer-Verlag, pp 131-132.

cells depress immune responses are not well understood, but the prognosis for cancer recovery is poorer when the immune system is depressed. Immune cells, including cytotoxic T cells and natural killer (NK) cells, actively detect and destroy cancer cells.

In addition to the general immunodepressive effects of cancer, some cancer cells have developed ways to elude immune system detection.[27] For example, cancer cells can internalize their immunoreactive cell surface antigens when antibodies attach to them. A reduction in antigenic sites decreases the likelihood of further stimulation of antibody production. Some tumors escape detection because they are coated with normal extracellular matrix molecules such as glycoproteins. The glycoproteins physically cover up the antigenic tumor markers. Tumor cells that closely resemble normal cells may trigger the production of regulatory T cells that suppress the activity of other immune cells. Regulatory T cells are a subclass of T lymphocytes. The conditions that activate them are as yet poorly understood, but they are probably important in keeping the immune system in check so that normal tissues are not attacked. Difficulty differentiating between the tumor cell and a normal cell may result in the production of regulatory T cells that actually aid tumor cell growth.

Bone marrow suppression contributes to the anemia, leukopenia, and thrombocytopenia that often accompany cancer. Bone marrow suppression may be due to invasion and destruction of blood-forming cells in the bone marrow, poor nutrition, and chemotherapeutic drugs. *Anemia* refers to a deficiency in circulating red cells. In addition to decreased production of blood cell precursors in the bone marrow, anemia may result from chronic or acute bleeding. The signs and symptoms of anemia, such as fatigue, increased heart rate, and increased respiratory rate, are related to a decrease in oxygen-carrying capacity.

Leukopenia refers to a decrease in circulating white blood cells (leukocytes). Malignant invasion of the bone marrow is a primary cause of leukopenia, with malnutrition and chemotherapy being contributing factors. A deficiency in white blood cells reduces the patient's ability to fight infection, which is a major cause of morbidity and mortality in cancer patients. Often the offending organism is *opportunistic;* it is unable to infect an immunocompetent host and becomes virulent only when a person is immunocompromised. Infections are very difficult to manage because the host is unable to mount an effective immune response. Infections are also difficult to prevent because the majority of the infecting organisms are

FIGURE 7-17 PET scan that detects uptake of radioactively labeled glucose is overlaid onto a CT scan background image. The yellow spots in the abdomen and mediastinum are indicative of multiple metastases of non-Hodgkin lymphoma. (From Alberts B et al, editors: *Molecular biology of the cell*, ed 5, New York, 2008, Garland Science, p 1206. Courtesy Dr. Sanjiv Sam Gambhir.)

BOX 7-1

Cancer's Seven Warning Signs

Change in bowel or bladder habits
A sore that does not heal
Unusual bleeding or discharge
Thickening or lump in breast or elsewhere
Indigestion or difficulty swallowing
Obvious change in wart or mole
Nagging cough or hoarseness

BOX 7-2

Cancer's Warning Signs in Children

Continued, unexplained weight loss
Headaches with vomiting in the morning
Increased swelling or persistent pain in bones or joints
Lump or mass in abdomen, neck, or elsewhere
Development of whitish appearance in pupil of the eye
Recurrent fevers not caused by infections
Excessive bleeding or bruising
Noticeable paleness or prolonged tiredness

FIGURE 7-18 General emaciated appearance in cancer cachexia. (From Jarvis C: *Physical examination and health assessment,* ed 2, Philadelphia, 1996, Saunders, p 297.)

from the patient's own endogenous flora (skin, gastrointestinal tract). The development of severe leukopenia or infection during treatment may necessitate changes in the chemotherapeutic regimen to allow bone marrow recovery.

Thrombocytopenia is a deficiency in circulating platelets, which are important mediators of blood clotting. Platelet deficiencies predispose to life-threatening hemorrhage. A platelet count of less than 20,000/mm^3 has been associated with spontaneous hemorrhage.

Anemia, leukopenia, and thrombocytopenia may be managed by administration of blood products containing red blood cells, white blood cells, and platelets, respectively. In fact, blood replacement therapy is used more often in cancer patients than in any other medical condition. When chemotherapy is terminated, stem cells in the bone marrow generally recover and the production of blood cells resumes. In some cases, the production of red and white blood cells can be enhanced by treating the patient with specific growth factors, such as erythropoietin (Epogen) or granulocyte-stimulating factors (Neupogen).

Hair loss and the sloughing of mucosal membranes are complications of radiation therapy and chemotherapy. Treatment is designed to kill the rapidly proliferating cancer cells, but normal cells with high growth rates such as mucosal epithelia and hair follicle cells are also damaged. Damaged mucosa is a primary source of cancer pain and anorexia, and may provide a portal for the invasion of organisms from the skin or gastrointestinal tract.

Paraneoplastic syndromes are symptom complexes that cannot be explained by obvious tumor properties and occur in 10% to 15% of patients with cancer. Many of the syndromes are associated with excessive production of hormones or cytokines by the tumor. Common paraneoplastic syndromes include (1) hypercalcemia, (2) Cushing syndrome secondary to excess adrenocorticotropic hormone (ACTH) secretion, and (3) hyponatremia and water overload secondary to excess antidiuretic hormone (SIADH, syndrome of inappropriate ADH) secretion. Small cell carcinoma of the lung is commonly the culprit for excess ACTH and ADH syndromes. Hypercalcemia (elevated serum calcium) is a paraneoplastic syndrome associated with abnormal production of parathyroid hormone–related protein (PTHrP) by the tumor cells. Unexplained hypercalcemia is regarded as evidence of cancer until proven otherwise. Hypercalcemia may be a consequence of metastatic bone cancer, and in this case it would be an expected finding rather than a paraneoplastic syndrome.

If left untreated, cancer has the potential to kill the host. The cause of death is multifactorial. Infection, hemorrhage, and organ failure are the primary causes of cancer death. The failure of cancer-ridden organs such as liver, kidney, brain, and lung results in the loss of life-sustaining functions. Treatment for cancer can also be detrimental to the host by contributing to immunosuppression and platelet deficiencies. The cumulative effects of one or more of these factors may lead to death.

KEY POINTS

- Regardless of the type of malignancy, affected individuals exhibit characteristic signs and symptoms, including pain, cachexia, bone marrow suppression, and infection.
- Bone marrow suppression is manifested as anemia, leukopenia, and thrombocytopenia.
- Immunosuppression with consequent infection is a primary cause of cancer-associated death.

CANCER THERAPY

The overall 5-year survival rate for patients with cancer is approximately 66%, with some types of cancer having much higher or lower rates.[3] Early detection of cancer, while it remains localized in the tissue of origin, is associated with the best prognosis for cure. Cure implies eradication of all cancer cells in the body and is different than the 5-year survival rate. Patients with metastatic invasion of regional lymph nodes still have a good opportunity for cure with appropriate therapy. Widespread invasion of multiple tissues and organs is associated with a poor prognosis, and therapy may be aimed at remission or palliation of symptoms rather than cure. The mainstays of cancer therapy are surgery, radiation therapy, and drug therapy. In some hormone-sensitive tumors (breast, prostate), hormonal blocking drugs may be used.

Immunotherapy and targeted molecular therapies have begun to emerge as important treatments for specific cancers. Traditional forms of treatment are not selective for cancer cells and result in unavoidable damage to normal tissue. The immune system, on the other hand, is noted for its ability to make subtle distinctions between normal and abnormal or foreign cells. Recognition of tumor cells as different from their normal counterparts is the basis of tumor immunology. Recognition depends on the expression of abnormal molecules or antigens on the cancer cell surface (Figure 7-19). Unfortunately, most tumor-associated antigens are also expressed to some degree on normal cells, which makes it difficult to develop strategies to target cancer cells selectively.

Transplantation of stem cells from the bone marrow or peripheral blood is an increasingly important aspect of cancer treatment for leukemia, lymphoma, and some solid tumors. The choice of treatment depends largely on the results of the staging procedure. A greater degree of metastasis generally requires a more aggressive therapeutic approach.

Surgery

The majority of patients with solid tumors are treated surgically, which can be curative in some localized cancers. The main benefit of surgery is removal of a tumor with minimal

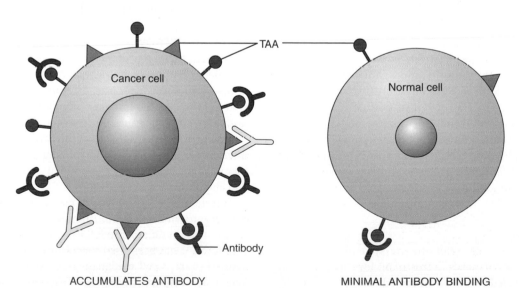

ACCUMULATES ANTIBODY   MINIMAL ANTIBODY BINDING

FIGURE 7-19 Cancer cells express abnormal antigens (tumor-associated antigens *[TAA]*) on their cell surface that can activate immune cells or be used as targets for monoclonal antibodies.

damage to other body cells. The surgeon generally removes a margin of normal-appearing tissue around the resected tumor to ensure complete tumor removal. Lymph nodes are subjected to biopsy and also removed if evidence of metastasis is present. Surgical resection of some tumors can be tricky if vital structures such as neurons or blood vessels are involved.

Surgery involves risks related to anesthesia, infection, and blood loss. The surgical procedure may be disfiguring or may result in loss of function. Surgical resection as the sole treatment for solid tumors is curative in a minority of patients because most patients already have undetectable metastases at the time of diagnosis.[28] There is evidence that tumor surgery can alter the behavior of the tumor and predispose the patient to recurrence.[28] Therefore, surgical resection is commonly accompanied by radiation therapy or chemotherapy. Even one remaining cancer cell could be sufficient to reinitiate tumor formation.

Radiation Therapy

Ionizing radiation is used for two principal reasons: to kill tumor cells that are not resectable because of location in a vital or inaccessible area and to kill tumor cells that may have escaped the surgeon's knife and remain undetected in the local area. Radiation kills cells by damaging their nuclear DNA. Cells that are rapidly cycling are more susceptible to radiation death because there is little time for DNA repair. Radiation may not kill cells directly; rather, it may initiate apoptosis. The *P53* tumor suppressor gene is an important mediator of this response. Many tumors have mutant *P53* and may be less susceptible to radiation-induced cell death.

It is difficult to kill all the cells of a large tumor by irradiation because they are heterogeneous; they are in different phases of mitosis and are cycling at different rates. A single radiation dose large enough to kill all the tumor cells would be sufficient to kill the normal cells as well. Radiation is often administered in smaller doses over several treatments and is most effective at eradicating small groups of tumor cells. It is often used in combination with surgery. Radiation is also useful for palliative reductions in tumor size. Pain from bone and brain tumors may be effectively managed with radiation therapy that shrinks the tumor. Tumors with bleeding surfaces may be coagulated with radiation to decrease blood loss.

A certain degree of destruction of normal cells in the irradiated field is expected with radiation therapy. Radiation is best used when tumor cells are regionally located. Total-body irradiation to kill tumor cells in disseminated locations is not recommended because of the likelihood of life-threatening tissue damage, although it may be used in preparation for bone marrow or peripheral stem cell transplantation.

Drug Therapy

Chemotherapy generally refers to the systemic administration of anticancer chemicals as treatment for cancers that are known or suspected to be disseminated in the body. Unlike surgery or radiation therapy, which is locally or regionally applied, parenterally administered chemotherapeutic drugs can find their cancer cell targets in areas throughout the entire body.

Most chemotherapeutic agents are cytotoxic because they interfere with some aspect of cell division. The more rapidly dividing cells are more susceptible to the killing effects of chemotherapeutic agents. In a large tumor mass, the rates of cell division are very diverse, with many slowly dividing cells. At any one time, only a portion of the tumor cells are in a cell cycle stage that is susceptible to chemotherapy. Several courses of chemotherapy are generally necessary to ensure that all tumor cells have been killed. It is difficult to kill slowly cycling tumor cells without also killing normal cells that are cycling at approximately the same rate. Small tumors are easier to eradicate because rates of cell division are generally faster. To prevent relapse, the "stem" cells that give rise to clones of malignant cells must be destroyed. Unfortunately, stem cells may not divide as rapidly as other cells. Resection or irradiation to reduce tumor size may prompt the stem cells to divide, thus making them more susceptible to chemotherapy. Tumor cells with mutations of the *P53* gene may be resistant to chemotherapeutic agents that work by damaging DNA, so drugs that work by interfering with the cancer cell cycle in other ways may be more effective.

Chemotherapeutic agents are not selective for tumor cells, and a certain amount of normal cell death also occurs. Rapidly dividing cells, particularly those of the bone marrow, intestinal epithelia, and hair follicles, are most affected. Bone marrow depression is a most serious side effect inasmuch as it predisposes the patient to anemia, bleeding, and infection.

New approaches to cancer drug therapy have emerged that indirectly inhibit tumors rather than seeking to kill tumor cells directly. A promising approach is to interrupt the tumor's blood supply. To proliferate, solid tumors must be supplied by a progressively expanding network of capillaries. The development of new capillaries, called *angiogenesis,* is accomplished by migration and growth of endothelial cells. Antiangiogenic drugs block the development of new capillaries.

Immunotherapy

Harnessing the power of the immune system to fight cancer is a particularly appealing idea because of the potential for *specificity.* Despite much progress in understanding the immune system in the last several years, the hope for effective immunotherapy for cancer has not yet been fully realized. Current modes of immunomodulation primarily involve the use of interferons, interleukins, and monoclonal antibodies. These therapies are generally used as adjuncts to surgery, irradiation, and chemotherapy.

Interferons are glycoproteins produced by immune cells in response to viral infection. Interferons inhibit cell proliferation and are stimulatory to NK cells, T cells, and macrophages. Interferon-α has been used successfully to treat hairy cell leukemia (a rare B-cell malignancy), chronic myelogenous leukemia, and multiple myeloma.[29] Interferon therapy produces symptoms similar to those of a viral infection: fever, chills, and muscle aches.

Interleukins are peptides produced and secreted by white blood cells. They are also called lymphokines or cytokines. Interleukin-2 (IL-2) is an important cytokine secreted by activated T-helper cells. It stimulates the proliferation of T cells, NK cells, and macrophages. IL-2 can be used to stimulate the growth of these immune cells in culture. Immune cells taken from a patient's blood can be grown in culture in the presence of IL-2. Then the greatly expanded number of immune cells can be given back to the patient, along with intravenous infusions of IL-2. Such treatment has been associated with regression of some tumors (melanoma, renal cell carcinoma).[30] Because IL-2 toxicity is high and many individuals have severe allergic reactions, the benefit of therapy must be weighed against the risks for each individual situation.

The use of monoclonal antibodies (antibodies having identical structure) in cancer therapy is currently the subject of intense investigation. Monoclonal antibodies specifically bind with target antigens and can therefore be used in several ways as treatment for cancer. Antibodies can be used to deliver a cytotoxic drug preferentially to the cancer cell and thus minimize drug interactions with normal cells. Similarly, antibodies can be used to direct other cytotoxic cells, such as NK and T cells, to tumor cells lurking in the body. Antibodies can be attached to a radioactive label and injected into a patient to screen for recurrence of tumor growth. Antibodies can also be directed against cells that support tumor growth.

Monoclonal antibodies have been developed for management of several cancers. For example, nearly 25% of breast cancers have overexpression of the HER2 receptor on the surface of malignant cells. The monoclonal antibody trastuzumab specifically binds to this HER2 protein and helps immune cells to find and kill the tumor cells.

Gene and Molecular Therapy

Because cancer is fundamentally a disorder of gene function, the use of gene therapy to alter the malignant behavior of cells may have high therapeutic potential. As specific gene derangements are identified for particular tumors, gene therapy may be used to suppress overactive oncogenes or replenish missing tumor suppressor function. Current uses of gene therapy for cancer include genetic alteration of tumor cells to make them more susceptible to cytotoxic agents or immune recognition, and genetic alteration of immune cells to make them more efficient killers of tumor cells. A number of these approaches to therapy have shown promise in clinical trials.

For example, human brain tumors have been managed by insertion of a viral gene for thymidine kinase. Introduction of this gene makes the tumor cells susceptible to subsequent treatment with the antiviral drug ganciclovir.[31] Tumor cells can also be made more recognizable to immune cells by insertion of genes that cause the tumor cells to express "foreign" proteins on their cell surface. This type of gene therapy has shown some benefit in melanoma and renal carcinoma. Replacement of genes for *P53* is an attractive therapy because tumor cells would be more susceptible to apoptosis.

Gene replacement of other tumor suppressors such as *pRb* or *APC* in those tumors that are deficient could help inhibit tumor proliferation.

Gene therapy can be directed at cells other than tumor cells to enhance the body's cancer defenses. One such approach involves harvesting immune cells from the cancer patient, inserting IL-2 genes, and then returning the genetically enhanced immune cells to the patient. The enhanced immune cells attack the tumor cells more vigorously than normal immune cells do and have been shown to persist in the body for 6 months or longer.

At present, gene therapy is limited by difficulty in delivering the new genes to the target cells. As methods improve, gene therapy will become an increasingly important part of cancer prevention and management.

Molecular therapies that target cytoplasmic signaling pathways have also been developed. For example, in chronic myelogenous leukemia a chromosomal rearrangement results in the abnormal production of an enzyme, BCR/ABL. This enzyme stimulates cell proliferation and contributes to the overproduction of leukemic cells. An agent that specifically inhibits this enzyme (Gleevec) has dramatically improved the management of this disease. Other drugs that specifically target abnormal tumor products are under development.

Stem Cell Transplantation

Transplantation of hematologic stem cells is used to manage life-threatening disorders in which the patient's bone marrow is incapable of manufacturing white blood cells, red blood cells, or platelets. Most often, nonfunctional marrow is a consequence of the high-dose chemotherapy and radiation used to manage hematologic malignancies such as leukemia and lymphoma. Stem cell transplantation also has been applied to other malignancies (e.g., breast cancer) and to nonmalignant disorders (e.g., aplastic anemia, sickle cell anemia, and thalassemia). Stem cells can be harvested from aspirates of bone marrow or from the donor's peripheral bloodstream. Bone marrow is rich in stem cells, but the peripheral blood is poor. The stem cell donor can be a tissue-matched individual (allogeneic), an identical twin (syngeneic), or the patient in question (autologous). A closer match between donor and recipient is associated with a better outcome.

Before infusion of donor stem cells, the patient's own immune cells must be suppressed to prevent transplant rejection. It is also necessary to eliminate any residual malignant cells from the body to avoid relapse of the cancer. Both of these objectives are accomplished through high-dose chemotherapy and total-body irradiation regimens, which leave the patient susceptible to severe anemia, infection, and bleeding. The therapeutic goal of stem cell transplantation is to restore immune and hematopoietic function. It may take weeks to months for the infused stem cells to set up housekeeping and begin to proliferate in their new host. During this time, the transplant recipient requires intensive monitoring and management of complications.

PART 3

Alterations in Immune and Inflammatory Response

Frontiers of Research

Immune System Responses

Sheila K. Smith • Peter A. Valen • Michael J. Kirkhorn

The human body is under constant attack by outside and, occasionally, unrecognized inside invaders. These invaders, including microbes, cancer cells, and abnormal protein fragments, may overcome recognition and establish a foothold. A large portion of the body's defense is provided by the immune system, which functions to recognize foreign invaders, mobilize protective forces, and remove or neutralize antigens. When the system fails to mount an adequate defense or mistakes our own healthy tissue as foreign, disease can result.

Today, largely through research into autoimmune disease, cancer, and the virus that causes acquired immunodeficiency syndrome (human immunodeficiency virus [HIV]), we are learning more about how the immune system works.

The immune system is an intricate network of organs, cells, and soluble proteins that functions to distinguish between "self" and "nonself." The immune system can be divided into innate immunity, with which we are born, and learned or adaptive immunity, which is acquired during life as we encounter foreign substances (antigens).

The components of the immune system involved in innate immunity—including macrophages, neutrophils, and complement—recognize a wide range of foreign antigens. Adaptive immunity, on the other hand, is specific to the particular antigen encountered. Because of adaptive immunity, the immune system can remember a previously encountered antigen and respond in a quick and vigorous way. This memory is carried by lymphocytes, which are long-lived cells. This immune response is why people generally have infectious diseases like chickenpox and measles only once, and it is also responsible for the success of vaccinations in preventing disease. Dwindling of immune memory over time accounts for the later development of herpes zoster (shingles) many years after a chicken pox infection.

The human immune system may be outsmarted by new forms of infection, such as viruses transmitted from another species, quickly evolving pathogens or viruses like HIV or cancer cells, exposure to novel pathogens as a result of rapid worldwide travel, or drug-resistant strains of organisms.

Occasionally the immune system malfunctions by misinterpreting the body's tissues as foreign, resulting in autoimmune disease. These diseases can be triggered in several ways. If tissue that is normally sequestered and therefore "hidden" from the immune system, such as fluid in the eyeball, escapes as a result of disease or injury, the immune system may react against it. Normal body tissues may be altered by viruses, drugs, sunlight, or radiation and therefore

Mast cell. This colorized micrograph shows a mast cell filled with dense red granules of the inflammation mediator called histamine. (*From Wilson SF, Thompson JM:* Respiratory disorders, *St Louis, 1990, Mosby.*)

Defense

become immunogenic. The immune system, responding to a foreign antigen, may mistakenly attack normal tissues that resemble the foreign antigen, as occurs in rheumatic fever following a streptococcal infection. Abnormal protein fragments may become entrapped or hidden within the complex lipoprotein structure of cell membranes, only much later resulting in an antigenic response when released from the cell membrane through normal physiologic processes. Finally, lymphocytes may be transformed by viruses or cancer and overproduce antibodies against normal human tissue. Examples of autoimmune diseases include multiple sclerosis, systemic lupus, Graves disease, rheumatoid arthritis, and type I diabetes mellitus. Other conditions that may represent autoimmune processes or include an autoimmune component include fibromyalgia, Crohn disease, scleroderma, and atherosclerosis. Autoimmune conditions are common, affecting about 5% of adults in Europe and North America, and predominate in women.

Research on the causes and treatment of these and other autoimmune diseases is proceeding rapidly. We are learning more about the precise genetic factors involved in the pathogenesis of these conditions. Research initiatives have led to information on gene markers and gene expression. Linkage studies can demonstrate whether a particular genetic variant is more often present in affected family members than in healthy family members. This methodology can identify areas of chromosomes associated with susceptibility to certain diseases. Ultimately, if a gene mutation responsible for a particular disease can be identified, as in severe combined immunodeficiency (SCID), for example, gene-transfer therapy may yield a cure.

Advances in genetic engineering and immunology are also leading to more effective vaccines. One such exciting development is the use of DNA vaccines. DNA coding for a foreign antigen is injected into an animal, resulting in direct production of the foreign antigen by host cells. These vaccines should result in fewer side effects because the foreign antigen is coming from the host itself. These vaccines should also be easier and less expensive to produce than conventional vaccines. Trials are under way using DNA vaccines against influenza, herpes simplex, T-cell lymphoma, and HIV. Potential risks include the possibility that the vaccine's DNA will be integrated into host chromosomes and turn on oncogenes or turn off suppressor genes or that prolonged immunostimulation by foreign antigens could lead to autoimmune disease.

Understanding the immune system and its various responses is critical to an understanding of not only the causes, but also the prevention, treatment, or even cure of human diseases.

Infectious Processes

Lorrie J. Dawson

KEY QUESTIONS

■ What is the role of epidemiology in the identification, definition, and prevention of infectious diseases?

■ What factors influence the transmission of infectious agents?

■ How do infectious microorganisms, including bacteria, viruses, fungi, and parasites, differ in structure, life cycle, and infectious processes?

■ What conditions compromise host defenses against microorganisms?

■ What are opportunistic infections, and when do they develop?

CHAPTER OUTLINE

I nfection is the cause of death for many people afflicted with a chronic or critical illness, with the very young and the very old being particularly susceptible to infection. Infections are caused by microorganisms that gain entry into the body. Once sufficient quantities of a microorganism adhere to or invade the human body, the signs and symptoms generally associated with infection are generated. The microorganisms that cause infection are called *pathogens,* and the major types of pathogens include bacteria, viruses, fungi, and parasites.

Different pathogens inhabit various environments such as hospitals, the food supply, water, and animal or human vectors. For example, many hospitalized patients are at risk for the development of sepsis, an overwhelming infection that may lead to shock, multiple organ failure, and death. The methods of preserving the food supply have an impact on transmission of infections, as do the location, density, and sanitary practices of a population. Globalization of the world's population, with the associated rapidity and extent of air travel, has major implications for the worldwide spread of infectious agents before the infected individual becomes symptomatic or identifiable.

Infection with pathogenic microorganisms has become a tool of war and terrorism in the world. "Weapons of mass destruction" are nuclear, chemical, and biological in nature. Whether it is anthrax spores sent through the mail or the threat of smallpox being introduced into a nonimmunized population, infection and the methods of preventing it have a key role in the defense of humanity. Health care professionals have a vital role in the prevention, early detection, and management of infections.

EPIDEMIOLOGIC CONCEPTS

Epidemiology is the study of health events and disease, their distribution, and associated causative factors in a defined population.[1] This science arose from the study of epidemics but now encompasses both infectious (e.g., human immunodeficiency virus [HIV] epidemic) and noninfectious (e.g., atherosclerosis) diseases. This chapter will confine its discussion to infectious disease, although some concepts are common to both.

The goals of epidemiology are to define the disease, identify outbreaks, assist in the development and evaluation of treatment protocols, and develop prevention strategies. This science attempts to attain these goals by conducting epidemiologic studies of disease. These studies can be broadly divided into observational studies, which describe events, exposures, and diseases occurring in a defined population, and experimental studies, which attempt to intervene in a controlled environment to study the effect of an intervention on the course of a disease.[2] Giving a randomly selected group of at-risk individuals educational programs about HIV prevention to determine the effect on risk-taking behavior is an example of an experimental study. Studying the natural history of the Ebola virus outbreak in Zaire in 1976 is an example of an observational study.

The U.S. Centers for Disease Control and Prevention and the World Health Organization have pivotal roles in identifying diseases, tracking their natural history, and defining protocols for their control and prevention. An example of how these organizations can control disease is the virtual eradication of smallpox. The World Health Organization, with the cooperation of other health organizations such as the Centers for Disease Control and Prevention, mandated immunizations for all those susceptible to the disease that were living in or traveling to areas where smallpox was prevalent. This immunization program, coupled with the lack of a viral host other than humans, led to the eradication of smallpox, except in the laboratory. Only the fear of the reintroduction of the virus into the population in a bioterrorism attack or biological warfare may mandate the continued immunization of susceptible populations such as health care workers, emergency personnel, and the military.

Transmission of Infection

Transmission of disease requires a chain of events that must occur unbroken to allow one human to infect another.[1,2] (Figure 8-1). The pathogenic organism must live and reproduce in a reservoir. The reservoir may be a human, as in the influenza virus; an animal, as in rabies; an insect, as in West Nile virus; or soil, as in enterobiasis (pinworm infestation).

The **pathogen** must have a portal of exit and a mode of transmission from the reservoir to a susceptible victim. The portal of exit is usually closest to the breeding site of the organism. For example, *Neisseria gonorrhoeae*, the organism that is responsible for gonorrhea, usually resides in the urethra of an infected male and in the vaginal canal of an infected female. The microorganism is transmitted to others by sexual contact.

Transmission of the pathogen can be either direct or indirect.[2-4] Direct transmission occurs when direct contact is made between the reservoir and the new host.[4] This contact can be physical or effected by fecal contamination or airborne droplets. Indirect contact occurs when the reservoir deposits the organism on an inanimate object (**fomite**), which then transmits the pathogen to the new host. An example of this mode of transmission is enterobiasis (pinworm) infestation, in which the eggs are deposited on soil, clothing, and bedding and ingested by hand-to-mouth transmissions. The pathogen gains entry to the victim through a portal, usually close to the breeding area in the body. If the skin barrier is broken as in

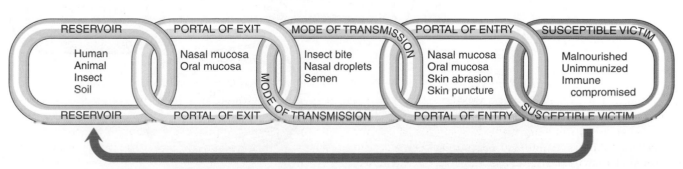

FIGURE 8-1 Chain of transmission of microorganisms from host to victim.

a surgical incision, microorganisms that normally reside on the skin can gain access to a rich environment for uncontrolled growth. If the host is susceptible to the pathogen, the microorganism grows in numbers to overwhelm the host's immune system and infection occurs. Thus the entire cycle repeats itself.

If a balance is established between the "person" and the microorganism to control the location of the pathogen and numbers of microorganisms on or in the body, pure *colonization* occurs. The microorganism does not cause infectious disease in that individual, but the organism continues to live and can be passed on to other victims. An example of this is *Staphylococcus aureus,* which can be found in the nasal passages of 25% to 30% of the population.[5] In these individuals, the bacteria does not cause disease but can be transmitted to another immunocompromised individual causing severe or life-threatening infection.

Control of disease occurrence depends on breaking this chain of transmission in one or more places[4] (Figure 8-2). A pathogen can be vulnerable in one or more links of the transmission chain. The goal of epidemiology is to identify these vulnerabilities and exploit them to stop disease transmission. Some pathogens are susceptible to direct attack by antimicrobials. Antibiotics are designed to directly kill bacteria or hold growth in check so that the body's defenses can eradicate them. Antiviral drugs work in different ways to limit viral infection.

Destroying nonhuman reservoirs and vectors of the pathogen can break the chain of transmission. For example, controlling the number of mosquitoes with insecticides and other biological means is a method used to curb the spread of malaria and West Nile virus. Immunization of domesticated animals against rabies eliminates one reservoir of potential rabies transmission. Distribution of clean needles in the intravenous drug user community is aimed at removing a common transmission vector (contaminated needles) for HIV, the causative pathogen responsible for acquired immunodeficiency syndrome (AIDS).

Blocking the portal of exit can also block transmission of the pathogen. Having patients with tuberculosis wear masks as they move through the hospital and implementing respiratory isolation techniques to stop transmission are interventions aimed at blocking the portal of exit. Standard precautions are infection-control guidelines designed to block the pathogen's portal of exit, route of transmission, and portal of entry.[2] Hand washing is one of the most effective ways to break the chain of transmission by blocking an important mode of transmission—contaminated hands.

Finally, susceptibility to infection is an important aspect of the transmission of a pathogen. Factors such as age, gender, ethnic group, and genetic makeup all affect the susceptibility of the host. Although these factors cannot be changed, improving the immune system by improving nutritional status, decreasing stress, and limiting fatigue can decrease the susceptibility to infection. Immunization has a key role in blocking the transmission of infection. Immune globulin can provide passive immunity to some infections.

Inappropriate antibiotic use has had a tremendous impact on the susceptibility of bacteria. Limiting inappropriate prescribing of antibiotics and instructing patients in the appropriate use of those antibiotics can limit the increase of antibiotic resistance. Limiting the use of antibiotics in the food supply can also limit the population's exposure and the development of antibiotic resistance.

Role of Host

The host defense system is multifaceted and consists of an **innate immune response** (Table 8-1) composed of mechanical and biochemical barriers, phagocytes, and chemical mediators, as well as a **specific immune response.**[3,6,7] (Host immune systems are discussed in greater detail in Chapter 9.) The body's skin and mucous membranes are effective mechanical and biochemical barriers to most organisms and infectious agents. The epithelium is difficult for organisms to penetrate because of its structure, pH, continual cell-sloughing process, attachment prevention, the passage of secretory IgA through the

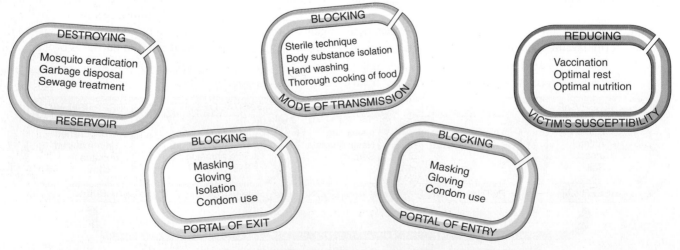

FIGURE 8-2 Breaking the chain of transmission of microorganisms from host to victim.

TABLE 8-1	
Mechanisms of Innate Defense	
Mechanism	**Description**
Species resistance	Genetic characteristics of the human species protect the body from certain pathogens
Mechanical and chemical barriers	Physical impediments to the entry of foreign cells or substances
Skin and mucosa	Forms a continuous wall that separates the internal environment from the external environment, preventing the entry of pathogens
Secretions	Secretions such as sebum, mucus, and enzymes chemically inhibit the activity of pathogens
Inflammation	The inflammatory response isolates the pathogens and stimulates the speedy arrival of large numbers of immune cells
Phagocytosis	Ingestion and destruction of pathogens by phagocytic cells
Neutrophils	Granular leukocytes that are usually the first phagocytic cell to arrive at the scene of an inflammatory response
Macrophages	Monocytes that have enlarged to become giant phagocytic cells capable of consuming many pathogens; often called by more specific names when found in specific tissues of the body
Natural killer cells	Group of lymphocytes that kill many different types of cancer cells and virus-infected cells
Interferon	Protein produced by cells after they become infected by a virus; inhibits the spread or further development of a viral infection
Complement	Group of plasma proteins (inactive enzymes) that produce a cascade of chemical reactions that ultimately cause lysis (rupture) of a foreign cell; the complement cascade can be triggered by adaptive or innate immune mechanisms

From Thibodeau GA, Patton KT: *Anatomy and physiology,* ed 6, St Louis, 2007, Mosby, p 804.

epithelium from lymphocytes, and the production of biochemical agents. These barriers may be interrupted or destroyed by medical interventions. For example, endotracheal tubes, urinary catheters, and intravenous catheters interfere with protective epithelial surfaces.[3]

Host Characteristics

Epithelial Barriers

Intact physical barriers (Figure 8-3) act as a blockade to foreign material entering the body. The epithelial cells of the skin provide multilayer protection from the many microorganisms with which the body comes in contact. The dry surface of the skin does not promote the growth of organisms because moisture is preferred. Constant shedding of the epidermis and mucosal membranes aids in the removal of any microorganisms that are attached to their surfaces. For example, an intestinal epithelial cell half-life is 30 hours, which limits the number of bacteria that could attach to the cell. The high fat content of the skin inhibits the growth of bacteria and fungi.[6,8]

The mucous membrane linings of the gastrointestinal and genitourinary tracts provide a barrier separating the sterile internal body from the external environment. The lungs are protected with a layer of mucous lining. The sticky consistency of mucus traps microorganisms, and the cilia sweep the microorganisms away. The mucociliary system and alveolar macrophages are important for ridding the lungs of trapped microorganisms.[6,8] Mechanisms such as coughing, sneezing, and urinating help to remove particles trapped on mucous membranes of the body.

Chemical barriers enhance the effectiveness of the mechanical barriers.[6,8] The acidic environment of the skin,

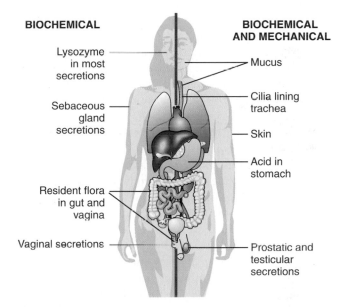

FIGURE 8-3 Some of the mechanical and biochemical barriers of the human body.

urine, and vagina inhibits bacterial growth. The secretion of hydrochloric acid with a pH of 1 to 2 by the stomach results in the killing of microorganisms. Saliva, mucus, tears, and sweat contain antimicrobial chemicals such as lysozyme, an enzyme that destroys bacterial cell walls.[6,8] Lactoferrin is another mucosal protein that keeps bacterial replication low by reducing the availability of free iron needed for bacterial growth. Sebaceous gland secretions act as antifungals. Immunoglobulins (IgA, IgG) are present in many of the body's secretions and prevent entry of bacteria and viruses through mucous membranes. (See Chapter 9 for a discussion about immunoglobulins.)

Removal or degradation of the body's mechanical and biochemical barriers creates a setting in which infection is likely. For example, burn victims who have lost portions of their skin barrier are at high risk for infection. Cellular changes induced by smoking reduce the number of cilia in the respiratory tract. Hospitalized patients who have incisions or intravenous and urinary catheters are at risk for infection because their skin barrier has been breached. The normal action of cilia in the respiratory tract in removing foreign particles is blocked by endotracheal tubes. When a urinary catheter is in place, flushing of bacteria from the urinary tract opening (meatus) is bypassed.

Risk Factors

Nutritional Status. Adequate nutrition is necessary to maintain a healthy immune system. It has long been recognized that malnutrition is a risk factor for the development of infection. Protein energy malnutrition (PEM) is associated with defects in cell-mediated immunity (specific), impaired intracellular destruction by neutrophils, reduced complement activity, and decreased levels of secretory IgA.[9]

Vitamin and trace element alterations have been associated with specific defects in the immune system. Severe iron deficiency alters the functioning of some of the cellular components of the immune system and is believed to increase the susceptibility to infection. Excess amounts of trace elements and fatty acids may also depress the immune system, which emphasizes the need for the intake of optimal amounts of nutrients.[9-11]

A host responding to an infection will need additional protein and nutrients to fight the microbial invasion. Decreased nutrition during this period can lead to a negative nitrogen balance. Anergy, or the failure to mount a localized response to a known antigen when given intradermally, can result from protein energy malnutrition. Anergy in a preoperative patient has been a marker for increased postoperative morbidity and sepsis.

Chronic Illness. Chronic illnesses such as diabetes, cancer, heart disease, and renal failure are associated with an increased risk of infection. Deaths in patients with chronic illnesses are frequently directly related to an infectious process. Infections are cited as the leading cause of death in patients with acute renal failure and diabetes.[12,13]

Diabetes alters the host's ability to resist infection. Phagocytosis is impaired with hyperglycemia, and detection of the pain of infection may be delayed because of neuropathies. The invasiveness of the microorganisms is increased when exposed to hyperglycemic environments. With increased glucose levels, *Candida* has been shown to flourish because of increased resistance to phagocytosis.[12]

Circulatory problems associated with heart failure or peripheral vascular disease are risk factors for infection. The cellular components of the immune system are dependent on the circulatory system to deliver them to the site of infection. In addition, antimicrobial agents need to be transported to the site of infection. Many pathogens thrive in areas with poor tissue perfusion.[6, 12]

Age. Age is also a variable in the ability to resist infections. Infants are at an increased risk for infection owing to an immature immune system. The lack of previous exposure to microorganisms makes the immune system naive and less efficient in mounting a defense. A newborn is susceptible to Gram-negative bacterial infections and sepsis because of the lack of IgM. Detection of infection in the newborn is based on a high level of suspicion and accurate recognition of the subtle signs of lethargy, feeding difficulties, temperature control problems, and changes in vital signs.[6]

The elderly are more susceptible to infection because of declining function of the immune system. Depressed cell-mediated immunity, changes in T-lymphocyte functioning, and atrophy of the thymus gland are some of the factors that may cause decreased immunity.[14] Greater morbidity and mortality are associated with infection in the elderly. The lungs and urinary tract are the most common sites of infection in the elderly.[14,15] The increased diversity and types of infections in the elderly in comparison with other age groups leads to a higher frequency of sepsis and bacteremia.[15] Infection may also be manifested atypically, with absence of fever and the sudden onset of confusion. The subtle changes and lack of fever obscure clinical recognition of the presence of an infectious process.[15,16]

Immunosuppression. Immunosuppression may result from a systemic disease involving the immune system, from the treatment for a disease, or from a genetic defect in the immune system. Defects may occur in one or more of the components of the immune response: phagocytic, complement, cellular, or humoral. A person is considered immunocompromised when such a defect is known to exist. The defect may be caused by a disease such as AIDS, by complement deficiencies, or by the absence of humoral antibody production. The defect may also be treatment induced or iatrogenic. Agents that can cause immunosuppression are antimetabolites, corticosteroids, chemotherapy, radiation, and antibiotics.[17] Immunocompromised hosts are highly susceptible to life-threatening infections, and so meticulous care in the prevention of infection is a high priority for such patients.

Stress has been implicated in predisposing an individual to an infectious process or the reactivation of an infection previously held in check. An example is the outbreak of a latent herpes simplex infection in response to stress. Stress hormones such as corticosteroids are known for their effect of depressing the immune system. Complex interactions exist between the immune system and the neuroendocrine system. Hormones such as corticosteroids, endorphins, and lymphokines participate in the regulatory loop between the two systems. (For further discussion, see Chapter 2.)

Abdominal trauma may result in splenic injury and possible therapeutic splenectomy. Patients with splenectomy are at high risk for overwhelming infection by *Streptococcus pneumoniae.* The spleen normally facilitates the phagocytosis of encapsulated bacteria. Prevention of life-threatening infections is aided by vaccination of all splenectomy patients with pneumococcal vaccine[18] as well as yearly influenza immunizations. The spleen is not removed except in extraordinary circumstances.

Role of Immunization

Immunization of a population is the most cost-effective method of altering susceptibility to a pathogen for which a vaccine has been developed.[1] There are two goals of immunization. The first is to confer immunity to a host by direct exposure to the altered pathogen. The second is to decrease the number of susceptible hosts in the population, thereby limiting the possibility of transmission of the disease. By this method, known as *herd immunity,* the disease can be controlled or eliminated without immunizing everyone, as long as a high enough percentage of the population is immunized. The number of susceptible hosts in the population decreases as immunization rates increase. When a critical percentage of the susceptible population is immunized, the chain of transmission is broken and the disease outbreak averted. If the percentage of adequately immunized individuals drops, epidemics may result.

Immunization exposes the potential host to altered bacteria, viruses, or their derivatives, which stimulates the body to produce antibodies against these pathogens without causing the disease. These antibodies allow the body to destroy the pathogen before it has a chance to cause disease when the potential host is exposed to the pathogen. Immunization often requires repeated exposure to the altered pathogens in the form of vaccines, such as those recommended by the American Academy of Pediatrics and the Centers for Disease Control and Prevention.[19]

Role of Environment

Multiple environmental factors affect the prevalence and transmission of various infections and infestations. To illustrate, parasitic infections are facilitated by hot and humid climates, overcrowded living conditions, the presence of insect vectors in bed linen or clothing, improper sewage disposal or treatment (such as the use of raw human sewage as fertilizer), the lack of clean water, and the consumption of contaminated raw or undercooked meat or vegetables.

Infections may be transmitted by inhalation of polluted dust or air. For example, the fungus *Coccidioides immitis,* which causes Valley Fever, is pandemic in the southwestern United States. Toxoplasmosis is caused by inhalation or ingestion of dirt, sand, or litter dust contaminated with cat feces that contain the causative protozoon *Toxoplasma gondii.*

Fecal contamination of meat and vegetables by improper cleaning or slaughtering techniques leads to many infections in the general population. *Salmonella* contamination of poultry during slaughter and dressing of the meat, coupled with improper preparation and incomplete cooking, leads to numerous *Salmonella* infections each year. In the early 1990s, fecal contamination of beef during the slaughter and dressing of the meat, coupled with incomplete cooking of the contaminated hamburger, led to *Escherichia coli 0157* infection of many people in the northwestern United States. Contamination of apples used in the processing of unpasteurized fruit juices also led to an *E. coli* outbreak.

Tuberculosis and poliomyelitis are known to occur in crowded living environments under conditions of poor nutrition and hygiene. Viral hepatitis type A is transmitted by the fecal-oral route, usually following consumption of contaminated food or water.[20]

Some infections occur only in certain regions of the world. African sleeping sickness, caused by the parasite *Trypanosoma brucei rhodesiense,* occurs only in woodland and savanna areas south and east of Lake Tanganyika. This environmental limitation is related to the environmental range of its vector, the tsetse fly, *Glossina morsitans.*[4]

Many infections are known to have seasonal patterns. For example, poliomyelitis occurs during the summer and fall in temperate zones and throughout the year in the tropics. Septic meningitis also tends to occur during the summer and fall. Epidemic typhus caused by *Rickettsia prowazekii* occurs in the winter or in cool climates under conditions of poor sanitation and poor hygiene. It is under these conditions that the human host is most likely to be wearing clothes and can be bitten by the human louse, which is the vector for this disease. Lyme disease is more prevalent in the summertime in wooded areas when people are more likely to be in the forest and be bitten by the deer tick, the insect vector of the disease.[2,4,21]

KEY POINTS

- Epidemiology is the study of health events and disease, their distribution, and associated causative factors in a defined population. Goals of epidemiology are to define a disease, identify outbreaks, assist in the development and evaluation of treatment protocols, and develop prevention strategies.
- Transmission of disease requires a chain of events that includes passing of the pathogen from the reservoir of the infection through a portal of exit to a susceptible host through a portal of entry by a circumscribed mode of transmission.
- The host has several lines of defense to prevent and fight infection. The skin and mucous membranes provide a first line of defense through mechanical and biochemical barriers. Shedding of epithelium, cilia action, acidic secretions, and enzymes help remove or destroy microorganisms before they gain access to the body.
- Malnutrition may depress immune function because many components require adequate proteins, vitamins, and minerals for synthesis. Immunoglobulins, complement factors, and clotting factors require adequate protein metabolism by the liver.

- Chronic illnesses such as diabetes and cardiovascular disease predispose to infection because circulation of immune components may be impaired and a high-glucose medium may enhance bacterial growth.
- Trauma, burns, invasive instrumentation, antibiotics, and immunosuppressive therapies, which may accompany acute illnesses, predispose an individual to infection by altering normal host defenses.
- The very young and very old are more susceptible to infection because of immature or degenerating immune function.
- Stress is associated with increased secretion of corticosteroids, which are believed to depress immune function. Exogenous steroids and other immunosuppressive therapies (radiation, antibiotics, anticancer drugs, and antirejection drugs) also increase the risk of infection.
- Immunizations alter the susceptibility of the host by stimulating the immune system to create antibodies to the pathogen.
- Environmental factors influence the likelihood of exposure and infection by microorganisms. Sanitation, air quality, living conditions, and climate are important factors.

HOST-PARASITE RELATIONSHIP

Normal Microbial Flora

The ability of the human body to resist infection requires an intact defense system. Host and environmental factors such as nutrition, age, illness, air quality, sanitation, and stress may alter the host's resistance to infection. In addition, characteristics of the pathogen such as virulence, toxins, adherence, and invasiveness may allow it to evade the human defense system and colonize.[4] This relationship between the host, the parasite, and the environment, as shown in Figure 8-4, is the framework for understanding infectious processes.[1]

The interactions between a host and the microorganisms that reside on or in it are referred to as the **host-parasite relationship.** Large numbers of microorganisms reside on the skin and in the gastrointestinal tract and vagina of the human host. These microbes normally cause no harm to the host. They obtain nutrients from the host in order to grow and reproduce. The host and these normal parasitic floras usually balance their interactions to the benefit of each in order to grow and survive—a symbiotic relationship.

Interestingly, these bacteria have a role in protecting the host from other pathogens thus preventing other microbial colonization. Normal bacterial flora also participate in metabolic processes such as the synthesis of vitamin K in the colon.[13] Harmless inhabitation of the skin or mucous membranes by these microorganisms is called **colonization.**

Resident floras are usually of specific types and occupy a certain environment in or on the host. These floras recolonize quickly if disturbed. For example, normal resident floras of the skin include bacteria such as *Corynebacterium, Staphylococcus epidermidis,* and *Streptococcus viridans,* as well as fungi, yeasts, and even mycobacteria.[6]

Normal floras and other microorganisms unlikely to cause infection can become pathogenic if the immune system is compromised. These infections are referred to as **opportunistic.** An increased number of people are at risk for opportunistic infections because of diseases of the immune system, such as AIDS, and because of therapies that depress the immune system, such as the use of steroids in the management of inflammatory conditions.

Microorganism Characteristics

Microorganisms possess certain characteristics that assist in their penetration and survival in the host despite the presence of an intact defense system. Virulence, toxin production, microbial adherence, and invasiveness are microorganism factors that influence the development of infection in the host.

Microbial adherence is the ability of the microorganism to latch onto and gain entrance into the host. Without the ability to either directly penetrate a host or stick to the host's tissue surface, pathogens are removed by normal host defenses. Entry into the host can occur directly, as with a surgical wound, arthropod bite, or direct penetration. For example, an infected female *Anopheles* mosquito can inject *Plasmodium vivax* with its bite and cause malaria.

Entry can also occur through the microorganism's ability to adhere to the host's epithelial cells because of adhesion molecules on the cell surface of certain microorganisms. The type of adhesion varies. For example, the mechanism of adhesion of *E. coli* is protein K88, and that for group A streptococci is lipoteichoic acids. Some bacteria, such as *E. coli,* have pili or fimbriae (hairlike structures) that enable them to attach to glycoproteins containing mannose on their hosts. Microbes are also attracted to and able to attach to certain cell surface proteins such as fibronectin or to the rough surfaces of intravascular or intracavity catheters.

Microbial development of a slime layer also facilitates adherence. The slime layer is the result of extracellular synthesis of a substance, usually a mucopolysaccharide, by enzymes on the surface of some bacteria. The slime layer, called *glycocalyx,* acts as glue or adhesive that sticks the bacteria to host surfaces. For example, the slime layer produced by *Streptococcus mutans* allows bacteria to adhere to tooth enamel and form plaque.[4]

Virulence and invasiveness factors include a variety of mechanisms that microorganisms have evolved to elude and block host defenses or assist in host invasion. These characteristics contribute to the pathogenicity of the microorganism by enabling it to penetrate natural barriers, resist death by phagocytosis, or survive antimicrobial therapy (e.g., methicillin-resistant *S. aureus*). Examples include bacterial enzymes, encapsulation, mutation, mobility, endospore formation, and resistance to phagocytosis and antimicrobial therapy.

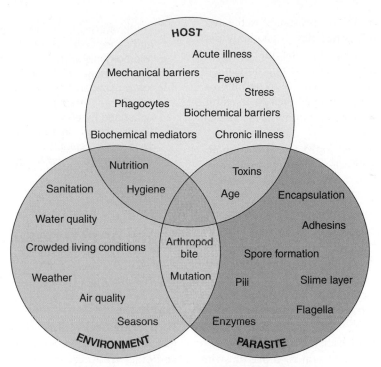

FIGURE 8-4 This depiction of the interactions of host, parasite, and environment provides a framework for understanding infectious processes.

Bacterial enzymes (such as fibrinolysin, coagulase, and hyaluronidase) aid in the microorganism's ability to spread or invade tissues. Most enzymes dissolve or hydrolyze blood, collagen, or connective tissue components. Fibrinolysin, produced by streptococci, dissolves coagulated plasma and allows local microbial spread into host tissues. Hyaluronidase is secreted by staphylococci, clostridia, streptococci, and other organisms.[21,22] This enzyme helps microbes to spread locally by dissolving a connective tissue component called hyaluronic acid.

Encapsulation prevents opsonization (recognition and binding) by antibodies and thus prevents the microorganism from being phagocytized. For example, *S. pneumoniae* (pneumococci) diplococci have a polysaccharide capsule that protects them from phagocytosis. The bacterial slime layer also protects bacteria from phagocytosis.

Other bacteria are capable of **endospore formation,** which allows the microorganism to survive under harsh environmental conditions. The endospore state is specifically triggered by bacterial genes under conditions of decreasing nutrients such as decreasing nitrogen or carbon in the environment. The endospore, which is capable of regeneration under favorable conditions, is a resting cell that is released when the microorganism dies. It is highly resistant to heat, lack of moisture, and chemicals. Examples of endospore-forming bacteria include *Clostridium, Bacillus,* and *Coxiella burnetii.*

Virulence is the characteristic of a microorganism in which that microorganism consistently causes disease in all infected hosts. It is the interaction between the host and the pathogen that results in harm to the host. *Staphylococcus*

TABLE 8-2

Historical Progression of *Staphylococcus aureus* Resistance to Antibiotics

Antibiotic and Year Introduced	Year Resistance Appeared
Penicillin, 1941	1940s
Streptomycin, 1944	Mid-1940s
Tetracycline, 1948	1950s
Erythromycin, 1952	1950s
Gentamicin, 1964	Mid-1970s
Methicillin, 1959	Late 1960s

Data from Morita MM: Methicillin-resistant *Staphylococcus aureus:* past, present and future, *Nurs Clin North Am* 28:625-637, 1993; and Rosenberg J: Methicillin-resistant *Staphylococcus aureus* (MRSA) in the community: who's watching? *Lancet* 346:132-133, 1995.

aureus in wounds, *E. coli* in urine, and pneumococcal pneumoniae in the lungs are examples of virulent organisms invading the host.[23,24,25]

Antimicrobial resistance is conferred to microorganisms that are able to mutate in response to changes in the host's environment in order to successfully infect the host.[7,26,27] For example, the development of methicillin-resistant *S. aureus* is the result of successful mutation of the organism and selection of resistant strains in response to antibiotic exposure. The ability of *S. aureus* to become antibiotic resistant was recognized with the introduction of penicillin (Table 8-2) and continues today.[7,26,28]

Another contributor to antibiotic resistance is the tendency for persons treated with antibiotics to take only part of their daily dose rather than completing the full course.[23,29] This practice may allow relatively resistant microorganisms that can survive a low-dose antibiotic course to become the dominant species. The resistant form may then be transmitted to other individuals and become common in the general population.

Some microorganisms have developed a resistance to antibiotics through repeated exposure to subtherapeutic doses and/or their indiscriminant use for nonbacterial infections. This "antimicrobial resistance" is a major threat to the successful management of bacterial infections. The emergence of vancomycin-resistant *Enterococcus* (VRE) and methicillin-resistant *S. aureus* (MRSA) among others is a very troubling development in infectious disease management. Multidrug-resistant tuberculosis has also emerged as a danger in the world. Viruses too have developed resistances to antiviral medications, requiring multidrug cocktails to keep the AIDS virus in check, for example.

Mobility is a characteristic of bacteria with **flagella,** motile appendages that allow the bacterium to move or swim toward nutrients in a favorable environment. This movement, called *chemotaxis,* is usually toward sugar or amino acid concentrations in the environment. Microorganisms may also produce toxins that can affect the host's cells systemically or locally. The toxins are classified as exotoxins or endotoxins. **Exotoxins** are polypeptide toxins that are produced and released by the organism. They are highly antigenic, highly toxic, and unstable when exposed to heat. They cause illness and death by binding to specific receptors in target organs and by interfering with vital metabolic pathways.[30] Some exotoxin-producing bacteria include *Clostridium botulinum, Clostridium tetani, S. aureus,* and *Shigella dysenteriae.*[4] For example, *C. tetani* produces an exotoxin called *tetanospasmin,* which is a powerful neurotoxin. Tetanospasmin interferes with synaptic transmission of inhibitory interneurons in the spinal cord, which leads to tetany, muscle spasms, characteristic "lockjaw" (trismus), and seizures.

Endotoxins are associated with Gram-negative bacteria such as enterobacteria, common causative agents of septic shock. Endotoxin is an immunogenic part of the bacterial cell wall (lipopolysaccharide) that triggers a massive immune response when the bacterium lyses.[30] The subsequent immune response leads to shock and multiple organ failure.[17] (See Chapter 20 for a further discussion of septic shock.)

KEY POINTS

- A number of microorganisms are considered resident flora because they live on or in the host without causing disease. Resident flora benefits the host by synthesizing molecules and inhibiting the growth of nonresident microorganisms. If the host's immune system is compromised, resident flora may become pathogenic and cause opportunistic infection.
- Microorganisms possess characteristics that enhance their pathogenic potential. Adherence is improved by the presence of adhesion molecules, slime layers, and pili. Escape from immune detection and destruction is enhanced by encapsulation, spore formation, mutation, flagella, and toxin production. Microorganisms that possess these characteristics are more virulent and thus more likely to cause disease.

TYPES OF PATHOGENIC ORGANISMS

Photographic examples of pathogenic organisms are shown in Figure 8-5.

Bacteria

Bacteria are single-celled organisms that have no internal organelles (Figure 8-6). Some live in the intestines of humans and other creatures, and participate in digestion. Others live in the soil and are responsible for its fertility. They degrade dead tissue and break it down for other organisms to use. Among the countless types of bacteria that exist, only a small percentage is known to be harmful to humans.[6,24]

Bacteria are classified into four major groups based on their cell wall shape and mechanism of movement: gliding bacteria (e.g., myxobacteria), spirochetes (e.g., *Treponema pallidum* [Figure 8-7]), mycoplasmas (e.g., *Mycoplasma pneumoniae*), and rigid bacteria. The rigid bacteria are further broken down into actinomycetes (e.g., *Mycobacterium tuberculosis*) and unicellular forms.

The unicellular forms of rigid bacteria include *intracellular obligate* parasites and *free-living* bacteria. Intracellular obligate parasites (e.g., *rickettsiae* and *chlamydiae*) must live within a host cell to survive.

Free-living bacteria are classified by morphology (shape) and their response to Gram staining. They have three basic shapes. **Cocci** are round and nonmotile. They may stick together in clumps that look like bunches of grapes (e.g., staphylococci), in pairs (e.g., diplococci), or in long strands (e.g., streptococci). **Bacilli,** by comparison, are rod shaped and about half are motile (e.g., *Pseudomonas aeruginosa*) (see Figure 8-6). The third shape is the **spiral** (e.g., *Spirillum*).

Bacteria are further differentiated by whether they retain a basic dye after iodine fixation, known as the **Gram stain** reaction. Gram staining separates bacteria into Gram-positive organisms, which look dark purple under the microscope; Gram-negative organisms, which look pink; or acid-fast organisms, which resist staining but, once stained, resist decoloration. Further differentiation of bacteria is based on nutritional requirements (such as whether the organism is anaerobic or aerobic), on colony characteristics, and on resistance.

Figure 8-8 classifies examples of pathogenic bacteria according to the part of the human body that they commonly

FIGURE 8-5 Examples of pathogenic organisms. **A,** Viruses (the human immunodeficiency virus [HIV] that causes AIDS). **B,** Bacteria (*Streptococcus* bacteria that cause strep throat and other infections). **C,** Fungi (yeast cells that commonly infect the urinary and reproductive tracts). **D,** Fungi (the mold that causes aspergillosis). **E,** Protozoans (the flagellated cells that cause traveler's diarrhea). **F,** Pathogenic animals (the parasitic worms that cause snail fever). (**A** and **F,** From Thibodeau GA, Patton KT: *Anatomy and physiology,* ed 6, St Louis, 2007, Mosby. **B-D,** Copyright Photographer/Visuals Unlimited. **E,** From Erlandsen SL, Magney J: *Color atlas of histology,* St Louis, 1992, Mosby.)

Microscopic Morphology of Bacteria

B

FIGURE 8-6 Types of microorganisms. **A,** Bacteria. **B,** Virus. **C,** Fungus. (**A,** From Mahon CR, Manuselis G: *Textbook of diagnostic microbiology,* ed 2, Philadelphia, 2000, Saunders. **B** and **C,** From Gould BE: *Pathophysiology for the health professions,* ed 3, Philadelphia, Saunders, 2006, p 78.)

FIGURE 8-7 Spirochetes (e.g., *Treponema pallidum*): immunohistochemistry of the muscular layer in the small intestine of a newborn with congenital syphilis. Multiple spirochetes are shown in red (both cross-sections and entire treponemes can be noted [100]). (Courtesy Jeannette Guarner, MD, and Sherif R. Zaki, MD, PhD, Centers for Disease Control and Prevention, Atlanta.)

infect. Once they have penetrated the initial defense mechanisms, the bacteria multiply and create a colony. In an attempt to contain and eliminate the invading bacteria, an acute inflammatory reaction in the body occurs. Phagocytic cells such as neutrophils and macrophages are recruited to the area, where they ingest and destroy the microorganisms. If these responses are insufficient to contain the infection, the bacteria move throughout the body through the natural currents of fluids (i.e., bloodstream, lymph system, or intrastitial fluids). Bacteria move through the lymph system to the lymph nodes where they stimulate an immune response. If they are present in sufficient numbers to overwhelm the lymph nodes, circulating clumps of bacteria (emboli) can cause bacteremia and microabscesses. In severe cases, sepsis, hypotension, organ system failure, and death can occur.

EYES
Chlamydia trachomatis
Streptococcus pneumoniae
Staphylococcus aureus
Neisseria gonorrhoeae

THROAT
Corynebacterium
diphtheriae
Streptococcus pyogenes
Bordetella pertussis

LUNGS
Mycoplasma pneumoniae
Legionella pneumophila
Streptococcus pneumoniae
Haemophilus influenzae
Mycobacterium tuberculosis

LIVER
Clostridium
Enterococci
Gram-negative bacilli

INTESTINES
Clostridium difficile
Clostridium perfringens
Salmonella
Shigella

VAGINA AND UTERUS
Neisseria gonorrhoeae
Chlamydia trachomatis
Gram-negative bacilli

SKIN
Staphylococcus aureus
Streptococcus pyogenes

BRAIN AND MENINGES
Haemophilus influenzae
Neisseria meningitidis
Streptococcus pneumoniae

EAR
Streptococcus pneumoniae
Haemophilus influenzae
Gram-negative enteric bacilli

HEART
Streptococcus viridans
Staphylococcus aureus
Enterococci

KIDNEY
Gram-negative bacilli
Escherichia coli

PROSTATE AND TESTES
Gram-negative bacilli
Neisseria gonorrhoeae

URETHRA
Neisseria gonorrhoeae
Chlamydia trachomatis
Gram-negative enteric bacilli

BONE
Staphylococcus aureus
Gram-negative enteric bacilli
Mycobacterium tuberculosis

JOINTS
Staphylococcus aureus
Neisseria gonorrhoeae
Streptococcus pyogenes

FIGURE 8-8 Examples of pathogenic bacteria classified according to the part of the human body that they commonly infect.

Box 8-1 summarizes primary pathogens associated with specific infections in the human host.[31] Numerous antibiotics have been developed to decrease the risk (prophylaxis) or severity of infection by specific bacteria. Table 8-3 summarizes antimicrobial selection based on the infecting organism.[29]

Viruses

Viruses, the smallest known infective agents, range in size from 20 to 300 nm.[22] They are composed of DNA or RNA and a capsule surrounding the genetic material. Viruses have only enough genetic information to code for 2 to 60 proteins. They are totally dependent on the host cell for energy and the "machinery" to replicate. A comparison of viruses and other microorganisms is presented in Table 8-4.

Viruses were once differentiated only by size. With advances in gene sequencing and use of the electron microscope, viruses can now be classified by the genetic makeup, the mode of replication, the structure of the viral capsule (also known as the *capsid*), and the specific host cell that the virus invades.

All viruses must enter a host cell to replicate, and invasion is accomplished by several methods. A virus can adhere to the cell membrane and cause phagocytosis. Once inside the host cell, the virus capsule is removed to expose viral genetic material to the cell's interior. Another way that a virus can invade a host cell is by sticking to the surface of the cell and injecting viral genetic material directly into the interior.

Some viruses direct the manufacture of an envelope that surrounds the viral capsid. The envelope is made of host cell membrane and viral proteins. The virus may be released from the host cells by budding from the cell's surface (Figure 8-9).

Viruses that do not manufacture an envelope are usually released by *lysing* the host cell, thus destroying it. The mechanism of lysis seems to be a progressive breakdown of the host cell's maintenance mechanisms with resultant buildup of waste products intracellularly and lack of nutrient transport into the cell. Ultimately, the cell membrane is disrupted and the cell lyses.

Two major categories of viruses exist: those that contain DNA and those that contain RNA (Table 8-5). RNA viruses are characterized either as **retroviruses** or as straight replicating viruses.

The DNA viruses (e.g., herpes simplex virus) must first produce messenger RNA in the host cell's nucleus with the host cell's enzymes. The proteins are then formed from

BOX 8-1

Examples of Primary Pathogens Associated with Specific Infections

Burns

Staphylococcus aureus
Streptococcus pyogenes (group A)
Pseudomonas aeruginosa
Gram-negative bacilli

Skin Infections

Staphylococcus aureus
Streptococcus pyogenes (group A)
Gram-negative bacilli
Treponema pallidum

Decubitus and Surgical Wounds

Staphylococcus aureus
Gram-negative enteric bacilli
Pseudomonas aeruginosa
Streptococcus pyogenes (group A)
Anaerobic streptococci
Clostridium spp.
Enterococcus
Bacteroides spp.

Meninges

Neisseria meningitidis
Haemophilus influenzae
Streptococcus pneumoniae
Streptococcus spp.
Escherichia coli
Gram-negative bacilli
Streptococcus pyogenes (group A)
Staphylococcus aureus
Mycobacterium tuberculosis
Listeria monocytogenes
Enterococcus (neonatal period)
Treponema pallidum
Leptospira

Brain Abscess

Streptococci (aerobic and anaerobic)
Bacteroides spp.
Staphylococcus aureus

Paranasal and Middle Ear

Streptococcus pneumoniae
Streptococcus pyogenes (group A)
Haemophilus influenzae
Gram-negative enteric bacilli
Pseudomonas aeruginosa
Anaerobic streptococci
Staphylococcus aureus

Throat

Streptococcus pyogenes (group A)
Neisseria gonorrhoeae
Bacteroides spp.
Fusobacterium
Spirochetes
Corynebacterium diphtheriae
Bordetella pertussis

Lungs

Mycoplasma pneumoniae
Streptococcus pneumoniae
Haemophilus influenzae
Staphylococcus aureus
Klebsiella
Pseudomonas aeruginosa
Gram-negative bacilli
Streptococcus pyogenes (group A)
Mycobacterium tuberculosis
Chlamydia psittaci
Legionella pneumophila
Anaerobic streptococci
Bacteroides spp.
Coxiella burnetii

Lung Abscess

Anaerobic streptococci
Bacteroides spp.
Fusobacterium
Staphylococcus aureus
Klebsiella
Gram-negative bacilli
Streptococcus pneumoniae
Enterococcus

Pleura

Staphylococcus aureus
Streptococcus pneumoniae
Haemophilus influenzae
Gram-negative bacilli
Anaerobic streptococci
Bacteroides spp.
Fusobacterium
Streptococcus pyogenes (group A)
Mycobacterium tuberculosis

Endocardium

Viridans group of streptococci
Staphylococcus aureus
Enterococcus
Other streptococci
Staphylococcus epidermidis
Gram-negative enteric bacilli
Pseudomonas aeruginosa

Peritoneum

Escherichia coli
Gram-negative bacilli
Enterococcus
Bacteroides fragilis
Anaerobic streptococci
Clostridium spp.
Streptococcus pneumoniae
Streptococcus pyogenes (group A)
Neisseria gonorrhoeae
Mycobacterium tuberculosis

Biliary Tract

Escherichia coli
Gram-negative bacilli
Enterococcus spp.
Staphylococcus aureus
Clostridium spp.
Streptococci (aerobic and anaerobic)

Kidney and Bladder

Escherichia coli
Gram-negative bacilli
Staphylococcus aureus
Staphylococcus epidermidis
Mycobacterium tuberculosis

Urethra

Neisseria gonorrhoeae
Chlamydia trachomatis
Trichomonas vaginalis
Gram-negative enteric bacilli
Ureaplasma urealyticum

Prostate

Gram-negative enteric bacilli
Neisseria gonorrhoeae
Staphylococcus aureus

Epididymis and Testes

Gram-negative bacilli
Neisseria gonorrhoeae
Chlamydia trachomatis
Mycobacterium tuberculosis

Bone (Osteomyelitis)

Staphylococcus aureus
Salmonella
Gram-negative enteric bacilli
Streptococcus pyogenes (group A)
Mycobacterium tuberculosis
Anaerobic streptococci
Pseudomonas aeruginosa

Joints

Staphylococcus aureus
Neisseria gonorrhoeae
Streptococcus pyogenes (group A)
Gram-negative enteric bacilli
Pseudomonas aeruginosa
Streptococcus pneumoniae
Neisseria meningitidis
Haemophilus influenzae (in children)
Mycobacterium tuberculosis

TABLE 8-3

Antimicrobial Selection Based on Organisms

Organism	First Drug of Choice	Alternative Drugs
Gram-Positive Cocci		
Staphylococcus aureus		
Non–penicillinase producing	Penicillin G or V	A cephalosporin, vancomycin, clindamycin, imipenem
Penicillinase producing	A penicillinase resistance penicillin	Vancomycin, cephalosporin, clindamycin, amoxicillin-clavulanic acid, ticarcillin-clavulanic acid, ampicillin-sulbactam, piperacillin tazobactam, imipenem, TMP-SMZ
Methicillin resistant	Vancomycin ± gentamicin Vancomycin ± rifampin	TMP-SMZ, minocycline, Quinupristin/Dalfopristin, Linezolid
Streptococcus, hemolytic groups A, B, C, G	Penicillin G or V	Erythromycin, cephalosporin, vancomycin, clindamycin, azithromycin, clarithromycin
Viridans	Penicillin G ± aminoglycoside	Cephalosporin, vancomycin
Anaerobic	Penicillin G	Clindamycin, cephalosporin
Enterococcus	Ampicillin + gentamicin	Vancomycin + gentamicin
Vancomycin resistant	Linezolid	
Pneumococcus	Penicillin G or V	Erythromycin, cephalosporin, vancomycin, TMP-SMZ, chloramphenicol, clindamycin, azithromycin, clarithromycin
Gram-Negative Cocci		
Neisseria meningitides (meningitis or septicemia)	Penicillin G	Cefotaxime, ceftizoxime, ceftriaxone, ampicillin, chloramphenicol
Neisseria gonorrhoeae (genital)	Ceftriaxone or cefixime	Ciprofloxacin, spectinomycin, ofloxacin, cefpodoxime proxetil
Moraxella catarrhalis	TMP-SMZ	Cefuroxime, cefotaxime, ceftizoxime, ceftriaxone, cefuroxime axetil, erythromycin, tetracycline, azithromycin, amoxicillin-clavulanic acid, clarithromycin
Gram-Positive Bacilli		
Bacillus anthracis	Penicillin G	Erythromycin, tetracycline
Listeria monocytogenes	TMP-SMZ	Ampicillin ± aminoglycoside
Clostridium tetani	Penicillin G	Metronidazole, chloramphenicol, clindamycin, imipenem
Clostridium perfringens	Penicillin	Cephalosporin
Corynebacterium diphtheriae	Erythromycin	Penicillin G
Gram-Negative Bacilli		
Escherichia coli (first UTI)	Sulfonamide, TMP-SMZ	Ampicillin, cephalosporin, ciprofloxacin, ofloxacin
Escherichia coli (sepsis)	Cefotaxime, ceftizoxime, ceftriaxone, ceftazidime	Ampicillin, TMP-SMZ, ciprofloxacin, imipenem, aminoglycoside, ofloxacin
Klebsiella pneumoniae	Cefotaxime, ceftizoxime, ceftriaxone, ceftazidime	TMP-SMZ, aminoglycoside, imipenem, ciprofloxacin, ofloxacin, piperacillin, mezlocillin
Enterobacter	TMP-SMZ, imipenem	Aminoglycoside, ciprofloxacin, ofloxacin, aztreonam
Legionella pneumophila	Erythromycin + rifampin	TMP-SMZ, clarithromycin, azithromycin, ciprofloxacin
Serratia	Cefotaxime, ceftizoxime, ceftriaxone, ceftazidime	TMP-SMZ, aminoglycoside, ciprofloxacin, ofloxacin, imipenem
Proteus mirabilis	Ampicillin	Aminoglycoside, TMP-SMZ, ciprofloxacin, ofloxacin
Pseudomonas aeruginosa	Aminoglycoside + antipseudomonal penicillin	Ceftazidime ± aminoglycoside, imipenem ± aminoglycoside, aztreonam ± aminoglycoside, ciprofloxacin ± piperacillin, ciprofloxacin ± ceftazidime
Pseudomonas cepacia	Ceftazidime	Chloramphenicol, tetracycline, TMP-SMZ, amoxicillin-clavulanic acid, imipenem
Helicobacter pylori	Tetracycline + metronidazole + bismuth subsalicylate	Amoxicillin + metronidazole + bismuth subsalicylate, tetracycline + clarithromycin + bismuth subsalicylate
Salmonella	Ceftriaxone, ciprofloxacin, ofloxacin	TMP-SMZ, ampicillin, chloramphenicol
Shigella	Ciprofloxacin, ofloxacin	Ampicillin, TMP-SMZ, ceftriaxone
Haemophilus influenzae		
Meningitis or epiglottiditis	Cefotaxime, ceftizoxime, ceftriaxone, ceftazidime	Chloramphenicol
Other sites	TMP-SMZ	Ampicillin, amoxicillin, doxycycline, azithromycin, clarithromycin, cefotaxime, ceftizoxime, ceftriaxone, cefuroxime, cefuroxime, axetil
Bordetella pertussis	Erythromycin	TMP-SMZ
Brucella	Tetracycline + gentamicin	TMP-SMZ ± gentamicin. Chloramphenicol ± gentamicin

(continued)

TABLE 8-3

Antimicrobial Selection Based on Organisms—cont'd

Organism	First Drug of Choice	Alternative Drugs
Gram-Negative Bacilli—cont'd		
Acinetobacter	Imipenem	Minocycline, TMP-SMZ, doxycycline, aminoglycosides, piperacillin, ciprofloxacin, ofloxacin, ceftazidime
Campylobacter	Erythromycin	Tetracycline, ciprofloxacin, ofloxacin
Pasteurella (plague)	Streptomycin	Chloramphenicol, tetracycline, gentamicin
Vibrio cholerae	Tetracycline	TMP-SMZ, ciprofloxacin, ofloxacin, ceftazidime
Spirochetes		
Treponema pallidum	Penicillin G	Tetracycline, ceftriaxone
Treponema pertenue	Penicillin G	Tetracycline
Leptospira	Penicillin G	Tetracycline
Borrelia burgdorferi (Lyme disease)	Tetracycline	Amoxicillin, ceftriaxone, cefuroxime axetil, azithromycin, clarithromycin, penicillin
Acid-Fast Bacilli		
Mycobacterium tuberculosis	Isoniazid + rifampin + pyrazinamide ± ethambutol or streptomycin	
Mycobacterium leprae	Dapsone + rifampin + clofazimine	Minocycline, ofloxacin, clarithromycin
Special Considerations		
Chlamydia psittaci	Tetracycline	Chloramphenicol
Chlamydia trachomatis	Doxycycline, azithromycin	Ofloxacin, sulfisoxazole
Mycoplasma pneumoniae	Tetracycline	Erythromycin, clarithromycin
Rickettsiae	Tetracycline	Chloramphenicol, ciprofloxacin, ofloxacin

Data from Tierney LM, McPhee SJ, Papadakis MA: *Current medical diagnosis and treatment,* ed 46, Stamford, Conn, 2006, McGraw-Hill. *TMP-SMZ,* Trimethoprim-sulfamethoxazole; *UTI,* urinary tract infection.

TABLE 8-4

Comparison of Viruses and Other Microorganisms

Organism	Grows in Nonliving Media	Contains Both DNA and RNA	Contains Ribosomes	Sensitive to Antibiotics
Bacteria	Yes	Yes	Yes	Yes
Mycoplasmas	Yes	Yes	Yes	Yes
Rickettsiae	No	Yes	Yes	Yes
Chlamydiae	No	Yes	Yes	Yes
Viruses	No	No	No	No

FIGURE 8-9 Scanning electron micrograph of HIV-1–infected T4 lymphocyte. Large numbers of HIV virions are budding from the plasma membrane of the lymphocytes. (Courtesy Centers for Disease Control and Prevention, Atlanta.)

the messenger RNA; the DNA of the virus is replicated by host polymerases, and new viruses are assembled in the host cell.

By comparison, RNA viruses, such as influenza virus (Figure 8-10), replicate their genetic information in one of two ways. Retroviruses contain encoding information for the enzyme **reverse transcriptase** so that they can create both messenger RNA and DNA from their own genome. The viral DNA is incorporated into the host cell's DNA, and when the host cell replicates, the viral DNA also replicates, thus perpetuating the viral genome as long as the host cell line survives. Viral proteins and RNA are manufactured by using the virus's messenger RNA and the host cell's organelles. HIV, the retrovirus that causes AIDS, is an example of a virus that causes permanent change in the genome (mutation) and function of the host cell.

TABLE 8-5

Examples of Primary Viral Pathogens Associated with Specific Infections

Family	Viral Example	Disease	Type of Nucleic Acid
RNA Viruses			
Astroviridae	Astrovirus		SS (+) RNA
Arenaviridae	Lymphocytic choriomeningitis virus	Meningitis	2 circular SS (antisense) RNA segments
Bunyaviridae	California encephalitis virus	California encephalitis	3 circular SS (antisense) RNA segments
Caliciviridae	Norwalk virus		SS (+) RNA
Coronaviridae	Coronaviruses		SS (+) RNA
Filoviridae	Ebola virus	Ebola virus	SS (−) RNA
Orthomyxoviridae	Influenza viruses	Influenza	8 SS (−) RNA*
Paramyxoviridae	Measles virus	Measles	SS (−) RNA
Picornaviridae	Poliovirus	Polio	SS (+) RNA
Reoviridae	Rotaviruses		10-12 DS RNA segments
Retroviridae	HIV-1	AIDS	2 identical SS (+) RNA segments
Rhabdoviridae	Rabies virus	Rabies	SS (−) RNA
Togaviridae	Rubella virus	Rubella	SS (+) RNA
DNA Viruses			
Adenoviridae	Human adenoviruses		DS DNA
Hepadnaviridae	Hepatitis B	Hepatitis B	DS DNA without SS portions
Herpesviridae	Herpes simplex virus	Herpes	DS DNA
Papovaviridae	JC virus	Warts	Circular DS DNA
Parvoviridae	Human parvovirus	Parvo	SS (+) or (−) DNA
Poxviridae	Vaccinia virus		DS DNA

Data from Mandell GL, Bennett JE, Dolan R, editors: *Principles and practice of infectious disease,* ed 5, New York, 2000, Churchill Livingstone.
DS, Double stranded; *SS,* single stranded; (+), message sense; (−), antimessage sense.
*Influenza C: seven segments.

FIGURE 8-10 Electron micrograph of influenza virus, an RNA virus (×150,000). (Courtesy FA Murphy, MD, Centers for Disease Control and Prevention, Atlanta.)

In contrast to RNA retroviruses, the straight replicating viruses reproduce in one of two ways, depending on whether the single-stranded RNA is a positive or a negative copy. Viruses in which the RNA is a single positive copy use the strand as a direct template to make viral proteins and a complementary RNA strand. The complementary strand then serves as a template for making more positive strands that can be packaged into new viruses. The RNA viruses that possess a negative copy replicate in a similar manner, except that the RNA must be transcribed to a positive complementary copy before it can produce proteins or viral RNA.

Most viral infections are self-limited, and few antiviral agents have been developed to treat them. Effective vaccines are available for some viruses, including polio, measles, rubella, and hepatitis A and B.

Fungi

Fungi are nonphotosynthetic, eukaryotic protists that are disseminated through the environment. They can reproduce by simply dividing (asexually) or by combining their genetic information before dividing (sexually). Infections caused by fungi are called mycotic infections, or **mycoses.** Fungi cause infection first by colonizing the area. The fungus adheres to and proliferates on the site of infection. The next phase requires invasion of the epithelium. Anything that breaks the integrity of the skin (e.g., maceration) facilitates the invasion. Polymorphonuclear leukocytes attempt to phagocytize and digest the invading fungi. Neutrophils, monocytes, and eosinophils can destroy fungi in the body, causing signs and symptoms of local inflammation i.e., edema, erythema, and itching at the site of infection.[1]

Certain fungi live in the body as normal flora (e.g., *Candida*). When the body's defense mechanisms are compromised, they can overgrow and cause local or systemic infections. Patients

TABLE 8-6

Fungal Infections

Infection	Distribution	Mode of Transmission	Vector
Cryptococcosis	Everywhere	Inhalation	Pigeon feces
Candidiasis	Normal flora	Ever present	N/A
Phycomycosis (mucormycosis)	Everywhere	Inhalation, ingestion, wound contamination	Decayed matter, soil
Histoplasmosis	River valleys (e.g., California), southwestern USA (Arizona, Nevada)	Inhalation	Bird and bat feces
Coccidioidomycosis (San Joaquin Valley fever)	Semiarid USA (e.g., California), southwestern USA (Arizona, Nevada)	Inhalation	Dust, dirt
Blastomycosis	Southeastern USA, south central USA, midwestern USA, Great Lakes region	Inhalation	Unknown
Aspergillosis	Everywhere	Inhalation	Decaying vegetation

who have been given antibiotics lose some of their normal flora along with the targeted pathogen. The fungi that are not affected by the antibiotic overgrow to fill that niche. Some patients suffering from AIDS, leukemia, alcoholism, drug abuse, and malnutrition, or those being treated with immunosuppressive agents lack the immune system to prevent fungi from overgrowing, and are therefore more susceptible to fungal infections (opportunistic fungi). When the environment contains more nutrients on which the fungi can grow, such as the hyperglycemic bloodstream of a diabetic or the vaginal tract of a female given antibiotics, fungi can overgrow and cause infections. Examples of opportunistic fungi are *Candida*, Phycomycetes, *Aspergillus*, and *C. immitis*.

Superficial mycoses, such as that caused by the dermatophytes (e.g., tinea pedis), occur only on superficial, dead, keratinized tissue like hair, epidermis, and nails.[6] Subcutaneous mycoses occur when fungi are introduced into subcutaneous tissue during trauma. These fungi, when present in tissue, cause chronic granulomatous disease. An example is *Sporothrix schenckii*. This fungus causes sporotrichosis, which may spread throughout the lymph system.[4]

Systemic mycoses may occur in both healthy and immunocompromised hosts. Because the fungi causing systemic infections are usually found in soil, these infections tend to be endemic to certain regions where the fungus is found.[1,4] Infection is caused by inhalation of dust containing the fungus. Because of the endemic nature of these fungi, large segments of the population in the area may have been exposed and infected without any symptoms. If symptoms develop, they are usually self-limiting and mild. However, for those with altered immune systems, the disease becomes severe and disseminated. Examples of systemic mycoses are histoplasmosis, blastomycosis, and coccidiomycosis.

To illustrate, *Histoplasma capsulatum* is a fungus that commonly occurs in soil in the central and eastern United States. *Histoplasma* also occurs in soil rich with chicken feces or bat guano. Humans and animals exposed to dust storms in endemic areas or contaminated with these feces are most likely to be infected. They may also have positive histoplasmin skin tests and may show calcified sites of infection in their lungs.[4, 17]

Generally, cultures of fungi are difficult to grow artificially in a laboratory. The most common method of identification is by visualizing their characteristic shapes on a slide of infected tissue.

Systemic treatment is used more commonly for the immune compromised patient or disseminated disease inasmuch as local infection is usually self-limited. Topical antifungal drugs may be used to treat superficial infections (e.g., athletes foot). Table 8-6 summarizes important aspects of the most common fungi.

Parasites

Parasites are representative of four families of the animal kingdom: protozoa, or single-celled animals (Figure 8-11); nemathelminths, or roundworms; platyhelminths, or flatworms; and arthropoda, or invertebrate animals with jointed appendages.[4, 21] These parasites live on or in the human body during some part of their life cycle. They depend on their human host for shelter and sustenance. Many parasites have very complicated life cycles that include a larval and adult stage. They rely on particular hosts and vectors to transmit the organisms from host to host. Host resistance depends on macrophages, neutrophils, eosinophils, and platelets, which kill both protozoa and worms. T cells are required to develop immunity against these organisms. This explains the high incidence

Symptoms	Location of Infection	
	Primary Site(s)	Secondary Site(s)
Fever, cough, weight loss, pleuritic pain, CNS disturbances	Pulmonary system	Meninges, skin, bone
Mucocutaneous pain and itching at site of infection	Fungemia, endocarditis	Kidneys, eyes, heart
Rhinocerebral mucormycosis: destruction of CN II, IV, V, VI; erosion of carotid artery; meningitis; brain abscess	Nose, brain, lung	Rare
Pulmonary mucormycosis: dyspnea, chest pain, hemoptysis		
Flulike: cough, fever, myalgias, weight loss, anemia, leukopenia, thrombocytopenia, painful oropharyngeal ulcers	Pulmonary system	Bone marrow
Cough, fever, pleuritic chest pain, weight loss, dyspnea, chest pain, CNS disturbances	Pulmonary system	Skin, bone, joints, meninges
Flulike: pleuritic chest pain, arthralgias, erythema nodosum, weight loss, fever, cough, chest pain	Pulmonary system	Skin, bone, joints, male GU tract
Dyspnea, chest pain, hemoptysis, wheezing	Pulmonary system	Brain, kidney, liver

FIGURE 8-11 Protozoa: mouse heart infected with *Trypanosoma cruzi.* Amastigotes are seen inside a muscle fiber (pseudocyst), as well as inside inflammatory cells (hematoxylin and eosin stain). (Courtesy Jeannette Guarner, MD, Centers for Disease Control and Prevention, Atlanta.)

of *Toxoplasma* infection in HIV patients with low CD4 T cell counts.[32]

The symptoms of parasitic infection depend on the area in which the infestation develops. Protozoan infestation of the gastrointestinal tract produces cramping, abdominal pain, and bloody diarrhea (amebiasis). Infestation of the blood produces fever, chills, rigor, and later anemia, all of which are associated with malaria (*Plasmodium* infection). Acute pruritus and rash occur after infection of the skin with *Sarcoptes scabiei* (scabies).[4]

Identification of the infectious agent is usually accomplished by visualizing either the adult parasite or its ova by direct observation of the area (inspection of the skin or hair) or by microscopic examination of blood, feces, or tissue samples. Table 8-7 summarizes various parasitic infections of humans, including the common name, location, symptoms, and mode of transmission.

KEY POINTS

- Microorganisms responsible for infections in humans include bacteria, viruses, fungi, and parasites.
- Bacteria are characterized according to shape (cocci, rods, spirals), reaction to stains (Gram negative, Gram positive, acid fast), and oxygen requirements (aerobic, anaerobic).
- Viruses are bits of genetic material (DNA, RNA) with associated proteins and lipids. The smallest infective agents known, viruses are intracellular pathogens that use the host's energy sources and enzymes to replicate. Viral replication may or may not destroy the host cell. DNA viruses may be incorporated directly into the host genome. RNA viruses serve as templates for the production of viral RNA and proteins.
- Retroviruses are RNA viruses that contain a special enzyme called *reverse transcriptase* that mediates the synthesis of a DNA copy of the RNA virus. The DNA can then be incorporated into the host genome and passed on to daughter cells when the cell divides.
- Fungal infections can be superficial (e.g., ringworm, athlete's foot), subcutaneous (e.g., sporotrichosis), or systemic (e.g., histoplasmosis). Systemic fungal infections tend to be more serious and usually do not occur unless the host's immune system is compromised.
- Parasites include protozoa, helminths (roundworms, flatworms), and arthropods. Manifestations of parasitic infections vary depending on the organism and site of infection. Common sites of parasitic infestation are the skin and gastrointestinal tract.

TABLE 8-7

Parasitic Infections

Parasitic Agent	Common Name of Disease	Location of Infection	Symptoms	Mode of Transmission
HELMINTHS (WORMS)				
Nematodes (Roundworms)				
Ancylostoma duodenale	Hookworm	Blood vessels of gut	Anemia	Skin penetration
Ascaris lumbricoides	Giant roundworm	Small intestine, lungs	Pneumonitis (rare), intestinal obstruction (rare)	Oral (fecal contamination), autoinfection
Enterobius vermicularis	Pinworm	Cecum	Anal pruritus	Oral
Onchocerca volvulus	River blindness	Skin, eye	Blindness	Insect inoculation
Strongyloides stercoralis	Strongyloidiasis	Small intestine, lungs	Eosinophilia, urticaria, rash, abdominal pain, pneumonitis	Skin penetration, autoinfection
Trichinella spiralis	Trichinosis	Muscles	Muscular pain, eosinophilia, fever, periorbital edema	Oral (infected meat)
Trichuris trichiura	Whipworm	Intestine	Rectal prolapse	Oral (fecal contamination)
Wuchereria bancrofti	Filariasis	Lymphatics	Elephantiasis	Insect (mosquito)
Trematodes (Flukes)				
Clonorchis sinensis	Liver fluke	Liver	Biliary obstruction (rare)	Oral (raw fish)
Fasciola hepatica	Liver fluke	Liver	Fever, right upper quadrant abdominal pain, eosinophilia	Oral
Fasciolopsis buski	Intestinal fluke	Liver	Abdominal pain, diarrhea	Oral
Paragonimus westermani	Lung fluke	Lung, intestine	Eosinophilia, cough, chest pain, bronchitis	Oral (poorly cooked freshwater crab or crayfish)
Schistosoma haematobium	Blood fluke	Urinary tract	Acute: rash, fever, cough, chest, chills	Skin inoculation
Schistosoma japonicum	Blood fluke	Mesenteric blood vessels	Hepatomegaly, splenomegaly	Skin inoculation
Schistosoma mansoni	Blood fluke	Mesenteric blood vessels	Lymphadenopathy, eosinophilia	Skin inoculation
Cestodes (Tapeworms)				
Diphyllobothrium latum	Fish tapeworm	Intestine	Megaloblastic anemia	Oral (poorly cooked fish)
Taenia saginata	Beef tapeworm	Intestine	Mild abdominal pain	Oral (poorly cooked beef)
Taenia solium	Pork tapeworm	Intestine	Mild abdominal pain	Oral (poorly cooked pork)
Echinococcus granulosus	Hydatid cyst	Lung, liver	Cholestasis, liver congestion and atrophy, biliary obstruction	Oral (inoculation with sheep, cattle, or dog feces)
PROTOZOA				
Entamoeba histolytica	Amebic dysentery	Intestine	Bloody, mucoid diarrhea; colicky abdominal pain	Contaminated water, raw vegetables
Plasmodium spp.	Malaria	Liver, erythrocytes	High fever, chills, rigor, anemia, headache, malaise, chest pain, abdominal pain	Female *Anopheles* mosquito
Leishmania spp.	Kala azar; cutaneous leishmaniasis	Reticuloendothelial cells of the body disseminates to spleen, liver, bone marrow, lymph glands	Chronic: abdominal discomfort, ascites, fever, weakness, pallor, weight loss, cough Acute: sudden fever, chills	All transmission accomplished through the bite of sandflies after biting specific infected mammals
Trypanosoma spp. T. cruzi	Chagas disease	Bloodstream	Local inflammation, lymphadenopathy, muscular necrosis including myocardium (heart failure), esophagus, and colon (dilation); fever, malaise, anorexia, edema of face	Insects—hematophagous (blood drinking) *Triatoma*

TABLE 8-7

Parasitic Infections—cont'd

Parasitic Agent	Common Name of Disease	Location of Infection	Symptoms	Mode of Transmission
PROTOZOA—cont'd				
T. brucei	African sleeping sickness	Bloodstream	Fever, malaise, headache, rash, CNS disturbances	Glossina flies (tsetse flies)
Toxoplasma gondii	Toxoplasmosis	Throughout body	Acute: usually asymptomatic Immunosuppressed: encephalitis, myocarditis, pneumonitis Newborn: impaired vision, neurologic disorders	Eating raw or undercooked meat, poultry, or dairy foods; oral inoculation with cat feces
Pneumocystis carinii	Pneumonitis	Lungs	Fever, cough, tachypnea, costal retractions, cyanosis	Inhalation
Giardia lamblia	Epidemic diarrhea	Intestine	Acute: self-limited diarrhea; occasionally malabsorption with weight loss	Fecal contamination of water; person to person
Trichomonas vaginalis	Trichomoniasis (vaginitis)	Vagina	Irritation, discharge	Sexually transmitted
ECTOPARASITES				
Pediculus humanus				
Var. corporis	Body louse	All hair-covered parts of body	Pruritus Nits at base of hair shaft	Person to person, by fomites
Var. capitis	Head louse	Head area		
Pediculus pubis	Pubic louse	Pubic area		
Sarcoptes scabiei (var. hominis)	Scabies	Skin	Pruritus, worse at night; linear burrows in folds of fingers, elbows, knees, axillae, pelvic girdle	Person to person
Maggots (larvae of dipterous flies)	Myiasis	Necrotic tissue	Depends on location of infestation	Dipterous flies
Chiggers (mites)		Skin	Intense pruritus, hemorrhagic papules	Inhabit dogs, rabbits, cats, rats; foul cheese, flour, house dust
Ticks		Skin	Can transmit tick paralysis, Lyme disease	Reside in wooded and grassy areas

SUMMARY

This chapter has described the infectious process, host defenses, and types and characteristics of microorganisms. The process of transmission of infection can be thought of as a chain with links that flow from the host or reservoir of the microorganism to the next susceptible victim. The goal of infection control is to block transmission of the microorganism to susceptible victims by severing the chain at one or more links.

Four basic types of microorganisms exist: bacteria, or single-celled organisms with cellular organelles that allow them to live independently in the environment; viruses, or tiny genetic parasites that require the host cell to replicate and spread; fungi, or nonphotosynthetic eukaryotic single- or multicellular creatures that are found throughout the environment; and parasites, which include protozoa, roundworms, flatworms, and arthropods. These organisms can be helpful or harmful to the host. When harmful, a microorganism is considered pathogenic. The study of pathogenic organisms and the way that they spread is called epidemiology.

The host-parasite relationship is determined by the characteristics of both the microorganism and the host. Microorganism factors that affect the relationship include whether the parasite must kill the host cell to propagate, the reaction of the host to the invading microorganism and its endotoxins, and the ability of the microorganism to live independently from the host in the environment. Host factors such as the integrity of barriers to transmission, nutritional status, age, and drug regimen all have an impact on this relationship.

Health care professionals have a key role in the prevention and early detection of infectious processes in hospital and community settings. The identification of high-risk individuals who are more susceptible to infection will assist in earlier detection of the manifestations of infection. Management of infections requires optimizing the client's host defense system and is supplemented by pharmacologic and nutritional interventions.

REFERENCES

1. Mandell GL, Bennett JE, Dolin R: *Principles and practice of infectious diseases,* ed 6, Philadelphia, 2004, Churchill Livingstone.
2. Garner JS: Guideline for isolation precautions: preventing transmission of infectious agents in healthcare settings, 2007, available at http://www.cdc.gov/ncidod/dhaqp/guidelines/isolation2007.pdf.
3. Chulay M, Burns S: *AACN essentials of critical care nursing,* ed 1, New York, 2005, McGraw-Hill Medical.
4. Heymann DL: *Control of communicable diseases manual,* ed 18, Washington DC, 2004, American Public Health Association.
5. U.S. Centers for Disease Control and Prevention: Boulder County Department of Health, 2002, available at http://www.cdc.gov/.
6. Price SA, Wilson LM: *Pathophysiology: clinical concepts of disease processes,* ed 6, St Louis, 2002, Mosby.
7. Guyton AC, Hall JE: *Textbook of medical physiology,* ed 11, Philadelphia, 2005, Saunders.
8. Widmaier EB, Raff H, Strang KT: *Vander's human physiology: the mechanisms of body function,* ed 10, New York, 2006, McGraw-Hill.
9. Schiable UE et al: Malnutrition and infection: complex mechanisms and global impacts, *PLoS Med* 4(5):115, 2007.
10. Artinian V, Hicham K, DiGiovene B et al: Effects of early enteral feeding on the outcome of critically ill mechanically ventilated medical patients, *Chest* 129:960-967, 2006.
11. Donahue R et al: Feeding the open abdomen: *J Parenter Enteral Nutr* 31(5):410-415, 2007.
12. Kahn CR: *Joslin's diabetes mellitus,* ed 14, Philadelphia, 2005, Lippincott Williams & Wilkins.
13. Esposito S et al: Antibiotic resistance in long-term care facilities, *New Microbiol* 30(3):326-331, 2007.
14. Gilbert DN et al: *The Sanford guide to antimicrobial therapy,* ed 37, Sperryville, 2007, Antimicrobial Therapy Inc.
15. Gleason PP et al: Associations between initial antimicrobial therapy and medical outcomes for hospitalized elderly patients with pneumonia, *Arch Intern Med* 159:2562-2572, 1999.
16. Benton TJ, Nixon LB: The aging urinary tract and asymptomatic bacteriuria, *Clin Geriatr* 15(2):17-22, 2007.
17. Gea-Banacloche JC et al: Sepsis associated with immuno-suppressive medicine, *Crit Care Med* 32(11), 2004.
18. Fitch SJ, Gossage JR: Optimal management of septic shock, *Postgrad Med* 111(3), 2002.
19. 2008 Child and Adolescent Immunization Schedule, available at http://www.cdc.gove/vaccines/recs/schedules/child-schedule.html, 2008.
20. Cooper RB: *Everything you needed to know about diseases,* Philadelphia, 2004, Springhouse.
21. Gorbach S, Bartlett JG, Blacklow NR: *Infectious diseases,* ed 3, Philadelphia, 2003, Lippincott Williams & Wilkins.
22. Donaldson TA: Immune responses to infection, *Crit Care Nurs Clin North Am* 19(1):1-8, 2007.
23. Iseman MD: *A clinician's guide to tuberculosis,* Philadelphia, 2000, Lippincott Williams & Wilkins.
24. Rakel RE, Bope ET: *Conn's current therapy 2008,* Philadelphia, 2008, Saunders.
25. George RB et al: *Chest medicine, essentials of pulmonary and critical care medicine,* ed 6, Philadelphia, 2006, Lippincott Williams & Wilkins.
26. Chadwick PR: Making real sense of methicillin-resistant, *Staphylococcus aureus, Lancet* 348:1525-1526, 1996.
27. Hooten TM, Levy SB: Antimicrobial resistance: a plan of action for community practice, *Am Fam Phys* 63:1087-1096, 2001.
28. Methicillin-resistant *Staphylococcus aureus* (MRSA), available at http://www.aap.org/new/mrsa.htm, 2007.
29. Tierney LM, McPhee SJ, Papadakis MA: *Current medical diagnosis and treatment,* ed 46, New York, 2006, McGraw-Hill Professional.
30. Cruz K, Hollenberg S: Update on septic shock: understanding the pathophysiology and recognizing disease: early recognition sets the stage for prompt therapy, *J Crit Illn* 18(4):151-157, 2003.
31. Cooper, DH et al, editors: *The Washington manual of medical therapeutics,* ed 32, Philadelphia, 2007, Lippincott Williams & Wilkins.
32. Roitt IM et al, editors: *Roitt's essential immunology,* ed 11, Boston, 2006, Blackwell Publishing Limited.

Inflammation and Immunity

Jacquelyn L. Banasik

MEDIA RESOURCES

Additional Material for Study, Review, and Further Exploration

 CD Companion ■ Review Questions and Answers
■ Glossary (with audio pronunciations for selected terms)
■ Disease Profiles ■ Animations

evolve **Website** at http://evolve.elsevier.com/Copstead/
■ Case Studies ■ Disease Profiles ■ WebLinks ■ Key Points Review

 Online Course (Modules 4, 5)

KEY QUESTIONS

■ What are the major organs and cellular components of the body's defense against foreign antigens?
■ How do immune cells communicate through cell-to-cell interactions and through secreted cytokines?
■ How do innate and adaptive immune mechanisms differ?
■ How do macrophages, granulocytes, and lymphocytes work together to locate, recognize, and eliminate pathogens?

■ What is the role of MHC class I and II proteins in cell-mediated immunity?
■ Why is an immune response usually more effective on subsequent exposure to an antigen than after the first exposure?
■ How do noncellular immune system components, including antibodies, complement, and clotting factors, aid the immune response?

CHAPTER OUTLINE

The immune system is a complex network of cells and tissues that work together to protect the body against foreign invaders. The wide variety of potential pathogens requires a defense system that is diversified and adaptable. Several types of white blood cells (WBCs) are of primary importance in localizing, recognizing, and eliminating foreign substances. These immune cells are strategically situated in diverse locations so that pathogens may be detected quickly. The dispersed nature of these defensive cells necessitates a complex system of intercellular communication to effectively mobilize reinforcements to areas of need. A tremendous amount of information has accumulated in the last 10 years about how immune cells communicate and the processes that enable them to migrate to particular locations. The impact of this research goes far beyond the traditional immune disorders such as immunodeficiency diseases and hypersensitivity reactions. Indeed, it is now difficult to identify many pathophysiologic processes that do not involve the immune system in some way. The immune system has been implicated in the pathogenesis of disorders as diverse as atherosclerosis, myocardial infarction, shock, diabetes, and stroke. Therefore, an understanding of immune function is fundamental to the study of a wide variety of diseases. This chapter describes the organs and cells that constitute the immune system, the mechanisms of action of innate and adaptive defenses, and the communication processes whereby immune cells achieve a coordinated response. Underreactions and overreactions of the immune system, immune system malignancies, and human immunodeficiency virus disease are described in Chapters 10, 11, and 12, respectively.

Components of the Immune System

The structures of the immune system include (1) skin and mucous membranes; (2) the mononuclear phagocyte system; (3) the lymphoid system, including spleen, thymus gland, and lymph nodes; and (4) bone marrow. All these structures are inhabited by different types of WBCs (leukocytes) that mediate **inflammation** and **immunity.** Leukocytes are responsible for locating and eliminating pathogens and foreign molecules.

They are aided in their task of bodily defense by a number of chemical mediators, including **complement, kinins,** clotting factors, **cytokines, and chemokines.**

Components of the immune system are often categorized into specific or innate defenses according to the mechanisms whereby antigens are recognized. Innate defenses require no previous exposure to mount an effective response against an **antigen,** and a wide variety of different antigens are recognized. Natural killer (NK) cells and phagocytic cells such as **neutrophils** and **macrophages** are mediators of innate defenses. In contrast, specific defenses respond more effectively on second exposure to an antigen (adaptive) and are highly restricted in the ability to recognize antigens. B lymphocytes (B cells) and T lymphocytes (T cells) are the agents of specific immunity.

Although separating immune components into specific and innate systems is helpful for studying inflammation and immunity, it is an artificial division because they function in a highly integrated manner. The approach used in this chapter is to first describe the major components of the immune system, discuss innate and specific adaptive defenses separately, and then summarize the integrated function of the entire system and its regulation.

EPITHELIAL BARRIERS

The skin and mucous membranes are sometimes called the "first line of defense" because they are frequently the initial sites of microbial invasion. Intact epithelia in skin and mucous membranes provide mechanical and chemical barriers that prevent microorganisms from gaining access to the body's tissues. The skin epithelium produces antimicrobial peptides called *defensins* that can kill a wide variety of bacteria and fungi. The intestinal epithelium produces another form of bactericidal peptide called *cryptocidins* that prevent bacteria from colonizing the intestinal wall.[1] Resident microorganisms may aid in providing this line of defense by making conditions inhospitable for pathogens (see Chapter 8). Disruption of the normal epithelial barriers increases the likelihood that pathogens will successfully establish an infection. Physical trauma (e.g., burns, lacerations, erosions) and biochemical alterations (e.g., pH changes, increased glucose concentration, decreased enzyme production) predispose to infection. Pathogens that breach the skin or mucous membranes are generally first detected by cells of the mononuclear phagocyte system. These cells are thought to derive from monocytes produced in the bone marrow. Specialized antibody-secreting cells also locate to the mucous membranes where they produce antibodies of the immunoglobulin A (IgA) class. IgA antibodies bind antigens on the mucosal surface and prevent them from entering more deeply into the tissues.

MONONUCLEAR PHAGOCYTE SYSTEM

The mononuclear phagocyte system (previously called the reticuloendothelial system) is composed of monocytes and macrophages that are widely distributed throughout the body. Monocytes from the circulating blood migrate to organs and tissues to become macrophages. Macrophages are found throughout the body and go by various names in different tissues, such as alveolar macrophages in the lungs, microglial cells in the brain, Kupffer cells in the liver, and histiocytes in connective tissue (Figure 9-1). Dendritic cells are a monocyte-derived cell type that specializes in capturing and presenting antigens to T cells. Dendritic cells are strategically located in subcutaneous and submucosal tissues.

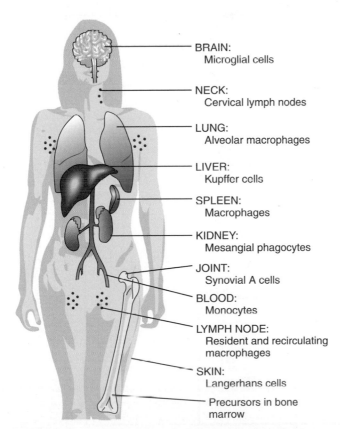

BRAIN:
Microglial cells

NECK:
Cervical lymph nodes

LUNG:
Alveolar macrophages

LIVER:
Kupffer cells

SPLEEN:
Macrophages

KIDNEY:
Mesangial phagocytes

JOINT:
Synovial A cells

BLOOD:
Monocytes

LYMPH NODE:
Resident and recirculating macrophages

SKIN:
Langerhans cells

Precursors in bone marrow

FIGURE 9-1 Cells of the mononuclear phagocyte system. (Redrawn from Schindler LW: *Understanding the immune system*, NIH Pub No 92-529, Bethesda, Md, 1991, U.S. Department of Health and Human Services, p 9.)

Macrophages and dendritic cells are often the first immune system cells to encounter a pathogen or foreign antigen after it has entered the body, and they are instrumental in communicating news of the invasion to other immune cells. This communication is accomplished through secretion of chemical signaling molecules called *cytokines* and by presentation of captured antigen to the specific, adaptive immune cells. Macrophages have many other roles in the immune response in addition to their sentry function. Macrophages are powerful phagocytes, each capable of ingesting numerous microbes. Macrophages are called on to clean up the area after an inflammatory reaction in which dead neutrophils and inflammatory debris have accumulated, and they have a role in wound healing.

LYMPHOID SYSTEM

The primary lymphoid organs are the bone marrow and thymus gland, which are the structures where lymphocytes develop. All types of lymphocytes are produced from stem cells in the bone marrow (Figure 9-2). T lymphocytes then migrate to the thymus for development, whereas B lymphocytes and NK cells stay in the marrow to develop. NK cells are a population of lymphocytes that lack both T-cell and B-cell markers. NK cells are produced and released from the bone marrow and function in innate immune responses. NK cells are found mainly in the circulation and spleen. Once mature, T and B lymphocytes migrate to the secondary lymphoid organs where they await activation by antigens. Secondary lymphoid organs include the tonsils, spleen, lymph nodes, and Peyer patches (Figure 9-3).

Primary Lymphoid Organs

Bone marrow is contained in all the bones of the body. The primary function of bone marrow is **hematopoiesis,** or the formation of blood cells. There are two kinds of bone marrow: red and yellow. Hematopoiesis is carried out by red (functioning) marrow. By adulthood, red marrow is confined to the pelvis, sternum, ribs, cranium, ends of the long bones, and vertebral spine. Yellow or fatty bone marrow is found in the remaining bones. It normally does not contribute to hematopoiesis in the adult, but can be recruited to become red marrow again under conditions of increased need for hematopoiesis.[2]

B lymphocytes (B cells) are produced and develop in the bone marrow. B cells migrate from the outer edges toward the center of the bone marrow as they develop. Pre-B cells are subjected to a highly selective quality control process, and less than 25% of the developing B cells are allowed to survive. During migration through the bone marrow, immature B cells are exposed to self antigens. B cells that do not bind to any antigens continue to develop into mature B cells. If immature B cells encounter antigens to which they bind while still in the bone marrow, a series of events is triggered to induce self-tolerance. The immature B cell is stimulated to reactivate the genetic recombination machinery in an attempt

FIGURE 9-2 Maturation of human blood cells showing pathways of cell differentiation from the pluripotent stem cell to mature granulocytes, monocytes, lymphocytes, thrombocytes, and erythrocytes. Production begins in embryo blood islands in the yolk sac. As the embryo matures, production shifts to the liver, spleen, and bone marrow. In an adult, nearly all hematopoiesis occurs in the bone marrow. The two major differentiation pathways are the myeloid pathway and the lymphoid pathway. The lymphoid pathway produces lymphocytes, whereas the myeloid pathway produces granulocytes, monocytes, platelets, and red cells.

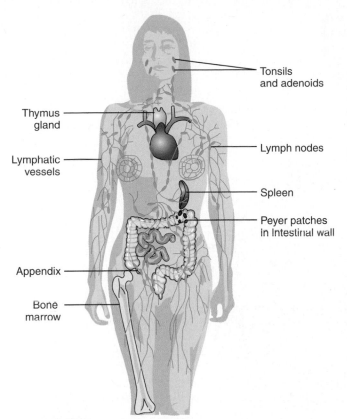

Tonsils
and adenoids

Thymus
gland

Lymphatic
vessels

Lymph nodes

Spleen

Peyer patches
in intestinal wall

Appendix

Bone
marrow

FIGURE 9-3 Principal organs of the lymphoid system.

to produce a new B-cell receptor (BCR) that does not bind to self antigen. If this receptor editing attempt fails to alter binding sufficiently, the immature B cell will undergo apoptosis in the bone marrow.[3] Mature B cells that leave the bone marrow to colonize secondary lymphoid organs are called *naive* B cells because they have not yet encountered antigen.

T lymphocytes (T cells) develop in the thymus, which is located in the anterior mediastinum overlying the heart. Pre-T cells initially enter the outer aspect (cortex) of the thymus lobules, and many die as they migrate to the center (medulla) of the thymus. The selection process for T cells is even more rigorous than that for B cells; only about 5% of the cells entering the thymus survive to reenter the circulation and colonize secondary lymphoid organs. The thymus is relatively large at birth and progressively increases in size until puberty. After puberty, the thymus steadily atrophies and only a low level of new T-cell development continues into adulthood.[4] The thymus produces interleukin-7 (IL-7), a cytokine that promotes T-cell proliferation.

Secondary Lymphoid Organs

Once mature, lymphocytes leave their primary lymphoid organs and travel through the blood to localize in peripheral, or secondary, lymphoid tissues, including lymph nodes, spleen, tonsils, and Peyer patches in the intestine. These naive T cells and B cells express specific receptor proteins on their cell surfaces that allow them to migrate or "home" to specific locations in lymph tissue. Most mature T lymphocytes are in constant

circulation through lymphatic tissues and the bloodstream. It has been estimated that a lymphocyte makes a circuit from the blood to tissues to lymphatics and back to the bloodstream once or twice per day.[3] Antigens can be carried to the naive cells in the lymph nodes by the specialized antigen-presenting dendritic cells. When exposed to an appropriate antigen, T cells and B cells migrate toward each other within the lymph nodes and begin to proliferate. Activated T cells may then migrate to lymph vessels and travel to the bloodstream, where they are dispersed throughout the system. The majority of B cells stay in the lymph node where they mature into antibody-secreting plasma cells. Lymphocyte recirculation and homing is regulated by binding interactions between various types of cell adhesion molecules (CAMs) including selectins, integrins, and addressins.[3]

Tonsils

Tonsils are aggregates of lymphoid tissue located in the mouth and pharynx. The tonsils are strategically located at the entrance to the digestive and respiratory systems, where they are likely to encounter microorganisms. Unlike lymph nodes, tonsils have no afferent (incoming) lymphatic vessels. They do have efferent lymphatic drainage so that activated lymphocytes from the tonsils can migrate to other lymphoid organs. Tonsils normally make an important contribution to immune function; however, they may occasionally become chronically infected, and surgical removal (tonsillectomy) is then necessary.

Spleen

The spleen is located under the diaphragm on the left side of the body. It measures about 12 cm in length, which makes it the largest of the lymphoid organs. The spleen provides an important filtering function for blood. The tissue structure of the spleen is similar to that of lymph nodes. It is surrounded by a capsule of connective tissue and filled with a meshwork of red pulp and localized masses of lymphocytes called *white pulp*. Within the red pulp are many blood-filled sinuses lined with macrophages. Macrophages filter out foreign substances and old red blood cells. Lymphocytes located in the white pulp are in a strategic position to come in contact with blood-borne antigens. Lymphocytes thus activated in the spleen can migrate to other lymphoid organs via efferent lymphatics. Like the tonsils, the spleen does not have afferent lymphatic vessels.

Lymph Nodes and Lymphatics

The lymphatic vessels begin with small, closed-ended lymphatic capillaries in direct contact with the interstitial fluid surrounding cells and tissues. Lymphatics pick up fluid and proteins that escape the bloodstream and return them to the circulation by way of the right lymphatic and thoracic ducts. Along the way from lymphatic capillaries to the thoracic ducts, lymph flows through specialized structures called *lymph nodes*. Lymph nodes are found primarily in the neck, axilla, thorax, abdomen, and groin. They often become tender and palpable

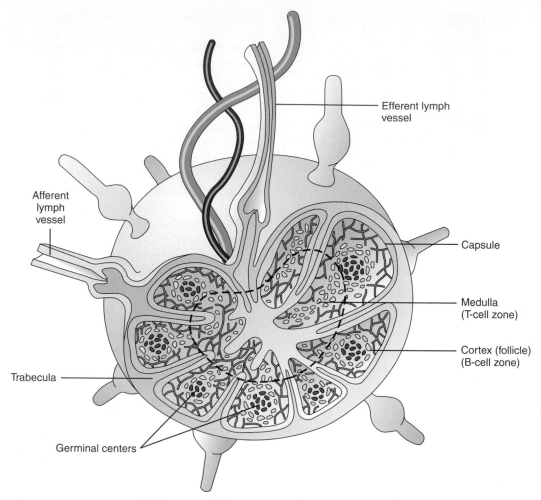

Efferent lymph
vessel

Afferent
lymph
vessel

Capsule

Medulla
(T-cell zone)

Cortex (follicle)
(B-cell zone)

Trabecula

Germinal centers

FIGURE 9-4 Schematic drawing of a typical lymph node showing afferent and efferent lymph vessels, as well as B-cell and T-cell zones.

when responding to foreign invaders. Projections of connective tissue called *trabeculae* divide the interior of the lymph node into compartments (Figure 9-4). Lymph nodes contain large numbers of B and T lymphocytes and macrophages. B cells are the predominant cell type in the cortical follicles, whereas T cells predominate in the area just under the cortex called the *paracortex*. The central region, or medulla, is populated by macrophages, B cells, and plasma cells (antibody-secreting B cells). Lymph fluid flows through the nodes in a way that allows these immune cells to filter, detect, and react to foreign material.

Peyer Patches

Aggregates of lymphoid tissue can be found scattered throughout the body, particularly in the gastrointestinal, respiratory, and urogenital tracts. These structures are analogous to lymph nodes, but they are not encapsulated and contain primarily B cells. Because of their location, these structures have been termed *mucosa-associated lymphoid tissue* (MALT) or *gut-associated lymphoid tissue* (GALT). These structures, also called *Peyer patches,* are of particular importance in producing antibodies to microorganisms that tend to invade mucosal tissue.

LEUKOCYTES

Leukocytes, or WBCs, are the primary effector cells of the immune system. Each of the different types of leukocytes found in blood has a special job to perform. All leukocytes, as well as red blood cells and platelets, are formed from stem cells in the bone marrow. Stem cells can produce daughter cells that differentiate along several different pathways to become mature cell types (see Figure 9-2). The first major differentiation step produces either a lymphoid stem cell or a myeloid stem cell. Lymphoid stem cells further differentiate to form B and T lymphocytes and NK cells. Myeloid stem cells can produce a variety of cell types, including red blood cells, platelets, monocytes, dendritic cells, and **granulocytes.** Monocytes that migrate from the blood into tissues are called *macrophages.* Granulocytes are further divided into neutrophils, eosinophils, and basophils. Basophils are precursors of the mast cells located in tissues.

Development of these cell types is influenced by hormonal signaling molecules called *cytokines*. Cytokines are produced locally in the bone marrow and by various other cells. Certain cytokines stimulate stem cell growth, proliferation,

TABLE 9-1

Leukocyte Proportions and Functions

Type	Percentage*	Role in Inflammation
Neutrophils	60-80	First to appear after injury, phagocytosis
Lymphocytes	20-30	Immune response
Monocytes (macrophages)	3-8	Phagocytosis
Eosinophils	1-6	Allergic reactions, parasite infection
Basophils	0-2	Contain histamine, mediate type I allergic reactions, initiate inflammation

*Total white cell count, 3500 to 10,000/µl.

and differentiation into particular cell types. The WBC count and differential are commonly measured laboratory tests used to evaluate white cell production. A normal WBC count and differential are shown in Table 9-1. The general features of each of the WBC types are summarized in the following sections.

Neutrophils

Neutrophils are circulating granulocytes that are also known as *polymorphonuclear leukocytes* (polys or PMNs). They account for 60% to 80% of the total WBC count. Neutrophils normally have two to five nuclear lobes and coarse, clumped chromatin. Neutrophils arise from bone marrow stem cells and undergo several stages of maturation. As illustrated in Figure 9-2, these stages, from least to most mature, are myeloblast, promyelocyte, metamyelocyte, band cell, and mature segmented neutrophil.

Neutrophils stored in the bone marrow outnumber, by about 10-fold, the quantity of circulating neutrophils. An adult produces more than 1×10^{11} neutrophils each day.[1] These stored neutrophils are released into the circulation, where they have a half-life of 4 to 10 hours. Neutrophils that are not recruited into tissues within about 6 hours undergo programmed cell death (apoptosis). Neutrophils are early responders to an acute bacterial infection and arrive in large numbers very quickly. They are phagocytes that engulf and degrade microorganisms. Circulating neutrophils have receptors on their cell surfaces that enable them to bind to endothelial cells in areas of inflammation. These receptors, called *L-selectins,* allow neutrophils to stick and roll along the capillary surface.[5] Other interactions between neutrophil integrin receptors and extracellular matrix then facilitate movement of neutrophils through the capillary wall and into the tissue. Neutrophils are attracted to areas of inflammation and bacterial products by **chemotactic** factors such as complement fragments and cytokines. This process is discussed in more depth in the section on Inflammation.

Initially during an acute infection, **neutrophilia,** or an increase in the number of circulating neutrophils, occurs as the bone marrow releases stored neutrophils. As neutrophils are consumed and demand exceeds production, an increase in the number of immature (band) neutrophils occurs. Bands are identified by their lack of nuclear segmentation. This increase in band cells is referred to as a "shift to the left of normal" (Figure 9-5). Traditionally, the band count has been used to differentiate bacterial from viral infections, and a greater shift to the left is viewed as a more severe infection. The utility of using the band count for these purposes has been called into question because the specificity is poor.[6]

Neutrophils produce potent chemical mediators that enable them to destroy microorganisms. More than 50 toxins released by neutrophils have been identified, including oxidizing free radicals, defensins, and proteolytic enzymes, such as elastase.[7] Because of the ability to generate free radicals and release enzymes, neutrophils can cause extensive damage to normal tissue during their inflammatory response.

Eosinophils

Eosinophils are circulating granulocytes that have two nuclear lobes and stain brilliant red-orange with eosin. They make up 1% to 6% of the total WBC count. Eosinophils mature in the bone marrow (3 to 6 days) and circulate in the blood for about 30 minutes. They have a half-life of 12 days in tissue. Eosinophils arise from myeloid stem cells and undergo a maturation process similar to that of neutrophils.

Eosinophils are particularly associated with and increase in number during allergic reactions and infection by intestinal parasites. The role of eosinophils in allergic reactions is less well characterized than that of mast cells. Eosinophils are recruited into areas of inflammation by the chemokine, eotaxin, which is produced by epithelial cells.[3] Eosinophils release inflammatory chemicals, such as lysosomal enzymes, peroxidase, major basic protein, and cationic protein. The triggers that stimulate eosinophil degranulation and their role in inflammation are not well understood. The primary function of eosinophils is to kill parasitic helminths (worms). Helminths are too large to be phagocytosed by neutrophils or macrophages, and their exterior is resistant to attack by complement or mast cell products. Eosinophils produce specialized molecules such as major basic protein and eosinophil cationic protein, which may be more effective against helminths.[1] Eosinophils recognize helminths that have been opsonized (coated) with IgE antibody. They bind to the IgE and then release their stored chemicals onto the surface of the opsonized helminth. Parasitic infections are a significant problem in much of the world, with one third of the population being affected.

Basophils and Mast Cells

Basophils are granulocytes characterized by granules that stain blue with basophilic dyes. Basophils account for 0% to 2% of the total leukocyte count. Basophils are structurally similar to mast cells. Mature basophils circulate in the vascular system, whereas mast cells are found in connective tissue, especially around blood vessels and under mucosal surfaces.

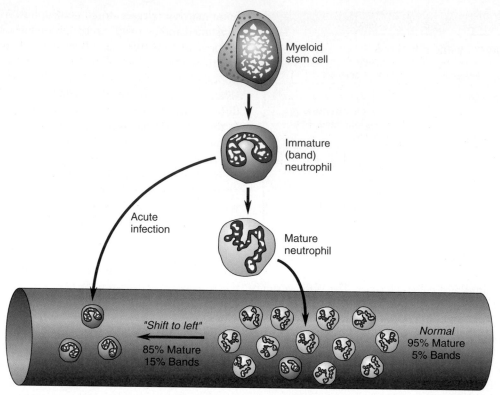

FIGURE 9-5 Inflammatory cytokines stimulate the release of more immature neutrophils, called *bands,* from the bone marrow. An increased ratio of bands to mature neutrophils is termed a "shift to the left." This clinical term evolved from the practice of listing bands to the left of mature cells on the laboratory report sheet. A shift to the left is commonly seen with acute bacterial infections.

When stimulated by cytokines, mature basophils can migrate to connective tissue, but once in the tissue, basophils (then called mast cells) do not reenter the circulation.

The average basophil life span is measured in days, whereas mast cells can live for weeks to months. Mast cells and basophils have IgE receptors that allow them to bind and display IgE antibodies on their cell surfaces. When an appropriate stimulus occurs, such as antigen binding to the IgE antibodies, mast cells and basophils release granules (**degranulate**) containing proinflammatory chemicals.

Mast cell and basophil granules contain histamine, platelet-activating factor, and other vasoactive amines that are important mediators of immediate hypersensitivity responses (Figure 9-6). Degranulation of mast cells and basophils begins the inflammatory response that is characteristically associated with allergic reactions. Mast cells and basophils are also involved in wound healing and chronic inflammatory conditions (see Chapter 10).

Monocytes and Macrophages

Monocytes and macrophages, like granulocytes, originate from bone marrow stem cells of the myeloid lineage. Monocytes are immature macrophages and account for about 5% of the total WBC count. Monocytes circulate in the bloodstream for about 3 days before they enter tissue to become macrophages. As described earlier, macrophages are found in widespread locations as part of the mononuclear phagocyte system.

FIGURE 9-6 Micrograph of a mast cell showing a large yellow nucleus and numerous packets containing histamine, which are colorized red. (From Thibodeau GA, Patton KT: *Anatomy & physiology,* ed 6, Mosby, 2007, p 805.)

Phagocytosis by macrophages is similar to that by neutrophils except that neutrophils are short lived and die in the process of fighting infection. Macrophages, in contrast, may live for months to years and can migrate in and out of tissue. Macrophages are more efficient phagocytes than neutrophils and can ingest several times as many microorganisms (Figure 9-7). Macrophages are capable of cell division and may proliferate at the site of inflammation.

Macrophages are covered with a variety of receptor proteins on their cell surface (Figure 9-8). Some of these receptors

FIGURE 9-7 Scanning electron micrograph of a macrophage (red) attaching to and phagocytizing bacteria (yellow). (From Nairn R, Helbert M: *Immunology for medical students,* ed 2, Mosby, 2007, p 3. With permission from Juergen Berger, Max-Planck Institute, and the Science Photo Library.)

help macrophages locate antigens that have been coated by antibodies. These receptors are called *Fc receptors* because they bind to the part of an antibody called the *constant fragment,* or *Fc.* Macrophages also have receptors for the complement component C3b. Complement, like antibodies, can coat an antigen and make it more recognizable to macrophages. Coating of antigen by antibodies or by complement is called **opsonization.** Macrophages have receptors that help them recognize bacteria directly. These innate pattern-recognition receptors bind to particular molecules prevalent in the bacterial cell wall. For example, mannose receptors and at least 10 different Toll-like receptors on macrophages allow them to recognize common microbial structures (see Figure 9-8). Other receptors, called *selectins* and *integrins,* help macrophages stick to capillary walls, and enter and move through tissue. Integrin receptors bind to proteins in the extracellular matrix and help macrophages target or "home" to certain areas.

In addition to their phagocytic function, macrophages have important secretory function. Some of the substances secreted by macrophages are cytokines, which help to coordinate the activities of other immune cells (Figure 9-9). Macrophage cytokines include IL-1, IL-6, IL-12, and tumor necrosis factor α (TNF-α). These cytokines promote inflammation, as well as the activity of other WBCs, including neutrophils and lymphocytes (see the section on Cytokines and Chemokines).

FIGURE 9-8 Macrophage surface receptors. Macrophages display receptors for a number of extracellular molecules that enhance their function such as cytokines, complement, selectins, integrins, and antibody *(Fc).* Toll-like receptors recognize patterns of microbial components and trigger intracellular signaling cascades in the macrophage. *IFN-γ,* interferon γ; *IL,* interleukin; *LPS,* lipopolysaccharide.

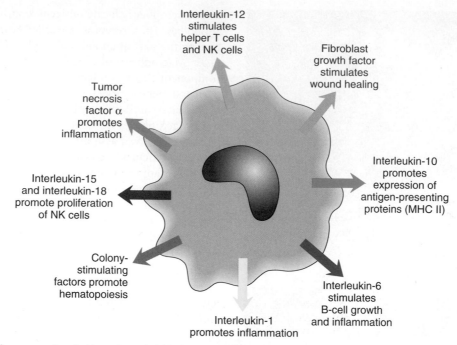

FIGURE 9-9 Macrophages are of central importance in initiating inflammation and recruitment of other leukocytes to areas of need. Macrophages secrete a variety of cytokines that induce inflammation and chemotaxis. Some macrophage cytokines stimulate the growth and differentiation of other white blood cell types.

Macrophages secrete a number of proteins that are important in wound healing. Some of these proteins are enzymes that break down tissue (collagenase, elastase, plasminogen activator), whereas others stimulate the growth of new granulation tissue (fibroblast growth factor, angiogenic factors).

A third function of macrophages, in addition to phagocytosis and secretion, is antigen presentation. For T cells to recognize antigens, these antigens must first be processed and presented on the surface of an antigen-presenting cell such as dendritic cells, macrophages, or B cells. Macrophages accomplish this task by first engulfing the antigen, then processing it into smaller pieces, and finally combining the antigen fragments with special membrane proteins. The antigen complexes are then displayed on the macrophage cell surface, where T lymphocytes (T helper cells) can recognize and become activated by them. Antigen presentation is explored in more detail in the section on Specific Adaptive Immunity.

Dendritic Cells

Dendritic cells are derived in the bone marrow from the same progenitor cells that produce monocytes and macrophages (Figure 9-10) and are structurally and functionally similar to macrophages (Figure 9-11). Dendritic cells derive their name from an unusual shape that has extensive projections from the surface. Dendritic cells are located throughout the body as part of the mononuclear phagocyte system. They function primarily as antigen-presenting cells, capturing antigen in tissues and then migrating to lymphoid areas to present antigen to T cells. Some types of dendritic cells produce chemical messengers called *type 1 interferon* (IFN α and IFN β) in response

to viral infections. Type 1 interferons suppress the viral replication machinery in nearby cells and help stop the local spread of the virus.

Lymphocytes

The three major types of lymphocytes are NK cells, T cells, and B cells. NK cells function in innate immunity, whereas B and T lymphocytes are the cells responsible for specific, adaptive immunity. B and T cells have the capacity to proliferate into "memory cells," which provide long-lasting immunity against specific antigens. NK, T, and B cells are derived from a common lymphoid stem cell in the bone marrow that is stimulated to proliferate by bone marrow–derived cytokines including IL-7. T cells then migrate to the thymus, where they mature. B cells remain in the bone marrow during their maturation phase. NK cells are released into the circulation. Together NK, B, and T lymphocytes compose approximately 20% of the total WBC count. Mature NK cells circulate and populate the spleen, whereas T and B cells migrate to secondary lymphoid organs.

Structurally, lymphocytes are small, round cells with a large, round nucleus. Despite their relatively uniform appearance, lymphocytes can be sorted into a number of subpopulations based on characteristic surface proteins called *cluster of differentiation (CD) markers.* More than 250 different CD markers have been identified thus far, with different immune cell types displaying different combinations on their cell surfaces. Lymphocytes have many complex and differentiated functions, and only the major lymphocyte subtypes are discussed in this chapter.

Myelomonocytic progenitor cell

IL-3, GM-CSF   GM-CSF, IL-3, M-CSF

G-CSF

Chemotaxis to sites
of bacterial infection.
Phagocytosis

Neutrophil

Blood-borne

GM-CSF
and TNF-α

Monocyte

M-CSF

Located in tissues.
Phagocytic and active
as an antigen-
presenting cell

Important as an antigen-
presenting cell in several
tissues, including skin,
thymus and lymphoid
follicles

Macrophage   Dendritic cell

FIGURE 9-10 Development of dendritic cells from a myelomonocytic progenitor cell and precursor cells in common with monocytes and macrophages. (Redrawn from Nairn R, Helbert M: *Immunology for medical students,* ed 2, Mosby, 2007, p 81).

FIGURE 9-11 Dendritic cell morphology. **A,** Light micrograph of resting dendritic cells from the bone marrow. **B,** Scanning electron micrograph of a mature dendritic cell showing extensive projections of the cell membrane. (From Thibodeau GA, Patton KT: *Anatomy & physiology,* ed 6, Mosby, 2007, p 808.)

Natural Killer Cells

NK cells have no B- or T-cell markers and are not dependent on the thymus for development. NK cells are considered to be innate immune cells because they can effectively kill tumor cells and virally infected cells without previous exposure. NK cells kill their target cells by a mechanism similar to that used by cytotoxic T cells. Unlike T and B cells, NK cells can respond to a variety of antigens and are therefore not specific for a particular antigen. Like neutrophils and macrophages, NK cells recognize antibody-coated target cells with their Fc receptors. This process is called *antibody-dependent cell-mediated cytotoxicity* (ADCC). NK cells also target virally infected cells and tumor cells. They are thought to be able to recognize virally infected

cells through innate pattern-recognition receptors, however only those cells that lack certain normal self proteins on their cell surface (major histocompatibility complex I, or MHC I, proteins) are targeted for killing.[3] Cells that display normal MHC I on their cell surfaces are protected from NK cell cytotoxicity, but will be susceptible to killing by cytotoxic T cells that recognize viral antigen displayed on the MHC I proteins.

T Lymphocytes

Two major classes of T lymphocytes can be differentiated by the presence or absence of CD4 and CD8 surface proteins (Figure 9-12). T cells that possess CD4 proteins (CD4+) are called T helper cells. T helper cells interact with antigens

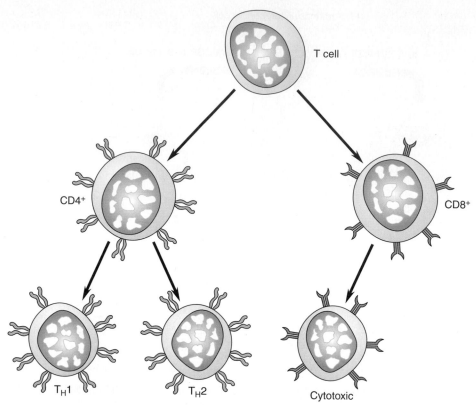

FIGURE 9-12 The two major classes of T lymphocytes can be differentiated by CD markers on the cell surface. T helper cells have CD4 markers, whereas cytotoxic T cells have CD8 markers. CD4 cells can be further differentiated into T_H1 and T_H2, which secrete different cytokines. CD8 cells are cytotoxic T cells.

presented on the surface of specialized antigen-presenting cells such as dendritic cells, macrophages, and B cells. T helper cells can be further divided into two subclasses called T_H1 and T_H2, based on the types of cytokines that they secrete (Figure 9-13). The T_H1 subset of T helper cells develops in response to IL-12 from macrophages and, when activated, secretes cytokines that activate other T cells (IL-2) and macrophages (interferon γ [IFN-γ]). T_H2 cells develop in response to IL-4 from activated T helper cells and secrete cytokines that stimulate B-cell proliferation and antibody production (e.g., IL-4, IL-5, IL-10, IL-13).[8]

The presence of CD8 protein ($CD8^+$) on a T lymphocyte characterizes it as a cytotoxic T cell. Cytotoxic T cells recognize antigen presented in association with surface proteins that can be found on all nucleated cells of the body (MHC I). When a $CD8^+$ T cell recognizes a foreign antigen on a cell, the antigen-presenting cell is killed; thus the name *cytotoxic T cell*. $CD8^+$ cells are particularly effective at destroying virally infected cells, foreign cells, and mutant cells (Figure 9-14). Proliferation of activated cytotoxic T cells is enhanced by T helper cell cytokines, particularly IL-2.

B Lymphocytes

B cells are distinguished from other lymphocytes by their ability to produce antibodies and by the presence of antibody-like receptors (B-cell receptors [BCRs]) on their cell surfaces. Each B cell carries many copies (100,000) of identical BCRs and is able to respond to only one antigen **epitope**[9] (Figure 9-15). B cells require "help" from T helper cells to respond efficiently

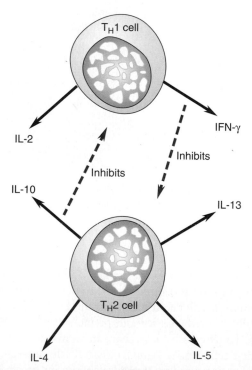

FIGURE 9-13 The two types of T helper cells, T_H1 and T_H2, secrete different cytokines. T_H1 cells secrete interleukin-2 and interferon γ, which stimulate T cells and macrophages. T_H2 cells secrete a number of cytokines that affect B cells. T_H1 and T_H2 cells inhibit the release of cytokines from one another and thus help regulate the immune response. *IFN-γ*, interferon γ; *IL*, interleukin.

FIGURE 9-14 Scanning electron micrograph of activated T cells (blue) and a tumor cell (red). (From Nairn R, Helbert M: *Immunology for medical students,* ed 2, Mosby, 2007, p 3. With permission from BSIP Lecaque and the Science Photo Library.)

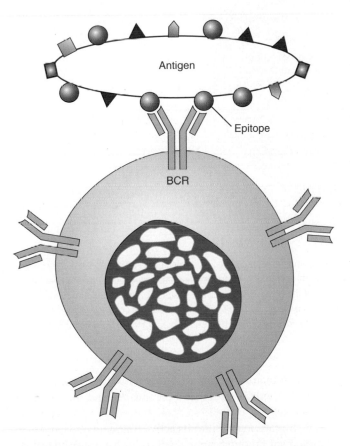

FIGURE 9-15 A typical B cell showing a number of identical B-cell receptors *(BCRs)* on the cell surface. Each BCR is capable of binding to two identical antigen epitopes.

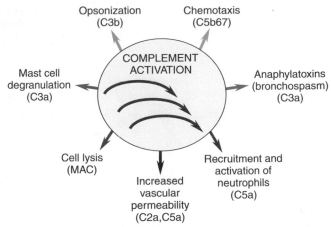

FIGURE 9-16 Activation of the complement cascade results in the production of products that perform a variety of functions to augment the immune response. *MAC,* membrane attack complex.

to nonprotein antigens such as bacterial sugar and lipid molecules. B-cell responses to nonprotein antigens are T-cell independent because T cells respond only to peptide antigens. Exposure to antigens stimulates B cells to mature into antibody-secreting plasma cells and memory cells. B cell memory cells form a reserve of cells that can quickly mount an immune response on subsequent exposure to the same antigen. Memory cells are able to survive for months to years, whereas most antibody-secreting plasma cells live for only a few days. Plasma cells are able to secrete antibodies at a rate of about 2000 per second per cell.[9] Memory B cells and plasma cells develop in germinal centers located in secondary lymphoid organs, including the lymph nodes and spleen. A few long-lived plasma cells inhabit the bone marrow and continue to produce a low level of antibody, which provides immediate protection on second exposure to the same antigen. The mechanisms of specific adaptive immunity are explored later in the chapter.

CHEMICAL MEDIATORS OF IMMUNE FUNCTION

Complement

The complement system consists of about 20 plasma proteins that interact to enhance inflammation, chemotaxis, and lysis of target cells. Complement proteins are synthesized in the liver and by macrophages and neutrophils. They circulate in the blood in an inactive form. Activation of the complement cascade occurs via three different pathways: classical, alternative, and lectin. In all three pathways, the inactive complement proteins are converted to their active form in a sequence of reactions. Major actions of complement proteins include cell lysis, facilitation of phagocytosis by opsonization, inflammation, and chemotaxis (Figure 9-16).

The classical pathway is usually triggered by IgG or IgM antibody-antigen complexes. The alternative pathway can be initiated on first exposure to an antigen. Lipopolysaccharide, in bacterial cell walls, and bacterial endotoxin are effective triggers of the alternative pathway. In the classical pathway,

to protein antigens. B cells bind and internalize the protein antigen, then process and present it to T helper cells. T cells that recognize the presented peptides bind to and are activated by the B cell. T-cell help is provided to the B cell by physical cell-to-cell contact through coreceptor binding, as well as through secreted cytokines. Some B cells can respond

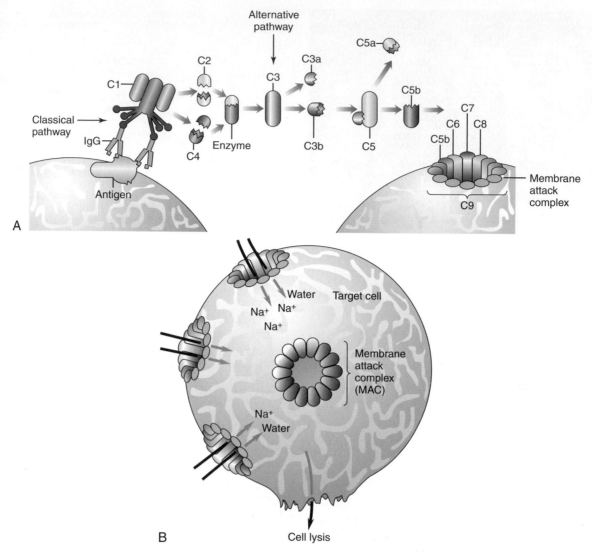

FIGURE 9-17 The complement cascade. **A,** The cascade is activated by the first complement molecule, C1, which binds an antigen-antibody complex. This event begins a domino effect, with each of the remaining complement proteins performing its part in the attack sequence. The end result is a hole in the membrane of the offending cell and destruction of the cell. **B,** Activation of the complement cascade results in the formation of membrane attack complexes that insert in the cell membrane. These porelike structures allow sodium and water influx, which causes the cell to swell and rupture. (**A,** Redrawn from Schindler LW: *Understanding the immune system,* NIH Pub No 92-529, Bethesda, Md, 1991, U.S. Department of Health and Human Services, p 11.)

an antibody hooked onto an antigen combines with C1, the first of the complement proteins. This step sets in motion a domino effect called the *complement cascade* (Figure 9-17). The alternative pathway begins with the activation of C3. The alternative pathway can be activated on first exposure and is part of the innate immune response.[10] The lectin pathway also can be triggered on first exposure. Lectin is a circulating biomolecule that binds mannose on bacterial cell walls and triggers complement activation at C2 and C4. C3 spontaneously degrades into active C3b fragments in plasma. If microbial cell surfaces are present, the C3b fragment can bind directly to the microbe. Two other complement proteins, factors B and D, combine with C3b to initiate the alternative pathway. C3 is the most important and plentiful of the complement proteins. C3 breaks down into two fragments called C3a and C3b. C3a is

a proinflammatory protein that causes histamine release from mast cells, contraction of smooth muscle, and increased endothelial cell permeability. C3b initiates the next step in the cascade by cleaving C5 into its active fragments C5a and C5b. Complement protein fragment C5a is both a powerful inflammatory chemical and a potent chemotactic agent. C5a chemotaxis stimulates neutrophils and monocytes to migrate to the inflamed tissue. C5a also activates neutrophils by triggering their oxidative activity and increasing their glucose uptake.

The C5b fragment combines with C6, C7, C8, and multiple units of C9 to form a large porelike structure (C5b6789) called the *membrane attack complex.* The membrane attack complex has a direct cytotoxic effect by attacking cell membranes and disrupting the lipid bilayer. This action allows free movement of sodium and water into the target cell, which causes it

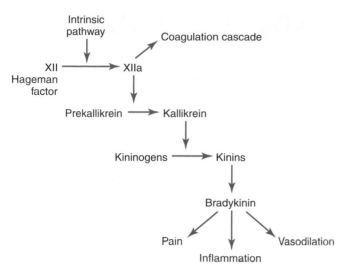

FIGURE 9-18 The common linkage of the kinin and coagulation systems through the activation of factor XII (Hageman factor). *XIIa,* Active factor XII.

to rupture (see Figure 9-17, *B*). The complement system is a potent inflammatory and cytotoxic system that is carefully regulated by eight known inhibitory factors.[3] Normal host cells produce membrane and inhibitory plasma proteins that prevent complement binding to their surface (e.g., C1 inhibitor, protein S).

Kinins

Bradykinin and kallidin are two of the many kinins present in the body. Kinins are small polypeptides that cause powerful vasodilation. They are especially active in the inflammatory process. The kinin system is linked to the clotting system via the Hageman factor (XII) and is activated with the activation of clotting.[1] The first step in this process is the conversion of factor XII to factor XIIa (Figure 9-18). Factor XIIa converts a substance known as prekallikrein to kallikrein. Kallikrein converts precursor substances known as kininogens to kinins. The most prevalent is kallidin, which is then converted to bradykinin. Activated kinins cause increased vascular permeability, vasodilation, and smooth muscle contraction. Kinins are also responsible for pain, which is one of the classic signs of inflammation.

Clotting Factors

The blood coagulation cascade's major purpose is to stop bleeding. It is also intimately involved in inflammation and triggering of the kinin system. The key linkage between the inflammatory response and clotting system is activated factor XII (Hageman factor) (see Figure 9-18). (The blood coagulation cascade is discussed in detail in Chapter 14.) Activation of the coagulation cascade results in the formation of insoluble fibrin strands, which provide an effective barrier to the spread of infection. Clot formation also activates the fibrinolytic cascade, which breaks down fibrin proteins. Some of the fibrin degradation products are chemotactic signals for neutrophils.

Cytokines and Chemokines

Cytokines are polypeptide signaling molecules that affect the function of other cells by stimulating surface receptors. Cytokines function in a complex intercellular communication network. WBC cytokines have gone by many names previously, including monokines, lymphokines, and interleukins, depending on their cell of origin. The number of known cytokines is large and growing; they can be grouped according to their source and function (Table 9-2).

Macrophages and T helper cells are the main sources of immune system cytokines. These cytokines generally function as chemotactic factors (chemokines), antiviral factors, mediators of inflammation, hematopoietic factors, or activation signals for specific types of WBCs. The major cytokines produced by macrophages are shown in Figure 9-9. T helper cells of the T_H1 subclass produce two main cytokines, IL-2 and IFN-γ, whereas T_H2 cells secrete a number of cytokines important to B-cell function (see Figure 9-13). Cytokines function to enhance and coordinate both innate and specific immune defenses. They are discussed in more detail in the sections that follow.

KEY POINTS

- The primary lymphoid organs are the thymus and bone marrow. T cells develop in the thymus, whereas B cells develop in the bone marrow. Mature lymphocytes then migrate to secondary lymphoid structures, including the spleen and lymph nodes.
- Blood cells are produced in the bone marrow in response to specific hematopoietic growth factors. Granulocytes (neutrophils, basophils, eosinophils) and monocytes (macrophages) are phagocytic cells that provide innate protection. Lymphocytes (B cells, T cells) are specific cells that react only to particular antigens. NK cells are lymphocytes that lack T-cell and B-cell markers and function in innate immune responses. Other blood components produced by bone marrow are erythrocytes and platelets.
- Neutrophils are the most numerous WBCs in blood. A large storage pool lies in the bone marrow and can be mobilized in response to antigen. Neutrophils are the predominant WBC type in early infection. They migrate to the area by following chemotactic factors and perform phagocytic functions. During acute bacterial infection, larger numbers of immature neutrophils (bands) are released into the blood, which is termed a "shift to the left." Chronic infections may produce a shift to the right with more segmented neutrophils than normal.
- Monocytes located in tissue are called *macrophages*. Monocytes and macrophages are distributed in strategic locations throughout the body, including the skin, lungs, gastrointestinal tract, liver, spleen, and lymph. Macrophages are powerful phagocytes and are predominant in late inflammation.
- T lymphocytes, the major effectors of cell-mediated immunity, interact with specific antigens on cell surfaces. They are important in immunity against foreign, infected,

TABLE 9-2

Selected Immune Cytokines and Their Functions

Cytokine	Origin	Function
IFN-α	Macrophages and induced by RNA or DNA viruses and by single- or double-stranded polyribonucleotide	Inhibits virus replication, toxic to cancer cells, stimulates leukocytes, facilitates NK cell activity, produces fever, increases B- and T-cell activity
IFN-β	Fibroblasts and induced by RNA or DNA viruses and by single- or double-stranded polyribonucleotide	Inhibits virus replication, toxic to cancer cells, facilitates NK cell activity, produces fever
IFN-γ	T cells (T_H1 and CD8$^+$) and NK cells	Inhibits virus replication, promotes antigen expression, activates macrophages, inhibits cell growth, induces myeloid cell lines, promotes B-cell switch to IgG
IL-1	Mononuclear phagocyte	Stimulates T cells and macrophages, induces acute phase reaction of inflammation, produces fever; similar to TNF and endogenous pyrogen
IL-2	T helper cells (T_H1)	Promotes growth of T cells, enhances function of NK cells, assists T-cell maturation in thymus, B-cell proliferation
IL-3	T cells, endothelial cells, fibroblasts, other cells	Induces proliferation and differentiation of other lymphocytes, pluripotent stem cells, mast cells, granulocytes
IL-4	T helper cells (T_H2)	Promotes T-cell/B-cell interactions, promotes synthesis of IgE by B cell and T_H2 cell growth, promotes mast cell and hematopoietic cell growth
IL-5	T helper cells (T_H2)	Promotes growth and differentiation of B cells to secrete IgA, induces differentiation of eosinophils
IL-6	Mononuclear phagocytes, T helper cells (T_H2), tumors, and nonlymphoid cells (e.g., endothelium)	Promotes immunoglobulin secretion by B cells, induces fever, promotes release of inflammation factors from liver cells, promotes differentiation of hematopoietic stem cells and nerve cells
IL-7	Stromal cells in bone marrow	Stimulates immature lymphocytes to divide to produce B and T cells
IL-8	Macrophages	Enhances inflammation and chemotaxis (CXCL chemokine)
IL-9	T_H2 cells	Enhances growth of T helper cells
IL-10	T cells and macrophages	Inhibits activation of macrophages and dendritic cells, inhibits IL-12 production
IL-11	Stromal cells in bone marrow	Stimulates platelet production
IL-12	Macrophages, dendritic cells	Enhances T_H1 cell activities and release of IFN-γ by T cells and NK cells
IL-13	T_H2 cells	Stimulates B-cell growth and IgE production, suppresses macrophages
IL-14	T cells	Induces B-cell proliferation
IL-15	Macrophages (esp. viral infection)	Similar actions to IL-2, enhances proliferation of T cells (CD8) and NK cells
IL-16	CD8$^+$ T cells	CD4$^+$ cell chemotaxis, suppresses viral replication of HIV
IL-17	CD4$^+$ T cells	Stimulates production of colony-stimulating factors, and chemokines
IL-18	Macrophages in response to microbes	Increases NK cell proliferation and secretion of IFN-γ by T_H1
IL-19	Uncertain	Similar to IL-10?
IL-20	Uncertain	Similar to IL-10?
IL-21	Uncertain	Similar to IL-15, stimulates production of NK cells
IL-22	Uncertain	Similar to IL-10?
IL-23	Macrophages and dendritic cells	Similar to IL-12, stimulates cell-mediated immunity
IL-24	Uncertain	Similar to IL-10?
IL-25	T_H2 cells	Stimulates production of cytokines by T_H2 cells
IL-26	Uncertain	Similar to IL-10?
IL-27	Macrophages and dendritic cells	Inhibits T_H1 cells
TNF-α	Macrophages	Induces leukocytosis, fever, weight loss, inflammation, necrosis of some tumors; stimulates lymphokine synthesis; activates macrophages; toxic to viruses and tumor cells
TNF-β	T cells	Inhibits B-cell and T-cell proliferation
G-CSF, M-CSF, GM-CSF	Macrophages, T cells, fibroblasts	Stimulates granulocyte and monocyte production in the bone marrow
TGF-β	T cells, macrophages	Inhibits T cells, B cells, and macrophages
Chemokines		
CXCL 1-16	Macrophages and various cells in tissues	Recruitment of neutrophils, macrophages, lymphocytes
CCL 1-28	Macrophages and various cells in tissues	Recruitment of neutrophils, macrophages, lymphocytes

GM-CSF, Granulocyte-macrophage colony-stimulating factor; *HIV,* human immunodeficiency virus; *IFN,* interferon; *IL,* interleukin; *NK,* natural killer; *TNF,* tumor necrosis factor; *TGF,* transforming growth factor.

or mutant cells. In addition, they secrete cytokines that boost the immune response of B cells and other cell types. T cells are composed of two main subtypes called CD4 (helper) and CD8 (cytotoxic). B lymphocytes are the major effectors of antibody-mediated immunity.

- The complement system consists of about 20 plasma proteins that interact in a cascade fashion to produce important mediators of inflammation and immunity. The cascade can be activated by microbial antigens (alternative pathway) or by antigen-antibody complexes (classical pathway).

- Cytokines are peptide factors released by immune cells. They have many functions, including as inflammatory mediators, chemotaxins, intercellular communication signals, growth factors, and growth inhibitors. Macrophages and lymphocytes are important sources of immune cytokines.

Innate Defenses and Inflammation

Inflammation occurs when cells are injured, regardless of the cause of the injury. It is a protective mechanism that also begins the healing process. The inflammatory response has three purposes: (1) to neutralize and destroy invading and harmful agents, (2) to limit the spread of harmful agents to other tissue, and (3) to prepare any damaged tissue for repair. Inflammatory reactions increase capillary permeability such that phagocytic cells, complement, and antibodies can leave the bloodstream and enter tissues where they are needed.

Five cardinal signs of inflammation have been described: (1) redness (rubor), (2) swelling (tumor), (3) heat (calor), (4) pain (dolor), and (5) loss of function (functio laesa). The suffix *itis* is commonly used to describe conditions associated with inflammation. For example, appendicitis, tendinitis, and nephritis refer to inflammation of the appendix, tendon, and kidney, respectively.

Inflammation can be caused by many conditions. Any injury to tissue will evoke an inflammatory response. Injury can arise from sources outside the body (exogenous) or from sources inside the body (endogenous). Surgery, trauma, burns, and skin injury from chemicals are all examples of exogenous injuries. Endogenous injuries may result from tissue ischemia such as myocardial infarction or pulmonary embolism.

Inflammation and infection are commonly confused because they often coexist. Under normal conditions, infection is always accompanied by inflammation; however, not all inflammation involves an infectious agent. For example, inflammation can occur with sprain injuries to joints, myocardial infarction, sterile surgical incisions, thrombophlebitis, and blister formation as a result of either temperature extremes or mechanical trauma.

Inflammation may be categorized as either acute or chronic. Acute inflammation is short in duration, lasting less than 2 weeks, and involves a discrete set of events. Chronic inflammation tends to be more diffuse, extends over a longer period, and may result in the formation of scar tissue and deformity.

INFLAMMATION

The inflammatory response is remarkably the same, regardless of the cause. Events in the inflammatory process include (1) increased vascular permeability, (2) recruitment and emigration of leukocytes, and (3) phagocytosis of antigens and debris. The inflammatory response is outlined in Figure 9-19.

Increased Vascular Permeability

Immediately after injury, the precapillary arterioles around the injured area contract briefly, which causes a short period of vasoconstriction. The amount of vasoconstriction depends on the degree of vascular injury and is usually of little significance.[11] Vasoconstriction is followed by a prolonged period of vasodilation caused by release of chemical mediators from injured tissues.

Vasoactive chemicals released during the inflammatory process include histamine, prostaglandins, and leukotrienes (Table 9-3). Mast cells are an important source of these inflammatory chemicals. Mast cells in the area of injury degranulate and release packets of histamine and other inflammatory chemicals. One of the early actions of these mediators is to vasodilate and cause endothelial cells to begin contraction and rounding up, thus increasing capillary permeability. The greater volume of blood increases the amount of pressure within the blood vessels (hydrostatic pressure). The increased pressure along with increased permeability pushes fluid out of

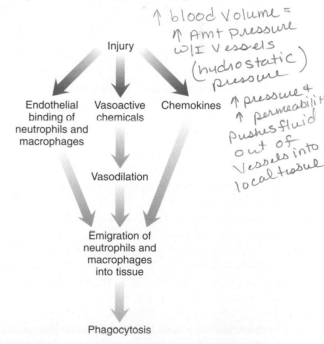

FIGURE 9-19 Tissue injury stimulates the release of a number of chemical mediators that promote vasodilation, chemotaxis, and binding of neutrophils and macrophages to area capillaries. These events facilitate the emigration of neutrophils and macrophages into the tissue, where they begin phagocytosis.

TABLE 9-3

Mediators of Acute Inflammation

Mediator	Vasodilation	Increased Permeability		Chemotaxis	Opsonin	Pain
		Immediate	Sustained			
Histamine	+	+++	−	−	−	−
Serotonin (5-HT)	+	+	−	−	−	−
Bradykinin	+	+	−	−	−	++
Complement 3a	−	+	−	−	−	−
Complement 3b	−	−	−	−	+++	−
Complement 5a	−	+	−	+++	−	−
Prostaglandin (E$_2$)	+++	+	+?	−	−	−
Leukotrienes (B$_4$, D$_4$)	−	+++	+?	+++	−	−
Lysosomal proteases	−	−	++*	−	−	−
Oxygen radicals	−	−	++*	−	−	−

Data from Roitt I, et al: *Immunology,* ed 6, St Louis, 2001, Mosby.
*Proteases and oxygen-based free radicals derived from neutrophils are believed to mediate a sustained increase in permeability by means of their damage to endothelial cells.

FIGURE 9-20 The cardinal signs of acute inflammation result mainly from vasodilation and increased vascular permeability.

the blood vessels and into the surrounding tissue contributing to local swelling. Because of the dilated blood vessels and open capillaries, more blood is carried to the injured area and contributes to the redness, pain, heat, and swelling of inflammation (Figure 9-20).

Histamine is an early mediator of this inflammatory response. It is such a potent vasodilator that it can cause significant reductions in blood pressure when released in excessive amounts. Histamine also causes bronchial constriction and mucus production. Histamine receptor blocking agents are widely used in allergic reactions, such as skin reactions and hay fever, to suppress these inflammatory actions of histamine.

Prostaglandins and leukotrienes are phospholipid compounds formed from arachidonic acid. The prostaglandins involved in inflammation contribute to vasodilation and increased permeability (Figure 9-21). Prostaglandin D$_2$ also acts as a chemotactic factor and stimulates neutrophil emigration. Prostaglandins cause pain by enhancing the sensitivity of

pain receptors.[11] They arise from the cyclooxygenase pathway and can be inhibited by drugs that block enzymes in this pathway, such as aspirin.

Five types of leukotrienes are generated from the lipoxygenase pathway: A$_4$, B$_4$, C$_4$, D$_4$, and E$_4$. Leukotriene B$_4$ is a potent chemotactic agent that causes aggregation of leukocytes; leukotrienes C$_4$, D$_4$, and E$_4$ are inflammatory and cause smooth muscle contraction, bronchospasm, and increased vascular permeability.[11] Leukotriene receptor blocking agents can be used to inhibit the inflammatory actions of these chemicals.

During the early phase of tissue inflammation, platelets move into the site and adhere to exposed vascular collagen. The platelets release fibronectin to form a meshwork trap and stimulate the intrinsic clotting cascade to help reduce bleeding. Platelets release a number of peptide growth factors, including platelet-derived growth factor and insulin-like growth factor.[12] Platelet-derived growth factor stimulates fibroblast cell proliferation, and insulin-like growth factor type 1 is a potent vascular endothelial cell chemotactic factor. Triggering of the blood coagulation cascade also occurs and leads to the formation of a fibrin clot. Usually, early clot formation occurs within several minutes. Fibrin is also deposited in the lymph system, where it causes lymphatic blockage. Lymphatic blockage "walls off" the area of inflammation from the surrounding tissue and delays the spread of toxins.

The vascular changes that occur soon after injury are beneficial to the injured tissue because irritating or toxic agents are diluted by the fluid that leaks out of the blood vessels into surrounding tissue. In addition, when the fluid leaves the blood vessels, the remaining blood becomes viscous (thick) and circulation is slowed, facilitating neutrophil emigration.

Emigration of Leukocytes

As blood flows through areas of inflammation, neutrophils move to the sides of the blood vessels and roll along the endothelium of the vessel wall. This process is referred

FIGURE 9-21 Generation of prostaglandins, thromboxane, and leukotrienes from arachidonic acid, and roles in inflammation. (From Kumar V et al: *Robbins basic pathology,* ed 8, Philadelphia, 2007, Saunders, p 48.)

to as *margination* or *pavementing.* Normally, neutrophils slide past the capillary endothelial cells and do not stick. Injured tissue triggers the expression of adhesion molecules on the surface of endothelial cells, and the adhesion molecules bind to receptors on neutrophils (Figure 9-22). These receptors, called *selectins,* help neutrophils stick and roll along the capillary endothelial surface.[5] Binding to and subsequent movement through the capillary wall are accomplished by another group of receptors called *integrins.* Chemokines present on the endothelium enhance the binding affinity of integrins so the neutrophil can attach firmly to the vessel wall. The process of passing through the blood vessel walls and migrating to the inflamed tissue is referred to as *emigration* or *diapedesis.* Diapedesis begins within a few minutes to hours of injury. Even though the spaces between endothelial cells lining the vessels are much smaller than the neutrophils, neutrophils are able to slide through a small portion at a time.

Neutrophils are attracted to the inflamed tissue by a process called **chemotaxis.** Biochemical mediators that attract neutrophils include bacterial toxins, degenerative products of the inflamed tissue, the C5a complement fragment, and other substances. Neutrophils are thus guided through the tissue to an area of injury by these chemicals. Because neutrophils are

highly mobile, they are first on the scene to begin phagocytosis and production of collagenase to break down dead tissue. Monocytes are slightly slower to arrive at an area of inflammation but use a similar process of emigration to gain entry to the area of tissue injury.

Eosinophils and NK cells also respond to the site of inflammation. Eosinophils are rich in chemical mediators such as hydrolases and peroxidases, which may contribute to the inflammatory process. NK cells are most effective in recognizing virally infected cells and opsonized microbes.

Phagocytosis

Once neutrophils and monocytes (macrophages) enter the tissue, they begin the process of phagocytosis (Figure 9-23). These cells produce a wide variety of enzymes that digest protein structures. Some of these enzymes include lysozyme, neutral proteases, collagenase, elastase, and acid hydrolases. Neutrophils and macrophages specialize in collagen and extracellular matrix degradation. Peptide bonds are cleaved in the extracellular matrix by collagenase, elastase, proteinase, and gelatinase. If the microbe is small enough to be internalized, it will be captured by the phagocyte and endocytosed into a phagosome. The phagosome then merges with a lysosome containing degradative enzymes. Large antigens may trigger

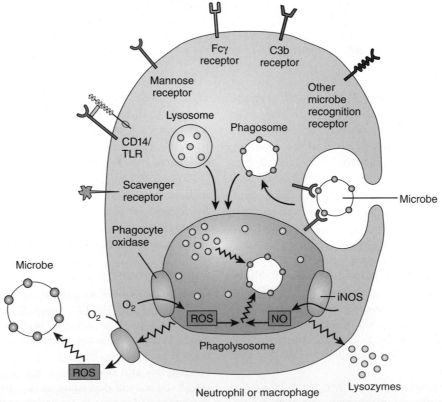

FIGURE 9-22 Emigration of neutrophils from the bloodstream into tissue is mediated by receptor interactions with the capillary endothelium. With inflammation and injury, endothelial cells begin to express binding molecules on their cell surfaces (selectins). Leukocytes also have selectins, which can bind to endothelial adhesion proteins. The selectin interactions cause the leukocytes to stick and roll. Chemokines on the surface of endothelial cells interact with neutrophils (and macrophages) to increase the binding affinity of integrin receptors on leukocytes. Firm attachment and diapedesis through the capillary wall is facilitated by integrins, which allow the neutrophils to bind to endothelial cells and extracellular matrix and then pull themselves into the tissue. *TNF,* Tumor necrosis factor; *IL,* interleukin.

FIGURE 9-23 Neutrophils and macrophages have a number of different receptors on their surface that enable them to bind to components of microbes or to opsonins like IgG and complement. Bound microbes are internalized into phagosomes that fuse with lysosomes containing numerous enzymes. Some of these enzymes degrade proteins (proteolytic), and others such as oxidase and inducible nitric oxide synthase *(iNOS)* produce free radicals that attack molecular bonds. When phagocytes are strongly stimulated or microbes are too large to internalize, the lysosomal enzymes may be activated or released at the cell surface causing tissue damage and inflammation. *ROS,* Reactive oxygen species.

the neutrophil to release its degradative enzymes extracellularly causing damage to local tissues.

Oxidizing agents, the most destructive of the inflammatory cell products, are formed as a result of the phagocyte oxidase enzyme system on the membrane of the lysosome. Neutrophils are capable of synthesizing and assailing microorganisms with these oxidizing agents, which include the following oxygen radicals: superoxide (O_2^-), hydrogen peroxide (H_2O_2), and hydroxyl ions (OH^-). Oxidizing agents directly attack cell membranes and thereby increase permeability. Nitric oxide products may also be produced by inducible nitric oxide synthase (iNOS) and function in concert with oxygen radicals to attack microbial molecules[1] (see Figure 9-23).

Because acute inflammation can cause severe tissue damage, it is not surprising that a system of inactivators is present. An important inhibitor of inflammatory damage is α_1-antiprotease. Antiproteases are made in the liver and circulate continuously in the bloodstream. α_1-antiprotease inhibits the destructive proteases released from activated neutrophils. A deficiency of antiproteases can predispose an individual to inflammatory tissue destruction.

Neutrophils have a limited capacity to phagocytose foreign and inflammatory debris. Once the neutrophil leaves the circulation to fight an infection, it is unable to return and will die at the site. When phagocytosis is incomplete, a collection of dead neutrophils, bacteria, and cellular debris, called *pus,* may form at the site. Macrophages are left with the job of removing spent neutrophils and preparing the site for healing. A predominance of monocytes and macrophages in an inflamed area signals the beginning of chronic inflammation.

Chronic Inflammation

Macrophages are essential for wound healing because of their phagocytic and debridement functions. Macrophages produce proteases that help in removing foreign protein from the wound. Macrophages also release tissue thromboplastin to facilitate hemostasis and stimulate fibroblast activity. Macrophages secrete other peptide growth factors such as angiogenic factor, which encourages the growth of new blood vessels. Macrophages also phagocytose spent neutrophils and their degradation products so they do not interfere with healing. Prolonged inflammation may impair healing and result in an accumulation of macrophages, fibroblasts, and collagen, called a *granuloma.* Granulomas are usually evident on examination of tissue biopsy as clusters of macrophages surrounding particulate matter or resistant microbes such as *Mycobacterium tuberculosis.* Fibrosis and scarring are evident because normal parenchyma is replaced with fibrous tissue.

HEALING

Healing of tissues following inflammation can occur in different ways over time. Usually the reconstructive phase begins 3 to 4 days after injury and persists for 2 weeks. The major cells involved in this phase include fibroblasts, endothelial cells, and myofibroblasts.

Fibroblasts are found all over the body and are thought to originate in mesenchymal primitive tissue. They synthesize connective tissue and are able to migrate. Fibroblasts are stimulated to make collagen, proteoglycans, and fibronectin by a variety of growth factors.[12] Macrophages secrete lactate and release growth factors that stimulate fibroblasts. Fibroblasts respond to contact and density inhibition and thereby facilitate orderly cellular growth. Myofibroblasts develop at the wound edge and induce wound contraction.

Endothelial cells grow into the connective tissue gel stimulated by angiogenic substances. They usually develop capillary beds from existing vessels. The new capillaries can bring in nutrients for tissue repair and wound healing. However, because the new capillaries are leaky, they contribute to continuing edema.

Regeneration of damaged tissue into the preexisting tissue type requires survival of the basement membrane and tissue stem cells. Some cell types regenerate constantly; among these types are the epithelial cells of the skin and mucous membranes, bone marrow cells, and lymphoid cells. Cells of the liver, pancreas, endocrine glands, and renal tubules are also able to regenerate when necessary. However, some cell types, such as neurons and muscle cells, regenerate poorly. The maturation phase of wound healing occurs several weeks after the injury and may last for 2 years or more. It is characterized by wound remodeling by fibroblasts, macrophages, neutrophils, and eosinophils. Wound remodeling is the process of collagen deposition and lysis with débridement of the wound edges. During this phase the wound changes color from bright red to pink to whitish. As long as a wound is pink, the maturation phase is not completed.

INFLAMMATORY EXUDATES

Exudate is fluid that leaks out of blood vessels, combined with neutrophils and the debris from phagocytosis. Exudates may vary in composition, but all types have similar functions, including (1) transport of leukocytes and antibodies, (2) dilution of toxins and irritating substances, and (3) transport of the nutrients necessary for tissue repair.

Serous exudate is watery, has a low protein content, and is similar to the fluid that collects under a blister. This type of exudate generally accompanies mild inflammation. With mild inflammation, the permeability of the blood vessels is not greatly changed. As a result, only some protein molecules escape from vessels, and serous exudate, with a low protein content, develops. Small amounts of red blood cells may leak into the serous fluid with capillary injury, resulting in a pink-tinged drainage called *serosanguineous* drainage.

With greater injury, more inflammation occurs and the blood vessels become more permeable. Because of this increased permeability, more protein can pass through the vessel walls. Fibrinogen, a large protein molecule, can pass through a highly permeable blood vessel wall. *Fibrinous exudate* is sticky and thick and may have to be removed to allow healing; otherwise, scar tissue and adhesions may develop. However, in some instances fibrinous exudate may be beneficial. In the case of acute appendicitis, fibrinous exudate may actually wall off and localize the infection and prevent its spread.

Purulent exudate is called pus. Purulent exudate generally occurs in severe inflammation accompanied by bacterial infection and is primarily composed of neutrophils, protein, and tissue debris. Large pockets of purulent exudate, called abscesses, must generally be removed or drained for healing to take place.

Hemorrhagic exudate has a large component of red blood cells. This type of exudate is usually present with the most severe inflammation. Hemorrhagic exudate occurs with severe leakage from blood vessels or after necrosis or breakdown of blood vessels.

SYSTEMIC MANIFESTATIONS OF INFLAMMATION

Inflammation is associated with both localized and systemic signs and symptoms. The localized symptoms, described previously, occur with both acute and chronic inflammation. Depending on the magnitude of injury and the resistance of the individual, localized inflammation can lead to systemic involvement. Systemic responses include fever, neutrophilia (increased blood neutrophil count), lethargy, and muscle catabolism. Three macrophage-derived cytokines—IL-1, IL-6, and TNF-α—are responsible for most of the systemic effects of inflammation.[11]

TNF-α and IL-1 act on the brain to raise body temperature, induce sleep, and suppress appetite. By raising the set point for body temperature, these cytokines induce conservation of heat through vasoconstriction, as well as increased heat production through shivering. An increase in body temperature is assumed to improve the immune response; however, the mechanism is unclear. IL-1 is responsible for stimulating the release of neutrophils from bone marrow storage sites, thus producing neutrophilia. All three cytokines act on skeletal muscle to enhance protein catabolism, which provides an available pool of amino acids for efficient antibody production by plasma cells.

The liver is an important target for IL-1, IL-6, and TNF-α. These cytokines induce the liver to release a number of proteins collectively called *acute phase proteins*, which include complement components, clotting factors, and protease inhibitors (Figure 9-24). Two of the most important acute phase proteins are C-reactive protein (CRP) and serum amyloid A. CRP binds to phospholipids on bacterial cell membranes and acts as an opsonin to facilitate phagocytosis.[3]

When the liver releases acute phase proteins, the level of fibrinogen in the serum is increased. Fibrinogen coats the surface of red blood cells and reduces their charge so that they aggregate more readily. A blood test called the *erythrocyte sedimentation rate* (ESR, "sed. rate") provides a simple measure of the level of inflammation in an individual. Thus an elevated ESR indicates the presence of inflammation in the body. The greater the inflammation, the faster the red blood cells settle

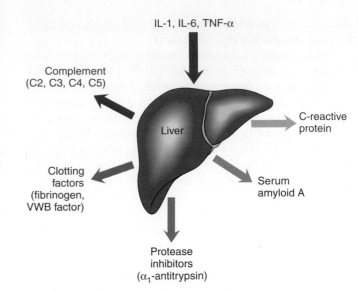

FIGURE 9-24 The liver is a target for three important cytokines, interleukin-1 *(IL-1)*, IL-6, and tumor necrosis factor α *(TNF-α)*. In response to these cytokines, the liver releases a number of proteins, collectively called *acute phase proteins*.

to the bottom of a test tube and the higher the ESR. The ESR is a nonspecific but clinically useful indicator of inflammation. Serum CRP activity is also used as a nonspecific indicator of inflammation in a manner similar to the ESR.

KEY POINTS

- Previous exposure to foreign antigens is not required for the activation of innate immune defenses. Inflammation is an important aspect of innate immunity that involves localization of harmful agents and the bringing of phagocytic cells to the area. Classic manifestations of inflammation are redness, swelling, heat, pain, and loss of function.
- Inflammatory chemicals such as histamine, prostaglandins, and leukotrienes are released from injured tissues, mast cells, macrophages, and neutrophils. These chemicals increase vascular permeability, vasodilate, and attract immune cells to the area (chemotaxis).
- Phagocytes migrate to the inflamed area, collect at the side of the vessel, and squeeze through into the tissue. Emigration of neutrophils and macrophages is facilitated by selectins and integrins present on the surface of endothelial cells and leukocytes. Neutrophils arrive in large numbers in acute bacterial infection and begin active phagocytosis. Neutrophils and macrophages produce proteolytic enzymes and oxidizing agents to destroy and digest antigens. With chronic inflammation, macrophages and lymphocytes predominate.
- Healing is mediated by growth factors released from platelets and immune cells that stimulate fibroblasts to divide and manufacture extracellular matrix proteins. Endothelial cells respond to angiogenic growth factors by forming capillary networks.

- Inflammatory exudate functions to transport immune cells, antibodies, and nutrients to the tissue and dilute the offending substances. Serous exudate is watery and low in protein; fibrinous exudate is thick, sticky, and high in protein; purulent exudate contains infective organisms, leukocytes, and cellular debris; and hemorrhagic exudate contains red blood cells.
- Systemic manifestations of inflammation include fever, neutrophilia, lethargy, muscle catabolism, increased acute phase proteins (CRP), and increased ESR. These responses are attributable to the IL-1, IL-6, and TNF-α released from macrophages and inflamed tissues.

Specific Adaptive Immunity

The specific immune system uses remarkably effective and adaptive defense mechanisms capable of recognizing foreign invaders, destroying them, and retaining a memory of the encounter such that an even more effective defense (adaptive) will be achieved after subsequent exposure. As previously described, B and T lymphocytes are the cellular mediators of specific adaptive immunity. B cells are said to provide "humoral" immunity because the antibodies they produce are found in body fluids, or "humors." T cells provide "cell-mediated" immunity because they recognize antigen presented on the surface of cells. To achieve immunity against specific antigens, B and T lymphocytes must be capable of recognizing an enormous range of foreign antigen yet not be reactive to self tissues.

Differentiation between self and nonself requires a complex lymphocyte development process in which self-reactive lymphocytes are destroyed and potentially useful lymphocytes are preserved. The MHC proteins have a primary role in enabling lymphocytes to react to foreign antigen while remaining tolerant to self antigen. Self tolerance is not always effectively maintained, and impairment in self tolerance can result in the development of autoimmune disorders (see Chapter 10).

MAJOR HISTOCOMPATIBILITY COMPLEX

A cluster of genes on chromosome 6 is known as the **major histocompatibility complex (MHC).** In humans, the MHC is also known as the **human leukocyte antigen (HLA)** complex. The proteins made by these genes are displayed on the surface of body cells and mark them as "self." The MHC contains three classes of genes: I, II, and III (Figure 9-25). Class I and II genes code for proteins that display or "present" antigens on the surface of cells. Antigen presentation is a vital first step in the initiation of an immune response. T lymphocytes cannot recognize foreign antigens unless they are displayed on MHC proteins on the surface of a cell. Class III genes code for a variety of proteins, many of which are of importance to inflammatory reactions, including several complement proteins.

A great deal of **polymorphism** is found in the MHC class I and II genes, which means that it is very unlikely that an individual will have exactly the same MHC genotype as another. For example, three gene loci for MHC class I proteins (A, B, C) are located on each chromosome 6, and an individual inherits one chromosome from each parent for a total of six MHC class I genes. Each of these genes has many different forms (alleles) such that each of the six is likely to be different (Figure 9-26). Related individuals will generally be more similar but not identical (unless identical twins). The "matching" of MHC gene expression is an important consideration for tissue and organ transplantation. The closer the match is,

FIGURE 9-25 Major histocompatibility complex genes are categorized into three main groups known as class I, II, and III. Class I and II genes code for antigen-presenting proteins, whereas class III genes code for a heterogeneous group of proteins, many of which serve immune functions.

Class I — Receptors for antigen presentation found on nucleated cells
Class II — Receptors for antigen presentation found on macrophages and B cells
Class III — Complement components and others

FIGURE 9-26 Each individual receives six class I major histocompatibility complex *(MHC)* genes including pairs of A, B, and C genes. One member of the pair is inherited from each parent. MHC class I genes are expressed in all nucleated cells of the body. Each individual also receives six class II MHC genes, three from each parent. However, class II proteins are composed of two polypeptide chains such that an individual may have 10 to 20 different MHC class II protein molecules. Class II MHC proteins are expressed on the surface of specialized antigen-presenting cells like macrophages, dendritic cells, and B cells. The structure of an individual's MHC proteins is assessed to determine the "tissue type" when matching for tissue transplantation procedures.

the less likely that the host will reject the transplant. An individual also receives six MHC class II genes that are expressed on specialized antigen-presenting cells, such as dendritic cells, macrophages, and B cells. Because of the potential for mixing and matching of class II MHC gene products, an individual may express 10 to 20 different MHC class II proteins.[1] It is the MHC class I and II proteins on the surface of cells that display both self and foreign antigens for inspection by T cells. Cells displaying foreign antigens stimulate an immune response, whereas those displaying self antigens do not. Genetic diversity in MHC gene expression is believed to be important to the preservation of a species because new pathogens are likely to encounter at least some individuals with MHC genotypes that can recognize and eliminate these pathogens.

ANTIGEN PRESENTATION BY MHC

Nucleated cells in the body are capable of expressing MHC class I proteins on their cell surfaces, whereas only certain specialized cells, primarily dendritic cells, macrophages, and B cells, are able to express MHC class II proteins. Cytotoxic T cells are able to recognize antigen bound to MHC class I proteins, whereas T helper cells recognize antigen bound to MHC class II proteins. T cells are screened during development in the thymus so that they recognize and are tolerant to self MHC proteins and do not react to self peptides displayed by self MHC proteins. This concept is explored further in the section on Mechanisms of Cell-Mediated Immunity.

The sources of antigen, mechanism of antigen processing, and T-cell response to antigen are quite different for MHC I and MHC II reactions.

MHC Class I Presentation

Nucleated cells continuously produce MHC class I proteins on the rough endoplasmic reticulum (ER) where they are combined with various peptide fragments that are present in the cytoplasm. These peptides come from degradation of normal intracellular proteins. The MHC I–peptide complexes are cycled to the cell surface for inspection by T cells. Normal MHCs displaying normal cellular proteins are ignored by T cells. If abnormal proteins are produced in the cell, then the MHC I–peptide complex will be recognized as foreign and an immune response will occur. The peptide antigens presented on MHC I are of intracellular origin. Because viruses are able to gain access to cells directly, viral protein is a common source of foreign MHC class I antigens. Abnormal intracellular proteins produced by mutant cells may also be presented on MHC I, thus targeting them for immune destruction. Before intracellular proteins can be presented at the cell surface, they must be processed and transported to the ER, where they are combined with newly synthesized MHC class I protein (Figure 9-27). Peptide fragments are generated in the cytoplasmic proteasomes and escorted through the ER by special transporters called *transporters associated with antigen processing* (TAPs). The TAPs are located near the MHC I complexes on the ER membrane and target the peptides to the MHC I binding cleft.

FIGURE 9-27 Nearly all nucleated cells of the body are able to process and display antigen in association with major histocompatibility complex *(MHC)* class I protein. The antigens come from the intracellular compartment, and a common source of foreign antigen is viral infection. The viral proteins made within the cell's cytoplasm are processed into peptide fragments in the proteasome and then enter the endoplasmic reticulum *(ER)* through TAP transporters. There they combine with MHC class I proteins. The MHC class I–antigen complex then shuttles to the cell surface within a vesicle. When the vesicle combines with the plasma membrane, the MHC class I–antigen complex is displayed on the cell surface. *TAP,* transporter associated with antigen processing; *CTL,* cytotoxic T lymphocyte. (From Abbas AK, Lichtman AH: *Cellular and molecular immunology,* ed 5, Philadelphia, 2003, Saunders, p 91.)

The MHC I binding cleft can accommodate peptide fragments of 8 to 11 amino acids[1] (Figure 9-28). The MHC I–antigen complexes then travel to the cell membrane, where they are displayed. Recognition of foreign antigen in association with the MHC I protein on the cell surface targets the presenting cell for destruction by cytotoxic T cells. When the cytotoxic T cell binds to the MHC I–antigen complex, it is stimulated to release enzymes and pore-forming proteins (perforins) that lyse the target cell. Cytotoxic T cells can only recognize an antigen if it is physically bound to an MHC class I molecule. Cytotoxic T cells are thus said to be MHC class I restricted.

MHC Class II Presentation

MHC class II proteins are used to present antigens obtained from extracellular sources. Extracellular antigens must first be engulfed by the antigen-presenting cell. Cells of the monocyte-macrophage lineage, dendritic cells, and B cells are responsible for presenting antigen by MHC II. Macrophages and dendritic cells obtain foreign antigens by phagocytosis and are thus able to process and present a large number of different antigens. They are said to be "nonspecific" for this reason. B cells, on the other hand, are very particular about the antigens that they engulf. The antigen must specifically bind to the BCR to be ingested by a B cell. Each B cell has only one type of BCR and therefore processes and presents only one specific antigen. The specificity of the BCR corresponds to the antibody that the activated B cell will produce. The process of

B-cell activation is explored in the section on Mechanisms of Humoral Immunity.

After the antigen-presenting cell has ingested an antigen, it is degraded into fragments within the cellular phagosomes (endocytic vesicle). MHC II proteins are synthesized on the rough ER and pick up an antigen from the phagosome on their way to the plasma membrane (Figure 9-29). The class II MHC molecule is formed by two protein chains, and the binding cleft is more flexible than that of MHC I proteins (Figure 9-30). Peptides displayed by MHC class II proteins range in size from 10 to 30 amino acids.[1] The MHC II–antigen complexes are then displayed at the cell surface where T helper cells can detect them. T helper cells can only recognize a foreign antigen if it is physically bound to an MHC II protein. T helper cells are thus said to be MHC II restricted. Naive T cells located in lymph nodes are usually presented with antigen by dendritic cells. Dendritic cells populate the body surfaces and mucous membranes. When they engulf antigen, they break their tissue attachments and migrate to lymph nodes where they interact with T helper cells.

MECHANISMS OF CELL-MEDIATED IMMUNITY

T cells are able to recognize foreign antigen displayed on the surface of antigen-presenting cells through specialized receptors called *T-cell receptors* (TCRs). Each T cell has tens of

FIGURE 9-28 Schematic **(A)** and ribbon **(B)** diagrams of the class I major histocompatibility complex molecule. Note that the peptide-binding cleft is formed from one polypeptide chain that restricts the size of peptide in the pocket to 8 to 11 amino acids. (From Abbas AK et al: *Cellular and molecular immunology*, ed 6, Philadelphia, 2007, Saunders, p 103.)

FIGURE 9-29 Only specialized cells are able to obtain extracellular antigen for processing and presentation in association with major histocompatibility complex *(MHC)* class II protein. These cells are primarily dendritic cells, macrophages, and B cells. The antigen is first engulfed into a vesicle called a *phagosome,* which fuses with a lysosome. Enzymes within the phagosome break the protein down into pieces. MHC II molecules are synthesized on the endoplasmic reticulum *(ER)* and then transported to the phagosome in a vesicle. The binding cleft of the MHC II protein is complexed with a blocking protein to prevent it from picking up peptide before it reaches the phagosome. The phagosome and vesicle fuse, and the MHC II loses its blocking protein and picks up an antigen peptide. The complex then migrates to the cell surface and combines with the cell membrane. The MHC II–antigen complex is then displayed on the cell surface. (From Abbas AK, Lichtman AH: *Cellular and molecular immunology,* ed 5, Philadelphia, 2003, Saunders, p 91.)

FIGURE 9-30 Schematic **(A)** and ribbon **(B)** diagrams of the class II major histocompatibility complex *(MHC)* molecule. Note that the peptide-binding cleft is formed from two separate polypeptide chains, which allows the size of peptide in the pocket to be 10 to 30 amino acids. (From Abbas AK et al: *Cellular and molecular immunology,* ed 6, Philadelphia, 2007, Saunders, p 104.)

[handwritten marginalia: TCRS are the same so can only respond to a single antigenic epitope. That's why T cells are specific]

thousands of identical TCRs on its cell surface.[9] Each T cell is thus able to recognize and respond to only a single antigenic epitope. This property is what makes T cells specific. The binding specificity of the TCR is randomly determined by recombination and rearrangement within the genes that code for the TCR-binding domain. Billions of different TCR amino acid sequences are possible, thus providing a tremendous diversity of potential antigen-binding specificities. This diversity increases the likelihood that one or more T cells will have the right TCRs to allow recognition of any of the various pathogens that may gain access to the body. The drawback to this random approach is that many TCRs will be useless or may bind self antigens. A rigorous selection process occurs in the thymus such that self-reactive T cells are eliminated. This selection process requires at least two steps. In the first, T cells must demonstrate an ability to recognize self MHC proteins displayed on the surface of specialized thymic cells. Portions of the TCR must make appropriate contact with the MHC protein, or the T cell will not be able to respond to antigens presented on the cell surface.[13] The expression of either CD4 or CD8 on the T cell helps determine which class of MHC the T cell must fit. T cells that do not have functional TCRs undergo apoptosis in the thymus. The second requirement is that the TCR does not bind tightly to MHC proteins that are displaying normal self-derived peptides. Tight binding to self peptides also triggers the cell to initiate apoptosis. T cells that pass these tests migrate to secondary lymphoid tissues to await foreign antigens. Exposure of a T cell to its corresponding antigen results in expansion of the T cell into a clone of cells that all recognize the same antigen. This process ensures that useful T cells are maintained in the body as memory cells, whereas T cells that do not encounter antigen will die out. Members of the T-cell clone migrate to lymphoid organs throughout the body, where they can respond rapidly should the same antigen reenter the system. The life span of mature T cells is long, but the numbers of memory cells in a clone will decline over time. However, intermittent exposure to the antigen is likely to occur and will stimulate proliferation and maintain immunity.

The two major types of T cells, T helper cells and cytotoxic T cells, react very differently to activation of their TCRs by antigen and are therefore described separately in the following sections.

T Helper Cells (CD4+)

[handwritten marginalia: TCR = T-cell Receptor]

T helper cells recognize antigen in association with MHC class II molecules. The CD4 protein is needed to enable T helper cells to bind the MHC II protein, whereas the TCR recognizes the specific antigen being presented (Figure 9-31). Binding of the TCR to its corresponding antigen generates a signaling cascade in the cytoplasm of the T helper cell (Figure 9-32). The TCR is linked to this signaling cascade through another protein called *CD3*. Stimulation of CD3 results in the activation of enzymes (kinases) in the cytoplasm that mediate the production of two second messengers, inositol trisphosphate and diacylglycerol (see Chapter 3). Inositol trisphosphate initiates a rise in the concentration of intracellular calcium ion,

FIGURE 9-31 T helper cells can recognize and bind antigen in association with major histocompatibility complex *(MHC)* class II molecules. The T-cell receptor *(TCR)* on the T helper cell binds to the antigen, and the CD4 protein recognizes the MHC class II protein. Binding is very specific because the TCR must match the antigen fragment precisely. Once binding is achieved, CD3 and ζ proteins associated with the TCR are activated to initiate intracellular enzyme cascades.

which also acts as a second messenger to change cell behavior. Other protein kinases turn on the genes for cytokines (e.g., IL-2, IFN-γ, and others), IL-2 receptors, and other cell surface proteins. As previously mentioned, the two subtypes of T helper cells, T_H1 and T_H2, secrete somewhat different amounts and types of cytokines. These cytokines provide the "help" that T helper cells give to other cells of the immune system. For example, IL-2 activates helper and cytotoxic T cells, NK cells, and macrophages, and IFN-γ is a potent activator of macrophages. IL-2 and IFN-γ are the main cytokines secreted by T_H1 cells. The cytokines secreted by T_H2 cells have stimulatory effects on B cells (e.g., IL-4, IL-5, IL-6, IL-13). In addition, when a B cell is serving as the antigen-presenting cell, T helper cells provide specific B cell help through direct cell-to-cell contact by receptor proteins.

Cytotoxic T Cells (CD8+)

Cytotoxic T cells recognize antigen displayed in association with MHC class I protein. The CD8 protein is needed to facilitate binding to the MHC I, whereas the TCR specifically recognizes the presented antigen (Figure 9-33). Binding of the TCR to its corresponding antigen triggers a number of responses in the cytotoxic T cell. This process is similar to that described for T helper cells and involves signal transduction through CD3

FIGURE 9-32 Major signaling pathways in activated T cells. *AP-1,* activation protein-1; *DAG,* diacylglycerol; *IP3,* inositol 1.4.5-trisphosphate; *MAP kinase,* mitogen-activated protein kinase; *NF-AT,* nuclear factor of activated T cells; *NF-kB,* nuclear factor kappa B; *PIP2,* phosphatidylinositol 4,5-bisphosphate; *PLC-γ,* phospholipase C-γ. (From Nairn R, Helbert M: *Immunology for medical students,* ed 2, Mosby, 2007, p 75.)

proteins. Antigen binding by cytotoxic T cells is not sufficient to activate them. Cytotoxic T cells also require costimulation by IL-2 cytokines. IL-2 is secreted primarily by activated T helper cells (T$_H$1). Thus, cytotoxic T cells require T helper cell "help" before they are effective. Cytokines are generally not enough to induce significant proliferation of target cells unless other costimulators are also present. This helps ensure that the cells that specifically recognize a particular antigen are the ones that get the help. Costimulators are often present on the surfaces of the presenting and responding cells (Figure 9-34). Once activated, cytotoxic T cells proliferate into memory cells as well as effector cells. Effector cells accomplish their cytotoxic functions in two ways: through perforins and through CD95.

Perforins are proteins manufactured in the cytotoxic T cell and stored in granules (vesicles) within the cytoplasm. A number of proteolytic enzymes (granzymes) are located in the granules along with the perforins. Binding to the target cell causes the granules to migrate to the contact site, where

they are released onto the target cell membrane (Figure 9-35). The perforins assemble into pores, which then allow the granzymes to move into the target cell. Granzymes degrade DNA and trigger target cell death (apoptosis).

Perforins function in a similar manner to the complement membrane attack complex previously described. It is not entirely clear how the cytotoxic T cell manages to escape injury in this process. Presumably, the perforins and granzymes are focused on the target cell in some controlled manner.

The CD95 protein on cytotoxic T cells is called the *CD95 ligand* (CD95L) or the *FAS ligand.*[14] It can bind specifically to complementary CD95 proteins (FAS) found on the surface of target cells. Normal, healthy cells do not express CD95 and are not recognized by cytotoxic cells. Binding of the CD95L to CD95 triggers programmed cell death (apoptosis) of the target cell (see Figure 9-35). This system is thought to be particularly important in culling senescent cells and self-reactive lymphocytes.

FIGURE 9-33 Cytotoxic T cells are able to recognize and bind antigen in association with major histocompatibility complex (MHC) class I molecules. The T-cell receptor on the cytotoxic T cell binds to the antigen, and the CD8 protein recognizes the MHC I protein. Binding is specific. Once binding is achieved, CD3 proteins initiate intracellular enzyme cascades.

FIGURE 9-34 Schematic diagram illustrating the formation of the "immunologic synapse." Numerous receptor-ligand interactions bind a T cell to an antigen-presenting cell *(APC)*. When the receptors and ligands interact in concert, the T cell and APC are activated. *ICAM*, Intercellular adhesion molecule; *MHC*, major histocompatibility complex; *LFA*, leukocyte function–associated antigen; *TCR*, T-cell receptor; *CTL*, cytotoxic T lymphocyte. (From Abbas AK et al: *Cellular and molecular immunology*, ed 6, Philadelphia, 2007, Saunders, p. 204.)

[handwritten note: Co-stimulators are often present on the surfaces of the presenting & responding cells (see above)]

FIGURE 9-35 Binding of a cytotoxic T cell to its target stimulates granules containing perforin and granzymes to migrate to the cell contact site. Perforins then assemble into pores on the target cell, through which the granzymes can enter the target cell cytoplasm. The granzymes interrupt the cellular DNA and trigger apoptosis. *ICAM*, Intercellular adhesion molecule; *MHC*, major histocompatibility complex; *LFA*, leukocyte function–associated antigen; *TCR*, T-cell receptor. *Fas ligand* (CD 95L).

MECHANISMS OF HUMORAL IMMUNITY

B cells are responsible for antibody-mediated (humoral) immunity. B cells have two major subpopulations: memory cells and plasma cells. Memory B cells contain antigen receptors and function in a manner similar to memory T cells. In other words, memory of exposure to an antigen is stored in a clone of memory B cells. When exposed to the same type of antigen in the future, these memory B cells are able to respond rapidly with appropriate antibodies.

Some B cells differentiate into short-lived antibody-producing factories called *plasma cells*. All of the plasma cells in a clone secrete antibodies with identical antigen-binding specificity (monoclonal antibody). The secreted antibodies circulate in the blood and body fluids and bind specifically to the antigen that triggered their production. Once antigen is cleared, the population of plasma cells declines and the antibody concentration (titer) falls. However, some long-lived plasma cells continue to secrete a level of antibody sufficient to provide immediate protection upon the next exposure to the same antigen.[1]

Antigen Recognition by B Cells

During their development in the bone marrow, B cells begin to express BCRs on their cell surfaces. The structure of the antigen-binding area on the BCR is randomly determined in a manner similar to that described for TCRs. Each BCR is coded for by two distinct types of genes: one for the variable region, which makes up the antigen-binding site, and one for the constant region, which is essentially the same for all antibodies of a given class (Figure 9-36). The structure of the BCR bound to the B-cell surface is similar to IgM. Rearrangement,

recombination, and selective splicing of variable-region genes allow for great diversity of BCR binding specificities. The potential number of different BCR structures is enormous. Some of these combinations are unsuitable for BCR assembly, and it has been estimated that a typical human B-cell population can recognize approximately 10^{11} different antigenic epitopes.[3] As is the case with T cells, useful B cells—ones activated by antigen—will be preserved in the body, whereas B cells that encounter no antigen will die out.

The growth and activity of B cells that recognize protein antigens are carefully regulated by T cells. Binding of antigen to the B cell's BCR is a necessary but insufficient stimulus to produce an effective B-cell clone. To be effectively activated, the B cell must engulf some of the antigen, process it, and present it to T helper cells. This activity will initiate cell-to-cell contact between the B cell and its complementary T-cell helper. A number of receptor interactions bind the T cells and B cells together, in addition to the main MHC II–TCR interaction, and include CD80-CD28 and CD154-CD40 (Figure 9-37). These cell-to-cell binding interactions stimulate intracellular signaling pathways in the B cell (and T helper cell) that promote clonal expansion and differentiation (see Figure 9-32). B cells also require certain cytokines to proliferate and begin antibody synthesis (Figure 9-38). B cells are quite dependent on T-cell help during the initial exposure to antigen (primary response), but less so on subsequent exposures. Some types of B cells have BCRs that bind nonprotein antigens, such as bacterial sugars and lipids. Since T cells only recognize peptides, these types of B-cell responses are T-cell independent. Other costimulatory signals, such as the complement fragment C3d on the antigen, may provide the necessary costimulation to achieve a B-cell response and antibody production. It is doubtful that memory cells are formed in this process[1] (Figure 9-39).

Antibody Structure

Each antibody (immunoglobulin) molecule contains two identical light polypeptide chains joined by disulfide bonds to two identical heavy polypeptide chains. The geometry of the relationship between the heavy (H) and light (L) chains forms a Y-like structure. The H chains form the stem of the Y, and the L chains are on the outside of the arms of the Y. The antigen-binding end of the antibody is often called the *Fab* (antigen-binding fragment), whereas the stem is called the *Fc* (constant fragment). It is the structure of the constant fragment that determines the antibody class.

Antibodies are differentiated into five classes: IgG, IgM, IgA, IgD, and IgE. The structure and properties of the immunoglobulin classes are listed in Table 9-4. IgG and IgE circulate as single molecules or monomers; IgA is a dimer (two antibodies joined together); and IgM consists of five antibody molecules joined together to form a pentamer. IgD is found mainly on the B-cell plasma membrane and does not circulate in significant quantity. IgD is thought to participate in signal transduction across the B cell membrane along with the BCR. Different antibody classes serve different immune functions in the body.

FIGURE 9-36 Two major classes of genes are responsible for coding for the variable (V) and constant (C) regions of an antibody. Variable genes code for the antibody region that binds to antigen. Constant genes form the stem of the antibody and are the same for any antibody of a given class.

Antigen presentation
to helper T cell

Activation of T helper
to release cytokines

FIGURE 9-37 Activation of a B cell requires T helper cell "help." This help is given through a number of cell-to-cell interactions via receptors, as well as through the secretion of cytokines that stimulate B-cell growth and differentiation.

FIGURE 9-38 Major signaling pathways in B-cells. AP-1, activation protein 1; DAG, diacylglycerol; Ip_3, inositol 1,4,5-trisphosphate; MAP kinase, mitogen-activated protein kinase; NF-AT, nuclear factor of activated T cells; NF-κB, nuclear factor-κB; PIP2, phosphatidylinositol 4,5-bisphosphate; PLC-γ, phospholipase $C_γ$. (From Nairn: *Immunology for medical students,* ed 2, Mosby, 2007.)

IgG, the most common type of immunoglobulin, accounts for 75% to 80% of all immunoglobulins. It is found in nearly equal proportions in the intravascular and interstitial compartments and has a long half-life of about 3 weeks.[15] IgG is the smallest of the immunoglobulins and can more easily escape the bloodstream to enter the interstitial fluid surrounding tissues.

IgM accounts for about 10% of circulating immunoglobulins and is predominantly found in the intravascular pool.[15] Its large pentamer structure prevents it from migrating through the capillary wall. IgM has a half-life of 10 days. It is the first immunoglobulin to be produced on exposure to antigens or after immunization and is the major antibody found on B-cell surfaces. IgM is the antibody class that works best to activate

FIGURE 9-39 In response to nonprotein antigens (T cell independent), B cells can be activated by complement opsonins on the microbial antigen. The complement-receptor *(CR)* interaction provides a costimulatory signal to the B-cell receptor–antigen signal. (Redrawn from Abbas AK et al: *Cellular and molecular immunology,* ed 6, Philadelphia, 2007, Saunders, p 221.)

complement, which is important for cytotoxic functions in the immune system. Only one molecule of IgM is needed to activate complement, whereas two molecules of IgG are needed to do the same.

IgA is produced by plasma cells located in the tissue under the skin and mucous membranes. IgA is primarily found in saliva, tears, tracheobronchial secretions, colostrum, breast milk, and gastrointestinal and genitourinary secretions. Transport of IgA into secretions is facilitated by binding to a secretory component produced by epithelial cells. This complex is called *secretory IgA* (Figure 9-40). The half-life of IgA is about 6 days.[15]

IgD is found in trace amounts in the serum (1%) and is located primarily on the membranes of B cells along with IgM. IgD has a half-life of 3 days.[15] Little is known about its function, but it is thought to be a cellular antigen receptor acting to stimulate the B cell to multiply, differentiate, and secrete other specific immunoglobulins.

IgE is found bound by its Fc tail to receptors on the surface of basophils and mast cells (Figure 9-41). Only trace amounts of IgE are identified in the serum. IgE has a half-life of 2 days.[13] It has a role in immunity against helminthic parasites (worms) and is responsible for initiating inflammatory and allergic reactions (e.g., asthma, hay fever). IgE functions as a signaling molecule and causes mast cell degranulation when antigen is detected at the mast cell surface (see Chapter 10).

Class Switching and Affinity Maturation

During the course of an antibody response, the class of antibody manufactured by a particular B cell usually changes. The antigen-binding site does not change significantly and remains specific for the particular antigen that initiated the response. To switch class, the B cell selects different constant region genes to splice to the antigen-binding fragment. Thus, most B cells begin by using genes that code for IgM and IgD. Then the B cell switches to produce IgG, IgE, or IgA.[16] The triggers that determine the class of antibody a particular B cell will produce are not completely understood. Some cytokines have a role in class switching. For example, IFN-γ promotes IgG production, IL-4 promotes IgE production, and transforming growth factor β (TGF-β) promotes IgA production[16] (Figure 9-42).

Knowledge about the normal progression of class switching may be helpful in determining whether an infectious process is acute or chronic. For example, a person newly infected with hepatitis B virus would be expected to have primarily IgM antihepatitis B, whereas in chronic or previous infection, B cells would switch class to produce mainly IgG. The relative concentrations of antihepatitis B IgM and IgG can help identify the time of onset of the infection.

Over the course of a B-cell antibody response, the affinity with which the antibodies bind to antigen often increases. This is thought to occur because of a process called *affinity*

TABLE 9-4

Diagram and Properties of Immunoglobulin Classes

PROPERTY	IgG	IgM	IgA	IgD	IgE
Half-life (days)	23-25	5	6	3	2.5
Percent total immunoglobulin	80	6	13	0-1	0.002
Molecular weight (daltons)	146,000	900,000	160,000	184,000	200,000
Complement fixation	++	+++	–	–	–
Placental transfer	+++	–	–	–	–
Receptor for macrophage	+++	–	–	–	–
Reaction with staph protein A	+++	–	–	–	–
Passive cutaneous anaphylaxis	+++	–	–	–	+
Transported across epithelium	–	Occasionally	+	–	–
Prominent antibody activity	Anti-Rh against infections	ABO isoaggulutinins, rheumatoid factor	Against infections	Binds to B cells in presence of IgM	Mast cells sensitization, cytophilic antibody skin sensitizing antibody
Cell-binding functions					
Mononuclear cells	+	–	–	–	?/+
Neutrophils	+	–	+	–	–
Mast cells/basophils	–	–	–	–	+++
T cells/B cells	+	+	+	+	+
Platelets	+	+	–	–	?

(IgM diagram labeled "J chain")

Data from Roitt I et al: *Immunology,* ed 6, St Louis, 2001, Mosby; and Abbas AK: *Cellular and molecular immunology,* ed 5, Philadelphia, 2003, Saunders.

FIGURE 9-40 IgA is often combined with a protein called *secretory component,* which helps bind two IgA molecules together at their F_c ends.

maturation during which B cells undergo a hypermutation response producing random changes in the antigen-binding pocket of the BCR.[17] Those that bind antigen most avidly are stimulated to proliferate to a greater extent. Thus, the antibodies formed later in an immune response are more efficient in binding antigen at lower and lower concentrations. Affinity maturation occurs in specialized germinal centers in the lymph nodes.

Antibody Functions

Antibodies function in a number of ways to enhance the localization and removal of antigens from the body. These functions can generally be summarized as precipitation, agglutination, neutralization, opsonization, and complement activation. Precipitation and agglutination occur because each arm of the immunoglobulin Y structure can bind an antigenic epitope. This structure allows the antibodies and antigens to bind together into large insoluble complexes that precipitate out of body fluids (Figure 9-43). Agglutination refers to the same process as applied to cellular antigens rather than soluble antigens. It is efficient for phagocytic cells to find the large complexes and clear them from the system.

Antibodies can function as antitoxins by neutralizing bacterial toxin. This role is accomplished by binding the toxins before they can interact with cells or by covering the active portions of the toxin and inactivating it. Some antibodies are effective opsonins. They coat the foreign antigen and thereby make it more recognizable to phagocytic cells. Macrophages, neutrophils, eosinophils, and NK cells have receptors for the Fc ends of the antibodies, which help them bind to opsonized antigens. Antibodies thus make the innate phagocytic processes more efficient. Antibodies (IgG and IgM) bound to foreign antigens on cell membranes also can activate the complement cascade and trigger release of chemotaxins, inflammatory mediators, and formation of the membrane attack complex.

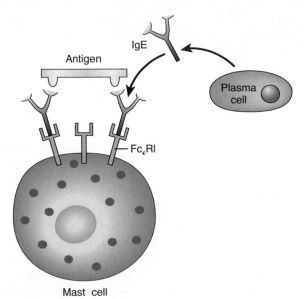

FIGURE 9-41 Mast cells bind IgE antibody with their Fc receptors *(FcεRI)* and display the IgE on the cell surface, where they are available to bind antigens.

FIGURE 9-42 Activated B cells undergo class switching from IgM to IgG, IgE, or IgA. Class switching is influenced by the presence of specific cytokines. *IFN,* Interferon; *IL,* interleukin; *TGF,* transforming growth factor. (Redrawn from Abbas AK et al: *Cellular and molecular immunology,* ed 6, Philadelphia, 2007, Saunders, p 230.)

FIGURE 9-43 Large antigen *(Ag)*-antibody complexes tend to precipitate out of solution, which makes it easier for phagocytic cells to find and eliminate the antigens.

PASSIVE AND ACTIVE IMMUNITY

Immunity is a state of resistance against infection from a particular pathogen. Immunity is provided primarily by adequate levels of circulating antibodies. Specific serum antibody concentrations can be measured by a blood test called an *antibody titer*. A sufficiently high antibody titer confers immunity by removing pathogens from the body before they cause signs and symptoms of illness. Immunity can be achieved passively or actively.

Passive Immunity

Passive immunity involves the transfer of plasma (sera) containing preformed antibodies against a specific antigen from a protected or immunized person to an unprotected or nonimmunized person. As a treatment, this is indicated in the following situations: (1) in B-cell immunodeficiencies; (2) following exposure of persons with high susceptibility to a disease without adequate time for active immunization; and (3) when antibody injection may alleviate or suppress the effects of an antigenic toxin.

Passive transfer of antibodies can occur in a variety of ways. In the fetus, certain maternal IgG antibodies can cross the placental barrier. Most of the time these antibodies are beneficial and assist the newborn in resisting pathogens. However, in some cases, these antibodies can be damaging to the fetus, as occurs in hemolytic disease of the newborn. In this disorder, maternal antibodies bind to and lyse fetal red blood cells (see Chapters 10 and 13).

Antibody, complement, and macrophage function is deficient at birth. Newborns who are breast fed may have improved immune function. Newborns receive IgA antibodies through breast milk. The infant's immature gastrointestinal tract and low proteolytic enzyme activity do not destroy all protein, which allows some of the IgA antibodies to be absorbed. These antibodies assist the infant in defending against bacterial and viral infections during infancy. It has been hypothesized by some researchers that IgA antibodies in breast milk may modify the ways that proteins cross the infant's highly permeable intestinal mucosa and help prevent food allergies in later life.[18]

Another method of passive immunity, called serotherapy, involves direct injection of antibodies into an unprotected person. The unprotected individual can receive a variety of substances, including immune globulin (human) such as IgG; specific immune globulins like hepatitis B immune globulin (human) or rabies immune globulin (human); plasma containing all human antibodies; or animal antibodies such as diphtheria antitoxin, tetanus antitoxin, botulism antitoxin, and antirabies serum.

Human immune globulin contains mostly IgG with traces of IgA and IgM. It is a sterile, concentrated protein solution that contains antibodies from the pooled plasma of many adults. It can be given intramuscularly or intravenously, depending on the product. Human immune globulins may be used as prophylaxis against hepatitis B and as therapy for the following conditions: antibody deficiency disorders, pediatric acquired immunodeficiency syndrome, and hypogammaglobulinemia after bone marrow transplantation.

Animal antibodies are given in specific situations only when necessary because of significant allergic risks with animal sera. Patients who have specific animal allergies or a history of asthma, allergic rhinitis, or other allergies are highly susceptible to serum sickness, anaphylaxis, or acute febrile reactions. Serum sickness occurs when antibodies bind to foreign proteins in the injected sera forming immune complexes that precipitate into capillaries and joints causing inflammation. Animal antibodies may be given to ameliorate toxins or venoms, including botulism, diphtheria, rabies, tetanus, snake bite, and spider bite.

Active Immunity

Active immunity confers a protected state owing to the body's immune response as a result of active infection or immunization. The development of active immunity requires the maturation and maintenance of memory B cells. On second exposure to antigen, the antibody response is much greater and more rapid (Figure 9-44). Exposure to antigen can be achieved through active infection or through immunization. The immune system must be exposed to the antigen long enough and in sufficient dose to stimulate an immune response.

Immunization tricks the immune system into responding to a perceived infection. Vaccines contain altered microorganisms or toxins that retain their ability to stimulate the immune system (antigenic properties) but do not have pathogenic properties. Vaccines can contain live and attenuated (altered) or killed infectious agents.

Vaccines that contain live altered virus or bacteria cause active infection but little injury to the vaccinated individual. These vaccines mimic a natural immune response, activating B and T cells, and provide good humoral and cellular immunity with longer lasting memory and often lifetime immunity. Examples of vaccines registered in the United States are listed in Box 9-1.

FIGURE 9-44 Time phases in the immune response. The primary response takes much longer to develop and falls off rapidly. On second exposure, a much quicker and greater antibody response is achieved.

BOX 9-1

Vaccines Licensed for Immunization and Distributed in the United States

Anthrax Vaccine Adsorbed
BCG Vaccine
Diphtheria and Tetanus Toxoids Adsorbed
Diphtheria and Tetanus Toxoids and Acellular Pertussis Vaccine Adsorbed
Diphtheria and Tetanus Toxoids and Acellular Pertussis Vaccine Adsorbed, Hepatitis B (recombinant) and Inactivated Poliovirus Vaccine Combined
Haemophilus b Conjugate Vaccine (Diphtheria CRM197 Protein Conjugate)
Haemophilus b Conjugate Vaccine (Meningococcal Protein Conjugate)
Haemophilus b Conjugate Vaccine (Tetanus Toxoid Conjugate)
Haemophilus b Conjugate Vaccine (Meningococcal Protein Conjugate) and Hepatitis B Vaccine (Recombinant)
Hepatitis A Vaccine, Inactivated
Hepatitis A Inactivated and Hepatitis B (Recombinant) Vaccine
Hepatitis B Vaccine (Recombinant)
Human Papillomavirus (Types 6, 11, 16, 18) Recombinant Vaccine
Influenza Virus Vaccine
Influenza Virus H5N1 (for National Stockpile)
Influenza Virus Vaccine, Live, Intranasal
Influenza Virus Vaccine, Trivalent, Types A and B
Japanese Encephalitis Virus Vaccine Inactivated
Measles Virus Vaccine, Live

Measles and Mumps Virus Vaccine, Live
Measles, Mumps, and Rubella Virus Vaccine, Live
Measles, Mumps, Rubella, and Varicella Virus Vaccine, Live
Meningococcal Polysaccharide Vaccine, Groups A, C, Y, and W-135 Combined
Mumps Virus Vaccine Live
Plague Vaccine
Pneumococcal Vaccine, Polyvalent
Pneumococcal 7-Valent Conjugate Vaccine (Diphtheria CRM197 Protein)
Poliovirus Vaccine Inactivated
Rabies Vaccine
Rotavirus Vaccine, Live, Oral, Pentavalent
Rubella Virus Vaccine Live
Smallpox (Vaccinia) Vaccine, Live
Smallpox Vaccine, Dried, Calf Lymph Type
Tetanus and Diphtheria Toxoids Adsorbed for Adult Use
Tetanus Toxoid
Tetanus Toxoid, Reduced Diphtheria Toxoid, and Acellular Pertussis Vaccine Adsorbed
Typhoid Vaccine Live Oral Ty21a
Typhoid Vi Polysaccharide Vaccine
Varicella Virus Vaccine Live
Yellow Fever Vaccine
Zoster Vaccine, Live

Updated October 15, 2007. FDA/Center for Biologics Evaluation and Research.

KEY POINTS

■ Specific immunity refers to functions of B and T lymphocytes. Each lymphocyte recognizes and reacts to only one particular antigen. On initial exposure to an antigen, lymphocytes undergo clonal expansion so that many lymphocytes are distributed throughout the body that can recognize and react to that particular antigen. These cells are called *memory cells*. Subsequent exposure results in a much faster and larger lymphocyte response.

■ T lymphocytes are able to bind antigens only when they are displayed on the surface of cells. Cytotoxic T cells (CD8+) react to cells that have foreign MHC class I proteins on their surface. T helper cells (CD4+) bind to cells that have MHC class II proteins on their surface. MHC class II proteins are found on antigen-presenting cells (B cells, dendritic cells, and macrophages). These cells engulf foreign antigens and combine the antigens with MHC class II proteins on their cell surface.

- T cells, which mature in the thymus, have two major subgroups: T helper cells and cytotoxic T cells. T helper cells perform a central role in specific immunity. Activation of T helper cells results in secretion of the cytokines necessary for clonal expansion of T and B lymphocytes. Cytotoxic T cells locate and lyse abnormal cells through the actions of perforins.

- B- and T-cell functions are interdependent. T cells cannot respond to soluble antigens. B cells can process free antigen and present it to T cells. On first exposure, B cells are minimally activated by antigen unless they are stimulated by cytokines and coreceptors from T cells.

- B lymphocytes mature in bone marrow and lymph tissue. B cells have receptors on their surfaces that can bind antigens. Each B cell binds only one particular antigen. With appropriate T helper cell "help," antigen binding causes the B cell to divide (clonal expansion). Some of the daughter cells become plasma cells, which actively produce and secrete antibodies. Other daughter cells (memory cells) resemble the original cell and are distributed in lymph throughout the body. On subsequent exposure to the antigen, antibody production is rapid.

- Antibodies are proteins that specifically bind a particular antigen. Antibodies have several functions, including precipitation, agglutination, neutralization, opsonization, and complement activation.

- The five major antibody classes are IgG, IgM, IgA, IgD, and IgE. Antibody class is determined by the structure of the Fc portion. IgG is the most prevalent antibody class (75%). IgM is the first kind to be produced on antigen exposure. IgA is found primarily in body secretions. IgD is present on the B-cell membrane and functions in signal transduction. IgE binds to basophil and mast cell membranes and mediates inflammation and allergy.

- Administration of preformed antibodies confers passive immunity. Passive immunity provides immediate but temporary protection. Active immunity occurs when individuals are exposed to antigen that stimulates their own lymphocytes to produce memory cells. Active immunity confers long-term protection but may take several weeks to develop.

GERIATRIC CONSIDERATIONS

Changes in the Immune System

In the elderly, immune system function is altered with a decreased ability to respond to antigenic stimulation. The elderly are able to respond to infections with previously produced "remembered" antibodies. However, they are less able to respond to new antigens. As a result of these changes, there is decreased speed of repair of tissue damage and increased vulnerability to disease. The cells of the immune system in elderly persons are not able to proliferate or reproduce as effectively as those in younger persons. Although the total number of T cells remains the same, T-cell function is decreased.

T cells are less able to proliferate and have decreased cytotoxicity. Antibody production also decreases, especially antibodies such as IgG. There is also a rise in autoantibody production, which may influence the increase in autoimmune disease in the elderly. Thymus size decreases after puberty, causing a decline in thymic hormone production, decreased T-cell differentiation, and reduced T-cell-related B-cell differentiation. Usually thymic hormone secretions stop after age 60 years. However, the role of thymus involution in elderly immune system changes is currently uncertain.

Integrated Function and Regulation of the Immune System

The innate and adaptive cells of the immune system work interdependently to protect the host from foreign antigens. Efficient interdependent function depends on a complex communication network that allows coordination of various immune components. One of the reasons that the immune system uses such a complex communication system is to ensure that normal healthy tissue is not injured. The destructive powers of the immune system must be tightly regulated to avoid undue tissue damage. These regulatory controls can be affected by aging and disease. The effects of aging on immune function are described in Geriatric Considerations: Changes in the Immune System. In the following sections, major events in the immune response to a new antigen are summarized and mechanisms of immune regulation are described.

INTEGRATED RESPONSE TO NEW ANTIGEN

A new antigen entering the body through the skin or mucous membranes will generally encounter tissue macrophages and dendritic cells stationed in strategic locations in the body as part of the mononuclear phagocyte system. Macrophages initiate activity of both the innate and specific immune components (Figure 9-45). First, activated macrophages release cytokines

Handwritten notes:
1) How do the cells recognize whats going on?
2) How do they mobilize to area?
3) What do they do when they get there?

Presented on MHC 2! must know → students often miss it up

using innate receptors to grab on + phago-cytose it then present it

Bacterial are extracellular
Viral intracellular
Thus PT is more relevant to c Helper? T + is more relevant to bacteria

Antigen is brought in on BCR.

How does the Antigen Show up

T cells proliferate

FIGURE 9-45 Diagram showing the integrated function of a number of immune components. Note that the macrophage is at the center of many immune functions, including chemotaxis and inflammation, presentation of antigen to T cells, and phagocytosis of antibody-antigen complexes. *NK,* Natural killer; *MHC,* major histocompatibility complex; *BCR,* B-cell receptor; *TCR,* T-cell receptor; *WBC,* white blood cell.

that initiate inflammation and chemotaxis. Some of these cytokines (TNF-α, IL-1) induce capillary endothelial cells to express selectins and integrin ligands that help circulating leukocytes to stick to the capillary wall (margination) and then move into the tissue locations of antigens (emigration). Neutrophils, macrophages, and NK cells are attracted to the infected area by chemotactic factors, some of which are released by macrophages, whereas others are products of the complement cascade and tissue injury. The complement cascade is activated by the alternative pathway on primary exposure to an antigen. Complement fragments C3a and C5a are potent inflammatory agents. Complement activation also results in the formation of membrane attack complexes that directly lyse cellular antigens.

Tissue injury associated with the infectious process also activates the coagulation cascade, which forms a fibrin meshwork to help entrap and localize the agent, and the kinin system, which promotes vasodilation to increase blood flow to the area. A number of other vasodilatory chemicals may be released from mast cells in the area when they degranulate. These inflammatory chemicals lead to the classic manifestations of inflammation: warmth, swelling, redness, pain, and loss of function. Neutrophils, macrophages, and NK cells that emigrate to the tissue find their targets through innate receptors on their cell surfaces. Thus, they are as effective on first exposure to an antigen as they are on subsequent exposures. These receptors bind to complement opsonins and molecules expressed on microbes such as lipopolysaccharide and mannose. NK cells release cytotoxins onto their targets; macrophages and neutrophils phagocytose and digest their targets.

Dendritic cells and macrophages ingest protein antigens to process and present them to T helper cells in association with MHC class II proteins. Dendritic cells move from the tissue and travel to the T cell zones of lymph nodes. Activation of T helper cells results in the secretion of a variety of cytokines that boost the growth and activity of many immune cells, including macrophages, neutrophils, NK cells, cytotoxic and T helper cells, and B cells. Some of the cytokines produced by activated T cells and macrophages stimulate stem cells in the bone marrow to produce more WBCs (neutrophilia). Other cytokines affect the brain (inducing fever, lethargy, and anorexia) and the liver (producing acute phase proteins).

Meanwhile, certain B cells that encounter the antigen in the lymph nodes will have the right BCR to bind and internalize it. Internalized antigen is then processed and presented to T helper cells in association with B cell MHC II proteins. Complementary T helper cells then bind the B cell (via MHC II–TCR–CD4 interactions) and provide help to the B cell through the secretion of cytokines and through coreceptor-mediated second-messenger signals. B cells thus activated proliferate into a clone of cells, some of which become memory cells, whereas others become plasma cells. Plasma cells synthesize and secrete antibodies that specifically bind the antigen. Significant antibody production takes 10 to 14 days to occur, and the infected individual may have signs and symptoms of illness during this time.

Antibodies enhance the function of innate phagocytic cells by collecting antigen into large complexes that are easier for nonspecific cells to locate and phagocytose. Activated T helper cells also secrete cytokines such as IL-2 and IFN-γ, which enhance the effectiveness of macrophages. After the antigen is cleared from the body, macrophages perform clean-up functions to remove inflammatory debris and dead neutrophils from the tissue. Macrophages also secrete enzymes and growth factors that stimulate tissue healing.

After the primary infection, B and T memory cells populate the body in much larger numbers and can mount an effective immune response very quickly on second exposure. The individual then has immunity for the particular pathogen because the antigen will usually be cleared from the system before significant illness occurs.

If the infectious agent is a virus, the story is somewhat different. Virally infected cells initiate cytotoxic T-cell activity, which serves to kill the infected cells. Natural killer cells are important for detecting and destroying virally infected cells that have down-regulated their MHC I proteins, making themselves invisible to cytotoxic T cells.[19] Helper T cell responses and B-cell production of antibody to the virus occur by the processes previously described. However, neutrophils are less important in the response to viral infection.

REGULATION OF IMMUNE FUNCTION *is important!*

The mechanisms that promote inflammation and enhance immune function are much better understood than those that negatively regulate these processes. However, the mechanisms for turning off an immune response and keeping inflammation in check are just as important. The destructive powers of the immune system can cause severe tissue damage unless carefully controlled.

Inhibition of immune responses occurs in a number of different ways. The process of inducing tolerance to self antigens is of primary importance. Because both T and B lymphocytes produce antigen-binding receptors by a random process, generation of self-reactive lymphocytes cannot be prevented. As previously mentioned, B and T cells are subjected to a rigorous selection process as they mature in the bone marrow or thymus. Several theories have been proposed to explain how self-reactive cells are detected and eliminated. The clonal deletion theory suggests that cells in the thymus process and present self antigens to developing T cells. Those lymphocytes that avidly bind self antigens are triggered to initiate programmed cell death (apoptosis).[20] There appears to be a critical time in fetal development when self antigens begin to be differentiated from foreign antigens. Before that time, antigens introduced into the fetus will be viewed as "self" and tolerance to them will develop. By the same token, self antigens that are not presented to T cells in the thymus may be viewed as foreign. This situation may occur with certain so-called sequestered antigens as would be found in the interior of the eye or testes. If these antigens are later released by trauma, an immune response may be directed against them.

Clonal deletion may not rid the body of all self-reactive lymphocytes; therefore many safeguards are in place to prevent

A number of T-cell theories of autoimmunity have been proposed, including thymus gland defects, decreased suppressor T-cell function, and altered T helper cell function. The theories attributing autoimmunity to thymus gland defects state that maturation and differentiation of T cells are affected by either decreased hormone secretion or failure of the thymus to expose T cells to all self products. In this theory, the thymus gland is responsible for exposing developing T cells to self products produced in the thymus or carried to the thymus gland. If some self products are not exposed to the developing T cells, the product will not be recognized as self and will subsequently be attacked. This lack of exposure to self products is thought to be a major factor in the development of generalized autoimmune diseases such as systemic lupus erythematosus (SLE). The theory attributing autoimmunity to decreased suppressor T-cell activity states that decreased numbers of suppressor T cells fail to repress immunoglobulin activity. This theory does not adequately explain tissue-specific or organ-specific autoimmune damage, but it may explain generalized autoimmunity as seen in SLE. The altered T helper cell function theory asserts that changed T helper cells lose their self tolerance through a variety of mechanisms, including disruption in the number of, or activity of, the T cells as a result of genetic mutations.[4] For example, a mutation of the transcription factor forkhead box p3(FOXP3) causes impaired development and function of CD4+ T cells, leading to autoimmune inflammation.[4]

A number of B-cell theories of autoimmunity also have been proposed. The theory attributing autoimmunity to escape of B-cell tolerance proposes that certain B cells lose their responsiveness to suppressor T-cell messages. The B-cell activation theories, which are well supported clinically and experimentally, suggest that extrinsic factors or intrinsic, genetic B-cell defects cause autoantibody production and an increase in the number and activity of B cells. A number of extrinsic factors, including viruses, bacteria, antibiotics, proteolytic enzymes, and lipopolysaccharides, have been found to be B-cell-activating factors that could trigger autoantibody production.

Research has linked mast cells to autoimmunity as well as hypersensitivity. Mast cells reside in most mucus membranes waiting for foreign proteins or bacteria to invade. Their cell membranes are studded with bacteria-sensing proteins, called Toll-like receptors, which cause release of up to 10,000 different chemicals in response to activation. Mast cells release the cytokine interleukin-1 (IL-1), attracting and enlisting inflammation-inducing cells to joints and leaking fluid into joints in the autoimmune disease of rheumatoid arthritis.[5] Other researchers believe that lymph or spleen mast cells may activate self-destructive T cells, which travel to the central nervous system to target myelin in multiple sclerosis.[5]

Genetic Factors

Genetic predisposition seems to be an important factor in the development of autoimmune disorders. Recent studies have shown that different cytokine profiles can be associated with autoimmunity. Those with genetically low levels of tumor necrosis factor α (TNF-α) and high levels of IL-10 may be more tolerant than those with normal levels.[3] The role of genetics is supported by the observation that certain MHC genes—also called human leukocyte antigen (HLA) genes—are frequently associated with certain autoimmune disorders (Table 10-1). Gender, which is genetically determined, also influences the expression of autoimmune disorders. The exact mechanisms of gender and genetic influence on autoimmune expression have not been established, but the relationship is significant. Females are at significantly higher risk for developing autoimmunity compared to males.

Certain MHC genes appear to increase the risk of development of autoimmune disease. One of the strongest correlations of MHC molecules with autoimmune disease is the linkage between the HLA-B27 phenotype and ankylosing spondylitis. In this case, 95% of all people with ankylosing spondylitis have a positive B27 phenotype. However, not everyone with a positive B27 phenotype develops ankylosing spondylitis, both because of differences in the way antigen is presented to the immune system and because of environmental factors. Other diseases are associated with different MHC phenotypes, but the correlation between risk for disease and presence of the disease marker is much lower. For example, Addison disease is associated with the DR3 phenotype, but it has only a 6% risk correlation. Juvenile rheumatoid arthritis is strongly associated with HLA-DR5.

TABLE 10-1				
Major Histocompatibility Genes and Autoimmune Disease				
Disease	**HLA (MHC) Antigen**	**Frequency in Patients (%)**	**Frequency in Controls (%)**	**Relative Risk**
Ankylosing spondylitis				
Caucasians	B27	89	43	69
Japanese	B27	85	<1	207
Rheumatoid arthritis	DR4	68	25	3.8
Graves disease	Dw3	56	25	3.7
Type 1 diabetes mellitus	DR3/DR4 heterozygous			33
Systemic lupus erythematosus	DR4	73	33	5
Narcolepsy	DR2	100	34	358

Data from Tierney LM, McPhee SJ, Papadakis MA, editors: *Current medical diagnosis and treatment,* ed 46, New York, 2007, Lange/McGraw-Hill.

There may also be disease-causing genotypes or genetic factors affecting expression of immune factors, such as "certain alleles of the cytotoxic T lymphocyte-associated antigen-4 gene (possibly a nonspecific exacerbating molecule of disease risk in several autoimmune diseases), the lymphoid protein tyrosine phosphatase nonreceptor type 22 gene (associated with type 1 diabetes and other autoimmune disease), TNF-α (involved in chronic inflammation, autoimmunity and malignancies) and the FOXP3 gene (expressed by CD4+ regulatory T cells), whose mutations can cause immune dysregulation, polyendocrinopathy and X-linked inheritance syndromes of systemic autoimmunity."[2] The FOXP3 deficiency is associated with both a primary immune deficiency disorder and an autoimmune disorder owing to its effect on regulatory T-cell immune function.[6]

Environmental Triggers

Chronic or multiple viral or bacterial infections may be associated with the development of autoimmune disease in susceptible persons; however, no clear explanatory model has been developed.[7] Viruses can activate B cells, decrease the function of T cells, contribute to the development of antigenic mimicry, or insert viral components on cell surfaces and trigger immune reactions. For example, Epstein-Barr virus, cytomegalovirus, and bacteria, such as *Helicobacter pylori*, have been frequently cited as potential triggers of autoimmune disease.[7]

Environmental and occupational stress can affect the immune system because of their relationship to the neuroendocrine system, leading to inflammation or lymphokine release that activates T cells. Neuroendocrine and immune system interaction during life stress, such as shift work or workplace stress, promotes the synthesis and overproduction of proinflammatory cytokines. In genetically susceptible persons, this increase in systemic and local proinflammatory cytokines may affect the system's balance enough to trigger autoimmune disease.[8] This relationship is so strong that some advocate identifying prone individuals early, modifying their lifestyle, and starting them on medication even before autoimmune disease symptoms occur.[9]

Although the etiology of autoimmunity continues to be investigated, the mechanisms whereby autoantibodies injure tissues are better understood. The autoantibodies produced by autoimmune disorders affect tissue by the mechanisms described for type II and type III hypersensitivity reactions found later in this chapter.

Pharmacotherapies

Few specific treatments for autoimmune disorders have been established, and immunosuppressive therapy is the treatment most often used. Because autoimmunity is expressed in different ways, the immunosuppressive treatment for each type of autoimmune disease is individualized, depending on disease expression. Immunosuppressive therapy, including corticosteroids and certain cytotoxic chemotherapeutic agents, has become an increasingly important treatment choice. These drugs are essential for inhibiting excessive or aberrant immune responses. The ideal immunosuppressive medication would be an agent that inhibits only the abnormal immune response without limiting the positive and protective functions of the immune system or causing any organ toxicity. Unfortunately, no immunosuppressive medications like that exist.

Immunosuppressive agents include corticosteroids and cytotoxins. Corticosteroids decrease the number of lymphocytes and decrease antibody formation, as well as alter the functional activities of lymphocytes. They also have many other activities as a result of their glucocorticoid function. Corticosteroids tend to be used in the treatment of many autoimmune diseases and are the oldest of the immunosuppressive drugs. Cytotoxins, such as methotrexate, are used to manage autoimmune disorders owing to their ability to kill actively proliferating lymphocytes after they are transformed from their resting G_0 state. The key to the use of cytotoxins is to effectively apply their killing activity without hurting the rest of the body. Cyclosporine (Sandimmune) is a more selective immunosuppressant that reversibly suppresses T helper cells in the G_0 or G_1 phase of the cell cycle without killing them. As a result, it inhibits the development of killer or cytotoxic T cells without decreasing the numbers of cells. It also impairs the ability of T cells to respond effectively to foreign antigens. It is used to suppress reactions during tissue or organ transplantation. Antirheumatic agents, such as etanercept (Enbrel) or infliximab (Remicade) are used as disease modifiers that bind to and block the activity of TNF-α and TNF-β. They may also modulate TNF-mediated responses, such as leukocyte migration and expression of adhesion molecules.

Therapeutic plasmapheresis is another type of therapy occasionally used in the management of autoimmune diseases. Plasmapheresis is analogous to dialysis and involves the selective filtering or removal of plasma or a plasma cell type. The patient's whole blood is filtered and the plasma component containing the autoantibodies removed and replaced with albumin or another colloid solution. This type of therapy has been effective in the management of myasthenia gravis, thrombocytopenic purpura, multiple sclerosis, and Rh-negative hemolytic disease of the newborn.

KEY POINTS

- Autoimmune disorders occur when the immune system erroneously reacts with "self" tissues. These disorders are thought to be polygenic and multifactorial; however, the exact etiologic process is unknown.
- The antigenic mimicry theory proposes that since self and foreign antigens are composed of the same basic building blocks—proteins, carbohydrates, nucleic acids, and lipids—small alterations in self tissue may lead to immunogenic attack.
- The theory involving release of sequestered antigens suggests that self antigens that do not come in direct contact with lymphocytes during fetal development may cause autoimmune reactions if they are subsequently released from sequestration.

- Abnormal production of subclasses of T lymphocytes, particularly suppressor T cells, has been proposed as a reason for the development of autoimmunity, as well as the development of abnormal B cells that do not respond to suppressor T cell signals.
- A genetic component is probable, inasmuch as certain autoimmune disorders are more commonly associated with particular MHC types and female gender.
- Viruses may also be causative in the development of autoimmune disorders. Viruses may alter self cells, thus precipitating an immune attack. Formed antibodies may then cross-react with similar but uninfected cells.
- Autoantibodies injure body tissues through the mechanisms described for type II and type III hypersensitivity reactions.

HYPERSENSITIVITY

Hypersensitivity is a normal immune response that is inappropriately triggered or excessive or produces undesirable effects on the body. The basic mechanism that triggers hypersensitivity is a specific antigen-antibody reaction or a specific antigen-lymphocyte interaction. Four classes or types of hypersensitivity are differentiated. Each type is characterized by a specific cellular or antibody response. Hypersensitivity types I, II, and III are mediated by antibodies produced by B lymphocytes. Type IV hypersensitivity is mediated by T cells. Hypersensitivity reactions are specific to a particular antigen and do not usually occur on first exposure to the antigen. Although the diseases or syndromes associated with each type differ in their clinical signs and symptoms, the underlying pathophysiologic process is similar within each type. In Table 10-2 the four major types of hypersensitivity are contrasted.

Type I Hypersensitivity

Etiology. Genetic mechanisms influence type I hypersensitivity with strong genetic or hereditary linkage regarding the IgE response to antigens (allergens). This genetic component involves both the ability to respond to an allergen and the general ability to produce an IgE antibody response. For example, children born to two allergic parents have a 50% chance of being allergic. Children born to one nonallergic and one allergic parent have a 30% chance of being allergic.

Researchers are currently exploring two genetic avenues that influence hyperresponsiveness and allergies: IgE levels and suppressor T-cell function. High IgE levels have been found in most but not all hypersensitive people. Although high IgE levels are associated with worse symptoms such as persistent

TABLE 10-2				
The Four Types of Hypersensitivity				
Characteristic	Type I: Atopic, Anaphylactic	Type II: Cytotoxic, Cytolytic	Type III: Immune Complex (Arthus Reaction)	Type IV: Delayed Hypersensitivity
Mediated by	IgE	IgM or IgG	IgG	T$_{DTH}$ lymphocytes
Complement activation	No	Yes	Yes	No
Immune response	Ag plus IgE, leading to mast cell degranulation	Surface Ag and Ab, leading to killer cell cytotoxic action or complement-mediated lysis	Ag-Ab complex in tissues; complement activated and PMNs attracted	Ag-sensitized T cells release lymphokines, leading to inflammatory reactions, and attract macrophages, which release mediator
Peak action	15-30 min	15-30 min	6 hr	24-48 hr
Serum transferability	Yes	Yes	Yes	No
Cell transferability	No	No	No	Yes (T cells)
Genetic mechanisms	Familial High IgE level HLA-linked *Ir* genes General hyperresponsiveness	HLA linked in some cases	Familial (autoimmune) HLA specificities	Unknown
Causes of reaction	T-cell deficiency Abnormal mediator feedback Environmental factors and Ag	Exposure to Ag or foreign tissue, cells, or graft	Persistent infection— microbe Ag Extrinsic environmental Ag Autoimmunity—self Ag	Intradermal Ag Epidermal Ag Dermal Ag
Manifestation (examples)	Asthma, rhinitis, atopic eczema, bee-sting reaction	ABO transfusions, hemolytic disease of newborn, myasthenia gravis	Glomerulonephritis, SLE, farmer's lung arthritis, vasculitis	Guillain-Barré disease, tuberculin test, contact dermatitis, multiple sclerosis

Ab, Antibody; *Ag,* Antigen; *Ig,* Immunoglobulin; *DTH,* Delayed-type hypersensitivity; *PMN,* Polymorphonuclear leukocyte; *HLA,* Human leukocyte antigen; *SLE,* Systemic lupus erythematosus.

wheezing, lower levels of IgE do not exclude type I hypersensitivity reactions.[10] It has also been found that low levels of suppressor T cells are associated with high IgE levels and the MHC genes *HLA-B8* and *HLA-Dw3*. *HLA-B8* may be linked to suppressor T-cell control of immune responses. These findings suggest that IgE production is under T-cell control. An individual's mix of T_H1 and T_H2 cells may contribute to allergic reactivity. T_H2 cells release IL-4 and IL-5, which stimulates B cells to produce IgE. T_H1 cells secrete interferon-γ and IL-2, which may inhibit IgE production by B cells. However, not all allergic people have high IgE levels.[10]

Several hypotheses regarding the mechanisms of allergic, type I hypersensitivity reactions have been proposed. It is hypothesized that a suppressor T-cell deficiency or abnormal mediator feedback increases mast cell degranulation and the inflammatory response. Environmental pollutants may play a role by increasing mucosal permeability and enhancing antigen (allergen) entry into the body. This increased entry would subsequently increase IgE responsiveness.

In addition, an allergic breakthrough hypothesis has been devised to explain type I hypersensitivity reactions. This hypothesis suggests that in both high-IgE and low-IgE responders, overt expression of clinical symptoms is seen only when some allergic breakthrough level is exceeded. Exceeding this hypothesized level may depend on the presence of concomitant factors, such as viral infections of the upper respiratory tract, transient IgA deficiency, or decreased suppressor T-cell activity.

Pathogenesis. Type I hypersensitivity is also known as immediate hypersensitivity, because the reaction is immediate. It is a sensitization reaction characterized by signs and symptoms of an allergic reaction that usually occurs 15 to 30 minutes after exposure to an antigen (allergen).

At the cellular level, immunoglobulin E (IgE) is the principal antibody mediating this reaction. IgE is produced by specialized plasma B cells and circulates in very small amounts in the blood. When an individual is exposed to an allergen, selected plasma B cells produce IgE. It usually takes repeated exposures to the allergen to cause significant levels of IgE to be present in the blood.

Mast cells and basophils are the principal effector cells, although there are many other cells with histamine and other inflammatory mediators that can be involved in the reaction. These may include neutrophils, eosinophils, lymphocytes, macrophages, epithelial cells, and endothelial cells. Mast cells are found throughout the body in all loose connective tissue. They are covered with IgE receptors—up to 500,000 on their cell surfaces—and they are filled with vesicles or granules containing potent vasoactive, proinflammatory chemical mediators (especially histamine) that produce inflammation when they are released. The IgE receptors on mast cells bind the Fc portion of an IgE antibody. The IgE antigen-binding sites are then displayed on the mast cell surface, where they can bind to antigens that pass by the mast cell (Figure 10-1). This process makes the mast cells responsive to particular antigens.

The initial incident during a type I hypersensitivity response is the cross-linking of two IgE receptors to one antigen on the mast cell located at the site of the allergen's entry into the body (see Figure 10-1). Cross-linking of IgE and the antigen causes an increase in intracellular calcium (Ca^{2+}) that

FIGURE 10-1 Type I hypersensitivity reaction.

results in immediate, massive, local mast cell degranulation of preformed and newly formed proinflammatory mediators. The release of mediators causes an inflammatory response.

Mast cells, basophils, and other effector cells release many chemicals. Some of the mediators are preformed and stored in vesicles, such as histamine, heparin, proteolytic enzymes, and chemotactic factors. Other mediators are formed during the degranulation process. Examples of newly formed mediators include superoxide, prostaglandins, thromboxanes, leukotrienes, bradykinin, and interleukins (see Chapter 9).

One of the most important mediators of type I hypersensitivity is histamine. Histamine binds to H_1 (histamine 1), H_2, and H_3 receptors, which are located on many types of cells. Mast cells have receptors for H_1, H_2, and H_3, with H_1 receptors being the most active. Basophils express predominantly H_2 receptors, whereas neutrophils and eosinophils have both H_1 and H_2 receptors. Recent evidence shows that H_1 and H_2 receptors are present on monocytes and macrophages, with an increase in H_1 receptors when monocytes differentiate into macrophages.[11] Histamine binding to H_1 receptors triggers increased vascular permeability, vasodilation (flushing), urticaria formation (hives), smooth muscle constriction (bronchoconstriction), increased mucus secretion and pruritus (increased itching), and increased gut permeability. The activation of H_2 receptors has opposing effects to H_1 receptors in some tissues and causes smooth muscle relaxation in the lower airways, augments gastric acid secretion from parietal cells, and in high concentrations has an inhibitory effect on inflammatory cells, decreasing degranulation and decreasing neutrophil chemotaxis. The H_3 receptors are located in postganglionic cholinergic nerves in lung bronchi.[11]

The proteolytic enzymes kininogenase and tryptase activate the kinin pathway and C3 activates the complement cascade via the alternative pathway. Heparin decreases clot formation. The chemotactic factors recruit or activate other inflammatory and immune cells. Leukotrienes cause smooth muscle contraction and increase vascular permeability.

Clinical Manifestations. Manifestations of an immediate hypersensitivity reaction vary in severity and intensity. For many people, type I hypersensitivity reactions are annoying, such as hives (urticaria), seasonal allergic rhinitis, eczema, or mild bronchoconstriction. In other people, the symptoms are more problematic, including tightening of the throat, localized edema, wheezing, and tachycardia, such as is associated with localized angioedema reactions or severe airway reactions. In a very small number of highly allergic people, the type I hypersensitivity reaction can be expressed as a life-threatening allergic reaction known as anaphylaxis such as that associated with bee sting, seafood, or peanut allergic reactions. Common allergenic medications, insects, and foods that can trigger type I hypersensitivity reactions are listed in Box 10-1.

Treatment. Treatment for type I hypersensitivity primarily involves pharmacologic management with antihistamines, β-adrenergics, corticosteroids, anticholinergics, and anti-immunoglobulin E therapy (IgE blocker therapy). Antihistamines such as diphenhydramine (Benadryl) are used

---

BOX 10-1

Possible Causes of Human Anaphylaxis

Medications
Penicillin, penicillin analogues, and other antibiotics
Radiographic contrast media
Aspirin, indomethacin, and other analgesics
Allergenic extracts

Biological Agents
Serum proteins, including γ-globulin
Insulin and other hormones
Vaccines
Enzymes such as penicillinase
Local anesthetics
Hymenoptera (stinging) insects
Polistes wasps
Honeybees
Fire ants
Hornets and yellow jackets

Foods
Nuts
Seafood, especially shellfish
Eggs
Fruit, especially citrus and strawberries
Tartrazine, yellow dye no. 5
Inorganic chemicals
Nickel
Aluminum
Zinc

---

to block the effect of histamine. This action decreases vascular permeability and bronchoconstriction. β-Adrenergic sympathomimetics are used to decrease bronchoconstriction and bronchospasm. **Epinephrine** is an adrenergic agent (α, $β_1$, and $β_2$) given subcutaneously or intravenously during acute allergic reactions, especially after food or bee sting reactions. Most patients with severe allergies to food or insect bites are given prescriptions for epinephrine in the form of EpiPen with an autoinjector. Corticosteroids are used to decrease the inflammatory response. Anticholinergics are used to block the parasympathetic system and thus allow greater sympathetic activity. This action indirectly causes bronchodilation. Anti-immunoglobulin E therapy (omalizumab) may be used for persons with severe persistent asthma. Omalizumab is a subcutaneously injected, monoclonal anti-IgE antibody that binds to the IgE molecule, thus inhibiting the binding of IgE to mast cells and basophils and promoting down-regulation of IgE receptors. It is used to improve asthma control in patients with moderate to severe persistent asthma.[10,12]

Prevention. Some protective, proactive actions taken during pregnancy are thought to decrease the likelihood that type I hypersensitivity will develop in children from families with a history of allergies. These actions include avoiding foods to which the mother is allergic, limiting excesses of one type of food during the last trimester of pregnancy, avoiding whole eggs during the last month before delivery and while breast-feeding, and limiting cow's milk to two glasses per day. Other actions that may be helpful during the child's infancy include avoiding exposure to environmental pollution, breast-feeding for a minimum of 6 months, supplementation with non-cow's milk products such as soy milk, giving solid foods only after the infant is 6 months old, keeping the infant's room as free of dust and molds as possible, and keeping pets (dogs, cats, birds) out of the home.

Pharmacotherapeutic Prevention. Another avenue for prevention of type 1 hypersensitivity reactions involves the use of desensitization therapy (immunotherapy). Desensitization, or immunotherapy, is more successful in patients with hay fever than in those with other types of allergies. It involves both environmental control of external allergens and titrated pharmacologic exposure to allergens. Environmental control involves a systematic plan to decrease exposure to house dust, molds, and animal dander. Pets are kept out of the house. The person must avoid food allergens, wool carpets, goose down or feather pillows, dried plants, and exposure to other animal and vegetable products. The person is urged to use air conditioning and electronic air filters.

Pharmacologic desensitization involves injecting a person with sufficient antigen (allergen) on a regular basis over a course of months or years, followed by periodic maintenance or booster therapy. Gradually the dose is increased until the person can tolerate the allergen without a type I hypersensitivity reaction. The goal of this therapy is a change in immunoglobulins so that there is an increase in IgG- and IgA-blocking antibodies, no increase in IgE during allergy season, decreased basophil reactivity, and decreased lymphocyte reactivity to allergens.

Type II Hypersensitivity

Etiology and Pathogenesis. Type II hypersensitivity, also known as tissue-specific, cytotoxic, or cytolytic hypersensitivity, is characterized by antibodies that attack antigens on the surface of specific cells or tissues. Often the reaction is immediate (15 to 30 minutes after exposure to the antigen). However, it can occur over time, such as in thyroiditis or myasthenia gravis. The mechanisms that encompass type II tissue-specific hypersensitivity all occur after the binding of antibody to tissue-specific antigens. The reaction is mediated by the complement system and a variety of effector cells, including tissue macrophages, platelets, natural killer cells, neutrophils, and eosinophils. IgG and IgM are the principal antibodies. Examples of this type of hypersensitivity reaction include ABO transfusion reactions, hemolytic disease of the newborn, myasthenia gravis, thyroiditis, hyperacute graft rejection, and autoimmune hemolytic anemia (Table 10-3). Transfusion reactions, hemolytic disease of the newborn, and graft rejection are examples of **isoimmunity (alloimmunity),** a condition in which the immune system reacts against antigens on tissues from other members of the same species.

The initial mechanism during a type II hypersensitivity response is exposure to antigen on the surface of foreign cells.

TABLE 10-3

Disease and Autoantibodies Associated with Type II Hypersensitivity

Disease	Antigen/Autoantibody
Type 1 diabetes	Islet cells
Insulin-resistant diabetic states	Insulin receptor
Myasthenia gravis	Acetylcholine receptor
Addison disease	Adrenal epithelial cells
Autoimmune hemolytic anemia	Red cell membrane
Immune thrombocytopenic purpura	Platelet membrane
Autoimmune neutropenia	Neutrophil antigens
Pernicious anemia	Intrinsic factor, gastric parietal cells
Lymphocytic thyroiditis	Thyroglobulin
Graves disease	Receptor for thyroid-stimulating hormone
Pemphigus vulgaris	Desmosomes
Hyperacute graft rejection	Donor antigens

The Fab portion of IgG or IgM antibodies binds to antigens on the target foreign cell to form an antigen-antibody complex (Figure 10-2). (Refer also to Chapter 9 for a discussion of IgG and IgM antibodies.) The Fc region of the IgG or IgM antibodies sticks out away from the cell membrane surface. The Fc region then acts as a bridge between the antigen and complement or the effector cells. This antigen-antibody binding with Fc bridging is the key and leads to lysis of the cell by one of several mechanisms. One mechanism is complement-mediated lysis. Complement-mediated lysis occurs through the classical pathway for activation of complement. The classical pathway of complement generates the activated complement component C3b via splitting of C4 and C2 by C1 (Chapter 9). The activated complement component C3b is bound to the target cell by the Fc region of IgG or IgM. C3b increases opsonization, which in turn increases the capacity of the system to allow lysis by other effector cells or by complement itself. Lysis of the foreign cell by complement occurs via the C5-C9 membrane attack complex (MAC), which disrupts the plasma membrane of the cell.

Transfusion Reaction. An example of this type of mechanism is a blood transfusion reaction. It occurs when a person receives blood from someone with a different blood group type (Table 10-4). If a person with type A blood having type A antigens and anti-B antibodies incorrectly receives type B blood with B antigens and anti-A antibodies, the anti-B antibodies will attach to the surface of the infused type B red blood cells and the anti-A antibodies in the infusion will attach to the surface of the circulating type A red blood cells. This event will stimulate the destruction of large numbers of red cells. The resulting signs and symptoms of this major blood group reaction include fever, chills, flushing, tachycardia, hypotension, low back pain, pleuritic chest pain, nausea, vomiting, restlessness, anxiety, oliguria, and headache. The reaction may progress to anaphylaxis, shock, and death.

FIGURE 10-2 Type II hypersensitivity reactions.

Hemolytic Disease of the Newborn. A second mechanism for antigen-antibody binding in type II hypersensitivity reactions is direct destruction by Fc-bearing effector cells, such as macrophages. The macrophage can link to exposed Fc antibody regions. Once this bridging occurs, the foreign cell is phagocytized and destroyed by lysosomes within the effector cell. This can be mediated with or without complement involvement. An example of this type of mechanism is hemolytic disease of the newborn (erythroblastosis fetalis).

This condition occurs during pregnancy when an Rh-negative mother is sensitized to her fetus's Rh-positive red cell group antigens because of exposure during her current or a previous pregnancy. The mother's IgG Rh-positive antibodies cross the placental barrier and attack the fetus's red blood cells. The mother's exposure occurs when mixing of fetal and maternal blood takes place—during an episode of antepartal bleeding, during birth, or during miscarriage of an Rh-positive child. After this exposure, Rh-positive antibodies develop in the mother and affect her subsequent children. It takes as little as 1 cm^3 of fetal blood exposure for antibodies to Rh-positive red cells to develop in the mother. Usually, the first Rh-positive child is not affected unless placental tearing or leakage into the mother's circulation occurs during pregnancy. Antibody screens are routinely performed during

TABLE 10-4
Major Blood Groups

Blood Group			
Phenotype	**Frequency (%)**	**Antigens**	**Antibodies in Serum**
A	42	A	Anti-B
B	8	B	Anti-A
AB	3	A and B	None
O	47	H	Anti-A, anti-B
Other Major Blood Group Systems			
Rhesus (Rh)		C, D, E, c, d, e	
	Rh$^+$	85	Cde, CDE
	Rh$^-$	15	Cde, CdE
Kell		K or k	
	K	9	K
	k	91	k
MN		M or N	
	MM	28	MM
	MN	50	MN
	NN	22	NN
Duffy		Fy^a, Fy^b, Fy	
	Fy^{a}Fy^b	46	Fy^a, Fy^b
	Fy^a	20	Fy^a
	Fy^b	34	Fy^b
	Fy	0.1	Fy

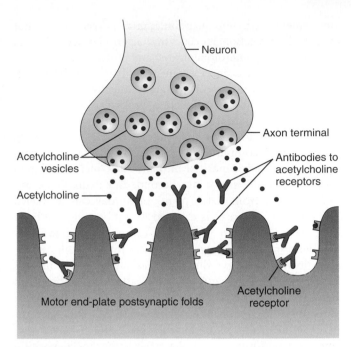

FIGURE 10-3 Type II hypersensitivity reaction in a person with myasthenia gravis. Having limited receptors available for acetylcholine impairs neuromuscular transmission.

pregnancy and RhoGAM administered at 28 weeks and at delivery for prevention of Rh-positive antibodies. RhoGAM contains antibodies against Rh antigens on fetal blood cells and is given to the mother to destroy fetal cells that may be present in her circulation before her immune system becomes activated and begins to produce anti-Rh antibodies. RhoGAM is not effective if the mother already has a positive antibody titer for fetal Rh antigens.

Myasthenia Gravis and Graves Disease. A third mechanism for antigen-antibody binding is seen in myasthenia gravis, an autoimmune disorder. In this case, antibodies form to the acetylcholine receptor on muscle membrane surfaces, primarily the motor end-plate (Figure 10-3). With antigen-antibody formation at the receptor site, complement disrupts the muscle cell membrane. Effector cells are not thought to be involved in this type II hypersensitivity reaction. The loss of acetylcholine stimulation at the motor end-plate causes the extreme muscular weakness associated with myasthenia gravis.

A fourth mechanism for antigen-antibody binding in type II hypersensitivity reactions is also mediated by effector cells. The effector cells in this case do not directly engulf and destroy the complex because the tissue is too large for the cells to engulf and destroy. Therefore, the effector cells, such as neutrophils, bind to the target cells and block the receptors from normal functioning, causing injury to or malfunction of the involved tissue. Lymphocytic thyroiditis and Graves disease are examples of this type of disorder.

Hyperacute Graft Rejection. Another type II hypersensitivity mechanism for antigen-antibody binding that involves both effector cells and complement is the hyperacute graft rejection that affects transplanted tissues. It occurs when the transplanted donor tissue has an antigen to which the recipient has preformed antibodies. For example, when tissue from a blood type A or B donor is transplanted into a blood type O recipient, the recipient has anti-A and anti-B antibodies. These antibodies will immediately attack the foreign transplanted tissue.

Onset begins immediately after revascularization of the transplanted tissue. At this time, the blood supply from the patient is established in the newly transplanted organ. The patient's antibodies attack the foreign protein antigens and form an antigen-antibody complex. Effector cell infiltration and complement-mediated lysis of donor tissues, inflammation, vascular thrombosis, and hemorrhage occur. The reaction happens so quickly that within 48 hours after transplantation the graft tissue is no longer functioning.

To prevent hyperacute graft rejection, tissue and blood typing of donors and recipients of transplanted tissue is extensive. Lists of potential recipients are matched to donors through organ donation laboratories both regionally and nationally. Only rarely has hyperacute graft rejection occurred because of an error in tissue or blood typing.

Type III Hypersensitivity

Etiology. Type III hypersensitivity results from failure of the immune and phagocytic systems to effectively remove antigen-antibody immune complexes and is not tissue specific. It is also known as an immune complex reaction. Type III hypersensitivity is characterized by antigen-antibody complex deposition into tissues, with consequent activation of complement and a subsequent inflammatory reaction. It is not an immediate reaction; it occurs over a period of several hours or longer (i.e., glomerulonephritis) and is often ongoing.

Three possible scenarios can precipitate type III hypersensitivity. First, persistent low-grade infection by a microbial or viral agent can stimulate a weak antibody response. The continuing nature of persistent infection and antibody response leads to chronic immune complex production. These immune complexes are not successfully removed from the blood and are deposited in many sites, including blood vessels, glomeruli, and joints. Second, an extrinsic environmental antigen from molds, plants, or animals can be inhaled into the lung, where it is exposed to antibody in the body fluid. This inhalation of antigen causes antigen-antibody complex formation in alveoli with immune complex deposition in the alveolar walls. Third, an autoimmune process can develop in which autoantibodies attack self antigens. In this case, the body forms both parts of the immune complex. Autoantibodies to either circulating or tissue-fixed self antigens may be produced. Because the self antigens persist over time, chronic immune complex production and deposition in tissues take place.

The mechanism of injury in type III hypersensitivity reactions is from activation of complement and other proinflammatory mediators in response to the antigen-antibody complex deposition. The antibody-antigen complex deposition does not cause the injury. The tissue injury is caused by an inflammatory reaction to the antibody-antigen complex. Therefore, it is not a tissue-specific reaction. The onset of this reaction occurs up to 6+ hours after exposure to the antigen. IgG and IgM are the principal antibodies. The principal effector cells are neutrophils and mast cells. The principal mediator of the reaction is complement. Examples of type III hypersensitivity reaction include systemic lupus erythematosus, immune complex glomerulonephritis, serum sickness, and drug-induced vasculitis. Diseases associated with type III hypersensitivity are listed in Table 10-5.

Pathogenesis. Type III hypersensitivity reactions tend to be ongoing with variations in symptoms based on changing antibody-antigen ratios, amount of complement available to mediate the inflammation, and the dynamic nature of the antibody-antigen reaction. It is sometimes difficult to differentiate between type II and type III hypersensitivity reactions. The key differences between a type II and a type III reaction are the location of antigen and the mechanism of injury. As previously described, type II reactions occur in response to tissue-specific antigen located on cell surfaces and involve direct cell death or malfunction from the antigen-antibody reaction. Type III hypersensitivity reactions involve antigens forming antigen-antibody complexes that precipitate out of the blood or body fluid and are deposited into tissues.

Type III hypersensitivity reactions involve a sequential process that begins with interaction between a circulating soluble antigen and soluble antibody or between an insoluble antigen and a soluble antibody. Depending on the concentration of antigen and antibody, multiple cross-linking of antigen and

TABLE 10-5	
Diseases Associated with Type III Hypersensitivity	
Disease	**Antigen**
Immune complex glomerulonephritis	GBM, exogenous antigens, drugs
SLE	Double-stranded DNA, DNA-histone complex, Sm, RNP, Ro:SSA, La:SSB, centromere
SLE-associated glomerulonephritis	Double-stranded DNA, DNA-histone complex, Sm, RNP, Ro:SSA, La:SSB
Acute allergic alveolitis	Various puffball spores from moldy dwellings
Farmer's lung disease	Thermophilic actinomycetes from contaminated hay or grains
Chemical worker's lung	Isocyanates
Still disease—postinfectious arthritis	RANA, or none identified
Rheumatoid arthritis	RANA
Serum sickness	Lymphocytes or thymocytes from heterologous serum
Henoch-Schönlein purpura	Upper respiratory viruses, drugs (antibiotics and thiazides), foods (milk, fish, eggs, rice, nuts, beans), and immunizations
Drug-induced vasculitis	Drugs (antibiotics and thiazides)
Polyarteritis nodosa	Antineutrophil cytoplasmic
Wegener granulomatosus	Antineutrophil cytoplasmic
Goodpasture syndrome	GBM

SLE, Systemic lupus erythematosus; GBM, Glomerular basement membrane; Sm, Smith; RNP, Ribonucleoprotein; Ro, Robert; La, Lane; SS, Single stranded; RANA, Rheumatoid arthritis nuclear antigen.

antibody occurs and immune complexes are formed. Most immune complexes are removed effectively before they can cause injury. In type III hypersensitivity, the immune complexes are not removed, which causes an inflammatory process and thus leads to tissue injury.

When both antigen and antibody are small or intermediate in size and soluble, the immune complex precipitates out of the body fluid and is deposited into tissues. When only the antibody is soluble, the antibody reacts with fixed antigen in the tissues. Then the antibody within the complex links with the complement system by its Fc receptors (Figure 10-4).

Activation of the classic complement cascade causes release of C3a and C5a, as well as the membrane attack complex. C3a stimulates the release of histamine from mast cells, indirectly increasing vascular permeability and vasodilation. Bronchial smooth muscle contraction occurs, resulting in bronchial constriction, wheezing, and coughing. C3a also causes the rounding up of endothelial cells, thereby increasing vascular permeability. The increased vascular permeability leads to edema formation, which allows cellular inflammatory components to move around more easily. It also dilutes and limits the duration of action of mediators. C5a is an even more powerful component than C3a. It causes a powerful release of proinflammatory mediators with actions the same as those of C3a. It is also a powerful chemotactic agent for neutrophils

FIGURE 10-4 Type III hypersensitivity reaction.

and causes a respiratory burst within neutrophils in which oxygen consumption is increased to 50 times normal along with increased glucose uptake and procoagulant activity.

As a result of the activation of complement, neutrophils, macrophages, and mast cells are attracted to the area and are activated. These cells begin lysis and destruction of tissue via the release of cytokines and the inflammatory response. The inflammation causes tissue destruction, scarring, and further reaction of the immune system against the damaged tissue (see Figure 10-4).

Tissue Deposition. Antigen-antibody complex deposition in tissues is affected by a number of factors, and size appears to be an important one. Smaller immune complexes are able to circulate for longer periods, which may increase the immune response. However, small complexes also can be removed more easily because they can pass through the glomerular basement membrane. The very large complexes can be phagocytized more easily because they are easily marked or fixed by complement and bound to red blood cells. The large complexes can then be transported to the liver, where they are phagocytized by the reticuloendothelial system—particularly the Kupffer cells in the liver—and easily removed from the system. However, large complexes can become stuck in the kidney where they are unable to cross the glomerular basement membrane.

Increased vascular permeability as a result of histamine or other vasoactive mediator release is also hypothesized to be an important factor in tissue deposition. Researchers have found that small immune complexes can be deposited in tissues treated with vasoactive mediators. Sites of increased turbulence and blood pressure tend to have increased immune complex deposition. These sites include the glomerular capillaries, joint linings, ciliary body, pulmonary alveolar membranes, and vascular endothelial linings, especially around curves or bifurcations.

Intermediate-sized immune complexes tend to be deposited because they do not fix complement well, do not bind with red blood cells well after fixation, and are not removed by the mononuclear phagocyte system well. Large numbers of any size immune complex can be deposited if they are so numerous that the phagocytic cells are overwhelmed. Deposition of immune complexes also depends on their immunoglobulin class and the affinity between the antigen and antibody. Finally, deposition may be affected by the type of antigen or by the relationship between the immune complex and sites with increased collagen. Because DNA and collagen have strong affinity, an increased quantity of DNA-anti-DNA immune complexes may be deposited in collagen membranes, such as in the kidney. The electrical charge of the immune complex may affect where it is deposited. For example, a positively charged immune complex may be attracted by a negatively charged basement membrane.

Immune Complex Glomerulonephritis

Etiology. Immune complex glomerulonephritis (an inflammatory renal disorder) is an example of a type III hypersensitivity reaction caused by persistent low-grade infection. It involves the interaction of soluble exogenous antigen with soluble antibody and is the cause of most glomerulonephritis cases. Glomerulonephritis typically occurs 10 days to 2 weeks after infection with a *Streptococcus* bacterial strain. The immune complex is deposited in the glomerular capillary wall and mesangium.

Clinical Manifestations and Treatment. This deposition causes damage to the glomerular basement membrane with resultant proteinuria, hematuria, hypertension, oliguria, and red cell casts in the urine (see Chapter 27). In some types of glomerulonephritis, the patient may have nephrotic syndrome and acute renal failure that may progress to chronic renal failure.

Treatment of glomerulonephritis involves the use of corticosteroids and other medications to decrease inflammation. Antihistamines and antiserotonins have been tried in attempts to decrease vasoactive mediators and vascular permeability. Anticoagulants and antiplatelet medications such as aspirin, as well as plasmapheresis, are currently being studied. In plasmapheresis, plasma is removed from the blood and fresh frozen plasma or albumin is used to replace the withdrawn plasma.

Systemic Lupus Erythematosus

Etiology. SLE is another example of a type III hypersensitivity reaction caused by autoantibody production. SLE tends to occur more frequently in women than in men, with an incidence of 7.6 per 100,000. It is primarily characterized by the development of antibodies against nuclear antigens such as DNA, deoxyribonucleohistone, and RNA. Production of autoantibodies to red blood cells, neutrophils, platelets, lymphocytes, and other organs or tissues may also occur.

In SLE, antinuclear (ANA) and anti-DNA autoantibodies attach to components of the nucleus to form immune complexes that are deposited on collagen-rich tissues, including the glomerular basement membrane and the dermal-epidermal junction. The exact mechanism causing cell damage and the release of nuclear components and subsequent development of antinuclear and anti-DNA antibodies is not known. However, once formed, the autoantibodies can react with DNA and nuclear components from damaged cells anywhere in the body. The resulting inflammatory response causes increased cell damage and further antigen-antibody immune complex formation, thus leading to a cyclic process. The immune complex deposition and resulting inflammatory response cause the signs and symptoms of SLE.

Clinical Manifestations. The disorder has a variety of signs and symptoms because any organ system can be involved. Because of the variable presentation, diagnosis may be difficult and specific criteria based on the presence of several signs, symptoms, and laboratory findings have been developed. Kidney involvement is common and may lead to nephritis and glomerulonephritis. Skin symptoms include an erythematous rash on exposed skin, purpura, alopecia, mucosal ulcerations, subcutaneous nodules, and splinter hemorrhages. The patient may have symptoms of arthritis or polyarthralgia, pleurisy, pericarditis, restrictive pulmonary disease, retinal changes, thrombocytopenia, anemia, and gastrointestinal ulceration. Central nervous system involvement includes neuritis, seizures, depression, or psychosis. A positive ANA test is usually present.

Treatment. Treatment of SLE ranges from administration of nonsteroidal antiinflammatory agents such as aspirin to systemic corticosteroids. Corticosteroids decrease inflammation and provide immunosuppression, which can decrease symptoms and add to the patient's quality of life. If the patient does not respond to corticosteroids, immunosuppressives or cytotoxic agents can be used.

Type IV Hypersensitivity

Type IV hypersensitivity is also known as delayed hypersensitivity. Delayed hypersensitivity is characterized by tissue damage resulting from a delayed cellular reaction to an antigen. Unlike other hypersensitivity reactions, primary antibody involvement is absent. The principal mediators are lymphocytes, including T helper cells (Td) that mediate the reaction by releasing lymphokines (cytokines) and/or antigen-sensitized cytotoxic T cells (Tc) that can directly kill cells. The principal effector cells are lymphocytes and macrophages, with mast cells involved in the early phases. Neutrophils are not involved in type IV hypersensitivity reactions. This reaction is slow in onset, beginning 24 hours after exposure and lasting up to 14 days after exposure. Clinical manifestations may linger for an even longer period.

Type IV hypersensitivity reactions involve a series of events evolving gradually. Mast cell degranulation occurs early in the evolution of a delayed hypersensitivity reaction, followed by lymphocyte and macrophage invasion. The mast cells are gatekeepers that regulate leukocyte migration in the microvasculature. Unlike that occurring in type I hypersensitivity reactions, the mast cell degranulation is more limited and localized. The reaction is also limited by the action of suppressor T cells, which inhibit other T-cell actions. Why and how the mast cells are activated in this type of hypersensitivity reaction is not well understood. However, the combined action of mast cell and T-cell mediators recruits other T cells and macrophages to the site.

Several types of delayed hypersensitivity reactions are recognized, including cutaneous basophil hypersensitivity (Jones-Mote sensitivity), contact hypersensitivity, tuberculin-type hypersensitivity, and granulomatous hypersensitivity.

Cutaneous Basophil Hypersensitivity. Cutaneous basophil is the most rapid type of delayed hypersensitivity reaction. It is a lymphocyte-mediated basophil reaction. Soluble antigen that has been injected intradermally or antigens introduced into the dermis trigger T-cell activation and subsequent release of cytokines and activation of basophils, which infiltrate the area. The reaction peaks with skin swelling in 24 hours and can last 7 to 10 days. An example of this type of hypersensitivity is skin graft reactions and rejection.

Contact Hypersensitivity. Contact hypersensitivity is the most familiar type IV hypersensitivity. It is an immune or inflammatory response to a wide variety of plant oils, chemicals, ointments, clothing, cosmetics, dyes, and adhesives. Contact hypersensitivity is an epidermal phenomenon. As a delayed reaction, it peaks in 48 to 72 hours. The reaction is slow because the skin-penetrating antigen is very small and in an incomplete form. This incomplete, lipid-soluble antigen is called a **hapten.** The hapten must first penetrate the epidermis, where it links with a normal body protein, called a *carrier,* in the epidermis. Only after the hapten combines with the carrier is it a complete antigen—often called a hapten conjugate.

The complete antigen is processed by dermal dendritic cells located in the suprabasal epidermis.[13] It has long been thought that epidermal macrophages, called Langerhans cells, also located in the suprabasal epidermis, were the cells that processed the complete antigen in type IV hypersensitivity reactions. However, new research demonstrates that the dermal dendritic cells, not the Langerhans cells, move to the local lymph channel, where they migrate to the regional lymph node.[13] Within the lymph node, the dermal dendritic cells display the now processed complete antigen to CD4+ T cells in the paracortex. Then the antigen-sensitized CD4+ T cells release lymphokines, which initiate an inflammatory response and attract other effector cells. The primary lymphokines include IL-2, IL-3, interferon, TNF, and macrophage-stimulating factors (Figure 10-5).

Lymphokines (cytokines) and prostaglandins are important in contact hypersensitivity. The presentation of antigen to T cells causes the lymphokine cascade of vasoactive and cytoactive substances. These substances cause inflammation as well as activation of other cells. After about 72 hours, the reaction begins to decrease because of degradation of the antigen and production of prostaglandin E, which inhibits IL-1 and IL-2 production.

After primary exposure or immunization, a cellular reaction takes place at each subsequent exposure site. Cross-reactivity with related substances also occurs in contact hypersensitivity. For example, a person with contact dermatitis to nickel will react when exposed to a variety of nickel alloys, including the metal in earrings, zippers, and belt buckles. Skin symptoms resulting from contact dermatitis include redness, edema, itching, and blisters. People with sensitivities may also experience respiratory symptoms if exposed to aerosolized hapten. This situation could occur when a person is downwind from burning poison ivy or burning tires.

Tuberculin-Type Hypersensitivity. Tuberculin-type hypersensitivity occurs when someone who has been previously infected by tuberculosis is exposed to tuberculin antigen in a tuberculin test. It is a dermal phenomenon that peaks in 48 to 72 hours. The person experiences redness, induration, and inflammation at the site of the intradermal injection. Because the amount injected is so small, the reaction disappears when

Hapten

Protein (carrier)

Epidermis

① Exposure to hapten with formation of complete antigen (hapten conjugate)

② Recognition and processing of antigen by antigen-processing cell (APC)

APC

③ Migration of APC to lymph node where antigens are presented to T cells

Helper T cell

④ Release of cytokines that stimulate proliferation of T cells and activate macrophages

Cytokines

Macrophage

T cells

⑤ Activated T cells and macrophages migrate to the epidermis, release inflammatory mediators, and cause cell destruction

FIGURE 10-5 Type IV hypersensitivity reaction.

TABLE 10-6

Granulomatous Disease Associated with Type IV Hypersensitivity

Disease	Bacterium
Tuberculosis	*Mycobacterium tuberculosis*
Leprosy	*Mycobacterium leprae*
Histoplasmosis	*Histoplasma capsulatum*
Coccidioidomycosis	*Coccidioides immitis*
Brucellosis	*Brucella abortus*
	Brucella suis (less common)
	Brucella melitensis (less common)
Tularemia	*Francisella (Pasteurella) tularensis*

the antigen has degraded. However, people with severe reactions may experience tissue necrosis at the site.

Granulomatous Hypersensitivity. Granulomatous hypersensitivity reaction is a primary defense against intracellular infections and represents a chronic type IV hypersensitivity reaction. It is a protective defense reaction that eventually causes tissue destruction because of persistence of the antigen. In this type of hypersensitivity, antigen is not destroyed within the macrophages, either because of failure of lysosome-phagosome fusion, as in tuberculosis and leprosy, or because of the resistance of various materials to internal lysozymes, as in retained suture material or talc. In an effort to protect the host, lymphocytes and macrophages actually cause the tissue damage by releasing cytokines and stimulating an inflammatory response.

Antigen is engulfed and ingested by macrophages attempting to destroy the antigen, but these actions are unsuccessful in type IV hypersensitivity. The macrophages form a core of inflammatory cells that include lymphocytes, tissue histiocytes, eosinophils, plasma cells, giant cells, and epithelioid cells. This collection of inflammatory cells develops into a ball-like mass called a granuloma. The predominant cell in the granuloma is the macrophage. Epithelioid cells come from macrophages and are large, flat cells with a large amount of endoplasmic reticulum. When epithelioid cells fuse, they form multinucleated giant cells. This core is surrounded by lymphocytes. Gradually, fibroblastic activity and increased collagen synthesis cause the granuloma to become fibrotic with scar formation. Often, central necrosis occurs within the granuloma and is called *caseous* or *cheesy necrosis*. Patients with granulomatous diseases have a variety of symptoms. Granulomatous diseases and the pathogens associated with them are listed in Table 10-6.

KEY POINTS

- Type I hypersensitivity is an immediate allergic or anaphylactic type of reaction mediated primarily by sensitized mast cells. The reaction is initiated when IgE antibodies located on the mast cell membrane are bound by antigen, with subsequent cross-linking of IgE

receptors. Mast cell degranulation releases chemicals that mediate the signs and symptoms of anaphylaxis. Released histamine, kinin, prostaglandins, interleukins, and leukotrienes cause increased vascular permeability, vasodilation, hypotension, urticaria, and bronchoconstriction. Examples of type I reactions include drug reactions, bee sting reactions, and asthma.
- Type II hypersensitivity occurs when antibodies are formed against antigens on cell surfaces, usually resulting in lysis of target cells. Cell lysis may be mediated by activated complement fragments (membrane attack complex) or by phagocytic cells that are attracted to target cells by the attached antibodies. Examples include transfusion reactions, erythroblastosis fetalis, myasthenia gravis, and hyperacute graft rejection.
- Type III hypersensitivity reactions occur when antigen-antibody complexes are deposited in tissues and result in the activation of complement and subsequent tissue inflammation and destruction. Antigen-antibody complexes activate the complement cascade and subsequently attract phagocytic cells to the tissue. Persistent low-grade infections, inhalation of antigens into alveoli, and autoimmune production of antibodies may result in chronic production of antigen-antibody complexes. Examples include glomerulonephritis and SLE.
- Type IV hypersensitivity reactions are T-cell mediated and do not require antibody production, in contrast to type I, II, and III reactions. Sensitized T cells react with altered or foreign cells and initiate inflammation. Contact dermatitis, tuberculin reactions, transplant rejection, and graft-versus-host disease are examples.

Deficient Immune Responses

Deficient immune responses result from a functional decrease in one or more components of the immune system. These disorders can affect lymphocytes, antibodies, phagocytes, and complement proteins. Two types of immune deficiency are differentiated: primary and secondary. Primary disorders are immune deficiencies not attributable to other causes; these may be congenital or acquired. Examples of primary immunodeficiency disorders include SCID syndrome, DiGeorge syndrome, selective IgA deficiency, and AIDS. Persons with a primary immunodeficiency can be predisposed to multiple deficiencies, as in agammaglobulinemia or SCID, or can have a single phenotype deficiency predisposing to a specific infection, such as disorders of the IL-12-interferon-γ (IFN-γ) circuit which predispose to infections caused by myocobacteria.[14] Secondary immunodeficiency disorders are a consequence of non-immune system disorders or treatments that secondarily affect immune function. Examples of secondary disorders include those associated with hyperlipidemia or malnutrition, medical treatments such as cancer chemotherapy, or biopsychosocial stress such as postsurgical immune system problems.

TABLE 10-7

Primary Immunodeficiency Disorders

Disorder	Functional Deficiency	Error
Bruton X-linked agammaglobulinemia	Antibody	*BTK gene mutant*
Common variable (acquired) hypogammaglobulinemia	Antibody	
Selective IgA deficiency	IgA antibody	
Secretory component deficiency—chronic mucocutaneous candidiasis	Secretory IgA	
Selective IgM deficiency	IgM antibody	
Selective deficiency of IgG subclasses	IgG antibody subclass	
Immunodeficiency with elevated IgM	IgG and IgA antibodies	
Transient hypogammaglobulinemia of infancy	Low antibodies	
Antibody deficiency with nearly normal immunoglobulins	Antibody	
Duncan X-linked lymphoproliferative disease	Anti–Epstein-Barr virus–linked antigen antibody	
DiGeorge syndrome (congenital thymic hypoplasia or aplasia)	Primarily T cells	Chromosome 22q11.2 deletion syndrome
Nezelof syndrome	T cells, antibody, neutropenia	
Autosomal recessive SCID	T cells, antibody	Defects of JAK3
Autosomal recessive SCID with ADA deficiency	T cells, antibody	
X-linked recessive SCID	T cells, antibody	Defects of *IL2RG* gene
Defective expression of MHC antigens	T cells, antibody	
SCID with leukopenia (reticular dysgenesis)	T cells, antibody, granulocytes	
Wiskott-Aldrich syndrome (immunodeficiency with eczema and thrombocytopenia)	Antibody, T cells	Defect of short arm of X chromosome at Xp11.3/mutation of *WASP* gene
Ataxia, telangiectasia	Antibody, T cells	
Cartilage-hair hypoplasia	T cells	
Immunodeficiency with thymoma	T cells, antibody	
Hyperimmunoglobulinemia E	Excessive IgE	
Lymphocyte function antigen 1 deficiency	Cytotoxic cells, phagocytic cells	
Chédiak-Higashi syndrome	Natural killer cells, phagocytic cells	
Chronic granulomatous disease of childhood	Phagocytic cells	
Acquired immunodeficiency syndrome	T cells, CD4 cells	

SCID, Severe combined immunodeficiency; *ADA*, adenosine deaminase; *BTK*, Bruton tyrosine kinase; *JAK*, Janus kinase; *MHC*, major histocompatibility complex; *WASP*, WAS protein.

PRIMARY IMMUNODEFICIENCY DISORDERS

Primary immunodeficiency disorders (PID) include congenital phenotypes that result from abnormal development or maturation of immune cells, as well as acquired primary disorders of immune cells such as HIV/AIDS. AIDS is described in Chapter 12 and only the congenital forms of primary immunodeficiency are included here. The classic view of primary congenital immunodeficiency disorders is that they are rare genetic disorders that are often sex linked. The most common primary disorders are listed in Table 10-7. However, there is strong genetic epidemiological data suggesting that most people have some inborn errors of immunity that may vary in clinical significance and severity. This observation has changed the view of congenital immunodeficiency (Table 10-8).[14]

The first clinical indicators of immunodeficiency disorders are the signs and symptoms of infection, and the disorders are often first suspected when an individual has severe recurrent, unusual, or unmanageable infections. It is thought that "given the strong epidemiological evidence documenting the importance of genetic background in predisposition to infections, any severe infectious illness may be considered a potential PID-defining phenotype."[14] Most people have the predisposition or clinical phenotype of at least one PID, the expression of which can occur at any age pending exposure to triggering agents, such as infectious disease or environmental factors.[14] Some PIDs can resolve spontaneously without relapse in childhood; or may be sporadic or may not manifest until adulthood, such as common variable immunodeficiency and dominant IFN-γR1 deficiency. Late onset may reflect impaired adaptive immunity, secondary infection, or exposure to microbes not encountered in childhood.[14]

B-Cell and T-Cell Combined Disorders
Severe Combined Immunodeficiency Disorders
Etiology and Pathogenesis. SCID disorders are the result of embryonic defects and are characterized by severe immune system dysfunction and a variety of clinical features. The most

TABLE 10-8

Paradigm Shift in Primary Immunodeficiencies

Primary Immunodeficiencies	Conventional View	Contemporary View
Patient and Population Levels		
Frequency	Rare	Common
Occurrence	Familial	Sporadic
Age at onset	Childhood	Adulthood
Prognosis	Spontaneously worsening	Spontaneously improving
Phenotype Level		
Disease-defining clinical phenotypes	Opportunistic infections	Other infections and phenotypes
Number of phenotypes per patient	High	Low (even single)
Number of episodes per patient	High	Low (even single)
Disease-causing cellular phenotypes	Hematopoietic	Nonhematopoietic
Genotype Level		
Disease-causing genes per patient	One (monogenic, Mendelian)	A few (oligogenic, major genes)
Mode of Mendelian inheritance	Autosomal and X-linked recessive	Autosomal dominant
Clinical penetrance	Complete	Incomplete
Mutations	Inherited from the parental genome	Germ line de novo or somatic

From Casanova JL, Abel L: Primary immunodeficiencies: a field in its infancy, *Science* 317(5838):618, 2007.

common SCID disorders are autosomal recessive (or Swiss type), autosomal recessive with deficiency of the enzyme adenosine deaminase, X-linked recessive, defective expression of MHC antigens, and SCID with leukopenia or reticular dysgenesis. Most of these disorders are caused by mutations of recombination activating genes *(RAG)* 1 or 2, both of which are involved in the process of antigen receptor gene assembly.[15]

The most severe form of SCID, called *reticular dysgenesis,* causes failure of all white blood cell development. Complete failure of lymphoid and myeloid stem cells during fetal development is not generally compatible with life—most infants die in utero or shortly after birth. Infants with reticular dysgenesis have failure of both lymphocyte and granulocyte development. Although the fetus grows normally, the infant is severely affected, with decreased numbers of lymphocytes, decreased antibodies, and decreased phagocytic cells. For those infants who survive birth, either umbilical cord blood or HLA-haploidentical (i.e., identical HLA-type) hematopoietic stem cell transplantation has been tried with mixed results.

The X-linked recessive type is caused by a defect of the *IL2RG* gene that is responsible for encoding common γ chain, which is needed by several cytokine receptors.[16] It is the most common type (50% of cases), affecting boys more often than girls. Infants with SCID caused by autosomal recessive or X-linked recessive disease lack circulating T cells and usually have a normal to increased number of B cells that do not function normally. The enzymes or other essential components necessary for immune cell functioning are deficient, particularly enzymes linked with purine nucleoside phosphorylase or adenosine deaminase metabolism. As a result, the infant accumulates toxic metabolites of purine or adenosine that affect lymphocytes. Antibody titers are decreased because of lack of antibody formation after immunization. T cells are low

in number (less than 1000/μl) or absent. Some infants have increased numbers of B cells, but they are unable to function normally. Generally, most patients have small, hypoplastic thymus glands indicative of poor or absent T-cell development.

Clinical Manifestations and Treatment. Infants with SCID caused by defective expression of MHC antigens have poor antibody production with decreased IgG, IgM, and IgA. Overall lymphocyte numbers are normal to slightly decreased, but T-cell number and function are decreased.

Infants with these syndromes are usually ill by 3 months of age and often have thrush, severe *Candida* diaper dermatitis, or infections such as otitis, pneumonia, and diarrhea. They are prone to sepsis, opportunistic infections with such pathogens as *Candida albicans* or *Pneumocystis jiroveci (carinii),* infections with such viruses as cytomegalovirus or herpesvirus, and common childhood diseases, such as varicella and measles. Because of their severity, infections in infants with SCID are medical emergencies.

Management of SCID includes bone marrow transplantation and gene therapy. In 2000, gene therapy with modified hematopoietic cells was used for the first time to successfully treat patients with SCID.[17]

Wiskott-Aldrich Syndrome

Etiology and Pathogenesis. Wiskott-Aldrich syndrome is an X-linked immunodeficiency disorder that affects both T cells and B cells. The gene deficiency is caused by a mutation of the WAS protein (WASP) gene and has been mapped to the short arm of the X chromosome at Xpll.23. The *WASP* gene is involved in cytoplasmic signaling and in reorganization of the actin cytoskeleton. In this syndrome, IgM is decreased. Other antibody concentrations are variable, with IgE and IgA usually elevated and IgG normal to low. This antibody variability is the result of increased antibody catabolism. Platelet deficiency is also associated with Wiskott-Aldrich syndrome. T cells are present but function deficiently. Affected infants have particular difficulty mounting immune responses to protein and polysaccharide antigens, including bacterial cell walls (e.g., *Pseudomonas aeruginosa, Staphylococcus pneumoniae*).

Clinical Manifestations and Treatment. Wiskott-Aldrich syndrome is clinically characterized by the presence of eczema, thrombocytopenic purpura, and infection. Affected children are prone to pneumococcal infections, including pneumonia, meningitis, otitis media, and sepsis. They are also subject to renal disease and malignancies. The average age of these infants at death is 3.5 years without treatment.

Infants with Wiskott-Aldrich syndrome are treated with antibody replacement therapy, and antibiotic therapy. Bone marrow transplantation, stem cell transplantation, and gene therapy are options used to manage this disorder in affected children.

T-Cell Disorders
DiGeorge Syndrome
Etiology and Pathogenesis. DiGeorge syndrome, or thymic hypoplasia, is a developmental T-cell disorder associated with total or partial loss of thymus gland function. The development of DiGeorge syndrome is caused by a chromosomal 22q 11.2 deletion (del 22q11). There may also be associated genetic modifiers that can vary in the clinical presentation. In this disorder, the aplastic or hypoplastic thymus is unable to assist in the maturation of T cells. Therefore, T cells are deficient. B cells are normal.

Clinical Manifestations and Treatment. Because this is a congenital disorder of fetal organ development, it is often associated with other congenital problems, such as cardiac and great vessel anomalies, hypoparathyroidism with hypocalcemia, esophageal atresia, genital anomalies, and unusual facial features, including mandibular hypoplasia and low set ears.

Infants with partial loss of thymus function may not have trouble with infections. However, infants with total loss of thymus function resemble children with SCID and rarely live to the age of 6 years without treatment. For these children, thymic transplantation has been helpful in reestablishing T-cell populations.

Chronic Mucocutaneous Candidiasis
Etiology and Pathogenesis. Chronic mucocutaneous candidiasis is an autosomal recessive T-cell disorder characterized by a selective deficiency of cell-mediated immunity against *C. albicans*. In this case, T cells do not produce the correct cytokines needed for the cell-mediated immunity to *Candida*. This causes persistent or recurrent severe skin, nail, and mucous membrane infections with *C. albicans*. B-cell and T-cell functions are usually normal, except for the inability of the T cells to respond to *Candida* infections. Occasionally IgA or other antibody levels may be affected.

Clinical Manifestations and Treatment. The goal of treatment is to reduce the severity of skin and mucous membrane infection and decrease the disfigurement from infection and scarring. This disorder is also associated with an autoimmune disorder called *autoimmune polyendocrinopathy-candidiasis-ectodermal dystrophy* (APECED).[18] The most common components of APECED are chronic mucocutaneous candidiasis, hypoparathyroidism, and Addison disease (see Chapter 40).

B-Cell Disorders
IgA Deficiency
Etiology and Pathogenesis. The most common B-cell primary immunodeficiency disorder is selective IgA deficiency. This disorder affects 1 in 400 persons. It is a B-cell disorder characterized by failure of IgA-bearing lymphocytes to become plasma cells, with resulting lack of serum and secretory IgA. Genetically, it can be an autosomal recessive or autosomal dominant disease.

Clinical Manifestations and Treatment. People with this disorder are prone to respiratory, gastrointestinal, and genitourinary tract infections. They tend to have many autoantibodies (including anti-IgA antibodies), with a high incidence of vascular and collagen autoimmune diseases. They often react to cow's milk, and inflammatory bowel conditions can develop. Because they have severe allergic reactions to blood or blood products containing IgA, exogenous IgA replacement is contraindicated. Treatment includes prevention of infection and management of infection with appropriate antibiotics.

Bruton X-Linked Agammaglobulinemia
Etiology and Pathogenesis. Bruton X-linked agammaglobulinemia, or congenital hypogammaglobulinemia, is a B-cell genetic disorder caused by a lack of normal B-cell development in the bone marrow. The disorder is linked to a mutation of a gene called *btk* (Bruton tyrosine kinase) located on the long arm of the X chromosome at position Xq21,1-11. In 1952 it was the first genetic immunodeficiency disorder identified. In this case, a mutation in a cytoplasmic signal-transducing molecule encoded by the *btk* gene results in B-cell deficiency with decreased serum concentrations of IgG and no detectable IgA or IgM. The number of T cells is increased and they function normally. The thymus also functions normally. The disease is characterized by recurrent bacterial infection and profound hypogammaglobulinemia resulting from decreased numbers of circulating B cells. Male infants are affected, but this disorder is not usually diagnosed until they are 9 to 12 months old because of passive maternal IgG protection.

Clinical Manifestations and Treatment. Frequent infections, most often caused by *Haemophilus influenzae* and *Streptococcus pneumoniae*, occur in these infants, causing pneumonia, otitis media, meningitis, sinusitis, and septicemia. The recurrent infections can lead to tissue destruction and injury.

Despite the infections, these infants can grow normally if treated with antibiotics and recurrent administration of human immune globulin. However, passive immunotherapy is not always effective. Many children die before the age of 6. If the child survives to adulthood, life expectancy is decreased and large joint arthritis is common.

Transient Hypogammaglobulinemia. Transient hypogammaglobulinemia of infancy is a self-limiting condition in which the infant is slow to acquire normal immunoglobulin levels. The infant experiences a lengthened period of low IgG levels after birth. Affected infants can demonstrate normal immunoglobulin levels and immune system function by approximately age 4. During the period of low antibody levels, they are more susceptible to infections, particularly respiratory tract infections.

SECONDARY IMMUNODEFICIENCY DISORDERS

A number of physical, psychosocial, nutritional, environmental, and pharmacologic factors can singly or in combination lead to the development of secondary immunodeficiency disorders. Many of these linkages are discussed in Chapter 8.

The direct and indirect linkages between the brain and the endocrine and immune systems are well known. As a result, excessive or defective neuroendocrine responses can lead to disease. For example, an excessive neuroendocrine response to stress with increased corticosteroids increases one's susceptibility to infectious agents and tumors but enhances resistance to autoimmune disease.[1] On the other hand, a defective neuroendocrine response to stress with low corticosteroid levels enhances autoimmune disease and inhibits infections and tumors.[2] Individuals experiencing physical and psychosocial stress, decreased social support, depression, and bereavement show decreased immune system functioning.

T-cell and B-cell numbers decrease after surgery. This temporary deficiency can last up to 1 month and is most likely a result of the stress of surgery. Some types of surgery, such as splenic surgery, actually reduce the effectiveness of the immune system. Removal of the spleen reduces serum IgM and the antibody response to encapsulated bacteria (e.g., *S. pneumoniae, H. influenzae, Staphylococcus aureus*). Disease states such as diabetes mellitus, drug- or alcohol-induced cirrhosis, severe burns, severe trauma, sickle cell anemia, malignancies, and severe infections are associated with secondary immune deficiencies. For example, when blood sugar rises in patients with diabetes mellitus, the white blood cell response to infection declines. Pregnancy and infancy are also associated with secondary immune dysfunction.

A number of pharmaceuticals affect the functioning of the immune system. Cytotoxins and other cancer pharmacotherapeutic drugs cause a state of generalized immunosuppression. For example, methotrexate is a phase-specific cytotoxin in which cells are killed only if they are in the S or DNA-synthetic phase. Cyclophosphamide is toxic to cells in any mitotic phase, although it is better at killing active cells. Anesthetics (halothane, cyclopropane, nitrous oxide, ether), alcohol, antibiotics, antithyroids, anticonvulsants, antihistamines, and steroids decrease cellular or humoral immunity by various methods. For example, chronic nitrous oxide toxicity leads to cell-mediated immune deficits. Therapeutic radiation (x-rays) also affects the immune system by destroying rapidly proliferating cells. In states when T-cell and B-cell clones are needed, irradiation eliminates these cells, thus blunting or reducing the effectiveness of the body's response.

A number of studies have linked immune system competency and nutritional status. Malnutritional states can lead to protein depletion, as well as carbohydrate, lipid, vitamin, and mineral deficiencies. Protein and calorie depletion leads to T-cell reductions and dysfunction. Antibodies are composed of proteins, levels of which are also low in a state of depletion. Low levels of zinc, an enzyme cofactor needed for lymphocyte function, as well as low levels of folic acid and vitamins B_6, A, and E, can lead to T-cell and B-cell dysfunction. Overnutrition, especially hyperlipidemia, can lead to lymphocyte and granulocyte dysfunction. Kinsella and Lokesh stated that deficiencies, imbalances, or excess nutritional factors may impair the development of all stem cells, alter the recognition and processing of antigens, hurt immune cell proliferation, reduce phagocytic and cytolytic capacity, and harm cooperative interactions between cells in the immune system.[19]

In the elderly, immune system function is altered. The response to antigenic stimulation is variable. The elderly are less able to respond to "new" antigenic stimuli. The cells of the immune system in the elderly are not able to proliferate or reproduce as effectively as in younger persons. Although the total number of T cells remains the same, T-cell function is decreased. T cells are less capable of proliferating and have decreased cytotoxicity. Antibody production also decreases. A rise also is seen in autoantibody production, which may influence the increase in autoimmune disease in the elderly.

KEY POINTS

- Primary deficiencies in immune function may be from congenital, genetic, or acquired defects that directly affect immune cell function.
- Secondary deficiencies are conditions that impair immune function as a result of other nonimmune system disorders, such as poor nutrition, stress, or drugs, that secondarily suppress immune function.
- Primary genetic immunodeficiency disorders are fairly common, with most causing moderate immune impairment that may not be diagnosed. Severe congenital immunodeficiency disorders are less common, but clinically significant. Impairment in T cells and B cells results in SCID. Functional B and T lymphocytes are lacking, and infants with SCID easily succumb to sepsis and opportunistic infections. Other types of primary immunodeficiency disorders affect a particular cell type: DiGeorge syndrome occurs with T-cell agenesis related to a lack of thymus function; chronic mucocutaneous candidiasis is caused by abnormal T cells that cannot respond to *Candida*; and selective IgA deficiency is caused by B-cell abnormality.
- Problems in neuroendocrine and immune system interactions are a cause of secondary immunodeficiencies. Excessive neuroendocrine response to stress with increased corticosteroid production increases susceptibility to infection.

- Medications such as cytotoxins and other cancer pharmacotherapeutic drugs cause generalized secondary immunosuppression. However, other medications, such as anesthetics, alcohol, antibiotics, and steroids, also affect the immune response and can lead to secondary immunosuppression.
- Malnutrition, a major cause of immune system dysfunction, leads to lymphocyte dysfunction and altered stem cell development.

SUMMARY

Human beings live in internal and external environments teeming with antigens capable of producing immunologic responses. Contact with an antigen or antigens usually leads to induction of a normal protective immune response. However, some individuals experience disease caused by either excessive or deficient immune responses.

Both excessive and deficient immune reactions are damaging to tissue. The tissues that are affected depend on the type of antigen, the type of antigen exposure, and the degree of immune responsiveness. In children with immune system dysfunction caused by embryonic defects, the lack or dysfunction of T cells, B cells, and antibodies can lead to lethal or recurrent infections that severely limit the child's ability to interact with the environment. As a result of their immune disorder, some of these children may never reach maturity. In the elderly, malnutrition, medications, and decreased immune system function as a result of aging, surgery, stress, decreased social support, depression, and bereavement lead to increased infections and autoimmune disease. Autoimmune disease is a type of excessive immune reaction in which the immune system reacts against the body's own cells.

Excessive immune reactions are common and involve a complex interplay between antigen and components of the immune system. Hypersensitivity disorders are differentiated by the cell type involved and the time course of the reaction. For example, type I hypersensitivity is a rapid response caused by a host of lethal chemicals generated by but involving only one antibody, IgE, and one effector cell, the mast cell. It is an antigen-antibody reaction causing the release of potent chemicals that can lead to extreme, even life-threatening reactions in susceptible individuals. Type II hypersensitivity is also immediate but is tissue specific involving IgG and IgM antibodies, a host of effector cells, and the complement system. It is a linkage between antigen on target cells and the Fab portion of IgG or IgM antibodies. Examples include blood transfusion reactions, hemolytic anemia, and myasthenia gravis.

Type III hypersensitivity reactions, which involve IgG as the major antibody and neutrophils and mast cells as the effector cells, take several hours to develop. These reactions involve the deposition of antigen-antibody immune complexes into tissue and activation of the complement system. This reaction is a deposition problem that depends on the solubility of the antigen-antibody complex and the vascular system. The tissues that have the antigen-antibody complex deposited into them become inflamed. SLE is the major example of type III hypersensitivity. Type IV hypersensitivity takes days to develop and involves cytotoxic T cells but no antibodies. Examples include poison ivy contact dermatitis, and organ transplant rejection.

REFERENCES

1. Calcagni E, Elenkov I: Stress system activity, innate and T helper cytokines, and susceptibility to immune-related diseases, *Ann NY Acad Sci* 1069:62-76, 2006.
2. Atassi MZ, Casali P: Molecular mechanisms of autoimmunity, *Autoimmunity* 41(2):123-132, 2008.
3. Check E: The virtue of tolerance, *Nature* 418:364-366, 2002.
4. Sakaguchi S, Powrie F: Emerging challenges in regulatory T cell function and biology, *Science* 317(5838):627-629, 2007.
5. Leslie M: Mast cells show their might, *Science* 317(5838):614-615, 2007.
6. Torgerson TR, Ochs HD: Regulatory T cells in primary immunodeficiency diseases, *Curr Opin Allergy Clin Immunol* 7(6):515-521, 2007.
7. Pordeus V et al: Infections and autoimmunity: a panorama, *Clin Rev Allergy Immunol,* Epub January 2008.
8. Boscolo P et al: Environmental and occupational stress and autoimmunity, *Autoimmun Rev* 7(4):340-343, 2008.
9. Shepsheleovich D, Shoenfeld Y: Prediction and prevention of autoimmune diseases: additional aspects of the mosaic of autoimmunity, *Lupus* 15(3):183-190, 2006.
10. Hayden ML: Immunoglobulin E-mediated airway inflammation is active in most patients with asthma, *J Am Acad Nurse Prac* 19(9):439-449, 2007.
11. Bachert C: The role of histamine in allergic disease: re-appraisal of its inflammatory potential, *Allergy* 57(4):287-296, 2002.
12. Hendeles L, Sorkness CA: Anti-immunoglobulin E therapy with omalizumab for asthma, *Ann Pharmacother* 41(9):1397-1410, 2007.
13. Fukunaga A et al: Dermal dendritic cells, and not Langerhans cells, play an essential role in inducing an immune response, *J Immunol* 180(5):3057-3064, 2008.
14. Casanova JL, Abel L: Primary immunodeficiencies: a field in its infancy, *Science* 317(5838):617-619, 2007.
15. Villa A et al: V(D)J recombination defects in lymphocytes due to RAG mutations: severe immunodeficiency with a spectrum of clinical presentations, *Blood* 97(1):81-88, 2001.
16. Notarangelo LD et al: Combined immunodeficiencies due to defects in signal transduction: defects of the gammac-JAK 3 signaling pathway as a model, *Immunobiology* 202(2):106-119, 2000.
17. Herzog RW, Hagstrom JN: Gene therapy for hereditary hematological disorders, *Am J Pharmacogenomics* 1(2):137-144, 2001.
18. Halonen M et al: AIRE mutations and human leukocyte antigen genotypes as determinants of the autoimmune polyendocrinopathy-candidiasis-ectodermal dystrophy phenotype, *J Clin Endocrinol Metab* 87(6):2568-2574, 2002.
19. Kinsella JE, Lokesh B: Dietary lipids, eicosanoids, and the immune system, *Crit Care Med* 18(suppl):S94-S113, 1990.

Malignant Disorders of White Blood Cells

Marie L. Kotter • Jacquelyn L. Banasik

MEDIA RESOURCES

Additional Material for Study, Review, and Further Exploration

CD Companion ■ Review Questions and Answers
■ Glossary (with audio pronunciations for selected terms)
■ Disease Profiles ■ Animations

ⓔvolve **Website** at http://evolve.elsevier.com/Copstead/
■ Case Studies ■ Disease Profiles ■ WebLinks ■ Key Points Review

 Online Course (Module 8)

KEY QUESTIONS

■ How do the various types of leukemia, lymphoma, and plasma cell myelomas differ based on the type of malignant transformation?
■ How do the clinical presentations, prognosis, and management of types of acute and chronic leukemia differ?
■ Why are malignant disorders of white blood cells commonly associated with bone marrow depression?

■ How is Hodgkin disease clinically and histologically differentiated from other types of lymphoma?
■ What is the purpose and process of staging procedures for lymphomas?
■ What clinical and laboratory findings would suggest a diagnosis of plasma cell myeloma?

CHAPTER OUTLINE

Leukemia, lymphoma, and plasma cell myeloma (multiple myeloma) are common neoplastic disorders of the bone marrow and lymphoid tissues. Depending on the location and specific types of white blood cells involved, these malignancies can be further divided into a number of specific subtypes. Leukemias can be conceptualized as circulating tumors that are disseminated from the beginning of the disease process and primarily involve the blood and bone marrow. Lymphoma tends to localize in lymph tissues but is often disseminated to other sites at the time of diagnosis. Plasma cell myeloma is a malignant transformation of B-cell plasma cells and has a predilection to form localized tumors in bony structures.

Malignancies of the blood-forming tissues and lymphatic structures often present with nonspecific symptoms. Malaise, weakness, unexplained fever, night sweats, and recurrent infections should raise suspicion of malignancy. Enlarged, nontender lymph nodes (lymphadenopathy) are a common finding in lymphoma and some leukemias. Often, white blood cell malignancies are found by chance during routine assessment of the complete blood cell count (CBC). A very high total white blood cell count or the presence of abnormal cell types should precipitate an assessment for hematologic cell malignancy. In general, earlier detection of malignancy is associated with a better prognosis for cure.

CLASSIFICATION OF HEMATOLOGIC NEOPLASMS

Various classification schemes have been used to group hematologic neoplasms, with clinicians favoring schemes that use clinical findings and pathologists preferring morphologic criteria. With the advent of technologies to identify specific genetic alterations and molecular characteristics of neoplastic cells, the traditional classification systems have become less useful. However, many clinicians and organizations, such as the American Cancer Society, continue to use traditional groupings to collect statistics and to provide information to the public. The approach used in this chapter incorporates the most recent World Health Organization (WHO) classifications for hematologic neoplasms and includes common clinical terminology. A major force behind the adoption of the WHO classification is the recognition that lymphoid leukemias and lymphomas are not separate disorders but represent different stages of the same biological disease. Thus, the major categories of the WHO system are based on the cell type of the neoplasm, rather than its location in the body.[1] Neoplasms involving cells of the myeloid lineage (Box 11-1) are separated from those of the lymphoid lineage (Box 11-2). The myeloid lineage includes red cells, platelets, monocytes, and granulocytes; the lymphoid lineage includes B cells, T cells, and natural killer (NK) cells (Figure 11-1). There are four major categories of myeloid neoplasms: myeloproliferative diseases; myelodysplastic/proliferative diseases; myelodysplastic syndromes; and acute myeloid leukemia (AML). There are three major categories of lymphoid neoplasms: B-cell neoplasm, T-cell and NK cell neoplasm, and Hodgkin disease. The term non-Hodgkin lymphoma is still in clinical usage and refers to lymphomas of

BOX 11-1

Proposed WHO Classification of Myeloid Neoplasms

Myeloproliferative Diseases (MPD)
Chronic myelogenous leukemia, Philadelphia chromosome
  (Ph1) (t[;22][qq34;q11], bcr/abl)+
Chronic neutrophilic leukemia
Chronic eosinophilic leukemia/hypereosinophilic syndrome
Chronic idiopathic myelofibrosis
Polycythemia vera
Essential thrombocythemia
Myeloproliferative disease, unclassifiable

Myelodysplastic/Myeloproliferative Diseases
Chronic myelomonocytic leukemia (CMML)
Atypical chronic myelogenous leukemia (aCML)
Juvenile myelomonocytic leukemia (JMML)

Myelodysplastic Syndromes
Refractory anemia (RA)
With ringed sideroblasts (RARS)
Without ringed sideroblasts
Refractory cytopenia (myelodysplastic syndrome) with
  multilineage dysplasia (RCMD)
Refractory anemia (myelodysplastic syndrome) with
  excess blasts (RAEB)
5q-syndrome
Myelodysplastic syndrome, unclassifiable

Acute Myeloid Leukemias (AML)
Acute myeloid leukemias with recurrent cytogenetic
  translocations
AML with t(8;21) (q22;q22), AML1(CBF)/ETO
Acute promyelocytic leukemia (AML with t(15;17)(q22;
  q11-12) and variants, PML/RAR_)
AML with abnormal bone marrow eosinophils
  (inv(16)(p13q22) or t(16;16)(p13;q11), CBF_/MYHIIX)
AML with 11q23 (MLL) abnormalities
Acute myeloid leukemia with multilineage dysplasia
  With prior myelodysplastic syndrome
  Without prior myelodysplastic syndrome
Acute myeloid leukemia and myelodysplastic syndrome,
  therapy related
  Alkylating agent related
  Epipodophyllotoxin related (some may be lymphoid)
  Other types

Acute Myeloid Leukemia (AML) Not Otherwise Categorized
AML minimally differentiated
AML without maturation
AML with maturation
Acute myelomonocytic leukemia
Acute monocytic leukemia
Acute erythroid leukemia
Acute megakaryocytic leukemia
Acute basophilic leukemia
Acute panmyelosis with myelofibrosis

Acute Biphenotypic Leukemias

From Jaffe ES et al, editors: World Health Organization classification of tumours: pathology and genetics of tumours of haematopoietic and lymphoid tissues, Lyon, France, 2001, IARC Press, p 194.

BOX 11-2

Proposed WHO Classification of Lymphoid Neoplasms

B-Cell Neoplasms
Precursor B-cell neoplasm
  Precursor B-lymphoblastic leukemia/lymphoma (precursor
    B-cell acute lymphoblastic leukemia)
Mature (peripheral) B-cell neoplasms
  B-cell chronic lymphocytic leukemia/small lymphocytic
    lymphoma
  B-cell prolymphocytic leukemia
  Lymphoplasmacytic lymphoma
  Splenic marginal zone B-cell lymphoma (6 villous
    lymphocytes)
  Hairy cell leukemia
  Plasma cell myeloma/plasmacytoma
  Extranodal marginal zone B-cell lymphoma of MALT type
  Nodal marginal zone B-cell lymphoma (6 monocytoid B cells)
  Follicular lymphoma
  Mantle cell lymphoma
  Diffuse large B-cell lymphoma
  Mediastinal large B-cell lymphoma
  Primary effusion lymphoma
  Burkitt lymphoma/Burkitt cell leukemia

T- and NK-Cell Neoplasms
Precursor T-cell neoplasm
  Precursor T-lymphoblastic lymphoma/leukemia
    (precursor T-cell acute lymphoblastic leukemia)

Mature (peripheral) T-cell neoplasms
  T-cell prolymphocytic leukemia
  T-cell granular lymphocytic leukemia
Aggressive NK-cell leukemia
Adult T-cell lymphoma/leukemia (HTLV1+)
Extranodal NK/T-cell lymphoma, nasal type
Enteropathy-type T-cell lymphoma
Hepatosplenic γδ T-cell lymphoma
Subcutaneous panniculitis-like T-cell lymphoma
Mycosis fungoides/Sézary syndrome
Anaplastic large cell lymphoma, T/null cell, primary
    cutaneous type
Peripheral T-cell lymphoma, not otherwise characterized
Angioimmunoblastic T-cell lymphoma
Anaplastic large cell lymphoma, T/null cell, primary
    systemic type

Hodgkin Lymphoma (Hodgkin Disease)
Nodular lymphocyte predominance Hodgkin lymphoma
Classical Hodgkin lymphoma
  Nodular sclerosis Hodgkin lymphoma (grades 1 and 2)
  Mixed cellularity Hodgkin lymphoma
  Lymphocyte depletion Hodgkin lymphoma

From Jaffe ES et al, editors: World Health Organization classification of tumours: pathology and genetics of tumours of haematopoietic and lymphoid tissues, Lyon, France, 2001, IARC Press, p 195.

More common entities are underlined.

*B and T/NK cell neoplasms are grouped according to major clinical presentations (predominantly disseminated/leukemic, primary extranodal, predominantly nodal)

FIGURE 11-1 Division of hematologic neoplasms into myeloid and lymphoid lineages. *PV,* Polycythemia vera.

TABLE 11-1

FAB Classification of Acute Myeloblastic (Myelocytic) Leukemias

Class	Morphology	Comments
M0: Minimally differentiated AML	Blasts lack definitive cytologic and cytochemical markers of myeloblasts but express myeloid lineage antigens	2% to 3% of AML
M1: AML without differentiation	Very immature myeloblasts predominate; few granules or Auer rods	20% of AML; Ph chromosome, present in 10% to 15% of cases, worsens prognosis
M2: AML with differentiation	Myeloblasts and promyelocytes predominate; Auer rods commonly present	30% of AML; presence of t(8;21) translocation associated with good prognosis
M3: Acute promyelocytic leukemia	Hypergranular promyelocytes, often with many Auer rods per cell; may have reniform or bilobed nuclei	5% to 10% of AML; disseminated intravascular coagulation common; presence of t(15;17) translocation is characteristic; responds to retinoic acid therapy
M4: Acute myelomonocytic leukemia	Myelocytic and monocytic differentiation evident; myeloid elements resemble M2; peripheral monocytosis	20% to 30% of AML; presence of Inv16 or del16q associated with better prognosis
M5: Acute monocytic leukemia	Monoblasts (peroxidase negative, esterase positive) and promonocytes predominate	10% of AML; usually in children and young adults; gum infiltration common; associated with abnormalities of chromosome 11q23
M6: Acute erythroleukemia	Bizarre, multinucleated, megaloblastoid erythroblasts predominate; myeloblasts also present	5% of AML; high blood counts and organ infiltration are rare; affected persons are of advanced age
M7: Acute megakaryocytic leukemia	Blasts of megakaryocytic lineage predominate; react with antiplatelet antibodies; myelofibrosis or increased bone marrow reticulin	

From Kumar V et al: *Basic pathology*, ed 7, Philadelphia, 2003, Saunders, p 437.
AML, Acute myeloblastic (myelocytic) leukemia; *Ph*, Philadelphia.

B-cell, T-cell, and NK cell origin. Non-Hodgkin lymphoma includes such a large and diverse group of malignancies that it has little relevance to prognosis or treatment. The WHO classification does not use this term. Other classification systems in current use include the FAB (French-American-British) system for subtypes of myeloid leukemia (Table 11-1). There are many etiologic, pathogenic, and treatment similarities among the hematologic malignancies, and these are addressed in a general way first, followed by sections on specific diseases.

ETIOLOGY OF MYELOID AND LYMPHOID NEOPLASMS

As in other malignant processes, the exact cause of hematologic neoplasms is unknown. The basic mechanism of malignant transformation involves mutation of cells, which disrupts growth control and differentiation pathways. These processes are thought to be similar to those described for solid tumors (see Chapter 7).

Viruses have long been suspected as mutagenic agents in some neoplasms, particularly retroviruses and herpesviruses. Close associations have been found between a small number of viruses and particular malignancies. For example, human T-cell leukemia virus (HTLV-1) is linked to the development of adult T-cell lymphoma/leukemia, and human immunodeficiency virus (HIV) is linked to B-cell lymphomas. Epstein-Barr virus (EBV) has been implicated in both Hodgkin disease and Burkitt lymphoma.[2] Effective immune surveillance is thought to keep proliferation in check and prevent progression in immunocompetent individuals.

Radiation exposure is an important etiologic factor for leukemia and lymphoma. Because of the relatively high turnover of hematologic cells, they are more susceptible to radiation-induced damage than most other cell types. An acute whole-body dose of radiation as occurs with nuclear explosions is known to increase the risk of leukemia. In Japanese survivors of the atomic bomb, the estimated lifetime risk of leukemia is 0.85%, sixfold higher than the norm.[3] There are substantial uncertainties about the risk of low-level, long-term exposure to radiation. The average annual exposure from usual sources including cosmic rays and medical procedures is very low and estimated to account for less than 5% of leukemia cases.

Despite intensive scrutiny, only a small number of chemicals have been shown unequivocally to increase the risk of hematologic malignancies. Benzene has been implicated in numerous studies, as has cigarette smoking. Other suggested carcinogens have failed to be confirmed, including exposure to hair dye, alcohol, and marijuana.[4] On the other hand, a study from the Children's Cancer Group found a link between high maternal intake of products high in bioflavonoids (beans, fresh vegetables, and fruit) and an increased incidence of infant leukemia.[5] These bioflavonoids were enzyme inhibitors (topoisomerase II inhibitors) that caused DNA cleavage and chromosome translocations. Many of the antineoplastic drugs used to treat cancers, especially the alkylating agents, are significant factors in the development of posttreatment hematologic neoplasia. Any drugs that suppress the bone marrow or immune function are also believed to predispose to the emergence of malignancies.

A number of disease conditions have been linked to the development of leukemia, although the mechanisms are unclear. A reduction or alteration in normal hematopoiesis, as occurs in such disorders as Fanconi anemia and aplastic anemia (see Chapter 13), is associated with a higher incidence of leukemia. A higher risk also has been noted in some genetic diseases, including Down syndrome and Klinefelter syndrome (see Chapter 6).

GENERAL PRINCIPLES OF MANAGEMENT

Diagnosis of Hematologic Neoplasms

Manifestations of hematologic neoplasms vary somewhat, depending upon the cell type involved. Common manifestations are shown in Box 11-3. Clinical symptoms are related to bone marrow suppression and organ dysfunction secondary to leukemic infiltration. Bone marrow suppression results in varying degrees of **leukopenia, anemia,** and **thrombocytopenia.** These three deficiencies cause the most common clinical manifestations and may prompt the patient to seek care.

Anemia, with a hematocrit of 25% to 30% or hemoglobin of 8 to 10 g/dl, may manifest with pallor, fatigue, malaise,

---

BOX 11-3

Common Manifestations of Hematologic Malignancies

History
Fever
Weight loss
Night sweats
Itching (pruritus)
Fatigue
Bone pain (sternum, tibia, femur, back)
Abdominal fullness
Bleeding episodes (epistaxis, menorrhagia)
Bruising, petechiae
Frequent infections
Headache, nausea, vomiting

Physical
Enlarged spleen
Enlarged liver
Enlarged lymph nodes
Hyperplasia of gums

Laboratory
Anemia or polycythemia
Thrombocytopenia or thrombocythemia
Leukopenia or leukocytosis
Blasts on peripheral blood smear
Elevated uric acid
Elevated alkaline phosphatase
Hypercalcemia

---

shortness of breath, and decreased activity tolerance. The severity of symptoms is determined by the rate of red blood cell decrease, as well as the absolute deficiency. Chronically low hemoglobin and hematocrit may be tolerated better than a drastic drop. Depending on symptoms, transfusion may be indicated when the hematocrit falls below 30%.

Thrombocytopenia, with a platelet count below 20,000 cells/μl, can manifest as petechiae, easy bruising, bleeding gums, occult hematuria, or retinal hemorrhages. Spontaneous intracranial bleeding can occur and may be fatal. In general, the risk of bleeding increases proportionately to the fall in platelet count. Platelet transfusion may be given when the risk of bleeding is high.

Insufficient numbers of functional leukocytes leaves the patient at high risk for development of infection, and the CBC is routinely monitored. **Neutropenia** is an absolute neutrophil count less than 500 cells/μl, and an affected patient requires protective isolation (neutropenic precautions) to prevent infection. Infections may be caused by bacterial, viral, fungal, or protozoal organisms. Often, the microorganisms are of the opportunistic variety; that is, they are part of the patient's own flora, which normally do not cause disease unless the host's immune system becomes incompetent. It is very difficult to protect patients from their own flora, and infection is the most common cause of death in the immunocompromised leukemic patient. The presence of infection is suspected if fever develops. Infections are managed aggressively with antibiotic agents to prevent development of life-threatening sepsis.

Infiltrative manifestations include lymphadenopathy, joint swelling and pain, weight loss, anorexia, hepatomegaly, and splenomegaly. Sternal tenderness is frequently present in chronic myeloid leukemia (CML). Gingival hyperplasia occurs in AML. Meningeal involvement is frequently encountered in children with acute lymphoid leukemia (ALL). Central nervous system (CNS) infiltration can occur with any type of leukemia and may be difficult to manage because of the poor ability of chemotherapeutic agents to cross the blood-brain barrier. CNS involvement can present with increased intracranial pressure, seizures, or changes in mental ability. Increased intracranial pressure should be suspected in the leukemia patient who complains of nausea, vomiting, headache, and visual changes.

A key aspect of diagnosis is the evaluation of a peripheral blood sample. Blood cell number and morphology is indicative; however, definitive diagnosis is usually made after bone marrow aspiration or lymph node biopsy. Malignant cells can be subtyped according to genetic and molecular characteristics to better determine prognosis and choice of treatment.[6]

Principles of Treatment

To make informed treatment decisions, the patient and family need information about the nature and prognosis of their disease, as well as about the risks and benefits of various treatment options. Many treatment protocols are experimental, and the outcomes may be uncertain. Sometimes the side effects of treatment and poor chance of effectiveness will weigh in favor of palliative care. Treatment decisions are complex and stressful for all concerned. A great deal of support must be available during the diagnostic, treatment, and monitoring phases.

The management of hematologic malignancies relies primarily on the use of combination chemotherapy to eradicate malignant cells and stem cell transplant to rescue and restore bone marrow function. In some cases radiation and tissue-specific drug therapy may be indicated. Unfortunately, the treatment regimen usually causes many serious side effects that must be monitored and treated.

The goal of chemotherapy is to induce long-term remission, that is, the absence of any detectable neoplastic cells in the body. A complete remission (CR) is defined as a return to normal hematopoiesis with normal red cell, neutrophil, and platelet count and no detectable neoplastic cells. For leukemia, the bone marrow must have less than 5% blasts, which are the most immature bone marrow cells, and be maintained for at least 4 weeks.[7] CR is not synonymous with cure. Therefore, most treatment protocols include several cycles of chemotherapy to eradicate the undetected cells. The choice of antineoplastic agents varies with the type of neoplasia and the stage of clinical disease. Most chemotherapeutic agents work by disrupting some aspect of DNA synthesis or cell replication and induce **apoptosis** (cell suicide; see Chapter 4). In general, rapidly dividing cells are more susceptible to apoptosis because they have less time for repair. Neoplasms with genetic defects that impair apoptotic pathways may be more difficult to eradicate and require more intense therapy. Unfortunately, these high doses are toxic to normal stem cells as well and can produce fatal bone marrow failure. Therefore, to effect a cure, high-dose chemotherapy is often followed by bone marrow "rescue" with transplantation of functional stem cells.

Chemotherapy usually includes two or three treatment phases: (1) remission induction phase, (2) postremission or consolidation phase, and (3) remission maintenance phase. The aim of treatment during the remission induction phase is to eliminate all detectable neoplastic cells and achieve a CR. Postremission consolidation therapy begins after CR is attained in an attempt to eliminate the population of undetected cells that may have escaped initial induction-phase treatment. Maintenance-phase treatment is used in the management of some neoplasms to prolong the remission interval. Intermittent chemotherapy may be continued for 2 to 3 years after initial induction of remission. Drugs that target the neoplastic cells specifically, such as monoclonal antibodies or molecular therapies, are generally less toxic than other agents and may be used for long-term maintenance in patients with residual disease.

In children and adults, the CNS can act as a sanctuary for neoplastic cells in diseases such as ALL and AML. This makes conventional routes of chemotherapy unsuccessful, because they do not permit drugs to cross the blood-brain barrier efficiently. Chemotherapeutic agents administered into the cerebrospinal fluid (CSF) via lumbar puncture (intrathecal route) can effectively eliminate leukemic cells in the CNS. This

therapy carries significant risk for temporary or permanent neurologic damage. A number of different chemotherapeutic agents can be administered safely by the intrathecal route, including methotrexate.[8]

Prevention and Management of Complications

Maintenance of adequate nutrition in patients with hematologic malignancy is a major challenge. Anorexia, weight loss, nausea, vomiting, and **stomatitis** are common findings, especially during the treatment phase. Children and adolescents on chemotherapy may experience significant growth delay, and measures to maintain protein and caloric intake are necessary. Newer antiemetic agents have been helpful in reducing nausea, vomiting, and anorexia associated with chemotherapy and should be considered in patients experiencing these symptoms.

Infection is the most troublesome of complications for the patient immunosuppressed by either disease or treatments. Constant vigilance in prevention, early detection, and rapid management of infections can profoundly affect the outcome of chemotherapy. The length of time that a patient remains neutropenic can be shortened with the use of growth factors to stimulate bone marrow production of granulocytes.

Bone marrow transplantation (BMT) has been an important part of the management of certain leukemias for many years. The intense chemotherapy used to induce remission can lead to bone marrow failure. Stem cells can be reintroduced into the host's bone marrow by bone marrow transplantation. The transplanted cells are given intravenously; they find their way to the host's bone marrow, where they establish residence and begin to produce functional white blood cells, red blood cells, and platelets. A close match between donor and host is necessary for a successful transplantation. Otherwise, the transplanted cells can mount an immune attack on the host's tissues—a life-threatening problem called *graft-versus-host disease* (see Chapter 10). In past years, bone marrow transplantation was obtained by aspiration from the marrow of a suitable donor and this is still appropriate in some cases. *Peripheral stem cell transplantation* allows stem cells to be harvested from the circulating blood stream. This procedure can be used to collect stem cells from the patient's own blood to be stored and then reinfused after chemotherapy and irradiation. This type of transplant is called *autologous*, whereas a transplant from a closely matched relative is called *allogeneic* (Figure 11-2). Use of autologous transplants eliminates the problem of graft-versus-host disease and reduces transplant-related mortality, but the potential for disease recurrence is higher than with allogeneic transplants.

It has been noted that in AML and CML, transplantation with allogeneic cells is much more successful in curing leukemia than is autologous transplantation. Transplanted cells in the allograft are thought to detect and kill leukemic cells in a process termed *graft versus leukemia*. Autologous transplants are appropriate in some cases, especially when a matched donor is not available, because they may extend life even though cure is unlikely. Autologous transplants are well tolerated and

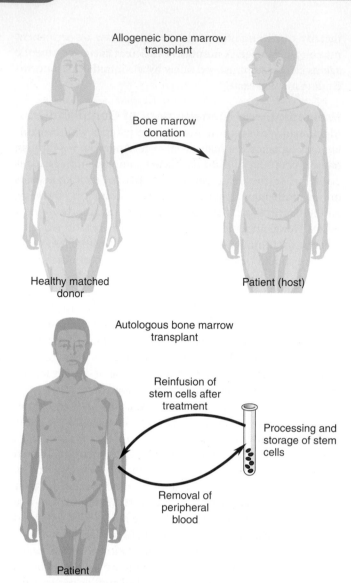

Allogeneic bone marrow transplant

Bone marrow donation

Healthy matched donor

Patient (host)

Autologous bone marrow transplant

Reinfusion of stem cells after treatment

Processing and storage of stem cells

Removal of peripheral blood

Patient

FIGURE 11-2 A comparison of allogeneic bone marrow transplant and autologous stem cell transplant.

cause fewer complications than allografts. Methods to purify a patient's collected peripheral blood by selectively removing neoplastic cells are available to reduce the risk of reintroducing malignant cells during autologous transplantation. Increased availability of stem cell transplants allows patients to undergo more intensive chemotherapy, aimed at cure rather than palliation, based on the knowledge that bone marrow rescue is possible.

Anemia is a common complication of leukemia and chemotherapy. Red blood cell production by the bone marrow is suppressed, but the size and shape of red cells present in the blood are normal. This is called *normocytic*, normochromic anemia. Administration of erythropoietin growth factors can enhance red blood cell production and moderate anemic episodes. However, patients frequently require red blood cell transfusion therapy to maintain adequate red blood cell counts. Patients with frequent or significant bleeding episodes

are also predisposed to severe anemia, and efforts to prevent bleeding will help to minimize anemia.

Platelet deficiency (thrombocytopenia) with resultant hemorrhage can be a life-threatening complication of leukemia and chemotherapy. In patients at high risk of bleeding, fresh frozen plasma or pooled platelets may be given to inhibit bleeding. Patients must be protected from trauma and may be placed on activity restrictions.

Pain is a common complication of the diagnostic and treatment protocols used in the cancer patient, as well as of the disease process itself. Pain most commonly involves the bones and joints and is the result of pressure caused by infiltration and accumulation of neoplastic cells in the bone marrow. *Hemarthrosis* (bleeding into joints) can cause acute episodes of joint pain. Chemotherapy may help reduce bone pain, as the number of neoplastic cells is reduced drastically. Patients are subjected to numerous painful procedures during diagnosis, treatment, and monitoring. Frequent blood and bone marrow sampling, placement of intravenous access lines for drug administration, and unpleasant drug side effects all contribute to the pain experience. Nausea and mouth pain (stomatitis) are frequent complaints during chemotherapy. Pain management with a variety of strategies, including narcotic and nonnarcotic drugs, distraction, and biofeedback, are generally helpful. (See Chapter 47 for a discussion of pain and pain management.)

Epithelial cells, with normally high rates of turnover, are particularly susceptible to damage by radiation and chemotherapy. Sloughing of skin and mucous membranes and hair loss are common. Loss of skin and mucous membrane integrity increases the risk of infection and can contribute significantly to the pain and discomfort of treatment. Abnormalities in growth, development, and fertility are complications of particular concern in children undergoing radiation and chemotherapy.

KEY POINTS

- Classification of the types of leukemia is based on cell type involved (lymphoid or myeloid) and degree of cell maturation. Common myeloid neoplasms include CML, polycythemia vera, essential thrombocythemia, and AML. Common lymphoid neoplasms include chronic lymphoid leukemia (CLL), acute lymphoblastic leukemia, plasma cell myeloma, Hodgkin disease, and various forms of non-Hodgkin lymphoma.
- Risk factors for the development of hematologic neoplasms include exposure to chemical, viral, and radiation mutagens; chemotherapy drugs; and immunodeficiency disorders.
- Common manifestations of hematologic neoplasia are the result of insufficient production of normal white blood cells, red blood cells, and platelets, as evidenced by leukopenia, anemia, and thrombocytopenia. Anemia manifests as pallor, fatigue, dyspnea, and decreased activity tolerance. Thrombocytopenia causes petechiae, bleeding gums, hematuria, and prolonged bleeding

time. Leukopenia manifests as frequent, recurrent infections. Other manifestations may occur with infiltration of tissues and organs. These include weight loss, anorexia, lymphadenopathy, bone pain, and CNS dysfunction.

- Chemotherapy is the mainstay of management for most hematologic neoplasms. Several courses may be needed to kill neoplastic stem cells. Most chemotherapeutic agents interfere with some aspect of DNA replication and cell division to induce apoptosis (cell suicide).

- Treatment is associated with a number of potential complications, including anemia, infection, and bleeding. Rapidly dividing hair cells and mucous membranes are also affected, leading to alopecia and stomatitis. Transfusion of blood products or stimulation of endogenous production with colony-stimulating factors and erythropoietin may be necessary. Bone marrow transplantation may be undertaken in some cases to restore stem cell function.

MYELOID NEOPLASMS

Myeloid neoplasms result from transformation and proliferation of a precursor stem cell in the bone marrow (Figure 11-3). The progeny of the aberrant stem cell clone accumulate in the bone marrow and are released into the circulation. In many cases, the abnormal stem cell is multipotent and causes the overproduction of more than one cell type,

resulting in myeloproliferative disease. The cells produced in myeloproliferative diseases are usually functional and have a normal morphologic appearance. The common myeloproliferative diseases are CML, polycythemia vera (PV), and essential thrombocythemia (ET), referring respectively to an excess of granulocytes, red blood cells, and platelets. These insidious and indolent disorders have few clinical symptoms and are commonly discovered on routine CBC analysis. Common features of CML, PV, and ET include involvement of a multipotent hematopoietic progenitor cell; marrow hypercellularity; overproduction of one or more functional blood cells; chromosomal abnormalities involving chromosomes 1, 8, 9, 13, and 20; eventual spontaneous conversion to AML, or development of marrow fibrosis.[9]

In contrast to the myeloproliferative diseases, the myelodysplastic syndromes and AML are characterized by neoplastic cells that are morphologically and functionally abnormal. The prognosis for myelodysplastic syndromes and AML is poor, and intensive treatment is necessary to extend life. AML and CML are described below. A discussion of PV and ET can be found in Chapters 13 and 14, respectively.

Chronic Myeloid Leukemia

Pathogenesis and Clinical Manifestations. CML represents approximately 15% of all cases of leukemia in the United States. The average age of onset is between 40 and 50 years, and CML occurs only occasionally in childhood and adolescence.[10] The majority of CML cases are characterized by malignant granulocytes that carry a unique chromosomal abnormality, the Philadelphia chromosome (Ph+). The Philadelphia chromosome is formed because of a balanced translocation between chromosomes 9 and 22 (Figure 11-4). The translocation causes two genes to be juxtaposed, resulting in a new fusion gene called *bcr/abl*. This mutation is thought to be critical in the development of CML. Molecular studies have revealed that the protein product of the fusion gene is a functional enzyme that spurs cell proliferation and reduces apoptotic cell death. CML is unusual among human

FIGURE 11-3 Maturation pathways of myeloid cells showing the different types of leukemia associated with various stages of development. M1, M2, and M3 types result in granulocytic leukemia; M4 has characteristics of monocytic and granulocytic leukemia; M5 is monocytic; M6 is associated with erythroid leukemia; and M7 is associated with megakaryocytic leukemia. *RBC*, Red blood cell.

FIGURE 11-4 A balanced translocation between chromosomes 9 and 22 results in the formation of a Philadelphia chromosome. The translocation causes two genes, *abl* and *bcr*, to become juxtaposed, resulting in a fusion gene. This fusion gene, *bcr-abl*, is thought to be essential for the development of chronic myeloid leukemia.

![A peripheral blood smear from a patient with CML showing segmented neutrophils among red blood cells.](placeholder)

FIGURE 11-5 A peripheral blood smear from a patient with CML. Note that a greater degree of neutrophil segmentation is found in CML than in acute myelogenous leukemia (see Figure 11-6), reflecting a more advanced stage of development. (From Kumar V et al: *Robbins basic pathology*, ed 8, Philadelphia, 2007, Saunders, p 464. Photograph courtesy Dr. Robert W. McKenna, Department of Pathology, University of Texas Southwestern Medical School, Dallas.)

FIGURE 11-6 A peripheral blood smear showing typical cells of acute myelogenous leukemia. (From Kumar V et al: *Robbins basic pathology*, ed 8, Philadelphia, 2007, Saunders, p 448.)

cancers because a single oncogene, *(bcr/abl),* is capable of conferring a malignant state.[11] Numerous mutations are necessary for development of most other cancers (see Chapter 7). The cells in CML are more mature than those found in AML, as noted by the greater degree of nuclear segmentation (Figure 11-5).

The usual clinical presentation of CML includes a high granulocyte count on the CBC and splenomegaly. Symptoms, when present, may include fatigue, weight loss, sweats, bleeding, and abdominal discomfort from the enlarged spleen.

Prognosis and Treatment. CML does not respond well to chemotherapy. Although most patients will achieve a temporary remission, the overall survival time is poor. In untreated patients the median survival is about 2 years.[12] After discovering the fusion protein (bcr/abl), drugs targeted to inhibit its action were developed (e.g., imatinib). The goal of anti-bcr/abl therapy is to reduce the number of leukemic cells with the bcr/abl phenotype to undetectable levels. It is not known whether imatinib can cure CML or what duration of treatment is necessary to permanently suppress the leukemic cell population. Some patients with CML have developed drug resistance against imatinib, and research is ongoing. The only known curative treatment is **allogeneic** bone marrow transplantation from a suitable donor. It is believed that the donor cells detect and kill the host's leukemic cells. Even with a human leukocyte antigen (HLA)-identical sibling donor, the probability of transplant-related mortality is about 25% and the likelihood of long-term disease-free survival is 50% to 60%.[11,12] Transplant-related mortality is about 50% if the HLA-matched donor is unrelated.[11] Bone marrow transplantation with cells harvested from the patient's own blood (autografting) during the early stages of CML also may be done, but it is less effective in curing the disease. For those not able to undergo stem cell transplantation, standard chemotherapy

during the chronic phase may be instituted. Chemotherapy may include hydroxyurea, interferon α (IFN-α), cytosine arabinoside (cytarabine, Ara-C), and imatinib. Once CML has progressed to the blast phase, essentially becoming AML, the prognosis is very poor, regardless of treatment, with an expected median survival of 3 to 4 months.

Acute Myeloid Leukemia

Pathogenesis and Clinical Manifestations. AML is primarily a disease of adults, comprising 80% of cases of acute leukemia in this population while accounting for only 20% of the cases of acute leukemia of childhood.[10] The median age at presentation is 64 years. Like CML, AML is a malignant disorder associated with transformation of a myeloid stem cell. The bone marrow aspirate must have more than 20% blasts to be classified as AML.[13] AML can present in a variety of ways because of the potential for myeloid stem cells to produce different cell types. Thus, AML has a number of subtypes. These are identified by the stage at which cell development stops (see Figure 11-3). The French, American, British (FAB) system for classifying AML as M0 through M7 is in common use (see Table 11-1). Acute granulocytic leukemia is the most common type of disorder, and the term is often used interchangeably with AML. Myeloblastic cells have a large, nonsegmented nucleus and fine chromatin (Figure 11-6). AML is also subtyped according to genetic abnormalities. Worse outcomes are noted with loss of the *P53* or *Rb* tumor suppressor gene function. The WHO classification of AML recognizes four common types of genetic abnormalities (see Box 11-1). Most are chromosomal translocations or inversions. If cytogenetic class is not apparent, then AML is classified by morphologic characteristics, including myeloid cell of origin and degree of differentiation or maturation. Correct classification increases the accuracy of prognosis and may influence the choice of treatment.

AML presents in a manner very similar to that of ALL, and the two are difficult to distinguish by clinical findings alone. Acute leukemia causes bone pain, anemia, thrombocytopenia, and increased susceptibility to infection. The skin, the genitourinary and gastrointestinal systems, and the respiratory tract are common infection sites. The onset of symptoms is abrupt, with most patients seeking care within a few weeks of disease onset. The prognosis is much worse for AML than for ALL, with fewer than 50% of children and only about 30% of adults achieving long-term survival.[6,14] An exception is the promyelocytic subtype of AML. Although it accounts for only 10% to 15% of AML cases, acute promyelocytic leukemia (APL) deserves special consideration because it is the most curable of all AML subtypes, with a 70% to 80% 5-year disease-free survival.[6] APL is characterized by a chromosomal translocation between 8 and 21, which forms a fusion gene called *PML/RARα*. The PML/RARα protein binds to a repressor complex in the cell nucleus and inhibits mycloid cell differentiation. RARα is a retinoic acid receptor that can be induced to release its inhibitory hold on differentiation when all-*trans* retinoic acid (ATRA) is administered. Addition of ATRA to the chemotherapy management of patients with APL significantly improves disease-free survival.[6] (See Box 11-4 for a comparison of acute and chronic leukemias.)

Prognosis and Treatment. Treatment protocols for AML are increasingly incorporating the cytogenetic profile of the leukemic cells to individualize therapy and monitor response. Traditionally the management of AML has two phases: remission induction and consolidation/postremission. A CR is attempted in the remission induction phase, with an attempt to eliminate any undetected residual leukemic cells during the consolidation/postremission phase. Patients with AML who are able to complete only one or two cycles of their chemotherapy because of toxicity almost invariably have recurrence of leukemia even when CR was achieved. To induce remission, most protocols use two cycles of a combination of agents (e.g., idarubicin + Ara-C + etoposide, called the ICE protocol; or daunorubicin + Ara-C + 6-thioguanine, called the DAT protocol). Postremission therapy commonly includes high-dose Ara-C in younger patients whereas the elderly require lower dose regimens. Drug treatment is constantly being evaluated and altered to obtain better outcomes. At present patients younger than age 60 years have a 4-year survival rate of 30% to 40%, whereas elderly patients have a 2-year survival rate of 20%.[6] With the advent of allogeneic stem cell transplantation, the chances for cure may improve; however, procedure-related mortality is 10% to 25%. New therapies using monoclonal antibodies to detect and destroy leukemic cells have been used and show promise for improving outcomes in AML.

KEY POINTS

- CML is a myeloproliferative disorder that affects adults primarily, has an insidious onset, and responds poorly to chemotherapy. CML is characterized by the presence of a gene translocation (Philadelphia chromosome) that produces a fusion gene called *bcr-abl*. The product of this gene is thought to be responsible for producing the malignancy. This molecular abnormality is the target of new drug therapies to eliminate neoplastic cells. The prognosis of CML remains relatively poor but may be improved with allogeneic BMT in which transplanted cells destroy leukemic cells.

- AML affects adults primarily, has an acute onset, responds fairly well to treatment, and has a prognosis somewhat worse than that of ALL. AML is usually a malignancy of granulocytes, although other myeloid cell types may be affected. Several gene abnormalities have been identified in AML that may indicate better or worse prognosis. The median survival of patients younger than age 60 years is 30% to 40% at 4 years.

LYMPHOID NEOPLASMS

The lymphoid neoplasms include malignant transformations of B cells, T cells, and NK cells. When present in blood and bone marrow, lymphoid neoplasms are called *leukemias,* and when they are localized in lymphoid tissues they are called *lymphomas.* The location of lymphoid neoplasms is a consequence of the stage of the disease. The WHO classification uses cell type rather than stage to classify the lymphoid neoplasms, resulting in some difficulty with the traditional conceptualization of leukemias and lymphomas. The factors that determine whether a particular neoplastic cell will present as leukemia or as lymphoma are not currently known. Subcategories of the B-cell and T-cell/NK groups are based on the maturity of the neoplastic cells (see Box 11-2). The *precursor cell* neoplasms are characterized by cells that have arrested development in the early blast stage, whereas the *mature cell* neoplasms are more differentiated and often located in peripheral sites (Figure 11-7).

Chronic Lymphoid Leukemia
Pathogenesis and Clinical Manifestations. CLL accounts for about 30% of all cases of leukemia in the United States. In 95% of cases, a malignant B-cell precursor is at fault.[15] Only

---

BOX 11-4

Comparison of Acute and Chronic Leukemias

	Acute	Chronic
Age	All ages	Adult
Clinical onset	Sudden	Insidious
Course of untreated disease	Weeks to months	Months to years
Predominant cell	Blasts, some mature forms	Mature forms
Anemia	Mild-severe	Mild
Thrombocytopenia	Mild-severe	Mild
WBC	Variable	Increased

Adapted from McKenzie S: Clinical laboratory hematology, Upper Saddle River, NJ, 2004, Pearson Ed., Inc, p 482.

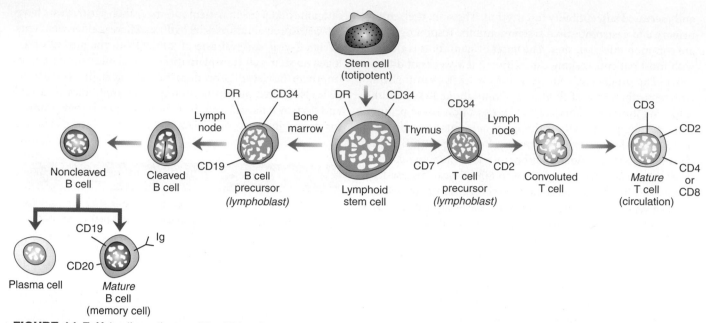

FIGURE 11-7 Maturation pathways of T and B lymphocytes showing the stages at which lymphocyte development is typically arrested in leukemia. Different markers are present on the surface of B cells and T cells at progressive stages of development, which are helpful in identifying the neoplastic cell type and maturity.

5% of cases of CLL are associated with T-cell transformation, but this type is more aggressive.[4] In general, B-cell CLL follows an indolent course, which is usually asymptomatic. Often CLL is found by accident on routine blood count examinations. When CLL becomes symptomatic, patients may experience fatigue, weight loss, and anorexia. Because the leukemic B cells do not produce antibodies normally, an increased susceptibility to certain types of infection may occur. Malignant lymphocytes invade lymphoid tissues and bone marrow, disrupting function. Lymphoid invasion often presents as enlarged, painless lymph nodes (lymphadenopathy) or enlarged spleen. Bone marrow infiltration reduces the production of other cells, including red blood cells and platelets. A typical slide of a bone marrow aspirate from a patient with CLL is shown in Figure 11-8. Note the preponderance of lymphoid cells. CLL cells are characterized by defective apoptosis and live longer than they should. They are derived from mature peripheral B cells. (See Box 11-4 for a comparison of acute and chronic leukemias)

Prognosis and Treatment. Certain genetic mutations confer better or worse prognosis. A mutation in the variable region of the immunoglobulin gene (IgV) is associated with a median survival of 24 years or more; those without this mutation have a median survival of less than 8 years.[15] CLL cell types demonstrating short telomere lengths and P53 dysfunction have poor outcomes. Because the average age of patients with CLL is about 65 to 70 years, those with indolent disease may not be treated; they are more likely to die of another disorder rather than CLL. Patients with cell types likely to progress rapidly may receive chemotherapy to induce remission. Those without complete response may

FIGURE 11-8 Bone marrow aspirate showing small lymphocytes with condensed nuclear chromatin typical of chronic lymphocytic leukemia, B-cell type. (From Henderson ES et al, editors: *Leukemia*, ed 7, Philadelphia, 2003, Saunders, color plate 11-28.)

consider stem cell transplantation to prolong the duration of remission.

Acute Lymphoblastic Leukemia/Lymphoma

Pathogenesis and Clinical Manifestations. ALL is a malignant disorder of the lymphoid cell lineage. The great majority of cases are the result of malignant transformation of B cells (80%), with the remainder involving T cells.[16] The abnormal cells resemble immature lymphocytes, called *lymphoblasts* (Figure 11-9). Most lymphoblastic neoplasms present as leukemias, but lymphoblastic lymphomas are thought to be the same disease at a different stage. B-cell leukemias are categorized into cytogenetic groups based on common chromosomal translocations. One of these transformations results in the *bcr/abl* fusion gene discussed previously in the context of CML. Three other types of translocations also form fusion genes that produce abnormal signaling components. These gene derangements have different prognoses and may respond differently to alternative treatment protocols.

Lymphoblasts do not mature and accumulate in large numbers in the blood and bone marrow. At least 20% of the bone marrow cells must be leukemic lymphoblasts to meet the diagnostic criteria for ALL.[16] Accumulation of leukemic cells in the bone marrow crowds out the production of normal red blood cells, platelets, and leukocytes. Circulating blasts are poorly functioning cells and do not provide effective immunocompetence. (See Box 11-5 for a comparison of ALL and acute nonlymphocytic leukemia [ANLL].)

ALL is primarily a disorder of children. It is the most common malignancy and the second leading cause of death in this population.[17,18] The peak incidence occurs between the ages of 3 and 7 years. A second peak occurs in middle age. The onset of symptoms is abrupt, with complaints of bone pain, bruising, fever, and infection being common. Children may refuse to walk and their parents may report loss of appetite, fatigue,

FIGURE 11-9 Peripheral blood smear showing typical cells of acute lymphocytic leukemia. (From Kumar V et al, editors: *Robbins basic pathology,* ed 8, Philadelphia, 2007, Saunders, p 448.)

and abdominal pain. The spleen, liver, and lymph nodes may be enlarged from leukemic infiltration. A small number of children (3%) may present with CNS signs from leukemic infiltration of brain tissues.[19]

Prognosis and Treatment. ALL is highly curable in the pediatric population, but less so in adults. The 5-year survival rate is 85% in children and 30% to 50% in adults.[19] Certain forms of ALL are more responsive to therapy. For example, children with pre–B-cell type have a 90% cure rate, whereas those with mature B-cell or immature T-cell leukemia have a poorer prognosis.

Chemotherapy is used for remission induction. Postremission chemotherapy with or without stem cell transplantation is indicated for most patients.[20] In general, adults with ALL require more intense therapy than children to achieve CR. Monoclonal antibodies may be used in patients whose tumors express specific antigens.

Hairy Cell Leukemia

Pathogenesis and Clinical Manifestations. Hairy cell leukemia is a rare, chronic type of leukemia. The disease represents about 2% of adult leukemias, but it is of interest because of its highly treatable nature. The median age at presentation is about 55 years and there is a 5-to-1 predominance of males.[21] Hairy cell leukemia has a B-cell phenotype and is characterized by the presence of peculiar cells with hairlike projections on their surface (Figure 11-10). At diagnosis, patients have hairy cells in the peripheral blood, as well as reduced numbers of granulocytes, platelets, and red blood cells. Splenomegaly is a common finding, being present in 90% of patients.

Prognosis and Treatment. Treatment may be instituted when a patient becomes symptomatic with an enlarged spleen, recurrent infection, bleeding disorder, or anemia. Appropriate chemotherapeutic protocol produces CR rates of 80%.[22]

Plasma Cell Myeloma (Multiple Myeloma)

Pathogenesis and Clinical Manifestations. Plasma cell myeloma, also known as multiple myeloma, is a malignant disorder of mature, antibody-secreting B lymphocytes, called *plasma cells.* Malignant plasma cells have a predilection to invade bone and form multiple tumor sites. Other tissues may be targeted also, including lymph nodes, liver, spleen, and kidneys. Plasma cell myeloma occurs exclusively in the adult population, usually affecting individuals older than age 40 years, with a median

---

BOX 11-5

Comparison of Acute Lymphocytic (ALL) and Acute Nonlymphocytic Leukemia (ANLL)

	ALL	ANLL
Age	Common in children	Common in adults
Hematology results	Anemia, neutropenia, thrombocytopenia	Anemia, neutropenia, thrombocytopenia
Cell morphology	Small to medium lymphoblasts, fine chromatin, indistinct nucleoli	Medium to large myeloblasts, distinct nucleoli, clear chromatin, Auer rods
Cytochemistry	PAS positive, peroxidase negative, Sudan black B negative	PAS negative, peroxidase positive, Sudan black B positive

Adapted from McKenzie S: *Clinical laboratory hematology,* Upper Saddle River, NJ, 2004, Pearson Ed. Inc., p 487.

age at presentation of 65 years.[23] Men are affected more often than women.

As with other forms of neoplasia, the exact etiologic process of plasma cell myeloma is unknown, but abnormalities in chromosome structure and number are commonly found.[23] The malignant plasma cells all belong to a single clone, and the excessive antibodies they produce are identical monoclonal antibodies. These accumulate in the bloodstream and can be detected by serum protein electrophoresis. Normally, serum antibodies are of many forms (polyclonal) and show a varied distribution of size on the electrophoresis test. In plasma cell myeloma, there is a large amount of one type of antibody, which forms a characteristic spike (Figure 11-11). Excessive production of light-chain antibody fragments by malignant

FIGURE 11-10 Peripheral blood smear showing cells typical of hairy cell leukemia. (From Henderson ES et al, editors: *Leukemia*, ed 7, Philadelphia, 2003, Saunders, color plate 11-29.)

plasma cells results in their accumulation in blood and urine. When found in urine, these light-chain fragments are called **Bence Jones protein.** In addition to helping to confirm the diagnosis, Bence Jones protein is important to the pathogenesis of plasma cell myeloma because it can accumulate in the kidneys and cause kidney damage. Malignant plasma cells tend to accumulate in bone, where they enhance osteoclastic activity and produce bone lesions.[23] Pathologic fractures, especially compression fractures of the vertebral column, are common. Bone destruction releases calcium into the bloodstream, with resultant hypercalcemia.

Most of the clinical manifestations of multiple myeloma are caused by bone and renal damage. The diagnosis of plasma cell myeloma is suspected based on the monoclonal antibody peak, the presence of Bence Jones protein, hypercalcemia, and evidence of bone lesions. The diagnosis is confirmed by bone marrow biopsy. Normally, the plasma cell component of the marrow comprises about 5%. In multiple myeloma, plasma cells may occupy 30% to 95% of the bone marrow (Figure 11-12). A minimum of at least 10% to 15% bone marrow plasma cells is necessary for the diagnosis of plasma cell myeloma.[23] The likelihood of bone marrow dysfunction increases as the plasma cell component increases. Normal production of erythrocytes, platelets, and leukocytes can be impaired to varying degrees.

The onset of plasma cell myeloma is generally slow and insidious. A premalignant stage of plasma cell myeloma is apparent in some individuals who have excess production of monoclonal antibodies but no evidence of bone lesions or Bence Jones protein in the urine. This stage is called monoclonal gammopathy of undetermined significance (MGUS). Approximately 25% of patients with MGUS progress to

FIGURE 11-11 Serum protein electrophoresis comparing abnormal myeloma protein in the γ region typical of benign monoclonal gammopathy **(A)** with the large quantity of monoclonal antibody (spike) γ typical of plasma cell myeloma **(B).** (From Skarin AT: *Atlas of diagnostic oncology*, Philadelphia, 2003, Mosby, pp 536-537.)

malignant disease.[17]Affected individuals remain asymptomatic until it is fairly advanced. The asymptomatic stage often lasts for many years after malignant transformation. During this time the only complaint may be frequent infections. Diagnosis during the asymptomatic phase is usually made because protein in the urine or high serum calcium levels are found on routine examination. Bone pain is usually the first symptom. Sometimes the evaluation of a fracture or back pain leads to the identification of myeloma. Anemia, recurrent infections, and bleeding tendencies are suggestive of bone marrow depression.

Renal insufficiency is a complication experienced by approximately 50% of patients with plasma cell myeloma.[23] Impairment of renal function is the result of a combination of factors, including hyperproteinemia, Bence Jones protein, hypercalcemia, and hyperuricemia. Renal function may continue to decline over time, culminating in end-stage renal disease (chronic renal failure).

Bone involvement is a consistent feature of plasma cell myeloma. Radiologic studies of ribs, spine, skull, and pelvis show a characteristic "honeycomb" appearance, owing to lucid areas of demineralized bone (Figure 11-13). Minimal trauma is likely to result in fractures. Sometimes fractures occur with no known trauma; these are called *pathologic* fractures.

Prognosis and Treatment. Antineoplastic agents may be used to induce and maintain a remission in plasma cell proliferation. The best chemotherapy regimen has not yet been determined. The remission induction rate with these agents is about 60%, with a median survival of about 3 years after initiation of therapy.[23] High-dose chemotherapy followed by allogeneic bone marrow transplantation is becoming more common and offers a better CR rate. However, the mortality rate associated with transplantation is high (approximately 40% to 50%).[17] Autologous stem cell transplantation is considered to be the optimal initial therapy for most patients. Pharmacologic management of renal dysfunction is often necessary.

Chronic bone pain is a common problem in the myeloma patient that may require use of multiple remedies. Narcotic and nonnarcotic pain relievers are often necessary. Localized application of radiation to bone lesions may reduce bone pain in some cases.

FIGURE 11-12 A bone marrow aspirate from a patient with multiple myeloma showing a large number of abnormal plasma cells with multiple nuclei and cytoplasmic droplets. (From Kumar V et al, editors: *Robbins basic pathology*, ed 8, Philadelphia, 2007, Saunders, p 455.)

KEY POINTS

- CLL is a neoplastic transformation of a mature, peripheral B cell that affects adults primarily and has an insidious onset. CLL is usually asymptomatic. Disease in certain genotypes is associated with long survival times and does not require therapy; in other cases, disease is

FIGURE 11-13 Vertebral body **(A)** and skull **(B)** radiographs showing the characteristic "honeycomb" appearance of demineralized bone associated with multiple myeloma. (Courtesy Marvin J. Stone, MD, Sammons Cancer Center, Baylor University Medical Center, Dallas.)

FIGURE 11-14 Schematic drawing showing the orderly, contiguous, and predictable spread of Hodgkin disease. (Redrawn and modified from Rosenberg SA: Hodgkin disease: no stage beyond cure, *Hosp Pract* 21[8]:97, 1986. After original illustrations by Bunji Tagawa.)

progressive and may be managed with stem cell transplantation or administration of monoclonal antibodies.

- ALL affects children primarily, has an acute onset, responds well to therapy, and has a good prognosis. ALL is associated with transformation of precursor "blasts" in the bone marrow. ALL often manifests with bone pain, infections, and a tendency to bleeding. A significant number of children with ALL have CNS involvement, and intrathecal chemotherapy is necessary.

- Plasma cell myeloma is caused by malignant transformation of antibody-secreting B lymphocytes. It primarily affects older adults. The onset of symptoms is insidious, with most patients experiencing a 4- to 10-year period of clinical latency. Some patients have a preneoplastic phase called MGUS. When present, symptoms include bone pain, pathologic fractures, anemia, thrombocytopenia, leukopenia, and renal insufficiency. Malignant plasma cells all secrete the same monoclonal antibody, and detection of this antibody in the blood or urine (Bence Jones protein) aids in diagnosis.

FIGURE 11-15 Histologic sample showing the typical binucleate Reed-Sternberg cells found in Hodgkin disease. An eosinophil can be seen below the Reed-Sternberg cell. (From Kumar V et al, editors: *Robbins basic pathology*, ed 8, Philadelphia, 2007, Saunders, p 457. Courtesy Dr. Robert W. McKenna, Department of Pathology, University of Texas Southwestern Medical School, Dallas.)

Hodgkin Disease. Hodgkin disease represents about 30% of all cases of malignant lymphoma, accounting for approximately 7000 new cases annually in the United States.[10] It occurs across the age continuum, with half of cases occurring in persons between the ages of 20 and 40 years. The overall incidence of Hodgkin disease is higher in males, who have a worse prognosis. The overall 5-year survival rate for treated Hodgkin disease, including all stages, is about 85%.[10]

Pathogenesis and Clinical Manifestations. Hodgkin disease is a malignant disorder of the lymph nodes characterized by the presence of **Reed-Sternberg** cells on histologic examination. Reed-Sternberg cells originate from B cells in the germinal

centers of lymph nodes.[24] Reed-Sternberg cells are malignant, but they tend to grow and spread in a very predictable manner. This predictability sets Hodgkin disease apart from other types of lymphoma. Hodgkin disease usually metastasizes along contiguous lymphatic pathways (Figure 11-14). Epstein-Barr virus is frequently found in the genome of transformed Reed-Sternberg cells and is thought to be important in the pathogenesis of Hodgkin disease. The malignant cells are clonal, originating from a single mutant precursor cell, and usually present in a single node or localized chain of nodes. In addition to malignant Reed-Sternberg cells, inflammatory cells accumulate within the node (Figure 11-15) such that

FIGURE 11-16 Hodgkin disease (stage IIA). Marked enlargement of cervical lymph nodes is present in this patient. It is usually painless and may be confined to only one area or may affect two or more areas. (From Skarin AT: *Atlas of diagnostic oncology*, London, 2003, Gower Medical, p 482.)

Reed-Sternberg cells constitute only a small minority (2%) of the cells in the lymph node tumor.[24]

There are two types of Hodgkin disease: (1) the rare lymphocyte predominance type, which accounts for 5% of cases, and (2) the classical type (cHD) representing the other 95%. The classical type can be divided further into four subtypes according to the relative number of reactive cells in the tumor. The histologic pattern does not seem to predict the prognosis. The stage of Hodgkin disease is more relevant.[24]

Clinical manifestations of Hodgkin disease are dependent on the site of origin as well as on the stage of dissemination. Lymphomas often are asymptomatic in the early stages. The usual clinical presentation includes painless lymphadenopathy that may be accompanied by fever, night sweats, pruritus, weight loss, and malaise. Usually enlargement occurs in lymph nodes above the diaphragm, the cervical nodes being the most common site. (Figure 11-16) Other supradiaphragmatic nodes are the supraclavicular, axillary, and mediastinal nodes. Less commonly, nodes below the diaphragm are the primary site. The inguinal nodes are the most common subdiaphragmatic site. As the disease spreads from the site of origin, other lymph nodes and lymphatic tissues may become involved, including the spleen and bone marrow. Staging procedures are performed to determine the extent of metastasis at the time of diagnosis. Staging dictates the treatment modality

best suited to provide the patient with the greatest chance for long-term survival.

Prognosis and Treatment. The staging protocol commonly used today was first adopted in 1971 at the Ann Arbor symposium and modified later in 1989 at the Cotswold meeting (Box 11-6).[25,26] The same procedure is also used for staging non-Hodgkin lymphomas. This protocol uses the presence or absence of certain clinical symptoms as well as the locations of affected nodes to determine the clinical stage of disease. The four stages are shown in Figure 11-17. The letter A denotes the absence of clinical symptoms, whereas the letter B is used when symptoms are present at the time of staging. These symptoms include loss of more than 10% of body weight, unexplained fevers, and night sweats. The clinical stage (CS) is based on history, physical examination, and noninvasive procedures, such as computed tomography (CT) scanning. The pathologic stage (PS) is determined by the results of invasive procedures, such as laparotomy and tissue biopsy. The stage dictates the treatment modalities used. In general, localized tumors are more amenable to application of radiation therapy, whereas disseminated disease responds better to systemic chemotherapeutic agents. Because Hodgkin disease often is detected while localized, radiation therapy is commonly used, with good results (Figure 11-18).

Patients with nonbulky stage IA or IIA disease may be candidates for radiation as sole therapy. However, a relatively high rate of relapse has been noted, and combined chemotherapy with limited field radiation is often used.[27] Patients with bulky disease, "B" symptoms, or stage III and IV disease require chemotherapy with or without radiation. In early-stage disease, appropriate treatment produces a 90% 10-year disease-free survival. More aggressive chemotherapy is indicated for patients with advanced Hodgkin disease.

B-Cell, T-Cell, and NK-Cell Lymphoma (Non-Hodgkin). The malignancies included in the classification of non-Hodgkin lymphoma are those that do not have the characteristic Reed-Sternberg cells found in Hodgkin disease. The majority of cases of non-Hodgkin lymphoma arise from lymph nodes, but they can originate in any lymphoid tissue. With the exception of a few subtypes, most cases of non-Hodgkin lymphoma occur in older adults (95%), and males are at a slightly higher risk than females. The incidence of non-Hodgkin lymphoma is on the rise, particularly in areas with large acquired immunodeficiency syndrome (AIDS) populations. More than 50,000 new cases of non-Hodgkin lymphoma are diagnosed annually in the United States.[9] The lifetime risk of developing the disease is about 1 in 50.

Most cases of non-Hodgkin lymphoma arise from B cells, T cells, or NK cells. Some of the more common types of non-Hodgkin lymphoma are summarized in Table 11-2. The prognosis and recommended treatment protocols vary according to type. A general schema for grouping non-Hodgkin lymphoma according to indolent or aggressive types is in common usage.[28] Generally, indolent disease is associated with longer survival times, whereas aggressive lymphomas tend to

BOX 11-6

Ann Arbor Staging System for Lymphomas with Cotswold Modifications

Stage I

Involvement of a single lymph node region or lymphoid structure (e.g., spleen, thymus, Waldeyer ring)

Stage II

Involvement of two or more lymph node regions on the same side of the diaphragm. The number of anatomic regions is indicated by a subscript (e.g., II_3)

Stage III

Involvement of lymph node regions or structures on both sides of the diaphragm

III_1: with or without splenic, hilar, celiac, or portal nodes

III_2: with para-aortic, iliac, mesenteric nodes

Stage IV

Involvement of extranodal site(s) beyond that designated "E"

The site is indicated by a letter code followed by a plus sign (+)

Modifying Characteristics

For Stages I to III

E: Involvement of a single, extranodal site contiguous or proximal to known nodal site

For All Stages

A: No symptoms

B: Fever (>38[C],) drenching sweats, weight loss (>10% body weight over 6 months)

X: Bulky disease

- >One third widening of mediastinum
- >10 cm maximal dimension of nodal mass

CS: Clinical stage is based on history, physical examination, laboratory studies, CT scans.

PS: Pathologic stage is based on tissue sampling obtained through invasive procedures such as laparotomy and biopsy.

Site notations: *N,* nodes; *H,* liver; *L,* lung; *M,* bone matter; *S,* spleen; *P,* pleura; *O,* bone; *D,* skin.

Stage I	Stage II	Stage III	Stage IV
• Involvement of single lymph node region *or* • Involvement of single extralymphatic site (stage I$_E$)	• Involvement of 2 lymph node regions on same side of diaphragm • May include localized extralymphatic involvement on same side of diaphragm (stage II$_E$)	• Involvement of lymph node regions on both sides of diaphragm • May include involvement of spleen (stage III$_S$) or localized extranodal disease (stage III$_E$) or both (III$_{E+S}$) For Hodgkin disease: III$_1$ • Disease limited to upper abdomen—spleen, splenic hilar, celiac, or porta hepatic nodes III$_2$ • Disease limited to lower abdomen—periaortic, pelvic, or inguinal nodes	• Disseminated (multifocal) extralymphatic disease involving one or more organs (e.g., liver, bone marrow, lung, skin), with or without associated lymph node involvement *or* • Isolated extralymphatic disease with distant (nonregional) lymph node involvement

NOTE: Stage designation "B" indicates unexplained weight loss >10% of body weight in preceding 6 months and/or fevers of >38C and/or night sweats. Stage designation "A" indicates the absence of the features characterizing "B."

FIGURE 11-17 Depiction of the locations of malignant cells in the various stages of lymphoma using the Ann Arbor staging system. (From Skarin AT: *Atlas of diagnostic oncology,* Philadelphia, 2003, Mosby, p 479.)

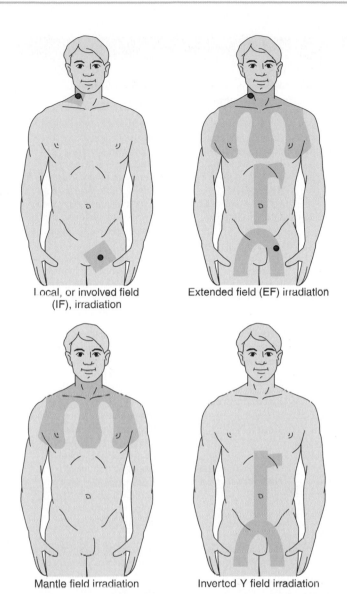

Local, or involved field (IF), irradiation

Extended field (EF) irradiation

Mantle field irradiation

Inverted Y field irradiation

FIGURE 11-18 Typical radiation fields for lymphoma. Different fields of radiation may be used depending on the location of disease.

be disseminated at presentation and carry a generally poorer prognosis. As a group, the non-Hodgkin types of lymphoma are more likely to spread early and unpredictably in comparison with Hodgkin disease.

Pathogenesis and Clinical Manifestations. The etiologic process of non-Hodgkin lymphoma is thought to be similar to that of other malignant transformations. The tumor cells are all derived from a single mutant precursor cell and are clonal. Viruses are suspected in the development of some types of lymphoma. In particular, Burkitt lymphoma is strongly associated with the presence of Epstein-Barr virus.[2] Adult T-cell lymphomas are associated with infection by human T-cell leukemia virus, type 1 (HTLV-1).[2] The overall 5-year survival rate for all types of non-Hodgkin lymphomas combined is about 50%.[10]

Most patients with non-Hodgkin lymphoma present with advanced disease (stage III or IV). Clinical manifestations may include painless lymphadenopathy, fever, night sweats, weight loss, malaise, and pruritus (similar to Hodgkin disease). A comparison of the features of Hodgkin disease and non-Hodgkin lymphoma is shown in Table 11-3. Extranodal involvement occurs early in the course of non-Hodgkin lymphoma, and patients may present with infiltrative disease of the skin, gastrointestinal tract, bone, or bone marrow. Complications occur more frequently than in Hodgkin disease. Two of the most serious oncology emergencies are obstruction of the superior vena cava and spinal cord compression. Infection, bone metastasis, and joint effusions also are common. Staging of non-Hodgkin lymphoma is done in the same way as for Hodgkin disease, and the classification system is the same as well. Earlier clinical stages are associated with the best prognosis for survival.

Prognosis and Treatment. The effectiveness of therapy for non-Hodgkin lymphoma is variable. Favorable outcomes are likely in stage I and II disease. However, non-Hodgkin lymphoma is likely to present as stage III or IV disease, which has a poor prognosis. Therapeutic management is determined by the clinical stage, histologic type, age of the patient, and bone marrow integrity at the time of diagnosis.[29] Radiation, chemotherapy, tissue-specific therapies, such as monoclonal antibodies and bone marrow transplants, may all be applicable.

KEY POINTS

- Hodgkin disease is characterized by malignant transformation of B cells in lymph nodes called *Reed-Sternberg cells.* Spread of malignant cells occurs along predictable, contiguous pathways. Most commonly, a single cervical lymph node is involved initially, with slow progression to nearby nodes.
- Non-Hodgkin lymphoma constitutes a diverse group of malignant diseases of lymphoid tissue. The characteristic Reed-Sternberg cell of Hodgkin disease is not present. Non-Hodgkin lymphoma is unpredictable in its spread and is often disseminated at diagnosis.
- Manifestations of Hodgkin disease and non-Hodgkin lymphoma are similar. These include painless lymph node enlargement, fever, night sweats, and weight loss. Early-stage disease is often asymptomatic.
- Staging is done to determine the degree of dissemination of disease. When affected lymph nodes are localized to one area (stage I) or one side of the diaphragm (stage II), the prognosis for cure is very good. Dissemination to lymph nodes above and below the diaphragm (stage III) or to extralymphatic organs or tissues (stage IV) carries a poorer prognosis.
- Radiation of the involved field is commonly used for malignant lymphoma in early stages. More disseminated disease may be treated with chemotherapeutic protocols. Non-Hodgkin lymphoma is routinely treated with chemotherapy because the disease is often well advanced at the time of diagnosis. Treatment may lead to bone marrow suppression and may predispose the patient to anemia, thrombocytopenia, and leukopenia.

TABLE 11-2

Summary of the More Common Lymphoid Neoplasms

Entity	Frequency	Salient Morphology	Immunophenotype	Comments
Precursor B-cell lymphoblastic leukemia/ lymphoma	85% of childhood acute leukemia	Lymphoblasts with irregular nuclear contours, condensed chromatin, small nucleoli, and scant agranular cytoplasm	TdT+ immature B cells (CD19+, variable expression of other B-cell markers)	Usually presents as acute leukemia; less common in adults; prognosis is predicted by karyotype
Precursor T-cell leukemia/ lymphoma	15% of childhood acute leukemia; 40% of childhood lymphomas	Identical to precursor B-cell lymphoblastic leukemia/lymphoma	TdT+ immature T cells (CD2+, CD7+, variable expression of other T-cell markers)	Most common in adolescent males; often presents as a mediastinal mass due to thymic involvement; highly associated with mutations in NOTCH1
Small lymphocytic lymphoma/chronic lymphocytic leukemia	3% to 4% of adult lymphomas; 30% of all leukemias	Small resting lymphocytes mixed with variable numbers of large activated cells; lymph nodes diffusely effaced	CD5+ B-cell expressing surface Ig	Occurs in older adults; usually involves nodes, marrow, and spleen; most patients have peripheral blood involvement; indolent
Follicular lymphoma	40% of adult lymphomas	Frequent small "cleaved" cells mixed with large cells; growth pattern is usually nodular (follicular)	CD10+ BCL2+ mature B cells that express surface Ig	Occurs in older adults; usually involves nodes, marrow, and spleen; associated with t(14;18); indolent
Mantle cell lymphoma	3% to 4% of adult lymphomas	Small to intermediate-sized irregular lymphocytes growing in a diffuse pattern	CD5+ mature B cells that express cyclin D1 and have surface Ig	Occurs mainly in older males; usually involves nodes, marrow, and spleen; GI tract also commonly affected; t(11;14) is characteristic; moderately aggressive
Extranodal marginal zone lymphoma	~5% of adult lymphomas	Variable cell size and differentiation; 40% show plasmacytic differentiation; B cells home to epithelium, creating "lymphoepithelial lesions"	CD5−, CD10− mature cells with surface Ig	Frequently occurs at extranodal sites involved by chronic inflammation; very indolent; may be cured by local excision
Diffuse large B-cell lymphoma	40% to 50% of adult lymphomas	Variable; most resemble large germinal center B cells; diffuse growth pattern	Mature B cells with variable expression of CD10 and surface Ig	Occurs in all ages, but most common in older adults; often arise at extranodal sites; aggressive
Burkitt lymphoma	<1% of lymphomas in the United States	Intermediate-sized round lymphoid cells with several nucleoli; diffuse tissue involvement associated with apoptosis products and "starry-sky" appearance	Mature CD10+ B cells expressing surface Ig	Endemic in Africa, sporadic elsewhere; increased frequency in immunosuppressed patients; predominantly affects children; often presents with visceral involvement; highly aggressive
Plasmacytoma/ plasma cell myeloma	Most common lymphoid neoplasm in older adults	Plasma cells in sheets, sometimes with prominent nucleoli or inclusions containing Ig	Terminally differentiated plasma cells containing cytoplasmic Ig	Myeloma presents as disseminated bone disease, often with destructive lytic lesions Hypercalcemia, renal insufficiency, and bacterial infections are common
Mycosis fungoides	Most common cutaneous lymphoid malignancy	In most cases, small lymphoid cells with markedly convoluted nuclei; cells often infiltrate the epidermis (Pautrier microabscesses)	CD4+ mature T cells	Presents with localized or more generalized skin involvement; generally indolent. Sézary syndrome, a more aggressive variant, is characterized by diffuse skin erythema and peripheral blood involvement

TABLE 11-2

Summary of the More Common Lymphoid Neoplasms—cont'd

Entity	Frequency	Salient Morphology	Immunophenotype	Comments
Peripheral T-cell lymphoma, not otherwise specified (NOS)	Most common adult T-cell lymphoma	Variable; usually a spectrum of small to large lymphoid cells with irregular nuclear contours	Mature T-cell phenotype (CD3$^+$)	Probably spans a diverse collection of rare tumors. Often disseminated, generally aggressive
Hodgkin lymphoma, modular sclerosis type	Most common type of Hodgkin lymphoma	Lacunar Reed-Sternberg cell variants in a mixed inflammatory background; broad sclerotic bands of collagen usually also present	CD15$^+$, CD30$^+$ Reed-Sternberg cells	Most common in young adults, often arises in the mediastinum or cervical lymph nodes
Hodgkin lymphoma, mixed cellularity type	Second most common form of Hodgkin lymphoma	Frequent classic Reed-Sternberg cells in a mixed inflammatory background	CD15$^+$, CD30$^+$ Reed-Sternberg cells	Most common in men, more likely to present at advanced stages than the nodular sclerosis type EBV[1] in 70% of cases

From Kumar V et al: *Robbins basic pathology*, ed 8, Philadelphia, 2007, Saunders, pp 448-449.

GI, Gastrointestinal; *Ig,* immunoglobulin.

TABLE 11-3

Clinical Differences in Hodgkin Disease and Non-Hodgkin Lymphoma

Characteristic	Hodgkin Disease	Non-Hodgkin Lymphoma
Pattern of spread	Contiguous spread	Noncontiguous spread
Extranodal disease	Uncommon	More common involvement of gastrointestinal tract, testes, bone marrow
Site of disease	Mediastinal involvement common	Mediastinal involvement less common
	Bone marrow involvement uncommon	Bone marrow involvement common
	Liver involvement uncommon	Liver involvement common
Extent of disease	Often localized	Rarely localized
B symptoms	Common	Uncommon

SUMMARY

Malignant disorders of white blood cells are classified according to cell type and fall into two major categories: myeloid neoplasms and lymphoid neoplasms. Myeloid neoplasms commonly present as leukemia and usually involve transformation of granulocytes. Lymphoid neoplasms may present as leukemia, lymphoma, or plasma cell myeloma. Leukemia is a malignant neoplasm of immature stem cells that is characterized by diffuse replacement of the bone marrow by neoplastic blasts. In most cases the leukemic cells spill over into the blood, where they may be seen in large numbers. These cells may also infiltrate the liver, spleen, lymph nodes, and other tissues throughout the body. Lymphoma is characterized by malignancy of cells found in lymphoid tissues and usually arises in the lymph nodes. Hodgkin disease is a special category of malignant lymphoma that is characterized by the presence of Reed-Sternberg cells. Hodgkin disease is more predictable in its spread than the non-Hodgkin types of lymphoma, and it is generally curable in the early stages. Non-Hodgkin lymphoma types comprise a large number of different disorders that involve malignant transformation of B cells, T cells, or NK cells. As with Hodgkin disease, earlier stages are more easily cured. However, the non-Hodgkin lymphomas tend to be unpredictable in their spread, and the prognosis is less certain. Plasma cell myeloma is a malignant transformation of mature, antibody-secreting B cells. Malignant plasma cells are monoclonal and all produce identical antibodies, which accumulate in the blood. These cells have a predilection to settle in skeletal structures, where they cause bone demineralization and destruction. Hypercalcemia, bone fractures, and renal damage are common complications of plasma cell myeloma. Treatment for the various types of hematologic neoplasms continues to evolve, and excellent disease-free survival is commonly achieved when the disease is caught in the early stages.

REFERENCES

1. Jaffe ES et al, editor: *Pathology and genetics of tumours of haematopoietic and lymphoid tissues*, Lyon, France, 2001, IARC Press.
2. Schulz TF, Neil JC: Viruses and leukemia. In Henderson ES, Lister TA, Greaves MF, editors: *Leukemia*, ed 7, Philadelphia, 2002, Saunders, pp 200-226.
3. Boice JD: Radiation-induced leukemia. In Henderson ES, Lister TA, Greaves MF, editors: *Leukemia*, ed 7, Philadelphia, 2002, Saunders, pp 152-170.
4. Pedersen-Bjergaard: Chemicals and leukemia. In Henderson ES, Lister TA, Greaves MF, editors: *Leukemia*, ed 7, Philadelphia, 2002, Saunders, pp 171-199.
5. Ross JA et al: Maternal exposure to potential inhibitors of DNA topoisomerase II and infant leukemia (United States): a report from the children's cancer group, *Cancer Causes Control* 7(6):581-590, 1996.
6. McKenzie SB: *Clinical laboratory hematology,* Upper Saddle River, NJ, 2004, Pearson Ed., p 487.
7. Löwenberg B, Griffin JD, Tallman MS: Acute myeloid leukemia and acute promyelocytic leukemia, *Hematology* (Am Soc Hematol Education Program):82-101, 2003.
8. Gaynon PS, Siegel SE: Childhood acute lymphoblastic leukemia. In Henderson ES, Lister TA, Greaves MF, editors: *Leukemia*, ed 7, Philadelphia, 2002, Saunders, pp 601-620.
9. Spivak JL et al: Chronic myeloproliferative disorders, *Hematology* (Am Soc Hematol Education Program):200-224, 2003.
10. *Cancer Facts and Figures 2003*, Dallas, 2003, American Cancer Society.
11. Melo JV, Hughes TP, Apperley JF: Chronic myeloid leukemia, *Hematology* (Am Soc Hematol Education Program):132-152, 2003.
12. Barnett MJ, Eaves CJ: Chronic myeloid leukemia. In Henderson ES, Lister TA, Greaves MF, editors: *Leukemia*, ed 7, Philadelphia, 2002, Saunders, pp 583-600.
13. Vardiman JW, Harris NL, Brunning RD: The World Health Organization (WHO) classification of the myeloid neoplasms, *Blood* 100:2292-2302, 2002.
14. Robatiner A, Lister TA: Acute myelogenous leukemia. In Henderson ES, Lister TA, Greaves MF, editors: *Leukemia*, ed 7, Philadelphia, 2002, Saunders, pp 485-517.
15. Keating MJ: Chronic lymphocytic leukemia. In Henderson ES, Lister TA, Greaves MF, editors: *Leukemia*, ed 7, Philadelphia, 2002, Saunders, pp 656-691.
16. Keating MJ et al: Biology and treatment of chronic lymphocytic leukemia, *Hematology* (Am Soc Hematol Education Program): 153-175, 2003.
17. Aster J: The hematopoietic and lymphoid systems. In Kumar V, Abbas AK, Fausto N, Mitchell, R, editors: *Robbins basic pathology,* ed 8, Philadelphia, 2007, Saunders, pp 421-478.
18. McKenzie SB: *Clinical laboratory hematology,* Upper Saddle River, NJ, 2004, Pearson Ed. p 487.
19. Gaynon PS, Siegel SI: Childhood acute lymphoblastic leukemia. In Henderson ES, Lister TA, Greaves MF, editors: *Leukemia*, ed 7, Philadelphia, 2002, Saunders, pp 601-620.
20. Joel SP, Robatiner A: Pharmacology of antileukemic drugs. In Henderson ES, Lister TA, Greaves MF, editors: *Leukemia,* ed 7, Philadelphia, 2002, Saunders, pp 394-440.
21. Hoffman M, Rai K: Hairy cell leukemia. In Henderson ES, Lister TA, Greaves MF, editors: *Leukemia*, ed 7, Philadelphia, 2002, Saunders, pp 693-703.
22. Linker CA: Blood. In Tierney LM, McPhee SJ, Papadakis MA, editors: *Current medical diagnosis and treatment,* ed 46, New York, 2007, McGraw-Hill, pp 493-547.
23. Barille-Nion S et al: Advances in biology and therapy of multiple myeloma, *Hematology* (Am Soc Hematol Education Program): 248-278, 2003.
24. Diehl V et al: Hodgkin's lymphoma: biology and treatment strategies for primary, refractory and relapsed disease, *Hematology* (Am Soc Hematol Education Program) 225-247, 2003.
25. Carbone PP et al: Report of the committee on Hodgkin's disease staging classification, *Cancer Res* 31:1860-1861, 1971.
26. Lister TA et al: Report of a committee convened to discuss the evaluation and staging of patients with Hodgkin's disease: Cotswold meeting, *J Clin Oncol* 7(11):1630-1636, 1989.
27. *Adult Hodgkin Lymphoma (PDQ):* National Cancer Institute, http://www.nci.nih/gov, 2007.
28. *Non-Hodgkin Lymphoma (PDQ):* National Cancer Institute, http://www.nci.nih/gov, 2007.
29. Vose JM et al: Update on epidemiology and therapeutics for non-Hodgkin's lymphoma, *Hematology* (Am Soc Hematol Education Program):241-262, 2003.

HIV Disease and AIDS

Faith Young Peterson

MEDIA RESOURCES

Additional Material for Study, Review, and Further Exploration

CD Companion ■ Review Questions and Answers
■ Glossary (with audio pronunciations for selected terms)
■ Disease Profiles ■ Animations

evolve **Website** at http://evolve.elsevier.com/Copstead/
■ Case Studies ■ Disease Profiles ■ WebLinks ■ Key Points Review

Online Course (Module 7)

KEY QUESTIONS

■ What are the common modes of HIV transmission and how can infection be prevented?
■ What is the scope of the HIV/AIDS epidemic in the United States and the world?
■ How does infection with HIV lead to progressive immunodeficiency and AIDS?
■ How has knowledge of the HIV lifecycle led to the development of multidrug treatment strategies?

■ How are CD4+ cell counts and various clinical findings used to classify the stages of HIV disease and AIDS?
■ What are the common systemic manifestations of AIDS and associated opportunistic infections?
■ What are the current treatment recommendations for HIV disease and AIDS?

CHAPTER OUTLINE

Human immunodeficiency virus (HIV) infection and acquired immunodeficiency syndrome (AIDS) are acquired immunodeficiency disorders resulting in defective immune functioning. The hallmark of HIV infection is defective cell-mediated immunity, especially the decrease in CD4+ or T-helper/inducer lymphocytes. CD4+ T cells are necessary for appropriate immune responsiveness because they are the cells that mediate between the antigen-presenting cells and other immune cells, such as B cells and other T cells. CD4+ lymphocytes are characterized by the presence of the CD4 receptor.

This chapter focuses on HIV disease and AIDS—from epidemiology to pathogenesis and management. HIV is the prototypical public health infectious disease of the late 20th century. HIV is an infectious organism. It was originally thought to be a rapid killer; however, it does not act like other infectious organisms that overwhelm the immune system. HIV infection is a chronic illness associated with widespread and diverse organ involvement with varying signs and symptoms, causing long-term suffering. It encompasses all of the armamentarium of a viral infection that has completed the evolutionary jump from animal to human. HIV has done more than just confuse and captivate scientists and health professionals; it also has mobilized risk groups and placed medicine and society at a crossroads of opinion. In this epidemic, the lines between privacy and public health and between morality and compassion have been debated. HIV disease is complex, but in its complexity it has opened the door to better understanding of the immune system.

EPIDEMIOLOGY

HIV infection is a primary immunodeficiency disease caused by the retroviruses, HIV type 1 and HIV type 2. The emergence of HIV worldwide has triggered major research efforts to better understand and combat its lethal effects on the immune system. Despite research and public health surveillance and prevention activities, the virus has continued mutating and spreading globally. HIV has caused a nondiscriminatory pandemic. It infects people worldwide without regard for age, race, gender, or social class. However, HIV infection is increasingly becoming a disease of poor, uneducated, or undereducated people of color.

Since its identification in the early 1980s, approximately 65 million people have been infected with HIV/AIDS and more than 25 million have died.[1] According to UNAIDS data in 2006, the global epidemic continues to grow and the numbers of persons with new HIV infections are increasing, particularly in third world countries. There are an estimated 38.6 million people living with HIV worldwide as of 2006.[1] Currently, two thirds or more of all cases occur in sub-Saharan Africa— approximately 24.5 million people as of 2005.[1] In Asia, Eastern Europe, and Latin America, it is spreading in epidemic proportions and may be underreported—approximately 8.3 million in Asia, 1.5 million in Eastern Europe and Central Asia, and 1.6 million in Latin America.[1] This means the adult prevalence percentage among all persons in the world is 1%.[1]

In third world countries, those infected with HIV have limited access to testing, medication for treatment, and dissemination of prevention information and education for the general public is limited.

In the United States, the Centers for Disease Control and Prevention (CDC) initially reported only persons diagnosed with AIDS, although since 1996, it is now reporting persons with HIV/AIDS. Approximately 1 million (980,000) people have been diagnosed with HIV/AIDS in the United States since the beginning of the epidemic.[2] It is estimated by the CDC that there are 432,325 persons living with HIV/AIDS in the United States, with 40,608 AIDS cases diagnosed in 2005. The numbers of deaths in the United States and other industrialized countries are stable or declining where access to medication, care, and prevention is greater (Figure 12-1).

Current statistics show that of the people diagnosed with HIV/AIDS in the United States, 49% are black, 31% white, 18% Hispanic, 1% Asian/Pacific Islanders, and less than 1% Native Americans and Alaska Natives.[3] Of these numbers, approximately one fourth are women and the rest are men.[3] In males living with HIV/AIDS, 67% contracted the disease through sex with other men (MSM), 13% were intravenous drug users (IVDs), 5% were combined MSM/IVDs, and 15% were exposed via heterosexual contact.[4] In women with HIV/AIDS, 64% are black, 19% are white, 15% are Hispanic, 1% are Asian/Pacific Islanders, and less than 1% are American Indian/Alaska Natives.[5] Approximately 80% of women with HIV/AIDS were exposed via high-risk heterosexual contact.[5] It is thought that non-injection drugs (such as crack cocaine or methamphetamine) may also contribute to the spread of HIV/AIDS because of sex trading for drugs, shelter, or money. Ninety percent of children younger than age 13 were infected perinatally. The number of HIV-infected individuals continues to increase despite prevention education. It is also disturbing that the number of men with HIV infection is still increasing, particularly in minority populations.

History

At the turn of the century, retroviruses were one of the first viruses discovered as the cause of cancer in chickens.[6] Originally, retroviruses were identified only in nonhuman species, where their presence was generally harmless or occasionally associated with tumors and slowly progressive cardiovascular, pulmonary, or neurologic diseases. Retroviruses have subsequently been identified in most animal species. HIV is very closely related to primate retroviruses. Researchers originally hypothesized that HIV was related to the green monkey virus and macaque monkey virus, termed *simian immunodeficiency virus* or *simian T-cell lymphotropic virus type III* (STLV-III). This primate retrovirus does not cause disease in monkeys. However, it was not until 1999 that HIV-1's natural reservoir was identified.[7] Researchers from the University of Alabama at Birmingham along with the National Institute of Allergy and Infectious Diseases (NIAID) and an international team of scientists found that HIV-1, subgroups M, N, and O, strongly resembled virus located in a subspecies of chimpanzees

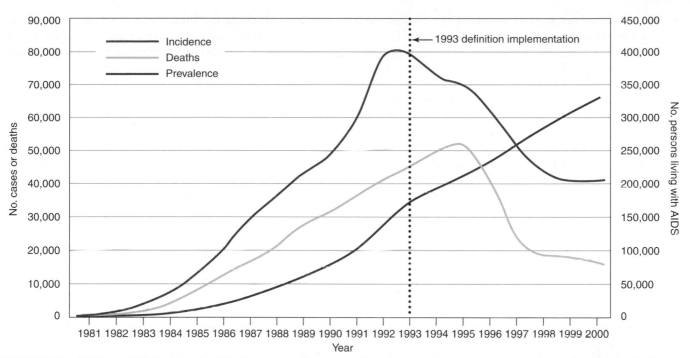

FIGURE 12-1 Estimated AIDS incidence and deaths among persons with AIDS, by year of diagnosis or death and year-end prevalence, United States, 1981 to 2000. Data were adjusted for delays in reporting of cases and deaths. (From Update: AIDS-United States, 2000, *MMWR Morb Mortal Wkly Rep* 51[27]:592-595, 2002.)

(Pan troglodytes troglodytes) native to west equatorial Africa.[7] As in the STLV-III viruses, the chimpanzees do not get sick from the HIV virus. The HIV-1 virus crossed species into humans, undergoing a series of mutations that became HIV-1 when humans contacted infected chimpanzee blood while hunting the chimpanzees for human consumption.[7] HIV then established itself in Africa as an epidemiologic disease after 1930.

In 1980 the first human retroviruses were found to affect T cells. Human T-cell lymphotropic virus type I (HTLV-I) was found to infect T cells and cause adult T-cell leukemia. HTLV-II was subsequently discovered and found to be associated with the development of hairy cell leukemias and T-cell leukemias. HTLV-IV is associated with chronic lymphomas, but this relationship is not well established. These transforming, cancer-causing viruses were originally thought to be closely linked to HIV. Such has proved not to be correct. However, their discovery enlightened Gallo, Essex, and Montagnier, who were able to narrow their search for the cause of AIDS.

In 1981 the first descriptions of immunodeficiency disease in previously healthy persons appeared in the medical literature. However, the specific retrovirus causing HIV infection and AIDS was not isolated until 1983 (Montagnier) and 1984 (Gallo).

HIV has been identified as a type of retrovirus from the subfamily Lentivirinae, with *Lentivirus* being its only genus. This subfamily is so named from the Latin (*lentus,* "slow") because infection develops gradually. It was originally labeled human HTLV-III (human T-cell lymphotropic virus-type III/lymphadenopathy-associated virus) by an international scientific committee, but was renamed HIV. HIV-2, a related

but distinct retrovirus, was later identified in 1986 and is most closely related to simian immunodeficiency virus. HIV-2 is differentiated from HIV-1 by a longer clinical latency period from the onset of infection to the development of symptoms.

Although the syndrome of AIDS was not reported until 1981, isolated cases of HIV or HIV-like infections were reported in the 1950s and 1960s. Positive tests on serum for HIV-1 antibodies were found in samples taken from a man in Leopoldville (now Kinshasa), Congo, a small region in Central Africa, in 1959 with implications that the virus emerged sometime in the 1930s to 1940s.[8,9] This infection appears to have remained localized before spreading to the rest of Central Africa during the late 1960s and early 1970s. It is commonly thought that HIV reached Haiti in the late 1970s and may have reached Europe and the Americas from there.

In the United States, the first suspected case occurred in 1968. A sexually active 15-year-old African-American male who was admitted to St. Louis City Hospital in 1968 had extensive lymphedema, chlamydial infection in most of his body fluids, and disseminated Kaposi sarcoma.[10] Tests on frozen autopsy tissue from 1969 confirm that he was infected with a virus closely related or identical to the AIDS virus. However, it was not until 1981 when previously healthy young homosexual men in increasing numbers contracted unusual diseases for their age group, such as *Pneumocystis jiroveci (carinii)* pneumonia (PCP) and Kaposi sarcoma, that researchers identified HIV. These young men in San Francisco, Los Angeles, and New York provided the basis of inquiry into the HIV infection. The first evidence of alternative forms of transmission of the virus by blood and blood products appeared in 1982. All these early patients were shown to have a type of HIV virus called HIV-1. It was at this time that the term *acquired immunodeficiency syndrome (AIDS)* was first used.

HIV-1 antibody testing technology was developed in 1985, at which time it was licensed by the Food and Drug Administration. In 1985, blood samples from Guinea-Bissau in West Africa revealed a new virus related to HIV-1 but distinctly different, called HIV-2. In the United States, HIV-2 was not identified until December 1987 in a visitor from West Africa. It is hypothesized that the independence wars and socioeconomic upheavals in the 1960s and 1970s led to its epidemic growth.[11] The first anti-HIV drug was approved in 1987. By 1988, the World Health Organization (WHO) declared December 1 as the first World AIDS Day, and in 2006 declared March 8 as National Women's and Girls HIV/AIDS Awareness Day. In 1999, international researchers discovered the origins of HIV-1, the predominant HIV stain. Since that time, there have been many new developments in the identification of how HIV causes abnormalities in the immune system, vaccination trials, and identification of key genetic factors in determining HIV/AIDS risk. In 2006, one of the major research trials, known as the Strategies for Management of Anti-Retroviral Therapies (SMART) trial found that episodic antiretroviral therapy more than doubles the risk of AIDS or death in people with HIV infection. The research into this epidemic continues with international researchers striving to find more effective medications as well as vaccines to prevent HIV infection.

Types of HIV

Both HIV-1 and HIV-2 are found worldwide. They are similar in structure and function but are differentiated from each other by their envelope glycoproteins, point of origin, and latency periods. HIV-1 is thought to have originated in Central Africa and HIV-2 is thought to have originated in West Africa. HIV-1 is the causative organism of most AIDS cases found in Central Africa, the United States, Europe, and Australia. HIV-2 is found primarily in West Africa.[11] HIV-2 produces a milder form of the disease and appears to be less virulent with a longer latency period than HIV-1.

Many subspecies or strains of HIV also exist because of the rapid rate of HIV virion mutation. The subspecies may exist in different hosts, as well as within an individual host. Currently, at least 10 subtypes of HIV-1 have been identified: group N (YBF30), group O, and group M with 8 subtypes (A, B, C, D, E, F, G, H). Research is currently focusing on the identification of HIV subtypes and strains in different populations and geographic areas. For example, in the United States, Europe, and Australia, most infected persons have HIV-1, subtype B, whereas in India, HIV-2 and HIV-1 strains A, B, and C are usually found.

Transmission

HIV-1 and HIV-2 are relatively weak viruses outside of the body. HIV viruses can infect people through three major types of transmission: sexual transmission via semen or vaginal and cervical secretions through homosexual, bisexual, or heterosexual intercourse; parenteral transmission via blood, blood products, or blood-contaminated needles or syringes; and perinatal transmission in utero, during delivery, or in breast milk. In very low titers, HIV is known to be present but has not been shown to be transmitted via urine, saliva, tears, cerebrospinal fluid, amniotic fluid, and feces. HIV is not known to be transmitted via saliva particulates or aerosol routes.

Common modes of transmission include needle/syringe sharing between intravenous drug users, unprotected sex with infected partners, receipt of HIV-contaminated blood or blood products or infected semen during artificial insemination, unanticipated needle or scalpel injury during care or surgical treatment of infected patients, and neonatal transmission from an infected mother to her infant. In men who have sex with men, having anal sex without a condom is the major cause of transmission. In both men and women, concomitant sexually transmitted diseases increase the risk of HIV infection. In women, high-risk heterosexual contact is influenced by lack of HIV knowledge, low perception of risk, concomitant drug or alcohol use, relationship dynamics such as fear of abuse or loss of relationship, and the increased biologic vulnerability of HIV contraction during vaginal intercourse, especially in the presence of other sexually transmitted diseases or vaginal inflammation. A study of black women in North Carolina found HIV-infected women were more likely to be poor, unemployed, having multiple sexual partners, to use crack/cocaine, to trade sex for money, shelter, or drugs or receive public assistance. In both men and women, noninjection drugs (such as crack cocaine) contribute by either decreasing inhibition to engage in risky sexual behaviors that would not be engaged in if sober or when users trade sex for drugs, money, or shelter.

Blood bank screening and testing procedures have nearly eliminated the transmission of HIV-contaminated blood in the United States. In the United States, all blood and blood products have been tested by HIV-1, HIV-2, and HIV-1 p24 antigen tests since 1996. However, this route of transmission remains high in third world countries, where there is a high number of HIV-infected persons, and much of the blood and blood products are not screened before use.

Health care workers who are exposed to blood or infected body fluids or needles/sharp instruments are at risk of contracting HIV. The risk of developing HIV is greatest for those health care workers who have a deep injury with visible blood from a contaminated needle or sharp instrument or who have a direct puncture into an artery or vein. They also are at risk if they have prolonged blood-skin contact, especially if extensive. The risk of infection is much lower with the use of universal precautions and postexposure prophylaxis.

Transmission from an infected mother to her infant may occur either in the intrauterine period, in the intrapartum period at the time of delivery, or postpartum via breast-feeding. Of these, intrapartum transmission at the time of delivery is thought to be the most common. HIV infection does not cause any specific congenital abnormalities, but there is an increased risk of spontaneous abortion. The overall risk to the fetus of HIV transmission is estimated to be between 15% and 40% for each pregnancy, with increasing risk in subsequent pregnancies for each HIV-positive fetus born. Increased risks of antepartum transmission include increased maternal viral load or high viremia during early infection; advanced maternal clinical disease as evidenced by low CD4$^+$ counts; and breaks in the placental barrier. Increased risks of intrapartum transmission include high maternal viral load at the time of delivery, prolonged ruptured membranes (more than 4 hours), infant exposure to blood/secretions, abruptio placentae, infant prematurity, and the presence of coinfections. The rate of HIV perinatal transmission is reduced with the use of antiretroviral therapy during pregnancy and during the first months of the infant's life. Currently, worldwide, 1800 children are infected with HIV daily, with most infected perinatally.[1]

In the United States, those at greatest risk of HIV infection include (1) MSM; (2) IVD who share needles or syringes; (3) sexual partners of those in high-risk groups, particularly heterosexual women; and (4) infants born to infected mothers. These are the areas that require preventive education and practices. Since the introduction of multiple drug therapy against HIV, the number of patients diagnosed with and dying from AIDS has declined in the United States. However, the number of HIV-infected persons continues to increase despite prevention education. The CDC estimates that up to one quarter of the people who are infected with HIV in the United States may be unaware that they are infected. Approximately 10% to 11% of all HIV cases involve people older than age 50, representing 15% of the total number of AIDS cases. The death rate in the older AIDS population is higher than in the younger AIDS population.

Heterosexual intercourse with infected partners, contaminated blood, and prenatal or perinatal transmission are the major routes of transmission of HIV in Africa, South and Southeast Asia, and developing countries.[1] In these countries an equal proportion of males and females are infected. The major risks for HIV transmission in third world countries include multiple sexual partners, sex with prostitutes, history of other sexually transmitted diseases, and genital lesions or abrasions of any kind.

Routine social contact with people who are HIV positive does not increase one's risk of HIV infection. For example, using public restrooms, swimming in public swimming pools, touching or hugging someone who is HIV positive, and eating with community utensils or in restaurants are safe practices. One cannot get HIV infection from insects such as mosquitoes.

Exposure to HIV does not mean that one will contract HIV or AIDS, and it does not mean rapid progression. The interacting forces between viral and host factors influence whether an individual will contract HIV infection, particularly the amount and virulence of the virus and the host's response by T-cell–mediated cytotoxicity or by cytokines. In studies of hemophiliacs who received tainted blood products, 10% to 25% of the individuals evaded infection. The risk of acquiring HIV also varies within populations owing to genetic difference that either increase or decrease susceptibility to the infection.

Researchers have identified an HIV resistance allele or deletion mutant of the *CCR5* gene in certain people.[12,13] When inherited from both parents, the mutant *CCR5* gene appears to protect individuals from infection even after multiple exposures. When only one gene is inherited, the progression to AIDS tends to be slower. The gene is not equally distributed among people. Persons of Caucasian-American and Caucasian-European descent have the highest number of mutant allele genes, and Native American, African, and East Asian people have the lowest number of mutant alleles.[12,13] Researchers have also found that stromal-derived factor (also known as pre-B–cell growth-stimulating factor) can downregulate cell factors important for HIV binding to lymphocytes (CXCR4) on cells effectively blocking HIV-1 infection.[14] Another recent study found that people who have fewer genes encoding CCL3L1, a potent HIV-blocking protein that interacts with CCR5, were more susceptible to HIV infection and had more rapid progression to AIDS.[15] Depending on the population, each additional CCL3L1 copy lowered the risk of acquiring HIV by between 4.5 and 10.5%.[15]

Prevention of Transmission

Because effective management of HIV is expensive and cure not yet possible, prevention is essential. However, one-time exposure to information or a single message is usually less successful than programs that teach prevention skills and reinforce positive behavior. The primary way to prevent transmission is to use safe sex practices. Safe sex practices include the following: abstaining from sex, using a condom (barrier protection) during sexual intercourse, avoiding multiple sexual partners, and knowing the HIV status of all sexual partners. In a recent study of young men who tested positive for HIV, 77% mistakenly believed that they were not infected or were at low or very low risk.[16] It is important that education regarding safe sex practices be tailored to appropriate age groups, ethnicity, culture, and sexual preference. Health care provider-patient dialogue may be helpful, but most providers do not use the visit to speak about HIV protection, leading to a missed opportunity.

Spermicides such as nonoxynol 9 or C31G do not inactivate HIV and other sexually transmitted microorganisms. No studies on the effects on the transmission of HIV of using progestins such as levonorgestrel (Norplant) or medroxyprogesterone (Depo-Provera), the diaphragm, or oral contraceptives suggest any benefit. The early use of antepartum and intrapartum antiretroviral therapy and avoidance of breast-feeding can prevent maternal-child HIV infection.

HIV infection in drug users can be prevented with the use of sterile needles via improved access to clean needles and avoidance of dirty or shared needles. Such intervention includes needle/syringe exchange programs for IVDs and cleaning of dirty needles with bleach before use. When using bleach, the user must rinse out all blood first; then fill the needle and syringe with full-strength bleach at least three times for 30 to 60 seconds.

Medical and health care personnel are at risk through occupational exposure to blood and body fluids. Self protection through the use of standard precautions can decrease risk by reducing exposure. Health care providers should carefully wash their hands before and immediately after patient contact. It is essential to wear disposable gloves for any actual or potential contact with blood or body secretions, when handling items contaminated with blood or body fluids, when performing fingersticks or heelsticks, or when the health care provider has scratches or cuts on the hand.

Gowns or plastic aprons, masks, goggles, or face shields should be worn to protect the face and clothing when there is risk of splashes and airborne droplets of blood or body fluids. Protective gear should be changed between patients. Careful prevention of parenteral exposure when using needles or other equipment should be emphasized. Needles and sharp implements should be disposed of in rigid, puncture-proof containers. Such implements should not be bent, broken, or recapped before disposal. In combative patients who must have blood drawn or injections given, careful use of humane and limited restraint devices may be necessary to prevent injury to the involved health care workers. Resuscitation bags and masks should be readily available to minimize the need for mouth-to-mouth procedures.

Unfortunately, accidents necessitating the development of postexposure prevention protocols do occur. If a health care worker sustains an injury with significant exposure to HIV-infected blood or body fluids such as a needlestick, a postexposure prevention protocol should be initiated as soon as possible and preferably before 72 hours. Such protocols involve the administration of two reverse transcriptase inhibitors. The length of administration of the agents depends on multiple factors and may be 4 weeks or longer. If the HIV-infected patient has advanced disease, the health care worker should take a protease inhibitor in addition to the reverse transcriptase inhibitors. This same protocol has been advocated for use as postsexual exposure prophylaxis.

KEY POINTS

- HIV disease is a primary immunodeficiency disorder caused by viral infection of CD4+ cells. It is a major health concern because it causes chronic, severe, long-term disease in the first world and very poor prognosis and death in the third world when therapy is not available.
- HIV types 1 and 2 are retroviruses that primarily infect CD4+ lymphocytes and macrophages. HIV-1 is the primary causative virus infecting persons in Central Africa, the United States, Europe, and Australia.
- HIV is acquired primarily through sexual transmission via semen and vaginal and cervical secretions; through parenteral transmission via blood, blood products, and contaminated needles/syringes; and through perinatal transmission from an infected mother to her infant antepartum, intrapartum, and postpartum via breast milk.

- HIV is known to be present in but is not believed to be transmitted via urine, saliva, tears, cerebrospinal fluid, amniotic fluid, feces, or aerosols.
- Those at greatest risk of HIV infection include homosexual and bisexual men, IVDs who share needles or syringes, sexual partners of those in high-risk groups, and infants born to infected mothers.
- The use of safe sex practices, such as condoms, and the use of safe parenteral practices, such as sterile needles/syringes, decrease the risk of infection.
- Exposure to blood and body fluids of infected individuals through skin, mucous membranes, and accidental needlesticks is the primary risk factor for health care workers. The universal use of standard precautions decreases the risk of infection.
- After significant accidental exposure to HIV-infected blood or body fluids, it is recommended that health care workers take postexposure antiretroviral medication as soon as possible after exposure and as needed for 4 weeks after exposure.

ETIOLOGY

HIV Structure

HIV is an RNA retrovirus that causes a defect in cell-mediated immunity that may progress to AIDS. The viral RNA must be converted to DNA before the viral genes can be expressed to make copies of the RNA virus. Like other retroviruses, HIV differs from DNA viruses in that the RNA genome cannot replicate without undergoing conversion into DNA.

HIV consists of a core or nucleocapsid containing two strands or chains of RNA, protein, and enzymes surrounded and protected by a spherical lipid bilayer viral envelope that is 0.0001 mm across. Between the envelope and core is a protein layer called p17. The nucleocapsid or core is composed of a protein called p24. Within the nucleocapsid, the two strands of RNA compose the HIV genome (Figure 12-2). The HIV

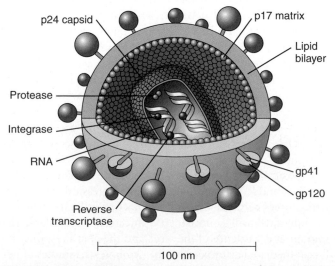

FIGURE 12-2 HIV particle showing the p24 capsid protein surrounding the two strands of viral RNA.

genome consists of at least nine genes. The *gag* gene encodes the core antigen proteins. The *pol* gene encodes reverse transcriptase proteins. The *env* gene encodes the viral envelope protein glycoprotein gp160, which is split into two fragments, gp120 and gp41, by cellular protease.

Several other genes have been identified, including *tat, rev, nef, vif, vpr,* and *vpu.* These genes are primarily regulatory genes. The *tat* gene encodes proteins that regulate HIV replication and can accelerate HIV viral protein production. It is controlled by *tat*-binding protein. The *rev* gene encodes proteins that regulate viral messenger RNA expression. Rev proteins inhibit regulatory proteins allowing the transport of HIV RNA from the nucleus. Rev proteins also enhance viral structural gene production. The *vif* (virion infectivity factor) gene appears to increase the ability of the virus to infect other cells. It suppresses the human protein (CEM 15) that inhibits HIV-1.

The HIV genome contains all the information regulating the virus's structural format and growth during its lifecycle. The enzymes within the core also are very important because they facilitate the conversion of RNA to DNA. This conversion is the means of information transfer with this virus. The enzymes include reverse transcriptase, integrase, and protease. Reverse transcriptase is composed of two associated enzymes called polymerase and ribonuclease. Reverse transcriptase is the unique enzyme in HIV that allows the virus to copy RNA into DNA. Protease is a complex enzyme that works as a "molecular scissors." It splits the other viral components by a process known as autocatalysis. Immature virions containing inactive gag/pol, a long precursor protein, are released in the plasma where they are cleaved by protease into smaller active units. Protease also clips p55, the core gag viral protein precursor, into smaller molecules and is needed to facilitate final mature viral assembly for HIV to be infectious.

The viral envelope consists of a membrane derived from the host cell. Viral glycoprotein studs protruding from the cell membrane make it look like a studded ball (Figure 12-3). Gp120 and gp41 are the two HIV envelope proteins that cover the viral particle surface. Gp120 is the most external and distal part of each "stud," whereas gp41 is the bridge that holds it onto the virion surface. The surface envelope also contains other cell surface proteins derived from the host cell containing adhesion molecules. Although the viral particle (virion) is roughly spherical, great diversity is found in size and shape, such as comet-shaped virions and virions with tails.

HIV Binding and Infection

Once inside the body, HIV particles are attracted to cells with receptors on their surface called CD4. The HIV envelope protein gp120 specifically binds to the CD4 receptor. Which CD4+ cells are attracted to the virus changes over time. The CD4 receptor is found on many types of cells, including T cells, microglial cells, monocyte-macrophages, follicular dendritic cells, immortalized B cells, retinal cells, Langerhans cells in the skin, bone marrow stem cells, cervical cells, bone marrow-derived circulating dendritic cells, and enterochromaffin cells in the colon, duodenum, and rectum. Of these cells, the CD4+ T-helper/inducer cells and macrophages are most often implicated and involved in the process of infection. Figure 12-4 illustrates a group of HIV-infected CD4+ cells imaged by scanning electron micrography. Initially the virus is attracted to macrophages and the virus is called "M tropic."[12] Later the virus becomes either dual tropic and affects both macrophages and T cells, or "T tropic" and affects primarily T cells.[12]

Usually T cells are infected before the onset of symptoms. CD4+ T cells are composed of two subsets: T-helper-1 (T_H1) and T-helper-2 (T_H2). The T_H1 subset produces interferon-γ and interleukin-2 (IL-2). The T_H2 subset produces IL-4, IL-6, and IL-10. Of these two subsets, the one that is markedly decreased in advanced disease is T_H1.

However, CD4 alone is not sufficient for fusion of the virion and host cell. A number of important coreceptors called chemokines are necessary for the virus to gain entry into cells. These important chemokine coreceptors must be present for the virion to fuse with the host cell. The chemokine called CCR5 must be present for the HIV particles to bind to the CD4+ cells in early infection during the M-tropic phase, and another chemokine receptor called CXCR4 must be present in later infection during the dual or T-tropic phase.[7] These coreceptors, particularly CCR5, are essential for HIV infection.

FIGURE 12-3 Schematic view of a retrovirus particle. The core is surrounded by an envelope that is derived from host membranes enriched with viral glycoproteins (gp120, gp41). Interaction of the envelope glycoproteins with a host-encoded cell surface receptor (CD4) is shown.

FIGURE 12-4 Scanning electron micrograph (low magnification) of a population of HIV-infected lymphocytes. (Courtesy Centers for Disease Control and Prevention, Atlanta.)

Since 1996 when the coreceptors were first discovered, a number of other coreceptors have been identified, including APJ, CCR2b, CCR3, CCR8, CCR9, CX3CR1, CXCR4, GPR1, GPR15, STRL33, US28, and V28.[17] The function of most of these coreceptors is unknown. It is hypothesized that some of the coreceptors may be needed for various strains of HIV, for HIV infection in babies and children, or for infection of the brain and nervous system.

The gp120 portion of the virion envelope must combine with the first receptor, CD4, and then change shape by refolding. In the second shape, it combines with the second receptor, either CCR5 or CXCR4, to fuse with the cell. Once the HIV particle is bound to both the CD4 receptor and the chemokine receptor on the host cell, gp41 implants itself in the cell membrane (Figure 12-5). This sequence of events causes the viral particle and the cell to fuse. The core of the virus is then injected into the cytoplasm of the host cell and infection is produced.

Once in the cytoplasm, a single-stranded DNA copy is made by reverse transcriptase from the viral RNA. Using the single-stranded DNA as a template, DNA polymerase copies it to make a second DNA strand and destroys the original RNA strands. The accuracy of DNA transcription is poor, with mutations occurring frequently. This tendency to mutate makes HIV highly resistant to antiviral medications.

Once formed, the new viral DNA migrates to the cell nucleus. Inside the nucleus, integrase splices the viral DNA, called HIV **provirus,** into the host cell's DNA. Once in the host cell's DNA, the viral DNA (provirus) is replicated together with the host cell's DNA during every cell division. Now the viral DNA is permanently part of the host cell's DNA (Figure 12-6). To cause further infection, the viral RNA must leave the nucleus and migrate to the cell surface. Rev proteins along with a human protein called CRM1 aid in the process of blocking the inhibition on transporting the viral RNA proteins from the cell nucleus. A human RNA helicase enzyme,

FIGURE 12-5 Early HIV infection, M tropic. In HIV infection, the virus must bind both a CD4 receptor and a coreceptor to fuse with the host cell. In the M-tropic phase, the key coreceptor is CCR5.

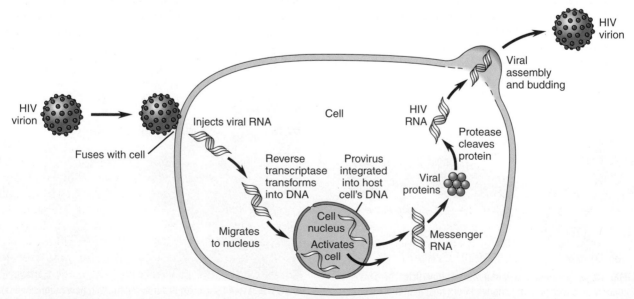

FIGURE 12-6 HIV lifecycle. A schematic representation from the time of initial HIV fusion with a host cell, integration into the host cell's DNA, and ending with the replication of a new virion.

DDX3, helps to straighten HIV's twisted strand of RNA before threading it through a small pore in the nucleus.[18]

When CD4+ cells decline, the diversity of CD4+ cells is affected. With antiretroviral therapy, the naïve T cells that can respond to new infections persist in low numbers despite an increase in memory T cells. Therefore, persons with HIV who are receiving antiretroviral therapy can respond to old but not new infections. This phase is indicative of deterioration in immune system function despite any temporary increase in CD4+ cell counts and decreased viral load from antiretroviral therapy.

Several researchers hypothesize that HIV-infected T cells can directly infect non-CD4–bearing epithelial cells.[19] From electron micrographic studies, they believe that infected T cells attracted to inflamed vaginal epithelial cells attach to the cells. The HIV virions are released from the bottom of the T cells, migrate through the cellular gap between the cells, and are ingested by the epithelial cells.[19] An opposing view is that infection in the presence of inflammation is caused by the presence of CD4+ macrophages or Langerhans cells that lie directly under the epithelial cells.[19] Macrophages may release tumor necrosis factor or other cytokines stimulating other antigen-presenting cells, or T cells.[20]

KEY POINTS

- HIV is an RNA virus known as a retrovirus. It must undergo reverse transcription within infected cells to form viral DNA.
- HIV consists of a nucleocapsid containing two strands of RNA, protein, and enzymes surrounded by a spherical lipid bilayer viral envelope. At least nine genes make up the HIV genome.
- The HIV genome contains all the information regulating the virus's structural format and growth, including the conversion of RNA to DNA.
- The enzymes needed to convert HIV RNA to DNA include reverse transcriptase, integrase, and protease.
- HIV gains access to CD4+ cells by attaching to the CD4 receptor on the cell surface. Viral envelope protein gp120 and coreceptor chemokines such as CCR5 or CXCR4 mediate attachment.

PATHOGENESIS

Effect of HIV on Immune Cells at the Cellular Level

The hallmark of HIV infection is the decrease in CD4+ T-helper/inducer lymphocytes. T-helper/inducer cells are necessary for appropriate immune responsiveness because they are the cells that mediate between the antigen-presenting cells and other immune cells such as B cells and other T cells. CD4+ lymphocytes are characterized by the presence of the CD4 receptor.

Macrophages have CD4 receptors and act as both targets and reservoirs for HIV. As the infection progresses, they become more functionally impaired with defective phagocytosis and chemotaxis, abnormal antigen presentation, and abnormal cytokine production. They also contribute to the T-cell decline by increasing CD4+ cell death.

Humoral immune system dysfunction is also present, although the effect of HIV on antibody-producing B cells is more poorly understood. There are some changes in B-cell structure as well as function. B-cell numbers usually remain normal. However, the B-cells are progressively dysfunctional with overproduction of nonessential antibodies, as well as failure to respond appropriately to normal immune system signals.[21] Immunoglobulin G_1 (IgG_1) and IgG_3 levels are usually elevated, causing hypergammaglobulinemia. IgM levels are elevated in early infection, whereas IgA levels are elevated in late infection. Despite these elevations, the responsiveness to polysaccharide (bacterial cell wall) antigens that require CD4+ cell activation of B cells is decreased. Immune complexes are increased, and B-cell differentiation and response to antigens are decreased. Autoantibodies, especially against erythrocytes, platelets, lymphocytes, neutrophils, nuclear proteins, myelin, and spermatozoa, occur either in association with disease processes (e.g., HIV-associated thrombocytopenia) or spontaneously. HIV antibodies are produced, but they are ineffective against the disease. Also B-cells have an increased risk of cell death through apoptosis.[21]

The envelope glycoproteins (gp120 and gp41) on the surface of virions are prime targets for antibody production. However, the success of the HIV infection is such that these viral envelope glycoproteins are not very antigenic or immunogenic. Several researchers believe that this property is due to the large amount of carbohydrate on the surface of gp120. Within the human body, high-carbohydrate substances look like "self" to the immune system. Therefore, the virus "hides" under the cover of the glycosylation. Another factor that allows HIV envelope proteins to escape the early antibodies is the way that gp120 and gp41 are bound together. Although the interface between gp120 and gp41 is an area that is highly immunogenic, the gp120 and gp41 molecules are noncovalently bonded together. Early antibodies cannot bind the assembled, functional envelope glycoprotein complex. Later, neutralizing antibodies are effective against the complex, but by that time the infection is well established.

Viral Production and Cell Death

Another key element in the success of HIV infection is that HIV replicates prolifically from the onset of infection. The high level of infection is characterized by a high level of virion turnover (HIV replication) and a high level of CD4+ cell turnover (host cell death). At least 10 billion HIV particles are produced and destroyed each day, with a plasma virus half-life of 6 hours and an acutely infected T-cell half-life of 1.1 days. The infection is successful because it generates so many virions that it overwhelms the body's defenses. HIV-infected CD4+ cells undergo viral budding to generate and produce new virions (Figure 12-7). In children infected with HIV, the virus is more aggressive and leads more rapidly to immune system dysfunction.

FIGURE 12-7 Scanning electron micrograph of HIV-1-infected CD4+ lymphocytes showing virus budding from the plasma membrane of the lymphocytes. (Courtesy Centers for Disease Control and Prevention, Atlanta.)

Despite its prolific virion generation, the production of new virus is variable between individuals and dependent on the host's cellular activity, as well as the interaction between HIV regulatory genes (*tat, nef, rev, vif*). In some cells, such as T cells, HIV can lie dormant until activated. In other cells, such as macrophages and monocytes, RNA copies of HIV are consistently being made and released, initially without destruction of the host cell. Other host cellular factors that influence viral production of HIV include inhibition by other proteins or low concentrations of initiation factors.

Sheehy et al have identified a human protein, CEM15, that is part of the innate antiviral defense system in the body.[22] It can repress or inhibit HIV-1 if present in the cell. However, not all cells produce CEM15. Those that do are called *nonpermissive* whereas those that do not are called *permissive*. *Vif* is needed by the HIV-1 virus to overcome the defense that CEM15 provides in nonpermissive cells. In permissive cells, the virus can reproduce freely without restriction whether *vif* is present or not.[22]

Several features associated with long-term survival of patients with HIV have been identified. Most importantly, long-term survivors have a low viral load and strong CD8+ killer T-cell activity. This CD8+ killer T-cell activity suppresses viral replication and thus slows progression of the disease, especially in the early stages of the disease. It is also thought that a strong immunologic defense preserves the manufacture of CD4+ T cells that especially recognize and react to HIV. If this ability is lost, these cells may not regenerate, even with treatment. Finally, the longer presence of a weaker strain of HIV, particularly when the virus is primarily attracted to macrophages (or M-tropic), may lead to longer survival.

The process of building new virus particles begins within the host cell's DNA. Segments at the end of the viral genome tell the host cell to make RNA copies of the viral DNA. Some of the genes direct the host cell to manufacture viral envelope proteins (gene name: *env*) and enzymes (gene name: *pol*),

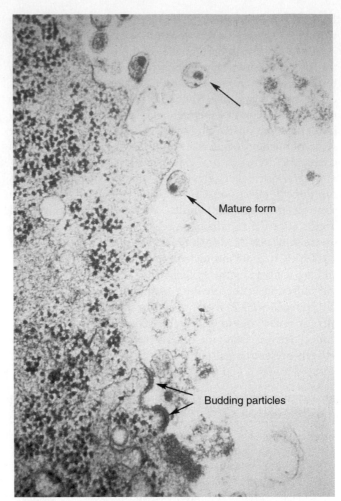

FIGURE 12-8 HIV-1/lymphadenopathy virus found in a hemophiliac patient with AIDS. Virus particles range in size from 90 to 120 nm. Viral budding and the production of new virions are facilitated by protease. (Courtesy Centers for Disease Control and Prevention, Atlanta.)

whereas other RNA strands become future genetic material (gene name: *gag*).

The assembly of new virus particles, called **virions,** occurs at the cell membrane. Three proteins are produced and migrate to the cell periphery, attach to the cell membrane, and cause the viral material to bud out from the membrane. The protein-cutting enzyme protease separates the envelope proteins from enzymes and RNA genetic material and binds the viral core (Figure 12-8). Therefore, the completed virion has a host cell membrane from which the envelope proteins gp120 and gp41 stick out like spikes.

During early infection, HIV is widespread throughout the body, with detectable viremia and viral seeding of lymph tissues. This process progresses to an asymptomatic phase of infection with little detectable virus in the blood. During this period, seeded HIV replicates in the lymph nodes and gradually destroys lymph tissue during the infection. The infection in the lymph nodes is more intense with higher HIV RNA expression in comparison with the low to moderate plasma concentration of virus. This phase of the infection is associated with chronic lymphadenopathy and a persistent, gradual decline in CD4+ T-cell numbers. The lymphadenopathy is caused by a vigorous immune response against HIV infection. After destruction of lymph tissue, viremia again occurs. It is hypothesized that the destroyed lymph nodes are no longer capable of removing or holding virus, thus allowing viral escape into the bloodstream. Even with combination antiretroviral treatment, HIV-1 can persist for several years in pools of resting, memory CD4+ T cells. This pool of memory CD4+ cells remains lost or unavailable to immune system attack inasmuch as such cells lack HIV surface antigens because they carry only provirus DNA.

Once viral production starts or restarts in activated cells, death of the infected cells may occur by a variety of mechanisms. Cells may die from the accumulation of intracellular viral DNA or the loss of normal cellular protein synthesis because of the infection. Most methods of host cell death involve the envelope protein gp120 or immune processes. Cross-linking of CD4 and gp120 can trigger automatic preprogrammed T-cell death (**apoptosis**). CD4 and gp120 cross-linking can also cause the cell to stop dividing and decreases the cell's ability to fight new infections—a condition called **anergy.** Profuse viral production with multiple CD4 receptors in close proximity can rip holes in the cell membrane and cause host cell death (Figure 12-9). Multiple virion buds with gp120 on their surfaces attach to the surrounding host cell membrane CD4 receptors. This attachment causes tearing of the host cell membrane with subsequent cellular edema and death.

Another process of cell death occurs when multiple uninfected cells become fused together with infected cells by the virus. This mass of cells, called a **syncytium,** can lead to a large number of cell deaths from a single event. When the virus affects primarily T cells (or T-tropic cells), there is a greater tendency to produce syncytia and cause even faster depletion of T cells.

New research shows that myeloid-derived dendritic cells (MDDCs) can aid in the formation of syncytia when they patrol the body, engulfing the virus and presenting the virus to T cells.[23] HIV is engulfed by the MDDCs, which are highly mobile. When an MDDC interacts with a T cell, there is a concentration of virus, receptor, and coreceptor that facilitates both infection of CD4+ T cells and the development of a syncytium.[22]

Cell death can occur when the immune system makes antibodies to the viral envelope protein. When gp120 is shed, it binds to uninfected CD4 receptors. Then the immune system attacks the uninfected but antibody-coated cells with the complement system or killer T cells and kills the uninfected host cells via antibody-dependent cellular cytotoxicity or natural killer cell cytotoxicity.

Cell death can be secondary to a type III hypersensitivity reaction. Gp120 and gp41 have characteristics similar to those of major histocompatibility class (MHC) antigens-carbohydrate-covered protein. In this case, immune cells may fail to recognize the difference between gp120 and "self MHC markers"

FIGURE 12-9 High magnification of a CD4+ lymphocyte infected with HIV-1. Note the large number of budding HIV virions, which can lead to host cell death by membrane tearing or syncytium formation. (Courtesy Centers for Disease Control and Prevention, Atlanta.)

and attack normal cells as nonself. This phenomenon causes the destruction of large numbers of T cells. Cells also may be affected by T-cell–mediated cytotoxicity or by cytokines and inflammation resulting from infection.

Progression of HIV Infection from Seroconversion to AIDS

HIV disease is an infectious state that progresses over time to AIDS with its many manifestations. AIDS is a syndrome, not a disease, which means that the virus can express itself in many ways. No one symptom typifies either HIV infection or AIDS. However, groups of signs and symptoms are useful in staging progress of the infection.

Once the HIV virion enters the body, it rapidly replicates (Figure 12-10). It is present in the blood and cerebrospinal fluid but is not detected by usual laboratory tests because no antibodies have formed yet. Usually no symptoms are present. It is a time of rapid virus replication. The person is infectious but does not know it.

Seroconversion occurs when sufficient antibodies are detected in the blood, usually between 3 weeks and 6 months

FIGURE 12-10 Progression of HIV infection. The clinical stages of HIV disease correlate with a progressive spread of HIV from the initial site of infection to lymphoid tissues throughout the body. The immune response of the host temporarily controls acute infection but does not prevent the establishment of chronic infection of cells in the lymphoid tissues. Cytokine stimuli induced by other microbes serve to enhance HIV production and progression to AIDS. CTLs, Cytotoxic T lymphocytes. (From Abbas AK et al: *Cellular and molecular immunology*, ed 6, Philadelphia, 2007, Saunders, p 481.)

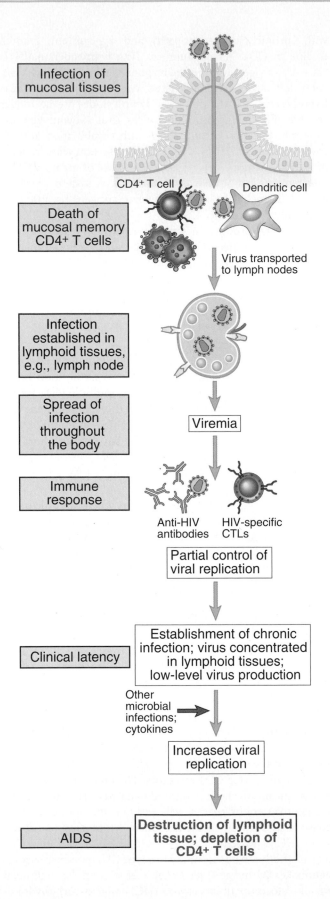

after exposure but rarely as long as 14 months. At the time of seroconversion, the person experiences signs and symptoms of acute retroviral syndrome or primary HIV infection. Up to 80% of people newly infected with HIV have flulike symptoms that can mimic other viral illnesses.[24] At this time, the symptoms of primary HIV infection include flulike or mononucleosis-like symptoms, such as fever, chills, headaches, nausea, vomiting, fatigue, weakness, arthralgias, sore throat, stiff neck, photophobia, irritability, and rash. The rash is not the same in everyone and may be maculopapular, vesicular, or urticarial. Encephalopathy may even develop. The CD4+ T-cell count is greater than 400 cells/μL. The number of white blood cells, including lymphocytes, is decreased except for an increased number of CD8+ T cells. Platelets also are decreased. The person has an elevated erythrocyte sedimentation rate. During this period, the HIV count in genital fluids is high and the individual is very infectious. Then, after 1 to 4 weeks, the symptoms disappear. However, HIV is still present and the person continues to be infectious throughout the rest of the course of the infection.

After this period of seroconversion, the patient experiences the clinical latency period, which may last for longer than 10 years (range: 3 to 12 years). Antiviral immune activity is ongoing. Production of virus is maintained or stabilized at a set level. The person feels well but may experience some chronic lymphadenopathy (enlargement of lymph nodes for more than 3 months) or mild general symptoms, including lack of energy, weight loss, frequent fevers, and sweats. The CD4+ T-cell count is greater than 400/μL. Stabilization of the serum level of virus at a certain point is attributable to the antiviral response, the number of CD4+ cells, and the virulence of the HIV strain. During this period of asymptomatic or mild infection, however, the provirus is producing large numbers of virions and destroying the body's immune system. Up to 2 million viral particles can be produced daily. The key point is that although the infection is clinically asymptomatic or mildly symptomatic, the virus is active, not latent.

Immediately after the latency period of infection, a period of rapid virus production occurs for up to 18 months. During this time, a persistent and continuous drop in the CD4+ T-cell count to less than 400 is taking place. The antiviral innate immune activity is less effective as the viral load (level of virus in the blood) increases.

As the viral loads increase and the immune system declines, the patient enters the stage of symptomatic, chronic

HIV infection. At this time, the patient goes from partially responding to skin testing (partial anergy) to complete anergy with no response to skin testing. Severe viral or fungal infections of the skin and mucous membranes develop. Oral and genital herpes simplex infections, including shingles or candidiasis (yeast) infections usually develop, as well as oral hairy leukoplakia. The patient also may have persistent skin rashes or flaky skin, short-term memory loss, or pelvic inflammatory disease that does not respond to treatment. Children tend to have growth delays or get sick frequently. The person may develop cytomegalovirus (CMV) infection, Epstein-Barr virus infection, or both, as well as other opportunistic infections.

A patient usually is not diagnosed with AIDS until the CD4$^+$ T-cell count is less than 200/μL. The person typically has one or more opportunistic infections, including PCP, *Toxoplasma gondii*-associated neural toxoplasmosis, cryptosporidiosis (gastroenteritis), and *Mycobacterium tuberculosis*. The person usually has one or more tumors or cancers, including Kaposi sarcoma (a connective tissue skin cancer), lymphomas, or cancer of the rectum or tongue. General symptoms of opportunistic infections include coughing or shortness of breath, difficult or painful swallowing, mental symptoms such as confusion, forgetfulness, or lack of coordination, seizures, severe and persistent diarrhea, fever, vision loss, nausea, abdominal cramps, vomiting, weight loss, extreme fatigue, and severe headaches.

Disease progression in infants and children is determined by when the child became infected (timing), viral load, the child's immune response, and viral virulence. In general, children with HIV progress more rapidly than adults. Most children fall into two distinct groups: those with rapid disease progression and those with slower disease progression. In those with rapidly progressing disease, symptoms develop within the first 6 months of life, sustained decreases in CD4$^+$ cell counts are noted, and AIDS develops within the first 2 years of life. Early aggressive treatment in perinatally infected infants may slow disease progression and prolong immune function. Children with AIDS generally get the same opportunistic infections as adults and also may get severe forms of common childhood diseases, such as conjunctivitis, otitis media, and tonsillitis.

CDC HIV Classification System

The CDC HIV classification system is a simple matrix classification system for adults and children and is the preferred method of staging. In this system, CD4$^+$ T-cell counts are linked with clinical symptomatology. The CDC has defined three CD4$^+$ T-cell categories and three clinical categories that are mutually exclusive. The CD4$^+$ T-cell categories define three T-cell ranges. In category 1, the CD4$^+$ T-cell count is greater than or equal to 500/μL; in category 2, the CD4$^+$ T-cell counts range from 200 to 499/μL; and in category 3, the CD4$^+$ T-cell count is less than 200/μL.[25]

In adults, the clinical categories are labeled A through C. Category A includes a variety of clinical conditions, such as asymptomatic, persistent generalized lymphadenopathy and a history of or current acute HIV infection with accompanying illness. Category B includes conditions that are secondary to impaired cell-mediated immunity, such as candidiasis (oral or vaginal), fever, persistent diarrhea, oral hairy leukoplakia, shingles, idiopathic thrombocytopenic purpura, pelvic inflammatory disease, listeriosis, and peripheral neuropathy. Category C includes conditions that are listed in the AIDS surveillance case definition. An individual in category C will remain in this category. The CDC classification matrix is shown in Table 12-1. An HIV-positive person with a CD4$^+$ count less than 200/μL or a category C AIDS indicator condition is diagnosed with AIDS. A list of AIDS indicator conditions is shown in Box 12-1.

In children, category N is an asymptomatic phase with no signs or symptoms of disease. Category A is a mildly symptomatic phase with two or more of the following conditions: lymphadenopathy, hepatomegaly, splenomegaly, dermatitis, parotitis, or recurrent/persistent upper respiratory infection, sinusitis, or otitis media. Category B is a moderately symptomatic phase in which the child exhibits some opportunistic infections as a result of impaired cell-mediated immunity or impaired bone marrow function. These conditions include anemia, thrombocytopenia, bacterial meningitis, pneumonia or sepsis, candidiasis, thrush, CMV, diarrhea, hepatitis, herpes simplex infection, herpes zoster infection, leiomyosarcoma, nephropathy, persistent fever, toxoplasmosis, and varicella. The category C phase is severely symptomatic with AIDS. The revised pediatric HIV classification system based on age-specific CD4$^+$ T-cell counts and percentage is shown in Table 12-2.

TABLE 12-1

CDC HIV/AIDS Classification Matrix

	Clinical Categories		
CD4$^+$ T-Cell Categories	A Asymptomatic Acute HIV	B Symptomatic, Not (A) or (C)	C AIDS Indicator
≥500/μL	A1	B1	C1
200-499/μL	A2	B2	C2
<200/μL AIDS indicator T-cell count	A3	B3	C3

From Centers for Disease Control and Prevention: 1993 Revised classification system for HIV infection and expanded surveillance case definition for AIDS among adolescents and adults, *MMWR Morb Mortal Wkly Rep* 41(RR-17):1-6, 1993.

BOX 12-1

Conditions Indicative of AIDS in HIV-Infected Persons

- Candidiasis of bronchi, trachea, or lungs
- Candidiasis, esophageal
- Cervical cancer, invasive*
- Coccidioidomycosis, disseminated or extrapulmonary
- Cryptococcosis, extrapulmonary
- Cryptosporidiosis, chronic intestinal (greater than 1 month's duration)
- Cytomegalovirus disease (other than liver, spleen, or nodes)
- Cytomegalovirus retinitis (with loss of vision)
- Encephalopathy, HIV-related
- Herpes simplex: chronic ulcer(s) (greater than 1 month's duration); or bronchitis, pneumonitis, or esophagitis
- Histoplasmosis, disseminated or extrapulmonary
- Isosporiasis, chronic intestinal (greater than 1 month's duration)
- Kaposi sarcoma
- Lymphoma, Burkitt's (or equivalent term)
- Lymphoma, immunoblastic (or equivalent term)
- Lymphoma, primary, of brain
- *Mycobacterium avium complex* or *M. kansasii,* disseminated or extrapulmonary
- *Mycobacterium tuberculosis,* any site (pulmonary* or extrapulmonary)
- *Mycobacterium,* other species or unidentified species, disseminated or extrapulmonary
- *Pneumocystis carinii* pneumonia
- Pneumonia, recurrent*
- Progressive multifocal leukoencephalopathy
- Salmonella septicemia, recurrent
- Toxoplasmosis of brain
- Wasting syndrome owing to HIV

From Appendix B of the 1993 Revised Classification System for HIV Infection and Expanded Surveillance Case Definition for AIDS Among Adolescents and Adults, MMWR 41(RR-17).
*Added in the 1993 expansion of the AIDS surveillance case definition.

DIAGNOSTIC TESTING

To diagnose HIV infection, laboratory tests such as the enzyme-linked immunosorbent assay (ELISA) and the Western blot are used to detect the presence of HIV antibodies, which in infected persons are found in measurable quantities. The ELISA test result is positive for HIV antibodies if the blood or oral mucosal transudate of an infected person reacts with the surface antigen of a killed HIV virus. The ELISA test uses purified viral proteins placed on plastic beads or in multiwell trays. When the test serum or oral mucosal transudate from a patient comes in contact with the purified viral proteins, an antigen-antibody reaction occurs. Antihuman antibody added to the reaction can be detected colorimetrically and indicates whether any antigen-antibody compounds have formed. This test is highly sensitive (more than 99%) and specific (more than 99%) in high-risk populations. For the test to be specific, however, it must be performed with both HIV-1 and HIV-2 viral antigens.

When the ELISA test result is positive, a second test, the Western blot, is used to confirm the presence of HIV antibodies. The Western blot test uses an expensive process called *electrophoresis,* so usually it is used only as a confirmatory test. This test identifies specific antibodies against the HIV protein antigens. The specificity of this test in combination with the ELISA is greater than 99.9%. The problem with this additional testing is that the patient must wait up to 1 to 2 weeks for confirmation.

A new, rapid, fingerstick-based HIV assay is being used as well: OraQuick Rapid HIV-1 Antibody test results can be obtained in about 20 minutes. However, positive results must be confirmed by a Western blot. It is also important to remember that false-negative tests can occur during the initial period of HIV infection before seroconversion.

Testing neonates for HIV is difficult because of maternal transmission of IgG antibodies against HIV. These passive maternal antibodies cross the placenta and can last as long as 15 months. Therefore, the best method to determine whether

TABLE 12-2

Revised Pediatric HIV Classification Matrix*

Immune Categories	CD4+ T-Cell Counts		
	<12 mo	1-5 yr	6-12 yr
Category 1: No suppression	>1500/μL >25%	>1000/μL >25%	>500/μL >25%
Category 2: Moderate suppression	750-1499/μL 15%-24%	500-999/ml 15%-24%	200-499/μL 15%-24%
Category 3: Severe suppression	<750/μL <15%	<500/μL <15%	<200/μL <15%

From Foundation for Care Management, Dunn JM, editor: Special considerations in treating HIV positive children, *HIV Hotline* 7(5):7-12, 1997.
*Based on age-specific CD4+ count per microliter and percentage.

a neonate has HIV is to culture the virus from blood and peripheral tissue.

MONITORING THE PROGRESSION OF HIV

An important test for monitoring HIV disease status is the absolute CD4+ cell count. The CD4+ count is a specific indicator of disease progression of HIV to AIDS. As the CD4+ cell count declines, the risk of progression to AIDS and the development of opportunistic infections and malignancies increase. Highly virulent communicable diseases can still occur when the CD4+ count is high. However, when the CD4+ cell count drops below 200 cells/μL, the number and severity of low-virulence diseases and opportunistic infections increase. It is at this level that many patients begin taking prophylactic medications to prevent opportunistic and other infections. Also used is the CD4+ lymphocyte percentage, which is more stable and has less variation over time. When the CD4+ lymphocyte percentage is less than 20%, the risk of developing AIDS is higher.

Another useful test is the plasma viral load, which indicates the amount of viral replication and the effectiveness of therapy and helps predict disease progression. The level of HIV RNA in plasma is the strongest predictor of outcome over time. When the plasma HIV RNA content is low, the risk of disease progression declines. The plasma viral load helps the clinician to assess the effectiveness of various therapies and is the basis for initiating more aggressive therapies to decrease the viral load. Usually, HIV RNA levels should drop after the onset of therapy and by 6 months should be undetectable in the plasma. The viral load assay counts copies of HIV RNA in 1 ml of plasma and is either a reverse transcriptase polymerase chain reaction (RT-PCR) or a branched DNA (bDNA) assay. Because each virion contains two strands of RNA, the actual virion level is half the HIV RNA counted. Tests are currently sensitive to 50 copies per milliliter. If the patient continues to have disease progression despite treatment, genotypic and phenotypic resistance tests may be ordered. These tests are expensive and have not been standardized or approved by the Food and Drug Administration. Genotypic testing identifies viral mutations, whereas phenotypic testing identifies the concentration of antiretroviral drug needed to inhibit viral replication in culture medium. Ideally this testing would allow the best drugs to be given to the patient.

Another common test is an anergy test or a delayed hypersensitivity (type IV) test for such organisms as *M. tuberculosis* or mumps or measles virus. In early HIV infection, these skin test results are normal. However, in advanced cases, the patient will have no response to testing because of the loss of macrophage and CD4+ T-cell functioning.

Two other tests may be used: β_2-microglobulin and p24 antigen. β_2-Microglobulin is a cell surface protein that indicates macrophage stimulation. Levels greater than 3.5 are associated with rapid progression of the disease. P24 antigen is indicative of active HIV replication and confirms the diagnosis of HIV infection. It is positive before seroconversion and may be used

before the ELISA result would be positive. It is also elevated in later stages of the disease, a period when antibody testing may be unreliable.

Other laboratory and diagnostic tests can assist in the identification, monitoring, and treatment of persons infected with HIV, including a complete blood cell count (CBC), a chemistry panel or screen, and chest radiographs. These tests are routinely used to detect infections and changes in a patient's physiologic status (Box 12-2). The CBC detects the development of anemia (as a result of infection or chronic illness or secondary to therapy) and neutropenia and thrombocytopenia, which may occur in advanced disease.

KEY POINTS

- HIV virions are attracted to cells with CD4 receptors such as T cells, microglial cells, monocyte-macrophages, follicular dendritic cells, immortalized B cells, retinal cells, Langerhans cells in the skin, bone marrow stem cells, cervical cells, bone marrow-derived circulating dendritic cells, and enterochromaffin cells in the colon, duodenum, and rectum.
- The hallmark of AIDS is a decrease in CD4+ cells, including T-helper lymphocytes and macrophages. B-cell responsiveness is decreased because of dependence on T-helper cell cytokines.
- The key element in HIV infection is the high level of virion production and the high level of CD4+ cell death.
- CD4+ cell death occurs via several mechanisms. Cross-linking of CD4 receptors by viruses may result in T-cell death, apoptosis, or anergy. Virions may cause the linkage of infected and uninfected cells, followed by cell fusion and death. B cells may form antibodies against infected T cells. Viral budding may cause excessive loss of cell membrane.
- Laboratory testing for HIV is accomplished by using either the ELISA or the Western blot test. Usually the ELISA test is performed first. If it is positive, the Western blot test is performed to confirm the presence of specific antibodies against HIV protein antigens.
- HIV is an infectious disease that progresses to AIDS and is characterized by different clinical manifestations at each stage. Individuals move through the stages at different rates.
- Flulike symptoms and the formation of anti-HIV antibodies (seroconversion) characterize the early stage of viral seeding. Next, symptoms of early immune dysfunction are present, including lymphadenopathy, fever, and night sweats. A surge in viral production and a drop in the CD4+ lymphocyte count follow this stage.
- In the later stages, CD4+ counts continue to fall and the person is subject to a number of opportunistic infections and tumor formation. An HIV-positive individual is diagnosed with AIDS when the CD4+ T-cell count is less than 200/μL or when a category C AIDS indicator condition is present.
- Children often have rapidly progressive disease, with onset of AIDS between ages 4 and 8 years.

CLINICAL MANIFESTATIONS

HIV affects all body systems, particularly the cutaneous, pulmonary, gastrointestinal (GI), neurologic, and ocular systems. GI manifestations develop in nearly all persons with HIV. Pulmonary and cutaneous symptoms develop in approximately 50% to 75% of all persons with HIV, and neurologic symptoms develop in 50% to 60%. Box 12-3 outlines the common agents of infection in patients with AIDS.

Systemic Manifestations

As implied in the classification systems presented earlier, the course of HIV infection parallels the functioning of the immune system. As immune function declines, the number of opportunistic infections and malignancies increases. The most significant systemic symptom is malnutrition or wasting syndrome. This is defined as unintended, involuntary loss of greater than 10% body weight due to HIV infection.[26] There is major muscle wasting, associated with the weight loss and malnutrition. The malnutrition is the result of a combination of factors, including an elevated metabolic rate, chronic inflammation, malabsorption, anorexia, decreased intake of food, and the effect of multiple opportunistic insults. In addition, tumor necrosis factor, which increases the breakdown of fat and decreases the synthesis of fatty acids, is elevated in HIV/AIDS patients with secondary infections. In Africa, HIV is known as "slim disease" because of the wasting. Malnutrition is a leading cause of death among AIDS patients in the United States. Prevention is key, involving assessment of nutritional parameters as well as nutritional education and exercise. A patient's body mass index, weight, calorie and protein intake, prealbumin, serum albumin, and triglyceride levels are frequently measured.

To prevent or delay the wasting process, several medications are being evaluated, including ketotifen, thalidomide, testosterone, anabolic steroids such as nandrolone (Deca-Durabolin) and oxandrolone, dehydroepiandrosterone, and a combination of medications. Ketotifen is a tumor necrosis factor inhibitor and antihistamine that is used because its side effects are appetite stimulation and weight gain. Thalidomide, which is also a tumor necrosis factor inhibitor, appears to be effective against wasting syndrome and increases fat-free mass.[15] Oxandrolone is an anabolic steroid designed specifically to promote weight gain, particularly lean body mass. Megestrol acetate (Megace), a progestational agent, and dronabinol, an antiemetic, are often used to decrease nausea and increase appetite. Use of human growth hormone (somatropin, Serostim) may also be given to increase lean body mass.[26]

Vitamins A, C, and E; the B vitamins; zinc; selenium; sulfur amino acids; and other antioxidants are also used. The use of these nutrients can prevent the up-regulation of inflammatory cytokines and thereby decrease inflammation. High-protein, high-calorie meals and snacks are recommended, along with nutritional supplements. High-fat foods should be avoided because they increase diarrhea, as can lactose-containing foods. Nutritional supplements (Ensure, Nitrofuel, Sustacal Plus, Advera, Lipisorb), which provide both protein and calories, are full of nutrients and can be formulated either with or without lactose and with or without medium-chain triglyceride oil (a more easily digested fat). Total parenteral nutrition as well as gastrostomy or jejunostomy tube feedings are reserved for those with severe malnutrition and GI manifestations.

Gastrointestinal Manifestations

GI manifestations are nearly universal in persons with HIV. In fact, the GI tract may be the major target organ in HIV infection. HIV may or may not be a significant direct pathogen in the GI tract. The major HIV GI complication is chronic diarrhea. The diarrhea, often watery or bloody, causes malabsorption and consequently severe weight loss. This complex of HIV-related malnutrition causes muscle loss leading to increased morbidity and risk of death. Antiemetics and antidiarrheals are often useful in controlling symptoms.

Whenever chronic diarrhea or other GI symptoms develop in a patient with HIV, it is important to determine the cause. GI symptoms can be the result of multiple opportunistic infectious agents and are rarely the result of tumors occurring in the GI tract. Some of the most significant infectious agents are viruses such as CMV and herpes simplex; fungi such as *Candida;* bacteria such as *Salmonella, Shigella, Clostridium difficile, Chlamydia trachomatis,* and *Campylobacter;* and parasites such as *Giardia, Isospora, Entamoeba histolytica,* and *Cryptosporidium.* GI symptoms include chronic diarrhea, oral candidiasis, anorexia, nausea, vomiting, mucous membrane ulcers, retrosternal pain on swallowing, abdominal pain, and low serum vitamin B_{12}. Ulcerations occur as a primary manifestation or secondary to the inflammation. Treatment involves the use of disease-appropriate antimicrobials, depending on the offending organism.

A common cause of diarrhea is the protozoa *Cryptosporidium.* It infects the intestinal epithelium lining the microvillus border. This organism is transmitted via water, food, animals, and other humans. The onset of cryptosporidiosis is generally acute and associated with explosive diarrhea within 4 to 14 days after infection. In nonimmunocompromised persons, the symptoms last up to 2 weeks, but in immunocompromised persons, the diarrhea and symptoms can persist indefinitely. Cryptosporidiosis causes nausea, vomiting, severe watery nonbloody diarrhea, abdominal pain, cramping, electrolyte disturbances, and dehydration. It is characterized by massive amounts of highly infectious diarrhea (more than 15 to 20 L).

Diagnosis is made by stool examination for ova and parasites and by bacterial culture and sensitivity. Antibiotic treatment is not always effective, but antimicrobials such as the macrolides have been used. In the acute phase, some patients must be given intravenous hydration for support. Thereafter, increased oral intake, along with low-residue, high-protein, high-calorie diets, and loperamide (Imodium) tablets, up to 16 to 18 per day, are used to help control the diarrhea.

Prevention of *Cryptosporidium* infection is most important. Preventive activities include routine testing of well water, using water filters at home, avoiding ice or unfiltered tap water both at home and in restaurants, and avoiding fresh fruit or vegetables rinsed with unfiltered water. Fruit and vegetables can be washed in bottled water, filtered water, or water with 20 drops of 2% iodine per gallon.

Oropharyngeal and esophageal *Candida albicans* infections occur in most patients with HIV at some time during the course of their disease. Most often, oral *candidiasis* is pseudomembranous in type, with white plaques that bleed when removed and leave an erythematous surface. *Candida* oropharyngeal lesions produce pain and discomfort during eating, loss of taste, and **xerostomia.** *Candida* esophageal lesions cause pain with swallowing, dysphagia, and a feeling of "throat swelling." These lesions lead to worsening wasting syndrome. Management of oropharyngeal *candidiasis* includes the use of topical antifungal agents (such as clotrimazole or nystatin) in a suspension or lozenges, whereas management of esophageal *candidiasis* includes antifungal agents by oral or intravenous routes of administration. Side effects include an unpleasant taste and GI side effects, with inconvenient dosing regimens (up to six times per day).

Pulmonary Manifestations

Pulmonary manifestations are a major source of morbidity and mortality in AIDS patients. Pulmonary diseases include opportunistic pneumonias, such as those associated with *P. jiroveci (carinii),* CMV, *M. tuberculosis, Histoplasma,* or *Staphylococcus,* as well as parenchymal lung diseases including Kaposi sarcoma, lymphoma, nonspecific pneumonitis, and adult respiratory distress syndrome. Infection with *M. tuberculosis* occurs in 4% of patients with HIV and is particularly problematic in third world countries where the tuberculosis comorbidity rates are up to 50%. Patients with HIV have an increased risk of being infected with a multidrug-resistant type of tuberculosis organism.

PCP is the most common initial opportunistic infection in AIDS. However, the incidence of *P. carinii* has decreased with the use of prophylaxis. *P. carinii* was classified as a protozoa, but recent research indicates that it is fungal and it was renamed *P. jiroveci.* This organism prefers alveolar environments and infects most people during early childhood. Children usually have *Pneumocystis* antibodies by 2 to 3 years of age, but the organism does not cause disease in immunocompetent persons. With immunodeficiency and $CD4^+$ cell counts below 200/μL, *Pneumocystis* becomes activated and causes PCP. The nonspecific symptoms of PCP resemble those of early HIV infection, including flulike fever, fatigue, and weight loss. The major pulmonary feature of PCP is severe hypoxemia with a PaO_2 less than 60 mm Hg. The most

FIGURE 12-11 *Pneumocystis jiroveci (carinii).* A chest radiograph shows bilateral lower lobe interstitial infiltrates. (Courtesy Dr. Paula Karvalho, Veterans Administration Medical Center, Boise, Idaho.)

severe pulmonary symptoms are similar to those of adult respiratory distress syndrome (Figure 12-11). These symptoms include decreased phospholipid (surfactant) production, early dry cough, dyspnea, tachypnea, chest discomfort, and marked pallor and cyanosis.

Diagnosis of PCP is by chest radiography, and organisms are identified in sputum with Wright-Giemsa stain. Sputum is induced by using 3% saline via nebulizer, and patients must avoid brushing their teeth, using mouthwash, or eating for 8 hours prior. Other tests that can be performed include bronchoalveolar lavage or biopsy and gallium scanning. Treatment usually includes the use of intravenous or oral trimethoprim-sulfamethoxazole (Bactrim, Septra) and parenteral and aerosolized pentamidine (NebuPent, Pentam 300).

To prevent PCP infections by prophylaxis, patients with $CD4^+$ counts of less than 200 cells/μL are given trimethoprim-sulfamethoxazole tablets either daily or three times per week to prevent the recurrence of infection. This is a very effective suppressive therapy that prevents life-threatening PCP. If patients cannot tolerate it, substitutes include aerosolized pentamidine, dapsone, or dapsone with pyrimethamine and leucovorin.

Mucocutaneous Manifestations

Mucocutaneous manifestations occur both early and late in the course of HIV infection. The viral exanthem of HIV infection, associated with seroconversion, is an erythematous, fine maculopapular rash found on the face, trunk, and

FIGURE 12-12 Herpes zoster in an HIV-infected individual. (From Callen JP: *Color atlas of dermatology*, Philadelphia, 1993, Saunders, p 382.)

arms. HIV viral exanthem is a self-limited manifestation that occurs in 40% to 60% of all HIV-infected persons. It is generally seen within 2 to 6 weeks of exposure and lasts up to 1 to 2 weeks. It is associated with mild pruritus, fever, malaise, night sweats, fatigue, pharyngitis, weight loss, diarrhea, headache, and lymphadenopathy.

Other mucocutaneous manifestations may be allergic, infectious, or neoplastic in origin. Cutaneous symptoms depend on the cause and location. Allergic causes may be the result of drug reactions or the development of seborrheic dermatitis, psoriasis, or skin-colored papular eruptions.

Viral causes include herpes simplex, varicella zoster, Epstein-Barr virus, and human papillomavirus (Figure 12-12). The development of genital warts (condylomata acuminata) from human papillomavirus is an early symptom of HIV disease in women. For mucocutaneous viral infections, acyclovir (Zovirax) or vidarabine is the recommended antiviral agent.

Oral hairy leukoplakia is an example of an oral mucous membrane viral infection thought to be caused by Epstein-Barr virus or human papillomavirus. Oral hairy leukoplakia is characterized by white to gray thickened, raised lesions with vertical folds, corrugations, or "hairs" that form on the tongue and buccal mucosa. Usually they form on the sides of the tongue (Figure 12-13). These lesions cannot be removed or scraped off with a tongue blade, which differentiates this infection from oral candidiasis or thrush. These lesions only occur as the $CD4^+$ count declines. They are not usually painful.

In HIV-infected persons, herpes simplex viruses 1 and 2 cause the formation of large groups of painful vesicles on an erythematous base; these vesicles rupture and crust and become large, ulcerative, and occasionally necrotic. They are chronic, painfully persistent, and usually occur on the genitalia, digits, and perianal or perioral areas. Herpes simplex virus may produce protein that enhances the replication of HIV.

Bacterial infectious causes of mucocutaneous manifestations include *M. avium* or *Staphylococcus aureus. Staphylococcus* is a common bacterial skin infection in patients with HIV associated with folliculitis, furuncles (boils), or bullous impetigo. Occasionally sepsis may occur. Treatment includes topical

FIGURE 12-13 Oral hairy leukoplakia, a manifestation of Epstein-Barr virus infection in HIV-infected individuals. (From Callen JP: *Color atlas of dermatology*, Philadelphia, 1993, Saunders, p 377.)

FIGURE 12-15 HIV-associated Kaposi sarcoma in the macular stage. (From Callen JP: *Color atlas of dermatology*, Philadelphia, 1993, Saunders, p 55.)

FIGURE 12-14 *Candida albicans* in an HIV-infected person. (From Callen JP: *Color atlas of dermatology*, Philadelphia, 1993, Saunders, p 386.)

FIGURE 12-16 HIV-associated Kaposi sarcoma in the nodular stage. (From Callen JP: *Color atlas of dermatology*, Philadelphia, 1993, Saunders, p 379.)

antibiotics, use of an antibacterial soap, and systemic antibiotics, either oral or intravenous, as needed. Abscesses usually are surgically opened and drained.

Fungal skin infectious agents include *Candida, Cryptococcus,* or *Histoplasma* (Figure 12-14). Vaginal candidiasis is the most common early skin symptom in HIV-positive women. Other infectious agents include parasites such as the mites that cause scabies. Treatment is with topical, oral, or intravenous antifungal or antiparasitic agents, depending on the severity of the infection.

Neoplasms can also occur, including Kaposi sarcoma, squamous cell carcinoma, basal cell carcinoma, or cutaneous lymphomas. Kaposi sarcoma is an AIDS-related malignancy that affects the skin and mucous membranes, lymphatics, and other internal organs. It is one of the few neoplasms indicative of immune system dysfunction.

Before 1981, Kaposi sarcoma was rarely found in the United States, except in elderly men of Mediterranean or Eastern European Jewish ancestry. With the AIDS epidemic, it is now found in young, formerly healthy persons who live in the United States, are homosexual or bisexual, and in whom AIDS develops. It rarely occurs in other high-risk groups or in women in the United States. Kaposi sarcoma is the most common tumor found in HIV-infected homosexual men.

The skin lesions of Kaposi sarcoma are individual tumors that begin as flat or macular subcutaneous patches. The patches initially range from light pink to deep purple and are painless, nonblanching, and nonpruritic (Figure 12-15). The lesions evolve from patches into thickened plaques or large nodules that may change to brown over time, especially in darkly pigmented persons. They may occur anywhere on the body, although they usually begin on the head—the face, eyelids, conjunctivae, pinnae, scalp, or buccal membranes (Figure 12-16). Lesions range in size from a few millimeters to coalesced patches covering large areas of the body. The lesions are highly vascular but do not bleed excessively. The lesions also may occur internally in either the lungs or intestines in approximately 40% of patients.

Kaposi sarcoma is managed with radiation therapy and medications, including chemotherapy. Surgery is rarely indicated except to remove large, uncomfortable lesions. Radiation therapy is used primarily for oral or cutaneous lesions. Mitotic inhibitors (e.g., Vinblastine, vincristine) or immunomodulators (e.g., interferon-α) have been useful chemotherapeutic agents in the management of Kaposi sarcoma. Smaller lesions may be managed with intralesional injections of a mitotic inhibitor. Persons with Kaposi sarcoma who have the best prognosis tend to have limited disease with no other opportunistic infections and no weight loss, fevers, or night sweats.

Gynecologic Manifestations

Gynecologic manifestations of HIV disease are marked by persistent monilial vaginitis secondary to *C. albicans*, cervical dysplasia, and neoplasia, as well as pelvic inflammatory disease. Cervical dysplasia affects 40% of HIV-infected women (Figure 12-17). Cervical dysplasia has no symptoms, but the cell changes can lead to neoplasia. Therefore, either Papanicolaou smears or colposcopic examinations should be performed every 6 months to detect cervical cancer early in HIV-positive women. Cervical cancer is particularly aggressive in women with HIV. Pelvic inflammatory disease is more common in HIV-positive women. Pelvic inflammatory disease is caused by the same type of organisms, including *C. trachomatis,* and is managed with the same antibiotics as used in non-HIV–infected women.

Neurologic Manifestations

Neurologic manifestations are often the reason that people with HIV seek treatment. HIV invades the neurologic system early in the course of its infection. It infects glial cells, endothelial cells, and brain macrophages. Central and peripheral nervous system manifestations may be caused by HIV infection directly or may be the result of infectious agents causing meningitis or neoplasms causing space-occupying lesions. Opportunistic infectious agents affecting the neurologic system include *Toxoplasma* and *Cryptococcus*. A variety of peripheral neuropathies can result from HIV infection directly, although some may be caused by herpes zoster infection.

HIV encephalopathy (AIDS dementia complex, subacute, or AIDS encephalopathy) is the most common neurologic encephalopathic manifestation. HIV encephalopathy is caused directly or indirectly by HIV infection or viral products, cytokine-related cellular damage, and the competition or interference between gp120 and neuroleukin, a nerve growth factor. This disorder can affect both adults and children. It occurs when other opportunistic infections begin to appear later in the disease process.

HIV encephalopathy is a syndrome characterized by progressive cognitive impairment or subcortical dementia. In other words, the patient is alert but demented and confused. Computed tomography shows diffuse atrophy in the cerebral cortex, widened sulci, ventricular enlargement, and shrinking of the basal ganglia. Cerebrospinal fluid analysis shows elevated protein and abnormal IgG levels. Symptoms may wax and wane over the course of a day, with intermittent periods of lucidity and confusion.

The cognitive neurologic symptoms associated with HIV encephalopathy include inattentiveness, confusion, forgetfulness, loss of concentration, slower verbal response, headache,

FIGURE 12-17 Cervical dysplasia. Women with AIDS require more frequent monitoring because cervical dysplasia commonly occurs and progresses rapidly.

apathy, and inability to complete or perform complex tasks. These symptoms can progress to global dementia associated with marked memory impairment and disorientation. Before the motor strength declines, the patient may forget time, place, person, and activities, which can lead to safety issues such as wandering, leaving appliances on, and forgetting to take medications.[27] The associated focal motor deficits include slower motor responses, clumsiness, weakness, loss of balance, handwriting changes, and slurred speech. As HIV encephalopathy progresses, the patient's motor strength declines with subsequent large muscle weakness that causes difficulty walking and moving. Associated generalized symptoms consist of fever and mild metabolic acidosis. Behavioral symptoms include personality changes, social withdrawal, depression, poor hygiene and grooming, lack of insight, apathy, agitation, and, less commonly, anxiety and hyperactivity. In children, head circumference does not increase with age.

As the disorder progresses, the neurologic symptoms become more severe. Ataxia, hypertonia, tremors, and incontinence appear. The person may be alert but cognitively impaired, mute, and paraplegic. Hemianopia (partial blindness), myoclonus, and seizures also may develop. The person may become comatose and lethargic with other systemic dysfunctions. Management of HIV encephalopathy includes treatment with antiretroviral agents. Other treatment includes coordinating home and environmental safety and patient/family support. Other medications, such as neuroleptics, are occasionally used to control agitation.

Ocular Manifestations

Ocular manifestations of HIV infection may be of infectious or noninfectious origin. Noninfectious causes of ocular problems include HIV retinopathy and malignancy. Infectious causes include bacteria such as *Treponema pallidum* (syphilis) and *Staphylococcus;* fungi including *Candida, Cryptococcus,* and *Histoplasma;* protozoa such as *Pneumocystis* and *Toxoplasma;* and viruses such as herpes simplex and CMV.

The most severe type of ocular infection is CMV retinitis. After an insidious onset, ocular CMV precipitates perivascular hemorrhages, fluffy exudates, and vasculitis in the retina. The CMV retinal infection leads to destruction and necrosis of the retina, with resulting blindness. Treatment of CMV retinitis involves the use of anti-CMV agents (e.g., ganciclovir) intravenously and the use of oral anti-CMV agents for prophylaxis. An intraocular sustained-release anti-CMV implant is also available for the management of acute and chronic CMV retinitis.

HIV-associated retinopathy causes the development of cotton-wool spots and microvascular retinal changes. Cotton-wool spots are small, indistinct white spots with associated hemorrhage. These changes are not as severe as CMV retinitis and may remit spontaneously.

Manifestations in Other Systems

A study by Bozzette et al in 2003 demonstrated no increased risk for cardiovascular or cerebrovascular events in patients with HIV.[28] However, the 2006 Strategies for Management of Antiretroviral Therapy (SMART) study, found that cardiovascular events, hyperglycemia, and hypertriglyceridemia and lipidemia were the result of HIV infection and not just caused by medications for HIV.[29] This study found that cardiovascular and renal disease were higher in HIV patients not treated effectively with antiretroviral medications. Therefore, evidence is increasing that immunosuppression and HIV viremia are involved in the pathophysiology of cardiovascular disease, and that HIV therapy may help protect patients from HIV-induced cardiovascular disease.[29]

Renal impairment can also occur with HIV infection. HIV can affect the kidneys and cause AIDS-associated nephropathy (AIDS-related glomerulopathy or HIV-associated nephropathy [HIVAN]), drug-induced ischemia, and renal failure. Hematologically, individuals with HIV have anemia, thrombocytopenia, and granulocytopenia.

Liver dysfunction is also a problem in persons with HIV because there is an increased risk of concomitant hepatitis C or B (HCV/HBV) infection. This comorbidity of HIV/HCV or HBV causes increased mortality from end-stage liver disease. Also compounding liver dysfunction in patients with HIV is the effect of multiple medications on the liver itself.

HIV-related endocrine dysfunction is usually associated with changes in hormone secretion secondary to the stress response; destruction of endocrine tissue from infection, cancer, or inflammation; or the use of pharmacologic agents. The adrenal gland is the organ most affected by HIV infection. Adrenal secretion of cortisol may be elevated with stress. Injury to the adrenal gland rarely leads to frank cortisol deficiencies. Most endocrine dysfunction is subtle, with few overt manifestations. Triiodothyronine, thyroxine, and thyroid-binding globulin levels may be elevated.

Rheumatologic manifestations of HIV infection are varied and include osteoporosis and osteopenia, along with musculoskeletal infections, such as infectious arthritis and osteomyelitis, which are caused by a decrease in the number of T cells. In patients with musculoskeletal infections, the most common organisms involved are *S. aureus, Streptococcus*

pneumoniae, C. albicans, Mycobacterium kansasii, and *Mycobacterium avium-intracellulare.* Other manifestations are caused by immune-mediated arthritis, such as Reiter disease, psoriatic arthritis, and undifferentiated spondyloarthropathy syndromes, or to disorders occurring as a direct result of the immune response to HIV, including polymyositis, vasculitis, and immune complex diseases related to the production of autoantibodies. The increasing incidence of osteopenia and osteoporosis in the HIV population is significant.[30] The actual cause for this increase is unclear but may be related to anti-retroviral therapy. Treatment includes using biphosphonate medications and selective estrogen receptor modulators.

Manifestations in Children

Children with HIV become symptomatic much faster than adults—usually within their first year of life. Because of the invasion of virus, children's growth and development are markedly affected, including physical growth retardation with failure to thrive, impaired intellectual development, and impaired motor functioning with decreased coordination. The infant develops normally until the virus begins its nervous system invasion. After that time, neurologic impairment is characterized by development of weakness, loss of previously accomplished developmental milestones, hypotonia, or hypertonia.

More serious bacterial and viral infections also develop in children who undergo repeated bouts of communicable diseases such as chickenpox. Extensive candidiasis without any relationship to antibiotic therapy may be an early symptom. Respiratory problems, including the development of PCP, are common.

Because lactose intolerance is common in these children, soy formulas are often used. Dairy products may be introduced into the diet gradually, as tolerated. Children need particular attention to their diet; increased calories and protein, as well as nutrient-rich snacks such as raisins and peanuts for growth and development, are advisable.

KEY POINTS

- All body systems are affected by HIV.
- Early HIV infection is characterized by fever, chills, headaches, nausea, vomiting, diarrhea, fatigue, weakness, arthralgia, sore throat, stiff neck, photophobia, irritability, and rash.
- The most significant systemic symptom is malnutrition or wasting, which is due to a combination of factors, including an elevated metabolic rate, chronic inflammation, malabsorption, anorexia, and the effect of multiple opportunistic insults.
- GI symptoms occur frequently in patients with HIV. Symptoms include diarrhea caused by *Cryptosporidium* or other agents, ulceration, and candidiasis, as well as multiple opportunistic infections.
- Pulmonary symptoms include opportunistic pneumonias (particularly PCP), tuberculosis, and adult respiratory distress syndrome.

- Mucocutaneous symptoms occur both early and late in the course of HIV infection. One of the first symptoms is the viral exanthem that occurs during the primary infection. Other manifestations may be allergic; infectious, such as candidiasis or herpes, human papillomavirus, and Epstein-Barr virus infections; or neoplastic, such as Kaposi sarcoma.
- Neurologic manifestations include peripheral neuropathy, encephalopathy with dementia, headache, apathy, and focal deficits.
- Gynecologic manifestations include persistent monilial vaginitis, cervical dysplasia, and pelvic inflammatory disease.
- Ocular manifestations include HIV-associated retinopathy, CMV retinitis, malignancy, and a variety of infectious causes.
- Children with HIV have growth and development problems, including impaired physical growth, intellectual development, and motor functioning.

TREATMENT

Antiretroviral Therapy Recommendations

The goal of medication and therapeutic management of HIV/AIDS is to delay disease progression, avoid drug resistance, minimize clinical manifestations, and ultimately prolong survival. Drug management of HIV infection has evolved from monotherapy, or therapy with one agent, to the use of multiple medications, called ART (antiretroviral therapy) or highly active antiretroviral therapy (HAART). This polydrug therapy approach involves the administration of multiple antiretroviral agents. It provides better viral suppression, thereby decreasing viral load, increasing CD4 counts, and decreasing resistance for a longer period. The objective of HAART is to provide the greatest viral suppression for the longest time to prevent viral mutations. This approach makes good sense. If one drug blocks 90% of viral replication, the others may eliminate the rest of the resistant virions. However, even with HAART, complete viral eradication is not possible with current treatment strategies.

The most important HIV treatment trial of 2006, called the SMART study, looked at whether "life would be better, if not longer, for HIV-infected individuals if they could reduce their exposure to antiretrovirals."[29] The study randomized two groups, one with continuous antiretroviral therapy and the other with episodic antiretroviral therapy based on CD4[+] cell count.[29] In the episodic arm of the study, antiretroviral therapy was started when CD4[+] cells dropped to 250 cells/μL and stopped when CD4[+] cells increased to 350 cells/μL. The study aimed to determine if complications from HIV antiretroviral therapy itself, such as drug toxicity, caused more harm and death than opportunistic infections. The study sponsored by NIH and started in 2002 involved 33 countries and 5472 participants. What shocked everyone were the unanticipated study results: "Rather than protect patients, the withdrawal of HIV therapy increased the risk of death from any cause, including that of opportunistic infection. In addition, the rates of cardiovascular, hepatic and renal disease—which are often considered antiretroviral-related—were greater in the treatment interruption group."[29] In summary, continuous HIV therapy was found to be more beneficial than treatment interruption with prolonged drug treatment holidays.

HIV drug treatment failures are the result of HIV resistance, which is a widespread problem and concern. Failure of HIV drug treatment is usually caused by poor adherence to HAART, poor toleration of the drugs, prior exposure to single or multiple antiretroviral drug therapy, or counteracting interactions among the drugs used. It is easy to see why persons taking the multidrug regimen may fail to comply with nutritional and drug therapy because of the sheer volume of drugs to be taken in a day. A person infected with HIV may take up to 13 to 30 pills per day; he or she must also remember which ones should be taken with food or on an empty stomach and which ones cannot be taken together at the same time. In addition, some persons with HIV/AIDS may be demented because of the disease, homeless, or addicted to intravenous drugs, any of which limits their ability to adhere to the strict treatment regimens. Finally, some of the treatments for opportunistic infection or cancer involve many other drugs: intravenous, oral, and intracavital.

Current recommendations for antiretroviral therapy for HIV per Department of Health and Human Services (DHHS) Guidelines, October 2006, include starting therapy for anyone with AIDS-defining illness or severe symptoms at any CD4[+] count or viral load and for all asymptomatic HIV-infected persons with a CD4[+] cell count less than 200/μL.[31] The DHHS Guidelines suggest that for asymptomatic HIV-infected persons with a CD4[+] cell count less than 350/μL but more than 200/μL, therapy be offered with full disclosure of all pros and cons.[31] In asymptomatic HIV-infected persons who have high viral loads of 100,000 copies/mL and a CD4[+] cell count more than 350/μL some clinicians may choose to treat after discussion with the patient.[31] There is increasing evidence that using viral load with CD4[+] cell counts to make treatment decisions may be advisable. Early antiretroviral treatment seems to be better tolerated by patients and helps to prolong life. In patients with low HIV RNA plasma levels (less than 500 copies per milliliter) and high CD4[+] counts, therapy may be withheld and the patient reevaluated every 3 to 6 months.

Some of the current medications available to adults with HIV have not been recommended for children younger than 13 years. In the past, treatment was often delayed weeks or months before starting therapy. Now it is recommended that multidrug therapy be begun at birth; however, virion levels are usually not detectable for up to 2 weeks after birth. Therefore, some physicians recommend intensive therapy for all infants born to HIV-positive women even though the infant may not have infection. This controversial method is not universal but does take into consideration the rapid progression of infection in infants.

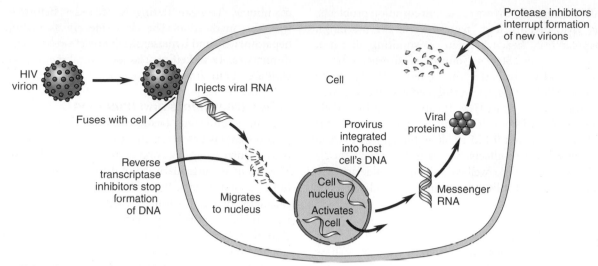

FIGURE 12-18 Antiretroviral therapy. The stages in the lifecycle of HIV in which antiretroviral therapy is effective are shown.

The major classes of antiretroviral medications are nucleoside reverse transcriptase inhibitors (NRTI) (nucleoside analogs), nonnucleoside reverse transcriptase inhibitors (NNRTIs) (nonnucleoside analogs), protease inhibitors, fusion inhibitors, and CCR5 antagonists. The current optimal combination of medications is multidrug therapy with two nucleoside analogs and one or two protease inhibitors (PIs) or two nucleosides and a nonnucleoside reverse transcriptase inhibitor, which is called *protease-sparing regimen*. Viral resistance to treatment is reduced by the complete suppression of virus (Figure 12-18). The fusion inhibitors and CCR5 antagonists are still new—the fusion inhibitors are used later as "salvage" therapy in combination with other therapies, whereas CCR5 antagonists are used for very early infections. In general, there are now a variety of antiretroviral medication choices available to meet patient needs, tolerance, and cost concerns.

Multidrug therapy retails at approximately $900 to $1400 per month. Patient compliance with complicated drug therapy that has many side effects is often variable. Virus resistance increases with treatment protocol noncompliance. In a 2006 study by Schackman et al, "the projected life expectancy from the time of entry into care for a hypothetical HIV-infected patient was found to be 24.2 years. The total lifetime care cost for a patient who initiated therapy at a CD4+ cell count of less than 350 cells/μL was $385,200 when rebates and other discounts of HIV medications were taken into consideration.... HAART cost made up 73% of the discounted cost..."[32] Therefore, the key appears to be encouraging patient compliance by tailoring medication regimens that improve tolerability and convenience.

Nucleoside Reverse Transcriptase Inhibitors

NRTIs resemble the natural substances used by the virus to build HIV DNA. NRTIs prevent HIV replication by preventing HIV DNA synthesis and have been found to slow progression of the disease. Nucleoside analogs include zidovudine, didanosine, zalcitabine, stavudine, lamivudine, and abacavir. All must be converted to an active state intracellularly. Class side effects include pancreatitis, bone marrow toxicity, peripheral neuropathy, and hepatic toxicity. They can also cause headache, nausea, vomiting, diarrhea, insomnia, malaise, myalgia, hypersensitivity reactions, lactic acidosis, and confusion. With this class of medications, liver function studies, CBC, and metabolic panel studies should be performed very frequently.

Of the NRTIs, the first is zidovudine (3-azido-3-deoxythymidine, AZT, Retrovir). Zidovudine is rapidly absorbed when taken orally and can penetrate the blood-brain barrier. Zidovudine is usually given to HIV-infected women during pregnancy as early as the 14th week of gestation. It is a pregnancy category C drug. Exactly how AZT blocks transmission to the fetus is unknown, but passive transplacental drug transport does occur. The long-term consequences of AZT use in pregnancy are unknown. Another medication in this class is lamivudine (3TC, Epivir), which is also used in patients with hepatitis B. It is approved for children and has the longest half-life. It is well absorbed and generally well tolerated. The combination of zidovudine/lamivudine (Combivir) is often used together. Didanosine (ddI, Videx) is the second oldest nucleoside analog. It is sometimes effective in patients resistant to zidovudine. It is usually combined with lamivudine as an alternative drug combination. Other combinations also may be used.

Nonnucleoside Reverse Transcriptase Inhibitors

NNRTIs also inhibit reverse transcriptase, but by a different mechanism. Drugs in this class include efavirenz (Sustiva), nevirapine (Viramune), and delavirdine (Rescriptor). These medications need not be converted intracellularly to be activated. The greatest benefit is that they are potent antiretrovirals. The biggest problem is that they affect the cytochrome P-450 system, which increases drug interactions and must be given cautiously. They can only be given in combination with other antiretrovirals. Class side effects include central nervous system effects (dizziness, drowsiness, concentration problems, insomnia, vivid dreams, and "hangover" in the morning), maculopapular rash, headache, nausea, vomiting, diarrhea, liver enzyme elevations, Stevens-Johnson syndrome, or hepatitis. Efavirenz (EFV, Sustiva) is the preferred NNRTI to be given with two NRTIs. It is a powerful medication that is very effective virologically against HIV. It can be given once daily in 600-mg capsules with meals or on an empty stomach. It is best taken between 6 and 9 PM to allow the patient to sleep through many of the side effects. Nevirapine is usually the alternative NNRTI and works well with the nucleoside analogs. It is important to monitor liver function, CBC, and metabolic panels frequently.

Protease Inhibitors

PIs attack at another phase in the viral life cycle. These medications inhibit the enzyme protease, whose action is to clip the viral protein precursors to the appropriate size. These precursors are essential for HIV maturation, infection, and replication. Protease inhibitor therapy is extremely expensive, with a retail price of approximately $6000 to $8000 per year. Protease inhibitors are never used as single agents because of the potential for a patient to develop resistance. They have poor CNS penetration and often cause lipid abnormalities and lipodystrophy, including development of "buffalo hump," increased abdominal girth, and increased breast size. They also interact with the cytochrome P-450 system and, as such, interact with many medications. Other side effects are related to plasma levels of the drug and can be severe, including asthenia, nausea, diarrhea, vomiting, anorexia, abdominal pain, taste perversion, and circumoral and peripheral paresthesias. Protease inhibitors include ritonavir (Norvir), atazanavir (Reyataz), fosamprenavir (Lexiva), lopinavir, indinavir, nelfinavir (Viracept), and amprenavir. There is also a combination medication of lopinavir-ritonavir (Kaletra). Ritonavir, atazanavir, and fosamprenavir are potent inhibitors of HIV that are found in high concentrations in serum and lymph nodes. Ritonavir and atazanavir must be taken with food to reduce side effects because they are often poorly tolerated. Liver function tests, CBC, and lipid panels should be monitored frequently.

Fusion Inhibitors

The fusion inhibitor enfuvirtide (Fuzeon, ENF) is the first of its class. These drugs work extracellularly by blocking fusion between the viral and target cell membranes. They are never used alone; rather they are used with other treatment regimens to decrease viral load. They are approved for use in children older than age 6.

CCR5 Antagonists

The CCR5 antagonist (Selzentry) is best suited for earlier infection when the CCR5 tropic virus (M-tropic phase) predominates (see Figure 12-5). At this phase, the key coreceptor is CCR5. This medication acts to block infection by blocking the coreceptor CCR5 and preventing HIV binding to the cell membrane. Tropism testing is necessary before treatment with this medication. The class side effects include strong hepatotoxicity and hypersensitivity reactions. Because of preliminary safety and efficacy issues, several medications in this class are still in clinical trials.

Other Treatments and Vaccines

Human granulocyte colony-stimulating factor (filgrastim [Neupogen]) is also being used to increase nonspecific immunity by increasing neutrophils in persons with neutropenia. This agent is particularly helpful in decreasing medication-induced neutropenia. It is given daily in a subcutaneous dose calculated by weight (usually 5 µg/kg). Epoetin alfa (erythropoietin) is also used to manage medication-induced anemia secondary to AZT use. The starting dosage is 8000 international units subcutaneously/week and may be increased to 48,000 international units/week until the hematocrit is 35% to 40%. An associated side effect is hypertension. Intravenous immunoglobulin can sometimes be used in HIV-infected children with T-cell counts above 200/µL. It can help to decrease the incidence of serious bacterial, minor bacterial, viral, and opportunistic infections.

Other studies are being conducted in an effort to find ways to rebuild the immune system. Researchers want to make sure that the T cells cloned after initiation of antiretroviral therapy will respond to both new and old infections. Currently, IL-2, a T-cell growth factor, is being infused intravenously or given subcutaneously intermittently for 5 days every 8 weeks. The strategy is effective in increasing populations of T cells, but it also increases the viral load transiently during treatment.

Prevention of HIV infection by active immunity conferred by vaccine is the ultimate goal of current research. This task is extremely difficult because of variability between strains of HIV and the frequency of HIV mutations. At this time, none of the vaccine trials have been successful and several have been stopped in phase II. A promising AIDS vaccine trial was stopped in September 2007 by Merck.[33] This vaccine focused on killer T cells rather than antibodies to HIV. However 24 of 741 patients actually became infected with HIV as a result of the vaccine.[33] Ongoing research is being carried out in an effort to quantify the effectiveness of other vaccines in stimulating both cellular and humoral responses to HIV.

KEY POINTS

- Management of HIV and AIDS includes the use of antiretroviral medications, including NRTIs, NNRTIs, and PIs.
- The current optimal combination of medications is triple therapy with two reverse transcriptase inhibitors and a PI.
- Efforts to stimulate immune function with peptide growth factors and the development of vaccines are under investigation.
- Aggressive treatment of opportunistic infections with appropriate antibiotics and antivirals is a large part of the treatment regimen.

SUMMARY

HIV is an RNA virus that primarily infects and destroys the immune system. In so doing, it destroys one of the basic foundations of human regulation and protection. HIV decreases the body's ability to fight organisms, opens the door to opportunistic infections, and allows neoplasms to emerge. HIV can infect anyone of any age. The ultimate intracellular pathogen, it slowly destroys the host while manufacturing billions of copies of itself. Study of this virus has improved our understanding of the immune system as well as of cellular function.

REFERENCES

1. UNAIDS: *Global AIDS epidemic continues to grow*, Geneva, 11/21/2006, WHO.
2. National Institutes of Health: *HIV infection and AIDS: an overview*, NIH, U.S. Department of Health and Human Services, 11/27/2007.
3. CDC: HIV/AIDS fact sheet: *HIV/AIDS among African Americans*, CDC, U.S. Department of Health and Human Services, June 2007.
4. CDC: *HIV/AIDS among men who have sex with men*, CDC, U.S. Department of Health and Human Services, June 2007.
5. CDC: *HIV/AIDS among women*, CDC, U.S. Department of Health and Human Services, June 2007.
6. Varmus H: Retroviruses, *Science* 240:1427-1435, 1988.
7. Gao F et al: Origin of HIV-1 in the chimpanzee *Pan troglodytes troglodytes, Nature* 397:436-441, 1999.
8. Balter M: Virus from 1959 sample marks early years of HIV, *Science* 279:801, 1998.
9. CDC: *Where did HIV come from?* CDC, U.S. Department of Health and Human Services, 11/27/2007.
10. Garry RF et al: Documentation of an AIDS virus infection in the United States in 1968, *JAMA* 260(14):2085-2087, 1988.
11. Lemey P et al: Tracing the origin and history of the HIV-2 epidemic, *Proc Natl Acad Sci USA* 10.1073/pnas.0936469100, 2003.
12. O'Brien SJ, Dean M: In search of AIDS-resistance genes, *Sci Am* 40(3):41-44, 1997.
13. Glass WG, et al: CCR5 deficiency increases risk of symptomatic West Nile Virus infection, *J Exper Med* (Published online January 17, 2006) DOI: 10.1084/jem.20051970. Accessed May 11, 2007.
14. Gonzalez E et al: The influence of CCL3L1 gene-containing segmental duplications on HIV-1/AIDS susceptibility, *Science* 307:1422-1424, 2005.
15. Winkler C et al: Genetic restriction of AIDS pathogenesis by an SDF-1 chemokine gene variant, *Science* 279:389-393, 1998.
16. MacKellar DA, Valleroy L, Secura G, et al: Unrecognized HIV infection, risk behaviors, and perceptions of risk among young men who have sex with men: opportunities for advancing HIV prevention in the third decade of HIV/AIDS, *J Acquir Immune Defic Syndr* 38:603-614, 2005.
17. Balter M: AIDS researchers negotiate tricky slopes of science, *Science* 280:825-826, 1998.
18. Yadavalli VSRK et al: Requirement of DDX3 dead box RNA helicase for HIV-1. Rev-RRE export function, *Cell* 199:381-392, 2004.
19. Cohen J: Women: absent term in the AIDS research equation, *Science* 269(5225):777-780, 1995.
20. Leslie M: Mast cells show their might, *Science* 317(5838):614-616, 2007.
21. Moir S et al: Decreased survival of B cells of HIV-viremic patients mediated by altered expression of receptors of the TNF superfamily. *J Exper Med* 200(5):587-599, 2004.
22. Sheehy AM et al: Isolation of a human gene that inhibits HIV-1 infection and is suppressed by the viral vif protein, *Nature* 48(6898):646-650, 2002.
23. McDonald D et al: Recruitment of HIV and its receptors to dendritic-cell-T-cell junctions, *Science* 300(5623):1295-1297, 2003.
24. Mahoney MR, Fogler JA: HIV infection: clues to timely diagnosis, *Consultant* 46(8):853-860, 2006.
25. Centers for Disease Control and Prevention: 1993 Revised classification system for HIV infection and expanded surveillance case definition for AIDS among adolescents and adults, *MMWR Morb Mortal Wkly Rep* 41(RR-17):1-6, 1992.
26. Wooland S: Wasting syndrome in HIV-AIDS patients: a guide to prevention and management, *Adv Nurse Practitioners* 9(9):42-48, 2001.
27. Coyne PJ, Lyne ME, Watson AC: Symptom management in people with AIDS, *Am J Nurs* 102(9):48-55, 2002.
28. Bozzette SA et al: Cardiovascular and cerebrovascular events in patients treated for human immunodeficiency virus infection, *N Engl J Med* 348:702-710, 2003.
29. El-Sadr WM et al: Strategies for Management of Antiretroviral Therapy (SMART) study group, *N Engl J Med* 355(22):2283-2296, 2006.
30. Greene MD: Older HIV patients face metabolic complications, *Nurse Practitioner* 28(66):17-28, 2003.
31. Department of Health and Human Services (DHHS) Panel on Antiretroviral Guidelines for Adults and Adolescents: *Guidelines for the use of antiretroviral agents in HIV-1 infected adults and adolescents*, Department of Health and Human Services, October 2006.
32. Schackman BR: The lifetime cost of current human immunodeficiency virus care in the United States, *Med Care* 44(11):990-997, 2006.
33. Cohen J: Promising AIDS vaccine's failure leaves field reeling, *Science* 318(5847):28-29, 2007.

PART 4

Alterations in Respiration and Tissue Oxygenation

Frontiers of Research

Blood and Circulatory Disorders

Sheila K. Smith • Ronald S. Go • Michael J. Kirkhorn

Voluntary blood donors are among the heroines and heroes of our time. They provide the precious fluid that allows the survival of accident victims and surgical patients. However, at times voluntarism is not enough. When blood replacement supplies run low, an additional concern is added to the multitude of worries that attend therapy and healing; such shortages revive one of the dreams of medicine: to find ways to bypass the donor. Gene therapy may eventually produce the means for therapeutic production of blood cells.

Donors donate, but the producers of blood cells are hormones—specifically, hematopoietic growth factors, or hemopoietins. They stimulate production of the variety of blood cell types that the body requires.

All of the many types of blood cells develop from a single type that originates in the bone marrow—stem cells, which have been called one of the most primitive cells known to exist in the body. Stem cells reside in the bone marrow—in adults, principally the marrow of membranous bones. The supply of red blood cells issuing from the marrow is regulated by a feedback cycle that ensures an adequate supply of cells for tissue oxygenation. When oxygen carried to the tissues decreases, the bone marrow immediately begins to produce more red blood cells, as it does in response to various forms of anemia. White blood cells, or leukocytes, which are indispensable to the immune system's ability to resist disease, are formed in the bone marrow and in lymph tissue.

In November 1998, scientists at the University of Wisconsin and Johns Hopkins University first announced that they had isolated and grown embryonic stem cells. The development of therapies from this discovery is requiring years of laboratory work, but the culturing of these cells is crucial because it places medical science at the bedrock of cell development, the gestational stage at which cells are differentiated for the development of body organs. Stem cell science is leading to therapies for previously untreatable diseases. New cells are being created from stem cells that could someday replace diseased cardiac, brain, or renal tissue. There is great hope that Stem-cell–generated tissues might repair tissue lost in spinal cord injury. Already stem cell therapies are used to restore bone marrow, to replace blood-forming cells damaged by disease or radiation.

The blood is contained within a dynamic system that is directly influenced by the ordinary details of daily life—whether we exercise and how much, what we eat, whether we maintain a normal body weight, and the state of our emotions. Because of this, learning about the health determinants of the vascular system is also a frontier of research. Nowhere is this frontier more evident than in our increasing understanding of the serious health consequences of high blood pressure and the simple daily choices that help us maintain vascular health and prevent illness.

The vascular system is a container of carefully balanced pressures. The flow of blood is monitored by pressure, volume, and chemical sensors. When pressures exceed the limits tolerated by monitoring systems, the body's controls may be activated. Blood flow to each tissue is monitored by microvessels that measure cell chemistry

Megaloblastic anemia (bone marrow aspirate). From Kumar V, Abbas AK, Fausto N:
Robbins and Cotran pathologic basis of disease, *ed 7, Philadelphia, 2005, Saunders.*
Courtesy Dr. Jose Hernandez, Department of Pathology, University of Texas Southwestern Medical School, Dallas.

Oxygen Transport, Blood Coagulation, Blood Flow, and Blood Pressure

indicating tissue metabolic needs, thus controlling local blood flow and nutrient delivery. Nervous system control of circulation also helps control tissue blood flow.

The heart pays attention to tissue metabolic demands by responding to the volume and forces of blood returning through the veins, and to nerve signals that trigger the heart to pump the required amounts of blood. The arterial pressure itself is carefully regulated: if arterial pressure falls below its normal mean level, immediate circulatory changes occur. The heart increases its contractile force, constricts venous reservoirs, and contracts the arterioles, all of which serve to provide more blood pressure for the arteriolar tree. Kidneys play their part by secreting pressure-controlling hormones and by regulating the amount of water within the vascular system, thus regulating blood volume.

Hypertension, or high blood pressure, is a concern because it directly causes a number of disorders and influences others, including stroke, coronary artery disease, atherosclerosis, heart attack, heart failure, renal disease, and renal failure. Adequately identifying and treating persons with hypertension considerably lowers mortality from cardiovascular disease.

Information from the National Institutes of Health, Clinical and Public Health Advisory from the National High Blood Pressure Education Program (2002) contributes to understanding the effects of lifestyle modifications, including engaging in moderate physical activity; maintaining a normal weight; limiting alcohol use; reducing sodium intake; maintaining adequate potassium intake; and consuming a diet rich in fruits, vegetables, and low-fat dairy products. These approaches have been found to prevent the development of high blood pressure in the general population, and to reduce blood pressure in persons with hypertension. As might be expected, the earlier in life that these prevention strategies are adopted, the greater their long-term potential for reducing the burden of high blood pressure complications.

The importance of lifestyle is substantiated by other recent findings that emphasize the significance of these behaviors for the health of the nation. In an analysis based on the Framingham Study (Cook, Cohen, Herbert, Taylor, & Hennekens, 1995), it was concluded that among Caucasian adults aged 35-64, decreasing the diastolic blood pressure by as little as 2 mmHg would result in a 17 percent reduction in the incidence of hypertension and a 14 percent decrease in the risk of cerebrovascular complications of high blood pressure. Unfortunately, comparable statistics are not yet available for groups with the highest risk for hypertension, namely persons with a strong family history, African Americans, persons who are overweight or obese, and those with a sedentary lifestyle. It can be predicted, however, that targeted intervention with higher risk populations can only serve to benefit individuals who are in greatest need of high blood pressure detection and treatment. Evidence on the efficacy of lifestyle modification is now so strong that the National Heart, Lung, and Blood Institute recommends the use of lifestyle modification as definitive or adjunctive therapy in all patients with hypertension.

Cook NR, Cohen J, Hebert PR, et al: *Implications of small reductions in diastolic blood pressure for primary prevention*, Arch Intern Med 155(7):701-709, 1995.

National Heart, Lung, and Blood Institute. National High Blood Pressure Education Program (November, 2002). *Primary prevention of hypertension: Clinical and public health advisory from the national high blood pressure education program.* NIH publication No. 02-5076. Bethesda, Maryland, 2002.

chapter

13

Alterations in Oxygen Transport

Marie L. Kotter • Susan G. Trevithick

MEDIA RESOURCES

Additional Material for Study, Review, and Further Exploration

CD Companion ■ Review Questions and Answers
■ Glossary (with audio pronunciations for selected terms)
■ Disease Profiles ■ Animations

evolve **Website** at http://evolve.elsevier.com/Copstead/
■ Case Studies ■ Disease Profiles ■ WebLinks ■ Key Points Review

  Online Course (Module 9)

KEY QUESTIONS

■ What factors are necessary for normal red blood cell production?
■ How are oxygen and carbon dioxide transported in the circulation?
■ How are laboratory tests used to detect anemia and polycythemia?
■ What are the general effects of anemia on body systems?

■ How are history, clinical manifestations, and laboratory studies used to differentiate the various forms of anemia?
■ How are history, clinical manifestations, and laboratory studies used to differentiate the various forms of polycythemia?
■ What are the appropriate treatment measures for each of the common types of anemia and polycythemia?

CHAPTER OUTLINE

Blood is a critical body fluid composed of formed elements and cells suspended in plasma that circulates through the cardiovascular system. As the primary transport system of the body, blood is involved in the physiologic and pathologic activities of all organs. The **red blood cell** (RBC), or **erythrocyte,** is essential to oxygen transport within the circulatory system. Red cells contain large numbers of hemoglobin molecules, which are designed to move oxygen efficiently from the lungs to other body tissues. Hemoglobin also aids in acid-base balance. In addition, RBCs carry carbon dioxide wastes away from the cells and back to the lungs for expiration.

COMPOSITION OF BLOOD

The total blood volume averages 75.5 ml/kg in men and 66.5 ml/kg in women, which is 5 to 6 L or 7% to 8% of body weight. The blood cells make up approximately 45%, and blood plasma 55%, of the blood volume. Blood **plasma** is composed of about 92% water and 7% plasma proteins (Figure 13-1). The arterial pH of normal blood is 7.35 to 7.45.

Organic and Inorganic Components

The plasma proteins are formed mainly in the liver. They are unable to leave the vascular space under normal circumstances and assist in regulating blood volume and the body's fluid balance. Plasma proteins contribute to colloid osmotic pressure, which is important in maintaining blood pressure. There are three general types of plasma proteins. The first is serum albumin, which is an essential factor in maintaining blood volume and pressure. The second is serum globulin, which is composed of three general fractions. The α fraction is associated with the transport of bilirubin, lipids, and steroids; the β fraction is associated with the transport of iron and copper in plasma; and the γ fraction contains the antibody molecules. Fibrinogen is the third major type of plasma protein. It is the inactive precursor of fibrin, which forms the framework of blood clots. Regulatory proteins, such as hormones and enzymes, are also present in the plasma. Diffusible nonorganic substances, such as sodium chloride, calcium, potassium, iodine, and iron, are used by body cells and make up 0.9% of plasma. Diffusible organic constituents, such as urea, uric acid, xanthine, creatine, creatinine, and ammonia, are products of tissue metabolism that are transported from the tissues to the kidneys and skin for excretion. Also included in this category are nutritive organic materials, such as amino acids, glucose, fats, and cholesterol, which are foodstuffs in solution absorbed from the gastrointestinal (GI) tract. They are transported to other body tissues for utilization and storage (Table 13-1).[1]

Cellular Components

The amounts of the different cellular components in the blood vary with age. Table 13-2 gives normal values from birth to 21 years.[2]

Erythrocytes

Of the cellular elements of blood (Table 13-3), **RBCs,** or **erythrocytes,** are the most numerous, with normal concentrations ranging from 4.2 to 6.2 million cells/mm³. RBCs are responsible for transporting oxygen to the tissues, and participate in both removing carbon dioxide from the tissues and buffering blood pH. They have no cytoplasmic organelles, nucleus, mitochondria, or ribosomes. Therefore, RBCs cannot synthesize protein or carry out oxidative reactions. Instead the erythrocyte's cytoplasm consists of a solution containing proteins, hemoglobin, and electrolytes that regulates diffusion through the cellular membrane. RBCs live for 80 to 120 days in the circulation; then they die and are replaced. Hemoglobin is the main functional constituent of the red cell. It is a protein that enables the blood to transport 100 times more oxygen than could be transported in plasma alone. An enzyme inside RBCs, carbonic anhydrase, is responsible for the buffering mechanism of red cells.[3]

The erythrocyte's size and shape also contribute to its function as a gas carrier (Figure 13-2). It is a small, biconcave disk, about 7.2 μm in diameter that must circulate through splenic sinusoids and capillaries, which are only 2 μm in diameter. This remarkable feat is accomplished through a property called *reversible deformability,* which allows the RBC to assume a torpedo-like conformation and then return to a biconcave disk shape.[3]

Leukocytes

White blood cells (WBCs), or **leukocytes,** protect the body by phagocytosis of microorganisms and other debris and participate in immune antibody formation. Leukocytes act primarily in the tissues but are also transported in the circulatory and lymphatic systems. The average adult has approximately 5000 to 10,000 leukocytes per cubic millimeter of blood. Monocytes and granulocytes are WBCs that share a common lineage with

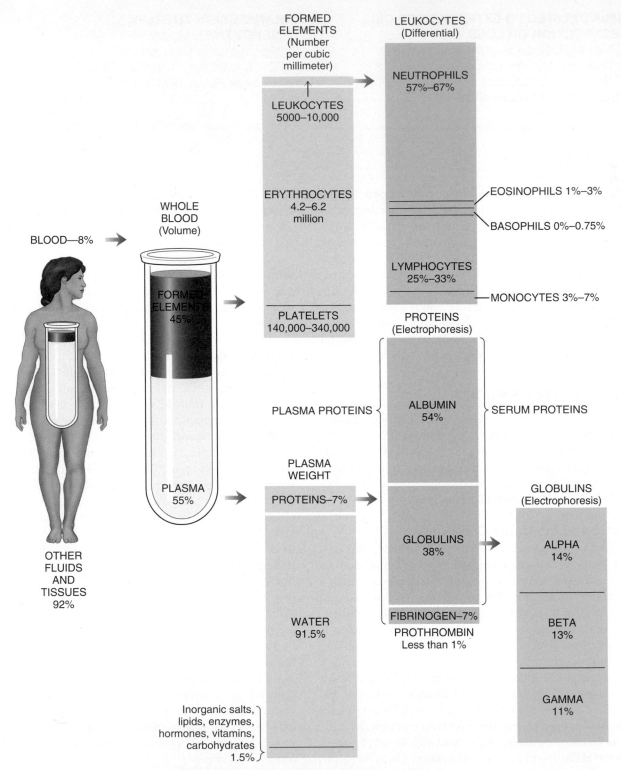

FIGURE 13-1 Composition of blood in the normal adult.

RBCs and platelets. Due to the interrelationship of RBCs, WBCs, and platelets, which are all derived from the myeloid stem cell (Figure 13-3), abnormalities in these cells are seen in some red cell diseases.[4] Leukocyte structure and function are discussed in detail in Chapter 9.

Platelets

Platelets are essential in the formation of blood clots and in the control of bleeding. They are not cells but are circulating cytoplasmic fragments of megakaryocytes and are incapable of mitotic division. They contain cytoplasmic granules that release

TABLE 13-1

Organic and Inorganic Components of Blood

Constituent	Amount/Concentration	Major Functions
Water	92% of plasma weight	Medium for carrying all other constituents
Electrolytes	Total <1% of plasma weight	Keep H_2O in extracellular compartment; act as buffers; function in membrane excitability
Na^+	136-145 mEq/L (142 mM)	
K^+	3.5-5 mEq/L (4 mM)	
Ca^{2+}	4.5-5.5 mEq/L (2.5 mM)	
Mg^{2+}	1.5-2.5 mEq/L (1.5 mM)	
Cl^-	100-106 mEq/L (103 mM)	
HCO_3^-	27 mEq/L (27 mM)	
Phosphate (mostly HPO_4^{2-})	3-4.5 mEq/L (1 mM)	
SO_4^{2-}	0.5-1.5 mEq/L (0.5 mM)	
Proteins	6-8 g/dl (2.5 mM)	
Albumin	3.5-5.5 g/dl	Provide colloid osmotic pressure of plasma; act as buffers; bind other plasma constituents (e.g., lipids, hormones, vitamins, metals)
Globulins	1.5-0.3 g/dl	Enzymes; enzyme precursors; antibodies (immune globulins); hormones
Fibrinogen	0.2-0.4 g/dl	Clotting factor
Gases, arterial plasma		
CO_2 content	22-30 mmol/L of plasma	By-product of metabolism; most CO_2 content is from HCO_3^- and acts as a buffer
O_2	PaO_2, 80 mm Hg or greater (arterial); $P\bar{v}O_2$ 30-40 mm Hg (venous)	Oxygenation
N_2	0.9 ml/dl	By-product of protein catabolism
Nutrients		Provide nutrition and substances for tissue repair
Glucose and other carbohydrates	70-105 mg/dl (5.6 mM)	
Total amino acids	40 mg/dl (2 mM)	
Total lipids	450 mg/dl (7.5 mM)	
Cholesterol	150-250 mg/dl (4-7 mM)	
Individual vitamins	0.0001-2.5 mg/dl	
Individual trace elements	0.001-0.3 mg/dl	
Waste products		
Urea (BUN)	10-20 mg/dl (5.7 mM)	End product of protein catabolism
Creatinine	0.7-1.5 mg/dl (0.09 mM)	End product of energy metabolism
Uric acid	2.5-8 mg/dl (0.3 mM)	End product of protein metabolism
Bilirubin	0.3-1.1 mg/dl	End product of red blood cell destruction
Direct conjugated	0.1-0.5 mg/dl	
Indirect unconjugated	0.1-0.7 mg/dl	
Individual hormones	0.000001-0.05 mg/dl	Functions specific to target tissue

Adapted with permission from Vander AJ et al: *Human physiology: the mechanisms of body function,* ed 7, New York, 1998, McGraw-Hill.

biochemical mediators involved in the hemostatic process. Normally, 150,000 to 400,000 platelets/mm^3 circulate freely in the blood. An additional one third of the body's platelets are in a reserve pool in the spleen. The average life span of platelets in the peripheral blood is approximately 4 to 5 days.[5]

KEY POINTS

- Of the 4 to 6 L of blood in the circulatory system, approximately 45% is blood cells and 55% is plasma. The plasma fraction contains dissolved substances, including nutrients, ions, plasma proteins, metabolic wastes, hormones, and enzymes.

- Red cells function to carry oxygen and carbon dioxide in the blood. They have a limited life span of 80 to 120 days because they contain no cytoplasmic organelles and thus are incapable of replacing lost or damaged cellular components. The normal red cell concentration is 4.2 to 6.2 million cells/mm^3.

- Leukocytes, or WBCs, are the other cell type present in blood. Leukocytes circulate in much lower numbers than RBCs (5000 to 10,000/mm^3). Leukocytes are important mediators of immunity.

- Platelets are not cells but are small fragments of megakaryocytes. The normal platelet count is 150,000 to 400,000 cells/mm^3.

TABLE 13-2

Age-Related Changes in Hematologic Values

Age	Hemoglobin (g)	Hematocrit (%)	RBC Count (millions/mm³)	Platelets (thousands/mm³)	Reticulocytes (%)	WBC Count (cells/mm³)	PMN Count Adult	Band Forms (%)	Eosinophils (%)	Basophils (%)	Lymphocytes (%)	Monocytes (%)
Birth	17.6	55	5.5	350.0	5.0	9000-30,000 (avg., 18,000)	9400 (52%)	9.1	2.2	0.6	31	5.8
24 hr	18.0	56	5.3	400.0	5.2	9400-34,000 (avg., 19,045)	9800 (52%)	9.2	2.4	0.5	31	5.8
1 wk	17.0	54	5.0	300.0	1.0	5000-21,000 (avg., 12,279)	4700 (39%)	6.8	4.1	0.4	41	9.1
2 mo	12.4	30	4.3	260.0	0.5	5500-18,000 (avg., 11,000)	3300 (30%)	4.4	2.7	0.5	57	5.9
6 mo	11.5	34	4.6	250.0	0.8	6000-17,500 (avg., 11,900)	3300 (28%)	3.8	2.5	0.4	61	4.8
2 yr	12.9	40	4.8	250.0	1.0	6000-17,000 (avg., 10,680)	3200 (30%)	3.0	2.6	0.5	59	5.0
6 yr	14.1	42	4.8	250.0	1.0	5000-14,500 (avg., 8500)	4000 (48%)	3.0	2.7	0.6	42	4.7
14 yr	15.0	M: 45 F: 42	5.1	250.0	1.0	4500-13,000 (avg., 7900)	4200 (53%)	3.0	2.5	0.5	37	4.7
21 yr	15.0	M: 45 F: 42	5.1	250.0	1.0	4500-11,000 (avg., 7400)	4200 (56%)	3.0	2.7	0.5	34	4.0

From Platt W: *Color atlas and textbook of hematology*, ed 2, Philadelphia, 1979, Lippincott, p 4.
Reproduced by permission of William R. Platt, MD.

TABLE 13-3

Characteristics of Blood Cells

Cell	Structural Characteristics	Normal Amounts in Circulating Blood*	Function	Life Span
Erythrocyte (red blood cell)	Nonnucleated biconcave disk containing hemoglobin	Males: $4.7\text{-}6.1 \times 10^{12}/L$ Females: $4.2\text{-}5.4 \times 10^{12}/L$	Gas transport to and from tissue cells and lungs	80-120 days
Leukocyte (white blood cell)	Nucleated cell	$4.8\text{-}10.8 \times 10^9/L$	Body defense mechanisms	See below
Lymphocyte	Mononuclear immunocyte	$1.2\text{-}3.4 \times 10^9/L$; 20%-44% leukocyte differential	Humoral and cell-mediated immunity	Days or years, depending on type
Neutrophil	Segmented poly-morphonuclear granulocyte with neutrophilic granules	$1.4\text{-}6.5 \times 10^9/L$; 50%-70% leukocyte differential	Phagocytosis, particularly during early phase of inflammation	5 days
Eosinophil	Segmented poly-morphonuclear granulocyte with eosinophilic granules	$0\text{-}0.7 \times 10^9/L$; 0%-4% leukocyte differential	Phagocytosis, antibody-mediated defense against parasites, participate in mucosal immune response	Unknown
Basophil	Segmented poly-morphonuclear granulocyte with basophilic granules	$0\text{-}0.2 \times 10^9/L$; 0%-2% leukocyte differential	Transport and release of heparin and histamine, involved in immune and inflammatory responses	Unknown
Monocyte-macrophage	Large mononuclear phagocyte	$0.11\text{-}0.59 \times 10^9/L$; 2%-9% leukocyte differential	Phagocytosis; process and present antigens	Months to years
Platelet	Discoid cytoplasmic fragment derived from megakaryocytes	$130\text{-}400 \times 10^9/L$	Hemostasis following vascular injury; forms hemostatic plug, provides cofactors, maintains vascular endothelium	9.5 days

Illustrations from GA Thibodeau, Patton KT: *Anatomy and physiology,* ed 6, St Louis, 2007, Mosby.
*Given in SI units.

FIGURE 13-2 Mature erythrocytes. A mature neutrophil is also shown. (Courtesy Beth Payne, Sacred Heart Medical Center, Spokane, Wash.)

STRUCTURE AND FUNCTION OF RED BLOOD CELLS

The cellular components of blood originate in the yolk sac mesenchyme, move to the liver and spleen during fetal life, and finally are limited to the marrow of the body skeleton (Figure 13-4). Bone marrow provides a special environment for hematopoietic cell proliferation and maturation. Developing cells are held in a fine reticular meshwork, which provides free access to plasma nutrients but retains developing cells until their maturity allows penetration of the endothelial barrier. In times of need, immature cells (reticulocytes and nucleated red blood cells, or NRBCs) are released early into the circulation; their presence in increased numbers is a sign that the hematopoietic system is stressed or is experiencing disease.[2]

Hematopoiesis

Hematopoiesis is the developmental process leading from pluripotential stem cells to mature, differentiated red cells, neutrophils, eosinophils, basophils, monocytes, and platelets. **Lymphopoiesis** describes this process for lymphocytes. Both hematopoietic and lymphopoietic stem cells probably derive from a single totipotent stem cell pool in fetal development, but it is uncertain if this is the functioning stem cell after birth (Figure 13-5). Research suggests that a pluripotential stem cell that is stimulated by erythropoietin and other poietins to cause further differentiation into separate cell lines may be the primary stem cell in adults.[6]

Hematopoiesis is a two-stage process that involves mitotic division (proliferation) and maturation (differentiation). Each type of blood cell has stem cells that undergo mitosis when stimulated by a specific biochemical signal, indicating that the number of circulating cells has decreased. Medullary or bone marrow hematopoiesis continues throughout life and can be accelerated by several mechanisms, including (1) an increase in differentiation of daughter cells, (2) an increase in number of stem cells, and (3) conversion of yellow (fatty) bone marrow (which does not produce cells) to red marrow (which does produce cells). Marrow conversion is stimulated by erythropoietin, which is the hormone from the kidney that stimulates erythrocyte production. In adults, extramedullary hematopoiesis, or production of blood cells in tissue other than bone, is usually due to disease.[7]

Erythrocyte development is shown in detail in Figure 13-3. During this process, the cell changes from a large nucleated cell, rich in ribosomes, to a reticulocyte, which is a small disk that has lost its nucleus. The reticulocyte (Figure 13-6) leaves the marrow, enters the bloodstream, and matures into an erythrocyte in 24 to 48 hours. During this period, mitochondria and ribosomes disappear; the cell can no longer synthesize hemoglobin, and it relies on glycolysis for adenosine triphosphate (ATP) production. The normal reticulocyte count is 1% of the total RBC count. This makes it a useful test to determine effective erythropoietic activity[7] as erythropoietin stimulates uncommitted stem cells to differentiate into proerythroblasts.

Hemoglobin Synthesis

The immature red cell can be viewed as a factory for hemoglobin synthesis. In a mature red cell, **hemoglobin,** the oxygen-carrying protein, composes about 90% of the cell's dry weight in the form of approximately 300 hemoglobin molecules.[3] Hemoglobin that is carrying oxygen is called oxyhemoglobin. Hemoglobin is composed of two pairs of polypeptide chains, the globins. Each globin has an attached heme molecule that is composed of iron plus a protoporphyrin molecule (Figure 13-7).[8]

After dietary iron is absorbed in the duodenum and proximal jejunum, it is transported through the plasma by the protein transferrin to transferrin iron receptors on the RBC membrane. The transferrin-receptor complex is engulfed by the cell into an invagination of the cell surface. The invagination becomes sealed off and forms an intracytoplasmic vacuole. Iron is then released and either stored as ferritin or used to synthesize heme (Figure 13-8).[2] About 67% of total body iron is bound to heme in erythrocytes and muscle cells, and 30% is stored bound to ferritin or hemosiderin-containing macrophages and hepatic parenchymal cells. The remaining 3% is lost daily in urine, sweat, bile, and epithelial cells that are shed in the intestines. The mitochondria are responsible for the synthesis of protoporphyrin. The final heme molecule consists of four porphyrin moieties assembled in a ring structure around a central iron molecule.[2]

Globin is assembled from two pairs of polypeptide chains produced on specific ribosomes. The protein chain produced in fetal life is altered after birth by sequential gene suppression and activation. At birth, red cells contain mainly fetal hemoglobin (hemoglobin F), which is composed of two α chains and two γ chains. Hemoglobin F is a more efficient gas carrier under decreased oxygen tension than hemoglobin A and releases CO_2 more readily. Within 120 days, fetal hemoglobin disappears and is replaced by adult hemoglobin

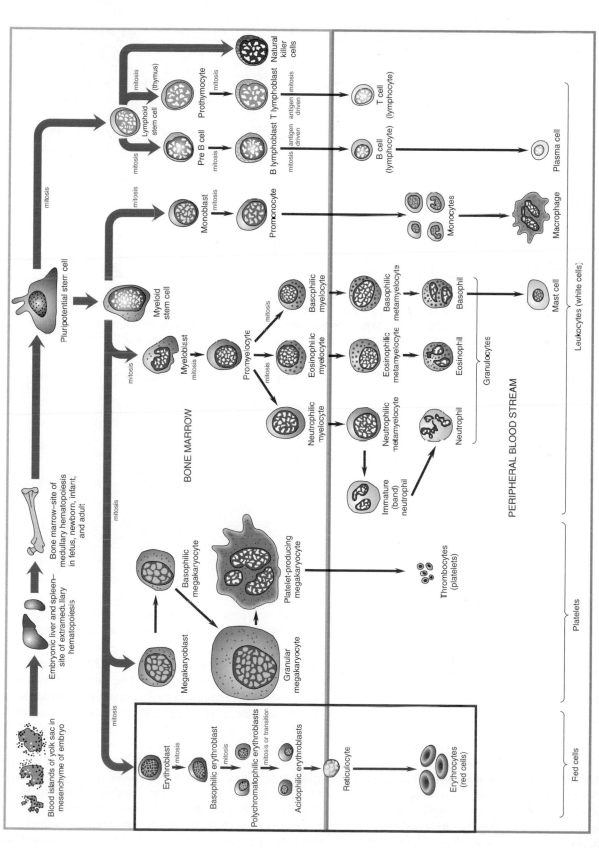

FIGURE 13-3 Maturation of human blood cells. Probable pathways of blood cell differentiation from the pluripotential stem cell to mature leukocytes, erythrocytes, and platelets. Production of cells begins in embryo blood islands in the yolk sac. As the embryo matures, production shifts to the liver and spleen (extramedullary hematopoiesis) and progresses to bone marrow (medullary hematopoiesis). In an adult, all production is in the bone marrow. Current thinking is that all cell production begins with a pluripotential stem cell, which differentiates into either a myeloid stem cell or a lymphoid stem cell, which then differentiates into a specific blast cell. For example, red cell differentiation begins with the proerythroblast, which matures into a basophilic erythroblast, to a polychromatophilic erythroblast, and to an acidophilic erythroblast, all of which are found in the bone marrow. Red cell differentiation concludes with production of reticulocytes and mature red cells (erythrocytes), which normally are found only in the peripheral blood.

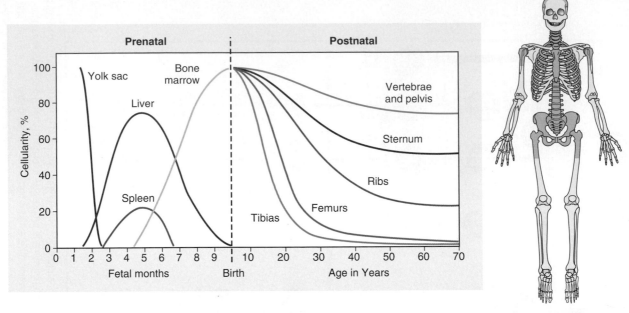

FIGURE 13-4 Location of active marrow growth in the fetus and adult. During fetal development, hematopoiesis is first established in the yolk sac mesenchyme, later moves to the liver and spleen, and finally is limited to the bony skeleton. From infancy to adulthood, there is progressive restriction of productive marrow to the axial skeleton and proximal ends of the long bones, which appear as shaded areas on the drawing of the skeleton.

FIGURE 13-5 Stem cells and normal hematopoiesis.

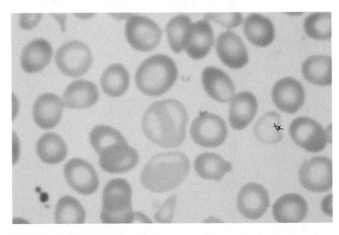

FIGURE 13-6 Reticulocytes seen on peripheral blood smear. The two reticulocytes in the center still contain remnants of intracellular organelles. (Courtesy Beth Payne, Sacred Heart Medical Center, Spokane, Wash.)

Nutritional Requirements for Erythropoiesis

In addition to iron, which is required for hemoglobin synthesis, the normal development of erythrocytes requires adequate supplies of protein, vitamins, and minerals. Erythropoiesis cannot proceed in the absence of vitamins, especially B_{12}, folate, B_6, riboflavin, pantothenic acid, niacin, ascorbic acid, and vitamin E. Folates and vitamin B_{12} (cobalamin) are absorbed from food by the ileal mucosa. Folate deficiencies or vitamin B_{12} deficiencies lead to impaired DNA synthesis in erythroid cells because the vitamins are coenzymes in a large number of key reactions in cellular metabolism. Absorption of vitamin B_{12} requires intrinsic factor in the gastric juice. Intrinsic factor is secreted by the stomach parietal cells and binds to vitamin B_{12}. The complex then moves down the gastrointestinal

(hemoglobin A) (Figure 13-9). This switch is the result of globin genes and is not well understood. Hemoglobin A is composed of two α chains and two β chains and makes up 97% of the hemoglobin found in adults. Hemoglobin A_2 makes up 2% to 3% of hemoglobin found in adults and is composed of $\alpha_2\delta_2$.[8,9]

Several hundred hemoglobinopathies have been described that have changes in the two α chains and two β chains. Most are characterized by the substitution of only one amino acid and are classified by the polypeptide chain in which the substitution occurs.[8]

FIGURE 13-7 Molecular structure of hemoglobin. The molecule is a spherical tetramer weighing approximately 64,500 daltons. It contains two α- and two β-polypeptide chains and four heme groups.

KEY

——— α chain   ——— γ chain (fetal)
——— β chain (adult)   ——— ε chain (embryonic)
——— δ chain (Hb-A$_2$)   ——— ξ (embryonic)

FIGURE 13-9 Changes in hemoglobin with development. Sequential suppression and activation of individual globin genes in the immediate postnatal period result in a switch from fetal hemoglobin (hemoglobin F: two α chains and two γ chains) to adult hemoglobin (hemoglobin A: two α chains and two β chains). A small amount of hemoglobin A$_2$ (two α chains and two δ chains) is also present in the adult. (From Young NS et al, editors, *Clinical Hematology,* Philadelphia, 2006, Mosby, p 24.)

FIGURE 13-8 Intracellular pathways for iron uptake and incorporation into hemoglobin in erythroblasts in the bone marrow. The iron-transferrin complex is picked up by a membrane-associated receptor and brought into the cell by invagination and formation of an intracytoplasmic vacuole. The iron is then released and stored as intracytoplasmic ferritin or used to synthesize heme, the precursor of hemoglobin. The transferrin-receptor complex is returned to the cell membrane, where the apotransferrin is expelled back into the circulation. (Redrawn from Hillman RS, Finch CA, editors: *Red cell manual,* ed 6, Philadelphia, 1992, FA Davis, p 8.)

tract to the ileum, where it attaches to specific receptor sites on the ileum mucosal cell. It is absorbed into the cell, released, and transported in the blood to the tissues and liver.[10,11]

Energy and Maintenance of Erythrocytes

For the RBC to perform efficiently and survive in the circulation for the full 120-day life span, it must have a source of energy. Without an energy source, ion pumps fail and the red cell becomes sodium logged and potassium depleted. The shape changes from a biconcave disk to a sphere, and it is

quickly removed from the circulation by the filtering action of the spleen and the mononuclear phagocyte system. The metabolism of the RBC is limited due to the absence of a nucleus, mitochondria, and other subcellular organelles. Although the binding, transport, and release of O_2 and CO_2 is a passive process that does not require energy, other energy-dependent metabolic processes occur that are essential to the RBC viability. The chief metabolic pathway, accounting for about 90% of the glucose used, is the anaerobic or Embden-Meyerhof pathway. The Embden-Meyerhof pathway provides ATP for regulation of intracellular Na^+, K^+, Ca^{2+}, and Mg^{2+} concentration via cation pumps. About 10% of the glucose undergoes aerobic glycolysis in the hexose monophosphate shunt. The hexose monophosphate shunt provides nicotinamide adenine dinucleotide phosphate (NADPH) and glutathione (GSH) to reduce cellular oxidants. This protects the cell from permanent oxidant injury. The methemoglobin reductase pathway protects hemoglobin from oxidation via NADH and methemoglobin reductase. Last, the Rapoport-Leubering pathway forms 2,3-diphosphoglycerate (DPG), which facilitates oxygen release to the tissues. These pathways contribute energy for maintaining (1) high intracellular K^+, low intracellular Na^+, and very low intracellular Ca^{2+} (cation pumps); (2) reduced hemoglobin; (3) high levels of reduced GSH; and (4) membrane integrity and deformability.[2] Deficiencies of enzymes that regulate these pathways can be due to natural causes, such as the normal aging process, or to an inherited deficiency of an enzyme.[3,12]

Stem cells → Nucleated erythrocytes 5 X 10⁹/kg → Marrow reticulocytes 5 X 10⁹/kg → Circulating reticulocytes 3.3 X 10⁹/kg → Circulating erythrocytes 330 X 10⁹/kg

FIGURE 13-10 Scale model of the erythron, showing the relative proportions of each component. The numbers below each box indicate the average number of cells per kilogram of body weight. (Redrawn from Wintrobe M et al, editors: *Clinical hematology,* ed 8, Philadelphia, 1981, Lea & Febiger, p 109.)

Red cell membrane structures are matrices formed from a double layer of phospholipids. In the red cell membrane, the globular proteins floating on the "sea of lipids" form a protein network on the cytoplasmic surface of the membrane. One half of the mass of the membrane is lipid, which is partially responsible for many of its physical characteristics. Both passive cation permeability and mechanical flexibility can be significantly influenced by changing the lipid composition of the membrane. Maintenance and renewal of membrane lipids in well-developed RBCs is important, and problems in these pathways result in premature cell death.[13]

Red Cell Production

When blood is described as a single body system, it is called the **erythron** (Figure 13-10). The erythron includes the blood cells and their bone marrow precursors. The size of the erythron increases or decreases based on the erythropoietic process and the pathologic changes in red cells seen in anemia.[14] **Erythropoiesis** is controlled by a system sensitive to alterations in the concentration of hemoglobin in the blood. A decrease in hemoglobin decreases the tissue oxygen tension in the kidney. In response to this hypoxia, the kidney secretes a hormone, **erythropoietin,** that stimulates primitive stem cells in the bone marrow to differentiate into proerythroblasts or pronormoblasts, thereby increasing the erythron (Figure 13-11).[3,15] Hypoxia from low hemoglobin level and other causes such as altitude, can also initiate this response.

Red Cell Destruction

As the red cell ages, the various enzyme activities decrease, membrane lipids decrease, hemoglobin A_2 and methemoglobin increase, and changes in cell size occur. **Methemoglobin** is formed when the iron of the hemoglobin molecule is oxidized to the ferric state (Fe^{3+}). The cell loses its ability to deform and becomes increasingly fragile. These aging red cells are then

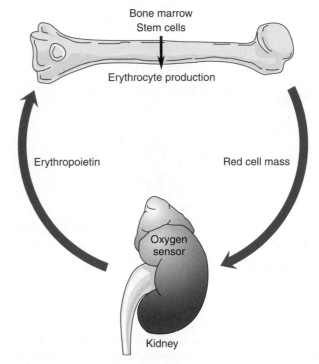

FIGURE 13-11 Feedback circuit illustrating the role of erythropoietin in the regulation of red cell mass.

removed by the mononuclear phagocytic system. The red cells are digested by proteolytic and lipolytic enzymes in phagolysosomes of macrophages. Some 80% to 90% of this process occurs in macrophages of the spleen and liver. Only 10% to 20% of normal destruction occurs intravascularly.[3,16]

Globin is broken down into amino acids, and the iron is recycled. Porphyrin is reduced to **bilirubin**, which is transported to the liver and conjugated by the enzyme glucuronyl transferase. Finally, conjugated bilirubin is excreted in the bile as glucuronide. Bacteria in the intestine convert conjugated

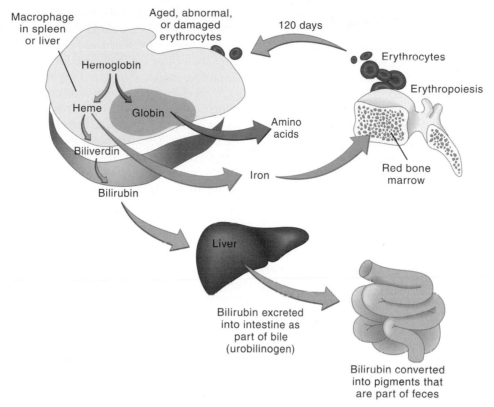

FIGURE 13-12 Most hemoglobin degradation occurs in the macrophages of the spleen. The globin and iron portions are conserved and reused. Heme is reduced to bilirubin, eventually degraded to urobilinogen, and excreted in the feces. Thus, indirect indicators of erythrocyte or erythrocyte destruction include the blood bilirubin level and urobilinogen concentration in the feces. (From Thibodeau GA, Patton KT: *Anatomy and physiology,* ed 6, St Louis, 2007, Mosby, p 654.)

bilirubin into urobilinogen, which is excreted primarily in the stool but also in the urine (Figure 13-12). Any condition causing increased red cell destruction increases the load of bilirubin to be cleared, which leads to increased serum levels of unconjugated bilirubin and increased excretion of urobilinogen. Increased levels of circulating bilirubin give the skin a yellow tone, which is called *jaundice.* In newborns, the albumin levels for bilirubin transport are low and liver glucuronidase for bilirubin conjugation is low, which may cause an accumulation of toxic unconjugated bilirubin. Unconjugated bilirubin is toxic because in this form it is lipid soluble and can easily cross cell membranes. This form of bilirubin has a high affinity for basal ganglia of the central nervous system. The conjugated form of bilirubin is water soluble but lipid insoluble so it cannot cross cell membranes.[3,16]

KEY POINTS

- Red cell development from pluripotential stem cells in the bone marrow is stimulated by a hormone growth factor called *erythropoietin.* Erythropoietin is secreted into the bloodstream by kidney cells in response to low oxygen tension in the blood.

- During development, red cells lose their nuclei and other cytoplasmic organelles. A reticulocyte is an immature red cell that still retains some cellular organelles. An increased blood reticulocyte count is a useful indicator of increased red cell production.

- Hemoglobin is the major component of red cells. It is composed of two pairs of polypeptide chains, each of which has a heme molecule attached. Oxygen can bind reversibly to an iron molecule at the center of each heme. When fully saturated, a hemoglobin molecule carries four oxygen molecules, and is referred to as *oxyhemoglobin.*

- Red cell production requires adequate amounts of several nutrients, particularly iron, vitamin B_{12}, and folate. Lack of intrinsic factor inhibits absorption of B_{12} from the small intestine and is a risk factor for anemia.

- Red cells rely on glycolysis for energy production because they do not contain mitochondria. As energy production declines due to red cell aging and loss of essential glycolytic enzymes, the cell swells, gets trapped in the spleen, and is removed from the circulation. Red cell degradation releases bilirubin, a toxic substance that is conjugated in the liver and excreted in urine and bile.

GAS TRANSPORT AND ACID-BASE BALANCE

RBCs have many important functions in the body related to gas transport and acid-base balance.[3,16,17] RBCs contain hemoglobin, which is responsible for oxygen transport to the body tissues.[3,16] Oxygen combines with the heme portion of hemoglobin to form oxyhemoglobin in a loose and reversible bond in the pulmonary capillary due to a high partial pressure of oxygen (PO_2) and is carried to the tissues with a low PO_2, where it is released.[17] Large quantities of carbonic anhydrase in RBCs catalyze the reaction between CO_2 produced by cellular metabolism in the tissues and water to form carbonic acid, which dissociates into hydrogen and bicarbonate ions for elimination by the lungs and kidneys. Approximately 90% of the CO_2 in the arterial blood and 60% of the CO_2 in the venous blood are transported as bicarbonate. Finally, the hemoglobin protein directly binds with the remaining CO_2 to form carbaminohemoglobin for CO_2 transport. Carbamino compounds are an acid-base buffer responsible for as much as 50% of the whole blood–buffering power.[3,16]

Oxygen Transport

Transport of oxygen to the body tissues and removal of carbon dioxide is a complex process involving interdependent function of the lungs, heart, and blood (Figure 13-13). Approximately 97% of oxygen in the blood is transported on red cells loosely and reversibly combined with hemoglobin (oxyhemoglobin), and 3% is dissolved in plasma. Each hemoglobin molecule can bind four atoms of oxygen. Despite a combining potential of 1.39 ml of oxygen per gram of hemoglobin in pure hemoglobin, a maximum of about 1.34 ml of oxygen per gram of hemoglobin is available, owing to a reduction of about 4% by impurities such as methemoglobin. The blood of an average person contains approximately 15 g of hemoglobin per 100 ml of blood. Therefore, in the average person, the hemoglobin in 100 ml of blood can combine with approximately 20 ml of oxygen if the hemoglobin is 100% saturated. This value is expressed as 20 vol%.[17,18]

$$\text{Oxygen } (O_2) \text{ capacity of hemoglobin (Hb)} =$$
$$\text{Hb (g/100 ml)} \times 1.34 \text{ ml } O_2/\text{g Hb} =$$
$$15 \text{g/100 ml} \times 1.34 \text{ml } O_2/\text{g Hb} =$$
$$20.1 \text{ml} O_2/100 \text{ml (or vol\%)}$$

The partial pressure of oxygen (PO_2) reflects the pressure or tension that oxygen exerts when it is dissolved in blood. Partial pressure is measured in millimeters of mercury (mm Hg). In the pulmonary capillaries, where PO_2 is high, oxygen binds efficiently with hemoglobin, but in the tissue capillaries,

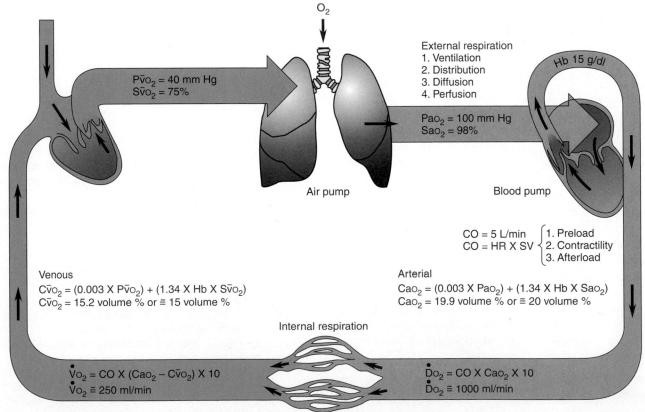

FIGURE 13-13 Oxygen transport. Diffusion of oxygen into the pulmonary capillaries occurs when alveolar PO_2 exceeds capillary PO_2. Maintenance of this gradient is dependent on adequate alveolar ventilation and perfusion. Delivery of oxygenated blood to the tissues *($\dot{D}O_2$)* is determined by the content of oxygen in the blood *(CaO_2)* and the cardiac output *(CO)*. The difference between arterial and venous oxygen is a reflection of oxygen consumption by tissues *($\dot{V}O_2$)*. *Hb*, Hemoglobin; *HR*, heart rate; *SV*, stroke volume.

where PO_2 is low, oxygen is released from hemoglobin. The partial pressure affects the tendency of oxygen to bind with hemoglobin.[19] The partial pressure of oxygen in arterial blood (PaO_2) is usually 80 to 100 mm Hg, whereas the partial pressure of oxygen in venous blood ($P\overline{v}O_2$) is usually 35 to 40 mm Hg. The amount of hemoglobin bound to oxygen relative to the total amount of hemoglobin is expressed as the oxygen saturation, in a percentage.[19,20] Saturation of arterial blood with oxygen (SaO_2) is normally 95% to 100%, whereas that of venous blood ($S\overline{v}O_2$) is 60% to 80%.[17-20]

The oxygen-hemoglobin dissociation curve (Figure 13-14) describes the relationship between PO_2 and SO_2. The upper part of the curve represents oxygen uptake in the lungs and demonstrates that significant changes in PO_2 result in only small changes in SO_2 to help ensure adequate oxygen delivery to the tissues.[18,19] On the steep lower portion of the curve, reflecting the venous blood, small changes in venous PO_2 result in large changes in $S\overline{v}O_2$.[19] Therefore, the tissues are protected with an available oxygen reserve as large quantities of oxygen are released from the blood for relatively small decreases in PO_2. Normally, tissue PO_2 does not rise above 40 mm Hg to enhance diffusion of oxygen from the blood to the tissues. The strength of the bond between hemoglobin and oxygen is called the *oxygen-hemoglobin affinity*. For any given PO_2, hemoglobin saturation will be higher when affinity is increased and saturation will be lower when affinity is decreased. Changes in hemoglobin affinity are represented by shifts in the oxyhemoglobin dissociation curve (see Figure 13-14). Shifts in the oxyhemoglobin

curve affect the ability of hemoglobin to pick up O_2 in the lungs and release it in the tissues. The ability of hemoglobin to release oxygen to the tissues is commonly assessed at point P_{50} on the oxygen-hemoglobin dissociation curve. The P_{50} is the PO_2 at which 50% of the hemoglobin is saturated. A decrease in oxygen affinity (shift to the right on the oxyhemoglobin dissociation curve) or an increase in oxygen affinity (shift to the left) can be caused by the conditions listed in Figure 13-14.[18]

A shift of the oxyhemoglobin dissociation curve due to changes in the blood levels of PCO_2 and the H^+ concentration is important to enhance oxygen uptake by the blood in the lungs and the release of oxygen from the hemoglobin to the body tissues. This is called the *Bohr effect*.[17]

A shift of the oxyhemoglobin dissociation curve to the right enhances oxygen release to the cell. The shift provides the increase in oxygen delivery that is needed during exercise and other types of stress, as well as in chronic disease states. A shift of the oxyhemoglobin dissociation curve to the left is seen with a decrease in H^+ ion concentration, with a decrease in PCO_2, with an increase in pH, with a decrease in temperature, with a decrease in 2,3-DPG, in some congenital hemoglobinopathies, and with carboxyhemoglobin.

Another important factor affecting O_2 delivery to tissues is the arterial oxygen content (CaO_2).[17,18,20] Arterial blood oxygen content (CaO_2) and venous blood oxygen content (CvO_2) can be calculated by adding the amount of oxygen combined with hemoglobin, and the amount of oxygen dissolved in plasma (Table 13-4).

FIGURE 13-14 Oxygen-hemoglobin dissociation curve: factors affecting hemoglobin's affinity for oxygen. Curve *B* is the standard oxyhemoglobin dissociation curve. Factors that shift the curve to the left are represented in curve *A*; factors that shift the curve to the right are represented in curve *C*. (Redrawn from Gottlieb JE: Breathing and gas exchange. 2,3-DPG, 2,3-diphosphoglycerate. In Kinney MR et al, editors: *AACN's clinical reference for critical care nursing*, ed 3, New York, 1993, McGraw-Hill, p 672.)

TABLE 13-4

Gas Values Significant to the Oxygenation of Blood

Gas Values	Description	Measurement/Reflection	Calculation/Formula	Normal Value/Formula
CaO_2	The arterial blood oxygen content is the amount of oxygen carried in the arterial blood	Measured in milliliters of oxygen per deciliter of blood (ml/dl), or vol%	The sum of oxyhemoglobin (15 Hb g/100 ml × 1.34 ml O_2/g Hb × 97.5% arterial saturation = 19.6 vol%) + the amount of oxygen dissolved in the plasma (PaO_2 = 100 mm Hg × 0.003 vol%/mm Hg = 0.3 vol%)	~20 vol% Formula: 19.6 vol% oxyhemoglobin + 0.3 vol% dissolved in plasma = 19.9 vol%
$C\bar{v}O_2$	The venous blood oxygen content is the amount of oxygen carried in the venous blood	Measured in milliliters of oxygen per deciliter of blood (ml/dl), or vol%	$C\bar{v}O_2$ = oxyhemoglobin (15 Hb/100 ml × 1.34 ml O_2/g Hb × 75% venous saturation = 15.0 vol%) + the amount of oxygen dissolved in the plasma ($P\bar{v}O_2$ = 40 mm Hg × 0.003 vol%/mm Hg = 0.12 vol%)	~15 vol% Formula: 15 vol% oxyhemoglobin + 0.12 vol% dissolved in plasma = approximately 15 vol%
$\dot{D}O_2$	Oxygen delivery or transport is the amount of oxygen delivered to the tissues	Measured in milliliters of oxygen per minute (ml/min)	*Normal arterial:* $\dot{D}O_2$ = cardiac output (L/min) × CaO_2 × 10 *Normal venous:* $\dot{D}O_2$ = cardiac output (L/min) × $C\bar{v}O_2$ × 10	*Normal arterial:* ~1000 ml of O_2/min *Normal venous:* ~750 ml of O_2/min
PaO_2	The partial pressure of oxygen in arterial blood	Measured in millimeters of mercury (mm Hg) Reflects the tension or pressure that is exerted by oxygen when it is dissolved in plasma		Normal PaO_2 is 80-100 mm Hg
$PaCO_2$	The partial pressure of carbon dioxide in arterial blood	Measured in millimeters of mercury (mm Hg) Reflects the tension or pressure that is exerted by carbon dioxide when it is dissolved in plasma		Normal $PaCO_2$ is 35-45 mm Hg
$P\bar{v}O_2$	The partial pressure of oxygen in venous blood	Measured in millimeters of mercury (mm Hg) Reflects the tension or pressure that is exerted by oxygen when it is dissolved in plasma		Normal PvO_2 is 35-40 mm Hg
$P\bar{v}CO_2$	The partial pressure of carbon dioxide in venous blood	Measured in millimeters of mercury (mm Hg) Reflects the tension or pressure that is exerted by carbon dioxide when it is dissolved in plasma		Normal PvO_2 is 41-51 mm Hg
SaO_2	The amount of hemoglobin bound to oxygen relative to the total amount of hemoglobin, both reduced and bound, in arterial blood	Expressed as a percentage		Normal SaO_2 is 95%-100%
$S\bar{v}O_2$	The amount of hemoglobin bound to oxygen relative to the total amount of hemoglobin, both reduced and bound, in venous blood	Expressed as a percentage		Normal $S\bar{v}O_2$ is 60%-80%

(continued)

TABLE 13-4				
Gas Values Significant to the Oxygenation of Blood—cont'd				
Gas Values	**Description**	**Measurement/Reflection**	**Calculation/Formula**	**Normal Value/Formula**
$\dot{V}O_2$	Oxygen consumption is the amount of oxygen consumed by the tissues	Measured in milliliters of oxygen per minute (ml/min) Oxygen consumption is derived from the difference between arterial oxygen transport and venous oxygen transport	$\dot{V}O_2 =$ cardiac output $\times$ $(CaO_2 - C\bar{v}O_2) \times 10$	Normal $\dot{V}O_2$ is 200-250 ml of O_2/min

Oxygen delivery, or $(\dot{D}O_2)$ is the amount of oxygen (in milliliters) delivered per minute to the tissues.[18] It is calculated by multiplying the arterial oxygen content (CaO_2) by the cardiac output (CO). Cardiac output is usually between 4 and 8 L/min. Therefore, oxygen delivery is approximately 1000 ml/min.

Oxygen consumption (VO_2) is the amount of oxygen consumed by the tissues and is measured in milliliters of oxygen per minute. Once the oxygen reaches the tissues, oxygen consumption is controlled by the rate of energy expenditure within the cells or the rate at which adenosine diphosphate (ADP) is formed from ATP to provide energy. The increasing concentration of ADP enhances the metabolic utilization of oxygen.[17] Oxygen consumption can be determined by subtracting the oxygen remaining in the venous blood (CvO_2) from the oxygen delivered to the tissues by the arteries (CaO_2), and is known as the *Fick equation*.[20]

Gas values (pressure and content) relative to the oxygenation of blood are summarized in Table 13-4.

Carbon Dioxide Transport

RBCs are also important in the transport of carbon dioxide in the blood. Carbon dioxide, a by-product of cellular metabolism, is transported in three forms in the blood: (1) as dissolved gas, (2) as bicarbonate ion (HCO_3^-), and (3) in association with hemoglobin (Figure 13-15).[17] The partial pressure of carbon dioxide (PCO_2) reflects the pressure or tension that carbon dioxide exerts when it is dissolved in the blood. Partial pressure is measured in millimeters of mercury (mm Hg). In the pulmonary capillaries, carbon dioxide easily dissociates from hemoglobin and then diffuses across the alveolar membrane into the alveolar sacs. In the body tissues, the carbon dioxide inside the cells diffuses into the blood and attaches to the hemoglobin as oxygen is released to the tissues. The partial pressure of carbon dioxide in the arterial blood $(PaCO_2)$ is usually 40 mm Hg and in the venous blood $(P\bar{v}CO_2)$ is usually 45 mm Hg.[17] These differences are much smaller than those of oxygen, but carbon dioxide diffuses much more readily. Dissolved carbon dioxide combines slowly with water in the plasma to form carbonic acid (H_2CO_3), but in the red cell the presence of carbonic anhydrase acting as a catalyst significantly accelerates this reaction.[17,20] Carbonic

FIGURE 13-15 Carbon dioxide is transported in three forms in the blood: (1) as dissolved gas, (2) as bicarbonate ion (HCO_3^-), and (3) in association with hemoglobin (Hb).

acid rapidly dissociates into hydrogen ions (H^+) and bicarbonate ions (HCO_3^-).[17,20] As the concentration of HCO_3^- in the red cell increases, it diffuses into the plasma, whereas the H^+ remains. This increase in intracellular cation concentration causes the anion chloride to diffuse from the plasma into the red cell to maintain electrical neutrality. This is referred to as the **chloride shift**.[18]

Hemoglobin provides an excellent acid-base buffer by reacting with the free hydrogen ions and directly with carbon dioxide to form carbaminohemoglobin $(Hb-CO_2)$, which is easily dissociated in the lungs as free carbon dioxide to be exhaled.[17] Unloading of oxygen in the tissue facilitates the loading of carbon dioxide and is referred to as the *Haldane effect*.[17,18]

Alterations in Oxygen Transport

There must be sufficient circulating hemoglobin mass to meet the metabolic needs of the body. A feedback mechanism ensures that when the oxygen reaching the tissues decreases, a compensatory increase occurs in the production of red cells.[3] The feedback mechanism regulating RBC production is under the control of erythropoietin. As stem cells differentiate into the erythroid committed line, the most primitive stem cell is referred to as the erythroid burst-forming unit (BFU-E), which is controlled by growth factors derived from T lymphocytes and macrophages and, to a lesser degree, by erythropoietin.[2,4] The BFU-E further differentiates into erythroid colony-forming units (CFU-E) more responsive to erythropoietin, and subsequently into normoblasts and mature RBCs.[2,3,4] The majority of erythropoietin is actively secreted by the kidney. Another 10% of erythropoietin is formed elsewhere in the body.[2,3,4]

Factors that decrease hemoglobin mass (such as anemia) or decrease arterial saturation (such as hypoxia from either cardiac or pulmonary conditions) impair oxygen delivery to the body tissues. This stimulates an increased release of erythropoietin and the production of RBCs.[3] Figure 13-16 illustrates the compensatory regulation of erythropoiesis that is seen in hypoxia, anemia, and polycythemia.

KEY POINTS

- Nearly all (97%) of the oxygen transported in blood is bound to hemoglobin within the red cells. Only 3% is dissolved in plasma. It is this 3% which is measured as PaO_2. At a normal PaO_2, hemoglobin is 95% to 100% saturated with oxygen. About 25% of the bound oxygen is unloaded to the tissues, resulting in a venous hemoglobin saturation of about 75%.
- The oxyhemoglobin dissociation curve describes the relationship between the partial pressure of oxygen and hemoglobin saturation. In the lung, where PO_2 is high (100 mm Hg), oxygen is loaded onto hemoglobin. In the tissues, where PO_2 is low (40 mm Hg), oxygen is unloaded from hemoglobin to tissues.
- The affinity of hemoglobin for oxygen is affected by temperature, acid-base status, 2,3-DPG levels, and carbon dioxide. Affinity decreases at the tissue level due to increased levels of acid, 2,3-DPG, and carbon dioxide. This shift to the right of the oxyhemoglobin dissociation curve enhances unloading of oxygen to the tissue. A shift to the left occurs in the lungs, where blood is more alkalotic and carbon dioxide levels are lower.

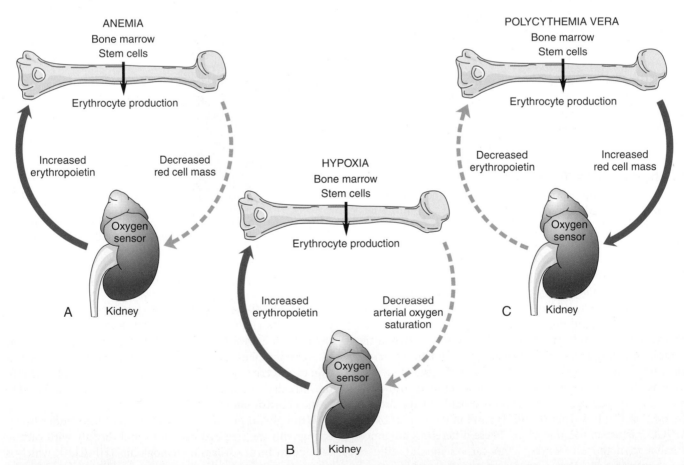

FIGURE 13-16 Alterations in the erythropoietin feedback circuit. Any factor decreasing oxygen delivery to the oxygen sensor cells results in increased secretion of erythropoietin and a compensatory increase in erythrocyte production as illustrated in **A** for anemia, with a decrease in erythrocyte mass, and in **B** for hypoxia, with a decrease in arterial oxygen saturation. An increase in erythrocyte mass, as occurs with polycythemia vera **(C)**, decreases erythropoietin production.

The increased affinity of hemoglobin for oxygen at the lung facilitates oxygen binding.

- The oxygen content of arterial blood is calculated by adding the amount bound to hemoglobin (Hb) plus the amount dissolved in plasma: $CaO_2 = (Hb \times 1.34 \times SaO_2) + (PaO_2 \times 0.003)$. Oxygen delivery to the body tissues is calculated by multiplying CaO_2 by cardiac output (CO): $\dot{D}O_2 = CaO_2 \times CO \times 10$.

- The consumption of oxygen by tissues can be estimated using the Fick equation: $\dot{V}O_2 = CO \times (CaO_2 - C\bar{v}O_2) \times 10$. Oxygen consumption increases with increased tissue metabolism.

- Hemoglobin is an important factor in carbon dioxide transport in the blood. In the tissues, hemoglobin binds carbon dioxide to form carbaminohemoglobin, which then releases carbon dioxide in the lungs. RBCs contain the enzyme carbonic anhydrase, which greatly increases conversion of carbon dioxide and water into HCO_3^- and H^+ at the tissue level. In the lungs, the reaction proceeds in reverse, producing carbon dioxide, which is eliminated by the lungs.

Anemia

Erythrocyte disorders are divided into two groups: (1) **anemia,** defined as a deficit of red cells, and (2) **polycythemia,** defined as an excess of red cells shown in Box 13-1.[21,22] An anemic patient has tissue hypoxia due to the low oxygen-carrying capacity of the blood. In contrast, a patient with polycythemia has increased blood viscosity and volume due to the increase in number of RBCs.[22] (Polycythemia is discussed in greater detail later in this chapter.) Table 13-5 presents the laboratory

---

BOX 13-1

Classification of Anemia and Polycythemia

I. Anemia
- A. Relative
  1. Macroglobulinemia
  2. Pregnancy
  3. Athletes
  4. Postflight astronauts
- B. Absolute
  1. Decreased red cell production
     (a) Acquired
        1) Pluripotent stem cell failure
           a) Aplastic anemia
              {1} Radiation induced
              {2} Drugs and chemicals
              {3} Viruses
              {4} Idiopathic
           b) Anemia of leukemia and myelodysplastic syndrome
           c) Anemia associated with marrow infiltration
           d) Anemia associated with chemotherapy
        2) Erythroid progenitor cell failure
           a) Pure red cell aplasia
           b) Endocrine disorders
           c) Acquired sideroblastic anemia
        3) Functional impairment of erythroid progenitors
           {1} Megaloblastic anemias
              a) B_{12} deficiency
              b) Folate deficiency
              c) Acute megaloblastic anemia due to nitrous oxide
              d) Drug induced megaloblastic anemia
           {2} Iron deficiency anemia
           {3} Anemia of chronic disease
           {4} Anemia of renal failure
           {5} Erythropoietin antibodies
     (b) Hereditary
        1) Pluripotential stem cell failure (Fanconi anemia)
        2) Erythroid progenitor cell failure (Diamond-Blackfan syndrome)

3) Hereditary sideroblastic anemia
4) Thalassemias
  2. Increased red cell destruction or loss
     (a) Acquired
        1) Mechanical
           a) Macroangiopathic (artificial heart valves)
           b) Microangiopathic (DIC)
           c) Parasites and microorganisms
        2) Antibody mediated
        3) Hypersplenism
        4) Chemical and physical injury
        5) Acute blood loss
     (b) Hereditary
        1) Hemoglobinopathies (sickle cell)
        2) Red cell membrane disorders
        3) Enzyme defects

II. Polycythemia (Erythrocytosis)
- A. Relative (decreased plasma volume)
  1. Dehydration
  2. Diuretics
  3. Stress or smoker's erythrocytosis
- B. Absolute (increased red cell volume)
  1. Primary polycythemia
     (a) Acquired (polycythemia vera)
     (b) Hereditary congenital polycythemia
  2. Secondary polycythemia
     (a) Appropriate
        1) Altitude
        2) Cardiopulmonary disorders
        3) Increased hemoglobin affinity for oxygen
     (b) Inappropriate
        1) Renal cysts and tumors
        2) Hepatoma
        3) Cerebellar hemangioblastoma
        4) Essential

Adapted from Lichtman MA et al, editors: *Williams' Hematology,* ed.7, New York, 2006, McGraw-Hill, pp 414-416.

TABLE 13-5

Laboratory Findings for Erythrocyte Disorders

Disease	Hct	Hb	MCV	MCH	MCHC	RETIC	RBC	WBC	PLT
Relative anemia	Low	Low	Normal	Low	Low	Normal	Low	Low	Low
Absolute Anemia Caused by Decreased Production									
Aplastic anemia	Low	Low	Normal	Low	Low	Low	Low	Low	Low
Chronic renal failure	Low	Low	Normal	Normal	Normal	Low	Low	Normal	Normal
Pernicious anemia	Low	Low	High	High	Normal	Low	Low	Low	Low
Folate deficiency	Low	Low	High	High	Normal	Low	Low	Low	Low
Iron deficiency	Low	Low	Low	Low	Low	Normal or high	Low	Normal	Normal
Thalassemia	Low	Low	Low	Low	Low	High	Low	Normal	Normal
Absolute Anemia Caused by Increased Destruction									
Intrinsic Abnormality									
Sickle cell	Low	Low	Normal	Normal	Normal	High	Low	Normal	Normal
Hereditary spherocytosis	Low	Low	Normal	Normal	Normal to high	High	Low	Normal	Normal
G6PD deficiency	Low	Low	Normal	Normal	Normal	High	Low	High	Normal
Extrinsic Abnormality									
HDNB	Low	Low	Normal	Normal	Normal	High	Low	High	Normal
Antibody-mediated drug reactions	Low	Low	Normal	Normal	Normal	High	Low	Normal	Normal
Acute blood loss	Normal to low	Normal to low	Normal	Normal	Normal	High	Normal to low	Normal to low	Normal to low
Polycythemias									
Relative polycythemia	High	High	Normal	Normal	Normal	Normal	High	High	High
Absolute polycythemia vera	High	High	Normal	Normal	Normal	High	High	High	High
Secondary polycythemia	High	High	Normal	Normal	Normal	High	High	Normal	Normal

Hct, Hematocrit; *Hb,* hemoglobin; *MCV,* mean corpuscular volume; *MCH,* mean corpuscular hemoglobin; *MCHC,* mean corpuscular hemoglobin concentration; *RETIC,* reticulocytosis; *RBC,* red blood cell; *WBC,* white blood cell; *PLT,* platelet; *G6PD,* glucose-6-phosphate dehydrogenase; *Segs,* segmented neutrophils; *HDNB,* hemolytic disease of the newborn; *NRBC,* nucleated red blood cell.

findings for erythrocyte disorders in terms of relative anemia, absolute anemia caused by decreased production, and absolute anemia caused by increased destruction.

Relative anemia is characterized by normal total red cell mass with disturbances in the regulation of plasma volume. For example, in pregnant women the average plasma volume is 43% greater than in nonpregnant women, which causes a "dilutional anemia."[21]

Absolute anemia includes those types of anemia with an actual decrease in numbers of red cells. This can be caused by decreased production of red cells or increased destruction of red cells.[21]

GENERAL EFFECTS OF ANEMIA

The clinical manifestations of anemia include a reduction in oxygen-carrying capacity, tissue hypoxia, and compensatory mechanisms to restore tissue oxygenation.[21,22] Increased pulmonary and cardiac function increases the oxygen supply, and an increase in oxygen extraction occurs to protect tissues. Specific adaptations to anemia to increase oxygenated blood flow include an increase in the heart rate, cardiac output, circulatory rate, and preferential increase in blood flow to vital organs. Specific adaptations to anemia to increase oxygen utilization by tissues include an increase in

Blood Smear	Other Laboratory Tests	Other Diagnostic Characteristics
Normal	Plasma volume increased, causing relative decrease in number of cells	Increased volume can be caused by pregnancy, splenomegaly, IV infusions
Normocytic, hypochromic RBCs; lack of neutrophils; increased lymphocytes	HbF may be increased; erythropoietin increased; bone marrow aplastic	Specific cause should be identified and removed from environment
Normocytic, normochromic RBCs; RBCs often have spicules	Erythropoietin decreased; bone marrow production suppressed	Kidney tests abnormal
Oval macrocytes; hypersegmented segs	Decreased B_{12} level; positive Schilling test	Neurologic symptoms; increased bilirubin
Oval macrocytes; hypersegmented segs	Decreased folic acid level; negative Schilling test	No neurologic symptoms
Microcytic, hypochromic RBCs	Serum iron decreased; iron-binding	Bone marrow iron decreased
Microcytic, hypochromic RBC	Decreased osmotic fragility; hemoglobin electrophoresis diagnostic; serum iron, TIBC, and ferritin normal	Hereditary disease
Normocytic, normochromic RBC target cells; sickle cells; NRBCs	HbS present on electrophoresis	Hereditary disease
Spherocytes present	Bilirubin elevated; haptoglobins reduced; abnormal RBC fragility	Hereditary disease
Heinz body smear positive	Tests only abnormal in hemolytic episodes	Hereditary disease
Spherocytes, NRBCs	Bilirubin elevated; Coombs test positive; urinary urobilinogen increased	Jaundice; edema; hepatosplenomegaly
Polychromatic RBCs due to increased reticulocytes	Bilirubin elevated; Coombs test positive; urinary urobilinogen increased	Jaundice
Appears normal until reticulocytes increase	Values depend on severity of hemorrhage and when blood is drawn	
Normal	Plasma volume decreased, causing relative increase in number of blood cells	Decrease in volume
Teardrops, macrocytes, and NRBCs may be present; shift to left on differential	O_2 saturation normal; bone marrow hypercellular; all three cell lines increased	
Normal	Hypoxemia may be evident; serum erythropoietin elevated	Lung disease may be present

2,3-DPG in erythrocytes and a decreased oxygen affinity of hemoglobin in tissues. Selective tissue perfusion provides shunting to vital organs in short-term compensation, and increased erythropoietic activity is stimulated to provide long-term compensation.[6] The extent of the physiologic adaptations is influenced by (1) the severity of the anemia; (2) the competency of the pulmonary and cardiac systems; (3) the oxygen requirements of the individual, which are dependent on physical and metabolic activity; (4) the duration of the anemia; (5) the underlying disease or condition; and (6) the presence and severity of coexisting disease.[21] Mild anemia is usually associated with no clinical symptoms, however early symptoms in patients with mild to moderate anemia include fatigue, generalized weakness, and loss of stamina, followed by tachycardia and exertional dyspnea. Healthy young patients may present with very few symptoms at hemoglobin levels of 7-8 g/dl; however, elderly patients and patients with cardiovascular or pulmonary disease may have symptoms with even modest degrees of anemia and hemoglobin levels of 9-11 g/dl. Specific symptoms related to moderate to severe anemia are orthostatic and nonorthostatic hypotension, vasoconstriction, pallor, tachypnea, dyspnea, tachycardia, transient murmurs, angina pectoris, heart failure, intermittent claudication, night cramps in muscles, headache, lightheadedness, tinnitus, roaring in the ears, and faintness.[6]

ANEMIA RELATED TO DECREASED RED CELL PRODUCTION

Aplastic Anemia

Etiology and Pathogenesis. Aplastic anemia is a stem cell disorder that is characterized by a reduction of hematopoietic tissue in the bone marrow, fatty marrow replacement, and pancytopenia. The decrease in functional bone marrow mass is usually caused by toxic, radiant, or immunologic injury to the bone marrow stem cells, which causes a decrease in red cells, white cells, and platelets, or **pancytopenia**.[23]

Aplastic anemia can be classified as acquired or familial. Acquired aplastic anemia can be caused by chemical and physical agents listed in Table 13-6. Other causes include certain viral infections (e.g., hepatitis, Epstein-Barr virus, human immunodeficiency virus [HIV], dengue), some mycobacterial infections, diffuse eosinophilic fasciitis, pregnancy, Simmonds disease, and sclerosis of the thyroid. Familial aplastic anemia is associated with Fanconi constitutional pancytopenia, pancreatic deficiency in children, and putative hereditary defect in cellular uptake of folate.[24]

Laboratory Features. Pancytopenia is characterized by low red cell, white cell, and platelet counts. The magnitude of the **granulocytopenia** is very important for the immediate prognosis. An absolute granulocyte count of less than 200/mm^3 results in immediate susceptibility to infectious complications. Coagulation tests are generally normal except for the bleeding time, which reflects the low platelet count.[24]

Clinical Manifestations. The onset is usually insidious, and patients often present only after the late manifestations of pancytopenia are evident. The symptoms due to the gradual fall of RBCs include weakness, fatigue, lethargy, pallor, dyspnea, palpitations, onset of transient murmurs, and the tachycardia of anemia. Fever, chills, and bacterial infections (particularly in the mouth or perirectal area) are seen secondary to **neutropenia**. Petechiae, bruising, nosebleeds, retinal hemorrhage, and increased menstrual flow are seen due to **thrombocytopenia**.[23]

Treatment. Treatment for aplastic anemia is multifaceted and dependent on the etiology and severity of the disease. Treatment includes (1) identification and avoidance of further toxin exposure; (2) human leukocyte antigen (HLA) and ABO typing of family members to identify serologically defined loci and potential bone marrow transplant donors; (3) maintenance of minimally essential levels of hemoglobin and platelets; (4) prevention and management of infection; (5) determination of efficacy of bone marrow transplantation; and (6) other forms of therapy, such as immunosuppressive therapy or stimulation of hematopoiesis and bone marrow regeneration in patients not suited to receive a transplant.[23-26] In patients with severe disease, the major curative approach is allogeneic bone marrow transplantation; however, only one third of all patients have compatible donors.[23-26] Preparative regimens using cyclophosphamide and antithymocyte globulin followed by post-transplant immunosuppression with cyclosporine and methyltrexate as prophylaxis

against graft versus host disease (GvHD) have resulted in a 90% disease-free survival rate at two years for patients with bone marrow transplants derived from an HLA-matched sibling donor.[27]

Course and Prognosis. Bone marrow transplantation is highly successful and curative for 80% to 85% of untransfused patients and 55% to 60% of patients with multiple previous transfusions. [27] Twenty to thirty percent of transplantation survivors with multiple previous transfusions experience severe GvHD, which can be significantly improved by immunosuppressive therapy in 50% to 70% of patients.[22] The risk of graft failure in patients who have not been transfused is less than 5%. Prognosis is related to the absolute neutrophil count and the platelet count. Children respond better than adults with both bone marrow transplantation and immunosuppression therapy, especially in patients with mild to moderate disease. Aplastic anemia is usually fatal unless managed with bone marrow transplantation.[23-27]

Anemia of Chronic Renal Failure

Etiology and Pathogenesis. The anemia of chronic renal failure occurs primarily from failure of the renal endocrine function, which causes impaired erythropoietin production and bone marrow compensation, and secondarily from failure of the renal excretory function, leading to hemolysis, bone marrow cell depression, and blood loss.[28]

Laboratory Features. This anemia is characterized by a decreased red cell count and low hemoglobin and hematocrit values. Some red cells appear grossly deformed with a few large spicules (Figure 13-17). The total leukocyte differential cell count, leukocyte counts, and platelet count are usually normal. The red cell indices—mean corpuscular volume (MCV), mean corpuscular hemoglobin (MCH), and mean corpuscular hemoglobin concentration (MCHC)—are also normal.[28,29]

Clinical Manifestations. Any of the clinical manifestations described earlier (see General Effects of Anemia) may be evident in chronic renal failure. The hematocrit falls in proportion to the degree of renal insufficiency, and uremia occurs as the glomerular filtration rate falls below 40 ml/min. Signs and symptoms of anemia usually manifest when the hematocrit falls to 20% or below.[29]

Treatment. Therapy consists of dialysis when the glomerular filtration rate is less than 15 mL/min, and erythropoietin is administered to achieve the target hematocrit of 33% to 36% and hemoglobin of 11 to 12 g/dl. The hematocrit and hemoglobin are monitored at least every 2 weeks to ensure adequate oxygen-carrying capacity and minimize an increased respiratory rate and heart rate. When the target hematocrit is achieved, adult patients can be maintained by administering 50 to 100 units per kilogram per week in divided doses. Pediatric patients younger than 5 years usually require higher initial and maintenance doses.[28-33] Patients with chronic renal failure are also prone to nutritional anemias (lack of iron, folate, and B$_{12}$) due to dietary restrictions and anorexia.

Course and Prognosis: More than 95% of patients respond to erythropoietin therapy. Patients who do not respond or

TABLE 13-6

Drugs Associated with Aplastic Anemia*

Category	High Risk	Moderate Risk	Low Risk
Analgesic			Phenacetin, aspirin, salicylamide
Antiarrhythmic			Quinidine, tocainide
Antiarthritic		Gold salts	Colchicine
Anticonvulsant		Carbamazepine, hydantoin, felbamate	Ethosuximide, phenacemide, primidone, trimethadione, sodium valproate
Antihistamine			Chlorpheniramine, pyrilamine, tripelennamine
Antihypertensive			Captopril, methyldopa
Anti-inflammatory		Penicillamine, phenylbutazone, oxyphenbutazone	Diclofenac, ibuprofen, indomethacin, naproxen, sulindac
Antimicrobial			
Antibacterial		Chloramphenicol	Dapsone, methicillin, penicillin, streptomycin, β-lactam antibiotics
Antifungal			Amphotericin, flucytosine
Antiprotozoal		Quinacrine	Chloroquine, mepacrine, pyrimethamine
Antineoplastic			
Alkylating agents	Busulfan, cyclophosphamide, melphalan, nitrogen mustard		
Antimetabolites	Fluorouracil, mercaptopurine, methotrexate		
Cytotoxic antibiotics	Daunorubicin, doxorubicin, mitoxantrone		
Antiplatelet			Ticlopidine
Antithyroid			Carbimazole, methimazole, methylthiouracil, potassium perchlorate, propylthiouracil, sodium thiocyanate
Sedative and tranquilizer			Chlordiazepoxide, chlorpromazine (and other phenothiazines), lithium, meprobamate, methyprylon
Sulfonamides and derivatives			
Antibacterial			Numerous sulfonamides
Diuretic		Acetazolamide	Chlorothiazide, furosemide
Hypoglycemic			Chlorpropamide, tolbutamide
Miscellaneous			Allopurinol, interferon, pentoxifylline

From Segel GB: Aplastic anemia. In Lichtman et al, editors: *Williams hematology,* ed 7, New York, 2006, McGraw-Hill, p 421. This list was compiled from the AMA Registry, Publications of the International Agranulocytosis and Aplastic Anemia Study, other reviews and studies, previous compilations of offending agents, and selected reports.

*Drugs that invariably cause marrow aplasia with high doses are termed high risk; drugs with 30 or more reported cases are listed as moderate risk; others are less often associated with aplastic anemia (low risk).

first respond when larger doses are given should be evaluated for an adequate iron supply, infection, or excessive splenic hemolysis.[28-33]

Anemia Related to Vitamin B$_{12}$ (Cobalamin) or Folate Deficiency

Etiology and Pathogenesis. The anemia resulting from a deficiency of either vitamin B$_{12}$ (cobalamin) or folate is caused by a disruption in DNA synthesis of the blast cells in the bone marrow. This disruption produces very large abnormal bone marrow cells called **megaloblasts.** In the peripheral blood, the red cells are larger than normal (**macrocytic**), the granulocytes are hypersegmented, and the numbers of red cells, white cells, and platelets are decreased.[34,35] All of these signs can be seen on the peripheral blood smear.

The classic anemia in this classification is pernicious anemia. The fundamental defect causing pernicious anemia is the lack of intrinsic factor. Without it, vitamin B$_{12}$ cannot be absorbed, thus leading to vitamin B$_{12}$ deficiency. This deficiency results in disordered nucleic acid metabolism, which causes **megaloblastic dysplasia,** a condition involving abnormal production and maturation of red cell, white cell, and platelet systems. There is strong evidence that pernicious anemia develops as a result of genetically determined autoimmune disease, which is manifested by serum and gastric juice antibodies against intrinsic factor and parietal cells.[34] The biochemical basis of the neurologic lesions in pernicious anemia is not known. There can be peripheral nerve degeneration, degeneration of the posterior columns of the spinal cord, or

FIGURE 13-17 Burr cells found in acute kidney disease. (Courtesy Beth Payne, Sacred Heart Medical Center, Spokane, Wash.)

both. There is some evidence of abnormal fatty acid metabolism in the peripheral nerves and degeneration of the white matter in the spinal cord in animals.[34,35]

Folate deficiencies resemble vitamin B_{12} deficiencies except for the neurologic disease, which is more characteristic of vitamin B_{12} deficiency. Folate deficiencies are usually the result of dietary deficiencies, alcoholism and cirrhosis, pregnancy, or infancy.

Laboratory Features. The peripheral blood shows low RBC counts of 500,000 to 750,000 cells/mm³, low WBC counts of 4000 to 5000 cells/mm³, and low platelet counts of 50,000 cells/mm³. These counts are usually not as low as those seen in aplastic anemia. The bone marrow shows megaloblastic dysplasia, which results in a peripheral blood picture of macrocytosis and hypersegmented neutrophils. The red cell indices show normal MCH and MCHC and increased MCV. The Schilling test, which measures excretion of radioactive vitamin B_{12}, indicates low levels, and the serum level of vitamin B_{12} is low. Gastric analysis reveals a lack of free hydrochloric acid in the gastric juice (achlorhydria).[34,35]

Clinical Manifestations. The clinical features of vitamin B_{12} deficiency include paranoid ideation, dementia, cognitive dysfunction, delusions, and hallucinations, often referred to as "megaloblastic madness."[34] The neurologic abnormalities include symmetric paresthesias of the feet and hands with vibratory sense and proprioception disturbances. The paresthesias progress to spastic ataxia owing to degenerative changes of the dorsal and lateral columns of the spinal cord. Cerebral signs include irritability, somnolence, memory impairment, and perversion of taste, smell, and vision.[34,35] Manifestations of pure folate deficiency include a blunted affect in general demeanor with evidence of depression, sleep deprivation, and irritability. History of circumstances likely to result in folic acid deficiency includes poor or fad diet, frank malabsorption, or alcoholism. In folate deficiency, cerebral symptoms, such as irritability, memory loss, and personality changes, are seen.[34,35] Clinical manifestations that are seen in both vitamin B_{12} and folate deficiencies include pedal edema, nocturia, tachypnea, dyspnea, and tachycardia associated with heart congestion;

glossitis, weight loss, malabsorption, and episodic or chronic diarrhea with steatorrhea are gastrointestinal manifestations. Musculoskeletal symptoms of arthralgia and frank arthritis are seen in autoimmune diseases; nocturnal pain and upper and/or lower extremity cramps often indicate spinothalamic tract involvement. Dermatologic symptoms include blotchy brown skin pigmentation, especially in nail beds and skin creases. When this is associated with vitiligo, autoimmune processes should be suspected.[34,35]

Recent research has reported an association between low folate levels and the risk of neural tube defects and abnormalities of the heart, urinary tract, and limbs in neonates. These data support the routine supplementation before pregnancy of all women who might become pregnant with 1.0 mg/day of folic acid.[34,35] This is the largest dose that will not mask vitamin B_{12} deficiency.

Treatment. Routine treatment with full doses of parenteral vitamin B_{12} (1 mg/day) and oral folate (1 to 5 mg/day) before the cause of the deficiency is identified should only be used in critically ill patients. In managing the anemia related to vitamin B_{12} or folate deficiency, it is important to (1) recognize that megaloblastic anemia is present, (2) ascertain if vitamin B_{12}, folate, or a combined deficiency is the cause, and (3) diagnose the underlying disease and mechanism responsible for the deficiency. In vitamin B_{12} and folic acid deficiency anemia, replacement therapy for vitamin B_{12} is oral cobalamin and folic acid. Transfusion therapy may be indicated in elderly or critically ill patients. Hypokalemia should be managed with potassium supplements to prevent sudden death, reportedly associated with a sharp drop in serum potassium level seen in vitamin B_{12} therapy.[34,35]

Course and Prognosis. The majority of patients respond well to replacement therapy; however, continued assessment and monitoring of these patients is essential to prevent hematologic or neurologic relapse secondary to inadequate therapy.[34,35] In patients with neurologic signs and symptoms, the reversibility of the neurologic damage is slow, with a maximal response requiring up to 6 months. Further substantial increases in recovery are unlikely after 12 months. In 90% of patients with subacute combined degeneration, major improvement is seen.[34] The degree of functional recovery is inversely related to the extent of the disease and duration of the signs and symptoms. Patients with signs and symptoms of less than 3 months duration may have complete reversal.[34,35]

Iron Deficiency Anemia

Etiology and Pathogenesis. Iron deficiency, the most common nutritional deficiency in the world, is the most common cause of anemia. Iron deficiency results in the unavailability of iron for hemoglobin synthesis. This may be due to low intake, diminished absorption (such as chronic disease), physiologic increase in requirements (such as pregnancy), excessive iron loss (such as acute or chronic hemorrhage), or chronic renal failure, hemodialysis, and idiopathic iron loss. The most common cause in men is occult gastrointestinal bleeding and in women is menorrhagia. Iron is one of the most carefully conserved body substances, and under normal conditions very little is lost except as a result of bleeding. Normal dietary requirements, if 10% is absorbed, are as follows: adult men, 12 mg/day; adult women aged 14 to 30 years, 15 mg/day; and adult women aged 60 years or more, 10 mg/day. Pregnant women require up to 30 mg/day, and children require 10 mg/day. A normal diet supplies the adult with about 10 to 15 mg/day.[36-40]

Laboratory Features. In latent iron deficiency there may be no anemia, but after receiving iron patients respond with a significant increase in blood hemoglobin level. In a typical case caused by chronic bleeding, the reduction in hemoglobin concentration is proportionately greater than the reduction in the red cell count. The red cells are smaller and paler than normal cells due to the decreased amount of hemoglobin and are described as **hypochromic, microcytic red cells.** Therefore, the red cell indices MCV, MCH, and MCHC are decreased. The white cell counts are usually normal. The platelet count varies, depending on the cause of the deficiency. In severely anemic children and infants, thrombocytopenia may be present. In patients who are bleeding, thrombocytosis may be present. The serum ferritin level is decreased to less than 10 ng/ml, the serum iron level is decreased, total iron binding capacity (TIBC) is increased, and tissue iron stores are decreased.[36-40]

Clinical Manifestations. In the majority of patients, anemia is asymptomatic; however, patients may experience general symptoms of anemia such as pallor, weakness, fatigue, dyspnea, palpitations, new and transient heart murmurs, irritability, headaches, lightheadedness, and pica (craving for nonfood substances such as dirt, clay, ice, laundry starch, cardboard, or hair). Restless legs are seen at night, especially in the elderly. In severe cases, gastrointestinal symptoms are seen, such as glossitis, dysphagia, erosions at the corners of the mouth, esophageal webbing, and atrophic gastritis, as well as changes in the fingernails, conjunctival pallor, and splenomegaly.[36-40]

Treatment. To maintain a normal iron balance in the body, men need to absorb 1.0-1.5 mg/day and women need to absorb 2-3 mg/day due to iron losses with menstruation. Iron deficiency anemia is managed with oral administration of ferrous sulfate (300 mg/day escalating to three times daily) until hematologic normality is reached. Infants may be given 50 to 100 mg daily in divided doses. Thereafter it is important to continue the treatment for 4 to 6 months to build iron stores. Urgent treatment may be accomplished with the administration to intravenous ferric gluconate following a test dose to determine possible hypersensitivity. Patients on dialysis should have a serum ferritin level greater than 100 µg/L to optimize their response to erythropoietin administration. Although iron therapy remediates the iron deficiency anemia, the underlying cause must be sought and corrected.[36-40]

Course and Prognosis. The symptoms may be alleviated in the first few days of treatment. The reticulocyte count is an index of erythropoiesis. The reticulocyte count increases as the RBC production increases and usually reaches maximal levels in 7 to 12 days, and the hemoglobin is usually normal by 2 months. The prognosis is excellent if the underlying cause is benign; however, even in patients with incurable disease states, management of iron deficiency anemia with iron therapy can increase the comfort level.[36-40]

ANEMIA RELATED TO INHERITED DISORDERS OF THE RED CELL

Thalassemia. Anemia can also be caused by increased RBC destruction, or **hemolysis.** Hemolytic anemias are characterized by decreased red cell survival rates. The thalassemias are examples of a type of anemia caused by decreased red cell survival rates. The red cells produced are abnormal and prone to destruction. This destruction is based on an intrinsic defect in the red cells.[41-44]

Etiology and Pathogenesis. The thalassemias are a group of diseases associated with the presence of mutant genes that suppress the rate of synthesis of globin chains. Thalassemias are classified according to the polypeptide chain or chains with deficient synthesis, such as α-thalassemia or β-thalassemia.[41-44]

A deficiency in one or more polypeptide chains causes decreased hemoglobin synthesis and an imbalance between α- and non–α-chain production. Because of the lack of hemoglobin, the anemia is severe, and the peripheral cells are microcytic and hypochromic. The disruption of the globin balance causes the normal chains to build up and precipitate within the cytoplasm. This damages the cell membranes, which leads to premature cell destruction. The most clinically severe form of the thalassemias is *thalassemia major,* which occurs in homozygous patients. *Thalassemia minor* is the term used to describe the heterozygous carrier state. For example, in homozygous β-thalassemia, the deficiency of β-chain synthesis results in the accumulation of α chains, which aggregate to form insoluble inclusions in bone marrow erythroid precursors (Figure 13-18). These inclusions cause early destruction of 70% to 85% of marrow erythroblasts. In response to this massive destruction, erythroid cell proliferation in homozygous β-thalassemia is significant.[41-44]

Patients who are significantly anemic have an increased intestinal iron absorption that is related to the degree of expansion of the RBC precursor population. This can be decreased with blood transfusions. The iron accumulates in the Kupffer cells of the liver, the macrophages in the spleen, and the parenchymal cells of the liver.[41]

Laboratory Features. Laboratory values vary, depending on the severity of the imbalance, which is determined by the genetic pattern. Due to the decrease in hemoglobin, the red cells are hypochromic and microcytic, and red cell indices—MCV, MCH, and MCHC—are decreased. Many target cells are present. In homozygous or major syndromes the hemoglobin is often less than 7 g/dl, and there are nucleated red cells in the peripheral blood. The leukocyte number is usually increased but the platelet number is normal. The bone marrow is hypercellular, with profound erythroblastic hyperplasia. There is evidence of hemolysis with increased unconjugated bilirubin levels and increased excretion of urobilin and urobilinogen. Hemoglobin electrophoresis is performed to determine the type of abnormal hemoglobin. An increased level of fetal

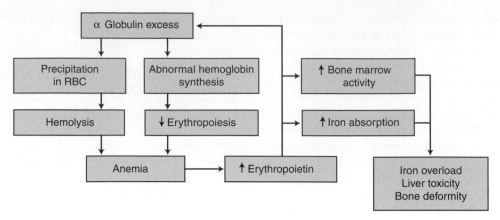

FIGURE 13-18 The pathophysiology of β-thalassemia. *HbF,* Hemoglobin F.

hemoglobin ranging from 10% to 90% is characteristic of homozygous α-thalassemia. No hemoglobin α is produced. Excess γ chains form γ4 homotetramers or Bart's hemoglobin. Excess β chains form β4 homotetramers or hemoglobin H.[41-44]

Clinical Manifestations. Patients may have any of the clinical manifestations described earlier (see General Effects of Anemia). The clinical findings are the result of deficient α-globin production in α-thalassemia or α-globin chain excess and persistent hemoglobin F production in β-thalassemia.[41-44]

α-Thalassemia is found primarily in Asian individuals; however, it has also been documented in increasing numbers in individuals of Mediterranean or African descent. Usually patients with α-thalassemia minor are silent carriers or present with mild to moderate anemia. They are identified during familial studies following the identification of a family member with Bart's hemoglobin hydrops fetalis or hemoglobin H disease (α-thalassemia major). Infants with Bart's hemoglobin hydrops fetalis are pale and edematous and have hepatomegaly, splenomegaly, and ascites. Individuals with hemoglobin H disease have typical facies and bone changes seen in β-thalassemia, splenomegaly, and hepatomegaly.[41-43]

β-Thalassemia occurs mainly in individuals of Mediterranean descent and presents as thalassemia major, intermedia, or minor. It is also seen in the Middle East, parts of India and Pakistan, and throughout Southeast Asia. Untreated patients with thalassemia major have skull bone deformities from intramedullary and extramedullary bone marrow expansion, mongoloid facies, bowing and **rarefaction** of long bones, extension of bone marrow into paraspinal or intra-abdominal tumors, **icterus,** hepatomegaly, splenomegaly, and cardiac failure or endocrinopathies, such as diabetes mellitus and hypogonadism from excessive intestinal iron absorption. Patients with thalassemia intermedia show fewer effects of iron overload, growth retardation, marrow expansion, and splenomegaly; however, deforming bone and joint disease, chronic leg ulceration, and infection are common in this form of thalassemia. Thalassemia minor is usually relatively asymptomatic.[41-44]

Treatment. Children with thalassemia are treated with blood transfusion therapy to maintain a hemoglobin level of 11 to 13 g/dl to ensure normal growth and development and to avoid skeletal deformities. Patients should be tested for presence of hepatitis B antibodies and immunized if they test negative. Splenectomy is recommended in children 6-7 years of age or in adolescents when their transfusion requirements exceed 1.5 times normal (>200/ml/kg/yr). Prior to the splenectomy, children should be immunized with polyvalent pneumococcal vaccine, Haemophilus influenzae and Neisseria meningitides. Iron supplements are avoided, and chelation therapy is started when the serum ferritin levels reach 1000 μg/dl. Vitamin C is required for management of iron overload. Bone marrow transplantation has been used with success in severe β-thalassemia. The best candidates are younger children, as older children have a high rejection and mortality rate.

Course and Prognosis. Infants with Bart's hemoglobin hydrops fetalis inherit an α-thalassemia gene from both parents who only have the α-thalassemia trait. These infants are usually stillborn or die within hours to days of birth. Some patients with hemoglobin H disease live a full life. Patients with β-thalassemia intermedia can expect to live until middle age; however, iron loading and crippling bone disease occur in the third and fourth decades. Children with adequate treatment with iron chelation prior to transplantation have disease-free survival rates up to 95%, while older patients and those exhibiting more than one risk factor have a rejection-free survival rate of less than 75%. Treatments under investigation include manipulation of the globin gene expression with drugs such as 5-azacytidine, hydroxyurea, erythropoietin, or butyrate analogues and gene therapy directed at replacing or compensating for the defective β-globin alleles. As this is a genetically transmitted disease, it is important for patients and parents to receive appropriate genetic counseling.[41-44]

Sickle Cell Anemia

Etiology and Pathogenesis. Sickle cell anemia is a genetically determined defect of hemoglobin synthesis. In hemoglobin S, valine is substituted for glutamic acid in the sixth position of the β chain, rather than the normal configuration. This apparently minor change in the molecular structure causes profound changes in hemoglobin stability and solubility. Under decreased oxygen tension, hemoglobin S undergoes polymerization, which causes the red cell to assume a sickled shape (Figure 13-19). Patients who are homozygous produce only hemoglobin S. No hemoglobin A is synthesized because all the β chains are S chains, which combine with normal α chains to form hemoglobin S. In heterozygous patients with sickle cell trait, both normal and S chains are formed. Because fewer abnormal chains are produced than normal ones, the amount of hemoglobin A usually exceeds that of hemoglobin S. It has been suggested that preferential sickling of cells with malarial parasites reduces the number of parasites and allows children with sickle cell trait who are infected with these parasites to reach reproductive age. This may have provided a selective advantage to the hemoglobin S trait, thereby preventing S from being genetically eliminated.[45-48]

The pathogenetic signs and symptoms of sickle cell disease all relate to the red cell sickling. Sickled red cells have a decreased survival time, which causes anemia. Sickled cells cause vascular occlusion, which results in capillary stasis, venous thrombosis, and arterial emboli. The most dangerous feature of sickle cell anemia is the occurrence of acute episodes of "crisis," which can be hemolytic or vascular (Box 13-2).[45-48]

Laboratory Features. The laboratory features in sickle cell anemia are distinctive. The anemia is usually severe, with red cells of different shapes and sizes. Target red cells are present, and occasionally sickled cells can be seen on smears (Figure 13-20). Red cell breakdown products are increased, which increases serum bilirubin, urobilinogen, and urobilin levels. Acute hemolytic crisis is characterized by hemoglobinuria, leukocytosis, and normoblastosis; diffuse intravascular coagulation may develop.[45-48]

Clinical Manifestations. Chronic hemolytic anemia, recurrent painful episodes, and acute and chronic organ dysfunction are the cardinal features of sickle cell anemia. Sickle cell anemia and sickle cell trait are found almost entirely in the black race.[45-48] Hemolysis of the sickle cells occurs in the spleen or vascular space, and vaso-occlusive events occur in the small

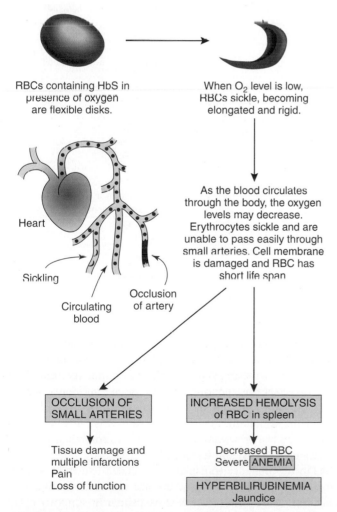

FIGURE 13-19 Sickle cell anemia: the effects of sickling. *RBC,* Red blood cell; *HbS,* hemoglobin S. (From Gould BE: *Pathophysiology for the health professions,* ed 2, Philadelphia, 2002, Saunders, p 247.)

BOX 13-2
Complications of Sickle Cell Anemia

Decreased RBC Survival
Anemia
Reticulocytosis
Hyperbilirubinemia
Increased pigment excretion
Cholelithiasis
Hyperplastic bone marrow
Osteoporosis
Osteosclerosis
Siderosis

Acute Hemolytic Crisis
Leukocytosis
Reticulocytosis
Hyperbilirubinemia
Hemoglobinuria
Normoblastosis
Diffuse intravascular coagulation (consumption coagulopathy)

Vascular Occlusion (Capillary Stasis, Venous Thrombosis, Arterial Emboli)
Splenomegaly
Splenic infarction
Splenic atrophy
Hepatomegaly
Cirrhosis
Hematuria
Sickle cell dactylitis
Aseptic necrosis of bones
Infarction of bone marrow
Infarction of various organs
Priapism
Skin ulcers
Pulmonary embolism

Painful Crisis (Occlusive Vascular Crisis)
Fever
Pain
Sudden death

Data from Miale J, editor: *Laboratory medicine hematology,* ed 6, St Louis, 1982, Mosby, p 637.

A   B

FIGURE 13-20 **A,** Blood smear showing sickle cells in sickle cell anemia. **B,** Scanning electron micrograph of deoxygenated sickled red cells. (**A,** Courtesy Beth Payne, Sacred Heart Medical Center, Spokane, Wash; **B,** from Young NS et al, editors, *Clinical hematology,* Philadelphia, 2006, Mosby, p 39.)

TABLE 13-7

Vasoocclusive Consequences of Sickle Cell Disease

Event	Incidence	Features
Acute		
Painful episodes	>50% of patients with HbSS and HbSβ-thalassemia	Mild to severe pain; one or several areas
Chest syndrome	10%-20% of adults	Difficult to distinguish from pneumonia; may involve entire lung
Priapism	10%-40% of males	Can have a more chronic form; causes impotence
Cerebrovascular accidents	1%-10% of children	Usually subarachnoid bleeding in adults
Hepatopathy	<2% of adults	Bilirubin may reach >80 mg/dl
Chronic		
Aseptic bone necrosis	10%-25% of adults	Hips and shoulders, common in HbSC
Proliferative retinopathy	50% of adults with HbSC; <5% HbSS 10%	Can lead to retinal detachment
Leg ulcers		Can be severe and disabling
Functional asplenia and autosplenectomy	Starts in infancy; >90% of adults with HbSS	Predispose to sepsis
Nephropathy	Renal failure in older patients	Nephritic syndrome, renal failure

Adapted from Sternberg MH: Hemoglobinopathies and thalassemias. In Stein JH et al, editors: *Internal medicine,* ed 5, St. Louis, 1998, Mosby, p 658.
HbS, Hemoglobin S (sickle hemoglobin); *HbSC,* hemoglobin SC disease; *HbSS,* hemoglobin SS (sickle cell anemia).

capillaries and venules caused by sickle cells.[45] The red cell life span is already shortened by the sickling and may precipitate a hemolytic crisis with jaundice. Sudden massive pooling of red cells, particularly in the spleen, can create a sequestration crisis, which is thought to result in the deaths that occur in the first years of life.[45-48] Infarctive crises or painful episodes are a result of obstruction of blood vessels, tissue hypoxia, and tissue death, and may occur throughout the body. Vaso-occlusive events are described in Table 13-7. Children with sickle cell anemia are shorter and experience delayed puberty, but they attain normal height with late adolescent growth. Bony abnormalities, "hand-foot" syndrome with periostitis of the metacarpal and metatarsal bones, splenomegaly, inability to concentrate urine, priapism with subsequent impotence,

underdeveloped genitalia and hypogonadism, hepatomegaly, jaundice, gallstones, tachycardia, acute chest syndrome (fever, chest pain, increasing WBC count, and pulmonary infiltrates), retinal vessel obstruction, cerebrovascular accidents, leg ulcers, and infections are all seen in sickle cell disease patients. Pregnant women may exhibit signs of pyelonephritis, pulmonary infarction, pneumonia, antepartum hemorrhage, premature fetal delivery, and fetal death.[45-48]

Treatment. Stem cell transplantation is curative and the treatment of choice. Currently there are no safe, effective antisickling agents, and treatment is primarily supportive. To avoid precipitation of a vaso-occlusive crisis, it is important to prevent dehydration, infection, fever, acidosis, hypoxemia, and cold exposure.[45-48] As salicylates impose an acid load, acetaminophen is the preferred antipyretic.[46] Vaccination for pneumococcal pneumonia should be done before 2 years of age in patients with sickle cell anemia and booster vaccinations given 3-5 years later. Penicillin prophylaxis is important to prevent streptococcal pneumonia and pneumococcal septicemia. Other vaccinations include *Haemophilus influenzae* type B and hepatitis B. Transfusions are used to restore normal hematocrit levels, and splenectomy is performed in children with sequestration syndrome. Treatment with oral hydroxyurea reduces leukocyte, PMN, reticulocyte, and sickle cell counts while increasing the hemoglobin and hematocrit and resulting in fewer acute painful episodes. Appropriate treatment of pain is important. During pregnancy, folic acid should be given to prevent neural tube defects. If iron deficiency is present, iron supplements should also be given. Transfusion should be used only when clinical and hematologic indicators are present.[45-48]

Course and Prognosis. Successful bone marrow stem cell transplantation cures sickle cell anemia. Bone marrow transplantation from a sibling matched donor has a 94% survival rate and an 84% event-free survival rate. Sickle cell anemia is a serious disorder, and without stem cell transplantation many patients die in childhood, especially in sequestration crisis. In young children with sickle cell anemia, there is a 30% incidence of splenic sequestration crisis with a 15% mortality rate. Functional hyposplenia predisposes individuals to infections, such as pneumonia and chronic pyelonephritis with renal failure. Heart failure, bone marrow and fat emboli, shock, and organ failure are common causes of death. In developed countries, patients who have not undergone stem cell transplantation may survive into the third and fourth decades, whereas survival past childhood in underdeveloped countries is unusual.[45-48] The survival rates have increased dramatically due to stem cell transplantation, newborn screening, early diagnosis, preventive measures to avoid sequestration crisis, and patient education.[45-48]

Hereditary Spherocytosis

Etiology and Pathogenesis. In hereditary spherocytosis, the red cells have defective red cell membrane skeletons, altered membrane properties, and altered cell metabolism. This causes them to have a decreased survival time in patients with an intact spleen. The disease is inherited as an autosomal dominant trait and is characterized by red cells that are fragile microspherocytes. In addition, there is increased destruction of **spherocytes** (abnormal spherical erythrocytes) in the spleen. Patients have anemia, intermittent jaundice, splenomegaly, and uniform responsiveness to splenectomy. The principal cellular defect is a loss of membrane surface area due to defects of several membrane proteins, including ankyrin, band 3, α-spectrin, and β-spectrin.[49-52]

Laboratory Features. The concentration of hemoglobin within the red cells is increased. Reticulocytosis is present, and microspherocytes are seen on the blood smear. Osmotic fragility is increased, and serum unconjugated bilirubin is increased. Following splenectomy, the hemoglobin is in the high-normal range.[49-52]

Clinical Manifestations. Hereditary spherocytosis is the most common hereditary hemolytic anemia and is most common in people with a northern European background. The major clinical manifestations are anemia, jaundice, splenomegaly, bile pigment gallstones, and chronic leg ulcers. The anemia is usually mild due to compensation by the erythropoietic bone marrow cells. Aplastic crisis precipitated by an infection may be seen with associated fever, abdominal discomfort, nausea, vomiting, rapidly increasing weakness, pallor, tachycardia, low blood pressure, and shock.[49-52]

Treatment. Treatment usually consists of splenectomy in children with severe cases (hemoglobin concentration <8 g/dl and reticulocyte count >10%) and children with moderate disease reflected (hemoglobin concentration 8-11 g/dl and reticulocyte count of 8% to 10%) when the anemia compromises physical activity. All children undergoing splenectomy should be immunized with polyvalent pneumococcal vaccine, Haemophilus influenzae and Neisseria meningitides. Oral penicillin should be given for several years after splenectomy to prevent pneumococcal sepsis. Folic acid therapy to prevent folate deficiency is necessary as well. Transfusion is usually indicated only in aplastic crisis.[49-52]

Course and Prognosis. Most patients have no or mild anemia, fluctuating degrees of jaundice, and episodes of aplastic or hemolytic anemia. Splenectomy is usually curative; however, the subsequent risk of acquiring a serious infection is significant.[49-52]

Glucose-6-Phosphate Dehydrogenase Deficiency

Etiology and Pathogenesis. An example of an RBC intracellular defect caused by an enzyme deficiency is glucose-6-phosphate dehydrogenase (G6PD) deficiency. The energy required for RBC membrane function and cellular integrity is derived from the anaerobic metabolism of glucose. Traditionally, hemolytic anemias caused by enzyme deficiencies have been called nonspherocytic to distinguish them from classic hereditary spherocytosis. When black soldiers receiving the antimalarial drug primaquine began suffering hemolytic episodes, a type of hemolytic anemia caused by a deficiency of G6PD (an enzyme in the red cell glycolytic pathway) was discovered. When G6PD-deficient RBCs are challenged by one of several drugs, glutathione is depleted and glucose utilization is inhibited. These events cause RBC membrane damage, which results in removal of the damaged cells by mononuclear phagocytes. Except in rare instances, G6PD-deficient persons do not have hemolytic anemia unless challenged by drugs.[53-58] G6PD deficiency is the most common metabolic disease of the RBC, and 130 million people are affected worldwide. This gene is found in 11% of African-American males and in Sephardic Jews. As the responsible gene is an X-linked recessive gene, close relatives of affected individuals should be screened. Because G6PD deficiency is found in areas where malaria was once endemic, G6PD deficiency is thought to have conferred selective advantage against *Plasmodium falciparum* malaria infection.[58]

Laboratory Features. Usually this anemia is first recognized during or after an infectious illness or following exposure to a suspect drug or chemical. The hematologic tests reflect the severity of the hemolytic episode. The diagnosis is made using a specific test that measures G6PD activity.[53-58]

Clinical Manifestations. Most individuals have no clinical manifestations of this disease. When such manifestations occur, hemolytic anemia is triggered by drug administration, infection, diabetic acidosis, the newborn period, and, in one subset, exposure to fava beans.[53-58]

Treatment. Treatment is usually preventive and consists of avoidance of drugs that trigger hemolytic episodes and aggressive infection management. Some patients may require transfusion therapy or exchange transfusion in the case of life-threatening hemolysis.[53-58]

Course and Prognosis. The prognosis is generally good as the episodes of hemolytic crisis are usually self-limiting, except in fava bean–susceptible individuals, in whom shock may develop in a short time.[55]

ANEMIA RELATED TO EXTRINSIC RED CELL DESTRUCTION OR LOSS

The final category of types of absolute anemia includes those caused by extrinsic abnormalities. The most important of these category types is immune hemolytic anemia caused by antibodies to red cells. Immune hemolytic anemias are further subdivided into those caused by isoantibodies, which may be the result of accidental immunization of individuals (e.g., hemolytic disease of the newborn), and those caused by autoantibodies (in individuals whose bodies create antibodies against their own red cells).[59-64]

Hemolytic Disease of the Newborn

Etiology and Pathogenesis. When fetal red cells cross the placenta, they may stimulate the production of maternal antibodies against antigens on the fetal red cell not inherited from the mother. These maternal antibodies cross into the fetal circulation and cause destruction of fetal cells. In severe cases, hydrops fetalis may result. Fetal-maternal ABO incompatibility is the most common cause of hemolytic disease of the newborn (HDNB), but Rh incompatibility is clinically more important because of the severity of the hemolytic disease in the fetus. With the introduction of Rh treatment, the total incidence of HDNB in Rh-negative women has been greatly reduced.[60,63]

Laboratory Features. Anemia, **reticulocytosis** (an increased number of circulating reticulocytes), and nucleated red cells are seen in the peripheral blood of the infant. There is a rough correlation between the hemoglobin levels and the severity of the disease. Untreated infants may experience a rapid fall in hemoglobin levels after birth. Leukocytosis is present, but platelet counts are usually normal. Infants with severe disease may have thrombocytopenia. Serum bilirubin, a hemolytic breakdown product, is readily transferred across the placenta. At birth, the baby's total bilirubin level reflects both the severity of the hemolytic process and the ability of the baby's liver enzyme system to conjugate and excrete bilirubin. Cord blood red cells show a characteristic positive direct antiglobulin test

(Coombs test), reflecting the maternal antibodies attached to the infant's red cells.[60,63]

During pregnancy, laboratory tests of amniotic fluid for bilirubin and antibodies and tests of the mother's peripheral blood for maternal sensitization are useful in predicting whether infants will be affected by HDNB.[60,63]

Clinical Manifestations. The clinical manifestations of HDNB are hemolytic anemia, extramedullary erythropoiesis, and hyperbilirubinemia. Jaundice, petechial hemorrhages, hepatomegaly, splenomegaly, heart failure (with pulmonary edema, pleural effusions, ascites, and edema), kernicterus (a condition in the newborn marked by severe neural symptoms, associated with high levels of bilirubin in the blood), and diffuse intravascular coagulation are seen in these infants. Many infants die in utero.[60,63]

Treatment. A standard dose of anti-Rh immunoglobulin (RhoGAM) is given to the mother before or after delivery. This immunoglobulin destroys the baby's RBCs before they can sensitize the mother. This dose protects the mother against 30 ml of Rh-positive blood. Amniocentesis and fetal blood sampling are used to evaluate the severity of the disease. In severe cases, in utero transfusion and early delivery have been performed on fetuses with severe **erythroblastosis.** Exchange transfusion lowers the serum bilirubin and the antibody content of the neonatal blood and removes cells susceptible to hemolysis. Phototherapy and phenobarbital are used to lower the bilirubin level.[60,63]

Course and Prognosis. The consequences of HDNB range from death, to possible retardation, to a barely perceptible hemolytic process. Severe anemia correlates with equally severe hyperbilirubinemia and high risk of central nervous system complications.[60,63] Many infants appear normal at birth, only to develop jaundice within 2 to 3 hours. Petechial hemorrhages develop soon after birth, and kernicterus is usually seen late in the second day of significant jaundice. Successful RhoGAM administration prevention programs have reduced the perinatal mortality rate to about 1% to 2%.[60,63]

Antibody-Mediated Drug Reactions

Etiology and Pathogenesis. Drug-induced immune hemolytic anemia is an example of a disease in which exposure to a drug causes destruction and lysis of the sensitized person's own red cells. Drugs can lead to red cell hemolysis by four different immune mechanisms (Table 13-8).[53,59,61,62,64]

Hapten Mechanisms. In the hapten mechanism, which is seen with penicillin, cephalosporins, and tetracycline, the drug combines with a component of the RBC membrane. An antibody is developed against the drug. When the drug is given again, it coats the red cells, and the antibody attaches to the drug–red cell complex. The antigen-antibody complex then causes hemolysis.[53,59,61,62,64]

Neoantigen Formation. The old terminology for neoantigen formation is *immune complex formation*. In this situation, the drug combines with the RBC membrane and the antibody reacts with the new antigenic sites created by the combination of the drug and membrane. The RBC is hemolyzed. The immune complex can also bind to platelet and leukocyte

TABLE 13-8

Mechanisms of Drug-Induced Hemolysis or Positive Direct Antiglobulin Test

	Drug Absorption	Neoantigen	Autoimmune	Nonimmune Adsorption
Prototype drug	Penicillin	Quinidine/stibophen	α-Methyldopa	First-generation cephalosporins
Role of drug	Cell-bound hapten	Antibody binds drug + RBC	Induces drug-independent RBC antibody	Modifies RBC membrane; adsorbs proteins non-antibody specifically
Typical DAT	IgG	C3	IgG	Nonimmunoglobulin
Antibody reactions	Reacts only with drug-coated cells	Reacts only with drug present	Drug independent; panagglutinin	No antibody present
Typical clinical presentation	Subacute onset; mild to severe hemolysis	Acute onset; severe hemolysis	Insidious onset; chronic mild hemolysis	No hemolysis

From Greer JP et al, editors: *Wintrobe's clinical hematology,* ed 11, Philadelphia, 2004, Lippincott Williams & Wilkins, p 1176.

RBC, Red blood cell; *DAT,* direct antiglobulin test; *C3,* complement third component.

membranes, causing anemia, leukopenia, and thrombocytopenia. Quinidine, hydrochlorothiazide, sulfonamides, isoniazid, tetracycline, and cephalosporin are common drugs that cause this type of reaction.[53,59,61,62,64]

Membrane Modification. In membrane modification, seen in cephalosporin sensitivity, the drug alters the RBC membrane protein. Plasma proteins attach to the altered RBC protein and cause a positive serologic test but no cell hemolysis.[61]

Autoantibody Induction. This mechanism was first studied in cases of hemolytic anemia with patients who were taking the antihypertensive agent methyldopa (Aldomet). The drug appears to induce antibody formation to red cell membrane Rh antigens. About 29% of the patients receiving this drug develop a positive antiglobulin test response.[53,59,61,62,64]

Laboratory Features. The laboratory features for all mechanisms show increased red cell turnover and anemia if hemolysis exceeds the rate of RBC production. Serologic tests, such as the direct antiglobulin test, will be positive. In hapten antibody–mediated drug reactions and in immune complex formation, the antiglobulin reaction is positive for immunoglobulins. In autoantibody induction, the antiglobulin reaction is positive for complement. Fragmented RBCs may be seen on the peripheral blood smear. These fragments are called *schistocytes* (Figure 13-21). Leukopenia and thrombocytopenia are sometimes seen with drug-induced platelet or leukocyte destruction.[53,59,61,62,64]

Clinical Manifestation. Types of immune drug-induced hemolytic anemia vary in symptoms and severity, depending on the mechanism involved. Hapten (e.g., penicillin) and autoimmune (e.g., methyldopa) drug-induced hemolytic anemias have an insidious onset of symptoms over a period of weeks. The neoantigen formation (e.g., quinine or quinidine) may present with sudden, severe hemolysis with hemoglobinuria and result in acute renal failure. Other clinical manifestations include acute respiratory distress syndrome and respiratory arrest.[53,59,61,62,64]

Treatment. Recognition and discontinuation of the responsible drug are usually the only treatment necessary. Steroid

FIGURE 13-21 Schistocytes are fragments of red blood cells produced by hemolytic pathologies. (Courtesy Beth Payne, Sacred Heart Medical Center, Spokane, Wash.)

therapy and transfusions may be required in cases of severe hemolysis.[53,59,61,62,64]

Course and Prognosis. Immune hemolytic anemia due to drugs is usually mild and the prognosis is good; however, with severe hemolysis, death can occur.[53,59,61,62,64] Laboratory findings for erythrocyte disorders are summarized in Table 13-5.

Acute Blood Loss

Etiology and Pathogenesis. Acute blood loss anemia may present after trauma or secondary to a disease process. Acute blood loss anemia rapidly decreases the overall blood volume and impairs oxygen delivery.[65,66]

Laboratory Features. A decrease occurs in both hematocrit and hemoglobin level due to blood loss. The hematocrit is less than 40% in men and 37% in women. The hemoglobin concentration is less than 14 g/dl in men and 12 g/dl in women.[65] Anemia may not be apparent in the early stages because the cells and plasma are diminishing simultaneously. As replacement fluids move into intravascular space, the anemia becomes apparent in later laboratory tests. The cells have normal MCV, MCH, and MCHC values.

Clinical Manifestations. In a normal 70-kg person with a 5000-ml total blood volume, 10% loss of blood (500 ml) rarely causes any clinical signs except occasional vasovagal syncope. A 20% loss (1000 ml) usually causes no clinical symptoms at rest, but tachycardia is seen with exercise, and a slight postural drop in blood pressure occurs.[65,66] A person with a 30% loss (1500 ml) usually presents with flat neck veins when supine, postural hypotension, and exercise tachycardia. A 40% loss (2000 ml) causes the central venous pressure, cardiac output, and arterial blood pressure to fall below normal while the patient is supine and at rest, with associated air hunger, tachycardia, and cold, clammy skin. A 50% loss of total blood volume (2500 ml) often causes shock and death.[65,66]

Treatment. Blood volume replacement therapy with crystalloid solutions, colloid solutions (plasma protein, albumin, or dextran), and fresh whole blood is essential in the early management of acute hemorrhage to restore blood volume and to prevent shock. Complete reliance on fresh whole blood for managing acute blood loss is contraindicated and should be reserved for patients with a low red cell mass, in whom tissue hypoxia is a threat. Replacement of red cell mass by increased red cell production is a gradual process, which occurs over 2-5 days as the marrow stem cells proliferate and mature. Maximal red cell production is seen by the 10th day after hemorrhage.[65,66]

Course and Prognosis. With adequate replacement therapy, the prognosis is excellent; however, the underlying cause must be identified and managed.

Other Extrinsic Abnormalities

Other *mechanisms,* such as mechanical heart valves or cardiopulmonary bypass machines, may cause physical damage to the red cells, resulting in hemolysis. Drugs and chemicals, physical agents (e.g., burns), or infectious diseases (e.g., malaria) may result in anemia. Venom from bee and wasp stings, spider and scorpion bites, and snake bites has been associated with hemolytic anemia. Finally, hypersplenism and splenomegaly can cause anemia, leukopenia, or thrombocytopenia severe enough to require splenectomy.[67]

TRANSFUSION THERAPY

Medical indications for transfusion therapy are restorations or maintenance of oxygen carrying capacity, blood volume, hemostasis, and leukocyte function. A summary of blood components, indications, actions, contraindications, precautions, and hazards is presented in Table 13-9.[66,68] Before transfusion therapy can occur, various donor tests are run on the blood unit sample. These include ABO and Rh(D); syphilis; HIV antigen and antibodies; hepatitis B and C antigens; and human T-cell lymphotropic virus. Blood centers, which are producing plasma for fractionation, also run a test for alanine aminotransferase.[68] Specific pretransfusion testing using blood samples from the recipient and the donor unit must be done to ensure that the blood component will not harm the recipient and the blood component will have an acceptable survival when transfused. ABO and Rh typing and RBC antibody

detection tests are run, and then a cross-match between the donor unit and the recipient is performed.[68] Types of transfusion reactions, signs and symptoms, usual causes, treatment, and precautions are summarized in Table 13-10.

KEY POINTS

- The general effects of anemia are due to tissue hypoxia and efforts to compensate for low oxygen carrying capacity. Vasoconstriction, pallor, tachypnea, dyspnea, tachycardia, ischemic pain, lethargy, and lightheadedness may be present. In addition, signs and symptoms relating to the specific cause of the anemia may be present. These accompanying manifestations are helpful in determining the cause of the anemia.

- Anemia may be due to abnormally low production of red cells and/or excessive loss or destruction. Decreased production of red cells may be due to stem cell failure (aplastic anemia), lack of erythropoietin (renal disease), or nutritional deficiencies of iron, vitamin B_{12}, or folate. Excessive red cell loss may be due to hemolysis (e.g., ABO and Rh incompatibility, drugs) or bleeding (e.g., surgery, trauma). Inherited disorders of red cells often impair production and increase destruction of red cells.

- Determination of the cause of anemia is based on the history, differential signs and symptoms, and results of laboratory studies. The important differentiating features of the major types of anemia are as follows:
    - *Aplastic anemia:* History of toxic or radiation injury to bone marrow. Accompanying leukopenia and thrombocytopenia. Red cells are normocytic and normochromic.
    - *Chronic renal failure:* History of renal disease. Decreased erythropoietin level and erythropoietin responsiveness. Red cells are normocytic and normochromic.
    - *Vitamin B_{12} and folate deficiency:* History of poor intake or gastrointestinal disease. Accompanying neurologic dysfunction. Red cells are megaloblastic (macrocytic).
    - *Iron deficiency:* History of poor intake or chronic blood loss. Decreased serum ferritin and iron levels. Red cells are microcytic and hypochromic.
    - *Hemolytic:* History of ABO or Rh incompatibility or drug exposure. Increased bilirubin, jaundice, positive direct antiglobulin. Red cells are normocytic and normochromic.
    - *Acute blood loss:* History of trauma, surgery, or known bleeding. Accompanying manifestations of volume depletion. Red cells are normal. Anemia may not be apparent until fluid loss is replaced.

- Inherited disorders of the red cell (thalassemia, sickle cell anemia, spherocytosis, G6PD deficiency) predispose red cells to early destruction because of abnormalities in hemoglobin structure, cell shape, membrane structure, or energy production. Manifestations of hemolysis (e.g., bilirubin, jaundice) are often present.

- The general management of anemia is aimed at removing the cause, if possible; restoring oxygen carrying capacity with blood transfusion when necessary; and preventing the complications of ischemia (e.g., with rest, oxygen therapy) and hemolysis (e.g., increased fluid intake, management of high bilirubin levels).

Polycythemia

In polycythemia, red cells are present in excess, increasing blood viscosity, which in turn causes clinical manifestations such as hypertension. The three types of polycythemia are classified according to cause. *Polycythemia vera* is associated with neoplastic transformation of bone marrow stem cells. *Secondary polycythemia* is due to chronic hypoxemia, with a resultant increase in erythropoietin production. *Relative polycythemia* is due to dehydration, which causes a spurious increase in the RBC count.

Polycythemia Vera

Etiology and Pathogenesis. Polycythemia vera or primary polycythemia is a type of chronic **panmyelosis** (See Chapter 11) and is part of the spectrum of myeloproliferative disorders. Polycythemia vera arises from the transformation of a single stem cell into a cell with a selective growth advantage that gradually becomes the predominant source of marrow precursors. There is an overproduction of normal red cells, white cells, and platelets. As with many malignancies, the cause is unknown. Possible mechanisms for the proliferation include (1) unregulated neoplastic proliferation of stem cells, (2) presence of abnormal myeloproliferative factor acting on normal stem cells, and (3) increase of stem cell sensitivity to erythropoietin and other hematopoietins.[69-73] Some researchers have postulated that it is damage to the undifferentiated stem cell by a virus, radiation, drugs, or other agents that causes mutation and subsequent neoplastic transformation.[69-73]

Laboratory Features. The diagnosis depends primarily on results of laboratory studies, which show an absolute increase in red cell mass and leukocytosis and thrombocytosis. The bone marrow shows **hyperplasia** of red cells, white cells, and platelets and extension of active hematopoietic marrow into bones of the extremities. Uric acid is increased due to excessive cell proliferation, which results in the destruction of an increased number of cells. Arterial oxygen saturation is normal, which differentiates polycythemia vera from the more common secondary (hypoxemic) polycythemia. Additional findings include elevated serum vitamin B_{12} and elevated leukocyte alkaline phosphatase levels (Figure 13-22).[69-73]

Clinical Manifestations. Symptoms include headache, backache, weakness, fatigue on exertion, pruritus, dizziness, sweating, visual disturbances, weight loss, paresthesias, dyspnea, joint complaints, and epigastric distress and pressure.[69-73] Common clinical manifestations include hypertension, thrombosis, and mucosal hemorrhage due to engorgement of retinal and sublingual veins, but each phase of the disease presents somewhat differently. Most of the clinical symptoms of polycythemia vera are related to the increased red cell mass, which gives rise to an increased blood viscosity. The liver and spleen become congested, which increases the risk of clots, acidosis, and organ infarction. The onset is insidious, with variable manifestations in virtually any organ system. Clinical symptoms appear between 60 and 80 years of age, and they appear more often in men and Caucasians. The disorder is rarely seen in children. In the pre-erythrocytic or developmental phase, hepatosplenomegaly, night sweats, and post-bathing pruritus are common. Other patients experience mild thrombohemorrhagic symptoms or **erythromelalgia** (painful erythematous palms and soles from an increased number of circulating platelets).[69-73]

The evolution of polycythemia vera is shown in Figure 13-23. The phases include an asymptomatic phase, a plethoric or erythrocytic phase, an inactive phase, and a spent phase when anemia develops. The final evolutionary phase of polycythemia vera is that of acute myeloid leukemia.[69-73]

In the erythrocytic phase, occlusive vascular lesions, such as transient ischemic attacks, cerebrovascular accidents (strokes), myocardial ischemia or infarctions, portal venous obstruction, or superficial venous thrombosis, occur and may be the first indication of the presence of the disease. The hyperviscosity produces symptoms of reduced cerebral blood flow, such as headaches, dizziness, and visual disturbances. Walking may induce leg pain and spasm, called *intermittent claudication*.[69-73]

Mucosal hemorrhagic manifestations include epistaxis, ecchymosis, and gastrointestinal and genitourinary bleeding. Progressive splenomegaly, intermittent claudication, peptic ulcer, hyperuricemia, and gout are often seen. The most striking feature is a ruddy or florid face, telangiectasis (chronic dilation of capillaries and small arterial branches producing small, reddish tumors of the skin) of the cheeks and nose, and purplish cyanosis of the lips and ears. Hypertension is seen in about half of patients. Distention of the retinal veins with a dark purple coloration is another important clinical finding. As the disease develops into the spent or postpolycythemia myeloid metaplasia phase, many patients complain only of **asthenia;** however, progressive hepatosplenomegaly, severe anemia, hemorrhage (particularly cutaneous), weight loss, and wasting often occur. The final phase is the development of acute myeloid leukemia.[69-73]

Treatment. There is no cure. Treatment is directed at reducing the increased blood volume, blood viscosity, red cell mass, and platelet counts by phlebotomy, radioactive phosphorus, and chemotherapeutic agents. Phlebotomy of 450-500 ml every 2-4 days until a normal hematocrit is reached alleviates many symptoms for most patients. Phlebotomy of only 200-300 ml should be considered for elderly patients or those with cardiovascular disease. In the past, a hematocrit of 50% was used as the upper limit of hematocrit tolerated before phlebotomy was used. Studies have found that increased vascular complications, decreased cerebral blood flow, and decreased mental alertness occurred when hematocrit levels exceeded 45%. Phlebotomy is effective in controlling red cell mass, but myelosuppressive therapy is needed when the platelet count increases to more than 800,000-1,000,000/μl to control hepatosplenomegaly and thrombocytosis. The agent of choice for myelosuppressive therapy is hydroxyurea, but radioactive phosphorus is also used. The efficacy of interferon remains to be determined.[69-73]

Course and Prognosis. Unmanaged polycythemia vera has a poor prognosis, with a survival of less than 2 years. The prognosis depends on the nature and severity of the complications,

TABLE 13-9

Summary of Blood Components

Component*	Major Indications	Action
Whole blood	Symptomatic anemia with large volume deficit	Restoration of oxygen-carrying capacity, restoration of blood volume
Whole blood irradiated	See *Whole blood;* risk for GVHD	See *Whole blood;* GVHD is reduced
RBCs; RBCs (adenine-saline added)†	Symptomatic anemia	Restoration of oxygen-carrying capacity
RBCs (deglycerolized)	See *RBCs;* IgA deficiency with anaphylactoid reactions	See *RBCs;* deglycerolization removes plasma protein; risk of allergic and febrile reactions reduced
RBCs irradiated	See *RBCs;* risk for GVHD	See *RBCs:* γ radiation inactivates donor lymphocytes; GVHD is reduced
RBCs (leukocyte-poor)	Symptomatic anemia, febrile reactions from leukocyte antibodies	Restoration of oxygen-carrying capacity
RBCs washed	See *RBCs;* IgA deficiency with anaphylactoid reactions; recurrent severe allergic reactions to unwashed red cell products	See *RBCs;* washing reduces plasma proteins; risk of allergic reactions may be reduced
Fresh-frozen plasma (FFP)	Deficit of labile and stable plasma coagulation factors and TTP	Source of labile and nonlabile plasma factors
Liquid plasma, plasma, and thawed plasma	Deficit of stable coagulation factors	Source of nonlabile factors
Plasma, cryoprecipitate reduced	TTP	See *FFP;* deficient in Factors I, VIII, vWF, and XIII; deficient in high molecular weight; vWF multimers as compared to FFP
Cryoprecipitated AHF; cryoprecipitated AHF, pooled	Hemophilia A,‡ von Willebrand disease,‡ hypofibrinogenemia, factor XIII deficiency	Provides factor VIII, fibrinogen, vWF, factor XIII
Platelets; platelets pooled	Bleeding from thrombocytopenia or platelet function abnormality	Improves hemostasis
Platelets, pheresis†	Bleeding from thrombocytopenia or platelet function abnormality	Improves hemostasis
Platelets irradiated; platelets pooled irradiated; platelets, pheresis irradiated	See *Platelets;* risk of GVHD	See *Platelets;* γ irradiation inactivates donor lymphocytes; reduced risk of GVHD
Platelets (leukocytes reduced); platelets, pheresis (leukocytes reduced)	See *Platelets;* febrile reactions; prevention of HLA alloimmunization	See *Platelets;* reduction of leukocytes reduces risk of febrile reactions, HLA alloimmunization, and CMV
Granulocytes, pheresis	Neutropenia with infection	Provides granulocytes
Granulocytes, pheresis irradiated; granulocytes platelets, irradiated	See *Granulocytes;* see *Platelets*	Provides granulocytes with or without platelets

AHF, Antihemophilic factor; *TTP,* thrombotic thrombocytopenic purpura; *GVHD,* graft-versus-host disease; *ITP,* idiopathic thrombocytopenic purpura; *vWF,* von Willebrand factor; *FFP,* fresh-frozen plasma; *CMV,* cytomegalovirus; *HLA,* human leukocyte antigen.
*For all cellular components, there is a risk that the recipient may become alloimmunized.
†RBCs and platelets may be processed in a manner that yields leukocyte-reduced components for which the main indications are prevention of febrile, nonhemolytic transfusion reactions and prevention of leukocyte alloimmunization. Risks are the same as for standard components, except for reduced risk of febrile reactions.
‡When virus-inactivated concentrates are not available.

Not Indicated for These Conditions	Special Precautions	Hazards	Rate of Infusion
Condition responsive to specific component	Must be ABO identical; labile coagulation factors deteriorate within 24 hours after collection	Infectious diseases; septic/toxic, allergic, febrile reactions; circulatory overload; GVHD	For massive loss, as fast as patient can tolerate
See *Whole blood*	See *Whole blood*	See *Whole blood*	See *Whole blood*
Pharmacologically treatable anemia; coagulation deficiency	Must be ABO compatible	Infectious diseases; septic/toxic, allergic, febrile reactions, GVHD	As patient can tolerate, but <4 hours
See *RBCs*	See *RBCs*		See *RBCs*
See *RBCs*	See *RBCs*	See *RBCs*	See *RBCs*
Pharmacologically treatable anemia; coagulation deficiency	Must be ABO compatible	Infectious diseases; septic/toxic, allergic reactions (unless plasma also removed [e.g., by washing]); GVHD	As patient can tolerate, but <4 hours
See *RBCs*	See *RBCs*	See *RBCs*	See *RBCs*
Condition responsive to volume replacement	Must be ABO compatible	Infectious diseases, allergic reactions, circulatory overload	<4 hours
Deficit of labile coagulation factors or volume replacement	Must be ABO compatible	Infectious diseases, allergic reactions	<4 hours
See *FFP*; deficiency of coagulation factors known to be depleted in this product, Factors I, VIII, vWF, XIII; volume replacement	Must be ABO compatible	See *FFP*	<4 hours
Deficit of any plasma protein other than those enriched in cryoprecipitated AHF	Frequent repeat doses may be necessary	Infectious diseases, allergic reactions	<4 hours
Plasma coagulation deficits; some conditions with rapid platelet destruction (e.g., ITP, TTP) unless life-threatening hemorrhage	Should not use some filters (check manufacturer's instructions); Must be ABO compatible with plasma	Infectious diseases; septic/toxic, allergic, febrile reaction; GVHD	<4 hours
Plasma coagulation deficits and some conditions with rapid platelet destruction (e.g., ITP)	Should not use some microaggregate filters (check manufacturer's instructions)	Infectious diseases; septic/toxic, allergic, febrile reactions; GVHD	<4 hours
See *Platelets*	See *Platelets*	See *Platelets*	See *Platelets*
See *Platelets*; leukocytes reduction; should not be used to prevent GVHD	See *Platelets*	See *Platelets*	See *Platelets*
Infection responsive to antibiotics	Must be ABO-compatible; do not use depth-type microaggregate filters	Infectious diseases; allergic, febrile reactions; GVHD	One unit over 2- to 4-hour period; observe closely for reactions
See *Granulocytes;* see *Platelets*	See *Granulocytes;* see *Platelets*	See *Granulocytes;* see *Platelets*	See *Granulocytes;* see *Platelets*

TABLE 13-10

Transfusion Reactions

Type	Signs and Symptoms	Usual Cause
Acute intravascular hemolytic (immune)	Hemoglobinemia and hemoglobinuria, fever, chills, anxiety, shock, disseminated intravascular coagulation (DIC), dyspnea, chest pain, flank pain, nausea/vomiting, headache, pain at needle site and along venous tract	Incompatibility due to clerical errors; involves ABO (primarily) or other erythrocyte antigen-antibody incompatibility
Delayed extravascular hemolytic (immune)	Fever, malaise, indirect hyperbilirubinemia, increased urine urobilinogen, falling hematocrit	Destruction of RBCs; usually involves non-ABO antigen-antibody incompatibility occurring 3-10 days post-transfusion
Graft versus host disease (GVHD)		Viable T lymphocytes react against tissue antigens in recipient. Immunocompromised recipients most at risk
Febrile	Fever, chills, rarely hypotension	Antibodies to leukocytes or plasma proteins
Allergic	Urticaria (hives), flushing, wheezing, laryngeal edema, rarely hypotension or anaphylaxis	Antibodies to plasma proteins
Hypervolemic	Dyspnea, rales, hypertension, pulmonary edema, cardiac arrhythmias, precordial pain, cyanosis, dry cough, distended neck veins	Too rapid or excessive blood transfusion
Noncardiogenic pulmonary edema	Dyspnea, pulmonary edema, normal cardiac pressures	Anti-HLA or antileukocyte antibodies
Hypothermia	Chills, low temperature, irregular heart rate, possible cardiac arrest	Rapid infusion of cold blood products
Electrolyte disturbances, hyperkalemia	Nausea, diarrhea, muscular weakness, flaccid paralysis, paresthesia of extremities, bradycardia, apprehension, cardiac arrest	Massive transfusions or in patients with renal problems
Citrate intoxication (hypocalcemia)	Tingling in fingers, tetany, muscular cramps, carpopedal spasm, hyperactive reflexes, convulsions	Massive transfusion of blood
Air emboli	Sudden difficulty in breathing, sharp pain in chest, apprehension, respiratory or cardiac arrest	Air emboli from blood administered under pressure
Bacterial sepsis	Shock, chills, fever	Contaminated blood component
Delayed reactions, transmission of infection	Signs of infection after transfusion (e.g., jaundice from hepatitis; bacterial or toxin contamination—high fever, severe headache or substernal pain, hypotension, intense flushing, vomiting/diarrhea)	Hepatitis, AIDS, malaria, syphilis, bacteria, viruses, other

Adapted with permission from Wong L, editor: *Nursing care of infants and children*, ed 8, St Louis, 2007, Mosby, p 1513-1514; and Pisciotto PT, Civarel Roberts SC, editors: *Blood transfusion therapy: a physician's handbook*, ed 3, Arlington, Va, 2000, American Association of Blood Banks.

the duration of the erythrocytotic phase, and the duration of the acute myeloid leukemia phase. Treatment in the erythrocytotic phase is essential, or the patients are at extremely high risk for thromboses. The development of thrombosis, hemorrhage, and myeloproliferative syndromes is common. Treated patients have a median survival of 10-15 years, with the most common causes of death being thrombosis, hemorrhage, leukemia, and other myeloproliferative conditions.[69-73]

Secondary Polycythemia

Etiology and Pathogenesis. Secondary polycythemia is absolute erythrocytosis caused by increased stimulation of RBC production, usually in response to tissue hypoxia caused by, for example, high altitude or lung disease. There are other less common types of secondary polycythemia that are caused by renal or other organ tumors, which cause an increase in erythropoietin production.[70,74]

Treatment	Precautions
Stop transfusion; hydrate; support blood pressure and respiration; induce diuresis; treat shock and DIC	Positively identify donor and recipient blood types and groups before transfusion is begun; verify with one other nurse or physician. Transfuse blood slowly for first 15-20 minutes and/or initial one-fifth volume of blood; remain with patient. In event of signs or symptoms, stop transfusion immediately, maintain patent IV line, and notify physician. Save donor blood to re–cross-match with patient's blood. Monitor blood pressure for shock. Insert urinary catheter and monitor hourly outputs. Send sample of patient's blood and urine to laboratory for presence of hemoglobin (indicates intravascular hemolysis). Observe for signs of hemorrhage resulting from DIC. Support medical therapies to reverse shock.
Monitor hematocrit, renal function, coagulation profile; no acute treatment generally required	Observe for post-transfusion anemia and decreasing benefit from successive transfusion
	Use γ-irradiated components to prevent GVHD
Stop transfusion; give antipyretics, acetaminophen (or aspirin if patient not thrombocytopenic)	Use of leukocyte-poor RBCs is less likely to cause reaction
Stop transfusion; give antihistamine; if severe, give epinephrine and/or steroids	Pretransfusion antihistamine; use of washed RBC components
Induce diuresis; phlebotomy; support cardio-respiratory system as needed	Transfuse blood slowly. Prevent overload by using packed RBCs or administering divided amounts of blood. Use infusion pump to regulate and maintain flow rate. If signs of overload, stop transfusion immediately. Place patient in semi-Fowler position to increase venous resistance
Support blood pressure and respiration (may require intubation)	Use washed RBCs; avoid unnecessary transfusion
Monitor temperature; if markedly subnormal, stop transfusion	Allow blood to warm at room temperature (<1 hour). Use an electric warming coil to rapidly warm blood
Kayexalate enemas if potassium >5.0 mEq/L	Use washed RBCs or fresh blood if patient at risk
Stop transfusion; administer IV calcium if severe	Infuse blood slowly (citrate reaction less likely to occur). If signs of tetany occur, clamp tubing immediately, maintain patent intravenous line, and notify physician
Stop transfusion; turn patient on left side; aspirate right atrial/ventricular air emboli	When infusing blood under pressure before container is empty: if air is observed in tubing, clamp tubing immediately below air bubble, clear tubing of air by aspirating air with syringe or disconnecting tubing and allowing blood to flow until air has escaped
Stop transfusion; support blood pressure; give antibiotics	Care in blood collection and storage
Stop transfusion; do culture and sensitivity tests; treat specific infection	Blood is tested for HBsAg (hepatitis B), syphilis, and, in most centers, HIV (AIDS); positive units are destroyed. Individuals at risk for carrying certain viruses are deferred from donation. Observe for signs of infection.

As this type of polycythemia demonstrates an increase in red cell mass with no involvement of other marrow elements, it is most commonly seen in association with a known hypoxic stimulus, increased erythropoietin, or excess adrenocortical steroids or androgens.[70,74]

Laboratory Features. The laboratory findings confirm increased red cell production with no increase in white cells or platelets. Erythropoietin levels are increased.[70,74]

Clinical Manifestations. The symptoms are those of the underlying disease state, such as cardiovascular disease with right-to-left shunt, chronic lung disease or alveolar hypoventilation, low barometric pressure, living at high altitudes, or abnormal hemoglobin concentration.[70,74]

Treatment. As this condition is a physiologic compensation, the clinical treatment is directed at identifying and managing the underlying cause. Phlebotomy has been used to reduce

FIGURE 13-22 Algorithm showing differentiating features of different forms of polycythemia. *Epo,* Erythropoietin; *BFU-E,* burst forming unit-erythroid; *2,3-BPG,* 2,3-bisphosphoglycerate; *EPOR,* erythropoietin receptor gene; *VHL,* von Hippel-Landau gene. (From Lichtman MA et al, editors: *Williams Hematology,* ed 7, New York, 2006, McGraw-Hill, p 791.)

cardiovascular work and appears to be helpful in both cardiovascular and chronic obstructive pulmonary disease. Oxygen administration is helpful in chronic lung diseases.

Course and Prognosis. The course and prognosis are influenced by the underlying disease process.

Relative Polycythemia

Etiology and Pathogenesis. **Relative** (spurious) **polycythemia** is characterized by an increased hematocrit in the presence of normal or decreased total RBC mass. Two types of patients manifest this characteristic. In the first group, the laboratory finding is secondary to an obvious disturbance in fluid balance such as is seen in severe dehydration or endocrinologic disorders. Patients in the other group, often described as having stress polycythemia, have hypertension, increased hematocrit levels, and no increase in total RBC mass or obvious fluid loss. Research is continuing on the etiologic process and pathogenesis.[69,74,75]

Laboratory Features. All hematologic tests are normal except for elevated hematocrit, hemoglobin level, and RBC count. The size and color of the red cell are normal. Increased levels of cholesterol and uric acid are common.[70,74,75]

Clinical Manifestations. The manifestations are contingent on the underlying cause. In dehydration, the patient will have flat neck veins, decreased skin turgor, thirst, tachycardia, and, in severe cases, low cardiac output and blood pressure. If the underlying condition is stress related, the symptoms are those of a catecholamine stress response. Patients are usually Caucasian middle-aged men. In patients with spurious polycythemia due to smoking, the problem is usually chronic, and the symptoms that are due to the hyperviscosity described for polycythemia vera are often found.[70,74,75]

Treatment. As this is a spurious form of polycythemia, it is important to recognize and manage the underlying cause. Fluid administration and management will resolve dehydration; however, spurious polycythemia is likely to be associated with a long-term condition that will require concurrent medical management. When the condition is a result of stress, identification of the stressors and stress management are indicated, with long-term follow-up. In spurious polycythemia due to smoking, the patient must stop smoking in order for the condition to resolve.[70,74,75]

Course and Prognosis. The long-term prognosis is excellent if the underlying condition is identified and resolved, but patients with chronic anxiety or an inability to quit smoking may experience the same complications related to erythrocytosis as are seen in polycythemia vera.[70,74,75]

Evolution of Polycythemia Vera

Asymptomatic
Splenomegaly
Isolated erythrocytosis
Isolated thrombocytosis

↓

Erythrocytotic phase
Erythrocytosis
Thrombocytosis
Leukocytosis
Splenomegaly
Thrombosis
Hemorrhage
Pruritus

↓

Inactive phase
No longer requires
phlebotomy or chemotherapy
Iron deficient

↓

Postpolycythemic myeloid metaplasia
Anemia
Leukoerythroblastosis
Thrombocytopenia or
thrombocytosis
Enlarging splenomegaly
Systematic symptoms
(fever, weight loss)

↓

Acute myeloid leukemia

FIGURE 13-23 Clinical evolution of polycythemia vera. (From Hoffman R et al, editors: *Hematology: basic principles and practice,* ed 4, New York, 2005, Churchill Livingstone, p 1216.)

KEY POINTS

- Three types of polycythemia have been identified, according to cause. Polycythemia vera is associated with neoplastic transformation of bone marrow stem cells. Secondary polycythemia is due to chronic hypoxemia, with a resultant increase in erythropoietin production. Relative polycythemia is due to dehydration, which causes a spurious increase in RBC count.
- Differential diagnosis of the type of polycythemia is based on the history and accompanying manifestations:
  - *Polycythemia vera*: Absence of hypoxemia and dehydration, accompanied by leukocytosis and thrombocytosis.
  - *Secondary polycythemia:* History of lung disease or living at high altitude. Hypoxemia evident on blood gas evaluation. Erythropoietin level is elevated.
  - *Relative polycythemia:* History of fluid loss or poor intake. Accompanying manifestations of dehydration.

- Treatment of polycythemia is aimed at removing the cause, if possible. Phlebotomy and bone marrow–suppressing agents may be used for polycythemia vera. Major complications of polycythemia are increased blood viscosity and the risk of thrombi.

SUMMARY

The purpose of the erythron is to ensure adequate oxygen delivery with respect to oxygen demand. This is enhanced by the unique ability of hemoglobin in RBCs to carry and release oxygen at a suitable tension to support energy-generating systems in the body tissues. Anemia, a deficit in RBCs, poses a serious threat to oxygen transport and to the ability of the body to receive adequate oxygenation. Intense research in RBC physiology and pathophysiology continually yields new information for a better understanding of erythrocyte disorders, improved treatment modalities, and improved prognoses.

REFERENCES

1. Platt W: Introduction to hematology. In Platt W, editor: *Color atlas and textbook of hematology,* Philadelphia, 1979, Lippincott, pp 1-6.
2. Hillman RS, Finch CA: General characteristics of the erythron. In Hillman RS, Finch CA, editors: *Red cell manual,* ed 7, Philadelphia, 1996, FA Davis, p 8.
3. Prchal JT: Production of erythrocytes. In Lichtman MA et al, editors: *Williams hematology,* ed 7, New York, 2006, McGraw-Hill, pp 393-403.
4. Ryan DH: Examination of the blood. In Lichtman MA et al, editors: *Williams hematology,* ed 7, New York, 2006, McGraw-Hill, pp 11-19.
5. Roberts HR, Monroe DM, Hoffman M: Molecular biology and biochemistry of the coagulation factors and pathways of hemostasis. In Lichtman MA et al, editors: *Williams hematology,* ed 7, New York, 2006, McGraw-Hill, pp 1665-1693.
6. Kaushansky K: Hematopoietic stem cells, progenitors, and cytokines. In Lichtman MA et al, editors: *Williams hematology,* ed 7, New York, 2006, McGraw-Hill, pp 201-220.
7. Diggs L, Sturm D, Bell A: *The morphology of human blood cells,* Abbott Park, Ill, 1985, Abbott Laboratories, pp 1-86.
8. Nagel RL: Disorders of hemoglobin function and stability. In Handin RL, Lux SE, Stossel TP, editors: *Blood: principles and practice of hematology,* ed 2, Philadelphia, 2003, Lippincott, pp 1597-1654.
9. Telen MJ, Kaufman RE: The mature erythrocyte. In Greer JP et al, editors: *Wintrobe's clinical hematology,* ed 11, Philadelphia, 2004, Lippincott Williams & Wilkins, pp 217-247.
10. McKenzie SB: Megaloblastic and nonmegaloblastic macrocytic anemias. *Textbook of hematology,* ed 2, Baltimore, 1996, Williams & Wilkins, pp 177-199.
11. Carmel R, Rosenblatt DS: Disorders of cobalamin and folate metabolism. In Handin RL, Lux SE, Stossel TP, editors: *Blood: principles and practice of hematology,* ed 2, Philadelphia, 2003, Lippincott, pp 1361-1398.
12. Beutler L: Composition of the erythrocyte. In Lichtman MA et al, editors: *Williams hematology,* ed 7, New York, 2006, McGraw-Hill, pp 387-391.
13. Bull BS: Morphology of the erython. In Lichtman MA et al, editors: *Williams hematology,* ed 7, New York, 2006, McGraw-Hill, pp 369-385.

14. Dessypris EN et al: Erythropoiesis. In Greer JP et al, editors: *Wintrobe's clinical hematology,* ed 11, Philadelphia, 2004, Lippincott Williams & Wilkins, pp 195-216.

15. Papayannopoulou T, D'Andrea A, Abkowitz J, et al: Biology of erythropoiesis erythroid differentiation, and maturation. In Hoffman RL et al, editors: *Hematology: basic principles and practice,* ed 4, New York, 2005, Churchill Livingstone, Accessed www.mdconsult.com September, 2007.

16. Guyton AC: Red blood cells, anemia, polycythemia. In Guyton AC, Hall JE, editors: *Textbook of medical physiology,* ed 11, Philadelphia, 2006, Saunders, pp 419-428.

17. Guyton AC: Transport of oxygen and carbon dioxide in the blood and body fluids. In Guyton AC, Hall JE, editors: *Textbook of medical physiology,* ed 11, Philadelphia, 2006, Saunders, pp 502-513.

18. Ellstrom K: The pulmonary system. In Alspach JG, editor: *Core curriculum for critical care nursing,* ed 6, St. Louis, 2006, Saunders, pp 45-183.

19. American Edwards Laboratories: *Continuous SvO$_2$ monitoring: theory and applications,* Irvine, Calif, n.d., The Laboratories.

20. Ahrens TS, Powers KC: Pulmonary clinical physiology. In Kinney MR, Packa DR, Dunbar SB, editors: *AACN's clinical reference for critical care nursing,* ed 4, St Louis, 1998, Mosby, pp 491-516.

21. Prchal JT: Clinical manifestations and classification of erythrocyte disorders. In Lichtman MA et al, editors: *Williams hematology,* ed 7, New York, 2006, McGraw-Hill, pp 411-418.

22. Prchal JT: Clinical manifestations and classification of erythrocyte disorders. In Lichtman MA et al, editors: *Williams hematology,* ed 7, New York, 2006, McGraw-Hill, pp 411-418.

23. Segal GB: Aplastic anemia. In Lichtman MA et al, editors: *Williams hematology,* ed 7, New York, 2006, McGraw-Hill, pp 419-436.

24. Guinan EC, Shimamura A: Aplastic anemia and acquired syndromes. In Greer JP et al, editors: *Wintrobe's clinical hematology,* ed 11, Philadelphia, 2004, Lippincott, Williams & Wilkins, pp 1397-1419.

25. Young NS, Maciejewski JP: Aplastic anemia. In Hoffman RL, et al, editors: *Hematology: basic principles and practice,* ed 4, New York, 2005, Churchill Livingstone. Accessed www.mdconsult.com September, 2007.

26. Castro-Malaspina H, O'Reilly RJ: Aplastic anemia and related disorders. In Goldman L, Ausiello D, editors: *Cecil textbook of medicine,* ed 22, Philadelphia, 2004, Saunders, pp 1044-1050.

27. Negrin RS, Blume KG: Principles of hematopoietic cell transplantation. In Lichtman MA et al, editors: *Williams hematology,* ed 7, New York, 2006, McGraw-Hill, pp 301-322.

28. Caro J: Anemia of chronic renal failure. In Lichtman MA et al, editors: *Williams hematology,* ed 7, New York, 2006, McGraw-Hill, pp 449-457.

29. Skorecki K, Green J, Brenner BM: Chronic renal failure. In Kasper DL et al, editors: *Harrison's principles of internal medicine,* ed 16, New York, 2005, McGraw-Hill, pp 1653-1663.

30. Rosovsky R, Marks PW: Hematologic manifestations of systemic disease: liver and renal disease. In Hoffman R et al, editors: *Hematology: basic principles and practice,* ed 4, New York, 2005, Churchill Livingstone. Accessed www.mdconsult.com, September 2007.

31. Tolkoff-Rubin N, Goes N: Treatment of irreversible renal failure. In Goldman L, Ausiello D, editors: *Cecil textbook of medicine,* ed 22, Philadelphia, 2004, Saunders, pp 716-726.

32. Means RT: Anemias secondary to chronic disease and systemic disorders. In Greer JP et al, editors: *Wintrobe's clinical hematology,* ed 11, Philadelphia, 2004, Lippincott Williams & Wilkins, pp 1445-1466.

33. Luke RG: Chronic renal failure. In Goldman L, Ausiello D , editors: *Cecil textbook of medicine,* ed 22, Philadelphia, 2004, Saunders, pp 708-716.

34. Antony AC: Megaloblastic anemias. In Hoffman R, et al, editors: *Hematology: basic principles and practice,* ed 4, New York, 2005, Churchill Livingstone. Accessed www.mdconsult.com, September, 2007.

35. Babior BM: Folate, cobalamin, and megaloblastic anemias. In Lichtman MA et al, editors: *Williams hematology,* ed 7, New York, 2006, McGraw-Hill, pp 477-509.

36. Andrews NC: Iron deficiency and related disorders. In Greer JP et al, editors: *Wintrobe's clinical hematology,* ed 11, Philadelphia, 2004, Lippincott Williams & Wilkins, pp 979-1009.

37. Adamson JW: Iron deficiency anemia and other hypoproliferative anemias. In Kasper DL et al, editors: *Harrison's principles of internal medicine,* ed 16, New York, 2005, McGraw-Hill, pp 586-592.

38. Beutler E et al: Disorders of iron metabolism. In Lichtman MA et al, editors: *Williams hematology,* ed 7, New York, 2006, McGraw-Hill, pp 511-553.

39. Brittenham GM: Disorders of iron metabolism: iron deficiency and overload. In Hoffman R et al, editors: *Hematology: basic principles and practice,* ed 4, New York, 2005, Churchill Livingstone. Accessed www.mdconsult.com, September, 2007.

40. Duffy TP: Microcytic and hypochromic anemias. In Goldman L, Ausiello D, editors: *Cecil textbook of medicine,* ed 22, Philadelphia, 2004, Saunders, pp 1003-1008.

41. Weatherall DJ: Disorders of globin synthesis: the thalassemias. In Lichtman MA et al, editors: *Williams hematology,* ed 7, New York, 2006, McGraw-Hill, pp 633-666.

42. Borgna-Pignatti C, Galanello R: The thalassemias and related disorders: quantitative disorders of hemoglobin synthesis. In Greer JP et al, editors: *Wintrobe's clinical hematology,* ed 11, Philadelphia, 2004, Lippincott Williams & Wilkins, pp 1319-1665.

43. Rodgers GP et al: Hemoglobinopathies: the thalassemias. In Goldman L, Ausiello D, editors: *Cecil textbook of medicine,* ed 22, Philadelphia, 2004, Saunders, pp 1009-1013.

44. Benz EJ: Hemoglobinopathies. In Kasper DL et al, editors: *Harrison's principles of internal medicine,* ed 16, New York, 2005, McGraw-Hill, pp 593-601.

45. Beutler E: Disorders of hemoglobin structure: sickle cell anemia. In Lichtman MA et al, editors: *Williams hematology,* ed 7, New York, 2006, McGraw-Hill, pp 667-700.

46. Lukens JN: Abnormal hemoglobins: general principles. In Greer JP et al, editors: *Wintrobe's clinical hematology,* ed 11, Philadelphia, 2004, Lippincott, Williams & Wilkins, pp 1247-1262.

47. Sauntharajah Y, Vichinsky EP, Embury SH: Sickle cell disease. In Hoffman R et al, editors: *Hematology: basic principles and practice,* ed 4, New York, 2005, Churchill Livingstone. Accessed www.mdconsult.com, September, 2007.

48. Embury SH: Sickle cell anemias and associated hemoglobinopathies. In Goldman L, Ausiello D, editors: *Cecil textbook of medicine,* ed 22, Philadelphia, 2004, Saunders, pp 1030-1039.

49. Gallagher PG: Disorders of the red blood cell membrane: hereditary spherocytosis, elliptocytosis, and related disorders. In Lichtman MA et al, editors: *Williams hematology,* ed 7, New York, 2006, McGraw-Hill, pp 571-601.

50. Golan DE: Hemolytic anemias: red cell membrane and metabolic defects. In Goldman L, Ausiello D, editors: *Cecil textbook of medicine,* ed 22, Philadelphia, 2004, Saunders, pp 1021-1030.

51. Mentzer WC, Glader BE: Hereditary spherocytosis and other anemias due to abnormalities of the red cell membrane. In Greer JP et al, editors: *Wintrobe's clinical hematology,* ed 11, Philadelphia, 2004, Lippincott Williams & Wilkins, pp 1089-1114.

52. Gallagher PG: Red blood cell membrane disorders. In Hoffman R et al, editors: *Hematology: basic principles and practice,* ed 4, New York, 2005, Churchill Livingstone. Accessed www.mdconsult.com, September 2007.

53. Bunn HF, Rosse W: Hemolytic anemia and acute blood loss. In Kasper DL et al, editors: *Harrison's principles of internal medicine,* ed 16, New York, 2005, McGraw-Hill, pp 607-617.

54. Vulliamy TJ, Luzzatto L: Glucose-6-phosphate dehydrogenase deficiency and related disorders. In Handin RL, Lux SE, Stossel TP, editors: *Blood: principles and practice of hematology,* ed 2, Philadelphia, 2003, Lippincott, pp 1921-1950.

55. Beutler E: Disorders of red cells resulting from enzyme abnormalities. In Lichtman MA et al, editors: *Williams hematology,* ed 7, New York, 2006, McGraw-Hill, pp 603-631.

56. Gregg XT, Prchal JT: Red cell enzymopathies. In Hoffman R, et al, editors: *Hematology: basic principles and practice,* ed 4, New York, 2005, Churchill Livingstone. Accessed www.mdconsult.com, September, 2007.

57. Golan DE: Hemolytic anemias: red cell membrane and metabolic defects. In Goldman L, Ausiello D, editors: *Cecil textbook of medicine,* ed 22, Philadelphia, 2004, Saunders, pp 1021-1030.

58. Glader BE: Hereditary hemolytic anemia due to enzyme disorders. In Greer JP et al, editors: *Wintrobe's clinical hematology,* ed 11, Philadelphia, 2004, Lippincott Williams & Wilkins, pp 1115-1140.

59. Neff AT: Autoimmune hemolytic anemias. In Greer JP et al, editors: *Wintrobe's clinical hematology,* ed 11, Philadelphia, 2004, Lippincott Williams & Wilkins, pp 1157-1182.

60. Ramasethu J, Luban NLC: Alloimmune hemolytic disease of the newborn. In Lichtman MA et al, editors: *Williams hematology,* ed 7, New York, 2006, McGraw-Hill, pp 751-765.

61. Packman CH: Hemolytic anemia resulting from immune injury. In Lichtman MA et al, editors: *Williams hematology,* ed 7, New York, 2006, McGraw-Hill, pp 729-750.

62. Weaver SJ, Johns TE: Drug-induced hematologic disorders. In Dipiro JT et al, editors: *Pharmacotherapy: a pathophysiologic approach,* ed 6, New York, 2005, McGraw-Hill, pp 1875-1889.

63. Eder AF, Manno CS: Alloimmune hemolytic disease of the fetus and newborn. In Greer JP et al, editors: *Wintrobe's clinical hematology,* ed 11, Philadelphia, 2004, Lippincott Williams & Wilkins, pp 1183-1202.

64. Cunningham MJ, Siberstein LE: Autoimmune hemolytic anemia. In Hoffman R et al, editors: *Hematology: basic principles and practice,* ed 4, New York, 2005, Churchill Livingstone. Accessed www.mdconsult.com, September 2007.

65. Hillman RS, Hershko C: Acute blood loss anemia. In Lichtman MA et al, editors: *Williams hematology,* ed 7, New York, 2006, McGraw-Hill, pp 767-771.

66. Galel S, Malone III JM, Viele MK: Transfusion medicine. In Greer JP et al, editors: *Wintrobe's clinical hematology,* ed 11, Philadelphia, 2004, Lippincott Williams & Wilkins, pp 831-882.

67. Beutler E: Hemolytic anemia due to chemical and physical agents. In Lichtman MA et al, editors: *Williams hematology,* ed 7, New York, 2006, McGraw-Hill, pp 717-721.

68. American Association of Blood Banks, America's Blood Centers: *Circular of information for the use of human blood and blood components (ARC 1751),* Arlington, Va, August 2002, American Red Cross.

69. Prchal JT, Beutler E: Primary and secondary polycythemias. In Lichtman MA et al, editors: *Williams hematology,* ed 7, New York, 2006, McGraw-Hill, pp 779-802.

70. Means RT: Erythrocytosis. In Greer JP et al, editors: *Wintrobe's clinical hematology,* ed 11, Philadelphia, 2004, Lippincott Williams & Wilkins, pp 1495-1500.

71. Hoffman R: Polycythemias. In Hoffman R et al, editors: *Hematology: basic principles and practice,* ed 4, New York, 2005, Churchill Livingstone. Accessed www.mdconsult.com, September 2007.

72. Gilliland DG, Dunbar CL: Myelodysplastic syndromes. In Handin RL, Lux SE, Stossel TP, editors: *Blood: principles and practice of hematology,* ed 2, Philadelphia, 2003, Lippincott, pp 335-377.

73. Spivak JL: Polycythemia vera and other myeloproliferative diseases. In Kasper DL et al, editors: *Harrison's principles of internal medicine,* ed 16, New York, 2005, McGraw-Hill, pp 626-631.

74. Means RT: Polycythemia: erythrocytosis. In Greer JP et al, editors: *Wintrobe's clinical hematology,* ed 11, Philadelphia, 2005, Lippincott Williams & Wilkins, pp 1538-1554.

75. Beutler E: Preservation and clinical use of erythrocytes and whole blood. In Lichtman MA et al, editors: *Williams hematology,* ed 7, New York, 2006, McGraw-Hill, pp 2159-2173.

Alterations in Hemostasis and Blood Coagulation

Naomi Lungstrom • Roberta J. Emerson

▌ MEDIA RESOURCES

Additional Material for Study, Review, and Further Exploration

 CD Companion ▪ Review Questions and Answers
▪ Glossary (with audio pronunciations for selected terms)
▪ Disease Profiles ▪ Animations

evolve **Website** at http://evolve.elsevier.com/Copstead/
▪ Case Studies ▪ Disease Profiles ▪ WebLinks ▪ Key Points Review

 Online Course (Module 9)

▌ KEY QUESTIONS

▪ How do platelets and factors of the clotting cascade contribute to hemostasis?
▪ What findings from the patient history, physical, or laboratory studies would indicate a potential bleeding disorder?
▪ How are laboratory tests used to differentiate the various coagulation disorders?

▪ What vascular alterations result in abnormalities of hemostasis?
▪ What are the common causes of platelet deficiencies, excesses, and dysfunction?
▪ What are the common causes of inherited and acquired disorders of coagulation?

▌ CHAPTER OUTLINE

The term **hemostasis** means arrest of bleeding or prevention of blood loss after a blood vessel is injured. Hemostasis is accomplished via a complex interaction involving the vessel wall, circulating platelets, and plasma coagulation proteins. If hemostasis is inadequate, bleeding results; if hemostasis is excessive, inappropriate clotting or thrombosis results.

This chapter reviews the process of hemostasis and how that process is evaluated by means of clinical assessment and laboratory tests. The focus of this chapter is disorders of hemostasis and coagulation that result in bleeding. Disorders that result in thrombosis are discussed in Chapter 15.

THE PROCESS OF HEMOSTASIS

Stages of Hemostasis

Primary hemostasis, the initial response to vascular injury, involves the interaction between platelets and the endothelium of the injured blood vessel. The immediate response of the vessel to trauma is vasoconstriction to reduce blood loss. Although nervous reflex may play a part, this vasoconstriction results primarily from local myogenic spasm that may last from minutes to hours. The more trauma to the vessel, the greater the degree of vascular spasm. More vasoconstriction occurs with a blunt or crushing injury (resulting in less bleeding) than with a sharp cut to a vessel.[1]

The second component of primary hemostasis is formation of a platelet plug. Platelets not only adhere to endothelial collagen exposed by injury, they also aggregate (clump together)

at the site of vessel injury. The formation of this platelet plug is usually completed within 3 to 7 minutes.

Secondary hemostasis involves the formation of a fibrin clot, or **coagulation,** at the site of injury to maintain the hemostasis already initiated. Clotting factors are activated via the **intrinsic pathway** or **extrinsic pathway,** and participate in a series of events that catalyze or facilitate the conversion of fibrinogen to fibrin. This process takes an average of 3 to 10 minutes.

Clot retraction, the final stage of clot formation, occurs when the components of the fibrin clot—the platelet plug, fibrin strands, and trapped red blood cells—are compressed or contracted to form a firm clot. This stage takes approximately 1 hour.

Platelets

Platelets have an integral role in hemostasis; thus, it is important to review their nature and function (Figure 14-1). A normal platelet count is between 150,000/mm³ and 350,000/mm³. Platelets, also known as *thrombocytes,* are the smallest of the formed elements in the blood. They are produced in the bone marrow from megakaryocytes, which are derived from the pluripotent stem cell. Approximately 70% of platelets are found in the circulation and 30% are sequestered in the spleen.[2] Factors such as the stress response, epinephrine, and exercise may stimulate platelet production. The average life span of a platelet is 10 days. On completion of its life span, a platelet is eliminated from the circulation by the tissue macrophage system.[1-3]

FIGURE 14-1 Platelets are complex cell fragments containing numerous chemical mediators that are released when platelets are activated. Platelets display a variety of cell surface receptors that mediate both adhesion to exposed subendothelium and aggregation with other platelets. *ADP,* Adenosine diphosphate; *VWF,* von Willebrand factor; *TxA₂,* thromboxane A₂; *Epi,* epinephrine.

FIGURE 14-2 A, Endothelial cells normally prevent platelet adhesion by releasing nitric oxide (NO) and prostaglandin I_2 (PGI_2), which increases platelet cGMP and cAMP levels, reducing the likelihood of their being activated. **B,** Injury to the vessel wall exposes collagen and von Willebrand factor (VWF), which are bound by specific receptors on platelets causing them to adhere and become activated. **C,** Activated platelets release numerous chemical mediators that bind to and stimulate other nearby platelets. Groups of platelets aggregate together by binding to fibrinogen molecules through their GpIIb/IIIa receptors. *ADP,* Adenosine diphosphate; *TxA₂,* thromboxane A_2.

Platelets play a complex role in the process of hemostasis. Initially, platelets adhere to subendothelial collagen exposed by trauma (Figure 14-2). After adhesion, the platelets become activated and initiate degranulation, the release of alpha granules and dense bodies. Alpha granules release platelet thrombospondin, fibrinogen, fibronectin, von Willebrand factor, and coagulation factors V and VIII. The dense granules release adenosine diphosphate (ADP), adenosine triphosphate (ATP), and serotonin. The presence of ADP and collagen encourages arachidonic acid formation, which leads to formation of thromboxane A_2 (a potent platelet aggregation agonist). Aspirin and other cyclooxygenase enzyme inhibitors can be used to block this cascade. Thromboxane A_2 stimulates the glycoprotein IIb/IIIa receptors on platelets to be expressed and further promotes platelet adhesion. The glycoprotein IIb/IIIa blockers (e.g., eptifibatide) are useful antiplatelet agents.[2-5]

In addition to the major role platelets play in primary hemostasis, they are also involved in secondary hemostasis and clot retraction. Platelets catalyze interactions between activated coagulation factors, accelerating the conversion of prothrombin to thrombin. Platelets also have a role in clot retraction.

Blood Coagulation Factors

With the exception of tissue factor (factor III; tissue thromboplastin) and calcium, blood coagulation factors are plasma proteins that circulate in the bloodstream in an inactive state. These factors are listed in Table 14-1 according to the internationally standardized nomenclature. The factors are numbered in the order of their discovery, not the order in which they participate in the clotting cascade. Factors with both active and inactive forms are differentiated with the letter "a" after the Roman numeral to designate the active form.

The liver is responsible for the synthesis of coagulation factors, with the exception of part of factor VIII. Factors II, VII, IX, X, protein C, and protein S are dependent on vitamin K for synthesis and normal activity. Some of the coagulation proteins also can be synthesized by other cells, such as megakaryocytes and endothelial cells.[4,5] Antithrombin III and protein C are protein complexes that promote anticoagulation. Antithrombin is a potent anticoagulant that binds to and inactivates free thrombin, preventing its binding and cleaving of fibrinogen. Protein C, a plasma protein that inactivates factors V and VIII, prevents clot formation. Protein S assists protein C in binding to phospholipase and stimulates release of tissue plasminogen activator, initiating fibrinolysis.[2,4,5] Low-molecular-weight heparins and heparin work by enhancing the activity of antithrombin III (Figure 14-3).

Fibrin Clot

In normal hemostasis, the fibrin clot is produced through activation of the intrinsic or extrinsic pathway and, in turn, the common final pathway. Effective hemostasis is the result of interactions between all of these pathways and is commonly referred to as the *coagulation cascade.*

Figure 14-4 illustrates the coagulation cascade. The intrinsic pathway of coagulation begins when blood comes into contact with altered vascular endothelium or another negatively charged surface, such as glass. This contact phase of coagulation involves four factors: (1) factor XII, (2) high-molecular-weight kininogen (HMWK), (3) prekallikrein, and (4) factor XI. Factor XII is activated to factor XIIa, which in turn activates XI to XIa and prekallikrein to its active form, kallikrein. Kallikrein liberates bradykinin from HMWK. The release of bradykinin produces an initial vasodilation followed by release of angiotensin II and vasoconstriction. The major role of factor XIa is activation of factor IX to factor IXa in the presence of calcium. Factor IXa then activates factor X to factor Xa in the presence of factor VIII, calcium, and phospholipid. This

TABLE 14-1

The Clotting Factors

Factor	Action
I: Fibrinogen	Factor I is converted to fibrin by the enzyme thrombin. Individual fibrin molecules form fibrin threads, which are the scaffold for clot formation and wound healing.
II: Prothrombin	Factor II is the inactive precursor of thrombin. Prothrombin is activated to thrombin by coagulation factor X (Stuart-Prower factor). After it is activated, thrombin converts fibrinogen (coagulation factor I) into fibrin and activates factors V and VIII.
III: Tissue thromboplastin	Factor III interacts with factor VII to initiate the extrinsic clotting cascade.
IV: Calcium	Calcium (Ca^{2+}), a divalent cation, is a cofactor for most of the enzyme-activated processes required in blood coagulation. Calcium also enhances platelet aggregation and makes red blood cells clump together.
V: Proaccelerin	Factor V is a cofactor for activated factor X, which is essential for converting prothrombin to thrombin.
VI: Discovered to be an artifact	No factor VI is involved in blood coagulation.
VII: Proconvertin	Factor VII activates factors IX and X, which are essential in converting prothrombin to thrombin. Synthesis is vitamin K dependent.
VIII: Antihemophilic factor	Factor VIII together with activated factor IX enzymatically activates factor X. In addition, factor VIII combines with another protein (von Willebrand factor) to help platelets adhere to capillary walls in areas of tissue injury.
IX: Plasma thromboplastin component (Christmas factor)	Factor IX, when activated, activates factor X to convert prothrombin to thrombin. This factor is essential in the common pathway of the intrinsic and extrinsic clotting cascades. A lack of factor IX is the basis for hemophilia B. Synthesis is vitamin K dependent.
X: Stuart-Prower factor	Factor X, when activated, converts prothrombin into thrombin. Synthesis is vitamin K dependent.
XI: Plasma thromboplastin antecedent	Factor XI, when activated, assists in the activation of factor IX. However, a similar factor must exist in tissues. People who are deficient in factor XI have mild bleeding problems after surgery but do not bleed excessively as a result of trauma.
XII: Hageman factor	Factor XII is critically important in the intrinsic pathway for the activation of factor XI.
XIII: Fibrin-stabilizing factor	Factor XIII assists in forming crosslinks among the fibrin threads to form a strong fibrin clot.

From Ignatavicus DD, Workman ML: *Medical surgical nursing: critical thinking for collaborative care*, ed 5, Philadelphia, 2006, Saunders, p 875.

FIGURE 14-3 Antithrombin III (ATIII) can bind and neutralize the activity of thrombin. Heparin is a catalyst that increases the activity of ATIII, making it more effective. Thrombin is a potent inducer of clot formation; thus, ATIII and heparin have significant anticoagulant properties.

activation usually takes place on the membrane of stimulated platelets. The common final pathway is initiated by factor Xa.

The extrinsic pathway of coagulation begins when the vascular wall is traumatized, as in a crush injury. Tissue factor (factor III) from injured tissue activates factor VII. Factor VIIa activates factor X to Xa, which in turn initiates the common final pathway. Factor VIIa also activates factor IX in the intrinsic system.

The common final pathway of coagulation is initiated by factor X, which is activated by both the intrinsic and extrinsic pathways. Factor Xa, in the presence of factor V, calcium, and phospholipid, converts prothrombin (factor II) to thrombin. This conversion is facilitated by the presence of activated platelets. Thrombin then cleaves fibrinogen to form an insoluble fibrin clot. Thrombin also activates factor XIII, which promotes fibrin stabilization. The clot is further stabilized by clot retraction. Thrombin also helps to perpetuate the clotting cascade by continuing to activate factors V and VIII.

Fibrinolysis

At the same time the fibrin clot is forming, the process of **fibrinolysis** or clot dissolution is initiated (Figure 14-5). Factor XII, HMWK, kallikrein, and thrombin are involved in the release of plasminogen activators. The plasminogen activators cleave plasminogen, a plasma protein that has been incorporated into the fibrin clot, to its active form, plasmin. Plasmin digests fibrinogen and fibrin and inactivates blood coagulation factors V and VIII. Fibrin split products, or fibrin degradation products, result from the dissolution of the fibrin clot.

The control of fibrinolysis is complex. The Kupffer cells of the liver and macrophages located in the spleen and bone marrow clear the circulation of activated clotting factors and fibrin degradation products. Antiplasmins that inhibit plasmin exist to prevent inappropriate fibrinolysis. All these factors and mechanisms are present to create a balance between clot production and clot dissolution.

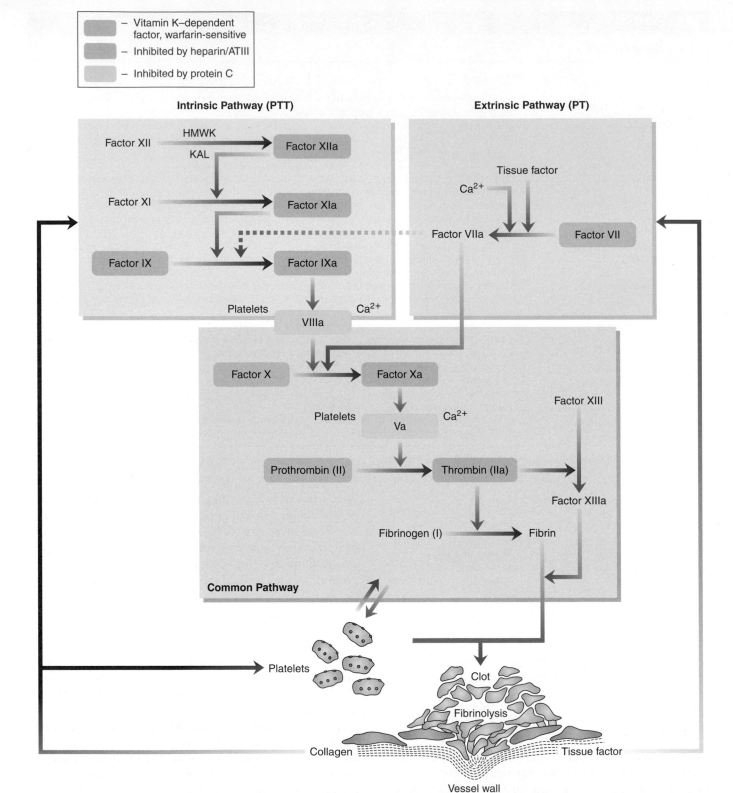

FIGURE 14-4 Coagulation cascade. *PTT,* Partial thromboplastin time; *PT,* prothrombin time.

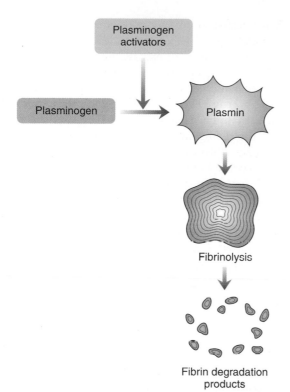

FIGURE 14-5 Fibrinolysis. Plasmin, activated from plasminogen, enzymatically cleaves fibrin proteins in the clot. This results in fibrin split products, which can be measured.

KEY POINTS

- Hemostasis involves several critical steps. These include vasospasm, formation of a platelet plug, and activation of the clotting cascade to form a fibrin clot.
- Factors released from platelets contribute to hemostasis by enhancing vasoconstriction, platelet aggregation, and vessel repair.
- Fibrin clot formation can be initiated by the intrinsic or extrinsic pathway. Each pathway requires the sequential activation of specific clotting factors, ultimately resulting in enzymatic cleavage of fibrinogen to form an insoluble fibrin clot.
- Initiation of fibrinolysis occurs simultaneously with clot formation to prevent excessive clotting and vessel occlusion.

EVALUATION OF HEMOSTASIS AND COAGULATION

Data obtained from clinical assessment and laboratory tests facilitate the identification and evaluation of a hemostatic abnormality. Evaluation of a patient for a bleeding tendency is indicated in the following circumstances: when there is a personal or family history of bleeding; during active bleeding that is unresponsive to standard interventions; as part of screening before surgery; and for ongoing evaluation of anticoagulation therapy. A bleeding tendency may be inherited or acquired, and may result from defects in blood vessels, platelets, or

TABLE 14-2

Clues from Patient History Regarding Bleeding Disorders

Clue from Patient History	Possible Cause
Family history of bleeding in both males and females	von Willebrand disease
Family history of bleeding in males	Hemophilia A or B
Newly acquired bruising	Drugs (especially aspirin and NSAIDs, anticoagulant therapy), thrombocytopenia
Excessive bleeding/bruising during/after surgery	Mild-severe deficiency of coagulation factors, von Willebrand disease; thrombocytopenia, drug ingestion
Bleeding following initial hemostasis	Factor XIII deficiency

coagulation factors. The purpose of the evaluation process is to determine if a problem exists and to ascertain the underlying cause so that appropriate management can be initiated.

Clinical Assessment

Both the family history and the personal history are important in the evaluation of a bleeding problem (Table 14-2). A family history of bleeding in males is often linked to one of the types of hemophilia, which accounts for the majority of serious inherited coagulation problems.[4,5] The location, severity, duration, and setting in which bleeding occurs are also important clues to the type of defect that is present. Bleeding associated with vascular or platelet defects usually occurs immediately after trauma (e.g., dental extraction), involves skin or mucous membranes, and is brief. Delayed bleeding or bleeding into muscles or joints is more typical of a coagulation defect.[5-8]

Systemic diseases, such as renal failure, liver disease, systemic lupus erythematosus, and malignancies may be associated with a bleeding problem. Medication history, including use of over-the-counter medications, is another important aspect in the evaluation of a hemostatic defect. A common cause of acquired bleeding problems is drug ingestion. Specific drugs that alter hemostasis include aspirin and aspirin-containing preparations, nonsteroidal antiinflammatory agents, some antibiotics, anticoagulants, alcohol, and chemotherapeutic and thrombolytic agents.

Many of the physical findings of bleeding are manifested in the skin and mucous membranes. The individual may appear pale or jaundiced. Pallor is associated with a marked decrease in hemoglobin; jaundice is associated with liver or gallbladder disease, possible coagulation disorders, and excessive red blood cell destruction.

Petechiae are flat, pinpoint, nonblanching red or purple spots caused by capillary hemorrhages in the skin and mucous membranes (Figure 14-6). Petechiae are commonly seen with vascular and platelet disorders. They are usually present on dependent areas of the body, such as the legs, or on areas constricted by tight clothing. Not all petechiae indicate a bleeding problem. Petechiae found on other body areas not constricted by tight clothing, such as the abdomen or thorax, may be associated with infectious disease or other pathophysiologic sources. Petechiae may be seen in the newborn as a result of the trauma of delivery, not as a result of a bleeding problem.

When petechiae occur in groups or patches, the term **purpura** is used (Figure 14-7). Purpuric lesions are often pruritic (itchy). Fever and malaise may be present, as may effusions into joints or viscera, manifested by joint or abdominal pain.

Ecchymosis occurs when blood escapes into the tissues, producing a bruise (Figure 14-8). If the area is raised, it is called a **hematoma. Hemarthrosis,** manifested by swelling and pain, is bleeding into a joint. Large ecchymoses, hematomas, and hemarthroses are seen in coagulation disorders.

Telangiectasia is a lesion created by dilation of capillaries and small arteries, typically on the lips, tongue, tips of the fingers and toes, and sometimes in visceral vessels (Figure 14-9). These thin, dilated, tortuous vessels are red to violet in color, blanch with pressure, and tend to bleed with minimal trauma. Spider telangiectasia branch into the subcutaneous and dermal layers of the skin and are often associated with liver disease.

FIGURE 14-6 Petechiae. (From Dockery GL: *Cutaneous disorders of the lower extremity,* Philadelphia, 1997, Saunders.)

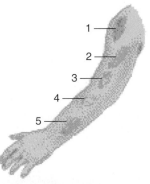

FIGURE 14-8 Ecchymosis. A large patch of capillary bleeding into tissues. Color in a light-skinned person is first red-blue or purple *(1)* immediately after or within 24 hours of trauma and generally progresses to blue to purple *(2),* blue-green *(3),* yellow *(4),* and brown to disappearing *(5).* (From Jarvis C: *Physical examination and health assessment,* ed 5, Philadelphia, 2008, Saunders, p 258.)

FIGURE 14-7 Purpura. (From Hurwitz S: *Clinical pediatric dermatology: a textbook of skin disorders of childhood and adolescence,* ed 2, Philadelphia, 1993, Saunders, p 269.)

FIGURE 14-9 Telangiectasia (spider or star angioma). A fiery red, star-shaped marking with a solid circular center. Capillary radiations extend from the central arterial body. With pressure, note a central pulsating body and blanching of extended legs. Develops on face, neck, or chest; may be associated with pregnancy, chronic liver disease, or estrogen therapy, or may be normal. (From Hurwitz S: *Clinical pediatric dermatology: a textbook of skin disorders in childhood and adolescence,* ed 2, Philadelphia, 1993, Saunders, p 266.)

TABLE 14-3

Select Laboratory Tests Used to Assess Bleeding

Test	Normal Value*	Purpose or Significance
Platelet count	150,000-350,000/mm^3	Determines number of platelets; decreased in ITP, anemias, DIC, infection, chemotherapy; increased in leukemia, cancer, splenectomy
Bleeding time	3-10 min	Assesses platelet and vascular response; increased in thrombocytopenia, vascular defects, severe liver disease, DIC, von Willebrand disease, aspirin ingestion
Prothrombin time	10-14 sec; 100%	Evaluates the extrinsic pathway of coagulation; increased in vitamin K deficiency, hemorrhagic disease of the newborn, liver disease, DIC, anticoagulant therapy. Evaluates all coagulation factors except VIII and XII
International normalized ratio	1.5 (low-level anticoagulation for atrial fibrillation) 2.0-3.0 (medium level anticoagulation for DVT, pulmonary embolism, MI, stroke prophylaxis) 2.5-3.5 (high level anticoagulation for mechanical heart valve)	Evaluates extrinsic pathway of coagulation (as prothrombin time); provides uniformity worldwide, independent of reagents
Activated partial thromboplastin time	33-45 sec	Evaluates the intrinsic pathway of coagulation; increased in hemophilia, vitamin K deficiency, liver disease, DIC, circulating anticoagulants, heparin therapy
Thrombin time	15 sec, or control + 5 sec	Measures conversion of fibrinogen to fibrin; increased in DIC, liver disease, low fibrinogen <100 mg/dl, multiple myeloma
Fibrinogen†	200-400 mg/dl	Measures fibrinogen level; decreased in liver disease, DIC
Fibrin split products or fibrin degradation products†	<3 μg/ml	Measures byproducts from breakdown of fibrin clot; increased in DIC, hypoxia, leukemia, thromboembolic disorders
Clot retraction†	1 hr: evidence of shrinking and increased firmness 24 hr: 50% of volume is clot, 50% is serum	Rough measure of platelet function; decreased in thrombocytopenia, von Willebrand disease
Platelet aggregation†	Visible aggregates form in <5 min	Measures rate and percentage of aggregation; decreased in mononucleosis, ITP, von Willebrand disease, leukemia, aspirin ingestion, thrombasthenia, Bernard-Soulier syndrome
Tourniquet test (Rumpel-Leede test, capillary fragility test)†	No petechiae or occasional petechiae	Evaluates vascular fragility and platelet function; positive test in thrombocytopenia, vascular purpuras, thrombasthenia
Euglobin lysis time†	No lysis of fibrin clot at 37° for 3 hr; clot is observed for 24 hr	Assesses fibrinolysis; increased lysis in DIC, incompatible blood transfusion, cirrhosis, cancer, obstetric complications
Plasma D-dimer assay	<200 ng/ml	Assesses fibrinolysis, increased in deep vein thrombosis, pulmonary embolism (highly nonspecific), DIC (high negative predictive value)

DIC, Disseminated intravascular coagulation; *DVT*, deep vein thrombosis; *ITP*, idiopathic thrombocytopenic purpura; *MI*, myocardial infarction.

*Value may vary, depending on source.

†Tests not included in a routine coagulation screen.

Other significant findings indicative of a bleeding disorder include blood (bright red, rusty, or black) in drainage or excreta, such as feces (**hematochezia** or **melena**), urine (**hematuria**), vomitus (**hematemesis**), nasal drainage (**epistaxis**), gastric drainage, or sputum (**hemoptysis**). Excessive menstrual bleeding may occur (**menorrhagia**). Acute abdominal or flank pain may indicate internal bleeding. Hypovolemia from bleeding may produce a shock state and present as hypotension, tachycardia, pallor, altered mentation, and decreased urine output. The two sites at which bleeding is most life threatening are the oropharynx (resulting in airway compromise) and within the brain tissue. One of the leading causes of death in patients experiencing severe disorders of coagulation is intracerebral hemorrhage.[5]

Laboratory Tests

Many laboratory tests are available to aid in the diagnosis of hemostasis problems (Table 14-3). Basic screening includes a complete blood cell count (CBC), including a platelet count and peripheral blood smear, bleeding time, prothrombin time (PT) or international normalized ratio (INR), activated partial thromboplastin time (aPTT), and thrombin time. These screening tests evaluate both primary and secondary hemostasis. The CBC determines if anemia is present, the platelet count

TABLE 14-4

Alterations in Laboratory Values Seen with Major Disorders of Hemostasis

Disorder	Platelet Count	Bleeding Time	PT/INR	aPTT	TT	FSP	FVIII	FIX
Idiopathic thrombocytopenic purpura	↓	Prolonged	N	N	N	N	N	N
Hemophilia A	N	N/Prolonged	N	↑	↑	N	↓	N
Hemophilia B	N	N/Prolonged	N	↑	↑	N	N	↓
Von Willebrand disease	N	Prolonged	N	↑	↑	N	↓	N
Vitamin K deficiency	N	Prolonged	↑	N/↑	↑	N	N	N/↓
Disseminated intravascular coagulation	↓	Prolonged	↑	↑	↑	↑	↓	↓
ASA/NSAIDs	N	Prolonged	N	N	N	N	N	N
Heparin	N/↓	Prolonged	N	↑	↑	N	N	N
Coumadin	N	Prolonged	↑	N/↑	↑	N	N	N
Vascular purpura	N	N/Prolonged	N	N	N	N	N	N
Liver disease	N/↓	Prolonged	↑	N/↑	N	N	N	N/↓

ASA, Acetylsalicylic acid; *NSAIDs*, nonsteroidal antiinflammatory drugs; *PT*, prothrombin time; *aPTT*, activated partial thromboplastin time; *TT*, thrombin time; *FSP*, fibrin split products; *FVIII*, factor VIII; *FIX*, factor IX; *N*, normal.

determines the number of platelets, and the peripheral smear indicates the number and gross morphologic characteristics of platelets. The bleeding time evaluates vascular status and platelet function. The PT and INR assess the extrinsic pathway of coagulation, and the aPTT assesses the intrinsic pathway. Reporting prothrombin activity as a percentage of PT in seconds can pose difficulty in the adjustment of anticoagulation therapy because the PT varies with each laboratory and the reagent used there. Laboratories have tried to compensate for this variation by using the ratio of the patient's value to the laboratory's control value, which again varied with the reagent. The INR is a standardized PT value used worldwide that controls for this reagent variability. Thrombin time measures the time needed to convert fibrinogen to fibrin; this reflects the quantity and quality of fibrinogen as well as the influence of any inhibitors. The D-dimer assay reflects fibrinolysis.

Further laboratory investigation is necessary if abnormalities are identified on the screening tests or if, despite normal screening test results, a bleeding problem obviously exists. Specific tests are available to assess abnormal platelet function, the presence of circulating anticoagulants, fibrin split products, and levels of individual coagulation factors. Table 14-4 reflects the alterations in laboratory values seen with the major disorders of hemostasis.

KEY POINTS

- Bleeding tendencies may be inherited or acquired. Abnormal bleeding, liver disease, and anticoagulant drug use may be important risk factors. Physical findings of petechiae, purpura, ecchymoses, telangiectasia, and occult or frank bleeding are indicative.
- Usual laboratory tests include platelet count, bleeding time, PT/INR (extrinsic pathway), and activated partial thromboplastin time (intrinsic pathway).

VASCULAR AND PLATELET DISORDERS

Vascular Disorders

Vascular disorders of hemostasis and coagulation are those in which the primary cause of bleeding is a problem with the vascular component of primary hemostasis. The vascular defect may be acquired (e.g., related to ingestion of a specific drug) or inherited.

Vascular Purpura

Etiology. Vascular purpura is a disorder in which purpura—patches of petechiae, or pinpoint hemorrhages, on the skin—are present. The primary cause of the purpura, or more extensive bleeding in some cases, is an abnormality of the vessels or the tissues that support them (see Figure 14-7).

Allergic purpura (anaphylactoid purpura, Henoch-Schönlein purpura) is most often seen in children between the ages of 4 and 7.[9-11] Drug-induced purpura may result from many drugs, including atropine, chloral hydrate, and other sedatives; sulfa drugs; procaine penicillin; and warfarin (Coumadin). Purpuric lesions and perhaps severe hemorrhage are components of the Ehlers-Danlos syndrome and osteogenesis imperfecta, both of which are inherited disorders of connective tissue.[12,13] Acquired disorders of connective tissue such as scurvy (vitamin C deficiency), senile purpura (seen in the elderly), and corticosteroid purpura (associated with chronic steroid drug therapy) may also result in purpuric lesions.

Pathogenesis. The allergic purpuras are thought to result from an autoimmune process that produces inflammation or vasculitis of small vessels. As a result, perivascular infiltration and serosanguineous effusion occur into surrounding tissues to produce the characteristic purpuric lesion. The pathophysiologic process of drug-induced purpura is not well understood. An autoimmune process has been proposed.

Structural abnormalities of vessels and perivascular supportive tissue provide the mechanism for bleeding in many of the vascular purpura. These abnormalities may be inherited or acquired. In Ehlers-Danlos syndrome and osteogenesis imperfecta, the vascular abnormality is thought to result from decreased amounts or poor quality of collagen and elastin; both are necessary for perivascular support. Vitamin C deficiency, which causes scurvy, results in defective collagen synthesis. The lack of proper collagen support for the vessels leads to bleeding. In the elderly (senile purpura), loss of subcutaneous fat and changes in connective tissue allow for more mobility of the skin. Shearing force then causes rupture of small vessels. Steroids induce catabolism of proteins in supportive tissues, decreasing the mechanical strength of the microvasculature.

Clinical Manifestations. The purpuric lesions characteristically appear and fade or disappear in groups. The lesions are not elevated and do not blanch with pressure.

With allergic purpura, the lesions tend to be palpable and are found on the proximal extremities, especially on the legs and buttocks; they may be accompanied by fever, itching, arthralgia, and paresthesia. Bleeding from the lesions themselves and generalized bleeding are uncommon. Usually, allergic purpura is self-limited, and the prognosis is good.

Generalized purpura is characteristic of drug-induced vascular purpura. The lesions quickly subside when the drug is discontinued. Other bleeding manifestations are uncommon.

The purpuric lesions associated with inherited connective tissue disorders, such as Ehlers-Danlos syndrome, often are accompanied by large ecchymoses and hematomas. Although not common, bleeding into the brain tissue may result in cerebrovascular accident (stroke).[12,13]

The purpuric lesions seen with scurvy typically occur around hair follicles and on the medial surfaces of the thighs and buttocks. Ecchymoses and large hematomas may also occur.

Senile purpura and corticosteroid purpura generally occur on the dorsum of the hands and forearms and are aggravated by trauma. Other bleeding is uncommon.

Diagnosis and Treatment. The diagnosis of vascular purpura is one of exclusion after platelet disorders and coagulation disorders have been ruled out. An abnormal tourniquet test (positive Rumpel-Leede test) in the setting of a normal or increased bleeding time, normal platelet count, and normal coagulation study results suggest a problem with the vascular component of hemostasis. The tourniquet test is an assessment for abnormal capillary fragility. To perform the test, a blood pressure cuff is applied and inflated to a point between the systolic and diastolic blood pressures for 5 minutes. The test is positive if there are more than 20 petechiae per square inch.

Treatment for vascular purpura includes removal or avoidance of the causative agent if one is identified (e.g., penicillin) and interventions to relieve symptoms such as itching. If more extensive bleeding accompanies the purpura, identification of the cause and interventions to control the bleeding are necessary.

Hereditary Hemorrhagic Telangiectasia

Etiology. A telangiectasia is a dilated or tortuous small blood vessel, found in the skin or mucous membranes, that has a tendency to bleed spontaneously or following minor trauma (see Figure 14-9). Hereditary hemorrhagic telangiectasia (Osler-Weber-Rendu disease) is transmitted as an autosomal dominant trait; the vascular abnormalities can be seen in children but become more prominent after puberty, peaking between the fourth and fifth decades. As the telangiectases—the skin spots resulting from the vascular lesion—become more prominent, the frequency and severity of the bleeding increase.[11,12]

Pathogenesis. The telangiectases result from an abnormality in vascular development. The vessel wall is composed of a single layer of endothelium; thus, support and contractile properties are deficient, leading to spontaneous bleeding or bleeding as a result of minor trauma.[12] Any mucosal surface (e.g., respiratory, gastrointestinal, and genitourinary tracts) may be involved. Arteriovenous malformations in the lung, liver, and brain are the most serious complications.[11]

Clinical Manifestations. Bright red or purple lesions, ranging from pinpoint to 3 mm in diameter, can be found on the nasal mucous membranes, lips, palate, tongue, face, trunk, palms of the hands, and the soles of the feet. Recurrent nosebleeds (epistaxis) is a hallmark, with increasing frequency as the patient ages. The severity of the disorder is linked to age of onset.[14,15] Typically the lesions are flat and blanch with pressure. The most common clinical problem is mucous membrane bleeding, especially epistaxis. However, bleeding may occur from telangiectases in any area. Frequent bleeding episodes may result in anemia.[14,15]

Diagnosis and Treatment. The diagnosis is confirmed by the presence of multiple telangiectases, repeated episodes of bleeding, or a family history of bleeding in both sexes. If telangiectases are not easily visible, the diagnosis is more difficult to make.

Treatment is primarily supportive and includes use of topical hemostatic agents or cauterization if the bleeding site is accessible; nasal tamponade; iron replacement; laser treatment for cutaneous lesions; embolization; and estrogen or estrogen with progesterone for epistaxis. Aminocaproic acid is used for controlling severe hemorrhage.[12] Blood transfusions or surgical intervention for uncontrolled bleeding or removal of an arteriovenous fistula may be considered in selected cases.[14,15]

Platelet Disorders

Platelet disorders of hemostasis and coagulation are those in which the primary cause of bleeding is an abnormality in the quantity or the quality of platelets.

Thrombocytopenia

Etiology. **Thrombocytopenia** is a common cause of generalized bleeding. Some of the many causes of thrombocytopenia are listed in Box 14-1.

Idiopathic thrombocytopenic purpura (ITP) is an immune-mediated thrombocytopenia that occurs in the absence of toxin or drug exposure or a disease known to be associated with decreased platelets. Acute ITP occurs at any age and in both sexes following an acute viral infection.[4,16-18] Resolution is usually spontaneous, and the prognosis is good. Chronic ITP is more common in adults 20 to 50 years of age. The onset is insidious, and women are affected most often. A pregnant woman with ITP can deliver a thrombocytopenic infant because the antiplatelet antibody crosses the placenta. Adult ITP

4. Anand M, Rajagopol K, Rajagopol KR: A model for the formation and lysis of blood clots, *Pathophys Haemost Thromb* 34 (2-3):109-120, 2005.
5. Fauci A: *Harrison's principles of internal medicine,* ed 17, New York, 2008, McGraw-Hill.
6. Hayward C, Rao A, Catttaneo M: Congenital platelet disorders: overview of their mechanisms, diagnostic evaluation and treatment, *Haemophilia 12* i:128-136, 2006.
7. Bolton-Maggs P, et al: A review of inherited platelet disorders with guidelines for their management, on behalf of the UKHCDO: *Br J Haemotol* 135:603-633, 2006.
8. George J: Platelets, *Lancet* 355:1531-1539, 2000.
9. Schneiderman P: Vascular purpuras, In Beutler E et al, editors: *Williams hematology,* ed 6, New York, 2001, McGraw-Hill.
10. Roberts P et al: Henoch-Schönlein purpura: a review article, *South Med J* 100(8):821-824, 2007.
11. Dillon M: Henoch-Schönlein purpura: recent advances, *Clin Exp Rheumatol* 25:566-558, 2007.
12. Germain D: Ehlers-Danlos syndrome type IV, *Orphanet J Rare Dis* 2:32-40, 2007.
13. Yen J, Lin S, Chen M, Niu D: Clinical feature of Ehlers-Danlos syndrome, *J Formos Med Assoc* 105(6):475-479, 2006.
14. Sadick H et al: Hereditary hemorrhagic telangiectasia: an update on clinical manifestations and diagnostic measures, *Wien Klin Wochenschr* 118(3-4):72-80, 2006.
15. Stuhrmann M, El-Harth A: Hereditary hemorrhagic telangiectasia: genetics, pathogenesis, clinical manifestation and management, *Saudi Med J* 28(1):11-21, 2007.
16. George J: Thrombocytopenia. In Beutler E et al, editors: *Williams hematology,* ed 6, New York, 2001, McGraw-Hill.
17. Briere J: Essential thrombocythemia, *Orphanet J Rare Dis* 2:3-19, 2007.
18. Stevens W, Koene H, Zwaginga J et al: Chronic idiopathic thrombocytopenic purpura: present strategy, guidelines and new insights, *Neth J Med* 64(10):356-363, 2006.
19. Sekhon S, Roy V: Thrombocytopenia in adults: a practical approach to evaluation and management, *South Med J* 99(5):491-498, 2006.
20. Bolton-Maggs P: Haemophilias A and B, *Lancet* 361(9371):1801-1809, 2003.
21. Kasper C, Lin C: Prevalence of sporadic and familial haemophilia, *Haemophilia* 13:90-92, 2007.
22. Meeks S, Josephson C: Should hemophilia treaters switch to albumin-free recombinant factor VIII concentrates, *Curr Opin Hematol* 13:457-461, 2006.
23. Riddel J, Aouizerat B: Genetics of von Willebrand disease type I, *Biol Res Nurs* 8(2):147-156, 2006.
24. James A: von Willebrand disease, *Obstet Gynecol Surv* 61(2): 136-145, 2006.
25. Humes HD: *Kelleys Textbook of Internal Medicine,* ed 4, Philadelphia, 2008, Lippincott Williams and Wilkins.
26. Ijland M, Pereira R, Corenelissen E: Incidence of late vitamin k deficiency bleeding in newborns in the Netherlands in 2005: evaluation of the current guideline, *Eur J Pediatr* 167:165-169, 2007.
27. Kumor D: Vitamin K status of premature infants: implications for current recommendations, *Pediatrics* 108(5):1117-1124, 2001.
28. Levi M: Disseminated intravascular coagulation, *Crit Care Med* 35(9): 2191-2195, 2007.

Alterations in Blood Flow

Roberta J. Emerson • Naomi Lungstrom

MEDIA RESOURCES

Additional Material for Study, Review, and Further Exploration

CD Companion ■ Review Questions and Answers
■ Glossary (with audio pronunciations for selected terms)
■ Disease Profiles ■ Animations

evolve **Website** at http://evolve.elsevier.com/Copstead/
■ Case Studies ■ Disease Profiles ■ WebLinks ■ Key Points Review

Online Course (Module 10)

KEY QUESTIONS

■ How do the structures of arteries, veins, capillaries, and lymphatics differ, and how do these differences reflect the functions of each?

■ What is the relationship among vessel resistance, blood pressure, and blood flow?

■ How is vascular resistance regulated centrally by the autonomic nervous system and locally by tissues?

■ What are the determinants of transcapillary exchange of fluids, electrolytes, and nutrients?

■ How do arterial and venous obstructions develop?

■ What are the clinical consequences of acute and chronic arterial obstruction?

■ What are the clinical consequences of superficial and deep venous obstructions?

CHAPTER OUTLINE

The primary functions of the circulatory system are the transportation of oxygen and nutrients and the removal of metabolic waste products within the body. To perform these functions, a complex circuitry of vessels traverses the body (Figure 15-1), powered by the pumping action of the heart. Propulsion of blood through the lungs is provided by the right ventricle, whereas systemic blood flow is driven by the left ventricle.

Nutrients are absorbed into the blood as it moves through the gastrointestinal tract via the splanchnic circulation. Oxygen uptake and the release of carbon dioxide occur in the specialized vascular bed of the pulmonary circulation. The liver, with its extensive blood supply, has a major role in metabolism and generation of metabolic waste products. These, and other metabolic byproducts, are carried by the blood to the kidneys for elimination. Inadequate circulation in the lungs, liver, or kidneys may interfere with the removal of metabolic wastes from the body. Effective transportation of oxygen and nutrients and the removal of waste materials depend on proper functioning of the circulatory system.

Aging produces significant changes in the circulatory system, altering the ability of the system to carry out its functions and increasing susceptibility to certain disease processes. The effects of the aging process on the circulatory system are summarized in Geriatric Considerations: Changes in the Circulatory System.

ORGANIZATION OF THE CIRCULATORY AND LYMPHATIC SYSTEMS

After passing through the pulmonary circulatory system and leaving the left ventricle, blood flows through a graduated series of tubes to tissues of the body before returning to the right side of the heart. The powerful left ventricle propels the blood to the aorta, arteries, arterioles, and, finally, to the capillary beds. Here the proximity of capillary endothelium to the other cells of the body facilitates movement of nutrients and oxygen into the cells and removal of cellular metabolic wastes. Capillary blood is then collected by venules, which flow into veins, returning blood to the vena cava and the right side of the heart (Figure 15-2). The complete process, moving approximately 5 L of blood through the entire circuit, takes only about a minute.

The lymphatic circulation is a specialized system of channels and tissues (nodes). It is not arranged in a circuit, as is the vascular system. Instead, the lymphatic vessels begin blindly, deep in the connective tissue. One of the functions of the lymphatic system is to reabsorb fluid that leaks out of the vascular network into the interstitium and return it to the general circulation. During the process of cellular exchange within the capillary bed, some fluid moves into the interstitium and fails to return to the vascular bed. This lost fluid can amount to as much as 2 to 4 L/day. At this circulatory level, lymphatic vessels lie in close proximity to the capillary vasculature. The fluid, now called *lymph*, is absorbed by the lymphatic vessels and returned to the venous circulation by way of the thoracic duct and the right lymphatic duct (Figure 15-3). Lymphatic drainage of the breast is illustrated in Figure 15-4.

Vessel Structure

To carry out their specialized functions, the blood and lymphatic vessels are different in their structure. Knowledge of the morphology of these vessels is essential for an understanding of the alterations in function produced by disease.

The primary differences between the smaller arterial and venous vessels are in terms of the quantities of muscle and connective tissue present. In arterioles, the principal tissue is smooth muscle, whereas in venules, smooth muscle is scarce and connective tissue dominates. The composition of the walls and the size and shape of the vessels also varies in larger arteries and veins. Capillary walls are composed of a single layer of endothelial cells. These simple structures carry out extraordinarily complex functions.

Anatomy of Arteries and Veins

The walls of both arteries and veins are composed of three microscopically distinct layers, or tunicae: the intima, the media, and the adventitia. The histologic constituents of these tunicae are similar in arteries and veins (Figure 15-5). Generally, the walls of veins are not as thick as the walls of arteries, but the lumina are larger.

The intima consists of a layer of endothelial cells that is in direct contact with the blood as it flows through the vessel. Periodically, the intimal layer of veins protrudes into the lumen, creating valves that prevent the backflow of blood. Arterial intima is characterized by an inner elastic membrane next to the endothelial cells. This elastic membrane is thickest in the aorta and decreases in density until only scattered elastic fibers can be identified in the smallest arterioles. With increasing age, the intimal arterial wall becomes thicker and less elastic. This interferes with diffusion of nutrients into the wall, causing the internal elastic membrane to degenerate and calcify.

The media, or middle layer, exhibits the greatest difference between arteries and veins. In arteries the media is the thickest of all the tunicae. Large arteries have smooth muscle fibers

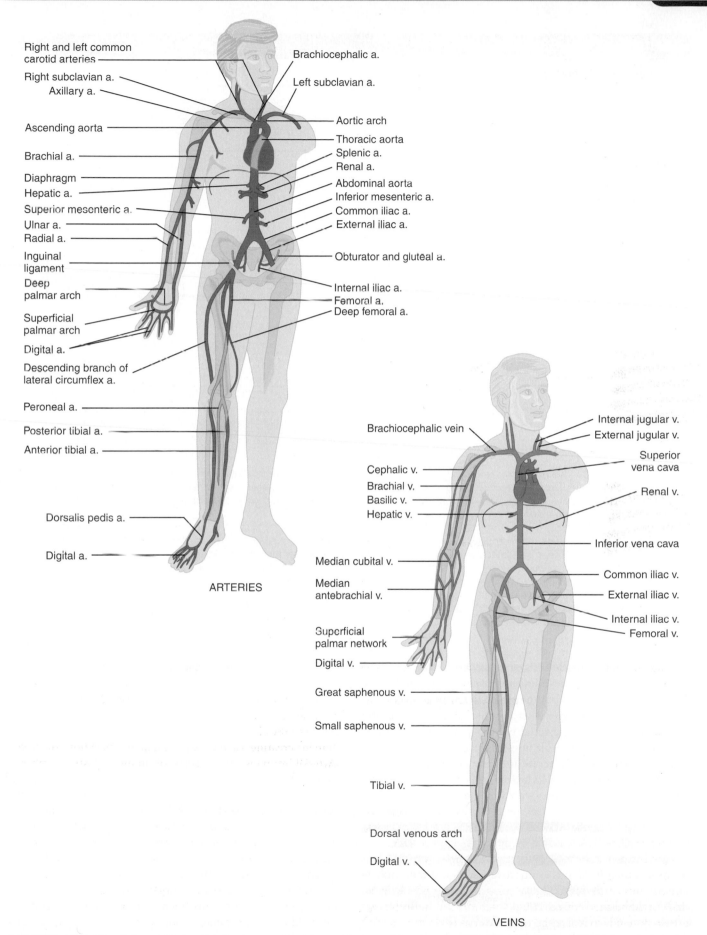

FIGURE 15-1 The primary systemic arterial and venous circulatory networks. *a.,* Artery; *v.,* vein. (From Black JM, Hawks J: *Medical-surgical nursing: clinical management for positive outcomes,* ed 8, Philadelphia, 2008, Saunders, p 1273.)

GERIATRIC CONSIDERATIONS

Changes in the Circulatory System

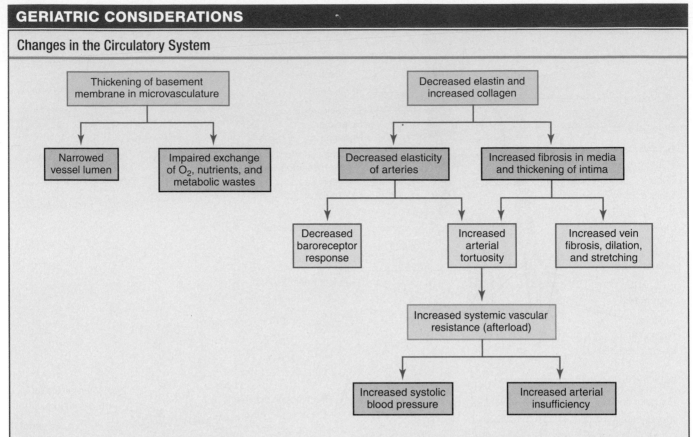

In the aging individual, changes occur throughout the vascular bed. The microvascular bed demonstrates thickening of the basement membrane. This change narrows the vessel lumen and impairs the free exchange of oxygen, nutrients, and metabolic wastes at the cellular level.

In both arteries and veins, the vascular changes occur first in the proximal portions. The intima becomes fibrotic and the endothelial cell variation increases. In the media, the amount of elastin and smooth muscle is reduced, whereas the amount of fibrotic and collagen tissue increases. With collagen cross-linking, the vessel walls lose elastic flexibility and recoil, becoming more stiff and less compliant. They become inflexible tubes with an increase in systemic vascular resistance (SVR). The increased SVR causes a reduction in tissue and organ blood flow and decreased perfusion.

Baroreceptor function is reduced because of decreased sensitivity of the receptors and diminished responsiveness of the vessels because of their rigidity. These factors decrease the body's ability to respond to hypotensive and hypertensive stimuli. The decreased compliance of the systemic vascular system increases afterload, forcing the left ventricle of the heart to work harder to meet the metabolic demands of the body.

arranged in a circular pattern and interspersed with elastic fibers. Progressing from arteries to ever-smaller arterioles, the smooth muscle remains but the elastic tissue disappears. This thick, smooth muscle layer is responsible for the firmness and limited distensibility of arterial vessels. With advancing age, changes in the intima result in decreased nutrition reaching the media, causing degeneration of the smooth muscle tissue. In veins, the media also has smooth muscle, usually arranged in a circular pattern with some longitudinal strands. The quantity of smooth muscle decreases as the veins become larger. Venous media also contains collagenous connective tissue, but elastic tissue is rare except in the largest veins.

In veins, the adventitia is the thickest of the tunicae. It is composed of collagenous connective tissue and longitudinal smooth muscle. In larger arteries there is a discernible external elastic membrane in the adventitia. This membrane disappears as the arteries decrease in diameter. Arterial adventitia consists predominantly of collagenous connective tissue. Some larger vessels also contain isolated, longitudinally arranged fibers of smooth muscle.

Anatomy of Capillaries

Capillaries are composed of a single thickness of endothelial cells attached to a protein network called the basement membrane. Moving from the end of an arteriole to the beginning of a venule, capillaries narrow to a diameter barely sufficient for a single red blood cell (RBC) to pass through the aperture. In some tissues, one or two smooth muscle cells form a precapillary sphincter that controls flow through the vessel (Figure 15-6).

There are spaces between the endothelial cells that vary in size from organ system to organ system. These spaces, or pores, permit certain constituents to pass in and out of the capillaries. For example, capillary beds in the brain have

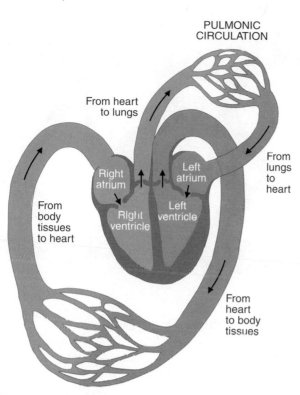

PULMONIC CIRCULATION

From heart to lungs

From lungs to heart

Right atrium

Left atrium

Right ventricle

Left ventricle

From body tissues to heart

From heart to body tissues

SYSTEMIC CIRCULATION

FIGURE 15-2 The circulatory system. Beginning from the body tissues, blood returns to the right side of the heart, through the right atria to the right ventricle, which propels it into the lungs. In the lungs, the metabolic waste carbon dioxide is removed and oxygen is replenished. Oxygenated blood leaves the pulmonic circulation and returns to the heart via the left atrium to the left ventricle. From the left side of the heart, the oxygenated blood enters the systemic circulation, where oxygen is delivered to the tissues in exchange for metabolic wastes. (From Black JM, Hawks J: *Medical-surgical nursing: clinical management for positive outcomes,* ed 8, Philadelphia, 2008, Saunders, p 1344.)

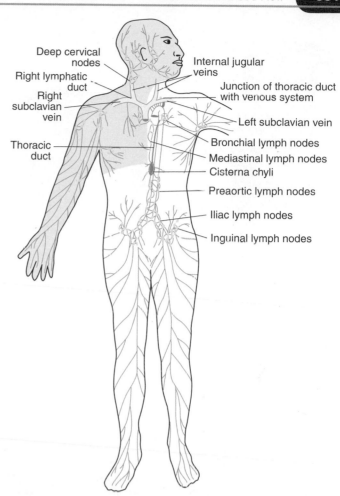

Deep cervical nodes

Right lymphatic duct

Right subclavian vein

Thoracic duct

Internal jugular veins

Junction of thoracic duct with venous system

Left subclavian vein

Bronchial lymph nodes

Mediastinal lymph nodes

Cisterna chyli

Preaortic lymph nodes

Iliac lymph nodes

Inguinal lymph nodes

FIGURE 15-3 Anatomy of the lymphatic system. Lymphatic capillaries collect the excess fluid from the vascular capillaries, returning it to the venous circulation at the junction of the internal jugular and subclavian veins. (From Monahan FD et al: *Phipp's medical-surgical nursing: health and illness perspectives,* ed 8, Philadelphia, 2007, Mosby, p 936.)

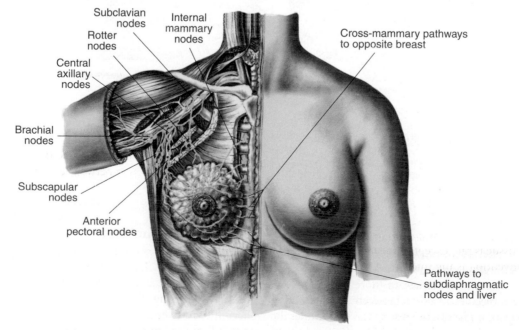

Subclavian nodes

Rotter nodes

Central axillary nodes

Brachial nodes

Subscapular nodes

Anterior pectoral nodes

Internal mammary nodes

Cross-mammary pathways to opposite breast

Pathways to subdiaphragmatic nodes and liver

FIGURE 15-4 Lymphatic drainage of the breast to the axillary and subclavian nodes, then to the jugular and subclavian veins. (From Monahan FD et al: *Phipp's medical-surgical nursing: health and illness perspectives,* ed 8, Philadelphia, 2007, Mosby, p 1661.)

FIGURE 15-5 Tunicae of arteries and veins showing the thicker walls of the arteries.

FIGURE 15-6 Capillary network.

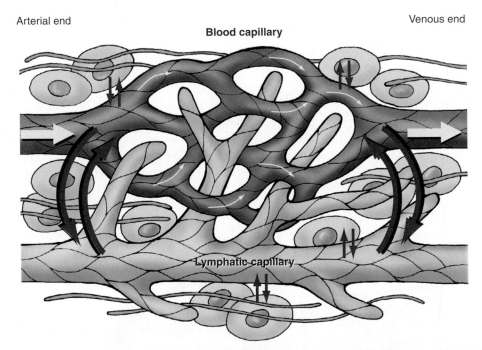

FIGURE 15-7 Lymphatic network. The lymphatic system is integrally related to the systemic vascular system. Excess fluid and plasma diffuse between the capillaries, interstitial spaces, and lymphatic vessels. Because lymphatic capillaries have larger spaces between endothelial cells, they can remove excess interstitial fluid or plasma that venous capillaries cannot reabsorb.

little or no spaces and permit only certain molecules to pass through. The space between endothelial cells of the brain is so small that it is referred to as the *blood-brain barrier*. In parts of the kidneys, however, capillaries are more porous, allowing much larger molecules to move between the circulation and the filtrate (urine). The size of these spaces determines the *capillary permeability* of a specific capillary bed.

Lymphatic Structure

Lymphatic vessels are thin walled and most resemble veins in their appearance. Like their counterparts in the circulatory system, they range in size from lymphatic capillaries to vessels of increasing diameter. Like veins, lymphatics have intermittent valves composed of folds of their inner layer that extend into the lumen (Figure 15-7). The walls of lymphatic capillaries contain contractile fibers that are stimulated when stretched, causing the vessels to contract and propel lymph along the vessel.

PRINCIPLES OF FLOW

Hemodynamics of the Circulatory System

The principles of blood flow are known as circulatory **hemodynamics.** These principles govern the quantity of blood passing by a given point in a specific period. Therefore, blood flow is measured as a given number of liters, milliliters, or cubic centimeters per second, minute, or hour. A discussion of the hemodynamics of the circulatory system includes the concepts of pressure, resistance, velocity, laminar and turbulent flows, wall tension, and compliance.

Blood Flow, Pressure, and Resistance

Blood flow is accomplished by movement along a pressure gradient within the vascular bed. This means that blood moves from an area of higher pressure to an area of lower pressure. The arterial and arteriolar walls with their muscular media coats provide the high-pressure end of the gradient. Seeking a lower pressure, blood moves toward the venous system. The thinner, more pliable walls of the venous bed furnish the low-pressure portion of the pressure gradient. The greater the pressure difference, the greater the rate of blood flow.

The movement of blood through the vascular system is opposed by the force of *resistance.* The relationship between blood flow and resistance is an inverse one: as resistance increases, blood flow decreases. This force has several determinants, each of which can change resistance considerably; these determinants are represented in physiology by *Poiseuille's law:*

$$\text{Resistance} = \frac{8nl}{\pi r^4}$$

The number 8 is a mathematical constant, as is the value of π. N represents blood viscosity; l represents the length of a given vessel; and r is the radius of the vessel. Using this formula, the effects of changes on the components of resistance are very predictable.

Two of the determinants of resistance are *vessel length* and *vessel radius.* As predicted by Poiseuille's law, resistance changes directly with the length of the vessel, and these changes in resistance significantly affect flow. As illustrated in Figure 15-8, given three vessels of the same radius, doubling the length increases the resistance and reduces the flow (*Q*) by 50%. Reducing the vessel length by half decreases resistance and increases the flow by 100%. These changes in flow occur when the pressure gradient remains constant and are caused solely by variations in vessel length. Resistance decreases as the radius of a vessel increases and resistance is inversely related to the fourth power of radius of a vessel, or r^4. Therefore, increasing a vessel's radius markedly reduces resistance and produces an exponential increase in blood flow. Figure 15-9 demonstrates the effect of doubling the radius of a vessel on the flow of blood if all other factors related to flow are held constant. The resulting flow of blood is 16 times greater in the greater diameter vessel.

Although there is variability in the length of vessels throughout the circulatory system, vessels are incapable of altering their own length. They do, however, possess a considerable ability to change their diameters, and many disease processes (e.g., arteriosclerosis) and drug therapies (e.g., vasopressors) are associated with changes in the size of the vessel

Q = 10 ml/sec

Q = 5 ml/sec

Q = 20 ml/sec

FIGURE 15-8 Relationship of vessel length to blood flow (*Q*) with a constant pressure gradient.

r = 2 cm

Q = 10 ml/sec

r = 4 cm

Q = 160 ml/sec

FIGURE 15-9 Relationship of vessel radius (*r*) to blood flow (*Q*) with a constant pressure gradient.

lumen. Even minor changes will produce major alterations in resistance and, hence, blood flow. This makes changes in diameter the most important determinant of resistance.

The third determinant of resistance is the *viscosity* of the blood itself, represented in Poiseuille's law as *n*. Viscosity is defined as the thickness of a fluid. When the blood is more viscous, the friction between the cells and the liquid increases, and an increase in resistance to flow is produced. Blood is composed of a suspension of cellular material and plasma. Roughly 99% of the cellular constituents of the blood are RBCs. The ratio of RBCs to plasma is presented in the laboratory value *hematocrit*. Increasing the number of RBCs or decreasing the plasma component results in more viscous blood (increased hematocrit), more resistance, and a slowing of blood flow. This is what occurs in dehydration, when the plasma component is relatively decreased, or in polycythemia, when the number of RBCs increases.

The relationship between the variables of driving pressure and resistance and their effect on blood flow is expressed by *Ohm's law*, as follows:

$$Q = P/R$$

Here, Q is the blood flow, P is the pressure difference between two points, and R is resistance. Altering any one of the determinants of resistance (vessel length, vessel radius, or blood viscosity) produces a change in flow. According to Ohm's law, a change in the pressure difference within the circulatory system also results in a change in the flow of blood. The arterioles are the major site of resistance in the vascular system and require a greater pressure to maintain blood flow. As the resistance decreases across the systemic vasculature, less pressure is necessary to maintain blood flow (Figure 15-10). *Total peripheral resistance* refers to the resistance throughout the entire vascular system. It can be calculated on the basis of the pressure difference between the arteries and the veins. Clinically, systemic vascular resistance (SVR) is used to specifically denote resistance peripheral to the heart and lungs. Because the primary determinant of SVR is the resistance vessels (arterioles), diseases or drug therapies that affect these vessels have the most profound impact on the SVR. Any condition that produces an increase in SVR, such as hypertension, requires more work for the heart to overcome the elevated resistance and eject its volume of blood (see Chapter 16). This increased workload means that the heart needs more oxygen and nutrients. When SVR is pathologically decreased, the blood is spread over a larger area and blood flow slows dramatically. Individual organs, such as the kidney and brain, may not obtain sufficient blood flow to meet metabolic needs. This is what occurs in distributive shock states (see Chapter 20).

Velocity and Laminar and Turbulent Flow

As previously discussed, blood flow is defined as the volume of blood that passes by a given point in a given unit of time. *Velocity* is a measure of the distance traveled in a given interval of time and is usually expressed in centimeters per second. Velocity is governed by the total cross-sectional area and

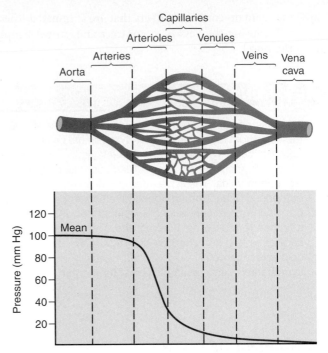

FIGURE 15-10 Mean pressure changes within the systemic vasculature. A significant decrease in pressure occurs as blood flows through the arterioles into the capillaries. The figure illustrates the role of the arterioles in the determination of vascular resistance. Because of the large number of capillaries, total resistance is not increased with the decreased radius of the capillaries.

varies inversely with it. An increase in the total cross-sectional area produces a decrease in velocity, whereas a decrease in the total cross-sectional area produces an increase in velocity. The total cross-sectional area of the aorta and vena cava is small and they have the most rapid rate of flow, whereas the capillary beds combine to produce the greatest total cross-sectional area and have the slowest flow rate. The dividing and subdividing of vessels within the circulatory system results in greater velocity in the arterial and venous beds than in the capillary bed (Figure 15-11). An understanding of the concept of velocity enhances discussion of laminar and turbulent flow.

When blood flows through a long, smooth-walled vessel, it does so in layers. The velocity of the layers varies, with blood in the center moving much faster than blood in the outer layers. The blood in the center layer moves the most quickly because it is in contact with blood only. The outermost layer is also in contact with the intima of the vessel wall, which exerts friction against the cellular components of the blood. Many blood cells stick to the intima; this layer may flow only minimally. Layers of blood between this outer layer and the central core of blood slide over one another with increasing velocity. This is referred to as the *parabolic profile of laminar flow* and is illustrated in Figure 15-12.

The streamlined nature of laminar flow is disrupted by normal anatomy and by pathologic processes creating turbulent flow. Turbulent flow is an interruption in the forward

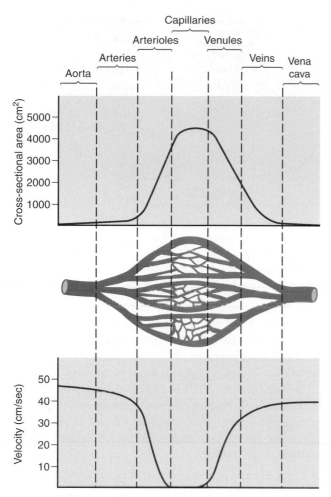

FIGURE 15-11 The effect of increasing cross-sectional area on the velocity of blood flow. Increased cross-sectional area in the capillary bed results in a significant decrease in velocity when compared to the arterial and venous networks.

FIGURE 15-12 Parabolic profile of laminar blood flow.

FIGURE 15-13 Turbulent flow generated at a blood vessel bifurcation.

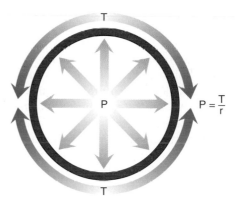

FIGURE 15-14 Law of Laplace as applied to a blood vessel. Distending pressure (P) is the difference between the pressures on either side of the vessel and is equal to the wall tension (T) divided by the radius of the blood vessel (r).

current of blood flow by crosswise flow (Figure 15-13). The propensity for turbulent flow increases with increasing velocity and increased vessel radius, so that some turbulence can be predicted at the aortic root and in the branches of major arteries. The same process can be seen in a river, where boulders interrupting the flow produce whirlpools and the characteristic roar of rapids. In the human body, turbulent flow through blood vessels can be auscultated as a **bruit.** Sometimes it can be palpated as well, and then it is called a **thrill.** This turbulence may be the result of a normal increase in velocity or blood moving through branching vessels at a sharp angle. Pathologically, turbulence results if blood flows around an obstruction in the vessel or over a roughened intimal surface. Regardless of cause, turbulent flow alters the parabolic profile seen with laminar flow, slowing velocity around the source of the turbulence. This slowing can cause cellular components of the blood to adhere to one another, the turbulent focus itself, and to the intimal wall, promoting the formation of a blood clot (**thrombus**).

Wall Tension and Compliance

The relationship between distending pressure and wall tension is expressed by the *law of Laplace* and is illustrated in Figure 15-14. This physical principle has broad applications in physiology; however, the present discussion focuses on its implications for blood vessels. The distending pressure (P) is the transmural pressure, or pressure on one side of the vessel wall minus the pressure on the other side of the blood vessel. It is equal to the wall tension (T) divided by the radius of the blood vessel (r). In summary, an increase in radius or distending pressure results in increased wall tension.

When the pressure of the blood in the vessel begins to fall, wall tension forces exceed distending forces, the radius decreases, flow declines, and resistance increases. The distending pressure may fall to a point at which it is no longer possible to hold the blood vessel open. If the pressure reaches 20 mm Hg, a point called the *critical* closing pressure, blood flow ceases entirely.

The smaller the radius of the blood vessel, as in a capillary when compared to an artery or a vein, the less tension is needed in the wall to balance out the distending pressure. Wall tensions fall rapidly from 170,000 dynes/cm in the aorta to 16 dynes/cm in the capillaries, rising to 21,000 dynes/cm in the vena cava.

Wall tension is a product of the elasticity of the vessel and is a force that opposes the distending pressure. How wall tension in a given vessel responds to changes in distending pressures is based on its compliance. Compliance reflects the distensibility of a blood vessel—its ability to accept an increased volume of blood. The large quantity of muscle tissue in much of the arterial system limits its distensibility. Veins, however, are highly distensible and compliant, capable of holding a large quantity of blood at a low pressure. Because of this quality, veins are referred to as *capacitance vessels*. When the body is at rest, 75% of the total blood volume is found in the systemic venous system.

Dynamics in the Microcirculation: Capillaries and Lymphatics

The smallest vessels of the vascular system and the lymphatic vessels are commonly referred to as the *microcirculation*. The primary function of the capillary bed is essentially the essence of the entire circulatory system: the exchange of gases and nutrients. Blood flow in the capillary bed is largely laminar, with minimal turbulence at bifurcations. Within each organ or tissue in the body, capillary blood flow is related to the driving force, which is the difference between arterial and venous pressures, and inversely related to resistance.

The exchange of materials across the capillary endothelium through the interstitial space, to or from the cells, occurs on an ongoing basis. Substances pass between tissue interstitial fluid and capillary blood by moving along a concentration gradient (diffusion), whereas fluid moves according to a pressure gradient (filtration). As fluid moves through the interstitial space, most of it returns to the capillary bed. Normally, approximately 10% of the fluid remains in the interstitium and is picked up by the adjacent lymphatic system to be returned to the general circulation. Alteration in the pressure gradient responsible for filtration can allow an excessive amount of fluid to escape into the interstitial space. Increased fluid accumulation in the interstitial space also can occur when the lymphatic flow is impaired or when capillaries become more permeable and "leak" fluid. These are the pathophysiologic mechanisms that result in **edema.**

The pressure gradient between the capillary and the interstitium is produced and maintained in accord with the balance of four distinct forces or pressures: (1) capillary hydrostatic

FIGURE 15-15 Components of the capillary pressure gradient. Filtration reflects the difference between the combined forces that push fluid out of the capillary (capillary pressure and interstitial fluid colloid osmotic pressure) and those that attempt to hold fluid in the capillary (plasma colloid osmotic pressure and interstitial fluid pressure).

pressure (P_{cap}), (2) interstitial fluid colloid osmotic pressure (π_{tissue}), (3) plasma colloid osmotic pressure (π_{cap}), and (4) interstitial fluid pressure (P_{tissue}) (Figure 15-15). This delicate balance of forces is summarized by *Starling's hypothesis,* which states that the net filtration is equal to the combined forces fostering filtration minus the combined forces opposing filtration. Using the normal values shown in Figure 15-15, each component of the formula and the resulting net filtration pressure is shown below:

$$\text{Pressures favoring filtration} = P_{cap} + \pi_{tissue}$$
$$(+17.3 \text{ mm Hg}) + (+8.0 \text{ mm Hg}) = 25.3 \text{ mm Hg}$$
$$\text{Pressures opposing filtration} = P_{tissue} + \pi_{cap}$$
$$(-3.0 \text{ mm Hg}) + (28 \text{ mm Hg}) = 25.0 \text{ mm Hg}$$
$$\text{Net filtration pressure} = (P_{cap} + \pi_{tissue}) - (P_{tissue} + \pi_{cap})$$
$$(+25.3 \text{ mm Hg}) - (+25.0 \text{ mm Hg}) = (+0.3 \text{ mm Hg})$$

Clinically, capillary fluid pressure and plasma colloid osmotic pressure are the most important concepts to a discussion of pathophysiology. Capillary fluid pressure is the blood pressure in the capillary. It is the force pushing fluid from the capillary into the interstitium and is often called the *hydrostatic pressure.* The strength of this force depends on the blood pressure and the resistance within the arterial and venous systems. Pathologic conditions resulting in an increase in either the blood pressure or the resistance to flow can alter this force, increasing it and propelling more fluid into the interstitial space, resulting in the formation of edema.

Plasma proteins are responsible for the plasma colloid osmotic pressure, the primary force resulting in fluid remaining in the capillary. Most plasma proteins normally remain in the capillaries because they are such large molecules that they cannot move through the capillary spaces. The vast majority of plasma protein, by weight, is albumin. Although globulins and fibrinogen have greater molecular weight, albumin is present in plasma in greater quantity. The number of dissolved molecules in the plasma determines the *plasma colloid osmotic pressure*. The number of dissolved molecules in the interstitial space establishes the interstitial fluid colloid osmotic pressure. Plasma has nearly four times the concentration of proteins than does the interstitium. For that reason, plasma colloid osmotic pressure normally exceeds that in the interstitium, favoring fluids remaining in the capillaries.

As previously illustrated, the net filtration pressure in a typical capillary is 0.3 mm Hg. This pressure difference is responsible for producing the fluid excess in the interstitial space, which is then normally picked up by the lymphatic system for eventual return to the systemic vascular circulation. If the pressures are altered, an even greater pressure gradient may be produced and more fluid moves from the capillaries into the interstitial space. Likewise, a change in the permeability *(K)* of the capillary wall that allows plasma proteins to leak out, or a reduction in lymphatic flow will allow fluid to collect in the interstitium. In each case, the result is **edema**, which can occur with many pathologic conditions. When the pathology is an impairment of lymphatic flow allowing fluid to collect in the interstitium, it is more specifically termed **lymphedema**.

Once absorbed into the lymphatic system, interstitial fluid is referred to as *lymph*. It is similar in composition to interstitial fluid but has a lower concentration of protein. Molecules of fat and bacteria are also found in lymph. Lymph circulates throughout the body at a rate of approximately 3 L/day. Lymphatic flow can be increased in several ways: by increasing the capillary pressure, decreasing the plasma colloid osmotic pressure, increasing the interstitial fluid colloid osmotic pressure, or increasing the permeability of the capillaries. The interstitial fluid hydrostatic pressure increases (becomes less negative) when any of these factors changes, producing an increase in lymphatic flow.[1]

KEY POINTS

- Physical laws govern the flow of blood through the circulatory system. Predictions regarding blood flow, blood pressure, and resistance to flow can be made using these laws. The important relationships may be summarized as follows:
    1. Flow = pressure/resistance
    2. Blood pressure = flow (cardiac output) × resistance
    3. Resistance = pressure/flow
- The main factors affecting resistance to flow are the radius and length of the vessels, and blood viscosity and turbulence. Usually, the radius of the vessel is the most important determinant of resistance. It affects resistance inversely and to the fourth power. A small decrease in radius results in a large increase in resistance.
- The velocity of blood flow varies inversely with the total cross-sectional area of the vascular bed. The capillaries have the greatest total cross-sectional area and, therefore, the slowest flow.
- Laplace's law describes the relationships among wall tension, distending pressure, and vessel radius *(P = T/r; T = Pr)*. An increase in radius or distending pressure

results in increased wall tension. At critical closing pressure, wall tension overwhelms distending pressure and blood flow ceases.
- The transcapillary exchange of fluid and nutrients is accomplished by the processes of diffusion and filtration. Diffusion refers to movement of solute and is determined by capillary permeability and the size of the concentration gradient. Filtration refers to movement of fluid and is affected in the following way:
    1. Increased capillary fluid pressure and interstitial fluid colloid osmotic pressure enhance filtration.
    2. Increased interstitial fluid pressure and plasma colloid osmotic pressure oppose filtration.
    3. Increased permeability (K) enhances filtration.

CONTROL OF FLOW

Blood flow throughout the periphery is controlled by central mechanisms that are mediated by the autonomic nervous system, the venous and thoracic pumps, and intrinsic autoregulatory mechanisms. Lymphatic flow is controlled by increasing interstitial fluid colloid osmotic pressure and by the stimulation of the contractile fibers (often called *lymphatic pumps*) as they are stretched. In healthy people, these mechanisms of control respond to changes in the internal and external environment and compensate rapidly and efficiently; however, during states of illness these mechanisms may be inadequate to compensate for alterations in flow.

Control of Blood Flow
Extrinsic Mechanisms
The autonomic nervous system provides the primary extrinsic control of blood flow through the sympathetic nervous system (SNS). Although parasympathetic nervous system (PSNS) innervation is important to the regulation of the heart, it is not important to the regulation of peripheral resistance. Within the medulla, groups of neurons form the *vasomotor center*. This area plays a major role in the maintenance of blood pressure (see Chapter 16). The vasomotor center responds to direct stimulation and to afferent stimuli of both an excitatory and inhibitory nature. A basal rate of discharge from the vasomotor center results in a continuous minimal level of contraction of vascular smooth muscle, referred to as *vasomotor tone*.

All blood vessels except the small venules and capillaries contain smooth muscle that is innervated by adrenergic fibers from the SNS. Because arteries have the most smooth muscle, they are most affected by SNS stimulation. Veins, by contrast, have little neural innervation, and venoconstriction has a minor role in controlling blood flow except in the skin and the splanchnic circulatory bed of the gut. In general, the release of norepinephrine, the SNS postganglionic neurotransmitter, results in arterial vasoconstriction via the α_1 receptors located on the vascular smooth muscle walls. Likewise, drugs that mimic the α_1-receptor response (α_1 agonists) produce vasoconstriction, increasing vasomotor tone and diastolic blood pressure. Administration of an α_1 antagonist results in the blockade of these receptors and results in vasodilation of the arterial bed, reducing blood pressure.

Although the β_2-adrenergic receptors located on blood vessels in skeletal muscle produce vasodilation when stimulated, they are only minimally affected by endogenous norepinephrine from the SNS. Epinephrine, the endogenous catecholamine released by the adrenal medulla, or its exogenous pharmacologic equivalent (adrenalin), stimulates these receptors, producing vasodilation. Therefore, their major role is not so much to maintain vasomotor tone but to increase nutrient and oxygen supplies to skeletal muscles during periods of increased demand.

Blood flow through the venous system into the right side of the heart is maintained by the pressure gradient from the veins and by the venous and thoracic pumps. Blood is propelled through the circuit, pushed by the force of left ventricular contraction, and moves forward toward the low-pressure side of the pump on the right side of the heart. In the peripheral veins, what is known as the *venous pump* is activated by skeletal muscle activity. Folds in the intimal wall of the veins create valves. Contraction of the skeletal muscles bordering the veins compresses them, forcing the valves open and propelling venous blood back toward the heart. Instigation of the venous pump significantly facilitates venous return. Patients who are immobilized by bed rest lose this valuable mechanism, which results in a decrease in cardiac preload to the right heart and increased work of the heart to maintain the cardiac output. The *thoracic pump* acts to increase venous return to the heart as intrathoracic pressure changes with breathing. Inspiration increases negative intrathoracic pressure, resulting in more venous return (see Chapter 17).

Intrinsic Mechanisms

Autoregulation refers to the ability of blood vessels within organs to maintain a relatively constant blood flow, regardless of changes in arterial pressure. This flow is *relatively* constant because it does have limits; there is a range within which it is maintained, and the range varies slightly from organ to organ. Several processes contribute to the autoregulation of perfusion to meet the needs of individual organs within the body.

It is known that as vascular smooth muscle is stretched, it contracts. Therefore, as arterial pressure rises and arterial walls stretch, contraction is stimulated, producing vasoconstriction. Resistance to flow is also increased with stretch by early closing of precapillary sphincters. This process certainly may contribute to autoregulation, but it is not the primary mechanism.

Over the past several decades, a great deal has been learned about the endothelium of blood vessels. Previously viewed as an inactive structure whose function was no more than the production of a barrier between the blood and the more functional layers of the vessel wall, those perceptions have fallen away.[2] We now understand that the endothelium is a major participant in vascular tone and growth of vascular smooth muscle.[2] The endothelium tissue plays an active role in the immune and inflammatory processes (see Chapter 9), platelet activity in normal coagulation and thrombus formation (see Chapter 14), and arteriosclerosis,[2-4] discussed later in this chapter. In a discussion of autoregulation, the key is the endothelial role in modulating vascular smooth muscle to produce vasoconstriction or vasodilation. The endothelium is capable of sensing alterations of a chemical or physical nature within the vessel and responding to these stimuli directly or through the release of signals that initiate change.[3] Almost all of the vasodilation occurs due to the effect of nitric oxide (NO). NO is a gas present in most body tissues and is produced by the cells of the vascular endothelium. As a gas, it diffuses from the endothelium to the smooth muscle cells, binding to intracellular receptors to impact cytoplasmic Ca^{++} and produce vasodilation.[3-5] Deficits of nitric oxide, or a decreased responsiveness, have been the focus of considerable recent research into the pathogenesis of hypertension (Chapter 16) and heart disease (Chapter 18).[2-7] Other relaxing factors produced by the endothelium include prostacyclin, and endothelium-derived hyperpolarizing factor.[6] Angiotensin II, endothelin, oxygen-derived free radicals, prostacyclin H_2, and thromboxane A_2 are among the constricting factors. The role of angiotensin II (AII) as a constricting factor has been the focus of considerable recent research.[7] Because drugs that block the effects of AII are available and in widespread use, the ability of these drugs to improve peripheral vascular blood flow has been an important finding.[7] In addition to substances produced by the endothelium itself, metabolic byproducts (metabolites) or substrates have been found to exert a direct effect, altering blood flow to the area.[1] Metabolites might include carbon dioxide or lactic acid. Histamine and prostaglandins are examples of metabolic substrates. Other substances such as acetylcholine, bradykinin, histamine, and substance P, exert their effect by increasing the formation of nitric oxide or are themselves generated by nitric oxide.[7] These various chemicals create a balance of forces in health. They may also be affected by aging, disease, or pharmacologic interventions.

A local increase in blood flow is referred to as **hyperemia.** The increase in local blood flow in response to increased metabolic demand is called *active* or *functional* hyperemia. *Reactive* hyperemia occurs when a temporary reduction in blood flow is reversed. The body responds by briefly increasing circulation to the area, resulting in the characteristic flushing seen, for instance, when a tourniquet is removed. The *tissue pressure hypothesis* of autoregulation postulates that an acute increase in the pressure within the arterial system causes an increase in interstitial volume and pressure. This increased tissue pressure, external to the vasculature, results in compression of small vessels, which increases resistance and reduces flow.

Control of Lymphatic Flow

The movement of lymph is expedited by lymphatic pumps. This is a general concept that encompasses the pumping action of the lymphatics themselves and the pumping effect on the lymphatic vessels produced by activity external to them. Like veins, lymphatic vessels have valves on their intimal surface that allow forward movement of fluid to join the venous return to the systemic circulation. Compression of lymphatic channels by adjacent skeletal muscles, the smooth muscle of organs, and the pulsatile movement of arteries force lymph forward. Intrathoracic pressure changes related to breathing increase lymphatic return as well as venous return. Lymphatic flow is therefore enhanced by increased physical activity, increased blood pressure, or increased respiratory rate. Lymphatic contractions are thought to be the primary factor in lymphatic flow. Lymph is propelled forward when lymphatic capillaries contract in response to being stretched. The rate of contractions increases as the volume of lymph increases.

KEY POINTS

- The blood flow through a particular vascular bed is regulated centrally by the autonomic nervous system and locally by the organ or tissue.
- In most vascular beds, the SNS causes constriction, which increases resistance and reduces flow. Smooth muscle cells in these vascular beds have α_1 receptors that bind the SNS neurotransmitter norepinephrine, causing contraction. There is no significant parasympathetic innervation of systemic vessels.
- Autoregulation refers to a tissue's ability to regulate its own flow. Autoregulation allows a tissue to maintain optimal flow despite changes in blood pressure or metabolic demands. In instances of high blood pressure or decreased metabolic demand, the arterioles and precapillary sphincters that control flow to the tissue constrict, reducing flow. In instances of low blood pressure or high demand, vessels dilate, increasing flow.
- Lymphatic vessels maintain flow by contracting when stretched with lymph. Intraluminal valves prevent backflow. External compression by contracting muscles enhances lymph flow.

GENERAL MECHANISMS THAT CAUSE ALTERED FLOW

A reduction in flow through the systemic vasculature results in the impaired ability to transport gases and nutrients to and from body tissues. Cells of the body vary in their oxygen demands. *Hypoxia,* an insufficient supply of oxygen, can occur for many reasons, such as a decrease in hemoglobin formation (see Chapter 13) or diminished oxygen transport in the lungs (see Chapter 21). When hypoxia is a result of a decrease in flow through the arterial system, it is called *ischemia.* Impairment in flow through the venous system interferes with the removal of metabolic waste products and causes fluid pressure to build up in the system, a condition known as *venous engorgement* or *venous obstruction.* When the lymphatic circulation is altered, the resulting fluid and pressure changes may be visible locally or systemically.

Blood Vessels: Obstructions

Pathologic processes affecting blood flow may involve impedance of the arterial or venous system. Some obstructions to flow are specific to either the arterial or venous portion of the system, but most can occur in some form in both. Obstructions to flow that may interfere with arterial or venous flow are presented in detail in the following discussion. Those that are specifically related to one or the other are detailed more fully later in the chapter.

Thrombosis. A **thrombus** is a stationary blood clot formed within a vessel or a chamber of the heart. Thrombosis is initiated by a change in the blood vessel resulting in localized stasis of flow. Inflammation of blood vessels may be the stimulus for thrombosis in either arteries or veins.

Etiology. Thrombosis refers to the pathologic formation of clots at these sites, to differentiate it from the clotting process that takes place as a homeostatic mechanism. Thrombi, blood clots, are composed of aggregated platelets, clotting factors, and fibrin that adhere to vessel walls.[1,8] Thrombi may form in the chambers of the heart in association with certain abnormal heart rhythms (see Chapter 19), following a myocardial infarction, damage to heart valves, or replacement of heart valves with artificial ones (see Chapter 18). More commonly, thrombi develop in either the arterial or the venous peripheral circulatory systems. Activation of the coagulation cascade within the vessel produces a hypercoagulable state resulting in thrombosis (see Chapter 14, Figure 14-4). Certain drugs, such as oral contraceptives, increase the tendency to form thrombi as well. Thrombosis is also more likely to occur when blood flow slows dramatically, becomes more turbulent, or if there is damage to intimal walls, creating a roughened surface.

Pathogenesis

Arterial. The significance of thrombosis rests in the ability of a clot within a blood vessel to reduce flow and increase turbulence, which enhances thrombus enlargement and the formation of more thrombi. The results of reduced blood flow vary depending on whether the arterial or venous system is involved. If the thrombus forms in the arterial system, decreased distal flow can result in **ischemia.** This is significant in several pathologic conditions, such as acute arterial occlusion (discussed in this chapter). Other examples of arterial thrombosis are explored elsewhere in this text (e.g., myocardial infarction, Chapter 18; stroke, Chapter 44).

Venous. In the venous system, thrombosis alters venous return, impairing removal of metabolic wastes and producing swelling (edema). When inflammation occurs in a vein (**phlebitis**) and is accompanied by the formation of a thrombus, it is called **thrombophlebitis.** The most common cause of thrombophlebitis is the inflammation produced by presence of a needle or catheter used for intravenous therapy. Thrombosis may also be initiated by a generalized reduction in flow and the accompanying release of vasoactive substances that occur in shock states (see Chapter 20). Systemic derangement in coagulation takes place in disseminated intravascular coagulation, resulting in thrombosis in the microcirculation throughout

BOX 15-1

Risk Factors Commonly Associated with Thrombosis

General (Arterial and Venous)
Hypercoagulable conditions
  ■ Polycythemia
  ■ Dehydration
  ■ Platelet aggregation
Pump failure
  ■ Heart failure
  ■ Shock
Dysrhythmias
Aging
Trauma, including surgery
Drugs
  ■ Anesthetic agents
  ■ Oral contraceptives
  ■ Tobacco

Arterial
Arteriosclerosis/atherosclerosis

Venous
Immobilization/sedentary lifestyle

the body (see Chapter 14). Risk factors associated with both arterial and venous thrombosis are listed in Box 15-1.

Clinical Manifestations and Treatment. Arterial thrombosis is usually manifested by intermittent claudication (pain with activity) in the affected limb that improves with rest. The limb might also be cool to touch and cyanotic. A late sign is a painful arterial ulcer found usually around one toe.[8]

Symptoms for venous thrombosis may be absent or may be life threatening secondary to pulmonary embolism. Other signs include calf or groin tenderness and swelling of the affected limb with associated increased skin temperature. Pain in the calf with dorsiflexion of the foot (Homan sign) appears in 10% of those with thrombophlebitis.

Interventions in the management of thrombus formation may be medical or surgical. Ideally, thrombosis is prevented in high-risk individuals through pharmacologic and other medical interventions. The prophylactic (preventive) interventions may include oral or parenteral anticoagulant therapy, or drugs to block platelet activation and/or aggregation.[9] Risk factors must be addressed. Once a thrombus has formed, anticoagulant therapy at a therapeutic level is initiated to prevent the enlargement of the thrombus and formation of further thrombi. But these drugs are not effective in dissolving an existing clot. These must be removed by the body's own fibrinolytic process, surgically removed, or dissolved by intravenous thrombolytic agents. These drugs are currently used for patients with thrombi in coronary and pulmonary arteries, peripheral arteries in the legs, and cerebral arteries. Their use must be closely supervised; patients receiving thrombolytic therapy are usually in critical care settings.[9] Additional medical prophylactic interventions may include the use of antiembolic stockings or sequential compression devices for immobilized patients, and initiation of ambulation as soon as possible. Surgical interventions, such as removal of the thrombus, may be an option.

Because thrombi partially or completely occlude flow through the involved vessel, they can produce ischemia distal to that point in an artery or congestion proximally in a vein. A thrombus that only partially occludes a vessel continues to be affected by the force of blood flow. Eventually, it may break free from the vessel wall and become an embolus.

Embolus. An **embolus** is a collection of material that forms a clot within the bloodstream. This traveling clot is propelled forward in the circulatory system by blood flow to a distant point, where it lodges to produce a new site of obstruction.

Etiology and Pathogenesis. An embolus is most often a blood clot, a **thromboembolus,** having begun as a thrombus that was subsequently dislodged from the vessel intima, valvular leaflets in the heart, or having formed within a chamber of the heart. Thromboemboli from the left side of the heart exit the aorta and most commonly lodge in a cerebral artery, resulting in a *stroke* (see Chapter 44). But most thromboemboli originate in the deep veins of the pelvis and lower extremities. They traverse the venous circulation and return to the right side of the heart, eventually lodging in the arterial side of the pulmonary vasculature and resulting in a pulmonary embolism (see Chapter 21). A thromboembolus from the right side of the heart will also result in a pulmonary embolism. Thromboemboli from the venous circulation are the most common cause of pulmonary emboli, but the cause may be nonthrombotic, as is the case for tumor, fat, air, amniotic fluid, or bacterial emboli; these are less frequent and are further examined later in this discussion.

Clinical Manifestations. An embolism exiting the left ventricle may lodge in the cerebral vasculature, leading to an ischemic stroke. Manifestations differ depending on the area of the brain affected. Symptoms include loss of cognitive function, motor changes, and different levels of sensory loss (see Chapter 44). More often, an embolism leaving the right ventricle lodges in the pulmonary vasculature. This pulmonary embolism may be asymptomatic or present with various signs and symptoms, many of which are vague and nonspecific.[10] Most common is the sudden onset of shortness of breath, increased respiratory rate, and chest pain. It may be a cause of sudden death.[10]

Treatment. *Embolectomy,* the surgical removal of an embolus, is usually confined to thromboemboli. The use of this surgical technique is contingent on the location of the embolus. In patients who experience repeated emboli, usually originating from the peripheral venous system, a filter (e.g., Greenfield filter) may be surgically implanted in the inferior vena cava.[10] As the blood passes through the filter, emboli are trapped and cannot progress into the pulmonary circulation. The body's own thrombolytic enzyme, plasmin, then destroys the trapped emboli.

Emboli Produced by Other Causes. Various other materials, some totally foreign to the bloodstream, can also form emboli if present in sufficient quantity. Fat emboli are aggregates of fat molecules released into the blood after trauma or surgery involving bone. Most frequently the long bones of the legs are the source of these emboli. Increased pressure generated within the traumatized bone by the inflammatory response forces molecules of fat from the interior of the bone into the bloodstream. Malignant neoplasms can metastasize by various means, one of which is via the blood as tumor emboli. Collections of bacteria and infectious exudate may break free from a source within the circulation, such as the leaflets of the valves of the heart in bacterial endocarditis. Once in the bloodstream, the bacterial emboli travel on, eventually occluding circulation and becoming a new site of infection. Air from the external environment is a foreign material when found in the bloodstream as air emboli. Bubbles of air, having most likely entered the blood through an intravenous catheter, come to rest in small blood vessels and obstruct perfusion. It is difficult to identify the specific volume of air that can sufficiently obstruct flow to result in deleterious effects in humans. In animal studies, the quantity of air needed to produce death varies, partially affected by the speed with which it is injected. Under some circumstances, a 5-ml injection of air will result in death of animal models. At other times, a 100-ml bolus of air will not produce adverse effects.[11]

Increased pressure in the abdomen generated during labor and delivery may force amniotic fluid into the bloodstream as emboli. Here the emboli cause a different set of problems. Amniotic fluid cannot perform the functions of the blood in carrying gases and nutrients, but as a fluid, it does not produce obstruction to flow. Instead, the proteins and cells in amniotic fluid act as antigens, initiating an immune response.

Vasospasm. **Vasospasm** is a sudden constriction of arterial smooth muscle that results in an obstruction to flow. In some cases, vasospasm is sufficient to produce hypoxia distally, as in variant (Prinzmetal) angina (see Chapter 18) or vasospasm of cerebral vessels following a hemorrhagic stroke (see Chapter 44). Frequently, the cause of vasospasm is unknown. Certain individuals may be unusually sensitive to hormonal changes or food additives, which may result in vasospasm of cerebral arteries. The vasodilation following cerebral vasospasm is thought to contribute to migraine headaches. Vasospasm may also be mediated by environmental factors, such as exposure to cold or emotional stress, producing a localized response.

Inflammation. **Vasculitis** is inflammation of the intima of an artery. Inflammation of the lining of a vein is called **phlebitis**. If superficial, these inflammations may be visible as reddened, tender streaks on the skin. Of more significance is their potential to serve as foci for the thrombotic process.

Arteritis *(angiitis)* is a specific term that identifies an inflammatory process of autoimmune origin in arteries. The initiating stimulus is frequently an infectious process that is viral or bacterial (especially streptococcal), or an adverse response to drugs such as sulfonamides or phenothiazines.

Mechanical Compression. A variety of forces external to the vascular system may result in partial or complete obstruction of blood flow. Trauma may produce direct pressure on a blood vessel, resulting in occlusion. This same effect may result from constriction from casts or tight dressings. Swelling secondary to bleeding or edema within a fascial compartment created by fascial tissue surrounding groups of muscle, or external compression of the compartment by a tight cast, eventually compromises the circulation distally, producing *compartment syndrome* (see Chapter 51). Prolonged occlusion produces neurovascular alterations that can be assessed before the ischemia is irreversible. These alterations are identical to those of acute arterial occlusion, discussed later in this chapter. In an untreated patient, compartment syndrome can result in prolonged hypoxia, ischemia, and necrosis of tissues.

Blood Vessels: Structural Alterations

An assortment of conditions affecting blood vessel structure will produce alterations in blood flow. The structure of arteries or veins may be changed secondary to congenital anomalies or pathologic processes triggered later in life.

Types of Structural Alterations

Valvular Incompetence. The intimal folds of veins that form the valves can be damaged, interfering with the effective flow of blood through a portion of the venous system (**valvular incompetence**). The subsequent pathologic processes may affect superficial veins (**varicose veins**) or deep veins (**chronic venous insufficiency**), resulting in severe tissue hypoxia and venous stasis ulcers.

Arteriosclerosis/Atherosclerosis. **Arteriosclerosis** is a complex condition that produces structural changes in arteries. **Atherosclerosis,** a specific type of arteriosclerosis, produces an increase in the number of smooth muscle cells and a collection of lipids within the intima of medium- and large-size arteries. This process eventually narrows the lumina and decreases their ability to dilate. Atherosclerotic changes are responsible for or contribute to many diseases throughout the body such as hypertension, renal failure, coronary artery disease (CAD), and cerebrovascular disease.

Aneurysms. An **aneurysm** is a localized dilation of an arterial wall. Aneurysms vary in the severity of their consequences, depending on their size, type, and location. All aneurysms produce an alteration in flow owing to the changes in vessel diameter. But more significant is the fact that the aneurysm represents a weakened area in the artery that may eventually rupture.

Arteriovenous Fistulas. An **arteriovenous fistula (AVF)** is an abnormal communication between arteries and veins. It is usually congenital in origin but may result from traumatic injury. Symptoms depend on the size and location of the fistula. Because AVFs provide a shortcut between the two vascular systems, they can result in alterations in oxygenation to the involved tissues and systemic hemodynamic changes. One of the most common and serious types of AVFs is **arteriovenous malformation (AVM).** An AVM is a tangled knot of arteries and veins found most commonly within the brain vasculature. AVMs may be the underlying cause of such conditions as headaches, hemorrhagic stroke, dementia, or seizures (see Chapters 44 and 45).

Lymphatic Vessels

The lymphatic collection system may be overwhelmed when changes in capillary or interstitial oncotic pressures increase filtration into tissues. The result is **edema,** the collection of an excessive amount of fluid in the interstitial spaces. A wide variety of conditions can result in edema.

When lymphatic flow is altered because of impairment in the circulation of lymph itself, the condition is called **lymphedema.** The result is also an excessive quantity of fluid in the interstitium, but the underlying cause is an obstruction to flow.

KEY POINTS

- Altered blood flow results from obstructive processes. Obstruction results in reduced flow beyond the obstruction (downstream) and increased pressure before the obstruction (upstream).
- In the arterial system, obstruction manifests primarily as distal ischemia. In the venous system, obstruction manifests as edema.
- The causes of vessel obstruction include thrombi, emboli, vasospasm, external compression (e.g., compartment syndrome), and structural alterations (e.g., atherosclerotic plaques, aneurysms).
- Alterations in pressures within the circulatory system or interstitium produce edema, whereas an impairment of the lymphatic system results in lymphedema.

ALTERATIONS IN ARTERIAL FLOW

Alterations in arterial flow result from obstruction (arteriosclerosis/atherosclerosis, inflammation, vasospasm, thrombi, emboli, and acute occlusion) or mechanical alterations (AVFs and aneurysms).

Arteriosclerosis/Atherosclerosis

Etiology and Pathogenesis. **Arteriosclerosis** is a generic term meaning "hardening of the arteries" and broadly includes three pathologic processes: Mönckeberg's sclerosis (medial calcific sclerosis), arteriolar sclerosis, and atherosclerosis. Mönckeberg's sclerosis is a noninflammatory, degenerative disorder in which the media of small and medium-size arteries becomes calcified.[12] The disease is a risk factor for cardiovascular disease, but the pathology is independent of atherosclerosis. The intimal layer is not a part of the pathogenesis; although the vessel becomes increasingly thickened and rigid, it remains patent because of the changes in the medial layer.[12] Arteriolar sclerosis is characterized by thickening and luminal narrowing of the small arteries that occurs in association with hypertension. However, because hypertension is primarily associated with atherosclerotic changes, this particular pathology is rarely addressed. Atherosclerosis, the most common arteriosclerotic process, affects intermediate-size and large arteries. Smooth muscle cells and lipids collect along the intimal surface, producing a narrowing of the luminal diameter and a reduction in flow (Figure 15-16).

Atherosclerosis is the dominant type of arteriosclerosis. The word is derived from two Greek words: *athero* (gruel or paste) and *sclerosis* (hardness).[13] It is the pathologic origin for the vast majority of arterial disease that is ultimately the leading cause of death in the United States and western Europe, and is increasing in developing countries.[14] Atherosclerosis tends to develop in large- and medium-size arteries, most frequently the coronary, cerebral, carotid, and femoral arteries and the aorta. Most of the mortality associated with atherosclerosis is the result of occlusion of coronary arteries (CAD), producing myocardial ischemia and infarction.[15] The remainder of atherosclerosis-related deaths is secondary to thrombotic or hemorrhagic processes, primarily in the brain (stroke) and extremities, although other organ systems including the kidneys, liver, and gastrointestinal tract are also affected. When

FIGURE 15-16 Atherosclerotic plaque rupture. **A,** Plaque rupture without superimposed thrombus, in a patient who died suddenly. **B,** Acute coronary thrombosis superimposed on an atherosclerotic plaque with focal disruption of the fibrous cap, triggering a fatal myocardial infarction. In both A and B, an *arrow* points to the site of plaque rupture. (**A,** From Kumar V et al: *Robbins basic pathology,* ed 8, Philadelphia, 2007, Saunders, p 351. **B,** Reproduced from Schoen FJ: *Interventional and surgical cardiovascular pathology: clinical correlations and basic principles,* Philadelphia, 1989, Saunders, p 61.)

BOX 15-2

Clinical Manifestations of Arterial Peripheral Vascular Disease

Skin assessment
- Cool or cold to touch
- Decreased or absent hair growth
- Dry, thin, glossy appearance
- Thickened nails
- Pallor when elevated, rubor when dependent
- Diminished or absent pulses

Pain assessment
- Sharp and stabbing
- Intensified with activity
- Relieved by rest or dependency

Ulcer assessment
- Severely painful
- Pale, gray base
- Well-defined edges
- Located on heels, lateral malleolus, between distal portions of phalanges, pretibial area

atherosclerosis involves the peripheral vascular system, it is most often the lower extremities, and the disease process may be called **atherosclerosis obliterans**.[8,16,17] Box 15-2 lists the manifestations of this arterial peripheral vascular disease. With arterial occlusion, patients may complain of pain with activity (*intermittent claudication*; Figure 15-17) and also have pain at rest with advanced disease. Peripheral pulses are diminished. Ulceration may occur (Figure 15-18).[8,17,18] Research results from the classic Framingham Study identified the development of lower extremity arterial disease in 5% of the subjects over the course of the 24-year data collection interval.[18]

Because of the breadth of diseases known to be associated with atherosclerosis, a great deal of research has been accomplished and an understanding of many of the significant aspects of its pathogenesis has evolved. These are summarized in Figure 15-19. The process is initiated by damage to the endothelial surface of the arterial intima, initiating an inflammatory response and an increase in the vessel wall permeability.[19] Many of the risk factors for atherosclerosis discussed later may be initiators of this vessel injury. The increased permeability of the vessel wall allows low-density serum lipoproteins to breach the intimal layer. Leukocytes also are drawn to the site, and along with the endothelial cells, they oxidize the lipids, producing further damage to the vessel wall. Simultaneously, platelets aggregate at the site of injury. They are activated, releasing platelet-derived growth factor (PDGF), which stimulates growth of smooth muscle cells. Media smooth muscle cells, normally confined to the other tunicas, are drawn to the intima where they proliferate. The result is an atherosclerotic *plaque*, primarily composed of smooth muscle cells, lipoproteins, and inflammatory debris. As the plaques slowly enlarge, the orifice of the artery is decreased and perfusion is diminished. In coronary artery disease, the plaque may also acutely rupture, initiating a thrombus formation and acute loss of perfusion (see Chapter 18).

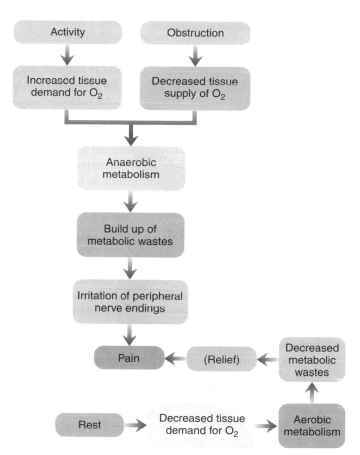

FIGURE 15-17 Pathophysiologic process of intermittent claudication and its relief.

FIGURE 15-18 Arterial ulcer. (From Zipes DP et al: *Braunwald heart disease: a textbook of cardiovascular medicine,* ed 7, Philadelphia, 2005, Saunders, p 1444).

S₁ = AV Valve closure

through the vessels of the systemic (body) circulation. The left atrium receives oxygenated blood from the lungs by way of the pulmonary veins and delivers it to the left ventricle. This oxygenated blood is pumped by the left ventricle into the aorta, which supplies the arteries of the systemic circulation. Venous blood is collected from capillary networks of the body and returned to the right atrium by way of the venae cavae. Blood from the head returns to the right atrium through the superior vena cava; blood from the body returns via the inferior vena cava. There are no valves between the venae cavae and the right atrium, and the characteristic right atrial pressure waves that are generated during the cardiac cycle are reflected into the jugular veins. An increased right atrial pressure may be observed as distention within the jugular veins.

The right side of the heart receives deoxygenated blood from the systemic circulation and pumps it through the lungs by way of the pulmonary artery. The pulmonary artery divides into left and right branches, which subdivide to supply blood to pulmonary capillary beds. Exchange of respiratory gases occurs at the pulmonary capillaries so that blood delivered to the left atrium by the pulmonary veins is well oxygenated.

Left and right heart circulations are connected in series such that the output of one becomes the input of the other. Thus, the functions of the right and left sides of the heart are interdependent. Failure of one side of the heart to pump efficiently soon leads to dysfunction of the other side.

Characteristic changes in the anatomy and physiologic functioning of the heart and circulatory systems occur with aging (see Geriatric Considerations: Changes in the Heart). In general, these changes result in a decreased cardiac reserve and a greater predisposition to cardiac muscle ischemia.

KEY POINTS

- Blood flows from the right atrium to the right ventricle through the tricuspid valve. The pulmonic valve lies between the right ventricle and the pulmonary artery. Blood flows from the left atrium to the left ventricle through the mitral valve. The aortic valve lies between the left ventricle and the aorta.
- Heart muscle (myocardium) is lined with endothelium on the inner surface and covered with epicardium on the outer surface.
- The pericardial sac envelops and protects the heart from friction.
- The right-sided heart chambers pump deoxygenated (venous) blood through the lungs. The left-sided heart chambers pump oxygenated blood through the systemic circulation.

CARDIAC CYCLE

Each heartbeat is composed of a period of ventricular contraction (**systole**) followed by a period of relaxation (**diastole**). The interval from one heartbeat to the next is called a **cardiac cycle**

and includes ventricular, atrial, and aortic (or pulmonic) events. Each of these events is associated with characteristic pressure changes within the cardiac chambers. Pressure changes result in valvular opening and closing and unidirectional movement of blood through the heart. The various events of the cardiac cycle are illustrated as a function of time in Figure 17-6. Another method of graphing ventricular function is the pressure-volume loop (Figure 17-7). Pressure-volume loops are useful for assessing the relationships between pressure and volume at various points in the cardiac cycle to evaluate left ventricular function. Abnormalities in these waveforms may occur with valvular disease, changes in blood volume, or pumping capacity of the heart (see Chapter 18). These waveforms are commonly monitored with specialized cardiac catheters in patients with cardiac or hemodynamic disorders.

The cardiac cycle can be described sequentially, beginning with ventricular filling. During diastole the ventricles are relaxed and blood flows in from the atria through open AV valves. Initially, ventricular filling occurs passively because of a pressure gradient between the atria and ventricles. Toward the end of ventricular diastole, the atria contract, squeezing more blood through the AV valves into the ventricles. Atrial contraction increases the ventricular blood volume by 15% to 20%.[2] This "atrial kick" is particularly important during fast heart rates, when the time for ventricular filling is shortened; the atrial contraction helps to load the ventricle quickly to prevent a reduction in stroke volume. Ventricular events include isovolumic contraction, ejection, and isovolumic relaxation. Each of these cycle events is further described in the following sections.

Isovolumic Contraction

Immediately following atrial systole the ventricles begin to contract, causing intraventricular pressure to rise and the AV valves to close. AV valve closure produces a sound that can be heard at the chest wall and is termed S_1. Ventricular pressure rises rapidly during isovolumic contraction because all four cardiac valves are closed, and the volume of blood within the ventricular chamber is forcefully compressed by the powerful ventricular myocardium (see Figure 17-6, *red tracing*). Volume remains constant during this phase. The rate of rise in pressure is an indication of the contractile state of the heart. The greater a change in pressure per unit time (dP/dT), the higher the contractile state. Sympathetic nervous system activation increases dP/dT whereas conditions such as heart failure are characterized by a slower rate of pressure development. The term *inotropy* is commonly used interchangeably with contractility and is reflected by the velocity and degree of cardiac muscle shortening during systole.

Ventricular Ejection

Ventricular contraction results in a rapid rise in ventricular pressure. As ventricular pressure exceeds aortic pressure (or pulmonic), the valve is forced open and a period of rapid ejection of blood from the ventricle follows. The rapid ejection phase is followed by a period of reduced ejection as aortic (or pulmonic) pressure rises and ventricular pressures and volumes fall.

GERIATRIC CONSIDERATIONS

Changes in the Heart

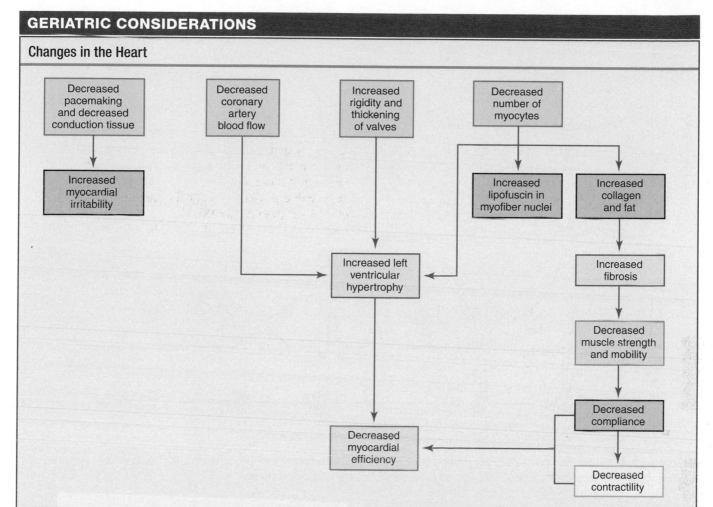

With aging, there is a decrease in the number of myocytes, but normally the heart size does not change appreciably. With the loss of overall cardiac muscle tissue, a corresponding expansion occurs in myocardial collagen and fat. The left ventricular muscle wall becomes thicker, with a resulting increase in oxygen demand. The endocardium becomes fibrotic and sclerosed. Cross-linking of the collagen tissue within the heart muscle increases myocardial stiffening, which causes decreased compliance. The decrease in compliance produces a decline in cardiac contractility, which reduces the heart's pumping ability. The rate of ventricular relaxation decreases.

Fibrotic changes in cardiac valves result from a combination of hemodynamic stress and generalized thickening. There is also a decrease in coronary artery blood flow to the myocardium, which affects myocardial oxygen and nutrient supply. The myocardial cells increase in size, with increased lipofuscin pigment and lipid deposition.

Within the specialized electrical conduction tissue, there is loss of myocytes in and fibrosis of conduction pathways, especially in the sinoatrial (SA) node, AV node, and bundle of His. There is a decreased number of pacemaker cells in the SA node resulting in less responsiveness of that node to adrenergic stimulation. Myocardial cell irritability increases. On the ECG, the P wave may be notched or slurred. The PR interval is longer, and the QRS amplitude decreases. The axis may shift left due to left ventricular muscle thickening (hypertrophy). The T wave may be notched, and the amplitude may decrease.

The changes previously noted affect cardiac function. The resting heart rate in the elderly is unchanged. During stress or exercise, the aging heart is unable to respond quickly with an elevated rate, and the maximal heart rate elevation is reduced. Once the heart rate is elevated, it takes a much longer time for the heart rate to return to the resting level. The cardiac stroke volume and cardiac output generally decrease with age. Oxygen consumption in the myocardium is reduced, resulting in less efficient function when stressed and an overall decreased cardiac reserve.

The amount of blood ejected with each contraction of the ventricle is called the *stroke volume* (SV). The volume of blood in the ventricle prior to ejection is the *end-diastolic volume* (EDV) and the amount of blood that remains in the ventricle after ejection is the *end-systolic volume* (ESV). Thus, stroke volume equals EDV minus ESV. An important and commonly used index of pumping effectiveness is the ejection fraction (EF), which is calculated by dividing SV by EDV. A normal EF is 60% to 80%; patients with systolic heart failure often have an EF of less than 40%.

Isovolumic Relaxation

The isovolumic relaxation phase begins with semilunar valve closure in response to falling ventricular pressures and ends when the AV valves open to allow ventricular filling. Ventricular

FIGURE 17-6 The events of the cardiac cycle showing relationships among left atrial and ventricular pressures, ventricular volume, and aortic pressure. An identical set of events occurs on the right side of the heart, although pressures are lower.

FIGURE 17-7 A pressure-volume loop showing changes in left ventricular volume and pressure over the cardiac cycle.

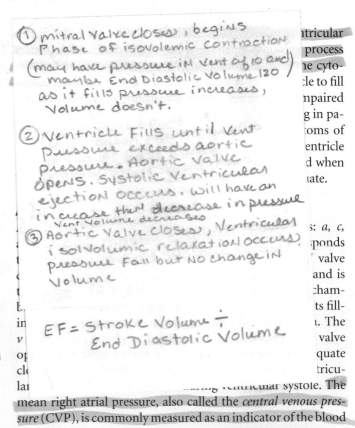

Handwritten notes (Fig 17-7): Aortic valve closed · Systolic Ejection by Ventricle · 2 (Aortic valve) opening Pressure increases · mitral valve opens · Filling · mitral valve closing · Isovolumic relaxation · SV · Isovolumic contraction · ESV · Volume (ml) · EDV

Handwritten notes (right):
1. mitral valve closes, begins Phase of isovolemic contraction (may have pressure in vent of 10 and) maybe End Diastolic Volume 120) as it fills pressure increases, Volume doesn't.
2. Ventricle Fills until vent Pressure exceeds aortic pressure. Aortic valve opens. Systolic Ventricular ejection occurs. Will have an increase then decrease in pressure vent volume decreases
3. Aortic valve closes, Ventricular isovolumic relaxation occurs) Pressure Fall but no change in Volume

EF = Stroke Volume ÷ End Diastolic Volume

blood volume remains constant during this period because all four cardiac valves remain closed. Closure of the semilunar valves causes the second heart sound, S_2. Opening of the AV valves signals the beginning of rapid ventricular filling and the start of another cardiac cycle. The rate of ventricular relaxation is indicated by the drop in ventricular pressure per unit time volume in the heart, which is dependent in part on the amount of blood being returned from the systemic circulation.

Aortic and Pulmonary Artery Events

Aortic and pulmonary artery pressures rise and fall in relation to the cardiac cycle. Arterial pressures fall to their lowest value just prior to semilunar valve opening. This lowest pressure is called *diastolic blood pressure*. Arterial pressure reaches its maximum during ventricular ejection and is called *systolic blood pressure*. A characteristic notch (*dicrotic notch*) in the arterial pressure curve may be seen as the semilunar valves close (see Figure 17-6, *blue tracing*).

The difference in aortic pressure between systole and diastole is partly dependent on the aorta's elastic characteristics. During systole, the aorta stretches to accommodate blood ejected by the ventricle. The stretched aorta has "stored" or potential energy that is released during diastole to maintain driving pressure and to keep blood flowing continuously through the circulation. Aortic stiffening, as occurs with aging or arteriosclerosis, may result in higher systolic and lower diastolic blood pressures due to loss of aortic elastic properties.[3] When aortic or pulmonic pressures are chronically elevated, the ventricles must generate more pressure to open the semilunar valves and eject the stroke volume. Over time this increase in pressure work can damage the heart muscle and lead to hypertrophy or failure.

KEY POINTS

- Characteristic pressure wave changes that occur during the cardiac cycle may be useful in diagnosing cardiac disease and volume status.
- The atria have three characteristic waves: *a, c,* and *v.* The *a* wave corresponds to atrial contraction, the *c* wave corresponds to the AV valve bulging during ventricular contraction, and the *v* wave corresponds to atrial filling.
- The ventricles have four important phases: isovolumic contraction, ejection, isovolumic relaxation, and diastolic filling. The rate and amplitude of these pressures reflect chamber volume, contractility, and valvular function. Left ventricular pressure/volume relationships are frequently used to diagnose heart failure.
- Pressure changes in the aorta during a cardiac cycle are partly dependent on the elasticity of the aorta. Differences between systolic and diastolic pressures are less with a compliant aorta. Aortic stiffness results in higher systolic and lower diastolic pressures.

CORONARY CIRCULATION

Anatomy of the Coronary Vessels

The blood supply to heart muscle is provided by the coronary arteries (Figure 17-8). Right and left coronary artery openings are located in the sinuses of Valsalva, in the aortic root, just beyond the aortic valve.[2] The right coronary artery originates near the aortic valve's anterior cusp and passes diagonally toward the right ventricle in the AV groove. In approximately 50% of the population, the right coronary artery gives rise to a posterior descending vessel that supplies blood to the heart's posterior aspect. In 20% of the population, the left coronary artery is dominant in supplying blood to the ventricles, and in 30% of the population the right and left coronary arteries deliver about the same amount of blood and neither is dominant.[4] The *left main coronary artery* arises

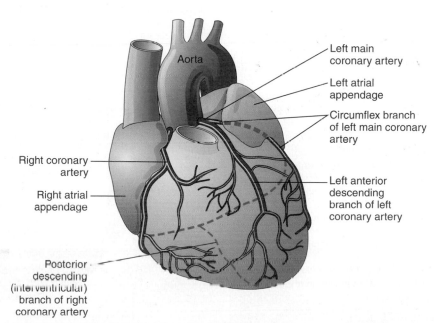

FIGURE 17-8 Coronary arteries supplying the heart. The right coronary artery supplies the right atrium, ventricle, and posterior aspect of the left ventricle in most individuals. The left coronary artery divides into the left anterior descending and circumflex arteries, which perfuse the left ventricle.

near the aortic posterior cusp and travels a short distance anteriorly before dividing into the *left anterior descending* and *circumflex* branches. The anterior descending branch supplies septal, anterior, and apical areas of the left ventricle, whereas the circumflex artery supplies the lateral and posterior left ventricle. The three major coronary arteries give rise to a number of smaller branches that penetrate the myocardium and branch into small arterioles and capillaries. Regular exercise and stable atherosclerotic plaques in the coronary arteries are thought to stimulate the development of more extensive collateral circulation in the heart. Collateral vessels may help limit infarct size in patients suffering acute coronary occlusions (see Chapter 18). Areas supplied by divisions of the coronary arteries are listed in Table 17-2. Most of the heart's capillary beds drain into the coronary veins, which then empty into the right atrium through the coronary sinus (Figure 17-9).

Regulation of Coronary Blood Flow

Blood flow through coronary vessels is determined by the same physical principles that govern flow through other vessels of the body, namely, driving pressure and vascular resistance to flow.[5] According to Ohm's law, an increase in driving pressure (P) increases blood flow (Q), whereas an increase in resistance (R) reduces blood flow: $Q = P/R$ (see Chapter 15). Driving pressure through the coronary arteries is determined by aortic blood pressure and right atrial pressure. This relationship can be expressed in the following equation:

Coronary driving pressure (P) = ABP − RAP, where ABP is aortic blood pressure and RAP is right atrial pressure. Thus, an increase in aortic pressure enhances coronary blood flow, whereas an increase in right atrial pressure opposes coronary flow.

Coronary vascular resistance (R) has two major determinants: (1) coronary artery diameter and (2) the varying degree of external compression due to myocardial contraction and relaxation. Coronary artery diameter is continuously adjusted to maintain blood flow at a level adequate for myocardial demands. **Autoregulation** is the term used to describe the intrinsic ability of the arteries to adjust blood flow according to tissue needs. Vessel dilation (*vasodilation*) occurs in response to increased tissue metabolism or reduced driving pressure, whereas decreased metabolic activity or increased driving pressure results in a decreased vessel diameter (*vasoconstriction*).

The mechanism of autoregulation can be explained by the metabolic hypothesis, which proposes that increased metabolism or decreased blood flow results in a buildup of vasodilatory chemicals in the vessel. Smooth muscle encircling the vessel relaxes in response to the presence of the chemicals, increasing vessel diameter. Several vasodilating substances have been proposed, including potassium ions, hydrogen ions, carbon dioxide, nitric oxide, prostaglandins, and adenosine. The endothelial cells that line vessels are known to secrete a variety of relaxing and constricting factors, which may contribute to autoregulation.[4] A low level of oxygen in the blood (*hypoxemia*) also may cause vasodilation of the coronary arteries. Vasodilatory substances are washed away as blood flow increases in response to increased vessel diameter. A declining level of vasodilatory chemicals results in vasoconstriction. Thus, vessel diameter is continuously adjusted according to concentrations of vasodilatory chemicals, which are directly related to the tissue's metabolic activity.

An ATP-sensitive potassium channel has been implicated in the regulation of coronary blood flow.[6] The concentration of ATP in vascular smooth muscle regulates a specific K^+ channel. As ATP levels rise in response to increased coronary flow, the channel closes, making it easier to depolarize the cell and contract vascular smooth muscle.

TABLE 17-2	
Areas Supplied by the Coronary Arteries	
Artery	**Area Supplied**
Right coronary	Right atrium (55% of persons)
	Right ventricle
	Intraventricular septum
	Sinus node (55% of persons)
	Atrioventricular node
	Bundle of His
Left anterior descending	Right atrium (45% of persons)
	Right ventricle (minor)
	Left ventricle (anterior, apex)
	Anterior papillary muscles
	Right and left bundle branches
	Intraventricular septum
Left circumflex	Left atrium
	Left ventricle (posterior, anterior)
	Sinus node (45% of persons)

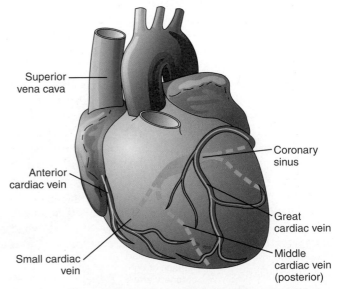

FIGURE 17-9 Venous drainage of the heart. Coronary veins drain blood from the myocardial capillary bed and deliver it into the right atrium.

Contraction of vascular smooth muscle reduces the diameter of the coronary arteries and reduces blood flow. The opposite also occurs: a reduction in ATP, due to low flow or increased metabolism, opens the K^+ channels. Potassium then leaks out of the vascular smooth muscle and short-circuits the depolarizing influences. This inhibits vascular contraction, leading to vasodilation and increased coronary blood flow. Substances other than ATP are believed to open and close these channels and may contribute to coronary regulation during periods of ischemia or increased metabolic demand.

Nitric oxide (NO) produced by endothelial cells lining the coronary arteries is an important regulator of coronary blood flow. NO is a diffusible gas produced by the enzyme, inducible nitric oxide synthase, in response to numerous stimuli including hypoxemia and platelet factors. NO is a potent vasodilator, and inhibition of its production is associated with reduced coronary blood flow. The majority of known risk factors for coronary heart disease have been shown to impair nitric oxide–dependent vasodilation of coronary arteries.[6]

Vessel diameter also is regulated by the autonomic nervous system. The coronary arteries are primarily innervated by sympathetic nerves, but they also receive a small amount of parasympathetic innervation. The sympathetic neurotransmitter norepinephrine (NE) binds to both α_1 and β_2 receptors in coronary arteries; α_1 stimulation results in vasoconstriction, whereas β_2 stimulation dilates. Under normal conditions the vasodilator response predominates, but in pathologic states, excessive α_1-mediated constriction can occur. The increased metabolic activity associated with sympathetic nervous system stimulation generally causes autoregulatory vasodilation and overrides the direct effect of norepinephrine on the vessels. Parasympathetic activity contributes to vasodilation by promoting the production of nitric oxide by coronary endothelial cells.

In addition to vessel diameter, coronary resistance is affected by myocardial contraction. During systole, cardiac muscle compression creates a marked rise in coronary resistance that reduces coronary blood flow (perfusion). Blood flow to the left ventricle is greatly decreased during systole because of the pressures generated by the thick muscular layer. Blood vessels that penetrate the myocardium to supply the innermost endocardial areas are more compressed during contraction than are outer epicardial vessels. Even though coronary artery driving pressure is greatest during ventricular systole, little blood flow reaches the ventricles because of the high external pressure applied to the coronary vessels as the myocardium contracts. Therefore, most myocardial blood flow occurs during the diastolic interval between ventricular contractions. The time the heart spends in diastole is directly related to heart rate. Faster heart rates reduce diastolic time and decrease coronary artery blood flow.

Cardiac muscle needs a continuous supply of oxygen and nutrients to perform its pumping functions. A disruption in cardiac blood flow (ischemia) generally results in some degree of pump failure and damage to cardiac tissues. Myocardial ischemia may be caused by conditions that reduce coronary blood flow or increase myocardial demands for oxygen. These include (1) reduced driving pressure (e.g., low aortic blood pressure or high right atrial pressure), (2) reduced vessel diameter (e.g., myocardial hypertrophy, arteriosclerosis, thrombosis, vasoconstricting chemicals), (3) reduced perfusion time (e.g., high heart rates, some dysrhythmias), and (4) increased metabolic demands (e.g., fever, sepsis, anemia).

KEY POINTS

- The right and left coronary arteries originate from the aortic root, within the sinuses of Valsalva. In most people the right coronary artery perfuses the right ventricle, AV node, sinoatrial (SA) node, and right atrium.
- The left coronary artery divides into the left circumflex artery and left anterior descending artery, which perfuse the left atrium and ventricle.
- Coronary blood flow is regulated centrally by the autonomic nervous system and locally by autoregulation. The amount of coronary flow depends on driving pressure and coronary resistance. Coronary resistance is dependent on vessel diameter.
- Adenosine and nitric oxide are two important vasodilating chemicals that are produced in response to inadequate oxygen delivery to the heart and help to increase blood flow so as to meet metabolic demands.
- Although driving pressure is highest during systole, there is little coronary flow because of vessel compression by the contracting myocardium. Most coronary blood flow occurs during diastole.

CARDIAC MYOCYTES

Cardiac muscle cells are divided into two general types: working cells, which have primarily mechanical pumping functions, and electrical cells, which primarily transmit electrical impulses. Both types are *excitable*: they are able to produce and transmit action potentials. Working myocardial cells are packed with contractile filaments and make up the bulk of the atrial and ventricular muscle. Electrical cells function to initiate and coordinate contraction of the working cells. Differentiated cardiac myocytes are unable to enter the cell cycle to proliferate; however, they can increase in size and synthesize more contractile proteins (hypertrophy). New myocardial cells can be formed from stem cells that have the potential to divide. Stem cells may be recruited from the circulation and stimulated to divide and mature into myocytes within the myocardium.[7] Conditions that increase myocardial cell death are thought to stimulate recruitment of stem cells into the myocardium. When the rate of myocardial cell loss exceeds replacement by stem cells, the condition of heart failure may ensue (see Chapter 19).

Myocyte Structure

Typical myocardial cells (myocytes) are illustrated in Figure 17-10. Cardiac myocytes are described as muscle "fibers" because of their long narrow shape. The plasma membrane (sarcolemma) of one cardiac cell is joined end to end with its neighbors by intercalated disks, which contain gap junctions that allow the rapid passage of electrical impulses from one cell to the next. The intercalated disks permit the many separate cells of the myocardium to function together in a coordinated manner. This arrangement is called a *functional syncytium*. The sarcolemma also forms membrane-lined channels that penetrate the cell and become the transverse tubules (T tubules) (Figure 17-11). The T tubules permit extracellular fluid and ions to diffuse near intracellular structures. Movement of ions across the sarcolemma is an essential part of cellular excitation and the subsequent contraction of intracellular elements. Cellular contractile elements are simultaneously activated because signals at the cell surface are rapidly transmitted internally by the T tubules.[8]

The sarcoplasmic reticulum (SR) is an extensive labyrinth of hollow membrane that stores significant amounts of intracellular calcium. It contains Ca^{2+}-sensitive channels that open briefly during depolarization and allow calcium ions to flow into the cytoplasm. An action potential traveling along the T tubule opens voltage-sensitive calcium ion channels (L type) in the plasma membrane. The Ca^{2+} ions that enter the cell through these channels interact with receptors on the SR membrane called *ryanodine receptors* (see Figure 17-11, *B*).

Activation of these receptors opens calcium gates on the SR, and Ca^{2+} rushes into the cytoplasm to initiate contraction. The SR also contains powerful sarcoplasmic endoplasmic reticulum calcium ATPase (SERCA) pumps that recover calcium ions from the cytoplasm and return them to the SR. Inside the SR, calcium is bound to specialized proteins including calsequestrin. This helps keep the free calcium concentration in the SR lower such that the calcium transporters have a lower gradient to pump against.

Cardiac muscle cells are packed with numerous mitochondria that are strategically positioned along the contractile fibers of the cell. The heart is also endowed with an extensive capillary network, approximately one capillary per muscle cell. The large number of mitochondria and abundant oxygen supply are necessary to keep pace with the high ATP requirements of the contractile elements and ion pumps.

Structure of the Contractile Apparatus

Microscopic inspection of the cardiac myocyte reveals a typical pattern of banding called *striation*.[9] This striated appearance is due to an organized structure of the proteins (myofibrils) of the contractile apparatus (Figure 17-12). The contractile proteins, actin and myosin, are called *filaments* because they are long and narrow. **Myosin** filaments are larger and referred to as *thick filaments*. *Thin filaments* are actually composed of several different types of protein bundled together. **Actin** is the primary constituent of thin filaments, with smaller amounts of the proteins **tropomyosin** and **troponin** bound to it.

The thick and thin filaments are specifically arranged in contractile units called *sarcomeres* (Figure 17-13). Sarcomeres are defined by dark bands called *Z disks* (also called Z lines), which lie perpendicular to actin and myosin filaments. A sarcomere extends from one Z disk to the next. Thin actin filaments are attached to Z disks and extend from them. The I bands (isotropic) are light in color and correspond to the position of thin actin filaments extending in both directions from the Z disk. Thick myosin filaments lie parallel to and between the thin filaments. They are held in place by a very large and elastic protein called *titin* that extends from the Z disk to the center of the sarcomere. Each myosin filament is surrounded by six thin filaments (see Figure 17-13). The dark A band corresponds to an area where the actin and myosin filaments overlap. An M line marks the center of the A band and the midpoint of the myosin filaments. One other zone, the H zone, corresponds to a region occupied solely by myosin filaments with no actin filament overlap. An efficient, synchronized contraction is enhanced by this precise arrangement of contractile elements.

Characteristics of Contractile Filaments

Myosin molecules are composed of six polypeptide chains, two heavy (H) chains and four light (L) chains. These light and heavy chains are organized into a tail region and two globular "head" areas (Figure 17-14). The myosin heads interact with actin filaments to produce muscle contraction. Thick filaments are made up of many myosin molecules with

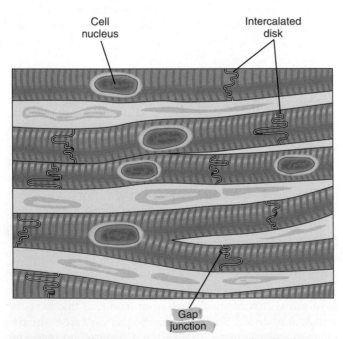

Cell nucleus

Intercalated disk

Gap junction

FIGURE 17-10 Myocardial cells, showing long narrow shape and interconnecting junctions, forming a functional syncytium. The end of one muscle cell is fused to the next by intercalated disks. Within these connections are specialized proteins that form a fluid-filled pore (gap junction) between the fused cells. Ions can travel through the gap junctions to transport changes in membrane potential from one cell to the next.

FIGURE 17-11 A, Schematic diagram of a portion of a cardiac myocyte showing the transverse tubules (T tubules), which extend horizontally from the plasma membrane into the cell interior. The T tubules are extensions of the plasma membrane that bring the extracellular fluid into juxtaposition with the terminal ends of the sarcoplasmic reticulum (SR). The T tubule with the SR on either side of it is called the *triad of the reticulum*. B, Calcium ions that enter the cytoplasm through voltage-gated L-type channels on the T-tubule membrane interact with the ryanodine receptors on the sarcoplasmic reticulum. The activated ryanodine receptors allow calcium ions to flow into the cell cytoplasm where they initiate contraction. As soon as they are released, calcium ions are rapidly captured by the sarcoplasmic endoplasmic reticulum calcium ATPase (*SERCA*) pumps on the SR membrane.

FIGURE 17-12 Electron micrograph of muscle fibrils showing characteristic banding pattern. The dark vertical lines are the Z disks. A sarcomere extends from one Z disk to the next. Compare with the schematic drawing in Figure 17-13. (From Fawcett DW: *The cell,* Philadelphia, 1981, Saunders.)

tail regions bundled together and heads sticking out at intervals along the bundle. The head regions are flexible and can bend and pull on actin filaments to accomplish muscle contraction. Myosin heads are oriented in opposite directions on either side of the center tail region (see Figure 17-14). Myosin heads have enzymatic properties and can cleave ATP to release energy necessary for muscle contraction. Different forms of myosin have varying rates of ATP hydrolysis, which affects how quickly the muscle contracts. The serum level of thyroid hormone is known to affect the type of myosin produced in heart cells. Hyperthyroidism is associated with a fast-cycling type and hypothyroidism with a slow type of myosin. The rate of myosin cycling can also be regulated at the light chain of the myosin protein. Cellular enzymes that attach a phosphate to the light chain speed up the rate of cycling. Phosphorylation is increased by activation of myocardial β_1 receptors and enhances contractility.[9]

As previously mentioned, thin filaments are composed of several different proteins, including actin, nebulette (nebulin), tropomyosin, and troponin. Actin filaments are actually polymers of many globular actin proteins that are attached end-to-end, like two strings of beads, and then twisted together to form a helix (Figure 17-15). Each of the actin beads has a site that can bind with myosin heads. Nebulette is a long protein that extends the entire length of the thin filament and is thought to regulate the length of the actin polymer such that all of the thin filaments are the same size. Tropomyosins are long, slender proteins that bind to a string of six or seven actin beads.[9] When myocardial muscle is relaxed, tropomyosin molecules inhibit the myosin-binding sites on the actin beads. A third protein complex, troponin, is attached to the thin filament and regulates the availability of binding sites on the actin filament by controlling the position of tropomyosin. Each troponin is composed of three subunits, called troponin T, I, and C. Troponin T binds to tropomyosin, troponin I participates in the inhibitory actions of tropomyosin, and troponin C binds up to four molecules of Ca^{2+}. As described below, tropomyosin and troponin are important regulatory proteins that control the activities of actin and myosin filaments. The specific isoforms (amino acid sequences) of troponin T and I present in heart tissue differ from those in other types of cells, and their presence in the serum can be used to detect myocardial infarction (see Chapter 18).

KEY POINTS

- The myocardial cells of the heart behave as a syncytium because they are joined by gap junctions within the intercalated disks that permit the flow of ions from one cell to the next.
- Myocytes are packed with actin and myosin proteins that form the contractile apparatus. The thick filaments are composed of myosin proteins. Myosin has enzymatic activity and splits ATP, releasing energy needed for movement of the filaments. Titin is a flexible protein that attaches the thick filament to the Z disk.
- The thin filament is composed of actin and two regulatory proteins, troponin and tropomyosin. At rest, tropomyosin inhibits myosin-binding sites on actin. The position of tropomyosin is regulated by the calcium-binding protein troponin. Nebulette is another actin-associated protein that helps regulate thin filament length.

Handwritten annotations:

Cytoskeletal structural / Cytopoxin

* myosin heads have enzamatic properties and can cleave ATP to release energy Necessary for muscle Contraction.

Actin is the thin Filament c̄ Proteins tropomyosin & troponin attached

The enzyme Head group that binds to Actin + Forms cross bridge. (uses ATP)

Head grabs Actin (this is the crossbridge each time it shortens.

* hyperthyroidism affects fast type, hypothyroidism affects slow type.
P horlation is increased by activation of myocardial B₁ receptors and increases Contractility.

* Dif forms of myocial have Varied Rates of ATP hydrolysis which affects Speed of contraction.

Actin Filaments are polymers of many globular Actin Proteins Attached end to end like beads) then twisted to form a helix

* each actin bead has a site that can bind c̄ a myocin head

* when relaxed the tropomycin molecules inhibit the myosin-binding sites on the actin beads.

FIGURE 17-13 Thick and thin filaments are organized into contractile units called *sarcomeres*. A sarcomere extends from one Z disk to the next and represents the fundamental unit of muscle contraction. See text for description of bands, zones, and lines. Overlap of thick and thin filaments in each area is shown in cross-section at the bottom. Each thick filament interacts with six thin filaments that surround it.

FIGURE 17-14 The thick filament of the sarcomere is composed of myosin proteins. Myosin head groups are oriented in opposite directions on either side of the center tail region. Phosphorylation *(P)* of the regulatory light chain increases myosin activity and rate of cross-bridge cycling.

FIGURE 17-15 Schematic drawing of the proteins that make up the thin filament. **A,** Globular actin proteins combine to form long double-helix filaments. **B** and **C,** The proteins troponin and tropomyosin combine with the actin helix to form the thin filament **(D).** Nebulin (nebulette) is a long cytoskeletal protein that extends the length of the thin filament and is thought to regulate filament length.

MOLECULAR BASIS OF CONTRACTION

Overview of Contraction

The heart's pumping action is accomplished by the additive contractions of the many myocytes that form the cardiac chambers. Because each myocyte contributes only a small amount to overall muscle shortening, all cells of the chamber must shorten simultaneously to produce a forceful contraction. The specialized cells of the conduction system function to stimulate myocardial contraction in a coordinated way. An action potential traveling down the conduction system is the usual trigger for contraction. Cardiac myocyte depolarization causes ion channels in the plasma membrane and T tubules to open, permitting sodium and calcium entry and release of calcium from the SR. The presence of free calcium in the sarcoplasm (muscle cytoplasm) results in contraction. These events describe the process of excitation-contraction coupling.

Sliding Filament/Cross-Bridge Theory of Muscle Contraction

The sliding filament, or cross-bridge, theory of muscle contraction is suggested by the anatomic configuration of the sarcomere described earlier. Muscle shortening is accomplished by increasing the amount of overlap of actin and myosin filaments. The Z disks at the ends of the sarcomere move closer together as overlapping actin and myosin filaments pull past one another. Myosin heads grip binding sites on the actin beads and pull the thin filaments toward the sarcomere's center.

Each time a myosin head binds an actin bead, it forms a so-called **cross-bridge.** Flexible myosin heads move in a ratchet-like manner to tug on the actin filaments (Figure 17-16). Each ratcheting motion moves actin filaments only minutely, and many sequential cross-bridge formations are required to shorten the entire sarcomere. Thus, myosin heads bend back and forth, binding and pulling on the actin filaments in a step-like fashion. Actin filaments are prevented from slipping back to their original position because some myosin-actin bonds are forming while others are releasing. The making and the subsequent breaking of each actin-myosin cross-bridge requires one molecule of ATP. Consequently, tremendous quantities of ATP are hydrolyzed with each cardiac contraction.

ATP hydrolysis, which occurs at the myosin head region, provides the energy for contraction and also affects the capability of myosin to bind actin.[9] Myosin has two functional states or conformations: (1) a low-affinity state in which it binds weakly and (2) a high-affinity state in which it avidly binds actin. The affinity of the myosin head for actin depends on whether ATP is bound (low affinity) or ADP and inorganic phosphate (P_i) are bound (high affinity). A proposed sequence of cross-bridge cycling is as follows (see Figure 17-16):

1. Free myosin heads bind ATP and hydrolyze it to ADP and P_i, which remain on the myosin. Myosin heads now have a high affinity for actin and are in a high-energy conformation.

2. If binding sites on actin are accessible, myosin binds to the actin.

*When there is No calcium troponin induces tropomycin to block myocin binding sites. When calcium comes in Troponin C binds with it and troponin complex induces tropomycin to move and expose the binding sites on actin.

Controls the position of tropomycin

When muscle Related tropomycin prevents myocin From binding to the actin head. During B,C+D it has a high affinity for Actin.

* muscle shortening is Accomplished by increasing the Amt of overlap of Actin and myocin Filaments

FIGURE 17-16 The cross-bridge cycle of muscle contraction. **A,** The myosin head has hydrolyzed its bound adenosine triphosphate *(ATP)* to adenosine diphosphate *(ADP)* and inorganic phosphate *(Pi)*, which remain on the myosin. In this state the myosin has high affinity for actin but cannot bind because the actin-binding sites are not accessible. **B,** When calcium ions enter the cell and bind to troponin, the tropomyosin-blocking protein moves to allow myosin to bind actin, forming a cross-bridge. **C,** The act of binding changes the shape of myosin so that ADP and Pi are released. The "power stroke" is accomplished by movement of the myosin neck region. **D,** When a new molecule of ATP binds to the myosin, it changes to a low-affinity state and releases from the actin. ATP is again hydrolyzed to ADP and Pi to start the cycle again. Each cross-bridge cycle uses one ATP molecule.

Handwritten figure annotations: Actin; Troponin; Tropomyosin; Thin filament; Thick filament (myocin); ADP Pi; myocin Head; Myosin binding sites; ADP Pi; Ca²⁺; ATP's Affinity provides energy ATP; → have to have ATP to break the bond.; ADP + Pi; * The more Crossbridges you make the more energy you use. (ATP) + increases O2 Consumption

3. Binding results in release of ADP and Pi and a ratchet movement of the myosin as it assumes its low-energy conformation, which shortens the sarcomere (power stroke).

4. With loss of ADP and Pi, myosin can bind another molecule of ATP. The myosin heads with ATP bound now have a low affinity for actin and release from the binding site. ATP is again hydrolyzed to ADP and Pi, and another cross-bridge cycle is initiated.

Continued cross-bridge cycling is dependent on the availability of ATP and calcium ions. A lack of ATP results in fewer cross-bridge cycles and inability of the muscle to shorten normally.

Role of Calcium in Muscle Contraction

Muscle contraction is dependent on the presence of an adequate amount of calcium ions in the cytoplasm. In the absence of free intracellular calcium, muscle contraction will not take place, even though myosin head groups have high affinity for actin-binding sites. This phenomenon can be explained in the following way. At rest, myosin heads are prevented from binding to actin by tropomyosin proteins, which inhibit actin-binding sites. The position of tropomyosin protein is controlled by troponin. When calcium is absent, troponin induces tropomyosin to inhibit the actin-binding sites. When calcium binds to troponin C, the troponin complex induces tropomyosin to move and expose the binding sites (see Figure 17-16, *A* and *B*). Cross-bridge formation immediately ensues because myosin heads have high affinity for these sites in the relaxed state. The concentration of free calcium ions in the myocardial cell determines how many actin sites are exposed and for how long, and therefore, determines the number of cross-bridges and extent of contraction. The release of Ca^{2+} into the cytoplasm is regulated by numerous neurotransmitters and hormones that affect contractility as described in later sections of this chapter.

Energy of Muscle Relaxation

Although muscle relaxation is generally viewed as a passive phenomenon, it actually requires significant energy to pump calcium ions out of the cytoplasm. As calcium levels fall, calcium diffuses away from the troponin molecules and tropomyosin is induced to cover the actin-binding sites. With actin-binding sites covered, myosin heads are unable to initiate cross-bridge formation, and thick and thin filaments slide back to their resting position. Removal of calcium ions is an energy-requiring process. Membrane pumps located in the sarcolemma and SR actively move calcium out of the sarcoplasm against a concentration gradient (Figure 17-17). The sarcolemma contains two different calcium pumps: one that requires ATP and one that uses the potential energy of the sodium gradient to remove calcium from the cell. Calcium pumps on the SR (SERCAs) require ATP. Thus energy deficiency due to myocardial ischemia can impair diastolic relaxation as well as systolic contraction of the heart muscle.

(handwritten margin note: Calcium levels fall, troponin induces tropomyocin to cover binding sites.)

Cardiac muscle cell

FIGURE 17-17 Calcium ions *(Ca²⁺)* are removed from the cardiac muscle cell cytoplasm by energy-dependent protein transporters in the plasma membrane and sarcoplasmic reticulum *(SR)* membrane. Thus cardiac relaxation is an energy-requiring process. *ADP,* adenosine diphosphate; *ATP,* adenosine triphosphate; *P_i,* inorganic phosphate.

CARDIAC ENERGY METABOLISM

The heart, like other tissues in the body, utilizes energy from ATP hydrolysis to drive its energy-requiring functions. Synthesis of ATP in cardiac muscle cells is accomplished by the same glycolytic and oxidative reactions described in detail in Chapter 3.

Oxygen Utilization

Because the heart is continuously active, its energy requirements are considerable. Very little ATP is stored in myocardial cells, so that a continuous supply of oxygen and nutrients is necessary to support ongoing ATP synthesis. Even under normal resting conditions, the heart extracts a large portion of oxygen from the blood perfusing it. Conditions of increased oxygen demand, therefore, must be met by increasing the rate of coronary blood flow. When oxygen delivery is insufficient to meet requirements for oxidative phosphorylation, the cell must rely on ATP produced by glycolysis. Unfortunately, glycolysis results in production of only enough ATP to maintain the cell for seconds to minutes. In addition, anaerobic glycolysis results in local buildup of lactic acid, which may further impair cardiac performance.

Under conditions of relative ATP excess, myocardial cells are able to transfer energy to a storage form called *creatine phosphate* (CP). This transfer is accomplished by the enzyme **creatine kinase** (CK or CPK), in the following reaction:

$$ATP + creatine \leftrightarrow ADP + CP$$

Although amounts of cellular CP are limited, they provide an immediate source of energy when cellular ATP levels drop acutely. Under conditions of ischemia, the enzymatic reaction would proceed in reverse, utilizing CP and adenosine diphosphate (ADP) to produce ATP, for immediate use by the cell. This phosphate transfer reaction is important during fluctuations in ATP supply because it does not require the presence of oxygen.

The enzyme CK is also useful in the diagnosis of myocardial cell damage. Myocardial cells that lose membrane integrity (necrosis) leak their enzymes into extracellular fluid and eventually into the bloodstream. Elevated levels of blood CK are indicative of the degree of acute myocardial cell death. Different types of tissue contain different forms of CK (isoenzymes). The MB form of CK is found in cardiac muscle, and elevated serum levels of this enzyme are indicative of myocardial infarction.[10] Other intracellular proteins, including troponin and myoglobin, are released during myocardial cell death and also can be used as markers of myocardial infarction (see Chapter 18).

Substrate Utilization

The primary foodstuffs that provide fuel for energy-producing enzymatic processes in cardiac muscle are glucose and fatty acids.[11] Amino acids are less important metabolic substrates for cardiac muscle except during states of starvation. The amount of fatty acids and glucose utilized by heart muscle cells depends on their relative concentrations in the blood. Fatty acids are the preferred fuel, particularly in a fasting state, when glucose levels are lower. Under fasting conditions, fatty acids account for approximately 85% of myocardial fuel and glucose contributes only 15%. After eating, when blood glucose levels rise, glucose utilization may increase to about 50%. Fatty acid metabolism requires oxygen and is therefore not useful under conditions of ischemia. The heart is also able to use lactate and ketones as sources of energy when they accumulate in the circulation. Lactate is derived from pyruvate under conditions of anaerobic metabolism, whereas ketones are formed from lipid metabolism when carbohydrate supplies are low. Thus, the heart is equipped to use a variety of substrates to produce ATP under varying metabolic conditions.

> ## KEY POINTS
>
> - CP is an immediately available storage form of energy. Under conditions of low ATP availability, CP is converted to ATP by the enzyme CK. (creatine phosphate)
> - The primary energy substrates for the heart are fatty acids and glucose, but the heart can utilize a variety of sources to produce energy depending on what is available in the circulation.

CARDIAC ELECTROPHYSIOLOGY

The plasma membranes of cardiac cells are endowed with special ion channels that make the cells excitable. Excitable tissues are capable of generating and conducting action potentials. The heart is rhythmically activated by action potentials, which are generated and transmitted by a specialized conduction system. Spread of an action potential over cardiac muscle cell surfaces results in myocardial contraction. An understanding of the electrophysiologic properties of the heart is important because many cardiac disorders result in disturbances in electrical function that produce abnormal conduction pathways, dysrhythmias, and conduction blocks.

Cardiac Resting Potential

Like other cells, resting cardiac cells are negatively charged on the inside with respect to the outside (see Chapter 3). A difference in potassium ion concentration across the cell membrane is the primary determinate of the resting membrane potential. Atrial and ventricular muscle cells generally have a resting membrane potential of −85 to −95 mV. Pacemaker cells in the SA node are less polarized having a resting membrane potential of about −60 mV. An increase in extracellular potassium ion tends to hypopolarize the cell (make it less negative), and a lower-than-normal extracellular potassium tends to hyperpolarize the cell (make it more negative). The degree of polarization is an important determinant of the ease with which an action potential can be initiated. Abnormalities in serum potassium level are a common source of cardiac dysrhythmias.

Cardiac Action Potential

Depolarization of cardiac cells to a threshold point results in activation of voltage sensitive ion channels in the membrane. A myocardial action potential (Figure 17-18) results from movement of ions through these open voltage-gated channels. The action potential in atrial and ventricular cells has five characteristic phases.[12] Atrial action potentials are shorter in duration because they have a reduced Phase 2 compared with ventricular cells.

Phase 0. Phase 0 begins when the membrane potential approaches threshold and voltage-gated "fast" sodium channels open momentarily. Due to a steep electrochemical gradient for sodium entry, rapid influx of sodium ions occurs. Sodium entry depolarizes the cell by neutralizing the difference in charge (polarity) across the membrane. A steep depolarizing deflection (upstroke) is recorded. Class I antiarrhythmic agents such as quinidine and lidocaine block voltage-gated sodium channels and interfere with phase 0 depolarization (see Chapter 19).[13]

Phase 1. Phase 1 is identified as a small repolarizing deflection that corresponds to closure of the fast sodium channels and beginning efflux of potassium from the cell. The interior of the cell is now more positively charged, which induces potassium ions to leave the cell.

Phase 2. Phase 2 is also called the *plateau phase* because little change in membrane potential occurs during this time, even though ions continue to move across the membrane. Phase 2 is primarily associated with an influx of calcium ions, which is offset by an efflux of potassium ions. The ability of K+ to leave the cell down its electrochemical gradient is inhibited during plateau phase by a relative inhibition of potassium channels.

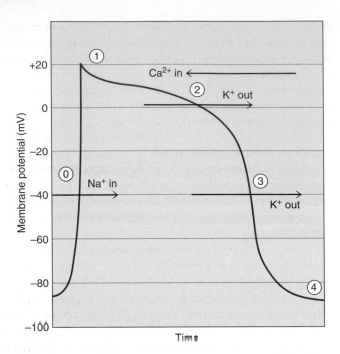

FIGURE 17-18 The ventricular myocardial action potential has five characteristic phases, representing changes in ion movement through the plasma membrane. *Phase 0:* Rapid upstroke due to sodium influx. *Phase 1:* Slight repolarization due to closure of sodium channels and beginning potassium efflux. *Phase 2:* Plateau due to offsetting influx of calcium and efflux of potassium. *Phase 3:* Rapid repolarization due to closure of calcium channels and increased potassium efflux. *Phase 4:* Resting membrane potential reestablished due to closure of all voltage-sensitive channels.

This is sometimes called potassium *rectification*. Chloride also may leave the cell during this phase. The voltage-gated calcium channels open and close slowly in comparison to fast sodium channels and are thus referred to as slow channels or L-type channels (long-lasting).

The calcium that enters the cell during phase 2 is linked to muscle contraction as previously described. The L-type calcium channels can be modified by agonists that prolong the open phase, such as catecholamines, and by antagonists that shorten the open phase, such as acetylcholine. Calcium channel–blocking agents (class IV antiarrhythmic agents) are used commonly in patients with cardiovascular diseases to inhibit calcium influx.[13] β-blockers (class II antiarrhythmics) also reduce calcium ion influx during phase 2 by indirectly inhibiting calcium channels.

Phase 3. Phase 3 is characterized by a rapid return to the resting membrane potential. This is accomplished by closure of the slow calcium channels and continued and even more rapid efflux of potassium ions from the cell through a variety of potassium channels. Sodium channels remain absolutely refractory during phases 1, 2, and early 3. The latter part of phase 3 represents a *relative refractory period,* when sodium channels may be induced to open, but a larger than normal depolarizing stimulus is required. If an abnormally early (premature) depolarization occurs during the relative refractory period, it

will be conducted more slowly than usual because few fast Na⁺ channels are ready to be activated. Slow conduction through the myocardium predisposes to cardiac dysrhythmias, such as ventricular fibrillation (see Chapter 19). Class III antiarrhythmic agents, like amiodarone, increase the refractory period by inhibiting opening of potassium channels during phase 3.[13]

Phase 4. Phase 4 of the ventricular myocyte action potential corresponds to the period of time between action potentials when no changes in membrane voltage are evident and the resting membrane potential is present. The resting membrane potential in ventricular myocardial cells is flat, and they do not spontaneously depolarize. In contrast, cells in the pacemaker and conduction system automatically depolarize and have a sloping phase 4. The Na⁺-K⁺ pump and Ca²⁺ pumps work continuously throughout all phases to maintain the internal and external concentrations of sodium, potassium, and calcium ions.

Rhythmicity of Myocardial Cells

Rhythmicity (automaticity) refers to intermittent, spontaneous generation of action potentials. A requirement for rhythmicity is that the cell membrane has channels that automatically open during phase 4. These channels open when the membrane potential becomes more negative during repolarization phase.[12] Progressive channel opening makes the pacemaker cells leaky to Na⁺, Ca²⁺, and K⁺. Gradually the flow of positive ions into a cell offsets the repolarizing currents and depolarizes the membrane, resulting in generation of an action potential. One contributor to the automatic depolarization during phase 4 is the I_f channel. The I_f channels originally were named for a "funny" current and later discovered to be sodium channels that are activated by membrane repolarization. Channels that allow calcium and potassium leak are also operative during phase 4 in pacemaker cells. Late in phase 4, an increase in calcium ion influx occurs through voltage-gated calcium channels called *T type* for "transient." These channels open and close more quickly than the L-type calcium channels that open during the action potential. Many of these channels can be regulated by various means, including autonomic neurotransmitters, in order to change heart rate. An action potential is initiated when phase 4 depolarization reaches the threshold for opening of voltage-gated, L-type, slow calcium channels. Repolarization is achieved in large part by an exodus of potassium ions from the cell. Rhythmic cells have a recognizable action potential that is characterized by a sloping phase 4 (Figure 17-19), in contrast to the flat phase 4 of ventricular muscle cells.

The rate of rhythmic discharge is determined by the relative influx of Na⁺ and Ca²⁺ versus the efflux of K⁺. In a normal heart, a cell with the fastest rate of spontaneous depolarization becomes the pacemaker for the rest of the heart. Cells in the SA node, located in the right atrium, generally function as the heart's pacemakers because they have the fastest rate of spontaneous depolarization. However, other cells in the conduction system are also capable of spontaneous

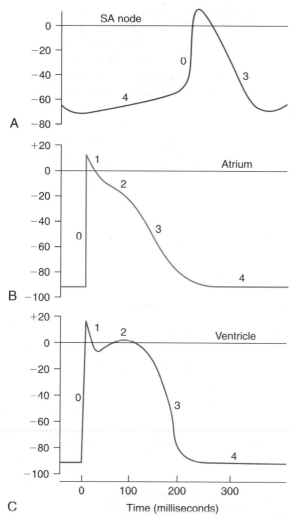

FIGURE 17-19 Rhythmic cells **(A)** have a sloping phase 4, in contrast to the flat phase 4 of the atrial **(B)** and ventricular **(C)** muscle cell. Spontaneous depolarization during phase 4 allows pacemaker cells to develop action potentials automatically. *SA,* Sinoatrial. (Adapted from Hoffman BF, Cranefield PF: *Electrophysiology of the heart,* New York, 1960, McGraw-Hill.)

depolarization and may initiate an action potential in certain circumstances.

The steepness of the slope of phase 4 depolarization determines the rate of action potential generation and therefore heart rate. Several factors determine the steepness of the slope, including membrane permeability to sodium, calcium, and potassium. For example, an increase in potassium ions leaving the cell would slow depolarization and result in a slower rate. Rhythmicity may be influenced by the autonomic nervous system, drugs, and electrolyte balance. These conditions are discussed in the following sections.

Specialized Conduction System of the Heart

Some myocardial cells are specialized to conduct action potentials throughout the heart in an organized and rapid manner. These cells make up the conduction system of the heart,

as shown in Figure 17-20. Normal excitation of the heart follows a pathway beginning with the SA node, atrial internodal pathways, AV node, bundle of His, ventricular bundle branches, and, finally, Purkinje fibers.

The SA node is located in the right atrium near the superior vena cava inlet. It receives innervation from sympathetic and parasympathetic branches of the autonomic nervous system. The SA node generally serves as a pacemaker for the heart, generating about 75 (range, 60 to 100) action potentials per minute in a resting adult. SA action potentials are spread contiguously through gap junctions to adjacent atrial cells at a rate of about 1.0 m/sec.[12] A fibrous skeleton separates atria from ventricles and prevents spread of impulses from atrial cells to ventricular cells. There are several small bundles of atrial muscle cells that conduct impulses slightly faster than the usual atrial cell. One such bundle, the anterior interatrial band (Bachmann bundle), conducts impulses from the SA node to the left atrium. The existence of three other bundles that conduct impulses from the SA node to the AV node has been suggested. Atrial depolarization results in atrial contraction, which increases the volume delivered to the still relaxed ventricular chambers.

After traversing the atria, the impulse initiated at the SA node arrives at the AV node (AV junction) located in the posterior septal wall of the right atrium just behind the tricuspid valve. There is a characteristic slowing of impulse conduction through the AV node, which allows for completion of atrial contraction prior to beginning ventricular systole. The AV node is actually composed of several different types of fibers that have somewhat different action potential conduction times. Overall, it normally takes about 0.13 second for an impulse to pass through the AV node. The slowness of conduction through AV fibers is mainly because there are few gap junctions between AV nodal cells so that cell-to-cell conduction of action potentials is more difficult due to high resistance.[12,14] The AV node is richly innervated by the autonomic nervous system. The AV node spontaneously depolarizes at a rate of 40 to 60 times per minute and usually becomes the heart's pacemaker if the SA node fails.

Purkinje cells (fibers), which lead from the AV node to ventricular myocardium, are vastly different from AV nodal cells. They are large and well structured to conduct impulses very rapidly. After penetrating the AV fibrous barrier, the bundle of Purkinje fibers travels 5 to 15 mm down the intraventricular septum toward the apex. The main bundle then divides into left and right bundle branches, which travel down the left and right sides of the intraventricular septum. Successive branches of Purkinje fibers penetrate the ventricular muscle mass from the endocardial side. Intraventricular septal areas are depolarized first, followed by apical muscle and finally the lateral walls (Figure 17-21). Early septal depolarization allows the septum to contract first and provide a stable wall for the left and right ventricles to contract against.[12] The total time elapsed between main bundle branch and terminal Purkinje fiber depolarization is only 0.03 second.[14] Therefore, the entire ventricular endocardium is activated almost simultaneously.

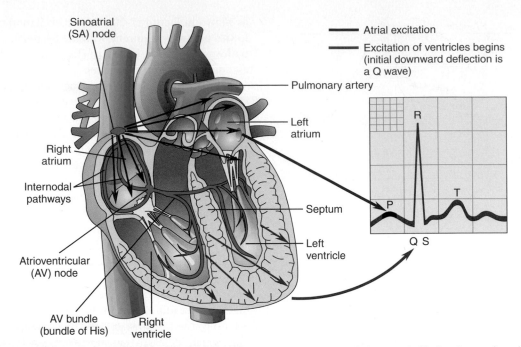

Atrial excitation

Excitation of ventricles begins (initial downward deflection is a Q wave)

FIGURE 17-20 Schematic drawing of the conducting system of the heart. An impulse normally is generated in the sinus node and travels through the atria to the AV node, down the bundle of His and Purkinje fibers, and to the ventricular myocardium. Recording of the depolarizing and repolarizing currents in the heart with electrodes on the surface of the body produces characteristic waveforms.

Purkinje fibers are capable of spontaneous depolarization at a rate of 15 to 40 times per minute and may become pacemakers for the heart if impulses from the SA and AV nodes are interrupted.

Action potentials are rapidly transmitted from the terminal Purkinje fibers to cardiac muscle fibers and then spread contiguously from cell to cell through gap junctions in the ventricular muscle. Approximately 0.03 second is required for the impulse to be transmitted through the ventricular myocardium.[14] Impulses normally travel from the terminations of Purkinje fibers at endocardial surfaces toward the epicardial surfaces. Depolarization of the right ventricle is accomplished slightly sooner than the left because of differences in muscle mass. Depolarization of the ventricular myocardium is followed by contraction and ejection of blood from the ventricles.

The capability of faster pacemakers to suppress the automatic discharge of slower pacemakers is called *overdrive suppression*. A slower pacemaker may be revealed if the normal pacemaker is suddenly interrupted. Sometimes it takes time for the slower pacemaker to "kick in" and begin pacing at its intrinsic rate. A previously rapid rate of depolarizations apparently enhances the activity of membrane Na+-K+ pumps, resulting in a period of hyperpolarization (more negative resting potential) when the faster pacemaker suddenly stops. Thus, it takes a bit longer to reach threshold and initiate the first action potential.

Autonomic Regulation of Rhythmicity

Both sympathetic and parasympathetic nerves supply the heart. Sympathetic innervation is widespread to all areas, including the ventricular myocardium. Parasympathetic innervation, by way of the vagus nerves, is localized primarily in SA and AV nodal areas. The right vagus nerve supplies the SA node, whereas the left vagus nerve supplies the AV node.[15] The autonomic nervous system exerts control over heart rate and velocity of impulse conduction. In general, sympathetic activation increases heart rate (*chronotropic effect*) and increases speed of conduction (*dromotropic effect*) as well as inducing heart muscle to contract more forcefully (*inotropic effect*). These effects are achieved by release of NE from sympathetic nerve endings. Binding of NE to β receptors on heart muscle cell membranes opens membrane channels, which allows more rapid sodium and calcium ion entry.

Parasympathetic stimulation primarily results in a reduction in heart rate and speed of action potential conduction. Acetylcholine is the neurotransmitter released by parasympathetic nerve endings. Acetylcholine binding to muscarinic receptors on heart cells increases membrane permeability to potassium ions, allowing them to leak from the cell. The resulting hyperpolarization makes it more difficult to reach threshold and initiate an action potential. The resting heart is normally under a predominant parasympathetic influence, which results in an SA discharge rate of about 75 beats/min. If parasympathetic activity is blocked, the spontaneous discharge rate of SA nodal cells increases to about 100 beats/min. An increase in vagal activity can reduce heart rate significantly. Breath holding, bearing down during defecation, and pressing on the carotid arteries may increase vagal tone and reduce heart rate. This is sometimes called a *vasovagal response* and may lead to dizziness and fainting.

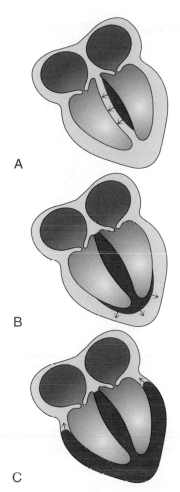

FIGURE 17-21 Sequence of ventricular depolarization showing septal depolarization in a left-to-right direction **(A),** followed by apical depolarization in an endocardial to epicardial direction **(B),** and finally, depolarization of the lateral walls **(C).** Repolarization proceeds in the opposite direction.

FIGURE 17-22 Comparison of the action potential from a single ventricular muscle cell, showing rapid depolarization and prolonged repolarization phases, against an electrocardiogram of potentials from the heart as a whole. Ventricular myocytes remain depolarized and refractory through the entire QT interval. (Redrawn from Guyton AC, Hall JE: *Textbook of medical physiology,* ed 11, Philadelphia, 2006, Saunders, p 125.)

KEY POINTS

- The cardiac resting membrane potential is about –90 mV. The resting membrane potential is determined by the ratio of intracellular to extracellular K+ concentration.
- The five phases of the cardiac action potential are due to changes in ion conductance through the plasma membrane. The main changes in ion conductance result from opening of the fast Na+ channels (phase 0), slow Ca²+ channels (plateau), and K+ channels (repolarization) in the plasma membrane.
- Spontaneous generation of action potentials in automatic cells is due to progressive leak of Na+ and Ca²+ into the cell via channels that automatically open during repolarization. The rate of cation leak determines the rate of pacemaker discharge. Parasympathetic influence increases K+ efflux and slows the rate. Sympathetic influence increases influx of Na+ and Ca²+ and increases the rate.
- The usual conduction pathway for depolarization of the heart begins at the SA node, progresses through the atria, enters the AV node, and activates the His Purkinje fibers. Purkinje fibers leave the AV node and divide into left and right branches that innervate the endocardial surface of the ventricular myocardium.

ELECTROCARDIOGRAPHY

As action potentials spread from cell to cell throughout the myocardium, an electrical current is transmitted to the body surface and can be detected by electrodes placed on the skin.[16] A recording of these electrical currents is called an *electrocardiogram* (ECG). The ECG is a useful indicator of abnormalities of the heart's conduction system. Irregularities in initiation of impulses, conduction rates, and conduction pathways can be identified. The ECG looks different from the cardiac action potential described previously because it registers depolarizing and repolarizing currents in the whole heart rather than the activity of individual myocytes (Figure 17-22).

Electrical currents traveling through the heart have both direction and magnitude and are often described as *vectors*. At any instant, electrical currents are moving in various directions through different regions of the heart. Waveforms recorded at the ECG electrodes are algebraic sums of all of these vectors. Patterns of electrical activity shown on the ECG vary according to the placement of electrodes on the body. In general, a wave of depolarization moving toward a positive recording electrode will register as an upward deflection on the ECG. A wave of repolarization moving away from a positive electrode also will register as an upward deflection on the ECG. A downward deflection results from a wave of depolarization moving away from a positive electrode (Figure 17-23). Placement of a recording electrode on the lower-left extremity (lead II) results in the typical ECG pattern shown in Figure 17-24. A description of the usual electrode placements is included in the section on diagnostic tests at the end of this chapter.

Each deflection on the ECG has a normal characteristic shape and time interval (see Figure 17-24). The three major wave complexes are the *P wave,* which corresponds to atrial depolarization, the *QRS complex,* which represents ventricular depolarization, and the *T wave,* which reflects ventricular repolarization. The PR interval, between the beginning of the P wave and the beginning of the QRS complex, includes atrial, AV node, and His Purkinje fiber depolarization. The normal sequence of ventricular depolarization begins with the septum, followed by the apex, and, finally, the base of the ventricular walls. Septal depolarization begins on the left septal surface and then travels toward the right, resulting in a small negative deflection, the *Q wave* in lead II (Figure 17-25). A large upright *R wave* corresponds to a wave of depolarization traveling down the ventricles toward the apex. Depolarization of the ventricular base, because it moves in a direction away from the lower limb electrode, is recorded as a negative *S wave.* The ST interval, between the S wave and the beginning of the T wave, is isoelectric (flat), as the entire ventricle is depolarized and no detectable current is flowing. The QT interval, from the beginning of the QRS complex to the end of the T wave, is commonly measured as an indicator of ventricular systole. The T wave is normally upright in lead II, representing a wave of repolarization moving away from a positive electrode. In some patients, particularly those with slow heart rates, the T wave is followed by a small positive deflection, called a *U wave.* Prominent U waves also are a sign of a low potassium level. Abnormalities in any time intervals may indicate abnormal conduction pathways and enhanced or slowed conduction times. Rhythm disturbances are discussed in detail in Chapter 19.

FIGURE 17-23 Electrocardiographic *(ECG)* waveforms may be positive (upward) or negative (downward), depending on the location of electrodes on the chest. **A,** A wave of depolarization moving toward a positive electrode results in a positive deflection. **B,** A wave of repolarization moving away from a positive electrode results in a positive deflection. **C,** A wave of depolarization moving away from a positive electrode results in a negative deflection.

KEY POINTS

- The ECG represents an algebraic sum of all depolarizing and repolarizing currents occurring in the heart. ECGs are useful for detecting conduction and rhythm disturbances.

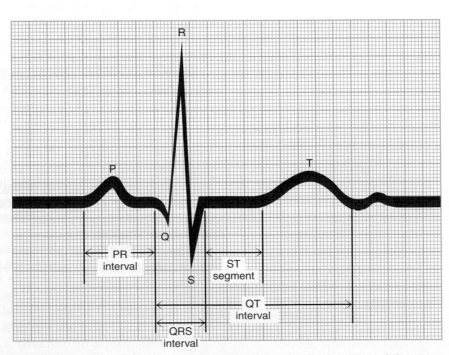

FIGURE 17-24 Usual electrocardiographic pattern recorded from lead II, showing characteristic waves and intervals.

- The major deflections of the ECG are:
  P wave: atrial depolarization
  PR interval: atrial, AV node, and Purkinje depolarization
  Q wave: septal depolarization
  R wave: apical depolarization
  S wave: depolarization of lateral walls (base)
  T wave: ventricular repolarization

DETERMINANTS OF CARDIAC OUTPUT

Cardiac output is a measure of the amount of blood pumped out of the heart each minute. Because the heart's primary function is to pump enough blood to circulate oxygen and nutrients to tissues, cardiac output is an extremely important indicator of cardiovascular health. The normal resting cardiac output is approximately 5 to 6 L/min, but it varies with body size and age. Cardiac output is often indexed to body surface area in an attempt to adjust for these differences (cardiac index = cardiac output/body surface area). A normal cardiac index ranges from 2.8 to 3.3 L/min/m². Regardless of the actual number of liters of blood pumped per minute, the adequacy of tissue perfusion is ultimately important.

Cardiac output is a product of heart rate and stroke volume (CO = HR × SV). **Stroke volume** refers to the amount of blood ejected from the ventricle with each contraction. An increase in heart rate (to a point) and/or an increase in stroke volume will result in a greater cardiac output. Conversely, a low heart rate and/or a decreased stroke volume will cause cardiac output to fall. To a certain extent, a change in one factor can be compensated for by a change in the other, thus maintaining cardiac output at a constant level. For example, it is common for an individual with limited stroke volume due to cardiac disease to have a high resting heart rate. Any physiologic, pharmacologic, or pathologic process that alters heart rate or stroke volume may affect cardiac output and therefore tissue perfusion.

Determinants of Heart Rate

Heart rate is primarily influenced by the autonomic nervous system. Release of norepinephrine by sympathetic nerve endings results in increased heart rate. A similar effect results from circulating norepinephrine and epinephrine released from the adrenal gland during sympathetic stimulation. Sympathetic activation of the heart is regulated by several reflex pathways that constantly monitor blood pressure and metabolic activity in the body. In general, detection of inadequate blood pressure, a lack of oxygen, or a buildup of metabolic end products results in activation of the sympathetic nervous system. Specialized sensory nerve endings, called *baroreceptors*, located in the aortic arch and carotid arteries respond to changes in blood pressure and transmit this information to the central nervous system by way of cranial nerves IX and X. A fall in blood pressure causes parasympathetic system inhibition and cardiac sympathetic nerve activation, resulting in a rise in heart rate. Conversely, a rise in blood pressure causes heart rate to fall because of parasympathetic activation and sympathetic inhibition. Under normal resting conditions, the heart rate is under parasympathetic influence, with a usual rate of 60 to 80 beats/min.

In addition to baroreceptors, other sensory fibers that detect pressure are located in the cardiac chambers. These sensory receptors respond to changes in intrachamber pressure, which reflect the volume of blood in the chamber. Atrial or ventricular overdistention suppresses parasympathetic influence and increases heart rate (Bainbridge reflex).[15] Heart rate may also be influenced by higher CNS activities that do not involve reflex pathways. Anxiety, fear, stress, excitement, trauma, and fever may activate the sympathetic system, for example. A variety of drugs can mimic or block the effects of both sympathetic and parasympathetic systems and therefore influence heart rate (see Chapter 18).

In general, an increase in heart rate results in an increase in cardiac output; however, at very high heart rates, cardiac

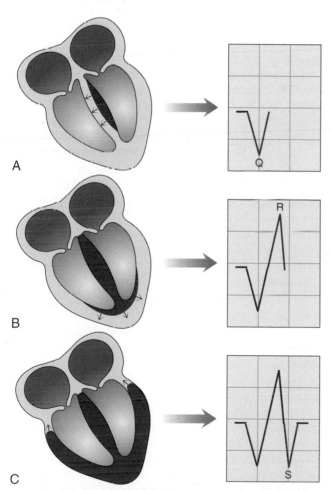

FIGURE 17-25 The QRS complex results from the sequence of ventricular depolarization. **A,** In lead II, septal depolarization is in a direction away from the positive electrode, resulting in a negative Q wave. **B,** Depolarization of the apex of the heart is in a direction toward the positive electrode, resulting in a large positive R wave. **C,** Depolarization of the lateral walls and base of the ventricles is in a direction away from the positive electrode, resulting in a negative S wave.

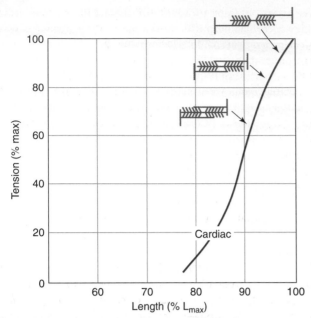

FIGURE 17-26 The force of muscle contraction depends in part on its resting length before activation. At short lengths, filaments may overlap and interfere with cross-bridge formation. At optimal length, the greatest tension is developed, and cross-bridge formation is enhanced.

FIGURE 17-27 Cardiac function curves showing the dependence of ventricular stroke volume on preload. Different hearts have different cardiac function curves and may respond differently to the same degree of preload. *SNS,* Sympathetic nervous system; *PSNS,* parasympathetic nervous system.

output may actually fall. At high heart rates (e.g., more than 200 beats/min in the young, even lower in the adult), the time for diastolic ventricular filling can be significantly reduced, resulting in a low stroke volume. The benefit of increased heart rate is therefore undermined by impaired pumping efficiency.

Determinants of Stroke Volume

Three major factors influence stroke volume: (1) the volume of blood in the heart (**preload**), (2) the contractile capabilities of heart muscle (**contractility**), and (3) impedance opposing ejection of blood from the ventricle (**afterload**). Each of these factors is in turn influenced by many other physiologic, pharmacologic, and sometimes pathologic variables.

Volume of Blood in the Heart (Preload)

The heart can only pump as much blood as is delivered to it by the circulatory system. Blood returning to the heart from the circulation is often called venous return. Normally, venous return is equal to cardiac output because the circulatory system is just that—a circuit. However, there may be inequalities over several heartbeats when changes in blood volume or blood distribution occur. The heart is well suited to adjust to these beat-to-beat changes in venous return such that the healthy heart pumps essentially whatever amount is delivered to it.

The amount of blood present in the ventricles just prior to contraction (end-diastolic volume) is an important determinant of stroke volume. The relationship between diastolic volume and the force of myocardial contraction is known as the **Frank-Starling law of the heart**.[2,17] In essence, this law states that an increase in resting muscle fiber length results in a greater development of muscle tension. Ventricular muscle

fiber length is determined by the volume of blood it contains, commonly called the *preload.* An increase in preload results in a greater force of contraction and a larger stroke volume. In this way, the ventricle is able to adjust its stroke volume, beat by beat, according to the amount of blood to be pumped.

The Frank-Starling law of the heart (also called the *length-tension relationship*) may be understood by recalling the molecular structure of contractile units of heart muscle. For contraction to occur, the actin and myosin filaments that make up the sarcomere must form cross-bridges and slide together. Stretching the muscle prior to contraction could optimize actin-myosin filament overlap and allow greater numbers of cross-bridges to form, resulting in a more forceful contraction (Figure 17-26). If sarcomere length is too short prior to contraction, further shortening is limited because actin filaments begin to abut the opposite Z disk. Stretching the muscle prior to contraction also appears to make the contractile apparatus more sensitive to calcium ions such that a greater contractile force occurs for a given calcium concentration.[2]

The cardiac function curve describes the effects of preload on ventricular stroke volume (Figure 17-27). In practice, stroke volume and ventricular end-diastolic volume are difficult to measure, and other indicators, such as ventricular pressure and cardiac output, may be used. Cardiac function curves can be measured in persons with poorly functioning hearts to determine the best filling volume (preload) for optimizing cardiac output. Often, the failing heart requires a higher than normal preload to maintain a normal cardiac output.

However, there are limits to the improvement in stroke volume with increased diastolic filling and beyond that point, the curve will flatten. On the flat part of the curve, an increase in preload increases the workload of the heart, but does not provide an improvement in output. The workload imposed on the heart chambers by preload is sometimes called the *volume work of the heart.* An increase in preload increases the volume work of the heart which must be met by increased oxygen uptake to maintain adequate ATP production.

Contractile Capabilities of the Heart (Contractility)

Heart muscle contractility depends on several factors, including (1) the amount of contractile proteins in the muscle cells, (2) the availability of ATP, and (3) the availability of free calcium ions in the cytoplasm. Contractility is, by definition, independent of fiber end-diastolic length and is therefore not affected by preload. Given an adequate ATP supply, the contractile state of the normal myocardium is primarily determined by factors that increase the availability of free calcium ions within the myocardial cell. In general, an increased intracellular free calcium level can be accomplished by enhanced release from internal stores, enhanced entry from extracellular fluid, and reduced rates of extrusion across the plasma membrane.

A variety of agents that increase contractility, called *positive inotropes,* are associated with increased intracellular calcium levels in the heart. These include the sympathetic neurotransmitters norepinephrine and epinephrine, thyroid hormone, caffeine, digitalis, and many others. Agents that depress contractility, called *negative inotropes,* achieve their effects by reducing intracellular calcium levels. These agents include L-type calcium channel blockers, parasympathomimetics, and sympathetic blocking drugs. The baroreceptor reflex, described previously in relation to heart rate, is also an important regulator of stroke volume through its effects on contractility. Positive inotropic agents increase ATP utilization by the myocardium, whereas negative inotropes decrease myocardial workload and reduce ATP requirements.

Cardiac disease may adversely affect contractility because of an inadequate oxygen supply or because of loss of myocardial pumping cells. These disorders are discussed in Chapter 18.

Impedance to Ejection from the Ventricle (Afterload)

The third major determinant of stroke volume is afterload, which refers to the impedance or resistance that must be overcome to eject blood from the chamber. Left ventricular afterload is determined primarily by aortic blood pressure. Because high blood pressure increases left ventricular afterload, vasodilating agents that reduce blood pressure can significantly decrease afterload. Normally the aortic valve offers little impedance to flow; however, aortic valve narrowing may significantly increase afterload. An increase in afterload will result in a decrease in stroke volume unless contractility or preload (or both) is adjusted to compensate. Conversely, a decrease in afterload will allow a larger than normal volume of blood to be ejected from the heart, requiring less myocardial work. The work done by the heart to overcome afterload is often called the *pressure work of the heart.* An increase in afterload increases pressure work and requires greater tension development within the walls of the chamber (wall stress). Increased wall stress not only increases myocardial workload and oxygen consumption, but if prolonged, it may trigger structural changes leading to hypertrophy of myocytes.

The ventricles normally eject only about 60% to 70% of their end-diastolic volume during contraction; the remaining 30% to 40% remains in the ventricle. **Ejection fraction** is influenced by afterload as well as preload and contractile state. A reduced ejection fraction is a common finding in persons suffering from myocardial infarction. Ejection fractions less than 20% indicate significant myocardial impairment and may be associated with systolic heart failure (see Chapter 19).

Cardiac Workload

The oxygen requirements of the heart are related to the amount of energy (ATP) exerted to perform its pumping function. The four determinants of cardiac output described in the previous section—heart rate, preload, contractility, and afterload—are also the major determinants of cardiac energy requirements. An increase in any of these four factors will increase ATP requirements and therefore cardiac cell oxygen requirements. High afterload is most detrimental, as it greatly increases cardiac work without producing a higher cardiac output. When oxygen supply to the heart is impaired, as in coronary atherosclerosis, it may be beneficial to reduce myocardial oxygen demand by reducing cardiac workload. This may be accomplished by reductions in heart rate, preload, afterload, and contractility.

KEY POINTS

- Cardiac output is the product of the heart rate times the stroke volume (CO = HR × SV). An increase in heart rate or stroke volume will increase cardiac output. An increase in heart rate can compensate for a decrease in stroke volume.
- Heart rate is controlled primarily by the autonomic nervous system. Factors that increase heart rate include low blood pressure (baroreceptors), acidemia (chemoreceptors), atrial and ventricular overdistention (Bainbridge reflex), and emotions. Activation of the vagus nerve will decrease heart rate.
- Stroke volume is influenced by preload. According to the Frank-Starling law, increased preload stretches the sarcomere, resulting in more forceful contraction.
- Increased contractility increases stroke volume by causing a greater percentage of the ventricular volume to be ejected. Any factor that enhances availability of cytoplasmic free Ca^{2+} will increase contractility.
- Increased afterload will decrease stroke volume. Afterload is determined primarily by the resistance of the arterial system. Vasoconstriction and high aortic pressure increase afterload.
- Any factor that increases heart rate, preload, contractility, or afterload will increase the workload of the heart.

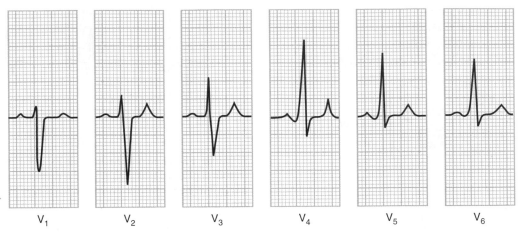

V_1 V_2 V_3 V_4 V_5 V_6

FIGURE 17-33 Normal electrocardiogram recorded from the six unipolar chest leads, V_1 through V_6. Note the R-wave progression across the precordial leads as the R waves become increasingly positive. (Redrawn from Guyton AC, Hall JE: *Textbook of medical physiology*, ed 11, Philadelphia, 2006, Saunders, p 129).

Echocardiography

Echocardiography uses reflected sound waves (ultrasound) to provide an image of cardiac structure and motion within the chest.[19] The cardiac echo is obtained by placing a blunt probe on the chest surface that transmits and receives high-frequency sound waves. Sound waves traveling through chest and heart structures are reflected back to the receiving probe. The time between sound wave emission and detection of reflected waves is used to calculate distances between the probe and reflecting tissue. The sound waves are not heard or felt by the subject and have no known detrimental effects on tissues. The probe is moved across the chest to assess cardiac structures of interest, and recordings are videotaped for later viewing.

Echocardiograms are particularly useful for diagnosis of heart enlargement, valvular disorders, collections of fluid in the pericardial space, cardiac tumors, and abnormalities in left ventricular motion. Estimations of ejection fraction and assessments of ventricular systolic and diastolic function can be made non-invasively by echocardiogram. An echocardiogram is shown in Figure 17-34.

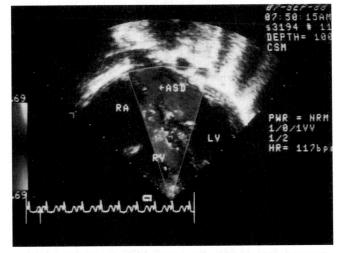

FIGURE 17-34 Color echocardiogram of a child with a large atrial septal defect *(ASD)*. The red indicates low-velocity blood flow through the defect toward the ultrasound transducer. The *yellow* indicates areas of turbulent blood flow. *ASD*, Atrial septum defect; *RA,* right atrium; *RV,* right ventricle; *LV,* left ventricle. (From Skorton DJ et al., editors: *Marcus cardiac imaging: a companion to Braunwald's heart disease*, ed 2, vol 1, Philadelphia, 1996, Saunders.)

Nuclear Cardiography

Radioactive substances injected into the bloodstream can be used to trace the patterns of blood flow in the heart.[19] Radiation exposure is minimal, as very small amounts of radioactive substances are used. Radioactive tracers can be linked to substances that accumulate in normal myocardial cells as the tracer is delivered by coronary blood flow. Areas with impaired perfusion will take up less radioactivity and appear as "cold spots" on the scan. Alternatively, a radioactive tracer can be linked to a substance that accumulates in recently infarcted tissue and is excluded from healthy cells. The infarct appears as a "hot spot" on the scan. Scanning usually is done using single-photon emission computed tomography (SPECT), which images numerous slices through the heart, or by planar imaging, which gives an overall picture in one plane only.

Thallium (^{201}Tl) and technetium-99 labeled compounds (^{99m}Tc sestamibi) are used to assess the adequacy of blood flow to cardiac tissues. After injection of the radioactive compound, the heart is scanned to visualize the amount of radioactivity taken up by cardiac tissues. Healthy cardiac tissues that receive adequate blood supply actively accumulate these isotopes. Areas of inadequate blood flow or infarcted tissue do not accumulate isotope and appear as cold spots on the scan.

Resting and exercise scanning are done to assess for exercise-induced perfusion defects. In recent years, scanning for the purpose of identifying infarcted tissue is uncommonly done. 99mTc-labeled Sn-pyrophosphate was traditionally used because it accumulates in recently infarcted tissue creating a hot spot of radioactivity.

Gated pool scanning (radionuclide ventriculogram) is used primarily to assess left ventricular motion and ejection fraction. Before it is injected intravenously, radioactive technetium is attached to albumin or red cells, and therefore it remains in the bloodstream and is not taken up by cells. Computer imaging is used to analyze blood flow through the chambers of the heart over many cardiac cycles. The dynamics of ventricular motion, such as hypercontractility or hypocontractility, may be visualized. Separate radionuclide ventriculogram evaluation has largely been replaced by SPECT scanning that allows simultaneous evaluation of perfusion and left ventricular function.

Cardiac Catheterization/Coronary Angiography

Cardiac catheterization/coronary angiography may be used to determine important structural and hemodynamic characteristics because it affords direct measurement of pressures within cardiac chambers; visualization of chamber size, shape, and movement; sampling for blood oxygen content in various heart regions; measurement of cardiac output and ejection fraction; and visualization and management of coronary artery obstructions.[19]

Cardiac catheterization angiography is associated with several serious risks, including bleeding, dysrhythmias, heart perforation, and coronary ischemia. The advent of noninvasive high-resolution MRI, echocardiograms, and SPECT scanning has replaced the need for cardiac catheterization in many instances; however, the value of information supplied is generally believed to outweigh the risks in certain cases. Catheterization is frequently used for interventions to rapidly improve coronary blood supply and to evaluate suspected or confirmed coronary artery disease, valvular dysfunction, congenital defects, left ventricular dysfunction, and coronary bypass graft patency.

Assessment of the left side of the heart, including the coronary arteries, is achieved by passing a catheter through a femoral or brachial artery into the aorta. The catheter is then manipulated into the left ventricle or left atrium to assess chamber pressures, and a ventriculogram is obtained. Contrast dye injected into the ventricular chamber is monitored fluoroscopically to assess ventricular function. The catheter is usually pulled back into the aorta and then advanced into one or more of the coronary arteries. The patency of the coronary arteries can be visualized by injecting contrast dye into them and monitoring by fluoroscopy (Figure 17-35). When contrast dye is in the coronary artery, a period of cardiac ischemia is produced during which the patient may experience angina, dysrhythmias, and coronary spasms. Coronary catheterization may also be done to insert

FIGURE 17-35 Coronary artery angiography. The *arrow* shows an area of obstruction of the right coronary artery. (From Johnson MR: Principles and practice of coronary angiography. In Skorton DJ et al., editors: *Marcus cardiac imaging: a companion to Braunwald's heart disease*, ed 2, vol 1, Philadelphia, 1996, Saunders.)

a probe for obtaining intracoronary ultrasounds. Ultrasounds are useful for assessing plaque morphologic characteristics (Figure 17-36).

Right-sided heart catheterization is done to evaluate right-sided heart structures. The catheter is introduced into a vein, usually femoral or antecubital, then threaded through the inferior vena cava and into the heart. Pressures and blood samples are obtained as the catheter is advanced into the right atrium, ventricle, and pulmonary artery. Right heart catheterization is useful in assessing tricuspid and pulmonary valve disorders, pulmonary hypertension, septal defects, and right ventricular function.

Coronary angiography is commonly followed by interventions to treat detected abnormalities. The coronary catheter can be used to direct thrombolytic agents to the site of coronary thrombosis and rapidly restore blood flow to ischemic areas. Laser therapy, coronary balloon angioplasty, and stent placement can also be performed during coronary angiography. These methods clear the coronary obstruction through thermal and mechanical means. The success of these approaches to management of coronary obstruction depends largely on how soon after an ischemic event they are done (Chapter 18).

FIGURE 17-36 Intracoronary ultrasonographic examples of plaque morphology. **A,** Concentric calcification of the left anterior descending artery. **B,** A normal vessel wall. **C,** Fibrous cap on coronary plaque. **D,** A soft plaque with rupture of the fibrous cap. (From Braunwald E, Zipes D, Libby P: *Heart disease: a textbook of cardiovascular medicine,* ed 6, Philadelphia, 2001, Saunders, p 416.)

SUMMARY

The heart's primary function is to pump sufficient blood to deliver oxygen and nutrients to the body. The heart may be viewed as two separate pumps: a right-sided pump that perfuses the lungs and a left-sided pump that perfuses the systemic circulation. The left ventricle must generate higher pressures and therefore has a thicker myocardial mass and higher energy requirements. Because little ATP storage in cardiac cells is possible, the coronary arteries must deliver a steady supply of oxygen and nutrients. Cardiac contraction can be described by the sliding filament/cross-bridge theory and occurs only in the presence of ATP and free calcium ions. Any factor that enhances intracellular calcium ion concentration will result in generation of a greater contractile force.

A coordinated cardiac contraction is possible because the heart's conduction system activates the chambers in a sequential manner. The sinoatrial node is the usual pacemaker because it has the highest intrinsic rate of diastolic depolarization. The diastolic depolarization rate is strongly influenced by the autonomic nervous system. The ECG shows the electrical activity of the heart and is a useful indicator of cardiac conduction abnormalities.

The ultimate indicator of cardiac function is the cardiac output, which is the product of heart rate and stroke volume. The autonomic nervous system is the main regulator of heart rate, whereas stroke volume is influenced by preload, afterload, and contractility. These factors are also the primary determinants of myocardial work and energy expenditure.

REFERENCES

1. Gray H: *Gray's anatomy*, ed 38, London, 1995, Churchill Livingstone.
2. Opie LH: Mechanisms of cardiac contraction and relaxation. In Libby P, Bonow R, Mann D et al, editors. *Braunwald's heart disease: a textbook of cardiovascular medicine,* ed 8, Philadelphia, 2008, Saunders, pp 509-540.
3. Levy MN, Pappano AJ: The arterial system. In Levy MN, Pappano AJ, editors: *Cardiovascular physiology,* ed 9, St Louis, 2007, Mosby, pp 125-140.
4. Ganong WF: Circulation through special regions. In Ganong WF, editor: *Review of medical physiology,* New York, 2003, McGraw-Hill, pp 614-632.
5. Levy MN, Pappano AJ: Hemodynamics. In Levy MN, Pappano AJ, editors: *Cardiovascular physiology,* ed 9, St Louis, 2007, Mosby, pp 107-124.

6. Canty JM: Coronary blood flow and myocardial ischemia. In Libby P, Bonow R, Mann D et al, editors. *Braunwald's heart disease: a textbook of cardiovascular medicine,* ed 8, Philadelphia, 2008, Saunders, pp 1167-1194.

7. Nadal-Ginard B et al: Myocyte death, growth, and regeneration in cardiac hypertrophy and failure, *Circ Res* 92:139-150, 2003.

8. Levy MN, Pappano AJ: The cardiac pump. In Levy MN, Pappano AJ, editors: *Cardiovascular physiology,* ed 9, St Louis, 2007, Mosby, pp 55-80.

9. Pollard TD, Earnshaw WC: Muscles. In Pollard TD, Earnshaw WC, editors: *Cell biology,* Philadelphia, 2008, Saunders, pp 705-725.

10. Panteghini M et al: Use of biochemical biomarkers in acute coronary syndromes. IFCC Scientific Division, Committee on standardization of markers of cardiac damage. International Federation of Clinical Chemistry, *Clin Chem Lab Med* 37: 683-693, 1999.

11. Ganong WF: Excitable tissue: muscle. In Ganong WF, editor: *Review of medical physiology,* New York, 2003, McGraw-Hill, p 82.

12. Levy MN, Pappano AJ: The cardiac action potential. In Levy MN, Pappano AJ, editors: *Cardiovascular physiology,* ed 9, St Louis, 2007, Mosby, pp 13-32.

13. Bauman JL, Schoen MD: Arrhythmias. In Dipiro JT et al, editors: *Pharmacotherapy: a pathophysiologic approach,* ed 6, New York, 2005, McGraw-Hill, pp 323-356.

14. Guyton AC, Hall JE: *Textbook of medical physiology,* ed 11, Philadelphia, 2006, Saunders, p 119.

15. Levy MN, Pappano AJ: Regulation of the heart beat. In Levy MN, Pappano AJ, editors: *Cardiovascular physiology,* ed 9, St Louis, 2007, Mosby, pp 81-106.

16. Conover MB: *Understanding electrocardiography,* ed 8, St Louis, 2003, Mosby.

17. Starling EH: *The Linacre lecture on the law of the heart,* London, 1918, Longmans Green.

18. Stoupakis G, Klapholz M: Natriuretic peptides: biochemistry, physiology, and therapeutic role in heart failure, *Heart Dis* 5(3):215-223, 2003.

19. Fang JC, O'Gara PT: The history and physical examination: an evidence-based approach. In Libby P, Bonow R, Mann D et al, editors: *Braunwald's heart disease: a textbook of cardiovascular medicine,* ed 8, Philadelphia, 2008, Saunders, pp 125-148.

chapter

18

Alterations in Cardiac Function

Jacquelyn L. Banasik

MEDIA RESOURCES

Additional Material for Study, Review, and Further Exploration

 CD Companionn ■ Review Questions and Answers
■ Glossary (with audio pronunciations for selected terms)
■ Disease Profiles ■ Animations

ⓔvolve **Website** at http://evolve.elsevier.com/Copstead/
■ Case Studies ■ Disease Profiles ■ WebLinks ■ Key Points Review

 Online Course (Module 11)

KEY QUESTIONS

■ What is the role of injury, inflammation, and lipid oxidation in coronary plaque initiation and progression?
■ What factors alter the balance between myocardial oxygen supply and demand?
■ How do the clinical features of the coronary heart disease syndromes differ?
■ How do valvular disorders alter cardiac pressure dynamics and workload?

■ What are the similarities and differences among the cardiomyopathies and myocarditis?
■ How do pericarditis and pericardial effusions differ in regard to cause and significance?
■ What factors determine whether a congenital heart defect will produce cyanosis?

CHAPTER OUTLINE

The incidence of cardiovascular disease increased rapidly in the United States during the last century, and it now claims the lives of approximately 875,000 people annually.[1] Approximately half of these deaths are due to coronary heart disease (CHD), whereas stroke, high blood pressure, heart failure, and others claim the remainder. Since the late 1960s, however, a decline in cardiac mortality has been achieved in the United States because of improvements in treatment and prevention. More than 16 million people living today have a history of angina pectoris or myocardial infarction (MI).[1] Men and women are equally represented, although women tend to be older when their heart disease becomes apparent. In 2008, the direct and indirect economic cost of cardiovascular diseases, including stroke, was estimated at $448.5 billion annually.[1] CHD is the most important cardiovascular disorder in terms of numbers affected and economic impact.

CORONARY HEART DISEASE

CHD is also called ischemic heart disease (IHD) and coronary artery disease (CAD) in some sources. These terms are related because CHD is characterized by insufficient delivery of oxygenated blood to the myocardium (ischemia) because of atherosclerotic coronary arteries (CAD). The American Heart Association compiles statistics under the heading of CHD, which includes the diagnoses of angina pectoris and myocardial infarction.[1] Other sequelae of CHD include dysrhythmias, sudden cardiac death, and heart failure. When metabolic demand for oxygen exceeds supply, the myocardium becomes ischemic, which leads to a dysfunction in cardiac pumping and predisposes to abnormal heart rhythms. If the ischemic episode is severe or prolonged, irreversible damage to myocardial cells may result in MI.

Etiology of Coronary Heart Disease

Atherosclerosis of coronary arteries is at the root of nearly all CHD. Atherosclerosis causes progressive narrowing of the arterial lumen and predisposes to a number of processes that can precipitate myocardial ischemia, including thrombus formation, coronary vasospasm, and endothelial cell dysfunction. Uncommon causes of cardiac ischemia include abnormalities of blood oxygen content (e.g., respiratory failure) and poor perfusion pressure through the coronary arteries

(e.g., hypotension, hypovolemia). Occasionally patients experience the signs and symptoms of cardiac ischemia but show no evidence of significant coronary artery atherosclerosis when evaluated by angiography. These patients are thought to have abnormalities of the microcirculation. Abnormal vascular regulation by endothelial cells in small vessels of the heart has been suggested as a probable mechanism. Endothelial cells secrete variable quantities of vascular relaxing and contracting factors and play a key role in controlling myocardial blood flow. Abnormalities of the microcirculation are more difficult to detect than coronary artery plaque, which is evident on coronary angiography. As evaluation methods improve, disorders of the microcirculation are likely to be more frequently recognized as factors contributing to CHD.

Mechanisms of Coronary Atherosclerosis

Knowledge about mechanisms of plaque formation in the coronary arteries has rapidly accumulated in recent years. Epidemiologic studies reported in the 1960s suggested associations among certain traits and habits and the development of CHD. More recent studies have confirmed and expanded on these *risk factors,* which include several major risks (age, family history, abnormal lipids, cigarette smoking, hypertension, diabetes, and obesity) and numerous probable risks (Box 18-1).[2] Although males and females succumb to heart disease in equal numbers, male gender is a risk factor for earlier development of heart disease (on average about 10 years earlier). The risk factors for CHD are the same as those for atherosclerosis in other arteries and are discussed in Chapter 15.

The observation that atherosclerotic plaque is composed primarily of lipid prompted the idea that abnormal lipid metabolism was a probable culprit in the development of CHD, and a great deal of attention has been focused on therapies to reduce serum cholesterol in individuals with dyslipidemia. Lipids are transported through the bloodstream in combination with specific proteins (**apoproteins**). Certain lipid-protein molecules (**lipoproteins**) are associated with a greater risk of atherosclerosis. The five major kinds of lipoproteins are shown in Figure 18-1. High levels of low-density lipoproteins (LDLs), which are high in cholesterol, have been associated with the highest risk. Very-low-density lipoproteins, which have large amounts of triglycerides, also appear to increase the risk. High-density lipoproteins, on the other hand, have been correlated with a decreased risk of atherosclerosis.[2]

BOX 18-1

Risk Factors for Coronary Heart Disease

Nonmodifiable Risks

Age: ≥45 years for men; ≥ 55 years for women
Gender: male
Family history of premature coronary heart disease
■ Myocardial infarction or sudden cardiac death in male
  first-degree relative at age less than 55 years or female
  first-degree relative at age less than 65 years

Lipid Risk Factors

Total cholesterol >200 mg/dl
LDL cholesterol >130 mg/dl
Triglycerides >150 mg/dl
HDL cholesterol <40 mg/dl

Nonlipid Risk Factors

Hypertension >140/90
Cigarette smoking
Thrombogenic state
Diabetes
Obesity
Physical inactivity
Poor diet (atherogenic)

Probable Risk Factors (Emerging)

Lipoprotein(a)
Small LDL particles (pattern B)
HDL subtypes
Apolipoprotein B
Homocysteine
Fibrinogen
High-sensitivity C-reactive protein
Impaired fasting glucose (100-125 mg/dl)

Data from NCEP III guidelines, 2002, NIH Publication No 02-5215.
LDL, Low-density lipoprotein; *HDL,* high-density lipoprotein.

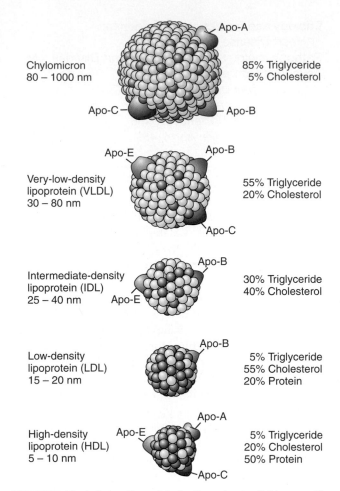

FIGURE 18-1 Serum lipoprotein fractions showing lipid composition and apoprotein components. Binding of lipoproteins to receptors is mediated through apoproteins.

High-density lipoproteins are thought to transport cholesterol from the peripheral tissues back to the liver, thus clearing away atheromatous plaque. The role of low-density and, indirectly, very-low–density lipoproteins is to bring cholesterol to the peripheral tissues (Figure 18-2). Cholesterol uptake by peripheral cells is mediated by LDL receptors on cell surfaces that bind and promote endocytosis of cholesterol. The liver normally binds and internalizes about 75% of the circulating LDL cholesterol.

Extreme cases of hyperlipidemia occur in individuals who have genetic derangements in lipid metabolism. These disorders run in families, and some are associated with the development of severe coronary atherosclerosis at a young age unless aggressively managed. The most common form of genetic hyperlipidemia (familial hypercholesterolemia) is associated with a defect in the LDL receptor on liver cells.[3] Inability of the liver to efficiently remove cholesterol from the bloodstream results in hyperlipidemia. Genetic disorders of lipid metabolism are described in Table 18-1. Even when lipid metabolism is normal, a high-fat diet can overwhelm the liver's ability to clear LDL cholesterol from the circulation and result

in hyperlipidemia. Dietary fat restriction may be beneficial in reducing cholesterol in this case.

Atherosclerotic plaque formation is initiated by injury to the coronary artery endothelium. The specific cause of endothelial dysfunction in the early stage of atherosclerosis is uncertain; however, several potential mechanisms have been described. These include chronic hemodynamic wall stress, which may explain the typical localization of plaques at arterial branch points and the role of hypertension as a risk factor; toxins from cigarette smoke; circulating inflammatory cytokines; and hyperlipidemia. Once the injury occurs, the endothelium may become more permeable and recruit leukocytes (Figure 18-3). LDLs leak through the endothelium and into the vessel wall (insudation) where they are oxidized by endothelial cells and macrophages.[4] Oxidized lipids are damaging to the endothelial and smooth muscle cells, and stimulate the recruitment of macrophages into the vessel wall where they engulf the lipids. Lipid-filled macrophages are called *foam cells.* The macrophages and foam cells release inflammatory mediators and growth factors that attract more leukocytes and stimulate smooth muscle proliferation. Excess lipid and

FIGURE 18-2 Schematic of lipoprotein metabolism in the body. Chylomicrons from dietary fat absorption are taken up by the liver and resynthesized into high-density lipoprotein *(HDL)* and very-low-density lipoprotein *(VLDL)*. HDL circulates to the peripheral tissues and takes up excess cholesterol for transport back to the liver. Triglycerides are removed for tissue use from VLDL, which becomes intermediate-density lipoprotein *(IDL)*. More triglyceride removal leads to the formation of low-density lipoprotein *(LDL)*. LDL is taken up by peripheral tissues to obtain cholesterol. About 70% of the circulating LDL returns to the liver.

TABLE 18-1	
Genetic Lipoprotein Disorders	
Disorder	**Gene**
LDL Particles	
Familial hypercholesterolemia	LDL-R
Familial defective Apo B-100	ApoB
Autosomal dominant hypercholesterolemia	PCSK9
Autosomal recessive hypercholesterolemia	ARH
Abetalipoproteinemia	MTP
Hypobetalipoproteinemia	ApoB
Familial sitosterolemia	ABCG5/ABCG8
Familial Lp(a) hyperlipoproteinemia	Apo(a)
Remnant Lipoproteins	
Dysbetalipoproteinemia type III	ApoE
Hepatic lipase deficiency	HL
Triglyceride-Rich Lipoproteins	
Lipoprotein lipase deficiency	LPL
ApoCII deficiency	ApoCII
Apo AV	ApoAV
Familial hypertriglyceridemia	Polygenic
Familial combined hyperlipidemia	Polygenic
HDL Particles	
ApoAI deficiency	ApoAI
Familial HDL deficiency/Tangier disease	ABCA1
Familial LCAT deficiency syndromes	LCAT
CETP deficiency	CETP
Niemann-Pick disease types A and B	SMPD1
Niemann-Pick disease type C	NPC1

Adapted from Genest J, Libby P: Lipoprotein disorders and cardiovascular disease. In Libby P, Bonow R, Mann D et al, editors: *Braunwald's heart disease: a textbook of cardiovascular medicine,* ed 8, Philadelphia, 2008, Saunders, p 1079.

LDL, Low density lipoprotein; *Lp(a),* lipoprotein a; *HDL,* high-density lipoprotein; *LCAT,* lecithin cholesterol acyltransferase; *CETP,* cholesteryl ester transfer protein.

factor modification, therapies to reduce plaque inflammation, inhibit lipid oxidation, and prevent thrombosis are in common use (Table 18-3). A major aim of therapy is to stabilize the plaques, making them less prone to rupture.

Atherosclerotic lesions generally increase in size over many years and progressively occlude the lumen of vessels. A significant reduction in blood flow can result when plaque occupies 75% or more of the arterial lumen. Clinically significant atherosclerotic plaque may be located anywhere within the three major coronary arteries or major secondary branches. All three coronary arteries are often simultaneously affected, although some individuals have only one or two diseased vessels. Surprisingly, the extent and severity of atherosclerotic lesions are not good predictors of the severity of ischemia.

Atherosclerotic coronary lesions have been characterized and attempts made to correlate the anatomic descriptions with plaque development and behavior. Typically atherosclerotic lesions begin as fatty streaks and progress to small regions of medial wall thickening with scattered macrophages at a young age. These lesions are considered to be precursor lesions and

debris begins to accumulate within the vessel wall and coalesce into a pool called the *lipid core* (Figure 18-4). Atherosclerotic plaques with large lipid cores are fragile and prone to rupture. Rupture of a plaque exposes subendothelial proteins and initiates platelet aggregation and thrombus formation. Thrombi may be asymptomatic if they are small and do not occlude the artery. Components of the thrombus may be incorporated into the plaque causing it to enlarge. Older plaques have significant collagen and fibrin, which form a cap and tend to make the plaque more stable. Numerous therapies aimed at stabilizing vulnerable plaques and preventing thrombus formation have been studied in clinical trials. Lipid-lowering therapy is a mainstay of treatment and prevention for atherosclerosis. Targets for serum LDL cholesterol have been developed by the National Cholesterol Education Program (NCEP) Adult Treatment Panel (NCEP III) based on the presence of known CHD or risk factors (Table 18-2).[5] In addition to risk

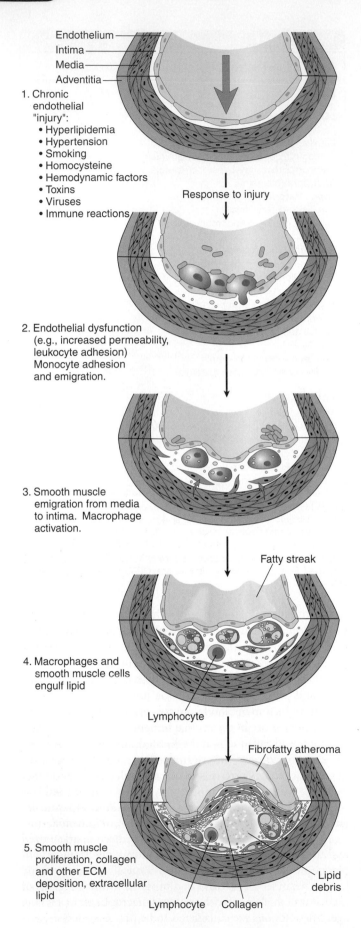

1. Chronic endothelial "injury":
   - Hyperlipidemia
   - Hypertension
   - Smoking
   - Homocysteine
   - Hemodynamic factors
   - Toxins
   - Viruses
   - Immune reactions

Endothelium
Intima
Media
Adventitia

Response to injury

2. Endothelial dysfunction (e.g., increased permeability, leukocyte adhesion) Monocyte adhesion and emigration.

3. Smooth muscle emigration from media to intima. Macrophage activation.

Fatty streak

4. Macrophages and smooth muscle cells engulf lipid

Lymphocyte

Fibrofatty atheroma

5. Smooth muscle proliferation, collagen and other ECM deposition, extracellular lipid

Lipid debris

Lymphocyte   Collagen

FIGURE 18-3 Pathogenesis of atherosclerosis. *1,* Chronic endothelial injury leads to *2. 2,* Endothelial dysfunction, permeability, and inflammation. *3,* Activated monocytes infiltrate the arterial wall and smooth muscle proliferates. *4,* Macrophages engulf lipid to become foam cells. *5,* A lipid core forms in the arterial wall and a fibrous cap evolves. (From Kumar V et al, editors: *Robbins basic pathology,* ed 8, Philadelphia, 2007, Saunders, p 347.)

are not symptomatic.[6] As the plaques acquire more free lipid within the arterial wall, they are more vulnerable to rupture, thrombus formation, and progressive plaque growth. These are considered to be advanced lesions and carry a significant risk of producing disruptions in coronary blood flow. Critical narrowing of the coronary lumen over time or sudden rupture of a plaque followed by thrombus formation cause the clinical syndromes of CHD, including angina, infarction, ischemic cardiomyopathy, and sudden cardiac death.

Stable plaques usually are asymptomatic or may be associated with exercise-induced angina pain (stable angina pectoris). However, plaques are vulnerable to rupture or erosion, which can initiate thrombosis formation and acute coronary occlusion. A variety of factors have been identified as markers of increased plaque vulnerability. These factors include (1) active inflammation within the plaque; (2) a large lipid core with a thin cap; (3) endothelial denudation (erosion) with superficial platelet adherence; (4) fissured or ruptured cap; and (5) severe stenosis predisposing to high shear stress.[7] Acute coronary syndrome (ACS, i.e., unstable angina or MI) and sudden cardiac death are nearly always associated with acute disruption of a vulnerable plaque. Because the types of plaques that are most vulnerable often do not significantly obstruct the lumen before they rupture, ACS frequently occurs in individuals whose disease had been asymptomatic. Patients with a high risk for or known presence of vulnerable plaques benefit from therapies such as lipid-lowering agents, to stabilize plaques and antiplatelet agents to prevent thrombosis.[8]

Pathophysiology of Ischemia

Ischemia of cardiac cells occurs when the oxygen supply is insufficient to meet metabolic demands. Myocardial cells are unable to store much energy in the form of adenosine triphosphate (ATP) and must therefore continuously receive a supply of oxygen for aerobic synthesis of ATP. ATP is essential for powering myocardial contraction as well as for cell maintenance. Because the heart is unable to slow its activity when ATP supplies dwindle, it is essential that a steady flow of oxygen be provided.

Factors that decrease myocardial oxygen supply or increase myocardial oxygen demand can upset the balance and result in cellular ischemia. Thus, the critical factors in meeting cellular demands for oxygen are (1) the rate of coronary perfusion and (2) the myocardial workload. Coronary perfusion can be impaired in several ways, including (1) large, stable atherosclerotic plaque, (2) acute platelet aggregation and thrombosis,

FIGURE 18-4 Sequence of events in the arteriolar wall associated with development of atherosclerosis. Note that smooth muscle cells migrate from the intima through the internal elastic membrane and into the intimal layer where they proliferate in response to growth factors. Macrophages in the intima release signals that alter the endothelial cell layer and induce expression of cell adhesion molecules that recruit monocytes into the tissue. (From Kumar V et al: *Robbins basic pathology,* ed 8, Philadelphia, 2007, Saunders, p 349.)

(3) vasospasm, (4) failure of autoregulation by the microcirculation, and (5) poor perfusion pressure.

Myocardial workload depends on heart rate, preload, afterload, and contractility (see Chapter 17). An increase in any of these variables increases myocardial oxygen requirements and may precipitate ischemia. However, even conditions resulting in very high myocardial oxygen consumption will seldom lead to ischemia unless some underlying impairment in coronary perfusion is present.

One or more of the aforementioned mechanisms are operative in producing clinically significant myocardial ischemia resulting in the acute or chronic coronary syndromes. Advanced fibrous plaque is thought to produce intermittent ischemia when 75% or more of the arterial lumen is occluded.[9] Because fibrous plaque progresses slowly over many years, the heart has time to develop alternative pathways for myocardial blood flow. This collateral circulation can preserve blood flow despite almost total occlusion of the coronary artery. Thus stable fibrous plaque may produce no symptoms of ischemia unless

the demand of the heart for oxygen is suddenly elevated, as occurs in exercise or stress. When the onset of ischemia is predictable with certain activities and subsides with rest, the patient is said to have a chronic coronary syndrome called *classic* or *stable angina pectoris.*

ACS occurs when sudden obstruction of coronary blood flow results in acute myocardial ischemia. Acute obstruction is usually associated with the formation of a clot in the coronary artery at the site of a vulnerable plaque. Rupture of the plaque exposes a rough area composed of collagen and other molecules that are thrombogenic. A high fibrinogen level, as occurs in smokers, and enhanced platelet adhesiveness, as occurs in hyperlipidemia, may enhance the risk of thrombus formation. Clot formation begins with adherence of platelets to the ruptured plaque. The platelets that initially attach release chemicals that attract more platelets, which aggregate and form a plug. The coagulation cascade may also be initiated and result in the formation of a platelet-fibrin clot that may occlude the vessel or break loose and travel farther along the

TABLE 18-2

Recommended Serum Low-Density Lipoprotein Targets to Reduce the Risk of Coronary Heart Disease

Patient Risk Category	LDL-C Cut Point for Initiating Drug Therapy mg/dl	LDL-C Goal mg/dl
High risk: CHD present or CHD risk equivalent (≥2 risks plus 10-year risk >20%)	>100	<100 (optional <70)
Moderately high risk ≥2 risks and 10-year risk 10%-20%	≥130	<130
Moderate risk ≥2 risks and 10- year risk <10%	≥160	<130
Lower risk ≤1 risk	≥190	<160

From National Cholesterol Education Program: Third Report of the Expert Panel on Detection, Evaluation, and Treatment of High Blood Cholesterol in Adults (Adult Treatment Panel III), *Circulation* 110:227-239, 2004.)

CHD, Coronary heart disease; *LDL-C,* low-density lipoprotein cholesterol.

TABLE 18-3

Actions of Therapies to Reduce Coronary Heart Disease

Therapy	Major Actions	Other Actions
Angiotensin inhibitors (ACEI, ARB)	Improves endothelial function	Antioxidant (LDL), antiinflammatory
Statins	Decreases LDL-C, increases HDL-C	Improves endothelial function, antiinflammatory, antioxidant (LDL)
Fish oil (omega-3)	Decreases LDL-C, increases HDL-C	Inhibits thrombosis
Fibrates	Improves endothelial function	Increases HDL
Aspirin	Inhibits thrombosis, antiinflammatory	
Exercise	Increases HDL	Improves endothelial function

ACEI, Angiotensin-converting enzyme inhibitor; *ARB,* angiotensin II receptor blocker; *LDL-C,* low-density lipoprotein cholesterol; *HDL-C,* high-density lipoprotein cholesterol.

vessel. Chemicals released by activated platelets include several vasoactive products (serotonin, thromboxane) that may contribute to spasm of the coronary vessel, further reducing blood flow.

Thrombosis occurs suddenly and may partially or completely obstruct the artery and cause acute ischemia. The ACS may present as unstable angina, MI, or sudden cardiac death. Appreciation of the role thrombus plays in coronary obstruction has resulted in the prophylactic use of antithrombotics, such as aspirin. Research indicates that the long-term use of small doses of aspirin reduces mortality from ischemic heart disease.[10]

Vasospasm usually occurs in areas of atherosclerotic plaque, but is also proposed as a mechanism of ischemia in patients who have anginal signs and symptoms but no significant amount of fibrous plaque in the coronary arteries. *Variant,* or *Prinzmetal,* angina is the term applied to vasospasm-initiated anginal symptoms. The etiology of spasm in vessels having no significant atherosclerotic plaques is unclear, but usually responds promptly to vasodilating agents. Intense vasospasm can occur in response to certain drugs, such as cocaine.

As previously mentioned, endothelial cells are important regulators of vascular tone. They secrete variable amounts of constricting and relaxing factors to control tissue perfusion. This autoregulation of blood flow allows the microvasculature to dilate when the need for oxygen in a particular area is increased. Failure of endothelial cells to appropriately regulate flow is a potential mechanism of myocardial ischemia.[11] Endothelial cells can be damaged by circulating toxins from cigarette smoke, immune cells, and infectious agents. Inflammatory disorders that may alter endothelial cell function include lupus erythematosus, Kawasaki syndrome, and polyarteritis nodosa. The importance of inflammatory processes in the pathogenesis of CHD has been recognized,

resulting in efforts to find markers (e.g., serum high-sensitivity C-reactive protein) and methods to reduce inflammation in those at risk.

Even if the coronary arteries and microcirculation are functioning properly, coronary perfusion may still be inadequate if perfusion pressure is low. Recall from Chapter 17 that coronary blood flow occurs primarily during diastole and depends on the driving pressure in the aorta. A fall in aortic blood pressure can significantly reduce coronary perfusion, particularly in vessels with high resistance to flow. Conditions such as shock, hemorrhage, and anesthesia may be associated with a fall in blood pressure, which decreases driving pressure and coronary perfusion and results in myocardial ischemia. However, the most common cause of cardiac ischemia is atherosclerotic coronary arteries.

KEY POINTS

- Cardiac ischemia occurs when the heart's demand for oxygenated blood exceeds its supply. In most cases, ischemia is a result of impaired blood flow through the coronary arteries.
- CHD is associated with coronary atherosclerosis. Risk factors for CHD are the same as for atherosclerosis of other arteries and include advancing age, male gender, family history, hyperlipidemia, diabetes, smoking, hypertension, and obesity. Endothelial injury and inflammation and lipid accumulation in the intima are thought to be the primary initiators of coronary atherosclerosis.
- Early atherosclerotic lesions are asymptomatic precursor lesions in which lipids begin to accumulate in the arterial wall. Advanced lesions may cause symptoms because of progressive arterial occlusion or acute plaque disruption and thrombus formation.

- Vulnerable plaques may rupture or become eroded, which stimulates clot formation on the plaque. Plaques with a large lipid core, thin cap, or high shear stress are vulnerable plaques.
- Chronic occlusion of a coronary vessel is associated with the clinical syndrome of stable angina. Acute occlusion is associated with plaque disruption and thrombus formation and results in ACS (unstable angina or MI).
- Myocardial ischemia may uncommonly be caused by coronary vasospasm, hypoxemia, or low perfusion pressure from volume depletion or shock.

Clinical Features and Management of Coronary Syndromes

Five syndromes can be differentiated according to the severity and onset of cardiac symptoms. Stable *angina pectoris* and *ischemic cardiomyopathy* are chronic syndromes that usually progress slowly and are a consequence of chronic obstruction from stable atherosclerotic plaques. The ACSs have an abrupt onset, life-threatening consequences, and are associated with acute changes in plaque morphology and thrombosis. The ACSs include *unstable angina* and *MI*. Unstable angina and MI are considered together because they are difficult to differentiate in the acute stage when therapeutic decisions must be made. Any of the coronary heart syndromes may precipitate *sudden cardiac death* and associated dysrhythmias.

Angina Pectoris. Angina pectoris literally means *chest pain* and is associated with intermittent myocardial ischemia. The length and the severity of the myocardial ischemia are insufficient to result in the acute death of cells. Bouts of chest pain and associated symptoms are generally recurrent and may be precipitated by conditions that increase myocardial oxygen demand, such as exercise, stress, sympathetic nervous system activation, and increased preload, afterload, heart rate, or muscle mass. Ischemic pain receptors from the myocardium travel to the central nervous system with the eighth cervical and first through fourth thoracic dorsal root ganglia. Sensory neurons from the jaw, neck, and arm also travel in these nerve trunks, so heart pain may be perceived as emanating from these body parts. This phenomenon is called *referred pain.* Anginal pain may be described as burning, crushing, squeezing, or choking. Pain is sometimes represented by expressions such as "an elephant is sitting on my chest" or by the patient placing a tight fist on the chest. Anginal pain may be mistakenly attributed to indigestion or dental pain. In some cases, patients have atypical symptoms of myocardial ischemia, such as back pain, fatigue, or weakness, rather than the classic symptom of chest pain.

Anginal ischemia, although temporary, may result in inefficient cardiac pumping with resultant pulmonary congestion and shortness of breath. Three patterns of angina pectoris have been described: (1) stable or typical angina, (2) Prinzmetal or variant angina, and (3) unstable or crescendo angina. All these patterns are associated with underlying coronary vessel disease and may be exhibited in a particular individual at different times and under different conditions. Unstable angina may progress to acute ischemia and is discussed in the Acute Coronary Syndrome section along with MI.

Stable Angina. *Stable angina* is the most common form and is therefore called *classic* or *typical angina.* Stable angina is characterized by stenotic atherosclerotic coronary vessels that reduce coronary blood flow to a critical level. The stenosed arteries dilate poorly in response to increased myocardial oxygen requirements. Under conditions of increased myocardial workload, such as during physical exertion or emotional strain, coronary perfusion is inadequate and ischemia results (Figure 18-5). The onset of anginal pain is generally predictable and elicited by similar stimuli each time. Stable angina is generally relieved by rest and nitroglycerin, a drug that causes coronary and peripheral vasodilation, reduces preload, and therefore reduces myocardial workload.

Prinzmetal Variant Angina. *Prinzmetal variant angina* is characterized by unpredictable attacks of anginal pain. Although most individuals with Prinzmetal angina have significant coronary atherosclerosis, the onset of ischemic symptoms is unrelated to physical or emotional exertion, heart rate, or other obvious causes of increased myocardial oxygen demand. Vasospasm has been identified as the probable mechanism leading to variant angina, although the cause of the vasospasm is unknown. Proposed mechanisms include atherosclerosis-induced hypercontractility, abnormal secretion of vasospastic chemicals by local mast cells, and abnormal calcium flux across vascular smooth muscle. Variant angina responds well to treatment with calcium channel–blocking drugs, which inhibit vascular smooth muscle contraction.

Patients with angina are at risk for developing ACS and need aggressive treatment for risk factor reduction and therapies to reduce the risk of plaque rupture, thrombosis, and dysrhythmia.

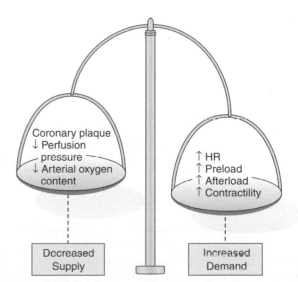

FIGURE 18-5 Factors that decrease coronary blood supply or increase myocardial oxygen demand can upset the balance and lead to ischemia and anginal pain.

Acute Coronary Syndrome. Unstable angina and MI are difficult to distinguish on the basis of clinical manifestations and are lumped together as ACS. Both are characterized by chest pain that may be more severe and lasts longer than the patient's typical angina and may occur in individuals whose disease was previously asymptomatic. In both cases, plaque rupture with subsequent acute thrombus development is thought to occur. In unstable angina, the occlusion is partial or the clot is broken down before the death of myocardial tissue. In MI, the occlusion is complete and the thrombus persists long enough for development of irreversible damage to myocardial cells resulting in necrosis. In the past, differentiation of unstable angina and MI was based on laboratory evaluation of serum biomarker levels (e.g., MB band of creatine kinase [CK-MB], troponins I and T). If cardiac biomarkers were elevated, which is indicative of necrosis, a diagnosis of MI was made; if not, a diagnosis of unstable angina was appropriate. In a time when monitoring and management of complications were the mainstay of treatment, this approach worked well. With the advent of reperfusion therapy, which is effective only if administered early in the course of infarction, the distinction between unstable angina and MI has become less clinically relevant. Because unstable angina and MI present a similar clinical picture in the acute phase, they have been lumped together in treatment protocols for ACS (Figure 18-6).[12] Patients with chest pain and evidence of acute ischemia on the electrocardiogram (ECG) (ST-segment elevation; STEMI) are candidates for acute reperfusion therapy. Patients presenting with symptoms of unstable angina and no ST elevation on the ECG (non-STEMI, NSTEMI) may not benefit from reperfusion strategies, and antiplatelet drugs are a cornerstone of therapy.[13] Differentiation between unstable angina and NSTEMI is made after obtaining cardiac necrosis markers; those with elevations are diagnosed with NSTEMI and those without elevations are diagnosed with unstable angina.

Etiology and Pathogenesis. MI results when prolonged or total disruption of blood flow to the myocardium causes cellular death by necrosis or apoptosis. Acute MI is an important form

of CHD resulting in more than 150,000 deaths annually in the United States.[1] It is estimated that an American male has a greater than 1 in 5 chance of sustaining an MI or fatal ischemic event before the age of 65. An MI may occur at any age, but the frequency rises with advancing age. Females younger than 45 years have a sixfold lesser risk of MI than men of the same age. After menopause, the rate of MI in women approaches that of their male counterparts and becomes essentially equal by age 80.[9]

As previously described, the initiating event in most MIs is believed to be development of a thrombus on top of an ulcerated or cracked atherosclerotic plaque. The initiating event is a sudden change in structure of the plaque. Platelets passing by the surface of the ruptured plaque adhere to it, initiate formation of a platelet plug, and activate the clotting cascade. The resultant thrombus grows until it occludes the vessel and triggers the transmural MI.

The thrombus theory of acute MI was controversial for many years because only 50% of persons dying of MI had a demonstrable thrombus at autopsy. Then DeWood and coworkers[14] demonstrated that about 90% of persons with acute MI had an intracoronary thrombus within 4 hours of the onset of symptoms, but only 60% had thrombi 12 to 24 hours later. This observation suggested that the thrombus was quickly dissolved by natural mechanisms after the occlusive event. Further support for the thrombus theory comes from the effectiveness of reperfusion therapies that successfully restore flow through obstructed coronary vessels and significantly reduce mortality.[15]

The cellular consequences of an acute interruption in blood flow to the myocardium do not occur instantaneously or uniformly. Acute occlusion causes a range of cellular events, depending on the availability and adequacy of collateral blood flow, the relative workload, and the length of time that flow is interrupted. A typical myocardial infarct has several zones composed of cells in various stages of ischemia and death.

Experiments in animal models indicate that complete occlusion of a coronary vessel results in a predictable pattern of cellular dysfunction and death.[9] Depletion of ATP in acutely ischemic

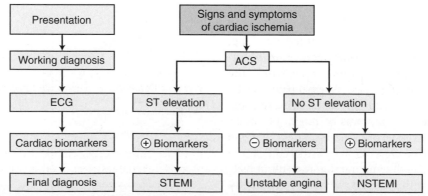

FIGURE 18-6 The acute coronary syndromes (ACS) are difficult to differentiate by presenting symptoms because all involve some degree of myocardial ischemia. The electrocardiogram (ECG) is used to determine those with ST elevation and those with no ST elevation. Serum levels of cardiac biomarkers are then used to make a final diagnosis. Most patients with ACS characterized by ST elevation are diagnosed with MI (STEMI), and a proportion of patients with no ST elevation also will have elevated serum markers and are diagnosed with MI (NSTEMI). Patients who do not exhibit serum enzyme elevations are usually diagnosed with unstable angina.

TABLE 18-4

Cellular Events After Myocardial Infarction

Time	Gross	Light Microscopic Findings	Electron Microscopic Findings
Reversible Injury			
0-½ hr	None	None	Relaxation of myofibrils; glycogen loss; mitochondrial swelling
Irreversible Injury			
½-4 hr	None	Usually none; variable waviness of fibers at border	Sarcolemmal disruption; mitochondrial amorphous densities
4-12 hr	Occasionally dark mottling	Beginning coagulation necrosis; edema; hemorrhage	
12-24 hr	Dark mottling	Ongoing coagulation necrosis; pyknosis of nuclei; myocyte hypereosinophilia; marginal contraction band necrosis; beginning neutrophilic infiltrate	
1-3 days	Mottling with yellow-tan infarct center	Coagulation necrosis, with loss of nuclei and striations; interstitial infiltrate of neutrophils	
3-7 days	Hyperemic border; central yellow-tan softening	Beginning disintegration of dead myofibers, with dying neutrophils; early phagocytosis of dead cells by macrophages at infarct border	
7-10 days	Maximally yellow-tan and soft, with depressed red-tan margins	Well-developed phagocytosis of dead cells; early formation of fibrovascular granulation tissue at margins	
10-14 days	Red-gray depressed infarct borders	Well-established granulation tissue with new blood vessels and collagen deposition	
2-8 weeks	Gray-white scar, progressive from border toward core of infarct	Increased collagen deposition, with decreased cellularity	
>2 mo	Scarring complete	Dense collagenous scar	

From Kumar V et al: *Robbins basic pathology,* ed 8, Philadelphia, 2007, Saunders, p 393.

cells begins immediately, followed within 1 to 2 minutes by an impaired ability to contract. Within 10 minutes, cellular concentrations of ATP fall to half of normal, and irreversible cell injury occurs after 30 to 40 minutes of complete occlusion (Table 18-4). Ischemic necrosis begins in the subendocardial zone and spreads across the ventricular wall toward epicardial surfaces. Epicardial areas are spared for longer periods because they have the greatest collateral network of arterial vessels. The ultimate size of the infarcted tissue depends on the extent, duration, and severity of ischemia. Areas of necrosis may be intermixed with or surrounded by zones of reversibly injured cells that are marginally perfused by collaterals. Injured cells die both from necrosis and from apoptosis.[16] Restoring perfusion to potentially salvageable cells is an important focus of treatment. (See Chapter 4 for a discussion of necrosis and apoptosis.)

Nearly all infarcts are located in the left ventricular walls. Isolated right ventricular infarction occurs in only 1% to 3% of MIs. Occlusion of the left anterior descending artery causes 40% to 50% of acute MIs, the right coronary artery contributes another 30% to 40%, and the left circumflex contributes 15% to 20%.[9] The locations of the resulting infarcts are shown in Table 18-5. It is common for individuals with coronary heart disease to suffer from more than one MI during their lifetime.

The area of necrosis resulting from MI undergoes a series of morphologic changes as the infarct ages.[9] These morphologic changes generally cannot be detected on gross examination

TABLE 18-5

Location of Myocardial Infarction According to Coronary Artery Affected

Arterial Obstruction	Location of Infarct
Left anterior descending (40%-50% of infarcts)	Anterior wall of LV near apex Anterior two thirds of interventricular septum
Right coronary (30%-40% of infarcts)	Posterior wall of LV Posterior one third of interventricular septum
Left circumflex (15%-20% of infarcts)	Lateral wall of LV

Data from Kumar V et al: *Robbins basic pathology,* ed 7, Philadelphia, 2003, Saunders, p 366.
LV, Left ventricle.

until 6 to 12 hours after infarct. After 18 to 24 hours, the area of infarction becomes paler than surrounding tissues. Thereafter, the area of infarction becomes obvious as it turns yellowish and soft with a rim of red vascular connective tissue (Figure 18-7). At 1 to 2 weeks, the necrotic tissue is progressively degraded and cleared away. Infarcted myocardium is particularly weakened and susceptible to rupture at this time. By 6 weeks, the necrotic tissue has been replaced by tough fibrous scar tissue.

FIGURE 18-7 This photograph of a 5- to 7-day-old posterolateral infarction clearly shows a large, pale yellow lesion surrounded by a dark red zone of inflammation. (From Kumar V et al: *Robbins basic pathology,* ed 7, Philadelphia, 2003, Saunders, p 369.)

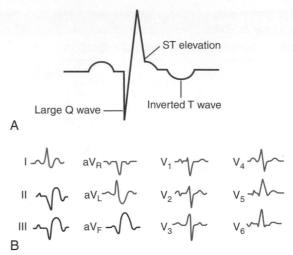

FIGURE 18-8 A, Typical ECG infarction pattern showing abnormally large Q wave, ST elevation, and inverted T wave. **B,** Typical ECG in acute inferior myocardial infarction. Note the Q waves and ST-segment elevation in leads II, III, and aV$_F$.

Diagnosis of MI. The diagnosis of MI is based on three primary indicators: signs and symptoms, electrocardiographic changes, and elevations of specific marker proteins in the blood. Other diagnostic examinations such as cardiac catheterization, echocardiography, and radionuclide scintigraphy may also be done to provide additional information (see Chapter 17).

Severe crushing, excruciating chest pain that may radiate to the arm, shoulder, jaw, or back is the harbinger of MI. Pain is commonly accompanied by nausea, vomiting, diaphoresis (sweating), and shortness of breath. In contrast to anginal pain, infarction pain generally lasts more than 15 minutes and is not relieved by rest or nitroglycerin. In some instances, however, the MI is entirely asymptomatic and may elude detection. Asymptomatic MI has been called *silent MI* and may be detected only serendipitously at a later date. Pain may be difficult to assess in individuals with atypical presentations or a tendency to ignore or deny their symptoms. Thus, although pain is an important indicator of acute ischemia, other clinical information is often needed to correctly distinguish between angina, infarction, and noncardiac sources of pain. Women, the elderly, and patients with diabetic neuropathies more commonly complain of atypical symptoms, including, fatigue, nausea, back pain, and abdominal discomfort. Atypical complaints in patients with CHD risk factors should prompt a high suspicion of MI.

Electrocardiographic Changes. Myocardial ischemia and infarction often result in characteristic changes on ECG waveforms. Injury and ischemia are indicated on the ECG by ST-segment changes. ST-segment elevation is thought to represent acute cell injury and ischemia. The presence of ST-segment elevation on the ECG indicates that the ischemic injury is ongoing and that efforts to improve perfusion or reduce oxygen demand may be effective in preserving myocardial muscle mass. Until measures of specific serum markers of infarction are obtained, these patients are regarded as having unstable angina/STEMI in treatment protocols for ACS. Infarcted muscle that is necrotic and no longer electrically active is indicated by the appearance of abnormally deep or wide Q waves and inverted T waves (Figure 18-8). These changes are very specific for MI and, when present, are diagnostic. Q waves are usually persistent findings, whereas ST-segment and T-wave changes may resolve over time. Q waves take time to develop and may not be present in the acute phase of an MI.

Dysrhythmias and the characteristic ST-segment changes that accompany MI are attributed to injured and ischemic cells that have not yet become necrotic. Reversibly injured cells have limited ATP supplies to power membrane pumps and are predisposed to leakage of ions across their cell membranes. Abnormal ion flux may result in continuous current flow even when the heart is at rest. This current leak may be seen on the ECG as ST-segment elevation.

The 12-lead ECG is used to localize the injured region of the left ventricle. Various leads of the 12-lead ECG "view" different regions of the heart. Abnormalities such as Q waves and ST-segment elevation in a particular lead or leads indicate that the damage is localized to the part of the left ventricle "seen" by that lead. MIs may thus be described as anterior, lateral, posterior, septal, inferior, or a combination of these. (The 12-lead ECG is described in Chapter 17.)

In some cases, patients presenting with ACS do not have ST elevation on the ECG. They may have ST depression or T-wave changes. Some of these patients will develop elevated serum markers indicating MI. These patients have NSTEMI. The infarct size is generally smaller, and the outcomes are better than those in patients with STEMI.[13]

Serum Markers. The appearance of certain proteins in the blood after myocardial cell death is a very sensitive and reliable indicator of MI. Myocardial cell death leads to elevated serum levels of myoglobin, troponin, lactate dehydrogenase, and creatine kinase.[9] Cardiac cells contain particular forms of these proteins called *isoforms*. An increase in these proteins suggests leakage from fatally damaged cells that have lost plasma membrane integrity. Cardiac biomarkers have a slightly different amino acid sequence than other cell types. In particular, myocytes contain the isoforms CK-MB, troponin I, and troponin T. An elevated level of serum CK-MB is a highly specific indicator of MI and considered to be diagnostic. However, CK-MB remains elevated for only 48 to 72 hours after MI. Two proteins that make up part of the cardiac cell contractile apparatus, troponins I and T, have become the markers of choice for detecting MI. Cardiac troponin levels become elevated in serum at about the same time as CK-MB, but they remain elevated for a longer period. Cardiac troponins I and T are highly sensitive and specific for cardiac cell death but less helpful in detecting new infarction (reinfarction) because levels remain elevated for a prolonged period (Figure 18-9). Cardiac myoglobin levels are elevated in serum very quickly after MI and may be helpful in early detection; however, cardiac myoglobin is less specific than the other markers. All serum markers are useful diagnostically only during the acute period of MI. Patients with ACS who do not develop elevations of these serum markers are diagnosed with unstable angina.

Clinical Course. In addition to chest pain, electrocardiographic abnormalities, and serum protein marker elevations, a person experiencing an MI may exhibit signs of cardiac inflammation, including fever, leukocytosis, and an elevated sedimentation rate. Symptoms of circulatory inadequacy, including fatigue, restlessness, anxiety, and weakness, may be present.

The events associated with MI are summarized in Figure 18-10. Note that totally ischemic cells, which die and become electrically silent, are the source of the clinical findings of Q waves and also release the indicative serum marker proteins (CK-MB, troponins). Partially ischemic cells are potentially salvageable but are unable to maintain normal ion flux across the cell membrane. Abnormal ion flux is responsible for the ST-segment changes in acute ischemia and also predisposes to a variety of cardiac dysrhythmias, including ventricular ectopy and conduction blocks (see Chapter 19).

Neither partially ischemic nor totally ischemic cells are able to contract effectively, and poor stroke volume leads to a drop in cardiac output. Decreased stroke volume triggers a number of compensatory actions designed to improve cardiac output. In particular, activation of the sympathetic nervous system increases the heart rate, contractility, blood pressure, and fluid retention by the kidney. Unfortunately, these compensatory efforts impose a greater workload on the heart and may contribute to further ischemic damage. Compensatory mechanisms are shown in Figure 18-11 and include sympathetic nervous system activation, enhanced preload, and hypertrophy of cardiac myocytes.

FIGURE 18-9 Time course of serum marker protein elevations after acute myocardial infarction. The MB band of creatine kinase (CK-MB) and troponin I are the most specific of the protein markers. Myoglobin is an early marker but is not very specific. (Redrawn from Antman EM: General hospital management. In Julian DG, Braunwald E, editors: *Management of acute myocardial infarction,* London, 1994, Saunders, p 631.)

Prognosis and Treatment. It is difficult to determine an overall prognosis for acute MI because many variables affect the outcome, including the extent and location of the infarct, previous cardiovascular health, age, and the presence of other disease processes. Of particular importance is the rapidity with which treatment is sought. Most deaths from MI occur before the victim reaches the hospital. The in-hospital mortality rate of MI is about 10%.[9] In approximately 25% of cases, an MI is not accompanied by any complications (uncomplicated MI) and the patient recovers rapidly. However, the remaining three-quarters of MIs are followed by one or more complications.[9] Potential complications include cardiac dysrhythmias, heart failure, cardiogenic shock, ventricular rupture, pericarditis, and thromboembolism.

Treatment for MI is directed at decreasing myocardial oxygen demand and increasing myocardial oxygen supply while monitoring and managing complications as they arise. Measures to reduce myocardial workload frequently include preload and afterload reduction, heart rate control, pain relief, and activity restriction. Sympathetic antagonists, nitrates, and morphine sulfate are the mainstays of drug therapy. Measures to increase oxygen delivery to ischemic areas include oxygen administration, antiplatelet therapy with aspirin and other antiplatelet agents, thrombolytic (fibrinolytic) drugs, anticoagulants, angioplasty, stent placement, and coronary artery bypass grafting (CABG) (Figure 18-12). Therapies aimed at opening the blocked coronary artery are called reperfusion therapies.

Early detection and management of dysrhythmias and conduction disorders are an important part of the immediate care of a patient with MI. Many dysrhythmias are life threatening and, at the very least, lead to decreased cardiac output or increased myocardial workload. Continuous electrocardiographic monitoring is generally the standard of care because of the high incidence of electrical disturbances after MI. Common dysrhythmias and conduction disorders are described in Chapter 19.

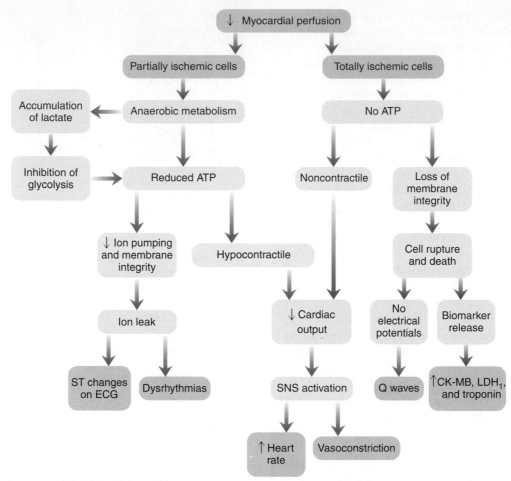

FIGURE 18-10 Summary of events after myocardial infarction. *ATP,* Adenosine triphosphate; *SNS,* sympathetic nervous system; *CK-MB,* MB band of creatine kinase; *LDH,* lactate dehydrogenase; *ECG,* electrocardiography.

Sudden Cardiac Death. Sudden cardiac death (SCD) is usually defined as unexpected death from cardiac causes within 1 hour of the onset of symptoms.[17] Successful resuscitation efforts by those trained in cardiopulmonary resuscitation (CPR) and use of the external defibrillators found in many public places has resulted in the increased survival of persons who experience SCD. Persons who survive SCD are at high risk for recurrence. Coronary heart disease is at the root of the vast majority of cases of sudden cardiac death. Rarely, sudden cardiac death may be a complication of hereditary or acquired structural or electrical abnormalities, such as long QT syndrome. It is estimated that 300,000 to 400,000 individuals experience SCD each year in the United States.[1] It is most often associated with coronary atherosclerosis and may be the initial manifestation of the disease. Acute MI occurs in only a small subset of cases of sudden cardiac death.[17] A lethal dysrhythmia such as ventricular fibrillation is usually the primary cause (see Chapter 19). Ischemia from multivessel atherosclerosis, diffuse myocardial atrophy, scarring and fibrosis of old MI tissue, and electrolyte imbalances are factors that may predispose the heart to the electrical abnormalities that lead to sudden cardiac death.

Chronic Ischemic Cardiomyopathy. Chronic ischemic cardiomyopathy refers to a disorder in which heart failure develops insidiously as a consequence of progressive ischemic myocardial damage. In most cases, individuals affected have a history of angina or MI, often many years before the onset of heart failure. Heart failure appears to be a consequence of slow, progressive apoptotic death of myocytes from chronic ischemia. The disease is usually found in elderly individuals. Atrophic and dead cells are scattered throughout the myocardium rather than being localized, as occurs with MI. The prognosis for patients with chronic ischemic cardiomyopathy is quite poor, with death from heart failure the common outcome. Heart failure is further discussed in Chapter 19.

KEY POINTS

- The clinical syndromes of CHD include angina pectoris, ACS (unstable angina, NSTEMI, STEMI), chronic ischemic cardiomyopathy, and sudden cardiac death. These conditions are all associated with advanced coronary atherosclerosis.

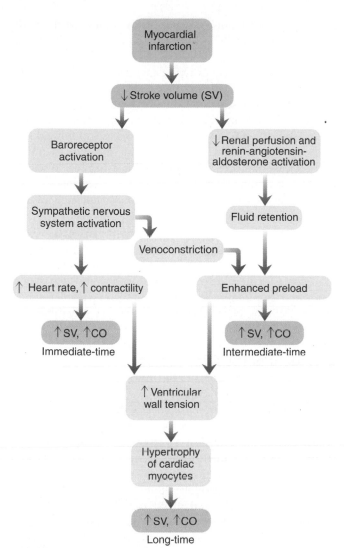

FIGURE 18-11 Compensatory responses to increase stroke volume *(SV)* and maintain cardiac output *(CO)* after myocardial infarction.

Thrombolysis

Enzymatic digestion of thrombus to open lumen

A

Percutaneous transluminal coronary angioplasty (PTCA)

Physical disruption of plaque to open lumen

B

Placement of a stent to prevent reocclusion

C

Coronary artery bypass grafting (CABG)

Surgical placement of a new conduit to bypass occlusion

D

FIGURE 18-12 Management of blocked coronary arteries includes **(A)** thrombolysis with drugs such as streptokinase and tissue plasminogen activator; **(B)** plaque disruption with percutaneous transluminal coronary angioplasty, followed by anticoagulation or stent placement; **(C)** placement of a stent to prevent reocclusion; and **(D)** coronary artery bypass grafting—surgical placement of a new conduit to bypass the occluded area of the artery.

- Angina is characterized by intermittent bouts of chest pain brought on by exertion and generally relieved by rest. No permanent myocardial damage occurs.
- Prolonged or severe ischemia results in MI that is characterized by severe, unrelieved chest pain, nausea and vomiting, diaphoresis, shortness of breath, and inflammation (fever, increased white blood cell count, increased sedimentation rate).
- Serum protein marker elevations and electrocardiographic changes are diagnostic of MI. The most specific and sensitive serum markers are increased CK-MB and troponin I and T. ECG changes include ST-segment elevation, large Q waves, and inverted T waves.
- A drop in cardiac output as a result of MI triggers a number of compensatory responses, including sympathetic activation. The sympathetic nervous system increases the heart rate, contractility, and blood pressure, all of which increase myocardial workload.

- Treatment of acute ischemia usually includes efforts to decrease myocardial oxygen demand (sympathetic antagonists, rest, heart rate control, pain relief, afterload reduction) and increase oxygen delivery (thrombolysis, angioplasty, coronary bypass grafting).

ENDOCARDIAL AND VALVULAR DISEASES

Endocardial and valvular structures may be damaged by inflammation and scarring, calcification, or congenital malformations. These processes interfere with the normal valvular property of unimpeded, unidirectional flow. Although congenital malformations may affect any valve, acquired valvular disorders generally involve the mitral or aortic valves. Abnormalities in valvular function cause altered hemodynamics in the heart and generally result in increased myocardial workload. Ultimately, heart failure may result from significant valvular dysfunction.

Normally, heart valves open completely, so blood flows through with little or no pressure difference across the valve. Failure of a valve to open completely is termed **stenosis.** Significant hemodynamic consequences generally begin to occur when the valve opening is reduced to half normal. The severity of stenosis can be estimated by the degree of pressure gradient across the valve (Figure 18-13). Stenosis results in extra pressure work for the heart because blood must be forced through the high resistance of a narrow valve opening. Stenosis generally progresses slowly over years to decades, which allows time for affected heart chambers to compensate through myocardial cell hypertrophy.

Regurgitation (insufficiency) refers to the inability of a valve to close completely, thereby allowing blood to flow backward across the valve when no flow should be occurring. Regurgitation may develop suddenly from valvular infection or rupture of a supporting papillary muscle. Sudden regurgitation is poorly tolerated inasmuch as little compensation is possible. Regurgitation results in extra volume work for the heart because more blood must be pumped to maintain adequate forward flow.

Diseased valves may exhibit elements of both stenosis and regurgitation, although one problem usually predominates. Postinflammatory scarring from rheumatic heart disease and valvular calcification with aging are the primary causes of stenosis (Figure 18-14). A wide variety of diseases of the endocardium may lead to valvular regurgitation, including rheumatic heart disease and infective endocarditis, which are discussed later in this chapter. Damaged valves are susceptible to infection, and antibiotic prophylaxis is therefore indicated for dental, surgical, and diagnostic procedures. The major causes of acquired mitral and aortic valvular diseases are listed in Table 18-6. Valvular disorders are often associated with abnormal turbulence of blood flow that produces heart sounds called *murmurs.* Careful assessment of the location and character of a murmur can help identify the underlying valvular abnormality. Defining characteristics of common valve disorders are described in Table 18-7.

Disorders of the Mitral Valve

Three important disorders of the mitral valve are stenosis, regurgitation, and mitral valve prolapse.

Mitral Stenosis. In *mitral stenosis* the flow of blood from the left atrium into the left ventricle is impaired. Mitral stenosis is therefore characterized by an abnormal left atrial–left ventricular pressure gradient during ventricular diastole (Figure 18-15). Normally the pressures in the atrium and ventricle are nearly equal during ventricular diastole when the mitral valve is open. Figure 18-15 shows that with mitral valve stenosis, atrial pressure remains higher than ventricular pressure throughout diastole. As the stenosis worsens, the pressure gradient often increases. In normal adults the area of the mitral valve orifice is 4 to 6 cm², and symptoms of stenosis do not appear until the orifice is narrowed to 2 cm². When the mitral valve orifice narrows to 1 cm², a critical stenosis is present and a pressure gradient of 20 mm Hg or more usually develops across the valve.[18] Increased pressure work of the left atrium leads to atrial chamber enlargement and hypertrophy. Progressive narrowing of the mitral valve may lead to markedly elevated left

Normal valve
(zero pressure gradient)

Stenosed valve
(6 mm Hg pressure gradient)

FIGURE 18-13 Development of a pressure gradient across a stenosed valve. The chamber behind the narrowed valve opening must work harder to force blood through.

FIGURE 18-14 Valvular degeneration and calcification. **A,** Calcific aortic stenosis of previously normal (three-cusp) valve. **B,** Calcific aortic stenosis of congenitally bicuspid valve. **C,** Mitral valve calcification. **D,** Cut section of valve from **C.** (From Kumar V et al: *Robbins basic pathology,* ed 8, Philadelphia, 2007, Saunders, p 402.)

TABLE 18-6

Major Causes of Acquired Valvular Heart Disease

Mitral Valve Disease	Aortic Valve Disease
Stenosis	
Postinflammatory scarring (rheumatic heart disease)	Postinflammatory scarring (rheumatic heart disease) Senile calcific aortic stenosis Calcification of a congenitally deformed valve
Regurgitation	
Abnormalities of leaflets and commissures: Postinflammatory scarring Infective endocarditis Mitral valve prolapse Fen-phen–induced valvular fibrosis Abnormalities of the tensor apparatus: Rupture of papillary muscle Papillary muscle dysfunction (fibrosis) Rupture of chordae tendineae Abnormalities of left ventricular cavity and/or annulus: LV enlargement (myocarditis, dilated cardiomyopathy) Calcification of mitral ring	Intrinsic valvular disease: Postinflammatory scarring (rheumatic heart disease) Infective endocarditis Aortic disease: Degenerative aortic dilation Syphilitic aortitis Ankylosing spondylitis Rheumatoid arthritis Marfan syndrome

Modified from Schoen FJ: Surgical pathology of removed natural and prosthetic heart valves, *Hum Pathol* 18(6):558-567, 1987; and from Schoen FJ, Mitchell R: The heart. In Kumar V et al: *Robbins basic pathology,* ed 8, Philadelphia, 2007, Saunders, p 401.
LV, Left ventricle.

TABLE 18-7

Defining Characteristics of Murmurs

Valve Disorder	Quality	Location, Radiation
Mitral stenosis	Low-pitched rumble, diastolic	At apex
Mitral regurgitation	Loud, pan-systolic, high pitched, blowing	Loudest at apex, transmitted to left axilla
Aortic stenosis	Harsh, midsystolic, crescendo-decrescendo	Right second intercostal space, transmitted to neck
Aortic regurgitation	Faint, blowing, diastolic	Left sternal border, aortic area, apex

atrial pressures and subsequent increased pulmonary vascular pressure. If uncorrected, mitral stenosis may result in chronic pulmonary hypertension, right ventricular hypertrophy, and right-sided heart failure.

The signs and symptoms of mitral stenosis are due to congestion of blood volume and increased pressure in the left atrium and pulmonary circulation, as well as decreased stroke volume of the left ventricle because of deficient filling. Symptoms are exacerbated by conditions that further decrease left ventricular filling such as an increased heart rate. Atrial dysrhythmias such as atrial fibrillation are common because of excessive atrial volume. Atrial enlargement and fibrillation also predispose to the development of atrial clots, which may dislodge and result in systemic embolization and stroke. Signs and symptoms of mitral stenosis secondary to pulmonary congestion may include orthopnea, cough, dyspnea on exertion, paroxysmal nocturnal dyspnea, abnormal breath sounds, and poor arterial oxygenation. Reduced left ventricular stroke volume may be apparent as fatigue, poor activity tolerance, and weakness. Exertional dyspnea is the most common complaint.

Blood rushing through the narrowed mitral valve during ventricular diastole can sometimes be heard as a low-pitched, rumbling diastolic murmur at the heart's apex. In many cases, an opening snap may also be heard.

Mitral Regurgitation. Mitral regurgitation is characterized by backflow of blood from the left ventricle to the left atrium during ventricular systole. Elevation of left atrial volume and pressure by regurgitant flow leads to characteristic giant V waves on the atrial pressure monitor (Figure 18-16). The severity of mitral insufficiency is related to the amount of left ventricular stroke volume that is regurgitant and depends, in part, on the aortic resistance to flow (afterload). A high afterload increases the amount of regurgitant flow. The left ventricle must pump a greater volume to compensate for the regurgitant flow and maintain an effective stroke volume. Both the left atrium and ventricle generally dilate and hypertrophy to compensate for the extra volume that they are required to pump. In most patients with mitral regurgitation, compensation is maintained for many years before symptoms occur.[18] If severe and uncorrected, mitral

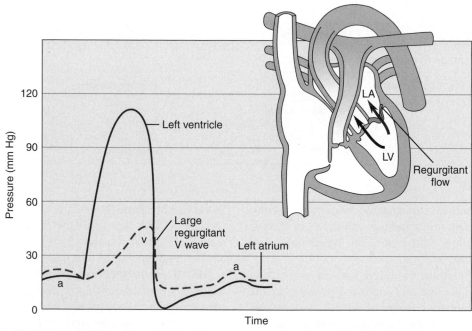

FIGURE 18-15 Mitral stenosis is characterized by an abnormal left atrial *(LA)*–to–left ventricular *(LV)* pressure gradient during ventricular diastole *(shaded area).*

FIGURE 18-16 Mitral regurgitation causes characteristic giant V waves on the left atrial *(LA)* pressure monitor. *LV,* Left ventricular.

regurgitation may eventually lead to left-sided heart failure. The signs and symptoms of mitral regurgitation are similar to those described for mitral stenosis and result from pulmonary congestion and poor cardiac output. Chronic weakness and fatigue are common complaints. The murmur of mitral regurgitation usually occurs throughout ventricular systole (pansystolic), radiates toward the left axilla, and has a high-pitched blowing character. The arterial pulse may be helpful in distinguishing the systolic murmur of mitral

regurgitation from that of aortic stenosis. The upstroke of the pulse is sharp and full in mitral regurgitation, whereas it is weaker and delayed in aortic stenosis.

Mitral Valve Prolapse. Approximately 2% to 3% of the population has mitral valves that balloon up into the left atrium during ventricular systole.[18] This condition is called *mitral valve prolapse* (Figure 18-17). Women between the ages of 20 and 40 years are most often affected. In a great majority of cases, the disorder is asymptomatic and diagnosed only incidentally on routine physical examination. In some cases, the prolapse is sufficient to cause a degree of mitral regurgitation. The cause of this valvular abnormality is uncertain, although it is commonly associated with other connective tissue disorders such as Marfan syndrome or scoliosis.

The finding of 2 mm or more displacement of the mitral valve leaflets above the annulus on echocardiogram is an important diagnostic criterion.[18] Mitral valve prolapse may be detected by a midsystolic click or systolic murmur. Individuals whose disease is symptomatic may experience palpitations, rhythm abnormalities, dizziness, fatigue, dyspnea, chest pain, or psychiatric manifestations such as depression and anxiety. The large majority of affected persons has no untoward effects and most are unaware of their condition. Complications of mitral valve prolapse are relatively rare and include infective endocarditis, sudden cardiac death, cerebral embolic events, and progression to mitral regurgitation.

Disorders of the Aortic Valve

The primary disorders of the aortic valve are stenosis and regurgitation.

Aortic Stenosis. With the decline in incidence of rheumatic fever, the predominant cause of aortic stenosis is age related calcification. The hallmark of this disorder is calcium deposits on the aortic cusps (see Figure 18-14). Calcification is particularly common in patients with a congenital bicuspid aortic valve. Aortic calcifications build up over several decades and generally become clinically apparent in individuals 70 to 90 years old. Rheumatic heart disease, on the other hand, occurs primarily in children and young adults and now accounts for only a small percentage of cases of acquired aortic stenosis in the United States.

Aortic stenosis results in obstruction to aortic outflow from the left ventricle into the aorta during systole. This condition is characterized by a left ventricular–aortic pressure gradient during ventricular ejection (Figure 18-18). The left ventricle produces high systolic pressure to overcome resistance of the stenotic aortic valve. The slow development of aortic stenosis allows the heart to maintain stroke volume by compensatory left ventricular hypertrophy. The combination of high left ventricular pressure and hypertrophy predisposes the heart

FIGURE 18-17 Appearance of mitral valve prolapse. Note how the valve balloons up into the left atrium. (From Kumar V et al: *Robbins basic pathology,* ed 8, Philadelphia, 2007, Saunders, p 403. Courtesy William D. Edwards, MD, Mayo Clinic, Rochester, Minn.)

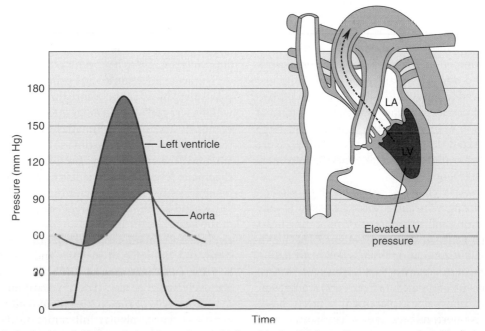

FIGURE 18-18 Aortic stenosis is characterized by an abnormal left ventricular *(LV)*–to–aortic pressure gradient *(shaded area). LA,* Left atrial.

to ischemia and attacks of anginal pain. Continued high left ventricular afterload from a stenotic aortic valve may lead to left-sided heart failure.

Critical obstruction is characterized by a mean systolic pressure gradient exceeding 40 mm Hg and an effective aortic valve orifice less than 25% of normal (< 1.0 cm² in an average-sized adult).[18] The symptoms of aortic stenosis are due to diminished cardiac output, with pulmonary complications occurring later as the left ventricle fails. Syncope, fatigue, low systolic blood pressure, and faint pulses are common signs and symptoms. Angina occurs in two thirds of patients with critical aortic stenosis and is often brought on by exertion and relieved by rest.[18] Angina is thought to occur because of thickening of the ventricular wall with reduced perfusion and high intraventricular wall tension. Syncope and "graying out" spells may occur when cerebral perfusion is inadequate. The onset of atrial fibrillation or heart block may precipitate worsening of symptoms. A characteristic murmur occurs during ventricular systole and varies in intensity, progressively getting louder and then diminishing (crescendo-decrescendo). The murmur of aortic stenosis generally radiates to the neck. The heart rate is usually slow to allow for a necessarily long ejection phase, and a prominent S_4 is usually present. Surgical correction is indicated for symptomatic aortic stenosis because medical therapy is not effective.

Aortic Regurgitation. Aortic regurgitation results from an incompetent aortic valve that allows blood to leak back from the aorta into the left ventricle during diastole. Causes of aortic regurgitation are similar to those of mitral regurgitation (see Table 18-6). Valvular incompetence may be secondary to an abnormal aortic valve or to aortic root dilation with widening of the aorta such that the valve leaflets no longer appose. Aortic root dilation is a more common cause of aortic regurgitation than primary valvular disease.[18] The aorta may dilate because of degenerative changes with aging or as a consequence of connective tissue disease. The left ventricle becomes volume overloaded because it contains its usual preload, received from the atrium, plus regurgitant blood from the aorta. The left ventricle compensates for this extra volume work with hypertrophy and dilation. A larger than normal stroke volume is thus achieved to produce a high systolic blood pressure. Diastolic blood pressure is generally lower than normal because of rapid runoff of blood into the ventricle. The large stroke volume and rapid decline in diastolic blood pressure result in a bounding peripheral pulsation, and the head may bob with each systole (Figure 18-19).

Aortic insufficiency is characterized by a high-pitched blowing murmur during ventricular diastole. Patients may complain of palpitations and a throbbing or pounding heart because of the large ventricular stroke volume. The major complication of aortic regurgitation is left-sided heart failure as a result of the high ventricular workload. However, chronic aortic regurgitation is well tolerated for years, and asymptomatic individuals can delay valve replacement surgery. Acute aortic regurgitation is poorly tolerated and necessitates immediate correction.

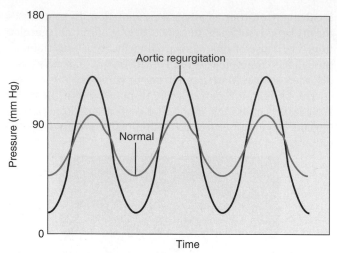

FIGURE 18-19 Typical arterial pressure fluctuation in aortic regurgitation showing a high systolic pressure and a low diastolic pressure.

Diseases of the Endocardium

Rheumatic Heart Disease. Rheumatic heart disease is an uncommon but serious consequence of rheumatic fever. The incidence of rheumatic fever has steadily declined in the United States, but the disease still affects an estimated 15 million people worldwide.[19] Rheumatic fever is an acute inflammatory disease that follows infection with group A β-hemolytic streptococci.

Damage is due to immune attack on the individual's own tissues. For incompletely understood reasons, antibodies against the streptococcal antigens are also directed against self tissues, possibly because of an immune hypersensitivity reaction resulting from cross-reactivity between streptococcal antigens and certain tissue molecules. Epitopes on the bacterial surface are similar to proteins on cardiac myosin, valve, skin, joint, and brain tissue. Most individuals with group A β-hemolytic streptococcal infection do not develop rheumatic fever, and a genetic predisposition to development of cross-reactive antibodies associated with certain human leukocyte antigen (HLA) types has been noted.[20]

The acute infection occurs primarily in children and is accompanied by fever and a sore throat. In only 3% of children with pharyngeal streptococcal infection does rheumatic fever eventually develop.[21] Rheumatic heart disease develops in 40% to 60% of persons with rheumatic fever.[21] Prompt initiation of antibiotic therapy is often effective in primary prevention of rheumatic fever. Rheumatic fever diffusely affects connective tissue in joints, the heart, and the skin. The central nervous system and kidney are also frequently involved. Inflammation of the heart usually includes all layers and results in carditis. Endocardial inflammation results in valvular swelling, erosions, and clumping of platelets and fibrin on valve leaflets. Scarring and shortening of valvular structures become progressively more severe. The myocardium and pericardium may show signs of rheumatic inflammation; however, if there is no associated valvular inflammation the diagnosis is unlikely to be rheumatic fever. Other hallmarks of rheumatic fever include joint inflammation, involuntary movements (Sydenham chorea), and a distinctive truncal rash. An elevated antibody titer against streptococcal products (antistreptolysin O, anti-DNase B) may help confirm the diagnosis. Unfortunately, individuals who experience rheumatic fever have a high chance of recurrence if they have another pharyngeal streptococcal infection.[21] Chronic prophylactic antibiotic therapy is recommended for individuals who develop rheumatic fever. There is no specific therapy for rheumatic fever and care is supportive. Anti-inflammatory medications may be given for symptom control, but there is no evidence that they alter the outcome.[21]

Infective Endocarditis. Infective endocarditis is caused by invasion and colonization of endocardial structures by microorganisms with resulting inflammation. A variety of organisms are known to have an affinity for the endocardium and for the cardiac valves in particular. Valvular lesions include growths of microorganisms enmeshed in fibrin deposits. These growths are called *vegetations.* They may become quite large, interfering with valvular function and predisposing to embolus formation. The most common bacterial culprits are several strains of *Streptococcus* and *Staphylococcus aureus.* A requisite for infective endocarditis is invasion of the bloodstream by infective organisms. The portal of entry may be obvious, as with an overt infection, intravenous drug addiction, or invasive surgical or dental procedures. Sometimes the source may be less obvious, such as the gastrointestinal tract or the oral cavity. Once the organism enters the circulation, several factors influence its ability to attack endocardial structures and cause disease.

Acute infective endocarditis may theoretically develop in any individual if host resistance is low, if the organism is highly virulent, and if the bacterial invasion is sufficiently large. Acute infective endocarditis usually affects individuals with previously normal valves and leads to death in a large percentage of patients. The overall mortality rate for infective endocarditis is between 16% and 27%.[21] Mortality rates vary with the type of infective organism. For example, the mortality associated with *Haemophilus* species is 10% to 15%, whereas *Pseudomonas aeruginosa* endocarditis carries a 50% to 89% mortality. Intravenous drug abusers are particularly susceptible to acute infective endocarditis. *Subacute* infective endocarditis has a more insidious onset and generally affects individuals with some preexisting propensity for valvular colonization. The offending organisms are less virulent. Rheumatic heart disease, congenital heart abnormalities, mitral valve prolapse, calcified valves, and prosthetic valves are important predisposing factors. Immunosuppression and repeated exposure through intravenous drug abuse are other predisposing influences. *S. aureus, Staphylococcus epidermidis,* and *Candida,* which colonize the skin, are common offenders in intravenous drug users. The valves on the right side of the heart commonly are infected in this population.

Organisms associated with subacute infective endocarditis usually are not virulent enough to attack normal healthy endocardium but are able to gain a foothold in hearts with some

underlying predisposition. Preexisting cardiac disease may allow the formation of platelet-fibrin deposits on the valves because of abnormal or stagnant blood flow patterns. These deposits become the site of organism attachment. Antibodies against the invader may further assist attachment by causing organisms to clump together.

The diagnostic findings in both acute and subacute infective endocarditis are much the same. Large, bulky, bacteria-laden vegetations hang from the heart valves and adjacent endocardial surfaces. In addition to the risk of embolization, vegetations may cause erosion or perforation of the underlying valve leaflet. In acute forms, adjacent myocardium may be eroded and abscessed. With time, valvular vegetations become fibrotic and calcified.

Unfortunately, the clinical features of subacute infective endocarditis are quite nonspecific, with low-grade fever the most consistent sign. Nonspecific fatigue, weight loss, and flu-like symptoms may be the only clues. Positive blood cultures may help confirm the diagnosis. In contrast, acute infective endocarditis has a more obvious onset with fever, chills, malaise, and, frequently, a heart murmur. Complications such as valvular insufficiency, myocardial abscess (Figure 18-20), embolization, and renal disease generally occur early in the course of the disease. The interval between initiation of bacteremia and the onset of symptoms is less than 2 weeks in the majority of cases.[21] Management of the acute and subacute types centers on antibiotic therapy, with surgical replacement of valves when indicated. Prevention through prophylactic antibiotic therapy in individuals at risk is an important consideration.

The endocardium is prey to many other disorders, such as systemic lupus erythematosus (an immunologic disease), calcium deposition secondary to renal disease, and nonbacterial thrombotic endocarditis secondary to hypercoagulable states associated with cancer.

FIGURE 18-20 Heart of a patient who died from acute bacterial endocarditis caused by *Staphylococcus aureus.* The left ventricle contains numerous abscesses formed by seeding from vegetations traveling in the coronary arteries. (From Kumar V et al: *Robbins basic pathology,* ed 7, Philadelphia, 2003, Saunders, p 382.)

KEY POINTS

- Valvular disorders are of two primary types. Failure of stenotic valves to open properly causes an abnormal pressure gradient across the valve and increases the pressure work of the heart. Regurgitant valves allow blood to flow backward across the valve and result in extra volume work for the heart.
- Mitral stenosis is characterized by a large left atrial–to–left ventricular pressure gradient during ventricular diastole. Mitral stenosis leads to left atrial and pulmonary congestion.
- Mitral regurgitation is characterized by large V waves in the left atrial pressure tracing and a loud systolic murmur that radiates to the left axilla. Mitral regurgitation increases the work of the left atrium and ventricle and can lead to left-sided heart failure.
- Aortic stenosis results in obstruction to the outflow of blood from the left ventricle. It is characterized by a large left ventricular–to–aortic pressure gradient and a crescendo-decrescendo murmur during systole that radiates to the neck. The extra pressure work can lead to left ventricular hypertrophy and failure.
- Aortic regurgitation is characterized by a high systolic and low diastolic blood pressure and a bounding pulse. The murmur of aortic regurgitation occurs during diastole. Left ventricular failure may result because of the high-volume work.
- Rheumatic heart disease results from immune-mediated damage to the endocardium after group A β-hemolytic streptococcal infection.
- Acute and subacute infective endocarditis results in the growth of bacteria-laden vegetations on heart valves. In addition to valvular erosion and scarring, embolization may occur.

BOX 18-2

Etiologic Agents of Myocarditis

Viral (Most Common)
Adenovirus
Coxsackie virus/Enterovirus
Cytomegalovirus
Parvovirus B19
Hepatitis C virus
Influenza
Human immunodeficiency virus
Herpes virus
Epstein-Barr virus
Mixed infections

Bacterial
Myobacterial species
Chlamydia pneumonia
Streptococcal species
Mycoplasma pneumoniae
Treponema pallidum

Fungal
Aspergillus
Candida
Coccidioides
Cryptococcus
Histoplasma

Protozoal
Trypanosoma cruzi

Parasitic
Schistosomiasis
Larva migrans

Toxins
Anthracyclines
Cocaine

Hypersensitivity
Clozapine
Sulfonamides
Cephalosporins
Penicillins
Tricyclic antidepressants

Autoimmune Activation
Smallpox vaccination
Giant cell myocarditis
Churg-Strauss syndrome
Sjögren syndrome
Inflammatory bowel disease
Celiac disease
Sarcoidosis
Systemic lupus erythematosus
Takayasu arteritis
Wegener granulomatosis

From Liu P, Schultheiss HP: Myocarditis. In Libby P, Bonow R, Mann D et al, editors: *Braunwald's heart disease: a textbook of cardiovascular medicine,* ed 8, Philadelphia, 2008, Saunders, p 1777.

MYOCARDIAL DISEASES

In addition to the diseases already discussed, which secondarily affect the myocardium as a consequence of inadequate blood supply or endocardial infection, two additional categories of diseases of heart muscle are *myocarditis* and *cardiomyopathy.* Myocarditis is an inflammatory disorder of the heart muscle characterized by necrosis and degeneration of heart muscle cells. Cardiomyopathy includes several disorders of the heart muscle that may be genetic or acquired but are noninflammatory. The division of these categories is somewhat arbitrary; however, the clinical course of myocarditis is generally acute and stormy, with recovery or death from cardiac failure occurring weeks to months after the onset of symptoms. In contrast, the cardiomyopathies generally evolve more insidiously over years, with few symptoms until the heart slips into failure.

Myocarditis

Myocarditis is characterized by inflammation, leukocyte infiltration, and necrosis of cardiac muscle cells. Causes of myocarditis are many and include microbial agents, several forms of immune-mediated disease, and several physical agents. The more common causes of myocarditis are listed in Box 18-2. The true incidence of myocarditis is unknown because the diagnosis relies largely on circumstantial evidence.

Most cases of myocarditis in North America are associated with viral infection, particularly Coxsackievirus, whereas Chagas disease from parasitic infection (*Trypanosoma cruzi*) is common in South America. Cardiac involvement generally appears days or weeks after a viral infection elsewhere in the body. Documenting a viral cause is often impossible, but a rising antibody titer supports the diagnosis. The mechanism of viral myocarditis is incompletely understood. Direct viral cytotoxicity may occur to some extent, and the virus may evoke an immune response directed against the heart. Most investigators currently believe the second mechanism to be most important. In countries other than the United States, nonviral organisms are more commonly associated with myocarditis. For example, the protozoan *T. cruzi*, which is endemic in areas of Central and South America, infects about 18 million persons worldwide.[22] A myocarditis called *Chagas disease* eventually develops in a large number of infected individuals. Chagas disease is a leading cause of cardiovascular death in endemic countries.[22]

In some cases of myocarditis, the immune system reaction against the myocardium appears to be the primary cause. Antibodies or activated lymphocytes are formed against heart tissue. Several drugs, including penicillin, tend to evoke a hyperactive immune response in some individuals and may cause an allergic-type reaction that affects the myocardium. Myocarditis accompanies some autoimmune disorders, such as systemic lupus erythematosus (SLE) and polymyositis. Toxins and chemical causes of myocarditis include cocaine, chemotherapeutic agents, snake bite and insect venoms, lead, and numerous others. Regardless of the specific cause, inflammation of cardiac muscle is characteristic.

Acute myocarditis is commonly characterized by left ventricular dysfunction or general dilation of all four heart chambers. The ventricular myocardium is "flabby" with patchy or diffuse necrotic lesions. The heart muscle appears inflamed and edematous with white blood cell infiltrates. Endocardial structures are usually normal. The clinical course of acute myocarditis varies in severity from asymptomatic to rapidly evolving heart failure. Generalized symptoms related to the inflammatory process may be present, as well as electrocardiographic changes caused by myocardial cell death. Common presenting symptoms include fatigue, dyspnea on exertion, and dysrhythmia with associated palpitations. Many persons recover completely, whereas others have progressive disease that is manifested years later as dilated cardiomyopathy. Thus myocarditis and the cardiomyopathic forms of myocardial disease overlap and are difficult to separate. Therapy is supportive and usually includes therapy for heart failure (see Chapter 19). Immunosuppressive therapy may be considered for myocarditis associated with autoimmune disease or hypersensitivity reactions.

Cardiomyopathy

Cardiomyopathies can be classified by cause or by functional impairments. Those with known causes have been classified as specific cardiomyopathy by the World Health Organization (Table 18-8).[23] Those cardiomyopathies with uncertain cause are classified based on their predominant pathophysiologic features. The major functional classes are the dilated, hypertrophic, and restrictive forms (Figure 18-21). The terms *primary cardiomyopathy* for dysfunction of unknown cause and *secondary cardiomyopathy* for myocardial dysfunction of known cause are also in clinical use. Definitions of primary cardiomyopathy usually exclude hypertensive, ischemic, congenital, valvular, pericardial, and inflammatory myocardial disorders, however classification of cardiomyopathy continues to evolve as understanding of genetic contributions to the condition are increasingly known.

TABLE 18-8

Classification of the Cardiomyopathies

Disorder	Description
Dilated cardiomyopathy	Dilatation and impaired contraction of the left or both ventricles. Caused by familial/genetic, viral and/or immune, alcoholic/toxic, or unknown factors, or is associated with recognized cardiovascular disease.
Hypertrophic cardiomyopathy	Left and/or right ventricular hypertrophy, often asymmetrical, which usually involves the interventricular septum. Mutations in sarcoplasmic proteins cause the disease in many patients.
Restrictive cardiomyopathy	Restricted filling and reduced diastolic size of either or both ventricles with normal or near-normal systolic function. Is idiopathic or associated with other disease (e.g., amyloidosis, endomyocardial disease).
Arrhythmogenic right ventricular	Progressive fibrofatty replacement of the right, and to some degree left, ventricular cardiomyopathy myocardium. Familial disease is common.
Unclassified cardiomyopathy	Diseases that do not fit readily into any category. Examples include systolic dysfunction with minimal dilatation, mitochondrial disease, and fibroelastosis.
Specific Cardiomyopathies	
Ischemic cardiomyopathy	Presents as dilated cardiomyopathy with depressed ventricular function not explained by the extent of coronary artery obstructions or ischemic damage.
Valvular cardiomyopathy	Presents as ventricular dysfunction that is out of proportion to the abnormal loading conditions produced by the valvular stenosis and/or regurgitation.
Hypertensive cardiomyopathy	Presents with left ventricular hypertrophy with features of cardiac failure due to systolic or diastolic dysfunction.
Inflammatory cardiomyopathy	Cardiac dysfunction as a consequence of myocarditis.
Metabolic cardiomyopathy	Includes a wide variety of causes, including endocrine abnormalities, glycogen storage disease, deficiencies (such as hypokalemia), and nutritional disorders.
General systemic disease	Includes connective tissue disorders and infiltrative diseases such as sarcoidosis and leukemia.
Muscular dystrophies	Includes Duchenne, Becker type, and myotonic dystrophies.
Neuromuscular disorders	Includes Friedreich ataxia, Noonan syndrome, and lentiginosis.
Sensitivity and toxic reactions	Includes reactions to alcohol, catecholamines, anthracyclines, irradiation, and others.
Peripartal cardiomyopathy	First becomes manifest in the peripartum period, but it is likely a heterogeneous group.

Derived from *Cirulation* 112;1825-1852, 2005. ACC/AHA 2005 Guideline Update for the Diagnosis and Management of Chronic Heart Failure in the Adult. Reprinted with permission. Table: Stages in the Development of HF/recommended therapy by stage. © 2007 American Heart Association.

A Normal   B Dilated cardiomyopathy

C Hypertrophic cardiomyopathy   D Restrictive cardiomyopathy

FIGURE 18-21 The three types of cardiomyopathy. **A,** Normal heart. **B,** Dilated cardiomyopathy demonstrating enlargement of all four chambers. **C,** Hypertrophic cardiomyopathy showing a thickened left ventricle. **D,** Restrictive cardiomyopathy characterized by a small left ventricular volume.

Dilated Cardiomyopathy. Dilated or congestive cardiomyopathy (DCM) is characterized by cardiac failure associated with dilation of one or both ventricular chambers. Numerous factors are suspected in the initiation of dilated cardiomyopathy, including alcohol toxicity, genetic abnormality, pregnancy, and postviral myocarditis. Alcohol and its metabolites are toxic to heart muscle cells and are associated with thiamine and other nutritional deficiencies. Peripartum cardiomyopathy is the term applied to cases of dilated cardiomyopathy discovered just before or just after delivery. The etiology is unclear; however inflammatory factors are implicated and a high incidence of lymphocytic activation has been reported. A risk of recurrence in subsequent pregnancies has been noted.

In some cases, dilated cardiomyopathy runs in families and has a presumed genetic basis. At least 20% of patients with DCM have a first-degree relative with signs of DCM.[24] Inherited genetic defects in the protein structure of myocardial cytoskeleton appear to be contributory in most genetic forms of DCM.

Postviral myocarditis is an attractive pathogenetic mechanism for dilated cardiomyopathy, as previously discussed. Myocardial biopsy specimens often reveal signs of inflammatory injury; however, progression from acute myocarditis to dilated cardiomyopathy has rarely been documented. A variety of other causes have been proposed as well. In fact, dilated cardiomyopathy is a bit of a catch-all term invoked to cover cases of dilated congestive failure having no well-defined origin.

Histologic examination of hearts with dilated cardiomyopathy reveals nonspecific changes in the majority of cases.[24] Hypertrophied or atrophied myocytes may be apparent, along with mild fibrosis. The clinical picture is one of slowly progressing biventricular heart failure with low ejection fraction (EF). Mortality rates are high, and about 50% of patients die within 2 years of diagnosis. In most cases, cardiac transplantation is the definitive treatment.

Hypertrophic Cardiomyopathy. In contrast to dilated cardiomyopathy, hypertrophic cardiomyopathy (HCM) is characterized by a thickened, hyperkinetic ventricular muscle mass. The hypertrophy is often not uniform throughout the heart, and in about 25% of patients the septum is most affected leading to the term *idiopathic hypertrophic subaortic stenosis.* The left ventricle is usually more involved than the right.

Substantial evidence suggests that this form of cardiomyopathy is transmitted genetically. Abnormalities of cardiac sarcomere proteins have been identified in several familial forms of the disease. Abnormalities in genes coding for myosin, tropomyosin, and troponin T have been linked to the development of HCM. It is estimated that about 35% of familial HCM cases are related to mutations of the myosin heavy chain gene, 15% to myosin-binding protein C mutations, and 15% to troponin T mutations.[9] The remaining third of cases are thought to have mutations in other cytoskeletal proteins. Although the genetic basis of hypertrophic cardiomyopathy is well established, the events leading from cytoskeletal protein mutations to clinical disease is poorly understood.

There is wide variation in the expression of HCM. It may be asymptomatic or may be associated with symptoms of ventricular outflow obstruction or impaired diastolic filling. Outflow obstruction is particularly problematic when the myocardial hypertrophy is localized in the subaortic septal region. Strenuous activity may precipitate profound outflow obstruction, negligible stroke volume, and sudden death. Other factors contributing to reduced stroke volume are the smaller intraventricular chamber size and a noncompliant ventricle characteristic of diastolic dysfunction with preserved EF. The most common symptoms of HCM are dyspnea (90%) and angina (75%). Microscopically, the hypertrophied muscle cells appear disorganized and haphazardly oriented into whorls rather than the usual linear arrangement.

The clinical course of HCM is variable, with most patients experiencing little change in cardiac function over many years. Surgery to thin the septal thickening (myectomy) is rarely performed any longer because this technique has been superseded by drug therapy. In general, drugs that increase myocardial contractility or heart rate are avoided because they further impair diastolic filling and worsen aortic outflow obstruction. β-Adrenergic antagonists and calcium channel–blocking drugs may be used to dampen the hypercontractility. Long-term survival is possible. Myocardial ischemia is common, and the risk of sudden cardiac death is high because of fatal dysrhythmias.

Patients who die from HCM usually do so suddenly and most often after or during vigorous physical exertion.[9]

Restrictive Cardiomyopathy. Restrictive cardiomyopathy (RCM) is the rarest form and is characterized by a stiff, fibrotic ventricle with impaired diastolic filling. In about 50% of cases, RCM can be attributed to specific clinical disorders, the most common being amyloidosis—abnormal deposition of amyloid protein in tissues. The mechanisms proposed for development of other cases include sarcoidosis, genetic inheritance (e.g., hemochromatosis), postviral syndrome, malnutrition, autoimmune disease, and exposure to agents containing serotonin.[24] Regardless of the specific cause, the myocardium becomes fibrosed, rigid, and noncompliant. The major difficulty is restricted diastolic filling with resultant low stroke volume and heart failure. Exercise intolerance, dyspnea, and weakness may be present. RCM is difficult to manage effectively because no specific therapy is available for most types.

Specific Cardiomyopathy. Cardiomyopathies of presumed known origin constitute the category of specific cardiomyopathy (see Table 18-8). The specific cardiomyopathies present functionally as dilated, hypertrophic, or restrictive disorders, and the symptoms are consistent with the functional categories described above.

KEY POINTS

- Myocarditis is an inflammatory disorder characterized by scattered necrotic and dead heart muscle cells. Most cases are associated with viral infection. The major complication of myocarditis is left ventricular dysfunction and dilation of the heart chambers, with reduced contractility.
- Cardiomyopathies encompass a number of disorders of heart muscle that may be genetic or acquired. In many cases the exact cause is unknown.
- Dilated cardiomyopathy is characterized by enlargement of both ventricular chambers, reduced contractility, and low EF.
- Hypertrophic cardiomyopathy primarily affects the left ventricle and ventricular septum. Genetic mutations in myosin proteins are suspected in most cases. Conditions that increase contractility of the heart (exercise, drugs) can result in obstruction of ventricular outflow and reduced cardiac output. EF is preserved, and diastolic dysfunction is predominant. Patients with HCM have a high risk of sudden cardiac death.
- Restrictive cardiomyopathy is characterized by a stiff, fibrotic left ventricle that resists diastolic filling. Decreased cardiac output and left-sided heart failure can result.

PERICARDIAL DISEASES

Pericardial disorders are rarely isolated processes of primary cause; rather, they are sequelae of other disorders such as systemic infection, trauma, metabolic derangement, or neoplasia. Despite the diversity of causative factors, pericardial involvement may be asymptomatic, manifested as an accumulation of fluid in the pericardial sac, or as painful inflammation of pericardial structures.

Pericardial Effusion

An accumulation of noninflammatory fluid in the pericardial sac is called *pericardial effusion.* Normally, the pericardial space contains only 30 to 50 ml of thin, clear fluid. Under pathologic conditions, as much as 500 ml may accumulate. The compositions of the usual types of effusions are as follows:

Serous—a transudate secondary to heart failure or hypoproteinemia

Serosanguineous—a mixture of serous fluid and blood that may follow blunt chest trauma, heart surgery, or cardiopulmonary resuscitation

Chylous—a collection of lymph from obstruction of lymphatic drainage

Blood—hemopericardium usually resulting from penetrating trauma to the heart

Cardiac Tamponade. The accumulation of pericardial fluid is generally without clinical significance except as an indicator of underlying disease processes. However, if the fluid accumulation is large or occurs suddenly, the life-threatening condition of cardiac tamponade may ensue. *Tamponade* refers to external compression of the heart chambers such that filling is impaired.

Signs and symptoms of cardiac tamponade include reduced stroke volume and compensatory increases in heart rate. Systemic venous congestion occurs because blood is prevented from entering the compressed heart by way of the superior and inferior venae cavae. Venous congestion may be apparent as distended neck veins. Changes in intrathoracic pressure during respiration may have exaggerated effects on cardiac filling. The presence of waxing and waning of blood pressure in synchrony with respiration is called *pulsus paradoxus.* Significant pulsus paradoxus is usually defined as a difference of 10 mm Hg or more in systolic blood pressure between inspiration and expiration. Other manifestations of tamponade include rising filling pressures in the heart chambers, muffled heart sounds, dull chest pain, diminished electrocardiographic amplitude, and a compressed cardiac silhouette on radiographs.

Treatment is aimed at relieving the pericardial pressure by aspirating the offending fluid (*pericardiocentesis*). Failure to manage tamponade may result in drastically reduced diastolic filling, cardiovascular collapse, and death. Pericardial effusions occasionally are detected by chance on chest x-rays being performed for other purposes. Nonsymptomatic pericardial effusions may be aspirated or merely monitored and allowed to resolve spontaneously. Treatment is directed at the underlying cause of the effusion.

Pericarditis

Inflammation of the pericardium originates from a variety of causes (Box 18-3). Rarely is the pericardium the primary site of disease. Pericarditis is often categorized as acute or chronic; however, these forms are morphologically and etiologically

BOX 18-3

Categories of Pericardial Disease and Selected Etiologies

Idiopathic*

Infectious
Viral* (echovirus, Coxsackievirus, adenovirus, cytomegalovirus, hepatitis B, infectious mononucleosis, HIV/AIDS)
Bacterial* (*Pneumococcus*, *Staphylococcus*, *Streptococcus*, mycoplasma, Lyme disease, *Haemophilus influenzae*, *Neisseria meningitidis*, and others)
Mycobacteria* (*Mycobacterium tuberculosis*, *Mycobacterium avium-intracellulare*)
Fungal (histoplasmosis, coccidiomycosis)
Protozoal

Immune-inflammatory
Connective tissue disease* (systemic lupus erythematosus, rheumatoid arthritis, scleroderma, mixed)
Arteritis (polyarteritis nodosa, temporal arteritis)
Inflammatory bowel disease
Early post-myocardial infarction
Late post-myocardial infarction (Dressler syndrome),* late postcardiotomy/thoracotomy,* late posttrauma*
Drug induced* (e.g., procainamide, hydralazine, isoniazid, cyclosporine)

Neoplastic disease
Primary: mesothelioma, fibrosarcoma, lipoma, and so on
Secondary*: breast and lung carcinoma, lymphomas, Kaposi sarcoma

Radiation induced*

Early postcardiac surgery

Hemopericardium
Trauma
Post-myocardial infarction free wall rupture
Device and procedure related: percutaneous coronary procedures, implantable defibrillators, pacemakers, post-arrhythmia ablation, post-atrial septal defect closure, post-valve repair/replacement
Dissecting aortic aneurysm

Trauma
Blunt and penetrating,* postcardiopulmonary resuscitation*

Congenital
Cysts, congenital absence

Miscellaneous
Cholesterol ("gold paint" pericarditis)
Chronic renal failure, dialysis related
Chylopericardium
Hypothyroidism and hyperthyroidism
Amyloidosis
Aortic dissection

From LeWinter M: Pericardial diseases. In Libby P et al, editors: *Braunwald's heart disease: a textbook of cardiovascular medicine,* ed 8, Philadelphia, 2008, Saunders, p 1831.
*Etiologies that can present as acute pericarditis.
HIV/AIDS, human immunodeficiency virus/acquired immunodeficiency syndrome.

similar.[9] Chronic pericarditis refers to a healed stage of the acute form that results in chronic pericardial dysfunction.

Acute Pericarditis. It is estimated that 80% to 90% of cases of acute pericarditis are idiopathic, and most of these are presumed to be viral.[25] Uncomplicated acute pericarditis typically resolves spontaneously and non-steroidal anti-inflammatory agents (NSAIDS) may be the only therapy used. A small number of cases may be complicated by significant pericardial effusion, persistent or recurrent inflammation, and may require hospitalization for more thorough diagnostic investigation to determine the specific etiology and more intensive therapy.

The symptoms of acute pericarditis are associated with the systemic effects of inflammation and pericardial damage and include fever, leukocytosis, malaise, and tachycardia. Acute pericarditis almost always presents with chest pain and may be confused with anginal pain. Sticking and rubbing of the visceral and parietal pericardial layers cause pain that may radiate to the back and be associated with esophageal discomfort and dysphagia (difficulty swallowing). Rubbing of the pericardial layers may be heard as a friction rub. The rub can be transient and intermittent and may sound squeaky or like scratchy sandpaper. Epicardial injury from pericarditis may be apparent on the ECG as ST-segment elevation. Treatment is generally symptom oriented and includes medications to relieve pain and minimize inflammation.

MI used to be a common cause of pericarditis, but the incidence of both acute post-MI pericarditis and the delayed pericarditis of Dressler syndrome have decreased in incidence by at least 50% with the advent of early reperfusion therapy for MI.[25] Acute post-MI pericarditis occurs within a few days of an MI in which the infarction involves the epicardial surfaces of the heart (transmural MI). The inflammation of the necrotic heart muscle extends to adjacent pericardial structures causing them to become inflamed as well. The degree of pericardial involvement reflects the size of the MI. In contrast, late pericarditis, occurring a week to a few months after the MI (Dressler syndrome) is believed to be an autoimmune reaction caused by exposure of the immune system to damaged myocardial tissue. Antimyocardial antibodies have been demonstrated, and the pericardial inflammation is diffuse and not localized to the area of myocardial injury.

Chronic Pericarditis. Healing of an acute form of pericardial inflammation may result in chronic (healed) pericardial dysfunction of two principal kinds: adhesive mediastinoperi-carditis and constrictive pericarditis. Adhesive mediastino-pericarditis is usually a consequence of suppurative or caseous pericarditis or a complication of previous cardiac surgery. It may also follow significant irradiation of the chest. The peri-cardial sac is destroyed and the external aspect of the heart ad-heres to surrounding mediastinal structures. The workload of the heart increases significantly because contraction is opposed by the attached surrounding structures.

Constrictive pericarditis may be a result of previous sup-purative or caseous pericarditis, commonly secondary to tu-berculosis. However, in many cases the cause of pericardial dysfunction is unknown. The pericardial sac becomes dense, nonelastic, fibrous, and scarred. It encases the heart like a stiff cage and impairs diastolic filling. The constrictive process generally occurs slowly and may be quite advanced by the time symptoms occur.

Symptoms may include exercise intolerance, weakness, fa-tigue, and systemic venous congestion. Treatment is aimed at relieving the constriction by removal of pericardium (pericar-dectomy) and administration of inotropic agents to improve cardiac contractility.

KEY POINTS

- Large accumulations of pericardial fluid can result in cardiac tamponade. External compression of the heart chambers impairs diastolic filling and results in de-creased stroke volume. Distended neck veins, pulsus paradoxus, elevated and equalized intrachamber pres-sures, and muffled heart sounds are indicative.
- Acute pericarditis causes sticking and rubbing of the visceral and parietal pericardial layers. A friction rub, pain radiating to the back, esophageal discomfort, and generalized signs of inflammation are usually present.
- Chronic pericarditis can lead to destruction of the peri-cardial sac with adhesion of the heart to surrounding mediastinal structures. Cardiac contraction may be im-paired.
- Constrictive pericarditis results in a fibrous, scarred pericardium that restricts cardiac filling.

CONGENITAL HEART DISEASES

Congenital heart disease is an abnormality of the heart that is present from birth. A wide variety of defects have been de-scribed, and only the pathophysiology of the most common defects will be included. A brief description of fetal cardiac de-velopment is a necessary prelude to a discussion of congenital heart diseases.

Embryologic Development

Development of the heart involves a complex orchestration of formation and resorption of structures. Abnormalities in the development of four important heart structures are at the root of most of the common heart defects: (1) development of the atrial septum, (2) development of the ventricular septum, (3) division of the main outflow tract (truncus arteriosus) into the pulmonary and aortic arteries, and (4) development of the valves. Each of these processes is briefly reviewed.

The primitive heart begins as an enlarged tube much like a blood vessel. The tube has three layers. The inner luminal layer is thin and composed of endothelial cells. This layer will eventually line the inner chambers of the heart and valves. The outermost layer is also thin and is called the *myoepicardial mantle*. The outer mantle will form the epicardial and mus-cular structures of the heart. In between these two thin layers of cells is a thick layer of gelatinous substance called *cardiac jelly*. Cardiac jelly is the precursor to endocardial cushion tis-sue, which is important in the formation of membranes in the heart, including the septa that separate the four chambers of the heart.

By day 23, the heart tube begins to beat. The tube folds on itself to form an asymmetric loop structure (Figure 18-22). One bulge of the loop forms a primitive single atrium, another forms the future left ventricle, and a third forms the future right ventricle and common ventricular outflow tract (trun-cus arteriosus). The common atrium is divided into right and left atria by growth of the interatrial septum. Atrial septation occurs in several steps. First, the *septum primum* is formed passively in the superior surface by an indentation caused by the overlying truncus arteriosus (Figure 18-23). Next, the superior and inferior endocardial cushions grow and extend toward each other. These flaps of tissue overlap but do not fuse so that blood can pass through from the right atrium to the left atrium. A reverse in the direction of flow, as occurs at birth, normally would push the flap shut and close the hole.

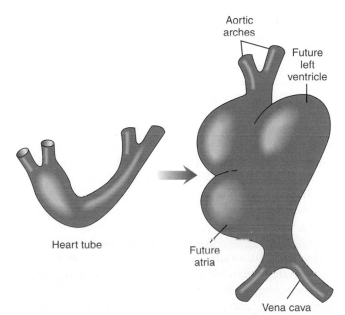

FIGURE 18-22 Asymmetric loop structure in early embryonic devel-opment of the heart.

FIGURE 18-23 Formation of the intracardiac septa.

FIGURE 18-24 Septation of the truncus arteriosus and formation of the semilunar valves.

This flaplike opening, called the *ostium secundum,* remains open throughout fetal life and is later called the *foramen ovale.*

Septal formation between the ventricles follows a similar pattern. The lower portion of the interventricular septum is formed by circular growth and fusing of the muscular ventricular walls. Then the muscular septum proliferates upward toward the atria. The inferior endocardial cushion tissue also grows downward to meet the uplifting muscular septum (see Figure 18-23).

At about the same time that the atrial and ventricular septal structures are being elaborated, the common ventricular outflow tract, the truncus arteriosus, is divided into the pulmonary and aortic channels. This process is accomplished by growth and eventual fusion of mounds of endocardial cushions located in the wall of the truncus arteriosus. The truncal endocardial cushions go on to form the semilunar valves as well (Figure 18-24).

The atrioventricular septum and valves are similarly formed by growth and fusion of the right and left lateral cushions. Superior and inferior cushions also contribute to formation of the septum between the atria and ventricles. Leaflets of the valves are initially formed by lumps of cushion material, which are replaced by muscle tissue from the ventricular wall. The muscle tissue also forms the chordae tendineae and papillary muscle structures. Eventually, the muscle cells of the leaflets and chordae tendineae are replaced by tough fibrous connective tissue.

When the embryonic heart is fully developed, two important passageways still permit bloodflow to bypass the lungs (Figure 18-25). The foramen ovale lies between the left and right atria and allows blood to bypass the right ventricle. Blood flows right to left through the atrial opening because the pres-

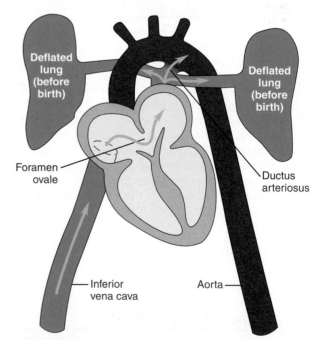

FIGURE 18-25 Fully developed embryonic heart showing the foramen ovale and ductus arteriosus. These structures allow blood to bypass the pulmonary circulation during fetal life.

sure in the left atrium is low. High resistance of the deflated lungs also causes right ventricular pressure to be high, which impedes right ventricular filling. The other important structure is the ductus arteriosus, a channel that connects the pulmonary artery and the aorta. Blood flows from the pulmonary artery into the aorta during fetal life because of high vascular resistance in the collapsed lungs. Both these communications

TABLE 18-9

Relative Frequency of Occurrence of Cardiac Malformations at Birth

Disease	Percentage
Ventricular septal defect	42
Atrial septal defect	10
Pulmonic stenosis	8
Patent ductus arteriosus	7
Tetralogy of Fallot	5
Coarctation of the aorta	5
Atrioventricular septal defect	4
Aortic stenosis	4
Complete transposition of the great arteries	4
Persistent truncus arteriosus	1
Anomalous pulmonary venous connection	1
Tricuspid atresia	1

Based on 44 published studies. Adapted from Hoffman JI, Kaplan S: The incidence of congenital heart disease, *J Am Coll Cardiol* 39(12):1890, 2002.

BOX 18-4

Features of Heart Failure in Infants

Poor feeding and failure to thrive
Respiratory distress (mainly tachypnea)
Rapid heart rate (160 to 180 beats/min)
Pulmonary rales or wheezing
Cardiomegaly and pulmonary edema on radiogram
Heptomegaly (peripheral edema unusual)
Gallop sounds
Color (ashen pale or faintly cyanotic)
Excessive perspiration
Diminished urine output

generally close after birth when the lungs inflate and the resistance on the right side of the heart falls. Clamping the umbilical cord also serves to increase systemic vascular resistance, which further augments the reverse in pressure gradient, with left heart pressures now exceeding those on the right.

Etiology and Incidence of Congenital Heart Disease

Congenital heart disease is the most common heart disorder in children, with an overall incidence of about 0.8% of all live births.[9] The most common heart defects are listed in Table 18-9, with approximate frequencies of occurrence. In more than 90% of cases, the cause of the heart defect is unknown.[9] Multifactorial inheritance with both genetic and environmental influences is probable. Very few cases of congenital malformation can be clearly attributed to environmental factors. Maternal rubella during the first trimester of pregnancy is the best documented environmental cause of heart defects. A large number of cardiac teratogens are suspected from animal studies, including hypoxia, ionizing radiation, and heavy alcohol consumption.

Several indications suggest that genetic influence is important in cardiac malformation. A twofold to tenfold increase in the incidence of congenital heart defects is seen in siblings. Several heart defects also occur more frequently in males. However, twin studies show that in only 10% of cases does a heart defect (ventricular septal defect) afflict both infants, even though their genotype is identical.[26] Thus a complex interplay between genetic and environmental influences is probable and as yet poorly understood.

Pathophysiology of Congenital Heart Disease

The many forms of congenital heart anomalies result in two primary pathologies: *shunts* and *obstructions*. A shunt denotes an abnormal path of blood flow through the heart or great vessels. The shunt may be further characterized as *right-to-left* or *left-to-right* to indicate the direction of abnormal blood flow. Right-to-left shunts allow unoxygenated blood from the right side of the heart to enter the left side and systemic circulation without first passing through the lungs. Infants with right-to-left shunting of blood generally have some degree of cyanosis because of the decreased oxygen content of the arterial blood (cyanotic defect). Conversely, a left-to-right shunt occurs when oxygenated blood from the left side of the heart or aorta flows back into the right side to be recirculated through the lungs. The blood reaching the systemic circulation is oxygenated and the infant is not cyanotic (acyanotic defect). However, the right side of the heart has an increased workload because of the extra shunt blood. In time, the overload of the right side of the heart can result in right ventricular hypertrophy and high right-sided heart pressures. A left-to-right shunt may then progress to a more dangerous right-to-left shunt when right heart pressures exceed left heart pressures. Congenital disorders causing abnormal blood flow through the heart include atrial septal defect, ventricular septal defect, patent ductus arteriosus, tetralogy of Fallot, transposition of the great arteries, truncus arteriosus, and tricuspid atresia.

Some heart anomalies produce obstructions to blood flow because of abnormal narrowings. Stenosis or atresia (failure to develop) of valves, and coarctation of the aorta are the most common obstructive defects. Obstructions do not result in cyanosis but generally increase the workload of the affected chamber. Heart failure is a potential consequence of congenital heart defects and presents differently in infants and children than in adults (Box 18-4).

In addition to being classified according to pathologic features as obstructions or shunts, heart defects are also classified according to the clinical manifestation of cyanosis. Acyanotic disorders include the obstructive disorders and left-to-right shunts. The cyanotic category includes abnormalities causing right-to-left shunts. Specific heart defects are described further and follow this categorization.

Acyanotic Congenital Defects

Atrial Septal Defect. During the third to fifth week of fetal development, the left and right atria are separated by flaps of tissue that become the atrial septum. The foramen ovale remains patent during intrauterine life such that blood may pass from the right to the left atrium and bypass the uninflated and nonfunctional lungs (Figure 18-26). The foramen ovale normally remains open in utero because pressure on the right side of the heart is higher than that on the left. With birth, however, the pressure gradient reverses as the lungs inflate and greatly reduce pulmonary vascular resistance. The higher left-sided pressure forces the flap shut, and fusion of the foramen ovale membrane normally occurs. The majority of atrial septal defects occur at the location of the foramen ovale. The abnormal septal opening may be of variable size. Small defects (1 cm) are well tolerated. Even larger atrial septal defects may be asymptomatic for many years as long as the shunt flow is left to right and therefore acyanotic.

The long-term increase in pulmonary blood flow may eventually lead to pulmonary hypertension, right ventricular hypertrophy, and a reversal of the shunt to a right-to-left pattern. Cyanosis, respiratory difficulty, and right-sided heart failure may ensue. Large or symptomatic atrial septal defects are commonly repaired surgically early in life, before pulmonary complications occur.

Ventricular Septal Defect. A ventricular septal defect is the most common congenital cardiac anomaly.[9] It is frequently associated with other cardiac defects such as tetralogy of Fallot, transposition of the great arteries, and atrial septal defects. The ventricular septum develops between the fifth and sixth weeks of fetal life as the membrane derived from the endocardial cushion fuses with the muscular septum (Figure 18-27).

The majority of ventricular septal defects are located in the membranous septum, very close to the bundle of His. As with atrial septal defects, the functional significance depends largely on the size of the defect. The shunt is initially left to right because left-sided heart pressures are higher. With the

increase in pulmonary blood flow, pulmonary hypertension and right ventricular hypertrophy may result and cause a reversal of the shunt.

Large ventricular septal defects may be apparent at birth because of rapidly developing right-sided heart failure and a loud systolic murmur. Large, symptomatic defects in infants or moderate defects in older children are repaired surgically to avoid progression to pulmonary vascular disease. Small ventricular septal defects in infants are generally not immediately repaired because of the tendency of such defects to close spontaneously.

Patent Ductus Arteriosus. The ductus arteriosus is a normal channel between the pulmonary artery and the aorta that remains open during intrauterine life (Figure 18-28). Within 1 to 2 days after birth, the ductus arteriosus closes functionally, and within a few weeks it closes permanently. The ductus arteriosus allows blood to flow from the pulmonary artery into the aorta, thus bypassing the lungs. Low oxygen tension and local production of prostaglandins appear to be important in maintaining patency of the channel during fetal life. After birth, flow through the ductus arteriosus switches to left to right because of the higher pressure in the aorta. This change in flow direction brings oxygenated blood through the ductus arteriosus and stimulates it to close. A reduction in prostaglandin E production after birth appears to contribute to constriction and closure. In many cases the reason for abnormal continued patency of the ductus arteriosus after birth is not well understood. Conditions that cause low blood oxygen tension may contribute to continued patency.

Most often a patent ductus arteriosus has no clinical significance early in life because the shunt is left to right and no cyanosis is evident. Surgical management is not usually immediately undertaken because these defects tend to close

FIGURE 18-26 Atrial septal defect. Blood flow through the defect is usually left to right and produces an acyanotic shunt.

FIGURE 18-27 Ventricular septal defect. Blood flow through the defect is usually left to right and produces an acyanotic shunt.

FIGURE 18-28 Patent ductus arteriosus. Blood flow through the ductus is usually from the aorta to the pulmonary artery and produces an acyanotic shunt.

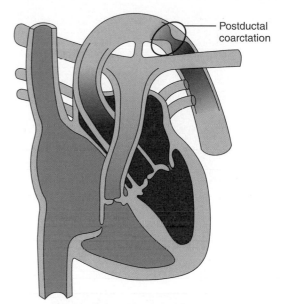

FIGURE 18-29 Coarctation of the aorta. The arterial narrowing can produce a weaker pulse in the lower extremities.

spontaneously. Prostaglandin inhibitors may be given to induce closure of the defect. Continued patency of the ductus arteriosus is usually obvious because of a harsh, grinding systolic murmur and often a systolic thrill (vibration). Surgical closure of the patent ductus arteriosus is done as soon as it becomes evident that spontaneous closure is unlikely. As with other left-to-right shunt disorders, uncorrected patent ductus arteriosus results in pulmonary hypertension complicated by respiratory and right-sided heart failure. Eventual reversal of the shunt to a right-to-left pattern results in cyanosis. Because the ductus is usually located distal to the origin of the subclavian artery, the lower extremities may show cyanosis whereas the upper extremities remain pink.

Coarctation of the Aorta. *Coarctation* refers to a narrowing or stricture that may impede blood flow. Coarctation of the aorta is a common heart defect that affects males 3 to 4 times more frequently than females. Narrowing of the aorta may occur anywhere along its length; however, in most cases the coarctation is located just before or just after the ductus arteriosus (Figure 18-29). Preductal coarctation (proximal to the ductus arteriosus) is usually more severe and often associated with other anomalies. In some instances, the aortic stricture is so severe that blood flow to the lower part of the body must be maintained solely through flow through the ductus arteriosus. This situation results in a very high workload for the right side of the heart and may lead to heart failure in the early neonatal period. Blood supply to the arms and head is unaffected because these arteries arise proximal to the stricture. Postductal coarctation is generally less severe and may go unrecognized until adulthood.

The upper extremities typically have an elevated blood pressure, with weak pulses and low blood pressure in the lower extremities. An important part of assessment of the newborn

is comparison of pulses in the upper and lower extremities to assess for symmetry. All types of coarctation are usually accompanied by systolic murmurs and ventricular hypertrophy. The stricture can be repaired surgically by resection of the narrowed region. If left untreated, significant coarctation may lead to congestive heart failure, intracranial hemorrhage, or aortic rupture.

Pulmonary Stenosis or Atresia. Isolated pulmonary stenosis and atresia are included in the category of acyanotic defects because they do not themselves result in cyanosis. However, they often occur in conjunction with other anomalies that allow survival into the neonatal period. The other defects may allow shunting of blood and result in cyanosis. In pulmonary atresia, no communication is found between the right ventricle and the lungs, so that blood must enter the lungs by first traveling through a septal opening and then through a patent ductus arteriosus. The right ventricle is typically underdeveloped (hypoplasia), and the atrial septal defect is large. Pulmonary stenosis can be mild to severe, depending on the extent of narrowing of the pulmonic valve. Pulmonary stenosis is usually due to abnormal fusion of the valvular cusps. Right ventricular hypertrophy occurs secondary to the high ventricular afterload caused by the narrowed outflow opening. Isolated pulmonary stenosis is easily corrected by surgery; however, the prognosis depends in large part on the health of the right ventricle.

Aortic Stenosis or Atresia. Congenital aortic atresia is rare and not compatible with survival. Depending on its severity, aortic stenosis is correctable and associated with a good prognosis. Aortic stenosis may involve the valvular cusps or the subvalvular fibrous ring just below the cusps. The narrowed aortic outflow tract results in a high left ventricular afterload, which causes the left ventricle to enlarge.

FIGURE 18-30 Tetralogy of Fallot showing the four characteristic abnormalities: pulmonary stenosis, ventricular septal defect, overriding aorta, and right ventricular hypertrophy. Tetralogy of Fallot is a cyanotic defect.

FIGURE 18-31 Transposition of the great arteries. Two separate circulations are formed, which is incompatible with life unless mixing of blood occurs through other defects. *ASD,* Atrial septal defect; *PDA,* patent ductus arteriosus.

A prominent systolic murmur is usually apparent. Surgical replacement is the definitive treatment if the stenosis is severe, progresses, or becomes symptomatic.

Cyanotic Congenital Defects

Tetralogy of Fallot. The four defining features of tetralogy of Fallot are (1) a ventricular septal defect; (2) an aorta positioned above the ventricular septal opening (overriding aorta); (3) pulmonary stenosis that obstructs right ventricular outflow; and (4) right ventricular hypertrophy (Figure 18-30).

The severity of the symptoms is related primarily to the degree of pulmonary stenosis. The heart is generally enlarged because of the extensive right ventricular hypertrophy. Even if the condition is untreated, individuals with tetralogy of Fallot may live into adulthood. The defect often results in cyanosis because the overriding aorta receives unoxygenated blood from the right side of the heart as well as oxygenated blood from the left side. The degree of cyanosis depends on the amount of blood received from the right side, which in turn depends on the degree of pulmonic obstruction. Surgical correction of the defects is usually recommended because prolonged non-corrective management carries the risk of infective endocarditis and secondary polycythemia.

Transposition of the Great Arteries. In the most common form of transposition of the great arteries, the aorta arises from the right ventricle and the pulmonary artery arises from the left ventricle (Figure 18-31). This anomaly results in the formation of two separate, noncommunicating circulations. The right side of the heart receives blood from the systemic circulation and recirculates it through the body by way

of the aorta. Blood reaching the body has not passed through the lungs and is therefore not oxygenated. The left side of the heart receives oxygenated blood from the lungs and then recirculates it through the lungs by way of the pulmonary artery. Unless some mixing of these separate circulations takes place through other heart defects, such as septal defects, transposition is not compatible with life.

Nearly all infants who survive the neonatal period have an interatrial opening, and most also have a patent ductus arteriosus. A good deal of mixing must be maintained after birth for the infant to survive. Surgery may be directed at improving the mixing of systemic and pulmonary blood by enlarging or creating openings in the heart. Corrective surgery in which the aorta and pulmonary arteries are cut from the heart and sewn to the opposite ventricular outflow tract is the treatment of choice. The coronary arteries must also be reimplanted into the new left ventricular outflow tract in this procedure.

Truncus Arteriosus. Truncus arteriosus is a congenital malformation in which failure of the pulmonary artery and aorta to separate results in formation of one large vessel that receives blood from both the right and left ventricles (Figure 18-32). A large ventricular septal defect and a single valvular structure are present and lead to the single large artery. Mixing of blood from the right and left sides of the heart results in systemic cyanosis. The amount of blood entering the systemic versus the pulmonary circulation depends on the degree of vascular resistance in the two systems. Abnormally high pulmonary blood flow may progress to pulmonary hypertension and right ventricular hypertrophy. Increased pulmonary resistance causes the cyanosis to become more severe as more

FIGURE 18-32 Truncus arteriosus is a cyanotic defect. Failure of septation results in a common outflow tract from the ventricles. A ventricular septal defect is also present.

blood enters the systemic circulation. Surgical correction is required for survival.

Tricuspid Atresia. Absence of the tricuspid valve is almost always associated with underdevelopment of the right ventricle and an atrial septal defect. Circulation is maintained by the defect, which allows blood to bypass the right ventricle. A patent ductus arteriosus is required to perfuse the lungs. In some cases, a concomitant ventricular septal defect is present and may allow some blood to pass into the right ventricle and enter the pulmonary circulation. Cyanosis is present from birth, and the mortality rate is high. Surgical correction is required for survival.

SUMMARY

A variety of disease processes may interfere with the heart's ability to provide the body with oxygenated blood. Among these processes are coronary heart disease, valvular and endocardial diseases, myocardial diseases, pericardial diseases, and congenital heart defects. Coronary heart disease includes several clinical forms: angina pectoris, acute coronary syndrome (unstable angina, MI), chronic ischemic heart disease, and sudden cardiac death. Stenotic coronary lesions obstruct blood flow to the myocardium and result in these ischemic clinical syndromes. Distinction between unstable angina and MI relies on the presence of serum markers of myocardial damage. Unstable angina is ischemia without cellular death and therefore does not result in biomarker elevation. MI, on the other hand, is associated with the death of myocardial cells and subsequent release of intracellular components. MI may be complicated by dysrhythmias and failure of the heart to pump efficiently.

Valvular disorders are of two types: those that impede flow because of stenosis and those that allow regurgitation because of failure to close completely. The general consequence of valvular disorders is increased myocardial workload secondary to high afterload (stenosis) or high preload (regurgitation). The heart may eventually decompensate and proceed to heart failure. The endocardial diseases rheumatic heart disease and infective endocarditis also primarily affect the heart valves and create stenosis and regurgitation.

Disorders of the myocardium include myocarditis, which is an inflammatory process, and cardiomyopathy, which is a noninflammatory process, usually of unknown cause. Most cases of myocarditis are viral; however, it is the immune system's response to the virus that appears to cause myocardial damage. Myocarditis results in a dilated, flabby heart with decreased pumping efficiency. The cardiomyopathies are a diverse group of disorders that may be classified as primary (having unknown cause) and specific (caused by a known disease process). Cardiomyopathies include a dilated form, a hypertrophic form, and a restrictive form. The primary problem in the dilated form is poor contractility of all heart chambers. The hypertrophic form may cause left ventricular outflow obstruction that interferes with cardiac output and increases left ventricular strain. Dysfunction in the restrictive form is caused by poor diastolic filling as a result of a stiff, fibrosed ventricular chamber.

Pericardial disorders include accumulations of fluid in the pericardial sac and acute and chronic forms of pericarditis. Pericardial fluid may be serous, serosanguineous, chylous, or frank blood. Pericardial accumulations are usually of little consequence except as indicators of underlying pathophysiologic processes. However, if the accumulation is large or rapid, it may compress the heart and interfere with diastolic filling—a process called *cardiac tamponade.* Pericarditis refers to inflammation of the pericardium. It is usually secondary to other disease processes. Pericardial inflammation generally causes pain and may be associated with a friction rub. Chronic pericarditis can cause erosion of the pericardial sac such that the epicardial layer of the heart may become fused to other mediastinal structures.

Alternatively, chronic pericarditis may cause the pericardial sac to become fibrotic and noncompliant such that it restricts expansion of the heart during diastolic filling.

A number of heart disorders may be present at birth and can be categorized as obstructions or shunts and as cyanotic or acyanotic. In general, disorders that allow unoxygenated blood from the right heart to enter the systemic circulation (right-to-left shunt) cause cyanosis. Examples of cyanotic defects include tetralogy of Fallot, transposition of the great arteries, truncus arteriosus, and tricuspid atresia. Examples of acyanotic defects are coarctation of the aorta, atrial and ventricular septal defects, and patent ductus arteriosus.

All heart diseases discussed in this chapter may be complicated by heart failure. Heart failure occurs when the pumping efficiency of the heart is decreased such that cardiac output is subnormal. It is often accompanied by congestion of the lungs or the systemic venous system. Heart failure is discussed in Chapter 19.

REFERENCES

1. American Heart Association: *Heart disease and stroke statistics—2008 update*, Dallas, 2008, The Association.
2. Third Report of the National Cholesterol Education Program (NCEP) Expert Panel on Detection, Evaluation, and Treatment of High Blood Cholesterol in Adults (Adult Treatment Panel III), Bethesda, 2002, National Heart, Lung, and Blood Institute, National Institutes of Health.
3. Libby P: The vascular biology of atherosclerosis. In Libby P, Bonow R, Mann D et al, editors: *Braunwald's heart disease: a textbook of cardiovascular medicine,* ed 8, Philadelphia, 2008, Saunders, pp 985-1002.
4. Schoen FJ, Cotran RS: Blood vessels. In Kumar V, Cotran R, Robbins S , editors: *Robbins basic pathology,* ed 7, Philadelphia, 2003, Saunders, pp 325-360.
5. Grundy SM et al: National Heart, Lung, and Blood Institute; American College of Cardiology Foundation; American Heart Association: Implications of recent clinical trials for the National Cholesterol Education Program Adult Treatment Panel III guidelines, *Circulation* 110(2):227-239, 2004.
6. Stary HC et al: A definition of initial, fatty streak, and intermediate lesions of atherosclerosis. A report from the Committee on Vascular Lesions of the Council on Arteriosclerosis, American Heart Association, *Circulation* 89(5):2462-2478, 1994.
7. Thim T, Hagensen MK, Bentzon JF et al: From vulnerable plaque to atherothrombosis, *J Intern Med* 263(5):506-516, 2008.
8. Wilensky RL, Hamamdzic D: The molecular basis of vulnerable plaque: potential therapeutic role for immunomodulation, *Curr Opin Cardiol* 22(6):545-551, 2007.
9. Schoen FJ, Mitchell R: The heart. In Kumar V, Abbas A, Fausto N et al, editors: *Robbins basic pathology,* ed 8, Philadelphia, 2007, Saunders, pp 379-419.
10. Eidelman RS, Hebert PR, Weisman SM et al: An update on aspirin in the primary prevention of cardiovascular disease, *Arch Intern Med* 163(17):2006-2010, 2003.
11. Hadi HA, Carr CS, Al Suwaidi J: Endothelial dysfunction: cardiovascular risk factors, therapy, and outcome, *Vasc Health Risk Manag* 1(3):183-198, 2005.
12. Body R: Emergent diagnosis of acute coronary syndromes: Today's challenges and tomorrow's possibilities, *Resuscitation* 2008 Apr 8 [Epub ahead of print].
13. Anderson JL et al: ACC/AHA 2007 guidelines for the management of patients with unstable angina/non–ST-elevation myocardial infarction: a report of the American College of Cardiology/American Heart Association Task Force on Practice Guidelines (Writing Committee to Revise the 2002 Guidelines for the Management of Patients With Unstable Angina/Non–ST-Elevation Myocardial Infarction): developed in collaboration with the American College of Emergency Physicians, American College of Physicians, Society for Academic Emergency Medicine, Society for Cardiovascular Angiography and Interventions, and Society of Thoracic Surgeons, *J Am Coll Cardiol* 50:e1-e157, 2007.
14. DeWood MA et al: Prevalence of total coronary occlusion during the early hours of transmural myocardial infarction, *N Engl J Med* 303(16):897-902, 1980.
15. Antman EM et al: 2007 Focused Update of the ACC/AHA 2004 Guidelines for the Management of Patients With ST-Elevation Myocardial Infarction: a report of the American College of Cardiology/American Heart Association Task Force on Practice Guidelines: developed in collaboration With the Canadian Cardiovascular Society endorsed by the American Academy of Family Physicians: 2007 Writing Group to Review New Evidence and Update the ACC/AHA 2004 Guidelines for the Management of Patients With ST-Elevation Myocardial Infarction, Writing on Behalf of the 2004 Writing Committee, *Circulation* 117(2): 296-329, 2008.
16. Nadal-Ginard B et al: Myocyte death, growth, and regeneration in cardiac hypertrophy and failure, *Circ Res* 92(2):139-150, 2003.
17. Antezano ES, Hong M: Sudden cardiac death, *J Intensive Care Med* 18(6):313-329, 2003.
18. Otto CM, Bonow RO: Valvular heart disease. In Libby P, Bonow R, Mann D et al, editors: *Braunwald's heart disease: a textbook of cardiovascular medicine,* ed 8, Philadelphia, 2008, Saunders, pp 1625-1693.
19. Carapetis JR, Steer AC, Mulholland EK et al: The global burden of group A streptococcal diseases, *Lancet Infect Dis* 5:685-694, 2005.
20. Raju BS, Turi ZG: Rheumatic fever. In Libby P, Bonow R, Mann D et al, editors: *Braunwald's heart disease: a textbook of cardiovascular medicine,* ed 8, Philadelphia, 2008, Saunders, pp 2079-2086.
21. Karchmer AW: Infective endocarditis. In Libby P, Bonow R, Mann D et al, editors: *Braunwald's heart disease: a textbook of cardiovascular medicine,* ed 8, Philadelphia, 2008, Saunders, pp 1713-1734.
22. Liu P, Schultheiss HP: Myocarditis. In Libby P, Bonow R, Mann D et al, editors: *Braunwald's heart disease: a textbook of cardiovascular medicine,* ed 8, Philadelphia, 2008, Saunders, pp 1775-1792.
23. Richardson P et al: Report of the 1995 World Health Organization/ International Society and Federation of Cardiology Task Force on the Definition and Classification of Cardiomyopathies, *Circulation* 93(5):841-842, 1996.
24. Hare J: The dilated, restrictive, and infiltrative cardiomyopathies. In Libby P, Bonow R, Mann D et al, editors: *Braunwald's heart disease: a textbook of cardiovascular medicine,* ed 8, Philadelphia, 2008, Saunders, pp 1739-1762.
25. LeWinter M: Pericardial diseases. In Libby P, Bonow R, Mann D et al, editors: *Braunwald's heart disease: a textbook of cardiovascular medicine,* ed 8, Philadelphia, 2008, Saunders, pp 1829-1853.
26. Newman TB: Etiology of ventricular septal defects: an epidemiologic approach, *Pediatrics* 76(5):741-749, 1985.

Heart Failure and Dysrhythmias: Common Sequelae of Cardiac Diseases

Jacquelyn L. Banasik

MEDIA RESOURCES

Additional Material for Study, Review, and Further Exploration

CD Companion ■ Review Questions and Answers
■ Glossary (with audio pronunciations for selected terms)
■ Disease Profiles ■ Animations

evolve **Website** at http://evolve.elsevier.com/Copstead/
■ Case Studies ■ Disease Profiles ■ WebLinks ■ Key Points Review

 Online Course (Module 11)

KEY QUESTIONS

■ What are the common predisposing factors for development of heart failure?
■ How does heart failure with primarily systolic dysfunction differ from heart failure with primarily diastolic dysfunction?
■ How do the compensatory responses triggered in heart failure work to restore cardiac output?

■ What are the clinical manifestations of heart failure?
■ How are preload, afterload, and contractility managed therapeutically in the patient with heart failure?
■ What are the characteristic electrocardiographic features of the common cardiac dysrhythmias?
■ What is the clinical significance and usual treatment of each of the common cardiac dysrhythmias?

CHAPTER OUTLINE

Heart failure (HF) and cardiac dysrhythmias (arrhythmias) may occur in association with cardiac diseases from a number of different causes. *Heart failure* refers to inability of the heart to maintain sufficient cardiac output to optimally meet metabolic demands of tissues and organs. Heart failure is the potential end point of all serious forms of heart disease. Many patients with heart failure exhibit symptoms of fluid overload, so the term *congestive heart failure* (CHF) may be used as a diagnosis in some cases. The term CHF may also be used to designate chronic heart failure as distinct from acute heart failure. This chapter includes the chronic forms of heart failure; acute failure is discussed in Chapter 20 because it commonly results in cardiogenic shock. Disturbances in electrical activity of the heart may signify underlying pathophysiologic processes and may also lead to insufficient cardiac output. Neither heart failure nor dysrhythmia is a primary medical disease, and underlying pathophysiologic processes must also be investigated.

Heart failure is defined as insufficient cardiac output due to cardiac dysfunction. Ineffectiveness of the cardiac pump often results in congestion of blood flow in the systemic or pulmonary venous circulation, as well as an inability to increase cardiac output to meet the demands of activity or increased tissue metabolism. HF is a clinical syndrome characterized by symptoms (dyspnea, fatigue) and signs (edema, rales) on physical examination.

Heart failure is an increasingly common disorder, affecting about 5.5 million Americans, with more than 550,000 new cases diagnosed in the United States each year.[1] Heart failure is the most common reason for hospitalization in patients older than 65 years.[2] The increasing incidence of HF reflects an improved survival rate after myocardial infarction (MI) as well as greater longevity of the population in general. The incidence of HF approaches 10 per 1000 population after age 65.[1]

HEART FAILURE

Etiology and Pathogenesis

A large number of disorders, including most of those discussed in Chapter 18, can lead to the development of heart failure. These disorders are often grouped into ischemic cardiomyopathies and nonischemic cardiomyopathies for comparison and research purposes. The majority of cases of HF are associated with ischemic cardiomyopathy due to coronary artery disease and hypertension.[2] Less common causes of HF include dilated cardiomyopathy, congenital heart defects, valvular disorders, respiratory diseases, anemia, and hyperthyroidism. The diagnosis of heart failure is based on the presence of a constellation of signs and symptoms that are characteristic of the syndrome, however, different sets of criteria are in use, including the Framingham Criteria and Minnesota Heart Failure Criteria.[3] Commonly used criteria for identifying heart failure include the presence of dyspnea, pulmonary rales, cardiomegaly, pulmonary edema, S_3 heart sound, and tachycardia (greater than 120 beats/min), although many other criteria may be applied.

Regardless of specific cause, the pathophysiologic state of heart failure results from impaired ability of myocardial fibers to contract (systolic failure), relax (diastolic failure), or both. Until the late 1980s, systolic dysfunction was thought to be the primary problem in all forms of HF. Now it is evident that about half of patients with chronic HF have preserved systolic function, but impaired diastolic function.[4] Differentiation of heart failure patients as having systolic failure or preserved systolic function is based primarily on the left ventricular ejection fraction (EF). Ejection fraction is calculated by dividing stroke volume by end-diastolic volume. A normal EF is 60% to 80%. Patients with systolic failure have characteristically low ejection fractions (<40%). Patients with EF greater than 50% do not have significant systolic dysfunction and are categorized as HF with normal EF (HFnlEF). The large majority of patients diagnosed with heart failure who have an EF greater than 50%, have diastolic dysfunction.[4] Many patients with low EF also have impaired diastolic function.

The overall mortality for heart failure is high, with about 50% (42% to 65% in various studies) of patients dying within 5 years of diagnosis.[2,5,6] Survival rates vary significantly between sexes, with men having a 35% survival rate at 5 years and women having a 53% survival rate.[5] The median survival time after diagnosis is 1.7 years in men and 3.2 years in women.[5] Patients with low EF but no congestive symptoms have a survival rate about the same as those with preserved EF who have congestive symptoms. The highest mortality occurs in patients with both low EF and congestive symptoms.

Systolic Dysfunction

Patients with systolic dysfunction have reduced myocardial contractility evidenced by a low EF and a reduced dP/dT during ventricular systole. The dP/dT is a measure of **inotropy,** how quickly the ventricle can develop a forceful contraction. The nature of the impaired contractility is only partially understood; however, myocyte loss, mechanical derangements of myocardial cells, and dysregulation of neurohormones are believed to be critical elements.[7]

Impaired contractility due to myocardial infarction (MI) is a common cause of heart failure. MI, with cell death and loss of contractile elements, reduces the heart's contractile force. The degree of pump failure is related to the amount of heart muscle lost. Myocardial cells are also subject to high rates of apoptosis (programmed cell death) in patients with heart failure. Apoptosis can be triggered by excessive stimulation by certain neurohormones and by ischemia. Over time, the loss of pumping cells contributes to reduced contractility.

Inadequate supplies of oxygen to the contracting cells may impair contractility because each myosin cross-bridge cycle requires a molecule of adenosine triphosphate (ATP). When ATP production is low, fewer cross-bridge cycles may be accomplished with each contraction, resulting in a reduced EF.

β-Receptor down-regulation is thought to be an important mechanism of impaired systolic function. Chronic overexcitation of cardiac β receptors by sympathetic neurotransmitters leads to a reduction in the number of β receptors and results in a myocardium that is less responsive to sympathetic stimulation and adrenergic drug therapy. β-Receptor–blocking agents have been shown to improve EF and also to reduce mortality, lending support to the view that chronic excessive sympathetic nervous system (SNS) activation is detrimental to cardiac function.[7]

The severity of systolic failure can be estimated by measuring the amount of blood that the ventricle is able to eject into the arterial system. A reduced stroke volume, reduced cardiac output, and lowered EF are associated with systolic heart failure. In severe systolic failure, the EF may fall below 15% or 20%. In general, the prognosis worsens as EF falls. Symptomatic patients with systolic heart failure often have impaired diastolic function also, which is associated with a higher mortality rate.[4]

Diastolic Dysfunction

Ischemic heart disease and hypertension are the two main causes of diastolic dysfunction, just as they are the primary causes of systolic failure. It is not clear why the same disease processes result in different cardiac dynamics in different individuals, with some having isolated systolic failure, some having isolated diastolic failure, and some exhibiting both abnormal systolic and diastolic function. HF with normal EF is more common in women, the elderly, and those with no history of MI.[4] Diastolic failure is a disorder of myocardial relaxation such that the ventricle is excessively noncompliant and does not fill effectively. Two separate functional processes occur during the diastolic relaxation phase: The first is an energy-requiring process (**lusitropy**) that removes free calcium ions from the cytoplasm by pumping them back into the sarcoplasmic reticulum and across the cell membrane into the extracellular fluid. Removal of calcium ions inhibits cross-bridge formation and allows the thick and thin filaments of the sarcomere to passively slide apart. Ischemia, with subsequent ATP deficiency, interferes with the efficiency of calcium ion removal and can impair the active phase of diastolic relaxation.

The second process is passive stretch of the ventricular myocardium to accommodate filling. Passive compliance of the ventricle can be decreased by deposition of fibrin and collagen during scar formation or by hypertrophic thickening of the ventricular wall. Impairment of both active and passive processes may occur together and are difficult to distinguish clinically.

The hallmark of HF with normal EF is that the patient exhibits clinical manifestations of HF, including low cardiac output, congestion, and edema formation, but has a normal EF (usually defined as greater than 50%), indicating absence of significant systolic impairment.[4] Because prognosis and treatment recommendations may differ, an echocardiogram to measure EF is recommended in all patients with HF to determine the presence of isolated diastolic dysfunction from systolic failure.[4] A comparison of the left ventricular pressure-volume loop in systolic and diastolic dysfunction is shown in Figure 19-1. Systolic failure is characterized by higher than normal diastolic volume and low EF, whereas the pressure-volume loop in diastolic failure indicates poor compliance with a lower diastolic volume at a higher than normal pressure.

KEY POINTS

- HF is a potential consequence of most cardiac disorders. HF occurs when the heart is unable to provide sufficient cardiac output to meet normal metabolic functions of the body.
- The most common cause of HF is myocardial ischemia from coronary artery disease, followed by hypertension and dilated cardiomyopathy.
- Impaired contractility resulting in systolic failure is frequently associated with HF. The biochemical basis of impaired contractility involves loss of cardiac muscle cells, β-receptor down-regulation, and reduced ATP production.

FIGURE 19-1 A comparison of the left ventricular pressure-volume loop in normal heart **(A)**, systolic dysfunction **(B)**, and diastolic dysfunction **(C)**. Note that end-diastolic *pressure* is higher than normal in both systolic and diastolic failure, but end-diastolic *volume* is lower in diastolic dysfunction. *EDV,* End-diastolic volume; *ESV,* end-systolic volume; *EF,* ejection fraction.

- In about half of HF patients, systolic function is preserved and diastolic dysfunction predominates. HF with normal EF is particularly likely to develop in the elderly, in women, and in those without history of MI.
- Left ventricular pressure-volume loops characterize the differences in systolic and diastolic dysfunction. High diastolic volume and reduced EF indicate systolic failure, whereas diastolic failure is characterized by higher diastolic pressure and low volume.

Compensatory Mechanisms and Remodeling

When the heart fails to provide adequate cardiac output to meet tissue demands, a number of compensatory mechanisms are triggered. These mechanisms are helpful in restoring cardiac output toward normal, but in the long term they are detrimental to the heart. Much of the current management of HF is aimed at attenuating the harmful consequences of these compensatory responses.[7] Three main compensatory mechanisms are activated in heart failure: SNS activation, increased preload, and myocardial hypertrophy (Figure 19-2).

Sympathetic Nervous System Activation

Sympathetic activation of the heart is primarily a result of baroreceptor reflex stimulation. The baroreceptors (pressoreceptors) located in the aorta and carotid arteries detect a fall in pressure due to diminished stroke volume and transmit this information to the central nervous system (CNS). The CNS increases activity in the sympathetic nerves to the heart, resulting in increased heart rate and contractility. However, because

of impaired contractile ability, the failing heart may have reduced responsiveness to sympathetic activation. Sympathetic activation also causes venoconstriction, which redistributes blood and increases cardiac preload. Sympathetic constriction of arterioles helps to maintain blood pressure when cardiac output is reduced. Specialized cells in the kidney called *juxtaglomerular cells* also receive SNS stimulation when cardiac output falls. The juxtaglomerular cells release renin and initiate the renin-angiotensin-aldosterone cascade, leading to salt and water retention by the kidney. Sympathetic activation is an early and immediate compensatory response to insufficient cardiac output.

Sympathetic activation is a very effective means for increasing cardiac output in an acute process, such as volume depletion. However, in heart failure, sympathetic activation becomes a chronic process that is ultimately deleterious. A major problem with excessive sympathetic activation is that afterload on the left ventricle can be increased significantly. A high afterload increases cardiac workload and may decrease stroke volume. Therefore, treatment of high blood pressure is important to improve cardiac function in patients with HF.[8]

β-Blocking agents have been advocated in the management of HF to block the cardiac effects of sympathetic activation. Many clinicians had been reluctant to utilize β-blockers in patients with HF because they are negative inotropes and have the potential to reduce cardiac output. In HF, where cardiac output is already low, the use of a negative inotrope would seem to be contraindicated. However, several randomized clinical trials have reported an improved mortality rate in patients receiving certain β-blockers and they are now recommended

FIGURE 19-2 The major compensatory mechanisms in heart failure that act to restore cardiac output. *RAS,* Renin-angiotensin-aldosterone system; *GFR,* glomerular filtration rate; *SNS,* sympathetic nervous system.

as standard therapy in most HF guidelines.[9] Long-term SNS stimulation of the heart may contribute to heart failure progression and remodeling of the cardiac tissue. Remodeling is a process of myocyte loss, hypertrophy of remaining cells, and interstitial fibrosis (Figure 19-3). The remodeled tissue is less functional and may predispose to worsening failure and cardiac dysrhythmias. Numerous other neurohormonal and cytokine derangements have been noted in HF and are under investigation to determine their potential roles in the myocardial remodeling that characterizes HF progression.[7]

Increased Preload

Increased **preload** in the cardiac chambers is initially a consequence of reduced EF with a resultant increase in residual end-systolic volume. Subsequently, decreased cardiac output to the kidney reduces glomerular filtration, resulting in fluid conservation. In addition, the renin-angiotensin-aldosterone cascade is activated because of reduced blood flow to the kidney and SNS activation of the juxtaglomerular cells. Angiotensin II and aldosterone enhance sodium and water reabsorption by the kidney, contributing to an elevated blood volume. Increased preload is a compensatory mechanism that enhances the ability of the myocardium to contract forcefully. An enlarged chamber volume causes the myocardial fibers to

lengthen during diastole, which results in greater fiber shortening during contraction (Frank-Starling mechanism).[10] The diastolic length of the muscle fibers is thought to determine the number of effective cross-bridge cycles that can be accomplished during systole.[10] Thus, up to a point, an increase in the volume or preload of the heart will result in a greater force of contraction (Figure 19-4). The cardiac function curve flattens out at a certain point, and little further benefit is obtained despite increasing preload. Patients with systolic failure have a cardiac function curve that is flat and shifted to the right of normal. Thus, they require a higher preload to achieve a given stroke volume. However, patients with HF often retain so much volume that their hearts are functioning on the flat part of the curve. These patients benefit from preload reduction, which will decrease systemic and pulmonary congestive symptoms and cardiac workload with little or no reduction in cardiac output. Diuretics are commonly used to achieve moderate preload reduction.

Myocardial Hypertrophy and Remodeling

Hypertrophy of cardiac muscle cells is the third mechanism of compensation and generally takes much longer to occur than preload enhancement or sympathetic activation. Hypertrophy appears to result, in part, from a chronic elevation of

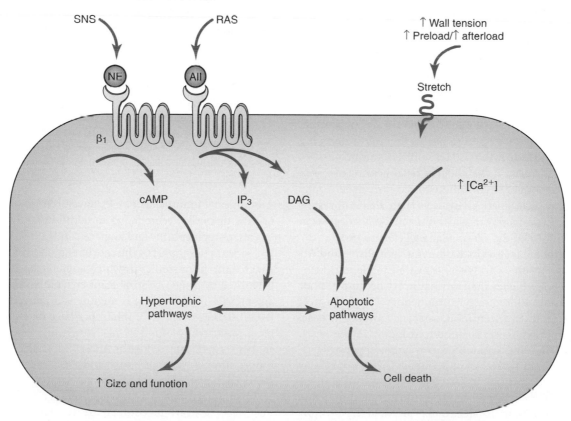

FIGURE 19-3 Mechanisms of ventricular remodeling in heart failure. Activation of β_1 receptors and AII receptors along with stretch of the cell membrane trigger signaling cascades. Under some conditions these triggers lead to effective hypertrophy and an increase in size and function, and in others they trigger apoptotic cell death. *SNS,* Sympathetic nervous system; *NE,* norepinephrine; *RAS,* renin-angiotensin-aldosterone system; *AII,* angiotensin II; *cAMP,* cyclic adenosine monophosphate; *IP₃,* 1,4,5-inositol trisphosphate; *DAG,* diacylglycerol.

FIGURE 19-4 Effect of increased preload on sarcomere length and stroke volume. Systolic failure results in a shift of the curve to the right and a dampening of maximal stroke volume. A greater preload is required to achieve a given stroke volume compared with the normal ventricle.

myocardial wall tension.[7] Wall tension may be high as a result of increased diastolic blood volume (high preload) or as a consequence of high systolic pressures generated in the chamber (to overcome high afterload). The relationship between myocardial wall tension and intrachamber pressure and diameter is described by the law of Laplace: tension = transmural pressure × radius/wall thickness. When the ventricular chamber enlarges and pressures increase, more tension is created in the ventricular muscle wall (Figure 19-5). The development of high systolic pressures in the ventricle may be necessary to overcome a high afterload, such as occurs with arterial hypertension and aortic valve stenosis. The hypertrophy of contractile elements in the myocardium boosts the heart's pumping force and helps to reduce the wall tension back toward normal. In general, an increase in chamber diameter because of excessive preload is thought to contribute to eccentric hypertrophy in which the muscle fibers elongate.[11] High afterload results in concentric hypertrophy in which the muscle fibers grow in diameter and thicken the ventricular wall (Figure 19-6).

Neurohormonal factors including norepinephrine and AII also have hypertrophic effects on the heart. Circulating angiotensin II levels are higher than normal in HF because of poor kidney perfusion, which triggers production of angiotensin II through the renin-angiotensin-aldosterone cascade. In heart failure, angiotensin II is also produced locally in the heart. Angiotensin II binding to its receptor on cardiac myocytes activates genes in the growth pathways. Initially, hypertrophy may help the heart compensate for acute loss of myocardial tissue from MI or help maintain cardiac function during chronic hypertension, but in time the signals that promote hypertrophy are thought to trigger a type of ventricular remodeling that contributes to progression of heart failure. Detrimental remodeling includes loss of myocardial cells through apoptosis and production of fibrous changes in the heart that stiffen the ventricles and contribute to diastolic failure (Figure 19-7).

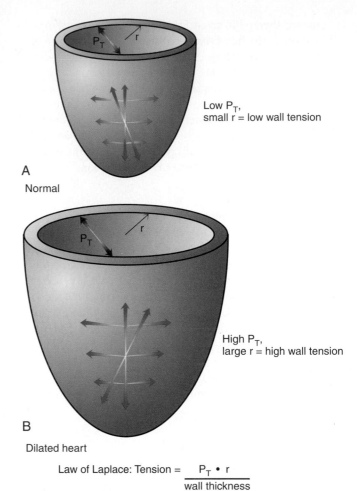

Law of Laplace: Tension = $\dfrac{P_T \cdot r}{\text{wall thickness}}$

FIGURE 19-5 Mechanism of myocardial hypertrophy due to increased ventricular wall tension. According to the law of Laplace, an increase in chamber radius or pressure will increase wall tension. The hypertrophic response increases wall thickness and helps to relieve wall tension. **A,** Heart with normal radius (r) and intraventricular pressure. **B,** Heart with enlarged chamber and high intraventricular pressure. P_T, Transmural pressure.

A number of immune cytokines have been implicated in the process of cardiac remodeling in addition to the neurohormones, norepinephrine and angiotensin II.[7,11]

Evidence in support of the role of angiotensin II in remodeling comes from studies in which angiotensin II production is blocked by drugs. An important enzyme in the pathway of angiotensin II production is angiotensin-converting enzyme (ACE). Drugs called ACE inhibitors have been developed to block the activity of this enzyme. Numerous clinical trials have shown a significant reduction in HF mortality with the administration of ACE inhibitors, and they are considered to be standard therapy.[12]

In summary, enhanced preload and cardiac hypertrophy may allow a heart to compensate for reduced ventricular function for an extended period. Unfortunately, these compensatory mechanisms, which serve to restore cardiac output to the tissues, also result in an increase in myocardial work and oxygen requirements and appear to cause detrimental remodeling. Progression and decompensation may occur

FIGURE 19-6 Forms of ventricular hypertrophy. **A,** Eccentric, in which muscle fibers grow in length and the chamber diameter increases. **B,** Concentric, in which muscle fibers grow in diameter and the ventricular wall becomes thicker. *RV,* Right ventricle; *LV,* left ventricle.

when the primary disease plus the superimposed burdens of compensation overwhelm the heart's ability to generate adequate contractile force. The focus of therapy for HF is to maintain a state of compensation by minimizing cardiac work while optimizing cardiac output and preventing or delaying ventricular remodeling.

KEY POINTS

- Compensatory mechanisms are activated in heart failure in an attempt to improve cardiac output. Unfortunately, these responses also increase myocardial workload and may perpetuate the heart failure. Treatment for HF is aimed at attenuating the harmful effects of the compensatory responses.
- Sympathetic activation is an early response to reduced cardiac output. Sympathetic nervous system activation increases heart rate, contractility, arterial vasoconstriction, and renin release. The failing heart generally has reduced responsiveness to SNS neurotransmitters due to β-receptor down-regulation.
- Decreased cardiac output reduces kidney perfusion and leads to activation of the renin-angiotensin-aldosterone

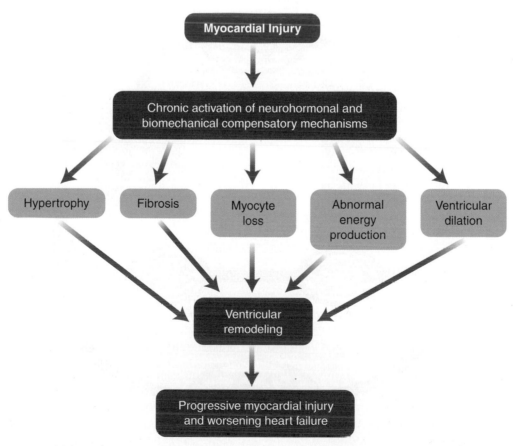

FIGURE 19-7 Mechanisms of cardiac remodeling that contribute to heart failure progression.

cascade and volume retention. Extra blood volume increases cardiac preload. Higher preload results in more forceful ejection of blood from the heart (Frank-Starling law) and improves cardiac output.

- Cardiac hypertrophy is stimulated by elevated myocardial wall tension and the growth-promoting actions of neurohormones, such as norepinephrine and angiotensin II. Hypertrophy adds contractile filaments and improves contractile force.

- The mechanisms that enable the heart to compensate for reduced stroke volume are detrimental in the long term. Excessive neurohormones, volume overload, and high wall tension contribute to abnormal ventricular remodeling. Gradually, the ventricle loses myocytes and accumulates fibrotic tissue. The remaining myocytes are usually hypertrophied. These processes lead to progression of HF over time.

Clinical Manifestations

The clinical presentation of HF differs depending on which ventricle (left, right, or both) is failing to pump blood adequately. Left ventricular failure is the most common presentation of HF. Because of circulatory dynamics, left ventricular failure often leads to right ventricular failure—a condition termed *biventricular failure.* The etiologic process, clinical manifestations, and management of isolated right ventricular failure differ substantially from left ventricular and biventricular failure. Recall that the right side of the heart receives blood from the systemic venous circulation and pumps it into the pulmonary system and the left side of the heart receives blood from the pulmonary circulation and delivers it to the systemic arterial system (Figure 19-8). Insufficient cardiac pumping is manifested by poor cardiac output, called *forward failure,* and by congestion of blood behind the pumping chamber, called *backward failure.* The clinical manifestations of left and right

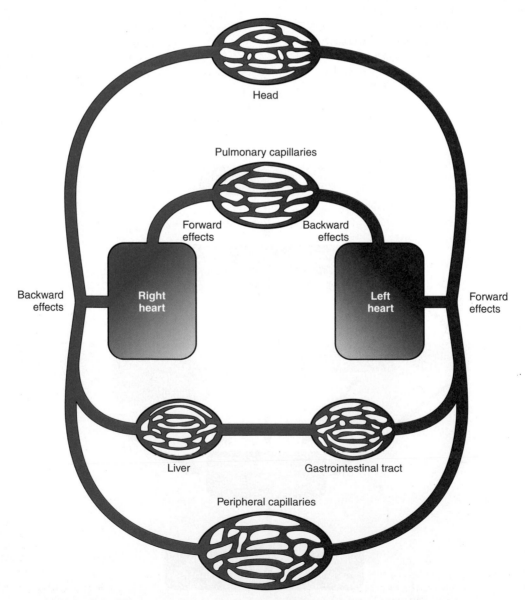

FIGURE 19-8 Systemic and pulmonary circulations viewed as separate but interdependent systems.

ventricular failure differ as a result of the anatomic location of the "backward" or congestive processes, but the forward effects of low cardiac output are the same.

The *forward* effects of HF are due to insufficient cardiac output with diminished delivery of oxygen and nutrients to peripheral tissues and organs. Inadequate perfusion of the brain may lead to restlessness, mental fatigue, confusion, anxiety, and impaired memory. Generalized fatigue, activity intolerance, and lethargy may be present.

Reduced perfusion of the kidney results in a decline in urine output (oliguria) with subsequent fluid retention. Activation of the renin-angiotensin-aldosterone cascade contributes to conservation of sodium and water by the kidney and may also cause vascular constriction. Vascular constriction serves to maintain blood pressure and redistribute reduced cardiac output to vital organs; however, it also increases the afterload against which the damaged left ventricle must pump. If renal blood flow becomes severely limited, the patient with left ventricular failure may develop kidney failure. Forward failure also results in activation of the SNS because of the baroreceptor reflex. Sympathetic activation contributes to vascular constriction and helps maintain blood pressure in the face of reduced cardiac output; however, as with angiotensin II, it increases left ventricular afterload. Sympathetic activation results in a compensatory increase in heart rate that may augment cardiac output to some extent but, again, raises myocardial ATP consumption.

Left-Sided Heart Failure

Left-sided heart failure is most often associated with left ventricular infarction, cardiomyopathy, aortic and mitral valvular disease, and systemic hypertension.[7] The *backward effects* of left-sided heart failure may produce dramatic clinical symptoms due to pulmonary dysfunction (Figure 19-9). Ineffective pumping of the left ventricle results in an accumulation of blood within the pulmonary circulation. As hydrostatic pressure builds within the pulmonary veins and capillaries, fluid is forced from the capillaries into interstitial and alveolar spaces, causing edema. Pulmonary congestion and edema are associated with a number of clinical findings (Figure 19-10). **Dyspnea,** or breathlessness, occurs early in the progression of left-sided heart failure and may be considered the cardinal symptom. Difficulty breathing may be exacerbated by activity (dyspnea on exertion), lying down (**orthopnea** and **paroxysmal nocturnal dyspnea),** and blood volume expansion from excessive salt or fluid intake. Orthopnea and paroxysmal nocturnal dyspnea are due in part to a redistribution of blood volume from the periphery to the heart when the individual lies down. The failing left ventricle is unable to effectively pump extra volume, and pulmonary congestion is worsened. The severity of orthopnea may be quantified by the degree of head elevation (e.g., number of pillows) used to relieve dyspnea. Paroxysmal nocturnal dyspnea refers to intermittent attacks of severe dyspnea during the night and is a most distressing form of orthopnea. The individual experiences

FIGURE 19-9 The pathophysiologic process of isolated left-sided heart failure, showing backward and forward effects. *RAS,* Renin-angiotensin-aldosterone system.

BACKWARD EFFECTS

- Dyspnea on exertion
- Orthopnea
- Cough
- Paroxysmal nocturnal dyspnea
- Cyanosis
- Basilar crackles

FORWARD EFFECTS

- Fatigue
- Oliguria
- ↑Heart rate
- Faint pulses
- Restlessness
- Confusion
- Anxiety

FIGURE 19-10 Clinical manifestations of isolated left-sided heart failure.

a feeling of suffocation and panic at not being able to overcome the dyspnea. Sitting or standing helps to relieve the dyspnea because blood pools in the extremities, reducing pulmonary hydrostatic pressure and congestion.

Clinical signs of pulmonary congestion include cough, respiratory crackles (rales), hypoxemia, high left atrial pressure (LAP), and typical findings on x-ray film. Cough results from bronchial irritation associated with congestion. In severe cases, sputum may be blood tinged, from breakage of fragile capillaries, and frothy, due to fluid buildup in the alveoli. The severity of pulmonary edema can be estimated from the location of crackles within the lung fields. Crackles are abnormal sounds caused by the movement of air through partially fluid-filled alveoli. Edema fluid collects in dependent lung fields because of gravity and progressively moves up the lung as more edema fluid accumulates. For example, in mild pulmonary edema, crackles might be heard with a stethoscope only at the base of the upright lung, but with increasing severity they become apparent in the lower third to half of the lung. Fluid in the alveoli and interstitial spaces also interferes with alveolar-capillary gas exchange and results in some degree of hypoxemia. Hypoxemia may be detected by arterial blood gas analysis or pulse oximetry and may be apparent clinically as cyanosis. **Cyanosis** refers to a blue coloration of the skin typically seen around the mouth (circumoral cyanosis) and results from the presence of significant amounts of desaturated hemoglobin in the blood. Cyanosis is a late sign and is clinically evident only when a large amount (about 5 g/dl) of hemoglobin is deoxygenated (less than or equal to 75% saturated).

Elevated LAP is a common finding in left-sided heart failure due to excessive blood volume and the compensatory responses of atrial dilation and hypertrophy. Atrial pressure can be estimated by inserting a balloon-tipped catheter (Swan-Ganz) into the pulmonary artery. If LAP acutely increases to 25 mm Hg (normal, 4 to 12 mm Hg), increased capillary filtration leads to pulmonary edema. Patients with chronic elevations in LAP associated with chronic HF are more resistant to developing acute pulmonary edema and may not experience symptoms until pressures approach 40 mm Hg.[13] Typical x-ray findings of fluid overload include an enlarged heart and engorged pulmonary capillaries and lymphatic vessels.

Acute cardiogenic pulmonary edema is a life-threatening condition associated with left ventricular failure that severely impairs gas exchange, producing dramatic signs and symptoms. The patient exhibits severe dyspnea and anxiety, and a bolt-upright posture is usually assumed in order to maximize respiratory effort. Bubbly crackles may be heard all the way up the lung from the bases to the apices, and pink frothy sputum may be expectorated or well up from the trachea into the nose and mouth. Anxiety and hypoxemia contribute to tachycardia, which may worsen the pumping efficiency of the failing heart. Cyanosis and symptoms of tissue hypoxia are usually apparent. The immediate treatment is aimed at reducing the fluid volume in the lungs and supporting oxygenation.

Right-Sided Heart Failure

Because the right and left ventricles function in series, left ventricular failure eventually increases the burden on the right ventricle and may cause it to fail as well. The causes of right ventricular failure must therefore include all the causes of left ventricular failure. Isolated right ventricular failure is rare and is usually a consequence of right ventricular infarction or pulmonary disease. Only 3% of MIs occur in the right ventricle; however, right ventricular infarctions are often poorly tolerated and difficult to manage.[7] Pulmonary disorders that result in increased pulmonary vascular resistance impose a high afterload against which the right ventricle must pump. The resultant right ventricular hypertrophy, called **cor pulmonale,** may progress to right ventricular failure as the lung disease worsens.

Any lung disorder that decreases the total cross-sectional area of the lung vasculature can increase pulmonary vascular resistance and produce right ventricular strain. Hypoxemia, for example, causes the pulmonary arterioles to constrict, which increases pulmonary resistance. Constriction or blockage of the vascular bed, such as occurs with pulmonary hypertension or pulmonary embolus, similarly reduces the cross-sectional area of the pulmonary vasculature and leads to increased pulmonary resistance. If the increase in pulmonary resistance and right ventricular workload occurs gradually, the right ventricle can compensate by increasing preload and hypertrophy. However, the thin musculature of the right ventricle has limited ability to adjust to acute changes in workload as would occur with a right ventricular infarction or large pulmonary embolus.

As with left-sided heart failure, congestion of blood occurs behind the failing right ventricle due to inefficiency of the pump. The *backward effects* of right-sided heart failure are due to congestion in the systemic venous system (Figure 19-11). Systemic venous congestion results in impaired function of the liver, portal system, spleen, kidneys, peripheral subcutaneous tissues, and brain (Figure 19-12).

The liver is usually somewhat increased in size and weight, but individual hepatocytes may show signs of atrophy and necrosis due to chronic passive congestion.[11] Impedance to blood flow through the liver may cause hydrostatic pressure to build in the portal system, leading to edema formation in the peritoneal cavity (ascites). Increased pressure in the portal system is reflected back to the spleen and gastrointestinal tract. The spleen is generally enlarged (congestive splenomegaly), and gastrointestinal symptoms such as anorexia and abdominal discomfort may be present.

Increased systemic venous pressure causes congestion of the kidneys, which contributes to the decreased glomerular filtration and fluid retention. Fluid retention may be perpetuated by the congested liver, which is unable to metabolize plasma aldosterone normally.[11] Excess fluid volume and venous congestion caused by right-sided heart failure result in subcutaneous edema. Edema is usually particularly apparent in the lower extremities or sacral area if the patient is supine.

FIGURE 19-11 The pathophysiologic process of isolated right-sided heart failure, showing backward and forward effects. *RAS*, Renin-angiotensin-aldosterone system.

BACKWARD EFFECTS

• Hepatomegaly
• Ascites
• Splenomegaly
• Anorexia
• Subcutaneous edema
• Jugular vein distention

FORWARD EFFECTS

• Fatigue
• Oliguria
• ↑ Heart rate
• Faint pulses
• Restlessness
• Confusion
• Anxiety

FIGURE 19-12 Clinical manifestations of isolated right-sided heart failure.

Drainage of venous blood from the head and neck by way of the superior vena cava is also impeded by right-sided heart failure. The jugular veins may be abnormally distended, and mental functioning may be impaired. The hepatojugular reflux test can be done to assess the severity of right-sided heart failure. The liver is manually compressed, causing a sudden increase in venous blood returning to the right heart, while jugular neck veins are observed for sudden distention. In the absence of right-sided heart failure, the sudden increase in venous return would enter the heart unimpeded and no neck vein distention would be apparent.

Biventricular Heart Failure

In many cases, heart failure is not isolated on one or the other side of the heart. Biventricular failure is most often a result of primary left ventricular failure that has progressed to right-sided heart failure. With biventricular failure, there is reduced cardiac output and there is pulmonary congestion due to left-sided heart failure as well as systemic venous congestion due to right-sided heart failure.

Class and Stage of Heart Failure

A variety of clinical criteria have been used to aid in the diagnosis of HF, but there is no universally accepted diagnostic test. A commonly suggested tool for detecting heart failure in previously undiagnosed individuals is called FACES of heart failure: *fatigue, activity limitation, congestion, edema, shortness of breath.* These are classic findings in HF and, if present, indicate a need for further diagnostic assessment. Traditionally, a patient with suspected HF would be diagnosed by x-ray and echocardiography. Echocardiography is a mainstay of evaluation for HF and is able to measure chamber size, volume, and dynamics during diastole and systole as well as determine ejection fraction. A blood test for B-type natriuretic peptide (BNP) may also be used to help identify patients with HF. BNP is similar to atrial natriuretic peptide (ANP) except that it is manufactured by the ventricular myocytes under conditions of volume overload. A significant correlation between the amount of BNP in the bloodstream and the severity of HF has been documented.[14]

The severity of symptoms can be used to assign a heart failure class (New York Heart Association classes [NYHA] I to IV).[15] Another classification scheme has been proposed by the American Heart Association (AHA) to allow inclusion of patients at high risk for heart failure but whose disease is not yet symptomatic. By including this pre–heart failure group, efforts aimed at prevention may be instituted in more patients. Class and stage are used to determine prognosis, therapy, and monitoring in HF. These two classification schemes are compared in Table 19-1.

KEY POINTS

- The clinical manifestations of HF are characterized by the effects of forward failure (reduced cardiac output) and backward failure (congestion behind the pumping chamber).
- Insufficient cardiac output may be manifested as confusion, fatigue, tachycardia, reduced urine output, and poor peripheral circulation.

TABLE 19-1

Comparison of ACC/AHA Stages of Heart Failure and NYHA Classes

ACC/AHA Stage	Description	Clinical Clues	NYHA Class
A	Patients at high risk of developing HF	Coronary artery disease, hypertension, diabetes, dyslipidemia, family history of cardiomyopathy	Not applicable
B	Patients who have structural heart disease but have never manifested signs or symptoms of HF	Left ventricular hypertrophy (by ECG or echo), valvular disease, past myocardial infarction	I
C	Patients who have current or previous symptoms of HF	Dyspnea, fatigue, exercise intolerance, prior HF hospitalization	II-III
D	Patients with advanced structural heart disease and marked symptoms of HF at rest	End-stage, awaiting transplant, receiving palliative care	IV

Adapted from Hunt SA et al: American College of Cardiology; American Heart Association: ACC/AHA 2005 guideline update for the evaluation and management of chronic heart failure in the adult: summary article, *Circulation* 112(12):1825-1852, 2005. *HF,* Heart failure.

- Left-sided heart failure is characterized by pulmonary congestion, which may manifest with dyspnea, orthopnea, crackles, cough, pulmonary edema, and hypoxemia.
- Right-sided heart failure is characterized by systemic venous congestion, which may manifest with jugular vein distention, hepatomegaly, splenomegaly, and peripheral edema.
- Left-sided heart failure frequently leads to development of right-sided heart failure. With biventricular failure, congestive signs and symptoms are found in both the pulmonary and systemic venous circulation.
- Heart failure is diagnosed by signs and symptoms, x-ray findings, and echocardiographic findings. A plasma BNP level may be used to diagnose HF in patients with shortness of breath.
- The severity of signs and symptoms is used to assign a heart failure class and stage.

Treatment

Therapy for HF is aimed at improving cardiac output while minimizing congestive symptoms and cardiac workload. These objectives are obtained by manipulating preload, afterload, and contractility. When possible, specific treatment is undertaken to correct the underlying cause of the heart failure.

Despite the large number of pharmacologic agents being used in the management of HF, only a few have been associated with significant improvement in mortality risk, particularly ACE inhibitors (and angiotensin-receptor blockers), aldosterone antagonists, and certain β-blockers (Table 19-2).[15] An algorithm proposed by the AHA and American College of Cardiology (ACC) suggests therapy goals and treatments for patients with HF and low EF according to stage of HF (Figure 19-13).

A clearer understanding of the underlying molecular mechanisms of HF is needed to improve pharmacologic management. Little research has been conducted to determine the

TABLE 19-2

Inhibitors of the Renin-Angiotensin-Aldosterone System and β-Blockers Commonly Used for the Treatment of Patients with HF with Low Ejection Fraction

Drug	Initial Daily Dose(s)	Maximum Dose(s)
ACE Inhibitors		
Captopril	6.25 mg 3 times	50 mg 3 times
Enalapril	2.5 mg twice	10 to 20 mg twice
Fosinopril	5 to 10 mg once	40 mg once
Lisinopril	2.5 to 5 mg once	20 to 40 mg once
Perindopil	2 mg once	8 to 16 mg once
Quinapril	5 mg twice	20 mg twice
Ramipril	1.25 to 2.5 mg once	10 mg once
Trandolapril	1 mg once	4 mg once
Angiotensin receptor blockers		
Candesartan	4 to 8 mg once	32 mg once
Losartan	25 to 50 mg once	50 to 100 mg once
Valsartan	20 to 40 mg twice	160 mg twice
Aldosterone antagonists		
Spironolactone	12.5 to 25 mg once	25 mg once or twice
Eplerenone	25 mg once	50 mg once
β-blockers		
Bisoprolol	1.25 mg once	10 mg once
Carvedilol	3.125 mg twice	25 mg twice (50 mg twice for patients > 85 kg)
Metoprolol succinate extended release (metoprolol CR/XL)	12.5 to 25 mg once	200 mg once

ACE, Angiotensin-converting enzyme; *kg,* kilograms; *mg,* milligrams.

From Hunt SA et al: American College of Cardiology; American Heart Association: ACC/AHA 2005 guideline update for the evaluation and management of chronic heart failure in the adult: summary article, *Circulation* 112(12):1825-1852, 2005.

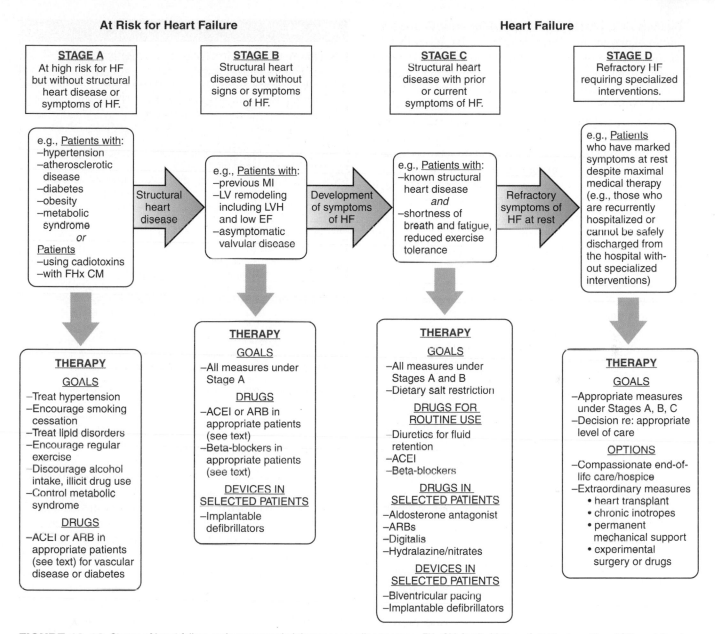

FIGURE 19-13 Stages of heart failure and recommended therapy according to stage. *FHx CM,* family history of cardiomyopathy; *ACEI,* angiotensin-converting enzyme inhibitors; *ARB,* angiotensin receptor blocker. (From Hunt SA et al: American College of Cardiology; American Heart Association: ACC/AHA 2005 guideline update for the evaluation and management of chronic heart failure in the adult: summary article, *Circulation* 112[12]:1825-1852, 2005.)

best treatment for patients with primarily diastolic failure, and treatment recommendations are similar.[3] Many patients with HF have signs and symptoms of elevated preload due to an expanded intravascular volume and a reduced EF. According to the Frank-Starling law, an elevated preload is desirable because it will enhance systolic shortening and improve cardiac output. Unfortunately, high preload exacerbates congestive symptoms and adds to the work of an already damaged heart. The aim of therapy, then, is to optimize preload such that congestive symptoms are minimized but cardiac output is not compromised. The right ventricle is particularly sensitive to reductions in preload, and care must be taken to avoid a significant drop in right ventricular output when intravascular volume is decreased. Drugs may be administered to reduce intravascular

volume, including diuretics and ACE inhibitors. Patients may be instructed to modify salt and fluid intake as well. Diuretics promote the excretion of fluid by increasing renal blood flow, blocking sodium and chloride reabsorption, or both.

With the exception of digitalis, positive inotropic agents are avoided in chronic heart failure because they are associated with higher mortality. However, when improving cardiac output is necessary to avoid shock, positive inotropic agents may be used. Positive inotropes work by increasing the availability of intracellular calcium ions during systole. Drugs that mimic SNS effects, such as norepinephrine, isoproterenol, dobutamine, and dopamine, may be used to improve cardiac output but have a potential for dramatically increasing myocardial oxygen consumption.

Digitalis or a related cardiac glycoside may be used for symptom management of heart failure. Cardiac glycosides directly inhibit the sodium-potassium pump present in the cell membrane of all cells. This results in an increase in intracellular sodium accumulation and a decrease in the gradient for sodium entry into the cell. A diminished sodium gradient slows the sodium-dependent calcium pump that normally removes intracellular calcium. This allows more calcium to remain in the cell, thus strengthening myocardial contraction. Digitalis also slows the heart rate through parasympathetic system activation and promotes sodium and water excretion through improved cardiac output to the kidney. Depletion of serum potassium (hypokalemia) may potentiate digitalis toxicity. Unlike the other positive inotropic agents, digitalis does not appear to increase mortality. Digitalis also does not improve mortality and is not recommended as routine therapy.[16]

Patients with enlarged hearts and conduction delays may benefit from pacemakers, which help to synchronize ventricular contraction. A wide QRS complex is the usual indication for resynchronization therapy in the HF patient. Pacing electrodes are placed in the atrium and both ventricles to allow coordinated depolarization of the heart muscle. Many patients experience significant improvement in congestive symptoms and activity tolerance with resynchronization.

Little research has been conducted to determine the best treatment for patients with HF and normal EF who have primarily diastolic failure. The effectiveness of renin-angiotensin-aldosterone system blocking agents, β-blockers, and digitalis in this population is not well established. Treatment goals are aimed at controlling etiologic factors, such as hypertension and rhythm abnormalities, as well as managing symptoms (Box 19-1).

KEY POINTS

- The primary aims of treatment are to improve cardiac output, minimize congestive symptoms, and prevent progression.
- ACE inhibitors and some β-blocking agents have been shown to improve mortality risk in patients with HF characterized by low EF.
- Diuretics alleviate congestive symptoms and reduce cardiac workload by reducing preload.
- Myocardial contractility may be improved acutely by positive inotropic drugs such as β agonists, however long-term use is associated with higher mortality. An exception is digitalis, which has positive inotropic effects, doesn't appear to alter mortality, and may improve symptoms in some patients.
- Resynchronization of ventricular depolarization with pacemakers may improve contraction in patients with wide QRS complexes.
- Few studies are available to guide therapy in patients with HF characterized by normal EF. Efforts to improve etiologic factors such as hypertension and atrial arrhythmias are recommended.

BOX 19-1

Recommendations for Treatment of Patients with Heart Failure with Normal Ejection Fraction

Physicians should control systolic and diastolic hypertension, in accordance with published guidelines.

Physicians should control ventricular rate in patients with atrial fibrillation.

Physicians should use diuretics to control pulmonary congestion and peripheral edema.

Coronary revascularization is reasonable in patients with coronary artery disease in whom symptomatic or demonstrable myocardial ischemia is judged to be having an adverse effect on cardiac function.

Restoration and maintenance of sinus rhythm in patients with atrial fibrillation might be useful to improve symptoms.

The use of β-adrenergic blocking agents, angiotensin-converting enzyme inhibitors, angiotensin II receptor blockers, or calcium antagonists in patients with controlled hypertension might be effective to minimize symptoms of heart failure.

The use of digitals to minimize symptoms of heart failure is not well established.

Adapted from Hunt SA et al: American College of Cardiology; American Heart Association: ACC/AHA 2005 guideline update for the evaluation and management of chronic heart failure in the adult: summary article, *Circulation* 112(12):1825-1852, 2005.

CARDIAC DYSRHYTHMIAS

Dysrhythmia or arrhythmia refers to an abnormality of the cardiac rhythm of impulse generation or conduction. A normal heartbeat is initiated at an appropriate rate in the sinoatrial (SA) node and follows a consistent pathway of depolarization through the atria, atrioventricular (AV) node, His-Purkinje system, and, finally, the ventricular myocardium (see Chapter 17). Electrical depolarization of the heart is normally followed by atrial and then ventricular muscular contraction. A number of factors may lead to disturbances in heartbeat, including hypoxia, electrolyte imbalance, trauma, inflammation, and drugs. Dysrhythmias are significant for two reasons: (1) they indicate an underlying pathophysiologic disorder and (2) they can impair normal cardiac output. Dysrhythmias can be categorized into three major types: abnormal rates of sinus rhythm, abnormal sites (ectopic) of impulse initiation, or disturbances in conduction pathways.

Dysrhythmia Mechanisms

Dysrhythmias are believed to arise from three mechanisms: inappropriate automaticity, triggered activity, or reentrant mechanisms.

Automaticity

Inappropriate automaticity implies that an atrial or ventricular cell that normally doesn't spontaneously depolarize acquires the ability to initiate action potentials. Failure to repolarize to normal resting membrane potential or plasma membrane leakiness to sodium or calcium ions at rest (phase 4) is thought to cause a shift in the resting membrane potential toward threshold, generating an action potential. Ischemia and subsequent ATP deficiency reduce the cell's ability to control electrolyte flux across the cell membrane. Electrolyte imbalance, particularly hypokalemia, contributes to abnormal automaticity.

Triggered Activity

Triggered activity occurs when an impulse is generated during or just after repolarization because of a depolarizing oscillation of the membrane potential (Figure 19-14). Early afterdepolarizations occur during the relative refractory period of phase 3 in patients with abnormally long repolarization times (prolonged QT syndrome). The prolonged action potential is thought to allow some of the voltage-gated calcium channels to reopen during phase 3 and trigger another impulse[17] (see Figure 19-14, *A*). Delayed or late afterdepolarizations occur after the repolarization phase is complete and are seen as oscillating depolarizing waves on the ECG (see Figure 19-14, *B*). If the delayed afterdepolarization reaches threshold, it will trigger an action potential. Digitalis toxicity and excessive catecholamine stimulation may contribute to this mechanism. Delayed afterdepolarizations are thought to occur because calcium ions are ineffectively removed from the cytoplasm during muscle relaxation. An increase in Ca^{2+} during phase 4 can trigger release of more Ca^{2+} from the sarcoplasmic reticulum and trigger an action potential.[17] A number of genetic abnormalities in intracellular calcium handling have been associated with triggered activity mechanisms.

Reentry

Reentry is thought to be the culprit in most tachydysrhythmias, including atrial and ventricular tachycardia, flutter, and fibrillation. Reentry is a complex process in which a cardiac impulse continues to depolarize in a part of the heart after the main impulse has finished its path and the majority of the fibers have repolarized. If the errant impulse proceeds slowly enough, it may eventually meet with nonrefractory cells and initiate an extra, ectopic cardiac depolarization. Reentry processes are produced when electrical conduction in a portion of the heart is abnormally slowed (functional) or has an unusually long pathway (anatomic). A number of theories have been proposed to describe the generation and conduction of reentry depolarizations including specific subsets of cells that continue to produce waves of activation or more general involvement of the myocardial tissue in propagating waves of conduction. Reentry depolarizations may occur as complex spiral waves in which the activating wavefront follows or "chases" its repolarizing tail (Figure 19-15). If the wavefront encounters only refractory tissue, the reentrant process suddenly terminates.[18] Myocardial ischemia and electrolyte abnormalities predispose to reentry mechanisms.

Dysrhythmia Analysis

ECG recording paper is specifically designed to allow easy measurement of waveform amplitude and duration (Figure 19-16). Each small box on the ECG paper represents an amplitude of 0.1 mV and a duration of 0.04 second (paper speed at 25 mm/sec).[19] Larger boxes are also marked on the paper and correspond to 0.5 mV in amplitude (five small boxes) and

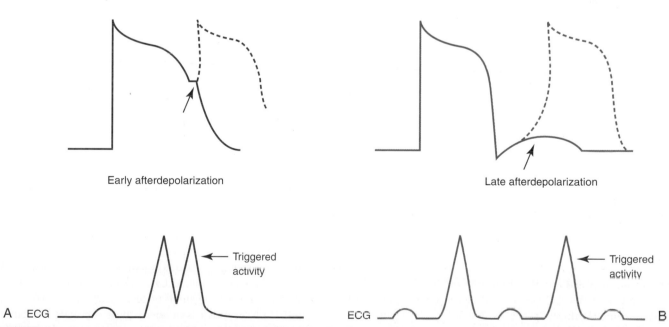

FIGURE 19-14 Mechanisms of triggered activity. **A,** Early afterdepolarization in ventricular cell showing triggered action potential during the repolarization phase. The electrocardiogram *(ECG)* shows an R wave occurring on top of the T wave (R-on-T phenomenon). **B,** Late or delayed afterdepolarization occurs after the repolarization phase has been completed and results in an early beat after the T wave. If the late afterdepolarization does not reach threshold, no triggered beat will occur.

FIGURE 19-15 Mechanism of reentry. **A,** A wave of depolarization that travels slowly or by an abnormal pathway may encounter myocardium that has had time to recover and can restimulate it. **B,** This may result in an extra beat, or the depolarization may continuously "chase its tail" in a circuit, causing defibrillation. The circuit can be relatively fixed or can wander into various "wavelets."

FIGURE 19-16 Electrocardiographic strip showing the markings for measuring amplitude and duration of waveforms, using a standard recording speed of 25 mm/sec.

0.2 second in duration (five small boxes). These markings allow measurement of waveform amplitude, duration, and heart rate. Rhythm strips presented in this chapter are from a single lead only (usually lead II), but it should be emphasized that thorough ECG interpretation often requires several leads to provide different views of electrical conduction through the heart. (Lead placement is discussed in Chapter 17.)

Normal Sinus Rhythm

Before one proceeds to the interpretation of dysrhythmias, the features of normal sinus rhythm must be understood. Normal sinus rhythm is generally defined as an impulse rate between 60 and 100 per minute that begins in the sinus node and follows the normal conduction pathway. Characteristics of normal sinus rhythm are listed in Table 19-3. The rhythm shown in Figure 19-17 is regular; there is a P wave for every

QRS complex; the PR, QRS, and QT intervals are of normal duration; and there are no "funny-looking" beats.

There are several methods for determining heart rate using the rhythm strip. The easiest but least accurate method is to count the number of QRS complexes within 6 seconds and multiply by 10. Electrocardiogram (ECG) paper has 3-second marks along the top that can be used to determine a 6-second interval. A more accurate method for determining heart rate is to count the number of small boxes between complexes. The number of boxes is divided by 1500 to determine heart rate because there are 1500 small boxes per minute (1500 × 0.04 second = 60 seconds). Neither of these methods is accurate with irregular rhythms, so heart rate must be calculated for a longer interval, usually 1 minute. With this understanding of rate calculation and methods to measure the duration and amplitude of waveforms, one can analyze dysrhythmias.

TABLE 19-3

Electrocardiographic Characteristics of Normal Sinus Rhythm

Characteristic	Findings
Rhythm	Regular, PP intervals and RR intervals may vary as much as 3 mm and still be considered regular
Rate	60 to 100 beats/min
P waves	One P wave preceding each QRS
PR interval	0.12 to 0.20 second, constant
QRS duration	0.04 to 0.10 second, constant
QT interval	0.40 second (varies with rate)

FIGURE 19-18 Sinus tachycardia (rate, 150/min).

FIGURE 19-19 Sinus bradycardia (rate, 35/min).

FIGURE 19-17 Normal sinus rhythm (rate, 64/min).

KEY POINTS

- Dysrhythmias are initiated by three types of depolarizing mechanisms: abnormal automaticity, triggered activity from afterdepolarizations, and reentrant circuits.
- Measurement of ECG waveform amplitude, duration, and frequency is necessary to analyze cardiac rhythms. ECG paper is marked in small boxes representing 0.1 mV of amplitude and 0.04 second of duration.
- Normal sinus rhythm is characterized by regular PP and RR intervals, a rate of 60 to 100 beats/min, and normal PR (0.12 to 0.20 second) and QRS (0.04 to 0.10 second) intervals.

Abnormal Rates of Sinus Rhythm

Sinus Tachycardia

Sinus tachycardia is an abnormally fast heart rate of greater than 100 beats/min (Figure 19-18). A number of factors, including sympathetic activation, decreased parasympathetic activity, fever, hyperthyroidism, pain, increased metabolism, low blood pressure, and hypoxia, can lead to sinus tachycardia, making it a very common dysrhythmia. Sinus tachycardia often is a compensatory response to increased demand for cardiac output or reduced stroke volume. Treatment is aimed at correcting the underlying cause. In some instances, however, the rate can become so high that ventricular filling is impaired and cardiac output is compromised. The heart rate at which this occurs will vary depending on age and cardiac

function. Sympatholytic agents or calcium channel–blocking agents may then be indicated.

Sinus Bradycardia

Traditionally a heart rate of less than 60 beats/min is called *bradycardia;* however, lower rates are commonly encountered in physically trained individuals. Sinus bradycardia results from slowed impulse generation by the sinus node in response to increased parasympathetic activity, sleep, drugs, increased stroke volume, or acute hypertension (baroreceptor reflex). Important features of sinus bradycardia are shown in Figure 19-19. Sinus bradycardia may be a normal finding in well-conditioned individuals who have large resting stroke volumes. Abnormal parasympathetic activation can result from pain (vasovagal), carotid sinus massage, endotracheal suctioning, and the Valsalva maneuver (bearing down). Slow heart rates may be well tolerated by some individuals and not require treatment. If the slow heart rate precipitates low cardiac output, it is usually treated with sympathomimetic or parasympatholytic drugs.

Sinus Arrhythmia

A degree of variability in the heart rate, or sinus arrhythmia, is a normal finding associated with fluctuations in autonomic influences and respiratory dynamics. Sinus arrhythmia can be particularly pronounced in children. Sinus arrhythmia must be differentiated from a sinus node irregularity called *sick sinus syndrome,* in which alternating periods of sinus bradycardia and tachycardia occur (Figure 19-20). Sick sinus syndrome may necessitate implantation of a permanent pacemaker. Sinus arrhythmia is a normal finding and thus requires no treatment.

FIGURE 19-20 A, Sinus arrhythmia is a normal finding that may be particularly pronounced in children. **B,** Sick sinus syndrome. The strip shows alternating periods of tachycardia and bradycardia.

Sinus Arrest

The absence of impulse initiation in the heart results in electrical *asystole*. It is characterized by a flat ECG lacking recognizable waveforms (Figure 19-21). Electrical asystole results in mechanical asystole and zero cardiac output. An escape rhythm from a slower pacemaker will generally begin to fire after several seconds of sinus arrest. Sinus arrest may result from MI, electrical shock, electrolyte disturbances, acidosis, and extreme parasympathetic activity. Prolonged complete electrical asystole is unlikely, and fine ventricular fibrillation may be the underlying rhythm. Sinus arrest may be treatable with a cardiac pacemaker.

FIGURE 19-21 Electrical asystole.

Abnormal Site of Impulse Initiation

Initiation of a cardiac impulse at a site other than the SA node occurs primarily for two reasons. First, SA node failure may allow a slower pacemaker to take over. Takeover by a slower pacemaker is called an *escape rhythm*. Second, enhanced excitability, triggered activity, or reentrant circuits may cause a premature depolarization and override the SA node.

Escape Rhythms

Escape beats can originate in the AV nodal region or in the ventricular Purkinje fibers. A junctional escape rhythm originates in the AV node, has a rate of 40 to 60 per minute, and has a normal QRS configuration (Figure 19-22). A ventricular escape rhythm originates in the Purkinje fibers, has a rate of 15 to 40, and is characterized by an abnormally wide QRS complex on the ECG (Figure 19-23). An important clue to identifying escape rhythms is the absence of normal P waves and PR intervals. After the impulse is generated in the Purkinje

---

KEY POINTS

- Sinus tachycardia (more than 100 beats/min) usually occurs from sympathetic activation of the heart. SNS activation may be compensatory (e.g., occurring in the setting of low blood pressure, low cardiac output, or hypoxemia) or may be due to pain and anxiety.
- Sinus bradycardia (less than 60 beats/min) usually occurs in response to parasympathetic activity. Bradycardia is treated if the slow heart rate precipitates inadequate cardiac output.
- Sinus arrhythmia is usually normal and more pronounced in young persons than in older adults.
- Sinus arrest may lead to prolonged intervals of electrical asystole and zero stroke volume until another pacemaker begins to fire. An artificial pacemaker may be required.

or nodal cell, it can be conducted backward to the atria (retrograde P wave). Thus, a P wave, if present, may be inverted and located before, during, or after the QRS complex. Escape rhythms are usually poorly tolerated because they are slow and associated with decreased cardiac output. Failure of the sinus node can be managed with a pacemaker.

Atrial Dysrhythmias

Premature Atrial Complexes and Tachycardia. Premature atrial complexes (PACs) originate in the atria but not at the SA node. The PAC occurs earlier than normal, is preceded by a P wave, and has a normal QRS configuration (Figure 19-24). P waves preceding the PAC usually have a different shape (morphology) than the sinus beats. Sometimes the PAC is not conducted through the AV node to the ventricle and is not followed by a QRS complex (nonconducted P wave). Isolated or rare PACs are not clinically significant. However, frequent PACs may indicate an underlying pathophysiologic process and may be precursors to more serious dysrhythmias. Paroxysmal focal

atrial tachycardia is a burst of atrial complexes resembling several PACs in a row (Figure 19-25). The rhythm is regular at a usual rate of 130 to 240 beats/min. It may be difficult to distinguish this rhythm from sinus tachycardia; however, differences in P-wave configuration are usually apparent. The period of atrial tachycardia may last for minutes, hours, or days and can result in ischemia. Patients may perceive atrial tachycardia as palpitations and may experience chest pain. Focal atrial tachycardia can occur in persons with no underlying heart disease in response to emotional stress or drugs. An episode may start as a PAC that has an abnormally slow conduction time through the atria and AV node. This is thought to allow the wave of depolarization to reexcite previously depolarized cells, resulting in reentry and perpetuation of the abnormal rhythm.

Atrial Flutter and Fibrillation. Atrial flutter is typically manifested by a rapid atrial rate of 240 to 350 beats/min and a characteristic saw-tooth pattern of atrial depolarizations (Figure 19-26). There is overlap in the mechanism of atrial tachycardia and atrial flutter, and several types of flutter have been described. These are commonly categorized according to atrial rate; type I (typical) has rates of 240 to 350 per minute, and type II has rates in excess of 350 per minute. The QRS configuration is normal; however, some of the atrial depolarizations do not conduct through the AV node, resulting in a slower ventricular rate. The ventricular rate may be irregular if there is a variable block or may be regular if there is a uniform block, such as 2:1 or 3:1. Reentry is the probable mechanism for typical atrial

FIGURE 19-22 Junctional escape rhythm (rate, 59/min).

FIGURE 19-23 Ventricular escape rhythm (rate, 33/min).

FIGURE 19-24 Premature atrial complex *(arrow)*. Note early P wave and different P-wave morphology.

FIGURE 19-25 Paroxysmal focal atrial tachycardia *(PFAT)* followed by transition to normal sinus rhythm *(NSR)*.

FIGURE 19-26 Atrial flutter with four atrial depolarizations to one ventricular depolarization.

flutter. Persons exhibiting atrial flutter usually have underlying heart disease, fluid overload, or atrial ischemia.

Atrial fibrillation is a completely disorganized and irregular atrial rhythm accompanied by an irregular ventricular rhythm of variable rate (Figure 19-27). The atrial impulses appear as small, squiggly waves of various sizes and shapes. Atrial fibrillation is sustained by multiple reentrant "wavelets" that continually change in size and direction. The majority of atrial depolarizations are blocked at the AV node, with few reaching the ventricles and initiating ventricular contraction. Atrial fibrillation causes the atria to quiver rather than to contract forcefully. This allows blood to become stagnant in the atria and may lead to formation of thrombi. Atrial fibrillation may occur intermittently or be sustained in the long term. Patients with chronic atrial fibrillation often are treated with anticoagulant medications to prevent atrial clot formation. Atrial fibrillation is a significant risk factor for cerebrovascular stroke. Patients with heart failure may experience more symptoms when they are in atrial fibrillation because the usual "atrial kick" that normally adds 15% to 20% more blood to the ventricle prior to systole is lost and therefore cardiac output may be reduced. Cardioversion with an electrical shock to the chest is commonly used to manage atrial fibrillation. Numerous antiarrhythmic agents can be used to convert atrial fibrillation to sinus rhythm or control the ventricular response rate, including calcium channel blockers, β-blockers, digitalis, and amiodarone.

Junctional Dysrhythmias

Premature junctional complexes can be initiated in two junctional zones: in the area just proximal to the AV node, where atrial fibers enter, or in the area just distal to the AV node, where nodal fibers enter the bundle of His. The impulse spreads upward into the atrium, causing a P wave, and downward into the ventricle, causing a normally configured QRS complex. The P wave may precede, follow, or be buried in the QRS complex. Premature junctional beats have the same clinical significance as PACs and are generally well tolerated.

Junctional tachycardia is a rapid junctional discharge in the range of 70 to 140 beats/min (Figure 19-28). The rhythm resembles a series of junctional premature beats, with P waves preceding, following, or buried in the QRS complexes. Differentiation of the electrocardiographic pattern produced by junctional tachycardia from that produced by atrial tachycardia is often difficult, and the term *supraventricular tachycardia* may be used for both.

Ventricular Dysrhythmias

Premature Ventricular Complexes. Premature ventricular complexes (PVCs) arise from the ventricular myocardium. The impulse depolarizes the ventricles but does not activate the atria or depolarize the sinus node. Thus, the normal rhythm of sinus discharge is not disturbed. The normal sinus impulse is generally buried in the bizarre-looking QRS from the premature ventricular beat. The sinus impulse does not result in a QRS complex because the ventricles are refractory from the premature depolarization. The next sinus beat occurs just when it would have occurred normally if there had been no premature beat. Thus, the interval between the sinus beat preceding the premature beat and the sinus beat following the premature beat is twice the regular interval (Figure 19-29). This is known as a *compensatory pause* and helps confirm the diagnosis of PVCs. The QRS of the premature complex is prolonged (more than 0.10 second) and bizarre in appearance. The T wave is usually in a direction opposite to the main QRS deflection. Premature ventricular beats are commonly associated with coronary artery disease, drug overdose, and electrolyte disturbances—particularly hypokalemia and hypomagnesemia. The clinical significance depends in part on the frequency of the premature beats. The PVCs may occur at regular intervals, such as bigeminy (every other beat) or trigeminy (every third beat). With high frequency, cardiac output may be compromised. Frequent PVCs may be managed with antiarrhythmic drugs, such as amiodarone.

FIGURE 19-28 Junctional tachycardia (rate, 108/min). Note that P waves follow the QRS waves because of retrograde depolarization spreading from the atrioventricular node to the atria. This rhythm may also be called supraventricular tachycardia.

FIGURE 19-29 Premature ventricular complex.

FIGURE 19-27 Atrial fibrillation showing an irregularly irregular ventricular response.

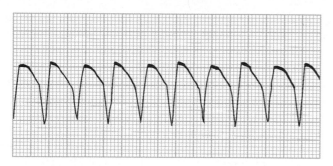

FIGURE 19-30 Ventricular tachycardia (rate, 178/min).

FIGURE 19-31 Ventricular fibrillation.

However, prophylactic use of antiarrhythmic drugs in patients with asymptomatic disease is not recommended. In some groups (e.g., after MI), certain antiarrhythmics have been linked to higher mortality.[18]

Ventricular Tachycardia. Ventricular tachycardia consists of three or more consecutive ventricular complexes at a rate greater than 100/min (Figure 19-30). The rhythm is fairly regular, and the complexes generally have the same configuration (monomorphic). With rapid rates, it may be difficult to distinguish the QRS complexes from the ST segments and T waves, and the ECG depicts a series of large, wide, undulating waves. The sinus node usually continues to discharge independently of the ventricular rhythm, and P waves, if seen, are not associated with the QRS complexes.

Reentry is the probable mechanism of ventricular tachycardia in most cases, although automaticity and triggered activity have also been implicated. Ventricular tachycardia is often associated with myocardial ischemia and infarction. Damage to the myocardium alters conduction times and conduction pathways, which sets the stage for reentry loops. High catecholamine levels and an abnormal electrolyte balance may contribute to the dysrhythmogenesis.

Ventricular tachycardia is a serious dysrhythmia that is nearly always indicative of significant heart disease. It may be fatal unless it is successfully and rapidly managed. Ventricular tachycardia may compromise cardiac output, resulting in loss of consciousness. Treatment consists of administration of antiarrhythmic drugs and, if necessary, cardiopulmonary resuscitation and electrical cardioversion.

Ventricular Fibrillation. Ventricular fibrillation is a rapid, uncoordinated cardiac rhythm that results in ventricular quivering and lack of effective contraction. The rhythm is generally easily identified, particularly when assessment of the patient indicates absence of pulse and loss of consciousness. The ECG is rapid and erratic, with no identifiable QRS complexes (Figure 19-31). Ventricular fibrillation results in death if not reversed within minutes.

The same conditions that result in ventricular tachycardia may cause ventricular fibrillation. A critically timed premature beat or accelerating ventricular tachycardia may be the precursor to ventricular fibrillation. The ventricular depolarization is thought to be fractionated into a number of localized reentrant currents within the myocardial mass.

The uncoordinated depolarizations are sustained because of variability in conduction velocities and refractory periods.

Ventricular fibrillation must be rapidly identified and managed with cardiopulmonary resuscitation and defibrillation with electrical current. Defibrillation differs from cardioversion in that the administration of current is not synchronized with the R wave and the amount of energy delivered is greater (200 to 350 J). The earlier the defibrillation is performed, the better is the chance for successful resuscitation. In some instances, the ventricular fibrillation pattern is very fine and is similar to the tracing seen in atrial arrest. Defibrillation is still indicated. Defibrillation and cardiopulmonary resuscitation are usually followed by administration of antiarrhythmic drugs.

KEY POINTS

- Failure of the SA node to generate impulses may result in a junctional or ventricular escape rhythm. These rhythms are slow and may be poorly tolerated. Absence of P waves is important in determination of escape rhythms.
- In most cases, premature beats and ectopic rhythms are attributed to reentry mechanisms. Reentry circuits may be established when portions of the heart have abnormal conduction rates or pathways. Enhanced automaticity and triggered activity are alternative mechanisms for generation of ectopic complexes.
- Atrial dysrhythmias include premature atrial complexes, tachycardia, flutter, and fibrillation. Atrial dysrhythmias are usually well tolerated unless the ventricular response rate is significantly altered.
- Junctional tachycardias are difficult to distinguish from atrial tachycardias and they are often regarded together as supraventricular tachycardias.
- Frequent PVCs, tachycardia, and ventricular fibrillation are associated with a significant fall in cardiac output and must be rapidly diagnosed and managed.

Conduction Pathway Disturbances

Disorders of cardiac impulse conduction include delays, blocks, and abnormal pathways. Cardiac ischemia and infarction commonly are associated with conduction blocks and delays, whereas abnormal pathways are usually congenital.

Disturbances of Atrioventricular Conduction

A disturbance in conduction between the sinus impulse and its associated ventricular response has been called *atrioventricular block*. The conduction may be abnormally slowed or completely blocked. The AV block results from a functional or pathologic defect in the AV node, bundle of His, or bundle branches. Three categories of AV block have traditionally been described: first-degree block, second-degree block (which includes types I and II), and third-degree (complete) block. These AV conduction disorders are associated with different pathologic processes and clinical implications.

First-degree block is generally identified by a prolonged PR interval (more than 0.20 second) on the ECG (Figure 19-32). The rhythm remains regular, and each P wave is associated with a QRS complex. First-degree block is a common finding and may occur in the absence of organic heart disease. Drugs and organic heart disorders, such as myocardial ischemia and congenital heart defects, may cause first-degree block. First-degree block is generally monitored but is not actively managed except to alleviate the underlying cause if possible.

Second-degree block is diagnosed when some of the atrial impulses are not conducted to the ventricles. Two types of second-degree block are identified by the pattern of nonconducted impulses. Type I (Mobitz type I, Wenckebach) is associated with progressively lengthening PR intervals until one P wave is not conducted (dropped beat). The pattern repeats, causing the QRS complexes to occur in groups. The PP intervals are constant, whereas the RR intervals vary (Figure 19-33). Type I second-degree block is usually due to reversible ischemia of the AV node, often associated with acute MI. The ischemic node is slow to recover after each depolarization, resulting in a longer and longer nodal delay until one impulse is not conducted. This gives the AV node time to recover, and the next atrial impulse is conducted more quickly, with a nearly normal PR interval, beginning the cycle again. Treatment is rarely required. If the block progresses to a type II block, a pacemaker may be required.

Type II second-degree block is identified by the presence of nonconducted P waves (dropped beats) with a consistent PR interval (Figure 19-34). The QRS complex is usually, but not always, wide (0.12 second or greater). Type II block is generally associated with pathologic lesion of the bundle of His, the right bundle branch, or both. It is the bundle branch block that causes the QRS complexes to be abnormally wide. Type II second-degree block is less common than type I but is more serious. It is usually associated with anterior septal MI or fibrosis of the conduction system. Type II block may

FIGURE 19-32 First-degree atrioventricular block; PR interval, 0.32 second.

FIGURE 19-33 Second-degree atrioventricular block, type I (Wenckebach, Mobitz type I). Note the progressive lengthening of the PR interval until one P wave is not conducted (dropped).

FIGURE 19-34 Second-degree atrioventricular (AV) block, type II (Mobitz type II). Every third P wave is followed by a QRS complex. The other P waves are not conducted through the AV node. The PR interval on conducted impulses is constant.

progress to complete heart block with slow ventricular escape rhythm and poor cardiac output. Type II block may also result in severe bradycardia due to the number of dropped beats. Symptomatic type II block may require implantation of a pacemaker.

Third-degree block may occur as a result of pathologic lesion of the AV node, bundle of His, or bundle branches. No impulses are conducted from the atria to the ventricles, and a junctional or ventricular escape rhythm is evident. The ECG shows regularly occurring P waves that are totally independent of the ventricular rhythm (Figure 19-35). If the QRS complex is narrow, the block is most likely in the AV node, proximal to the bundle of His. A prolonged QRS interval (more than 0.12 second) indicates pathology distal to the bundle of His, within the bundle branches. The severity of symptoms is determined primarily by the heart rate, with slower rhythms being more serious. A pacemaker is generally required.

Abnormal Conduction Pathways

Some individuals have congenital abnormalities of the cardiac conduction system called *accessory pathways*. These extra conduction tracts provide alternative pathways for depolarization of the heart, resulting in abnormally early ventricular depolarizations following atrial depolarizations. The best known of these preexcitation syndromes is Wolff-Parkinson-White syndrome. This syndrome is caused by accessory pathways that originate in the atria, bypass the AV node, and enter a site in the ventricular myocardium. This results in more rapid activation of the ventricle, a short PR interval, initial slurring of the QRS (δ wave), and a wide QRS complex (Figure 19-36). The accessory pathway may provide a mechanism for reentry and the development of supraventricular tachycardia. Identification and treatment of individuals with preexcitation syndromes is desirable to prevent

symptoms of supraventricular tachycardia and to reduce the possibility of deterioration of the rhythm to atrial or ventricular fibrillation. Antidysrhythmic agents and measures to interrupt the pathway, such as vagal stimulation, may be used.

Intraventricular Conduction Defects

Abnormal conduction of impulses through the intraventricular bundle branches is called *bundle branch block*. The two primary bundles are the right bundle branch, which supplies the right ventricle, and the left bundle branch, which supplies the left ventricle. The left bundle branch is further divided into three fascicles: anterior, posterior, and septal (Figure 19-37). These supply the anterior, posterior, and septal portions of the left ventricle, respectively. Slowed or obstructed conduction occurring in one or more of these bundles results in abnormal ventricular depolarization and wide, bizarre-appearing QRS complexes. Bundle branch blocks are best detected with ECG leads V_1 and V_6.

Right bundle branch block may be present in almost any form of heart disease. It is occasionally found in individuals having no clinical evidence of heart disease. Right bundle branch block can progress to complete heart block in some cases. The electrocardiographic pattern is indicative of blocked conduction to the right ventricle such that the left ventricle depolarizes first, then spreads to the right ventricle. Right bundle branch block is classically associated with a late R wave in lead V_1 and an S wave in V_6. These changes are compared with the normal V_1 and V_6 in Figure 19-38.

Left bundle branch block causes a delay in left ventricular depolarization. The right ventricle is activated first through the right bundle branch, followed by right to-left activation of the septum and, finally, left ventricular activation. The QRS complex is abnormally wide (more than 0.12 second) but has a nearly normal deflection pattern in V_1 and V_6. In V_1, the

FIGURE 19-35   Complete third-degree atrioventricular block. Note that there is no relationship between P waves and QRS complexes because the atria and ventricles are depolarizing independently.

FIGURE 19-36   Electrocardiogram in lead II from a patient with Wolff-Parkinson-White syndrome. Note the slurred upstroke of the R wave (delta wave). (From Conover MB: *Understanding electrocardiography*, ed 8, St Louis, 2003, Mosby, p 288.)

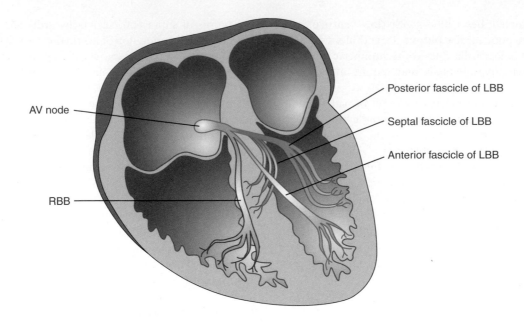

FIGURE 19-37 The right bundle branch *(RBB)* innervates the right ventricle. The left bundle branch *(LBB)* has three divisions: the posterior, septal, and anterior fascicles. *AV,* Atrioventricular.

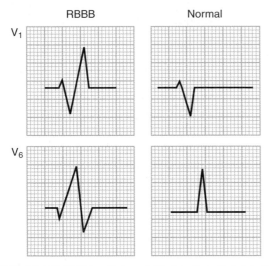

FIGURE 19-38 Right bundle branch block pattern. Note late R wave in V_1 and abnormal S wave in V_6.

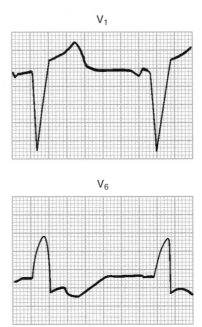

FIGURE 19-39 Left bundle branch block pattern. Note wide S wave in V_1 and wide R wave in V_6.

small R wave normally associated with septal depolarization is absent, and V_6 consists of a wide R wave (Figure 19-39).

Left anterior fascicular block is also called *anterior hemiblock.* Impaired conduction in the anterior fascicle causes the posterior aspect of the left ventricle to be activated first, followed by spread through the left ventricular myocardium in an upward and leftward direction. The electrocardiographic pattern shows small initial R waves followed by large S waves in leads II and III. The duration of the QRS complex is within normal limits.

Left posterior fascicular block (hemiblock) is due to a block in the posterior fascicle of the left bundle, which causes the anterior left ventricle to be activated first, followed by spread in a downward and rightward direction. The electrocardiographic findings include Q wave in leads II, III, and aV_F and

R wave in leads I and aV_L. These electrocardiographic findings may mimic ventricular hypertrophy or inferolateral MI, making recognition difficult.

Slowed or obstructed conduction may occur simultaneously in more than one bundle or fascicle, leading to the terms *bifascicular block* and *trifascicular block.* For example, a right bundle branch block occurring in conjunction with a left posterior hemiblock is called a *bilateral* or *bifascicular block.* Trifascicular block refers to a bifascicular bundle block (most commonly right bundle branch block with left anterior hemiblock) in addition to a first-degree block (prolonged PR interval). The prolonged PR interval is usually due to incomplete block in the left posterior fascicle. Complete trifascicular block would make it impossible for a supraventricular depolarization to activate the ventricles and would be a third-degree or complete heart block.

a rhythm showing a consistent PR interval with some nonconducted P waves. This block is more serious because it has a tendency to progress to complete AV (third-degree) block.

KEY POINTS

- Disturbances of AV conduction are generally referred to as AV blocks. First-degree block is characterized by a prolonged PR interval and usually requires no treatment.
- Two types of second-degree block have been identified. Type I (Wenckebach) is characterized by progressive prolongation of the PR interval until one P wave is not conducted. Type I block is associated with AV nodal ischemia. Type II second-degree block is identified by

- Third-degree or complete heart block is diagnosed when there is no apparent association between atrial and ventricular conduction. This rhythm is serious, as it is typically associated with slow ventricular rhythm and poor cardiac output.
- Accessory conduction pathways are suspected in persons exhibiting preexcitation syndromes such as Wolff-Parkinson-White syndrome. Severe tachycardias and other reentrant rhythms may occur.
- Disturbances of intraventricular conduction (bundle branch blocks) are characterized by wide, bizarre-looking QRS complexes. Any of the three ventricular fascicles may be affected (right bundle, left anterior fascicle, or left posterior fascicle).

TABLE 19-4

Major Electrophysiologic Classes of Antidysrhythmic Compounds

Type	Drug	Conduction Velocity*	Refractory Period	Automaticity	Ion Block
Ia	Quinidine Procainamide Disopyramide	↓	↑	↓	Sodium (intermediate)
Ib	Lidocaine Mexiletine Tocainide	0/↓	↓	↓	Sodium (fast on-off)
Ic	Flecainide Propafenone[†] Moricizine[‡]	↓↓	0	↓	Sodium (slow on-off)
II[§]	β-Blockers Acebutolol Atenolol Esmolol Metoprolol Nadolol Pindolol Propranolol Timolol	↓	↑	↓	Calcium (indirect)
III	Amiodarone[†¶] Bretylium[†] Dofetilide[†] Sotalol Ibutilide	0	↑↑	0	Potassium
IV[§]	Verapamil Diltiazem	↓	↑	↓	Calcium
Other	Digitalis	—	—	—	Enhances vagal tone, slows heart rate and AV node conduction
	Adenosine	0	↑	↓	Binds A_1 receptors and ↑ K^+ efflux, slows heart rate and AV conduction

*Variables for normal tissue models in ventricular tissue.
[†]Also has type II, β-blocking actions.
[‡]Classification controversial.
[§]Variables for sinoatrial and atrioventricular nodal tissue only.
[¶]Amiodarone also blocks calcium and sodium channels (fast on-off).

Treatment

Dysrhythmias are generally treated if they produce significant symptoms or are expected to progress to a more serious level. A number of antiarrhythmic drugs have proved effective in managing many dysrhythmias; however, most have also been shown to cause dysrhythmias (proarrhythmic).[18] These drugs alter the properties of ion movement across cardiac membranes and affect automaticity as well as the rate and duration of depolarization and repolarization. The major electrophysiologic classes of antidysrhythmic (antiarrhythmic) compounds are summarized in Table 19-4. Treatment may also include measures to improve cardiac output, including pacemakers and drugs to improve contractility and blood pressure. Dysrhythmias causing severely reduced cardiac output, such as severe bradycardia, asystole, ventricular tachycardia, and ventricular fibrillation, require cardiopulmonary resuscitation until an effective cardiac rhythm is established.

Ablation procedures may be effective in eliminating a focus of dysrhythmia generation if one can be identified. An electrophysiologic study is done to evoke and analyze the dysrhythmia, followed by interruption (ablation) of the area generating it. Ablation is accomplished with high-frequency radio waves (radioablation) or by surgical excision. The electrophysiologic study requires insertion of electrodes directly into the heart by way of a venous or arterial catheter. The electrodes are used to record activity in specific locations and to deliver electric shocks to initiate or terminate an abnormal rhythm.[20] This test is useful in assessing responses to drug therapy and in identifying risk for sudden cardiac death. Those at high risk may benefit from insertion of implantable defibrillators that detect lethal rhythms and apply an electric shock to convert the rhythm.

described as having systolic failure. Those with normal EF, usually defined as greater than 50%, usually have diastolic failure. Many patients with low EF have both systolic and diastolic dysfunction.

Three major compensatory mechanisms operate to maintain cardiac output in the failing heart: (1) sympathetic activation, (2) increased preload, and (3) cardiac muscle cell hypertrophy. Unfortunately, these mechanisms also increase myocardial workload and oxygen requirements and may trigger neurohormonal dysregulation and ventricular remodeling associated with HF progression and decompensation. Heart failure is a progressive disorder that leads to death within about 5 years of diagnosis for about 50% of patients. Progression of HF is related to myocardial remodeling characterized by myocyte loss and myocardial fibrosis. Therapies that slow the remodeling process may slow the progression of heart failure. The primary aims of therapy are to improve cardiac output, minimize congestive symptoms and cardiac workload, and slow the detrimental remodeling process.

Dysrhythmia refers to an abnormality of electrical impulse generation or conduction. Dysrhythmias may occur in association with a number of cardiac and noncardiac disorders. Disturbances in electrical activity of the heart can indicate underlying pathophysiologic processes but are not themselves primary medical diseases. Dysrhythmias are significant because they can signal underlying pathophysiologic disorders and can disrupt normal cardiac output. Dysrhythmias can be categorized into three major types: (1) abnormal rates of sinus rhythm, (2) abnormal sites of impulse initiation, and (3) disturbances in conduction pathways. Treatment for dysrhythmias centers on maintaining adequate cardiac output, providing antiarrhythmic drugs as needed, and diagnosing and managing the underlying pathologic process.

SUMMARY

Heart failure may result from a number of cardiac and noncardiac disorders that diminish myocardial contractility or impose an excessive workload on the heart. Heart failure is a clinical diagnosis based on characteristic signs and symptoms. Decreased cardiac output to the tissues results in decreased renal blood flow, fluid retention, activity intolerance, and mental fatigue. Backward effects are due to congestion of blood behind the ineffectively pumping ventricle. With left-sided heart failure, the congestion is located in the lungs and produces a number of signs and symptoms, including dyspnea, orthopnea, hypoxemia, crackles, and frank pulmonary edema. Isolated right-sided heart failure causes congestion in the systemic venous system leading to congestion and dysfunction of the liver, spleen, and kidney, as well as peripheral subcutaneous edema and distended neck veins. In the early stages HF may be asymptomatic, and attention to risk factors and early structural abnormalities of the heart may allow early intervention. Two types of HF have been described based on EF. Those with low ejection fraction are commonly

REFERENCES

1. American Heart Association: *Heart disease and stroke statistics—2008 update,* Dallas, 2008, The Association.
2. National Heart Lung and Blood Institute: *Congestive heart failure data fact sheet,* Bethesda, National Institutes of Health, 1996, The Institute.
3. Kim J, Jacobs DR Jr, Luepker RV, et al: Prognostic value of a novel classification scheme for heart failure: the Minnesota Heart Failure Criteria, *Am J Epidemiol* 164(2):184-193, 2006.
4. Bursi F, Weston SA, Redfield MM, et al: Systolic and diastolic heart failure: differences and similarities, *JAMA* 296(18):2209-2216, 2007.
5. Ho KK, et al: The epidemiology of heart failure: the Framingham Study, *J Am Coll Cardiol* 22(suppl A):6A-13A, 1993.
6. Loehr LR, Rosamond WD, Chang PP, et al: Heart failure incidence and survival (from the Atherosclerosis Risk in Communities Study), *Am J Cardiol* 101(7):1016-1022, 2008.
7. Mann DL: Pathophysiology of heart failure. In Libby P, Bonow R, Mann D, et al, editors: *Braunwald's heart disease: a textbook of cardiovascular medicine,* ed 8, Philadelphia, 2008, Saunders, pp 541-560.
8. Parker RB, Patterson JH, Johnson JA: Heart failure. In Dipiro JT, et al, editors: *Pharmacotherapy: a pathophysiologic approach,* ed 6, New York, 2005, McGraw-Hill, pp 219-260.
9. Fowler MB, Lottes SR, Nelson JJ, et al: β-Blocker dosing in community-based treatment of heart failure, *Am Heart J* 153(6):1029-1036, 2007.

10. Levy MN, Pappano AJ: The cardiac pump. In Levy MN, Pappano AJ, editors: *Cardiovascular physiology,* ed 9, St Louis, 2007, Mosby, pp 55-80.

11. Schoen FJ, Mitchell R: The heart. In Kumar V, Abbas A, Fausto N, et al, editors: *Robbins basic pathology,* ed 8, Philadelphia, 2007, Saunders, pp 379-420.

12. Kazi D, Deswal A: Role and optimal dosing of angiotensin-converting enzyme inhibitors in heart failure, *Cardiol Clin* 26(1): 1-14, 2008.

13. Gehlbach BK, Geppert E: The pulmonary manifestations of left heart failure, *Chest* 125(2):669-682, 2004.

14. Stoupakis G, Klapholz M: Natriuretic peptides: biochemistry, physiology, and therapeutic role in heart failure, *Heart Dis* 5(3):215-223, 2003.

15. Hunt SA, et al: American College of Cardiology; American Heart Association: ACC/AHA 2005 guideline update for the evaluation and management of chronic heart failure in the adult: summary article, *Circulation* 112(12):1825-1852, 2005.

16. The effect of digoxin on mortality and morbidity in patients with heart failure. The Digitalis Investigation Group, *N Engl J Med* 336(8):525-533, 1997.

17. Rubart M, Zipes DP: Genesis of cardiac arrhythmias: electrophysiological considerations. In Libby P, Bonow R, Mann D, et al, editors: *Braunwald's heart disease: a textbook of cardiovascular medicine*, ed 8, Philadelphia, 2008, Saunders, pp 727-762.

18. Bauman JL, Schoen MD: Arrhythmias. In Dipiro JT, et al, editors: *Pharmacotherapy: a pathophysiologic approach,* ed 6, New York, 2005, McGraw-Hill, pp 321-356.

19. Conover MB: *Understanding electrocardiography,* ed 8, St Louis, 2003, Mosby.

20. Miller JM, Zipes DP: Therapy for cardiac arrhythmias. In Libby P, Bonow R, Mann D, et al, editors: *Braunwald's heart disease: a textbook of cardiovascular medicine,* ed 8, Philadelphia, 2008, Saunders, pp 799-822.

chapter

20

Shock

Jacquelyn L. Banasik

MEDIA RESOURCES

Additional Material for Study, Review, and Further Exploration

CD Companion ■ Review Questions and Answers
■ Glossary (with audio pronunciations for selected terms)
■ Disease Profiles ■ Animations

evolve **Website** at http://evolve.elsevier.com/Copstead/
■ Case Studies ■ Disease Profiles ■ WebLinks ■ Key Points Review

 Online Course (Module 11)

KEY QUESTIONS

■ What are the common causes of cardiogenic, hypovolemic, obstructive, and distributive shock?
■ What are the common cellular and tissue responses to shock of any cause?
■ How does the body try to compensate for insufficient cardiac output during shock states?

■ How do clinical and hemodynamic findings differ among types of shock?
■ What is the role of the immune system in septic shock and the progressive stage of other types of shock?
■ How is shock managed, and why does it have such a high mortality?

CHAPTER OUTLINE

Shock is a life-threatening condition characterized by insufficient delivery of oxygenated blood to the microcirculation, resulting in tissue hypoxia and cellular dysfunction. In 1895, John Collins Warren described shock as a momentary pause in the act of death.[1] Despite advances in the understanding and management, shock still has a high rate of mortality. This chapter presents an overview of circulatory shock, including the major causes, cellular and systemic pathogenesis, clinical manifestations, and general therapeutic management.

PATHOGENESIS OF SHOCK

Shock is characterized by an imbalance between oxygen supply and oxygen requirements at the cellular level.[2] When the cell does not have adequate amounts of oxygen and nutrients, it is unable to meet its metabolic demands. Cellular hypoxia results in impaired cellular function and may progress to irreversible organ damage and death. The causes of circulatory shock classically are divided into four general types: cardiogenic, obstructive, hypovolemic, and distributive.[3] Each of these types is associated with a number of primary causes (Box 20-1). Cardiogenic shock results from heart disorders that result in inadequate cardiac output despite sufficient vascular volume. Obstructive shock develops when circulatory blockage disrupts cardiac output, such as a large pulmonary embolus or cardiac tamponade. Because the causes of obstructive shock are associated with failure of the heart to pump sufficiently, some sources include obstructive shock within the category of cardiogenic shock. Hypovolemic shock is associated with loss of blood volume as a result of hemorrhage or excessive loss of extracellular fluids, such as through vomiting, diarrhea, or excessive diuresis. Distributive shock is characterized by a greatly expanded vascular space because of inappropriate vasodilation. Vasodilation leads to hypotension and altered perfusion of tissues. Anaphylactic, neurogenic, and septic are forms of distributive shock. Each type of shock has certain unique features (Table 20-1), but all are associated with impaired tissue oxygenation that can progress to refractory shock and organ failure.

Impaired Tissue Oxygenation

The common denominator of all forms of shock is impaired oxygen utilization by cells, which disrupts function and, if ongoing or severe, may lead to cell death, organ dysfunction, and stimulation of inflammatory reactions. Recent discoveries about the contribution of inflammatory reactions in the pathogenesis of shock have provided new insight into this complicated syndrome.

The reason for impaired oxygen utilization by cells differs with the various types of shock, but the outcomes are similar. A continuous supply of oxygen is needed by cells to allow sufficient production of energy in the form of adenosine triphosphate (ATP). Inadequate oxygen availability at the cellular level quickly impairs aerobic metabolism of glucose, fatty acids, and amino acids and causes the cells to rely on the relatively inefficient processes of glycolysis to produce cellular ATP. (A review of ATP synthesis can be found in Chapter 3.) Glycolysis is the enzymatic process of converting glucose to pyruvate, with the net production of two ATP molecules per glucose molecule. If oxygen were available, pyruvate would normally enter the mitochondria and proceed through the citric acid cycle. In the absence of cellular oxygen, the citric acid cycle is inhibited and pyruvate accumulates in the cytoplasm. Pyruvate accumulation would quickly inhibit further glycolysis and shut down ATP production entirely except that it can be converted to a substance called *lactate*, which diffuses from the cell and into the extracellular fluid. Accumulation of lactate in the bloodstream (more than 5 to 6 mmol/L) is considered a sign of significant tissue hypoxia.[4,5]

An inadequate supply of cellular ATP inhibits energy-requiring cellular functions, including maintenance of ion concentrations across the plasma membrane. Because of their steep electrochemical gradients, extracellular sodium and calcium ions tend to leak into the cell. ATP-dependent pumps in the cell membrane are needed to continuously pump these ions back out. Failure of ion pumps leads to sodium and water

---

BOX 20-1

Etiology of Circulatory Shock

Cardiogenic Shock
Myocardial infarction
Cardiomyopathy
Valvular heart disease
Ventricular rupture
Congenital heart defects
Papillary muscle rupture

Obstructive Shock
Pulmonary embolism
Cardiac tamponade
Tension pneumothorax
Dissecting aortic aneurysm

Hypovolemic Shock
Acute hemorrhage
Dehydration from vomiting, diarrhea
Overuse of diuretics
Burns
Pancreatitis

Distributive Shock
Anaphylaxis
Neurotrauma
Spinal cord trauma
Spinal anesthesia
Sepsis

TABLE 20-1

Comparison of Clinical Findings in Different Types of Shock

Parameter	Cardiogenic	Hypovolemic	Septic
Hypotension	Yes	Yes	Yes
Systemic vascular resistance	High	High	Low
Cardiac output	Low	Low	High
Cardiac preload	High	Low	Low
Venous oxygen saturation	Low	Low	High
Urine output	Low	Low	Low
Skin temperature	Cool	Cool	Warm

accumulation in the cell (hydropic swelling) and an excess of intracellular free calcium. Intracellular calcium ions trigger a cascade of cellular events that further impair energy production and plasma membrane integrity. Cell death from oxygen deprivation takes from minutes to several hours, depending on the rate of cellular metabolic activity. However, even a short period of oxygen deprivation often sets in motion a complex cascade of events that lead to further cell damage (Figure 20-1). Two important aspects of this cascade are (1) formation of oxygen radicals and (2) induction of inflammatory cytokines.

Ischemic cells may produce oxygen-free radicals when oxygen supplies are restored. This process has been called *reperfusion injury*. Reactive oxygen molecules include superoxide (O_2^-), peroxide (H_2O_2), hydroxyl radicals (OH^-), and singlet oxygen (O). These molecules are unstable and will attack membrane structures, denature proteins, and break apart cell DNA. Another source of oxygen radicals is immune cells, particularly neutrophils, which are recruited to the area of tissue injury. Thus cellular injury may continue and progress long after the initial hypoxic insult has been resolved.

The role that immune cytokines play in shock has been studied extensively in septic shock but is thought to be similar in the late stages of other types of shock as well. Macrophages and tissue cells are stimulated to release inflammatory cytokines in response to hypoxic tissue injury and, in the case of septic shock, in response to endotoxin or other microorganism antigens.[6] The tumor necrosis factor-α (TNF-α) and interleukin-1 (IL-1) cytokines in particular have been shown to increase in the bloodstream of patients with septic shock and are thought to be important mediators of vascular failure and progressive organ damage.[6] Numerous other immune cytokines and neurohormonal mediators have been implicated in the pathogenesis of shock (Table 20-2). These mediators represent potential therapeutic targets for a disorder that is notoriously difficult to manage effectively.

A hallmark of shock is failure of the microcirculation to appropriately autoregulate blood flow. Normal tissues are able

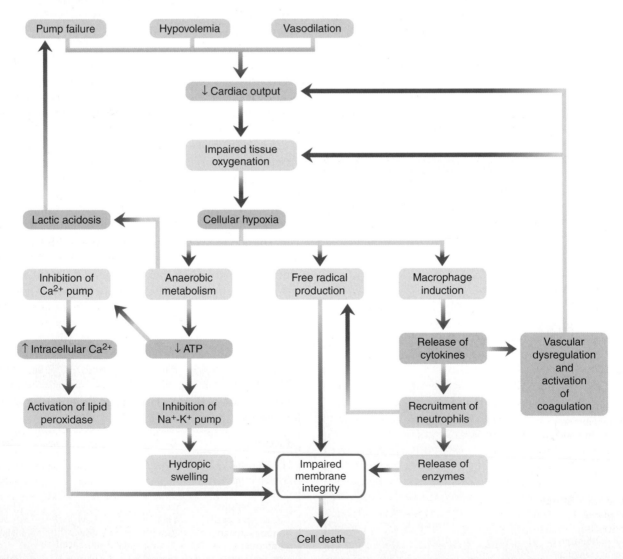

FIGURE 20-1 Shock is a complex process involving cellular hypoxia, free radical formation, and systemic inflammation. All forms of shock are associated with impaired tissue oxygenation, which triggers a cascade of events leading to tissue injury and death. *ATP,* Adenosine triphosphate.

TABLE 20-2

Immune Cytokines and Neurohormones Associated with Circulatory Shock

Mediator	Associated Dysfunction
IL-1α	Inflammation, vasodilation, vascular leakiness
IL-1β	Inflammation, vasodilation, vascular leakiness
IL-6	Fever, increased acute phase protein
TNF-α	Inflammation, neutrophil activation
IL-10	Antiinflammatory, may suppress shock
TGF-β	Fibrosis, pulmonary edema
PAF	Platelet activation, chemotaxis
PAI-1	Increased clotting, thrombosis
Substance P	Proinflammatory
Chemokines	Neutrophil recruitment and binding to vessel endothelium
Nitric oxide	Vasodilator
C5a	Chemotactic
Protein C	Inhibits thrombus formation
Vasopressin	Improves vascular tone and responsiveness to NE/E
Cortisol	Antiinflammatory, improves vascular response to NE/E
Endothelin	Vasoconstriction
Adrenomedullin	Vasodilation
Norepinephrine	Vasoconstriction
Epinephrine	Inotropic, bronchodilation
Leukotrienes	Inflammation, bronchospasm
Histamine	Increased vascular permeability, edema
Heparin	Inhibits action of histamine
Angiotensin II	Vasoconstriction
Heat-shock proteins	Protect protein structure and function, inhibits apoptosis

IL, Interleukin; *TNF,* tumor necrosis factor; *TGF,* transforming growth factor; *PAF,* platelet-activating factor; *PAI,* plasminogen activator inhibitor; *NE,* norepinephrine; *E,* epinephrine.

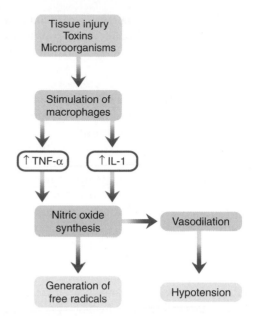

FIGURE 20-2 Excess production of nitric oxide is an important mechanism of vascular failure in shock. The tumor necrosis factor-α and interleukin-1 cytokines are promoters of inducible nitric oxide synthase. These cytokines are released from macrophages that have been activated by tissue injury or toxins. *TNF-α,* Tumor necrosis factor-α; *IL-1,* interleukin-1.

the venules and the degree of microcirculatory dysfunction is poorly correlated with systemic hemodynamics. Overall, this imbalance leads to a so-called *oxygen debt* in the tissues. It has been suggested that the overall oxygen debt can be estimated clinically by the serum lactate level and degree of metabolic acidosis, both of which imply a switch to anaerobic metabolism by oxygen-deprived tissues.[5]

In septic shock, immune cytokines are believed to be at the root of the microcirculatory maldistribution problem. TNF-α, IL-1, and other inflammatory mediators induce vascular cells to produce excessive amounts of the vasodilator nitric oxide.[6] Nitric oxide in normal quantity is thought to be protective for tissues during shock, whereas excessive production is detrimental. Nitric oxide is produced in endothelial cells and vascular smooth muscle by two enzymes, nitric oxide synthase (NOS) and inducible nitric oxide synthase (iNOS). TNF-α and IL-1 increase the activity of iNOS and thereby cause excessive production of nitric oxide (Figure 20-2). Efforts to minimize the microcirculatory oxygen debt in early shock and to quickly restore adequate microcirculatory blood flow distribution, as evidenced by normalized serum lactate and acid-base balance, is an important focus of therapy for all types of shock.

Compensatory Mechanisms and Stages of Shock

A number of compensatory responses are set in motion to restore tissue perfusion and oxygenation in the early stage of shock. Historically, these responses to shock have been divided into three clinical stages: compensated shock, progressive shock, and refractory shock. Although these stages may be useful for determining prognosis and the likelihood of the

to match blood flow with metabolic needs across a wide range of blood pressures. This property ensures that blood flow is evenly distributed to tissues according to metabolic needs. In shock, autoregulation fails leading to an abnormal distribution of blood flow.[7] Some capillary beds receive inadequate flow and become progressively more hypoxic, whereas other vascular routes are excessively dilated and receive too much flow. Advances in technology have allowed direct visualization of capillary flow through tissue beds and confirmed the presence of perfusion abnormalities in the microcirculation. These abnormalities differ depending on the primary cause of shock.[7] In cases of reduced cardiac output resulting from hypovolemic or cardiogenic shock, there is a homogeneous reduction in blood flow through a given tissue's arterioles, capillaries, and venules that is directly related to the severity of cardiac output reduction. In distributive shock states, such as septic shock, the degree of microcirculatory flow is heterogeneous within a tissue with some capillaries being closed and others open. Often there is high flow rate through some of patient's recovering, shock is viewed as a continuum in which compensatory mechanisms become progressively less effective as function of the microcirculation becomes increasingly impaired.

Insufficient cardiac output and decreased effective tissue perfusion are early defects in all types of shock. Insufficient cardiac output may be a consequence of an ineffective cardiac pump (cardiogenic, obstructive) or insufficient blood volume to fill the vascular space (hypovolemic, distributive). A number of compensatory mechanisms are triggered in response to inadequate cardiac output in an attempt to restore adequate perfusion pressure (Figure 20-3). Baroreceptors located in the aorta and carotid arteries quickly sense the decrease in pressure and transmit signals to the vasomotor center in the brainstem medulla. Stimulation of the sympathetic nervous system (SNS) results in increased cardiac output and vascular resistance. Because blood pressure is determined by the product of cardiac output and vascular resistance, an increase in one or both of these factors will help restore blood pressure. The SNS increases cardiac output through several mechanisms. The adrenal medulla is stimulated to release increased amounts of the catecholamines epinephrine and norepinephrine (NE), which circulate to the heart and stimulate β_1 receptors. The β_1 receptors respond by increasing the heart rate and force of contraction in an attempt to increase cardiac output. The SNS also enhances venous return to the heart by constricting systemic arterioles and venules. Arterial vasoconstriction reduces flow through the capillary bed, which causes hydrostatic pressure in the capillaries to fall. Fluid reabsorption from interstitial spaces helps increase blood volume and improve preload. Blood vessels in the skin, kidneys, and gastrointestinal tract constrict and shunt blood to the heart and brain.

The SNS stimulates cells in the kidney to release renin, which triggers the renin-angiotensin-aldosterone cascade. Renin is also secreted from the kidneys in response to decreased blood flow and pressure in the afferent arterioles. Renin triggers the formation of angiotensin II, which is a potent vasoconstrictor and also stimulates kidney nephrons to conserve sodium and water. Conservation of volume by the kidney is further enhanced by aldosterone, which is secreted from the adrenal cortex in response to angiotensin II. Reabsorption of fluid from the kidney helps increase blood volume and enhances venous return to the heart. Another hormone, antidiuretic hormone (vasopressin), is secreted from the posterior pituitary in response to reduced blood volume. Antidiuretic hormone stimulates the kidney tubules to reabsorb water and improves the vascular response to catecholamines. In shock, urine output may fall to zero as the kidneys attempt to conserve fluid to maintain blood volume and cardiac output. Unfortunately, the kidney tubules often sustain damage because of the low-flow state, which may result in the complication of acute renal failure.

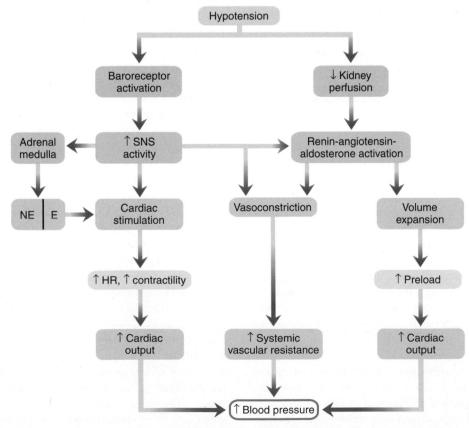

FIGURE 20-3 Compensatory mechanisms are triggered in shock to help maintain arterial blood pressure despite a fall in cardiac output. *NE,* Norepinephrine; *E,* epinephrine; *SNS,* sympathetic nervous system; *HR,* heart rate.

These compensatory mechanisms work well in the early stage of hypovolemic shock and may maintain blood pressure within the normal range until the volume of blood loss becomes too great (Figure 20-4). In other forms of shock, compensatory mechanisms are less effective in restoring cardiac output. In cardiogenic shock, the compensatory responses may worsen the already high preload and impose a greater workload on the failing heart. In distributive shock, the vasculature is not responsive to SNS signals to constrict. Blood pools in the peripheral tissues, which makes it difficult for the heart to maintain cardiac output despite sympathetic stimulation to increase the heart rate and contractility.

The early, compensated stage of shock may be difficult to detect clinically (Figure 20-5). A high index of suspicion is needed in patients with heart failure, trauma, blood loss, and severe infection. In addition, the following clinical findings may be present:

- A narrow pulse pressure with or without hypotension
- Tachycardia greater than 100 beats/min
- Fast and deep respirations
- Decreased urinary output
- Increased urine specific gravity
- Cool, clammy skin
- Altered mentation
- Dilated pupils

At some point, which is highly variable and differs among individuals depending on age, comorbidities, and specific etiology, the compensatory mechanisms can no longer sustain adequate perfusion to tissues and cells begin to suffer significant hypoxic injury. This condition is sometimes called the *progressive stage of shock*. Active therapeutic intervention is required at this stage or the patient will probably not survive. As previously described, reduced delivery of oxygen to tissues results in hypoxic injury, free radical damage, and stimulation of the inflammatory response. Lactic acidosis may occur during the progressive stage of shock. In addition to being a marker of anaerobic metabolism, lactate can alter the acid-base balance of the blood and create a metabolic acidosis. Metabolic acidosis places a greater burden on the respiratory and renal systems and may contribute to further dysfunction. Metabolic acidosis can affect electrolyte balance and contribute to cardiac dysrhythmias and conduction disturbances. In addition, myocardial depressant factors are released that impair myocardial contractility.[8] These factors contribute to reduced cardiac output and a progressive cycle of worsening tissue hypoxia.

As shock continues to progress, the vascular system begins to fail. Arterioles become unresponsive to catecholamines and previously constricted vascular beds begin to dilate. Widespread dilation and low cardiac output combine to

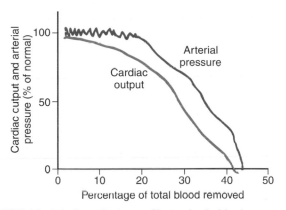

FIGURE 20-4 In the early stages of hypovolemia, blood pressure is stable even though cardiac output is falling. When volume losses equal about 25% of the total blood volume, blood pressure falls precipitously. (Redrawn from Guyton AC, Hall JE: *Textbook of medical physiology*, ed 11, Philadelphia, 2006, Saunders, p 279.)

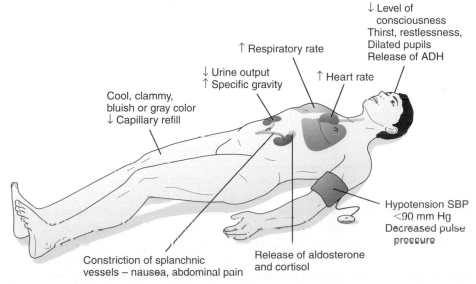

FIGURE 20-5 Classical manifestations of shock. *ADH*, Antidiuretic hormone; *SBP*, systolic blood pressure.

produce severe hypotension. The low blood pressure is not sufficient for organ perfusion. At this stage the effects of shock produce more shock processes. Tissue damage often activates the clotting cascade, which contributes to sluggish blood flow, vascular thrombosis, and more severe tissue ischemia. Release of inflammatory mediators, along with vascular occlusion, may precipitate organ failure. The kidney, liver, and lung are particularly susceptible. At some point, the stage of refractory shock occurs and the patient becomes unresponsive to therapeutic interventions.

The progressive stage of shock is characterized by the following:

- Low blood pressure, usually lower than 90 mm Hg
- Narrow pulse pressure
- Tachycardia
- Acute renal failure (oliguria, increased blood urea nitrogen and serum creatinine)
- Decreased level of consciousness
- Increased respiratory rates
- Metabolic and respiratory acidosis with hypoxemia

KEY POINTS

- Shock represents a diverse group of life-threatening circulatory conditions. The common factor among all types of shock is hypoperfusion and impaired cellular oxygen utilization. Inadequate cellular oxygenation may result from decreased cardiac output, maldistribution of blood flow, or reduced blood oxygen content.
- During the compensatory stage of shock, homeostatic mechanisms are sufficient to maintain adequate tissue perfusion despite a reduction in cardiac output. Manifestations of SNS activation are an elevated heart rate, increased myocardial stimulation, bronchodilation, vasoconstriction, cool clammy skin, dilated pupils, and decreased urine output. Blood pressure is maintained even though cardiac output has fallen.
- During the progressive stage of shock, compensatory mechanisms begin to fail and hypotension and progressive tissue hypoxia result. Shift of cells to anaerobic metabolism results in lactate production and metabolic acidosis. A lack of cellular ATP production leads to cellular swelling, dysfunction, and death. Generation of oxygen-free radicals, release of inflammatory cytokines, and activation of the clotting cascade lead to further cellular and organ dysfunction.

TYPES OF SHOCK

In addition to the general pathophysiology of shock described above, each type of shock has special features that affect prevention, diagnosis, and treatment. These features are briefly reviewed here, and the reader is referred to the specific chapters that describe the primary disorders that predispose to shock, including cardiogenic (Chapters 18 and 19), hypovolemic (Chapter 24), anaphylactic (Chapter 10), neurogenic (Chapter 44), and septic (Chapter 8).

Cardiogenic Shock

Etiology and Pathogenesis. Cardiogenic shock occurs primarily as a result of severe dysfunction of the left, right, or both ventricles that results in inadequate cardiac pumping. The most common cause of cardiogenic shock is myocardial infarction resulting in a significant dysfunction or loss (greater than 40%) of left ventricular myocardium.[9] Other causes of cardiogenic shock include right ventricular myocardial infarction, end-stage cardiomyopathy, papillary muscle dysfunction, free wall rupture, and congenital heart defects.

The low cardiac output state is associated with a high left ventricular diastolic filling pressure (preload), a finding that differentiates cardiogenic from hypovolemic forms of shock (Figure 20-6). High left ventricular preload leads to movement of fluid from the pulmonary vascular beds into the pulmonary interstitial space, which initially results in interstitial pulmonary edema and later in alveolar pulmonary edema.

The SNS is stimulated as a compensatory mechanism to increase cardiac output. The result is an increase in heart rate and systemic vascular resistance. The increase in systemic vascular resistance makes it even more difficult for the heart to pump. Activation of the renin-angiotensin-aldosterone system results in further increases in resistance and preload. The net result of the activation of compensatory mechanisms is to increase myocardial workload and oxygen demand. Thus the compensatory responses can precipitate further myocardial damage and cause a progressive decline in cardiac output.

Clinical Manifestations. Sympathetic nervous stimulation increases the heart rate and vascular resistance, which maintain blood pressure even though cardiac output has decreased. As compensatory mechanisms fail, systolic blood pressure falls and diastolic pressure increases (as a result of the sympathetic stimulation), thus narrowing the pulse pressure. Heart rates exceed 100 beats/min. Peripheral vasoconstriction occurs and produces cool, clammy skin. Auscultation of the lungs reveals coarse crackles resulting from pulmonary edema. An S_3 summation gallop may be audible over the left apex as a result of increased preload in the left ventricle.

Frequent assessments of cardiac output and cardiac index are helpful in the clinical treatment of a patient in cardiogenic shock. A pulmonary artery catheter may be inserted to measure cardiac index and left heart filling pressures (pulmonary capillary occlusion pressure). Pulmonary artery pressures are increased, with the pulmonary capillary occlusion pressure typically being greater than 15 mm Hg (normal, less than 12 mm Hg).[9] When pulmonary capillary occlusion pressure acutely increases, pulmonary congestion may develop because fluid shifts from the capillary into the interstitial and alveolar spaces. Patients with chronic congestive heart failure may not develop pulmonary edema until pulmonary occlusion pressures exceed 20 to 40 mm Hg. Arterial blood gas values initially demonstrate a respiratory alkalosis secondary to hyperventilation. As pulmonary edema progresses, respiratory acidosis with hypoxemia may occur. Hypoxemia further impairs myocardial function.

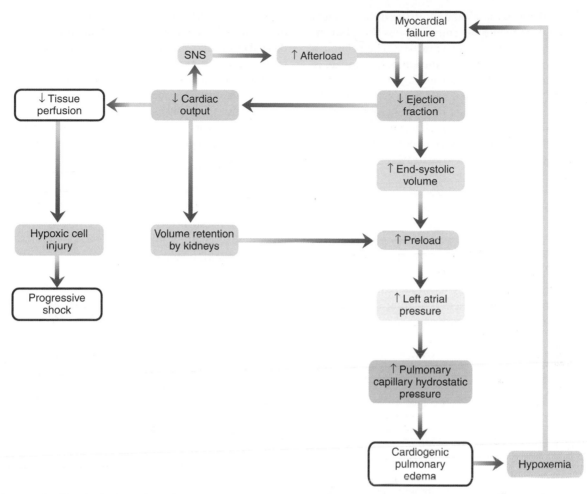

FIGURE 20-6 Cardiogenic shock results in decreased tissue perfusion and cardiogenic pulmonary edema because of reduced myocardial function, usually associated with left ventricular failure. *SNS,* Sympathetic nervous system.

Determination of mixed venous oxygen levels in blood samples obtained from the pulmonary artery catheter is helpful in assessing the adequacy of cardiac output. Decreased tissue oxygen delivery because of low cardiac output increases the degree of oxygen extraction. Mixed venous blood samples show decreased venous oxygen saturation with a decreased cardiac output. An increase in mixed venous oxygenation would be expected with improved cardiac output.

Treatment. Cardiogenic shock is difficult to manage because the underlying myocardial damage is often not reversible. Prevention of cardiogenic shock through measures to limit infarct size during acute myocardial ischemia is desirable. Early efforts to restore coronary perfusion are associated with a decrease in the incidence of cardiogenic shock after myocardial infarction.[9,10] (A discussion of reperfusion therapy can be found in Chapter 18.)

The goal of treatment for cardiogenic shock is to decrease myocardial oxygen demands, increase myocardial oxygen delivery, and increase cardiac output. It is difficult to achieve these goals because interventions to increase cardiac output tend to increase myocardial oxygen demands.

Pharmacotherapy. Positive inotropic drugs are frequently used in the management of cardiogenic shock to increase contractility. Positive inotropes include β-adrenergic agonists such as NE, dobutamine, and dopamine and phosphodiesterase inhibitors that prevent the degradation of cyclic adenosine monophosphate (cAMP). These drugs have the ability to increase contractility, increase cardiac output, and increase tissue perfusion; however, they all increase myocardial oxygen demand. NE is the natural neurotransmitter of the sympathetic nerves and its administration mimics SNS activation by increasing heart rate, contractility, and vascular resistance. Dobutamine increases contractility by stimulating β-receptors but, unlike NE or dopamine, has minimal α-receptor activity. The major effect of dobutamine is on contractility rather than heart rate. Dobutamine may contribute to a decrease in vascular resistance and must be used with caution in hypotensive patients.[11] Vasodilators may be used to decrease the workload of the heart by decreasing left ventricular afterload. Examples of commonly used vasodilators include nitroprusside and nitroglycerin.

Mechanical Assist Devices. Cardiogenic shock is sometimes managed by mechanical assist devices. For temporary management, **intraaortic** balloon counterpulsation may be indicated.[12] A catheter with a balloon at the distal segment is inserted through the femoral artery and positioned in the aorta just distal to the left subclavian artery. The balloon is connected to a console that triggers the balloon to inflate in diastole and deflate in systole. The effect of balloon inflation during diastole is to increase perfusion pressure of the coronary arteries. Sudden deflation of the balloon just before ventricular systole creates a vacuum effect in the aorta that reduces left ventricular afterload. A reduction in afterload decreases left ventricular workload and increases stroke volume. Balloon counterpulsation restricts mobility and is associated with a number of vascular complications. Long-term management of patients with low cardiac output can be achieved with mechanical pumps that take over the function of the ventricle or ventricles (ventricular assist devices). Ventricular assist devices are commonly used in patients awaiting heart transplantation. In some cases, the temporary decrease in cardiac workload afforded by the ventricular assist device is associated with significant improvement in cardiac structure and function and the device can be removed.

KEY POINTS

- Cardiogenic shock is usually a result of severe ventricular dysfunction associated with myocardial infarction. Other causes include cardiomyopathy, ventricular rupture, and congenital heart defects.
- Diagnostic features of cardiogenic shock include decreased cardiac output as a result of left ventricular dysfunction, along with elevated left ventricular end-diastolic pressure, S_3 heart sounds, and pulmonary edema. Sympathetic activation leads to an increased heart rate, vasoconstriction, and a narrow pulse pressure.
- Low cardiac output leads to reduced oxygen delivery to tissues. Tissues extract a greater percentage of oxygen from the delivered blood, which leads to reduced SvO_2.
- Therapy is aimed at improving cardiac output and myocardial oxygen delivery while reducing cardiac workload. Pharmacologic treatment often includes the use of inotropic agents, afterload-reducing agents (vasodilators), and preload-reducing agents (venodilators, diuretics). Intraaortic balloon counterpulsation may be used to reduce afterload and improve coronary artery perfusion. Ventricular assist devices may be used for longer-term circulatory support, whereas heart transplantation provides definitive treatment.

Obstructive Shock

Etiology. Obstructive shock develops when the heart is prevented from pumping because of a mechanical obstruction to blood flow. Impaired ventricular filling leads to reduced cardiac output and signs and symptoms similar to cardiogenic shock, and it is considered by many to be a form of cardiogenic shock. Causes of mechanical obstruction include pulmonary embolism, cardiac tamponade, and tension pneumothorax.

Prompt relief of the obstruction is necessary to restore cardiac output and prevent cardiovascular collapse.

Clinical Manifestations. Obstructive shock is usually characterized by manifestations of right-sided heart failure. Depending on the location of the obstruction, elevated pressures in the cardiac chambers may be evident.

Pulmonary embolism results in elevated right-sided heart pressures, but left-sided pressures remain normal to low. Pulmonary emboli are usually generated in the veins of the lower extremities in patients with immobility, trauma, or hypercoagulable states. Pulmonary embolism is manifested as sudden, severe dyspnea and deteriorating arterial blood gas values. A perfusion scan of the lung may demonstrate an area of reduced blood flow. Pulmonary emboli are not generally detectable by chest radiographs.

Cardiac tamponade, which results from an accumulation of fluid in the pericardial sac, causes elevation of pressures on both the right and left side of the heart. Despite the elevated pressure, preload in the heart chambers is low, as is stroke volume. The elevated pressure is due to external compression of the heart chambers. Risks for the development of cardiac tamponade include pericarditis, blunt trauma to the chest, and cardiac surgical procedures. In pericarditis, a pericardial friction rub can sometimes be heard and may help with the diagnosis.

Tension pneumothorax results in shifting and compression of mediastinal structures, including the heart, which compromises left ventricular filling. Accumulation of air in the pleural space may occur because of trauma or spontaneous rupture of lung parenchyma. A tension pneumothorax develops when the air in the pleural space begins to exert a positive pressure on lung and mediastinal structures. A deviated trachea and decreased or absent breath sounds may occur. Arterial blood gas values can deteriorate rapidly. Tension pneumothorax is detectable by chest radiography.

Treatment. Management of obstructive shock is aimed at identifying and removing the offending obstruction. Compensatory mechanisms are generally ineffective in obstructive shock, and the patient's condition may deteriorate rapidly.

KEY POINTS

- Obstructive shock results from mechanical obstructions that prevent effective cardiac filling and stroke volume.
- Pulmonary embolism, cardiac tamponade, and tension pneumothorax are common causes of obstructive shock.
- Prompt management of the underlying obstruction is necessary to prevent cardiovascular collapse.

Hypovolemic Shock

Etiology and Classification. Hypovolemic shock results when circulating blood volume is inadequate to perfuse tissues.[13] The pathogenesis of early stage hypovolemic shock is straightforward: decreased intravascular volume leads to a decrease in venous return, which causes a decrease in cardiac output (Figure 20-7). The decrease in cardiac output results in decreased tissue perfusion and decreased oxygen delivery.

Circulatory volume deficits may be the result of internal or external losses. Internal losses can result from internal hemorrhage, fracture of long bones, or leakage of fluid into the interstitial spaces. External losses can result from external hemorrhage, burns, severe vomiting and diarrhea, or diuresis. External hemorrhage is the most common cause of hypovolemic shock.

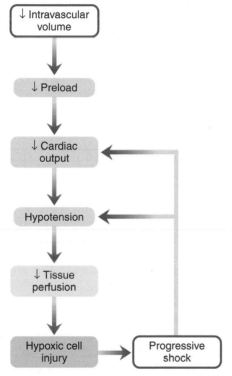

FIGURE 20-7 Pathogenesis of hypovolemic shock.

The American College of Surgeons stratifies hemorrhagic shock into four classes according to the degree of blood volume lost (Table 20-3).[3] These values are based on a 70 kg adult and are guidelines that may not apply to all patients with hemorrhage, depending on etiology, rate of blood loss, and comorbidities.

The initial stage hemorrhage (class 1) occurs with blood loss up to 750 ml or 15% of total blood volume. Compensatory mechanisms maintain cardiac output, and the patient's vital signs remain within the normal range. Class II compensated hemorrhage is categorized as blood loss between 750 and 1500 ml (15% to 30%). The patient becomes anxious and restless. Blood pressure remains normal when the patient is supine but decreases upon standing (orthostatic hypotension). The heart rate is between 100 and 120 beats/min. The respiratory rate is normal to mildly increased. Urine output is between 20 and 30 ml/hr. The capillary refill time may be prolonged. (The capillary blanch test is performed by depressing a patient's fingernail and observing how long after release the skin color takes to return to normal. Normal capillary refill times are less than 2 seconds.)

Class III hemorrhage (progressive stage) is blood loss between 30% to 40% of total blood volume (1500 to 2000 mL). The patient is anxious and confused. Blood pressure is decreased with a narrow pulse pressure. The heart rate is greater than 120 beats/min. Respiratory rates are between 30 and 40 respirations/min. Urine output is 5 to 20 ml/hr. The capillary refill test is prolonged.

Severe Class IV hemorrhage (refractory stage) occurs when more than 40% of total blood volume is lost (2000 ml or more). The patient is lethargic and has severe hypotension with a narrow pulse pressure. The heart rate usually exceeds 140 beats/min, and the respiratory rate is markedly increased. Urine output is negligible. The capillary refill test is prolonged.

The clinical features of other forms of hypovolemic shock are similar to those of hemorrhagic shock, although the volume loss has usually occurred more gradually.

TABLE 20-3

Classification of Hemorrhagic Shock

	Class I (Initial Stage)	Class II (Compensated Stage)	Class III (Progressive Stage)	Class IV (Refractory Stage)
Blood loss (ml)	≤750 (15%)	750-1500 (15%-30%)	1500-2000 (30%-40%)	>2000 (>40%)
Clinical features	Minimal tachycardia Normal or increased pulse pressure	Tachycardia Tachypnea Decreased pulse pressure Cool clammy skin Delayed capillary refill Slight anxiety	Tachycardia Tachypnea Decreased systolic blood pressure Oliguria Changes in mental status such as confusion and agitation	Marked tachycardia Decreased systolic blood pressure Narrowed pulse pressure Markedly decreased urinary output Loss of consciousness Cold, pale skin

Clinical Manifestations. The cardiac output and cardiac index are found to be decreased. Pulmonary artery pressures and pulmonary capillary wedge pressures are decreased because of the decreased preload. The finding of a low preload distinguishes hypovolemic shock from cardiogenic shock. In cardiogenic shock, preload is high and cardiac output is low. In hypovolemic shock, preload and cardiac output are both low.

Systemic vascular resistance is increased as a result of sympathetic activation. This increase is a compensatory mechanism in hypovolemia to maintain perfusion pressure. SvO_2 may be decreased because of decreased oxygen delivery and increased oxygen extraction.

Treatment. The first intervention for hemorrhagic shock is to control the source of blood loss. Second, volume losses are replaced with appropriate fluids to normalize blood pressure, cardiac output, and perfusion of the microvasculature. In severe, uncontrolled hemorrhage, efforts to increase blood pressure should be postponed until the hemorrhage is under control.[13] Otherwise the increased blood pressure may worsen the hemorrhage. In all types of hypovolemic shock, fluid replacement is the primary therapy. The three main types of fluid therapy agents are colloids, crystalloids, and blood products. There continues to be controversy about which type of fluid is the most appropriate for resuscitation of hypovolemic shock.

Colloids are solutions that increase the serum colloid osmotic pressure within the vascular compartment. Increased colloid pressure pulls fluid from the interstitium into the vascular space. Examples of colloid solutions are normal human serum albumin, dextran, and hetastarch. Colloids generally are not recommended for hypovolemic shock unless the patient has significant interstitial edema.

Crystalloids are solutions that contain electrolytes. Isotonic solutions such as lactated Ringer solution or normal saline solution are commonly used crystalloid solutions. Isotonic fluids are preferred over glucose or hypotonic electrolyte solutions because isotonic solutions remain in the extracellular space and are more effective in increasing blood volume. Isotonic crystalloid fluids are preferred for volume resuscitation in hypovolemic shock that is not associated with severe anemia.[14]

When significant anemia accompanies hypovolemia, *blood products* may be the treatment of choice. In hemorrhagic shock, whole blood or packed red blood cells (RBCs) with saline may be given to replace blood volume loss. Significant anemia may contribute to tissue hypoxia simply because of reduced oxygen-carrying capacity, however recent research suggests that RBCs may also regulate capillary blood flow by releasing vasodilating substances, including ATP, into the microcirculation under conditions of hypoxia. Significant reductions in RBC flow through capillaries has been suggested as a mechanism for further impairing microcirculatory function.[2]

In general, pharmacologic agents are not indicated for hypovolemia. Restoration of blood volume is essential. However, in some cases of shock, blood pressure remains low despite large amounts of fluid replacement, so vasoconstrictor agents must be used to support blood pressure.

Distributive Shock

Distributive shock is characterized by an abnormally expanded vascular space caused by excessive vasodilation. Vasodilation results in peripheral pooling of blood in the venous capacitance vessels and creates a relative hypovolemia. Preload and stroke volume are insufficient to maintain perfusion of the brain and tissues. Anaphylactic, neurogenic, and septic are the types of distributive shock. All are characterized by vasodilation and profound hypotension, but the cause and pathogenesis of each type differ significantly.

Anaphylactic Shock

Etiology and Pathogenesis. Type I anaphylactic reactions involve an antigen/IgE antibody reaction on the surface of mast cells and basophils. IgE antibodies attach to receptor sites on these cells, where they await activation by specific antigens. Exposure to that antigen causes receptors on mast cells and basophils to cross-link and become activated. A host of vasoactive chemicals are released, including histamines, leukotrienes, bradykinins, and prostaglandins.[15,16] These substances result in bronchoconstriction, peripheral vasodilation, and increased capillary permeability. (A detailed discussion of type I anaphylaxis can be found in Chapter 10.) In some cases, mast cell degranulation is triggered by a mechanism that does not involve IgE. These reactions may be called *anaphylactoid* (Box 20-2).

Most type I anaphylactic reactions are mild and do not result in shock. Even in more severe anaphylaxis, prompt treatment can prevent the shock syndrome. Shock occurs when peripheral dilation is massive, and a type of hypovolemic shock is precipitated. In this case, blood volume may be normal but the sudden enlargement of the vascular space causes blood to pool in the periphery. In some cases, there is also significant leakage of fluid from the bloodstream into the interstitial spaces.[16] Both of these conditions cause cardiac preload to drop, followed by a decrease in cardiac output.

dial depressant facto
k. Contractility can
myocardial perfusi
tropic agents.
ntions aimed at inc
ardial workload and
cially in cardiogenic
y monitored and m
romise.

mined by multiplyi
ntent (CaO_2). CaO_2
en bound to hemo
monary capillaries
n with oxygen. In
d CaO_2 and impai
mental oxygen adm
ial oxygen saturati
d transfusion may

2 is **oxygen consu**
of the oxygen deliv
amount of oxyge
gen delivered is ta
In a normal phys
6 of the oxygen to
then DO_2 falls bec
t a greater percen
amount returning
ution of blood fl
aired, as in septic
mount of oxygen
r than it should
he heart in venou
ter in the pulmor
ration (SvO_2). Ou
assessed by mor
mple, one would
alue back toward
shock, one would
alue back toward
tabolically active

t is available to as
shock. A flow-
serted through th
surement of intr
(Figure 20-9). A
easurement of rig
ed to indicate rig
eload. The prima
is in the manage
ressure is associat

All these immune responses are normal reactions to microbial invasion and are necessary for eradicating infections. In overabundance, however, these mechanisms constitute a systemic inflammatory response that can result in shock. The major components of the complex pathophysiologic processes of septic shock are illustrated in Figure 20-8.

Septic shock is associated with profound peripheral vasodilation. Systemic vascular resistance is decreased, and despite the increased cardiac output, blood pressure falls. The veins also dilate, and intravascular pooling occurs in the venous capacitance system. Because of maldistribution of blood flow, some portions of the tissue are underperfused and some are overperfused. Excessive flow to areas of lower metabolic demand limits oxygen extraction, which contributes to a common finding of lower overall oxygen consumption. In the initial stage of septic shock, a relative hypovolemia is present because of the increased size of the vascular compartment. Fluid administration to increase preload to a central venous pressure between 8 and 12 mm Hg is advocated at this stage, even though cardiac output may already be quite high.[21] Cardiac output between 8 and 12 L/min is common in early septic shock. Even this level of cardiac output may be inadequate to perfuse the expanded vascular bed.

The generalized inflammatory response triggered in septic shock affects capillary permeability. Increased capillary permeability results in fluid movement out of the vascular beds into the interstitial space. Generalized soft-tissue edema occurs and can interfere with tissue oxygenation and organ function.

Clinical Manifestations. In contrast to other forms of shock, the clinical manifestation of early septic shock is a hyperdynamic state characterized by high cardiac output and warm extremities (see Table 20-1).

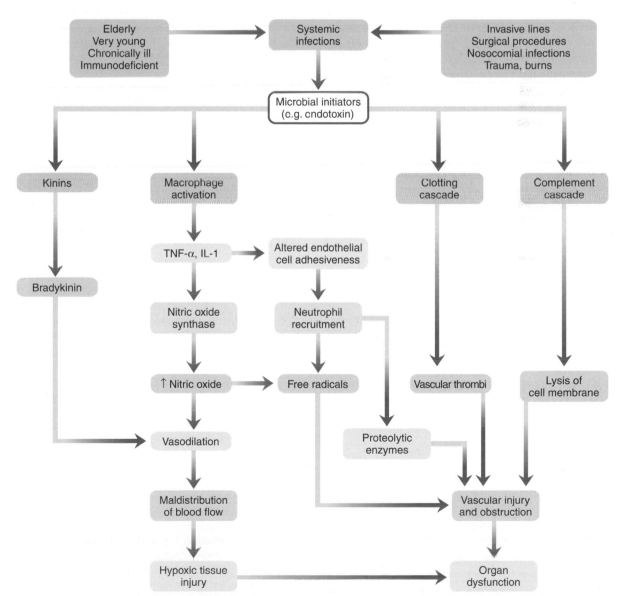

FIGURE 20-8 Pathophysiologic process of septic shock. Septic shock is characterized by immune-mediated mechanisms of cellular injury and organ dysfunction. *TNF-α,* Tumor necrosis factor-α; *IL-1,* interleukin-1.

BOX 20-2

Common Triggers of Anaphylaxis

Anaphylactic (IgE-Dependent)
Foods
- Peanuts
- Tree nuts
- Crustaceans (crab, shrimp)

Medications
- β-Lactam antibiotics
- Other antibiotics
- Aspirin and other nonsteroidal antiinflammatory drugs

Venoms
- Bee sting
- Snake bite

Animal proteins
- Cat
- Dog
- Horse

Anaphylactoid (IgE-Independent)
Radiocontrast media
Opioids
Muscle relaxants
Temperature
- Cold
- Heat

Transfusion reactions
- IgG
- IgM

Unidentified Triggers
Idiopathic

Clinical Manifestations. The onset of symptoms is usually within 2 to 30 minutes of exposure to the antigen; however, symptoms may not develop for several hours.[15] The clinical presentation can vary widely in severity depending on the stimulus and rapidity of therapy. Initially the patient appears very anxious, with an increased heart rate and respiratory rate. Hypotension, urticaria, pruritus, and angioedema then develop. Often the patient has a sense of impending doom. Bronchoconstriction causes wheezing and cyanosis, and laryngeal edema results in hoarseness and stridor.

Prevention and Treatment. Prevention of anaphylactic shock is achieved by avoidance of precipitating allergens. Anaphylactic shock is most frequently associated with antibiotic therapy, in particular β-lactams.[15] Other common causes include other types of drugs, peanuts and tree nuts, insect stings, and snake bites (see Box 20-2). More than one third of cases are of unknown cause. Anaphylaxis is not a reportable disease, and the incidence is unknown; however, the estimated risk of occurrence is 1% to 3% per person in the United States.[15]

Initial therapy for anaphylactic shock is directed to removing the inciting antigen if possible. Airway management and circulatory support are critical. Tracheal intubation and assisted ventilation may be needed. Bronchodilators can be used to manage bronchospasm. Epinephrine is helpful in stabilizing mast cells to prevent further release of inflammatory mediators and increasing blood pressure.[15] Intravenous fluid therapy is used to increase intravascular volume and fill the enlarged vascular space. Increased preload will enhance cardiac output. A vasopressor may be given in an attempt to constrict the arterioles and raise blood pressure. Steroids may be given for their antiinflammatory effects, but the onset of action tends to be slow. Antihistamines may be administered to block histamine receptors, although their effectiveness is reduced once symptoms are present and the inflammatory mediators have been released.[15] Response to therapy for anaphylactic shock is usually rapid with a good outcome if instituted early; however, approximately 1% of anaphylactic episodes are fatal, and the majority of these are associated with antibiotics and nut allergies.[15]

Neurogenic Shock. Neurogenic shock is often transitory. It may result from depression of the vasomotor center in the medulla or from interruption of sympathetic nerve fibers in the spinal cord. Causes of neurogenic shock include brain trauma that results in depression of the vasomotor center, spinal cord injury, high spinal anesthesia, and drug overdose.

Interruption of the neural pathway for the baroreceptor reflex results in loss of sympathetic tone in the vasculature. Profound peripheral vasodilation of both arterioles and veins occurs and leads to peripheral pooling of blood and hypotension. Decreased venous return to the heart results in decreased cardiac output and hypotension. Body position greatly influences the development of neurogenic shock. When the body is horizontal, venous return may be adequate and cardiac output and blood pressure are sufficient. However, when an upright position is assumed, peripheral pooling from gravitational effects causes a severe drop in cardiac output and blood pressure. Syncope and fainting will follow unless measures are taken to redistribute the blood. Elevation of the legs, slow position changes, and the use of pressure stockings on the legs may help prevent peripheral pooling. Vasoconstricting drugs and fluid expansion may sometimes be used to increase blood pressure if mechanical measures are ineffective. The outcome of neurogenic shock depends in large part on the severity of neurologic injury. Shock resulting from head trauma has a poor prognosis, whereas acute neurogenic shock associated with spinal cord injuries may resolve as spinal cord reflexes return in the weeks following the injury.

Septic Shock. Septic shock is a common cause of death in intensive care units in the United States, and the incidence continues to increase. Large numbers of immunocompromised individuals in the population and extensive use of invasive technology contribute to the high rates of septic shock. The mortality associated with septic shock averages between 30% and 50% in various clinical trial registries.[17,18] High mortality is in part because of the underlying diseases that often accompany sepsis, such as trauma, peritonitis, cancer, and immune deficiency diseases.

Etiology. Sepsis results from the presence of microorganisms in the bloodstream (bacteremia). However, most cases of bacteremia do not result in shock. Normally, the body's defense systems effectively destroy the bacteria and prevent widespread dissemination of the infection. Immunocompromised individuals are prone to disseminated infections called *bacteremia* (the term *septicemia* is still in clinical use, but is discouraged because of imprecise meaning). When the body's response to infection or other insults results in systemic signs and symptoms of widespread inflammation, the term *systemic inflammatory response syndrome* (SIRS) is applied. Septic shock is a severe systemic inflammatory reaction to infection that results in abnormal vasodilation, hypotension, and tissue hypoxia owing to the maldistribution of blood flow. Confusion about the meaning of the terms bacteremia, sepsis, septic shock, and SIRS prompted a consensus conference to provide definitions for clinical and research purposes (Table 20-4).[19]

Patients at high risk for septic shock include the very young and the elderly. Patients in these age groups are less likely to be able to destroy invading microorganisms. Patients who are debilitated, malnourished, or immunocompromised by acquired immunodeficiency syndrome or chemotherapy or have chronic health problems are also at increased risk. Medical interventions that predispose a patient to septic shock include the use of invasive lines, catheters, and procedures; surgery; and immunosuppressive therapy.

Pathogenesis. Septic shock commonly is associated with Gram-negative infections. Gram-negative bacteria include *Escherichia coli, Klebsiella pneumoniae, Enterobacter aerogenes, Serratia marcescens, Pseudomonas aeruginosa,* and *Proteus* species.[20] Gram-positive organisms *(Staphylococcus aureus, Staphylococcus epidermidis, Streptococcus pneumoniae)* and fungi *(Candida* species) are also important causes of septic shock. A frequent portal of entry is the genitourinary tract. Other entry sites include the gastrointestinal tract, the respiratory tract, and the skin.

Gram-negative bacteria have within their cell walls a lipopolysaccharide or **endotoxin.** It is composed of an O antigen side chain, an R core, and an inner lipid A, which is the toxic component of the endotoxin.[20] Endotoxins are released into the blood during bacterial cell lysis and initiate a chain of pathophysiologic events. Macrophages are stimulated by endotoxin to release inflammatory cytokines, including TNF-α and IL-1.[6] As previously described, TNF-α and IL-1 are thought to be major factors in the pathogenesis of septic shock because they stimulate release of more immune cytokines and the overproduction of nitric oxide.

Macrophage cytokines activate neutrophils and platelets, which release many toxic mediators such as platelet-activating factor, oxygen free radicals, and proteolytic enzymes.[6] Activation of the arachidonic acid cascade in neutrophils and platelets results in prostaglandin, leukotriene, thromboxane, and prostacyclin release, all of which have profound effects on vascular smooth muscle. Increased levels of thromboxane A_2 and B_2 produce pulmonary vasoconstriction, mediate bronchoconstriction, and act as potent platelet aggregators. Prostacyclin is a potent vasodilator and may contribute to the development of hypotension.

A number of other inflammatory cascades are activated in septic shock. The complement system is activated with release of C5a and C3a, and can produce microemboli and endothelial cell destruction. Histamine, a potent vasodilator, is released by mast cells. Histamine also increases capillary permeability, which enhances edema formation. The coagulation system is activated and may enhance the development of thrombi. The kinin system is activated and bradykinin is released, which results in vasodilation and increased capillary permeability.

TABLE 20-4

Definitions Related to Sepsis

Condition	Definition
Bacteremia (fungemia)	Presence of viable bacteria (fungi) in the bloodstream
Infection	Inflammatory response to invasion of normally sterile host tissue by the microorganisms
Systemic inflammatory response syndrome (SIRS)	Systemic inflammatory response to a variety of clinical insults that can be infectious or noninfectious etiology. The response is manifested by two or more of the following conditions: T >38° C (100.4° F) or <36° C (96.8° F); HR >90 beats/min; RR >20 breaths/min or Pa_{CO_2} <32 torr; WBC >12,000 cells/mm³, <4000 cells/mm³, or >10% immature (band) forms; positive fluid balance (>20 mL/kg over 24 h); hyperglycemia; plasma C-reactive protein/procalcitonin >2 SD above normal value; arterial hypotension; cardiac index >3.5 L/min; arterial hypoxemia; acute oliguria; creatinine increase >0.5 mg/dL; coagulation abnormalities; ileus; platelets <100,000 mcL; bilirubin >4 mg/dL; hyperlactatemia; decreased capillary refill
Sepsis	The SIRS secondary to infection
Severe sepsis	Sepsis associated with organ dysfunction, hypoperfusion, or hypotension. Hypoperfusion and perfusion abnormalities can include, but are not limited to, lactic acidosis, oliguria, or acute alteration in mental status.
Septic shock	Sepsis with persistent hypotension despite fluid resuscitation, along with the presence of perfusion abnormalities. Patients who are on inotropic or vasopressor agents may not be hypotensive at the time perfusion abnormalities are measured.
Multiple-organ dysfunction syndrome (MODS)	Presence of altered organ function requiring intervention to maintain homeostasis

From Dipiro JT et al, editors: *Pharmacotherapy: a pathophysiologic approach,* ed 7, New York, 2008, McGraw-Hill, p 1944.
HR, Heart rate; *Pa$_{CO_2}$,* arterial carbon dioxide tension; *RR,* respiratory rate; *SD,* standard deviation; *T,* temperature; *WBC,* white blood cell count; *Torr,* mm Hg.

In the hyperdynamic stage of septic shock, blood pressure falls because of the decreased systemic vascular resistance and decreased venous return. Diastolic pressure falls because of a lack of sympathetic tone, and a widened pulse pressure results. The heart rate and stroke volume increase and cardiac output is higher than normal, but the patient remains hypotensive. The patient is usually febrile and may have associated chills. In contrast to cardiogenic and hypovolemic shock in which the peripheral circulation is reduced and extremities are cool and constricted, the skin is pink and warm to the touch in sepsis as a result of peripheral vasodilation. The patient's level of consciousness may be altered as a result of cerebral ischemia. In septic shock, SvO_2 levels may be higher than normal because of the maldistribution of blood flow. Abnormal vasodilation causes greater flow through areas with low metabolic activity. Oxygen consumption by tissues is decreased because metabolically active tissues do not receive enough flow. Lactic acidosis may be present because of tissue hypoxemia.

In the progressive stage of septic shock, some patients deteriorate to a hypodynamic phase. The hypodynamic phase is characterized by decreased cardiac output and the development of organ ischemia. The pulse pressure narrows and the skin becomes cool and clammy. Profound hypotension unresponsive to catecholamines generally occurs. Arterial blood gas analysis reveals a metabolic and respiratory acidosis with hypoxemia. Myocardial depression either from ischemia or toxins acting as myocardial depressants contributes to a falling cardiac output, deteriorating tissue perfusion, and refractory shock.

Treatment. The primary treatment in early septic shock is isotonic fluid administration to restore adequate ventricular preload.[21] If fluid administration does not restore hemodynamic stability, inotropic treatment may be indicated to increase cardiac output and oxygen delivery to tissues.[21] Vascular unresponsiveness to these agents may improve with administration of glucocorticoids. In some cases the normal adrenal production of cortisol may be insufficient and glucocorticoid replacement is helpful. High-dose and high-potency glucocorticoids are not recommended because of their immunosuppressive activity.[21]

Appropriate broad-spectrum antibiotic therapy is started as soon as septic shock is suspected and after quickly obtaining appropriate cultures. Positive blood cultures can be used to narrow the antibiotic regimen to cover the specific microbes, however blood cultures are negative in about 50% of cases despite the probable presence of systemic microorganisms.[21] Eradication of the inciting organism reduces the stimulus perpetuating SIRS. Shock itself may propagate sepsis by impairing circulation to the intestinal wall and allowing resident microorganisms to traverse from the colon to the bloodstream. Antibiotic selection for septic shock must be modified as new infective organisms are detected.

Because the inflammatory response is believed to be a critical aspect of septic shock, numerous agents designed to inhibit various components of SIRS have been investigated. Unfortunately, nearly all of these agents have failed to provide significant benefit. Some subgroups of septic patients [are] helped by these agents, but overall the trials have be[en disap]pointing. Activated protein C is currently recomm[ended for] those with severe sepsis and a high-risk score for m[ortality.] Protein C has both anti-inflammatory and antithro[mbotic ac]tions, which may be helpful in sepsis, but the comp[lication of] bleeding is common. Therapy for septic shock is co[mplex] and requires intensive monitoring and treatment of [complica]tions. These aspects are discussed in the next sec[tion of this] chapter.

KEY POINTS

- Anaphylactic, neurogenic, and septic shock are [forms of] distributive shock characterized by excessive [vasodila]tion and peripheral pooling of blood. Cardiac [output is] inadequate because of reduced preload.
- Anaphylactic shock is a result of excessive m[ast cell] degranulation in response to antigen. Mast cell [stim]ulation usually is mediated by IgE antibodies. [Release] of vasodilatory mediators such as histamine [into the] circulation by mast cells results in severe hypo[tension.] Urticaria, bronchoconstriction, stridor, wheez[ing, and] itching are usually present. Treatment includes [mainte]nance of airway patency and the use of epinep[hrine, an]tihistamines, vasopressors, and fluids to resto[re blood] pressure.
- Neurogenic shock results from loss of sympath[etic inner]vation of arteriolar smooth muscle. Medullary de[pression] (brain injury, drug overdose) or lesions of sym[pathetic] nerve fibers (spinal cord injury) are the usual ca[uses.]
- Septic shock results from a severe system[ic inflam]matory response to infection. Gram-negative [bacteria,] Gram-positive bacteria, and fungal infections [are com]mon causes of septic shock. In Gram-negativ[e sepsis,] endotoxins in bacterial cell walls stimulate [the host] immune system activation. Septic shock from [any or]ganism is characterized by release of large nu[mbers of] immune mediators (cytokines) resulting in wi[despread] inflammation. The clotting cascade, complem[ent sys]tem, and kinin system are activated as part o[f the im]mune response.
- Widespread inflammation leads to profound p[eripheral] vasodilation with hypotension, maldistribution [of blood] flow with cellular hypoxia, and increased capi[llary per]meability with edema formation.
- Initially, septic shock is characterized by ab[normally] high cardiac output resulting from immune-med[iated va]sodilation and sympathetic activation of the h[eart. The] patient is usually febrile, pink, and warm. Eve[n though] cardiac output is high, cellular hypoxia is pre[sent be]cause of maldistribution of blood flow. Reduce[d tissue] oxygen utilization is manifested as a high SvO_2.
- Therapy for septic shock is aimed at improving [the dis]tribution of blood flow and managing infection [with an]tibiotics. Administration of fluid and drugs to [improve] cardiac and vascular performance is done to [improve] the distribution of blood flow.

FIGURE 20-9 A properly po[sitioned] artery. Cardiac output determina[tion...] the distal port. A balloon at the e[nd...] is inflated, it will float into a sma[ller...] atrial pressure.

a low preload and may in[dicate the need for vol]ume replacement to enha[nce...] high right atrial pressure m[ay indicate the need for] volume reduction to decr[ease...] tive symptoms.

Another catheter lum[en...] tery allows measuremen[t of...] Measurement of pulmona[ry...] sessing pulmonary comp[liance...] pulmonary artery pressur[e...] as the lungs react to inf[lammation and become] edematous. In the absenc[e...] diastolic pressure reflects [the...] left atrial pressure is impo[rtant...] tricular preload—an imp[ortant determinant of out]put. A more accurate asse[ssment...] obtained by using a sma[ll...] to obtain a pulmonary c[apillary wedge pressure.] the balloon is inflated, the [catheter floats into the pul]monary artery and wedge[s...] arterial pressure events be[...] pressure in the capillary. [...] sure is a direct reflection [of...] pressure indicates reduce[d...] indicate the need for extra[...]

Frontiers of Research

Advances in Treatment of Respiratory Disorders

Sheila K. Smith • Gregory P. Thompson • Michael J. Kirkhorn

I nhale • Exhale • Hold your breath • Gasp in surprise or fright • Catch your breath • Sigh in relief • Breathe easier

Our breathing reveals us. We may conceal moments of strong emotion by taking deep breaths. We quiet and center ourselves by slowing the breath. The need for conscious control only proves how meaningful breathing is. Breathing even reveals the content of our collaboration with others: to conspire is to breathe together. Anyone who inspires you is infusing or enkindling you, as though responsive breathing could fill or fire a spirit. The practice of yoga teaches us to "just breathe." The breath is the universe moving through us, becoming of us, giving us sustenance, energy, and life.

Our lives are sustained by respiration. Alternative medicine experts might argue that many of our common illnesses are brought on by the simple fact that most of us are shallow inhalers. Whether or not this statement is true, without doubt we jeopardize our respiration in ways that are either careless or deliberate. An estimated 46.2 million adults in the United States smoke cigarettes. Cigarette smoking is responsible for more than 440,000 deaths annually and costs more than $75 billion per year in medical expenditures. Others suffer lifelong illness from exposure to uranium dust, coal dust, asbestos, volatile organic compounds, urban particulates, and other contaminants encountered either at work or at large in the environment.

We are slowly learning the value of prevention. In 1950, cigarette manufacturers were conspicuous advertisers in the Journal of the American Medical Association. One ad presented the testimonial of a "throat expert," who reported "not one single case of throat irritation due to smoking Camels." Another recommended that for "utmost enjoyment" physicians and patients alike should try Parliament cigarettes, with the "built-in filter mouthpiece."

The cost of cigarette smoking is, of course, disease —lung cancer, heart disease, and chronic obstructive pulmonary disease. A quick scan of the diseases and combinations of diseases of the respiratory system shows that tobacco smoking is a constant threat. Smoking causes disease or worsens any existing respiratory condition, a fact confirmed by many studies. The value of quitting permanently is clear from findings of the Lung Health Study of the National Heart, Lung, and Blood Institute of the National Institutes of Health, which concluded that quitting smoking is the only effective measure for improving chronic obstructive pulmonary disease.

Often we inflict respiratory diseases on one another or allow our habits to aggravate allergies or illnesses in otherwise healthy people. The body has no adequate means to filter out the disease-causing ingredients of tobacco smoke or other contaminants. The nose does its complicated work of warming, humidifying, and filtering the air we breathe, but this efficient appendage cannot save those who subject themselves or are subjected to lethal contamination. Particles too small to be filtered by the nose settle into small bronchioles, which is a cause of lung disease among miners. Tiny particles of cigarette smoke, as well as the chemicals

Lung section from a patient who had nosocomial Pseudomonas pneumonia. High-powered photomicrograph demonstrates abundant bacteria (deep blue) invading the wall of the blood vessel. (From Kumar V et al: Robbins basic pathology, ed 7, Philadelphia, 2003, Saunders.)

Respiratory Function

used in manufacturing cigarettes, also escape the body's filters and cause lung disease or lung cancer.

Disease caused or aggravated by outside contaminants is only some of the pathology found in the respiratory system. Researchers say that asthma now affects 1 in 15 people in the United States and Europe. While asthma can generally be effectively controlled with inhaled corticosteroids and bronchodilators, the epidemic of asthma is of great concern. Acute irreversible asthma causes thousands of deaths each year, and severe asthma contributes to worsening consequences of otherwise less severe illnesses such as upper respiratory infections. In the United States, asthma-related morbidity and mortality is rising among African Americans, Hispanics, and children living in urban areas. In rapidly developing Asian countries, which frequently lag behind in industrial and environmental controls, risks for developing asthma are profound. Some advocate immunization against the contaminants that set off asthma attacks, such as dust mites, cat dander, molds, and cockroaches. Partly because asthma sufferers are usually allergic to multiple aeroallergens, immunization—with a purified extract of ragweed, for example—is recommended by the National Institutes of Health only when drugs fail or when it is impossible to avoid allergens; the British Thoracic Society does not recommend it at all.

Other respiratory disorders that we thought were reasonably well controlled are again becoming significant threats to public health. Tuberculosis is once again increasingly prevalent, and a multidrug-resistant form is extremely dangerous to persons with compromised immune systems; avian influenza threatens to become one of the next major and potentially deadly epidemics of airborne viral contaminants; and acquisition of common childhood viruses such as respiratory syncytial virus (RSV) or rhinovirus infections (common colds), can trigger the development of long-term asthma.

In the acute care environment, health professionals have learned to watch alertly for signs of acute respiratory distress syndrome (ARDS), which can develop slowly or suddenly, often with devastating results. Researchers report that acute lung injury and ARDS play pivotal roles in most occurrences of systemic inflammatory response syndrome and multiple organ system dysfunction. Understanding the pathophysiology of this severe lung disorder has guided researchers and practitioners in their approach to often fatal respiratory system failure.

When the endothelial lining of alveolar capillary membranes is damaged in ARDS, fluid molecules that normally remain inside the capillaries leak into surrounding tissues. The result is pulmonary edema, which significantly disrupts normal gas exchange. Blood passes through saturated and collapsed alveoli without receiving oxygen. Supplemental oxygen cannot reach the damaged alveoli, affecting whole body tissue oxygenation and vital system functioning.

ARDS presents a combination of exacting responsibilities for the health care professional. Patients with ARDS require careful detection of changes in respiratory status, gas exchange, and oxygen absorption, as well as adequate nourishment. Twenty-five years ago, 9 in 10 ARDS patients died. The mortality is still above 50%, but a high-quality clinical response can now offer the patient a good possibility for recovery.

chapter

21

Respiratory Function and Alterations in Gas Exchange

Lorna Schumann

MEDIA RESOURCES

Additional Material for Study, Review, and Further Exploration

CD Companion ▪ Review Questions and Answers
▪ Glossary (with audio pronunciations for selected terms)
▪ Disease Profiles ▪ Animations

evolve **Website** at http://evolve.elsevier.com/Copstead/
▪ Case Studies ▪ Disease Profiles ▪ WebLinks ▪ Key Points Review

Online Course (Module 12)

KEY QUESTIONS

▪ How do the structures involved in gas exchange in the lungs differ from conducting structures?
▪ What factors determine the work of breathing?
▪ How are alveolar ventilation and oxygenation estimated and assessed?
▪ What factors affect the distribution of ventilation and perfusion in the lungs?

▪ How are oxygen and carbon dioxide transported in the circulation?
▪ What pathophysiologic factors might alter ventilation-perfusion matching in the lungs?
▪ What are the risk factors and complications of pulmonary venous thromboembolism and hypertension?
▪ What are the various types of pulmonary malignancies?

CHAPTER OUTLINE

The primary function of the lungs is gas exchange. Oxygen is transported to the body tissues, and carbon dioxide, a waste product, is transported out of the body. The exchange of these gases takes place at the alveolar-capillary membrane. For effective gas exchange to occur, the processes of ventilation, perfusion, and diffusion must occur simultaneously at the alveolar-capillary interface. Problems with any of these three processes can result in hypoxemia (low arterial oxygen) or hypercarbia (high arterial carbon dioxide). An understanding of the anatomy and physiology of pulmonary gas exchange is necessary for learning about the pathophysiologic processes that follow.

FUNCTIONAL ANATOMY

Development of the Pulmonary System

Initially, the laryngotracheal diverticulum includes the esophagus and the trachea as a single tube. Then longitudinal ridges begin to develop along the tubular wall and form a septum (wall), which separates the esophagus from the trachea. Failure of this septum to develop leads to a tracheoesophageal fistula (abnormal opening), leaving a communication between the esophagus and the trachea. This abnormality occurs about once in every 2500 births. Approximately 90% of the cases of esophageal atresia (blind pouch) are of the type seen in Figure 21-1, *A*. Figures 21-1, *B* through *D*, show variations of tracheoesophageal fistulas.[1]

As the laryngotracheal tube continues to elongate, the lung bud divides into two bronchial buds, which become the bronchi and the right and left lung. The right bronchus becomes larger than the left. The right mainstem bronchus is normally more vertical than the left because it is the main continuation

of the laryngotracheal tube and branches off the trachea at a 20-degree angle. The left bronchus branches off the trachea at an angle of 40 to 60 degrees. This normal anatomic development increases the chances that an inhaled foreign body will lodge in the right mainstem bronchus rather than the left.

Fetal lung development can be divided into four periods:

1. During the pseudoglandular period (5 to 17 weeks) when the bronchial divisions are differentiated, and the major elements of lung tissue are present except for those involved in gas exchange: the respiratory bronchioles and alveoli.

2. During the canalicular period (16 to 25 weeks) when the bronchi and bronchioles enlarge and vascularization of lung tissue takes place. At the end of this period, respiration is possible because of the development of respiratory bronchioles and primitive alveoli. Alveoli are grapelike sacs in which gas exchange occurs. Type II pneumocytes (epithelial cells that are on the internal surface of alveoli) begin to secrete surfactant at the end of this period. Surfactant is a phospholipid essential for maintaining alveolar patency.

3. During the terminal sac period (24 weeks to birth) terminal sacs become thinner, preparing the lung tissue for gas exchange. Proliferation of pulmonary capillaries is also prominent during this period. Infants born prematurely in the early weeks of this period (25 to 28 weeks) are susceptible to the development of respiratory distress syndrome (RDS) due to the immaturity of the pulmonary structures.

4. The alveolar period (late fetal life to 8 years) is the final period of lung development when alveolar ducts form from terminal sacs and alveoli mature by increasing in size and in number. Approximately one eighth to one sixth of the adult number of alveoli are present at birth.[1] During this growth period, there is a lack of structural collateral

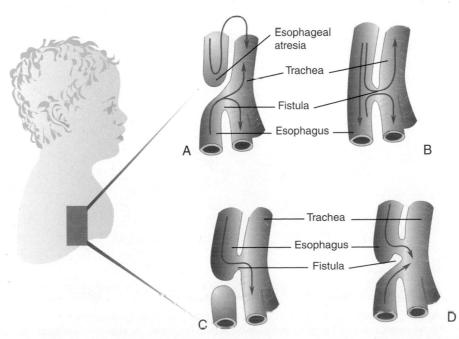

FIGURE 21-1 The four primary types of tracheoesophageal fistulas. **A,** The most common type, with complete atresia (blind pouch) of the esophagus. **B,** A common opening between the trachea and esophagus. **C,** An opening from an esophageal pouch into the trachea. **D,** A double opening from two unconnected ends of the esophagus. *Arrows* indicate flow of fluid from the esophagus to the trachea.

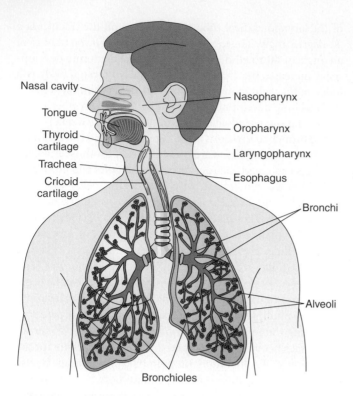

FIGURE 21-2 Sagittal view diagram of the nasopharyngeal cavity (nasal cavity, nasopharynx, oropharynx, and laryngopharynx) and the respiratory passages beginning at the trachea and ending at the alveoli.

pathways necessary for maintaining open airways. This may make the individual more susceptible to atelectasis (incomplete expansion) and obstruction. Lung damage during this period may cause permanent defects in lung development.[1]

Upper Airway Structures

The respiratory system can be divided into two major anatomic areas: the upper airway and the lower airway. The upper airway consists of the nasopharyngeal cavity (nasopharynx, oropharynx, laryngopharynx) (Figure 21-2). The lower airway contains the larynx, trachea, bronchi, bronchopulmonary segments, terminal bronchioles, and the acinus (the alveolar region supplied by one terminal bronchiole, which includes numerous alveoli) (see Figure 21-2).

The nasal cavity conducts gases to and from the lungs, and filters, warms, and humidifies the air. It is a rigid box composed of two thirds cartilage and one third bone, which prevents collapse during movement of air. The convoluted turbinates (cone-shaped bones) of the nasal cavity are highly vascular, and their blood flow forms an efficient heat exchanger. Evaporation of water from the turbinate surface and from the mucus secreted by mucosal glands raises the water vapor of the inspired air to normal saturation. Therefore, air is warmed to body temperature and humidified to approximately 80% saturation.

Air is filtered by the large hairs (vibrissae) of the nasal cavity and cilia that line the nasal cavity. The cilia sweep foreign particles trapped by mucus into the nasopharynx, where they are swallowed or expectorated. An electron micrograph of the tracheobronchial lining is shown in Figure 21-3.

FIGURE 21-3 Cells composing the bronchial epithelium are ciliated epithelial cells *(CE)*, goblet cells *(G)*, and basal cells *(B)*. Goblet cells have abundant mucus granules in the cytoplasm, and their apical surface is devoid of cilia. Basal cells, as their name indicates, are located along the abluminal portion of the lining epithelium, adjacent to the basal lamina. The arrows at the apical surface of the airway cells indicate the location of junctional complexes between contiguous epithelial cells. (Human lung surgical specimen, transmission electron microscopy.) (From Murray JF, Nadel JA: *Textbook of respiratory medicine*, ed 4, Philadelphia, 2005, Elsevier.)

FIGURE 21-4 A, Electron micrograph shows the ultrastructural characteristics of cilia *(Ci)* on airway epithelial cells *(E)*. Each cilium has a long slender shaft that ends with a conical tip. The base of the cilium is anchored in the cell's apical cytoplasm by a curved and tapered basal foot (modified centriole; arrowhead). Also extending from the apical surface of ciliated airway epithelial cells are microvilli *(Mv)*. The two horizontal arrows in **A** represent the cross-sectional planes illustrated in **B** and **C. B** and **C,** Airway cilia have the classic microtubular arrangement of motile cilia, namely, nine peripheral doublets and two central singlets. Microvilli are randomly distributed among the cilia. (Human lung surgical specimen, transmission electron microscopy.) (From Murray JF, Nadel JA: *Textbook of respiratory medicine*, ed 4, Philadelphia, 2005, Elsevier.)

Pseudostratified ciliated columnar epithelium lines the trachea and bronchi. Goblet cells and mucus-producing glands are contained in this area and are responsible for producing approximately 100 ml/day in the adult. The composition of mucus is 95% water plus mucopolysaccharides, mucoproteins, and lipids. Maintenance of water content and fluid balance is important to the mobilization of secretions. A child has more mucus-producing glands and therefore produces more mucus than an adult. In the disease state of a child, an overproduction of mucus in combination with small airway size may precipitate tracheobronchial obstruction.[2,3]

Cilia (Figure 21-4) beat in a sweeping motion like oars rowing a boat at approximately 1000 to 1500 strokes per minute.[2,3] Mucociliary transport (movement of mucus upward) is a primary defense mechanism of the tracheobronchial tree. Inhaled particles, bacteria, and macrophages are removed from the respiratory tract by ciliary clearance and cough reflex. Ciliary function is impaired by smoking, alcohol ingestion, hypothermia, hyperthermia, cold air, low humidity, starvation, anesthetics, corticosteroids, noxious gases, the common cold, and increased mucus production.[2,3]

The four paranasal sinuses are air-containing spaces adjacent to the nasal passages that provide speech resonance and increase the heat and water vapor exchange surfaces. The sinuses are swept clean by mucociliary action when the communicating passages that connect them with the nasal passages remain open.

The eustachian tube between the middle ear and the posterior nasopharynx maintains the air in the middle ear at atmospheric pressure. To prevent secretions or food from entering the middle ear during swallowing, the pharyngeal muscles close the eustachian tube briefly. The nasal end of the eustachian tube is surrounded by flexible cartilage arranged in a spiral configuration. The muscles surrounding the eustachian cartilage close the opening by pulling the cartilage tighter. Because the tube is shorter in children, the potential for otitis media (infection of the middle ear) is increased.[2,3]

Lower Airway Structures

After air passes through the nasal cavity or oral cavity into the pharynx, it passes to the larynx and finally into the tracheobronchial tree. The acinus (Figure 21-5) is located at the end of the tracheobronchial tree and is composed of bronchioles, alveolar ducts, and alveoli.

The larynx is the transition area between the upper and lower airways. Anatomically it is considered part of the lower airway, but functionally it is similar to the upper airway. The larynx contains the epiglottis, vocal cords, and cartilages. The anatomic arrangement of the larynx functions to prevent aspiration during swallowing and to assist in phonation and coughing. Each vocal cord is attached anteriorly to the thyroid cartilage and posteriorly to the arytenoid cartilage. Vibration of the cords leads to phonation. Food is prevented from entering the trachea during swallowing by closure of the epiglottis. If food or fluid should bypass the epiglottis and enter the tracheobronchial tree, the cough reflex is initiated. A cough reflex is produced when the epiglottis and vocal cords close tightly against air entrapped in the lungs. When the expiratory muscles contract forcefully against the closed epiglottis and vocal cords, a pressure of approximately 100 mm Hg is created. When the cords and epiglottis suddenly open, the high-pressure buildup is allowed to escape. This reflex rapidly removes foreign matter from the tracheobronchial tree.[2,3]

The major cartilages of the larynx are the thyroid, cricoid, and arytenoid. The thyroid cartilage is a large shield-shaped cartilage often referred to as the *Adam's apple.* Immediately below the thyroid cartilage is the site for emergency opening (cricothyroidotomy) of the tracheal passageway. The cricoid cartilage lies below the thyroid cartilage and is the narrowest point in the airway of a child. It is the only complete tracheal ring, and because of its narrowness in the small child's airway, an endotracheal tube cuff is not necessary for required intubation of the airway.

The trachea, bronchi, and bronchioles make up the conducting airways that allow passage of gases to and from the gas exchange units (alveoli). These conducting airways make up a proportionately larger amount of the total airway system in the infant and child than in the adult. The trachea (Figure 21-6) contains incomplete cartilaginous rings; it is approximately 11 to 13 cm long and lies between the cricoid cartilage and the carina (ridge located at the lower end of the trachea). Individual variations in tracheal shape include U, circular, D, C, triangular, and elliptical (Figure 21-7). Of 111 adult tracheas studied, the incidence of shapes in order of frequency was 48.6%, C; 27%, U; 12.6%, D; 8.2%, elliptical; 1.8%, circular; and 1.8%, triangular.[4] These tracheal variations may affect ventilation of patients who have endotracheal tubes in their airways and require mechanical ventilation.

The majority of cough receptors lie at the carina. There the trachea divides into two mainstem (primary) bronchi, which contain cartilage and smooth muscle. Viewing the body anteriorly, the carina is located at the angle of Louis, between the sternum and manubrium at the second intercostal space.

The small size of the conducting airway in the infant and child makes even a small decrease in the size of the lumen from an obstruction critical to airway conduction.[5] Primary bronchi further divide into five (secondary) lobar branches, three to the right lung and two to the left lung. Each lobar branch enters a lobe of the lung and further divides into bronchopulmonary segments (ten segments in the right lung, nine segments in the left lung) (Figure 21-8).[2,3] Each bronchopulmonary segment is composed of 50 or more terminal

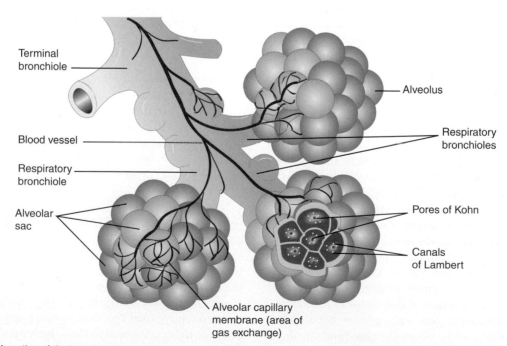

FIGURE 21-5 A portion of the lower respiratory tract, including a terminal bronchiole, respiratory bronchioles, and alveoli, where interchange of O_2 and CO_2 occurs between the thin walls of the alveoli and the capillary membrane.

Structure of Trachea and Major Bronchi

FIGURE 21-6 Anterior diagram of the trachea and major bronchi. *R,* Right; *L,* left. (From Netter FH: *Respiratory system,* vol 7, Summit, NJ, 1979, CIBA Pharmaceutical, p 23.)

bronchioles (conducting airways), which branch into respiratory bronchioles where gas exchange begins.

Nervous system control of the bronchi and bronchioles is mediated by the autonomic nervous system. Stimulation of the parasympathetic nervous system via the vagus nerve leads to constriction (by means of acetylcholine receptors) of bronchial smooth muscle. Stimulation of the sympathetic nervous system leads to relaxation of bronchial smooth muscle. Sympathetic stimulation is mediated by β_2-adrenergic receptors, which are under the control of circulating catecholamines.[5] (See the discussion in the Neurologic Control of Ventilation section later in this chapter for additional information.)

Terminal bronchioles, which include the conducting airways, further subdivide into two or more respiratory bronchioles in which gas exchange begins. The respiratory bronchioles divide into two or more alveolar ducts, which in turn supply several alveoli.

The lung is fully developed by the eighth year of life.[1,2] The large alveolar surface area in conjunction with pulmonary surfactant, a phospholipid produced by type II alveolar cells, lowers surface tension and facilitates gas exchange. Two other types of cells are found: type I alveolar cells (type I pneumocytes), which are the epithelial structural cells of the alveoli, and alveolar macrophages, which act as a defense mechanism by phagocytizing particles in the alveoli. Alveolar macrophages can be damaged by smoking and by inhalation of silica (SiO_2).

Adult lungs contain approximately 300 million alveoli, and the newborn lung contains one eighth to one sixth the adult number.[1-3] An elderly person may also have a reduction in the number of alveoli as part of the normal aging process, but many elderly people retain the same number of alveoli they had as a younger adult.

Gas exchange occurs in the alveolar units (see Figure 21-5) where oxygen (O_2) and carbon dioxide (CO_2) transfer across the alveolar-capillary membrane. The partial pressures of gases in the alveoli are termed P_{AO_2} for oxygen and P_{ACO_2} for

U shape   D shape   Triangular

Circular   C shape   Elliptical

FIGURE 21-7 Examples of variation in tracheal shape.

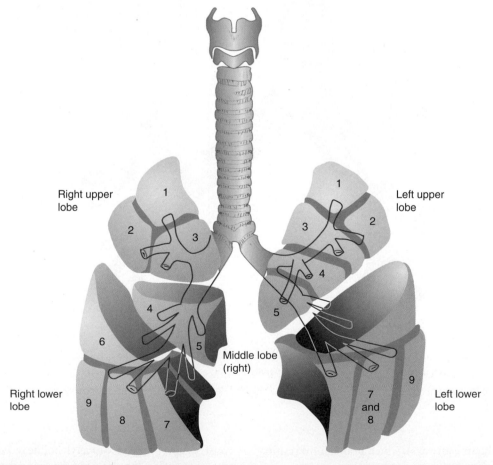

Right upper lobe

Left upper lobe

Middle lobe (right)

Right lower lobe

Left lower lobe

FIGURE 21-8 Bronchopulmonary segments of the human lung. Right and left upper lobes: *1,* apical segment; *2,* posterior segment; *3,* anterior segment. Left upper lobe: *4,* superior segment; *5,* inferior segment. Middle lobe (right): *4,* lateral segment; *5,* medial segment. Right and left lower lobes: *6,* superior (apical) segment; *7,* medial basal segment; *8,* anterior basal segment (on left, *7* and *8* combine to form the anteromedial basal segment); *9,* lateral basal segment. (*10,* posterior basal segment visible in medial view, not shown here).

carbon dioxide. The partial pressures of gases in the blood are termed Pa_{O_2} for oxygen and Pa_{CO_2} for carbon dioxide. Collateral alveolar ventilation can also occur through holes in the alveolar walls, called the pores of Kohn or canals of Lambert. A small child has less collateral ventilation because of fewer pores of Kohn.[6] The alveolar membrane is thicker in the neonate and reaches the adult thinness of 0.5 mm by the age of 8 years. This thinner membrane may allow increased transfer of O_2. The healthy older adult has very thin-walled, enlarged air sacs and fewer capillaries than a younger adult.[2,7] Respiratory system changes associated with normal aging are described in Geriatric Considerations: Changes in the Respiratory System.

Pulmonary Circulation

Blood supply to the lungs comes from two sources: the bronchial artery system, which supplies a small amount of oxygenated blood to the pleura and lung tissues, and the pulmonary artery system, which provides a vast capillary network for O_2 and CO_2 exchange. The capillary networks of the neonate, young child, and elderly person are less than those in the average healthy adult. Oxygen-depleted (unoxygenated)

GERIATRIC CONSIDERATIONS

Changes in the Respiratory System

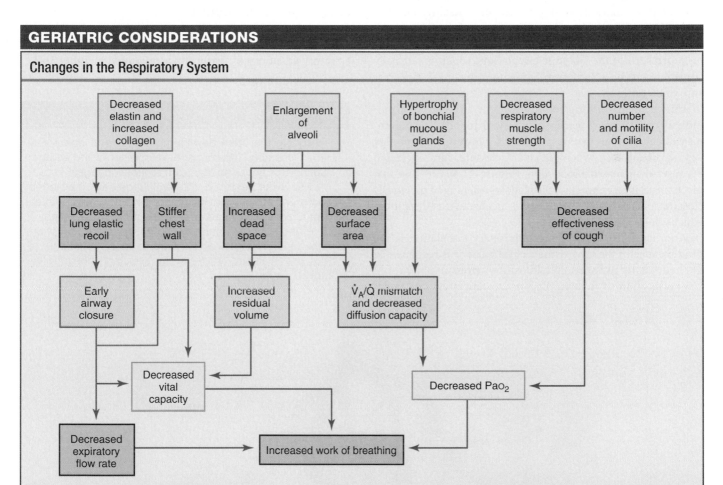

With aging, the result of all pulmonary changes is an increase in the work of breathing. The lungs show a reduction in elastin and a rise in collagen, leading to decreased elastic recoil and increased compliance. These changes give rise to increased residual volume and early airway closure. The chest wall becomes stiffer or more rigid due to rib and cartilaginous calcification. The strength of the diaphragm, intercostal muscles, and accessory muscles declines. The stiff chest wall and diminished respiratory muscle strength cause other functional changes, including an increase in dead space and decreased expiratory flow rates and vital capacity.

There is a reduction in the number and motility of cilia resulting in a decrease in respiratory clearance. There is an increase in and hypertrophy of bronchial mucous glands. The decreased respiratory muscle strength, increased mucus, chest wall stiffness, and cilia loss together reduce cough effectiveness.

Within the lungs, there is enlargement of alveoli and respiratory bronchioles with subsequent decreased surface area. The arterial blood flow through the pulmonary vessels decreases proportionally with changes in cardiac output. The loss of elastic recoil causes the enlarged respiratory bronchioles to collapse or close before the alveoli empty. Alveoli enlargement, along with reduced pulmonary artery blood flow and early airway closure, lowers diffusion capacity and the amount of gas exchange. It also increases air trapping and residual volume.

Owing to chest wall stiffness and lung rigidity, apical ventilation increases in the elderly, whereas basilar ventilation decreases. Ventilation-perfusion ($\dot{V}_A/\dot{Q}$) mismatch occurs as a result of increasing apical ventilation with poor apical capillary blood flow. The result of these changes leads to reduced arterial oxygen pressure (Pa_{O_2}). Because of increased ($\dot{V}_A/\dot{Q}$) mismatch, the Pa_{O_2} may decrease when the elderly individual reclines.

blood leaves the right ventricle by way of the pulmonary artery trunk, which branches into the right and left pulmonary arteries. The pulmonary arteries further divide into smaller arteries and arterioles that feed into the capillary network where gas exchange occurs from the alveolar-capillary membrane. Pulmonary artery blood is unoxygenated, and blood in the pulmonary veins is oxygenated. The opposite is true in the rest of the body, where the arterial blood is oxygenated and the venous blood is unoxygenated.

The capillary network is a low-pressure system that can expand two to three times normal size before a significant increase in pulmonary capillary pressures is detectable. The normal pulmonary arterial pressure in a healthy adult is about 22/8 to 25/8 mm Hg. The mean pulmonary arterial pressure is approximately 15 mm Hg. This compares with the high pressure of the systemic circulation, which is normally considered to be 120/80 mm Hg, with a mean arterial pressure of 96 mm Hg.

Under normal resting conditions, only about 25% of pulmonary capillaries are perfused (filled with blood). The pulmonary circulation has two mechanisms for lowering pulmonary vascular resistance when vascular pressures are increased because of increased blood flow (Figure 21-9).[2,3,5] The first mechanism is recruitment, which allows opening of previously closed capillary vessels. The second mechanism is distention, which allows for widening of capillary vessels.

Another factor influencing pulmonary circulation is the fluid balance of the lung tissues. Fluid balance is regulated by the hydrostatic pressure, colloid osmotic pressure, and capillary permeability. When capillary hydrostatic pressure exceeds colloid osmotic pressure, fluid moves from the capillary to the interstitium. If the fluid shift is not controlled, the fluid volume will continue to increase until fluid is moved into the alveoli. Alveolar edema is more serious than interstitial edema (fluid in the interstitial space) because of its negative effects on gas exchange. Pulmonary interstitial and alveolar edema is common in disease processes such as congestive heart failure and infectious diseases of the lung. Other disease processes that also increase capillary permeability are acute respiratory distress syndrome (ARDS) and infant respiratory distress syndrome. (See Chapter 23 for further discussion.)

Age-Related Variations

Structural and physiologic variations occur at each end of the age continuum. A summary of anatomic and physiologic respiratory variations by age group is presented in Table 21-1.[8]

KEY POINTS

- Respiratory system development begins at about day 26 of gestation. Abnormal development of the septum during this time can lead to tracheoesophageal fistula. At 25 weeks gestation, the fetal lungs have developed sufficiently to allow respiration, although alveolar development and surfactant production are just beginning.
- The upper airway includes the nasopharynx, oropharynx, and laryngopharynx. The primary functions of the upper airway are to warm, filter, and humidify inspired air.

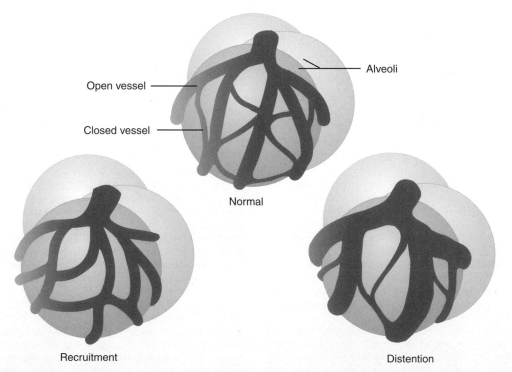

Open vessel
Closed vessel
Alveoli
Normal
Recruitment
Distention

FIGURE 21-9 Two mechanisms for lowering pulmonary vascular resistance in capillary vessels. Recruitment allows for opening of previously closed capillaries. Distention allows for widening of capillary vessels.

TABLE 21-1

Variations in Anatomy and Physiology of the Respiratory System by Age Group

	Young Newborns	Children	Adults	Elderly (over 60 years old)
Pao_2 (mm Hg)	60-70	90-100	90-100	70-80
$Paco_2$ (mm Hg)	45-50	35-45	35-45	35-45
pH	7.3-7.4 (depends on Apgar score)	7.35-7.45	7.35-7.45	7.30-7.45
Bicarbonate (mEq/L)	20-26	22-28	24-30	24-30
Anatomic dead space	Proportional to size	Proportional to size	~150 ml	~150-200 ml
Number of alveoli	12.5% to 16.5% of adult number	Adult number by 8 years old	300,000/lung	≤300,000/lung
Thickness of alveolar membrane	Thicker than adult	Adult by 8 years old	<0.5 μm	Thinner than adult
Number of capillaries	Less than adult	Adult by 8 years old	Adult	Less than adult
Vital capacity	Proportionately less than adult	Proportional to size	4.7 L	Less than adult
Tidal volume	Proportional to size	Proportional to size	500 ml	Less than adult (30% less by age 80 years)
Compliance	More compliant than adult	Similar to adult	Static compliance (90-100 ml/cm H_2O)	Less compliant
Airway resistance	Greater than adult	Greater than adult	1.0-1.5 cm H_2O/L/sec	Adult level or less

Data from Fretwell ME: Aging changes in structure and function. In Carnevali DL, Patrick M, editors: *Nursing management for the elderly*, ed 3, Philadelphia, 1993, Lippincott.

- The lower airway includes structures below the larynx—the trachea, bronchi, bronchioles, and alveoli. The larynx functions to prevent aspiration during swallowing and is the location of the vocal cords.
- The trachea, bronchi, and bronchioles serve as conducting passageways for air. They do not engage in gas exchange. Sympathetic influence on these airways causes relaxation (by means of β_2-adrenergic receptors), and parasympathetic influence causes constriction (by means of acetylcholine receptors).
- Exchange of respiratory gases occurs in the alveoli. The epithelial cells that make up the alveoli are called *type I cells* (type I pneumocytes). Type II pneumocytes produce surfactant in the alveoli. The grapelike structure of the alveoli provides a huge surface area for gas exchange.
- The upper and lower airways are lined with cilia, which move rhythmically to transport mucus and trapped debris out of the respiratory tree. Ciliary function is impaired by a number of factors, including smoking, alcohol consumption, low humidity, and anesthesia.
- The lungs are perfused by two sources: bronchial arteries bring a small amount of oxygenated blood to nourish lung tissues; pulmonary arteries bring the entire cardiac output of the right ventricle to the alveoli for gas exchange.
- The lung has a large reserve capacity for gas exchange. At rest, only about 25% of the pulmonary capillaries are perfused. During periods of high lung blood flow (such as high cardiac output during exercise), previously unperfused capillaries are recruited, and already perfused capillaries become distended.
- Filtration of fluid through pulmonary capillaries is influenced by hydrostatic pressure and colloid osmotic pressure in the same way as other capillaries. Excessive filtration can lead to pulmonary edema, which interferes with normal gas exchange.

VENTILATION

Lung Volumes and Capacities

Ventilation is the process of moving air into the lungs and distributing air within the lungs to gas exchange units (alveoli) for maintenance of oxygenation and removal of CO_2.[5] Measures of ventilation (amount of air moved) include four lung volumes and four lung capacities. Figure 21-10 schematically presents the various lung volumes and capacities; Table 21-2 defines each term and provides further details.

Lung volumes and capacities vary with individual body size, age (decreased in the neonate, young child, and the elderly),[7-9] and the individual's body position (supine versus upright). Testing of pulmonary function to measure these volumes and capacities is covered under the "Diagnostic Tests" section in Chapter 22. Other measures important to ventilation are dead space, minute ventilation, and alveolar ventilation.

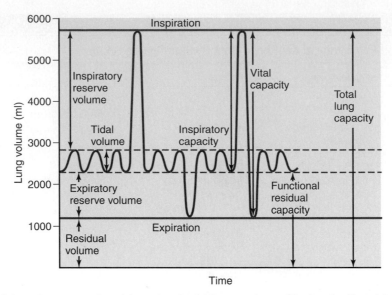

FIGURE 21-10 Schematic representation of the various lung volumes and capacities for a healthy adult (see also Table 21-2).

TABLE 21-2	
Lung Volumes and Capacities	
Term	**Definition (Typical Volume)**
Lung Volumes	
Tidal volume	A normal breath (~500 ml) or the amount of gas entering or leaving the lung during normal breathing
Inspiratory reserve volume	The amount of gas a person is able to inspire above a normal breath (e.g., maximal deep breath, ~3 L)
Expiratory reserve volume	The amount of gas expired beyond tidal volume (~1.2 L)
Residual volume	The volume of gas left in the lungs at the end of a maximal expiration (~1.2 L)
Lung Capacities	
Vital capacity	The total volume of gas that can be exhaled during maximal expiration (~4.8 L)
Inspiratory capacity	The amount of gas that can be inspired from a resting expiration (~3.5 L)
Functional residual capacity	The amount of gas left in the lungs at the end of a normal expiration (~2.4 L)
Total lung capacity	The amount of gas contained in the lungs at maximal inspiration (~6.0 L)

Dead Space

Dead space includes three dimensions: anatomic dead space, alveolar dead space, and physiologic dead space. Anatomic dead space includes the volume of nonusable gas (not used in gas exchange) in the conducting airways from the nose down to the respiratory bronchioles.[5,10,11] Generally in adults this area is equal to 1 ml per pound of *ideal* body weight, or approximately 150 ml. In newborns and young children, the anatomic dead space is proportionately larger for their size.[6] The anatomic dead space of elderly persons may increase slightly over that of healthy young adults because of the loss of alveolar sacs. Alveolar dead space is composed of ventilated, but unperfused or underperfused areas of the lung, and is often referred to as *wasted ventilation*.[5] Alveolar dead space increases with the development of pulmonary emboli owing to decreased perfusion. Physiologic dead space (functional dead space) is the sum of the anatomic dead space and alveolar dead space.[7,11] Approximately one third of each breath occupies dead space.

Minute Ventilation

Minute ventilation or expired volume ($\dot{V}_E$) is the product of tidal volume times respiratory rate per minute. For example, a person with a tidal volume (milliliters of air inhaled with each breath) of 500 ml who is breathing at a rate of 15 breaths/minute has a minute ventilation of 7500 ml (see Table 21-2 for typical volumes).

Alveolar Ventilation/Oxygenation

By comparison, alveolar ventilation ($\dot{V}_A$) equals the difference between tidal volume (V_T) and anatomic dead space volume (V_D) multiplied by the respiratory rate (RR) per minute.[10]

$$\text{Alveolar ventilation } (\dot{V}_A) = (V_T - V_D) \times RR$$

Because alveolar ventilation is affected by both anatomic dead space and the respiratory rate, slow deep breathing yields a greater alveolar ventilation than rapid shallow respiration.

The patient breathing 25 times/minute at a V_T of 200 ml would have an alveolar ventilation as follows:

$$(200\ ml - 150\ ml) \times 25\ breaths/minute = 1250\ ml$$

A patient breathing 10 times/minute at a V_T of 600 ml would have an alveolar ventilation of:

$$(600\ ml - 150\ ml) \times 10 = 4500\ ml$$

The partial pressure of oxygen in the alveoli (P_{AO_2}) is the driving force to move O_2 into the blood and is estimated with the following equation:

$$P_{AO_2} = F_{IO_2}\,(P_B - 47) - (Pa_{CO_2} \div 0.8)$$

where F_{IO_2} is the fraction of inspired oxygen; P_B is the barometric pressure; 47 is the constant for water vapor pressure (mm Hg); 0.8 is the respiratory quotient; and Pa_{CO_2} is the laboratory measurement of arterial CO_2 (mm Hg).

The value for P_{AO_2} is normally very close to that for Pa_{O_2}. The difference between alveolar and arterial oxygen tensions is called $A - aD_{O_2}$. A large $A - aD_{O_2}$ indicates poor matching of alveolar ventilation with alveolar blood flow ($\dot{V}_A/\dot{Q}$ matching).

For example, the calculation of $A - aD_{O_2}$ for a person at sea level ($P_B = 760$ mm Hg) breathing room air ($F_{IO_2} = 0.21$) with $Pa_{O_2} = 75$ mm Hg and $Pa_{CO_2} = 40$ mm Hg:

$$P_{AO_2} = 0.21\,(760 - 47) - (40/0.8) = 150 - 50 = 100$$

Therefore, using the arterial blood gas value obtained for the Pa_{O_2} and the calculated P_{AO_2} of 100, a difference of 25 mm Hg is determined:

$$A - aD_{O_2} = 100 - 75 = 25\ mm\ Hg$$

This large of a difference indicates a significant problem with gas exchange.

In critical care settings, it is often useful to calculate the $A - aD_{O_2}$ value to monitor the efficacy of oxygen exchange across the lung. The normal $A - a$ gradient is less than 10 mm Hg at room air, but it increases with age and increasing F_{IO_2}. A rising $A - aD_{O_2}$ value indicates worsening lung function, even though hypoxemia (Pa_{O_2} lower than 80 mm Hg at sea level) may not necessarily be present.

Hypoxemia that is primarily caused by hypoventilation suggests that the lung is normal, and treatment that increases ventilation will remedy the problem. This type of hypoxemia is characterized by a normal $A - aD_{O_2}$ value.

A simple method of calculating expected Pa_{O_2} is the "law of 5's." By multiplying the F_{IO_2} (%) by 5, the care provider has an estimate of what the oxygen level should be under normal, healthy conditions (e.g., $5 \times 21\%$ room air = 105).

Mechanics of Breathing

The mechanics of breathing include the concepts of airway resistance, lung compliance, and opposing lung forces (elastic recoil versus chest wall expansion) of the lung. These factors affect the overall performance of gas exchange and the work of breathing.

The lungs have a natural recoil tendency, whereas the chest wall favors the expanded state. During inspiration, the chest wall muscles (external intercostals) contract, elevating the ribs as the diaphragm moves downward. These two actions create a negative intrapleural pressure that causes the lung to expand. During expiration, the lung deflates passively because of the elastic recoil (elastic fibers in the lung tissue), relaxation of the diaphragm, and the surface tension of the alveoli. Figure 21-11 shows the interaction of lung forces during inspiration and expiration. In the normal resting individual, expiration is accomplished almost entirely by relaxation of the diaphragm.[5] At the end of a normal expiration, the alveoli still contain some air volume, known as the *functional residual capacity*. If the alveoli were allowed to empty completely, the high surface tension in the alveoli would make it more difficult to reinflate

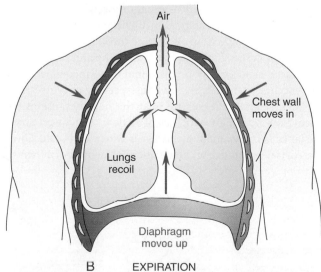

FIGURE 21-11 Lung forces during inspiration and expiration. **A,** During inspiration, the respiratory muscles contract, the chest wall expands, and air flows into the lungs. **B,** During expiration, the respiratory muscles relax, the lungs recoil, and air flows passively out of the lungs.

them and add significantly to the work of breathing. In the absence of surfactant, which reduces alveolar surface tension, the alveoli tend to collapse—a condition called *atelectasis*. Excessive surface tension can increase the work of breathing so much that mechanical ventilation may be required. This is often the case in ARDS and in infant respiratory distress syndrome (see Chapter 23).

Airway Resistance

Airway resistance is determined by the relationship between pressure and flow. It is influenced by airway radius and the pattern of gas flow. Resistance increases as the radius of the airway tube decreases. Resistance is calculated by the following formula:

Resistance = pressure difference ÷ rate of airflow

The radius of the airway decreases from the trachea to the terminal bronchioles. As mucus builds up in the airway, the passage is narrowed, and resistance to airflow increases. Other factors affecting airway resistance include stress, pulmonary conditioning, and age.

The trachea and bronchi contain cartilage and small amounts of muscle. The cartilage assists in maintaining airway passage stability, thus preventing airway collapse. The bronchioles and terminal bronchioles do not contain cartilage but have increased amounts of smooth muscle that are innervated by the autonomic nervous system. Stimulation of cholinergic fibers leads to bronchoconstriction. Stimulation of the β_2-adrenergic receptors leads to bronchodilation. The bronchial muscles function to maintain an even distribution of ventilation. A circadian rhythm is associated with bronchial tone, with maximal bronchodilation occurring at about 6 PM and maximal bronchoconstriction occurring at 6 AM.[2]

Airway resistance is also affected by the pattern of gas flow (Figure 21-12). Air movement from the nasal cavity through the large bronchi occurs by turbulent flow, which creates friction and increases resistance. Bronchospasm in the smaller airways and high gas flow also create turbulent flow. Laminar flow occurs in the small airways of the lung and creates minimal resistance to airflow. Transitional flow (mixed pattern of flow) occurs in the larger airways, especially at bifurcations. The highest airway resistance is at the nose because of turbulent flow with high velocities of airflow. The lowest airway resistance is in the small bronchioles where turbulent flow is low. Airway resistance is even higher in the newborn than the

adult and continues to be greater than that of the adult up to the age of 5 years. Resistance changes very little in the elderly lung.[6,12,13]

Lung Compliance

Lung compliance is another factor that influences the work of breathing. Compliance represents lung expandability and the ease of lung inflation. It is best illustrated by the effort required to blow up a new balloon as compared to blowing up a balloon that has been inflated many times before. It is a measure of the relationship between pressure and volume. It is represented by the formula:

Compliance = change in volume ÷ change in pressure

Two factors associated with compliance are chest wall expandability (not usually measured) and lung expandability. Lung compliance can be measured in the static (motionless) or dynamic state. Effective static compliance is determined by dividing the pressure required to deliver a volume of gas by the tidal volume as delivered by a ventilator. A more accurate measurement of compliance requires the insertion of an esophageal balloon. Normal static compliance in a healthy young adult would be 90 to 100 ml/cm H_2O.

Compliance provides an estimate of airway resistance and elasticity. Lung compliance is increased in neonates and children younger than 3.5 years because of their chest wall flexibility.[6] Lung compliance may decrease in the elderly because of increasing chest wall rigidity from calcification of costal cartilages, reduced mobility of ribs, and partial contraction of inspiratory muscles.[11,12] Compliance may be further compromised by loss in the elastic fibers of the lung that occurs with age.[11,12] There appears to be a reduction in number and thickness of elastic fibers with advancing age. Changes in the thoracic vertebrae and intervertebral disks also lead to decreased expansion of the chest wall in the elderly.[7,8,12] Disease processes that make the lung stiffer and decrease respiratory function include pneumonia, pulmonary edema, atelectasis, ARDS, and pulmonary fibrosis. Other factors that decrease compliance by decreasing chest wall distensibility are obesity, abdominal distention, kyphoscoliosis, and abdominal surgery (due to decreased respiratory effort from surgical pain). Lung compliance is increased in patients with emphysema owing to loss of alveoli and elastic tissue (see Chapter 22).

Distribution of Ventilation

Distribution of ventilation is affected by body position. In the upright individual, the alveoli at the apices of the lung are much larger than those at the base. Figure 21-13 shows the variation in structural size of alveoli at the apex compared with that at the base. In the normal upright individual, ventilation is greatest near the bottom of the lung and decreases toward the apices.[5] These regional differences are less in a supine person. The greater lung expansion at the bases results from a greater compliance of the alveoli at the bases and the downward displacement of the diaphragm, which expands the lower lobes more than the upper lobes. When an individual is

Laminar   Turbulent   Transitional

FIGURE 21-12 Patterns of gas flow.

FIGURE 21-13 Sections of lung from the apex *(upper panel)* and 20 cm below the apex *(lower panel)* obtained from a greyhound dog lung; specimens frozen in a vertical position. The upper panel shows what alveoli in the apex *(zone 1)* of the lung look like in the upright position: the air sacs are large, and blood flow is diminished. The lower panel represents the base of the lung zone with optimal ventilation and perfusion (×188). (From Murray JF: *The normal lung,* ed 2, Philadelphia, 1986, Saunders, p 110.) (Courtesy Jon B. Glazier, MD.)

in the supine lateral position, ventilation is best in the dependent part of the lung fields, but the difference is not as great as that seen in the upright lung.

Neurologic Control of Ventilation

Respiration is influenced by a number of factors. These include neural control centers, chemoreceptors, lung receptors, proprioceptors, and pressure receptors. The factors that regulate respiration are reviewed in this section.

Neural control of the respiratory system is located in the medulla oblongata and the pons, which is commonly referred to as the *respiratory center.* Efferent nerve impulses travel from the brainstem by way of the phrenic nerve to the diaphragm to stimulate muscular contractions for inspiration.

The medullary respiratory center within the brainstem consists of two groups of widely dispersed neurons that function as a unit to regulate breathing. The dorsal respiratory group of neurons sends out impulses that stimulate inspiratory muscles (in the intercostals and diaphragm). The impulses are generated in increasing fashion, termed a *ramp signal.* Impulses begin slowly and increase steadily for about 2 seconds. Abrupt cessation of signals for 3 seconds allows for expiration, and then the cycle begins again.[2,3,5] This system establishes the basic respiratory rhythm. Figure 21-14 provides a schematic diagram of these interactive mechanisms on respiratory control.

The pneumotaxic center of the upper pons (see Figure 21-14) appears to influence the rate of respiration and ends inspiration by inhibition of the inspiratory ramp, with increasing action potentials in a crescendo fashion. In addition, input from the spinal cord, cortex, and midbrain contributes to the normal smooth pattern of respiration. The apneustic center of the lower pons (demonstrated to exist in dogs) influences the pattern of respiration and probably prevents the "switching off" of the inspiratory ramp. It may function to provide an extra driving force for the inspiratory neurons, thus prolonging inspiration.

Sensory inputs to the respiratory control center include central chemoreceptors, peripheral chemoreceptors, Hering-Breuer stretch receptors, proprioceptors, baroreceptors, and environmental sensations.

The central chemoreceptors within the medullary center respond to changes in CO_2 and pH. A person's normal stimulus to breathe occurs when a small increase in arterial carbon dioxide tension ($Paco_2$) leads to stimulation of respiration. Alveolar ventilation can increase 10-fold with an acute rise in $Paco_2$. Acidosis (decrease in pH) can also increase alveolar ventilation.

The peripheral chemoreceptors located in the aortic arch and carotid bodies respond primarily to decreases in arterial O_2. Increases in the hydrogen ion concentration (decreased pH) or the $Paco_2$ also stimulate peripheral chemoreceptors, but these effects are less important than the response of central chemoreceptors.

The Hering-Breuer reflex involves stretch receptors located in the alveolar septa, bronchi, and bronchioles. Inflation of the lung initiates the response that sends neuronal impulses up the vagus nerve to the medulla to cause inhibition of inspiration. Therefore, the rate and duration of inspiration are affected. This reflex is seen primarily in neonates (less so in adults) and at high tidal volumes (greater than 1500 ml) and prevents overdistention of the lung.[2,3,5]

Proprioceptors located in the muscles and tendons of movable joints respond to body movement (exercise). The stimulus of body movement leads to stimulation of respiration (rate and depth) to maintain oxygen levels during exercise.[3]

Baroreceptors located in the aortic arch and carotid arteries respond to changes in blood pressure. The aortic arch transmits impulses through the vagus nerve, and the carotid bodies transmit impulses through the glossopharyngeal nerve. An increase in arterial blood pressure leads to inhibition of

FIGURE 21-14 Interactive mechanisms influencing control of respiration.

respiration. A decrease in mean arterial blood pressure below 80 mm Hg leads to stimulation of respiration.

Environmental factors also influence respiration. Individuals demonstrate changes in respiration related to such factors as a cold shower, a pin prick, stress, or airway irritation from air pollution and smoking. Infection and fever also increase the respiratory rate.

KEY POINTS

- Approximately one third of each breath occupies areas of the lung that do not engage in gas exchange. Total (physiologic) dead space includes the anatomic dead space of the bronchial tree and the dead space of unperfused alveoli.
- Alveolar ventilation may be severely compromised in persons with small tidal volumes or increased dead space. When tidal volume is not significantly greater than dead space, increased respiratory rate is not effective in restoring alveolar minute ventilation.
- To move air into the lungs, the respiratory muscles generate a negative intrapleural pressure that causes air inflow, owing to the pressure gradient between the atmospheric pressure at the mouth (zero pressure) and the alveolar pressure (negative pressure).
- Airways and tissues of the lung resist inflation. Resistance is provided by the airways, elastic fibers in the lung, and surface tension in the alveoli. The degree of resistance can be estimated by measuring overall lung compliance. A compliant lung requires minimal pressure to accomplish a large increase in volume; a noncompliant (stiff) lung requires the generation of high pressure to inflate the lung.
- Airway resistance is primarily determined by the diameter of the airways. Airway constriction greatly increases airway resistance. Parasympathetic stimulation of the airways results in constriction; sympathetic (β_2) stimulation results in dilation.
- Elastic fibers in the lung are stretched during inspiration, then recoil passively to achieve expiration. Destruction of elastic fibers increases lung compliance; excessive fiber production (fibrosis) decreases lung compliance.
- High surface tension in the alveoli causes the surfaces to stick together, making inflation more difficult. Surfactant functions to reduce surface tension. A lack of surfactant makes the lungs more difficult to inflate (decreased compliance).
- The medulla oblongata and pons contain the neurons that integrate information regarding the ventilatory status of the body from chemoreceptors, proprioceptors, and stretch receptors. Respiratory neurons in the medulla initiate inspiration and establish the basic inspiratory-expiratory pattern. Pneumotactic center neurons in the pons primarily influence the rate and depth of respiration.

■ Central chemoreceptors located within the medulla detect changes in pH and P_{CO_2}. Peripheral chemoreceptors are located in the aorta and carotids and detect changes in arterial pH, P_{CO_2}, and P_{O_2}. An increase in P_{CO_2} or a decrease in pH or P_{O_2} stimulates ventilation.

PULMONARY BLOOD FLOW

Pulmonary Vasculature

Perfusion (blood flow) is the second process of respiration, the first being alveolar ventilation. The pulmonary circulation is a low-pressure system (25/8 mm Hg). Unoxygenated blood from the right ventricle is pumped into the main pulmonary artery and then into its branches, which divide into capillary beds throughout lung tissue. The capillary beds surround the alveoli and allow for easy exchange of O_2 and CO_2.

Distribution of Blood Flow

Distribution of blood flow (perfusion) is uneven and is affected by body position and exercise. When a person is upright, blood flow is decreased in the upper regions of the lungs (apices) when compared to the lower regions (bases). When a person assumes the supine position, blood flow to the posterior dependent portion of the lung is higher. Blood flow to the anterior nondependent portions is lower, although the redistribution of blood flow is less dramatic than that seen in the upright lung.

The effect of gravity on the lung has led to the concept of lung zones.[5] Figure 21-15 depicts three lung zones. Zone 1

reflects blood flow in the apices of the lung. Blood flow is minimal because the enlarged alveolar sacs create an alveolar pressure that is higher than capillary pressure, leading to pulmonary capillary collapse. Zone 2, the middle region of the lung, has a pulmonary arterial pressure greater than the pressure inside the alveoli during ventricular systole, but this may fall below alveolar pressure during diastole. Thus, zone 2 is characterized by intermittent perfusion, which increases moving from the upper region of the zone to the lower region of the zone in the upright position.

Zone 3 is continuously perfused throughout the entire cardiac cycle. Pulmonary arterial pressure is greater than pulmonary venous pressure, which in turn is greater than alveolar pressure. In this zone, capillary vessels are distended and vascular resistance is low.[5,6]

Normally, 1% to 2% of the cardiac output bypasses (right-to-left shunt) alveolar ventilation, creating a decrease in arterial oxygen by 3 to 5 mm Hg.[10] In bronchial anastomotic diseases, the amount of shunting may rise to 10% to 20%.[10]

Ventilation-Perfusion Ratios

The discussion about distribution of ventilation and perfusion indicates that the best overall ventilation and perfusion occurs in the dependent lung fields. A factor important to the concepts of ventilation and perfusion is the matching of an adequate volume of air in the alveoli to adequate pulmonary blood flow. In the ideal state, 4 L/min of alveolar ventilation is matched to 5 L/min of capillary blood flow in the lungs, creating a normal alveolar ventilation-to-perfusion ratio ($\dot{V}_A/\dot{Q}$) of 0.8 (Box 21-1). Two major factors that affect this normal

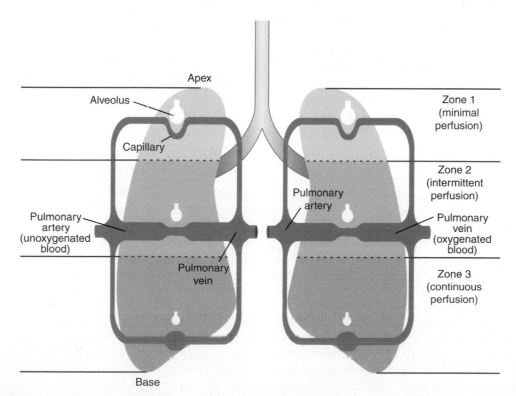

Apex

Alveolus

Capillary

Pulmonary artery (unoxygenated blood)

Pulmonary vein

Pulmonary artery

Zone 1 (minimal perfusion)

Zone 2 (intermittent perfusion)

Pulmonary vein (oxygenated blood)

Zone 3 (continuous perfusion)

Base

FIGURE 21-15 Schematic representation of the three lung zones in which different hemodynamic conditions govern blood flow (see text for discussion).

BOX 21-1

Ventilation-Perfusion ($\dot{V}_A/\dot{Q}$)* Equations

Low ($\dot{V}_A/\dot{Q}$) (underventilated):

$$\frac{2\,L/min\ alveolar\ ventilation}{5\,L/min\ blood\ flow}$$

Normal $\dot{V}_A/\dot{Q}$:

$$\frac{4\,L/min\ alveolar\ ventilation}{5\,L/min\ blood\ flow}$$

High ($\dot{V}_A/\dot{Q}$) (underperfused):

$$\frac{4\,L/min\ alveolar\ ventilation}{2\,L/min\ blood\ flow}$$

*$\dot{V}_A/\dot{Q}$, where $\dot{V}_A$ = alveolar ventilation and $\dot{Q}$ = blood flow.

$\dot{V}_A/\dot{Q}$ ratio are right-to-left shunt, and regional ventilation and perfusion changes. Other factors influencing the ratio are position changes, exercise, bed rest, and lung disease.

In a normal person in the upright position, ventilation and perfusion are lower in the upper lung (apex) than the lower lung (base). In the apex, alveoli are large and receive limited blood flow, whereas in the base, alveoli are smaller and allow for greater expansion of capillaries and thus more blood flow. In the apex, $\dot{V}_A/\dot{Q}$ is as much as 2.5 times the ideal value, causing a moderate degree of physiologic dead space. In the base, $\dot{V}_A/\dot{Q}$ is as low as 0.6 times the ideal value, representing low $\dot{V}_A/\dot{Q}$, where the blood flow exceeds ventilation. During exercise, blood flow to the upper lung region increases dramatically, thus decreasing physiologic dead space. With bed rest, the dependent area of the lungs becomes the back region in the supine position, so that blood flow is increased to that region and alveoli are smaller.

The three types of $\dot{V}_A/\dot{Q}$ imbalances are (1) high $\dot{V}_A/\dot{Q}$, (2) low $\dot{V}_A/\dot{Q}$, and (3) shunt. High $\dot{V}_A/\dot{Q}$ is conceptually related to physiologic dead space, in which the alveolar unit is ventilated, but not perfused. High $\dot{V}_A/\dot{Q}$ units have a low P_{CO_2} and normal P_{AO_2} and can be viewed as a respiratory reserve, which can be used if perfusion is restored.

Low $\dot{V}_A/\dot{Q}$ is conceptually related to lower P_{aO_2} (hypoxemia). Low $\dot{V}_A/\dot{Q}$ occurs regionally in areas where the airways are partially obstructed and airflow rates are low. Although an increase in total ventilation results in a decrease in alveolar CO_2, the increment in P_{AO_2} and O_2 content in end-capillary blood is minimal.[5,13,14] Low $\dot{V}_A/\dot{Q}$ is responsive to treatment with oxygen because the airways are only partially obstructed, so it is possible for oxygen to enter the alveoli by diffusion.

Physiologic shunt, which is functionally equivalent to right-to-left shunt, contributes to lowering of P_{aO_2}. Normally, in a healthy person, physiologic shunt is less than 5% of cardiac output. In patients with acute respiratory failure (ARF), physiologic shunt may rise to more than 50%.[14] Although physiologic shunt is similar to low $\dot{V}_A/\dot{Q}$ in affecting low oxygen

levels, shunt is not responsive to oxygen therapy because the alveoli are collapsed or consolidated and oxygen cannot gain entry into them. See the Acute Respiratory Failure section for details.

Hypoxic Vasoconstriction

Alveolar hypoxia leads to a normal compensatory hypoxic vasoconstriction of the pulmonary vessels passing through poorly ventilated portions of the lungs. Blood is diverted from areas of low alveolar oxygen to areas of higher oxygen as a means of compensatory adaptation. By diverting blood flow to areas of higher oxygen concentration, the negative effects on gas exchange are reduced. Low alveolar oxygen leads to contraction of smooth muscle in the walls of the small pulmonary arterioles. One hypothesis for this reaction is that cells in the perivascular tissue release an unknown vasoconstrictor substance in response to hypoxia.[5]

KEY POINTS

- Distribution of blood flow is affected by gravity such that perfusion is greatest in dependent lung fields.
- Zones of the lung describe regional differences in perfusion. Zone 1 has no perfusion and is equivalent to dead space; zone 2 is intermittently perfused; zone 3 is continuously perfused throughout the cardiac cycle.
- Optimal alveolar-capillary gas exchange depends on matching of ventilation and perfusion at the alveolus. Abnormalities in $\dot{V}_A/\dot{Q}$ matching can result in inadequate oxygenation of the blood and insufficient CO_2 removal. Three types of regional $\dot{V}_A/\dot{Q}$ imbalance have been described: high $\dot{V}_A/\dot{Q}$ (dead space), low $\dot{V}_A/\dot{Q}$ (poor ventilation), and intrapulmonary shunt (no ventilation).
- Vessels in lung areas that are poorly ventilated, and therefore hypoxic, will constrict to minimize $\dot{V}_A/\dot{Q}$ imbalances by diverting blood to better ventilated areas. This is termed *hypoxic vasoconstriction.*

DIFFUSION AND TRANSPORT OF RESPIRATORY GASES

Barriers to Diffusion

Diffusion is the movement of gas from a high-concentration area to a low-concentration area. The alveolar-capillary membrane through which O_2 and CO_2 must diffuse consists of six barriers (Figure 21-16). For O_2 to reach the hemoglobin molecule, it must pass through surfactant, the alveolar membrane, interstitial fluid, the capillary membrane, plasma, and the red blood cell (RBC) membrane. The rate of diffusion of a gas is proportional to the tissue area and the difference in gas partial pressure between the two sides of alveoli, and inversely proportional to the tissue thickness through which the gas must move. Oxygen diffuses into the blood from the alveoli, and CO_2 diffuses out of the blood into the alveoli. Under normal conditions, O_2 and CO_2 move across the alveolar-capillary

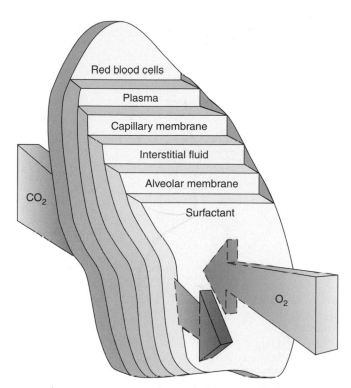

FIGURE 21-16 Schematic representing the six barriers through which O_2 and CO_2 must diffuse for gas exchange to occur.

membrane in only 0.25 second. The RBC spends about 0.75 second within the pulmonary capillary system surrounding the alveoli, thus allowing an extra 0.50 second of exchange time. Even with mild disease processes, O_2 and CO_2 have adequate time for transfer.

Under abnormal conditions, such as thickening of the alveolar-capillary membrane (pneumonia, pulmonary edema, and interstitial lung disease) and decreased available surface area (emphysema), the diffusion capacity of the lung tissue is impaired. Diffusion capacity may be further impaired by increased physical activity because of the decreased time spent by the RBCs in the pulmonary capillary system. Thickening of the alveolar-capillary membrane also occurs with aging.

CO_2 is more diffusible than O_2 because of its greater solubility.[5] Factors that determine the ability and the speed of a gas to diffuse include the available surface area of alveoli and capillaries, the integrity of the capillary and alveolar membranes, the availability of hemoglobin to transport oxygen, the solubility of the gas, the diffusion coefficient of the gas, and the differences in partial pressure of the gases on each side of the alveolar membrane. For example, because CO_2 is 24 times more soluble than O_2, it diffuses more rapidly and requires a lower partial pressure.

Conditions that cause $\dot{V}_A/\dot{Q}$ mismatch impair diffusion of gases. The decreased diffusing capacity seen in the aged person is further compromised by a decrease in the number of pulmonary capillaries and decreased lung volume and capacities. The end result is a decreased Pao_2 and increased $\dot{V}_A/\dot{Q}$ mismatch. The Pao_2 drops about 3 to 5 mm Hg for each decade

after age 30 years.[5] Therefore, an 80-year-old individual could be expected to have a Pao_2 of 75 mm Hg. Diffusion is also decreased in the newborn because of the thickness of the alveolar membrane.[6] In a healthy adult, the Pao_2 value would be 90 to 100 mm Hg (see Table 21-1 for variations in respiratory anatomy and physiology by age grouping).

The difference between Pao_2 and Pao_2 is a good indicator of diffusion and $\dot{V}_A/\dot{Q}$ matching. Pao_2 is alveolar oxygen, and Pao_2 is arterial oxygen.

Oxygen Transport

Oxygen is transported to the tissues by two mechanisms: (1) dissolved in plasma and (2) bound to the hemoglobin molecule. Only about 0.3 ml of O_2 per 100 ml is carried dissolved in the plasma.[5] The remaining O_2 is transported on the hemoglobin molecule. A high concentration (partial pressure) of O_2 in the pulmonary capillaries causes O_2 to bind to the hemoglobin molecule. Heme is an iron-porphyrin compound that joins with the four polypeptide chains of the protein globin. Oxygen binds to each of the four heme sites to form oxyhemoglobin. At the tissue level where the partial pressure of O_2 is low, O_2 is released from the hemoglobin molecule. Depending on tissue needs, one fourth of the oxygen is normally unloaded at the tissues in a resting individual, which results in venous blood being 75% saturated with oxygen.

Fully bound O_2 is considered to be 100% saturated and yields a Pao_2 of 95 to 100 mm Hg. Increasing alveolar O_2 above this level will have no further effect on increasing the amount of O_2 carried on the hemoglobin molecule (Figure 21-17). Oxygen binds to the hemoglobin molecule in the lungs and is delivered to tissues. Oxygen binds when there is a high affinity of hemoglobin for oxygen (at the lungs) and releases when the affinity is decreased at the tissue level to maintain adequate metabolic processes. When Pao_2 is less than 60 mm Hg, saturation of hemoglobin with oxygen (Sao_2) falls steeply (see Figure 21-17). The oxyhemoglobin dissociation curve schematic diagram shows the effects of increases and decreases in O_2 affinity at any Pao_2. Decreased O_2 affinity, also termed a *shift to the right*, aids in the release of O_2 from the hemoglobin molecule, thus facilitating movement of O_2 from the blood to the tissues.

Increased O_2 affinity, termed a *shift to the left*, represents a tighter binding of O_2 to the hemoglobin molecule, thus decreasing its delivery to the tissues. Although an increased affinity for O_2 reflects a higher percentage of saturated hemoglobin, its ineffective release in the tissues may be profound. Factors that affect hemoglobin affinity and shift the curve to the left (increased affinity) include alkalosis, hypothermia, decreased $Paco_2$, and decreased 2,3-diphosphoglycerate (2,3-DPG), an end product of RBC metabolism. Factors that shift the curve to the right (decreased affinity) include acidosis, hyperthermia, increased $Paco_2$, and increased 2,3-DPG. The availability of O_2 is also decreased by decreased cardiac output and anemia.

Cao_2 is the sum of dissolved oxygen in the plasma plus the oxygen carried on the hemoglobin (Hb) molecule. (See

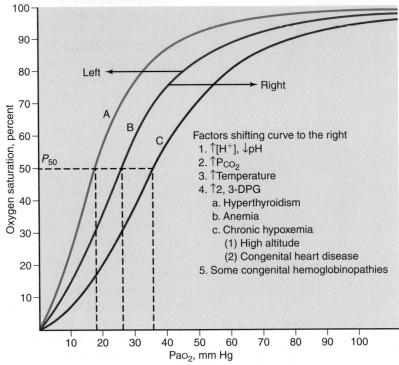

Factors shifting curve to the left
1. $\downarrow[H^+]$, $\uparrow$pH
2. $\downarrow P_{CO_2}$
3. $\downarrow$Temperature
4. $\downarrow$2, 3-DPG
   a. Hypothyroidism
   b. Bank blood
5. Some congenital hemoglobinopathies
6. Carboxyhemoglobin

Factors shifting curve to the right
1. $\uparrow[H^+]$, $\downarrow$pH
2. $\uparrow P_{CO_2}$
3. $\uparrow$Temperature
4. $\uparrow$2, 3-DPG
   a. Hyperthyroidism
   b. Anemia
   c. Chronic hypoxemia
      (1) High altitude
      (2) Congenital heart disease
5. Some congenital hemoglobinopathies

FIGURE 21-17 Oxyhemoglobin dissociation curve showing factors affecting hemoglobin's affinity for oxygen. Curve *B* is the standard curve under normal conditions. Curve *A* shows a shift to the left, which represents an increased affinity of hemoglobin for oxygen. Curve *C* demonstrates a shift to the right, which represents a decreased affinity. (From Gottlieb JE: Breathing and gas exchange. In Kinney MR, Packa DR, Dunbar SB, editors: *AACN's clinical reference for critical care nursing*, ed 4, New York, 1998, McGraw-Hill, p 672.)

Chapter 13 for a more detailed discussion of oxygen carriage and transport.) Normal arterial blood oxygen content (CaO_2) is 20 ml of O_2 per 100 ml of blood (vol%) and can be calculated by the following formula:

CaO_2 (vol%) =
   [Hb (g/dl) × 1.34 (ml of O_2/g of Hb) × (SaO_2)] + (PaO_2 × 0.003)

Carbon Dioxide Transport

Carbon dioxide, a byproduct of cell metabolism, is transported in the blood in four ways: dissolved in plasma (5% to 10% of the total CO_2 transport); as carbonic acid in the plasma (insignificant amount); as bicarbonate (60% to 70%); and as carbamino compounds on the hemoglobin molecule (20% to 30%). The greatest bulk of CO_2 transport is in the bicarbonate form. In the presence of the RBC enzyme carbonic anhydrase, CO_2 combines with water to form carbonic acid, which in turn almost instantaneously breaks down into bicarbonate ions and hydrogen ions. The released hydrogen ions attach to

the hemoglobin molecule, while the bicarbonate ion diffuses into the plasma and combines with sodium. Chloride ions in the surrounding plasma shift into the RBC (chloride shift). This chemical process is reversed when the venous blood reaches the lungs, so that CO_2 can diffuse across the alveolar membrane to be exhaled.

KEY POINTS

■ Oxygen and CO_2 diffuse quickly across alveolar-capillary membranes. Complete equilibration of gases occurs in the first third of the capillary under normal conditions. Diffusion may be incomplete when the alveolar-capillary membrane is abnormally thickened or capillary blood flow is extremely rapid.

■ Carbon dioxide is more soluble and diffuses more quickly than O_2. Disorders of diffusion often affect O_2 transfer earlier and more significantly than CO_2 transfer.

- Oxygen is carried in the blood in two forms: dissolved in solution ($Pao_2 \times 0.003$); and bound to hemoglobin ($Hb \times Sao_2 \times 1.34$). Significantly more O_2 is bound than dissolved. Low hemoglobin and low hemoglobin saturation profoundly affect the O_2 content in the blood.

- The oxyhemoglobin saturation curve describes the relationship between Pao_2 and hemoglobin saturation. At a Pao_2 of 90 to 100 mm Hg, hemoglobin is fully saturated. An increase in Pao_2 above this level does not significantly improve O_2 content.

- The affinity of hemoglobin for O_2 is affected by temperature, acid-base status, 2,3-DPG levels, and CO_2. Affinity decreases at the tissue level because of increased acid, 2,3-DPG, and CO_2. This "shift to the right" enhances the unloading of O_2 at the tissue. A "shift to the left" occurs at the lung, where the blood is more alkalotic and CO_2 levels are lower. Increased affinity of hemoglobin in the lung enhances oxygen binding.

- Carbon dioxide is transported in the blood in three major forms: dissolved, as carbaminohemoglobin, and as the bicarbonate ion. The most important of these is bicarbonate ion, which is formed from the combination of CO_2 and H_2O, forming carbonic acid (H_2CO_3). Carbonic acid breaks into HCO_3^- and H^+. At the lung, the reaction proceeds in the reverse to form CO_2, which diffuses into the alveoli.

ALTERATIONS IN PULMONARY FUNCTION

Hypoventilation and Hyperventilation. Hypoventilation occurs when delivery of air to the alveoli is insufficient to meet the need to provide oxygen and remove carbon dioxide. It is influenced by decreased rate and depth of respiration. Hypoventilation results in increased $Paco_2$ (>45 mm Hg) and resultant hypoxemia due to increased alveolar carbon dioxide, which displaces oxygen.[12] Causes may be drugs such as morphine or barbiturates (which depress the central respiratory drive), disorders such as obesity (pickwickian syndrome), myasthenia gravis, obstructive sleep apnea, chest wall damage, or paralysis of respiratory muscles (especially the diaphragm).[5] Pain related to surgery of the thorax or abdomen often results in hypoventilation secondary to decreased inspiration.

Hyperventilation is an increase in the amount of air entering the alveoli, leading to hypocapnia ($Paco_2$ <35 mm Hg).[5,13] A physiologic cause of hyperventilation is hypoxic stimulation of peripheral chemoreceptors. Causes such as pain, fever, and anxiety are common. Less common causes include obstructive and restrictive lung diseases, sepsis, and brainstem injury (central neurogenic hyperventilation). Hyperventilation is a normal physiologic response to high altitude as a compensatory mechanism to decrease $Paco_2$. Low $Paco_2$ leads to a greater ability to bind oxygen to hemoglobin (shift to the left) despite low oxygen pressure in the inspired air at high altitude.

Ineffective gas exchange from ventilatory failure occurs when an adequate volume of gas is maldistributed, minute ventilation is decreased, and/or alveolar hypoventilation

occurs. Maldistribution of gas occurs in patients with emphysema, in which gas exchange occurs only in some alveolar units.[5] In the healthy lung, some maldistribution of gas occurs because of gravitational forces on the lung, as previously discussed. In addition to the gravitational forces, airway resistance affects distribution of gases. In obstructive pulmonary diseases, the increased airway resistance develops in localized regions because of (1) plugging of airways from increased sputum production, (2) mucosal hypertrophy and edema, (3) loss of structural integrity of the airway, and (4) airway narrowing from bronchial smooth muscle contraction when there is hyperactivity of the airways.[5] During expiration, air leaves the areas of least resistance first, thus creating areas of maldistribution of gas.

Hypoxemia and Hypoxia. Two terms frequently used in discussing decreased Pao_2 are *hypoxemia* and *hypoxia*. Hypoxemia refers to deficient blood oxygen as measured by low arterial O_2 and low hemoglobin saturation as measured by arterial blood gases or pulse oximetry (O_2 saturation). Hypoxia refers to a decrease in tissue oxygenation. Tissue hypoxia is difficult to measure, but may be assumed when either blood flow or Pao_2 is abnormally low. A decrease in blood flow leads to a decrease in oxygen delivery.

Resultant types of hypoxia can be classified into four categories: hypoxic hypoxia, anemic hypoxia, circulatory hypoxia, and histotoxic hypoxia. Hypoxic hypoxia occurs when the Pao_2 is decreased despite normal O_2-carrying capacity.[6] Causes include high altitude, hypoventilation, and airway obstruction. Oxygen therapy usually provides adequate treatment.

Anemic hypoxia results from a decrease in O_2-carrying capacity. Any disorder resulting in low hemoglobin can cause anemic hypoxia, including sickle cell anemia, carbon monoxide poisoning, and other anemias.

Circulatory hypoxia results from a low cardiac output state in which the O_2-carrying capacity is normal, but blood flow is reduced. Examples of circulatory hypoxia include shock, cardiac arrest, severe blood loss, thyrotoxicosis, and congestive heart failure.

The final classification is histotoxic hypoxia, which occurs when interference of a toxic substance leads to the inability of tissues to utilize available oxygen. Cyanide poisoning is an example of this hypoxic classification.

Ineffective gas exchange occurs when ventilation and perfusion are mismatched, when diffusion abnormalities exist, and when right-to-left shunt exists. During periods of normal perfusion not all capillaries are open; however, the capillary system has the ability to recruit (open up) more capillaries and to distend (expand) capillaries already in use (see Figure 21-9) to increase alveolar blood flow when it is needed as a compensatory mechanism. In addition, 1% to 3% of the total blood flow in the lung is not oxygenated because the thebesian, pleural, and bronchial veins drain unoxygenated blood into the left side of the heart and into the pulmonary veins.

Areas of low $\dot{V}A/\dot{Q}$ (see Box 21-1) may have normal perfusion but receive inadequate alveolar ventilation (Figure 21-18, *A*). Areas of low $\dot{V}A/\dot{Q}$ are similar to shunting of

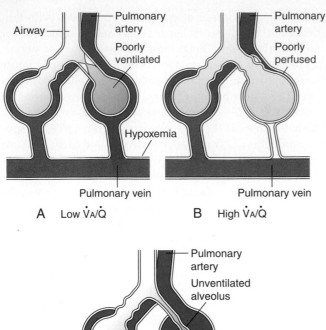

A Low $\dot{V}_A/\dot{Q}$ — Airway, Pulmonary artery, Poorly ventilated, Hypoxemia, Pulmonary vein

B High $\dot{V}_A/\dot{Q}$ — Pulmonary artery, Poorly perfused, Pulmonary vein

C Shunt — Pulmonary artery, Unventilated alveolus, Pulmonary vein

FIGURE 21-18 Ventilation-perfusion abnormalities. **A,** Low ($\dot{V}_A/\dot{Q}$) areas that are well perfused but underventilated. **B,** High ($\dot{V}_A/\dot{Q}$) areas that are well ventilated but underperfused. **C,** Shunt areas that have no ventilation but are perfused (blood flow passes unventilated alveoli).

unoxygenated pulmonary arterial blood through totally unventilated units. Areas of high $\dot{V}_A/\dot{Q}$ (see Figure 21-18, *B*) may have adequate ventilation (high oxygen level in the alveoli), but have areas of decreased perfusion. This effect is similar to having increased dead space, clinically represented by areas of ventilation without blood flow, as seen in the patient with a pulmonary embolus (PE). Although it is difficult clinically to differentiate diffusion defects from shunt effect, abnormalities occur in patients who have thickening of the alveolar-capillary membrane. Examples of diseases with thickened membranes include Goodpasture syndrome, systemic lupus erythematosus, sarcoidosis, diffuse interstitial fibrosis, and alveolar cell carcinoma.[3]

Ineffective gas exchange is also seen in patients with pulmonary shunt (see Figure 21-18, C). A shunt effect results from blood passing from the right side to the left side of the heart without passing through ventilated areas of the lung. Anatomic shunts may occur in patients with ventricular septal defects, atrial septal defects, and patent ductus arteriosus. Localized pneumonia and ARDS result in intrapulmonary shunts because of $\dot{V}_A/\dot{Q}$ mismatch, in which alveoli are perfused but not ventilated.

Partial pressures of arterial O_2 in the newborn (60 to 70 mm Hg) and elderly (70 to 80 mm Hg) are less than those in the adult. The lower O_2 pressure is well tolerated in the newborn because of the presence of fetal hemoglobin, which has a decreased binding of 2,3-DPG, thus facilitating oxygen transfer by shifting the oxygen dissociation curve to the left. The newborn also has a higher hemoglobin concentration (20 to 21 g/dl) for the first few weeks after birth. Therefore, oxygenation is not normally a problem. The lower Pao_2 of the newborn is also associated with an increased $Paco_2$. Other blood gas values (see Table 21-1) show little difference from those of adults unless an oxygenation problem is present, such as infant respiratory distress syndrome or congenital heart disease.

Acute Respiratory Failure. Acute respiratory failure is defined as a state of disturbed gas exchange resulting in abnormal arterial blood gas values, a Pao_2 value less than 60 mm Hg (hypoxemia), and a $Paco_2$ value greater than 50 mm Hg (hypercapnia) with a pH less than 7.30 when the patient is breathing room air.[1,13-15] Patients with respiratory failure can be divided into three categories: (1) those with failure of respiration or oxygenation leading to hypoxemia and normal or low carbon dioxide levels; (2) those with failure of ventilation leading to hypercapnia; and (3) those with a combination of respiratory and ventilatory failure.

Etiology. The precise pathophysiologic mechanism of ARF depends on the cause or causes of the disease process. A number of conditions may cause respiratory failure (Box 21-2), including disorders of the neuromuscular chest apparatus (poliomyelitis, Guillain-Barré syndrome, quadriplegia, hemiplegia), disorders affecting the chest skeletal system (kyphoscoliosis), and chest trauma (rib and sternal fractures). Shock (e.g., septic, hypovolemic), PE, and pulmonary edema may also lead to respiratory failure. Extreme obesity may lead to alveolar hypoventilation, resulting in respiratory failure. The most common lung diseases causing ARF are advanced emphysema, pneumonia, asthma, and ARDS.

In general, the development of hypoxemia is related to poor matching of ventilation and perfusion. The development of hypercapnia is related to inadequate alveolar ventilation in relation to production of carbon dioxide.

Clinical Manifestations. Clinical features of ARF vary with the cause. General features of hypoxia and hypercapnia include headache, dyspnea, confusion, decreased level of consciousness, restlessness, agitation, dizziness, tremors, and initial hypertension, followed by hypotension and tachycardia.[13] Early signs include rapid, shallow breathing with increased inspiratory muscle movement. Late findings include cyanosis, nasal flaring, and sternal and intercostal retractions.[1,5,7,12] The increased work of breathing may lead to cool, clammy skin, dysrhythmias, and decreased capillary refill.

Diagnosis. Diagnostic tests include measurement of arterial blood gases and chest radiography. A Pao_2 of less than 60 mm Hg and a $Paco_2$ of greater than 50 mm Hg on room air are common findings.[12,13] Chest radiographic findings depend on the disease process. Other supporting tests include an electrolyte panel with evidence of electrolyte imbalance such as low

BOX 21-2

Causes of Acute Respiratory Failure

Central Nervous System
Drug overdose (sedative, hypnotic, opioid, anesthetic)
Cerebral vascular accident (stroke)
Hypothyroidism
Central nervous system infections
Brain trauma
Brain tumor

Neuromuscular Diseases and Related Disorders
Guillain-Barré syndrome
Myasthenia gravis
Multiple sclerosis
Muscular dystrophy
Myxedema
Poliomyelitis
Polymyositis
Drug or toxin induced
- Botulism
- Aminoglycosides
- Organophosphates
- Neuromuscular blocking agents
Tetanus
Amyotrophic lateral sclerosis
Quadriplegia
Hemiplegia

Chest Wall and Diaphragm
Trauma (thoracic/abdominal)
Kyphoscoliosis
Upper abdominal or thoracic surgery
Pleural effusion
Hemothorax/pneumothorax/chylothorax
Massive ascites

Airways
Laryngospasm
Foreign body aspiration
Asthma
Acute exacerbation of chronic bronchitis or emphysema

Pulmonary Parenchyma Diseases
Lung contusion
Aspiration
Pneumonia
Interstitial lung diseases
Emphysema
Pulmonary fibrosis
Acute respiratory distress syndrome
Infant respiratory distress syndrome
Pulmonary emboli (blood, fat, air, amniotic fluid)
Cardiac and noncardiac pulmonary edema
Shock
Increased CO_2 production
- Fever
- Infection
- Hyperthyroidism
- Drugs

---

potassium and low sodium, and a complete blood cell count with evidence of increased white blood cells associated with infection or decreased red blood cells and hemoglobin due to anemia.

Treatment. Maintaining ventilatory support by maintaining airway patency and ensuring adequate alveolar ventilation is the primary goal of therapy. Mechanical ventilation may be the initial treatment, followed by management of the underlying cause. If a neuromuscular problem or skeletal weakness is present, assisted ventilation with a positive-pressure volume ventilator is indicated to maintain airway patency and ensure adequate alveolar ventilation.

The primary goal of therapy is to provide adequate oxygenation at the cellular level by maintaining a Pao_2 greater than 60 mm Hg (oxygen saturation, 90%). Specific interventions depend on the cause. If acute respiratory failure is caused by chronic obstructive pulmonary disease, then vigorous management of bronchospasm and possible infection is required using a combination of methylxanthines, β_2 agonists, corticosteroids (controversial), and antibiotics. Heart failure or hypotension may require drug therapy. Diuretics may be given for volume reduction depending on the fluid volume status of the patient. Hypotension should be managed promptly with

volume replacement and/or vasopressors. The use of corticosteroids in high doses for the first 24 to 48 hours of the disease process is controversial, because no conclusive evidence of efficacy is available.[12-14]

General supportive care consists of providing adequate nutrition to maintain fluid and electrolyte balance, pain management and emotional support, and preventing complications of gastrointestinal stress and bed rest. Developing a method of communication with ventilated patients is also very important. High-calorie, high-protein, low-carbohydrate nutritional support is recommended. A diet high in carbohydrates should be avoided because of its tendency to increase carbon dioxide production.[13] See Chapter 23 for specific treatments for ARDS and infant respiratory distress syndrome.

KEY POINTS

- Ventilatory failure occurs when alveolar ventilation is insufficient to accomplish adequate gas exchange. Ventilatory failure may result from decreased respiratory rate, decreased tidal volume, or increased dead space.

Arterial blood gas analyses demonstrate hypercarbia and hypoxemia.

- A general deficiency of O_2 in the blood (hypoxemia) results from poor diffusion at the alveoli (hypoxic hypoxia) or anemia (anemic hypoxia). Tissue hypoxia may be due to general hypoxemia or poor perfusion (circulatory hypoxia) or poor uptake of O_2 by the tissue (histotoxic hypoxia).

- Oxygenation failure occurs when diffusion of gases across the alveolar-capillary interface is impaired. Oxygenation failure may be due to $\dot{V}_A/\dot{Q}$ mismatching, right-to-left shunt, or excessive barriers to diffusion. Arterial blood gas values demonstrate hypoxemia but not necessarily hypercarbia.

- Acute respiratory failure is generally diagnosed from arterial blood gas disturbances. The usual defining values are a Pao_2 less than 60 mm Hg and a $Paco_2$ greater than 50 mm Hg when the subject is breathing room air.

- Conditions that predispose an individual to hypoventilation, ventilation-perfusion mismatch, or right-to-left shunt may lead to respiratory failure (e.g., drugs, neuromuscular weakness, chest wall deformities or trauma, and parenchymal lung diseases).

- Manifestations of respiratory failure are due to tissue hypoxia and compensatory responses and include confusion, tremors, hypotension, depressed consciousness, tachypnea, and tachycardia.

- The goal of therapy is to reduce tissue hypoxia by maintaining Pao_2 above 60 mm Hg. Depending on the underlying disease process, this may require mechanical ventilation, supplemental oxygen, nutritional supplementation, bronchodilators, and antibiotics.

BOX 21-3

Mechanisms of Secondary Pulmonary Hypertension

Increased Pulmonary Vascular Resistance
Vasoconstrictive
- Alveolar hypoxia due to bronchitis or emphysema
- Acidosis
- High altitude
- Thromboembolic causes from obstruction or release of histamine, serotonin, or catecholamines
- Hypoxia due to neuromuscular disease, obesity, obstructive sleep apnea, or kyphoscoliosis

Obstructive
- Embolism (blood clots, fat emboli, amniotic emboli, tumor cells, or foreign body)

Obliterative (loss of capillary bed)
- Emphysema
- Lung resection
- Pulmonary fibrosis
- Collagen vascular disease
- Vasculitis

Increased Left Atrial Pressure
Mitral stenosis, mitral regurgitation
Left ventricular failure
Constrictive pericarditis

Increased Pulmonary Blood Flow/Viscosity
Atrial septal defects
Ventricular septal defects
Polycythemia
Patent ductus arteriosus
Congenital heart disease

ALTERATIONS IN PULMONARY VASCULATURE

Pulmonary Hypertension

Etiology. Normally the pulmonary circulation is a high-flow, low-pressure system. Pulmonary hypertension is defined as a sustained increase in pulmonary arterial pressure above 30 mm Hg systolic. In some cases of pulmonary hypertension, systolic pressures may be as high as 60 to 110 mm Hg. Two broad types of pulmonary hypertension exist: primary (idiopathic) and secondary. Primary pulmonary hypertension (PPH) is rapidly progressive and more common in women than men (1.7:1 ratio). PPH usually presents in the third to fourth decade of life.[16] The cause is unknown but can be associated with portal hypertension of cirrhosis, appetite-suppressant drugs, and human immunodeficiency virus infection. It may be familial.[14] The long-term prognosis is poor, and medical management is usually ineffective.

Secondary pulmonary hypertension results from a known disease process or pathophysiologic condition. Increased pulmonary blood flow, increased resistance to blood flow, and increased left atrial pressure are the three major mechanisms resulting in pulmonary hypertension. Of these, increased resistance to blood flow is the most common cause due to hypoxic vasoconstriction seen in chronic bronchitis and advanced emphysema.[15,16] Box 21-3 lists the major causes of secondary pulmonary hypertension.

Pathogenesis. Chronic exposure to the mechanisms listed in Box 21-3 (except PPH) results in morphologic changes within the arterial lumen. Initially, the walls of the small pulmonary vessels thicken because of an increase in the muscle mass of the media. This initial response is thought to occur as a result of local tissue hypoxia, acidosis, or both.

As the underlying pathologic process intensifies, the internal layer of the pulmonary artery wall becomes fibrotic, with further muscle thickening. In addition, muscle development occurs in vessels that are normally nonmuscular. Pulmonary atherosclerosis is present in major pulmonary vessels as well.

Sustained pulmonary hypertension (mean pulmonary arterial pressure of 27 to 60 mm Hg) results in the formation of plexiform (network of blood vessels) lesions. These nodular lesions are composed of irregular, interconnecting blood channels that further impede an already compromised pulmonary vasculature. Tissue necrosis and hemorrhage often result.

Clinical Manifestations. The clinical manifestations of pulmonary hypertension vary according to the severity and duration of the underlying pathologic process. Because of the normal distensibility of pulmonary capillaries and the ability of the lung to recruit additional reserve capillary beds with increased pressure or flow, the condition often remains asymptomatic until significant damage to pulmonary vasculature has occurred. Exercise intolerance (because of progressive loss of pulmonary capillary distention and recruitment capabilities) is often one of the earliest clinical symptoms. Patients may also experience syncope, increasing dyspnea, chest pain on exertion, fatigue, hemoptysis, and pulmonary edema. Eventually, cor pulmonale (right-sided heart enlargement secondary to primary lung disease) and right ventricular failure will develop if persistent, severe pulmonary hypertension continues because of persistent back pressure to the right-sided heart chambers. (See the discussion of cor pulmonale and heart failure in Chapter 19.) Common signs and symptoms of pulmonary hypertension are dyspnea (60% of cases); syncope; chest pain; jugular vein distention; a systolic ejection click; narrowing or a splitting of S_2, S_4; and accentuation of the pulmonary component of the second heart sound (P_2).[11,14,16,17] In advanced cases, tricuspid and pulmonary valve insufficiency are present.[14,16]

Diagnosis. Ideally, pulmonary artery catheters would be used to obtain accurate pulmonary arterial pressures in patients at rest and during exercise. Unfortunately, even if mild pulmonary hypertension is present, pulmonary arterial pressures are usually normal at rest. Pulmonary arterial pressures measured in the exercising subject would be the optimal diagnostic tool. However, the feasibility of exercising a patient with invasive central line monitoring is problematic. The pulmonary artery catheter could become wedged and necrosis could occur, or the catheter could slip back into the ventricle and irritate the myocardium, causing ventricular dysrhythmias. Stress testing without exercise may be done in the cardiac catheterization laboratory by using medications to increase cardiac output.

A chest radiograph, although usually normal in cases of mild pulmonary hypertension, is one of the earliest diagnostic tools to suggest the presence of moderate to severe hypertension. Enlargement of the pulmonary arteries and right ventricle, as well as abnormal vessel contours, is indicative of hypertensive disease. The 12-lead electrocardiogram (ECG) shows evidence of right ventricular hypertrophy. The two-dimensional echocardiogram (a noninvasive technique) can also provide evidence of pulmonary hypertension. Echocardiography may reveal mitral stenosis, left atrial myxoma, and right heart enlargement. Further diagnostic tests should be done to exclude causes of secondary pulmonary hypertension.

Treatment. The major treatment for pulmonary hypertension is early identification and control of the underlying disease process. In the case of left-to-right shunts, surgical closure of an atrial septal defect or patent ductus arteriosus may be indicated. Because the most common cause of pulmonary hypertension is related to increased pulmonary vascular resistance, treatment is often directed at reversing vasoconstriction by administering supplemental oxygen and avoiding vigorous exercise. Depending on the stage of hypertension, vasodilators and diuretics are commonly used in an attempt to control the symptoms. These medical regimens have produced inconsistent results.[15,16]

Advanced stages of primary pulmonary hypertension are irreversible. The only feasible intervention is lung or heart-lung transplantation. Continuous long-term infusion of prostacyclin (epoprostenol) is being used for its potent vasodilatory effect on the pulmonary vessels. It improves exercise capacity, quality of life, and long-term survival.[16]

Pulmonary Venous Thromboembolism

Etiology. A pulmonary embolus is undissolved detached material that occludes blood vessels of the pulmonary vasculature. As a result, circulation distal to the obstructed area is impaired. Approximately 650,000 patients are affected annually, with an estimated mortality of 50,000 annually. Of those who experience fatal PE, 8% to 10% die within 1 hour of the onset of initial symptoms.[18-20]

More than 90% of pulmonary thromboemboli originate in the deep veins of the lower extremities.[17] Other sources of PE include fat, air, and amniotic fluid. The types of emboli and their causes are summarized in Table 21-3.

Virchow, a pathologist of the 1800s, discovered three physiologic factors that predispose patients to thrombus formation, increasing the risk of PE. The three factors, commonly referred to as *Virchow's triad*, are venous stasis/sluggish blood flow, hypercoagulability, and damage to the venous wall (intimal injury). Several predisposing factors enhance the probability of thrombus development and the subsequent risk for PE. Using Virchow's triad, predisposing factors have been categorized under each of the three components (Box 21-4). The most common risk factors for venous thromboembolus formation are immobility, trauma, pregnancy, cancer, heart failure, and estrogen use.[19,20]

Pathogenesis. Thrombi are dislodged from their point of origin by multiple mechanisms, including direct trauma, exercise and muscle action, and changes in blood flow. Once released into the venous system, thrombi are referred to as emboli and travel toward the heart and lungs. Regardless of whether the emboli are actual blood clots or an alternative type of material (see Table 21-3), the undissolved material travels to the

TABLE 21-3

Embolism Types and Causes

Embolism Type	Cause
Thrombotic	Blood clots develop in the venous system, predominantly in the thighs and legs
Fat	Globules of fat secondary to fractures of the pelvis or long bones
Amniotic fluid	Collections of fluid, hair, or other debris related to complicated labor, especially in older, multiparous women
Air	Venous access through IV catheters
Tumor	Fragments from malignant tissue
Foreign material	Foreign bodies (bullets, sutures, catheter tips, orally prepared medications injected IV)
Septic	Infected tissue or related substances (fungal/bacterial)
Parasitic	Parasites present in lung vasculature

Factors Predisposing to Pulmonary Embolism of Virchow's Triad

Venous Stasis

Extended bed rest (delayed venous removal of activated clotting factors)
Immobility (activated clotting factors)
Vascular disorders (thrombophlebitis of the lower extremities and pelvic area)
Congestive heart failure (venous backflow/stasis)
Cardiac arrhythmias (atrial fibrillation)
Dehydration
Prolonged air travel
Obesity

Hypercoagulability

Oral contraceptives (estrogen therapy), hormone replacement therapy
Pregnancy
Polycythemia (chronic high altitude; chronic pulmonary disease with decreased Pao_2 and increased $Paco_2$)
Malignant pathologic processes
Cigarette smoking
Inherited resistance to activated protein C
Deficiency of protein S
Deficiency of antithrombin III
Prothrombin gene mutation
Presence of antiphospholipid antibodies (lupus), anticoagulant and anticardiolipin antibodies

Damage to Vessel Wall (Intimal Injury)

Blunt trauma
Penetrating wounds
Bone fractures with soft-tissue injury
Surgical procedures (hip, pelvic, abdominal, cardiovascular)
Obstetric manipulations during labor and delivery
Burns

---

pulmonary vasculature.[13] The lower lobes are frequently involved because of high blood flow.[14] The impact of pulmonary emboli on the cardiopulmonary circulation depends on the size and cross-sectional area of circulatory impairment. If the embolus occludes less than 25% of the pulmonary vessels in a healthy individual, no physiologic changes may be seen. When the occlusive area approaches 25% to 30%, pulmonary arterial pressures may begin to rise, with potential right-sided heart failure.[16,17] In the patient without any underlying pulmonary pathology, 50% of the cross-sectional pulmonary circulation must be impaired before dangerously high pulmonary arterial pressures are generated. Because of the large pulmonary capillary reserve, significant damage is necessary before pulmonary decompensation occurs.[14]

Pulmonary arterial pressures increase because of vasoconstriction from actual mechanical obstruction of blood vessels and the release of serotonin and neural sympathetic stimulation in a combined neurohormonal response. Right-sided heart failure occurs because of the high resistance generated by the pulmonary vasculature. Eventually, hypotension occurs as a result of diminished cardiac output.[16]

Actual pulmonary infarction (death of lung parenchyma) occurs only in about 10% to 15% of cases of PE.[16] Pulmonary necrosis is rare because three sources are available for oxygen supply: the pulmonary arterial circulation, the bronchial arterial circulation, and the airways. Significant underlying pulmonary or cardiac impairment (chronic obstructive pulmonary disease, mitral stenosis) increases the risk for occurrence of pulmonary infarctions.[14,16]

Clinical Manifestations. Presenting symptoms depend on the size of the embolus, as well as on any underlying cardiopulmonary pathologic conditions. Initial symptoms may include restlessness, apprehension, and anxiety. The most common symptom is dyspnea (75% to 85% of patients).[14] In addition, tachycardia and tachypnea are often present. Sudden dyspnea and severe chest pain are usually associated with medium-sized to massive pulmonary emboli. Chest pain may be nonpleuritic or pleuritic (infarction).[18] Pain on inspiration is seen in 65% to 75% of patients.[15] Hemoptysis may or may not occur. As the clinical picture worsens, patients experience heart failure, shock, and respiratory arrest.

Diagnosis. Because PE is often misdiagnosed, the clinician should have a high index of suspicion when clinical manifestations, combined with factors predisposing to pulmonary embolism (see Box 21-4), are noted.[19,20] Although no simple noninvasive test has both high specificity and high sensitivity, the $\dot{V}a/\dot{Q}$ lung scan is one of the primary tests performed to determine the presence of a PE. The lung-scanning device determines if a mismatch exists between ventilation and perfusion. Adequate ventilation with impaired perfusion (blood flow) to the pulmonary vasculature (mismatch) is indicative of PE if the scan is performed within 8 hours of symptom onset. Helical angiography is replacing $\dot{V}a/\dot{Q}$ lung scans as the initial test for pulmonary thromboembolism. This noninvasive test requires administration of radiocontrast dye.[13]

Other screening tools, such as arterial blood gas analyses, ECGs, chest radiographs, and cardiac enzyme determinations, are valuable for ruling out related pathologic processes. Arterial blood gases generally reveal decreased Pao_2 and $Paco_2$ and increased pH. A chest radiograph may be normal or show elevated diaphragm, pleural effusion, infiltrates, or atelectasis. An ECG is abnormal in 70% to 85% of cases with acute PE.[14,18] Common electrocardiographic findings are sinus tachycardia, nonspecific T-wave and ST-segment changes, and T-wave inversion.[18]

However, the only conclusive diagnostic test for PE is pulmonary arteriography, but is rarely done. This invasive procedure involves the injection of radiopaque material into the pulmonary artery. If an intraluminal filling deficit can be identified, the test is considered diagnostic for PE. A duplex ultrasonography of the lower extremities to determine the site of deep vein thrombosis should also be performed.

Treatment. The primary intervention for PE is prevention. Patients who are at risk for developing one of the factors of Virchow's triad must be treated prophylactically. In the case of prolonged bed rest, active range-of-motion exercises, as well as prophylactic low-dose subcutaneous sodium heparin or low-molecular-weight heparins may be used. Intraoperative and postoperative graded compression stockings and intermittent pneumatic leg compression are beneficial in reducing the risk of PE.[13]

Patients with suspected or confirmed PE are given supplemental oxygen or ventilator support with immediate activity limitations to decrease oxygen demand. A continuous heparin IV drip is used as a mainstay of therapy.[13] Although heparin does not dissolve the clot, formation of new clots is prevented. Heparin may also stimulate the intrinsic fibrinolytic system, enhancing the degradation of the PE. Thrombolytic therapy may be used to dissolve the emboli. However, thrombolytics create an increased risk of bleeding, and unless the patient has a massive embolism and is hemodynamically unstable, they are not used.[17]

If patients are thought to be releasing multiple emboli despite adequate heparin therapy, an umbrella filter (Mobin-Uddin) or a "bird's nest" filter may be placed in the inferior vena cava to trap emboli as they migrate toward the pulmonary vasculature.[13,19] Inferior vena cava filters reliably prevent recurrent PE with a recurrence rate of about 1% at 12 days.[19] An embolectomy may be performed on an emergency basis if the hemodynamic consequences of the emboli are life threatening and the patient has refractory hypotension.

KEY POINTS

- Pulmonary hypertension usually results from conditions that increase the resistance of the pulmonary vasculature. Disorders that reduce the total cross-sectional area of the lung increase resistance and promote pulmonary hypertension. Destruction of capillaries (emphysema), blockage of vessels (emboli), and vasoconstriction (hypoxemia) are common examples.
- Pulmonary hypertension may occur when left atrial pressure is elevated. Pulmonary arterial pressure must increase to maintain the driving pressure necessary to propel blood through the pulmonary circulation. The excessive pulmonary blood flow that accompanies left-to-right shunting of blood through heart defects may also lead to pulmonary hypertension.
- Cor pulmonale (right ventricular hypertrophy) and right-sided heart failure may develop with sustained high pulmonary vascular resistance. Symptoms of pulmonary hypertension are few until the right side of the heart is affected.
- Treatment centers on efforts to ameliorate the underlying cause if possible (e.g., closure of heart defects, administration of oxygen to reduce hypoxic vasoconstriction). Vasodilators and diuretics may be used to reduce pulmonary arterial pressure and reduce strain on the right side of the heart.
- Pulmonary emboli result in obstruction of blood flow through part of the pulmonary system. When emboli are large or multiple, a significant increase in pulmonary pressure may result, causing right ventricular failure.

- Emboli may be composed of fat, air, amniotic fluid, or thrombi (blood clot). Thrombi are the most common cause. Thrombi generally form in the leg under conditions of venous stasis, enhanced coagulation, or vascular trauma.
- Pulmonary embolism is suspected with sudden dyspnea and chest pain. Symptoms of right-sided heart failure may be present when emboli are large. A ventilation-perfusion scan may be done to confirm the diagnosis.
- Prophylactic anticoagulation in persons at risk for thrombus formation is important to prevent PE. Postoperative pneumatic leg compression also reduces the risk of thrombus formation. Bed rest, oxygen, thrombolytic therapy, and anticoagulation are the mainstays of therapy for acute PE. Ventilator support and measures to improve the functioning of the right side of the heart may be necessary in severe cases.

PULMONARY MALIGNANCIES

Etiology

The incidence of lung cancer in the United States has been increasing in recent years, with greater than 180,000 new cases per year.[21,22] The four major types of lung cancer are large cell carcinoma, small cell carcinoma, squamous cell carcinoma, and adenocarcinoma. Lung cancer is responsible for more than 32% of cancer deaths in men and greater than 25% of cancer deaths in women.[13] Tobacco smoking is the major cause (85%) of lung cancer, with approximately 160,000 deaths reported per year. About 3800 deaths per year are reported in nonsmokers who receive secondary smoke from the environment.[21-24] The remaining percentage of lung cancer is not attributable to smoking. Individuals at highest risk for developing lung cancer are those who started smoking before the age of 25 years, have smoked one or more packs of cigarettes a day for 20 years, work under conditions of asbestos exposure, and are older than 50 years.[21-24] (See Chapter 7 for further discussion of cancer.)

Pathogenesis

Squamous cell carcinoma (20% to 35% of cases) usually originates (in two thirds of cases) in the central bronchi near the hilus as an intraluminal growth.[13,21,22] Cytologic examination of sputum reveals the squamous cell carcinoma, leading to earlier detection of this cancer than with other lung neoplasms. The tumor normally doubles its volume in 100 days and, as it advances, metastasizes to regional lymph nodes in the area.[13]

Adenocarcinomas (35% to 40% cases) usually appear in the periphery of the lung and are not as amenable to early detection as squamous cell carcinoma. Adenocarcinomas are characterized by acinar bronchoalveolar and papillary tumors. Doubling time is about 180 days, with metastasis occurring to distant organs, which may be due to aerosol transmission in the case of bronchoalveolar (2% of cases) carcinoma.[13,21,22]

Large cell carcinomas (5% to 10% of cases) develop in the lung periphery and are similar to adenocarcinoma. The tumor cells are large and are arranged in nests or clusters. The tumor doubles in size about every 100 days and metastasizes to distant organs.[13,21,22]

Small cell (oat cell) carcinoma (15% to 20% of cases) tends to originate extrinsically in the central bronchus region, thus compressing and narrowing the bronchi. The narrowing may lead to signs and symptoms of obstruction of a central airway, leading to wheezing. This type of tumor grows rapidly and doubles in about 33 days.[13] Widespread metastasis is common with small cell carcinomas and they are the most resistant to therapy.

Clinical Manifestations

Clinical features vary according to the type and the location of the tumor, and whether it has metastasized. Approximately 10% to 25% of cases are asymptomatic.[13] Signs and symptoms can be classified as intrathoracic or extrathoracic.

Extrathoracic manifestations are weight loss, anemia, and clubbing. Facial and upper extremity edema is noted in cases of tumor compression of the superior vena cava.

Intrathoracic manifestations include dyspnea, cough, chest pain, hemoptysis, and increased sputum production (with bronchoalveolar carcinoma). Hoarseness may be evident and is caused by pressure of the tumor on the recurrent laryngeal nerve. Phrenic nerve involvement (1% of lung cancer patients) leads to paralysis of the hemidiaphragm on the affected side and the potential for development of atelectasis and pneumonia. Clinical findings of endobronchial obstruction include atelectasis, postobstructive pneumonia, pleural effusion (12% to 33%), and Horner syndrome (miosis, ipsilateral ptosis, and dyshidrosis).[13] Abdominal breathing measures are taught to the patient who does not recover diaphragmatic function from damage to the phrenic nerve.[13] Extension of the cancer cells to the pleural cavity may cause pleural effusion.

Diagnosis

Pulmonary function tests may show increased volumes in moderately advanced cases of bronchial carcinoma.[14] As the tumor blocks the airway, an obstructive pattern of pulmonary disease may lead to increased or decreased functional residual capacity due to the effect of the mass lesion.

The definitive diagnosis of cancer requires positive cytologic or histologic findings. Bronchoscopy washings are a common method of diagnosing lung cancer in patients whose lesions are centrally located. Pleural fluid samples show positive findings in 50% to 65% of patients with malignant pleural effusion.[13] Histologic examination of tissue after biopsy of the pleura, lung tissue, or mediastinal lymph nodes may also be helpful in diagnosing lung cancer. (See Chapter 7 for discussion of tumor classification.)

Chest radiographs show abnormal findings in nearly all patients with lung cancer. Common findings are hilar (squamous cell) and/or peripheral (adenocarcinoma) masses, atelectasis, mediastinal widening, infiltrates, pleural effusions, and cavitation (squamous cell carcinoma). Chest studies are helpful in evaluating tumor size and nodal involvement. Computed tomography scans of the chest are used for staging and for follow-up study after treatment.

Treatment

Primary treatment options for pulmonary neoplasms are surgery, chemotherapy, radiation therapy, laser therapy, and tissue-specific therapies for airway lesions. Patients are also strongly encouraged to stop smoking.[21,23]

The treatment of choice for non–small cell carcinoma is surgery. For nonoperable neoplasms, radiation therapy is the secondary choice. Radiotherapy improves survival in patients with nonresectable non–small cell carcinoma.[13,21] Combination chemotherapy is the therapy of choice in patients with extensive small cell carcinoma.[13,21] Combined chemotherapy and chest radiation therapy has proved effective as a cure for patients in whom disease was detected early. Radiation therapy is also used for palliation of symptoms.

KEY POINTS

- Cigarette smoking is the major cause of lung cancer. Lung cancer is usually disseminated at the time of diagnosis and is associated with a high mortality.
- Lung cancers can develop in the bronchial tree (small cell, squamous cell) or in the parenchyma (large cell, adenocarcinoma).
- Lung cancer may be advanced before symptoms become troublesome. Manifestations include cough, hemoptysis, hoarseness, chest pain, and pleural effusion. The diagnosis is based on examination of cells from bronchial secretions or tissue biopsy. Pulmonary masses may be detected by plain radiography or computed tomography of the chest.
- As with other cancers, treatment includes surgical removal of resectable tumors followed by radiation therapy and/or chemotherapy.

SUMMARY

The primary function of the respiratory system is oxygenation of the tissues. This function is accomplished by the movement of O_2 from the atmosphere through the airways to alveolar sacs. The inhaled air is warmed, humidified, and filtered in the upper airway on its way to the alveoli. Once in the alveoli, O_2 is exchanged for CO_2, a gaseous waste product, and is transported by means of hemoglobin molecules to the tissues. The respiratory system has numerous control mechanisms that influence its function. For example, the respiratory control centers may be inhibited when a person has a brain injury, thus producing inadequate respiration. Failure of oxygenation is seen in acute respiratory failure. Acute respiratory failure, defined as a Pao_2 less than 60 mm Hg and a $Paco_2$ greater than 50 mm Hg at room air, occurs in individuals who have developed

$\dot{V}_A/\dot{Q}$ mismatching, right-to-left shunt, or hypoventilation. Diseases affecting the pulmonary vasculature include pulmonary hypertension and pulmonary embolism. Pulmonary hypertension is associated with disease processes (e.g., emphysema, PE, hypoxemia) that increase pulmonary vascular resistance. Pulmonary emboli result in obstruction to blood flow in the pulmonary vasculature. The health or disease of a patient's cardiovascular, renal, and hematologic systems also affects the functioning of the respiratory system. Health care professionals have a key role in the prevention and management of respiratory disease and in patient and family education.

REFERENCES

1. Moore KL, Persaud TVN: *The developing human: clinically oriented embryology,* ed 8, Philadelphia, 2007, Saunders.
2. Ganong WF: *Review of medical physiology,* ed 21, Los Altos, Calif, 2005, Lange.
3. Guyton AC, Hall JE: *Textbook of medical physiology,* ed 11, Philadelphia, 2005, Saunders.
4. Mackenzie CF: Compromises in the choice of orotracheal or nasotracheal intubation and tracheostomy, *Heart Lung* 12:485-492, 1983.
5. West JB: *Respiratory physiology: the essentials,* ed 7, Philadelphia, 2004, Lippincott Williams & Wilkins.
6. In Kliegman RM, Behrman RE, Jenson HB et al, editors: *Nelson textbook of pediatrics,* ed 17, Philadelphia, 2007, Saunders.
7. Kumar V, Cotran RS, Robbins SL: *Robbins basic pathology,* ed 7, Philadelphia, 2007, Saunders.
8. Fretwell ME: Aging changes in structure and function. In Carnevali DL, Patrick M , editors: *Nursing management for the elderly,* ed 3, Philadelphia, 1993, Lippincott.
9. Allen SC: The respiratory system. In Tallis R, Fillit HM, editors: *Brocklehurst's textbook of geriatric medicine and gerontology,* ed 6, New York, 2003, Churchill Livingstone.
10. Chernlack NS, Altose MG, Kelsen SD: The respiratory system. In Berne RM, Levy MN, editors: *Physiology,* ed 6, St Louis, 2008, Mosby.
11. Rossi A et al: Aging and the respiratory system, *Aging* 8(3):143-161, 1996.
12. Cooper DH, Krainik AJ, Lubner SJ et al, editors: *The Washington manual of medical therapeutics,* ed 32, Philadelphia, 2007, Lippincott Williams & Wilkins.
13. Chestnutt MS, Prendergast TJ: Lung. In Tierney LM, McPhee SJ, Papadakis MA, editors: *Current medical diagnosis and treatment,* ed 46, New York, 2007, Lange/McGraw-Hill, pp 222-315.
14. West JB: *Pulmonary pathophysiology: the essentials,* ed 7, Philadelphia, 2007, Lippincott Williams & Wilkins.
15. West JB: *Pulmonary physiology and pathophysiology: an integrated case-based approach,* ed 2, Philadelphia, 2007, Lippincott Williams & Wilkins.
16. Petropoulos P: Pulmonary hypertension. In Ferri FF, editor: *Ferri's clinical advisor: instant diagnosis and treatment,* St Louis, 2007, Mosby, pp 750-752.
17. Whelan CA: Pulmonary hypertension. In Buttaro TM, Trybulski J, Polgar-Bailey P et al, editors: *Primary care: A collaborative practice,* ed 3, St Louis, 2008, Mosby, pp 477-480.
18. Ferri FF: Pulmonary embolism. In Ferri FF, editor: *Ferri's clinical advisor: instant diagnosis and treatment,* St Louis, 2007, Mosby, pp 748-749.
19. Gossage JR: Pulmonary embolism. In Rakel RE, Bope ET, editors: *Conn's current therapy 2008,* Philadelphia, 2008, Saunders, pp 262-265.
20. Smiley CM, Polgar-Bailey P: Chest pain (non-cardiac). In Buttaro TM, Trybulski J, Polgar-Bailey P et al, editors: *Primary care: A collaborative practice,* ed 3, St Louis, 2008, Mosby, pp 425-427.
21. Ferri FF: Lung neoplasm. In Ferri FF, editor: *Ferri's clinical advisor: instant diagnosis and treatment,* St Louis, 2007, Mosby, pp 514-516.
22. Theodore PR, Jablons D: Thoracic wall, pleura, mediastinum, and diaphragm. In Doherty GM , editor: *Current surgical diagnosis and treatment,* ed 12, New York, 2005, Lange/McGraw-Hill, pp 325-379.
23. Winland-Brown JE, Porter BO, Moody LE et al: Respiratory problems. In Dunphy LM, Winland-Brown JE, Porter BO et al, editors: *Primary care: the art and science of advanced practice nursing,* ed 2, Philadelphia, 2007, FA Davis, pp 304-393.
24. Lara PN, Gandara DR, Edelman MJ: Primary lung cancer. In Rakel RE, Bope ET, editors: *Conn's current therapy 2008,* Philadelphia, 2008, Saunders, pp 231-236.

chapter

22

Obstructive Pulmonary Disorders

Lorna Schumann

MEDIA RESOURCES

Additional Material for Study, Review, and Further Exploration

 CD Companion ■ Review Questions and Answers
■ Glossary (with audio pronunciations for selected terms)
■ Disease Profiles ■ Animations

 evolve **Website** at http://evolve.elsevier.com/Copstead/
■ Case Studies ■ Disease Profiles ■ WebLinks ■ Key Points Review

■ **Online Course (Module 12)**

KEY QUESTIONS

■ What are the clinical manifestations and common causes of acute airway obstruction?
■ What is the role of inflammation in the development of asthma?
■ How does the underlying genetic defect in cystic fibrosis lead to pulmonary and exocrine gland dysfunction?
■ How does smoking cause both the alveolar destruction of emphysema and the bronchial damage of chronic bronchitis?

■ What is the rationale for using drugs such as β_2 agonists, acetylcholine antagonists, leukotriene inhibitors, corticosteroids, and mast cell stabilizers to manage obstructive pulmonary disorders?
■ What pulmonary function test abnormalities are characteristic of obstructive pulmonary disorders?

CHAPTER OUTLINE

O bstructive lung diseases are manifested by increased resistance to airflow. Obstructive diseases of the lung can be classified into those involving (1) obstruction from conditions in the wall of the lumen (e.g., asthma, bronchitis), (2) obstruction resulting from increasing pressure around the outside of the airway lumen (e.g., emphysema secondary to loss of lung tissue and elasticity, enlarged lymph node, or tumor), and (3) obstruction of the airway lumen (e.g., presence of a foreign body, excessive secretions, aspiration of fluids).[1,2]

These classifications are mainly terms of convenience, as many respiratory disease processes involve several areas of the pulmonary system. This chapter presents obstructive lung diseases in the order listed above. Involvement of the airways produces narrowing of the passages so that airflow obstruction occurs. The major obstructive airway diseases are asthma, bronchitis, and emphysema.

OBSTRUCTION FROM CONDITIONS IN THE WALL OF THE LUMEN

Asthma

Etiology. Asthma is a lung disease characterized by (a) airway obstruction that is reversible (but not completely in some patients); (b) airway inflammation; and (c) increased airway responsiveness to a variety of stimuli.[2,3] In terms of symptoms, asthma is defined by paroxysms of diffuse wheezing, dyspnea, and cough, resulting from spasmodic contractions of the bronchi. Airway inflammation leads to epithelial denudation, collagen deposition beneath the basement membrane, mast cell activation, mucosal edema, increased viscid secretions, and smooth muscle contraction. With proper treatment, most asthmatics can control the disease and prevent development of emphysema or bronchitis. Asthma occurs in about 5% to 12% of the U.S. population and is common among children and adults alike.[2-6] Asthma is the most common chronic disease of childhood.[6,7] High-risk populations include African Americans, inner-city dwellers, and premature or low-birth-weight children.[3,7] Pathophysiology of both intrinsic (non-allergic, sometimes referred to as *adult-onset*) and extrinsic (allergic, sometimes referred to as *pediatric onset*) asthma is thought to involve inflammation of the airways. Most cases of asthma can be triggered both by allergens and by stimuli, such as exercise and exposure to cold air. The terms *intrinsic* and *extrinsic* are still used, but many prefer the terms *non-allergic* and *allergic*. The clinical features of all forms are similar.

Asthma is associated with release of inflammatory chemicals from mast cells in the airways. The mechanisms stimulating mast cell release are allergic, immunoglobulin E (IgE)-mediated triggers for extrinsic/allergic asthma (Figure 22-1). Intrinsic/non-allergic asthma occurs in patients who have no history of allergy.[8] Allergic asthma (extrinsic) makes up approximately one third to one half of all cases.[8,9] Asthma is often associated with a history of hay fever or eczema (atopy), a positive family history of the disease, and positive skin test reactions to allergens (dust mites, cat/dog dander, industrial chemicals).[8,10] Pharmacologic therapy, allergen-specific immunotherapy, and environmental control are usually beneficial.[6,9] Refer to Chapter 10 for details on IgE-mediated mechanisms and hyposensitization methods.

Intrinsic/non-allergic asthma frequently develops in middle age and has a less favorable prognosis. Respiratory infections or psychological factors appear to be contributory, whereas antigen-antibody reactions appear to have less of a role in the disease process, although IgE levels may be elevated.[8-10] Attacks are often severe, and patients have a variable response to medical therapy.[10] Allergen-specific immunotherapy and environmental control measures are *not* usually helpful. Airways are hyperreactive, and patients may present with extreme dyspnea, orthopnea, and agitation.

Exercise-induced asthma is common, especially in children and adolescents.[8,9] Bronchospasm often occurs within 3 minutes after the end of exercise and usually resolves in 60 minutes.[9,10] Heat loss, water loss, and increased osmolarity of the lower respiratory mucosa are believed to stimulate mediator release from basophils and tissue mast cells. This mediator release is then thought to produce airway smooth muscle contraction. Running, jogging, and tennis are the most common instigators of exercise-induced asthma. Bicycling and swimming are much less likely to induce symptoms.

Occupational asthma may be accompanied by positive skin test reactions to protein allergens in the work environment. Occupational exposures to allergens, such as fumes from plastic, formaldehyde, isocyanates, some metals, textiles, engine exhaust, sulfur dioxide, fluoride, and western red cedar dust, *do not* provoke skin reactions.[10,11] To prove hypersensitivity, it may be necessary to conduct challenge tests in the patient by inhalation of the suspected dust or fumes in a controlled environment. The individual affected by occupational asthma tends to have progressively more severe attacks with subsequent exposures. Symptoms may clear over a weekend or vacation and recur when the individual is back at work.[10] This repeated history often is sufficient to establish the diagnosis. Hyposensitization in most cases of occupational asthma is ineffective because of lack of an IgE antibody reaction and because the chemicals that cause symptoms usually are toxic when injected.[10,11]

Drug-induced asthma can produce symptoms ranging from mild rhinorrhea to respiratory arrest requiring mechanical ventilation. In patients with nasal polyps, sinusitis, and asthma, ingestion of aspirin may induce severe or occasionally fatal asthmatic attacks. Sometimes anaphylactoid reactions cause a decrease in blood pressure, itching, rhinorrhea, or a rash after aspirin ingestion. Aspirin intolerance with asthma usually occurs in adults. Attacks may occur within minutes of ingestion or may be delayed up to 12 hours. Nonsteroidal antiinflammatory drugs such as indomethacin (Indocin), ibuprofen (Motrin, Advil), and related drugs may also induce asthma in the aspirin-intolerant patient. Aspirin reactions are not immunologically mediated. Therefore, skin testing is not useful for diagnosing aspirin intolerance. Because aspirin and nonsteroidal antiinflammatory drugs inhibit the conversion of arachidonic acid to prostaglandins, it may be that aspirin shunts arachidonic acid breakdown products to the leukotriene system. Leukotrienes, released from mast cells, are slow-reacting substances of anaphylaxis with powerful bronchoconstriction activity (see Figure 22-1). Avoidance is the most practical approach to this problem because testing can be dangerous.

Asthma can occur from ingestion of food additives. Tartrazine (yellow dye no. 5), which is used to color pharmaceuticals, hair products, and food products, may also produce

A SENSITIZATION TO ALLERGEN

NORMAL AIRWAY

B ALLERGEN-TRIGGERED ASTHMA

CONSTRICTED AIRWAY IN ASTHMA

IMMEDIATE PHASE (MINUTES)

C LATE PHASE (HOURS)

FIGURE 22-1 A, Sensitization to allergen. Inhaled allergens elicit a T_H2-dominated response favoring IgE production and eosinophil recruitment. **B,** Allergen-triggered asthma. On re-exposure to antigen, the immediate reaction is triggered by cross-linking of IgE bound to receptors on mast cells in the airways. These cells release preformed mediators that inflame epithelial cells. Antigen then enters the mucosa to activate mucosal mast cells and eosinophils, which in turn release additional inflammatory mediators. **C,** Late phase. The arrival of recruited leukocytes signals the initiation of the late phase of asthma and more mediator release, which cause damage to epithelium. (From Kumar V et al, editors: *Robbins basic pathology,* ed 8, Philadelphia, 2007, Saunders, p 491.)

severe asthma in susceptible persons. A complete list of drugs containing tartrazine can be obtained from the Food and Drug Administration.

Monosodium glutamate (MSG), used as a flavor enhancer in foods, can produce faintness, nausea, sweating, a fall in blood pressure, and, occasionally, asthma. Sodium or potassium metabisulfite, used to preserve fruits, vegetables, and meats, can cause anaphylactoid reactions. A challenge with the chemical may be necessary to establish a diagnosis, as metabisulfites are widespread in our society.

Hops in beer have also been implicated in causing severe bronchospasm. Skin reactivity does not occur, and the mechanism of the problem is not IgE mediated. The diagnosis involves a history of exposure followed by symptoms.

Pathogenesis. The immunohistopathologic features of asthma include denudation of airway epithelium, collagen deposition beneath the basement membrane, edema, mast cell activation, and inflammatory cell infiltration by neutrophils, eosinophils, and lymphocytes.[1,3] Inflammation of the airway contributes to acute bronchospasm (bronchoconstriction), mucosal edema, mucous plug formation, and airway wall remodeling (Figure 22-2). Genetic predisposition (chromosomes 5, 11, 14) for atopy and structural predisposition (smaller airways) are the strongest predisposing factors for developing asthma.[3,5] There is a strong association of the ADAM 33 gene with asthma bronchial hyperresponsiveness.[8]

With allergic asthma, an IgE-mediated response is common and is manifested by elevated IgE levels, allergic rhinitis, eczema, a positive family history of allergy, and attacks associated with seasonal, environmental, or occupational exposure. The mechanism of action is initiated by exposure to a specific antigen that has previously sensitized mast cells in airway mucosa. When the antigen reacts with the antibody on the surface of the mast cell, packets of chemical mediator substances stored in

the cell are released. The chemical mediators that are released include histamine, slow-reacting substances of anaphylaxis (leukotrienes), prostaglandins, bradykinins, eosinophilic chemotactic factor, serotonin, and others.[1-3,7] Figure 22-1 depicts common chemicals that are released by the mast cell and the physiologic effect of these chemicals. Cytokines are probably the most important inflammatory mediators, particularly those associated with T_H2 helper T-cell activation (granulocyte-macrophage colony–stimulating factor and interleukins 3, 4, 5, and 13). These cytokines may be responsible for modulating inflammatory and immune cell function.[1,2] Other inflammatory mediators are arachidonic acid metabolites such as leukotrienes and prostaglandins, platelet activating factor (PAF), neuropeptides, reactive oxygen species, histamine, and adenosine. With the release of chemical mediators, the normal respiratory epithelium is denuded and replaced by goblet cells, resulting in mucosal edema, inflammatory exudates, and hyperresponsiveness of the airway (bronchoconstriction and leakage).[2,12,13] Alterations in epithelial integrity lead to increased microvascular permeability. A secondary mediator response occurs 6 to 12 hours after the primary asthma attack and is more refractory to treatment. Neutrophil chemotactic factor may be the cause of this secondary response.[10]

Histologic changes in the epithelial basement membrane occur over time. The basement membrane is a complex structure that separates endothelial cells from underlying stroma. The membrane provides tensile strength and physical support to surrounding structures.[8] It also functions as a filter and as a site for cell attachment. In a classic study by Hogg in 1982, the width of the basement membrane was shown to thicken in asthmatics over time.[12] The width seen in asthmatics is 17.5 μm, whereas that seen in healthy subjects is 7 μm. Airway remodeling has been detected pathologically. Declines in pulmonary function over time can progress to chronic

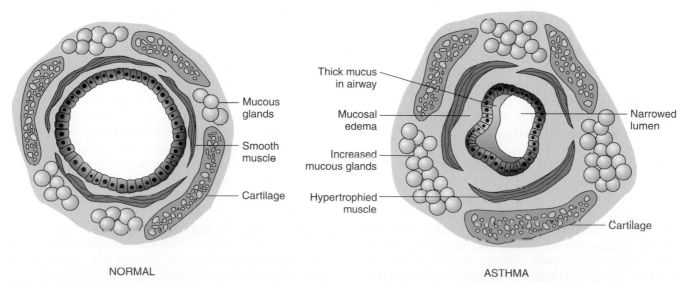

NORMAL　　　　　　　　　　　　ASTHMA

Thick mucus in airway
Mucosal edema
Increased mucous glands
Hypertrophied muscle
Mucous glands
Smooth muscle
Cartilage
Narrowed lumen
Cartilage

FIGURE 22-2 Common bronchial wall remodeling changes in asthma are hypertrophied smooth muscle, edema, mucous gland hypertrophy, and mucus in the lumen.

obstructive pulmonary disease (COPD).[10] Figure 22-1 depicts the pathogenesis of asthma in relation to mast cell release and parasympathetic stimulation by way of the vagus nerve. Vagal stimulation leads to edema, mucus hypersecretion, and bronchoconstriction. The nerve endings of asthmatic patients have been found to be devoid of the bronchodilator neuropeptide vasoactive intestinal peptide.[10]

Clinical Manifestations. Common symptoms are wheezing, feelings of tightness of the chest, dyspnea, cough, and increased sputum production.[10] Some patients have only a chronic dry cough, and others have a productive cough.[9] Especially in children, cough is often the earliest sign of exacerbation of asthma. Wheezing is caused by vibration in narrowed airways, which act like the vibrating reed of a wind instrument, yielding a musical sound.[14] Because airways naturally widen with inspiration, inspiratory wheezes reflect increased constriction. Sputum is often thick, tenacious, scant, and viscid (sticky). Physical findings vary with the severity of the attack. A mild attack may be associated with a random monophonic expiratory wheezing associated with airway narrowing, tachycardia, and tachypnea. Random monophonic wheezes are located throughout the chest and come and go on examination. The area in which they are heard best is indicative of the area of obstruction (e.g., if they are heard best at the mouth, this is indicative of large airway obstruction).[14,15] Tachycardia is an early sign of hypoxemia. A more severe attack requiring medical assistance may be accompanied by the use of accessory muscles of respiration, intercostal retractions, distant breath sounds with inspiratory wheezing, orthopnea, agitation, tachypnea, and tachycardia. In the severe state, the patient may appear cyanotic, agitated, restless, and confused. The intensity of wheezing is *not* a reliable indicator of blockage of airflow. The measurement of peak expiratory flow rate (PEFR) is the best indicator of reduction in airflow (see discussion under Diagnosis). PEFRs are adjusted for weight, height, age, gender, ethnicity, posture, effort, smoking, and circadian rhythm. A PEFR of less than 80 L/min indicates severe obstruction.[9,16] When obstruction is the tightest, the patient cannot move enough air with enough velocity to make wheezing sounds. Isolated inspiratory wheezing may be an indicator of upper airway obstruction caused by mucus or laryngeal obstruction.[4] A patient with severe respiratory distress, prolonged expiration (indicating that the person is having difficulty moving air out of the lungs), neck and intercostal retractions, and minimal air sounds is critically ill and requires emergency intervention.

Diagnosis. The diagnosis of asthma is based on physical findings, sputum examination, pulmonary function tests, blood gas analysis, and chest radiography. Radiographic findings may be normal or may show evidence of hyperinflation with flattening of the diaphragm in progressive disease.[8] Abnormal physical findings include cough, wheezing, a hyperinflated chest, and decreased breath sounds. Asthmatic sputum samples reveal Charcot-Leyden crystals (formed from crystallized enzymes from eosinophilic membranes), eosinophils, and Curschmann spirals (mucous casts of bronchioles).

Forced expiratory volumes decrease during asthma attacks. PEFR is measured to determine the index of airway function. The PEFR is the maximal flow of expired air attained during a forced vital capacity (FVC) procedure.[15] The evaluation of asthma should include the measurement of forced expiratory volume over 1 second (FEV_1), FVC, and the ratio FEV_1/FVC before and after administration of a short-acting bronchodilator.[8] Airflow obstruction is indicated by a FEV_1/FVC ratio of less than 75%.[9] Classification of asthma severity and control (Figures 22-3 and 22-4) is based on presenting symptoms, frequency of nighttime symptoms, and lung function.[2] Figure 22-5 shows stepped therapy for asthma based on classification.

Arterial blood gas values may be normal during a mild attack, but as the bronchospasm increases in intensity, respiratory alkalosis and hypoxemia become prominent findings. Elevation of arterial partial pressure of carbon dioxide ($Paco_2$) is a poor prognostic sign, indicating that the patient's ability to continue breathing at a rapid rate has diminished and that exhaustion is imminent.

Respiratory failure may be evidenced by severe respiratory distress in a patient who shows no radiographic evidence of pneumothorax. As the patient improves, the wheezing becomes louder. When wheezing is no longer heard after an asthma attack, pulmonary function tests may continue to show obstructive changes for several weeks. Some patients have a slight monophonic wheeze continuously between asthma bouts and still are comfortable and functional.[14]

Determination of allergens is done by skin testing or inhalation of suspected allergens. Skin testing is usually more helpful in young patients who have extrinsic asthma. Bronchial provocation testing with histamine or methacholine[9] may be useful in confirming the diagnosis of asthma in certain cases (see the Diagnostic Tests section later in the chapter).

A complete blood cell count can show an elevated number of white blood cells (WBCs) with increased eosinophils. Eosinophils are prominent in the cellular infiltrate of the bronchioles, the sputum, and the peripheral blood. A fall in the total eosinophil count is a valuable measure of effectiveness of corticosteroid treatment. With effective treatment, the total eosinophil count is depressed below 10/μl.[1,9]

Treatment. Patients should be taught to avoid the things in the environment that trigger asthma attacks. Environmental control includes dust control; removal of allergens such as feathers, molds, and animal danders; and, in some cases, removal of rugs and carpets. Other environmental control factors that help some patients include the use of air purifiers and air conditioners. The patient should also be taught preventive therapy in regard to smoking cessation, and avoidance of passive smoke, aerosols, and odors. Patients should seek early treatment for respiratory infections.[17]

Pharmacologic therapy for all three major obstructive disorders is similar, and focuses on decreasing inflammation and bronchoconstriction including β_2 agonists, corticosteroids, leukotriene modifiers, and mast cell inhibitors (Figure 22-6). Other therapies used in more severe asthmatics include home oxygen therapy and home administration of small-volume

Components of Severity		Classification of Asthma Severity ≥12 years of age			
			Persistent		
		Intermittent	**Mild**	**Moderate**	**Severe**
Impairment Normal FEV$_1$/FVC: 8–19 yr 85% 20–39 yr 80% 40–59 yr 75% 60–80 yr 70%	Symptoms	≤2 days/week	>2 days/week but not daily	Daily	Throughout the day
	Nighttime awakenings	≤2x/month	3–4x/month	>1x/week but not nightly	Often 7x/week
	Short-acting beta$_2$-agonist use for symptoms control (not prevention of EIB)	≤2 days/week	>2 days/week but not daily, and not more than 1x on any day	Daily	Several times per day
	Interference with normal activity	None	Minor limitation	Some limitation	Extremely limited
	Lung function	• Normal FEV$_1$ between exacerbations • FEV$_1$ >80% predicted • FEV$_1$/FVC normal	• FEV$_1$ >80% predicted • FEV$_1$/FVC normal	• FEV$_1$ >60% but <80% predicted • FEV$_1$/FVC reduced 5%	• FEV$_1$ <60% predicted • FEV$_1$/FVC reduced >5%
Risk	Exacerbations requiring oral systemic corticosteroids	0–1 year (see note)	≥2/year (see note) ⟶		
		⟵ Consider severity and interval since last exacerbation. ⟶ Frequency and severity may fluctuate over time for patients in any severity category. Relative annual risk of exacerbations may be related to FEV$_1$.			
Recommended Step for Initiating Treatment (See Figure 22-5 for treatment steps.)		Step 1	Step 2	Step 3	Step 4 or 5 and consider short course of oral systemic corticosteroids
		In 2–6 weeks, evaluate level of asthma control that is achieved and adjust therapy accordingly.			

Key: FEV$_1$, forced expiratory volume in 1 second; FVC, forced vital capacity; ICU, intensive care unit

Notes:

- The stepwise approach is meant to assist, not replace, the clinical decisionmaking required to meet individual patient needs.
- Level of severity is determined by assessment of both impairment and risk. Assess impairment domain by patient's/caregiver's recall of previous 2-4 weeks and spirometry. Assign severity to the most severe category in which any feature occurs.
- At present, there are inadequate data to correspond frequencies of exacerbations with different levels of asthma severity. In general, more frequent and intense exacerbations (e.g., requiring urgent, unscheduled care, hospitalization, or ICU admission) indicate greater underlying disease severity. For treatment purposes, patients who had ≥2 exacerbations requiring oral systematic corticosteroids in the past year may be considered the same as patients who have persistent asthma.

FIGURE 22-3 Classifying asthma severity and initiating treatment in youths ≥12 years of age and adults who are not currently taking long-term control medicines. (From National Institute of Health's National Heart, Lung, and Blood Institute. 2007 National Asthma Education and Prevention Program "Expert Panel Report 3: Guidelines for the Diagnosis and Management of Asthma," p 344, Figure 4-6.)

nebulizer treatments via intermittent positive-pressure ventilation. At home, peak flow monitoring is helpful to parents or patients in determining a treatment plan and when to seek medical assistance. Peak flow meters are also helpful in monitoring progress of the patient with around-the-clock therapy.[10]

Allergen-specific immunotherapy (hyposensitization) may be used as an adjunct to other therapies. The allergen is first identified by testing with purified allergens using the scratch, prick, or intradermal method. Desensitization therapy has been shown in controlled study to reduce the frequency and severity of asthmatic episodes when a single offending allergen can be identified.[10]

Status asthmaticus (severe attack unresponsive to routine therapy) requires more rapid and intense therapy, which may include epinephrine, subcutaneous terbutaline, and/or aminophylline. Once airflow has improved, aerosol bronchodilating inhalers may be used. Intravenous corticosteroids are the mainstay of therapy. Oxygen therapy with or without mechanical ventilation may be necessary in severe cases.

The more patients understand about their asthma, the better they are at self-managing their symptoms. Educational materials are available from the American Lung Association, the Asthma and Allergy Foundation of America, and the National Institute of Allergy and Infectious Diseases.

Components of Control		Classification of Asthma Control ($\geq$12 years of age)		
		Well Controlled	**Not Well Controlled**	**Very Poorly Controlled**
Impairment	Symptoms	$\leq$2 days/week	>2 days/week	Throughout the day
	Nighttime awakenings	$\leq$2x/month	1–3x/week	$\geq$4x/week
	Interference with normal activity	None	Some limitation	Extremely limited
	Short-acting beta$_2$-agonist use for symptom control (not prevention of EIB)	$\leq$2 days/week	>2 days/week	Several times per day
	FEV$_1$ or peak flow	>80% predicted/ personal best	60–80% predicted/ personal best	<60% predicted/ personal best
	Validated questionnaires ATAQ ACQ ACT	0 $\leq$0.75* $\geq$20	1–2 $\geq$1.5 16–19	3–4 N/A $\leq$15
Risk	Exacerbations requiring oral systemic corticosteroids	0–1 year	$\geq$2/year (see note)	
		Consider severity and interval since last exacerbation		
	Progressive loss of lung function	Evaluation requires long-term followup care		
	Treatment-related adverse effects	Medication side effects can vary in intensity from none to very troublesome and worrisome. The level of intensity does not correlate to specific levels of control but should be considered in the overall assessment of risk.		
Recommended Action for Treatment (See Figure 22-5 for treatment steps.)		• Maintain current step. • Regular followups every 1–6 months to maintain control. • Consider step down if well controlled for at least 3 months	• Step up 1 step and • Reevaluate in 2–6 weeks. • For side effects, consider alternative treatment options.	• Consider short course of oral systemic corticosteroids, • Step up 1–2 steps, and • Reevaluate in 2 weeks. • For side effects, consider alternative treatment options.

*ACQ values of 0.76–1.4 are indeterminate regarding well-controlled asthma.
Key: EIB, exercise-induced bronchospasm; ICU, intensive care unit

Notes:

■ The stepwise approach is meant to assist, not replace, the clinical decisionmaking required to meet individual patient needs.
■ The level of control is based on the most severe impairment or risk category. Assess impairment domain by patient's recall of previous 2-4 weeks and by spirometry/or peak flow measures. Symptom assessment for longer periods should reflect a global assessment, such as inquiring whether the patient's asthma is better or worse since the last visit.
■ At present, there are inadequate data to correspond frequencies of exacerbations with different levels of asthma control. In general, more frequent and intense exacerbations (e.g., requiring urgent, unscheduled care, hospitalization, or ICU admission) indicate poorer disease control. For treatment purposes, patients who had $\geq$2 exacerbations requiring oral systemic corticosteroids in the past year may be considered the same as patients who have not-well-controlled asthma, even in the absence of impairment levels consistent with not-well-controlled asthma.
■ Check NIH website for information on ATAQ, ACQ and ACT questionnaires.
■ Before step up in therapy:
— Review adherence to medication, inhaler technique, environmental control, and comorbid conditions.
— If an alternative treatment option was used in a step, discontinue and use the preferred treatment for that step.

FIGURE 22-4 Assessing asthma control and adjusting therapy in youths $\geq$12 years of age and adults. (From National Institute of Health's National Heart, Lung, and Blood Institute. 2007 National Asthma Education and Prevention Program "Expert Panel Report 3: Guidelines for the Diagnosis and Management of Asthma," p 345, Figure 4-7.)

KEY POINTS

■ An asthma episode may range in severity from mild to life threatening, depending on the degree of airway obstruction. With intense narrowing of the bronchi, severe hypoxemia may result.
■ Several types of asthma have been identified. Nonallergic (intrinsic) asthma is precipitated by exercise, stress, and exposure to pulmonary irritants, but no specific allergen can be identified. Drugs such as aspirin and exposure to occupational allergens have also been identified as etiologic agents.

■ Allergic (extrinsic) asthma is mediated by IgE, which is produced in response to specific antigens. The IgE binds to mast cells and causes them to release inflammatory chemicals in response to antigen. Skin testing may be helpful in identifying suspected allergens.
■ Prevention of asthma attacks is an important part of therapy. Avoidance of precipitating factors and prophylactic drug therapy are recommended. Bronchodilators, corticosteroids, and oxygen therapy are mainstays of treatment for an acute attack.

FIGURE 22-5 Stepwise approach for managing asthma in youths ≥12 years of age and adults. (From National Institute of Health's National Heart, Lung, and Blood Institute. 2007 National Asthma Education and Prevention Program "Expert Panel Report 3: Guidelines for the Diagnosis and Management of Asthma," p 343, Figure 4-5.)

Acute Bronchitis

Etiology. Acute inflammation of the trachea and bronchi is produced most commonly (80% of the 12 million cases per year in the U.S.) by a variety of viruses such as influenza virus A or B, parainfluenza virus, respiratory syncytial virus, coronavirus, rhinovirus, Coxsackie virus, and adenovirus. Nonviral causes include *Streptococcus pneumoniae, Haemophilus influenzae, Mycoplasma, moraxella,* and *Chlamydia pneumoniae.*[7,8] Numerous other pathogens, as well as heat, smoke inhalation, inhalation of irritant chemicals (e.g., sulfur dioxide or chlorine, bromine, or fluorine gases), and allergic reactions have also been identified.[18] Highest incidences are noted in smokers, young children, the

elderly, and in the winter months.[8,19] The swelling of bronchial mucosa in children associated with obstruction, respiratory distress, and wheezing is known as *asthmatic bronchitis.* Acute bronchitis differs from bronchiolitis in the size of the airways affected (i.e., trachea and bronchi as opposed to the small bronchioli).[20]

Pathogenesis. The airways become inflamed and narrowed from capillary dilation, swelling from exudation of fluid, infiltration with inflammatory cells, increased mucus production, loss of ciliary function, and loss of portions of the ciliated epithelium. Many viruses and mycoplasmal bacteria inhibit macrophages and lymphocytes, temporarily promoting secondary bacterial invasion. Microorganisms may also induce

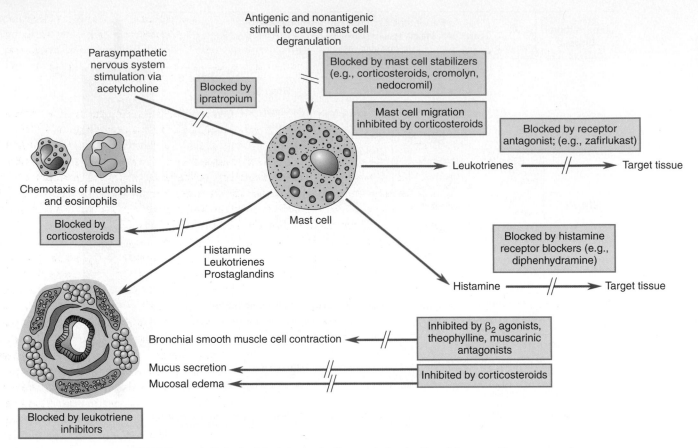

FIGURE 22-6 Pathophysiologic basis of asthma and site of action of drugs used in management.

long-lasting hyperirritability of the respiratory tract with associated episodes of bronchospasm.

Clinical Manifestations. The presentation of acute bronchitis is usually mild and self-limited, requiring only supportive treatment. Cough may be productive or nonproductive. Associated symptoms include low-grade fever, substernal chest discomfort, sore throat, postnasal drip, and fatigue. In children, the smaller airways are easily obstructed by inflammation, so that severe obstruction may occur.[8] The smallness of airways in proportion to body size is due to a smaller lumen in relation to the vessel wall. Associated inflammation of the larynx and trachea produces croup (see Croup Syndrome section in this chapter for further details).

Diagnosis. Diagnosis of acute bronchitis is usually based on the clinical presentation, with recent onset of cough being the distinctive hallmark. Neither the appearance of purulent sputum nor a WBC count is a reliable diagnostic indicator. A chest radiograph is required to distinguish acute bronchitis (normal radiograph) from pneumonia (pulmonary infiltrates on radiograph).

Treatment. Acute bronchitis is predominantly caused by viruses (rhinovirus, coronavirus, adenovirus, influenza virus). Viral infections do not respond to antimicrobial therapy, and symptoms resolve spontaneously in most normal, otherwise healthy individuals. Acute bronchitis caused by bacterial organisms responds well to antibiotic therapy. Codeine-containing medications are helpful in relieving the cough associated with bronchitis that interferes with sleep. Nonpharmacologic recommendations are to increase fluid intake, avoid smoke, and use a vaporizer in the bedroom.

The dangers of acute bronchitis include the potential for bacterial invasion, which can worsen symptoms in patients with chronic obstructive pulmonary disease (COPD) and precipitate serious infections in the aged or those with debilitating disease.

Chronic Bronchitis

Etiology. The next two sections of this chapter present chronic bronchitis and emphysema. Characteristic pathologic and clinical findings are described for each of these classifications. Clinically, pure forms of emphysema and chronic bronchitis are rare, and most patients present a combination of both of these obstructive processes. Patients with emphysema and chronic bronchitis make up most cases of COPD.

The major causes of chronic bronchitis are cigarette smoking (90% cases),[12] repeated airway infections, genetic predisposition, and inhalation of physical or chemical irritants.[8,9,21,22]

Chronic bronchitis (also referred to as type B COPD or the "blue bloater"[8,9,21]) is diagnosed *symptomatically* by hypersecretion of bronchial mucus and a chronic or recurrent productive cough of more than 3 months duration and occurring each year for two or more successive years in patients

FIGURE 22-7 Histologic features of chronic bronchitis. (Lumen of bronchus is above.) Note slight desquamation of mucosal epithelial cells and marked thickening (approximately twice normal thickness) of mucous gland layer. Vascular congestion is evident. (From Kumar V et al: *Robbins basic pathology,* ed 8, Philadelphia, 2007, Saunders, p 489.)

FIGURE 22-8 Structure of a normal bronchial wall. In chronic bronchitis, the thickness of the mucous glands increases and can be expressed as the Reid index, given by the following formula: $(b - c)/(a - d)$. The ratio is normally less than 0.4. A ratio of 0.7 indicates severe bronchitis.

in whom other causes have been excluded.[9] For patients with chronic bronchitis and emphysema, airway obstruction is persistent and irreversible. The National Center for Health Statistics reports a 3:1 ratio of annual cases of chronic bronchitis to emphysema.[23]

Pathogenesis. Pathologic changes in the airway include chronic inflammation and swelling of the bronchial mucosa resulting in scarring, increased fibrosis of the mucous membrane, hyperplasia of bronchial mucous glands and goblet cells, hypertrophy of bronchial glands and goblet cells, and increased bronchial wall thickness, which potentiates obstruction to airflow. Inflammation appears to predominantly be the result of neutrophil activity.[21] Interleukin-8 levels are elevated indicating sustained attraction of neutrophils to the site of inflammation. CD8 T-lymphocyte levels are also elevated. During acute exacerbations, bronchial biopsy specimens have a 30-fold increase in eosinophils.[21] Figures 22-7 and 22-8 show the histologic changes seen in chronic bronchitis. Hypertrophy of mucosal glands and goblet cells leads to increased mucus production; the mucus then combines with purulent exudate to form bronchial plugs. Chronic bronchitis patients often display bacterial colonization with *H. influenzae* and *S. pneumoniae.*[21] The mucociliary clearance action is impaired or lost, and some areas of ciliated columnar epithelium are replaced by squamous cells.[21] Ciliary dysfunction occurs due to a decreased number of cilia and decreased action of available cilia.

Often the inflammatory and fibrotic changes extend into the surrounding alveoli. The narrowed airways and the mucous plugs prevent proper oxygenation and potentiate airway obstruction. High airflow resistance increases the work of breathing, leading to increased oxygen demands. In areas of greater obstruction to airflow, alveoli empty and fill more slowly, leading to ventilation-perfusion $\dot{V}_A/\dot{Q}$ mismatch, thus lowering arterial oxygenation. The chronic bronchitis patient may appear as the blue bloater (Figure 22-9), reflecting the pathophysiologic process of oxygen desaturation (cyanosis) and edema associated with right-sided heart failure in advanced disease or exacerbations; hence, patients appear "blue and bloated."

Involvement of small pulmonary arteries related to inflammation in the bronchial walls and the compensatory vasoconstriction of pulmonary blood vessels from hypoxia produce pulmonary hypertension. In addition, widespread bronchial narrowing and mucous plugging produce ventilation-perfusion mismatch with hypoxemia and hypercarbia from impeded ventilation. The combination of hypoxia and hypercarbia increases pulmonary artery resistance and pulmonary hypertension.[21] As the process of pulmonary hypertension continues, right ventricular end-diastolic pressures increase, leading to right ventricular dilation (cor pulmonale) and right-sided heart failure. An enlarged right heart results in increased venous pressure, liver engorgement, and dependent edema. Manifestations of heart failure may occur during exacerbations of bronchitis and subside with appropriate treatment.[9,21]

Destruction of bronchial walls results in dilation of airway sacs. This is termed *bronchiectasis.* Causes of bronchial wall destruction include severe streptococcal or staphylococcal pneumonia, repeated bouts of acute bronchitis, infection with the mold *Aspergillus fumigatus,* mucous plugs, foreign bodies, or immunologic deficiencies. (Refer to the Bronchiectasis section later in this chapter for a more detailed description of this disease process.) The dilated sacs contain pools of infected secretion that do not clear themselves and serve as sources of further infection that can spread to adjacent lung fields by the lymphatics or venous drainage to other areas of the body, commonly the brain. If bronchiectatic lesions are localized, surgical resection of the affected portions of lung may be helpful. Narrowing of the airways and turbulent airflow from mucous obstruction produce bronchoconstriction.

Clinical Manifestations. The typical patient is an overweight man or woman (1:2 ratio) in his or her thirties or forties[9,21,22,24] or older with shortness of breath on exertion, excessive

CLINICAL
MANIFESTATIONS

- Excess body fluids
  (edemal plethora)

- Chronic cough

- Shortness of breath
  on exertion

- Increased sputum

- Cyanosis (late sign)

A

B

FIGURE 22-9 A, A "blue bloater" with edema from right-sided heart failure. **B,** A patient with chronic obstructive bronchitis. Note the stocky build and the presence of pursed-lip breathing and barrel chest. The slight gynecomastia is a side effect of corticosteroid therapy. The patient's shoulders are raised because of shortness of breath and increased work of breathing. (**B,** From Black JM et al: *Medical-surgical nursing: clinical management for positive outcomes,* ed 8, Philadelphia, 2008, Saunders, p 1581.)

amounts of sputum, chronic cough, evidence of excess body fluids (edema, hypervolemia), and a history of smoking. In addition, the patient often complains of chills, malaise, muscle aches, fatigue, loss of libido, and insomnia.

Sputum production may be variable and worsens with respiratory infection. Cough and sputum production are most severe in the mornings. Gradually, patients develop progressive shortness of breath on exertion. Most patients do not seek help until dyspnea becomes troublesome. By the time dyspnea on exertion is present, the disease is well advanced.[21,22]

In the end-stage disease process, the patient presents with signs of right-sided heart failure (distended neck veins, a right ventricular heave, a right ventricular gallop, and peripheral edema).[21] Hypoxia leads to pulmonary hypertension. Cyanosis is a late sign.

Diagnosis. Measures used to confirm the diagnosis include chest radiography, which may show increased bronchial vascular markings, congested lung fields, an enlarged horizontal cardiac silhouette, and evidence of previous pulmonary infection. Pulmonary function tests show normal total lung capacity (TLC), increased residual volume (RV), and decreased FEV_1. Early pulmonary function testing prior to the onset of symptoms shows increased closing volume and a decrease in the maximal midexpiratory flow rate.[21] Arterial blood gas evaluation may show elevated $PaCO_2$ and decreased PaO_2 (often below 65 mm Hg); abnormal ABGs develop early in the disease process. The electrocardiogram may reveal atrial arrhythmias and evidence of right ventricular hypertrophy. Secondary polycythemia (increased numbers of red blood

cells) related to continuous or nocturnal hypoxemia is common.[9,21] Hypoxemia leads to a compensatory production of red blood cells in an attempt to carry more oxygen to the body tissues.

Depending on the severity of the disease, the physical examination may reveal scattered crackles, rhonchi, and wheezes; use of accessory muscles to breathe; jugular vein distention; clubbing; and pedal and ankle edema. Table 22-1 lists the distinguishing features of both emphysema and chronic bronchitis.

Treatment. Because bronchitis and emphysema are most frequently seen in combination, the therapies are similar. The overall goals are to (1) block the progression of the disease, (2) return the patient to optimal respiratory function, and (3) return the patient to usual activities of daily living.

Pharmacologic treatment involves the use of inhaled short-acting β_2 agonists and inhaled anticholinergic bronchodilators, cough suppressants, and antimicrobial agents for infections. Inhaled or oral corticosteroids may also be used in the treatment of some patients for acute exacerbations. Theophylline products are used less frequently due to their narrow therapeutic range and toxicity. However, many patients derive significant benefits from theophylline.[21,22]

Low-dose oxygen therapy is recommended for patients with PaO_2 levels less than 55 mm Hg.[21,22] Mechanical ventilation may become necessary to get the patient over a crisis period of acute exacerbation. Although traditionally the mechanism of carbon dioxide retention with oxygen therapy was thought to be related to a diminished ventilatory drive,

TABLE 22-1

Common Distinguishing Features of Emphysema and Chronic Bronchitis*

Patient Data	Emphysema (Type A: Pink Puffer)	Bronchitis (Type B: Blue Bloater)
History		
Lifestyle	Smoker	Smoker
Weight	Weight loss	Overweight
Onset of symptoms	Usually after age 50 years	Usually after age 40 years
Sputum	Mild, mucoid	Excessive, purulent
Cough	Minimal or absent	Chronic; more severe in mornings
Dyspnea	Progressive exertional dyspnea	Mild to moderate, but may gradually progress to severe exertional dyspnea
Patient complaints	Dyspnea on exertion, fatigue, insomnia	Chronic cough with mucopurulent sputum, chills, malaise, muscle aches, fatigue, insomnia, loss of libido
Physical Signs		
Edema	Absent	Present
Central cyanosis	Absent	Present in advanced disease
Use of accessory muscles to breathe	Present	Absent until end stage
Body build	Thin, wasted	Stocky, overweight
Anteroposterior chest diameter	"Barrel chest," 1:1 ratio anteroposterior chest diameter	Normal
Auscultation of chest	Decreased breath sounds, decreased heart sounds, prolonged expiration	Wheezes, crackles, rhonchi, depending on the severity of disease
Percussion	Hyperresonance	Normal
Jugular vein distention	Absent	Present
Other	Pursed-lip breathing	Evidence of right-sided heart failure (cor pulmonale)
General Diagnostic Tests		
Chest radiography	Narrowed mediastinum; normal or small vertical heart; hyperinflation; low, flat diaphragm; presence of blebs or bullae	Congested lung fields, increased bronchial vascular markings, enlarged horizontal heart
Arterial blood gas analysis	Decreased Pao_2 (60-80 mm Hg); increased $Paco_2$ with advancing disease	Decreased Pao_2 (<65 mm Hg); increased $Paco_2$
Electrocardiography	Normal or tall symmetrical P waves; tachycardia, if hypoxic	Right axis deviation, right ventricular hypertrophy, atrial arrhythmias
Hematocrit	Normal	Polycythemia
Pulmonary Function Tests		
Functional residual capacity	Increased	Normal or slight increase
Residual volume	Increased	Increased
Total lung capacity	Increased	Normal
Forced expiratory volume	Decreased	Decreased
Vital capacity	Decreased	Normal or slight decrease
Static lung compliance	Increased	Normal

*Clinically, features of bronchitis and emphysema are not always clear-cut because many patients have a combined disease process.

current research suggests that oxygen therapy may instead cause increased $\dot{V}_A/\dot{Q}$ imbalance, precipitating a rise in carbon dioxide. It is important to remember that not all patients with a history of COPD are carbon dioxide retainers. Home oxygen therapy has been demonstrated to retard the development of pulmonary hypertension and cor pulmonale in chronic bronchitis.[9,21] Portable oxygen saturation monitors for evaluating the effectiveness of oxygen administration at home may also be used.

Smoking cessation is essential to decreasing the progression of the disease. A reduction in exposure to inhaled pulmonary irritants is also advised.[22] Supportive therapies include adequate rest, proper hydration (8 to 12 glasses of water per day unless the patient has congestive heart failure), and physical reconditioning programs using a treadmill or stationary bicycle. Alternating rest and exercise improves results on pulmonary function tests. Walking has proved to be the best form of exercise for increasing duration and intensity of activity.

All COPD patients also benefit from yearly influenza vaccine and pneumococcal vaccine.

OBSTRUCTION RELATED TO LOSS OF LUNG PARENCHYMA

Emphysema

Etiology. Emphysema (also referred to as type A COPD or the "pink puffer") is defined *pathologically* by destructive changes of the alveolar walls without fibrosis and abnormal enlargement of the distal air sacs.[8,9,21,22] Emphysema is frequently associated with chronic bronchitis. According to the National Center for Health Statistics (2005 data), of the 12.7 million Americans with COPD, 8.9 million primarily have chronic bronchitis and 3.8 million primarily have emphysema.[24] The etiologies of emphysema include smoking, air pollution, certain occupations (e.g., welding, mining, and working with or near asbestos), and alpha-1 antitrypsin deficiency (1%). Emphysema tends to develop over a long period and thus is seen more frequently in persons older than 50. Cigarette smoking in excess of 70 pack-years is highly predictive of

COPD.[21] The normal aging process, starting at about age 30, reflects changes similar to those seen in emphysema, including a loss of alveoli, an increase in the size of alveolar ducts, a loss of gas-exchanging surface area (4% per decade), and a decrease in bronchiolar musculature.[21]

When emphysema occurs in young to middle-aged adults or before the age of 50 in a smoker, it may be associated with a deficiency of α_1-antitrypsin activity in the lung. α_1-Antitrypsin deficiency is a hereditary disorder characterized by low serum levels (25 to 50 mg/dl) of α_1-antitrypsin.[21,22] α_1-Antitrypsin is a protective enzyme that inhibits proteolytic breakdown of alveolar tissue. The protease enzymes (neutrophil-derived elastase) that break down lung protein are released from neutrophils that migrate to the lung during inflammation causing alveolar wall destruction.[21]

Emphysema may follow bacterial lung infections, which involve secretion of proteases that destroy the elastin proteins responsible for the normal elasticity of the lung tissue. Bacterial infections block mechanisms that normally inhibit the release of proteolytic enzymes from degenerating neutrophilic granulocytes.

Pathogenesis. The pathologic changes leading to alveolar destruction are associated with the release of proteolytic enzymes from inflammatory cells such as neutrophils and macrophages. Smoking is commonly associated with emphysema. Smoking causes alveolar damage in two ways: (1) it leads to inflammation in the lung tissue (parenchyma), thus initiating a chain of events leading to the release of proteolytic enzymes that directly damages alveolar tissue; and (2) it inactivates α_1-antitrypsin, which normally acts to protect the lung parenchyma.[21,22] Figure 22-10 illustrates the pathogenesis of emphysema.

With the loss of alveolar walls, there is also a marked reduction in the pulmonary capillary bed, which is essential for exchange of oxygen and carbon dioxide between the alveolar air and capillary blood. There is also a loss of elastic tissue in the lung, which leads to a decrease in the size of the smaller bronchioles. The loss of lung tissue leads to a loss of *radial traction,* which normally holds the airway open, and to increasing pressure around the outside of the airway lumen, which in turn increases airway resistance and decreases airflow. Figure 22-11 shows the effect of decreased radial traction on the size of small bronchioles. Air then becomes trapped in distal alveoli, leading to distended air sacs, which adds to the collapsing pressure on more proximal bronchi and increases airway obstruction. Loss of alveolar walls and air trapping lead to the formation of bullae (large, thin-walled cysts in the lung) that further rob the lung of its gas transport function. The appearance of the lung and lung tissue from typical emphysematous patients is shown in Figures 22-12 and 22-13.

Three major classifications of emphysema exist: (1) centriacinar (also called *centrilobular*), which is associated with both smoking and chronic bronchitis and destroys the respiratory bronchioles; (2) panacinar (also called *panlobular*), which destroys the alveoli; and (3) paraseptal, which affects the peripheral lobules. Some of the classifications of emphysema

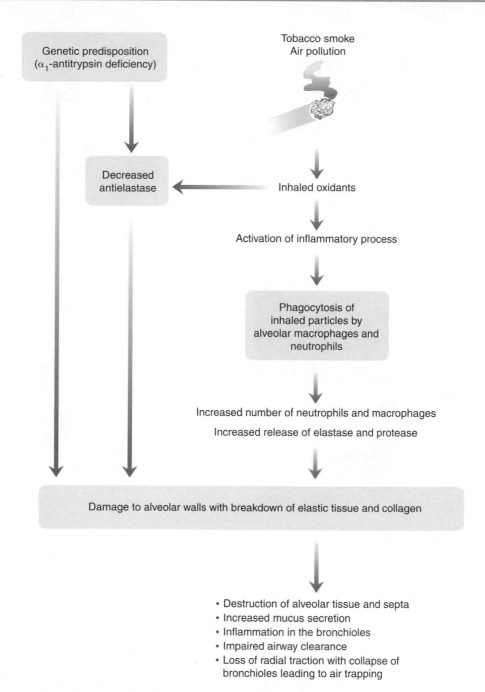

FIGURE 22-10 Pathogenesis of smoke-induced emphysema.

and the topographic distribution of emphysema in lung tissue are shown in Figure 22-14.

Clinical Manifestations. Patients with emphysema commonly seek help because of progressive exertional dyspnea. The typical patient with advanced disease is a thin man or woman in his or her middle 50s who has had increasing shortness of breath for the past 3 to 4 years. As with chronic bronchitis, the incidence of emphysema is increasing in women who smoke. Patients become thin due to increased respiratory effort and resulting caloric expenditure with decreased ability to consume adequate calories. The difficulty in breathing is evidenced by the use of accessory muscles to breathe, progressive

dyspnea, and the use of pursed-lip breathing in an effort to get more air out over a longer period of time before the small airways collapse. Cough may be minimal or absent. Digital clubbing is common. The appearance of overinflation (barrel chest) shows an increase in lung volume, which can be confirmed by pulmonary function testing. With the loss of alveolar walls and formation of bullae, the patient is at risk for developing a pneumothorax and may present with chest pain on the affected side and dyspnea. Decreased arterial oxygen saturation remains minor until late in the course of the disease. Late in the disease process, the major symptom is dyspnea on exertion. These patients may be referred to as "pink puffers"

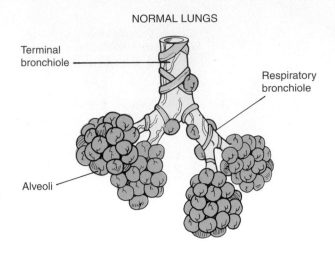

FIGURE 22-11 Loss of radial traction in emphysema leads to airway collapse. **A,** Terminal bronchiole in cross-section. **B,** Terminal bronchiole with narrowed lumen resulting from loss of surrounding alveoli, leading to decreased radial traction and airway collapse.

FIGURE 22-12 Gross appearance of emphysematous lung. *Left,* Normal lung tissue from a nonsmoker. *Right,* Lung tissue from a smoker who has developed emphysema.

FIGURE 22-13 Pulmonary emphysema. There is a marked enlargement of airspaces with thinning and destruction of alveolar septa. (From Kumar V et al: *Robbins basic pathology,* ed 8, Philadelphia, 2007, Saunders, p 487.)

FIGURE 22-14 Types of emphysema. (From Black JM et al: *Medical-surgical nursing: clinical management for positive outcomes,* ed 8, Philadelphia, 2008, Saunders, p 1580.)

CLINICAL
MANIFESTATIONS

- Use of accessory muscles to breathe

- Pursed-lip breathing

- Minimal or absent cough

- Leaning forward to breathe

- Barrel chest

- Digital clubbing

- Dyspnea on exertion (late sign)

A

B

FIGURE 22-15 A, The "pink puffer." Note the use of accessory muscles and pursed-lip breathing in an effort to get more air out of the lungs. **B,** A patient with emphysema. Note the thin appearance and the presence of continuous oxygen therapy. The use of accessory muscles of respiration (neck and shoulder muscles) reflects the patient's shortness of breath and increased work of breathing necessary to increase minute ventilation and to maintain adequate arterial blood gas values. (**B,** From Black JM et al: *Medical surgical nursing: clinical management for positive outcomes*, ed 8, Philadelphia, 2008, Saunders, p 1581.)

(Figure 22-15), a term related to the physiologic matching of ventilation and perfusion. They tend to have more areas of high ventilation in relation to perfusion. Ventilation-perfusion matching and a sustained high respiratory effort produce a relatively normal arterial oxygen level until late stages of the disease.[1,2,9,21,22]

Diagnosis. The diagnosis of emphysema is based on the patient's history and physical findings, pulmonary function tests, chest radiographs, arterial blood gases, and electrocardiogram. Changes seen on pulmonary function tests include an increased functional residual capacity, increased RV, increased TLC, decreased FEV_1, and decreased FVC.[9,21] Chest radiographs show hyperinflation; a low, flat diaphragm; the presence of blebs or bullae; a narrow mediastinum; and a normal or small "vertical" heart (see Table 22-1). Electrocardiographic findings may be normal or show tall P waves. Sinus tachycardia may be the first sign of decreased oxygenation. Supraventricular arrhythmias (atrial tachycardia, atrial flutter, and atrial fibrillation) and ventricular irregularities may also occur.[9] Arterial blood gas values typically reveal a normal mild decrease in Pao_2 (65 to 75 mm Hg) and a normal (or, in late stages, elevated) $Paco_2$.[23]

Physical examination reveals a thin, wasted individual who is using accessory muscles to breathe and sits slightly hunched forward in an effort to breathe better. Auscultation and percussion of the lung fields reveal decreased breath sounds and lack of crackles and rhonchi, decreased heart sounds, prolonged expiration, decreased diaphragmatic excursion, and

hyperresonance of the chest. Pursed-lip breathing, chronic morning cough because of mucus buildup at night, and an increased anteroposterior chest diameter (barrel chest) are also common findings. Weight loss occurs because of anorexia and lack of energy to eat. Bronchoconstriction leads to wheezing.

Treatment. Refer to the treatment section under "Chronic Bronchitis" earlier in this chapter for detailed treatment modalities common to both obstructive lung diseases. An excellent patient teaching manual called *Better Breathing: A Self-Teaching Manual* is available from PAL Medical, Inc., Maitland, Florida. Poor prognosis is associated with weight loss, so treatment is focused on maintaining proper nutrition.

KEY POINTS

- Emphysema is a form of chronic obstructive pulmonary disease (COPD) that results from destruction of alveoli and small airways. Emphysema occurs primarily in cigarette smokers and is often seen in association with chronic bronchitis.

- Alveolar destruction is due to release of inflammatory proteolytic enzymes that degrade lung proteins. Smoking also inhibits a protective enzyme, α_1-antitrypsin, that normally keeps the proteolytic enzymes in check. Genetic deficiency of α_1-antitrypsin is an uncommon cause of emphysema.

- Emphysema causes two major problems with respiration: (1) a decrease in surface area for gas exchange and (2) airway collapse due to loss of radial traction. Airway collapse is greater on expiration, resulting in air trapping and hyperinflation.
- Emphysema is characterized by dyspnea, weight loss, use of accessory muscles to breathe, a low, flat diaphragm, and a barrel chest. Cyanosis is not present until late stages of the disease. By sustaining high ventilatory effort, a patient can have blood oxygen levels that are generally maintained near normal. Carbon dioxide levels may be normal or low due to hyperventilation.
- Therapy for emphysema is similar to that for chronic bronchitis. Cessation of smoking is necessary to prevent progression of the disease. Present damage is irreversible. Oxygen therapy improves activity tolerance and quality of life.

OBSTRUCTION OF THE AIRWAY LUMEN

Bronchiectasis

Etiology. Bronchiectasis means dilation of bronchi. It is either acquired or congenital, and is classified as both an obstructive and a suppurative (pus-forming) disorder. Acquired bronchiectasis is now rare in the United States because of rapid diagnosis and management of bronchopulmonary infections. Fifty percent of the cases of bronchiectasis are associated with cystic fibrosis.[26] Children are at higher risk for development of bronchiectasis because of anatomic factors such as small, soft, elastic bronchi. Bronchi in children are easily damaged by overinflation and distention from inflammation and infection.

Bronchiectasis can be classified according to bronchial shape: saccular (with cavity-like dilatations) or cylindrical, and with widening of the bronchial walls. A fusiform shape is a combination of saccular and cylindrical changes. These anatomic changes are shown in Figure 22-16. Little clinical or pathophysiologic difference in the three types has been demonstrated.

Pathogenesis. Bronchiectasis is characterized by recurrent infection and inflammation of bronchial walls, which leads to persistent dilation of the medium-sized bronchi and bronchioles. Inflammation results in destruction of the walls of central bronchi and obliteration of peripheral bronchi and bronchioles.[23] *H. influenzae* is the most common cause of bacterial infections.[23,26] The destructive process leads to loss of ciliated columnar epithelium, with transformation to a squamous cell and pus formation, which in turn leads to obstruction of airflow. Lung tissue of a patient with cystic fibrosis complicated by varicose bronchiectasis is shown in Figure 22-17.

Clinical Manifestations. The child usually presents with a chronic productive cough with copious amounts of purulent, foul-smelling, green or yellow sputum. The sputum has the characteristic of separating into three distinct layers in a sputum cup.[23,26] Other clinical features are hemoptysis, fever,

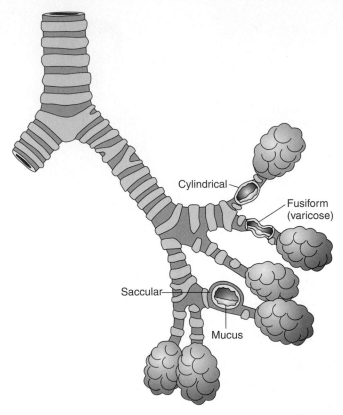

FIGURE 22-16 Bronchial dilatations due to bronchiectasis. The saccular form occurs in the segmental bronchi, which are severely dilated and end blindly. The varicose form resembles varicose veins with irregular dilatations and constriction. The cylindrical form shows uniform slight dilatation.

night sweats, moist crackles including bases, rhonchi, halitosis (bad breath), skin pallor, and, infrequently, digital clubbing. Clubbing is caused by prolonged decreased oxygenation, which leads to fibrous tissue hyperplasia in the area between the nail and distal portion of each digit. Clubbing is associated with lymphocytic extravasation, increased vascularity, and edema. The severity of clubbing parallels the severity of pulmonary disease.[20] Digital clubbing can be identified by two methods, as seen in Figure 22-18. Hypoxemia is seen in severe cases. Complications of bronchiectasis are malnutrition, recurrent pneumonia, right ventricular failure, and secondary visceral abscesses.[9]

Diagnosis. Generally, the diagnosis of bronchiectasis is based on a history of chronic productive cough. The patient complains about producing copious amounts of foul-smelling, purulent sputum. Radiographic abnormalities may reveal small cysts, thickening of bronchial walls, and increased bronchial markings (areas of intensity showing bronchi, which are usually not distinct). Pulmonary function tests show decreased airflow and vital capacity in advanced cases. Arterial blood gas analyses reveal decreased Pao_2 and increased $Paco_2$ from obstruction to airflow. High-resolution computed tomography is the test of choice for diagnosing bronchiectasis.[9]

FIGURE 22-17 Bronchographic features of varicose and cystic bronchiectasis. **A,** A left tracheobronchogram in a shallow posterior oblique projection reveals mildly dilated and slightly irregular bronchi that terminate after four to six generations of branchings from the trachea in a squared or bulbous appearance (arrowheads). The findings are those of varicose bronchiectasis. **B,** A bilateral tracheobronchogram in the anteroposterior projection demonstrates a multitude of contrast material–filled cystic spaces resembling a cluster of grapes (arrowheads), a characteristic feature of cystic bronchiectasis. Note that the cystic spaces appear after only two to three bronchial generations. Less severe bronchiectasis of the varicose type is present in the right lower lobe (open arrows). (From Fraser RG et al: *Diagnosis of diseases of the chest,* ed 3, vol 3, Philadelphia, 1990, Saunders, p 2199.)

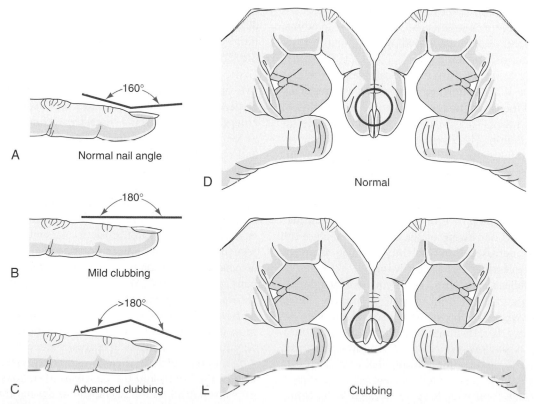

FIGURE 22-18 Clubbing. **A,** Normal fingernail angle is 160 degrees. **B,** Early mild clubbing appears as flattened angle between nail and skin (180 degrees). **C,** Advanced clubbing shows a rounded (clubbed) fingertip and nail. To assess clubbing by Schamroth's diagnostic method **(D and E),** place the nails of the second digits together. Obliteration of the normal diamond-shaped space between the nails is an abnormal finding, signifying clubbing.

Treatment. Antibiotic therapy accompanied by inhalation of bronchodilators followed by vigorous chest percussion and postural drainage is the mainstay of therapy. Proper hydration and nutrition are important in promoting liquefaction of secretions and preventing increased susceptibility to infection resulting from malnutrition. Maintaining adequate nutrition is problematic due to fatigue and the energy required to eat. (Refer to the Cystic Fibrosis section later in the chapter for further discussion on treatment.) In severe cases, when other measures fail, bronchoscopy with bronchial lavage may be necessary to remove thick, purulent secretions. In the child with severe saccular bronchiectasis, removal of the affected area of the lung may be necessary. Patient education materials can be obtained from the Cystic Fibrosis Foundation.[27] Childhood immunizations have led to a decrease incidence of bronchiectasis due to pertussis.[28]

Bronchiolitis

Etiology. Bronchiolitis is characterized by widespread inflammation of bronchioles due to infectious agents such as respiratory syncytial virus (RSV) (50% of cases),[28] influenza virus (type A, B, or C), or bacteria (*H. influenzae*, pneumococci, or hemolytic streptococci), and occasionally is produced by allergic reactions. RSV infection is a common cause of hospitalization in infants.[23] Other organisms that may cause bronchiolitis include *Mycoplasma, Chlamydia, Ureaplasma,* and *Pneumocystis (carinii) jiroveci.*[29] RSV occurs in yearly epidemics in winter to spring, usually in children younger than 2 years.[30] The average incubation period is 5 days, with inoculation occurring through the nose and eyes.[9,29] In adults, bronchiolitis is commonly associated with smoking, toxic fumes, and immunosuppression.[9]

Pathogenesis. Once initiated by the causal agent, proliferation and necrosis of bronchiolar epithelium occur, producing obstruction and increased mucus production.[9] Production of thick, tenacious mucus leads to airway obstruction, atelectasis, and hyperinflation. Three possible mechanisms of airway obstruction may follow the inflammatory process. They include (1) development of inflammatory exudate, which may displace surfactant, leading to airway obstruction; (2) release of chemical mediators, which may produce bronchiolar constriction; and (3) development of inflammation, which may induce fibrosis and narrowing of the airway.[1,23] Goblet cell metaplasia and increased bronchial muscle mass may also occur, resulting in further airway narrowing.

Clinical Manifestations. The severity and course of the disease are variable, ranging from mild to fatal. Common clinical features include wheezing due to bronchospasm, crackles, decreased breath sounds, retractions, increased sputum, dyspnea, tachypnea (rapid, shallow respirations), and low-grade fever. Otitis media is a common complication often associated with *S. pneumoniae.*[29]

Diagnosis. Patients commonly have an elevated WBC count. The chest radiograph may show enlarged air sacs, interstitial infiltrates, atelectasis, or severe hyperinflation. Pulmonary function tests reveal severe obstruction to airflow. Rapid diagnosis of RSV may be made by identifying the viral antigen from nasal washings or nasal swab culture of secretions, using an enzyme-linked immunosorbent assay or immunofluorescent assay.

Treatment. Adequate oxygenation is maintained by providing humidified oxygen; monitoring blood gases or oxygen saturation; and providing oral, inhaled, or intravenous bronchodilator agents and, in selected cases, corticosteroids.[23] General information about pharmacologic agents commonly used in the management of various respiratory disorders is listed in other texts. Use of these agents depends on the severity of the diagnosis and prescriber preference.

Other therapies include sedation for anxiety, hydration, and the administration of appropriate antivirals and antibiotics. Patients are encouraged to stop smoking and to avoid passive smoke exposure. The use of eye-nose goggles by health care workers is recommended to control the spread of RSV. The virus is spread through the air or by contact with secretions from the eye, nose, or mouth, and transmission may not be prevented by the use of masks and gowns.

Cystic Fibrosis

Etiology. Cystic fibrosis (mucoviscidosis) is an autosomal recessive disorder of the exocrine glands. It is the most common genetic lung disease in the United States, with an incidence of 1 in 2000 to 3300 Caucasian births.[9,23,26,31] One in 25 Caucasians are heterozygous carriers of the cystic fibrosis gene.[9] The incidence in African Americans is rare (1 in 17,000 live births), and in Native Americans the incidence is 1 in 80,000 births.[31,32] It is almost never seen in the Asian population.[16,32] About 35% of the 30,000 cases of cystic fibrosis in the United States involve individuals older than 18 years.[9,16] Cystic fibrosis can be classified either as an airflow obstructive disorder or as a suppurative (pus-forming) disorder. Hypersecretion of abnormal, thick mucus that obstructs exocrine glands and ducts is a characteristic finding in the disease.[8]

With advances in antibiotic therapy and early recognition and management of complications, patients with cystic fibrosis are living longer into adulthood. The median survival age is now 31 years.[9,23,26] Some patients are now having families.

Pathogenesis. Cystic fibrosis is classified as an autosomal recessive disorder. More than 800 mutations in the gene that encodes for the cystic fibrosis transmembrane conductance regulator (CFTR) have been described.[9,23] One genetic defect associated with cystic fibrosis involves deletion of three base pairs in codon 508 (AF508) that code for phenylalanine on chromosome 7 (band q31).[16] With the loss of these three base pairs, the *CFTR* gene is dysfunctional.[9,23] This is the most common genetic mutation causing cystic fibrosis and occurs in 60% to 75% of cystic fibrosis patients tested.[9,23] *CFTR* encodes a membrane chloride channel and is expressed in the sweat glands, the lungs, and the pancreas. Mutations in the *CFTR* gene result in alteration in chloride and water transport across the apical surface of epithelial cells.[9,23] Cystic fibrosis primarily affects the pancreas, intestinal tract, sweat glands, and lungs, and in males causes infertility.[28] The mucus-producing glands in the gastrointestinal tract enlarge generating excessive secretions. The thick eosinophilic mucous secretions plug the glands and ducts of the pancreatic acini, intestinal glands, intrahepatic bile ducts, and the gallbladder, causing dilation and fibrosis.[31,32] These changes result in decreased production of pancreatic enzymes necessary for digestion of fats, carbohydrates, and proteins, thus leading to increased fat and protein in the stool.[31,32]

The bronchopulmonary system is also affected by the thick, tenacious mucus that results from failure of chloride channels to function in the apical membranes of mucosal cells. Decreased flow of ions and water results in viscid mucus.[9,32] High concentrations of DNA in airway secretions (due to inflammation and lysis of neutrophils) increase sputum viscosity.[9,31,32] The thick mucus causes airway obstruction, atelectasis, and hyperinflation and also decreases ciliary action, thus contributing to mucus stasis, which provides a medium for pulmonary infection. Sweat glands, salivary glands, and lacrimal glands are also affected, leading to high concentrations of sodium and chloride in these secretions.[9,31,32]

Clinical Manifestations. Typical findings include a history of cough in a young adult or child; thick, tenacious sputum; recurrent pulmonary infections (commonly *Pseudomonas aeruginosa*); and recurrent episodes of bronchitis. These processes ultimately progress to pneumonia and bronchiectasis, right-sided heart failure (cor pulmonale), and exercise intolerance.

Physical examination may reveal digital clubbing (late sign), dyspnea, tachypnea, sternal retractions, unequal breath sounds, moist basilar crackles and rhonchi, and a barrel chest that is hyperresonant to percussion.[9] Other findings that may be present are pancreatic insufficiency (85% to 90%), cirrhosis of the liver (15% to 20%), diabetes mellitus (8% to 15%), gallstones (30% to 35%), nasal polyps (15%), and failure of development of the vas deferens in males.[9,16,23,31-33] Infants frequently present with a history of multiple respiratory infections, meconium ileus, failure to thrive, jaundice, salt depletion, and edema.[9,16,23]

Nutritional assessment reveals depleted fat stores, steatorrhea (fatty stools), anorexia, decreased growth rate in children (weight, height, head circumference), and decreased midarm indices.[16,23]

Diagnosis. The diagnosis of cystic fibrosis is based on clinical and laboratory findings. Diagnostic studies that are routinely done include arterial blood gas measurement, pulmonary function tests, sputum culture and sensitivity with Gram stain, and chest radiography. Specific diagnostic tests for cystic fibrosis include stool examination for fat, pilocarpine iontophoresis (sweat test), and genetic testing. A 72-hour stool collection combined with the dietary history during that time is used to determine fat absorption and fecal fat excretion. A coefficient of fat absorption of less than 95% (85% in infants) can be used to define steatorrhea (fatty stools).[34] Arterial blood gas analyses commonly show hypoxemia and hypercapnia because of airway obstruction. Pulmonary function tests reveal decreased vital capacity, decreased airflow rates, increased airway resistance, increased functional residual capacity, and decreased

tidal volume. Chest radiographs show evidence of patchy atelectasis, bronchiectasis, obstructive emphysema, cystic lung fields, and peribronchial thickening.[1,16,23,31-33]

The quantitative pilocarpine iontophoresis sweat test reveals elevated sodium and chloride levels, with more than 98% of patients having levels greater than 60 mEq/L in children and greater than 80 mEq/L in adults.[8,33] A diagnostic blood test for the genetic marker AF-508 may be useful for confirming the diagnosis and providing genetic information to the family.[8]

Treatment. Management of cystic fibrosis involves an interdisciplinary approach. A comprehensive program that focuses on multiorgan derangements is recommended. Because pulmonary disease accounts for the majority of morbidity and mortality associated with cystic fibrosis, treatment is aimed at aggressive pharmacologic management of pulmonary infection. Treatment includes the use of bronchodilators, and mobilization of the thick mucus by postural drainage and chest physiotherapy (percussion and vibration) is a priority. Alternative methods for mucus removal include the forced expiratory technique, which involves coughing (huffing) with an open glottis.[33] Recombinant human deoxyribonuclease I (Dornase alfa) acts by digesting extracellular DNA (released from lysed neutrophils) present in the viscid sputum of cystic fibrosis patients to decrease the viscoelasticity of sputum, thus improving pulmonary function and decreasing the risk of infection.[8,9,33,35]

High-dose antibiotic therapy is used for acute exacerbations of respiratory infections to decrease bacterial growth in the lungs. An annual influenza vaccine is recommended because of the increased risk of complications associated with infection.[9,31]

Nutritional therapy includes unrestricted fat consumption (approximately 30% of caloric intake), a high-protein diet, and vitamin supplements (especially the fat-soluble vitamins A, D, E, and K). Other pharmacologic therapy related to nutrition is aimed at replacement of pancreatic enzymes (pancreatin or pancrelipase). Maintenance of weight in children with cystic fibrosis often requires an intake of 150% of the normal calories recommended for healthy children.[31] In some cases, enteral feedings or intravenous nutrition may be necessary on a short-term basis. Salt supplementation may be necessary in hot weather.

Heart-lung or lung transplantation is currently the only definitive treatment.[9] More than 200 cystic fibrosis patients worldwide have undergone transplantation, with a 3-year survival of 55%.[9] Patients receiving transplants showed marked improvement in mobility, energy, and quality of life.

Identification of the disease-related gene, the cystic fibrosis transmembrane conductance regulator (*CFTR*), has advanced prospects for corrective gene therapy. One limiting factor is that the therapeutic gene has a short-term expression.

Acute Tracheobronchial Obstruction

Etiology. Acute tracheobronchial obstruction requires immediate treatment. Causes frequently include aspiration of a foreign body (e.g., a piece of meat, peanut, coin), malpositioned endotracheal tube, laryngospasm, epiglottitis, trauma, swelling from smoke inhalation, postsurgical blood clot, and compression of the bronchus or trachea by tumors or enlarged lymph nodes. With inhaled foreign bodies, the right side of the lung is affected more often than the left because of the angle of the anatomic extension of the right main bronchus from the trachea.

Pathogenesis. Obstruction by one of the etiologic agents listed earlier can be partial or complete. The health care worker must be prepared to assess the situation rapidly and act immediately to clear the airway.

Clinical Manifestations. With complete obstruction, no air movement will be heard on auscultation, but the patient may still be making inspiratory chest movements. Other clinical features of complete obstruction include inability to talk, tachycardia, cyanosis, and rapid progression to unconsciousness unless the problem is quickly reversed.

With partial obstruction of the airway, the patient usually presents with stridor, sternal and intercostal retractions, wheezing, nasal flaring, tachypnea, dyspnea, tachycardia, and use of accessory muscles to breathe. Cyanosis is a late sign that usually indicates exhaustion or complete obstruction.

Diagnosis. The diagnosis of airway obstruction is based on clinical features and arterial blood gas analyses. Arterial blood gas values frequently show hypoxemia and hypercarbia. Chest radiographs may reveal the location of the obstruction.

Treatment. Treatment involves opening the obstructed airway as quickly as possible. Blows to the patient's back or use of the Heimlich maneuver may be necessary for the foreign body to be expelled. Aspirated contents occluding the airway are suctioned to relieve obstruction. If these methods are unsuccessful, an emergency tracheostomy should be performed in the case of a suspected upper airway obstruction in the subglottic region or above.

Epiglottitis

Etiology. Epiglottitis is a rapidly progressive cellulitis of the epiglottis and adjacent soft tissues. Acute epiglottitis is suspected when odynophagia (pain with swallowing) seems out of proportion to pharyngeal findings. Inability to swallow saliva with evidence of drooling is common. Epiglottitis is classified as a subtype of croup. The causative organism is primarily *H. influenzae* type B (Hib). It is most often seen in children 2 to 4 years old. Pneumococci, streptococci, and staphylococci are also causal agents.[23,36] The role of viruses in epiglottitis is unclear.[36]

Pathogenesis. The infecting agent localizes in the supraglottic area in the epiglottis and pharyngeal structures, causing rapid and potentially fatal inflammation with swelling and airway obstruction.

Clinical Manifestations. The patient frequently presents with acute respiratory difficulty that has progressed rapidly over several hours. Common signs and symptoms include drooling, dysphagia, rapid onset of fever, dysphonia, inspiratory stridor, and inspiratory retractions. The child often sits in a "sniffing dog" position, which provides the best airway patency. The oropharynx is edematous and cherry red.[28,36]

Diagnosis. Definitive diagnosis is obtained by direct or fiberoptic visualization of the epiglottis. Lateral neck radiographs assist in making a definitive diagnosis and reveal a classic "thumbprint sign" (swollen epiglottis that looks like a thumbprint). A complete blood count may reveal leukocytosis with a shift to the left.[36]

Treatment. This condition is a true medical emergency and may necessitate intubation. Antibiotic therapy should be started immediately. Preventive treatment with the Hib vaccine is the key to decreasing the incidence of this disease.

Croup Syndrome

Etiology. Croup syndrome describes a number of acute viral inflammatory diseases of the larynx. Croup diseases include laryngotracheobronchitis (viral croup), epiglottitis (discussed previously), and bacterial tracheitis. Viral croup affects the larynx, trachea, and bronchi. It is often caused by parainfluenza virus type 1. Other potential infecting organisms include parainfluenza types 2 and 3, RSV, influenza virus, adenovirus, and *Mycoplasma pneumoniae*.[23] Croup usually occurs in the fall and early winter, affecting children ages 6 months to 3 years.[35]

Pathogenesis. The infectious agent causes inflammation along the entire airway, leading to edema formation in the subglottic area.[1,2]

Clinical Manifestations. The child presents with a history of upper respiratory infection or cold that has developed into a barking cough with stridor. Fever is low grade or absent. In severe cases the child may present with stridor at rest, retractions, and cyanosis.

Diagnosis. Diagnosis is based on clinical manifestations and lateral neck films to rule out epiglottitis. Direct laryngoscopy is also used to confirm the presence of epiglottitis because the clinical presentation is similar to that of croup. Lateral neck radiographs show subglottic narrowing and a normal epiglottis. The classic steeple sign associated with viral croup shows narrowing below the vocal cords.[23,37]

Treatment. Supportive treatment is used for viral croup. Mist therapy, oral hydration, and avoidance of stimulation are used in outpatient therapy. Hospitalized children are managed with oxygen therapy and pulse oximetry. Nebulized epinephrine is effective in relieving airway obstruction. Endotracheal intubation may be required for children with respiratory failure.

KEY POINTS

- Obstructive disorders are associated with increased resistance to airflow.
- Bronchiectasis is associated with recurrent inflammation of the bronchial walls, chronic cough, and aneurysm-like dilatations of the bronchioles. These bronchiolar dilatations serve as pockets of infection, producing purulent, foul-smelling sputum. Treatment centers on antibiotic therapy and removal of secretions.

- Bronchiolitis refers to widespread bronchiolar inflammation, often associated with smoking and a number of infectious agents. Inflammation results in mucosal swelling, excessive mucus production, and bronchial muscle constriction—all of which narrow the airway lumen and may lead to wheezing and dyspnea. Treatment centers on bronchodilating agents and management of the underlying cause.
- Cystic fibrosis is an autosomal recessive disorder of exocrine glands and mucus cells. Secretions are excessively thick because of insufficient chloride and water transport. Thick secretions cause airway obstruction, atelectasis, and air trapping. Associated symptoms resulting from dysfunction of the exocrine pancreas are apparent. Treatment centers on removal of secretions and providing antibiotic therapy for complicating respiratory infections.
- Obstruction of the trachea or large bronchi may occur acutely, requiring immediate treatment. Usual causes include foreign body aspiration, trauma, and inflammation. With complete obstruction, no movement of air occurs, even though inspiratory efforts may be observed. Partial airway obstruction is associated with wheezing, retractions, and stridor. Treatment centers on removing the obstruction, if possible, or creating a patent airway by a tracheostomy.
- Epiglottitis is a medical emergency. *Haemophilus influenzae* type B, the primary organism associated with epiglottitis, invades the supraglottic structures (epiglottis and arytenoids), causing inflammation and edema, leading to obstruction. Key points in the clinical diagnosis are rapid onset of fever, pain and difficulty swallowing, and drooling. Lateral neck x-ray films reveal a classic thumbprint sign, which is indicative of epiglottal swelling. Airway maintenance via endotracheal intubation or tracheostomy and antibiotic therapy are the primary treatments. The Hib vaccine has greatly decreased the number of cases seen in the pediatric population.
- Croup is usually from a viral infection of the subglottic area. Children ages 6 months to 3 years present with cough and stridor following an upper respiratory infection. Humidification, oxygenation, and inhaled epinephrine are the primary treatment modalities.

DIAGNOSTIC TESTS

Pulmonary Function Testing

The primary criterion in diagnosing obstructive disease is the demonstration of obstruction to airflow in the lungs. Table 22-2 lists common ventilatory parameters referred to in spirometry.

Spirometry is performed by asking the patient to inhale deeply and then to exhale as quickly as possible until maximal air is exhaled. The total volume of air exhaled is known as the *forced vital capacity.* To determine flow, the time required for exhaling the air is also measured. The volume exhaled in the first second is a reliable and reproducible index of obstructive airway disease. This value is the *forced expiratory volume in 1 second.* Figure 22-19 presents spirogram examples of normal, restrictive, and obstructive graphs for FEV_1 and FVC. For all spirometric studies, normal values are based on large population studies of healthy volunteers and are adjusted for height, weight, age, and gender data that are available for comparison.

A simple formula has been developed to define and quantify airflow obstruction. If the FEV_1/FVC ratio is 75% or greater, no significant obstruction of airflow is present. If the value obtained is between 60% and 70%, then mild obstruction of airflow is present. Moderate obstruction is defined as a value of 50% to 60%; and severe obstruction is present when the FEV_1/FVC ratio is less than 50%. Therefore, using a spirometer and measuring both volume and time, the diagnosis of chronic obstructive pulmonary disease can be made and the severity quantified.

From the spirometric ventilatory measurements (see Table 22-2), other determinations of airflow can be made from the middle to later parts of a FVC maneuver. These measures are

TABLE 22-2

Common Ventilatory Parameters Measured by Spirometry

Parameter	Definition
Tidal volume	Volume of air inspired and expired with a normal breath (400-500 ml or 5 ml/kg of body weight)
Residual volume	Volume of gas left in lung after maximal expiration; stabilizes alveoli
Vital capacity or forced vital capacity	Maximal air that can be expired after a maximal inspiratory effort; includes inspiratory reserve volume, tidal volume, and expiratory reserve volume
Functional residual capacity	Volume of air left in lungs after a normal expiration; includes expiratory reserve volume and residual volume
Forced expiratory flow rate (FEF_{25}, FEF_{50}, FEF_{75})	Volume of air forcibly exhaled per unit time (liters per second or liters per minute) at 25%, 50%, and 75% of the FVC
Peak expiratory flow rate	Highest rate of flow sustained for 10 msec or more at which air can be expelled from the lungs

See Figure 21-10 for normal values.

helpful in determining the presence of small airway disease. Some investigators believe that small airway disease may be a precursor to the development of chronic bronchitis and emphysema.[1,21]

Frequently, an inhaled bronchodilator, such as albuterol or metaproterenol, may be given, with testing repeated in 15 to 20 minutes. If the FEV_1 improves by 15% or more, the patient is considered to have a positive bronchodilator response, indicative of partially reversible bronchospasm of the smooth muscles of the airways. This is most often the case with asthma or asthmatic bronchitis.

A second pulmonary function test known as the *diffusion capacity* measures the ability of the alveolar gases to diffuse into the capillary blood. The technical details of this test are beyond the scope of this book, but it is a valuable test for determining either thickening (fibrosis) of the alveolocapillary membrane or destruction (emphysema) of the membrane.

By breathing mixtures of an inert gas, such as helium, the TLC can be determined. This volume is composed of the FVC and the RV. The RV is the volume of air that remains in the lung after a person has voluntarily exhaled all of the air from the lungs (see Figure 21-10). RV/TLC is normally 30% to 35%. In some patients with airflow obstruction, air tends to get trapped in the lungs, thereby increasing the RV and resulting in overinflation of lung tissue.

Arterial blood gases are also useful as a pulmonary function measurement. Using these values, a careful assessment of both the oxygenation and the acid-base status can be determined. The normal pH is 7.40, the normal $Paco_2$ is 40 mm Hg, and the normal Pao_2, at sea level, is 80 to 100 mm Hg. In COPD, especially in severe stage, Pao_2 falls and $Paco_2$ rises. Table 22-3 lists normal arterial blood gas values for various groups. A thorough discussion of arterial blood gas analysis can be found in Chapter 25.

Bronchial Provocation Tests

The controlled induction of bronchospasm by inhalation of various agents is occasionally used to identify patients with hyperreactive airways and to prove whether certain inhaled substances can produce bronchospasm. Usually a series of inhalations is administered, followed by a series of ventilation measurements. Generally the test is stopped when the FEV_1 falls at least 20% more than the control measurement. This should only be done where emergency support services are available. Bronchoprovocation is contraindicated if the patient is already exhibiting symptoms or requires continual asthma medication. Allergens can be administered as solutions, dusts, or fumes. The amount administered should be no more than the patient would normally encounter in the environment. If symptoms occur, they can be readily reversed by two to four inhalations of albuterol or metaproterenol.

General hyperreactivity of the bronchi can be detected by having the patient inhale histamine phosphate solutions or methacholine (related to acetylcholine) or nebulized distilled water. A fall of more than 20% in the FEV_1 is indicative of hyperreactivity.

FIGURE 22-19 Comparison of spirograms for normal lungs, restrictive lung disease, and obstructive lung disease. FEV1, Forced expiratory volume in 1 second; FVC, forced vital capacity.

TABLE 22-3				
Normal Arterial Blood Gas Values				
Parameter	**Adult***	**Pregnancy**	**Newborn**	**COPD (Late Findings)**
Pao_2 (mm Hg)	80-100	75-100	60-70	Decreased
$Paco_2$ (mm Hg)	34-45	30-37	35-45	Increased
pH	7.35-7.45	7.35-7.45	7.30-7.40	Decreased
HCO_3^- (mEq/L)	24-30	20-26	20-26	Increased
Base excess (mEq/L)	±2	—	—	—
O_2 saturation (%)	96-100	95-100	90-100	Decreased

COPD, Chronic obstructive pulmonary disease.

*For elderly, Pao_2 can be estimated by the following formulas[24]: 104 – (patient's age × 0.42) for patients lying supine; and 104 – (patient's age × 0.27) for patients sitting.

KEY POINTS

Obstructive disorders are associated with characteristic abnormalities on pulmonary function testing. These include

- Decreased FEV_1
- Low FEV_1/FVC ratio (<70%)
- Improvement in FEV_1 after use of a bronchodilator (asthma)
- Increased residual volume
- Increased functional residual capacity

SUMMARY

Health care professionals have a key role in the management of respiratory disorders in the hospital and in the community. Obstructive pulmonary diseases presented in this chapter include airway obstruction, obstruction from conditions affecting the tracheobronchial walls, and loss of lung parenchyma (emphysema). Obstructive pulmonary disorders are characterized by increased resistance to airflow. With bronchiectasis, obstruction is due to inflammation, infection, and dilation of the bronchioles. Similarly, bronchiolitis is associated with inflammation; however, in this situation, inflammation leads to mucosal edema and excessive mucus production. Airway obstruction from cystic fibrosis is related to production of excessive, thick secretions. Obstruction of the airway in croup is the result of edema and increased secretions caused by viral infection. Similarly, epiglottitis is an infectious process requiring emergency treatment. The primary organism causing epiglottitis is *H. influenzae*. The incidence of epiglottitis has been greatly reduced with the advent of the Hib vaccine.

An inflammatory process is also seen in asthma and bronchitis. The inflammation is associated with increased mucus production and edema of the tracheal bronchial mucosa in asthma and bronchitis. Bronchospasm of the tracheobronchial tree due to exposure to allergens, pulmonary irritants, stress, and exercise may result in hypoxemia. Obstruction to airflow in emphysema is due to loss of alveoli and small airways. The most common cause is cigarette smoking.

REFERENCES

1. West JB: *Pulmonary pathophysiology: the essentials*, ed 7, Philadelphia, 2008, Lippincott Williams & Wilkins.
2. West JB: *Pulmonary physiology and pathophysiology: an integrated case-based approach*, ed 2, Philadelphia, 2007, Lippincott Williams & Wilkins.
3. *National Asthma Education and Prevention Program Expert Panel Report II Guidelines for Diagnosis and Management of Asthma*, Washington, DC, 2006 Update, US Department of Health and Human Services.
4. Vura-Weis DL: Allergies and asthma. In Sloane PD, Slatt LM et al, editors: *Essentials of family medicine*, ed 5, Philadelphia, 2008, Lippincott Williams & Wilkins, pp 745-768.
5. Brooks AM: Asthma. In Garfunkel LC, Kaczorowski J, Christy C, editors: *Mosby's pediatric clinical advisor: instant diagnosis and treatment*, St Louis, 2002, Mosby, pp 171-173.
6. Kolski GB: Asthma in children. In Rakel RE, Bope ET, editors: *Conn's current therapy, 2008*, Philadelphia, 2008, Saunders, pp 759-765.
7. Lester MR: Asthma in children. In Rakel RE, Bope ET, editors: *Conn's current therapy 2008*, Philadelphia, 2007, Saunders.
8. Ferri FF: Asthma. In Ferri FF, editor: *Ferri's clinical advisor: instant diagnosis and treatment*, St Louis, 2007, Mosby, pp 89-91.
9. Chesnutt MS, Prendergast TJ: Lung. In Tierney LM, McPhee SJ, Papdakis MA , editors: *Current medical diagnosis and treatment*, ed 46, New York, 2007, Lange/McGraw-Hill, pp 222-315.
10. Goroll AH, Mulley AG: Management of asthma. In Goroll AH, Mulley AG, editors: *Primary care medicine: office evaluation and management of the adult patient*, ed 5, Philadelphia, 2006, Lippincott Williams & Wilkins, pp 357-370.
11. Binstadt BA, Schneider L: Allergic disorders and immunodeficiency. In Graef JW, editor: *Manual of pediatric therapeutics*, ed 7, Philadelphia, 2007, Lippincott-Raven, pp 500-516.
12. Hogg JC: The pathophysiology of asthma, *Chest* 82:8s-11s, 1982.
13. Guyton AC, Hall JE: *Textbook of medical physiology*, ed 11, Philadelphia, 2005, Saunders.
14. Prendergast TJ et al: Pulmonary disease. In McPhee S, Lingappa VA, Ganong WF et al, *Pathophysiology of disease: an introduction to clinical medicine*, ed 5, New York, 2005, McGraw Hill.
15. Williams PV: Management of asthma, *Clin Symp* 49(3):2-32, 1997.
16. Jaskiewicz J: Cystic Fibrosis. In Garfunkel LC, Kaczorowski J, Christy C, editors: *Mosby's pediatric clinical advisor: instant diagnosis and treatment*, St Louis, 2002, Mosby, pp 263-264.
17. Boguniewicz M, Leung DYM: Allergic disorders. In Hay WW et al, editors: *Current pediatric diagnosis and treatment*, ed 18, New York, 2007, Lange/McGraw-Hill, pp 1049-1077.
18. Mainous AG, Hueston WJ: Acute respiratory infections. In Sloane PD et al, editors: *Essentials of family medicine*, ed 5, Philadelphia, 2007, Lippincott Williams & Wilkins, pp 769-785.
19. Kormis WA: Approach to the patient with acute bronchitis or pneumonia in the ambulatory setting. In Goroll AH, Mulloy AG, editors: *Primary care medicine: office evaluation and management of the adult patient*, ed 5, Philadelphia, 2006, Lippincott Williams & Wilkins, pp 388-397.
20. Weiss EF: Clubbing. In Greene HL et al, editors: *Clinical medicine*, ed 2, St Louis, 1996, Mosby, pp 563-566.
21. Goroll AJ, Mulley AG: Management of chronic obstructive pulmonary disease. In Goroll AH, May LA, Mulley AG, editors: *Primary care medicine: office evaluation and management of the adult patient*, ed 5, Philadelphia, 2006, Lippincott Williams & Wilkins, pp 345-356.
22. Garcia JA, Jenkinson SG: Management of chronic obstructive pulmonary disease. In Rakel RE, Bope ET, editors: *Conn's current therapy, 2008*, Philadelphia, 2008, Saunders, pp 225-230.
23. Kerby GS et al: Respiratory tract and mediastinum. In Hay WW et al, editors: *Current pediatric diagnosis and treatment*, New York, 2007, Lange/McGraw-Hill, pp 493-541.
24. National Center for Health Statistics: Chronic obstructive pulmonary disease (COPD), website, www.cdc.gov/nchs/fastats/copd.htm, February 2007.
25. Johnston CB et al: Geriatric medicine. In Tierney LM, McPhee SJ, Papadalos MA, editors: *Current medical diagnosis and treatment*, ed 46, Norwalk, Conn, 2007, Appleton & Lange, pp 51-67.
26. Ferri FF: Bronchiectasis. In Ferri FF, editor: *Ferri's clinical advisor: instant diagnosis and treatment*, St Louis, 2007, Mosby, p 138.
27. Cystic Fibrosis Foundation, 6931 Arlington Rd, Suite 2000, Bethesda, MD 20814; 800-344-4823, www.cff.org.
28. Behrman RE, Kliegman RM, Jenson HB: *Pocket companion to accompany Nelson textbook of pediatrics*, ed 16, Philadelphia, 2001, Saunders, pp 505-506.
29. Shandera WX, Koo H: Infectious diseases: viral and rickettsial. In Tierney LM, McPhee SJ, Papadakis MA, editors: *Current medical diagnosis and treatment*, ed 46, New York, 2007, Lange/McGraw-Hill, pp 1378-1430.
30. Chen S: Respiratory syncytial virus/bronchiolitis. In Garfunkel LC, Kaczorowski J, Christy C, editors: *Mosby's pediatric clinical advisor: instant diagnosis and treatment*, St Louis, 2002, Mosby, pp 635-636.

31. Froh DK: Cystic fibrosis. In Rakel RE, Bope ET, editors: *Conn's current therapy, 2008,* Philadelphia, 2008, Saunders, pp 230-233.

32. Fishman DS, Bousuares A: Management of nutritional gastrointestinal and hepatic disorders. In Graef JW, editor: *Manual of pediatric therapeutics,* ed 7, Philadelphia, 2007, Lippincott-Raven, p 359.

33. Yusen RD et al: Pulmonary diseases. In Ahya SN, Flood K, Paranjothi S, editors: *Washington manual of medical therapeutics,* ed 32, Philadelphia, 2007, Lippincott Williams & Wilkins, pp 245-289.

34. Bluth MG, Hardin RE, Tenner S et al: Laboratory diagnosis of gastrointestinal and pancreatic disorders. In McPherson RA, Pincus MR, editors: *Henry's clinical diagnosis and management by laboratory methods,* ed 21, Philadelphia, 2006, Saunders, p 291.

35. Yusen RD, Lefrak SS: Pulmonary II: Diseases. In Lin TL, Rypkema SW, editors: *The Washington manual of ambulatory therapeutics,* ed 31, Philadelphia, 2002, Lippincott Williams & Wilkins, pp 202-226.

36. Opal SM, Lieber JJ: Epiglottitis. In Ferri FF, editor: *Ferri's clinical advisor: instant diagnosis and treatment,* St Louis, 2007, Mosby, pp 309-310.

37. Jackson MA, Vahle H: Croup. In Garfunkel LC, Kaczorowski J, Christy C, editors: *Mosby's pediatric clinical advisor: instant diagnosis and treatment.* St Louis, 2002, Mosby, pp 259-260.

chapter

23

Restrictive Pulmonary Disorders

Lorna Schumann

MEDIA RESOURCES

Additional Material for Study, Review, and Further Exploration

CD Companion ■ Review Questions and Answers
■ Glossary (with audio pronunciations for selected terms)
■ Disease Profiles ■ Animations

ⓔvolve **Website** at http://evolve.elsevier.com/Copstead/
■ Case Studies ■ Disease Profiles ■ WebLinks ■ Key Points Review

Online Course (Module 12)

KEY QUESTIONS

■ How do fibrotic lung disorders develop?
■ How is the pathogenesis of acute (adult) respiratory distress syndrome similar to that of infant respiratory distress syndrome?
■ How do abnormal accumulations in the pleural space affect lung function?

■ What neuromuscular disorders are associated with reduced lung compliance?
■ What is the pathogenesis of tuberculosis?
■ What pulmonary function test abnormalities are characteristic of restrictive pulmonary disorders?

CHAPTER OUTLINE

Restrictive pulmonary diseases are the result of decreased expansion of the lungs due to alterations in the lung parenchyma, pleura, chest wall, or neuromuscular function. These disorders may be classified as pulmonary or extrapulmonary and represent acute or chronic patterns of lung dysfunction rather than a single clinical disease. Table 23-1 lists the various disease processes that can be classified as restrictive. These diseases are characterized by a decrease in total lung capacity (TLC), vital capacity (VC), functional residual capacity (FRC), and residual volume (RV). The greater the decrease in lung volume, the greater the severity of the disease.[1] Blood gas analysis often shows decreased arterial partial pressure of oxygen (Pao_2) and normal or decreased arterial partial pressure of carbon dioxide ($Paco_2$), resulting in increased pH (respiratory alkalosis).

This chapter presents information related to restrictive pulmonary diseases, including lung parenchyma disorders, pleural space disorders, neuromuscular and chest wall disorders, pneumonia, and tuberculosis. Specific lung parenchyma disorders including interstitial fibrosis, sarcoidosis, hypersensitivity pneumonitis, and pneumoconiosis, as well as atelectatic

disorders, including acute (adult) respiratory distress syndrome (ARDS) and infant respiratory distress syndrome (IRDS), are presented. Pleural space disorders, divided into pneumothorax and pleural effusions, are discussed. The section on neuromuscular and chest wall disorders is divided into neuromuscular weakness, chest wall deformities, and obesity. The final section presents the etiologic factors, pathogenesis, clinical manifestations, diagnosis, and management of pneumonia, tuberculosis, and severe acute respiratory syndrome (SARS). Table 23-2 describes variations in respiratory parameters that affect restrictive lung disease in infant and elderly populations.

Lung Parenchyma Disorders

FIBROTIC INTERSTITIAL LUNG DISEASES

The term *interstitial lung disease* describes a group of disorders (more than 180 disease entities) that are characterized by acute, subacute, or chronic infiltration of alveolar walls by cells, fluid, and connective tissue.[1-4] If left untreated, the inflammatory process may progress to irreversible fibrosis.[4] The incidence of interstitial lung disease is 5 cases per 100,000 persons.[3]

Diffuse Interstitial Lung Disease

Etiology. Diffuse interstitial lung disease (also known as *diffuse interstitial pulmonary fibrosis*) is the name typically used for restrictive diseases characterized by thickening of the alveolar interstitium.[2] Synonyms frequently presented in the literature include *interstitial pneumonia, diffuse parenchymal lung disease, Hamman-Rich syndrome, intrinsic fibrosing alveolitis, cryptogenic fibrosing alveolitis,* and *idiopathic pulmonary fibrosis.*

Pathogenesis. Pathogenesis of the disease is not well understood, but is possibly related to an immune reaction that usually begins with injury to the alveolar epithelial or capillary endothelial cells.[1,2] Pathophysiologic changes may include interstitial and alveolar wall thickening and increased collagen bundles in the interstitium (Figure 23-1). Lung tissue becomes infiltrated by lymphocytes, macrophages, and plasma cells. Persistent alveolitis may lead to obliteration of alveolar capillaries, reorganization of the lung parenchyma, and irreversible fibrosis.[2] These changes in turn lead to large air-filled sacs (cysts) accompanied by dilated terminal and respiratory bronchioles.

The immune response noted in interstitial lung disease is characterized by three pathologic patterns in the alveoli: inflammation, fibrosis, and destruction.

The inflammatory pattern occurs early and is potentially reversible.[4,5] The triggering event (e.g., occupational exposure, drug ingestion, connective tissue disease) causes an inflammatory response leading to increased numbers of inflammatory cells (i.e., neutrophils, lymphocytes, macrophages).[1,2,4] An associated injury to the alveolar capillary basement membrane from the triggering event leads to increased membrane permeability and movement of fluid and debris into the alveoli. The initial injury, in association with the inflammatory pattern, leads to fibroblastic proliferation and deposition of

TABLE 23-1

Restrictive Pulmonary Disorders

Disorder Type	Representative Examples
Diseases of the Lung Parenchyma	
Neoplastic disease	—
Pneumonia	Pneumonia (viral, bacterial, fungal), hypersensitivity pneumonitis
Granulomatous disease	Sarcoidosis, tuberculosis, coccidioidomycosis, blastomycosis
Pneumoconioses	Occupational lung disease
Acute interstitial pneumonitis	—
Collagen disease	Rheumatoid arthritis, scleroderma, systemic lupus erythematosus
Atelectasis	—
Pulmonary resection	—
Vascular Diseases	
	Pulmonary edema, pulmonary embolism
Acute respiratory distress syndrome	—
Diseases of Extrapulmonary Restriction	
Chest wall disease	Kyphoscoliosis, ankylosing spondylitis, obesity
Neuromuscular disease	Quadriplegia, hemiplegia, Guillain-Barré syndrome, myasthenia gravis, amyotrophic lateral sclerosis, muscular dystrophy
Pleural diseases	Pleural effusion, hemothorax, pneumothorax, chylothorax
Other	Abdominal distention, surgery, pregnancy

TABLE 23-2

Age-Related Features Contributing to Restrictive Lung Disease

Anatomic Site	Impact on Restrictive Disease
Infant	
Sternum and ribs are cartilaginous with soft chest wall	Diminishes effect of restrictive disease in infants
Ribs are horizontally oriented so that ribs move in and out easily	Diminishes effect of restrictive disease in infants
Accessory muscles of respiration are poorly developed	Majority of respiratory movement relies on diaphragm; restrictive diseases that compromise diaphragmatic excursion affect respiratory status; e.g., thoracic or abdominal surgery, paralysis, and abdominal masses all affect diaphragmatic excursion
Diaphragm rests horizontally and draws lower ribs inward in supine position so that diaphragmatic excursion is decreased	Leads to compromised effort of breathing
Cartilage of infant larynx is soft, so airway is compressed when neck is flexed or hyperextended	Increases airway resistance
During first month of life, neonate is obligate nose breather	Nasal obstruction may lead to respiratory distress from decreased airflow
Small diameter of airway leads to increased resistance to airflow	Mucus or edema in the airway may lead to significant increase in resistance and a decrease in airway diameter
Fewer alveoli than in adults, leading to decreased radial traction applied to the airways	Increased tendency of airways to collapse
Pores of Kohn and channels of Lambert are underdeveloped, leading to fewer collateral ventilation pathways	May lead to respiratory compromise, reducing ventilatory support with restrictive diseases
Elderly	
Decreased ciliary activity	Increased incidence of infection; decreased mucus clearance in all types of respiratory disorders
Decreased chest wall compliance and decreased lung elasticity in some areas of the lung	Leads to a reduction in lung volume; leads to decreased expansion of the lungs and to decreased matching of ventilation and perfusion
Decreased stress tolerance	Increased incidence of disease and trauma with age
Decreased muscle tone	Decreased physical conditioning
Impaired immunity as evidenced by decreased T-cell function; increased autoantibodies	Decreased resistance to infection
Decreased oxygen uptake	Decreased oxygen level in the blood
Decreased vital capacity	Decreased alveolar expansion
Decreased cough reflex	Impaired ability to clear secretions and inhaled particulate matter

large amounts of collagen. The fibrotic pattern is manifested by increases in mesenchymal cells and fibroblasts in the interstitium, and alveolar walls become thickened with increased amounts of fibrous tissue.[5,6]

The lung destruction pattern is manifested by loss of alveolar walls. Radiographically, this appears as a "honeycomb lung" and indicates end-stage disease.[2] Ground-glass appearance on chest radiograph is often an early finding.[3] The fibrotic and honeycomb patterns respond poorly to treatment.[5]

Clinical Manifestations. The most common patient complaint is progressive dyspnea with nonproductive cough.[3,5] Clinical features include rapid, shallow breathing; dyspnea; irritating, nonproductive cough; clubbing of the nail beds (40% to 80% cases)[4]; bibasilar end-expiratory[3,4] crackles (Velcro rales); and marked dyspnea with exercise. Cyanosis is a late finding. Anorexia and weight loss are noted on physical exam. As the disease progresses, patients exhibit an inability to increase cardiac output with exercise as evidenced by low maximal heart rate and high peripheral vascular resistance. Arterial oxygen desaturation occurs with exercise.[4]

Diagnosis. The chest radiograph shows a honeycomb appearance and a coarse reticular pattern indicating late stage of disease.[2,3,5,6] Ground-glass haziness is indicative of the presence of infiltrates. Open lung biopsy or transbronchial biopsy, gallium-67 scanning, and bronchoalveolar lavage may be used for diagnostic evaluation.[3] Pulmonary function testing findings are usually consistent with restrictive lung disease (decreased vital capacity, total lung capacity, and diffusing capacity).[3]

Treatment. The patient should be encouraged to avoid tobacco use and environmental exposure to the offending cause.[2-4] Primary therapy consists of administration of antiinflammatory and immunosuppressive agents. Immunosuppressive agents have been useful in reducing the dosage of corticosteroids. Lung transplantation has been used successfully in selected patients.[3,5,7]

Sarcoidosis

Etiology. Sarcoidosis is categorized as an acute or chronic systemic disease of unknown cause, although an immunologic basis appears likely.[1] Activation of the alveolar macrophage due to an unknown antigen trigger is a possible cause.[1]

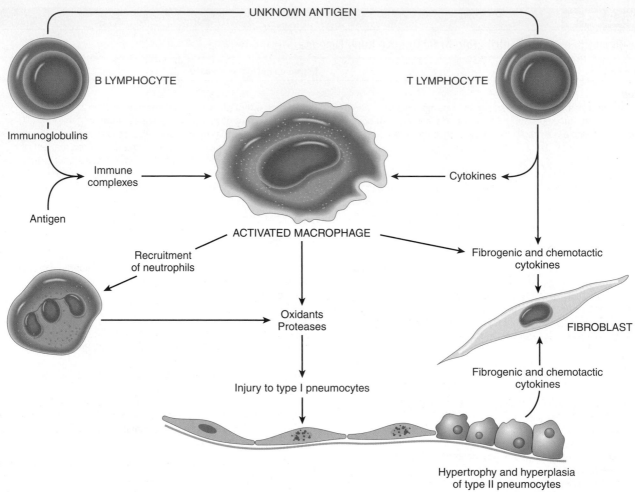

FIGURE 23-1 Possible schema of the pathogenesis of idiopathic pulmonary fibrosis. (From Kumar V et al: *Robbin's basic pathology,* ed 8, Philadelphia, 2007, Saunders, p 483.)

The acute process occurs more commonly in women in the second or third decade of life.[1,2] The chronic form is seen more commonly in the third to fourth decades of life, with the highest incidence seen in North American blacks (35.5/100,000) and northern European whites (10.9/100,000).[2]

Pathogenesis. The disease is characterized by the development of multiple, uniform, noncaseating epithelioid granulomas that affect multiple organ systems, most commonly the lymph nodes and lung tissue. The noncaseating granulomas are fibrotic and are surrounded by large histiocytes.[1,2,7] Sarcoid granulomas may also occur in the bronchial airways. Abnormal T-cell function is noted with this disease.[7] Other systems and/or organs frequently involved are the skin, eyes, spleen, liver, kidney, and bone marrow.[1,7]

Clinical Manifestations. Sarcoidosis is characterized by malaise, fatigue, weight loss, fever, dyspnea of insidious onset, and a dry, nonproductive cough.[2,7] Other features include erythema nodosum (lesions marked by the formation of painful nodes on the lower extremities); macules, papules, hyperpigmentation and subcutaneous nodules; hepatosplenomegaly; and lymphadenopathy. Patients with the acute disease usually present with enlarged lymph nodes and arthritis, although some patients experience no symptoms.[7] Skin lesions and lacrimal and parotid gland involvement are also noted in the acute process.[1] Iritis, uveitis, blurred vision, conjunctivitis, and ocular discomfort may develop.[7]

Diagnosis. Common laboratory findings in patients with sarcoidosis include leukopenia, anemia, increased eosinophil count, elevated sedimentation rate, and increased calcium levels (seen in 5% of patients).[2,7] Serum levels of liver enzymes may also be elevated. Approximately 70% of patients exhibit anergy (decreased sensitivity to specific antigens such as *Trichophyton, Candida,* mumps virus, and tuberculin).[2] Patients with active disease also demonstrate elevated levels of angiotensin-converting enzyme (40% to 80% of cases).[2]

Chest radiographs can be used to differentiate stages of the disease process: stage 0, normal; stage I, hilar adenopathy alone; stage II, hilar adenopathy and bilateral pulmonary infiltrates; and stage III, pulmonary infiltrates without adenopathy. Stage IV is characterized by advanced fibrosis with evidence of honeycombing, hilar retraction, bullae, cysts, and emphysema.[7] Gallium-67 scans will localize areas of granulomatous infiltrates. Pleural effusion is noted in 10% of cases of sarcoidosis.[1,2,7] Pulmonary function test results may be normal or may show evidence of restrictive disease and/or obstructive disease.[7]

Transbronchial lung biopsy demonstrates noncaseating granulomas, thus providing a definitive diagnosis (75% to 90% cases). Bronchoalveolar lavage may be used to monitor cell content in patients with sarcoidosis.[1,7] The lavage fluid is characterized by increased lymphocytes and a high CD4/CD8 cell ratio.[2]

Treatment. Administration of corticosteroids and management of symptoms is the mainstay of treatment for patients whose disease process does not resolve spontaneously and in whom progressive lung disease or evidence of extrapulmonary sarcoidosis develops. For patients with progressive disease that does not respond to corticosteroids, immunosuppressive agents may be used.[7] The prognosis is best for stage I disease. Death due to pulmonary insufficiency occurs in about 5% to 7% of patients.[2,7]

Hypersensitivity Pneumonitis

Etiology. Hypersensitivity pneumonitis, also called *extrinsic allergic alveolitis,* is classified as both a restrictive disease and an occupational disease. Numerous (greater than 300) inhaled organic agents are responsible for the inflammatory process.[8] Table 23-3 lists various allergens related to the disease. Unlike other pulmonary diseases, hypersensitivity pneumonitis has a predominance in nonsmokers (80% to 95% of cases).[8]

Pathogenesis. The causative agent is suggested by the patient's history and confirmed by demonstration of precipitating antibodies in the serum directed to the causative antigen. The causative antigen combines with the serum antibody in the alveolar walls, leading to a type III hypersensitivity reaction. Type III hypersensitivity diseases are caused by the formation of antigen-antibody complexes[1,8] (see Chapter 10). These antigen-antibody complexes then elicit the granulomatous inflammation that leads to lung tissue injury, as evidenced by thickened alveolar walls; formation of exudate in the bronchiolar lumen; and infiltration by lymphocytes, plasma cells, and eosinophils.[1,8,9] Fibrotic lung changes occur in advanced cases.

Many individuals develop precipitating antibodies (precipitin) from organic dust exposure, but only a few develop pneumonitis.[9] Genetic predisposition may be involved in an exaggerated response to the offending agent. Experiments in animals show that a delayed hypersensitivity (type IV) reaction to the antigen is also required before pneumonitis can occur.[9]

Clinical Manifestations. In the acute disease, symptoms start 4 to 6 hours after exposure and resolve in 18 to 24 hours.[8] General symptoms may include chills, sweating, shivering, myalgias, nausea, lethargy, headache, and malaise.[1,9,10] The patient may or may not have a fever. Respiratory symptoms may include dyspnea at rest, dry cough, tachypnea, and chest discomfort. Physical findings may include cyanosis (a late sign) and crackles (rales) in the lung bases.[1,3]

In the chronic form, progressive diffuse pulmonary fibrosis develops in the upper lobes—the hallmark of the disease.[1] In the intermediate form, the disease may manifest with acute febrile episodes and progressive pulmonary fibrosis with cough, dyspnea, fatigue, and, eventually, cor pulmonale (right-sided heart enlargement due to lung disorders).[8]

Diagnosis. During the acute/subacute phase, transient bilateral pulmonary infiltrates or increased bronchial markings with alveolar nodular infiltrates may be found on chest radiographs. In the chronic phase, diffuse reticulonodular infiltrates and fibrosis are present.[9]

Skin testing with the causative antigen may produce a red, indurated, hemorrhagic reaction 4 to 12 hours after injection that lasts several days.[1] This reaction suggests precipitin-mediated sensitivity. Skin testing for most precipitating antigens is impractical because most produce irritating reactions before the precipitin reaction occurs, and many individuals without the disease have precipitating antibodies.

Common laboratory findings include an increased white blood cell count and a decreased Pa_{O_2}. Hypoxemia worsens with exercise. Pulmonary function tests show decreased lung volumes, diffusing capacity, and compliance.[1,8]

Treatment. The goal of therapy is to identify the offending agent and prevent further exposure. This may require a change in environment or occupation. Oral corticosteroids may be used to decrease the inflammatory process.[8,10]

TABLE 23-3

Causes of Hypersensitivity Pneumonitis

Disease	Antigen	Allergen Source
Farmer's lung	*Thermophilia, Actinomyces*	Moldy hay, silage
Bird fancier's lung	Parakeet, pigeon, chicken	Bird excreta, feathers, and animal protein
Bagassosis	Thermophilic bacteria	Moldy sugarcane pulp
Mushroom, cork, maple bark, or malt hypersensitivity, cheese maker's lung, redwood lung	Various fungi	Handling moldy products
Grain handler's lung	Wheat weevil	Insect-infected grain
Pituitary extract hypersensitivity	Heterologous pituitary and serum proteins	—
Fish-meat worker's lung	Protein, fungi	Animal food
Humidifier lung (fever)	Thermophilic bacteria, amoebae, and fungi	Humidifiers and evaporative air coolers

KEY POINTS

- Diffuse interstitial pulmonary fibrosis is a restrictive disorder characterized by thickening of the alveolar interstitium. The disorder is an immune-mediated disorder that follows an initial lung injury.
- Lung tissues are characteristically infiltrated by immune cells (macrophages and lymphocytes). Excess fibrin deposition results in stiff, noncompliant lungs. Vital capacity, tidal volume, FRC, and diffusion capacity are generally reduced. Respiratory rate increases to compensate for the small tidal volume.
- Treatment centers on administration of drugs to depress immune system activity, such as corticosteroids.
- Sarcoidosis is a restrictive disorder associated with abnormal protein deposits (granulomas) in the lung. Granulomas are fibrotic and are associated with immune cells (histiocytes). The cause is unknown.
- Symptoms include progressive dyspnea, fever, enlarged lymph nodes, and generalized symptoms of inflammation. Pulmonary lymph nodes may be primarily affected, with progression to parenchymal involvement. Pulmonary function test results are consistent with a restrictive disorder, demonstrating reduced lung volumes and increased respiratory rate.
- Treatment centers on alleviation or relief of the symptoms. Corticosteroids may be used to reduce inflammation.
- Hypersensitivity pneumonitis includes a group of inflammatory lung disorders associated with inhalation of organic particles. Antibodies are produced in response to the inhaled particles; then antigen-antibody complexes deposit in the lung, initiating inflammation and granuloma production.
- Hypersensitivity pneumonitis is characterized by general symptoms of inflammation (e.g., fever, chills, malaise), dyspnea, dry cough, and tachypnea. Chronic exposure leads to progressive fibrosis and pulmonary dysfunction characteristic of restrictive parenchymal disease.

Occupational Lung Diseases

Etiology. Occupational lung diseases result from the inhalation of toxic gases or foreign particles. Traditionally, occupational lung diseases included pathologic conditions that were associated with the effects of exposure to inhaled dusts. However, a holistic approach to these diseases requires consideration of atmospheric pollutants as well as natural genetic resistance and compliance with health maintenance behaviors. The distinction between occupational and environmental respiratory diseases is becoming increasingly difficult. The integration of multiple environmental areas (home, work, and leisure) further compounds the complexity of defining occupational respiratory diseases.

Although atmospheric pollutants (toxic gases) are not discussed in detail here, their impact on occupational respiratory diseases must not be minimized. The sources, potential clinical manifestations, and potential pathologic processes associated with common atmospheric pollutants are presented in Table 23-4.

Pneumoconiosis is defined as parenchymal lung disease caused by the inhalation of inorganic dust particles. Commonly, the greater the exposure to the dust, the worse the pathologic consequences. Anthracosis (coal miner's lung or black lung), silicosis (silica inhalation), and asbestosis (asbestos inhalation) are common examples of occupational lung diseases. However, exposure to several other dusts may also impair respiratory function. Included in this list are antimony ore, barium, iron, tin, fuller's earth (clay), kaolin (china clay), and talc.

Many workers are exposed to "pathogenic dust" through their jobs and the processing, packaging, or manufacturing of a specific product.[8,11] Predisposing factors such as preexisting lung disease, exposure to atmospheric pollutants, duration of dust exposure, amount of dust concentration, and particle size affect the onset and severity of the respiratory impairment.

TABLE 23-4

Common Atmospheric Pollutants Contributing to Lung Disease

Pollutant	Source	Clinical Manifestations	Potential Disease Processes
Carbon monoxide	Automobile exhaust (incomplete fossil fuel combustion)	Lethargy, impairs mental skills, cherry-red mucous membranes, headache	Hypoxemia, respiratory failure
Sulfur oxides	Factories (corrosive, poisonous by-products of combustion of sulfur-containing fuels)	Inflamed mucous membranes, eyes, upper respiratory tract, bronchial mucosa; cough	Pulmonary edema, bronchitis
Photochemical oxidants (ozone, hydrocarbons, or nitrogen oxides)	Byproduct of exposure of hydrocarbons and/or nitrogen oxides (from fossil fuel combustion with high temperatures) to sunlight	Inflammation of eyes, upper respiratory tract; cough	Tracheitis, bronchitis, pulmonary edema
Cigarette smoke	Cigarettes (carbon monoxide, nicotine, "tars")	Impaired exercise tolerance, decreased mental activity, tachycardia, hypertension, sweating	Bronchial carcinoma, chronic bronchitis, emphysema, coronary heart disease
Particulate matter	Factories/power stations; small particles, visible smoke and soot	Cough; dyspnea; itchy, watery eyes; irritated mucous membranes	Bronchitis, tracheitis, asthma

Pathogenesis. The respiratory tract is protected by two inter-related systems: the mucociliary system and alveolar macrophages. The inhalation of inorganic particles has little effect on the mucociliary system. However, atmospheric pollutants (sulfur oxides, nitrogen oxides, and tobacco smoke) interfere with and can paralyze ciliary action.[1] As a result, the clearance effect is impaired, and inorganic particles cannot be removed.

Alveolar macrophages attempt to engulf and remove inorganic dust by one of the following methods: (1) migrating to small airways to use the mucociliary escalator; (2) engulfing dust and exiting through the lymph and/or blood system; (3) migrating through bronchial walls, depositing dust particles in extraalveolar tissue; or (4) destroying the particle (silica).[1,11]

Macrophage impairment is the primary mechanism through which inorganic particles initiate lung diseases. In an attempt to maintain a sterile alveolar environment, macrophages secrete lysozymes to control foreign particle activity. These enzymes, released in response to the particulate stimuli, eventually damage the alveolar walls, which may cause deposition of fibrous materials.

Although the type of inorganic particle inhaled individualizes the pathophysiologic response, the general response is similar in the context of occupational lung diseases. Silica is one of the most toxic particles to alveolar macrophages. Dense deposits of collagen material are formed around the silica particles, resulting in marked fibrotic tissue deposition and restrictive lung disease. Coal dust and asbestos initiate a similar, although less severe, response. The pathologic processes and clinical features for each of the major occupational lung diseases are summarized in Table 23-5.

Clinical Manifestations. Pneumoconioses (anthracosis, asbestosis, silicosis) generally produce no symptoms in the early stages. Physical evidence of the disease occurs when the pulmonary circulation is impaired due to increased pulmonary vascular resistance or a pulmonary infection develops. Workers may remain symptom free for up to 10 to 20 years with chronic exposure.[1,2,11] Once again, symptom manifestation is dependent on the predisposing factors.

As pneumoconioses progress, patients present with a progressive, productive cough and dyspnea, especially with exercise. In addition, patients may complain of progressive weakness and fatigue. Clubbing of fingers may also be present. Late clinical features include chronic hypoxemia, cor pulmonale, and respiratory failure.

Diagnosis. The reliability of pulmonary changes noted on chest radiographs varies with the severity of the disease. When the patient is symptom free, no changes may be noted. However, as the pneumoconioses progress, micronodular mottling and haziness become apparent.[1] In addition, nodules, fibroses, and calcifications resulting from dust particle deposition are noted. Pneumoconioses usually produce one of three radiographic findings: nodular, reticular, or linear. However, because of the insidious progression of occupational lung diseases, radiographs negative for lung disease do not exclude the presence of the disease process.

Changes in pulmonary function tests demonstrate predominantly restrictive impairment (see Figure 22-19) with a component of obstructive functional impairment, depending on the severity and type of dust inhalation.[1]

Finally, hypoxemia is evident from arterial blood gas measurements in the late disease stages. Falling Pao_2 levels are accompanied by decreased $Paco_2$ levels as the body initially compensates for the hypoxemia with an increased respiratory drive. However, as the disease progresses, both hypoxemia and hypercapnia are evident.

Treatment. Preventive measures are the key to limiting the onset and severity of occupational lung diseases. Adherence to federal standards for dust and particulate matter, as well as continuing education of workers and employers, will have a dramatic impact on the incidence of respiratory diseases. The use of respirators for miners and the use of water sprays to decrease airborne particles in mines are two common examples of prevention techniques. Early evaluation of a work environment predisposed to occupational lung diseases is where "treatment" must begin.[11]

Two primary goals in the management of active occupational lung diseases are to prevent further parenchymal

TABLE 23-5

Major Occupational Lung Pneumoconioses

Pneumoconioses	Pathologic Findings	Clinical Features
Anthracosis (coal miner's lung)	*Early:* Collection of coal particles with small amount of dilation of airway	*Early:* Minimal to no symptoms; may be seen with dyspnea with cough but often due to unrelated bronchitis or emphysema
	Late: Progressive, massive fibrosis, with condensed areas of black fibrous tissue	*Late:* Worsening dyspnea on exertion, productive cough, respiratory failure
Silicosis	Dense collagen deposits in respiratory bronchioles and alveoli and along lymphatics	*Early:* No symptoms noted *Late:* Productive cough, dyspnea, especially with exercise; increased risk for tuberculosis
Asbestosis	Fibrous deposits secondary to long, thin fibers, allowing deep lung penetration	Progressive dyspnea on exertion, weakness, clubbing of fingers; pleural thickening with plaque development

damage and to relieve signs and symptoms, when possible. Ideally, if the problematic dust can be identified, the individual should be removed from the environment. However, if a job change is unrealistic, every possible measure must be implemented to prevent further inhalation of dust particles. Included in this treatment is the evaluation of current health maintenance behaviors.

Treatment consists of corticosteroids, inhaled bronchodilators, oxygen therapy, and respiratory treatments (intermittent positive-pressure ventilation, postural drainage, and deep breathing exercises). The effectiveness and utilization of these therapies depend on the patient's condition and the stage of disease. Rarely are those pathologic conditions reversed with medical treatment. The primary goal is to halt symptom progression.

KEY POINTS

- Occupational lung diseases result from chronic inhalation of gases and inert particles. Commonly identified particles include coal, silica, and asbestos. Smoking and environmental pollutants may be contributing factors because they depress the ciliary function necessary to remove inhaled particles.
- The presence of inert particles in the alveoli initiates macrophage activity and inflammation. Inert particles cannot be digested by phagocytes, so they are walled off by deposition of fibrous proteins.
- Manifestations of pneumoconioses are related to the restrictive nature of the pulmonary dysfunction. Progressive dyspnea, decreased vital capacity and FRC, and increased respiratory rate are common. Blood gas analyses show progressive hypoxemia; carbon dioxide levels may remain normal or low until late in the disease.
- Treatment includes prevention of further exposure and administration of corticosteroids, bronchodilators, and oxygen therapy.

ATELECTATIC DISORDERS

Acute (Adult) Respiratory Distress Syndrome

Etiology. Acute (adult) respiratory distress syndrome is characterized by damage to the alveolar-capillary membrane. In the U.S. there are 125,000 to 150,000 cases per year. Mortality statistics range from 30% to 63%.[1,2,12,13] Clinically, ARDS is associated with a decline in the Pao_2 that is refractory (does not respond) to supplemental oxygen therapy. Damage to the alveolar-capillary membrane causes widespread alveolar infiltrates (visible on chest radiographs) and severe dyspnea. Patients who recover from the acute injury can expect to return to relatively normal lung function.[1,12] Follow-up studies (9 months to 4 years) in ARDS survivors show a mild restrictive pulmonary function accompanied by cough, dyspnea, and sputum production.[2,4] Some individuals continue to have abnormalities in diffusing capacity, oxygenation, and lung mechanics.[2,4] ARDS is associated with severe trauma, sepsis (greater than 40% of cases), aspiration of gastric acid (greater than 30% of cases), fat emboli syndrome, and shock from any cause (Box 23-1).

BOX 23-1

Major Disorders Associated with ARDS

Shock (any process leading to a low blood flow state)
Infectious causes
- Sepsis syndrome (primarily from gram-negative bacteria) with or without sustained hypotension (>40% cases)
- Pneumonia (viral, bacterial, fungal, mycobacterial)
- Miliary tuberculosis
- *Bronchiolitis obliterans*—organizing pneumonia
Trauma: pulmonary contusion
Embolism
- Fat emboli
- Air emboli
- Thrombus formation
- Amniotic fluid embolism
Head injury (increased intracranial pressure)
Aspiration (>30% of cases)
- Gastric contents
- Drowning (fresh/salt water)
Drug overdose
- Heroin
- Methadone
- Propoxyphene
- Barbiturates, salicylates, thiazides, colchicine

Inhaled toxins
- Smoke inhalation
- High concentrations of oxygen (iatrogenic)
- Corrosive chemicals (ammonia, sulfur dioxide, chlorine, nitrogen dioxide)
- Free-base cocaine smoking
Radiation
Hematologic disorders
- Disseminated intravascular coagulation
- Massive blood transfusion
- Post–cardiopulmonary bypass
- Thrombotic thrombocytopenic purpura
Metabolic disorders
- Pancreatitis
- Uremia
- Paraquat ingestion
Burns
Cancer
Anaphylaxis
Eclampsia
Radiation pneumonitis
High-altitude exposure

The precise mechanism of lung injury is not known, but the common denominator appears to be increased permeability of the pulmonary vasculature and flooding of the alveoli with proteinaceous fluid, leading to the development of protein-rich pulmonary edema (noncardiogenic pulmonary edema). The acute lung injury triggers the immune system to activate the complement system and to initiate neutrophil sequestration in the lung (Figure 23-2).

Pathogenesis. The pathogenetic sequence of events in ARDS is shown in Figure 23-2. The initial injury to the alveolar-capillary membrane may be caused by direct damage, as seen in aspiration of acidic gastric contents, or by indirect damage,

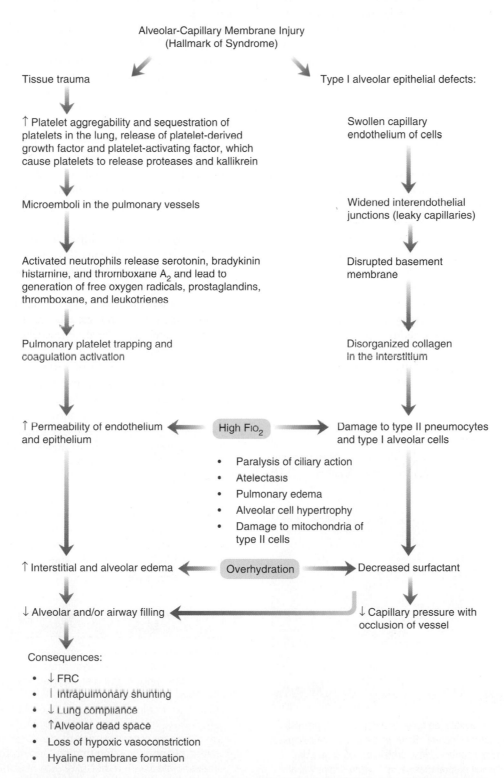

FIGURE 23-2 Pathogenesis of acute respiratory distress syndrome. *FRC,* Functional residual capacity.

as occurs in shock from any cause. Therapeutic interventions (shown in the center boxes of Figure 23-2) may act to compound the effects of the initial lung injury. The resulting injury leads to an increase in alveolar-capillary permeability, which results in interstitial and alveolar edema.

The four characteristic pathophysiologic abnormalities of ARDS involve (1) injury to the alveoli from a wide variety of disorders, (2) changes in alveolar diameter, (3) injury to the pulmonary circulation, and (4) disruptions in oxygen transport and utilization.[12,13] Common findings in this type of injury include (1) severe hypoxemia caused by intrapulmonary shunting of blood; (2) a decrease in lung compliance; (3) a decrease in FRC; (4) diffuse, fluffy alveolar infiltrates on the chest radiograph; and (5) non-cardiogenic pulmonary edema.[1,9,12,13]

The mechanism by which the FRC is decreased appears to be the result of very stiff, noncompliant lungs associated with alveolar edema and exudate, which exaggerate surface tension forces.[1,2,12,13] Early alveolar closure and continued closure lead to atelectasis and loss of lung volume.[1] The decrease in lung compliance, often severe in ARDS, is reflected in the high ventilatory pressures required to deliver an adequate volume of gas. It is thought that this decrease in lung compliance is due to loss or inactivation of surfactant with subsequent increased recoil pressure of the lungs.[1,2,12,13] In addition, proteinaceous fluid fills the alveoli and impairs ventilation. Figure 23-3 shows alveolar damage due to ARDS. Alveoli contain dense proteinaceous debris, desquamated cells, and hyaline membranes. The decrease in Pa_{O_2} is a result of perfusion of large numbers of alveoli that are poorly ventilated (areas of low ventilation-perfusion) or not ventilated (areas of shunt).

FIGURE 23-3 Diffuse alveolar damage (acute respiratory distress syndrome), shown in photomicrograph. Some of the alveoli are collapsed; others are distended. Many contain dense proteinaceous debris, desquamated cells, and hyaline membranes *(arrow)*. (From Kumar V et al: *Robbin's basic pathology*, ed 8, Philadelphia, 2007, Saunders, p 483.)

Clinical Manifestations. The clinical features of ARDS usually include a history of a precipitating event that has led to a low blood volume state ("shock" state) 1 or 2 days prior to the onset of respiratory failure. The patient may complain of sudden marked respiratory distress.[1,2] Early signs and symptoms include a slight increase in pulse rate, dyspnea, and a low Pa_{O_2}. The initial presenting sign may be shallow, rapid breathing.

With progression of the disease, the patient demonstrates tachycardia, tachypnea, hypotension, marked restlessness, decreased mental status, and frothy secretions. On auscultation of lung fields, crackles and rhonchi are heard. The patient may be using accessory muscles to breathe and demonstrating intercostal and sternal retractions. A late sign is cyanosis.

Diagnosis. The hallmark of ARDS is hypoxemia that is refractory to increasing levels of supplemental oxygen. Uncorrected hypoxemia is associated with hypotension, decreased urine output, respiratory and metabolic acidosis, and eventual cardiopulmonary arrest. Arterial blood gas determinations reveal hypoxia, acidosis, and hypercapnia.[13] The chest radiograph may initially be normal but progresses to a diffuse "whiteout" (Figure 23-4) indicative of diffuse alveolar infiltrates. The infiltrates characteristically spare the costophrenic angles.[2]

Pulmonary function tests show a marked decreased in FRC, decreased lung volumes, decreased lung compliance, and a ventilation-perfusion ($\dot{V}_A/\dot{Q}$) mismatch with a large right-to-left shunt.[1] Histologic changes found on open lung biopsy reveal atelectasis, hyaline membranes, cellular debris, and interstitial and alveolar edema[1,12,13] (see Figure 23-3).

Treatment. The management of ARDS entails identifying the underlying cause, addressing the cause (e.g., sepsis), maintaining fluid and electrolyte balance, and providing adequate oxygenation with the use of a volume ventilator utilizing pressure support, and positive end-expiratory pressure (PEEP). Patients may require fraction of inspired oxygen (F_{IO_2}) levels of 1.0. The goal is to keep the Pa_{O_2} above 60 mm Hg. Because of increased permeability of the alveolar-capillary membrane, excessive fluid administration can produce or intensify pulmonary edema. High-frequency jet ventilation (HFJV), inverse ratio ventilation (IRV) and inhaled nitric oxide have also been used to treat ARDS.[4,13] ARDS can be prevented experimentally by blocking systemic inflammatory cells. Numerous agents have been investigated.[13]

KEY POINTS

- ARDS causes profound hypoxemia and a greatly increased work of breathing, often requiring mechanical ventilation and high-level oxygen therapy to maintain the Pa_{O_2} above 60 mm Hg.
- ARDS occurs in association with other pathophysiologic processes, such as trauma, sepsis, or shock. These disorders increase the risk of development of disseminated pulmonary inflammation leading to ARDS. ARDS is associated with a mortality rate of about 50%.

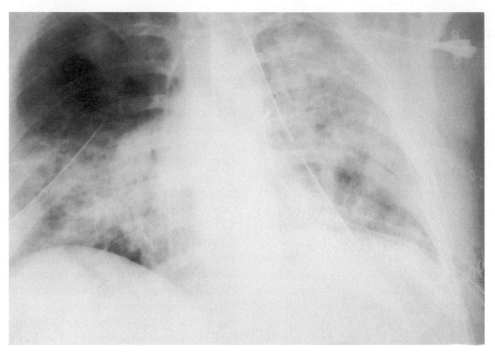

FIGURE 23-4 Chest radiograph of a 28-year-old man who was involved in an automobile accident. The patient presented with multiple bilateral rib fractures and bilateral pneumothorax. Within 24 hours, severe acute respiratory distress syndrome developed (note diffuse "whiteout").

- ARDS is a consequence of widespread pulmonary inflammation leading to three major pathophysiologic processes:
  1. Noncardiogenic pulmonary edema associated with "leaky" pulmonary capillaries.
  2. Atelectasis associated with lack of surfactant (surfactant normally decreases surface tension in small alveoli and prevents them from collapsing).
  3. Fibrosis (hyaline membranes) associated with inflammatory deposition of proteins.
- ARDS is associated with profound alterations in pulmonary function, including decreased vital capacity, decreased FRC, decreased compliance, and decreased tidal volume. Respiratory rate is increased, and symptoms of tissue hypoxia may be apparent.
- Noncardiogenic pulmonary edema is evident as "whiteout" on chest radiograph. Crackles and wheezing may be heard throughout the chest. Profound dyspnea and the use of accessory muscles are common. Atelectasis and pulmonary edema result in right-to-left pulmonary shunting. Blood gas determinations show hypercarbia and hypoxemia, which do not improve much with oxygen therapy.
- Therapy is mostly supportive, i.e., to enhance tissue oxygenation until the inflammatory process resolves. Mechanical ventilation with PEEP and supplemental oxygen is the mainstay of therapy. PEEP is used to increase FRC and prevent alveolar collapse at end-expiration. PEEP may also force edema fluid out of the alveoli. High levels of oxygen (>60%) may contribute to ARDS because of absorption atelectasis. F_{IO_2} should be reduced as soon as possible.

Infant Respiratory Distress Syndrome

Etiology. Infant respiratory distress syndrome, also known as *hyaline membrane disease*, has features similar to those of ARDS. It is a syndrome of premature neonates, characterized by hemorrhagic pulmonary edema, patchy atelectasis, and hyaline (glassy) membranes.[1] Hypoxemia that is refractory to increasing levels of oxygen supplementation is the hallmark of the syndrome. The incidence is 60% in infants born at less than 30 weeks who are not treated with corticosteroids and decreases to 35% for infants receiving antenatal steroids.[14] The incidence in infants older than 34 weeks is 5%.[14,15] High-risk factors include birth prior to 25 weeks gestation, birth at advanced gestational age, poorly controlled diabetes in the mother, deliveries after antepartum hemorrhage, cesarean section without antecedent labor, perinatal asphyxia, second twin, previous infant with RDS, and Rh factor incompatibility.[14]

Pathogenesis. The primary cause of IRDS is a lack of pulmonary surfactant, leading to increased alveolar surface tension and decreased lung compliance.[14] Surfactant, a phospholipid, is produced by type II alveolar cells in increasing quantities after 32 weeks gestation. With IRDS, lung compliance is decreased to one fifth to one tenth of normal.[1,14,15]

The neonate with IRDS must generate high intrathoracic pressures (25 to 30 mm Hg) to maintain patent alveoli. The premature neonate has a soft, compliant chest that is drawn inward with each inspiratory contraction of the diaphragm, making it difficult to maintain the high pressures needed to maintain adequate oxygenation. The end result from increased work of breathing and decreased ventilation is progressive atelectasis, increased pulmonary vascular resistance, profound hypoxemia, and acidosis.[1]

Surfactant also functions to maintain pulmonary fluid balance. Alteration of surface tension forces, normally maintained by surfactant, causes further leakage of proteinaceous fluid into the alveoli. This fluid contains fibrin and cellular debris, which causes hyaline membrane formation. Surfactant normally decreases surface tension in the alveolus during expiration, allowing the alveolus to remain partially open, thus maintaining FRC.[15]

A secondary cause of IRDS is immaturity of the capillary blood supply, which leads to $\dot{V}A/\dot{Q}$ mismatch, thus adding to the problems of hypoxemia and metabolic acidosis. In addition, a right-to-left shunt from an open foramen ovale or patent ductus arteriosus may increase the hypoxemia.[2]

Histologically, there is progressive damage to the basement membrane and respiratory epithelial cells. With increasing edema and loss of epithelial cells, patchy areas of atelectasis develop. Cellular damage from the disease process, excess fluid administration, and high levels of FIO$_2$ lead to increased capillary permeability and leakage of high-protein fluid into the alveoli.

Clinical Manifestations. The typical neonate presents with shallow respirations; intercostal, subcostal, or sternal retractions; diminished breath sounds; flaring of nares; hypotension; peripheral edema; low body temperature; oliguria; tachypnea (60 to 120 breaths/min); and bradycardia.[14,15] Late findings include frothy sputum, central cyanosis, and an expiratory grunting sound. Nasal flaring is a physiologic response mechanism used to increase airway diameter in an attempt to overcome airway resistance. An expiratory grunt is a physiologic response mechanism reflecting an attempt to create a physiologic PEEP by exhaling against a partially closed glottis. Paradoxical respirations ("seesaw" movement of the chest wall) may also be noted, indicating increased work of breathing.

During the first 48 to 72 hours of life, neonates with IRDS need progressively higher levels of FIO$_2$ to maintain adequate (60 to 80 mm Hg) oxygen levels.[14-16] As the work of breathing increases and oxygen levels decrease, metabolic acidosis occurs.[17]

Diagnosis. Initial arterial blood gas determinations reveal hypoxemia and metabolic acidosis due to lactic acid formation by hypoxic tissues. As the disease progresses, hypercapnia and respiratory acidosis develop. The chest radiographic appearance progresses from normal, shortly after birth, to a diffuse whiteout or ground glass indicative of diffuse bilateral atelectasis and alveolar edema. Generalized hypoinflation of the lungs is also seen on the chest study.

Measurement of the lecithin-sphingomyelin (L/S) ratio and desaturated phosphatidylcholine concentration in amniotic fluid may be done to determine the ability of the fetus to secrete surfactant. If the L/S ratio is ≥2:1 (3:1 in mothers with diabetes), the incidence of RDS is less than 5%.[18] The presence of phosphatidylglycerol in the amniotic fluid is indicative of pulmonary maturity.[18] Administration of glucocorticoids prior to delivery may stimulate lung maturation and improve the L/S ratio.

Treatment. The mainstay of therapy is mechanical ventilation with PEEP or continuous positive-airway pressure. Prevention is a primary goal. The therapeutic goal, as in the adult with ARDS, is to maintain adequate oxygen levels between 50 and 90 mm Hg.[1,2,16] The lowest FIO$_2$ settings should be used to maintain adequate arterial oxygen levels. High FIO$_2$ (100%) delivered for extended periods of time may result in further alveolar damage, primary persistent pulmonary hypertension, and retrolental fibroplasia (failure of the peripheral retina to vascularize, leading to blindness).[16]

Exogenous surfactant (bovine, porcine, or synthetic) administration to premature infants has decreased the mortality rate in IRDS by 50%.[17] Surfactant decreases surface tension, thereby reducing the amount of pressure required to open the alveoli. High-frequency ventilation has proved to be effective in infants with severe IRDS by providing more uniform lung inflation, improving lung mechanics and improving gas exchange. Infants ventilated with high-frequency ventilation require lower mean airway pressures and have better gas exchange than those ventilated conventionally.[17]

General supportive therapy of adequate intravenous nutrition, fluid and electrolyte balance, minimal handling, and a neutral thermal environment should be maintained. Broad-spectrum antibiotics are prescribed for infections after cultures have been done or prophylactically until blood cultures prove negative.[16]

KEY POINTS

- The symptoms of IRDS are very similar to those of ARDS. IRDS occurs most commonly in premature infants born prior to adequate development of their surfactant-producing pneumocytes (25 weeks gestation). Maturity of surfactant-producing cells can be estimated from the L/S ratio in amniotic fluid. An L/S ratio of less than 2:1 is associated with a higher risk of IRDS.
- Lack of surfactant causes atelectasis and increased work of breathing due to high alveolar surface tension. Leakage of inflammatory exudate into the alveoli results in formation of hyaline membranes.
- Symptoms of IRDS include nasal flaring, expiratory grunt, thoracic retractions, and rapid shallow respirations. Chest radiographs demonstrate a "whiteout." As in ARDS, blood gas values are poor, indicating severe hypoxemia and acidosis.
- Therapy for IRDS includes supportive measures, such as mechanical ventilation with PEEP or continuous positive airway pressure, and supplemental oxygen as well as specific measures to increase alveolar surfactant levels.

Pleural Space Disorders

Pneumothorax

Etiology. Pneumothorax is characterized by the accumulation of air in the pleural space. A primary pneumothorax is classified as spontaneous, occurring mainly in tall, thin men between ages 20 and 40 years without underlying disease factors.[1,2,19] Cigarette smoking increases the risk of spontaneous pneumothorax.[19] A secondary pneumothorax occurs as a result of complications from pre-existing pulmonary disease (such as asthma, emphysema, cystic fibrosis, infectious disease [pneumonia or tuberculosis], or interstitial lung disease). In the U.S., there are approximately 20,000 new cases annually. A specific category of secondary pneumothorax associated with menstruation is called *catamenial pneumothorax* (pathogenesis unknown). A catamenial pneumothorax occurs primarily in the right hemothorax, and is associated with endometriosis.[20] A third classification (tension pneumothorax) is traumatic in origin, resulting from penetrating or nonpenetrating injury. Other examples of traumatic pneumothorax have iatrogenic causes, such as placement of central lines, percutaneous lung biopsy, and mechanical ventilation.[2]

Pathogenesis. Primary spontaneous pneumothorax (Figure 23-5) results from rupture of small subpleural blebs in the apices.[1] When air enters the pleural space, the lung collapses and the rib cage springs out.[1] The subpleural blebs are believed to occur in the apices as a result of negative mechanical pressures

in the upper third of the upright lung field. Secondary pneumothorax occurs as a result of complications from an underlying lung problem and may be due to rupture of a cyst or bleb.[1,2] Tension pneumothorax (see Figure 23-5) results from the buildup of air under pressure in the pleural space. Air enters the pleural space during inspiration but cannot escape during expiration.[1] The lung on the ipsilateral (same) side collapses and forces the mediastinum toward the contralateral (opposite) side, thus decreasing venous return and cardiac output (see Figure 23-5). With an open, "sucking" chest wall wound, air enters during inspiration but cannot escape during expiration, leading to shift of the mediastinum (contents of the septum between the two lungs) and trachea.

Clinical Manifestations. The clinical features of pneumothorax include tachycardia, decreased or absent breath sounds on the affected side, hyperresonance, sudden chest pain on the affected side (90%), and dyspnea (80%).[19] Small pneumothoraces (less than 20%) are usually not detectable on physical examination.[20] Tension pneumothorax and a large spontaneous pneumothorax are emergency situations, with patients presenting with severe tachycardia, hypotension, a tracheal

SPONTANEOUS PNEUMOTHORAX

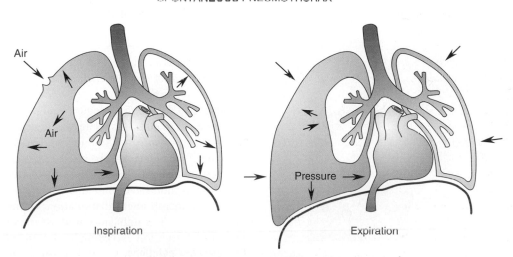

Inspiration   Expiration

TENSION PNEUMOTHORAX

FIGURE 23-5 *Top,* Spontaneous pneumothorax. *Bottom,* Tension pneumothorax: air builds up under pressure, leading to collapse of the ipsilateral lung and shift of the mediastinum to the contralateral side.

shift to the contralateral side, neck vein distention, hyperresonance, and subcutaneous emphysema. Figure 23-6 shows severe subcutaneous emphysema (air in the tissues due to tracheobronchial rupture).

Diagnosis. Arterial blood gas analysis shows a decreased Pao_2 and acute respiratory alkalosis. The chest radiograph shows depression of the hemidiaphragm on the side of the pneumothorax and a pleural line with absence of vessel markings peripheral to this line.[2,19,20] Chest radiography should be done with the patient standing. Expiratory films show a better demarcation of the pleural line than inspiratory films. The diagnosis may be based on clinical features without radiographic confirmation. However, a chest radiograph is usually obtained. A chest radiograph in tension pneumothorax shows a mediastinal shift (Figure 23-7). The electrocardiogram may show axis deviations, nonspecific ST-segment changes, and T-wave inversion.[21]

Treatment. The management of pneumothorax depends on the severity of the problem and the cause of the air leak. If the lung collapse is less than 15% to 25%, the patient may or may not be hospitalized. Typically, the patient is treated symptomatically.[2,20] A nonhospitalized patient should be monitored closely.[21,22] The expectation is for complete resolution within several weeks. If the collapse is greater than 15% to 25%, chest tube placement with water seal and suction is recommended.[1,2,19-22]

Chemical pleurodesis may be indicated for patients with recurrent spontaneous pneumothorax to promote adhesion

FIGURE 23-6 Subcutaneous emphysema (air in the tissues) from tracheobronchial disruption and injuries of the esophagus. (From Kirsh MM, Sloan H: *Blunt chest trauma: general principles and management,* Boston, 1977, Little, Brown, p 109.)

of the visceral pleura to the parietal pleura to prevent further ruptures.[1,2,21,22] Patients with a previous pneumothorax should be warned about exposure to high altitude, scuba diving, and smoking. A thoracotomy may be performed in patients in whom further spontaneous pneumothorax and blebs develop. Surgery permits stapling or laser pleurodesis of ruptured blebs.[1,2,22]

Pleural Effusion

Etiology. Pleural effusion is not a disease, but rather a pathologic collection of fluid or pus in the pleural cavity as a result of another disease process. Normally, 5 to 15 ml of serous fluid is contained in the pleural space.[2] There is a constant movement of pleural fluid from parietal pleural capillaries to the pleural space, which is then reabsorbed into the parietal pleural lymphatics. The pleural membrane is a porous mesenchymal serous membrane that allows for movement of interstitial fluid. The fluid has a mucoid characteristic allowing for easy movement of the lungs.[23] The five major types of pleural effusion are (1) transudates, (2) exudates, (3) empyema due to infection in the pleural space, (4) hemothorax or hemorrhagic pleural effusions, and (5) chylothorax or lymphatic pleural effusions.[2] Transudates are low in protein (ratio of pleural fluid protein to serum protein is less than 0.5), low in lactate dehydrogenase (LDH; pleural fluid LDH/serum ratio less than 0.6), and have a specific gravity below 1.016.[24,25] Transudates are frequently associated with severe heart failure or other edematous states, such as cirrhosis with ascites, nephrotic syndrome, and myxedema.[2] Exudates are high in protein (>0.5 mg/dl) and high in LDH (pleural fluid LDH/serum ratio >0.6).[22,24-26] Common causes of exudates are malignancies, infections (especially pneumonia), pulmonary embolism, sarcoidosis, post–myocardial infarction syndrome, and pancreatic disease. Empyema is a high-protein exudative effusion resulting from infection in the pleural space. Hemothorax (the presence of blood in the pleural space) is often the result of chest trauma. Hemorrhagic pleural effusion contains a mixture of blood and pleural fluid. If the hematocrit of the fluid is greater than 50% of the hematocrit of peripheral blood, the fluid collection is called a *hemothorax.*[1,2] Chylothorax or chylous pleural effusion is an exudative process that develops from trauma as a result of leakage of chyle (lymph fluid) from the thoracic duct or from rheumatoid pleural effusion or tuberculous pleuritis.[1,2]

Pathogenesis. Pathophysiologic changes associated with the various types of effusions relate to changes in pleural capillary hydrostatic pressure, colloid oncotic pressure, or intrapleural pressure. Transudates can be caused by increased hydrostatic or decreased oncotic pressure. Exudates are associated with increased production of fluid due to increased permeability of the pleural membrane (inflammation) or impaired lymphatic drainage.[2,24,25] The imbalance in these pressures is associated with fluid formation exceeding fluid removal.

Clinical Manifestations. Clinical features vary depending on the cause and size of the effusion. Small effusions may be asymptomatic (which is common) in patients with less than 300 ml of fluid in the pleural cavity.[22,24] General features

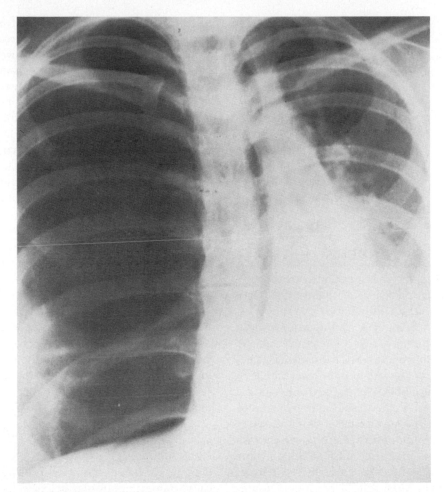

FIGURE 23-7 Upright posteroanterior chest radiograph showing a right-sided tension pneumothorax. Note marked deviation of trachea and cardiac silhouette into the left side of the chest. There is also depression of the right hemidiaphragm. (From Kirsh MM, Sloan H: *Blunt chest trauma: general principles and management,* Boston, 1977, Little, Brown, p 62.)

include dyspnea, pleuritic pain that is sharp and worsens with inspiration, dry cough, decreased chest wall movement, absence of breath sounds, dullness to percussion, and decreased tactile fremitus over the affected area.[22-26] A massive pleural effusion may lead to a contralateral tracheal shift.[22]

Diagnosis. Thoracentesis should be done to analyze the fluid and to reduce the amount of fluid in the pleural cavity. Evaluation of the pleural fluid is done to determine the characteristics of the fluid, as an additional indicator of origin. Pleural fluid should be analyzed for chemistry (pH, LDH, and glucose) and presence of pathogenic bacteria. Chest radiography should be done to detect pleural-based densities, infiltrates, signs of CHF, hilar adenopathy, and loculation of fluid. Computed tomography and ultrasonographic tests assist in complicated effusions and distinguish a mass from a large effusion.[22,24-26] Ultrasonography is also useful for thoracentesis guidance.

Treatment. Treatment is directed at the underlying cause of the effusion and relief of symptoms. Closed chest tube drainage in adults or thoracentesis is indicated if the effusion is large. Closed chest drainage in pediatric cases is controversial.[25]

A thoracotomy to control bleeding may be required in patients with excessive bleeding (greater than 200 ml/hr).[27]

KEY POINTS

- The pleural space is usually a potential space, containing only a small amount of fluid for lubrication. Accumulations of air (pneumothorax), pus (empyema), blood (hemothorax), lymph (chylothorax), or transudate in the pleural space can restrict lung expansion.
- Tension pneumothorax occurs when pleural air progressively accumulates and develops a positive pressure in the pleura. The ipsilateral (same side) lung collapses, and mediastinal structures (trachea, heart) are shifted to the opposite side. Breath sounds are diminished or absent on the affected side.
- Tension pneumothorax and a large, simple (spontaneous) pneumothorax are medical emergencies requiring treatment to remove pleural air and re-expand the lung. This usually requires insertion of a chest tube. Chemical

- pleurodesis may be done in persons prone to spontaneous pneumothorax.
- A number of disease processes may result in accumulation of fluid in the pleural space. Analysis of the type of fluid (e.g., transudate, exudates, blood, pus) indicates the underlying disease process. General manifestations include dyspnea, cough, pleuritic pain, and, over the effusion, diminished breath sounds and dullness to percussion.

Neuromuscular, Chest Wall, and Obesity Disorders

NEUROMUSCULAR DISORDERS

Diseases affecting the muscles of respiration or their nerve supply can lead to dyspnea and respiratory failure. Table 23-6 summarizes the features of these disorders.

Poliomyelitis. Poliomyelitis is a viral disease in which the poliovirus attacks motor nerve cells of the spinal cord and brainstem. The incidence of poliomyelitis in the United States is approximately 8 cases per year. All of these cases have been related to the oral polio vaccine (OPV).[28] The diaphragm and intercostal muscles can be affected, resulting in weakness or paralysis and respiratory failure. At least 95% of infections are asymptomatic.[28] Patients with minor symptoms present with fever, headache, vomiting, diarrhea, constipation, and sore throat.[29] Respiratory muscle function generally recovers, although occasionally patients have chronic respiratory insufficiency from previous disease. As the result of mass vaccination of the population, new cases are quite rare and usually occur in unvaccinated immigrants.[28]

Amyotrophic Lateral Sclerosis. Amyotrophic lateral sclerosis (ALS) is a degenerative disease of the nervous system that involves both upper and lower motor neurons. ALS occurs in males more than females (2:1) and has a prevalence of 5 in 100,000 persons. Commonly, muscles innervated by both spinal nerves and cranial nerves are affected. Clinically, progressive muscle weakness and wasting develop, eventually leading to profound weakness of respiratory muscles and death. Although the course of the disease is variable from patient to patient, the natural history is one of irreversibility and progressive deterioration.[2,30] (see Chapter 45).

Muscular Dystrophies. Duchenne muscular dystrophy is a hereditary disease, passed from mothers to sons (X-linked recessive) and occurs in 1/3500 male births. The disease is characterized by progressive muscular weakness, initially in the lower extremities, and wasting. In later years (twenties to thirties), respiratory muscles become involved, leading to hypoxia, hypercapnia, and frequent respiratory infections (see Chapter 51).[2]

Guillain-Barré Syndrome. Guillain-Barré syndrome, also called *acute polyneuritis,* is a disorder that is presumed to have an immunologic basis. Infection involving *Campylobacter jejuni* often precedes the diagnosis. Guillain-Barré syndrome is characterized by demyelination of peripheral nerves. Frequently, patients have a history of recent viral or bacterial illness (66% of cases) followed by development of ascending paralysis. Clinically, weakness and paralysis begin symmetrically in the lower extremities and progress or ascend proximally to the upper extremities and trunk. In severe cases, respiratory muscle weakness accompanies limb and trunk symptoms. Generally, the natural history of the disease leads to recovery, with minor residual motor deficits occurring in 15% to 20% of patients. Mortality is about 3% (see Chapter 45).[31]

Myasthenia Gravis. Patients with myasthenia gravis experience weakness and fatigue of voluntary muscles, most frequently those innervated by cranial nerves, but peripheral and respiratory muscles can also be affected. The hallmark of the disorder is weakness made worse by exercise and improved by rest. The incidence in the U.S. is 2 to 5 cases/year/million persons. The primary abnormality is found at the neuromuscular junction, where transmission of impulses from nerve to muscle is impaired by a decreased number of receptors on the muscle. Although myasthenia gravis is a chronic illness, the manifestations can often be managed by appropriate therapy, and individual episodes of respiratory failure are potentially reversible.[2] Respiratory failure in this disorder can be due to increasing severity of illness or overmedication (see Chapter 51).

CHEST WALL DEFORMITIES

Kyphoscoliosis

Etiology. Kyphoscoliosis may develop from an unknown cause (idiopathic) or may be related to congenital (Pott disease) or neuromuscular disease (muscular dystrophy, Marfan syndrome, neurofibromatosis, Friedreich ataxia, or poliomyelitis).[32] Most idiopathic cases of scoliosis are found in adolescents (11 years or older). The female-to-male ratio is 7:1.[33]

Pathogenesis. Commonly, a bony deformity of the chest wall occurs as a result of kyphosis (hunchback appearance; posterior curvature deformity) and scoliosis (lateral curvature deformity) (Figure 23-8). The higher the deformity in the vertebral column, the greater the compromise of respiratory status. Lung volumes are compressed, leading to atelectasis, $\dot{V}_A/\dot{Q}$ mismatch, and hypoxemia.[2]

Clinical Manifestations. Common clinical features include dyspnea on exertion; rapid, shallow breathing; and chest wall deformity as evidenced by ribs protruding backward, flaring on the convex side, and being crowded on the concave side. Hypoxemia develops later, and eventually carbon dioxide retention occurs.[1]

Diagnosis. Diagnostic findings include hypercapnia, hypoxemia (due to $\dot{V}_A/\dot{Q}$ mismatch), and decreased lung volumes and lung capacities as evidenced by decreased values on pulmonary function tests. Also noted are increased pulmonary arterial pressures because of the associated pulmonary hypoxemia. Radiographs show accentuated bony curves.[1,32,33] Screening for scoliosis and kyphoscoliosis in school-aged children has proved to be an excellent method of early diagnosis of these conditions.

Clinical Manifes
paradoxical mo
eral. The injury
tion and palpat
of breath, pain
poxemia. Arteri
appear.[35] Pneu
physema are co

Diagnosis and
termine the tre
segments, result
mechanical ven
by positive pres
the flail section,
Pain manageme
dural anesthesia

Disorders of C
Etiology. *Obesity*
mass index (BM
and height. Over
Obesity results f
caloric expenditi
survey reported
overweight. The
25.1% of women
in blacks than in
than in those wi
risk for a variety
diabetes mellitus
disease, gallstone
men; uterus, bili
pulmonary impa
more have an all
of those with a B
Pathogenesis. En
thyroidism, the
lesions all can lea
of obesity is exce
Several hormone
and metabolism.
release of neurop
metabolic rate. G
such as familial pa
Laurence-Moon
Cohen syndrome

Obesity may
mechanisms of o
tory drive and inc
thought to have a
tem.[1] In addition,
thoracic contents
ing lung expansio
hypoventilation is
obese boy in Cha
syndrome is asso
obstruction.[1]

TABLE 23-6

Neuromuscular Disorders Affecting the Respiratory System

Disease	Etiology	Pathophysiology	Clinical Features
Poliomyelitis (myelitis is inflammation of the spinal cord)	Develops from an enteral virus acquired by ingestion or respiratory droplet	After a 1- to 3-week period, the virus invades the intestinal blood supply; once in the circulation the virus invades all areas of the body; invasion of the central nervous system leads to neural damage and initiation of an inflammatory reaction	General symptoms are tremors, muscle weakness; bulbar poliomyelitis affects the respiratory muscle nerves, leading to respiratory paralysis; patients usually exhibit shoulder girdle paralysis first, followed by intercostal and diaphragm muscle paralysis; paralysis may be rapid or slowly progressive; also seen are diplopia, facial weakness, dysphagia, difficulty chewing, nasal voice, and loss of gag reflex
Amyotrophic lateral sclerosis	Cause unknown; current theories include autoimmune disease and a slow virus	Affects the anterior horn cells of both upper and lower motor neurons	Progressive weakness affecting distal more than proximal muscles; atrophy, fasciculations, and spasticity are noted; involvement of the respiratory muscles leads to respiratory dysfunction requiring mechanical ventilation
Muscular dystrophies (most common is Duchenne type)	Hereditary disease (X-linked recessive) passed from mothers to sons	Progressive muscular weakness noted initially in lower extremity muscles; in later years (twenties and thirties) respiratory muscles become involved; patients are at risk for respiratory infections	Progressive muscular weakness and wasting; skeletal deformities are also common; involvement of the respiratory muscles (diaphragm, intercostals, and accessory muscles) leads to hypoxia and hypercapnia
Guillain-Barré syndrome (acute idiopathic polyneuropathy)	Exact cause unknown, but thought to be an auto-immune disease triggered by a viral infection	The disease usually follows an infection or vaccination, peripheral nerves are affected, leading to neural inflammation, demyelination, and axon destruction	Progressive weakness and loss of motor function beginning in the feet and legs and ascending upward; sensory loss may also be noted but is not as dramatic as motor loss; loss of respiratory muscle control leads to respiratory failure, which frequently requires mechanical ventilation; autonomic nervous system symptoms may also be noted (tachycardia, arrhythmias, hypotension or hypertension, loss of ability to sweat)
Myasthenia gravis	Considered an autoimmune disease with both humoral (B cell) and cell-mediated (T cell) components	Autoantibodies and T cells bind to and damage acetylcholine receptors, leading to decreased functioning of receptors	Common symptoms are diplopia, ptosis, difficulty swallowing, increased weakness with activity, nasal voice, slurred speech, and weakness of proximal extremities; as the disease progresses, respiratory muscles become involved, leading to respiratory failure; pneumonia may result from respiratory failure and immobility

FIGURE 23-8
Major's physical

Treatment. Tre
ty and the age
cially women,
less than 20 de
A postural ex
braces for moc
vanced cases v
cal stimulation
spinal instrum
cal stabilizatio
greater than 60
tion in later lif

Ankylosing S

Etiology. Anky
female ratio 10
decade of life.[1]
at the site of l
iliac joints. Th
patients with
(Chapter 10).[3]
chest expansion
the upper lobe
cavitation.[34] Tr
occurs in abou

Pathogenesis. /
matory disease
and fixation of
articular proce:
by inducing a
ligament ossifi

Clinical Manifes
back pain and
rest. With exer
ease process ad
leading to restr

Chest wall n
ther restriction

Infection or Inflammation of the Lung

Pneumonia

Etiology. The term *pneumonia* (from the Greek *pneuma*, "breath") refers to an inflammatory reaction in the alveoli and interstitium of the lung, usually caused by an infectious agent. Pneumonia can result from three different sources: (1) aspiration of oropharyngeal secretions composed of normal bacterial flora and/or gastric contents (25% to 35% of all pneumonias); (2) inhalation of contaminants (virus, *Mycoplasma*); or (3) contamination from the systemic circulation.[2,40-42]

There are several ways to classify pneumonia. Pneumonias are typically classified as community acquired or hospital acquired. They are further classified as bacterial, atypical, and viral. The bacterial pneumonias may be grouped as either gram positive or gram negative, based on the staining characteristics of the organism. *Staphylococcus* and *Streptococcus* (including pneumococci) are the predominant gram-positive organisms. Gram-negative bacteria that may cause pneumonia include *Haemophilus influenzae*, *Klebsiella* species, *Pseudomonas aeruginosa*, *Serratia marcescens*, *Escherichia coli*, and *Proteus* species.

Anaerobic bacteria may present clinically as a lung abscess, necrotizing pneumonia, or empyema. These diseases are usually caused by aspiration of normal oral bacteria (such as *Bacteroides* and *Fusobacterium*) into the lung.[2] Mycoplasmal pneumonia is more commonly seen in the summer and fall in young adults. Other causes of pneumonia occur less frequently in the general population. Legionnaires disease, for example, is a severe systemic illness characterized by fever, diarrhea, abdominal pain, liver and kidney failure, and pulmonary infiltrates. The organism lives in water and is transmitted by means of potable water, condensers, and cooling towers.[2] The current treatment of choice is a macrolide antibiotic.

Patients whose immune systems have been compromised by disease or by drug therapy may be susceptible to the development of opportunistic pneumonia. For example, *Pneumocystis (carinii) jiroveci* pneumonia, an opportunistic infection, is commonly found in patients with cancer or with human immunodeficiency virus (HIV). (See Chapter 12 for further discussion of acquired immunodeficiency syndrome [AIDS].)

Aspergillus, an opportunistic fungus that is widespread in nature, may cause progressive pneumonia. *Aspergillus* is released from walls of old buildings under reconstruction. Attention should be given to the renovation of old hospitals and avoiding placement of susceptible patients in a reconstruction area.[42]

To assist the reader in differentiating among the various types of pneumonia, Table 23-7 presents the etiologic factors, common clinical features with age-related characteristics, radiologic findings, and antibiotic therapies for 11 forms of the disease.[2] There are many other types of pneumonia that are not listed.

Pathogenesis. Normally, pulmonary defense mechanisms (immune responses, cough reflex, sneezing, mucociliary clearance) protect individuals from pneumonia. Community-acquired pneumonia occurs when defense mechanisms are compromised.[2,40] A highly virulent organism may also overwhelm a person's defense mechanisms. Community-acquired pneumonias are commonly bacterial in origin.[40] After microbial agents enter the lung, they multiply and trigger pulmonary inflammation. Alveolar air spaces fill with an exudative fluid, and inflammatory cells invade the alveolar septa. Acute bacterial pneumonia may be associated with significant $\dot{V}_A/\dot{Q}$ mismatching and hypoxemia because inflammatory exudate collects in the alveolar spaces. Alveolar exudate tends to consolidate and becomes difficult to expectorate. Viral pneumonia does not produce exudative fluids.[2] Figure 23-9 shows the histologic progression of acute bacterial pneumonia. Patients with chronic illnesses and those who are immobile or immunosuppressed or have decreased level of consciousness are at highest risk for developing pneumonia.[21] Disruption of the body's normal defense mechanisms leads to increased risk of pneumonia. Other patients at risk are those who have undergone thoracic or abdominal surgery or anesthesia.

Clinical Manifestations. Clinically, the pathogenic cause, severity of the disease, and age of the patient may cause variations in the presentation of pneumonia. Some patients present with fever only.[25] Crackles (rales) and bronchial breath sounds may be heard over the affected lung tissue. Patients may present with chills, cough, purulent sputum, and an abnormal chest radiograph. Patients with viral pneumonia may present with an upper respiratory prodrome (fever, coryza, cough, hoarseness) accompanied by wheezing and/or rales.[21] Typical features of *Chlamydia* pneumonia are cough, tachypnea, rales, wheezes, and no fever. *Mycoplasma* pneumonia is a common cause of pneumonia in older children and adults.[21] Signs and symptoms include fever, cough, headache, and malaise.

Diagnosis. The chest radiograph demonstrates parenchymal infiltrates (white shadows) in the involved area, indicative of inflammatory alveolar processes.[2,21,41] In a patient with symptoms and clinical findings of pneumonia, a Gram stain of expectorated sputum from deep in the lungs may be obtained to distinguish bacterial from viral pneumonia and gram-negative from gram-positive organisms. If the patient had been previously healthy, the cause of the majority of these infections would either be viral, mycoplasmal, or the gram-positive pneumococcal bacterium. However, if the patient had been hospitalized or has other illnesses such as emphysema, diabetes, or alcoholism, then gram-negative organisms should be suspected. Because 24 to 48 hours may be required for culture of the etiologic agent, antibiotic therapy should be started empirically.[2] Once culture and sensitivity results are obtained, antibiotic therapy may be changed. Diagnosis is based on the chest radiograph, white blood cell count (greater than 15,000/µl for acute bacterial pneumonia[21]), and sputum culture, coupled with clinical features of fever with recurrent chills, cough, dyspnea, and rales.

Treatment. Once the organism has been cultured, specific antibiotic selection is based on sensitivity of the organism to different antibiotics. Table 23-7 presents treatment options.

TABLE 23-7

Differentiating Features of Types of Pneumonia

Etiologic Organism	Common Clinical Features	Chest Radiograph	Antibiotic Treatment
Staphylococcus aureus; Gram-positive cocci in clumps	Follows upper respiratory infection; fever, chills, pleuritic chest pain, cough, yellow purulent sputum; seen in patients in chronic care facilities	Consolidation, may have cavitation	Methicillin-susceptible strains: nafcillin or oxacillin with or without rifampin; methicillin-resistant strains: vancomycin with or without rifampin; alternative choice: cephalosporins, clindamycin, vancomycin
Streptococcus pneumoniae (pneumococcus); gram-positive diplococci	More common in alcoholics, also seen with chronic cardio-pulmonary disease; fever, chills, pleuritic chest pain, cough, rust-colored sputum	Patchy infiltrates	Procaine penicillin G or aqueous penicillin G, amoxicillin; alternative choice: macrolides, cephalosporins, doxycycline, quinolones; prophylactic vaccine available
Haemophilus influenzae; pleomorphic gram-negative coccobacilli	Upper respiratory symptoms, fever, vomiting, irritability, cough, purulent sputum, dyspnea; affects children and older adults, affects people with chronic cardiorespiratory problems	Consolidation	Cefotaxime, ceftriaxone, doxycycline, azithromycin, TMP-SMX; alternative choice: quinolones or clarithromycin
Klebsiella pneumoniae; gram-negative encapsulated rods	Seen frequently in middle-aged men and associated with alcoholism and diabetes mellitus; rust-colored sputum	Consolidation	Aminoglycoside plus third-generation cephalosporin; alternative: aztreonam, imipenem, quinolone
Pseudomonas aeruginosa; gram-negative rods	Chronic obstructive pulmonary disease, cystic fibrosis, and mechanical ventilation; fever, chills, and copious greenish, foul-smelling sputum	Infiltrates, small pleural effusion	Aminoglycoside plus ticarcillin/clavulanate or piperacillin/tazobactam or aztreonam or imipenem
Escherichia coli; gram-negative rods	Complication of gastrointestinal surgery	Infiltrates, may have pleural effusion	Aminoglycoside plus third-generation cephalosporin; alternative: aztreonam, imipenem, quinolone
Virus	Fever, malaise, headache, nonproductive cough	Patchy infiltrates	Amantadine, rimantadine
Legionella species; no bacteria	Acute onset with fever, diarrhea, myalgia, and abdominal pain	Consolidation	Macrolides with or without rifampin; alternative: TMP-SMX, quinolone
Mycoplasma pneumoniae (atypical pneumonia) monocytes and neutrophils; no bacteria	Ages 5 to 25 years; most common in young adults; associated with otitis media and myringitis; sore throat, headache, myalgia, dry cough, fatigue, low-grade fever	Infiltrates	Erythromycin, doxycycline; alternative: quinolone or other macrolide
Pneumocystis (carinii) jiroveci (fungus)	Immunosuppressed patients (infants, children, and adults); 60% of patients have AIDS	Diffuse infiltrates, or chest x-ray may appear normal	TMP-SMX or pentamidine; isethionate plus prednisone; alternative: dapsone plus TMP-SMX, clindamycin plus primaquine
Anaerobic pneumonia (aspiration pneumonia), mixed flora	Predisposition to aspiration, fever, weight loss, malaise; risk increases with decreased level of consciousness, artificial airway, and sedation; seen in individuals with poor dental hygiene	Infiltrates in dependent lung fields	Penicillin G; alternative choices: clindamycin, metronidazole, cefoxitin

TMP-SMX, Trimethoprim-sulfamethoxazole; *AIDS*, acquired immunodeficiency syndrome.

and process the microorganisms. The organisms either are destroyed or persist and multiply. Once the infection becomes established, lymphatic and hematogenous dissemination occur. T cells and macrophages surround the organisms in granulomas that limit multiplication and spread.[46] Dormant organisms persist for years. Reactivation may occur if the patient's immune system becomes impaired.[2,46]

The pathologic manifestation of pulmonary tuberculosis is the Ghon tubercle or complex, which has parenchymal and lymph components. The parenchymal component is composed of a well-circumscribed necrotic nodule that later becomes fibrotic and calcified. The lymph component is found in the lymph nodes. Primary pulmonary tuberculosis is shown in Figure 23-10.

Clinical Manifestations. Clinical features of reactivated disease include a history of contact with an infected person, low-grade fever, cough, night sweats, fatigue, weight loss, malaise, and anorexia. Chronic cough is the most common symptom.[2,46] As the disease progresses, the patient develops a productive cough with purulent sputum. Physical examination of the lung fields reveals apical crackles (rales) (*M. tuberculosis* organisms prefer lung apices due to the higher concentration of oxygen in the apices) or bronchial breath sounds over the region of lung consolidation. The patient appears malnourished and chronically ill.[2] Common sites of extrapulmonary tuberculosis are peritoneum, gastrointestinal tract, liver, spleen, bone, joints, lymph nodes, central nervous system, and genitourinary system.[46] (Refer to Chapter 12 for a discussion of

FIGURE 23-10 The morphologic spectrum of tuberculosis. A characteristic tubercle at low magnification **(A)** and in detail **(B)** illustrates central granular caseation surrounded by epithelioid and multinucleated giant cells. This is the usual response seen in patients who have developed cell-mediated immunity to the organism. Occasionally, even in immunocompetent individuals, tubercular granulomas may not show central caseation **(C)**; hence, irrespective of the presence or absence of caseous necrosis, special stains for acid-fast organisms need to be performed when granulomas are present in histologic sections. In immunosuppressed individuals, tuberculosis may not elicit a granulomatous response ("nonreactive tuberculosis"); instead, sheets of foamy histiocytes are seen, packed with mycobacteria that are demonstrable with acid-fast stains **(D)**. (From Kumar V et al: *Robbin's basic pathology,* ed 8, Philadelphia, 2007, Saunders, p 519. **D,** Courtesy Dr. Dominick Cavuoti, Department of Pathology, University of Texas Southwestern Medical School, Dallas.)

tuberculosis in HIV-infected patients.) Pulmonary function tests are characteristic of restrictive diseases, with decreased lung volumes and decreased compliance.

Diagnosis. Definitive diagnosis is made by results of sputum culture or identification of the organism by DNA or RNA amplification techniques.[46] Three consecutive morning sputum specimens are obtained to identify the slow-growing acid-fast bacillus. Expectoration of sputum in the early morning is ideal because the sputum is more concentrated and more plentiful. Cultures require 1 to 3 weeks for determination.[46] Gastric washings or bronchial washings may also be used for diagnostic culturing.

Chest radiographs usually show nodules with infiltrates in the lung apex and posterior segments of the upper lobes. Elderly patients may present with lower lobe infiltrates with or without pleural effusion. Figure 23-11 shows the radiographic appearance of cavitary tuberculosis in a 23-year-old man. A miliary pattern (diffuse small nodular densities) is seen with dissemination of the organism in miliary tuberculosis.[2]

Another diagnostic test is the tuberculin (Mantoux test) skin test (5 tuberculin units/0.1 ml of purified protein derivative injected intradermally). This test does not distinguish between current disease and past infection. If the induration in a person with HIV infection is 5 mm or greater, if the patient has close contact with individuals with tuberculosis, and if the patient has a chest radiograph consistent with tuberculosis, the likelihood of active disease is high.[1] An induration of 10 mm or greater is the reaction size for other high-risk individuals, such as intravenous drug abusers, individuals who are debilitated, children younger than 4 years or with immunosuppression, and individuals living in countries with a high incidence of the disease

(Asia, Africa, Latin America). An induration of 15 mm or greater is considered positive for tuberculosis in all other persons.[2,46]

False-positive results may occur in persons with other mycobacterial infections or if they have received bacille Calmette-Guérin, a live attenuated strain of *Mycobacterium bovis* that provides active immunity against tuberculosis. False-negative results may also occur in patients who are malnourished, elderly, or immunocompromised.[2] Immunocompromised patients may not be able to mount a response (wheal) to injection of the organism.

Treatment. Primary therapy for active tuberculosis consists of (1) administering multiple drugs to which the organism is susceptible; (2) adding at least two new agents to the drug regimen when treatment failure is suspected; (3) providing the safest, most effective therapy for the shortest period of time; and (4) ensuring adherence to therapy by utilizing directly observed therapy.[2] Nonadherence to therapy due to adverse drug reactions is a major cause of treatment failure. HIV-negative individuals without MDR-TB are typically treated for 6 to 9 months.

KEY POINTS

- Tuberculosis is caused by inhalation or ingestion of the bacterium *Mycobacterium tuberculosis*. The organism spreads through the lymph and blood. Bacteria are ingested by macrophages and walled off by inflammatory proteins (granulomas). The organisms may not be killed and can persist in a dormant state for years. These walled-off areas of inflammatory cells and bacteria become fibrotic and calcified, forming Ghon tubercles—the hallmark of tuberculosis.
- Symptoms are somewhat nonspecific: low-grade fever, cough, night sweats, fatigue, and weight loss. With progression of the disease, the cough is productive of purulent sputum.
- The diagnosis is based on a positive purified protein derivative skin test for tuberculosis, positive sputum cultures, and characteristic nodules on chest radiographs.
- Antibiotics are used for managing tuberculosis. Drug therapy continues for 9 to 12 months for active disease and may be used for shorter periods in persons exposed to tuberculosis but having no active disease.

FIGURE 23-11 Cavitary pulmonary tuberculosis in a 23-year-old man. (From Kersten LD: *Comprehensive Respiratory Nursing*, Philadelphia, 1989, Saunders, p 146.)

SUMMARY

Restrictive pulmonary disorders are those in which lung expansion is restricted. Restrictions are commonly caused by diseases that affect the lung parenchyma (e.g., diffuse interstitial pulmonary fibrosis), chest wall disorders, neuromuscular disorders, pleural space disorders, pneumonia, and tuberculosis. These diseases are characterized by a reduced vital capacity and a small residual lung volume. They differ from obstructive diseases, covered in Chapter 22, in that airway resistance is not increased.

REFERENCES

1. West JB: *Pulmonary pathophysiology: the essentials*, ed 7, Philadelphia, 2008, Lippincott Williams & Wilkins.
2. Chesnutt MS, Prendergart TJ: Lung. In Tierney LM, McPhee SI, Papadakis MA, editors: *Current medical diagnosis and treatment*, ed 46, New York, 2007, Lange/McGraw-Hill, pp 222-315.
3. Ferri FF: Diffuse interstitial lung disease. In Ferri FF, editor: *Ferri's clinical advisor: instant diagnosis and treatment*, St Louis, 2007, Mosby, p 264.
4. Yusen RD, Mayse ML, Chakinala M, et al: Pulmonary diseases. In Cooper DH et al, editors: *The Washington manual of medical therapeutics*, ed 32, Philadelphia, 2007, Lippincott Williams & Wilkins, pp 245-289.
5. Goroll AH, Mulley AG: Management of sarcoidosis: evaluation of interstitial lung disease. In Goroll AH, Mulley AG, editors: *Primary care medicine: office evaluation and management of the adult patient*, ed 5, Philadelphia, 2006, Lippincott Williams & Wilkins, pp 384-387.
6. Schwartz MJ, King TE, Cherniack RM: Infiltrative and interstitial lung diseases. In Mason RJ, Broaddus VC, Murray JF et al: *Textbook of respiratory medicine*, ed 4, Philadelphia, 2004, Saunders, pp 1571-1734.
7. Ferri FF: Sarcoidosis. In Ferri FF, editor: *Ferri's clinical advisor: instant diagnosis and treatment*, St Louis, 2007, Mosby, pp 799-800.
8. Zacharisen, MC: Hypersensitivity pneumonitis. In Rakel RE, Bope ET, editors: *Conn's current therapy*, Philadelphia, 2008, Elsevier, pp 276-278.
9. Thurlbeck WM, Miller RR: The respiratory system. In Rubin E, Farber JL, editors: *Essential pathology*, ed 3, Philadelphia, 2001, Lippincott Williams & Wilkins, pp 542-627.
10. O'Conner CJ: Hypersensitivity pneumonitis. In Ferri FF, editor: *Ferri's clinical advisor: instant diagnosis and treatment*, St Louis, 2007, Mosby, pp 441-442.
11. Oliver LC, Stoeckle JD: Evaluation and prevention of occupational and environmental respiratory disease. In Goroll AH, Mulley AG, editors: *Primary care medicine: office evaluation and management of the adult patient*, ed 5, Philadelphia, 2006, Lippincott Williams & Wilkins, pp 309-314.
12. West JB: *Pulmonary physiology and pathophysiology: an integrated, case-based approach*, ed 2, Philadelphia, 2007, Lippincott Williams & Wilkins.
13. Ferri FF: Acute respiratory distress syndrome. In Ferri FF, editor: *Ferri's clinical advisor: instant diagnosis and treatment*, St Louis, 2007, Mosby, pp 30-31.
14. Irvine LA: Neonatology. In Gunn VL, Nochyba C, editor: *The Harriet Lane handbook*, ed 17, Philadelphia, 2005, Mosby.
15. Carpenter TC, Dobyns EL, Grayck EN et al: Critical care. In Hay WW et al, editors. *Current pediatrics: diagnosis and treatment*, ed 18, New York, 2007, Lange/McGraw-Hill, pp 368-372.
16. Neonatal handbook: respiratory distress syndrome. Available at: www.netsvic.org.au/nets/handbook/index.cfm. Accessed June 2007.
17. Pramanik A: Respiratory distress syndrome. Available at www.emedicine.com/ped/topic1993.htm. Accessed October 2006.
18. Pagana KD, Pagana TJ: *Mosby's diagnostic and laboratory test reference*, ed 8, St Louis, 2007, Elsevier.
19. Ramberan H: Pneumothorax, spontaneous. In Ferri FF, editor: *Ferri's clinical advisor: instant diagnosis and treatment*, St Louis, 2007, Mosby, pp 702-703.
20. Thilo EN, Rosenberg AA: The newborn infant. In Hay WW et al, editors: *Current pediatrics: diagnosis and treatment*, ed 18, New York, 2007, Lange/McGraw-Hill, pp 1-64.
21. Kerby GS, Accurso FJ, Deterding RR et al: Respiratory tract and mediastinum. In Hay WW et al, editors: *Current pediatrics: diagnosis and treatment*, ed 18, New York, 2007, Lange/McGraw-Hill, pp 493-541.
22. Theodore PR, Jablons D: Thoracic wall, pleura, mediastinum and lung. In Doherty GM, editor: *Current surgical diagnosis and treatment*, ed 12, New York, 2005, Lange/McGraw-Hill, pp 325-389.
23. Guyton AC, Hall JE: *Textbook of medical physiology*, ed 11, Philadelphia, 2006, Elsevier.
24. Goroll AH, Mulley AG: Evaluation of pleural effusions. In Goroll AH, Mulley AG, editors: *Primary care medicine: office evaluation and management of the adult patient*, ed 5, Philadelphia, 2006, Lippincott Williams & Wilkins, pp 329-334.
25. Kerby GS, Accurso FJ, Deterding RR et al: Disorders of the pleura and pleural cavity. In Hay WW et al, editors: *Current pediatrics: diagnosis and treatment*, ed 18, New York, 2007, Lange/McGraw-Hill, pp 534-535.
26. Cassivi SD, McKellar SH: Pleural effusion and empyema thoracic. In Rakel RE, Bope ET, editors: *Conn's current therapy*, Philadelphia, 2008, Elsevier, pp 248-250.
27. Light RW: Disorders of the pleura and mediastinum. In Fauci AS et al, editors: *Harrison's principles of internal medicine*, ed 17, New York, 2008, McGraw-Hill, pp 1658-1661.
28. Opal SM, Policar M: Poliomyelitis. In Ferri FF, editor: *Ferri's clinical advisor: instant diagnosis and treatment*, St Louis, 2007, Mosby, p 704.
29. Shandera WX, Koo H: Infectious diseases: viral and rickettsial. In Tierney LM, McPhee SI, Papadakis MA, editors: *Current medical diagnosis and treatment*, ed 46, New York, 2007, Lange/McGraw-Hill, pp 1378-1430.
30. Harrison T: Amyotrophic lateral sclerosis. In Ferri FF, editor: *Ferri's clinical advisor: instant diagnosis and treatment*, St Louis, 2007, Mosby, p 47.
31. Ubogu EE: Guillain-Barré syndrome. In Ferri FF, editor: *Ferri's clinical advisor: instant diagnosis and treatment*, St Louis, 2007, Mosby, pp 367-368.
32. Eilert RE: Orthopedics. In Hay WW et al, editors. *Current pediatrics: diagnosis and treatment*, ed 18, New York, 2007, Lange/McGraw-Hill, pp 787-805.
33. Mercier LR: Scoliosis. In Ferri FF, editor: *Ferri's clinical advisor: instant diagnosis and treatment*, St Louis, 2007, Mosby, p 808.
34. Hellmann DB, Stone JH: Arthritis and musculoskeletal disorders. In Tierney LM, McPhee SI, Papadakis MA, editors: *Current medical diagnosis and treatment*, New York, 2007, Lange/McGraw-Hill, pp 807-825.
35. Hemmila MR, Wahl WL: Management of the injured patient. In Doherty GM, editor: *Current surgical diagnosis and treatment*, ed 12, New York, 2006, Lange/McGraw-Hill, pp 207-244.
36. Iannuccilli J: Obesity. In Ferri FF, editor: *Ferri's clinical advisor: instant diagnosis and treatment*, St Louis, 2007, Mosby, pp 615-617.
37. Baron RB: Nutrition. In Tierney LM, McPhee SI, Papadakis MA, editors: *Current medical diagnosis and treatment*, ed 46, New York, Lange/McGraw-Hill, 2007, pp 1279-1310.
38. The National Health and Nutrition Examination Survey (NHANES): Analytic and Reporting Guidelines. Available at: www.cdc.gov/nchs/data/nhanes_20_04/nhanes_analytic_guidelines_dec_2005.pdf
39. Fitzgerald PA: Endocrinology. In Tierney LM, McPhee SI, Papadakis MA, editors: *Current medical diagnosis and treatment*, ed 46, New York, 2007, Lange/McGraw-Hill, pp 1123-1218.
40. Manden LA, Wanderink R: Pneumonia. In Fauci AS et al, editors: *Harrison's principles of internal medicine*, ed 17, New York, 2008, McGraw-Hill, pp 16-19, 1629.
41. Hatipoglu U, Rubinstein I: Bacterial pneumonia. In Rakel RE, Bope ET, editors: *Conn's current therapy*, Philadelphia, 2008, Elsevier, pp 253-260.
42. Kerby GS, Accurso FJ, Deterding RR, et al: Acquired disorders involving the alveoli. In Hay WW et al, editors: *Current pediatrics: diagnosis and treatment*, ed 18, New York, 2007, Lange/McGraw-Hill, pp 517-521.
43. Centers for Disease Control and Prevention: Severe acute respiratory syndrome. Available at www.cdc.gov/ncidod/sars/2007.
44. Ferri FF: Severe acute respiratory syndrome. In Ferri FF, editor: *Ferri's clinical advisor: instant diagnosis and treatment*, St Louis, 2007, Mosby, pp 818-819.
45. Opal SM, Alonso GO: Tuberculosis, pulmonary. In Ferri FF, editor: *Ferri's clinical advisor: instant diagnosis and treatment*, St Louis, 2007, Mosby, pp 923-926.
46. Sharma SK, Mohan A: Tuberculosis and other mycobacterial diseases. In Rakel RE, Bope ET, editors: *Conn's current therapy*, Philadelphia, 2008, Elsevier, pp 278-287.

PART 5

Alterations in Fluid Balance, Excretion, and Reproduction

Frontiers of Research

The Sea Within Us

Sheila K. Smith   Linda Felver   Michael J. Kirkhorn

Humans are awash in fluids. This "sea within us" flows through our blood and lymph vessels, surrounds our cells, and even resides within them. Like the sea, our body fluids are salt water. In this salt water are sodium, chloride, potassium, calcium, magnesium, phosphate, and other electrolytes. The fluid outside of the cells (extracellular fluid) normally has different concentrations of these electrolytes than does the fluid inside cells (intracellular fluid). Many physiologic mechanisms combine to keep the volume, concentration, electrolyte composition, and degree of acidity (pH) of body fluids within their normal homeostatic ranges.

Persons who have chronic diseases often have risk factors for imbalances that make managing fluid and electrolytes a necessary part of their lives. Persons who have type 1 diabetes have increased risk for low plasma magnesium, extracellular fluid volume (ECV) deficit, diabetic ketoacidosis, low plasma phosphate, and either high or low plasma potassium, depending on their medications. Persons who have chronic renal failure have high risk of ECV excess; high plasma potassium, magnesium, and phosphate; and metabolic acidosis. Persons with heart failure risk fluid volume overload, pulmonary edema, and respiratory distress. Nurses teach individuals who have chronic diseases

how to prevent imbalances and how to recognize them if they occur. Acute pathophysiologic processes bring additional needs for nursing care.

Many medications alter electrolyte homeostasis. For example, persons who take most kinds of diuretics on a long-term basis should learn to increase their intake of potassium and magnesium. They need to know which foods are rich in these electrolytes and how to recognize the muscle weakness of low plasma potassium.

Current research indicates that many persons use herbal preparations and other supplements that can cause fluid, electrolyte, or acid-base imbalances. For example, licorice root (licorice extract; *Glycyrrhiza*) causes the kidneys to excrete more potassium. In the presence of other risk factors or with excessive use, this increased potassium excretion causes symptomatic low plasma potassium. Licorice root also causes the kidneys to retain sodium and water, leading to ECV excess.

Chronic alcohol abuse frequently causes low plasma magnesium due to poor magnesium intake and absorption, diarrhea, vomiting, and alcohol-induced increased renal excretion of magnesium. Low plasma magnesium decreases plasma potassium by increasing potassium excretion in the urine. Low magnesium

Transmission electron micrograph of glycogen granules (green) in a liver cell. Glycogen (a polysaccharide) is the form in which human cells store glucose (a monosaccharide). (From Thibodeau GA, Patton KT: Anatomy & physiology, ed 5, St Louis, 2003, Mosby. Courtesy Brenda Russell, PhD, University of Illinois at Chicago.)

Fluid, Electrolyte, and Acid-Base Homeostasis

suppresses parathyroid hormone, causing low plasma calcium. Chronic alcohol abuse also carries high risk for alcoholic ketoacidosis, low plasma phosphate, and ECV deficit. Alcohol-related diseases such as pancreatitis bring risk of additional imbalances. Clinicians who encounter persons who abuse alcohol need considerable knowledge of prevention, assessment, and management of these imbalances.

Assessment for fluid and electrolyte imbalances occurs in many settings. Home health nurses assess for ECV deficit in adults by measuring postural blood pressures and pulse and examining other physical signs. Telephone advice nurses can assess for the same imbalance by asking whether the person feels lightheaded when rising from a sitting or lying position. Hospital clinicians look for low serum potassium or increased urine specific gravity on a laboratory report. Practitioners in community settings can assess for low potassium by asking patients whether their legs feel heavy when they climb stairs. Other electrolyte abnormalities may be detected through abnormal cardiac rhythms. In the setting of nausea, vomiting, or diarrhea, significant dehydration and electrolyte imbalance can occur within a short time.

Assessments can be adapted for persons of different ages. In adults, assessment of postural blood pressure and filling of neck veins gives useful information about ECV. These assessments are not reliable in infants and small children. Recent research on assessment of ECV deficit in children indicates that testing skin turgor and capillary refill is important. However, in older adults, poor skin turgor is not a reliable indicator.

Safe therapy for specific imbalances depends on thorough knowledge of fluid, electrolyte, and acid-base homeostasis. Nurses teach parents whose children have vomiting and diarrhea how to replace body fluids with salty liquids containing a small amount of sugar, based on research into the best composition of oral rehydration solutions. Other research has taught nurses who add potassium to flexible intravenous bags to mix them carefully end-to-end before hanging them. The medication injection port is located near the infusion outlet port on these containers. Without mixing, the potassium is delivered in a bolus, which has caused severe cardiac dysrhythmias.

Fluid, electrolyte, and acid-base imbalances may cause death. Clinicians can do much to prevent, assess, and manage these imbalances. Keeping the volume, concentration, electrolyte composition, and pH of the "sea within us" within homeostatic ranges provides the optimal environment for our cells, organ systems, and the complex biochemistry of life.

chapter

24

Fluid and Electrolyte Homeostasis and Imbalances

Linda Felver

MEDIA RESOURCES

Additional Material for Study, Review, and Further Exploration

CD Companion ■ Review Questions and Answers ■ Glossary (with audio pronunciations for selected terms) ■ Disease Profiles ■ Animations

evolve **Website** at http://evolve.elsevier.com/Copstead/
   ■ Case Studies ■ Disease Profiles ■ WebLinks ■ Key Points Review

 Online Course (Module 13)

KEY QUESTIONS

- What physiologic and pathophysiologic conditions predispose an individual to disturbances in fluid intake?
- How do the compositions of plasma and interstitial fluids differ? How are they similar?
- How is water and electrolyte movement across cell membranes regulated?
- What are the usual and pathologic routes of fluid exit from the body?
- Under what conditions are extracellular volume deficit and excess likely to occur, and what are the characteristic clinical findings?

- Under what conditions are water excess (hyponatremia) and water deficit (hypernatremia) likely to occur, and what are the characteristic clinical findings?
- What physiologic and pathophysiologic conditions can lead to alterations in electrolyte intake, absorption, distribution, or excretion?
- What are the characteristic clinical findings of plasma excesses and deficits of potassium, calcium, magnesium, and phosphate ions?

CHAPTER OUTLINE

The fluid of the body flows in arteries, veins, and lymph vessels; it is secreted into specialized compartments as diverse as joints, cerebral ventricles, and the intestinal lumen; it both surrounds and permeates the cells. Body fluid serves as a lubricant and as a solvent for the chemical reactions that we call *metabolism;* it transports oxygen, nutrients, chemical messengers, and waste products to their destinations; it plays an important role in the regulation of body temperature. Because the fluid within the body is so widespread and serves so many functions, it is not surprising that abnormalities in the volume, concentration, or electrolyte composition of body fluid cause clinical problems.

Disorders of fluid or electrolyte homeostasis occur as a result of many different pathophysiologic conditions. In severe cases, these disorders cause death. Although these disorders arise from many specific causes in different patient populations, these specific causes fall into general categories that arise from the principles of normal fluid and electrolyte homeostasis. This chapter first presents the principles of normal fluid homeostasis and then, building on that foundation, continues with a discussion of fluid imbalances. Similarly, it explains the principles of electrolyte homeostasis before presenting plasma electrolyte imbalances.

BODY FLUID HOMEOSTASIS

The term **body fluid,** as used in this chapter, pertains to water within the body and the particles dissolved in it. The body fluid is contained in two major compartments: **extracellular** (outside the cells) and **intracellular** (inside the cells). In all age groups except infants, approximately two thirds of body fluid is intracellular.[1] The other one third of body fluid is extracellular. Infants have more extracellular fluid than intracellular fluid; this proportion reverses within a few months as the infant grows. The extracellular fluid lies between the cells (**interstitial** compartment), in the blood vessels (**vascular** compartment), in dense connective tissue and bone, and in several minor compartments that are collectively termed the **transcellular** fluids (e.g., synovial, cerebrospinal, and gastrointestinal fluids). The major body fluid compartments are depicted in Figure 24-1.

The fluids in the various body compartments have different compositions, although their total particle concentration is equal. The intracellular fluid is relatively rich in potassium and magnesium ions, inorganic and organic phosphates, and proteins. It is relatively low in sodium and chloride ions. In contrast, the extracellular fluid in the vascular and interstitial

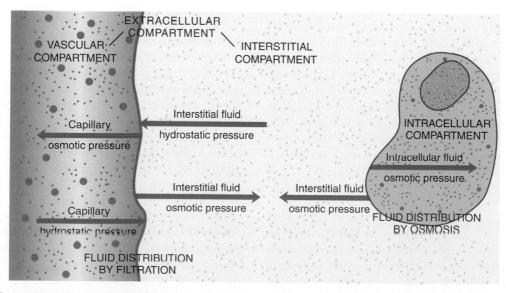

FIGURE 24-1 Factors that influence body fluid distribution. Fluid distribution between the vascular and interstitial compartments is the net result of filtration across permeable capillaries. The distribution of fluid between the interstitial and intracellular compartments occurs by osmosis rather than by filtration.

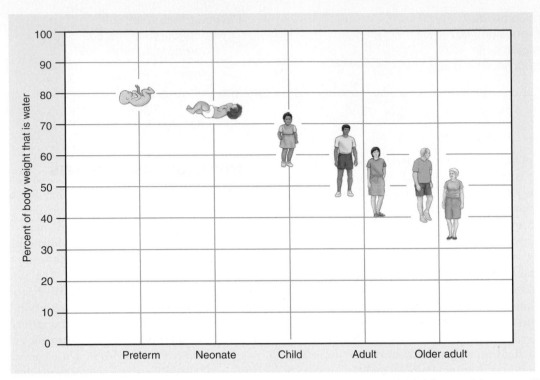

FIGURE 24-2 Percentage of total body water by age. The percentage of body weight that is water is high in infancy and decreases with increasing age.

compartments is relatively rich in sodium, chloride, and bicarbonate ions and relatively low in potassium, magnesium, and phosphate ions. The vascular portion of the extracellular fluid contains many proteins, whereas the interstitial and transcellular portions of the extracellular fluid contain very few proteins. Most transcellular fluids are secreted by epithelial cells; their composition varies according to their function.

Total body water is the total of the water in all fluid compartments. The percentage of body weight that is water varies according to a person's age and proportion of body fat (Figure 24-2). A full-term newborn infant is about 75% water by weight. (Preterm infants have an even higher percentage of water.) This percentage decreases with age. In a standard adult man, body water is about 60% of body weight. The percentage is less (about 50%) in women because they have a greater proportion of body fat than men of the same weight. In obese adults, with a much larger proportion of body fat, less of the body weight is water. In older men, 50% of the body weight is typically composed of water; in older women, it is even less. The decrease in this percentage with increased age is due primarily to the relative increase in body fat that occurs with normal aging.

One liter of water weighs 1 kg (2.2 lb). Thus, a lean, middle-aged, healthy adult man who weighs 70 kg (154 lb) has approximately 42 liters of body water. Of this amount, approximately 25 liters is intracellular water. The approximately 17 liters of extracellular water is distributed as 3 liters of plasma water, 8 liters of interstitial and lymph water, 5 liters of water trapped in dense connective tissue and bone, and 1 liter of transcellular water.

Fluid homeostasis is a dynamic process. This process may be viewed as the net result of four subprocesses: *fluid intake, fluid absorption, fluid distribution,* and *fluid excretion.* In some individuals who have pathophysiologic conditions, loss of fluid through abnormal routes also occurs. The interplay of these subprocesses is fluid homeostasis (Figure 24-3).

Fluid Intake and Absorption

Fluid intake is entry of fluid into the body by any route. Healthy people ingest fluids orally, both by drinking and by eating (water contained in food). They also synthesize a small amount of water through cellular metabolism of the foods they eat. Fluid intake by drinking is influenced by habit, social factors, and thirst. Physiologic triggers of thirst include increased **osmolality** (concentratedness) of extracellular fluid (osmoreceptor-mediated thirst); decreased circulating blood volume (baroreceptor-mediated and angiotensin II and III–mediated thirst); and dryness of the mucous membranes of the mouth and possibly other visceral signals.[2] In older adults, cerebral osmoreceptor-mediated thirst diminishes; thus, older adults who do not have a habit of drinking fluids throughout the day may not have sufficient fluid intake to meet their needs.[3]

Additional routes of fluid intake that may occur in patients who have various pathophysiologic conditions include intravenous intake; intake tubes into the gastrointestinal tract, other body cavities, subcutaneous tissue or bone marrow; rectal intake (such as tap water enema); and, occasionally, intake through the lungs (such as near-drowning). Fluid intake by many of these routes often is controlled by health care professionals.

FIGURE 24-3 Fluid homeostasis. Fluid homeostasis is the interplay of fluid intake and absorption, fluid distribution, fluid excretion, and fluid loss through abnormal routes.

Unless fluid intake occurs intravenously, the fluid must be absorbed before it reaches the vascular compartment. Fluid absorption from the gastrointestinal tract partially depends on osmotic forces generated by absorption of electrolytes and other particles.

Fluid Distribution

Much of the fluid that reaches the vascular compartment then distributes into other fluid compartments. Fluid distribution between the vascular and interstitial compartments is the net result of filtration across permeable capillaries. At the capillary level, two forces tend to move fluid from the capillaries into the interstitial compartment: capillary hydrostatic pressure (the outward push of vascular fluid against the capillary walls) and interstitial fluid osmotic pressure (the inward-pulling force of particles in the interstitial fluid). Concurrently, two forces tend to move fluid from the interstitial compartment into the capillaries: capillary osmotic pressure (the inward-pulling force of particles in vascular fluid) and interstitial fluid hydrostatic pressure (the outward push of interstitial fluid against the outside of the capillary walls).[3]

The distribution of fluid between the vascular and interstitial compartments is analogous to two groups of people pushing on opposite sides of a swinging door—the strongest "push" will determine in which direction the door will swing. Thus, at any one point along a capillary, the direction and amount of fluid flow between the vascular and interstitial compartments are determined by the net result of opposing forces. These forces are illustrated in Figure 24-1.

In contrast, *the distribution of fluid between the interstitial and intracellular compartments occurs by* **osmosis,** *rather than by filtration.* Cell membranes are semipermeable membranes. This means that they are permeable to water but not to electrolytes, many of which require specialized transport mechanisms to cross a cell membrane. Thus, water can move freely through a cell membrane, but electrolytes and other particles cannot. When there is a difference in particle concentration (osmolality) inside and outside cells because the particles cannot move freely, the *water* crosses the membrane rapidly to equalize the osmolality.

The direction of movement of water by osmosis is determined by the particle concentrations on the two sides of the semipermeable cell membrane. If, on the one hand, the particle concentration (osmolality) of the interstitial fluid becomes higher than the particle concentration inside cells, water will move by osmosis from the cells to the interstitial fluid to equalize the osmolality in the two compartments. If, on the other hand, the osmolality of the interstitial fluid becomes lower than the osmolality of the intracellular fluid, then water will move from the interstitial compartment to the intracellular compartment to equalize the osmolality. In this way, changes in the osmolality of the interstitial and intracellular compartments control the distribution of water between them.[4]

Distribution of fluid between the intracellular and transcellular compartments is controlled by processes within the epithelial cells that secrete these fluids.

Fluid Excretion

The fourth component of fluid homeostasis is fluid excretion. Fluid excretion normally occurs through the urinary tract, bowels, lungs, and skin. Fluid is excreted through the skin as visible sweat (which may or may not occur) and as insensible perspiration (which always occurs). Another obligatory route of excretion of water is through the lungs as a person exhales. Fecal excretion of fluid occurs with normal bowel function and increases dramatically in a person who has diarrhea. In a healthy person, the largest volume of fluid is excreted in the urine.

The amount of fluid excreted in the urine is controlled primarily by the hormones antidiuretic hormone (ADH), aldosterone, and natriuretic peptides (e.g., atrial or A-type natriuretic peptide [ANP] or atrial natriuretic factor [ANF]), and to a lesser degree by minor hormones such as renal prostaglandins, and by the renal sympathetic nerves. ADH is synthesized by cells in the supraoptic and paraventricular nuclei of the hypothalamus. The axons of these cells extend down the median eminence of the pituitary stalk. The release of ADH thus occurs from the posterior pituitary gland. Factors that increase release of ADH into the blood include increased osmolality (concentratedness) of the extracellular fluid, decreased circulating fluid volume, pain, nausea, and physiologic and psychological stressors. The hormone circulates to the distal tubules and collecting ducts in the kidneys where, consistent with its name, ADH causes reabsorption of water. Reabsorption of water decreases the urine volume and makes the urine concentrated, thus decreasing fluid excretion. Factors that decrease ADH release (such as decreased osmolality of the extracellular fluid and ethanol intake) allow a large dilute urine volume.

Aldosterone is another hormone that influences urine volume. Aldosterone is synthesized and secreted by cells in the adrenal cortex. The major stimuli for its release are angiotensin II (from the renin-angiotensin system, which is activated by decreased circulating blood volume) and an increased concentration of potassium ions in the plasma. Aldosterone causes the renal tubules to reabsorb sodium and water (saline), so that it also decreases fluid excretion, although by a different mechanism than ADH. When more aldosterone is secreted, the urine volume is smaller; decreased secretion of aldosterone causes a larger urine volume.

A comparison of ADH and aldosterone is useful to remember their actions. ADH is the tap water hormone. It causes the kidneys to reabsorb water. Renal reabsorption of water due to ADH makes a smaller volume of more concentrated urine. Aldosterone is the salt water hormone. It causes the kidneys to reabsorb sodium and water. Renal reabsorption of sodium and water due to aldosterone makes a smaller volume of urine.

ANP normally is secreted from cells in the heart when the atria are stretched. B-type natriuretic peptide (BNP) is released from ventricular cells when ventricular diastolic pressure increases abnormally, as in heart failure. ANP and BNP cause natriuresis (sodium excretion in the urine), which is accompanied by water excretion. Thus, these natriuretic peptides (NPs) promote fluid excretion in the urine. When the vascular volume increases, the heart is stretched, and more NPs are released to cause renal excretion of the excess.[5] When the vascular volume is decreased, the heart is less stretched; therefore, fewer NPs are released and the kidneys excrete less fluid. NPs oppose the action of aldosterone, but they are not as strong as aldosterone.

The urine volume that an individual produces also is highly dependent on having adequate blood pressure to perfuse the kidneys and on the glomerular filtration rate. Thus, renal excretion of fluid is the end result of several factors, including hormones that respond to different stimuli and have different actions on the renal tubules.

Fluid Loss Through Abnormal Routes

People who have pathophysiologic conditions often experience loss of fluid through abnormal routes. Examples of these routes are emesis; tubes in the gastrointestinal tract or other body cavities; hemorrhage; drainage from fistulas, wounds, or open areas of skin; and paracentesis. Fluid lost through abnormal routes may be a significant factor in disturbing fluid homeostasis.

If the body's physiologic mechanisms are functioning well, the processes of fluid homeostasis maintain normal body fluid status. If fluid intake is large, fluid excretion increases by the mechanisms described previously that increase urine volume

(large volume of dilute urine). If fluid intake is diminished or if fluid is lost through abnormal routes, fluid excretion decreases (small volume of concentrated urine), and thirst may cause an increase in fluid intake.

If pathophysiologic processes interfere with normal fluid homeostasis or if the normal processes become overwhelmed, then fluid imbalances result. For example, a person who has a pathophysiologic process that prevents the kidneys from excreting much fluid may accumulate too much fluid unless the fluid intake is reduced. The opposite problem will occur in a person whose fluid intake is too small to replace a large amount of fluid excreted or lost through abnormal routes.

KEY POINTS

- Fluid homeostasis is a dynamic process that includes fluid intake and absorption, fluid distribution across body fluid compartments, fluid excretion, and, in some individuals, fluid loss through abnormal routes.
- Habit and thirst are important regulators of fluid intake. Individuals who are unable to control their own fluid intake (such as those receiving fluids intravenously and immobile or unconscious patients) are at high risk for fluid imbalance.
- Fluid (water and small particles) moves back and forth between the vascular and interstitial areas by filtration at the capillaries. Capillary hydrostatic pressure is the primary force promoting fluid movement from the capillaries to the interstitial fluid. Plasma colloid osmotic pressure is the primary force that causes interstitial fluid to move back into the capillaries.
- Water moves in and out of cells by osmosis. Electrolytes do not move freely across cell membranes but are transported by membrane channels and carriers.
- Fluid excretion may be visible (urine, feces, sweat) or invisible (respiration and insensible perspiration). Fluid loss may occur through abnormal routes such as emesis and wound drainage. To maintain fluid balance, fluid intake must counterbalance fluid excretion and loss through abnormal routes.
- Healthy kidneys adjust fluid excretion in response to blood pressure and several hormones. Aldosterone induces the kidneys to conserve saline (salt and water); natriuretic peptides (ANP and BNP) promote saline excretion. ADH causes the kidneys to retain water, thus concentrating the urine. Urine volume and concentration are important indicators of body fluid balance.

FLUID IMBALANCES

If fluid homeostasis is disturbed by pathophysiologic processes or other factors (such as medications), fluid imbalances may occur. Fluid imbalances fall into two major categories: imbalances of extracellular fluid volume (**saline imbalances**) and imbalances of body fluid concentration (**water imbalances**).

Extracellular Fluid Volume

In some circumstances, individuals have too much or too little extracellular fluid. These disorders are called **extracellular fluid volume (ECV) imbalances** because they involve a change in the *amount* (volume) of the extracellular fluid. These disorders also are termed *saline imbalances* because they are disorders of **isotonic** salt water. (Isotonic saline is salt water in the same concentration as the normal plasma concentration.) In an ECV imbalance, the *concentration* of the extracellular fluid may be normal; there is simply too much or too little of it. Some individuals have an ECV imbalance and an imbalance of body fluid concentration at the same time. In this case, both the volume and serum sodium concentration of the extracellular fluid are abnormal. This section discusses only the volume imbalances; the concentration imbalances are discussed separately because they may occur separately.

Volume Deficit. ECV deficit is caused by removal of a sodium-containing fluid from the body. It is a decrease in saline (salt water) in the same concentration as the normal extracellular fluid, which is why the condition sometimes is termed **saline deficit.** In an uncomplicated ECV deficit, the serum sodium concentration is normal. The *concentration* of the extracellular fluid is normal; the *amount* of the extracellular fluid is abnormally decreased (Figure 24-4).

Etiology. Specific causes of ECV deficit are listed in Box 24-1. All causes of ECV deficit involve removal of a sodium-containing fluid from the extracellular compartment. The sodium-containing fluid usually is removed from the body; however, it may be sequestered in a "third space" in the body that is outside the extracellular compartment. For example, ascites (fluid in the peritoneal cavity) that develops rapidly may deplete the ECV. Another example is fluid that accumulates rapidly in the bowel during an acute intestinal obstruction. Although the fluid in these examples remains in the body, it no longer is part of the extracellular fluid, and signs and symptoms of ECV deficit occur.

Clinical Manifestations. Signs and symptoms of ECV deficit are the result of decreased fluid volume in the vascular and interstitial areas. These clinical manifestations include sudden weight loss, postural blood pressure decrease with concurrent increased heart rate, flat neck veins (or veins collapsing with inspiration) when a patient is supine, prolonged small-vein filling time, prolonged capillary refill time, lightheadedness, dizziness, syncope, and oliguria. If the kidneys are responding normally, the small volume of urine will be concentrated (and thus quite yellow). An ECV deficit that develops slowly also may be manifested by decreased skin turgor (skin tenting when it is pinched up over the sternum), dryness of oral mucous membranes between cheek and gum, hard stools, soft sunken eyeballs, longitudinal furrows in the tongue, and absence of tears and sweat. An infant who develops ECV deficit has a sunken fontanel; neck veins are not reliably assessed in infants.

Sudden weight loss is a sensitive measure of ECV deficit. One liter of saline weighs 1 kg; therefore, a person who loses 1 kg in 24 hours has excreted 1 liter of fluid or lost it through an abnormal route. It is not possible to lose a kilogram of fat overnight; a sudden weight loss of this magnitude results only from fluid loss, if the body weight is measured accurately. An ECV deficit may occur without a weight loss if fluid is sequestered in a third space somewhere in the body, as with ascites or intestinal obstruction.

A postural blood pressure decrease with concurrent increased heart rate that is measured when a previously supine person stands, or sits with legs dependent, is a good indicator of fluid volume depletion in the vascular compartment. Severe ECV deficit may lead to hypovolemic shock, which can be fatal if not treated effectively with fluid replacement.

FIGURE 24-4 Extracellular fluid volume deficit. Decreased volume of extracellular fluid in vascular and interstitial compartments is characteristic of extracellular fluid volume deficit.

BOX 24-1

Causes of Extracellular Fluid Volume Deficit

Gastrointestinal Excretion or Loss of Sodium-Containing Fluid
Emesis
Diarrhea (includes laxative abuse)
Gastric suction or intestinal decompression
Fistula drainage

Renal Excretion of Sodium-Containing Fluid
Adrenal insufficiency
Salt-wasting renal disorders
Extensive diuretic use
Bed rest

Other Loss of a Sodium-Containing Fluid
Hemorrhage
Massive diaphoresis
Third-space fluid accumulation
Paracentesis and similar procedures
Burns

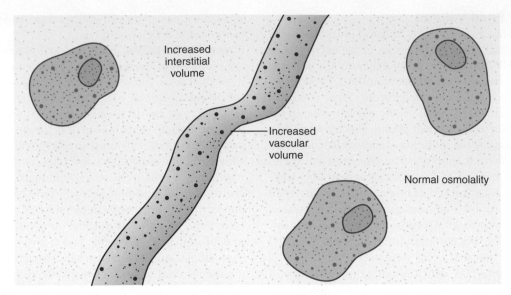

FIGURE 24-5 Extracellular fluid volume excess. Increased volume of extracellular fluid in vascular and interstitial compartments is characteristic of extracellular fluid volume excess.

Volume Excess. ECV excess is essentially the opposite of an ECV deficit. It is the condition in which the amount of extracellular fluid is abnormally increased. Both the vascular and the interstitial areas have too much fluid (Figure 24-5). In an uncomplicated ECV excess, the *concentration* of the extracellular fluid is normal, but an excessive *amount* of that fluid is present.

Etiology. ECV excess is caused by addition or retention of saline (salt water in the same concentration as normal plasma). For this reason, it sometimes is termed **saline excess.** As mentioned previously, the hormone aldosterone causes the kidneys to retain saline. ECV excess, therefore, may be caused by conditions that involve excessive aldosterone secretion. For example, increased aldosterone secretion is a compensatory mechanism that commonly accompanies chronic heart failure and eventually leads to ECV excess.[6] Additional causes of ECV excess are presented in Box 24-2.

Clinical Manifestations. Signs and symptoms of ECV excess are sudden weight gain, edema, and manifestations of circulatory overload: bounding pulse, neck vein distention in a person in the upright position, crackles in the dependent portions of the lungs, dyspnea, orthopnea, and even the frothy sputum of pulmonary edema. An infant who develops ECV excess has a bulging fontanel; assessment of neck veins is not effective in infants.

Sudden weight gain is a sensitive measure of ECV excess. It is impossible to gain a kilogram of fat overnight; such a sudden weight gain is an accumulation of saline. People who eat salty food in a restaurant weigh more the next day because the water they drank combined with the salt in the food to make isotonic saline. The isotonic saline expands the extracellular fluid, causing a mild saline excess until it is excreted by the kidneys. This is the reason that low-sodium diets are prescribed for people who have pathophysiologic processes that cause saline excess (e.g., compensated heart failure).

BOX 24-2

Causes of Extracellular Fluid Volume Excess

Excessive Intravenous Infusion of Sodium-Containing Isotonic Solutions
Normal saline (0.9% sodium chloride)
Ringer injection
Lactated Ringer injection

Renal Retention of Sodium and Water
Primary hyperaldosteronism
Chronic heart failure
Cirrhosis
Acute glomerulonephritis
Chronic renal failure
Cushing disease
Corticosteroid therapy

Body Fluid Concentration

In contrast to the ECV disorders just discussed, imbalances of body fluid concentration are disorders of the *concentration* rather than of the *amount* of extracellular fluid. Body fluid concentration disorders also are called **water imbalances.** The serum sodium concentration reflects the osmolality (concentratedness) of the blood. Imbalances of body fluid concentration are recognized by abnormal serum sodium concentration. The normal serum sodium concentration is 135 to 145 mEq/L (may vary slightly with different laboratories). Many individuals develop imbalances of both ECV and serum sodium concentration at the same time. Isolated imbalances of serum sodium concentration may also occur. This section discusses the concentration imbalances separately.

BOX 24-3

Causes of Hyponatremia

Gain of Relatively More Water Than Salt
Excessive antidiuretic hormone
Excessive intravenous infusion of 5% dextrose in water (D5W)
Hypotonic irrigating solutions
Tap water enemas
Psychogenic polydipsia (compulsive water drinking)
Forced excessive water ingestion (child abuse or club initiation)
Excessive beer ingestion (beer potomania)
Near-drowning in fresh water
Selective serotonin reuptake inhibitors (SSRIs)

Loss of Relatively More Salt Than Water
Diuretics, especially thiazides
Salt-wasting renal disease
Replacement of water but not salt lost through emesis, diarrhea, gastric suction, diaphoresis, or burns

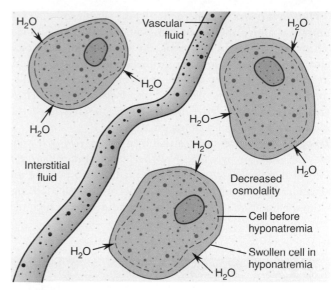

FIGURE 24-6 Cell swelling in hyponatremia. Decreased osmolality (concentration) of extracellular fluid in hyponatremia causes water to move into cells by osmosis.

Hyponatremia. *Natrium* is the Latin word for sodium. A serum sodium concentration below the lower limit of normal indicates hyponatremia. When hyponatremia is present, the extracellular fluid contains relatively too much water for the amount of sodium ions present; it is more dilute than normal.

Etiology. Hyponatremia is caused by factors that produce a relative excess of water in proportion to salt in the extracellular fluid. Because the serum sodium concentration reflects the osmolality of the blood, the reduced serum sodium of hyponatremia indicates that the extracellular fluid has a reduced osmolality; it is too dilute. Hyponatremia also is called *hypotonic syndrome, hypoosmolality,* and *water intoxication.* All of these terms reflect the abnormal concentration of the extracellular fluid that results when the normal proportion of salt to water in the extracellular fluid is disrupted.

A *gain of relatively more water than salt* will cause hyponatremia. As mentioned previously, the hormone ADH causes the kidneys to retain water (not sodium and water) in the body. This hormone is part of the system that normally regulates the osmolality of extracellular fluid. However, circumstances that cause prolonged or excessive release of ADH cause the kidneys to retain too much water, which effectively dilutes the blood; hyponatremia is the result. ADH is elevated in the syndrome of inappropriate secretion of ADH (SIADH). It also may be produced **ectopically.** For example, small cell (oat cell) carcinoma is a type of lung tumor that frequently synthesizes and releases ADH. This ectopic production of ADH from a tumor is not subject to the feedback inhibition of normal ADH release, so inappropriate amounts of ADH are released. With continually high levels of ADH being produced by the tumor, the kidneys retain excessive amounts of water—a gain of water relative to salt. Pain, nausea, and other physical and psychological stressors also increase ADH release, which can be significant in hospitalized patients, especially in the postoperative period.[7] Although it is difficult to drink enough

water to cause hyponatremia, water intake that exceeds renal excretory capacity is seen in some situations. For example, the hyponatremia of beer potomania arises when people habitually drink 14 or more cans of beer daily with very little food intake.[8] Factors that cause hyponatremia by gain of water relative to salt are presented in Box 24-3.

Hyponatremia also may be caused by a *loss of relatively more salt than water.* If salt is removed from the body while water remains, then the extracellular fluid once again will become too dilute; hyponatremia results. Factors that cause hyponatremia by loss of salt relative to water also are presented in Box 24-3. Although Box 24-3 separates causes of hyponatremia into two categories, some types of hyponatremia are due to simultaneous gain of water and loss of salt. For example, hyponatremia in marathon runners occurs from loss of salt through heavy sweating and gain of water from excessive water intake plus a poorly understood inappropriate renal water retention.[9]

Clinical Manifestations. Clinical manifestations of hyponatremia are nonspecific manifestations of central nervous system dysfunction.[3] They vary from malaise, anorexia, nausea, vomiting, and headache to confusion, lethargy, seizures, and coma. Profound hyponatremia causes fatal cerebral herniation. The signs and symptoms are caused by swelling of neurons and glial cells as a result of the decreased osmolality of extracellular fluid. When the extracellular fluid becomes too dilute, the intracellular fluid initially is more concentrated. Therefore, water moves into cells by osmosis (Figure 24-6). The severity of the signs and symptoms depends on how rapidly hyponatremia develops as well as on the absolute value of the serum sodium concentration. A rapid decrease in osmolality produces more severe manifestations than a slow decline, other factors being equal.

Hypernatremia. Hypernatremia is a serum sodium concentration above the upper limit of normal (145 mEq/L). When hypernatremia is present, the extracellular fluid contains relatively too little water for the amount of sodium ions present; it is too concentrated. Hypernatremia also is called *water deficit, hypertonic syndrome,* and *hyperosmolality.* These terms all reflect the relative deficit of water to salt in the extracellular fluid that occurs in hypernatremia.

Etiology. Hypernatremia is caused by a *gain of relatively more salt than water* or by a *loss of relatively more water than salt.* Both of these processes cause the body fluids to become too concentrated. Patients who receive concentrated tube feedings without enough water, especially older adults, are at high risk

for hypernatremia because they gain relatively more solute than water, which causes an obligatory loss of relatively more water than salt in the urine. Hypernatremia can be prevented in these individuals by administering water between feedings. Other specific factors that cause hypernatremia are presented in Box 24-4 under the two major categories.

Clinical Manifestations. Signs and symptoms of hypernatremia are similar to those of hyponatremia in that they are nonspecific manifestations of central nervous system dysfunction.[3] In hypernatremia, the increased osmolality of the extracellular fluid causes neurons and glial cells to shrivel because water moves from the cells to the interstitial fluid by osmosis (Figure 24-7). The dysfunction ranges from confusion and lethargy to seizures and coma. Thirst and oliguria (except for hypernatremia of renal origin) are common. Severe hypernatremia may cause death.

BOX 24-4

Causes of Hypernatremia

Gain of Relatively More Salt Than Water
Tube feeding
Intravenous infusion of hypertonic solution
Near-drowning in salt water
Overuse of salt tablets
Food intake with reduced fluid intake
Difficulty swallowing fluids
No access to water
Inability to respond to thirst

Loss of Relatively More Water Than Salt
Diabetes insipidus (deficient antidiuretic hormone)
Tube feeding (causes obligate water loss in urine)
Osmotic diuresis
Prolonged emesis, diarrhea or diaphoresis without water
 replacement

Both Volume and Concentration

Clinical Dehydration. Clinical dehydration is a combination of two fluid disorders: ECV deficit and hypernatremia. A person who has clinical dehydration has too small a volume of fluid in the extracellular compartment (vascular and interstitial), and the body fluids are too concentrated (Figure 24-8).

Etiology. Clinical dehydration occurs commonly in individuals who have vomiting and diarrhea and do not know how (or are unable) to replace the salt and the water that is exiting the body. Fluid excreted in diarrhea and lost by vomiting, plus the normal daily respiratory, skin, and urine excretion, is the equivalent of hypotonic saline (isotonic saline with extra water added). Removal of the saline portion of this fluid from the body causes ECV deficit, and removal of the extra water from

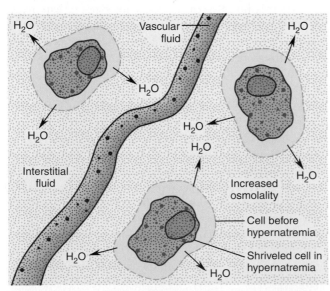

FIGURE 24-7 Cell shriveling in hypernatremia. Increased osmolality (concentration) of extracellular fluid in hypernatremia causes water to move from cells by osmosis.

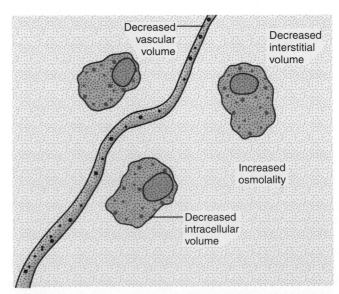

FIGURE 24-8 Clinical dehydration. Decreased volume of extracellular fluid in vascular and interstitial compartments plus cell shriveling from increased osmolality of extracellular fluid are combined in clinical dehydration.

the body causes hypernatremia. The combination of these two imbalances is clinical dehydration.

Clinical Manifestations. Signs and symptoms of clinical dehydration are the combination of the signs and symptoms of the two separate disorders. Therefore, a person who is clinically dehydrated will have clinical manifestations as listed in Box 24-5. Infants and older adults are at highest risk for clinical dehydration, although it can occur at any age.[10]

Interstitial Fluid Volume

Edema. Edema is an excess of fluid in the interstitial compartment. It may be a manifestation of ECV excess or it may arise from other mechanisms. Forces that determine the distribution of fluid between the vascular and interstitial compartments are described previously in this chapter (see the Fluid Distribution section). An increase in the forces that tend to move fluid from the capillaries into the interstitial compartment or a decrease in forces that tend to move fluid from the interstitial compartment into the capillaries will cause edema by altering normal fluid distribution between the vascular and interstitial compartments. Thus, edema may arise from increased capillary hydrostatic pressure, increased interstitial fluid osmotic pressure, blockage of lymphatic drainage, or decreased capillary osmotic pressure (Figure 24-9).

Increased capillary hydrostatic pressure is caused by increased ECV, by the increased local capillary flow that accompanies inflammation, and by venous congestion. *Increased interstitial fluid osmotic pressure* occurs when inflammation increases vascular permeability and proteins leak into the interstitial fluid. Lymphatic drainage normally removes minute

amounts of protein that enter the interstitial fluid. *Blockage of lymphatic drainage* (e.g., by a tumor, parasites, fibrosis from radiation therapy, or surgical removal of lymph nodes) also causes edema when the interstitial accumulation of protein increases interstitial fluid osmotic pressure.[11] Edema resulting from increased interstitial fluid osmotic pressure or blockage of lymphatic drainage is frequently localized. *Decreased capillary osmotic pressure* occurs when the plasma proteins are decreased, as in malnutrition or liver disease (decreased protein synthesis). Edema from this cause may be extensive.

In summary, edema represents increased interstitial fluid volume, a condition that may be local or generalized. Edema may be a sign of ECV excess (which causes increased capillary hydrostatic pressure), or it may be caused by other factors that alter the distribution of fluid between the vascular and interstitial compartments.

KEY POINTS

- ECV deficit (saline deficit) occurs when sodium-containing fluids are lost from the body (e.g., emesis). It is an abnormally reduced volume of the vascular and interstitial fluids. ECV deficit is characterized by normal serum sodium and manifestations of volume deficit (weight loss, poor skin turgor, postural hypotension, oliguria).
- ECV excess (saline excess) commonly is due to processes that cause the kidneys to retain sodium and water. It is an abnormally increased volume of the vascular and interstitial fluids. ECV excess is characterized by a normal serum sodium level and manifestations of volume excess (weight gain, peripheral edema, distended neck veins, dyspnea).
- Hyponatremia (water excess) is associated with excessive ADH secretion or hypotonic fluid intake. It is characterized by a low serum sodium concentration, which indicates that body fluids are abnormally dilute. Clinical manifestations (confusion, lethargy, seizure, coma) occur because of cell swelling.
- Hypernatremia (water deficit) is associated with inadequate water intake or excessive water excretion or loss. It is characterized by a high serum sodium level, which indicates that body fluids are too concentrated. Clinical manifestations (confusion, lethargy, seizure, coma) occur because of cell shriveling.
- Clinical dehydration occurs commonly in individuals who have gastroenteritis or other conditions that remove hypotonic sodium-containing fluids from the body. It is the combination of ECV deficit and hypernatremia. The clinical manifestations are those of both fluid disorders.
- Edema occurs when there is too much fluid in the interstitial compartment. It may be localized or generalized. The causes of edema at the capillary level are increased capillary hydrostatic pressure, increased interstitial fluid osmotic pressure, blockage of lymphatic drainage, and decreased capillary osmotic pressure.

FIGURE 24-9 Causes of edema. **A,** Normal capillary filtration without edema. **B,** Edema due to increased capillary hydrostatic pressure. **C,** Edema due to increased interstitial fluid osmotic pressure from increased capillary permeability. **D,** Edema due to blocked lymphatic drainage. **E,** Edema due to decreased capillary osmotic pressure from hypoalbuminemia.

PRINCIPLES OF ELECTROLYTE HOMEOSTASIS

Electrolytes are ionized salts dissolved in water. The most clinically important electrolytes are the ions sodium, potassium, calcium, magnesium, chloride, bicarbonate, and phosphate. Although sodium ions are electrolytes, serum sodium imbalances are osmolality (concentration) imbalances, as explained previously in this chapter. This section discusses homeostasis and imbalances of potassium, calcium, magnesium, and phosphate ions. Bicarbonate is discussed in Chapter 25 because it is important in acid-base balance and imbalances.

The concentration of an electrolyte in the plasma is different from its concentration inside cells. For normal body function, the electrolyte concentration must be normal in both areas. In clinical situations, the plasma (or serum) concentration of an electrolyte is measured. Normal serum electrolyte concentrations are listed in Table 24-1. The concentration of an electrolyte in the plasma is the net result of four processes: *electrolyte intake, electrolyte absorption, electrolyte distribution,* and *electrolyte excretion.* These processes work together in a dynamic fashion to maintain electrolyte concentrations within their normal limits (Figure 24-10). Thus, if intake of a specific electrolyte increases, excretion of that electrolyte also may increase and normalize the plasma levels. Similarly, if electrolyte intake decreases dramatically, electrolytes may be redistributed into the plasma to maintain the normal plasma concentration.

Electrolyte Intake and Absorption

Electrolyte intake normally occurs orally, through food and drink. It is important to remember that oral medications (e.g., magnesium antacids) also may be an important source of electrolyte intake. Intravenous fluids and nutritional solutions are common sources of parenteral intake of electrolytes. Blood transfusions may provide significant amounts of electrolytes. Less common, but important if it occurs, is intramuscular injection of the electrolyte magnesium.

Some patients have electrolyte intake through tubes into body cavities. The most obvious examples are nasogastric and gastrointestinal feeding tubes, but more unusual situations may cause significant electrolyte intake in specific individuals (e.g., irrigation of the renal pelvis with magnesium-rich solutions). Rarely, electrolyte intake may occur through such unusual routes as the lungs (e.g., near-drowning in salt water, which is rich in magnesium) or the skin (e.g., through application of ointments to large areas of broken or burned skin). Electrolyte intake is controlled by the individual and by health care providers.

If electrolyte intake occurs orally, the electrolyte must be absorbed before it is physiologically useful. Absorption of some electrolytes, such as potassium ions, depends on concentration gradients. Absorption of other electrolytes, such as calcium, depends on the availability of binding proteins, which is influenced by the activity of vitamin D.[1] The contents of the gastrointestinal tract may influence electrolyte absorption. Many agents bind electrolytes and prevent them from being absorbed. For example, undigested fat in the intestines binds calcium and magnesium ions contained in food and prevents them from being absorbed. The pH of intestinal contents also influences the absorption of certain electrolytes, especially calcium ions. Medications often alter electrolyte absorption. Surgical removal of portions of the gastrointestinal tract can decrease electrolyte absorption.

TABLE 24-1	
Normal Serum Electrolyte Concentrations	
Electrolyte	**Normal Concentration Range**
Calcium (total)	9-11 mg/dl (4.5 to 5.5 mEq/L)
Magnesium	1.5-2.5 mEq/L
Phosphate	2.5-4.5 mg/dl (adults and older children)
	4.5-6.5 mg/dl (children)
	4.3-9.3 mg/dl (neonates)
Potassium	3.5-5.0 mEq/L
	3.9-5.9 mEq/L (neonates)
Sodium	135-145 mEq/L
	135-162 mEq/L (neonates)

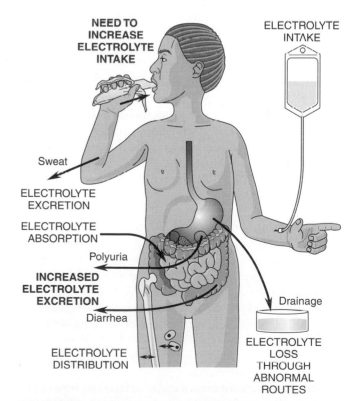

FIGURE 24-10 Electrolyte homeostasis. Electrolyte homeostasis is the interplay of electrolyte intake and absorption, electrolyte distribution, electrolyte excretion, and electrolyte loss through abnormal routes. If electrolyte excretion or loss through abnormal routes increases, electrolyte intake also must increase to prevent electrolyte imbalance.

Electrolyte Distribution

Every fluid compartment contains electrolytes. However, the electrolyte composition differs in these various compartments. The concentrations of potassium, magnesium, and phosphate ions are higher inside cells than in the fluid outside the cells. Although calcium ion concentration is higher inside cells, much of the intracellular calcium is bound to other molecules; the concentration of physiologically active ionized calcium ions is higher in the extracellular fluid. The bones serve as an important reservoir of calcium, magnesium, and phosphate ions. The cells and the bones are often called the *electrolyte pools.*

Distribution of electrolytes between the extracellular fluid and the electrolyte pools is influenced primarily by hormones such as epinephrine (potassium ions), insulin (potassium and phosphate ions), and parathyroid hormone (calcium ions). Certain medications also influence electrolyte distribution. Significant movement of electrolytes between the cells and the extracellular fluid may occur within minutes.[1] In the absence of changes in electrolyte intake and excretion, a shift of electrolytes from the extracellular fluid into the electrolyte pools will decrease the plasma electrolyte concentration. Conversely, a shift of electrolyte from an electrolyte pool into the extracellular fluid will increase the plasma electrolyte concentration.

Electrolyte Excretion

Electrolyte excretion occurs through urine, feces, and sweat. Urinary excretion of some electrolytes is influenced by hormones (e.g., aldosterone increases potassium ion excretion), although factors such as the flow rate of renal tubular fluid are also influential. Many different medications alter the rate of urinary excretion of electrolytes.[12]

Fecal excretion of electrolytes is influenced by the type of feces produced. Diarrhea increases the excretion of potassium and magnesium ions in particular. The composition of the feces also influences the amount of electrolyte excretion. Undigested fat in the intestines binds calcium and magnesium ions that are secreted into the gastrointestinal tract and prevents them from being reabsorbed. Thus, these electrolytes are excreted in the feces.

Electrolyte Loss Through Abnormal Routes

When electrolytes exit the body through routes other than the normal urine, feces, and sweat, this may be termed *electrolyte loss through abnormal routes.* This factor alters electrolyte homeostasis in patients who have diverse pathophysiologic conditions. Examples of electrolyte loss through abnormal routes are vomiting, nasogastric suction, paracentesis, hemodialysis, wound drainage, and fistula drainage. Loss of electrolytes through abnormal routes may be uncontrollable or may result from therapeutic procedures.

Electrolyte homeostasis is a dynamic interplay between the processes of electrolyte intake, electrolyte absorption, electrolyte distribution, and electrolyte excretion. In some people, electrolyte loss through abnormal routes becomes an important factor that requires adjustment of electrolyte intake and/or electrolyte excretion to prevent development of electrolyte imbalances. Individuals who have acute or chronic illnesses have many factors that tend to cause electrolyte imbalances by disrupting or interfering with electrolyte intake, absorption, distribution, or excretion. As a result, they may develop single or multiple electrolyte imbalances.[13]

KEY POINTS

- The electrolyte composition of the body is maintained by a careful balance of electrolyte intake, absorption, distribution, and excretion. Electrolyte imbalances result from disruption of one or more of these processes or from electrolyte loss through abnormal routes.
- The plasma concentration of an electrolyte may not reflect the intracellular concentration. Cells contain higher concentrations of potassium, calcium, magnesium, and phosphate ions, whereas the extracellular fluid contains higher concentrations of sodium, chloride, and bicarbonate ions.

ELECTROLYTE IMBALANCES

Electrolyte imbalances are widespread in many pathophysiologic conditions. An electrolyte imbalance may be a total body imbalance or it may be an imbalance in distribution of electrolytes within compartments, with the total body amount remaining normal. Based on the principles of electrolyte homeostasis explained in the previous section of this chapter, an excess of electrolytes in the extracellular fluid may be caused by increased electrolyte intake or absorption, shift of electrolytes from an electrolyte pool into the extracellular fluid, and decreased electrolyte excretion, either singly or in combination. Conversely, a deficit of electrolytes in the extracellular fluid may be caused by decreased electrolyte intake or absorption, shift of electrolytes from the extracellular fluid to an electrolyte pool, increased electrolyte excretion, loss of electrolytes through abnormal routes, or some combination of these factors.

Plasma Potassium

The normal concentration of potassium ions in serum is 3.5 to 5.0 mEq/L (may vary slightly with different laboratories), except in neonates, in whom it may be higher. Most of the potassium ions in the body are inside cells; the standard serum potassium measurement gives only the concentration of the small portion of potassium ions in the extracellular fluid. Because a number of factors cause potassium ions to move into or out of body cells, concentration of potassium in the plasma and total body potassium content are not necessarily correlated. Whether or not they are accompanied by total body potassium imbalances, plasma potassium imbalances may cause clinically significant signs and symptoms.

Hypokalemia. Hypokalemia denotes a decreased potassium ion concentration in the extracellular fluid. A decrease in the plasma potassium concentration does not necessarily denote a decrease in total body potassium. Thus, hypokalemia may coexist with a total body potassium deficit, a total body potassium excess, or a normal total body potassium ion concentration.

Etiology. Hypokalemia is caused by factors that decrease potassium intake, shift potassium from the extracellular fluid into the cells, increase potassium excretion through the normal routes, and cause potassium loss from the body by some abnormal route. Potassium-wasting diuretics and corticosteroids such as prednisone are well-known causes of hypokalemia from increased renal potassium excretion. The hormone aldosterone increases potassium excretion in urine; hypokalemia is associated with pathophysiologies such as compensated heart failure and cirrhosis that are accompanied by increased aldosterone levels. Black licorice contains substances that act like aldosterone in the body. Many traditional Chinese medicines and other herbal preparations contain black licorice, and excessive ingestion of these agents or black licorice candy leads to hypokalemia.[14] In many cases, several factors lead to hypokalemia. For example, some people follow a fad diet (decreased potassium intake) and abuse diuretics (increased potassium excretion) in an attempt to lose weight. Specific causes of hypokalemia are listed in Box 24-6.

Clinical Manifestations. The resting membrane potential of muscle cells is determined by the ratio of intracellular to extracellular potassium ion concentration. For this reason, potassium imbalances cause altered function of muscles (skeletal, smooth, and cardiac). In hypokalemia, both smooth and skeletal muscle cells are hyperpolarized (more electrical charge than usual across the cell membrane).[15] Therefore, these muscles are less reactive to stimuli. The resulting clinical manifestations include abdominal distention, diminished bowel sounds, paralytic ileus, postural hypotension, skeletal muscle weakness, and flaccid paralysis. The skeletal muscle weakness of hypokalemia is bilateral weakness that typically begins in the lower extremities and ascends. It may involve the respiratory muscles, causing respiratory paralysis more commonly than does hyperkalemia.

Many types of cardiac dysrhythmias arise from hypokalemia. Cardiac muscle cells usually become hyperpolarized with hypokalemia. However, with very low plasma potassium concentrations, hypopolarization of cardiac muscle occurs, most likely because of decreased potassium conductance. Hypokalemia also increases the rate of diastolic depolarization, which may give rise to ectopic beats, decreases conduction velocity in the atrioventricular node, prolongs cardiac action potentials by decreasing the rate of repolarization, shortens the absolute refractory period, and prolongs the relative refractory period.[16] Cardiac dysrhythmias in severe hypokalemia may cause sudden cardiac death.[17]

Hypokalemia also may cause polyuria by interfering with the action of ADH at the renal tubules. The plasma potassium concentration at which the various clinical manifestations of hypokalemia appear depends on individual responsiveness and the presence of other concurrent electrolyte and acid-base disorders. Chronic hypokalemia can cause rhabdomyolysis

---

BOX 24-6

Causes of Hypokalemia

Decreased Potassium Intake
Anorexia
NPO (nothing by mouth) orders and intravenous solutions without potassium
Fasting
Unbalanced diet

Shift of Potassium from Extracellular Fluid to Cells
Alkalosis
Rapid correction of acidosis
Excess insulin (e.g., during total parenteral nutrition)
Excess β-adrenergic stimulation
Hypokalemic familial periodic paralysis

Increased Potassium Excretion Through Normal Routes
Renal Route
Potassium-wasting diuretics
Corticosteroid therapy
Cushing disease
Hyperaldosteronism
Excessive ingestion of black licorice (glycyrrhizin)
Hypomagnesemia
Parenteral carbenicillin or similar agents
Amphotericin B, cisplatin, and many other drugs
Fecal Route
Diarrhea (includes laxative abuse)
Skin Route
Excessive diaphoresis

Loss of Potassium Through Abnormal Routes
Emesis
Gastric suction
Fistula drainage

(skeletal muscle breakdown), selective myocardial cell necrosis, and nephropathy.[18]

Hyperkalemia. If the serum potassium concentration rises above 5.0 mEq/L (the upper limit of normal), hyperkalemia is present. Hyperkalemia denotes an elevation of potassium ion concentration in the extracellular fluid. As mentioned previously, most of the potassium ions in the body are inside cells, and many factors cause potassium ions to move into or out of the cells. Thus, total body potassium may be increased, normal, or decreased in hyperkalemia, depending on its cause.

Etiology. Hyperkalemia is caused by factors that increase potassium intake, shift potassium from the cells into the extracellular fluid, and decrease potassium excretion. For example, large numbers of potassium ions shifting from cells into the extracellular fluid after a crushing injury or massive cell death from cytotoxic chemotherapy will cause hyperkalemia.[19] Several factors together can cause hyperkalemia, such as when an individual who develops decreased potassium excretion due to oliguric renal failure continues to have a normal dietary potassium intake. Specific causes of hyperkalemia are summarized by category in Box 24-7.

BOX 24-7

Causes of Hyperkalemia

Increased Potassium Intake
Excessive or too-rapid intravenous potassium infusion
Insufficiently mixed intravenous potassium
Large transfusion of stored blood
Massive doses of potassium penicillin G

Shift of Potassium from Cells to Extracellular Fluid
Acidosis caused by nonorganic acids
Insufficient insulin
Crushing injury
Cytotoxic drugs (tumor lysis syndrome)
Hyperkalemic periodic paralysis
β-Adrenergic blockade and prolonged strenuous exercise

Decreased Potassium Excretion
Oliguria (such as in hypovolemia or renal failure)
Potassium-sparing diuretics
Adrenal insufficiency
Renin-deficient states
Drugs that reduce aldosterone effects (angiotensin-converting enzyme [ACE] inhibitors, angiotensin II receptor antagonists, and selective aldosterone blockers)
Nephrotoxic drugs

Clinical Manifestations. As might be expected from the role of potassium ions in establishment of the resting membrane potential of muscle cells, hyperkalemia causes muscle dysfunction. As hyperkalemia develops, smooth muscle and skeletal muscle cells become hypopolarized. The main clinical manifestation at this stage is mild intestinal cramping and diarrhea, which occurs only in some individuals. As hyperkalemia worsens, skeletal muscle cells become hypopolarized to the extent that their resting membrane potentials lie above their threshold potential; once they have discharged, they are unable to contract again. This situation causes the typical skeletal muscle weakness and flaccid paralysis of hyperkalemia. The skeletal muscle weakness is an ascending weakness that appears first in the lower extremities. Both hypokalemia and hyperkalemia cause skeletal muscle weakness and/or paralysis, but the underlying alterations in the resting membrane potentials are different.

Cardiac muscle undergoes the same changes in resting membrane potential as skeletal muscle in hyperkalemia. In addition, hyperkalemia decreases the duration and rate of rise of cardiac action potentials and decreases conduction velocity in the heart. These pathophysiologic mechanisms underlie the cardiac dysrhythmias of hyperkalemia.[16] Severe hyperkalemia causes cardiac arrest.

The plasma potassium concentration at which each of these clinical manifestations occurs varies, depending on the rapidity of rise of the potassium concentration, the causes of the hyperkalemia, and other concurrent electrolyte or acid-base imbalances. Patients who have chronic renal failure often undergo potassium adaptation and have relatively mild symptoms at high plasma potassium concentrations that would be disabling in other persons. The mechanisms of potassium adaptation include increased aldosterone levels that increase potassium excretion by the colon and shift potassium ions from extracellular fluid into cells, helping to normalize resting membrane potentials.[20]

Plasma Calcium

Calcium in the plasma is present in three forms: some calcium ions are bound to plasma proteins (such as albumin); some are bound to small organic ions (such as citrate); and the rest are unbound. Only the free ionized calcium is physiologically active. Two laboratory measurements are available for calcium: total serum calcium and ionized calcium. The *total serum calcium* measures all of the calcium (bound plus unbound). The normal range of total serum calcium in adults is 9 to 11 mg/dl or 4.5 to 5.5 mEq/L (may vary slightly with different laboratories). Unless a calcium value specifies ionized calcium, it is total calcium. The *ionized calcium* measures only the unbound ionized form. The normal range of ionized calcium in adults is 4.0 to 5.0 mg/dl, about half of the total calcium (varies with different laboratories). Clinically significant calcium imbalances are caused by alterations in the plasma concentration of unbound ionized calcium.

Hypocalcemia. Hypocalcemia occurs if the serum calcium concentration drops below the lower limit of normal. If the fraction of unbound ionized calcium in the blood is decreased by more calcium binding to plasma proteins or other organic ions, the total serum calcium (the usual laboratory measurement) may be normal, but *ionized* hypocalcemia is present and may cause signs and symptoms.

Etiology. Hypocalcemia is caused by factors that decrease calcium intake or absorption, decrease the physiologic availability of calcium, and increase calcium excretion. For example, hypocalcemia in pancreatitis arises from impaired fat digestion caused by lack of pancreatic lipase in the intestines. Both dietary calcium and calcium ions secreted into the intestine from the extracellular fluid bind to undigested fat in the intestine and are excreted in the feces. Thus, both decreased calcium absorption and increased calcium excretion play a part in hypocalcemia associated with pancreatitis. Ionized hypocalcemia is common in intensive care unit patients, again due to multiple factors.[21] Box 24-8 lists specific causes of hypocalcemia organized according to the general etiologic factors.

Clinical Manifestations. Calcium ions play an important role in determining the speed of ion fluxes through nerve and muscle cell membranes. Thus, calcium imbalances alter normal neuromuscular excitability. Clinical manifestations of hypocalcemia are those of increased neuromuscular excitability: positive Trousseau sign; positive Chvostek sign; paresthesias; muscle twitching and cramping; hyperactive reflexes; carpal spasm; pedal spasm; tetany; laryngospasm; seizures; and cardiac dysrhythmias. The increased neuromuscular excitability of hypocalcemia is caused by a decrease in the threshold potential of excitable cells, so that action potentials are generated more easily. Cardiac effects of hypocalcemia arise from prolonged

---

BOX 24-8

Causes of Hypocalcemia

Decreased Calcium Intake or Absorption
Diet with insufficient calcium and vitamin D
Chronic kidney disease (deficient activated vitamin D)
Excessive dietary phytates or oxalates
Steatorrhea
Pancreatitis
Chronic diarrhea (includes laxative abuse)
Malabsorption syndromes

Decreased Physiologic Availability of Calcium
Hypoparathyroidism
Excessive phosphate intake
Tumor lysis syndrome (high phosphate)
Hypomagnesemia
Alkalosis
Large transfusion of citrated blood
Rapid infusion of plasma expanders that bind calcium
Elevated plasma free fatty acids
Chronic kidney disease

Increased Calcium Excretion Through Normal Routes
Steatorrhea
Pancreatitis

BOX 24-9

Causes of Hypercalcemia

Increased Calcium Intake or Absorption
Milk-alkali syndrome
Vitamin D overdose (includes shark cartilage supplements)

Shift of Calcium from Bone to Extracellular Fluid
Hyperparathyroidism
Immobilization
Paget disease
Bone tumors
Multiple myeloma
Leukemia
Nonosseous malignancies that produce bone-resorbing factors

Decreased Calcium Excretion
Thiazide diuretics
Familial hypocalciuric hypercalcemia

---

plateau phase of the cardiac action potential, impaired atrioventricular and intraventricular conduction, and impaired myocardial contractility, which can cause heart failure.[16,22]

Positive Trousseau sign is occurrence of a carpal spasm after occlusion of arterial blood flow to the hand for approximately 3 minutes. Positive Chvostek sign is spasm of muscles in the cheek and corner of the mouth produced by tapping the facial nerve in front of the ear. Positive Trousseau and Chvostek signs are general indicators of increased neuromuscular excitability from any cause, so they must be interpreted in the context of other clinical manifestations and specific risk factors for hypocalcemia. Chvostek sign may be positive in neonates without electrolyte imbalances.

Hypercalcemia. Hypercalcemia occurs when the serum calcium concentration rises above the upper limit of normal (11 mg/dl or 5.5 mEq/L). It indicates an elevation of the calcium concentration of the extracellular fluid.

Etiology. Hypercalcemia is caused by factors that increase calcium intake or absorption, cause a shift of calcium from bone to extracellular fluid, and decrease calcium excretion. For example, many malignant tumors produce chemicals that circulate in the blood and shift calcium from bones into extracellular fluid.[23] These bone-resorbing factors include parathyroid hormone–related peptide and prostaglandins. In addition, circulating factors in malignancy may decrease renal excretion of calcium ions, which also contributes to hypercalcemia. Specific causes of hypercalcemia are listed by category in Box 24-9.

Clinical Manifestations. Hypercalcemia causes decreased neuromuscular excitability. Clinical manifestations of hypercalcemia include anorexia, nausea, emesis, constipation, fatigue, polyuria, muscle weakness, diminished reflexes, headache, confusion, lethargy, personality change, and cardiac dysrhythmias. The decreased neuromuscular excitability is caused by elevation of the threshold potential of excitable cells. Cardiac effects of hypercalcemia include shortened plateau phase of the action potential, increased rate of diastolic depolarization of sinus node cells, and delayed atrioventricular conduction.[16] Renal calculi may occur due to the high calcium concentration of the urine. Hypercalcemia caused by bone resorption may give rise to pathologic fractures.

Plasma Magnesium

The normal serum magnesium concentration is 1.5 to 2.5 mEq/L (may vary slightly with different laboratories). Similarly to calcium, magnesium ions also are present in the blood as bound (physiologically inactive) and unbound ionized (physiologically active) forms. Ionized magnesium levels are available in some research settings. Plasma magnesium imbalances may occur concurrent with or in the absence of total body magnesium imbalances.

Hypomagnesemia. If the serum magnesium concentration decreases below the lower limit of normal (1.5 mEq/L), hypomagnesemia is present. Hypomagnesemia indicates a decreased magnesium concentration of the extracellular fluid and does not necessarily indicate a total body magnesium deficit (although the two may occur concurrently).

Etiology. Causes of hypomagnesemia are decreased magnesium intake or absorption, decreased physiologic availability of magnesium, increased magnesium excretion, and loss of magnesium by an abnormal route. Chronic alcoholism is a major risk factor for hypomagnesemia because it is associated with decreased magnesium intake, decreased physiologic availability of magnesium, increased urinary and fecal magnesium excretion, and magnesium loss through emesis.[24] Hypomagnesemia often causes hypokalemia by increasing urinary excretion of potassium.[25] In such cases, correction of hypomagnesemia is necessary before the hypokalemia can be corrected. Specific causes of hypomagnesemia are listed in Box 24-10.

Clinical Manifestations. Magnesium ions in the extracellular fluid normally depress the release of acetylcholine at neuromuscular junctions. If too few magnesium ions are present, excessive amounts of acetylcholine are released (Figure 24-11). Therefore, the clinical manifestations of hypomagnesemia are those of increased neuromuscular excitability. Such manifestations may include insomnia, hyperactive reflexes, muscle cramps, muscle twitching, grimacing, positive Chvostek sign, positive Trousseau sign, nystagmus, dysphagia, ataxia, tetany, and seizures. Cardiac dysrhythmias also occur.

Hypomagnesemia causes decreased activity of the enzyme that drives the Na^+-K^+ pump in cell membranes, so that intracellular potassium decreases in the myocardium. Increased spontaneous firing in the sinus node, shortening of the absolute refractory period, and lengthening of the relative refractory period contribute to cardiac dysrhythmias in hypomagnesemia.[16]

Hypermagnesemia. If the serum magnesium concentration rises above the upper limit of normal (2.5 mEq/L), hypermagnesemia is present. Hypermagnesemia indicates an excess of magnesium in the extracellular fluid.

Etiology. The major causes of hypermagnesemia are increased magnesium intake and decreased magnesium excretion. Shift of magnesium from bones to extracellular fluid is seen transiently in some stages of hyperparathyroidism. More commonly, hypermagnesemia from excessive intake of magnesium in laxatives and antacids occurs in people of any age who have unrecognized renal impairment. Older adults are at highest risk from these magnesium-containing medications.[26] Individuals who have oliguria, as in chronic renal failure, are another high-risk group for development of hypermagnesemia. Specific causes of hypermagnesemia are summarized in Box 24-11.

Clinical Manifestations. Too many magnesium ions in the extracellular fluid depress neuromuscular function by decreasing the release of acetylcholine at neuromuscular junctions (see Figure 24-11). Thus manifestations of hypermagnesemia include decreased deep tendon reflexes, lethargy, hypotension, flushing, diaphoresis, drowsiness, flaccid paralysis,

---

BOX 24-10

Causes of Hypomagnesemia

Decreased Magnesium Intake or Absorption
Chronic alcoholism
Malnutrition
Prolonged intravenous therapy without magnesium
Ileal resection
Chronic diarrhea (includes laxative abuse)
Malabsorption syndromes
Steatorrhea
Pancreatitis

Decreased Physiologic Availability of Magnesium
Elevated plasma free fatty acids

Increased Magnesium Excretion Through Normal Routes
Renal Route
Diabetic ketoacidosis
Chronic alcoholism
Hyperaldosteronism
Diuretic therapy
Aminoglycoside (e.g., gentamicin) toxicity
Amphotericin B, cisplatin, and many other drugs
Fecal Route
Steatorrhea
Pancreatitis

Magnesium Loss Through Abnormal Routes
Emesis
Gastric suction
Fistula drainage

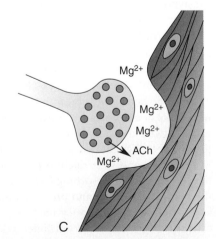

FIGURE 24-11 Acetylcholine (ACh) release at neuromuscular junctions is altered in magnesium imbalances. **A,** Normal magnesium concentration suppresses the release of acetylcholine at neuromuscular junctions to normal levels. **B,** In hypomagnesemia, more acetylcholine is released at neuromuscular junctions, causing increased neuromuscular excitability. **C,** In hypermagnesemia, less acetylcholine is released at neuromuscular junctions, causing decreased neuromuscular excitability.

BOX 24-11

Causes of Hypermagnesemia

Increased Magnesium Intake or Absorption
Ingestion or aspiration of seawater
Excessive ingestion of magnesium-containing medications
  (e.g., laxatives, antacids)
Excessive intravenous infusion of magnesium

Decreased Magnesium Excretion
Oliguric renal failure
Adrenal insufficiency

BOX 24-12

Causes of Hypophosphatemia

Decreased Phosphate Intake or Absorption
Chronic alcoholism
Chronic diarrhea
Malabsorption syndromes
Excessive or long-term use of antacids that bind phosphate

Shift of Phosphate from Extracellular Fluid to Cells
Refeeding after starvation (includes anorexia nervosa)
Total parenteral nutrition
Hyperventilation (respiratory alkalosis)
Insulin
Epinephrine
Intravenous glucose, fructose, bicarbonate, or lactate

Increased Phosphate Excretion Through the Normal Renal Route
Alcohol withdrawal
Diuretic phase after extensive burns
Diabetic ketoacidosis
Diuretic therapy

Phosphate Loss Through Abnormal Routes
Emesis
Hemodialysis

BOX 24-13

Causes of Hyperphosphatemia

Increased Phosphate Intake or Absorption
Overzealous phosphate therapy
Excessive use of phosphate-containing enemas or laxatives

Shift of Phosphate from Cells to Extracellular Fluid
Tumor lysis syndrome
Crushing injury
Rhabdomyolysis

Decreased Phosphate Excretion
Chronic kidney disease
Oliguric renal failure
Adrenal insufficiency

---

respiratory depression, bradycardia, cardiac dysrhythmias, and even cardiac arrest. Mechanisms that cause the cardiac effects of hypermagnesemia include decreased cardiac conduction and depression of membrane excitability.[16]

Plasma Phosphate

The normal range of phosphate concentration in adult plasma is 2.5 to 4.5 mg/dl (may vary slightly with different laboratories). Symptomatic phosphate imbalances are less common than other electrolyte imbalances, but, like other electrolyte imbalances, they may be fatal if untreated.

Hypophosphatemia. Hypophosphatemia is present when the phosphate concentration in the plasma decreases below the lower limit of normal (2.5 mg/dl). However, the clinical manifestations of hypophosphatemia are often not observed unless the plasma phosphate concentration is less than 1.0 mg/dl. Persons whose plasma phosphate concentration is less than 1.0 mg/dl are said to have *severe symptomatic hypophosphatemia.*

Etiology. Hypophosphatemia is caused by factors that decrease phosphate intake, shift phosphate from extracellular fluid to cells, increase phosphate excretion, and cause loss of phosphate through abnormal routes. Frequently, many factors combine to produce severe symptomatic hypophosphatemia. Any factor that causes a rapid increase in cellular metabolism will cause phosphate to shift from extracellular fluid into cells. Patients who are severely malnourished (such as cancer patients with advanced disease) are at high risk for severe symptomatic hypophosphatemia after nutritional replacement is started because of their increased cellular metabolism and previously depleted phosphate stores.[27] Specific factors that cause hypophosphatemia are summarized in Box 24-12.

Clinical Manifestations. Phosphate is an important component of adenosine triphosphate (ATP), the major source of energy for many cellular processes. The signs and symptoms of severe symptomatic hypophosphatemia are due, in part, to decreased ATP within the cells. Another contributing mechanism is tissue hypoxia caused by decreased 2,3-biphosphoglycerate in the red blood cells. Signs and symptoms include anorexia, malaise, paresthesias, hemolysis, diminished reflexes, muscle aches, muscle weakness, respiratory failure, confusion, stupor, seizures, coma, and impaired cardiac function. The impaired cardiac function of severe hypophosphatemia results from decreased cardiac contractility and stroke work concurrent with increased left ventricular end-diastolic pressure and may cause congestive cardiomyopathy.[16]

Hyperphosphatemia. Hyperphosphatemia is an increase of the serum phosphate concentration above the upper limit of normal (4.5 mg/dl).

Etiology. Hyperphosphatemia may be caused by increased phosphate intake, shift of phosphate from cells or bones to extracellular fluid, and decreased phosphate excretion. Examples of specific causes in these categories are listed in Box 24-13. Hyperphosphatemia is common in people who have oliguric renal failure, either acute or chronic. In chronic kidney disease, renal phosphate excretion is severely decreased but intestinal absorption of dietary phosphate continues. In addition, elevated parathyroid hormone in chronic kidney disease shifts phosphate from bones into extracellular fluid.[28]

Clinical Manifestations. Clinical manifestations of hyperphosphatemia depend on the effect of the elevated phosphate ion concentration on calcium ions. Typically, hyperphosphatemia causes hypocalcemia. The signs and symptoms are thus the manifestations of increased neuromuscular excitability that were presented in the discussion of hypocalcemia. However, in some patients, especially those who have chronic kidney disease, hyperphosphatemia causes deposition of calcium phosphate salts in the soft tissues of the body. These patients develop signs and symptoms such as aching and stiffness of joints, itching, and conjunctivitis, depending on the areas in which these salts precipitate.

- Manifestations of calcium imbalances are caused by changes in threshold potential of nerve and muscle cells. Hypocalcemia decreases the threshold potential, causing hyperexcitability (twitching, tetany); hypercalcemia increases the threshold potential, causing neuromuscular depression (hyporeflexia).
- Manifestations of magnesium imbalances are similar to those of calcium imbalances. Magnesium ions normally inhibit release of acetylcholine at neuromuscular junctions. Hypomagnesemia increases neuromuscular excitability (hyperreflexia and twitching), and hypermagnesemia depresses neuromuscular excitability (hyporeflexia and flaccid paralysis).
- Severe symptomatic hypophosphatemia is characterized by manifestations of generalized cellular ATP deficiency. Hyperphosphatemia may cause hypocalcemia, with resulting increased neuromuscular excitability, or it may be associated with precipitation of calcium phosphate into soft tissues of the body.

KEY POINTS

- Plasma electrolyte deficits are caused by factors that decrease electrolyte intake or absorption, shift electrolytes from the extracellular fluid to an electrolyte pool, increase electrolyte excretion, and cause loss of electrolytes through abnormal routes.
- Plasma electrolyte excesses are caused by factors that increase electrolyte intake or absorption, shift electrolytes from an electrolyte pool to the extracellular fluid, and decrease electrolyte excretion.
- Abnormalities in plasma electrolyte concentrations may profoundly affect cellular function. Excitable cells, such as nerve and muscle, are particularly sensitive to electrolyte imbalances.
- Manifestations of potassium imbalances are due to changes in resting membrane potentials. Hypokalemia causes hyperpolarization; hyperkalemia causes hypopolarization. Both hyperkalemia and hypokalemia cause skeletal muscle weakness, flaccid paralysis, and cardiac dysrhythmias.

SUMMARY

This chapter presents the principles of fluid and electrolyte homeostasis and imbalances. Boxes 24-14 and 24-15 summarize pediatric and geriatric variations, respectively. Fluid and electrolyte homeostasis involves the continuous interplay of intake, absorption, distribution, and excretion of fluid and electrolytes. Loss of fluid and electrolytes through abnormal routes may also occur. When the normal mechanisms are impaired or overwhelmed, fluid and electrolyte imbalances occur. Fluid imbalances may involve the volume or the concentration of body fluid. Plasma electrolyte imbalances may be deficits or excesses and may not reflect total body electrolyte deficits or excesses. Signs and symptoms of fluid and electrolyte imbalances are summarized in Table 24-2. The pathophysiology of specific fluid and electrolyte imbalances can be derived from a working knowledge of normal fluid and electrolyte homeostasis.

BOX 24-14

Pediatric Variations

- Infants have more extracellular fluid than intracellular fluid; this proportion reverses by a few months of age.
- About 75% of the body weight of a term infant is water; this percentage is even higher in preterm infants. The percentage of body weight that is water decreases as the child grows older.
- In the first few days after birth, an infant loses fluid equal to 5% to 10% of its body weight; this is a normal process during adjustment to extrauterine life.
- Neonates have a high metabolic rate and thus a high turnover rate of water.
- Infants have increased insensible water excretion due to proportionately large body surface area, proportionately large respiratory mucosa surface area, vasomotor immaturity, and increased skin permeability. Preterm infants have even greater insensible water excretion through the skin due to flaccid extended posture (and thus greater exposed body surface area) and greater vasomotor immaturity.
- Use of phototherapy and radiant heat warmers increases insensible water excretion.
- Glomerular filtration rate is lower in infants than adults.
- The kidneys of infants have limited ability to concentrate urine or to dilute it; thus, infants are unable to excrete a large load of water effectively or to conserve fluid when needed.
- Infants communicate thirst by crying, which may not be understood by their caregivers.
- Infants and toddlers are a high-risk group for clinical dehydration.
- Assessment of extracellular volume imbalances in infants should focus on tension of fontanel rather than degree of filling of neck veins.
- Infants whose caregivers use powdered formula are at high risk for hypernatremia if the formula is reconstituted with extra powder to "strengthen" the baby.
- Laboratory normal ranges of electrolytes generally are wider for infants than older children and adults.
- Neonatal hypocalcemia may occur in infants who needed resuscitation at birth or have high-risk conditions.
- Preterm infants may have reduced body calcium stores because fetal calcium stores are built during the last trimester of pregnancy; these infants have increased incidence of neonatal hypocalcemia.
- Assessment of increased neuromuscular excitability (hypocalcemia and hypomagnesemia) in infants should not include Chvostek sign; this sign is often positive in normal neonates. Increased neuromuscular excitability in infants includes jitteriness, hyperactive reflexes, and a high-pitched cry.
- Neonates whose mothers were given magnesium sulfate for eclampsia in the 24 hours before birth may be born with hypermagnesemia. Hypermagnesemic infants lie in a flaccid, extended posture.

BOX 24-15

Geriatric Variations

- Older adults have less body water than middle-aged adults because body composition changes with increasing age (decreased muscle mass, increased fat in internal organs). About 50% of the body weight of a lean older man is water and about 45% of the body weight of a lean older woman is water; the percentage is lower in obese older adults.
- Glomerular filtration rate is lower in older adults than in middle-aged adults.
- The kidneys of older adults are less able to concentrate urine and thus less able to conserve fluid when needed. This decreased ability to concentrate urine is also responsible for nocturia, since a larger than normal volume of urine is produced at night.
- Older adults have a reduced thirst response when the osmolality of body fluids increases; thus, they may not be aware that they are becoming dehydrated.
- Older adults are a high-risk group for clinical dehydration.
- Decreased skin turgor is not reliable as a sign of extracellular fluid volume depletion in older adults, due to age-related changes in collagen and elastin. Decreased skin turgor (skin tenting when pinched) may occur in older adults who have normal fluid volume.
- Older adults who receive tube feedings are at higher risk for hypernatremia than middle-aged adults.
- Older adults probably absorb more magnesium from antacids and cathartics than do middle-aged adults. With age-related changes in renal excretion, older adults who use oral magnesium laxatives or antacids regularly are at high risk for hypermagnesemia.

TABLE 24-2

Summary of Signs and Symptoms of Fluid and Electrolyte Imbalances

Imbalance	Heart	Blood Vessels	Interstitial Area	CNS	Lungs
↓ Extracellular volume	Tachycardia	Postural blood pressure decrease with concurrent heart rate increase, flat neck veins, ↑ small-vein filling time, thready pulse	↓ Skin turgor; soft, sunken eyeballs; longitudinal furrows in tongue	Dizziness	
↑ Extracellular volume		Distended neck veins, bounding pulse	Edema		Crackles, dyspnea, orthopnea, frothy sputum
↓ Na⁺				Confusion, lethargy, coma, seizures	
↑ Na⁺				Confusion, lethargy, coma, seizures	
↓ K⁺	Dysrhythmias	Postural hypotension			
↑ K⁺	Dysrhythmias, cardiac arrest				
↓ Ca⁺⁺	Dysrhythmias, impaired myocardial contractility			Seizures	
↑ Ca⁺⁺	Dysrhythmias			Confusion, lethargy, personality change	
↓ Mg⁺⁺	Dysrhythmias			Insomnia, seizures	
↑ Mg⁺⁺	Bradycardia, dysrhythmias, cardiac arrest	Hypotension, flushing		Drowsiness, lethargy	Respiratory depression
↓ Pᵢ	Impaired cardiac function, decreased cardiac output			Confusion, stupor, coma, seizures	Respiratory failure
↑ Pᵢ (may cause ↓ Ca⁺⁺)					

ECV, Extracellular fluid volume; P_i, inorganic phosphate.

Skeletal Muscle	Neuromuscular Excitability	Gastrointestinal Tract	Kidneys	Other
		Dry oral mucous membranes, hard stools	Oliguria	Sudden weight loss, sunken fontanel (infants), no tears or sweat, thirst with severe ↓ ECV
		Hepatomegaly		Sudden weight gain, bulging fontanel (infants)
		Anorexia, nausea, emesis		Malaise, headache
			Oliguria	Thirst
Ascending weakness, flaccid paralysis		Abdominal distention, bloating, ↓ bowel sounds, constipation, paralytic ileus	Polyuria	
Ascending weakness, flaccid paralysis		Cramping, diarrhea		
Twitching, cramping, carpal spasm, pedal spasm	Increased excitability, Trousseau sign, Chvostek sign, paresthesias, hyperactive reflexes, tetany			Laryngospasm
Weakness	Decreased excitability, depressed reflexes	Anorexia, nausea, emesis, constipation	Polyuria	Fatigue, headache
Twitching, cramping, grimacing, tremors	Increased excitability, Trousseau sign, Chvostek sign, hyperactive reflexes, tetany	Dysphagia		Nystagmus, ataxia
Flaccid paralysis	Depressed reflexes			Diaphoresis
Aching, weakness	Paresthesias, depressed reflexes	Anorexia		Malaise, hemolysis
			If Ca⁺⁺ remains high, damage from deposition of crystals	If Ca⁺⁺ remains high, pruritus, conjunctivitis, arthritis

REFERENCES

1. Guyton AC, Hall AE: *Textbook of medical physiology*, ed 11, Philadelphia, 2006, Saunders.
2. Johnson A: Psychobiology of thirst and salt appetite, *Med Sci Sports Exercise* 39:1388-1400, 2007.
3. Rose BD, Post TW: *Clinical physiology of acid-base and electrolyte disorders*, ed 5, New York, 2001, McGraw-Hill.
4. Stein WD: Cell volume homeostasis: ionic and nonionic mechanisms. The sodium pump in the emergence of animal cells, *Int Rev Cytol* 215:231-258, 2002.
5. Potter L, Abbey-Hosch S, Dickey D: Natriuretic peptides, their receptors, and cyclic guanosine monophosphate-dependent signaling functions, *Endo Rev* 27:47-72, 2006.
6. Kasper D et al (eds): *Harrison's principles of internal medicine*, ed 16, New York, 2005, McGraw-Hill.
7. Paut O, Lacroix F: Recent developments in the perioperative fluid management for the paediatric patient, *Curr Opin Anaesthesiol* 19(3):268-277, 2006.
8. Sanghvi S, Kellerman P, Nanovic L: Beer potomania: an unusual cause of hyponatremia at high risk of complications from rapid correction, *Am J Kidney Dis* 50:673-680, 2007.
9. Sanchez L, Corwell B, Berkoff D: Medical problems of marathon runners, *Am J Emer Med* 24:608-615, 2006.
10. Mentes J: Oral hydration in older adults: greater awareness is needed in preventing, recognizing, and treating dehydration, *Am J Nurs* 106(6):40-50, 2006.
11. Chang D, Feigenberg S, Indelicato D et al: Long-term outcomes in breast cancer patients with ten or more positive axillary nodes treated with combined-modality therapy: the importance of radiation field selection, *Intl J Radiat Oncol Biol Phys* 67(4):1043-1051, 2007.
12. Schaefer T, Wolford R: Disorders of potassium, *Emer Med Clin N Am* 23:723-747, 2005.
13. Liamis G, Mitrogianni Z, Liberopoulos E et al: Electrolyte disturbances in patients with hyponatremia, *Int Med* 46:685-690, 2007.
14. Yasue H, Itoh T, Mizuno Y et al: Severe hypokalemia, rhabdomyolysis, muscle paralysis, and respiratory impairment in a hypertensive patient taking herbal medicines containing licorice, *Int Med* 46:575-578, 2007.
15. Krishnan A, Colebach J, Kiernan M: Hypokalemic weakness in hyperaldosteronism: activity-dependent conduction block, *Neurol* 65(8):1309-1312, 2005.
16. Felver L: Fluid and electrolyte balance and imbalances. In Woods SL et al, editors: *Cardiac nursing*, ed 5, Philadelphia, 2005, Lippincott, pp 173-188.
17. Faccini M, Sala L, Malfatto G et al: Low-K^+ dependent QT prolongation and risk for ventricular arrhythmia in anorexia nervosa, *Intl J Cardiol* 106:170-176, 2006.
18. Van den Bosch A, van der Klooster J, Zuidgeest D et al: Severe hypokaelemic paralysis and rhabdomyolysis due to ingestion of liquorice, *Neth J Med* 63:146-148, 2005.
19. Karagiannis A, Tsorlalis I, Kakafika A et al: Acute renal failure due to tumor lysis syndrome in a patient with non-Hodgkin's lymphoma, *Ann Hematol* 84:343-346, 2005.
20. Musso C: Potassium metabolism in patients with chronic kidney disease (CKD), part I: patients not on dialysis (stages 3-4), *Intl Urol Nephrol* 36:465-468, 2004.
21. Sedlacek M, Schoolwerth A, Remillard B: Electrolyte disturbances in the intensive care unit, *Semin Dial* 19(6):496-501, 2006.
22. Iwazu Y, Muto S, Ikeuchi S et al: Reversible hypocalcemic heart failure with T wave alternans and increased QTc dispersion in a patient with chronic renal failure after parathyroidectomy, *Clin Nephrol* 65:65-70, 2006.
23. Van Poznak C: Hypercalcemia of malignancy remains a clinically relevant problem, *Cancer J* 12:21-23, 2006.
24. Gonzalez M, Cavalcanti T, Vianna C et al: Hypomagnesaemia causing QT interval prolongation and torsade de pointes in an alcoholic patient, *Resuscitation* 70:346-347, 2006.
25. Odvina C, Mason R, Pak C: Prevention of thiazide-induced hypokalemia without magnesium depletion by potassium-magnesium-citrate, *Am J Ther* 13:101-108, 2006.
26. Onishi S, Yoshino S: Cathartic-induced fatal hypermagnesemia in the elderly, *Int Med* 45:207-210, 2006.
27. Korbonits M, Blaine D, Elia M et al: Metabolic and hormonal changes during the refeeding period of prolonged fasting, *Eur J Endocrinol* 157:157-166, 2007.
28. Kestenbaum B: Mineral metabolism disturbances in patients with chronic kidney disease, *Eur J Clin Invest* 37:607-622, 2007.

Acid-Base Homeostasis and Imbalances

Linda Felver

MEDIA RESOURCES

Additional Material for Study, Review, and Further Exploration

CD Companion ■ Review Questions and Answers
■ Glossary (with audio pronunciations for selected terms)
■ Disease Profiles ■ Animations

evolve **Website** at http://evolve.elsevier.com/Copstead/
■ Case Studies ■ Disease Profiles ■ WebLinks ■ Key Points Review

 Online Course (Module 13)

KEY QUESTIONS

■ What are the chemistry and functional importance of the bicarbonate buffer system?
■ What is the role of the respiratory system in regulating carbonic acid (carbon dioxide)?
■ What is the role of the kidneys in regulating bicarbonate ion and acids other than carbonic acid?
■ How do the lungs compensate for acid-base imbalances resulting from altered levels of metabolic acids?

■ How do the kidneys compensate for acid-base imbalances resulting from altered levels of carbonic acid?
■ How are arterial blood gas values used to categorize an acid-base disorder as acidosis or alkalosis, respiratory or metabolic, compensated or not?
■ What pathophysiologic conditions predispose an individual to each of the four primary acid-base imbalances?

CHAPTER OUTLINE

When the pH of body fluids becomes abnormal, cellular function is impaired. The pH of a fluid reflects its degree of acidity or alkalinity. Technically, pH is the negative logarithm of the hydrogen ion (H^+) concentration. The normal hydrogen ion concentration of the blood is about 40 nmol/L (40×10^{-9} mol/L)—a very small number.[1] The pH (negative logarithm) of this number is 7.40, which is easier to use in clinical settings. An alteration in pH is a change in the hydrogen ion concentration.

An acid releases hydrogen ions. The more hydrogen ions present, the more acidic the solution. The normal pH of adult blood ranges from 7.35 to 7.45 (may vary slightly with different laboratories). The range is somewhat wider in infants and children. Table 25-1 lists normal laboratory values for pH and other acid-base parameters. If the blood and other body fluids become too acidic (reflected by pH decreased below the lower limit of the normal range), dysfunction occurs; if the pH of the blood falls below 6.9, death is likely to result.

TABLE 25-1

Normal Laboratory Values for Acid-Base Parameters

Characteristic	Normal Range
Pa_{CO_2} (arterial blood)	36-44 mm Hg (adults)
	30-34 mm Hg (infants)
HCO_3^- (serum)	22-26 mEq/L (adults)
	19-23 mEq/L (infants)
pH (arterial blood)	7.35-7.45 (adults)
	7.11-7.36 (neonates)
	7.36-7.41 (infants)

Similarly, if the body fluids become too alkaline, as reflected by pH increased above the upper limit of the normal range, dysfunction also occurs. If the pH of the blood rises above 7.8, death again is likely.

Normal cellular metabolism continually releases acids (carbonic and metabolic) that must be excreted from the body to prevent body fluids from becoming too acidic. This chapter discusses the normal mechanisms of acid-base homeostasis and the acid-base imbalances that arise when these homeostatic mechanisms become dysfunctional or overwhelmed.

ACID-BASE HOMEOSTASIS

Three major mechanisms regulate the acid-base status of the body: buffers, the respiratory system, and the renal system. Laboratory measurements such as arterial blood gas values are useful indicators of the acid-base status of extracellular fluids. The partial pressure of carbon dioxide in arterial blood (Pa_{CO_2}) is an indicator of the respiratory component of acid-base balance. The plasma bicarbonate ion (HCO_3^-) concentration is an indicator of the renal (metabolic) component of acid-base balance.[1] The pH of the blood indicates the net result of normal acid-base regulation, any acid-base imbalance, and the body's compensatory responses. It is important to remember that the pH measured clinically is that of the blood and may not reflect the pH inside cells or in cerebrospinal fluid.

Buffers

Buffers are chemicals that help control the pH of body fluids. Each buffer system consists of a weak acid, which releases hydrogen ions when the fluid is too alkaline, and a base, which takes up hydrogen ions when the fluid is too acidic. In this way, potential changes in pH are adjusted immediately by the action of buffers. All body fluids contain buffers. Chief among them are bicarbonate buffers (in the extracellular fluid), phosphate buffers (in intracellular fluid and urine), hemoglobin buffers (inside erythrocytes), and protein buffers (in intracellular fluid and the blood). These buffers are the first line of defense against pH imbalances.

The bicarbonate buffer system is the most important buffer in the extracellular fluid. Bicarbonate ions (HCO_3^-) and carbonic acid (H_2CO_3), the two components of the

bicarbonate buffer system, are in chemical equilibrium in the extracellular fluid.[2] If too much acid (e.g., lactic acid) is present, the bicarbonate ions take up hydrogen ions (H^+) released by the acid and become carbonic acid. Through the action of the enzyme carbonic anhydrase, the carbonic acid then is excreted through the respiratory system in the form of carbon dioxide and water. Thus the excess acid is neutralized when bicarbonate ions are used in the buffering process.

$$HCO_3^- + H^+ \rightleftharpoons H_2CO_3 \xrightarrow{\text{carbonic anhydrase}} CO_2 + H_2O$$

Conversely, if too little acid is present in the extracellular fluid, the carbonic acid portion of the bicarbonate buffer system releases hydrogen ions.

$$H_2CO_3 \rightleftharpoons HCO_3^- + H^+$$

The pH of any fluid is determined by the relative amounts of acids and bases contained in it. For the pH of the blood to be within the normal range, the ratio of bicarbonate ions to carbonic acid must be 20:1, which means that 20 bicarbonate ions must be present for every carbonic acid molecule. This relationship is explained formally by the Henderson-Hasselbalch equation, which is a mathematical description of the pH of a buffered solution, here written specifically for the bicarbonate buffer system.

$$pH = pK_a + \log \frac{[HCO_3^-]}{[H_2CO_3]}$$

Square brackets, used throughout this chapter, are a standard notation for concentration. pK_a is the dissociation constant for any particular acid; it equals 6.1 for carbonic acid.[2] If the normal 20:1 ratio of bicarbonate ions to carbonic acid is present, the pH will be 7.4.

$$pH = 6.1 + \log 20$$
$$pH = 6.1 + 1.3$$
$$pH = 7.4$$

The 20:1 ratio of bicarbonate ions to carbonic acid necessary for a normal pH is an important concept in understanding the compensatory mechanisms for acid-base imbalances that are discussed later in this chapter.

Respiratory Contribution

The respiratory system is the second defense against acid-base disorders. Body cells continuously produce carbon dioxide (CO_2). Together, CO_2 and water (H_2O) make carbonic acid (H_2CO_3). The lungs excrete carbon dioxide and water from the body. Therefore, during the process of exhalation the lungs effectively excrete carbonic acid. The respiratory system adjusts the amount of carbonic acid that remains in the body by altering rate and depth of respiration.

The rate and depth of respiration are influenced strongly by chemoreceptors that sense the Pa_{CO_2} and pH of the blood. If too much carbonic acid begins to accumulate in the blood of a healthy person, the rate and depth of respiration increase and excess carbonic acid is removed. This response corrects the imbalance and restores blood chemistry to normal. If, on the other hand, too little carbonic acid is present in the blood, the rate and depth of respiration decrease to retain carbonic acid until it once more is present in normal amounts. Again, the imbalance is corrected and the blood chemistry returns to normal. Thus the body's correction of a carbonic acid excess or deficit is dependent on normal function of all components of the respiratory system, including the chemoreceptors, respiratory neurons in the brainstem, motor nerves to respiratory muscles, diaphragm and other respiratory muscles, chest wall, and, of course, the airways, lungs, and pulmonary circulation. In older adults, the chemoreceptor response to increased $Paco_2$ may occur more slowly.

The $Paco_2$ indicates how effectively the respiratory system is excreting carbonic acid. If the $Paco_2$ is elevated above the upper limit of the normal range, carbonic acid has accumulated in the blood. In other words, the respiratory rate and depth have been too small or lung disease has prevented sufficient carbonic acid (carbon dioxide and water) excretion.[3] Similarly, if the $Paco_2$ is decreased below the lower limit of the normal range, the lungs have excreted more carbonic acid than usual. In other words, the respiratory rate and depth have been excessive.[4]

Carbonic acid is known as a volatile acid because it can be excreted as gases (CO_2 and H_2O). It is the only volatile acid in the body. Other acids that accumulate in the body, such as lactic acid and acetoacetic acid, are nonvolatile. They are organic acids that have no gaseous form. The lungs can excrete only carbonic acid; they cannot excrete nonvolatile acids that may accumulate in the body. If a nonvolatile acid (such as lactic acid) accumulates in the blood, rate and depth of respiration will increase because the excess hydrogen ions stimulate the chemoreceptors. This hyperventilation does not excrete lactic acid (which would correct the problem), but it does remove carbonic acid from the blood. Removing carbonic acid from the blood when another acid is present in excess helps keep the pH from dropping too low.[5] However, this response makes other values abnormal. The respiratory response to an imbalance of any acid except carbonic acid is called *compensation*. A compensatory response does not correct a pH disorder but it does compensate for it by adjusting the pH back toward normal, even though other blood chemistry values are made abnormal in the process.

The compensatory response to a deficit of any acid except carbonic acid is hypoventilation.[1] By decreasing rate and depth of respiration, the body retains carbonic acid. This carbonic acid accumulation helps keep blood pH from rising to a fatal level when another acid is deficient in the body. Respiratory compensation for an imbalance of metabolic acid begins in minutes but requires at least several hours for full effectiveness. Respiratory responses to changes in carbonic and metabolic acids are summarized in Table 25-2.

Renal Contribution

The third defense against acid-base disorders is the kidneys. The kidneys can excrete any acid from the body except carbonic acid (which is excreted by the lungs). Cells continuously produce metabolic acids during normal metabolism. The kidneys excrete these metabolic acids. If a metabolic acid begins to accumulate in the blood, the kidneys increase their acid excretion mechanisms to correct the problem. If a metabolic acid is deficient in the blood, the kidneys slow their acid excretion mechanisms to allow acid to accumulate to normal levels. The body's ability to correct an excess or deficit of a metabolic acid depends on normal function of the renal system. Infants excrete more bicarbonate in their urine than do older children or adults; their kidneys are less effective in excreting acid. The renal response to a large acid load also is less efficient in older adults.

The kidneys have several mechanisms that accomplish acid excretion.[2] Understanding these mechanisms requires a knowledge of basic renal physiology. Briefly, at the glomerulus, fluid filtered from the blood enters the glomerular (Bowman) capsule, which is the beginning of the nephron. The fluid inside the nephron (renal tubular fluid) is modified by the cells that line the lumen of the renal tubule. Renal tubular fluid that passes through the entire nephron becomes the urine. Renal tubular epithelial cells have different membrane structures on opposite sides of the cells. The luminal membrane (next to the renal tubular fluid) contains different transporter proteins than the basolateral membrane (next to the interstitial fluid). This structure allows these cells to secrete certain substances into the renal tubular fluid and move other substances into the interstitial fluid.

In the proximal tubules, renal tubular epithelial cells excrete metabolic acid by secreting hydrogen ions into the tubule lumen. For every hydrogen ion (H^+) that is secreted into the renal tubular fluid, one bicarbonate ion (HCO_3^-) is moved into the interstitial fluid.[6] The fluid filtered from the blood at the glomerulus contains many bicarbonate ions and most or all of that bicarbonate is reabsorbed (returned to the blood) during secretion of hydrogen ions. Renal tubular cells are able to secrete additional hydrogen ions into the tubular fluid to remove large amounts of hydrogen ions from metabolic acid.

Once the H^+ are in the renal tubular fluid, most of them combine with other chemicals: bicarbonate ions, which were

---

TABLE 25-2

Respiratory Responses to Changes in Carbonic and Metabolic Acids

Stimulus	Respiratory Response	Result
Increased $Paco_2$, decreased pH	Hyperventilation	Correction of imbalance
Decreased $Paco_2$, increased pH	Hypoventilation	Correction of imbalance
Decreased pH from excess of metabolic acids	Hyperventilation	Compensation for imbalance
Increased pH from deficit of metabolic acids	Hypoventilation	Compensation for imbalance

filtered at the glomerulus, as described previously; urine buffers, such as phosphate, which were filtered at the glomerulus; or ammonia (NH_3), which is produced by renal tubular cells. Net H^+ excretion occurs after HCO_3^- has been reabsorbed in the amount that was filtered at the glomerulus. Thus net H^+ excretion is accomplished in the form of buffered H^+ (called *titratable acidity*) and H^+ attached to ammonia (ammonium ions, NH_4^+). Figure 25-1 illustrates these processes. These processes operate also in the thick ascending limb of the loop of Henle and the distal nephron, where the intracellular chemistry differs slightly but the overall processes are the same.

When the kidneys need to excrete more hydrogen ions, renal tubular cells increase their production of ammonia (NH_3). Ammonia, a gas, moves easily into the renal tubular fluid where it combines with hydrogen ions to become ammonium ions (NH_4^+). Ammonium ions are not lipid soluble, so they do not cross easily from the renal tubular fluid back to the blood. Only free hydrogen ions contribute to the acidity of the urine, not those that are part of ammonium ions. Consequently, increased production of ammonia is an effective way of excreting more hydrogen ions in the renal tubular fluid without making the urine too acidic.

The concentration of HCO_3^- in plasma reflects the effectiveness of renal regulation of metabolic acids. If metabolic acids are accumulating in the blood, they will be buffered by HCO_3^- and the HCO_3^- concentration will drop below normal. Thus, a decreased concentration of HCO_3^- in plasma indicates a relative excess of metabolic acids. An increased HCO_3^- concentration in plasma indicates a relative deficit of metabolic acids (in other words, a relative excess of base).

Although the kidneys are unable to excrete carbonic acid, they can compensate for carbonic acid imbalances by adjusting the excretion of metabolic acids. For example, if carbonic acid accumulates in the blood, the kidneys can increase the excretion of metabolic acids. This compensatory action helps keep the pH of the blood from becoming too abnormal. Similarly, if a deficit of carbonic acid in the blood is prolonged, the kidneys will decrease the excretion of metabolic acids. As these metabolic acids accumulate in the blood, they will compensate for the lack of carbonic acid and return the pH of the blood toward normal. The body's compensatory response to an imbalance of one kind of acid thus returns the pH of the blood toward normal by creating an imbalance of another kind of acid. The renal compensatory response to an imbalance of carbonic acid requires several days to be fully operative.[7] Renal responses to changes in metabolic and carbonic acids are summarized in Table 25-3.

KEY POINTS

- During normal cellular metabolism, both carbon dioxide and metabolic acids are produced. Carbon dioxide (CO_2) combines with water (H_2O) to form carbonic acid (H_2CO_3). Both carbonic and metabolic acids must be excreted to maintain acid-base homeostasis.

- Buffers are chemicals (a weak acid plus its base) that prevent large changes in pH by releasing or taking up hydrogen ions (H^+). The bicarbonate buffer system is the most important buffer in the extracellular fluid. The normal ratio of bicarbonate to carbonic acid is 20:1. Any deviation from this ratio alters the pH of the blood.

- The lungs excrete carbon dioxide. Rate and depth of respiration normally are adjusted by chemoreceptors in response to acid-base and oxygen status. Increased ventilation (hyperventilation) decreases the amount of carbon dioxide in blood and thus reduces the amount of carbonic acid. Decreased ventilation (hypoventilation) allows carbon dioxide to accumulate and thus increases the amount of carbonic acid in the blood.

- The kidneys excrete metabolic acids. They can secrete H^+ into the renal tubular fluid and retain HCO_3^- in the body or may allow some HCO_3^- to be excreted, depending on homeostatic demands. Most H^+ in the urine is buffered (titratable acidity) or in the form of ammonium ions. The concentration of HCO_3^- in plasma reflects the relative amount of metabolic acid in the blood.

- The lungs compensate for acid-base imbalances resulting from altered levels of metabolic acids; the kidneys compensate for acid-base imbalances resulting from altered levels of carbonic acid. With compensation, the pH returns toward normal but $Paco_2$ and HCO_3^- levels are abnormal.

ACID-BASE IMBALANCES

The four primary acid-base disorders are metabolic acidosis, respiratory acidosis, metabolic alkalosis, and respiratory alkalosis. Acidosis is the presence of a condition that tends to decrease the pH of the blood below normal (make the blood relatively more acidic). If blood pH actually is decreased, *acidemia* also is present. Alkalosis is the presence of any factor that tends to increase the pH of the blood above normal (make the blood relatively more alkaline). The term *alkalemia* denotes an increased blood pH. The pathophysiology of the four primary acid-base disorders can be reasoned logically from the principles of acid-base homeostasis.

Metabolic Acidosis

Etiology. Metabolic acidosis is a condition that tends to cause a relative excess of any acid except carbonic acid.[8] Metabolic acidosis may be caused by an increase in acid (not carbonic), by a decrease in base, or by a combination of the two. These mechanisms decrease the normal 20:1 ratio of HCO_3^- to H_2CO_3.

An increase of any acid except carbonic acid will decrease the normal ratio of bicarbonate to carbonic acid because the bicarbonate ions are used up in buffering the excess acid. For example, when caloric intake is insufficient, as with prolonged fasting, the body begins to use its fat stores for energy. If too little glucose is ingested, the fat is metabolized incompletely and ketoacids accumulate in the blood. This condition is termed *starvation ketoacidosis.*[9]

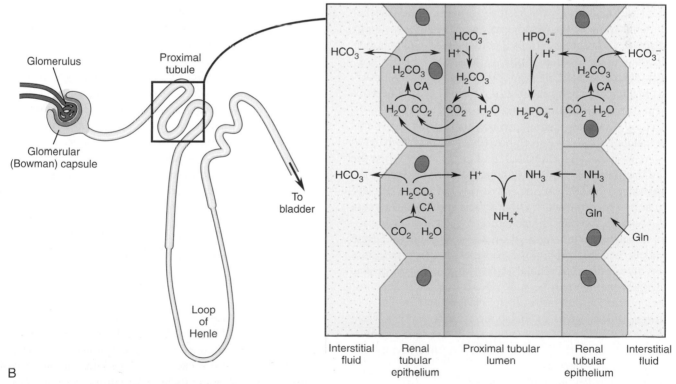

FIGURE 25-1 A, Diagram of a nephron. **B,** Renal proximal tubule mechanisms for excretion of metabolic acid. Hydrogen ions secreted into the renal tubular lumen combine with filtered bicarbonate (which then is reabsorbed), buffers (phosphate buffer illustrated here), or ammonia (forming ammonium ions). *CA,* Carbonic anhydrase, an enzyme; *Gln,* glutamine, an amino acid. (**A,** From Solomon EP: *Introduction to human anatomy and physiology,* ed 3, St. Louis, 2009, Mosby, p 266.)

TABLE 25-3

Renal Responses to Changes in Metabolic and Carbonic Acids

Stimulus	Renal Response	Result
Decreased pH from excess of metabolic acids	Secrete more H$^+$ Make more ammonia	Correction of imbalance
Increased pH from deficit of metabolic acids	Secrete fewer H$^+$ Make less ammonia Excrete HCO$_3^-$	Correction of imbalance
Decreased pH from excess of carbonic acid	Secrete more H$^+$ Make more ammonia	Compensation for imbalance
Increased pH from deficit of carbonic acid	Secrete fewer H$^+$ Make less ammonia Excrete HCO$_3^-$	Compensation for imbalance

BOX 25-1

Common Causes of Metabolic Acidosis

Increase in Acid
Ketoacidosis (diabetes mellitus, starvation, alcoholism)
Severe hyperthyroidism
Severe infection
Burns
Circulatory shock
Tissue anoxia
Oliguric renal failure
Intake of acids or acid precursors (e.g., salicylates, methanol, ethylene glycol)

Decrease in Base
Diarrhea
Gastrointestinal fistula that drains intestinal or pancreatic secretions
Intestinal decompression
Renal tubular acidosis

Bicarbonate ions are a type of base. Any condition that causes excessive removal of bicarbonate ions from the body may cause metabolic acidosis. For example, the intestinal fluid is rich in bicarbonate ions, which originate from pancreatic secretions. Diarrhea causes removal of this base from the body and thus contributes to the development of metabolic acidosis.[10]

Other causes of metabolic acidosis are listed in Box 25-1 under the two general mechanisms discussed: increase in acid (except carbonic acid) and decrease in base. Either mechanism tends to make the blood overly acidic. Pathophysiology of diarrhea and other disorders that may cause metabolic acidosis is discussed in other chapters of this text.

Clinical Manifestations. Signs and symptoms of metabolic acidosis include headache, abdominal pain, and central nervous system depression (confusion, lethargy, stupor, coma).

Central nervous system depression that occurs in patients with metabolic acidosis is due primarily to the decreased pH of the cerebrospinal and interstitial fluid in the brain. When the pH of the interstitial fluid falls, intracellular pH decreases, the protein structure and enzyme activity in cells are altered, and cellular dysfunction results. Other factors specific to the cause of the acidosis also may induce central nervous system depression, such as hyperosmolality with diabetic ketoacidosis. Severe metabolic acidosis predisposes to ventricular dysrhythmias (from myocardial intracellular acidity) and decreased cardiac contractility, which may be fatal.[8] Death from brainstem dysfunction usually occurs when the pH falls below 6.9.

Arterial blood gases in metabolic acidosis show a bicarbonate concentration below normal. If metabolic acidosis is uncompensated, the pH also is below normal because the usual 20:1 ratio is decreased.

Uncompensated metabolic acidosis:

$$\frac{\text{Decreased [HCO}_3^-]}{\text{Unchanged [H}_2\text{CO}_3]} = \text{pH low}$$

Compensatory Response. The respiratory compensation for metabolic acidosis is hyperventilation. The low blood pH stimulates the peripheral chemoreceptors, which then stimulate ventilatory neurons in the brainstem.[2] The end result is increased rate and depth of respiration. As the rate and depth of respiration increase, more carbonic acid (carbon dioxide and water) is excreted. Although hyperventilation does not remove metabolic acid from the body, it does change the ratio of bicarbonate ions to carbonic acid in a favorable direction. Because the bicarbonate ion concentration already is decreased by the metabolic acidosis, the compensatory decrease in carbonic acid brings the ratio (and thus the pH) back toward normal.

The arterial blood gases of a person who has compensated metabolic acidosis show decreased bicarbonate concentration (the primary imbalance), decreased Paco$_2$ (compensation), and slightly decreased or even normal pH, depending on the degree of compensation. A flowchart for interpreting laboratory measures specific to acid-base imbalances is presented in Figure 25-2. Sample laboratory values for people with metabolic acidosis are presented in Table 25-4.

Compensated metabolic acidosis:

$$\frac{\text{Decreased [HCO}_3^-]\text{ (primary)}}{\text{Decreased [H}_2\text{CO}_3]\text{ (compensatory)}} = \begin{array}{l}\text{pH slightly low}\\\text{(partially compensated)}\\\textit{or }\text{pH in the normal range}\\\text{(fully compensated)}\end{array}$$

Respiratory Acidosis

Etiology. Respiratory acidosis is a condition that tends to cause an excess of carbonic acid.[8] This condition is aptly named because carbonic acid is excreted by the lungs in the form of carbon dioxide and water during exhalation.

Respiratory acidosis is caused by factors that impair the respiratory excretion of carbonic acid. Such factors include impaired gas exchange, inadequate neuromuscular function, and

*To differentiate between possible fully compensated imbalances with the pH in the normal range, look at the previous laboratory values for the patient. If no previous values are available, choose the acidosis if the pH is below 7.40 and the alkalosis if the pH is above 7.40.

FIGURE 25-2 Flowchart for interpretation of laboratory measurements specific for acid-base imbalances. Use this flowchart to determine the primary acid-base imbalance from a set of laboratory values. Begin on the left with $Paco_2$ and follow the *arrows*. This flowchart does not include mixed acid-base imbalances.

impairment of respiratory control in the brainstem. Box 25-2 provides examples of factors that may cause respiratory acidosis. These factors all decrease the normal 20:1 ratio of bicarbonate ion to carbonic acid (and thus decrease the pH of the blood) by increasing the carbonic acid portion of the ratio. Chronic respiratory acidosis often develops in people who have chronic obstructive pulmonary disease (COPD), especially Type B COPD. If an acute respiratory infection also develops, their acidosis may become worse.[3] Such a condition may be termed *acute-on-chronic respiratory acidosis.* Pathophysiology of COPD and other disorders that may cause respiratory acidosis is discussed in other chapters of this text.

Clinical Manifestations Signs and symptoms of respiratory acidosis are headache, tachycardia, cardiac dysrhythmias, and neurologic abnormalities such as blurred vision, tremors, vertigo, disorientation, lethargy, or somnolence.

Headache occurs because of dilation of blood vessels in the brain. This cerebral vasodilation increases cerebrospinal fluid pressure; papilledema may result. Neurologic manifestations may be more prominent in patients with respiratory acidosis than in those with metabolic acidosis because carbonic acid (in the form of carbon dioxide and water) crosses the blood-brain barrier relatively easily. The neurologic manifestations are due to the decreased pH of the cerebrospinal and interstitial fluid in the brain. This decreased interstitial fluid pH causes decreased intracellular pH, with resulting cellular dysfunction. Cardiac dysrhythmias in patients with respiratory acidosis occur due to decreased pH inside myocardial cells.[8,11] Severe respiratory acidosis causes peripheral vasodilation and hypotension may result, especially if cardiac dysrhythmias also are present.

Arterial blood gases in patients with respiratory acidosis show $Paco_2$ above normal. If respiratory acidosis is

TABLE 25-4

Sample Laboratory Values for People with Acid-Base Imbalances

Laboratory Value for Imbalance	Explanation
Partially Compensated Metabolic Acidosis (Diabetic Ketoacidosis)	
Pa_{CO_2} 30 mm Hg	Decreased because of compensatory hyperventilation
HCO_3^- 12 mEq/L	Decreased because of buffering of ketoacids
pH 7.22	Decreased because of excess metabolic acids; would be even lower without respiratory compensation
Uncompensated Respiratory Acidosis (Acute Asthma Episode)	
Pa_{CO_2} 55 mm Hg	Increased because of impaired gas exchange
HCO_3^- 24 mEq/L	Normal; renal compensation has not yet occurred in this acute condition
pH 7.26	Decreased because of excess carbonic acid
Fully Compensated Respiratory Acidosis (Type B COPD)	
Pa_{CO_2} 60 mm Hg	Increased because of impaired gas exchange
HCO_3^- 36 mEq/L	Increased because of renal compensation in this chronic condition
pH 7.35	Normal because of renal compensation, but below 7.4
Uncompensated Metabolic Alkalosis (Repeated Emesis and ECV Depletion)	
Pa_{CO_2} 42 mm Hg	Normal, but increasing because of compensatory hypoventilation
HCO_3^- 36 mEq/L	Increased because of loss of H^+ from emesis and renal retention of HCO_3^- from ECV depletion
pH 7.52	Increased because of metabolic acid deficit
Uncompensated Respiratory Alkalosis (Hypoxemia from Pulmonary Embolism)	
Pa_{CO_2} 28 mm Hg	Decreased because of hyperventilation caused by chemoreceptor response to decreased Pa_{O_2}
HCO_3^- 24 mEq/L	Normal; renal compensation has not yet occurred in this acute condition
pH 7.52	Increased because of carbonic acid deficit

ECV, Extracellular fluid volume

BOX 25-2

Common Causes of Respiratory Acidosis

Impaired Gas Exchange
Chronic obstructive pulmonary disease (COPD)
Pneumonia
Severe asthma
Pulmonary edema
Acute (adult) respiratory distress syndrome
Obstructive sleep apnea

Impaired Neuromuscular Function
Guillain-Barré syndrome
Chest injury or surgery (pain limits ventilation)
Hypokalemic respiratory muscle weakness
Severe kyphoscoliosis
Respiratory muscle fatigue

Impaired Respiratory Control (Brainstem)
Respiratory depressant drugs (opioids, barbiturates)
Central sleep apnea

uncompensated, the pH is below normal because the usual 20:1 ratio is decreased.[1]

Uncompensated respiratory acidosis:

$$\frac{\text{Unchanged [HCO}_3\text{]}}{\text{Increased [H}_2\text{CO}_3\text{]}} = \text{pH low}$$

Compensatory Response. The compensatory response to respiratory acidosis is increased renal excretion of metabolic acid. This mechanism requires several days to be effective. Although the kidneys cannot excrete carbonic acid, their ability to excrete more metabolic acid changes the ratio of bicarbonate ions to carbonic acid in a favorable direction so that the pH moves toward normal. As the kidneys excrete more metabolic acid, the bicarbonate concentration increases because fewer bicarbonate ions are used for buffering. Because carbonic acid concentration already is increased, the compensatory increase in bicarbonate concentration tends to normalize the ratio of HCO_3^- to H_2CO_3. The arterial blood gases of a person who has compensated respiratory acidosis show increased Pa_{CO_2} (the primary imbalance), increased bicarbonate concentration (compensation), and slightly decreased or even normal pH, depending on the degree of compensation. Table 25-4 presents sample laboratory values for people with respiratory acidosis.

Compensated respiratory acidosis:

$$\frac{\text{Increased [HCO}_3\text{]}}{\text{(compensatory)}} = \begin{array}{l} \text{pH slightly low} \\ \text{(partially compensated)} \\ \textit{or} \text{ pH in the normal range} \\ \text{(fully compensated)} \end{array}$$
$$\text{Increased [H}_2\text{CO}_3\text{]}$$
$$\text{(primary)}$$

Metabolic Alkalosis

Etiology. Metabolic alkalosis is a condition that tends to cause a relative deficit of any acid except carbonic acid.[8] Metabolic

BOX 25-3

Common Causes of Metabolic Alkalosis

Increase in Base
Intake of bicarbonate or bicarbonate precursors (acetate, citrate, lactate)
Massive transfusion with citrated blood
Mild or moderate extracellular fluid volume deficit

Decrease in Acid
Emesis
Gastric suction
Mild or moderate extracellular fluid volume deficit
Hyperaldosteronism
Hypokalemia

alkalosis may be caused by an increase in base (bicarbonate), by a decrease in acid, or by a combination of the two. Bicarbonate may be ingested in antacids such as baking soda and over-the-counter bicarbonate products (e.g., effervescent antacids). With overuse of these agents, enough bicarbonate is absorbed from the gastrointestinal tract to increase the blood bicarbonate concentration, thus increasing the pH.[12]

In addition to a gain in bicarbonate, metabolic alkalosis also may be caused by a decrease in acid. The stomach is a major reservoir of acid. Emesis and gastric suction remove acid from the body and create a relative excess of base; this situation is, by definition, metabolic alkalosis. Increased renal excretion of acid with retention of bicarbonate occurs in extracellular fluid volume deficit.[13] Metabolic alkalosis due to mild or moderate extracellular fluid volume deficit often is called *contraction alkalosis* and is common during diuretic therapy. (Severe extracellular fluid volume deficit is associated with tissue anoxia, circulatory shock, and metabolic acidosis.) Hypokalemia causes metabolic alkalosis by shifting hydrogen ions into cells and increasing renal excretion of acid.

Causes of metabolic alkalosis are summarized in Box 25-3. Pathophysiology of the disorders that may cause metabolic alkalosis is discussed in other chapters of this text.

Clinical Manifestations. Signs and symptoms in patients who have metabolic alkalosis may arise from the extracellular fluid volume depletion that caused the alkalosis. Thus postural hypotension may be present. Hypokalemia frequently coexists with metabolic alkalosis.[14] As described previously, hypokalemia may cause metabolic alkalosis. In addition, metabolic alkalosis that arises from another cause frequently induces hypokalemia by shifting potassium ions into cells. Regardless of whether the hypokalemia preceded or followed the metabolic alkalosis, the bilateral muscle weakness of hypokalemia frequently is evident in individuals who have metabolic alkalosis.

In people who experience signs and symptoms from the metabolic alkalosis itself, the initial manifestations are those of increased neuromuscular excitability.[16] Fingers and toes may tingle; signs of tetany may progress to seizures. Increased interstitial pH causes increased excitability of nerve cell membranes. In addition, alkalosis causes more ionized calcium

to bind to albumin, thus causing an ionized hypocalcemia that contributes to increased neuromuscular excitability. People who develop metabolic alkalosis may become quite belligerent. With severe metabolic alkalosis, initial excitation may change to central nervous system depression. Confusion, lethargy, and coma may ensue from dysfunction of brain cells. Death occurs when the pH is around 7.8. The plasma bicarbonate concentration is elevated in people with metabolic alkalosis.

Uncompensated metabolic alkalosis:

$$\frac{\text{Increased [HCO}_3^-]}{\text{Unchanged [H}_2\text{CO}_3]} = \text{pH high}$$

Compensatory Response. The compensatory response to metabolic alkalosis is hypoventilation. This shallow breathing retains carbonic acid within the body, thus increasing the lower portion of the bicarbonate ion–to–carbonic acid ratio. Because the upper portion of the ratio has been increased by the elevated bicarbonate concentration of metabolic alkalosis, the respiratory compensation tends to move the pH toward normal. However, respiratory compensation for metabolic alkalosis usually is incomplete. The need for oxygen drives ventilation, even though the increased pH tends to depress it. Thus the arterial blood gases of a person who has compensated metabolic alkalosis usually show increased bicarbonate concentration (the primary imbalance), increased $Paco_2$ (compensation), and slightly increased pH. Table 25-4 presents sample laboratory values for people with metabolic alkalosis.

Compensated metabolic alkalosis:

$$\frac{\text{Increased [HCO}_3^-] \text{ (primary)}}{\text{Increased [H}_2\text{CO}_3] \text{ (compensatory)}} = \begin{array}{c}\text{pH slightly high}\\ \text{(partially compensated)}\end{array}$$

Respiratory Alkalosis

Etiology. Respiratory alkalosis is a condition that tends to cause a carbonic acid deficit.[8] With a deficit of carbonic acid, the blood is relatively too alkaline.

Respiratory alkalosis is caused by hyperventilation.[4] Carbonic acid is excreted during exhalation; when respirations are excessively rapid and deep (hyperventilation), too much carbonic acid is excreted. The resulting deficit of carbonic acid is respiratory alkalosis. For example, in gram-negative sepsis, respiratory neurons in the brainstem often are stimulated abnormally, causing hyperventilation. Other causes of hyperventilation (and thus of respiratory alkalosis) are listed in Box 25-4.

Clinical Manifestations. Clinical manifestations of respiratory alkalosis arise from increased neuromuscular excitability. Paresthesias (numbness and tingling) often occur in the fingers and around the mouth; carpal and pedal spasm may occur. Increased extracellular pH has a direct effect of increasing membrane excitability in both central and peripheral neurons. In addition, increased pH of the cerebrospinal fluid and cerebral interstitial fluid alters brain cell function, causing confusion in some people. Respiratory alkalosis causes cerebral vasoconstriction, which reduces blood flow in the brain.

Common Causes of Respiratory Alkalosis (Hyperventilation)

Hypoxemia
Acute pain
Anxiety, psychological distress
Prolonged sobbing
Alcohol withdrawal
Stimulation of the brainstem (salicylate overdose, meningitis, head injury, gram-negative sepsis)

The alkalosis also decreases the availability of ionized calcium, which contributes to increased neuromuscular excitability.

The increased excretion of carbonic acid in people with respiratory alkalosis causes the Pa_{CO_2} to be abnormally low. If the imbalance is uncompensated, the pH is abnormally high.

Uncompensated respiratory alkalosis:

$$\frac{\text{Unchanged } [HCO_3^-]}{\text{Decreased } [H_2CO_3]} = \text{pH high}$$

Compensatory Response. The compensatory response to respiratory alkalosis is decreased renal excretion of metabolic acid. As metabolic acids accumulate in the blood, the bicarbonate ion concentration decreases because bicarbonate ions are used for buffering. Because the carbonic acid concentration already is decreased, renal compensation for respiratory alkalosis tends to return the ratio of bicarbonate ions to carbonic acid, and thus the pH, toward normal. Renal compensatory mechanisms take several days to be fully effective. Many of the causes of respiratory alkalosis are short lived and, for that reason, may not be compensated renally. Arterial blood gases of a person who has compensated respiratory alkalosis show decreased Pa_{CO_2} (the primary imbalance), decreased bicarbonate concentration (compensation), and slightly increased or perhaps normal pH, depending on the degree of compensation. Table 25-4 presents sample laboratory values for people with respiratory alkalosis.

Compensated respiratory alkalosis:

$$\frac{\begin{array}{c}\text{Decreased } [HCO_3^-] \\ \text{(compensatory)}\end{array}}{\begin{array}{c}\text{Decreased } [H_2CO_3] \\ \text{(primary)}\end{array}} = \begin{array}{c}\text{pH slightly high} \\ \text{(partially compensated)} \\ \textit{or } \text{pH in the normal range} \\ \text{(fully compensated)}\end{array}$$

Mixed Acid-Base Imbalances

In most people, only one of the four primary imbalances discussed in this chapter arises at a time. If the imbalance persists, a compensatory imbalance arises as well. This situation was discussed previously in this chapter. Occasionally, however, two primary imbalances arise in the same person.[17] This latter situation is termed a *mixed acid-base imbalance*.[1] For example, a patient who has bacterial pneumonia may develop respiratory acidosis. If severe *C. difficile*–associated diarrhea develops during antibiotic therapy for the pneumonia, a concurrent metabolic acidosis may arise. In this mixed imbalance, the pH is likely to be very low because the two types of primary acidosis impair the effectiveness of the usual compensatory mechanisms. Specifically, the usual compensatory mechanism for metabolic acidosis is hyperventilation, which causes increased excretion of carbonic acid from the body. With bacterial pneumonia, however, the effectiveness of alveolar ventilation is already impaired and carbonic acid is being retained in the blood. Analogously, patients who have both types of primary alkalosis often have a very high pH because their usual compensatory mechanisms are impeded by the concurrent acid-base disorders.

Mixed acid-base disorders may also occur with a nearly normal pH if a primary acidosis and a primary alkalosis are involved. An example of this type of mixed disorder is a head-injured patient whose treatment includes hyperventilation by mechanical ventilation to reduce intracranial pressure (respiratory alkalosis) but who at the same time has a metabolic acidosis from acute renal failure. In this situation, the Pa_{CO_2} is decreased (respiratory alkalosis), the plasma bicarbonate concentration is decreased (metabolic acidosis), and the pH depends on the relative severity of the two imbalances.

KEY POINTS

- Acidosis is a condition that tends to cause a relative excess of acid. Alkalosis is a condition that tends to cause a relative excess of base.
- Metabolic acidosis is characterized by pH below 7.40 and abnormally low HCO_3^-. It is caused by processes that lead to metabolic acid accumulation (e.g., lactic acidosis) or loss of HCO_3^- (e.g., diarrhea). Compensatory hyperventilation decreases the Pa_{CO_2}.
- Metabolic alkalosis is characterized by pH above 7.40 and abnormally high HCO_3^-. It is caused by processes that lead to metabolic acid loss (e.g., vomiting) or gain of HCO_3^- (e.g., bicarbonate antacids). Compensatory hypoventilation increases the Pa_{CO_2}.
- Respiratory acidosis is characterized by pH below 7.40 and abnormally high Pa_{CO_2}. It is caused by processes that lead to hypoventilation by impairing gas exchange (e.g., lung diseases), neuromuscular function of the chest (e.g., hypokalemic muscle paralysis), or respiratory control mechanisms in the brainstem (e.g., opioid overdose). Compensatory excretion of H^+ and retention of HCO_3^- by the kidneys increase the HCO_3^- concentration.
- Respiratory alkalosis is characterized by pH above 7.40 and abnormally low Pa_{CO_2}. It is caused by processes that lead to hyperventilation (e.g., hypoxemia, pain, anxiety). Compensatory retention of H^+ and excretion of HCO_3^- by the kidneys decrease the HCO_3^- concentration.
- Mixed acid-base disorders occur when two primary acid-base disorders are present independently. They may arise from simultaneous dysfunction of the respiratory system and kidneys. Depending on the combination of disorders, the pH may be nearly normal or grossly abnormal.

SUMMARY

Acid-base homeostasis involves the interplay of buffers, the respiratory system, and renal mechanisms. Metabolic acids are produced continually by cellular metabolism. These metabolic acids enter the blood, where they are buffered, and eventually are excreted by the kidneys. In healthy people, the kidneys adjust the rate of excretion of metabolic acids to meet the demands of the acid load being produced. The concentration of bicarbonate ions in the blood indicates the effectiveness of renal excretion of metabolic acids. Carbon dioxide and water (carbonic acid) that also are produced by cellular metabolism are excreted by the lungs. In healthy people, changes in the respiratory rate and depth adjust the rate of excretion of carbonic acid appropriately. The $Paco_2$ indicates the effectiveness of respiratory excretion of carbonic acid.

If one of the acid-base regulatory mechanisms becomes dysfunctional or overwhelmed, another mechanism can produce a compensatory response that will help normalize the pH of the extracellular fluid, even though it will not correct the acid-base imbalance. Thus the kidneys adjust their excretion of metabolic acids when respiratory excretion of carbonic acid is altered abnormally. Similarly, the respiratory system adjusts the rate of excretion of carbonic acid if renal regulation of metabolic acids is impaired or overwhelmed. The pH of the blood at any time is the net result of the operation of these regulatory and compensatory mechanisms.

Primary acid-base imbalances arise when the normal regulatory mechanisms for acid-base homeostasis become impaired or are overwhelmed by a large acid or alkaline load. Pediatric and geriatric variations are summarized in Boxes 25-5 and 25-6, respectively. Primary metabolic acidosis arises when the kidneys are unable to excrete enough metabolic acid, or bicarbonate is lost from the body. The compensatory response to metabolic acidosis is hyperventilation. Primary respiratory acidosis arises when the lungs are unable to excrete enough carbonic acid. The compensatory response to respiratory acidosis is increased renal excretion of metabolic acid.

Primary metabolic alkalosis arises when the kidneys excrete too much metabolic acid or there is a gain of bicarbonate. The compensatory response to metabolic alkalosis is hypoventilation. Primary respiratory alkalosis arises when the lungs excrete too much carbonic acid. The compensatory response to sustained respiratory alkalosis is decreased renal excretion of metabolic acid. The $Paco_2$ reflects the respiratory component of an acid-base imbalance, and the plasma bicarbonate concentration reflects the metabolic (renal) component of an acid-base imbalance.

A mixed acid-base imbalance occurs when two primary imbalances exist at the same time. The two primary imbalances may drive the pH to an extremely abnormal value or may nearly cancel each other's effect on the pH, although the $Paco_2$ and plasma bicarbonate concentration may still be very abnormal.

BOX 25-5

Pediatric Variations

- Neonates often have mild metabolic acidosis. Infants younger than 1 month have a reduced ability to excrete a large acid load; their kidneys are less able to reabsorb bicarbonate, they produce less ammonia, and urinary buffers are limited in quantity. These factors increase the risk of metabolic acidosis from acid accumulation.
- Adolescents with eating disorders may develop metabolic alkalosis from repeated emesis or metabolic acidosis from starvation and laxative-induced chronic diarrhea.

BOX 25-6

Geriatric Variations

- The chemoreceptor response to increased $Paco_2$ (hyperventilation) is delayed in older adults, which may delay their ability to correct respiratory acidosis.
- Older adults are at increased risk of respiratory depression (and thus respiratory acidosis) from barbiturates because of increased drug half-life.
- Older adults' kidneys are less able to excrete a large acid load, which increases the risk for metabolic acidosis from acid accumulation.
- Diarrhea from chronic laxative overuse may contribute to metabolic acidosis.

REFERENCES

1. Rose BD, Post TW: *Clinical physiology of acid-base and electrolyte disorders,* ed 5, New York, 2001, McGraw-Hill.
2. Guyton AC, Hall AE: *Textbook of medical physiology,* ed 11, Philadelphia, 2006, Saunders.
3. Ucgun I, Metintas M, Moral H et al: Predictors of hospital outcome and intubation in COPD patients admitted to the respiratory ICU for acute hypercapnic respiratory failure, *Resp Med* 100:66-74, 2006.
4. Abbiss C, Nosaka K, Laursen P: Hyperthermic-induced hyperventilation and associated respiratory alkalosis in humans, *Eur J Appl Physiol* 100:63-69, 2007.
5. Ward S: Ventilatory control in humans: constraints and limitations, *Exp Physiol* 92:357-366, 2007.
6. Boron WF: Acid-base transport by the renal proximal tubule, *J Am Soc Nephrol* 17:2368-2382, 2006.
7. de Seigneux S, Malte H, Dimke H et al: Renal compensation to chronic hypoxic hypercapnia: downregulation of pendrin and adaptation of the proximal tubule, *Am J Physiol* 292:F1256-F1266, 2007.
8. Felver L: Acid-base balance and imbalances. In Woods SL et al, editors: *Cardiac nursing,* ed 5, Philadelphia, 2005, Lippincott, pp 189-196.
9. Ensminger SA, Regner KR, Froehling DA: 35-year-old woman with cough, fever, and anorexia, *Mayo Clin Proc* 78:753-756, 2003.
10. Bar A, Riskin A, Iancu T et al: A newborn infant with protracted diarrhea and metabolic acidosis, *J Pediatr* 150:198-201, 2007.
11. Crampin E, Smith N, Langham A et al: Acidosis in models of cardiac ventricular myocytes, *Phil Trans Royal Soc London, Series A* 364:1171-1186, 2006.

12. Grotegut C, Dandolu V, Katari S et al: Baking soda pica: a case of hypokalemic metabolic alkalosis and rhabdomyolysis in pregnancy, *Obstet Gynecol* 107(2 Pt 2):484-486, 2006.

13. Schoolwerth A, Kaneko T, Sedlacek M et al: Acid-base disturbances in the intensive care unit: metabolic acidosis, *Semin Dial* 19:492-495, 2006.

14. McCauley M, Gunawardane M, Cowan M: Severe metabolic alkalosis due to pyloric obstruction: case presentation, evaluation, and management, *Am J Med Sci* 332:346-350, 2006.

15. Gawarammana I, Coburn J, Greene S et al: Severe hypokalaemic metabolic alkalosis following ingestion of gaviscon, *Clin Toxicol* 45(2):176-178, 2007.

16. Chou C, Chen Y, Chau T et al: Acquired bartter-like syndrome associated with gentamicin administration, *Am J Med Sci* 329(3):144-149, 2005.

17. Al-Jubouri M, Inkster G, Nee P et al: Thyrotoxicosis presenting as hypokalaemic paralysis and hyperlactataemia in an oriental man, *Ann Clin Biochem* 43(Pt 4):323-325, 2006.

Renal Failure and Dialysis

Sheila K. Smith • Fadi Ghandour • Michael J. Kirkhorn

The kidney has multiple functions. Kidneys excrete urine through the activity of about 2 million nephrons, each of which is able to filter the urine from the blood. After the urine is filtered in the glomerulus, part is reabsorbed and another part passes to the renal pelvis. In this way, kidneys clean unwanted substances—metabolic end products or excess ions of sodium, potassium, chloride, or hydrogen—from the blood plasma.

The kidneys are important blood pressure regulators. The rate at which they dispose of extracellular fluid helps keep the arterial pressure at normal levels. Kidneys are endocrine organs as well; they secrete erythropoietin, the hormone that regulates red blood cell production and converts vitamin D to its active form.

Elevated blood pressure, if not well controlled, can lead to congestive heart failure, adverse cardiovascular events, and kidney failure. When diseased, the kidney can cause hypertension, and if hypertension is not controlled, it can cause kidney damage.

Chronic kidney disease is a worldwide public health problem. In the United States, the incidence and prevalence of chronic kidney disease are increasing. End-stage kidney (renal) disease (ESRD), the point at which renal dialysis or transplant is required, is a drastic end point of kidney failure. Since 1972 federal Medicare funding has covered the costs of treatment for approximately 90% of persons in the U.S. with ESRD. Current estimates for the total cost of Medicare-funded ESRD programs exceed $28 billion, for 661,330 patients. The incidence of ESRD disease has been increasing almost 8% to 10% each year. The severity of this disease is suggested by the fact that more than 60% of ESRD patients die within 5 years.

Fibrin stain showing platelet-fibrin thrombi (red) in the glomerular capillaries, characteristic of microangiopathic disorders. (From Kumar V et al: Robbins and Cotran pathologic basis of disease, ed 7, Philadelphia, 2005, Saunders.)

Renal and Bladder Function

Diabetes is the most common cause of ESRD, followed by hypertension. There are striking racial and ethnic differences in the incidence and prevalence of ESRD. African Americans, American Indians, Alaskan Natives, Native Hawaiians, and Hispanic persons have a disproportionately high incidence and prevalence of ESRD. It is possible that differential access to health care and attention to the adequate management of chronic kidney disease for minority groups may be a cause of concern. Few studies have shown a correlation between environmental factors and the development and progression of chronic renal disease.

Transplantation is the best treatment for patients with ESRD. Transplantation prolongs and improves the quality of life. Patients need lifelong medications to prevent rejection of the transplant kidney. These medications have major side effects and can cause a variety of complications. Hemodialysis is used in patients with severely impaired kidney function. It can be inconvenient and time consuming, as hemodialysis at a dialysis center requires three sessions each week for 3 to 4 hours per session. Peritoneal dialysis, on the other hand, offers a lifestyle alternative in that the patient undergoes dialysis at home through a catheter placed in the abdomen. Both methods of dialysis are effective, but carry their own risks and complications.

Chronic kidney disease of differing etiologies is managed with blood pressure management, using at times several antihypertensive medications. These patients are followed up closely by their nephrologist to help them avoid dialysis as much as possible. Disease issues faced by chronic kidney disease patients include fluid overload, elevated potassium levels, bone disease, anemia, acid management, infection control, and special diet control.

chapter 26

Renal Function

Jacquelyn L. Banasik

MEDIA RESOURCES

Additional Material for Study, Review, and Further Exploration

CD Companion ■ Review Questions and Answers ■ Glossary (with audio pronunciations for selected terms) ■ Disease Profiles ■ Animations

Website at http://evolve.elsevier.com/Copstead/
■ Case Studies ■ Disease Profiles ■ WebLinks ■ Key Points Review

Online Course (Module 14)

KEY QUESTIONS

- How does the structure of the glomerulus determine the composition of the tubular filtrate?
- What factors determine glomerular filtration rate?
- How do individual nephrons regulate their glomerular filtration rates?
- How are solutes and water transported across the renal tubular epithelium?
- What is the role of the kidney in fluid, electrolyte, and acid-base balance?
- How does renal function change across the life span?
- How are laboratory and diagnostic tests used to evaluate renal function and disease?

CHAPTER OUTLINE

The kidneys are responsible for maintaining fluid and electrolyte homeostasis and ridding the body of water-soluble wastes. To accomplish these functions, the kidneys filter more than 7 L of fluid per hour, then reabsorb about 99%, producing a small amount of urine containing a high concentration of wastes.[1] The kidneys can alter the amount and composition of urine to keep blood volume and electrolyte composition within normal limits. In addition, the kidneys perform two important endocrine functions: production of erythropoietin, which is a regulator of red blood cell quantity, and activation of vitamin D, which is a cofactor for intestinal calcium absorption.

Most individuals have two kidneys, each containing more than a million **nephrons,** which provide a large renal reserve. The nephron is the functional unit of the kidney, performing all filtration, reabsorption, and secretory functions. Removal of 50% of a person's nephrons, as occurs with kidney donation, results in no significant impairment of renal function, although renal reserve is reduced.[2] Serious renal impairment generally does not occur until between 75% and 90% of the total nephrons have been damaged. Thus, clinical findings may not be evident until late in the course of kidney disease. A number of laboratory and diagnostic tests are used to assess renal structure and function and to identify disease processes. These are briefly described at the end of this chapter. Kidney diseases, renal failure, and abnormalities of the bladder are discussed in Chapters 27, 28, and 29, respectively. A discussion of fluid and electrolyte imbalances and acid-base disturbances can be found in Chapters 24 and 25, respectively. The essentials of kidney structure and nephron function are presented in this chapter.

RENAL ANATOMY

The urinary system consists of the kidneys, ureters, urinary bladder, and urethra (Figure 26-1). The kidneys are located in the **retroperitoneal** space in the posterior abdomen. One kidney is on each side of the vertebral column between the level of the twelfth thoracic and third lumbar vertebrae. The costovertebral angle (CVA), the point at which the bottom of the rib cage meets the spine, is commonly used as an external landmark for finding kidney position during physical examination.[3] The right kidney is located beneath the liver and is placed slightly lower than the left kidney.

The kidneys are protected and surrounded by strong back and flank muscles, fascia, and fat. The kidneys are somewhat mobile and can be injured by high-impact activities, such as bouncing along on horseback or on a mountain bike, or by direct trauma, as might occur from falls or blunt trauma. Kidney hemorrhage results in bleeding into the retroperitoneal space but not into the peritoneal cavity.

The kidneys drain urine into the ureters by gravity flow. The ureters provide peristaltic action to move urine along to the bladder where it is stored. The two principal parts of the bladder are the body and the neck. The body stores urine and is made up of smooth muscle known as detrusor muscle. Detrusor muscle extends in all directions throughout the bladder and contracts as a unit in response to initiation of action potentials. The urinary bladder collects 300 to 500 ml before stretch receptors signal a need for bladder emptying. Urine is drained from the bladder by the urethra when

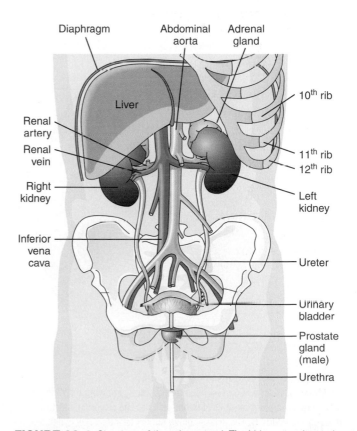

FIGURE 26-1 Structure of the urinary tract. The kidneys are located in the retroperitoneal space in the posterior abdominal cavity, in contact with the diaphragm and covered on the upper portions by ribs.

the internal and external sphincters are relaxed. Innervation and control of bladder function are discussed in detail in Chapter 29.

An adult kidney weighs approximately 115 to 170 g; is 11 cm long, 6 cm wide, and 3 cm thick; and is shaped like a red kidney bean, with the concave portion, termed the **hilum,** facing the vertebral column.[1] A thin, fibrous capsule covers each kidney and encloses blood vessels, lymphatic vessels, and nerve fibers, including pain receptors. Lymphatic vessels, blood vessels, and nerves enter and exit the kidney through the hilum.

Renal Parenchyma

On cross-section, the kidney is seen to contain three principal areas: the pelvis, the medulla, and the cortex (Figure 26-2). The renal pelvis is a large collecting area for the urine that drains from the many collecting ducts of the nephrons. The minor (smaller) calices collect urine as it drains from the papilla of the renal pyramids. The normal kidney has 8 to 18 minor calices and 2 to 3 major calices.[1] The major calices are large collecting spaces located between the minor calices and the upper part of the ureter.

The medulla contains 8 to 18 renal pyramids, the bases of which are adjacent to the outer cortex, whereas the apices open into the minor calices. The pyramids consist of collecting tubules, collecting ducts, long loops of Henle, and vasa recta. The papillae are the openings at the tips of the renal pyramids through which urine exits the collecting ducts.

The renal cortex, which is the outer rim of the kidney, is about 1 cm thick. The cortex contains all of the glomeruli as well as 85% of the nephron tubules. Fifteen percent of nephrons send their loops of Henle deep into the medulla and are called **juxtamedullary nephrons.** Columns of cortical tissue are found between the medullary pyramids and provide the passageway for the interlobar arteries.

Renal Lymphatics and Innervation

There are two lymphatic systems in the kidney. One system is composed of vessels that are located both in the renal capsule and immediately under the capsule in the outer cortex. The other lymphatic system is composed of vessels that accompany and wrap around the arterial blood vessels. All the lymphatic vessels, as well as blood vessels and nerves, exit the kidney through the hilum, and lymph drains into the para-aortic lymph nodes.

The kidneys are innervated by the sympathetic division of the autonomic nervous system. The lesser splanchnic nerves come from the renal plexuses, which are located next to the renal arteries. These nerve fibers travel with the renal arterial blood vessels and terminate in smooth muscle of the afferent and efferent arterioles, proximal and distal tubules, and the renin-secreting juxtaglomerular cells.[4,5] Stimulation of the sympathetic nervous system results in renal vasoconstriction and renin release. The renal capsule and all structures between the renal pelvis and urinary meatus are innervated with pain receptors (see Chapter 27).

FIGURE 26-2 A, Cross-section of the kidney showing the renal pelvis, medullary pyramids, and cortex. Normal kidneys have 8 to 18 renal pyramids and a corresponding number of minor calices. The major calices drain urine into the ureter. Blood vessels, lymphatic vessels, and nerves enter and exit through the hilum. **B,** The arterial blood supply to the kidney is derived from the renal arteries, which branch from the abdominal aorta and enter the kidney through the hilus. The renal artery branches to form several interlobar arteries, which travel toward the cortex in the renal columns. The interlobar arteries branch to form the arcuate arteries, which divide further to form the interlobular arteries. Interlobular arteries branch multiple times to provide the afferent arterioles for each of the kidney's million nephrons.

Renal Blood Supply

Approximately 25% of the cardiac output is delivered to the kidneys, the majority of which circulates through the cortex, while only 1% to 2% perfuses the medulla.[5] Total renal blood flow in both kidneys is approximately 1200 ml/min. Blood flows to the kidneys from the abdominal aorta through the renal arteries, which then divide into several interlobar arteries.[5] The interlobar arteries travel in the renal columns adjacent to the pyramids (see Figure 26-2). When the interlobar arteries reach the border of the medulla and the cortex, they branch into the arcuate arteries. The arcuate arteries then travel along the cortical medullary border parallel to the renal capsule. The arcuate arteries branch further to form small interlobular arteries, which penetrate the cortex and branch extensively to form the afferent arterioles. The afferent arterioles divide to form glomerular capillaries, which coalesce to form the efferent arterioles (Figure 26-3). The efferent arterioles branch again to form a second capillary bed. The peritubular capillaries wrap around the proximal and distal convoluted tubules (Figure 26-4). Some capillaries, called *vasa recta,* dip down into the medulla to surround the loops of Henle and collecting ducts. The vasa recta have

FIGURE 26-3 Scanning electron micrograph showing branching of an interlobular artery into two afferent arterioles (af), with associated glomerular tufts and efferent arterioles (ef). (From Kimura K et al: Effects of atrial natriuretic peptide on renal arterioles: morphometric analysis using microvascular casts, *Am J Physiol* 259:F936, 1990. Used with permission.)

FIGURE 26-4 The nephron tubule is covered by peritubular capillaries and vasa recta, which pick up the fluid and solutes that have been reabsorbed by the tubular epithelium and return them to the general circulation.

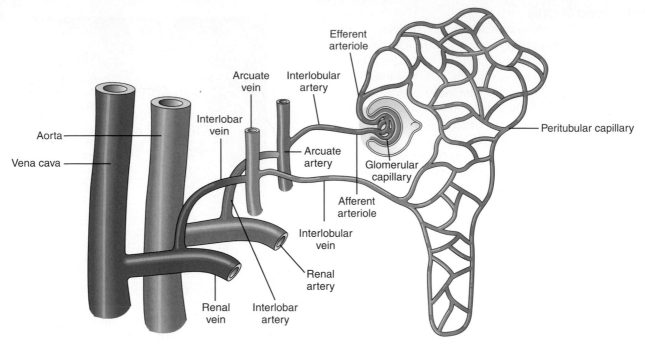

FIGURE 26-5 The venous vessels of the kidney parallel the arterial vessels and are similarly named.

a specialized loop structure that enables them to pick up interstitial fluid without excessive removal of interstitial solutes. Solutes and water move into and out of the vasa recta passively such that the descending limb gains solute as it dips into the highly concentrated medulla, but then most of the solute is lost as the ascending loop makes its way back up to the cortex.

The capillaries of the peritubular system and the vasa recta join together and drain into interlobular venules. The veins that drain blood from the kidney run parallel to the arteries and are similarly named (Figure 26-5).

KEY POINTS

- The kidneys are located in the retroperitoneal space, just under the diaphragm. The right kidney is slightly lower than the left. The costovertebral angle is an external landmark useful for locating the kidneys.
- The kidney can be divided into three principal anatomic sections: the pelvis, the medulla, and the cortex. The pelvis is composed of urinary collecting structures, called *calices*. The medulla is the middle portion and contains the renal pyramids. The cortex is the outer portion and contains glomeruli and nephron tubules.
- The kidneys are supplied with lymphatics to drain excess interstitial fluid and proteins and with sympathetic neurons to regulate blood supply and renin release.
- Blood is supplied to the kidneys by the renal artery, which divides several times to form the interlobar, arcuate, and interlobular arteries. The interlobular arteries branch multiple times to form afferent arterioles for each of the millions of kidney glomeruli.

- Each nephron has its own afferent arteriole, capillary tuft, and efferent arteriole. Efferent arterioles continue on to form peritubular capillaries, or vasa recta, which wrap around nephron structures and eventually drain into the renal veins. The loop structure of the vasa recta enables them to pick up interstitial fluid without removing excessive solute.

OVERVIEW OF NEPHRON STRUCTURE AND FUNCTION

Most of the physiologic functioning of the kidney can be understood by examining the function of an individual nephron. Thus, the nephron is said to be the functional unit of the kidney. Nephrons are organized in parallel such that each must accomplish all the necessary processing before releasing urine into the collecting ducts. Complex autoregulatory mechanisms ensure that the workload is evenly distributed among the kidneys' many nephrons.

As the unit of kidney function, a nephron must accomplish three major functions: (1) filtration of water-soluble substances from the blood; (2) reabsorption of filtered nutrients, water, and electrolytes; and (3) secretion of wastes or excess substances into the filtrate. Different segments of the nephron are specialized to accomplish each of these processes. Each nephron is composed of a glomerulus, which includes the capillary tuft and Bowman capsule, and a tubule, which includes the proximal convoluted tubule, loop of Henle, distal convoluted tubule, and collecting tubule (Figure 26-6). The nephron tubule is composed of a single layer of epithelial cells with an apical side facing the lumen and a basolateral side

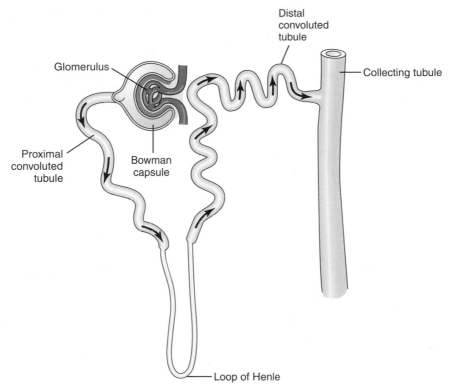

FIGURE 26-6 The nephron is composed of a glomerulus, proximal convoluted tubule, loop of Henle, distal convoluted tubule, and collecting tubule. Filtration occurs at the glomerulus, and the remaining tubule segments perform reabsorption and secretion functions.

facing the interstitial space and capillaries (Figure 26-7). The epithelial cells in each segment of the tubule are specialized for certain functions (Table 26-1). Nearly all cells in the nephron have a single cilium that protrudes from the apical surface into the lumen of the tubule. These cilia are mechanoreceptors and chemoreceptors that sense flow rate and composition of the tubular filtrate. Stimulation of the cilium triggers signaling cascades within the tubule cells that regulate cell proliferation, differentiation, and apoptosis. Abnormalities in cilia signaling function have been found in patients with polycystic kidney disease, associated with mutations in genes (polycystin, PKD1, PKD2) that code for cilia membrane proteins (see Chapter 27).

Glomerulus

The glomerulus is the site of fluid filtration from the blood to the nephron tubule. It is formed by a capillary tuft, which lies between the afferent and efferent arterioles, and by the surrounding epithelial cells of Bowman capsule. The outer layer of the glomerular capsule is called the *parietal layer* and consists of a single thickness of epithelial cells resting on a layer of basement membrane (Figure 26-8). The inner (visceral) layer of the capsule is composed of specialized epithelial cells called *podocytes*. Podocytes have foot processes that surround the glomerular capillary walls (Figure 26-9). Between the podocyte and the capillary endothelium is a layer of extracellular matrix called *basement membrane* (see Figure 26-8).

Spaces between the endothelial cells are called *fenestra*, and spaces between the podocyte foot processes are called *slit pores.* These intercellular spaces provide the surface area for glomerular filtration and make the glomeruli considerably more permeable than other capillaries in the body (Figure 26-10). The basement membrane is an important selectivity barrier of the glomerulus, preventing plasma proteins, erythrocytes, leukocytes, and platelets from passing through. Cells are too large to pass through pores, and plasma proteins are negatively charged and repelled to some extent by the basement membrane. Slit pores have a thin diaphragm of protein that restricts the filtration of plasma proteins that make it through the basement membrane.[6] *Nephrin* is an important protein in the slit pores as demonstrated by the massive proteinuria (protein in urine) that occurs when it is genetically mutated.[1] Proteins and blood cells are not usually present in the urine. If the glomerulus is injured, blood cells and proteins may filter through and be found in urine. Proteinuria is an important sign of basement membrane dysfunction. Except for the lack of proteins and cells, the glomerular filtrate is very similar in composition to plasma. The **glomerular filtration rate (GFR)** averages about 125 ml/min.

Another important component of the glomerulus is the mesangium, which includes mesangial cells and mesangial matrix. Mesangial cells have a number of functions including provision of structural support for glomerular capillaries, secretion of matrix proteins, phagocytosis, and regulating GFR.

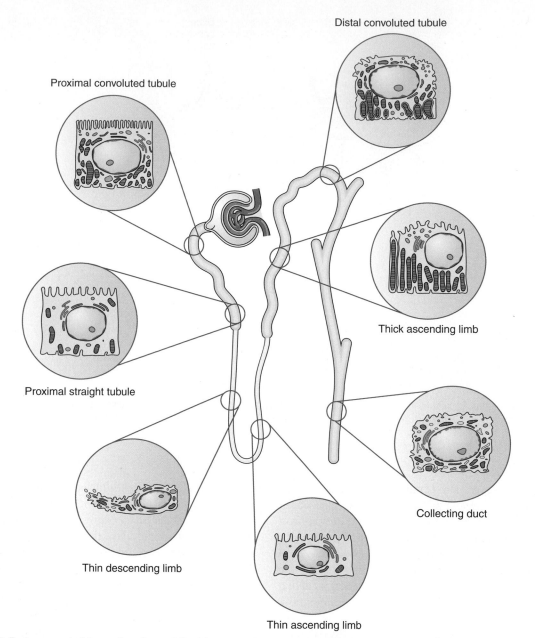

FIGURE 26-7 Each segment of the nephron is specialized for certain functions, which is reflected in the type of epithelial cells that make up the tubules.

By contracting and relaxing, mesangial cells can alter available surface area for filtration and affect GFR.

Proximal Convoluted Tubule

Bowman capsule drains the glomerular filtrate directly into the proximal tubule segment, where two thirds of the water and electrolytes are rapidly transported from the filtrate to the interstitium for reabsorption by peritubular capillaries[7] (Figure 26-11). Nutrients, vitamins, and small proteins normally are reabsorbed completely in the early proximal tubule. The early proximal tubule is the site of most bicarbonate ion reabsorption, whereas chloride ion is reabsorbed in the late proximal tubule. The proximal tubule is made up of cuboidal epithelium and convoluted to provide a greater surface area for reabsorption. The epithelial cells in this segment have microvilli that form a brush border next to the filtrate and substantially increase the apical surface area. Proximal tubule cells have high adenosine triphosphate (ATP) requirements because most reabsorption utilizes active transport mechanisms that are dependent on Na^+-K^+ ion pumps in the basolateral membrane. The specifics of some of these transport mechanisms are discussed in subsequent sections. Water is reabsorbed passively through paracellular transport between the tubular cells and through water channels in the tubule cell membranes made of proteins called *aquaporin 1*. Reabsorption of solutes creates the osmotic force for passive water reabsorption.

TABLE 26-1

Functions of the Nephron Segments

Nephron Segment	Functions
Glomerulus	Filters fluid from the blood into Bowman capsule; prevents the passage of blood cells and proteins
Proximal convoluted tubule	Transports two thirds of the filtered water and electrolytes and all of the filtered bicarbonate, glucose, amino acids, and vitamins from filtrate to interstitium
Descending loop of Henle	Transports water, delivers a concentrated filtrate to the ascending loop of Henle
Ascending loop of Henle	Actively transports Na^+, K^+, Cl^- to produce a hypo-osmotic filtrate and a high interstitial osmolality
Distal convoluted tubule	Transports Na^+, Cl^-, water, and urea; responsive to aldosterone; site of macula densa regulation of GFR; secretes H^+ and K^+
Collecting tubule	Passive transport of water under the influence of ADH; secretes H^+ and K^+

GFR, Glomerular filtration rate; *ADH,* antidiuretic hormone.

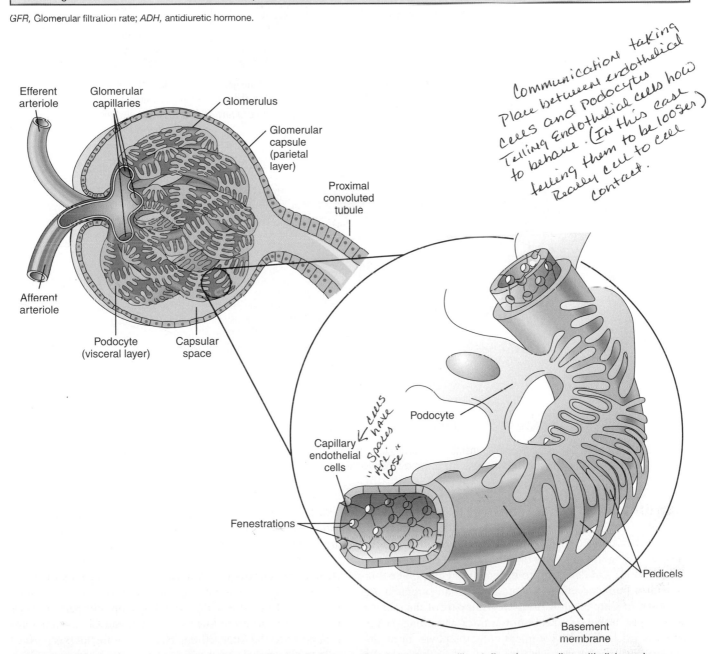

Communication taking place between endothelial cells and podocytes Telling Endothelial cells how to behave. (In this case telling them to be looser) Really cell to cell contact.

cells have spaces "ARE" "loose"

FIGURE 26-8 The structure of the glomerulus, including the afferent and efferent arterioles, capillary tuft, and surrounding epithelial membrane of Bowman capsule, is shown. The enlargement shows the glomerular membrane to be composed of the endothelial cells of the capillary, the podocytes of Bowman capsule, and the basement membrane between them.

FIGURE 26-9 An electron micrograph showing a close-up view of podocyte foot processes of the glomerular capillary. Note the spaces between the podocyte foot processes that contribute to a highly permeable glomerular membrane. *CB,* Podocyte cell body; *PB,* primary branch; *SB,* secondary branch; *TB,* tertiary branch; *Pe,* pedicles; *FS,* filtration slits. (From Kessel RG, Kardon RH: *Tissues and organs: a text-atlas of scanning electron microscopy,* San Francisco, 1979, WH Freeman.)

FIGURE 26-10 A section of the glomerular membrane showing the large spaces between the endothelial cells and podocyte foot processes. Filtration occurs through the fenestra and slit pores. The basement membrane provides the principal selectivity barrier of the glomerulus.

Loop of Henle

The loop of Henle is divided into the descending and ascending limbs, which differ significantly in structure and function. The descending limb receives filtrate from the proximal convoluted tubule and delivers it to the ascending limb. The thin descending limb and initial part of the ascending segment are composed of simple epithelium. The thin part of the loop of Henle is permeable to water, but the thick ascending part is not.[4] The thick ascending segment contains powerful membrane pumps that cotransport ions (Na^+, K^+, $2Cl^-$) from the filtrate and deposit them in the interstitial fluid surrounding the loops of Henle and collecting ducts (Figure 26-12). About 15% of nephrons have extra long loops of Henle that dip down into the medulla (juxtamedullary nephrons). These nephrons are vital for creating concentrated urine.

The loop formation of the loop of Henle creates a countercurrent mechanism, which allows the ascending loop of Henle to create a high interstitial gradient in the medulla of the kidney (Figure 26-13). Because the ascending loop is impermeable to water, water cannot follow the Na^+, K^+, and Cl^- ions that are pumped into the interstitium. The descending loop is permeable to water, and water will be drawn out by the extra ions that were pumped into the interstitium by the ascending limb. Thus, the filtrate that reaches the ascending limb will be more

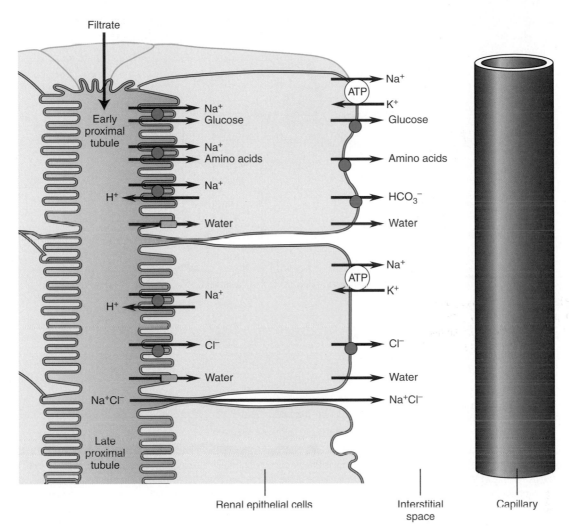

FIGURE 26-11 The proximal convoluted tubule has numerous membrane transporters that function to reabsorb filtered glucose, amino acids, water, and electrolytes. The early proximal tubule reabsorbs nearly all of the filtered bicarbonate ions, whereas the late proximal tubule reabsorbs chloride ions.

FIGURE 26-12 The epithelial cells of the thick ascending loop of Henle possess powerful ion pumps that cotransport Na^+, K^+, and $2Cl^-$ ions from the filtrate into the cell. The Na^+ is then pumped out of the basolateral membrane and into the interstitium. The loop of Henle ion cotransporter is responsible for creating a highly concentrated medullary interstitium.

concentrated than the original filtrate. Delivery of a more concentrated filtrate to the ascending limb allows the Na^+-K^+-$2Cl^-$ cotransporter to pump out a greater number of ions and reach an even higher interstitial gradient. This countercurrent mechanism creates a maximal osmolarity of about 600 mOsm/L at the tip of the loop of Henle as compared with the usual extracellular osmolarity of 280 to 300 mOsm/L at the cortex. Another 600 mOsm/L is contributed by the accumulation of urea particles in the interstitium.[8] Urea moves passively from the filtrate into the interstitium down its concentration gradient. Urea becomes concentrated in the tubule filtrate when electrolytes and water are removed in the proximal tubule and loop of Henle. An overall interstitial osmolarity is generated that begins in the cortex at about 300 mOsm/L and increases progressively to about 1200 mOsm/L at a point deep in the medulla. This high interstitial osmolarity provides a gradient for water reabsorption from the collecting ducts as they pass through the medulla on their way to the renal pelvis. The maximal interstitial gradient attained is dependent on the length

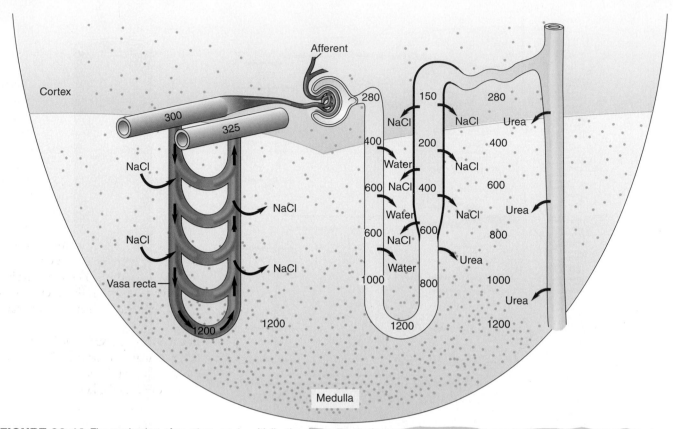

FIGURE 26-13 The mechanism of countercurrent multiplication. Ion pumps in the ascending loop of Henle create a gradient for removal of water from the descending loop. The filtrate reaching the ascending loop is then more concentrated, allowing the ascending loop to pump even more ions to further increase the osmolarity of the interstitial fluid. NaCl accumulation in the interstitium contributes about half of the total osmolality. Urea particles in the interstitium contribute the other half of the particles that produce the interstitial gradient in the medulla. As water is removed from the collecting duct, urea becomes more concentrated and moves passively down its gradient into the interstitium. The specialized loop structure of the vasa recta allows it to pick up interstitial water without significant solute removal. Although solutes are acquired in the descending segment, they passively diffuse back out as the ascending segment reaches the cortex. This process is called *countercurrent exchange.*

of the loops of Henle. In some animals, such as desert rats and camels, very long loops of Henle create a much higher interstitial osmolarity, which allows formation of extremely concentrated urine. Fluid that is reabsorbed from collecting tubules into the medullary interstitium is picked up by the specialized capillary network called the vasa recta and returned to the venous circulation. Like other capillaries, the vasa recta passively exchange ions according to concentration gradients and passively reabsorb fluid by filtration forces. The loop structure of the vasa recta allows the capillary to passively leak accumulated solute back into the interstitium as the capillary makes its way back to the cortex from the medulla. This process minimizes the washout of the interstitial osmolality and has been called the *countercurrent exchange mechanism.*

Distal Convoluted Tubule

The filtrate that reaches the distal tubule is normally hypoosmotic (150 mOsm/L) in comparison with plasma (280 mOsm/L) because electrolytes have been removed by the pumps in the ascending loop of Henle.[8] At this point in the nephron, only 10% of the original glomerular filtrate remains,

and further reabsorption in the distal tubule is largely under hormonal control. Aldosterone and angiotensin II (AII) stimulate the tubule cells to reabsorb sodium and water, whereas atrial natriuretic peptide (ANP) and urodilatin inhibit reabsorption.

Collecting Duct

The distal tubules of several nephrons empty into a single collecting tubule, which then merges into progressively larger and fewer collecting ducts that run parallel to the loops of Henle. Eventually the collecting ducts form the medullary pyramids, which empty into the minor calices through the papilla. The collecting ducts travel through the high interstitial gradient of the medulla on their way to the renal pelvis. The collecting ducts have two cell types called *principle cells (P cells)* and *intercalated cells (I cells).* The majority of cells are the P type that responds to antidiuretic hormone. In the presence of antidiuretic hormone (ADH), more than 99% of the original filtrate is reabsorbed by the time it reaches the renal pelvis, creating 30 to 60 ml of concentrated urine per hour. The I cells participate in acid-base balance by regulating the secretion of acid.

$$GFR = 12.5[(50 + 0) - (10 + 30)]$$

$$GFR = 125\,ml/min$$

The main driving force for filtration is hydrostatic pressure in the glomerular capillaries. The glomerular capillary hydrostatic pressure exerts a force against the glomerular capillary walls. As blood circulates through the capillaries, the hydrostatic pressure pushes blood against the walls, and fluid is filtered out. The hydrostatic pressure remains fairly constant along the length of the capillary and exerts an average force of approximately 50 mm Hg.

The glomerular capillary oncotic (colloid osmotic) pressure exists because proteins are present in the blood. Plasma proteins are negatively charged and attract positive ions, which subsequently attract water. Because ions and water are attracted to the proteins and are not pushed against the capillary wall, the glomerular capillary colloidal osmotic pressure opposes filtration by holding water and ions in the capillaries. The glomerular oncotic pressure is lower at the afferent end and becomes progressively higher along the length of the capillary (see Figure 26-14).

The hydrostatic pressure in Bowman capsule is determined by the volume of filtrate present in the capsule. This pressure exerts a force against the walls of Bowman capsule and the glomerular capillaries and opposes filtration. The normal Bowman capsule hydrostatic pressure is about 10 mm Hg. Normally plasma proteins do not filter into Bowman capsule. If they did filter, then they would create Bowman capsule oncotic pressure. This pressure would enhance glomerular

KEY POINTS

- The nephron is the structural and functional unit of the kidney that performs all filtration, secretion, and reabsorption functions.
- Filtration occurs at the glomerulus, a structure formed by the glomerular capillary tuft, the podocytes of Bowman capsule, and the basement membrane.
- The selectivity barrier for glomerular filtration includes the basement membrane and proteins in the slit pores of podocytes, which prevent the passage of cells and large proteins. The filtrate in Bowman capsule is otherwise very similar in composition to plasma.
- The proximal tubule reabsorbs about two thirds of the filtered water and electrolytes and all of the glucose, amino acids, proteins, and vitamins.
- The loop of Henle contains powerful Na^+-K^+-$2Cl^-$ cotransporters, which pump ions into the interstitium to create a high interstitial osmolarity in the renal medulla. The loop formation of the loop of Henle is essential for the countercurrent mechanism, which creates the high interstitial osmolarity.
- The distal and collecting tubules "fine-tune" sodium and water reabsorption under the influence of endocrine hormones, including aldosterone, AII, ANP, ADH, and urodilatin to create dilute or concentrated urine as needed to maintain fluid balance.

REGULATION OF GLOMERULAR FILTRATION

The GFR is determined by the filtration pressure in the glomeruli and by the permeable surface area of the glomerular membrane (K_f). Filtration pressure varies considerably from the afferent end of the glomerulus to the efferent end and is difficult to measure directly. The average net filtration pressure for the capillary as a whole is about 10 mm Hg, and the permeability constant K_f is about 12.5 ml/min per mm Hg. GFR is the product of filtration pressure and K_f (10 mm Hg × 12.5 ml/min per mm Hg = 125 ml/min).[5] The GFR is determined by the physical principles of filtration across a capillary membrane (Figure 26-14).

Physics of Filtration

Filtration rate is affected by factors that alter hydrostatic and oncotic pressure on either side of the glomerular membrane, as shown by the following filtration equation:

$$GFR = K_f[(P_{GC} + \pi_{BC}) - (P_{BC} + \pi_{GC})]$$

where P_{GC} is glomerular capillary hydrostatic pressure (mm Hg); π_{BC} is oncotic pressure in Bowman capsule (mm Hg); P_{BC} is Bowman capsule hydrostatic pressure (mm Hg); and π_{GC} is oncotic pressure in the glomerular capillary (mm Hg). The following is an illustrative example resulting in a normal GFR of 125 ml/min:

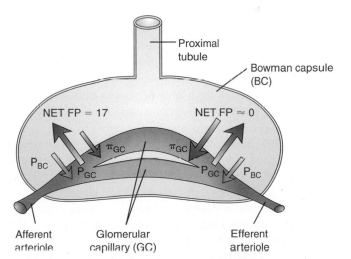

FIGURE 26-14 Net filtration is higher at the afferent end of the glomerular capillary because the hydrostatic blood pressure in the capillary exceeds the pressure in Bowman capsule and the oncotic pressure in the capillary. Toward the efferent end of the capillary, the filtration pressure is low because the oncotic pressure of the blood is high and offsets the hydrostatic blood pressure. Capillary oncotic pressure gets progressively higher along the capillary because fluid is filtering out of the blood into Bowman capsule and leaving the proteins behind so they become more concentrated and exert a greater oncotic pressure. *FP,* Filtration pressure; π, oncotic pressure; *P,* hydrostatic pressure.

filtration because proteins attract cations and water. In a healthy kidney, this pressure is negligible.

In summary, the net filtration pressure across the glomerular membrane is approximately 10 mm Hg. The filtration pressure is higher at the afferent arteriole side of the capillary and diminishes as the blood reaches the efferent end. This occurs because the capillary oncotic pressure is lower at the afferent end. As blood passes through the capillaries, continued filtration leaves a greater concentration of proteins in the capillaries, which raises the oncotic pressure. As blood reaches the efferent arterioles, filtration may cease.

Factors Affecting Filtration Pressure

One of the most important physiologic regulators of GFR is blood volume.[5] When blood volume increases because of fluid intake, the blood pressure rises slightly and causes glomerular hydrostatic pressure to increase. GFR increases, and the extra fluid is pushed into the filtrate to be excreted from the body. The opposite also occurs: when blood volume is decreased, capillary hydrostatic pressure falls, resulting in a lower GFR, and fluid is conserved. The glomerular capillary is protected from large swings in blood pressure by autoregulation. Autoregulation adjusts the arteriolar resistance to maintain a relatively steady rate of blood flow despite changes in perfusion pressure. Autoregulation is effective when arterial blood pressure varies between 90 and 180 mm Hg.[5] Autoregulation of renal blood flow is achieved in part by a stretch response in the vascular smooth muscle of the afferent arterioles. When blood pressure increases, the vascular smooth muscle cells reflexively constrict to keep blood flow at about the same rate. This mechanism is called *myogenic autoregulation.*

Other factors can affect GFR by altering the pressure within Bowman capsule or affecting plasma oncotic pressure. Obstruction in the tubules or collecting ducts can significantly elevate the pressure in Bowman capsule. According to the filtration equation, GFR would fall because filtration pressure would be reduced. Because plasma oncotic pressure is determined primarily by the concentration of plasma proteins, a low serum albumin would increase GFR.

Although K_f is called a constant, it is subject to change for physiologic and pathologic reasons. Specialized mesangial cells located in the glomerulus are thought to be important regulators of K_f. These cells contract and relax in response to various stimuli and alter the surface area for filtration.[9] Contraction squeezes the capillary cells together and reduces GFR, whereas relaxation allows the permeable surface area to expand. Disease processes that damage the glomerular membrane also can affect permeability. Sclerotic processes reduce K_f, whereas some inflammatory injuries may increase it.

Tubuloglomerular Feedback

Each nephron is able to regulate its own individual GFR through a process termed *tubuloglomerular feedback.* A specialized group of cells forms the regulatory structure, called the **juxtaglomerular apparatus.** The juxtaglomerular apparatus is composed of the glomerulus, the macula densa, and

specialized juxtaglomerular cells, which are located around the glomerular arterioles (Figure 26-15). The macula densa cells are located near the end of the thick ascending loop of Henle, which loops up to come in contact with the glomerulus and juxtaglomerular cells.

Macula densa cells sense changes in the NaCl delivered to the tubule. When glomerular filtration is too high, an excessive load is delivered to the distal tubule. The mechanism whereby macula densa cells sense GFR is not completely understood. Some researchers suggest that it is the NaCl delivery to the macula densa cells that is sensed. A high tubule NaCl level means that transport processes in the previous nephron segments have been overwhelmed because GFR is too high; the macula densa sends signals to the glomerulus to reduce GFR. Conversely, a low NaCl level at the macula densa indicates that the nephron transporters are being underutilized, and GFR can be increased. Macula densa cells possess the same Na/Cl/K transporters as other cells in the thick ascending limb and when NaCl delivery is high, more is transported into the cells through this transporter. Tubuloglomerular feedback helps to distribute GFR evenly among the kidneys' 2 million nephrons.

The mechanisms whereby macula densa cells are able to alter GFR are only partially understood. Glomerular filtration can be regulated by altering filtration pressure or by altering the filtration constant, K_f. The macula densa could alter GFR by regulating the resistance of the afferent and efferent arterioles and by stimulating mesangial cells to contract or relax.

Afferent dilation and efferent constriction would increase the hydrostatic pressure within the glomerulus and increase GFR. Conversely, afferent constriction and efferent dilation would reduce filtration pressure and decrease GFR. Macula densa cells release adenosine and ATP in response to high NaCl in the tubule, both of which have been shown to bind to smooth muscle cells in the afferent arterioles and cause constriction.[10] The juxtaglomerular cells that surround the afferent arteriole are also thought to be mediators of tubuloglomerular feedback. The juxtaglomerular cells produce and release **renin,** an enzyme that converts angiotensinogen to angiotensin I (AI). Angiotensin I is then converted to AII by endothelial cells in the glomerular capillary, which possesses angiotensin-converting enzyme (ACE) activity. AII is a potent vasoconstrictor that constricts both afferent and efferent arterioles.[11] The signals that pass from the macula densa to the glomerulus to regulate tubuloglomerular feedback are not completely known; however, in addition to roles for adenosine and ATP, release of prostaglandins and nitric oxide have been demonstrated.[11] Some prostaglandins have vasodilating activities, whereas others are vasoconstrictors.

The importance of prostaglandins and AII in regulating GFR is supported by the observation that drugs that inhibit their activity interfere with tubuloglomerular feedback in some persons. For example, ACE inhibitors block AII production and may interfere with constriction of the efferent arteriole. This can be particularly detrimental to renal function in patients who require high filtration pressures, such as those with polycystic kidney disease or collecting system obstructions. Drugs that inhibit cyclooxygenase, such as aspirin and

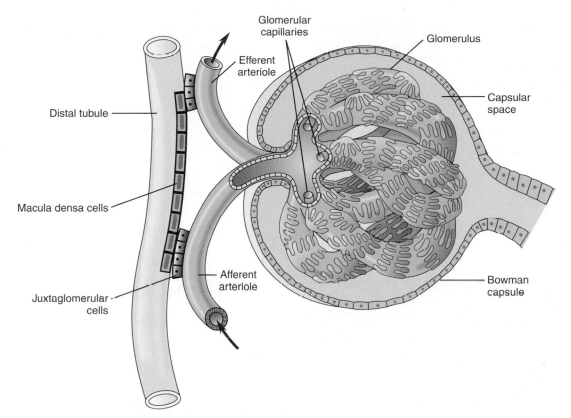

FIGURE 26-15 The juxtaglomerular apparatus is composed of the macula densa cells of the distal tubule, the afferent and efferent arterioles, and the renin-secreting juxtaglomerular cells. Macula densa cells sample the distal filtrate for NaCl content and send signals to the glomerulus to adjust glomerular filtration rate.

nonsteroidal anti-inflammatory drugs, interfere with prostaglandin production and may precipitate excessive renovascular constriction in some patients.[12]

Effects of Glucose and Amino Acids

The amount of glucose and amino acids filtered into the tubular fluid may alter GFR through the tubuloglomerular feedback mechanism. Both glucose and amino acids are filtered freely through the glomerular membrane and then are reabsorbed by active transport processes in the proximal tubule. Reabsorption occurs through transporters that use sodium ion entry into the cell to actively cotransport glucose and amino acids. The greater the load of tubular glucose and amino acids, the greater the amount of sodium reabsorbed by the proximal tubule. Fewer sodium ions are transported to the macula densa cells in the distal tubule, and the macula densa perceives this as a need to increase GFR.[5] In addition, chronically high serum glucose as occurs in poorly controlled diabetes mellitus may induce excessive nitric oxide production, producing hyperfiltration, excessive GFR, and damage to the glomerulus.

Role of Mesangial Cells

Mesangial cells are located around the glomerular capillaries and are thought to regulate the surface area available for glomerular filtration.[9] Contraction of the mesangial cells reduces surface area, and relaxation increases it. Mesangial cells are responsive to glomerular stretch and are stimulated to contract when more blood enters the glomerulus. This response provides a negative feedback that decreases surface area when filtration pressure is increased. In addition, mesangial cells respond to a number of chemical mediators, including AII and endothelin (peptides that favor mesangial contraction) and ANP and nitric oxide (substances that favor relaxation). Mesangial cells thus may regulate GFR by altering the filtration constant K_f.

> ### KEY POINTS
>
> - GFR is determined by the permeable surface area (K_f) and by capillary hydrostatic pressure and Bowman capsule oncotic pressure, which favor filtration, and by plasma oncotic pressure and Bowman capsule hydrostatic pressure, which oppose filtration. Normal GFR is about 125 ml/min.
> - The filtration rate in an individual nephron is regulated by tubuloglomerular feedback in which macula densa cells sample the NaCl content (or other constituents) in the distal tubule and signal the juxtaglomerular apparatus to make appropriate adjustments in GFR.

- Afferent constriction and efferent dilation decrease GFR, whereas afferent dilation and efferent constriction increase GFR. AII and prostaglandins are important chemical mediators of arteriolar resistance.
- Excessive filtration of glucose and amino acids can result in increased GFR because their reabsorption in the proximal tubule requires cotransport of sodium ions. Fewer sodium ions are delivered to the macula densa, and GFR is increased.
- Mesangial cells respond to glomerular capillary stretch by contracting to reduce the surface area for filtration. Mesangial cells also respond to chemical signals that induce them to contract and relax, which alters GFR accordingly.

TRANSPORT ACROSS RENAL TUBULES

Reabsorption and secretion of substances across the nephron tubule are accomplished by two routes; the *transcellular* and the *paracellular* routes. Transcellular transport uses specific transporter proteins in the membranes of the tubular epithelial cells to move substances between the tubular filtrate and the interstitial fluid. Most of these transport processes are dependent on Na^+ reabsorption and made possible by the Na^+-K^+ pump in the basolateral membrane. Paracellular transport refers to movement of substances through the tight junctions that hold the tubular epithelial cells together. Substances using the paracellular route therefore do not traverse the cell membrane and instead move passively through the spaces between cells. *Reabsorption* is the process of transporting a substance from the filtrate into the renal capillaries and requires several transport steps. First the substance is moved from the filtrate into the tubular cell through transporters on the apical surface of the cell; then it passes through another transporter on the basolateral side of the tubular cell and into the interstitium. From the interstitium it moves passively by diffusion or filtration into the capillary. In general, the reabsorption of cations, especially sodium, provides an electrical gradient to pull anions across the tubule and into the interstitium. Reabsorption of ions and solutes creates an osmotic force to pull water passively across the renal epithelium. A summary of transport in the various tubule segments is shown in Figure 26-16. The details of glucose, bicarbonate, H^+, and K^+ transport are described as important representative examples.

Reabsorption of Glucose

Glucose is filtered freely across the glomerular membrane such that the tubular load (in milligrams per minute) is determined by the product of serum glucose (in milligrams per milliliter) and GFR (in milliliters per minute). Normally, all of the filtered glucose is reabsorbed in the proximal tubule by a sodium-dependent cotransporter called SGLT 2 (Figure 26-17). The transport proteins have a maximal rate of transport that can be exceeded if the tubular load of glucose is too great. The transport maximum for normal kidneys is about 375 mg/min in men

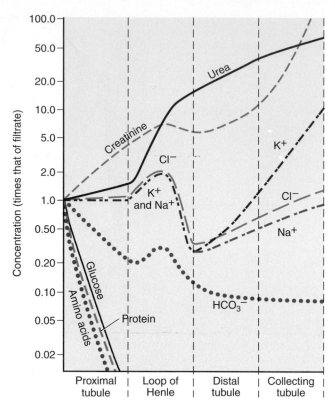

FIGURE 26-16 Summary of nutrient and electrolyte composition of the filtrate in each segment of the nephron. Two thirds of the filtrate is reabsorbed in the proximal tubule. (Adapted from Guyton AC, Hall JE, editors: *Textbook of medical physiology,* ed 11, Philadelphia, 2006, Saunders, p 338.)

and 300 mg/min in women.[4] A tubular load of glucose in excess of this amount results in glycosuria. In fact, some spillage of glucose begins at a much lower tubular load because of uneven distribution of GFR to individual nephrons or differences in the number of transporters in different nephrons. Some nephrons with higher GFR or fewer transporters may exceed their transport maximums, while other nephrons are working below capacity. The point at which glucose begins to spill into the urine is called the *renal threshold*. In normal kidneys with a GFR of 125 ml/min, the renal threshold will be reached when serum glucose approaches 180 mg/dl, but significant glycosuria will not occur until the transport maximum is reached at a serum glucose level of about 300 mg/dl. Persons with low GFR associated with renal disease may not experience spillage of glucose until the serum glucose level is much higher, and glycosuria is not a reliable indicator of serum glucose level in these individuals. For example, a patient with a GFR of 50 ml/min and a serum glucose of 300 mg/dl will have a tubular glucose load of only 150 mg/min, which is well below the normal renal threshold. No glycosuria would occur despite the high serum glucose level.

Regulation of Acid-Base Balance

The kidney tubules have an important role in maintaining the pH of the blood. In addition to excreting excess H^+, the kidneys also regulate the concentration of bicarbonate (HCO_3^-)

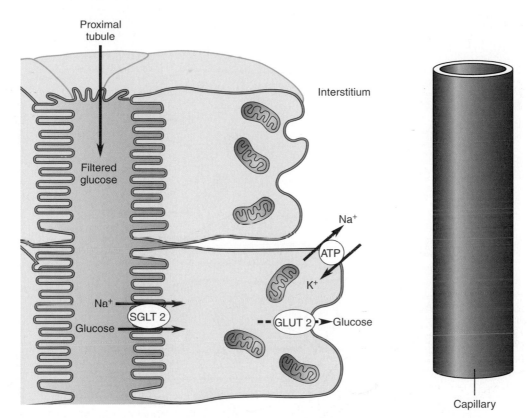

FIGURE 26-17 The glucose transporter in the proximal tubule *(SGLT 2)* is dependent on sodium reabsorption from the filtrate. The Na^+-K^+ pump in the basolateral membrane keeps the intracellular sodium level low and maintains a gradient for sodium and glucose reabsorption. Glucose diffuses out of the tubule cell and back into the interstitial fluid through passive carrier proteins *(GLUT 2)*. *ATP*, Adenosine triphosphate.

in the blood. The pH of the blood normally ranges between 7.35 and 7.45 and is determined by the ratio of acid (H_2CO_3) to base (HCO_3^-). The lungs and kidneys work together to maintain this balance. Metabolic processes create an excess of acid, which is excreted by the lungs in the form of CO_2 and by the kidneys in the form of H^+. In addition, HCO_3^- is filtered freely through the glomerulus and must be efficiently reabsorbed to maintain acid-base balance. Most HCO_3^- is reabsorbed in the proximal tubule; however, the distal segment also participates in regulating HCO_3^- and H^+ transport.

Reabsorption of HCO_3^- is complex because it is not directly transported across the apical membrane; rather, it is combined with H^+ in the tubule to form H_2CO_3, which dissociates into CO_2 and water (Figure 26-18). The H^+ for this reaction is secreted into the filtrate in exchange for Na^+. Carbonic anhydrase present in the brush border of the proximal tubule cell catalyzes the reaction. Carbon dioxide is lipid soluble and diffuses passively into the tubular cell. Once inside, intracellular carbonic anhydrase catalyzes the reverse reaction to once again form HCO_3^- and H^+. The HCO_3^- is transported out through the basolateral membrane, whereas the H^+ is recycled to the tubular fluid to bind with another HCO_3^-. The energy to power this reabsorptive process is provided by the Na^+-K^+ pump, which keeps intracellular Na^+ low so that the sodium gradient can continue to move H^+ into the tubule lumen through the Na^+-H^+ exchanger.

Normally, all of the filtered HCO_3^- is reabsorbed by this mechanism to help maintain acid-base balance.[13] Excess H^+ ions that find no HCO_3^- in the filtrate with which to bind are excreted in the urine, and urine is normally acidic. The number of H^+ ions that can be excreted in urine is limited to a pH of about 4.0. However, urine buffers, including HPO_4^{2-} and NH_3, are secreted into the filtrate and bind with excess H^+, greatly increasing the ability of the kidney to excrete an acid load (see Figure 26-18). Ammonia (NH_3) is produced by the renal epithelium via metabolism of the amino acid glutamine. Ammonia binds to H^+ to form ammonium ion (NH_4^+), whereas HPO_4^{2-} binds to H^+ to form $H_2PO_4^-$.

Renal Compensation Process

In some cases, the kidneys are called on to compensate for an abnormality in lung function. The lungs normally regulate the amount of carbon dioxide in the blood ($Paco_2$). When $Paco_2$ is high, more carbonic acid is formed, and the blood pH becomes acidic. The kidneys compensate by excreting more H^+ and by creating new HCO_3^- to enhance the buffering capacity of the blood. These HCO_3^- ions are additional to those already being reabsorbed from the filtrate and are, thus, new.

New HCO_3^- is created within the renal tubule cell by two processes. First, excess circulating CO_2 from respiratory acidosis diffuses into the renal cell and is converted to HCO_3^- and H^+ by the enzyme carbonic anhydrase. The new HCO_3^- is

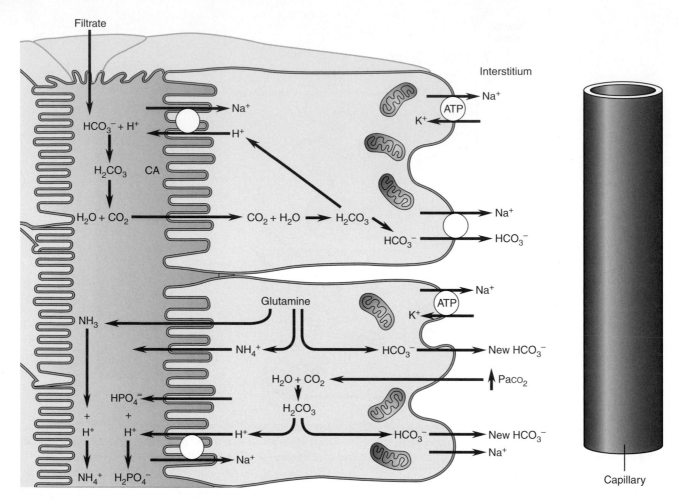

FIGURE 26-18 Bicarbonate ion reabsorption across the renal tubule. Filtered HCO_3^- is combined with secreted H^+ to form carbonic acid, which dissociates into water and carbon dioxide. Carbon dioxide is lipid soluble and diffuses into the cells, where the reverse reaction converts it back to HCO_3^- and H^+. The bicarbonate ion moves out of the basolateral membrane and returns to the bloodstream, whereas the H^+ is returned to the lumen to bind with another HCO_3^- ion. Excess H^+ ions are excreted in the urine in combination with phosphate and ammonia buffers. The kidney is able to create new bicarbonate as needed to maintain pH balance. *CA*, Carbonic anhydrase; *ATP*, adenosine triphosphate.

sent back to the bloodstream, and the new H^+ is secreted into the urine filtrate, where it binds with a renal buffer and is excreted. The second process involves the production of ammonium ions within the tubule cell. New HCO_3^- can be formed by the metabolism of glutamine, which also produces NH_4^+ within the tubule cell.[13] The NH_4^+ is excreted in the urine, and the new HCO_3^- is sent back to the bloodstream (see Figure 26-18). Gradually, the creation of new HCO_3^- in this way increases the serum HCO_3^- concentration and restores the pH toward normal. This process may take hours to days.

The kidneys are also able to compensate for respiratory alkalosis by excreting some of the filtered HCO_3^-. Alkalosis reduces the number of H^+ ions available for transport into the filtrate. Some of the filtered HCO_3^- escapes the proximal tubule without being converted to CO_2 and is excreted in the urine.

Secretion of Potassium

There is normally a net excess of potassium from dietary sources that must be excreted by the kidneys. The primary transporter responsible for this process is the Na^+-K^+ pump in the basolateral cell membrane. The Na^+-K^+ pump moves K^+ into the tubular cell and increases the gradient for diffusion of K^+ through the apical membrane and into the filtrate (Figure 26-19). Principle cells in the distal tubule and collecting duct are the site of potassium excretion. The activity of Na^+-K^+ pumps in these segments is sensitive to aldosterone, a steroid hormone secreted by the adrenal cortex. Aldosterone increases reabsorption of Na^+ and water and excretion of K^+. Potassium excretion also is affected by the activity of the K^+-H^+ exchanger and by the plasma K+ concentration.

KEY POINTS

- Reabsorption across the tubular epithelium occurs by transcellular and paracellular routes. The transcellular route utilizes transporters in the apical and basolateral membranes of tubular cells to move substances from the filtrate, through the cell, to the interstitium. The paracellular route allows passive transport of substances

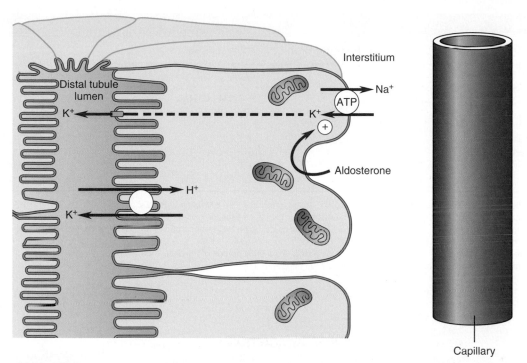

FIGURE 26-19 Tubular secretion of potassium ion. Increased serum potassium and aldosterone increase the activity of the Na⁺-K⁺ pump and enhance K⁺ secretion into the filtrate. The H⁺-K⁺ exchanger also regulates the secretion of K⁺ ions. *ATP,* Adenosine triphosphate.

in between the tubular cells. Renal capillaries passing through the interstitium passively take up substances through filtration and diffusion and return them to the venous circulation.

- Reabsorption of glucose is accomplished by proximal tubule cell sodium-dependent transporters. These transporters have transport maximums that can be overwhelmed by excessive tubular loads of glucose, in which case glycosuria results.

- The kidneys participate in acid-base regulation through secretion of excess H⁺ and by reabsorption and creation of HCO_3^-. Urine buffers HPO_4^{2-} and NH_3 bind excess H⁺ and increase the ability of the kidney to excrete an acid load.

- HCO_3^- is not directly reabsorbed across the renal epithelium; it is first converted to CO_2 by the enzyme carbonic anhydrase. The H⁺ ions needed for this reaction are provided by Na⁺-H⁺ pumps on the apical cell membrane.

- Secretion of potassium ions is promoted by activity of the Na⁺-K⁺ pump on the basolateral cell membrane. In the distal tubule, these pumps are regulated by aldosterone, which increases potassium excretion.

REGULATION OF BLOOD VOLUME AND OSMOLALITY

The kidneys play a vital role in maintaining normal blood volume and osmolality. As previously discussed, changes in blood volume alter the pressure in the glomerulus and affect GFR. An increase in blood volume results in a pressure diuresis, whereas a fall in blood volume reduces urine output. The kidney tubules are responsive to a number of hormonal signals that fine-tune tubular reabsorption (Table 26-2). These hormones include ADH, aldosterone, AII, ANP, urodilatin, uroguanylin, and guanylin. Antidiuretic hormone is the principal regulator of osmolality, and the others regulate extracellular volume through increasing or decreasing NaCl and water reabsorption.

Antidiuretic Hormone

ADH (also called vasopressin) is secreted from the posterior pituitary when osmoreceptors located in the hypothalamus detect a high osmolality of the extracellular fluid. Principle cells in the collecting tubules respond to ADH by translocating water pores called *aquaporin 2* to the apical membrane (Figure 26-20). These pores make the tubule permeable to water and allow water to be reabsorbed from the urinary filtrate. The high interstitial gradient of the medulla provides the osmotic force for water reabsorption. Recall that this gradient was formed by the action of powerful ion pumps in the thick ascending limb of the loop of Henle.

As water is reabsorbed into the medullary interstitium, it creates a high tissue pressure that pushes fluid into the vasa recta. The vasa recta return the reabsorbed water to the general circulation. The reabsorbed water dilutes the blood and reduces osmolality. Osmoreceptors in the brain detect the reduced osmolality and inhibit further production of ADH. When blood osmolality is too low, ADH secretion is completely inhibited, and the collecting tubules become impermeable to water. Water is not reabsorbed from the filtrate, and a large

TABLE 26-2

Hormones That Regulate NaCl and Water Reabsorption

Hormone*	Major Stimulus	Nephron Site of Action	Effects on Transport
Angiotensin II	↑Renin	PT, TAL, DT/CD	↑NaCl and H_2O reabsorption
Aldosterone	↑Angiotensin II, ↑ [K⁺]p	TAL, DT/CD	↑NaCl and H_2O reabsorption†
ANP, BNP, urodilatin	↑ECFV	CD	↓H_2O and NaCl reabsorption
Uroguanylin, guanylin	Oral ingestion of NaCl	PT, CD	↓H_2O and NaCl reabsorption
Sympathetic nerves	↓ECFV	PT, TAL, DT/CD	↑NaCl and H_2O reabsorption†
Dopamine	↑ECFV	PT	↓H_2O and NaCl reabsorption
ADH	↑P_{osm}, ↓ECFV	DT/CD	↑H_2O reabsorption†

ANP, atrial natriuretic peptide; *BNP*, brain natriuretic peptide; *BP*, blood pressure; *CD*, collecting duct; *DT*, distule tubule; *ECFV*, extracellular fluid volume, *[K⁺]p*, plasma K concentration; *P_{osm}*, plasma osmolality; *PT*, proximal tubule; *TAL*, thick ascending limb.

*All of these hormones act within minutes, except aldosterone, which exerts its action on NaCl reabsorption with a delay of 1 hour. Aldosterone exhibits its maximum effect after a few days.

†The effect on H_2O reabsorption does not include the thick ascending limb or the early portion of the distal tube.

From Koeppen B, Stanton B: *Renal physiology*, ed 4, Philadelphia, 2007, Mosby, p. 65.

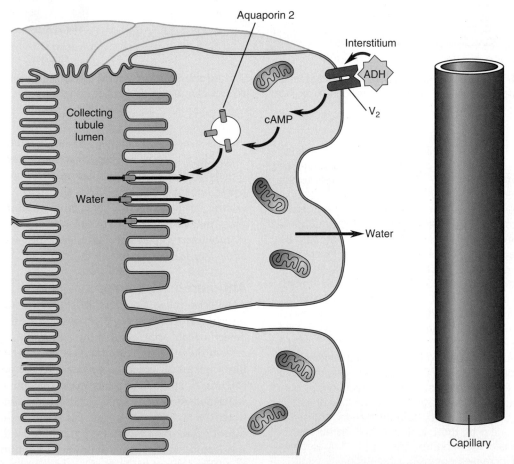

FIGURE 26-20 Antidiuretic hormone *(ADH)* action on the collecting tubule epithelium. ADH binds to receptors on the basolateral cell membrane, resulting in translocation of water pores (aquaporin 2) to the apical surface. Increased water permeability results in reabsorption of water from the filtrate and into the interstitium. *cAMP*, Cyclic adenosine monophosphate; *V_2*, vasopressin-2 receptor.

quantity of dilute urine is produced. Loss of water in excess of solute returns the blood osmolality toward normal.

An insufficiency of ADH secondary to pituitary damage results in the condition of *diabetes insipidus* in which large volumes of dilute urine are excreted leading to severe fluid imbalances. A similar problem occurs when the collecting tubules are unresponsive to ADH. This condition is called *nephrogenic diabetes insipidus* and usually results from genetic defects in either the ADH receptor (V_2) or the aquaporin 2 genes.[4]

Aldosterone, Angiotensin II, Natriuretic Peptides, Urodilatin, Uroguanylin, and Guanylin

Aldosterone, AII, ANP, urodilatin, uroguanylin, and guanylin alter blood volume without affecting its concentration. Aldosterone and AII increase reabsorption of Na^+, which provides a gradient for water reabsorption. Because salt and water are reabsorbed together, the osmolality of the reabsorbed fluid is isosmotic with plasma.

AII and aldosterone are produced when the juxtaglomerular cells in the kidney are stimulated to release renin. Renin is released in response to (1) decreased blood flow to the kidney, (2) reduced serum sodium levels, and (3) activation of sympathetic nerves to the juxtaglomerular cells.[4] Renin begins a cascade of reactions that result in the production of AII and aldosterone. When AII and aldosterone restore blood volume and blood pressure to normal, the stimuli for renin release are removed and the concentrations of AII and aldosterone fall.

ANP is released from atrial cells in the heart when the chamber is overstretched by excessive blood volume. ANP inhibits all of the actions of AII and results in loss of sodium and water in the urine. Thus, ANP reduces extracellular volume, but the fluid losses are isosmotic with plasma, and blood osmolality remains unchanged. Urodilatin is a peptide that is secreted by distal and collecting tubule cells in response to increased circulating volume.[7] It is very similar in structure and function to ANP and inhibits Na^+ and water reabsorption by the collecting duct.

Uroguanylin and guanylin are peptide hormones produced by neuroendocrine cells in the intestine in response to NaCl ingestion. The target for these hormones are guanylyl cyclase receptors located on cells in the proximal tubule and collecting duct. Binding to these receptors generates cGMP, which inhibits Na^+, Cl^-, and water reabsorption and produces an effect similar to that of natriuretic peptides and urodilatin.

Diuretic Agents

The ability of the kidneys to reabsorb fluid can be inhibited by drugs that block sodium and water reabsorption. These agents are called *diuretics* and include osmotic diuretics, ACE inhibitors, loop diuretics, thiazide-like diuretics, and inhibitors of aldosterone activity (Table 26-3).[14] Diuretics work by altering osmotic gradients in the kidney tubules so that reabsorption of water is inhibited. Recall that water always moves passively according to an osmotic gradient. When the solute content of the filtrate is elevated, reabsorption of water is inhibited, resulting in a larger output of urine.

Osmotic diuretics (e.g., mannitol) are filtered through the glomerulus and are not reabsorbed by the tubules. The osmolality of the filtrate is increased by the presence of the solute, and more water remains in the tubule and is excreted in the urine. ACE inhibitors (e.g., captopril) inhibit the formation of AII and aldosterone, which normally stimulate the kidney tubules to reabsorb Na^+. In the absence of these hormones, more Na^+ stays in the urinary filtrate, resulting in less reabsorption of water.

Loop diuretics (e.g., furosemide) block the Na^+-K^+-$2Cl^-$ pumps in the ascending loop of Henle. The ions that would normally have been pumped into the interstitium stay in the filtrate and hold water with them. In addition, the maintenance of the high interstitial gradient in the medulla may be impaired. Washout of the gradient reduces the force for water reabsorption from the collecting ducts.

Thiazide-like diuretics (e.g., hydrochlorothiazide) block Na^+ reabsorption in the distal tubule. Sodium ions remain in the filtrate and oppose the action of the interstitial osmotic gradient.

All of these agents also increase the excretion of K^+ and are called *potassium-wasting diuretics*. Patients receiving chronic diuretic therapy with these agents usually require potassium replacement therapy.

In contrast, the aldosterone-blocking agents (e.g., spironolactone) are potassium sparing. Recall that aldosterone increases activity of the Na^+-K^+ pumps on the basolateral membrane of the distal tubule cells. These pumps promote Na^+ and water reabsorption and potassium secretion. Blockage of aldosterone reduces the activity of these pumps and results in less sodium and water reabsorption as well as less potassium excretion. Significant elevations in serum K^+ can occur with these agents.

Diuretics are used primarily in the management of high blood pressure (see Chapter 16) and congestive heart failure (see Chapter 19), but they also may be used in the diagnostic phase of acute renal failure or to manage potassium overload.

TABLE 26-3

Commonly Used Diuretics

Diuretic	Action
Osmotic diuretics	Increase solute load in tubule
ACE inhibitors	Block production of AII and aldosterone
Loop diuretics	Block the Na^+/K^+/$2Cl^-$ transporter in the ascending loop of Henle
Thiazide-like diuretics	Block Na^+ reabsorption in the distal tubule
Aldosterone inhibitors	Block the action of aldosterone on the distal tubule Na^+/K^+ transporters

KEY POINTS

- The kidneys regulate blood volume and osmolality by altering GFR and reabsorption from the urinary filtrate.
- Changes in blood volume alter the filtration pressure in the glomerulus, resulting in a pressure diuresis when blood volume is high and in reduced filtration and fluid conservation when blood volume is low.
- The kidney tubules are responsive to hormones that alter their reabsorptive properties. ADH increases the

permeability of the collecting tubule to water, resulting in increased reabsorption and reduced blood osmolality.

- Aldosterone, AII, ANP, and urodilatin alter blood volume without affecting blood osmolality. Aldosterone and AII increase sodium and water reabsorption, whereas ANP and urodilatin inhibit their reabsorption.
- Diuretics alter the osmolality of the urinary filtrate and oppose the reabsorption of water, resulting in an increase in urine volume.

KEY POINTS

- The kidney secretes two important endocrine hormones: erythropoietin, a growth factor for red cells, and active vitamin D, a necessary cofactor for calcium absorption from the intestine.
- In chronic renal failure, impaired production of these hormones results in anemia and osteodystrophy.

ENDOCRINE FUNCTIONS

The kidney is the source of two important endocrine hormones: erythropoietin and active vitamin D. Secretion of these hormones is impaired in chronic renal failure and contributes to the anemia and osteodystrophy found in this disorder (see Chapter 28).

Erythropoietin

Erythropoietin is a peptide growth factor that stimulates erythrocyte development in the bone marrow. The regulation of erythropoietin secretion is not completely understood; however, hypoxemia and decreased circulating red cell mass are known to increase its release. Hypoxia stimulates a transcription factor (hypoxia-inducible factor, HIF) that activates erythropoietin gene transcription.[15] Presumably, an increase in red cell production results in increased delivery of oxygen to the kidney and inhibits further production of erythropoietin. Erythropoietin is commercially available in a recombinant form that can be given parenterally. The anemia of chronic renal failure usually responds well to erythropoietin replacement therapy.

Vitamin D

Synthesis of active vitamin D is an interdependent function of the skin, liver, and kidney. The precursors to active vitamin D can be formed in the skin in response to the ultraviolet rays in sunlight, or they can be ingested in fortified food products. These precursors (cholecalciferol) then must undergo a series of two hydroxylations to become active. The first occurs in the liver, resulting in the formation of 25-hydroxycholecalciferol. The kidney performs the second hydroxylation to form 1,25-hydroxycholecalciferol, which is the active form of vitamin D.[16] Vitamin D is a necessary cofactor for calcium absorption from the intestine. It may also facilitate calcium reabsorption in the kidney tubules.

In chronic renal failure, the production of active vitamin D is impaired, resulting in poor calcium absorption from the intestine and low serum calcium levels. A low serum calcium level is the stimulus for parathyroid hormone release, resulting in removal of calcium and phosphate from the bones. Eventually excessive parathyroid hormone activity leads to the condition of osteodystrophy and predisposes to skeletal fractures (see Chapter 28).

AGE-RELATED CHANGES IN RENAL FUNCTION

Fetus

The fetal kidney begins to excrete urine between the 11th and 12th weeks of development.[17] Fetal urine is hypotonic to plasma because despite the fact that ADH is present and the volume receptors and osmoreceptors are functional, the renal distal tubule is less sensitive to ADH than the adult nephron. Perhaps this is related to the immaturity of the distal tubule, with inadequate binding sites for ADH and a low osmolality in the renal medulla. In addition, the placenta serves as a pseudokidney in regulating fetal fluid and electrolyte balance.

Infant

In the early postnatal period, the GFR is approximately 40 ml/1.73 m^2, compared to the normal adult value of 110 ml/1.73 m^2.[17] Renal blood flow is slow, the reabsorption of amino acids is limited, the ability to concentrate urine is minimal, and autoregulation is not fully achieved. Owing to an immature ability of the infant kidneys to regulate urine osmolality, infants are predisposed to volume depletion during fluid losses, such as those that occur with diarrhea, fever, fluid restrictions, or decreased intake. Volume regulation improves as the kidney matures. In addition, the glomerular and tubular basement membranes thicken, the glomeruli become increasingly permeable, and the loops of Henle lengthen. Systemic changes, such as increased cardiac output and increased plasma proteins, also influence the improvement in renal function. Between the first and second years of life, renal function essentially reaches maturity. Thereafter the kidney grows in proportion to overall body growth, reaching maximal size between 35 and 40 years of age.

Adult and Elderly

As part of the normal aging process, the kidney begins to diminish in size and function after the fourth decade and significantly by the middle of the sixth decade. The effects of aging on renal function are described in Geriatric Considerations: Changes in the Renal System. By the sixth decade the kidney has shrunk by 7%, and by the eighth decade it has shrunk by 20%.[18] The shrinkage occurs mostly in the cortex and is primarily due to loss of glomeruli. After age 40 years, the number of glomeruli begins to decrease, and by age 70 years it is estimated that as many as 30% to 50% of the glomeruli have been lost. Renal

GERIATRIC CONSIDERATIONS

Changes in the Renal System

Decreased renal blood flow	Decreased size and weight of nephrons	Decreased bladder innervation	Decreased bladder capacity	Increased urinary muscle weakness	Change in structure of female urethra	Loss of diurnal excretory pattern

Decreased GFR

Decreased size and weight of kidney

Decreased sensation of filling

Decreased sphincter tone

Nocturia

Decreased excretory and reabsorptive capabilities of tubules

Increased risk of incontinence

Difficulty starting urinary stream

Decreased excretion of drugs and metabolites	Decreased secretion of H$^+$	Decreased urine concentration	Increased renal threshold of glucose	Decreased glycosuria

In the aging individual, there is a 30% to 50% decrease in the number, size, weight, and function of the nephrons, with an accompanying reduction in the size and weight of the kidney. There is increasing interstitial fibrosis of the renal afferent arterioles. Loss of nephrons and diminished renal blood flow contribute to a decrease in the glomerular filtration rate (GFR).

There is also a decrease in the length and the excretory and reabsorptive capabilities of the tubules. The tubule changes affect the countercurrent mechanism, leading to significant changes in urine concentration, excretion, and absorption. Specifically, the changes include reduced urine concentration, decreased sodium retention, diminished drug and metabolite excretion, decreased hydrogen ion (H$^+$) secretion, and increased renal threshold for glucose. With aging, the kidney does not respond quickly to correct pH or sodium imbalances.

With aging, urinary muscles weaken, and sphincter tone and bladder capacity decrease. This increased muscular weakness can lead to a rise in the residual volume in the bladder and difficulty in starting the urinary stream. The length of the urethra decreases. There is also less bladder innervation and a reduced sensation of filling. A loss of the diurnal excretory pattern induces nocturia.

---

blood flow decreases after the fourth decade at an approximate rate of 10% per decade because of vascular changes, especially in the cortical blood vessels. After age 30 years the GFR declines by approximately 7.5 to 8 ml/min per decade of life.[18] By age 80 years, creatinine clearance is less than 100 ml/min.

As the number of functional nephrons decreases with aging, there is less renal reserve. Under normal conditions, the kidney functions adequately; however, elderly people are much more susceptible to fluid and electrolyte imbalances and renal damage. The elderly are also very susceptible to kidney damage from drugs and medications, including contrast media. Consequently, it is essential that renal function be evaluated before, during, and after they receive these agents or substances.

KEY POINTS

- Renal function is impaired at both ends of the life span. Infants have reduced ability to make concentrated urine due to kidney immaturity. Aged individuals have reduced numbers of functioning nephrons, reduced renal blood flow and GFR, and decreased ability to conserve salt and water.
- The very young and very old are at increased risk for fluid and electrolyte imbalances and drug toxicity.

TESTS OF RENAL STRUCTURE AND FUNCTION

Urinalysis, serum **creatinine**, blood urea nitrogen (BUN) levels, and tests of GFR are most helpful in evaluating kidney function, whereas other diagnostic tests are best for evaluating kidney structure.

Urine and Blood Studies

Routine assessment of urine is commonly performed to screen for a variety of kidney and metabolic disorders. Serum creatinine and BUN levels are used to monitor the progression of renal disease or to screen for occult renal insufficiency.

TABLE 26-4

Normal Composition of Urine

Characteristics	Normal Value
Color	Light yellow to amber
PH	Acidic
Specific gravity	1.003-1.030
Red cells	<5/HPF
White cells	<5/HPF
Protein	Negative
Glucose	Negative
Ketones	Negative
Nitrites	Negative
Casts	None
Crystals	None

HPF, High-powered field.

Urinalysis

Most often urinalysis is done on a single voided sample; however, longer collections may be done for quantitative analysis. Urinalysis assesses urine color, clarity, odor, specific gravity, pH, glucose, ketones, protein, and sediment (including cells, crystals, **casts,** and bacteria or other organisms). The first urine voided in the morning is the most concentrated, due to overnight fasting, and therefore is the best specimen to use for a routine or baseline urinalysis, especially to assess pH, osmolality, and sediment (Table 26-4).

A 24-hour urine collection measures the total quantity of a substance or substances excreted in a day. This is helpful for evaluating substances that are excreted in varying concentrations throughout the day, such as hormones, creatinine, protein, urea, and glucose.

Urine microscopy and culture and sensitivity tests assess the urine for presence of microorganisms and accompanying cells and to determine the medications or drugs to which the organisms are most sensitive. For these tests, a few milliliters of urine is collected by the clean-catch method and placed into a sterile container.

Urine is approximately 95% water and contains varying amounts of water-soluble waste products. Freshly voided urine has a slight odor due to the breakdown of urea to ammonia. If urine stands for a period of time or has a large bacteria population, it will have a strong ammonia smell. The ingestion and excretion of certain foods, such as asparagus, or of certain medications, such as vitamins, may cause urine to have a different odor.

The pale yellow to amber color of urine is due to the presence of urochrome pigments. Urine color can change because of the presence of cells or with an increased urine concentration. The presence of red blood cells (RBCs), or hematuria, can cause urine color to range from brown to bright red. White blood cells (WBCs) can make urine look cloudy. Concentrated urine is usually dark yellow to orange. Certain foods and drugs can change urine color. For instance, if beets

have been eaten, the urine may be burgundy, and if the individual has taken phenazopyridine (Pyridium), the urine may be orange.

Normally, urine is clear and slightly acidic, although the pH range is 4.5 to 8.0. Urine allowed to stand undisturbed will become cloudy and alkaline because of the breakdown of urea to ammonia, which increases the pH. Cloudiness can result from the presence of cells, bacteria, crystals, casts, or fat substances.

Urine specific gravity and urine osmolality are measures of the concentration of solute in the urine. Urine specific gravity varies with the amount of solids in the urine, such as cells, casts, and microorganisms, but urine osmolality is not affected by these substances. Thus, urine osmolality is a more accurate measure of the kidneys' ability to concentrate and dilute the urine. The range for specific gravity is 1.003 to 1.030, with the higher number indicating a more concentrated urine. Usually urine osmolality and specific gravity vary throughout the day and from day to day. Results that remain fixed over consecutive voidings and days could be an indicator of renal disease.

Normal urine contains little or no protein. A small amount of protein in the urine is insignificant, but excretion of more than 150 mg per 24 hours should be investigated, as it could indicate glomerular capillary disease. Proteinuria can cause urine to be foamy.

Glycosuria, or glucose in the urine, is abnormal and usually indicates hyperglycemia (elevated blood glucose), which can occur with diabetes mellitus or following an excessive ingestion of sugar. Rarely does glycosuria indicate renal disease.

A few epithelial cells, erythrocytes, leukocytes, and bacteria are normally found in urine. Fewer than 5 RBCs or WBCs per high-powered field is considered to be within normal limits. An excess of any of these cells may indicate a pathologic process; however, collection technique and presence of menstrual blood may be confounding factors.

Crystals and stones are not usually found in the urine. Either can originate anywhere along the urinary tract. If found in the urine, their composition should be identified and the urinary tract assessed for more crystals and stones (see Chapter 27).

When urinary casts are present, they provide important clues for differentiating renal diseases. Casts are formed in the nephron tubule and are composed of a protein meshwork with entrapped cells or cell fragments. Cells in the thick ascending loop of Henle produce and secrete small amounts of a glycoprotein, called *Tamm-Horsfall* (also called *uromodulin*) into the tubular lumen. This protein forms the meshwork that entraps cells in the tubule to form casts and is found in normal urine. Normal protein casts that do not have cells in them are called agranular casts. There are many types of abnormal casts, each associated with certain renal pathologic conditions. For example, WBC casts are associated with renal infections (pyelonephritis); RBC casts indicate inflammation of the glomerulus (glomerulonephritis); and epithelial cell casts indicate sloughing of tubular cells (acute tubular necrosis).

Serum Creatinine and Blood Urea Nitrogen

Creatinine is an end product of muscle metabolism that is excreted exclusively by the kidney. The serum creatinine level averages approximately 0.7 to 1.5 mg/dl and is relatively constant throughout the day and from day to day. Creatinine levels are slightly higher in men than in women because of men's larger muscle mass.

Serum creatinine is a fairly reliable indicator of renal function because it is affected by only two factors: (1) the rate of creatinine produced from muscle, which is relatively constant in the absence of muscle breakdown; and (2) the rate of creatinine excreted by the kidney, which is determined primarily by the GFR. Therefore, the GFR is reflected in the serum creatinine level. For instance, when GFR decreases by half, the concentration of creatinine in the serum doubles. A rise in serum creatinine indicates a decrease in renal function.

Urea is an end product of protein metabolism. It is excreted primarily by the kidney and measured in the blood as **blood urea nitrogen** (BUN). The BUN averages approximately 10 to 20 mg/dl and rises with a decrease in renal function, a decrease in fluid volume, and an increase in catabolism and dietary protein intake. When a change in renal function occurs, the BUN tends to change more rapidly than creatinine does; however, BUN is less specific. Often BUN and creatinine are measured together, and the ratio is determined. Acute changes in GFR are reflected in a higher BUN-to-creatinine ratio, usually greater than 20:1.

Measures of Glomerular Filtration Rate

GFR is an important parameter in the assessment of renal function. GFR is commonly measured by evaluating the clearance of a filterable substance from the plasma. Creatinine clearance is frequently used to assess GFR, but it is not completely accurate because some secretion and reabsorption occurs in the nephron tubules. At low GFR, creatinine clearance is quite unreliable. The accuracy of creatinine clearance tests can be improved by administration of cimetidine, a drug that blocks the tubular secretion of creatinine.[19]

More accurate measurement of GFR is obtained by using inulin, an inert substance that is filtered freely at the glomerulus and is completely unaffected by tubular secretion and reabsorption. The use of inulin is more expensive and cumbersome than creatinine clearance because it must be injected. The formula for measuring clearance is the same regardless of the marker substance used. Creatinine clearance is used in the following example, but the corresponding values for inulin can be substituted in the equation.

Creatinine clearance estimates the GFR by measuring the amount of blood that is cleared of creatinine each minute. Usually a 24-hour urine specimen and a blood specimen at the midpoint of the urine collection are used to determine creatinine clearance; however, shorter intervals can be used. The measured values are calculated in the following formula:

$$\text{Clearance} = \frac{\text{urine volume (ml/min)} \times \text{urinary creatinine (mg/dl)}}{\text{Plasma creatinine (mg/dl)}}$$

An estimate of GFR called the *Modification of Diet in Renal Disease study equation* (MDRD) can be made using only patient demographics and serum creatinine (S_{cr}).[20] This estimate is based on an average body surface area for an adult of 1.73 m^2. It does not require urine collection, making it simple compared to other measures of clearance:

$$\text{GFR (ml/min/1.73 m}^2\text{)} = 186 \times (S_{cr})^{-1.154} \times (\text{Age})^{-0.203}$$
$$\times (0.742 \text{ if female}) \times (1.210 \text{ if African American})$$

Diagnostic Tests

Although studies of urine and blood are good indicators of renal function, they often are not adequate to determine the underlying pathologic process. Diagnostic tests are helpful in assessing structural abnormalities, such as tumors, obstructions, congenital anomalies, perfusion defects, and histologic abnormalities. Sometimes a combination of diagnostic tests is necessary.

Kidney, Ureter, and Bladder Roentgenography

A kidney, ureter, and bladder (KUB) roentgenography is a plain radiograph (x-ray) taken of the abdomen to visualize the kidneys, ureters, and bladder. A KUB study shows the position, shape, size, and number of macroscopic or gross renal, ureteral, and bladder structures and surrounding bones. In addition, foreign bodies, radiopaque objects, stones, and neoplasms can be seen on KUB. The KUB may serve as a screening examination to inform further diagnostic testing.

Intravenous Urography/Pyelography

During intravenous urography, also called intravenous pyelography (IVP), an iodine-containing radiopaque dye is injected into a vein; it circulates through the kidney and is excreted in the urine. A rapid series of radiographs is made as the dye is being excreted. This test shows the size, shape, and location of urinary tract structures and can be used to evaluate renal excretory function. The dye is **nephrotoxic**, meaning poisonous to the kidney, and allergenic to some people. A state of hydration helps the dye to pass through the kidney and prevents renal damage. Because fecal matter and gas in the intestinal tract will interfere with visualization of the kidneys and ureters on the radiographs, a laxative or enema may be indicated before IVP.

Retrograde pyelography, also called *retrograde urography*, is an invasive procedure during which a catheter or cystoscope is passed into the bladder and ureters. A radiopaque dye is injected into the urinary tract, and x-ray films are made. Additional films are obtained as the catheters are removed, and more should be obtained approximately 15 to 30 minutes after the initial set to make sure all the dye has been excreted. This test provides anatomic information about the urinary tract from the renal pelvis through the urinary meatus and is often done when an obstruction is suspected. If desired, separate urine specimens may be obtained from each kidney before the dye is injected. Retrograde urography is often done in conjunction with cystoscopy (visualization of the bladder).

Complications associated with retrograde pyelography are urinary tract infection from retrograde movement of organisms with catheter insertion and dye injection. Hematuria can be associated with urinary tract infection or can result from injury to the urinary tract mucosa from the catheter or cystoscope. Ureteral edema can result from manipulation of the catheters and obstruct urine flow. Signs and symptoms of ureteral edema include decreased urine output and possibly pain.

Radionuclide Studies

Renograms and renal scans are diagnostic studies that use radioactive isotopes to assess kidney structure and function. In general, the renogram is more useful for assessing function, whereas the renal scan is better at detecting structural anomalies. During a renogram procedure, a small amount of filterable radioactive material is administered intravenously. It circulates through the kidney and is excreted in the urine. As the radionuclide circulates through the renal vessels and nephrons, a radiation detection probe counts the activity of the radioactive substance and simultaneously creates a graphic record of the activity. This test assesses renal function by measuring renal blood flow, glomerular filtration, and tubular secretion.

The renal scan uses a radionuclide that tends to accumulate in areas that are well perfused by blood. The renal scan images depict concentration of the radionuclide in the kidney and provide anatomic and some physiologic information. In the presence of tumors or nonfunctioning areas, the radioactive material will not be detected by the scan.

A more dynamic assessment of renal physiology can be obtained using positron emission tomography (PET) or single-photon emission computed tomography (SPECT). These modalities use scintigraphic imaging to view the kidney and can pick up subtle, dynamic changes. Regional differences in GFR, for example, can be detected by PET scan.

Radionuclide studies are safe to use with young children and when a client is allergic to radiopaque dye. There is a low incidence of allergic reactions to radiopharmaceuticals. In addition, because these substances are low-dose radiation, radionuclide studies can be repeated without deleterious effects.

Ultrasonography

Ultrasonography is a noninvasive, painless procedure that uses high-frequency sound waves to image renal structures. The sound waves are at a frequency above the limit of human hearing. Ultrasound is used because its short wavelength produces a more detailed picture or image than other types of sound waves. A probe with a transducer inside is held against the back and emits ultrasound waves that travel through tissue to the kidney and reflect off the kidney, back to the probe. The reflective waves are echoes. The returning echoes are converted by the transducer to electrical signals that a computer plots as points of light on a screen. Eventually the points build into lines, which form a picture or image.

Ultrasonography demonstrates gross renal anatomy, true kidney depth, structural abnormalities, and perirenal masses, and it can be used to distinguish between a fluid-filled cyst and a solid tumor.

Computed Tomography

Computed tomography (CT) combines roentgenography with computer technology and is a noninvasive, painless procedure. Instead of using broad x-ray beams, CT uses thin x-ray beams, each about 10 degrees apart. The information obtained during scanning is transmitted to a computer, which constructs a tomograph and calculates its density. Because the kidneys are located deep within the abdominal cavity, they opacify better after an IV injection of a contrast agent. CT shows more detail than ultrasonography. CT can demonstrate perirenal and renal masses, renal vascular disorders, and filling defects of the collecting system.

Magnetic Resonance Imaging

Magnetic resonance imaging (MRI) is a painless, noninvasive procedure that does not use x-rays or radioactive markers. The imager applies a strong magnetic field that causes protons to align themselves with the magnetic field. Pulses of radio waves are emitted that cause the magnetic fields to rotate or resonate. The rotating fields induce electrical signals that the computer analyzes and uses to create images or pictures on a screen. The renal images are available in all planes and show more detail than the images achievable with CT. Newer methods of MRI have been developed to obtain dynamic images using the movement of contrast dye through the kidney. Sequential fast-pulse imaging (functional MRI) allows assessment of obstructions, vascular disorders, and renal insufficiency.

Renal Biopsy

The purpose of a kidney biopsy is to obtain renal tissue that may be studied to determine the nature and extent of renal disease for diagnosis, management, and prognosis. Tissue obtained during a renal biopsy is taken from the outer or cortical region of the kidney. The renal tissue is studied histologically by light and electron microscopy and immunofluorescence. Some indications for a kidney biopsy are persistent proteinuria, hematuria originating from the kidney, unexplained acute renal failure, glomerular disease, renal mass, rejection of a transplanted kidney, and renal involvement in systemic disease.

Biopsy of the kidney may be accomplished by the open or closed method. Both are invasive procedures that require sterile technique. An *open renal biopsy* is rarely performed any longer and requires an operation with the subject under general anesthesia. An incision is made, the kidney is exposed, the biopsy needle is inserted into the kidney, a piece of tissue is extracted, and the area is closed and sutured. A closed renal biopsy, also called a **percutaneous** renal biopsy (percutaneous means "through the skin"), is usually done in a radiology suite, although it can be done at the bedside. The client is instructed to hold his or her breath as the biopsy needle is inserted through the skin and into the kidney. The movement of the needle as the client breathes is proof that it is in the kidney because the kidneys are in contact with the diaphragm and move with ventilation. Needle position in the kidney can also be confirmed with imaging techniques such as ultrasonography or fluoroscopy. In addition, the client usually complains of intense pressure or dull pain as the needle enters the kidney because the renal capsule is innervated by pain receptors. A small fragment of tissue is obtained, and the needle is withdrawn.

With either method of renal biopsy, hemorrhage is the most common complication. Hemorrhage may occur in the kidney, around the kidney, or into the urine. Other complications are infection, pain, clot formation in the kidney that could obstruct urine flow, aneurysm, intrarenal arteriovenous fistula, and laceration of adjacent organs or blood vessels.

Some contraindications to renal biopsy are hypertension, bleeding tendencies, documented renal neoplasm, gross sepsis, and frequent coughing or sneezing.

KEY POINTS

- Urinalysis provides important information about kidney function. Normal urine is clear, pale yellow to amber, and slightly acidic, and it may contain a few cells. Urine osmolality and specific gravity normally vary over the course of the day, depending on fluid intake. Urine is abnormal if it is cloudy or malodorous or contains protein, RBCs, crystals, stones, or casts. A fixed osmolality or specific gravity may indicate renal impairment.
- Serum creatinine and BUN are useful indicators of renal function. Serum creatinine is a more reliable indicator of renal function than BUN. In conditions of reduced GFR, serum creatinine and BUN levels increase.
- GFR can be estimated by measuring the clearance of a filterable substance from the urine. Creatinine clearance is frequently used for this purpose, but it is not completely accurate because of some tubular processing. Inulin clearance provides a more accurate measurement of GFR. The MDRD is a simple calculated method of estimating GFR using serum creatinine values.
- Diagnostic studies used to evaluate kidney structure and function include plain radiography, pyelography, radionuclide studies, ultrasound, CT, and MRI. Renal biopsy may be performed to obtain tissue for histologic examination.

SUMMARY

The kidneys have a vital role in excreting water-soluble waste products and maintaining fluid, electrolyte, and acid-base homeostasis. To perform these functions, the kidneys must have a sufficient GFR. Most waste products are removed by filtration rather than by secretion; thus, a reduced GFR results in accumulation of wastes in the blood.

The kidney has a large renal reserve and accomplishes its functions well until more than 75% of the nephron mass is dysfunctional.

The nephron is the structural and functional unit of the kidney. It performs three essential functions: filtration, secretion, and reabsorption. Filtration occurs at the glomerulus at a rate of about 125 ml/min. The composition of filtrate is similar to that of blood except that proteins and blood cells are absent. Normally 99% of the filtrate is reabsorbed along the nephron tubules, resulting in the elimination of 30 to 60 ml/hr of concentrated urine. Each nephron regulates its own GFR through tubuloglomerular feedback to prevent overloading its reabsorptive capacities.

The kidneys are responsive to a number of endocrine hormones that regulate blood osmolality and volume, including ADH, aldosterone, AII, ANP, urodilatin, uroguanylin, and guanylin. In addition, the kidneys produce two important endocrine hormones: erythropoietin and vitamin D. Urinalysis, serum creatinine and BUN levels, and tests of GFR are important indicators of renal function. Structural abnormalities can be assessed by a variety of imaging techniques.

REFERENCES

1. Koeppen BM, Stanton BA: Structure and function of the kidneys. In Koeppen BM, Stanton BA, editors: *Renal physiology*, ed 4, St Louis, 2007, Mosby, pp 19-30.
2. Ramcharan T, Matas AJ: Long-term (20-37 years) follow-up of living kidney donors, *Am J Transplant* 2(10):959-964, 2002.
3. Jarvis C: *Physical examination and health assessment*, ed 4, Philadelphia, 2004, Saunders, p 564.
4. Ganong WF: Renal function and micturition. In Ganong WF, editor: *Review of medical physiology*, ed 21, New York, 2003, Lange/McGraw-Hill, pp 702-732.
5. Guyton AC, Hall JE: Urine formation by the kidneys: II. Tubular processing of the glomerular filtrate. In Guyton AC, Hall JE, editors: *Textbook of medical physiology*, ed 11, Philadelphia, 2006, Saunders, pp 327-347.
6. Haraldsson B, Nyström J, Deen WM: Properties of the glomerular barrier and mechanisms of proteinuria, *Physiol Rev* 88(2):451-487, 2008.
7. Guyton AC, Hall JE: Urine formation by the kidneys: I. Glomerular filtration, renal blood flow, and their control. In Guyton AC, Hall JE, editors: *Textbook of medical physiology*, ed 11, Philadelphia, 2006, Saunders, pp 307-326.
8. Koeppen BM, Stanton BA: Regulation of extracellular fluid volume and NaCl balance. In Koeppen BM, Stanton BA, editors: *Renal physiology*, ed 4, St Louis, 2007, Mosby, pp 91-112.
9. Stockand JD, Sansom SC: Glomerular mesangial cells: electrophysiology and regulation of contraction, *Physiol Rev* 78:723-744, 1998.
10. Castrop H: Mediators of tubuloglomerular feedback regulation of glomerular filtration: ATP and adenosine, *Acta Physiol (Oxf)* 189(1):3-14, 2007.
11. Schnermann J, Levine DZ: Paracrine factors in tubuloglomerular feedback: adenosine, ATP, and nitric oxide, *Annu Rev Physiol* 65:501-529, 2003.
12. Harris RC: COX-2 and the kidney, *J Cardiovasc Pharmacol*, 47(Suppl. 1):S37-S42, 2006.
13. Koeppen BM, Stanton BA: Regulation of acid-base balance. In Koeppen BM, Stanton BA, editors: *Renal physiology*, ed 4, St Louis, 2007, Mosby, pp 129-148.
14. Saseen JJ, Carter BL: Hypertension. In Dipiro JT et al, editors: *Pharmacotherapy: a pathophysiologic approach*, ed 6, New York, 2005, McGraw-Hill, pp 185-217.

15. Fisher JW: Erythropoietin: physiology and pharmacology update, *Exp Biol Med* 228(1):1-14, 2003.
16. Mondry A, Wang Z, Dhar PK: Bone and the kidney: a systems biology approach to the molecular mechanisms of renal osteodystrophy, *Curr Mol Med* 5(5):489-496, 2005.
17. Davis ID, Avner ED: Glomerular disease. In Behrman RE, Kliegman RM, Jenson HB, editors: *Textbook of pediatrics,* ed 17, Philadelphia, 2004, Saunders, pp 1731-1735.
18. Choudhury D et al: Effect of aging on renal function and disease. In Brenner BM, editor: *Brenner and Rector's the kidney,* ed 6, Philadelphia, 2000, Saunders, pp 2187-2216.
19. Kabat-Koperska J, Safranow K, Gołembiewska E et al: Creatinine clearance after cimetidine administration: is it useful in the monitoring of the function of transplanted kidney? *Ren Fail* 29(6):667-672, 2007.
20. Levey AS, Bosch JP, Lewis JB et al: A more accurate method to estimate glomerular filtration rate from serum creatinine: a new prediction equation. Modification of Diet in Renal Disease Study Group, *Ann Intern Med* 130(6):461-470, 1999.

Intrarenal Disorders

Roberta J. Emerson

MEDIA RESOURCES

Additional Material for Study, Review, and Further Exploration

CD Companion ▪ Review Questions and Answers
▪ Glossary (with audio pronunciations for selected terms)
▪ Disease Profiles ▪ Animations

ⓔvolve **Website** at http://evolve.elsevier.com/Copstead/
▪ Case Studies ▪ Disease Profiles ▪ WebLinks ▪ Key Points Review

 Online Course (Module 14)

KEY QUESTIONS

▪ How are the locations of renal pain, findings on urinalysis, and other diagnostic test results used to differentiate the causes of kidney disease?
▪ How are renal tumors differentiated, detected, and managed?
▪ How do autosomal dominant and recessive forms of polycystic kidney disease differ?
▪ What risk factors and clinical findings are associated with pyelonephritis?

▪ What physiologic and pathophysiologic disorders predispose to the formation of renal calculi of differing compositions?
▪ How are the various forms of glomerulonephritis differentiated?
▪ What laboratory and clinical findings suggest a diagnosis of nephrotic syndrome?

CHAPTER OUTLINE

Functional kidneys are necessary for the removal of waste products from the blood and the maintenance of fluid, electrolyte, and acid-base balance despite wide variations in intake and losses. Systemic disorders that alter the delivery of blood flow to the kidney may adversely affect the kidney's ability to perform its filtering and homeostatic functions. In addition, many disorders occur primarily within the kidney and have the potential to result in renal insufficiency or failure. In general, these disorders can be categorized as (1) congenital, (2) neoplastic, (3) infectious, (4) obstructive, and (5) glomerular.

COMMON MANIFESTATIONS OF KIDNEY DISEASE

Pain

Thorough pain assessment is an essential component of the history and physical examination of any patient. The results can be useful in localizing the etiology of the pain, but assessment is also challenging because pain perceived as coming from the abdomen can originate from so many varied organs and tissues within the abdomen or extra-abdominally (see Chapter 47). Pain associated with the urinary tract may originate from the lower urinary tract (ureters, bladder or urethra) or the kidney itself. Renal or kidney pain is also referred to as nephralgia (-algia is from the Greek *algos,* meaning pain). Extensive damage to a kidney can occur without nephralgia because most of the kidney lacks pain receptors. However, the renal capsule is innervated by nociceptors, and when a disease process causes it to be distended, inflamed, or punctured, a dull to sharp pain is felt. Distention or inflammation produces a dull, constant pain. This may be the result of intrarenal fluid accumulation such as occurs with inflammation, infected or bleeding cysts, hemorrhage from blunt trauma, or neoplastic expansion. In addition, whenever the renal capsule is penetrated (e.g., during biopsy or trauma), a dull pain or intense pressure may be felt. The renal pelvis and the rest of the urinary tract are innervated by many pain receptors. Obstruction of the intrarenal collecting system causes pain if the obstruction leads to distention of the renal pelvis or capsule. Large calculi, however, can develop insidiously in the renal pelvis or calices and may be painless until they start to move into the ureteral junction. Ischemia caused by the occlusion of renal blood vessels (e.g., from an embolus, atherosclerotic disease, or tumor) results in a constant dull or sharp pain.

Pain associated with intrarenal disorders affecting the capsule is classically assessed by palpation or light percussion over the costovertebral angle posteriorly and is recorded as **CVA tenderness** or **flank pain.** Sympathetic nerves transmit information from renal and ureteral nociceptors to the spinal cord between the T10 and L1 levels. Because these sympathetic nerves enter the spinal cord at this level, the pain can be felt throughout the corresponding T10-L1 dermatomes. A **dermatome** is an area of skin innervated by a specific spinal cord segment (Figure 27-1). Visceral and cutaneous afferent fibers enter the spinal cord in close proximity and converge on some of the same neurons at the spinal, thalamic, and cortical levels of

FIGURE 27-1 Dermatomes T10 (thoracic) to L1 (lumbar) correspond to areas that innervate the renal structures.

the central nervous system. When visceral pain fibers are stimulated, concurrent stimulation of cutaneous fibers occurs and the visceral pain is perceived as though it had originated in the skin. Nerve fibers from the renal plexus communicate with the spermatic plexus, and because of this association, scrotal pain in males and labial pain in females may accompany renal pain.

Abnormal Urinalysis Findings

Urinalysis is an essential laboratory test for all suspected problems of the genitourinary system[1] (See Chapter 26). After history taking and a physical examination, urinalysis generally serves as a starting point for the differential diagnosis. First, urine is examined grossly, encompassing both the solvent and solutes. The color, odor, and turbidity of the urine offer the first clues. Dark, strong-smelling urine may be an indicator of decreased renal function. Cloudy pungent urine generally indicates an infectious process, the turbidity being a result of leukocytes in the urine. Dipstick tests and microscopic analysis provide a great deal of additional information. Microscopic examination entails the assessment of the urine sediment, the portion that remains after the urine specimen is centrifuged.[1] Table 27-1 lists major kidney disorders that are associated with abnormalities identified by urine dipstick testing. Table 27-2 provides abnormal microscopic urinalysis results indicative of kidney disorders.

Other Diagnostic Tests

Many of the diagnostic tests presented in Chapter 26 are applicable to intrarenal disorders. The simple KUB identifies gross abnormalities of the kidney related to position, size, and shape as well as renal calculi that are radiopaque.[1] Renal vasculature can be examined by renogram or renal scan; renal scans will also identify tumors in the kidney. Ultrasonography differentiates the solid mass of a tumor from fluid-filled cysts. Computerized tomography and MRI provide detailed information regarding multiple pathologies including thrombi or other vascular occlusions, masses, and obstructions involving the kidney. In situations in which these diagnostic tests are insufficient and actual tissue examination is necessary (e.g., tumor assessment), a renal biopsy may be required.[1]

TABLE 27-1

Urine Dipstick Findings Associated with Kidney Disorders*

Urine Dipstick Finding	Associated Kidney Disorders
Specific Gravity	
■ Decreased	Chronic kidney disease (decreased concentrating ability)
	Diabetes insipidus
■ Increased	Diabetes mellitus
	Syndrome of inappropriate secretion of antidiuretic hormone
pH	
■ Increased (6.5-8.0)	>7.5 Urinary tract infection with urea-splitting bacteria (e.g., *Proteus*)
	Renal tubular acidosis
	Calcium or struvite calculi
■ Decreased (4.5-5.5)	Uric acid or cystine calculi
Hematuria	Renal cell carcinoma
	Tubulointerstitial renal disease
	Urinary tract infection
	Trauma
	Glomerulonephritis
	Obstructive processes (e.g., calculi, neoplasms)
Proteinuria	Diabetic nephropathy
	Renal hypertension
	Glomerulopathies
	Nephrotic syndrome
	Renal arterial or venous obstruction
Glycosuria and Ketones	Diabetes mellitus
	Protein-energy malnutrition
White Blood Cells/ Leukocyte Esterase	Urinary tract infection
Nitrites	Urinary tract infection (especially with Gram-negative bacteria)

*Data derived from Gerber GS, Brendler CB: Evaluation of the urologic patient: history, physical examination, and urinalysis. In Wein JA et al, editors: *Campbell-Walsh Urology*, ed 9, Philadelphia, 2007, Saunders, pp 97-105.

KEY POINTS

- Renal pain is generally perceived at the costovertebral angle. Pain is transmitted to the spinal cord between T10 and L1 by sympathetic afferent neurons. Pain may be felt throughout the dermatomes corresponding to T10-L1. Renal pain is usually due to distention and inflammation of the renal capsule and has a dull, constant character.
- Urinalysis provides a foundation for the differential diagnosis of renal dysfunction. Dipstick and microscopic urinalysis results provide clues to intrarenal pathologies.
- Other diagnostic tests provide information related to abnormal kidney anatomy and function.

CONGENITAL ABNORMALITIES

A wide variety of anomalies in the development of the kidneys have been documented in the literature. One or both kidneys may be involved. In some cases, findings are associated with other abnormalities, while in others the renal abnormalities are isolated. Congenital kidney abnormalities may be exceptionally rare or may occur with considerable frequency. They may be identified prenatally during ultrasound assessment of the developing fetus, noted at birth, or manifest only in later life. Discussion here will focus on the more common congenital anomalies as a complete discussion of all these pathologies is beyond the scope of this text.

TABLE 27-2

Microscopic Urinalysis Findings and Associated Kidney Disorders*

Microscopic Urinalysis Finding	Associated Kidney Disorders
Cells	
■ RBCs (circular shaped)	Urinary tract infection
	Trauma
	Obstructive disorders (e.g., calculi, neoplasm)
■ RBCs (irregularly shaped)	Glomerulopathies
■ WBCs (>1-2/HPF)	Infection or inflammation (e.g., urinary tract infection, neoplasm, calculi)
■ Irregular transitional epithelial cells	Malignancy
Casts	
■ Hyaline	Usually no pathologic significance
	Chronic kidney disease
	Pyelonephritis
■ Fatty	Nephrotic syndrome
	Nephrosis
■ RBC	Glomerulonephritis
■ WBC	Acute glomerulonephritis
	Acute pyelonephritis
	Acute tubulointerstitial nephritis
■ Waxy	Chronic kidney disease
	Diabetic nephropathy
	Glomerulonephritis
Crystals	
■ Cystine	Cystinuria
	Acidic urine
■ Uric acid	Uric acid calculi
	Acidic urine
■ Calcium oxalate	Calcium calculi
	Acidic urine
■ Calcium phosphate	Calcium calculi
	Alkaline urine
■ Triple phosphate/struvite	Struvite calculi
	Alkaline urine
■ Bacteria ≥5/HPF	Bacterial urinary tract infection
■ Yeast	Yeast urinary tract infection
■ Parasites (e.g., *Trichomonas vaginalis*)	Vaginitis in women
	Urethritis in men

*Data derived from: Gerber GS, Brendler CB: Evaluation of the urologic patient: history, physical examination, and urinalysis. In Wein JA et al, editors: *Campbell-Walsh urology*, ed 9, Philadelphia, 2007, Saunders, pp 105-109.

Pagana KD, Pagana TJ: *Mosby's manual of diagnostic and laboratory tests*, ed 3, St Louis, 2006, Mosby, pp 1007-1014.

Renal Agenesis and Hypoplasia

Renal agenesis means a failure of one or both kidneys to embryonically develop at all.[2,3] On the other hand, **renal hypoplasia** describes a condition in which some fetal development of the kidneys has occurred. Hypoplasia may be insufficient for extrauterine life if both kidneys are involved or impact later renal functioning. Probably it is most accurate to conceptualize renal hypoplasia as existing on a continuum of agenesis on one extreme and slight decreases in the number of nephrons on the other.[2,4] They both can be found as a single entity or in combination with other congenital malformations.

Bilateral renal agenesis (BRA) is found in approximately 1 in 5,000 fetuses and results from failure of the metanephros (renal buds) to develop in the fetus.[2] It is incompatible with extrauterine life and results in stillbirth or death shortly thereafter.[2,4] It is usually found in Potter syndrome, where severely inadequate quantities of amniotic fluid result in compression of the fetus within the uterus.[2] This pathology is characterized by a collection of associated anomalies that includes wide-spaced eyes with epicanthal folds, low-set ears with insufficient cartilage, a nose that is beaked, and receding chin.[4]

Unilateral renal agenesis (URA) is more common than bilateral renal agenesis, although the actual incidence is more difficult to discern.[3] It has been estimated to occur approximately 1:1000 based upon more than 9000 postnatal autopsies, but actual diagnosis may not occur until much later in life. Under these circumstances, overall incidence is more accurately estimated at 1:500. It has been suggested this estimate is excessive because some of those diagnosed with URA could have involuted, malformed kidneys. URA is often associated with concurrent congenital anomalies, both within the urinary tract and beyond it. Nonurological anomalies are usually cardiac or gastrointestinal in nature. These findings have facilitated the identification of specific genetic mutations associated with URA. Sometimes renal agenesis has been found to be familial and inherited as a dominant trait; screening by ultrasound of parents and siblings has been recommended when infants with agenesis or dysgenesis are involved. Poorly controlled diabetes and exposure to certain drugs (e.g., those affecting angiotensin II) and chemicals have been implicated as teratogens. In URA, the remaining kidney usually enlarges as a compensatory mechanism. Animal studies indicate an increased risk of hypertension, proteinuria, glomerulosclerosis, and chronic kidney disease, but such data in humans are limited. Lifelong monitoring of renal function is recommended.[3]

It has been estimated that 40% to 60% of the cases of end-stage renal failure in the pediatric population is due to congenital renal hypoplasia.[2] It is associated with low birth weight, and, although other environmental factors have been explored, it is more likely that mutations of genes responsible for the process of kidney fetal development are accountable. Likely, there are key genes that are ultimately responsible for the number of nephrons that develop in the kidneys. Studies have suggested that, even in the presence of compensatory hypertrophy, when the number of functioning nephrons is reduced to approximately 53% of normal, glomerulosclerosis and hypertension are initiated. Again, when renal hypoplasia has been identified, lifelong monitoring is recommended.[2]

In some cases, cysts have been identified in the remaining kidney tissue in both URA and renal dysgenesis, adding these conditions to the long list of cystic kidney diseases.[5]

Cystic Kidney Diseases

Cystic disease of the kidneys incorporates a wide range of hereditary, developmental, and acquired conditions.[5] Including renal neoplasms with cystic changes, more than 40 classifications and subtypes have been identified in the literature. Depending on the classification, these fluid-filled craters may be present at birth or only visible later in life. They may involve one or both kidneys and be accompanied by other anomalies, or they may be the only pathology present.[5] More commonly found in men, and increasing in prevalence with aging, renal cysts have been reportedly identified in more than half of patients over the age of 50.[6] Cysts may be found in other organs, or limited to the kidneys, depending on the disorder. Within the kidney, cysts may be diffuse or confined to one anatomic area.[5] They may be isolated findings, or there may be many within a single kidney.[6] With a growth rate of 2.8 mm/year, cysts may achieve significant size, producing flank pain and hemorrhage.[6]

The two most common forms of renal cystic disease are the autosomal recessive and autosomal dominant polycystic diseases;[5] discussion will be limited to these classifications and their subtypes. Autosomal recessive polycystic kidney disease (ARPKD) is usually diagnosed in infants and young children, whereas autosomal dominant polycystic kidney disease (ADPKD) is generally diagnosed in adulthood.[5] In individuals with a family history of polycystic disease, diagnosis can usually be accomplished through renal sonography.[7] Although the pathogenesis is similar, the ARPKD and ADPKD forms of the disease are genetically different, and their clinical courses are usually distinct (Table 27-3).

Autosomal Recessive Polycystic Kidney Disease.

The incidence of ARPKD is 1:20,000 live births, and it is often identified in the neonatal period when an accompanying pulmonary hypoplasia results in the death of 30%.[5] In ARPKD, the kidneys retain their shape but are uniformly enlarged, and collecting ducts are dilated from the medulla to the cortex. The classic presentation of ARPKD for 20% to 40%

of those affected is the development of systemic hypertension and progression to end-stage kidney disease by the age of 15. Those who live to reach adulthood typically retain some renal function, but experience a progressive decline in liver function.[5] The *polycystic kidney and hepatic disease* gene (PKHD1), which is located on chromosome 6p, has been identified in association with ARPKD.[5,8] The gene is so named due to the inclusion of liver pathology with the disease. Abnormal portal ducts are found in neonates, and portal fibrosis is noted in older patients.[5,8] There has been no documented evidence of ARPKD being linked with renal neoplasia.[5] A recessive pattern of inheritance within the family and pathology on liver biopsy are the best diagnostic data because both the clinical presentation and the results of sonograms, CT, or MRI can be similar to those of the autosomal dominant form of polycystic disease.[5]

Autosomal Dominant Polycystic Kidney Disease.

ADPKD is the most common of all the hereditary cystic kidney diseases,[5,7,9,10] with an incidence of 1 to 2:1,000 live births.[5,9,10] For 10% of the end-stage kidney disease patients receiving hemodialysis in Europe and the United States, the etiology of their disease is ADPKD.[5] It is documented in all ethnic groups worldwide.[7,9]

There are three genetically distinct but phenotypically similar forms of ADPKD. Gene PKD1, located on chromosome 16, codes for a protein involved in the regulation of the cell cycle and intracellular calcium transport in epithelial cells; a group of voltage-linked calcium channels are coded for by gene PKD2 on chromosome 4; and the PDK3 gene is postulated but not currently identified.[5,7,9] Distribution of these genotypes is such that 85% of the cases are associated with PDK1 and just under 15% with PDK2, while only a few are believed to be linked to PDK3.[5,7,9] Mutations of these genes add further complexity to ADPKD.[7] Approximately 10% of the cases of ADPKD are not familial in origin and appear sporadically.[5,9] Because of significant variability in clinical presentation within families, environmental modifying factors have been

---

TABLE 27-3

Comparison of Autosomal Recessive and Autosomal Dominant Polycystic Kidney Disease

Feature	Autosomal Recessive	Autosomal Dominant
Gene defect	Chromosome 6p	Gene PKD1 on chromosome 16, or gene PKD2 on chromosome 4, or gene PDK3 location unknown
Incidence	1:20,000	1-2:1000
Age at diagnosis	Usually neonate to childhood	Usually fourth to fifth decade
Imaging findings	Symmetrically enlarged kidneys	Enlarged kidneys, often asymmetrical
Histologic findings	Cysts derived from epithelial cells of collecting ducts	Entire nephron involved
Liver involvement	Abnormal portal ducts progressing to fibrosis	Multiple cysts
Other systemic findings	Usually none	Cysts in other abdominal organs, aneurysms, abnormal cardiac valves, hernias, and diverticuli

suggested, though not yet documented.[7] It does seem that the specific gene is responsible for the initiation of cystic development, but not necessarily their expansion.[7]

The result of these genetic abnormalities is a reduction of intracellular calcium and excessive concentrations of intracellular cAMP; the development of the cysts seems to be related to the increased quantities of cAMP.[7] It appears that cells lose their normal physical orientation and mechanisms of communication with one another; the precise mechanisms of this process at a molecular level remain unknown.[10] As the cysts multiply and expand, the overall size of the kidneys increases and there is a progressive decline in glomerular filtration rate (GFR) as the amount of normally functioning tissue is slowly reduced.[7] Figure 27-2 provides a comparison of normal and polycystic kidneys. Kidneys may increase to four times their normal size, and weight of the organs can increase by a factor of 10 to 12.[9] Renal perfusion decreases, and significant remodeling occurs in the renal circulation.[7] Expansion of the cysts compacts and distorts the vascular system, and the resulting local ischemia activates the intrarenal renin-angiotensin system. The progressive reduction in renal function appears to be primarily associated with an increase in the size of the kidney and the overall volume of the cysts.[7]

Typically, both kidneys are involved, but 17% of the cases have been found to be unilateral; these are most likely to be pediatric cases, and the other kidney is often affected by the time the child reaches adulthood.[5] There are a few cases of unilateral ADPKD with agenesis of the other kidney reported in the literature. Many round cysts of varying sizes from <0.01 to several centimeters are dispersed throughout the medulla and cortex, and any portion of the nephron may be involved.[5] By the time the disease is identified, patients with ADPKD have hundreds of thousands of cysts.[9]

In contrast to its recessive form, ADPKD is associated with pathologies in other body systems.[5] In 50% of cases there are cysts in other abdominal organs (liver, pancreas, spleen, lung, seminal vesicles, and ovaries), while 10% to 30% have Berry aneurysms in the Circle of Willis cerebral circulation.[5,7] By far, the most common of all the extrarenal presentations is liver cyst development.[7] Subcutaneous cysts; aneurysms of the coronary arteries; and abnormal cardiac valves, hernias, and diverticuli are all documented.[5,7] Prolapse of the mitral valve is present in 25% of ADPKD cases.[7] There is a significant risk of uncontrolled renal cellular proliferation resulting in neoplasms for the individual with ADPKD, but benign adenomas occur more frequently than carcinomas.[5] The incidence of renal cell carcinoma is no greater in ADPKD than in the general population, but it does occur at an earlier age.[7]

Although prenatal and neonatal cases have been reported and ADPKD can present at any age, it usually manifests during the patient's 40s or 50s.[5] In less than 1% of cases, ADPKD is identified in the neonate or in utero.[7] ADPKD is marked by a great deal of variability in the rate of decline in renal function.[9] By the age of 70, half of the patients with the PKD2 gene still have satisfactory renal function, while the majority of patients with the PKD1 gene have progressed to end-stage renal disease.[7] The disease process appears to advance more rapidly in men than in women.[7]

In the early phases of the disease, the ability to concentrate urine is decreased.[7] Approximately 50% of the patients 20 to 34 years of age have hypertension before their renal function is significantly affected; by the time the disease has progressed to end-stage renal disease, this number approaches 100%. Unfortunately, the diagnosis of hypertension is often made late in the disease process; early interventions for hypertension are urged because death from ADPKD is most often due to cardiovascular disease. Hypertension also increases the likelihood of escalated loss of renal function, proteinuria, and hematuria.[7]

In 60% of adult patients with ADPKD, pain is the most frequent complaint.[7] Pain may be due to bleeding within the kidney, movement of kidney stones, or the development of urinary tract infections. Kidney stones develop in 20% of the cases and are usually uric acid–based or calcium oxalate–based. Urinary tract infections are most often due to *Enterobacter* organisms. Infection of the cysts themselves may also develop; these infections are more difficult to treat, and many cases require months of antimicrobial therapy. When it occurs, hemorrhage of cysts is usually self-limited.[7]

Concomitant cystic liver involvement is usually asymptomatic until the patient with ADPKD reaches end-stage renal disease.[7] At this time, the increased size of the liver may cause dyspnea, gastrointestinal reflux, and back pain. Involvement of other organs and tissues results in additional manifestations; each of these requires attention by healthcare providers.[7]

Diagnosis is based on genetic history and imaging techniques, most often ultrasonography.[7,9] When there is no family history of ADPKD, a presumption of the disease is made if imaging identifies cysts and bilaterally enlarged kidneys, or cysts in the liver and both kidneys. Genetic testing is then performed to substantiate the diagnosis.[7,9]

FIGURE 27-2 Comparison of normal and polycystic kidneys. (From Lewis SL: *Medical-surgical nursing: assessment and management of clinical problems,* ed 7, St. Louis, 2007, Mosby, p 1176.)

Treatment of ADPKD is primarily supportive, emphasizing the control of blood pressure and management of whatever associated pathologies are present.[7] Once end-stage renal disease is reached, dialysis is initiated. Patients with ADPKD seem to have fewer problems with dialysis than do patients with other pathologies. Ultimately, the treatment of choice is renal transplantation, and the results are equivalent to those of others undergoing this procedure.[7]

NEOPLASMS

Neoplasms found in the kidney may be benign or malignant primary tumors, or they may be secondary metastases from extrarenal sites. Since the kidney is encased in a tough, fibrous capsule, as they grow, all renal neoplasms will distort the architecture of the kidney and ultimately hinder renal function. As a characteristic of the malignant cell phenotype, malignant renal neoplasms also carry the threat of metastasis to distant sites.

Benign Renal Neoplasms. Several benign tumors may be found in the kidney, developing from the renal cortex, medulla, or capsule, but they are less common than malignant neoplasms.[6] Contrary to most benign tumors, those in the kidney are not truly encapsulated.[6]

Etiology and Pathogenesis. **Renal cortical adenomas** are small, solid growths that develop from cortical tissue.[6] These tumors have been documented to occur at incidences of less than 1% up to 23%, depending on the study. They typically remain small (<1 cm), and the patient is asymptomatic. **Metanephric adenoma** appears to be histologically related to nephroblastoma (Wilms tumor).[6] **Oncocytoma** is the most difficult to differentiate from renal cell carcinoma,[6,11,12] especially the chromophobe subtype.[12] They are light brown to tan in color with well-defined borders.[6] Numerous histologic variations have been identified, further complicating diagnosis. **Angiomyolipoma** of the kidney is a benign growth composed of adipose and smooth muscle tissue and blood vessels. It is believed to be hormone-dependent because it is primarily found in postpubescent women. **Nephroma** is a benign cystic neoplasm that cannot be reliably differentiated from renal cell carcinoma in adults or nephroblastoma in children. **Mixed epithelial stromal tumor of the kidney** has only recently been identified and may be related to cystic nephromas. This tumor is most often found in perimenopausal women, most of whom are taking estrogen replacement therapy. The specific characteristics of this benign tumor are in the process of being determined, and it may incorporate several distinct lesions. **Leiomyomas** are benign growths evolving from the renal capsule, pelvis, or even the renal vein. Other benign tumors have been identified in the kidney, but most of these are exceedingly rare, according to the available literature. These include hemangiomas, fibromas, lipomas, lymphangiomas, and even reninomas—benign neoplasms of the juxtaglomerular cells responsible for the secretion of renin.[6]

Diagnosis and Treatment. Differentiating benign from malignant growths is extremely difficult, both from radiologic and clinical findings.[6] They may attain sufficient size as to be palpable abdominal masses, produce flank pain, and hemorrhage; these findings are the same as those associated with malignant renal tumors. Generally, benign renal neoplasms are treated by removal of the kidney (**nephrectomy**) since they are space-occupying lesions and because of a propensity to undergo malignant changes.[6] More recently, laparoscopic and tissue-sparing approaches have been developed, allowing the retention of more functioning renal tissue.[13]

Renal Cell Carcinoma. The vast majority of renal cancer is due to renal cell carcinoma (RCC) (85%)[14-16]; transitional cell cancers of the pelvis and soft-tissue malignancies such as sarcomas account for the remainder, at about 11% and 2%, respectively.[14] Figure 27-3 illustrates a cross-sectional view of RCC. In the United States, the number of new cases of RCC is more than 39,000 annually, with 13,000 deaths.[17] This represents only 2% to 3% of all malignancies.[15,17] Since the early 1970s, the incidence has progressively risen at an annual rate of 3% in the United States and most of Europe.[13-15]

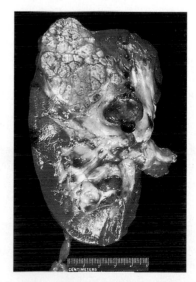

FIGURE 27-3 Cross-sectional view of renal cell carcinoma. (From Lewis SL: *Medical-surgical nursing: assessment and management of clinical problems,* ed 7, St. Louis, 2007, Mosby, p 1178.)

Although occurring in men at twice the frequency of women,[6,14] the rise in incidence is more rapid among women in the United States.[14] Incident rates among African Americans are 20% higher[6] and continue to increase more rapidly than Caucasians.[14] Rates among Hispanics are also rising.[15] Taken as a whole, these trends are gradually altering the overall distribution of the disease. Age at diagnosis averages the early sixties.[14] Survival rate at 5 years for those with advanced metastatic RCC is less than 10%.[16]

Etiology and Pathogenesis. Although only a small portion of the cases of RCC are attributed to genetic factors, the risk of its development is increased 2 to 4 times when there is a first-degree relative with the disease.[14] These inherited cases of RCC are typically diagnosed in younger patients, and are more often both bilateral and multifocal.[12] These hereditary kidney cancers have been the source of most of the knowledge regarding RCC. Several specific genes have been identified in these cases and are associated with specific subtypes.[15,18] The inherited forms of RCC that have been the best described are von Hippel-Lindau, hereditary papillary renal carcinoma, Birt-Hogg-Dubé syndrome, and hereditary leiomyomatosis renal cell carcinoma.[18,19] Now that their genetic basis has been identified, current research is exploring mechanisms of carcinogenesis.[18,19] The von Hippel-Lindau (VHL) gene is also implicated in the nonfamilial, sporadic cases of RCC.[13]

The identification of risk factors has been derived from pooled data from a large number of studies worldwide,[14,15] and these are listed in Box 27-1. The primary risk factors are obesity and cigarette smoking, with risk reduction documented with both weight loss and smoking cessation. A number of previously identified risks have been disproven from these meta-analyses (e.g., acetaminophen, aspirin, and alcohol use),[14] while others (e.g., low fruit/vegetable intake) have simply been inadequately substantiated.[15]

Renal cell carcinoma actually encompasses several subtypes, histologically differentiated from one another. This variability in histology complicates diagnosis.[16] The World Health Organization (WHO) has established a system of terminology and differentiation of these subtypes.[16] The most common of these (approximately 80%) is **clear cell RCC,**[11,16] so named because the cells contain clear cytoplasm.[12] These tumors originate in the renal cortex from cells of the proximal tubule and are usually unilateral and random in occurrence with rare cases of familial patterns of inheritance.[11] In nearly every case of clear cell RCC, there is an omission or unbalanced chromosomal translocation responsible for the loss of the smallest overlapping region of chromosome 3.[19] The tumors themselves are spherical, with clearly defined margins of bright yellow to grey-white tissue.[19] Tumors often invade the renal vein and then the inferior vena cava. Clear cell RCC is most frequently associated with metastatic disease.[12] The tumor enters adjacent lymph nodes and metastasizes via the lymphatics as well as the vascular system. The lung is the primary site of metastasis, followed by the liver, bone, adrenal glands, and the contralateral kidney.[12] Next in frequency is **papillary RCC,** representing 10% to 15% of all renal cell carcinomas.[11,16] Papillary RCC evolves from cells of the distal tubule, and affects men much more often than women (5:1). This type of RCC may also be sporadic or hereditary, and two subtypes of familial papillary RCC have been identified.[11] It is not associated with chromosome 3 deletions.[19] Papillary RCC may be multifocal and bilateral. Papillae may be seen grossly as yellow flakes. Tumors may protrude into the renal calyces and pelvis, ultimately invading the collecting tubules and often the renal vein.[19] When compared to clear cell RCC, papillary RCC is less likely to metastasize so has a better prognosis; however, if it does metastasize, the prognosis is poorer than that of clear cell RCC.[11] Some references describe **translocation-associated RCC** as a separate subtype that retains features of papillary RCC but is unique both genetically and clinically.[12] **Chromophobe RCC** represents 5% to 6% of all RCC cases.[11,12,16] This subtype originates from the renal parenchyma.[11] Because of slow growth and infrequent metastasis, 5-year survival rates exceed 90%.[11] It is associated with multiple chromosomal losses.[19] Cell membranes are prominent. Finally, **medullary** and **collecting duct carcinomas** are the least common, representing less than 1% of all RCC cases.[11] Unfortunately, they occur in younger patients, develop rapidly, and carry only a 30% 5-year survival rate.[11,12] Medullary RCC has been found to be associated with the sickle cell trait.[11] A final group of RCC is **unclassified;** these renal carcinomas that fail to conform to any delineated category represent 7% of renal epithelial tumors.[12]

Based upon the considerable research involving the function and dysfunction of the von Hippel-Lindau gene, the pathophysiologic basis of clear cell RCC has been clarified.[13,16,20] The mutation or inhibition of the VHL gene, a tumor suppressor gene, results in the accumulation of a number of factors that activate genes for vascular endothelial growth factor, platelet-derived growth factor, and erythropoietin. An environment conducive to tumor growth is created.[13,20] Understanding of these pathways has lead to new therapeutic interventions for RCC.[13,20]

Clinical Manifestations. RCC is often asymptomatic until it is quite advanced. When it does present with signs and symptoms, the most common are CVA tenderness, hematuria, and a palpable abdominal mass. Dyspnea, cough, and bone pain develop secondary to metastasis.

BOX 27-1

Risk Factors for Renal Cell Carcinoma

- Cigarette smoking
- Obesity
- Hypertension
- Diabetes mellitus
- Asbestos exposure
- Prior oophorectomy or hysterectomy
- Long-term renal dialysis
- Kidney transplantation

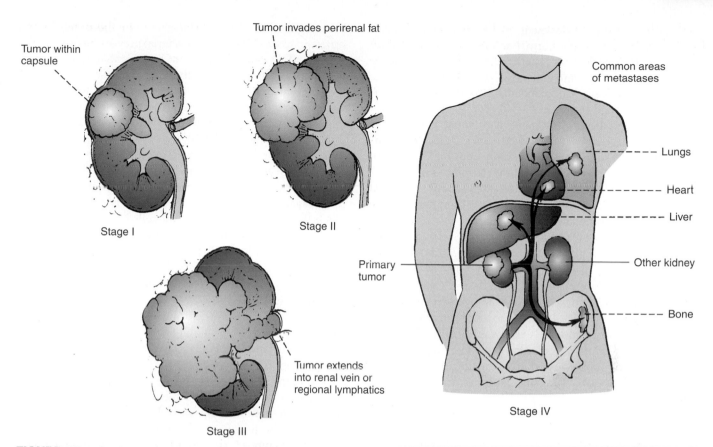

FIGURE 27-4 Staging system for renal cell carcinoma. (From Black JM, Matassarin-Jacobs E: *Medical-surgical nursing: clinical management for continuity of care,* ed 7, Philadelphia, 2005, Saunders, p 923.)

Diagnosis and Treatment. Renal ultrasound and CT of the abdomen may be of value. If cysts accompany RCC, renal ultrasound is 98% accurate in discerning them. Figure 27-4 illustrates the staging system used with RCC. When RCC is localized, it can be surgically removed in a nephrectomy, and this is the standard of treatment.[11,16] Unfortunately, metastasis occurs in more than one third of cases,[11,13] even following nephrectomy,[16] and metastatic RCC has been found to be unresponsive to cytotoxic chemotherapy.[13,18] The standard nephrectomy is a major surgery, necessitating a large lateral incision. Other less radical approaches include nephron-sparing interventions and laparoscopic nephrectomy. In metastatic disease, spontaneous regression of metastases following nephrectomy occurs in less than 1% of cases. Conventional chemotherapeutic interventions have been found to elicit a poor response in advanced RCC. Interferon-α and interleukin-2 are cytokines used as tissue-specific therapies in these situations with clear cell RCC, with 15% to 25% response rates.[13,16] Systemic, nonsurgical interventions for the other subtypes of RCC have not been established.[16] More targeted therapies, specifically angiogenetic inhibitors, have been in clinical trials or are now available for selected patient situations.[13,16,21]

Nephroblastoma (Wilms Tumor). Nephroblastoma is the fourth most frequently occurring pediatric malignancy and the most common childhood kidney cancer, affecting 1:10,000 children.[22,23] Eighty percent of the cases are diagnosed prior to the age of 5 years,[22,23] with a median of 3 to 4 years of age.[23] Wilms tumor is very rarely found in children older than 15 years of age.[23] Incidence is equally distributed between the genders,[22] and it is primarily unilateral and sporadic with only 1% to 2% of those with Wilms tumor having a relative with one.[23] In 5% to 10% of cases, the tumor presents bilaterally or multifocally.[22,23] It is believed that these cases are the result of a germline mutation that provides a genetic predisposition to Wilms tumor.[22] Bilateral presentation is often associated with cysts in combination with the tumor.

Etiology and Pathogenesis. Nephroblastomas develop from embryonic pluripotent kidney precursor cells.[22] Precursor lesions called *nephrogenic rests,* persistent clusters of embryonic cells, are notable histologic findings.[23] The first gene found to be associated with Wilms tumor was WT1, located on the short arm of chromosome 11.[22] WT1 codes for a protein that functions as a transcription factor in embryonic kidneys and plays a key role in their development.[22] Germline mutations or deletions of this protein are associated with Wilms tumor and a wide variety of other genitourinary abnormalities, mental retardation, and syndromes of congenital anomalies in approximately 10% of cases,[22,23] but the genetic defects responsible for most cases remain unknown.[22]

Nephroblastomas are typically large, well encapsulated tumors that grow rapidly. They undergo hemorrhage and cystic changes; necrosis that occurs due to the hemorrhaging is responsible for the development of the cysts. As the malignant cells proliferate, the normal architecture of the kidney is altered. The renal pelvis becomes compressed, and locally the tumor infiltrates into the renal veins and hilar nodes. Metastasis is typically via the bloodstream to the brain, liver, adrenal glands, and bone.

Clinical Manifestations. A palpable abdominal mass is evident in about 80% of cases. Abdominal pain, hypertension, and hematuria are also common local manifestations. Nephroblastoma may produce a tumor thrombus in the inferior vena cava, which can lead to decreased venous return and lower-extremity edema. Additional signs or symptoms may be noted reflective of the sites of metastasis.

Diagnosis and Treatment. Most often the tumor is identified by the parents or during a routine physical examination. Renal ultrasound and/or CT scan will usually identify anatomical abnormalities associated with the tumor. Over the past 20 years, treatment protocols have improved to the point that what was previously a lethal disease now has a cure rate of 85%.[22] Key to treatment is the removal of the involved kidney (nephrectomy). Radiation and chemotherapy are routine following surgery. Radiation therapy may also be administered preoperatively to shrink tumors and reduce their vascularity.

KEY POINTS

- A number of benign and malignant primary tumors may develop in the kidney. Symptoms depend on the size of the tumor and whether metastasis has occurred. Tumors may be asymptomatic until quite large. At that time, a palpable abdominal mass, hematuria, and flank pain may be noted.

- Tumors are usually detected with renal ultrasound and/or CT scan. Nephrectomy remains the initial treatment of choice for both benign and malignant renal tumors. Nephron-sparing approaches are increasingly utilized.

- RCC is particularly resistant to radiation, immunotherapy, and chemotherapy. This combined with the advanced stage at diagnosis make the prognosis for late-stage disease and recurrent cancer quite poor. Recent advances based upon gene pathways hold future promise.

- Nephroblastoma, or Wilms tumor, is the most common kidney cancer in children. Nephrectomy, radiation therapy, and chemotherapy are used in the management of nephroblastomas. Cure rates are excellent.

INFECTION

Normally, a number of host defense mechanisms serve to protect the renal system from infection. Chemically, the acidic pH and the presence of urea in the urine produce a relatively hostile environment for bacterial growth. Bacteriostatic prostatic secretions in men also act as a protective mechanism against bacterial invasion. In women, glands in the distal urethra secrete mucous that captures bacteria, preventing progression to the bladder. Small numbers of bacteria that may enter the system are washed out by micturition. Normal unidirectional flow prevents **reflux** of urine from the bladder to the kidney via the ureter by contraction of the vesicoureteral junction that occurs when the bladder fills. In children, urinary tract infections may be associated with vesico-ureteral reflux or other anatomical malformations of the urinary tract[24] (see discussion of vesicoureteral reflux in Chapter 29). Epithelial cells of the urinary tract provide a physical barrier to infectious organisms, and indigenous proteins trap bacteria or block their adhesion to epithelial cells.[24] The inflammatory response to bacterial attachment encourages their destruction and removal. As is so often the case with the inflammatory response, it is the secondary injury associated with this response that is ultimately responsible for subsequent damage to urinary structures.[24]

Infection of the kidney is known as **pyelonephritis** or upper urinary tract infection and affects the renal parenchyma, pelvis, and calices. Of all the urinary tract structures, infection of the kidney is the most severe.[25] Although infectious organisms responsible for upper urinary tract infections may be delivered to the kidney via the bloodstream or lymphatic system, they most commonly reach the kidneys as an ascending infection from the lower urinary tract (urethra, bladder, and ureters)[26] (Figure 27-5). Infection of the lower urinary tract is discussed in Chapter 29.

The most common causative agents of renal system infection are serogroups of *Escherichia coli,* while *Enterobacter, Enterococcus, Proteus mirabilis,* and strains of *Klebseilla* are responsible for most of the other infections.[25,26] Most often, infections with these other organisms is linked to calculi or with anatomic abnormalities of the urinary tract. In certain populations, *Staphylococcus saprophyticus* and group B *Streptococcus* have been identified. Fungal infections, mycoplasmas, and other anaerobic bacteria are occasionally responsible. Infections due to *Neisseria gonorhoeae* or *Chlamydia trachomatis* are associated with sexually transmitted diseases and are typically limited to the urethra.[26] Uropathogenic bacteria possess adhesins to facilitate binding to epithelial cells of the urinary tract.[26-28] Enhanced adhesion in some individuals may be associated with impaired secretion of cytokines and impeded inflammatory response of leukocytes. Some organisms secrete proteins that aid in protecting the bacteria from phagocytosis by cells of the immune system.[26] Bacterial virulence is further enhanced in some cases by the secretion of toxins and the protection from the immune cells afforded by a bacterial capsule.[25,27] At the same time, the organisms responsible for urinary tract infections undergo continuous mutation in an effort to overcome both host defenses and antimicrobials used in their treatment.[24]

Risk factors for urinary tract infections are listed in Box 27-2. One of the most significant preventive interventions is the early removal of urinary catheters.[25] Anatomically, women are at increased risk due to their shortened urethras, but the

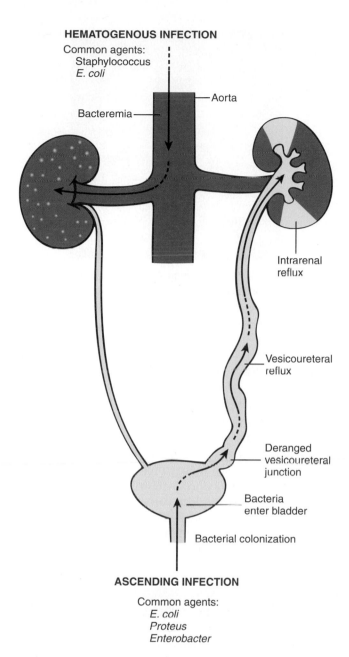

HEMATOGENOUS INFECTION

Common agents:
  Staphylococcus
  E. coli

Aorta

Bacteremia

Intrarenal
reflux

Vesicoureteral
reflux

Deranged
vesicoureteral
junction

Bacteria
enter bladder

Bacterial colonization

ASCENDING INFECTION

Common agents:
  E. coli
  Proteus
  Enterobacter

FIGURE 27-5 Pathways of renal infection. (From Kumar V et al: *Robbins basic pathology,* ed 8, Philadelphia, 2007, Saunders, p 560.)

BOX 27-2

Risk Factors for Urinary Tract Infections

- Increasing age
- Vesicoureteral reflux
- Congenital anatomic anomalies of the urinary tract
- Female gender
- Pregnancy
- Diaphragms with spermicidal agents for contraception
- Neurogenic bladder
- Instrumentation of the urinary tract (catheterization, cystoscopy)
- Urinary obstruction (calculi, benign prostatic hyperplasia)
- Glucocorticoids, radiation, or cytotoxic chemotherapy
- Immunodeficiency conditions such as AIDS
- Diabetes mellitus
- Obesity
- Sickle cell trait

Acute Pyelonephritis

Etiology and Pathogenesis. Recent research results suggest that there is an inherited susceptibility to acute pyelonephritis.[31] Pregnancy is the major risk factor for acute pyelonephritis in women due to the physiologic alterations that occur in the urinary tract.[26] In nonpregnant women, men, and children, the most common risk factors for acute pyelonephritis are diabetes mellitus, anatomical abnormalities of the urinary tract (especially vesicoureteral reflux in children[27]), and obstructive causes.[26] Annual incidence among hospitalized women has been documented in one study as 3 to 4:10,000, while that of women in the community was 12 to 13:10,000.[32] For men, the same study reported that nosocomial acute pyelonephritis had an annual incidence of 1 to 2:10,000, and community-based infection occurred at a rate of 2 to 3:10,000. The populations with the highest incidence were young women, infants, and the elderly. *E. coli* is the causative organism in 80% of acute pyelonephritis cases involving women and 70% of those involving men.[32] Pyelonephritis is usually unilateral, involving the right kidney (>50%); 25% of the cases involve the left kidney, and pyelonephritis is bilateral 25% of the time.[26]

Acute infection of the kidney usually originates as an ascending infection but may arrive at the kidney via the bloodstream. Once in the kidney, adhesins on the bacteria bind to epithelial cell receptors, initiating an inflammatory response. Different organisms possess a variety of mechanisms to assist binding. Inflammatory chemokines facilitate the movement of leukocytes into the urine. Inflammatory mediators and bacterial toxins are responsible for the parenchymal damage to the kidney.

Clinical Manifestations. The onset of acute pyelonephritis is sudden; patients are acutely ill and present with fever, chills, CVA tenderness, as well as symptoms of lower urinary tract infection (dysuria, urgency, and frequency).[26] Nausea, vomiting, and anorexia are frequent accompaniments, increasing the fever-induced dehydration.[26]

Complications of acute pyelonephritis include abscesses, septic shock, acute respiratory distress syndrome, recurrent/chronic

---

resulting infections are most often confined to the lower urinary tract.[26] More than 7 million Americans experience a urinary tract infection every year.[25] Bacterial infections of the urinary tract in children are second in frequency to middle ear infections (otitis media).[24] From birth to 7 years, 7.8% of girls and 1.7% of boys have a urinary tract infection.[29] The majority of these occur in the first 12 months. Male children who are uncircumcised experience these infections 10 times more frequently than those who are circumcised.[29] Twenty percent of elderly women, 10% of elderly men, and 4% to 7% of pregnant women have been found to have asymptomatic urinary tract infections.[30]

pyelonephritis, and chronic kidney disease due to scarring produced by recurrent infections.[24,26] Renal scarring and the subsequent development of chronic kidney disease are more likely when there are pre-existing anatomic or functional urinary tract abnormalities.[25] Chronic kidney disease has been found to progress more rapidly following acute pyelonephritis. Pre-existing chronic kidney disease can also increase the severity of an infection. Overall, however, the risk of decreased renal function subsequent to acute pyelonephritis is low, occurring in only 3% to 4% of cases. The term **urosepsis** describes organisms in the bloodstream originating from a urinary tract infection. Urinary tract infections are the cause of more than 40% of cases of nosocomial sepsis.[25] Figure 27-6 illustrates acute pyelonephritis complicated by abscess formation.

Diagnosis and Treatment. In addition to the clinical manifestations, diagnosis of acute pyelonephritis is confirmed by urinalysis results illustrating significant bacteria.[26] White and red blood cells and leukocyte esterase are also noted. The urinalysis dipstick may be positive for nitrites, especially if Gram-negative organisms are involved. White blood cell casts are common findings.[26] The literature suggests that proteinuria may be evident in 63% to 83% of urinary tract infections; however the specific relationship between the two has not been thoroughly elucidated.[30] Barring complications, patients are treated with empiric antimicrobial therapy on an outpatient basis for 7 to 10 days.[26] If improvement is not noted within 48 to 72 hours or the patient's condition deteriorates, urine is cultured to allow targeted therapy and the patient may be further assessed for such problems as urinary obstruction or an extra-urinary focus of infection. In cases of complicated acute pyelonephritis, such as septicemia, patients are hospitalized and treated with intravenous antimicrobials and fluids.[26]

Chronic Pyelonephritis. Chronic pyelonephritis is characterized by small atrophied kidneys with diffuse scarring and blunting of the calices secondary to persistent or recurrent infection of the kidney.

Etiology and Pathogenesis. As a result of recurrent or inadequately managed infections, chronic interstitial inflammation develops, with lymphocyte and plasma cell infiltration of the renal parenchyma.[25] Fibrosis of the interstitium, including the renal tubules, decreases the number of functional nephrons.[24] Individuals at risk for developing chronic pyelonephritis have bacteriuria associated with obstructive disorders such as renal calculi, neurogenic bladder, vesicoureteral reflux, or underlying intrarenal disease. Chronic or recurrent pyelonephritis is one potential cause of chronic kidney disease (see Chapter 28).

Clinical Manifestations. The symptoms of chronic pyelonephritis may be minimal or similar to those of acute pyelonephritis.[24,25] Flank pain is often less intense than that associated with acute disease. It is often diagnosed incidentally during the diagnostic evaluation and management of such conditions as hypertension, urinary tract infection, or elevated serum creatinine levels reflecting decreased GFR.[24,25]

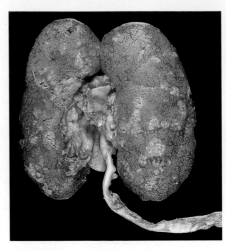

FIGURE 27-6 Acute pyelonephritis. Cortical surface shows grayish-white areas of inflammation and abscess formation. (From Lewis SL: *Medical-surgical nursing: assessment and management of clinical problems,* ed 7, St Louis, 2007, Mosby, p 1161.)

Diagnosis and Treatment. Urinalysis results typically parallel the findings of acute pyelonephritis, but may not be as profound. Diagnostic testing includes renal ultrasound and other imaging tests that show one or both kidneys to be smaller than normal with distorted architecture and significant scarring. Renal tubules may be dilated or atrophied. Other diagnostic tests may be performed to determine underlying pathologies such as vesicoureteral reflux or obstruction due to renal calculi. Treatment is based on the correction of these underlying causes, antimicrobial therapy that may continue for several months, and support of compromised renal function, if it exists.

KEY POINTS

- Pyelonephritis is an infection of the renal pelvis and parenchyma that is usually due to an ascending urinary tract infection. Costovertebral angle tenderness is the classic symptom. It is frequently accompanied by fever, chills, nausea, vomiting, and anorexia. Urinalysis generally shows evidence of an infective process. The presence of WBC casts is specifically indicative of an upper urinary tract infection as opposed to a lower urinary tract infection. When managed promptly and effectively, acute pyelonephritis does not generally result in decreased renal function.

- Chronic pyelonephritis can potentially result in chronic kidney disease. It is usually associated with vesicoureteral reflux or obstructive processes leading to persistent urine stasis. Ongoing inflammation causes fibrosis and scarring and loss of functional nephrons. The diagnosis is confirmed by renal imaging. Urinalysis results mirror those of acute pyelonephritis, but may not be as significant. Treatment includes correction of the underlying processes and often extended antimicrobial therapy.

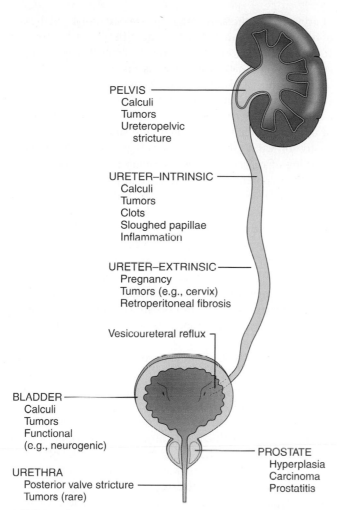

PELVIS
  Calculi
  Tumors
  Ureteropelvic
    stricture

URETER–INTRINSIC
  Calculi
  Tumors
  Clots
  Sloughed papillae
  Inflammation

URETER–EXTRINSIC
  Pregnancy
  Tumors (e.g., cervix)
  Retroperitoneal fibrosis

Vesicoureteral reflux

BLADDER
  Calculi
  Tumors
  Functional
  (e.g., neurogenic)

URETHRA
  Posterior valve stricture
  Tumors (rare)

PROSTATE
  Hyperplasia
  Carcinoma
  Prostatitis

FIGURE 27-7 Obstructions of the urinary tract. (From Cotran RS et al: *Robbins pathologic basis of disease,* ed 6, Philadelphia, 1999, Saunders, p 988.)

TABLE 27-4	
Causes of Renal System Obstruction	
Type of Obstruction	**Cause**
Intraluminal	Calculi, clot
	Tumor: bladder, urethra, kidney
	Papillary necrosis
Extrinsic	Prostatic hypertrophy
	Retroperitoneal fibrosis
	Tumor: pelvic, retroperitoneal
Acquired	Neurogenic bladder
	Ureteral stricture
	Urethral stricture

OBSTRUCTION

Obstructive disorders of the urinary tract interfere with the flow of urine. Obstruction can occur at any point in the system from the renal pelvis to the urethral meatus (Figure 27-7). In general, it causes dilation of the tract proximal to the obstruction. Stasis of urine occurs and predisposes to urinary tract infection and structural damage. Prolonged obstruction results in postrenal acute renal failure and can ultimately lead to acute tubular necrosis (intrarenal acute renal failure) (Chapter 28).

Disorders resulting in urinary tract obstruction may be congenital or acquired. In children, urinary tract obstruction is usually due to anatomic abnormalities such as ureteral valves, strictures of the urethral meatus, and stenosis at the ureterovesical or ureteral pelvic junction. Obstruction in adults predominantly occurs as a result of acquired disorders and may be either intraluminal (e.g., renal calculi) or secondary to extrinsic compression (e.g., tumors). Acquired obstructions are due to anatomical anomalies of the urinary tract

(Table 27-4). Complications of urinary obstruction include infection, sepsis, acute renal failure, and potentially, chronic kidney disease.

Changes that occur within the urinary tract as a result of obstruction are dependent on (1) location and degree of obstruction (i.e., partial or complete, unilateral or bilateral) and (2) the duration and timing (acute onset or chronic) of the obstruction. Initially, in complete or significant partial obstruction, hydrostatic pressure increases proximal to the obstruction as a consequence of continued glomerular filtration and simultaneous obstruction to the flow of urine. Other structures proximal to the obstruction then begin to dilate. The more distal to the kidney the obstruction is located, the less dilation is seen because the pressure is distributed over a greater surface area. Complete obstruction of a ureter results in its dilation (**hydroureter**). The renal pelvis and tubules enlarge with the increased pressure, and the renal papillae flatten. The enlarged kidney is called **hydronephrosis.** Glomerular filtration rate (GFR) and renal perfusion decline, and eventually portions of the kidney become ischemic. Over the course of several weeks, if the obstruction is not corrected, tubular atrophy and destruction of the medulla result in scar tissue and nonfunctioning or poorly functioning glomeruli. Postrenal acute renal failure is discussed in detail in Chapter 28.

Partial obstruction is much more common. In this situation, the renal pelvis may become very dilated but the structural or functional disruption of the kidney may be minimal. If the obstruction is bilateral, however, clinical manifestations of fluid retention will be present. Patients often complain of symptoms such as weight gain, nausea, anorexia, malaise, headaches, increased abdominal girth, and ankle edema. Functionally, partial obstruction can produce a slight to moderate decrease in blood flow and GFR and an inability to concentrate urine or secrete potassium and hydrogen ions. Compensatory hypertrophy occurs in the unaffected kidney. Renal calculi are the most common cause of urinary tract obstruction.[32]

Renal Calculi (Nephrolithiasis). Renal calculi or lithiasis are crystal aggregates composed of organic and inorganic materials located within the urinary tract. These calculi are thought to form within the kidney, in the tubules or the collecting system, and may then migrate to more distal structures. Occasionally, terminology is used to identify where these calculi are found (e.g., *ureterolithiasis* located in the ureters), but more commonly, the terms *renal calculi* or **nephrolithiasis** are used to describe the formation and passage of calculi anywhere within the urinary tract.[33] The term *lithiasis* comes from the Greek and means *stone*, so renal calculi are also referred to as *kidney stones*.

Nephrolithiasis affects individuals throughout the world[34,35] and has been traced back as far as Egyptian mummies.[33,35] The annual incidence in North America and Europe is approximately 0.5%.[34] It is estimated that 10% to 15% of Americans will experience a kidney stone during their lifetimes,[32-34] but the incidence is even higher in the Middle East (20% to 25%).[33] The United States has been shown to have a greater incidence of calculi in the upper urinary tract (kidney) than elsewhere in the world,[33,36] where stones in the bladder are a more common finding.[36,37] Historically, kidney stones have been more common in men than women,[33,35] but rates in women are increasing.[35] Examining incidence according to race/ethnicity, renal calculi occur most often among Caucasians, followed by Hispanics, Asians, and African Americans in decreasing frequency[35]; however, African Americans have the highest incidence of calculi associated with infection.[33] Although little is currently known about genetic predisposition, it is clearly a factor given the ethnic distribution and the increased risk associated with family history[36] and the fact that some stones are associated with congenital metabolic abnormalities. The rate with which renal calculi recur varies from 3.6% to 67% and appears to be highest when metabolic abnormalities are key to their etiology.[34,37] The peak incidence of renal stone formation corresponds to the period of peak mean temperature for the specific area; in the United States that is July through September.[35, 36] It has been postulated that this is due to increased fluid loss through perspiration and increased sunlight-induced levels of Vitamin D.[35] Occupations where there is increased exposure to high temperatures or sedentary levels of activity are also associated with an increased incidence of stone formation. There appears to be an increased prevalence of calculi in areas of the United States characterized by mountains, desert, or tropical climates. Prevalence increases moving from the north to the south and from west to east; the southeastern United States therefore has the highest rates of all. Stone formation is also correlated with increased weight and body mass index, especially in women.[35] Nephrolithiasis has been found to be uncommon prior to the age of 20,[35] with the greatest prevalence in the 20 to 30 age range.[33] Incidence in children has been increasing worldwide; most recent available data indicate nephrolithiasis is the cause for hospitalization in 1:1000-7600 children.[36,37] Thirty percent of the children found to have renal calculi have some sort of genitourinary abnormality.[37]

Etiology and Pathogenesis. Crystallization and stone formation occurs with many solutes found in urine and may be promoted or inhibited by a number of factors.[37] Some of these factors are inherent to the urinary tract and the characteristics of urine, while others are unique to the individual and the type of renal calculi formed. Box 27-3 identifies general factors that contribute to the formation of renal calculi. The general process of stone formation, however, is a physiologic constant.

The pathogenesis of nephrolithiasis begins with urine becoming supersaturated with the specific solute.[34-36] Urine is a solution of solvent (water) and solutes (particles). Certain of these solutes have a tendency to form crystals if their concentration within the urine becomes great enough; this is the meaning of *supersaturation*.[34] Urinary supersaturation is an essential requirement for stone formation.[33-36] These crystals begin their development somewhere in the nephron's loop of Henle, distal tubule, or collecting duct.[38] Crystallization is enhanced when a person is dehydrated (decreased solvent).[34,36] Crystals are unable to aggregate into a calculus of sufficient size to obstruct the urinary tract if urine is moving freely through the system.[36] Adequate fluid intake is therefore an inhibitor to stone formation, and since urine flows by gravity, urinary stasis as may occur with immobility and a sedentary lifestyle facilitate calculus formation. This is true for all types of renal calculi.[36]

In addition to a crystalline component, nephrolithiasis also consists of a noncrystalline, organic component termed the calculus *matrix*.[35] The matrix represents approximately 2.5% of the overall weight of the calculus. For some stones, the matrix is the dominant component; this is primarily true for stones that form with chronic urinary tract infections, where 65% of the stone is matrix. Matrix itself is made up of protein, sugar, glucosamine, bound water, and organic ash. The specific role matrix plays in genesis of calculi is unclear.[35]

The types of renal calculi are shown in Table 27-5, along with their relative incidence in adults, and primary risk factors. Calcium oxalate–based stones are by far the most common in both children and adults.[33-37] Calcium-based calculi less

---

BOX 27-3

General Contributing Factors to Nephrolithiasis

- Hyperparathyroidism
- Gout
- Certain medications
- Hypertension
- Urinary tract infections
- Chronic inflammatory bowel disease; irritable bowel disease; chronic diarrhea
- Excess dietary meat
- Excess dietary sodium
- Excess dietary oxalate
- Past medical history or family history of nephrolithiasis
- Obesity
- Insulin resistance/Type 2 diabetes mellitus
- Dehydration
- Prolonged immobility
- Congenital kidney defects/Anatomic alterations (e.g., abnormal kidney shape)
- Vesicoureteral reflux

TABLE 27-5

Types of Nephrolithiasis, Relative Incidence, and Specific Risk Factors

Constituent of Stone	Incidence	Specific risks
Calcium oxalate (primarily)	75%	Genetic predisposition; idiopathic; hypercalcemia and/or hypercalciuria (hyperparathyroidism; prolonged immobility; increased gastrointestinal absorption; impaired renal reabsorption); hyperuricosuria (see risks below); hyperoxaluria
Struvite	7%-10%	Urinary tract infection with urea-splitting bacteria (e.g., *Proteus*, *Klebsiella*, *Pseudomonas*)
Uric acid	7%-10%	Genetic predisposition; hyperuricosuria associated with gout, acute leukemia, glycogen storage disease, malignancy; excessive intake of meat, fish, poultry; obesity; type 2 diabetes; urine pH <5.5
Cystine	1%-3%	Genetic defect in renal cystine reabsorption
Ephedrine, guaifenesin, indinavir, xanthine	All <1%	Secondary to specific medications

frequently incorporate other constituents such as phosphate, hydroxyapatite, or brushite.[35] Calcium-based nephrolithiasis is primarily idiopathic in etiology (unknown cause), but a genetic component is implicated.[33,37,39] Primary risk factors for calcium-based calculi are hypercalciuria and/or hypercalcemia, hyperoxaluria, and hyperuricosuria.[33,34,37] Hypercalciuria and/or hypercalcemia is commonly due to increased gastrointestinal absorption, impaired renal tubular reabsorption, primary hyperparathyroidism, and, less often, prolonged immobility, metastatic bone cancer, multiple myeloma, prolonged metabolic acidosis, hypocitraturia, and excessive amounts of vitamin D.[33,34,37] Hyperoxaluria can increase the urinary saturation of calcium oxalate.[34] It may be due to a genetic defect that increases urinary oxalate excretion, a defect in liver metabolism, or increased gastrointestinal absorption of an oxalate-rich diet (rhubarb, spinach, chocolate, nuts, beer, coffee, tea, cocoa, or excessive vitamin C).[33,34,39] Hyperuricosuria facilitates precipitation of calcium-oxalate or may produce uric acid stones.[33-35] There is a genetic predisposition for hyperuricosuria, which may be found in association with gouty arthritis or secondary purine excess due to overproduction in myeloproliferative disorders, excess purine-rich foods, or errors of purine metabolism.[33,34,39] Foods high in purine include organ meats like liver and kidney, sardines, anchovies, salmon,

and foods high in yeast such as beer and bread. Uric acid and struvite calculi are the second most frequently occurring stones, following calcium oxalate stones. In addition to the risk factors previously identified for hyperuricosuria, an increased body-mass index, and glucose intolerance or type 2 diabetes are frequently associated with uric acid stones.[34] Calculi are uric acid–based in diabetics 30% to 40% of the time compared with 10% or less in the nondiabetic population.[34] The basis of struvite stones is not metabolic, but rather is changes that occur within the urinary tract with some infectious processes, and often assisted by some underlying anatomic or functional abnormalities that facilitate urinary stasis.[33,34] Struvite stones are composed of magnesium, ammonium, and phosphate. Urinary tract infection with certain bacterial species capable of splitting urea into two ammonium ions and one bicarbonate ion neutralize the urine and support bacterial proliferation as well as stone formation. Struvite stones form around a bacterial nucleus, producing an antimicrobial barrier. They grow rapidly and assume a jagged formation known as *staghorn*.[33,34] Other types of nephrolithiasis are less common and are associated with familial defects in renal transport[34,37] or are produced as adverse effects of certain drugs (e.g., ephedrine, guaifenesin, indinavir, and xanthine).[33]

Clinical Manifestations. Signs and symptoms of renal calculi differ with their size and location[33,36] and may mimic any number of other causes of abdominal pain.[33] Pain may be vague, or more commonly, acute renal colic or flank pain.[33,36] Stones within the kidney are responsible for flank pain that may be dull and localized. As the stone moves to the ureteropelvic junction and down into the ureter, spasmodic, intermittent sharp pain known as renal colic develops. The pain may radiate into the ipsilateral groin area, testicle, or labia. The pain induced by nephrolithiasis makes the patient acutely uncomfortable and will usually result in continuous movement. Pain is often accompanied by nausea and vomiting, diaphoresis, tachycardia, and tachypnea. When the stone reaches the bladder, there is often a noticeable reduction in the pain; if it results in a partial obstruction at the urethra, dysuria, urgency, and frequency are common findings. These findings may present earlier if there is a concomitant urinary tract infection.[33,36] Renal calculi may develop as a result of a urinary tract infection (struvite stones), or increase the risk of its development.[33,36] If the infection reaches the kidney itself (pyelonephritis), the patient will become acutely ill[33] (see Acute Pyelonephritis section). Prolonged or repeated nephrolithiasis may result in scarring of the kidney, and if bilateral, chronic kidney disease.[33]

Diagnosis and Treatment. In addition to the clinical manifestations, other data are considered during the diagnostic process. A thorough family history should be obtained, risk factors for nephrolithiasis should be assessed, and any anatomic or functional urinary tract anomalies identified.[33,36] Urinalysis permits the identification of a concomitant infection, levels of specific stone-forming constituents (e.g., hypercalciuria), and urinary pH, which affects crystallization. Hematuria (gross or microscopic) may be present persistently or intermittently

---

BOX 27-4

General Interventions for Nephrolithiasis

- Narcotic analgesics for pain management
- Increased fluid intake (>2 liters/day; oral and/or IV)
- Antimicrobials for urinary tract infection
- Shock wave lithotripsy, ureteral stenting, ureteroscopy for removal of large stones unable to pass spontaneously
- Dietary modifications unique to stone composition
- Medications unique to stone composition (e.g., allopurinol for uric acid stones)

BOX 27-5

Dietary Modifications for Nephrolithiasis

- Increased water intake (minimum of 2 liters/day)
- Adequate dietary calcium intake
- Avoid calcium supplementation
- Avoid foods with additional vitamin D (and C, if recommended)
- Avoid calcium-based antacids
- Limit intake of coffee, tea, or colas to ≤2/day
- Reduce protein intake from meat, fish, and poultry
- Limit dietary sodium and oxalate intake
- Avoid high-purine foods for uric acid stones (and if recommended, for calcium)

---

with or without other manifestations.[33,36,38] If a stone has been passed and is available, it is sent for analysis of its composition. Complete blood count, serum electrolytes, serum creatinine and BUN, and assessment of parathormone level provide information related to risk factors and renal function.

The traditional gold standard for the assessment of renal calculi has been intravenous pyelogram (IVP),[33,36] but it has been effectively replaced by computerized tomography (CT scans).[36] Basic abdominal x-rays identify only those stones that are radiopaque and in the diagnosis of renal calculi have only a 62% sensitivity and 67% specificity.[36] Only calcium-containing calculi can be expected to be seen by x-ray; the other types of stones are either radiolucent or inadequately visualized.[40] Ultrasonography is considered as effective as IVP, but provides limited data relative to renal function. It is second in choice for diagnosis to the CT scan.[36] CT scanning can identify renal calculi, other potential sources of flank pain, and anatomic anomalies.[33,36] When combined with contrast, the same level of assessment of renal function as an IVP provides can be obtained.[36]

Treatment of nephrolithiasis may be medical or surgical and is determined by the size and position of the calculus, its composition, presence of urinary tract infection, and whether one or both kidneys are involved. Interventions are generally summarized in Box 27-4, and dietary changes are listed in Box 27-5. The goal is not only treatment of existing stones, but prevention of their recurrence.[33] Acutely, pain requires intervention with opiates. Morphine is especially useful as it reduces spasms as well as affecting both transmission and perception of painful stimuli. With increased fluid intake, most stones pass out of the urinary tract spontaneously in both children and adults.[33,36] Stones 4 mm or less in size pass spontaneously for about 90% of adult patients[33] and up to 67% of the time in children.[36] Stones larger than 4 mm in children require interventions such as ureteral stenting, lithotripsy, or endoscopic removal.[36] In adults, 50% of patients are able to pass stones of 4 to 6 mm in size, and 20% of patients pass stones larger than 6 mm without other interventions.[33] Other interventions that may be required include extracorporeal shock-wave lithotripsy, where the stone is broken into smaller pieces for passage, or percutaneous approaches to stone removal by endoscopy with basket retrieval, ultrasonic, or laser lithotripsy.[36] Open surgical approaches are required when

no other intervention is successful, but are usually avoidable and therefore uncommon. Unfortunately, depending upon the type of renal calculus, 30% to 50% of adults can expect a recurrence within 5 to 10 years.[36,40] Thirty-three percent of children can be expected to have another episode of nephrolithiasis in a mean of 7.2 years.[36] Dietary modifications can decrease this risk.[40] Recommendations are designed for each individual patient, based upon the type of stone and specific risk factors.[40]

KEY POINTS

- Obstructive processes result in urine stasis, which predisposes to infection and structural damage. Common causes of obstruction include stones, tumors, prostatic hypertrophy, and strictures of the ureters or urethra. Of all potential causes, renal stones are the most common.
- Complete obstruction results in hydronephrosis, decreased GFR, and ischemic kidney damage because of increased intraluminal pressure. Prolonged postrenal acute renal failure due to the obstruction may result in acute tubular necrosis (intrarenal acute renal failure) and chronic kidney disease.
- Stones tend to form in the urinary tract under conditions of solute supersaturation, low urine volume, and abnormal urine pH. Certain factors increase the risk of stone formation, while others act as inhibitors.
- Most stones are composed of calcium crystals. Other forms include uric acid, struvite, cystine, and stones that form in association with certain medications.
- Stationary stones in the renal pelvis are generally asymptomatic. When the stone migrates to the junction with the ureters and beyond, intense renal colic pain ensues. Pain is usually abrupt in onset and may radiate. Additional signs and symptoms include nausea, vomiting, and diaphoresis.
- Most stones pass spontaneously, but other interventions may be necessary including lithotripsy or endoscopic approaches. Stones tend to recur, and prevention is enhanced by a high fluid intake to dilute the urine and dietary changes based upon the type of stone.

GLOMERULAR DISORDERS (GLOMERULOPATHIES)

Glomerular disorders result from alterations in the structure and function of the glomerular capillary circulation and are broadly delineated as **glomerulopathies.** The membranes of glomerular capillaries have three layers: endothelium, basement membrane, and a layer of specialized epithelial cells with footlike projections (podocytes) that encircle the basement membrane[41] (Figure 27-8). Together, this triple layer comprises the filtration barrier of the glomerulus. The glomerular filtrate passes through gaps (slit pores) between these podocytes, enters the space in Bowman's capsule, and progresses into the proximal tubule. Glomerulopathies are responsible for 90% of the cases of end-stage renal disease.[42]

Pathologic changes to nephron glomeruli may occur insidiously, altering function over the course of months or years, or they may have an acute onset, with rapidly developing

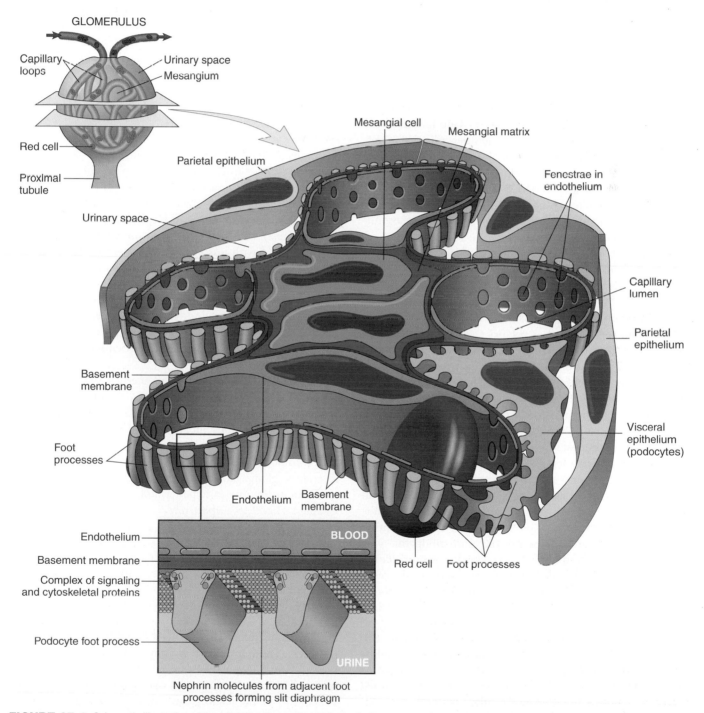

FIGURE 27-8 Schematic illustration of the lobe of a glomerulus. Note the foot processes of the podocytes, basement membrane, and endothelium of the glomerular capillary. (From Kumar V et al: *Robbins basic pathology,* ed 8, Philadelphia, 2007, Saunders, p 543.)

impairment. In some cases, there are no apparent signs or symptoms and glomerular dysfunction is identified serendipitously during routine physical examination or evaluation of some other health concern. The specific etiologies of glomerulopathies are often unknown. Hereditary and environmental factors are implicated; metabolic, infectious, hemodynamic, toxic, immune, genetic, and other mechanisms of injury are involved.[42] Immune or inflammatory processes are most often implicated.[42]

The challenge in any discussion of glomerulopathies lies in the often confusing range of clinical and pathological approaches to their classification. One approach is to classify glomerular disorders according to primary and secondary etiologies.[43] *Primary glomerulopathies* are disease states in which the kidney is the only or the predominant organ involved, and *secondary glomerulopathies* result from drug exposure, infection, or glomerular injury in the setting of multisystem or vascular abnormalities. Goodpasture syndrome is an example of a secondary glomerulopathy, affecting the basement membranes of both the glomeruli of the kidney and the alveoli of the lung.[44] Systemic lupus erythematosus also causes a secondary glomerulopathy.[45] Diabetic nephropathy and renal damage due to undiagnosed or inadequately managed hypertension are also examples of secondary glomerulopathies.

The specific location and features of glomerular injury is another method of classification that has been used. Glomerular involvement may be characterized as *diffuse* (all glomeruli) or *focal* (some but not all glomeruli).[43,45,46] Within the affected glomeruli, lesions may be *global,* affecting all parts of the glomerulus, or present as patches *(segmental)* when only specific parts of the glomerulus are involved.[42,46,47] At a cellular level, the pathology is said to be *proliferative* if there is hyperplasia,[48] and if there are accumulated neutrophils, it may be termed *exudative.* If thickening of glomerular capillary walls is present, the glomerulopathy is *membranous.* Membranous changes involve the basement membrane and are usually due to accumulated deposition of immunoglobulins (IgG) and complement components (C5).[43,44,48-51] *Sclerotic* changes refer to scarring due to persistent or recurrent injury and may occur within the capillaries, the capillary space, or at the point of initiation of the proximal tubule. Some references use the term *fibrosis* to describe this process.[52] The site of deposition of noncellular materials as part of the glomerulopathic process may be described specifically as *mesangial, subendothelial,* or *subepithelial.*[43] Efforts to specify the glomerulopathy often result in combinations of terminology such as *focal segmental,*[46,47] or *membranoproliferative.*[48] Various glomerulopathies may be linked to more than one type of injury however, so this lack of specificity makes absolute classification by this criterion less beneficial. Its primary value rests in providing a common vocabulary for the description of glomerulopathic lesions. Renal biopsy and histologic examination are required for this level of specificity. More recently, a method of classification according to the degree and type of dysfunction, injury, or loss of the glomerular podocytes has been proposed.[42]

Glomerulopathies may result in proteinuria, hematuria, abnormal urinary casts, decreased GFR, and hypertension, however these manifestations may not all be present in a single pathology and/or they may present along a continuum of degree. Proteinuria is classically the clinical manifestation associated with glomerulopathy; other urinary or systemic conditions may present with hematuria, urinary casts, reduced GFR, or hypertension. Damage to the glomerulus will result in protein loss from the bloodstream into the urine.[1] Under normal circumstances, protein molecules are too large to pass through the slit pores of the glomerulus, so they are retained in the bloodstream. The very small Bence-Jones protein associated with multiple myeloma is easily filtered and will appear in the urine in that condition. Transient proteinuria may be seen with diets high in protein, or excessive exercise or emotional stress. Normally, protein lost in the urine amounts to less than 100 mg in 24 hours.[1] Glomerulopathies may be classified according to the degree of proteinuria.[43] **Nephrotic syndrome** is specifically characterized by protein loss ≥3 to 3.5 grams in 24 hours[1] and is most commonly associated with minimal change disease/lipoid nephrosis, focal segmental glomerulosclerosis, and membranous nephropathy, but can occur with any glomerulopathy if the injury is sufficient to allow significant protein loss.[53] **Nephrosis** is frequently used synonymously with nephrotic syndrome, but in other cases it is correlated with less proteinuria—usually approximately 2.0 grams in a day.[1] **Nephritic syndrome** is also a reflection of glomerular inflammation. In this case, hematuria is seen on gross urinalysis, and RBC casts are present in the sediment. Mild to moderate proteinuria, edema, hypertension, oliguria, and decreased GFR producing an elevation in serum creatinine may also be noted. It is most often seen in acute and chronic glomerulonephritis.[1,53]

The most common types of glomerular disease are acute postinfectious glomerulonephritis, IgA nephropathy, rapidly progressive/crescentic glomerulonephritis, nephrotic syndrome (includes membranous glomerulonephritis, focal segmental glomerulosclerosis, minimal change disease/lipoid nephrosis), and chronic glomerulonephritis. By far the most common secondary glomerulopathies are diabetic nephropathy and glomerulopathy due to hypertension. These are addressed in Chapters 41 and 16, respectively.

Glomerulonephritis

Glomerulonephritis includes an assortment of immune-mediated conditions that produce inflammation of glomeruli and other areas of the kidney.[43] It may have a primary etiology, which is commonly believed to be autoimmune, or a secondary one in which it is associated with a number of autoimmune, metabolic, malignant, or infectious systemic disorders. Although there is some variation, for the most part, glomerulonephritis is more common among men than women.[43] More than 20 years ago, glomerulonephritis was believed to be the leading cause of the end-stage of chronic renal disease.[41] While worldwide it remains the second most common cause,[43] in the United States the glomerulopathies associated with diabetes mellitus and hypertension hold that distinction.[41,43]

Acute Glomerulonephritis

The term *acute glomerulonephritis* encompasses a constellation of inflammatory glomerulopathies that are characterized by the abrupt onset of varying degrees of hematuria, proteinuria, oliguria and azotemia, edema, and hypertension.[43] A wide variety of triggers may initiate the process (Box 27-6). The pathophysiologic process is summarized in Figure 27-9.

Postinfectious acute glomerulonephritis is historically most well known to follow skin (impetigo) and throat infections with specific strains of group A β-hemolytic streptococci.[43,53] This etiology is common today only among children in impoverished areas of developed countries and developing countries,[43,53] where it is the basis of 4.6% to 51.6% of pediatric acute renal failure admissions.[53] The reduction in incidence of this etiology elsewhere is most likely due to early diagnosis and treatment of streptococcal infections.[53] At the same time, other etiologies are increasing in incidence, notably hepatitis C.[48] The infectious organism acts as the antigen, initiating an antibody-antigen reaction. The onset of glomerular inflammation varies; in the case of a streptococcal etiology, damage to the glomerulus is initiated 1 to 3 weeks following the initial infection.[41]

BOX 27-6

Triggers of Acute Glomerulonephritis

Infectious
Poststreptococcal glomerulonephritis
Nonstreptococcal/postinfectious glomerulonephritis

Bacterial
Infective endocarditis
Meningococcemia
Pneumococcal pneumonia
Sepsis

Viral
Hepatitis B
Hepatitis C (associated cryoglobinemia)
Mononucleosis
Mumps/measles
Varicella

Parasitic
Malaria
Toxoplasmosis

Primary Disease
Berger disease (IgA nephropathy)
Mesangial proliferative
Mesangiocapillary glomerulonephritis

Multisystem Disease
Goodpasture syndrome
Henoch-Schönlein purpura
Polyarteritis nodosa
Systemic lupus erythematosus
Vasculitis

Miscellaneous
Guillain-Barré syndrome
Serum sickness
Irradiation for Wilms tumor

FIGURE 27-9 Summary of the pathophysiologic process of acute glomerulonephritis and associated clinical manifestations.

As with most other forms of glomerulonephritis, antibody deposition leading to inflammation is the key pathologic event[43]; in this case, IgG is the immunoglobulin involved.[53] Proliferation of mesangial cells is initiated following immune complex deposition[41] resulting in characteristic proliferative lesions. It has been hypothesized that there are variations in glomerular pathology related to the type of infection.[48] Autoimmune mechanisms in poststreptococcal glomerulonephritis have also been suggested.[53] Complement is activated, primarily by the alternate pathway.[53] It is deposited within the glomerulus; this is a major aspect of most forms of glomerulonephritis.[43] In response to complement chemotaxic factors, macrophages, neutrophils and T helper cells infiltrate the glomerular capillary walls.[53] Elevated levels of IL-6, IL-8, and tumor necrosis factor-α are noted in the serum. Lysosomal enzymes are released and attack glomerular walls. The resulting changes in the structure of the glomerular wall results in a decrease in the surface area for filtering and allows substances that were previously restricted to enter the glomerular space. Locally-acting vasoactive compounds such as angiotensin and leukotrienes contract mesangial cells and reduce perfusion to glomerular capillaries, decreasing GFR.[53] In severe cases, the coagulation cascade is activated and fibrin is deposited within capillaries, further impairing perfusion.[43]

Clinical manifestations of postinfectious acute glomerulonephritis vary in severity.[53] Smoky or coffee-colored urine due to hematuria and red cell casts (nephritic syndrome) are the most common findings. White cell casts may also be present. The degree of proteinuria is variable, and may reach nephrotic syndrome level. Reduced GFR presents as increased circulating volume producing edema and hypertension, and oliguria with increasing serum levels of creatinine and nitrogenous wastes (BUN).[53]

Diagnosis is based on the patient's history, clinical manifestations, and urinalysis results. Renal function is evaluated by BUN and creatinine levels. A renal biopsy may be indicated. Care is supportive and symptomatic. Dialysis may be needed to support renal function. Especially in children, resolution of the inflammatory process may occur within about 2 weeks (poststreptococcal) with no sequela or complications, or the deterioration of renal function may continue, resulting in chronic glomerulonephritis, nephrotic syndrome (glomerulosclerosis), and chronic kidney disease.[41]

IgA nephropathy (Berger disease) is the most commonly diagnosed type of acute glomerulonephritis in developed countries,[43,54] more common in the adult population than among pediatric patients.[43] Upper respiratory or gastrointestinal viral infections appear to be the triggers, initiating the deposition of IgA in the glomerular mesangium.[54] Complement is activated, and inflammatory cells are released resulting in varying degrees of glomerular injury. Involvement of specific T regulatory cells has been implicated. Hematuria is usually apparent within 1 to 2 days, but the proteinuria, edema, and hypertension common with other glomerulopathies are generally not evident. Prognosis is variable; as many as half the patients develop glomerulosclerosis and end-stage renal disease.[54]

Crescentic Glomerulonephritis/Rapidly Progressive Glomerulonephritis (RPGN)

The condition previously known as *rapidly progressive glomerulonephritis* is now more often called *crescentic glomerulonephritis* because of its characteristic lesions.[43] The lesions are proliferative in nature and composed of crescent-shaped depositions of accumulated epithelial cells, fibrin, and macrophages that are found in Bowman space.[43] Podocytes that are progressively losing their markers of differentiation are also a part of the process.[42] This form of glomerulonephritis has an acute onset, with hematuria, proteinuria, and red cell casts followed by a swift decline in renal function. Its identification is considered a medical emergency.[43] It primarily affects adults in their sixth or seventh decade. When not idiopathic, causes of crescentic glomerulonephritis fall into four general categories: (1) complication of an acute or subacute infection; (2) complication of a multisystem disease; (3) drug exposure; and (4) as a primary disorder in the absence of other systemic disease. The most common infections associated with this disorder are poststreptococcal glomerulonephritis and infective endocarditis. Multisystem diseases associated with it are systemic lupus erythematosus, Henoch-Schönlein purpura, systemic necrotizing vasculitis, and Goodpasture syndrome. Examples of drugs identified as causative are penicillamine, hydralazine, allopurinol in the presence of vasculitis, and rifampin.[43]

Goodpasture syndrome is a type II hypersensitivity reaction resulting in IgG antibody formation against the basement membranes of the glomeruli and alveoli.[44] It is rare, with an annual incidence of 1:1 million individuals in a bimodal fashion; risk is greatest in the mid-twenties and late fifties. Survival through the acute period reaches 90% with current treatment interventions, but drops to less than 50% at 2 years, and for the 40% to 50% of patients who progress to chronic kidney disease mortality rates increase even further. Patients suffer with the clinical manifestations of glomerulonephritis and also shortness of breath and hemoptysis due to pulmonary involvement. Manifestations of pulmonary involvement may appear prior to those associated with glomerulonephritis. Treatment is based on system support; plasmapheresis (therapeutic plasma exchange to decrease circulating antibodies) and immunosuppression are the most common interventions.[44]

Chronic Glomerulonephritis

Glomerular diseases that assume a progressive course ultimately develop into chronic kidney disease.[43] These patients present with persistent proteinuria, with or without hematuria, and slowly declining renal function. In many cases, patients appear to have recovered from the initial insult. Proteinuria and hypertension are both capable of advancing renal damage. The pathophysiology is an extension of that seen in acute glomerulonephritis. Proliferative and membranous lesions are present, but sclerotic injury dominates resulting in ongoing fibrotic changes. Tubulointerstitial damage contributes to the reduction in renal function. Nephrons atrophy and ultimately the kidneys become small, scarred, and nonfunctional.

As the chronic kidney disease progresses, supportive interventions may retard the process (see Chapter 28) but the patient ultimately reaches end-stage renal disease and dialysis or transplantation is required.[43]

Nephrotic Syndrome

Nephrotic syndrome is a glomerulopathy in which there is a urinary elimination of >3 to 3.5 grams of protein per day due to glomerular damage.[55] Ultimately, most patients will develop the full constellation of nephrotic syndrome manifestations: hypoalbuminemia, hyperlipidemia, edema, and a propensity for thrombus formation. The most common primary causes are minimal change disease (lipoid nephrosis), idiopathic focal segmental glomerulosclerosis, and membranous nephropathy. Several systemic diseases such as systemic lupus erythematosus and Henoch-Schönlein purpura, as well as infections, malignancies, and vasculitis have been found to be associated with nephrotic syndrome, but the most common cause in adults is diabetes mellitus.[55] Mutations of the NPHS1, NPHS2, WT1, and LAMB2 genes result in congenital nephrotic syndrome in children.[56] Together, mutations of these four genes are responsible for two-thirds of the nephrotic syndrome cases diagnosed in children ≤1 year of age.[56]

The pathophysiology of nephrotic syndrome is shown in Figure 27-10. The increased permeability of the glomerular membrane allows large quantities of protein to leave the bloodstream and exit the body in the urine. This produces hypoalbuminemia and proteinuria. Urine is characteristically frothy or foamy in appearance.[55] The low serum albumin serves to stimulate the liver to increase production of cholesterol and lipoproteins, producing hyperlipidemia.[55-57] The actual mechanism has not been fully elucidated but is clearly multifactorial and complex.[55-57] Cholesterol and low-density lipoproteins (LDL) are elevated; cholesterol levels are consistently over 200 mg/dl, and levels of 600-700 are not uncommon.[55] Lipid casts or fat droplets may appear in the urine.[1,55] Oval fat bodies, epithelial cells from the tubules, may also be sloughed.[1,55] Levels of free fat-soluble hormones and drugs normally traveling in the circulation bound to globulins may be increased.[55] The increased risk of thrombotic events in nephrotic syndrome is due to a hypercoagulable state.[58,59] This complication has many possible etiologics, but most likely the proteins required for hemostasis are lost in the urine, stimulating hepatic synthesis of clotting factors.[59] Renal vein thrombosis, deep vein thrombosis, pulmonary embolism, and transient ischemic attacks have all been documented.[58,59] Arterial thrombosis is less frequent than venous, and may be related to the correlation of hypoalbuminemia with decreased levels of antithrombin.[59] Edema is the most common clinical manifestation of nephrotic syndrome. Two theories have been proposed to explain its development.[55] Both theories are well substantiated by anecdotal clinical evidence and animal

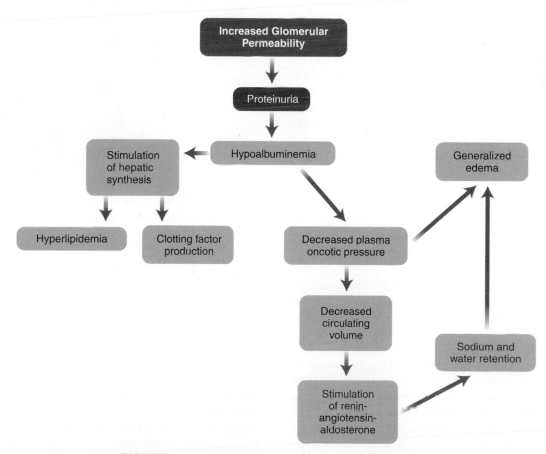

FIGURE 27-10 Pathophysiologic process of nephrotic syndrome.

models. As the serum albumin is lost, the oncotic pressure within the blood vessels declines and the hydrostatic pressure is relatively increased, forcing fluid into the interstitial spaces. Reduction in circulating volume results in the activation of the renin-angiotensin-aldosterone system, causing sodium and then water retention and promoting more protein loss and edema. The second theory holds that the kidneys' intrinsic sodium-retaining mechanism is activated prior to the loss of protein, expanding circulating volume, and increasing capillary filtration and edema formation. Research has found that although levels of atrial natriuretic peptide are within normal limits, a postreceptor defect inhibits normal response.[55] A vicious cycle of protein loss, fluid retention, and edema is initiated.

Treatment of nephrotic syndrome, regardless of causation, includes gradual removal of fluid with diuretics to treat edema.[55] Elevated lipids are routinely treated with lipid-lowering therapy, if rapid recovery from nephrotic syndrome is not anticipated.[55,57] Once in remission, the hyperlipidemia typically resolves spontaneously.[55] Hypertension is treated with angiotensin II receptor blockers and/or angiotensinogen-converting enzyme inhibition, as is recommended for chronic kidney disease. Treatment with immunosuppression or immunomodulation is standard for most primary etiologies, although response is variable.[55]

Membranous Nephropathy (MN)

MN is the most common cause of idiopathic nephrotic syndrome among Caucasian adults—about 20% of all cases.[49,50] Twenty percent of these MN cases have secondary causes such as infections, autoimmune diseases, and malignancies. For lack of any concrete evidence, the remaining 80% are said to be idiopathic.[49,50] Figure 27-11 illustrates the histologic findings with MN and the pathologic changes in the glomerulus. Immune deposits of IgG, frequently IgG4, membrane attack complex of complement C5b-9, and yet-to-be-identified antigens collect in the subepithelium of the distal portion of the basement membrane and produce a membranous thickening[49,50] as the podocytes are damaged by the immune response.[51] Spontaneous remission occurs in approximately one third of cases; within 10 years, 40% of the individuals with MN have end-stage renal disease.[49,50] This is most likely to occur in men over the age of 50.[55]

Focal Segmental Glomerulosclerosis (FSGS)

FSGS is a major cause of idiopathic steroid-resistant nephrotic syndrome in adults[46] and the incidence in children is increasing so that it now represents between 8% and 10% of their cases of nephrotic syndrome.[60] Disproportionately, more blacks than other ethnic groups develop FSGS.[55] Mutations of the NPHS2 gene have been found to be associated with both the sporadic and familial forms of the disease.[61] Autosomal dominant FSGS has a later onset and is slower to progress than the recessive forms.[47] FSGS may be a primary glomerulopathy or may develop secondarily to a number of immunologic, metabolic, interstitial, hemodynamic, or other conditions.

FIGURE 27-11 Membranous nephropathy. **A,** Diffuse thickening of the glomerular basement membrane. **B,** Schematic diagram illustrating subepithelial deposits, effacement of foot processes, and the presence of "spikes" of basement membrane material between the immune deposits. (From Kumar V et al: *Robbins basic pathology,* ed 8, Philadelphia, 2007, Saunders, p 552.)

Only a portion of the glomeruli are affected (segmental), and glomeruli within the kidney are not uniformly impacted (focal). This is a disease of glomeruli podocytes that over time progresses to scarred lesions. Epithelial and endothelial cellular injury initiate the protein loss across the glomerular membrane, and proteins collect within the mesangial cells causing their hyperplasia. Phagocytic immune cells, IL1 and TNF cytokines, complement, nitric oxide, angiotensin, the coagulation cascade, and numerous growth factors all play a role in chronic glomerular injury. Only 5% of patients will experience complete remission. Once proteinuria reaches nephrotic syndrome levels, 50% of those with FSGS will reach end-stage renal disease within 6 to 8 years.[47]

Minimal Change Disease (MCD)

Previously called *lipoid nephrosis,* MCD is due to a phenotypic alteration in glomerular podocytes, whereby the foot processes fuse together.[42] It is usually initiated by an allergic or immune condition, including lymphomas. The result of the altered structure of the podocytes is a less effective glomerular filtration and the loss of copious amounts of albumin in the urine. This is the only pathologic feature in the glomerulus.[42] Onset of edema, nephrotic levels of protein loss, and hypoalbuminemia is sudden.[55] It is the primary cause of idiopathic nephrotic syndrome in children, accounting for 77% of nephrotic syndrome diagnoses by biopsy in children and adolescents.[60] Although a longer course is usually needed in children, MCD responds well to treatment with corticosteroids.[55] Fewer patients progress to end-stage renal disease with MCD than the other common forms of nephrotic syndrome.

KEY POINTS

- Glomerulopathies alter glomerular capillary structure and function. Damage is mediated by immune processes. The glomerular damage may result in some combination of hematuria, proteinuria, abnormal casts, decreased GFR, edema, and hypertension.
- Glomerulonephritis is due to an immune response to a variety of potential triggers and may have a primary or secondary etiology. Attraction of immune cells to the area of inflammation results in lysosomal degradation of the basement membrane. The GFR may fall, in part because of contraction of mesangial cells resulting in decreased surface area for filtration.
- Glomerulonephritis may be classified as acute, crescentic, or chronic. Acute forms are usually triggered by infection. The cause of the crescentic form is often unknown, but it may be secondary to other disease processes such as Goodpasture syndrome. Chronic forms are those that progress to chronic kidney disease.
- Treatment of glomerulonephritis may include steroids, plasmapheresis, and supportive measures such as dietary and fluid management and management of systemic and renal hypertension. End-stage renal disease is a common outcome of chronic glomerulonephritis, necessitating dialysis or kidney transplantation.
- Nephrotic syndrome occurs because of increased glomerular permeability to proteins, which results in a urinary loss of 3 to 3.5 g of protein or more per day. Proteinuria leads to hypoalbuminemia and generalized edema as a result of decreased blood colloid osmotic pressure. Hyperlipidemia and hypercoagulability are thought to occur because of a generalized increase in liver activity stimulated by hypoalbuminemia.

- Treatment of nephrotic syndrome is conservative, consisting of management of symptoms and the underlying process that initiated the syndrome, when possible. Although many cases resolve spontaneously, others progress to end-stage renal disease.

SUMMARY

Many diseases can cause damage to the kidney. Any process that disrupts the normal architecture of the kidney will cause altered function, whether in the glomeruli, the vascular tree, or the collecting/draining system. Despite the kidney's resiliency and capacity to respond to treatment, ultimately any abnormality in the system has the potential to progress to chronic kidney disease. Glomerulopathies are the primary contributors to chronic renal disease.

REFERENCES

1. Pagana KD, Pagana TJ: *Mosby's manual of diagnostic and laboratory tests,* ed 3, St. Louis, 2006, Mosby.
2. Dziarmaga A, Quinlan J, Goodyer P: Renal hypoplasia: lessons from Pax2, *Pediatr Nephrol* 21:26-31, 2006.
3. Woolf AS, Hillman KA: Unilateral renal agenesis and the congenital solitary functioning kidney: developmental, genetic and clinical perspectives, *BJU International* 99:17-21, 2006.
4. Schwaderer AL et al: Renal anomalies in family members of infants with bilateral renal agenesis/adysplasia, *Pediatr Nephrol* 22:52-56, 2007.
5. Bisceglia M et al: Renal cystic diseases: a review, *Adv Anat Pathol* 13:26-56, 2006.
6. Campbell SC, Novick AC, Bukowski RM: Neoplasms of the upper urinary tract. In Wein JA et al, editors: *Campbell-Walsh urology,* ed 9, Philadelphia, 2007, Saunders, pp 1575-1582.
7. Torres WE, Harris PC, Pirson Y: Autosomal dominant polycystic kidney disease, *Lancet* 369:1287-301, 2007.
8. Sweeney WE, Avner ED: Molecular and cellular pathophysiology of autosomal recessive polycystic kidney disease (ARPDK), *Cell Tissue Research* 326:671-685, 2006.
9. Pei Y: Diagnostic approach in autosomal dominant polycystic kidney disease, *Clin J Am Soc Nephrol* 1:1108-1114, 2006.
10. Simons M, Walz G: Polycystic kidney disease: cell division with a c(l)ue? *Kidney International* 70:854-864, 2006.
11. Nelson EC, Evans CP, Lara PN: Renal cell carcinoma: Current status and emerging therapies, *Cancer Treatment Reviews* 33:299-313, 2007.
12. Reuter VE: The pathology of renal epithelial neoplasm, *Semin Oncol* 33:534-543, 2006.
13. Novick AC: Kidney cancer: past, present, and future, *Urol Oncol* 23:188-195, 2007.
14. McLaughlin JK, Lipworth L, Tarone RE: Epidemiologic aspects of renal cell carcinoma, *Semin Oncol* 33:527-533, 2006.
15. Moore LE, Wilson RT, Campleman SL: Lifestyle factors, exposures, genetic susceptibility, and renal cell cancer risk: an overview, *Cancer Investigation* 23:240-255, 2005.
16. Young AN et al: Current trends in molecular classification of adult renal tumors, *Urology* 67:873-880, 2006.
17. Jemal A et al: Cancer statistics, 2006, *CA Cancer J Clin* 56:106-130, 2006.
18. Sudarshan S, Linehan WM: Genetic basis of cancer of the kidney, *Semin Oncol* 22:544-551, 2006.
19. Linehan WM et al: Identification of the genes for kidney cancer: Opportunity for disease-specific targeted therapeutics, *Clin Cancer Res* 13(2 Suppl):671s-679s, 2007.

20. Bratslavsky et al: Pseudohypoxic pathways in renal cell carcinoma, *Clin Cancer Res* 13(16):4667-4671, 2007.

21. Vira MA et al: Genetic basis of kidney cancer: a model for developing molecular-targeted therapies, *BJU International* 99:1223-1229, 2007.

22. Rivera MN, Haber DA: Wilms' tumour: connecting tumorigenesis and organ development in the kidney, *Nat Rev Cancer* 5(9):699-712, 2005.

23. Scott RH et al: Syndromes and constitutional chromosomal abnormalities associated with Wilms tumour, *J Med Genet* 43:705-715, 2006.

24. Mak RH, Kuo H: Pathogenesis of urinary tract infection: an update, *Curr Opin Pediatr* 18:148-152, 2006.

25. Fünfstück R, Ott U, Naber KG: The interaction of urinary tract infection and renal insufficiency, *Int J Antimicrob Agents* 28S:S72-S77, 2006.

26. Sheffield JS, Cunningham FG: Urinary tract infection in women, *Obstet Gynecol* 106(5 Pt 1):1085-1092, 2005.

27. Choi YD et al: Vesicoureteral reflux in adult women with uncomplicated acute pyelonephritis, *Urology* 66:55-58, 2005.

28. Lane MC, Mobley HLT: Role of p-fimbrial-mediated adherence in pyelonephritis and persistence of uropathogenic *Escherichia coli* (UPEC) in the mammalian kidney, *Kidney International* 72:19-25, 2007.

29. Blumenthal I: Vesicoureteric reflex and urinary tract infection in children, *Postgrad Med J* 82:31-35, 2005.

30. Carter JL et al: Does urinary tract infection cause proteinuria or microalbuminuria? *Nephrol Dial Transplant* 21:3031-3037, 2006.

31. Lundstedt A et al: Inherited susceptibility to acute pyelonephritis: a family study of urinary tract infection, *J Infect Dis* 195(8):1227-1234, 2007.

32. Czaja CA et al: Population-based epidemiologic analysis of acute pyelonephritis, *Clin Infect Dis* 45(3):273-280, 2007.

33. Colella J: Urolithiasis/nephrolithiasis: what's it all about? *Urol Nurs* 25(6):427-448, 475, 2005.

34. Moe OW: Kidney stones: pathophysiology and medical management, *The Lancet* 367:333-344, 2006.

35. Pearle MS, Lotan Y: Urinary lithiasis: Etiology, epidemiology, and pathogenesis. In Wein JA et al, editors: *Campbell-Walsh urology,* ed 9, Philadelphia, 2007, Saunders, pp 1363-1373.

36. Srivastava T, Alon US: Urolithiasis in adolescent children, *Adolesc Med Clin* 16(1):87-109, 2005.

37. Sarica K: Pediatric urolithiasis: etiology, specific pathogenesis and medical treatment, *Urol Res* 34:96-101, 2006.

38. Pietrow PK, Karellas ME: Medical management of common urinary calculi, *Am Fam Physician* 74(1):86-94, 2006.

39. Moe OW, Bonny O: Genetic hypercalciuria, *J Am Soc Nephrol* 16:729-745, 2005.

40. Taylor EN, Curhan GC: Diet and fluid prescription in stone disease, *Kidney Int* 70(5):835-839, 2006.

41. Guyton AC, Hall JE: *Textbook of medical physiology,* ed 11, Philadelphia, 2006, Saunders.

42. Wiggins RC: The spectrum of podocytopathies: a unifying view of glomerular diseases, *Kidney Int* 71:1205-1214, 2007.

43. Chadban RC, Atkins RC: Glomerulonephritis, *The Lancet* 365:1797-1806, 2005.

44. Bergs L: Goodpasture syndrome, *Crit Care Nurse* 25(5):50-58, 2005.

45. Davidson A, Aranow C: Pathogenesis and treatment of systemic lupus erythematosus nephritis, *Curr Opin Rheumatol* 18(5):468-475, 2006.

46. Reidy K, Kaskel FJ: Pathophysiology of focal segmental glomerulosclerosis, *Pediatr Nephrol* 22:350-354, 2007.

47. Glick AM: Focal segmental glomerulosclerosis: a case study with review of pathophysiology, *Nephrol Nurs J* 34(2):176-182, 2007.

48. Smith KD, Alpers CE: Pathogenic mechanisms in membranoproliferative glomerulonephritis, *Curr Opin Nephrol Hypertens* 14:396-403, 2005.

49. Ronco P, Debiec H: Molecular pathomechanisms of membranous nephropathy: from Heymann nephritis to alloimmunization, *J Am Soc Nephrol* 16:1205-1213, 2005.

50. Ronco P, Debiec H: new insights into the pathogenesis of membranous glomerulonephritis, *Curr Opin Nephrol Hypertens* 15:258-263, 2006.

51. Nangaku M, Shankland SJ, Couser WG: Cellular response to injury in membranous nephropathy, *J Am Soc Nephrol* 16:1195-1204, 2005.

52. Liu Y: Renal fibrosis: new insights into the pathogenesis and therapeutics, *Kidney Int* 69:213-217, 2006.

53. Rodriguez-Iturbe B, Batsford S: Pathogenesis of poststreptococcal glomerulonephritis a century after Clemens von Pirquet, *Kidney Int* 71:1094-1104, 2007.

54. Huang H et al: Is IgA nephropathy induced by abnormalities of CD4 and CD25 Treg cells in the tonsils? *Med Hypotheses* 69:410-413, 2006.

55. Appel GB: Improved outcomes in nephrotic syndrome, *Cleve Clin J Med* 73:161-167, 2006.

56. Hinkes BG et al: Nephrotic syndrome in the first year of life: two thirds of cases are caused by mutations in 4 genes (NPHS1, NPHS2, WT1, and LAMB2), *Pediatrics* 119:907-919, 2007.

57. Buemi M et al: Statins in nephrotic syndrome: a new weapon against tissue injury, *Med Res Rev* 25:587-609, 2005.

58. Nandish SS, Khardori R, Elamin EM: Transient ischemic attack and nephrotic syndrome: case report and review of literature, *Am J Med Sci* 332:32-35, 2006.

59. Signhai R, Brinble KS: Thromboembolic complications in the nephrotic syndrome: pathophysiology and clinical management, *Thromb Res* 118:397-407, 2006.

60. Borges FF et al: Is focal segmental glomerulosclerosis increasing in patients with nephrotic syndrome? *Pediatr Nephrol* 22:1309-1313, 2007.

61. Franceschini N et al: NPHS2 gene, nephrotic syndrome and focal segmental glomerulosclerosis: a HuGE review, *Genet Med* 8:63-75, 2006.

Acute Renal Failure and Chronic Kidney Disease

Roberta J. Emerson

MEDIA RESOURCES

Additional Material for Study, Review, and Further Exploration

CD Companion ■ Review Questions and Answers
■ Glossary (with audio pronunciations for selected terms)
■ Disease Profiles ■ Animations

ⓔvolve **Website** at http://evolve.elsevier.com/Copstead/
■ Case Studies ■ Disease Profiles ■ WebLinks ■ Key Points Review

 Online Course (Module 14)

KEY QUESTIONS

■ How do the prerenal, intrarenal, and postrenal types of acute renal failure differ in etiology, prognosis, clinical manifestations, and management?

■ What are the characteristic clinical and laboratory findings in each of the three stages of acute tubular necrosis (acute intrarenal renal failure)?

■ What is the relationship between the degree of nephron loss, reductions in glomerular filtration rate, and the stages of chronic kidney disease?

■ What are the similarities and differences between acute renal failure and end-stage chronic kidney disease?

■ What are the characteristic findings of uremic syndrome?

■ How can acute renal failure be prevented, and how is it treated?

■ How is the progression of chronic kidney disease retarded?

■ How is end-stage chronic kidney disease treated?

CHAPTER OUTLINE

The kidneys have a number of regulatory roles within the body.[1] These key functions include the regulation of body fluid volume and osmolality, of electrolyte balance, and of acid-base balance. Additionally, the kidneys produce and secrete hormones, and excrete metabolic waste products and foreign materials.[1] When the kidneys are unable to carry out these functions on a temporary or permanent basis, the ramifications are significant to every body system.

ACUTE RENAL FAILURE

Lacking a precise definition, acute renal failure (ARF) is generally accepted as a generic term for a potentially reversible syndrome characterized by the abrupt deterioration of renal function, occurring over hours to weeks, that results in the retention of nitrogenous waste products.[2-5] Diagnostic criteria for ARF likewise vary, but an acute increase in the serum creatinine level of 0.5 mg/dl (44.2 µmol) appears quite universal.[2,3] Although unaffected for some patients, most patients with ARF experience marked alterations in urinary output during the course of illness. *Oliguria* is defined as an output of <400 ml in a 24-hour period; if the output is <100 ml in that same period of time, it is termed *anuria.* Varying with the severity and duration of presentation, ARF may also be accompanied by disruptions in fluid, electrolyte, and acid-base balance.[2,3,5] Serum creatinine and the calculated glomerular filtration rate (GFR) are monitored as a reflection of renal function. Retention of nitrogenous metabolic waste products also occurs, termed *azotemia* or *uremia,* and is tracked by changes in blood urea nitrogen (BUN) levels.

Acute renal failure is present at the time of admission for 1% to 5% of patients[3] but more frequently develops when patients are hospitalized. Mortality in critical care units, where 15% to 20% of the patients may be affected, can reach 70%.[3] Over the past 50 years, mortality from ARF has remained unchanged, despite advancement in clinical management.[5] Acute renal failure uncomplicated by concomitant illness has a mortality rate of 7% to 23%, depending on the report.[6] Mortality rates can also be stratified for particular populations. For postoperative patients, mortality rates are higher than the 50% rate reported for medical patients. Probably because of the development of multiple organ failure, mortality in trauma patients may reach 83%.[5]

Etiology and Pathophysiology

The risk of developing acute renal failure is increased by certain pre-existing conditions. These comorbidities include pre-existing kidney impairment, atherosclerosis, hypertension, diabetes mellitus, heart failure, and liver impairment/failure.[3-5] Not only are the elderly more likely to have one or more of these conditions, aging itself results in changes within the kidney making it more susceptible to damage. These alterations in function increase the risk of ARF and can negatively impact overall prognosis. The aging kidney is less capable of autoregulating perfusion pressure, has a decreased urine-concentrating ability, a reduced ability to conserve sodium, and a diminished

response to ADH. The elimination of potassium is decreased due to reduced levels of aldosterone. Awareness of thirst is decreased, and fluid and electrolyte imbalances are both more common and more severe. The GFR at the age of 80 is half what it was at age 30. By age 70, the number of nephrons is diminished by 50%, markedly reducing renal resilience. Older tubular cells may also be more susceptible to damage because cellular antioxidant defenses dwindle with age. See Chapter 26 for a discussion of the effects of aging on renal function.

Acute loss of renal function is attributable to conditions that affect renal perfusion (prerenal), obstruct urine flow distal to the kidney (postrenal), or circumstances within the kidney blood vessels, tubules, glomeruli, or interstitium (intrarenal).[2,3,7] These anatomic delineations are broadly seen as the types or causes of ARF, but the specific etiology must also be identified. Determination of the specific etiology as well as the type of ARF is essential for effective management. Box 28-1 shows the types of ARF and some of their etiologies. When acute renal failure develops in hospitalized patients, it is frequently due to a combination of pre-existing risk factors and multiple insults, often involving more than one etiology.[4]

Prerenal Acute Renal Failure

When acute renal failure develops because of diminished perfusion of the kidney, it is termed *prerenal* acute renal failure because the etiology occurs before the kidney itself.[7] As seen in Box 28-1, this can be due to an absolute or relative decrease in circulating volume, or abnormalities of renal hemodynamics. Actual or relative depletion of volume are the most common etiologies.[2,3,8] Prerenal causes are responsible for 70% of the ARF acquired in the community and for 40% of the cases that develop in the hospital.[4] Fever, vomiting, diarrhea, burns, hemorrhage, and overuse of diuretic therapy produce fluid volume deficits that can lead to prerenal ARF. In distributive shock the vascular bed is so enlarged that adequate renal tissue perfusion is impaired. The same problem results if large volumes of fluid collect in extravascular spaces as in edema (interstitial space) or ascites (peritoneal space). Any number of conditions reduces the ability of the heart to generate a cardiac output sufficient to meet the needs of body organ systems. Even though the kidney receives 20% to 25% of the cardiac output[7], that volume may be inadequate when the cardiac output is markedly decreased by cardiogenic shock, heart failure, or lethal ventricular dysrhythmias.

Although most patients who develop prerenal acute renal failure have an episode of decreased blood pressure that results in decreased perfusion to the kidney, in some cases perfusion drops without the blood pressure falling below normal.[9] These "normotensive" cases of prerenal ARF arise in susceptible individuals with very modest reductions in blood pressure who have pre-existing impairments in renal autoregulation. Use of nonsteroidal anti-inflammatory drugs (NSAIDs), angiotensin-converting enzyme (ACE) inhibitors, and angiotensin II (AII) receptor blockers are known to interfere with renal vascular autoregulation and can precipitate prerenal ARF in certain populations of patients; this includes

BOX 28-1

Types of Acute Renal Failure

Prerenal
- Absolute decrease in circulating volume
  - Hemorrhage
  - Dehydration
  - Burns
- Relative decrease in circulating volume
  - Distributive shock (neurogenic, anaphylactic, septic)
  - Third-spacing and edema
  - Decreased cardiac output
    - Cardiogenic shock
    - Dysrhythmias
    - Cardiac tamponade
    - Heart failure
    - Myocardial infarction
- Primary renal hemodynamic abnormalities
  - Occlusion or stenosis of renal artery*
  - Drug-induced impairment of renal autoregulation in susceptive persons[t]

Postrenal
- Benign prostatic hyperplasia
- Kinked or obstructed catheters
- Intra-abdominal tumors
- Strictures
- Calculi

Intrarenal/Intrinsic
- Tubular (acute tubular necrosis)
  - Ischemic
    - Prolonged prerenal failure
    - Transfusion reactions
    - Rhabdomyolysis
  - Nephrotoxic
    - Prolonged postrenal failure
    - Certain antimicrobials (antibiotics; antifungal and antiviral drugs)
    - Radiographic contrast media
    - Certain cytotoxic chemotherapy agents
    - Recreational drugs (amphetamines, heroin)
    - Environmental agents (heavy metals, carbon tetrachloride, insecticides)
    - Snake and insect venom
- Glomerular
  - Acute glomerulonephritis
- Interstitial
  - Acute allergic interstitial nephritis
  - Acute pyelonephritis
- Vascular
  - Vasculitis
  - Emboli
  - Nephrosclerosis (due to primary hypertension, hypertensive emergencies, and urgency)

*Use of ACE inhibitors or A-II receptor blockers increase the risk.

[t]Pre-existing chronic renal insufficiency, cirrhosis, heart failure, elderly (>60 years) with atherosclerotic cardiovascular disease, hypotension, diuretic use, nephritic syndrome.[2]

those who are older than 60 years of age with atherosclerotic cardiovascular disease, pre-existing renal insufficiency (elevated serum creatinine), heart failure, advanced liver disease, or nephrotic syndrome.[2,9] These drugs cause either vasoconstriction of afferent arterioles (NSAIDs) or vasodilation of efferent arterioles (ACE inhibitors and AII blockers); either of these actions results in a decrease in glomerular perfusion pressure.[3,9] Thrombosis, embolus, dissection, or stenosis of the renal arteries will also result in prerenal ARF [2,3,9] and the risk increases significantly if ACE inhibitors or AII blockers are being used.[2,9]

Prerenal oliguria is the kidney's normal physiologic response to a decrease in perfusion [2,7,9], and at least for a time, the renal tissue is unharmed. The sensed decrease in renal blood flow results in a decrease in GFR and urine output. Neurohumoral mechanisms of local autoregulation are activated as the kidneys endeavor to autoregulate perfusion and maintain GFR, and systemic mechanisms such as RAAS act to increase the total circulating volume.[2,7] Because of the kidney's ability to tolerate significant reduction in perfusion as long as it is not greater than about 20% to 25% of normal, if the hypoperfusion etiology is identified and corrected, prerenal oliguria will not affect the parenchyma of the kidney.[2,7] Efforts to restore adequate perfusion should be fully effective in restoring completely normal renal function within 1 to 2

days.[9] In the case of normotensive patients who have impaired perfusion, by far the smallest subset of prerenal ARF, interventions must be targeted to the specific etiology.[9] Regardless of the etiology, persistent prerenal ARF will result in hypoxic renal cells; if hypoxia continues and ischemia lasts more than a few hours, prerenal ARF will progress to acute tubular necrosis (intrarenal acute renal failure).[7,8]

Postrenal Acute Renal Failure

Obstruction of the normal outflow of urine from the kidneys can result in postrenal ARF.[3,7,8] Box 28-1 lists the most common etiologies of this type of acute renal failure. Drugs such as acyclovir, indinavir, and topiramate may lead to obstruction by forming precipitates in the urine.[10] If only one kidney is affected, activity of the remaining kidney will increase to maintain fluid and electrolyte balance.[7] Obstruction of the renal pelvis or ureters of both kidneys, of the bladder outlet, or the urethra will result in discernable postrenal acute renal failure. This type of ARF is the least common and the most amenable to intervention. Normalization of renal function depends on the length of time the obstruction persists.[3] Should obstruction persist, the increasing retrograde pressure of urine will result in acute tubular necrosis (intrarenal acute renal failure), and if the obstruction continues over several days or weeks, irreversible damage to the kidney will result.[7,8]

Intrarenal Acute Renal Failure

Acute renal failure intrinsic to the kidney itself is further classified by the specific anatomical area involved: vascular, interstitial, glomerular, or tubular[2,3] (see Box 28-1). Some references incorporate the vascular and tubular classifications together since damage to one ultimately leads to damage of the other.[7] All of these etiologies are capable of producing the potentially reversible rapid decline in renal function that is acute renal failure. When the small vessels within the kidney are inflamed, obstructed, or damaged by an acute hypertensive episode, the injury may be sufficient to impair nephron functioning. Acute glomerulonephritis is due to a Type III immune reaction; immune complexes are deposited in the basement membrane of the glomerulus.[3,7] Normal renal function is disrupted to some degree during this acute inflammatory process, usually lasting about 2 weeks. Acute glomerulonephritis is discussed in detail in Chapter 27. Inflammation of interstitial tissues may be sufficient to result in intrarenal acute renal failure; this is usually due to an infection of the kidney (pyelonephritis), an allergic reaction most commonly to drugs, or an autoimmune disease.[2,3] Drug-induced intrarenal acute renal failure may be the result of damage to the renal tubules, glomeruli, interstitium, or vasculature.[10]

By far the most common cause of intrarenal acute renal failure is acute tubular necrosis (ATN), which itself has many potential etiologies.[2-4,7] Acute tubular necrosis is the result of tubular cell injury due to either an ischemic pathology or a toxin. Interestingly, the diversity of potential etiologies of ATN is highly variable across world populations.[2] In Africa, Latin America, southeast Asia, and India, snakebites and tropical diseases are prevalent. Crushing injuries resulting in the release of large quantities of myoglobin that obstruct tubules (rhabdomylosis) develop in earthquake-prone areas of the world.[2] Acute tubular necrosis is the dominant cause of ARF among hospitalized patients in the United States.[4] Thirty-five to fifty percent of the ATN cases that develop in critical care units are associated with sepsis, and the concurrent failure of at least one other organ system is common. Postsurgical ATN is responsible for 20% to 25% of the cases that develop in the hospital; most of these are due to prolonged prerenal ARF.[2]

The most common source of ischemic ATN is prolonged prerenal ARF that results in renal cellular hypoxia.[4] Indeed, prerenal ischemia and ischemic ATN are a matter of degree, points on a continuum of hypoxic tubular injury.[3] The medulla is less vascular than the cortex, so it is particularly vulnerable to ischemic injury.[11]

The list of chemicals that are toxic to the kidney is expansive,[2,3,7] each one inducing a specific toxic reaction in the tubular cells and resulting in the death of many of them.[7] Of all of these nephrotoxins, the most widespread is contrast media.[2,7] It is responsible for 12% of the cases of ARF in the hospital and can develop within 48 hours of administration.[6] ATN due to contrast media results in prolonged hospitalization, increased healthcare costs, and an increased risk of death.[2,6] Results of experimental research suggest that the ATN resulting from contrast media is a product of both tubular cell toxicity and ischemia.[6] The ascending limb of the nephron in the renal medulla seems to be particularly susceptible to contrast media-induced injury.[6] Nephrotoxic injury without ischemia results in less tubular damage. In this case, only the epithelial cells are affected and they are capable of rapid and effective regeneration. In ATN secondary to ischemia, or if ischemia accompanies the toxic damage, injury is more profound and both the course of illness and recovery are prolonged.

In ATN, there are two pathophysiologic processes that result in the rapid decrease in glomerular filtration rate: a vascular process and a tubular one.[2] The two processes are interrelated, and the severity of one contributes to the severity of the other. Renal blood flow is decreased by 30% to 50% in ATN, and blood is shunted from the medulla to the cortex, further compromising the medullary cells.[2,6] Local vasoconstrictors such as prostaglandins and leukotrienes are released, and the effects of sympathetic nervous system (SNS) stimulation contribute further to the vasoconstriction.[6] Hypoxia or direct tubular damage due to toxins initiates an inflammatory response, activating the cascade of inflammatory mediators. When perfusion is restored, more inflammatory cells are enlisted and reperfusion injury perpetuates damage in some areas. Cells in part of the proximal tubule and outer cortex begin the repair process when perfusion is returned, but endothelial cells and those in the ascending limb continue to be injured, necrose, and commit apoptosis, resulting in a further decline in GFR.[2,6]

The pathogenesis of the tubular process is a reflection of the ischemia[2] and the inflammatory process (Figure 28-1). If the renal insult results in a more minor injury, the cells that are unable to recover will commit apoptosis; severe injury results in frank necrosis.[4] The distal tubule is the site of most of the apoptotic cells.[2] Damaged tubular epithelial cells, both viable and nonviable, are shed from the basement membrane and accumulate in the tubular filtrate where they obstruct filtrate flow.[2,7] These cells combine with inflammatory cells and debris[2] to form casts that contribute further to the urinary obstruction.[2] Obstructed urinary flow produces an increased pressure within the nephron that is communicated backwards to the glomerulus, further reducing the GFR. The increasing pressure generated by the tubular obstruction forces filtrate through the partially denuded tubular basement membrane into the interstitial space and even into the bloodstream, a process known as *tubular backleak*. Half of the already limited quantity of glomerular filtrate may be lost to the interstitium by this process.

Recovery following ATN is highly dependent on the extent of injury and slower than in the other two types of ARF.[3,6,7] If sufficient destruction of the basement membrane occurs, there may be no recovery and the patient develops end-stage chronic renal disease, the final stage of chronic kidney disease. But the tubules can repair themselves within 10 to 20 days when the basement membrane is intact and new epithelial cells are produced on that surface.[7] As with the other types of renal failure, the clinical presentation of ATN is primarily

FIGURE 28-1 Pathogenesis of acute tubular necrosis.

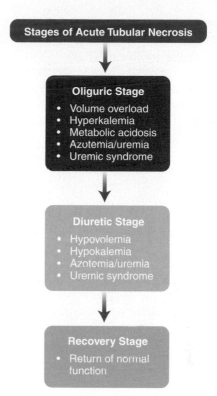

FIGURE 28-2 Stages of acute tubular necrosis and primary clinical issues.

TABLE 28-1

Laboratory Value Differences in Prerenal and Intrarenal Acute Renal Failure*

Laboratory Test	Prerenal Findings	Intrarenal Findings
FENa %	<1	>2
Proteinuria	Absent	Possible
Urine specific gravity	>1.020	1.010-1.020
Urine osmolality (mOsm/kg)	>500	300-500
BUN:creatinine ratio	>20:1	10-20:1
Urine sodium concentration (mmol/L)	<10	>20
Urinary sediment	Few hyaline casts	Tubular, RBC, and WBC casts

*Derived from Gammill HS, Jeyabalan A: Acute renal failure in pregnancy, *Crit Care Med* 33(10):S372-S384, 2005; Needham E: Management of acute renal failure, *Am Fam Physician* 72(9):1739-1746, 2005; Lameire N, Van Biesen W, Vanholder R: Acute renal failure, *The Lancet* 365:417-430, 2005.

FENa %, Fraction of excreted sodium, percent.

a reflection of the loss of the normal functions performed by the kidney.

Clinical Presentation of Acute Tubular Necrosis

Prerenal ARF can be reversed before perfusion drops to about 20% of normal and ischemia results.[7] It is at this point that ATN develops. Prerenal or postrenal renal failure will ultimately progress to intrarenal ARF if not corrected within a few hours.[7] The course of ATN is roughly divided into three stages, and the clinical presentation varies with the stage[3] (Figure 28-2). The laboratory findings that differentiate prerenal from intrarenal renal failure are shown in Table 28-1. Table 28-2 provides the laboratory profile associated with renal failure; some of these findings are more likely to be noted in end-stage chronic kidney disease than in acute renal failure. Serum creatinine levels begin to increase within 24 hours.[6] As with other aspects of the clinical presentation, laboratory findings are affected by the stage of ATN.

Oliguric Stage

Most patients with ATN develop oliguria; those with severe injury often become anuric.[2,3,7] As urine output drops, metabolic waste products are retained and fluid and electrolyte balance is disrupted.[7] These alterations are reflected in the results of physical assessment and in laboratory data.

Renal function is monitored according to fluctuations in the serum creatinine[2] and the calculated GFR that is derived from it.[12,13] Normal GFR declines with age. The preferred formula for calculating GFR utilizes the serum creatinine and is adjusted for gender, age, and race[12] (Box 28-2). The correction for blacks reflects the fact that they have higher glomerular filtration rates at the same level of serum creatinine as do Caucasians. This formula has not been substantiated with those <18 or >70 years of age or ethnic subgroups other than Caucasians and blacks. For

TABLE 28-2

Laboratory Profile for Renal Failure

Test	Normal Range for Adults	Values in Renal Failure	Comments
Test to Evaluate Removal of Nitrogenous Wastes			
Serum creatinine	*Male:* 0.6-1.2 mg/dl *Female:* 0.5-1.1 mg/dl *Older adults:* Decreased	**In Chronic Renal Failure** May increase by 0.5-1.0 mg/dl every 1-2 yr May be as high as 15-30 mg/dl *before* symptoms of CRF are present **In Acute Renal Failure** Gradual increase of 1-2 mg/dl every 24-48 hr May increase 1-6 mg/dl; in 1 wk or less	Consistently elevated levels indicate decreased renal function. Serum creatinine levels are used to evaluate the effectiveness of dialysis treatments.
Blood urea nitrogen	10-20 mg/dl *Older adults:* May be slightly increased	**In Chronic Renal Failure** May reach 180-200 mg/dl *before* symptoms develop **In Acute Renal Failure** Often increases by 1-20 mg/dl at same pace as serum creatinine level May reach 80-100 mg/dl within 1 wk	Increases depend on protein intake and other factors. Rate of increase is controlled by limiting protein intake. This intervention is believed to decrease the rate of onset of systemic symptoms, such as anorexia, nausea, and vomiting. Elevations have multiple causes, including diminished renal function, excessive protein intake, sepsis, GI bleeding, dehydration, and tissue catabolism.
Electrolyte Studies			
Serum sodium	136-145 mEq/L; 136-145 mmol/L (SI units)	Normal or decreased	Clients with renal failure retain sodium. With associated water retention, serum sodium levels seem normal. With excessive water retention, serum sodium levels seem decreased owing to hemodilution. Assess the client for evidence of fluid volume excess: edema, weight increase, or elevation of diastolic blood pressure. Limit fluid intake as directed. Avoid excessive sodium intake. Monitor for signs of hypernatremia: dry skin, excessive thirst, dry mucous membranes, elevated body temperature, and flushed skin. Client may need diuretics or dialysis.
Serum potassium	3.5-5.0 mmol/L (SI units)	Increased	Advise the client to avoid salt substitutes and to limit potassium-containing foods. Monitor for rapidly increasing serum potassium levels in ARF. ECG changes occur with serum potassium levels ≥6.5. Monitor for signs of hyperkalemia: dizziness, weakness, cardiac irregularities, muscle cramps, diarrhea, and nausea. May require administration of sodium polystyrene sulfonate (Kayexalate) or other treatment.
Serum phosphorus (phosphate)	3.0-4.5 mg/dl, 0.97-1.45 mmol/L (SI units) *Older adults:* May be slightly decreased	Increased	Short-term increases have potential to cause rapid decrease in serum calcium level and cardiac rhythm disturbances. Long-term increases demineralize bones of calcium and enhance fracture potential. Phosphate-binding medications help control hyperphosphatemia and prevent calcium depletion from the bones.

TABLE 28-2

Laboratory Profile for Renal Failure—cont'd

Test	Normal Range for Adults	Values in Renal Failure	Comments
Electrolyte studies—cont'd			
Serum calcium	Total calcium: 9.0-10.5 mg/dl; 2.25-2.75 mmol/L (SI units) Ionized calcium: 4.5-5.6 mg/dl; 1.05-1.3 mmol/L (SI units) *Older adults:* slightly decreased	Decreased	Decreases in ARF may necessitate replacement. Decreases in CRF may only be slight and may or may not necessitate replacement. As the serum phosphate level increases, the serum calcium level decreases. Chronic calcium deficiency leads to renal osteodystrophy. Control of phosphate excess is usually essential before calcium replacement is initiated. Monitor for manifestations of hypocalcemia: abdominal cramps, hyperactive reflexes, tingling fingertips, and spasms in feet and wrists.
Serum magnesium	1.3-2.1 mEq/L; 0.65-1.05 mmol/L (SI units)	Increased	Advise the patient to avoid compounds containing magnesium (e.g., laxatives).
Serum carbon dioxide combining power (bicarbonate)	23-30 mEq/L (venous); 23-30 mmol/L (SI units)	Decreased	Replace bicarbonate. Monitor respiratory rate and depth. Monitor for decreased orientation.
Arterial blood pH	7.35-7.45	Decreased (in metabolic acidosis) or normal	The respiratory system attempts to compensate by hyperventilation (increased rate and depth of respiration). Values are within the normal range if blood buffers and lungs can compensate. Monitor breathing rate and depth. Monitor level of consciousness.
Arterial blood bicarbonate (HCO_3^-)	21-38 mEq/L	Decreased	Provide replacement PO, IV, or by hemodialysis or peritoneal dialysis.
Arterial blood $Paco_2$	35-45 mm Hg	Decreased	Monitor for respiratory fatigue (the client breathes more rapidly and deeply to "blow off" carbon dioxide).
Other Blood Studies			
Hemoglobin	*Female:* 12-16 g/dl, 7.4-9.9 mmol/L (SI units) *Male:* 14-18 g/dl, 8.7-11.2 mmol/L (SI units) *Older adults:* Slightly decreased	Decreased	Decreased levels indicate anemia. Monitor for pallor, weakness, lethargy, dizziness, possible shortness of breath, and activity intolerance.
Hematocrit	*Female:* 37%-47% *Male:* 42%-52% *Older adults:* May be slightly decreased	Decreased to 20%	Same as for hemoglobin. With erythropoietin therapy, may be able to obtain levels as high as 36%.
Urinalysis*			
Specific gravity	Usually 1.010-1.025 Possible range: 1.005-1.030	Usually decreased and fixed	Reflects inability of the tubules to produce a concentrated or diluted urine in response to changes in plasma osmolarity. Monitor for fluid volume deficit or excess.
pH	Average: 5.5-6 Possible range: 4.6-8	May be fixed; pH does not change with dietary changes	Collect a freshly voided specimen for testing.
Glucose	None or <15 mg/dl Usually detectable in urine of nondiabetic clients when blood level is 160-180 mg/dl	Increased	The renal threshold is often increased; therefore the blood glucose level may be >160–180 mg/dl before glucose is detectable in the urine. Monitor *blood* glucose levels.

(continued)

TABLE 28-2

Laboratory Profile for Renal Failure—cont'd

Test	Normal Range for Adults	Values in Renal Failure	Comments
Urinalysis*—cont'd			
Protein	0-8 mg/dl	Increased when there is glomerular damage or disease	Increases may be an incidental and benign finding. Transient increases occur with extreme exercise, fever, stress, or infection. Persistent proteinuria requires 24-hr collection for determination of total quantity excreted. Persistent proteinuria may indicate a serious renal problem. Instruct the client about the need for follow-up. Instruct the client in the correct procedure for collection of 24-hr specimen.
Occult blood	No RBCs or occasionally 2 or 3 RBCs per high-power field No hemoglobin	More than 2 or 3 RBCs per high-power field Detectable hemoglobin	Hemoglobin is detectable when hemolysis of RBCs has occurred. Intact RBCs are detectable only with microscopic examination. Collect a freshly voided specimen for testing.
WBCs	0-5 per high-power field	Increased in urinary tract infection	Often indicates need for urine culture.
Bacteria	Fewer than 1000 colonies/ml	Increased in the presence of infection, with or without an increase in WBCs	Obtain urine culture.
Casts	None or a few; composed of RBCs, WBCs, protein, or tubular cell casts such as hyaline	Casts present	Casts may be a benign occurrence or may signify that some renal injury or disease is present. Collect a freshly voided specimen for direct microscopic examination.
Creatinine clearance	*Male:* 107-109 ml/min *Female:* 87-107 ml/min *Older adults:* Progressively decreased with advancing age	Decreased	Change reflects decreases in GFR. Creatinine clearance is determined from a 24-hr urine collection and a serum creatinine value.

Arf, Acute renal failure; *ECG,* electrocardiogram; *CRF,* chronic renal failure; *GI,* gastrointestinal; *GFR,* glomerular filtration rate; *RBCs,* red blood cells; *SI,* Systeme Internationale; *WBCs,* white blood cells.

*Urine may become cloudy with heavy sediment. Urine output and appearance vary, depending on remaining renal function.
Adapted from Ignatavicius DD, Workman ML: *Medical-surgical nursing: critical thinking for collaborative care,* ed 5, Philadelphia, 2006, Saunders, pp 1733-1735.

BOX 28-2

Modification of Diet in Renal Disease (MDRD) Study Equation for Estimating GFR*

$$GFR\ (ml/min/1.73m^2) = 186 \times (P_{cr})^{-1.154} \times (age)^{-0.203} \times (0.742\ if\ female) \times (1.210\ if\ black)$$

P_{Cr}, Plasma creatinine

*National Kidney Foundation. Available at http://www.kidney.org/professionals/KLS/GFR.CFM#4

pregnant women; those at the extremes of age or weight; those with malnutrition, skeletal muscle disease, paraplegia, or tetraplegia; or vegetarians with rapidly changing renal function, a 24-hour urine collection for creatinine clearance is the preferable method of assessing renal function.[12] A GFR calculator for adults and another for pediatric patients is available from the National Kidney Foundation at: http://www.kidney.org/professionals/KLS/GFR.CFM#4.

Organic metabolic waste products are retained as the GFR declines. Historically, this has been monitored by changes in serum BUN (azotemia or uremia). Although urea represents the largest amount of these wastes, other uremic solutes are involved and have been found to be responsible for many of the collection of signs and symptoms termed uremic syndrome[14] (Table 28-3). Although these manifestations are classically much more severe in end-stage chronic kidney disease, there is no identifiable point at which uremia presents so some may be present in ARF. A GFR that is only slightly less than 50% of the normal for age may produce mild manifestations.[14] Metabolic wastes are acidic and the renal system is unable to excrete H^+ ions or form bicarbonate, so acidosis develops.[7] This, combined with the direct toxic effects of azotemia on the myocytes, is responsible for a negative inotropic effect

TABLE 28-3

Pathophysiology of Manifestations of Uremic Syndrome

System	Manifestation	Pathophysiologic Basis
Central nervous system	Uremic encephalopathy ■ Disorientation ■ Lethargy ■ Coma	Brain cells shrink due to osmotic gradient
Peripheral nervous system	Motor neuropathies ■ Weakness Sensory neuropathies ■ Numbness ■ Tingling	Toxin interference with nerve transmission
Cardiovascular system	Bleeding Anemia Decreased cardiac output Ischemic syndromes Pericarditis*	Decreased platelet function and coagulation factor production Decreased RBC lifespan; blood loss Negative inotropic effect Escalated coronary heart disease Uremic crystals deposited in the pericardium
Immune system	Infections	Decreased immune cell production and immune response
Gastrointestinal system	Anorexia Nausea and vomiting	Direct effect of toxins
Skin	Impaired healing* Pruritus; dermatitis* Uremic frost*	Decreased collagen production Deposition of uremic crystals on the skin
Acid-base	Metabolic acidosis	Accumulation of acidic metabolic wastes

*More likely to occur with chronic renal failure

on the heart. Decreased myocyte functioning can be significant in elderly patients, especially if there is pre-existing heart failure. Level of consciousness may be altered and peripheral neuropathies may be disconcerting to the patient. Appetite suppression, nausea, and/or vomiting are uncomfortable and make meeting nutritional needs a challenge.[15] Impaired healing and the increased risk of infection are especially concerning postoperatively, but increase the possibility of nosocomial infection for all patients. Development of uremia in ARF necessitates temporarily replacing renal function with dialysis.[14]

Since it cannot be excreted, body water is retained. This hypervolemia results in the development of edema and hypertension.[7] Other signs and symptoms of fluid volume overload include distended neck veins (JVD), weight gain, and possibly additional manifestations of heart failure, which may be precipitated in susceptible patients due to the acute onset of volume excess. Normally, as renal perfusion is reduced, the kidney responds by increasing the reabsorption of sodium and reducing its elimination; in ATN, this mechanism is impaired and sodium is lost in the reduced volume of urine that is produced.[8] Tubular casts are present in the urine, and white blood cells, red blood cells, and protein are also likely to appear.[8] Other electrolytes are typically retained in the blood (K^+, Mg^{++}, and $PO4^=$), and their levels in the urine are decreased (see Table 28-2). Of all the potential electrolyte problems, hyperkalemia is of greatest concern since the normal range is narrow (3.5 to 5 mEq/liter) and levels of less than

double the normal values can be fatal.[7] The hyperkalemia and metabolic acidosis can exacerbate one another, as intracellular potassium ions are exchanged for intravascular hydrogen ions (see Chapter 25). Changes in the other electrolytes may not be seen unless the oliguric stage is prolonged. This stage is a reflection of the decreased perfusion within the kidney and may persist up to two weeks.

Diuretic Stage

Termination of the oliguric stage is marked by the beginning of renal recovery: the diuretic stage. Unfortunately, not all patients recover; in about 5% of cases ARF is not reversible.[2] In the elderly, 16% of those with ARF do not regain renal function. This diuretic stage reflects the return of tubular patency; urine is excreted in large volumes because mechanisms for concentrating filtrate have not recovered. Typically, urine output is more than a liter per day, but may be as much as 4 to 5 liters. The elevated levels of BUN contribute an osmotic diuresis, as the large molecules are filtered and draw more water into the tubules. Renal perfusion begins to increase, slowly advancing filtration ability and tubular function. During this stage, the voluminous diuresis will produce a fluid volume deficit without rapid replacement. Electrolytes initially retained, especially potassium, may now be lost and require replacement as well. Over the course of several days, the quantity of urine output normalizes and the patient enters the final stage of ATN: recovery.

Recovery Stage

Full recovery of renal function, if it does occur, may take only a week but more often as much as a year. Full recovery is indicated when the serum creatinine returns to within the normal range. This variation in recovery time is due to the diversity of ATN causes and degree of damage, but also the quality of interventions provided and patients' concomitant conditions. Even after recovery, progressive loss of renal function following ARF is a frequent finding, even in pediatric cases. The lingering damage to renal function following ARF in childhood has been found to result in progressive deterioration by adolescence or early adulthood.[2] In 30% of the cases, some degree of renal insufficiency persists and recovery is incomplete.

KEY POINTS

- ARF is an abrupt reduction in renal function producing an accumulation of waste materials in the blood. Oliguria is usually present. ARF is classified into three types according to the site of disruption: prerenal, intrarenal, and postrenal. Distinction between the types of ARF is necessary to determine appropriate therapy.
- Prerenal renal failure is due to conditions that impair renal blood flow, such as hypovolemia, hypotension, cardiac failure, and renal artery obstruction. It is characterized by clinical manifestations of a low GFR, usually including oliguria, high urine specific gravity and osmolality, and low urinary sodium. Signs and symptoms of fluid volume overload are present. Prolonged prerenal renal failure results in intrarenal renal failure.
- Postrenal ARF is due to obstruction within the urinary collecting system distal to the kidney. Obstruction results in elevated pressure in Bowman's capsule, which impedes glomerular filtration. Clinical findings vary, based on the duration of the obstruction. Prolonged postrenal renal failure results in intrarenal renal failure.
- Intrarenal failure is due to a primary dysfunction of the nephrons. Although it may be due to glomerular, vascular, or interstitial etiologies, most often the problem is within the renal tubules, resulting in acute tubular necrosis. ATN may occur with nephrotoxic or ischemic insults. Clinical manifestations depend upon the stage of ATN.
- ATN has three characteristic stages. The first stage, characterized by oliguria and progressive uremia, may last 1 to 2 weeks. Dialysis may be necessary at this time. Oliguria is followed by a diuretic stage that lasts 2 to 10 days. During the diuretic phase, urine volume increases, but tubular function remains impaired and azotemia continues. The recovery phase, lasting up to 12 months, is characterized by gradual normalization of serum creatinine and BUN. Often a degree of renal insufficiency persists.
- ARF results in characteristic alterations in laboratory tests of the blood and urine. Renal function is monitored by serum creatinine and calculated creatinine clearance. The retention of metabolic wastes (azotemia/uremia), which is monitored by the BUN, produces widespread systemic effects (uremic syndrome).

CHRONIC KIDNEY DISEASE

Chronic renal failure is the outcome of the progressive and irrevocable loss of nephrons.[7,12,13] The normal resiliency of the kidney means that more than 75% of the total number of nephrons must be lost before clinical manifestations appear.[7] What is termed *chronic renal failure* is the final outcome of chronic kidney disease (CKD). More commonly, this point is called *end-stage renal disease* (ESRD) in acknowledgement of the progressive process of deterioration of renal function. At some point in the CKD process, renal disease will proceed to ESRD progressively, irreversibly, and for the most part, unrelated to the initial cause.[16,17]

Chronic kidney disease is a global health problem. Historically the majority of the overall morbidity and mortality throughout the world was due to infectious disease; today, chronic diseases are responsible for most of the world's illness and death.[18] More than 4 million people throughout the world have end-stage renal disease[18,19] and depend on dialysis, while many of them await renal transplantations that may not be available in time to save their lives. Every year, this number increases by roughly 250,000.[18] The highest incidence of untreated ESRD is found in North America, Japan, and Europe.[18] Mortality rates in the United States are 22%, 16% in Europe, and 7% in Japan.[17] Nearly 20 million people have CKD in the United States; about 8 million of these are in the moderate to severe stages of the disease, while another 450,000 or more have reached ESRD.[13,20] Because of the rapidly escalating incidence of the two primary risk factors—diabetes and hypertension, CKD is likely to increase in the years to come.[18]

Risk Factors

Chronic kidney disease is defined as either decreased kidney function or kidney damage of 3 months or more duration based on blood tests, urinalysis, and imaging studies.[12,20] Alternatively, it may be defined as a glomerular filtration rate (GFR) <60 ml/minute/1.73 m^2 for 3 months with or without indication of damage to the kidney.[12] CKD is a syndrome in that it can occur as a complication of many other conditions; this means that the etiologies and/or risk factors of these conditions are also risk factors for the development of chronic kidney disease. Although some of the conditions and risk factors have been identified for many years, new research findings have added to the list and altered perceptions of their relative importance (Box 28-3).

From a worldwide perspective, in developed and developing countries, the major condition putting people at risk for ESRD is now diabetes mellitus.[18,21] Diabetic nephropathy is diagnosed in 20% to 30% of diabetics.[21] Currently, roughly 50% of the cases of ESRD are attributed to diabetes,[12,18,20] while the prevalence of glomerulonephritis, cystic kidney disease, and hypertension as the causes of ESRD have remained relatively level in the past 10 years.[20] Type 2 diabetes is projected to double in incidence worldwide within the next 25 years; diabetic nephropathy is a major complication of that disease.

BOX 28-3

Risk Factors for Chronic Kidney Disease

- Acute tubular necrosis (not progressing beyond the oliguric stage)
- Developmental/congenital conditions
  - Renal agenesis
  - Aplastic kidneys
  - Renal hypoplasia
  - Ectopic/displaced kidneys
  - Fused kidneys
- Cystic disorders
  - Polycystic kidney disease
  - Medullary cystic disease
- Neoplasms
  - Benign tumors of the kidney
  - Malignant tumors of the kidney (including Wilms tumor)
- Infections
  - Recurrent pyelonephritis
  - Renal tuberculosis
- Glomerulonephritis

- Systemic conditions
  - Diabetes mellitus
  - Diabetes insipidus
  - Hypertension
  - Hyperparathyroidism
  - Liver failure/cirrhosis
  - Gout
  - Amyloidosis
  - Scleroderma
  - Goodpasture syndrome
  - Systemic lupus erythematosus (produces glomerulonephritis)
- Other
  - Genetics
  - Increasing age
  - Ethnicity
  - Overweight/obesity
  - Dyslipidemia
  - Family history of cardiovascular disease
  - Smoking

Of those who develop diabetic nephropathy, about 30% ultimately reach ESRD while the remainder most often dies from cardiovascular disease before that point.[20]

Hypertension is a major risk factor for CKD, and it also develops as a complication of it.[17] Currently, 20% to 30% of the incidence of kidney failure is attributed to hypertension.[12,20] The aging of the population in the United States is predicted to escalate the incidence of systolic hypertension and resulting renal disease.[22] Together, hypertension and diabetes account for >70% of patients with ESRD who are undergoing dialysis.[21]

Other contributions to the development of CKD are made by glomerulonephritis (<10%) and cystic kidney disease (2% to 3%).[12] Some of the risk factors for CKD are not amenable to modification. These include a family history of CKD, a history of exposure to toxins (heavy metals, tobacco smoke, radiopaque dyes), age over 60 years, and ethnicity (black, Hispanic, American Indian, Asian, Pacific Islander).[21] It has been recommended that high-risk groups be screened for CKD (those with family histories, diabetes mellitus, hypertension, recurrent urinary tract infections, urinary obstructions, or other systemic conditions affecting the kidney) and that screening be extended to those without any other identified risks but who are over 60 years old.[12] The role of genetic factors in CKD has received increased attention in research, and specific chromosomal loci associated with both disease and regenerative implications have been identified.[19] Although there are genetic mutations responsible for the development of some CKD, more frequently genetic factors are evident only with conditions such as hypertension or diabetes where they impact the progression of the disease process.[19]

Cardiovascular disease and CKD have many risk factors in common: increasing age, male gender, black race, hypertension, diabetes mellitus, smoking, decreased GFR, proteinuria, and RAAS over activity.[23] Along with other cardiovascular

risks, BMI at the level of overweight (BMI 25 to 29.9 kg/m^2) and obesity (>30 kg/m^2) has been found to increase risk for CKD.[21,24] Obesity-related glomerulopathy is associated with progressively worsening proteinuria, attaining the level of nephrotic syndrome (see Chapter 27), which precedes a decline in the GFR by several years. Although these individuals do not develop the edema, hypoalbuminemia, or radical hyperlipidemia usually seen in nephrotic syndrome, protein loss is equivalent. Alterations in glomerular perfusion and filtration, sodium reabsorption, renal sympathetic activity, and activity of the RAAS have all been identified as pathologic features of obesity-related glomerulopathy. Visceral adipose tissue is a known supply of all the elements of the RAAS.[24] Obesity itself is a significant risk factor for both diabetes and hypertension, the primary causes of CKD.

Pathophysiology of Progression of Chronic Kidney Disease

Regardless of the origin of CKD, the decline in renal function is progressive and irreversible. The pathophysiology of this progression is complex, and new research findings have identified a variety of contributory factors. There are treatment implications for retarding CKD progression for all of these factors, although in many cases, application is yet to be achieved. Progression of CKD is monitored by changes in GFR, presence and degree of proteinuria, examination of urinary sediment for white or red blood cells, serum creatinine levels, and imaging studies with renal ultrasonography to document kidney size.[25]

Pathophysiologic progression of CKD is characterized histologically by glomerulosclerosis and interstitial inflammation and fibrosis.[26-28] Proximal tubular cells have been found in *in vitro* studies to have altered their phenotype, but this has not been confirmed in human models. Clearly, interstitial damage is significant, and complement activation as part of the inflammatory response plays a major role in this process.[26] Proteinuria has historically been seen as reflective of renal damage; new research suggests the inability of the glomerular membrane to inhibit protein passing into the filtrate may actually produce further tubular injury.[16,26] Disproportionate proteinuria produces injury to the lysosomal pathways within cells; damage to tubules may result from burst lysosomes.[28] However, in certain diseases, most notably hypertensive nephrosclerosis, interstitial injury advances to ESRD without significant proteinuria.[16] In the case of primary hypertension, histologic changes to the renal vasculature are believed to facilitate glomerular injury including glomerulosclerosis, interstitial fibrosis and tubular atrophy.[29] Functional impairment of the kidneys is not so much correlated with the degree of glomerular damage as it is to tubulointerstitial injury.[16] Interstitial fibrosis may initially be the result of any of the sources of tubular damage producing ATN [30] as well as all of the other conditions responsible for CKD.[31] Glomerular injury and tubulointerstitial injury are interdependent.[31] Glomerular damage extends the tubulointerstitial process; degenerative and inflammatory lesions of the glomerulus increase filtrate leak into the interstitial tissues, contributing to further inflammation, and ultimately, nephron loss.[30] Tubulointerstitial damage has been identified as the final common pathway of CKD.[16] The decline in GFR is due to the effects of tubulointerstitial damage: tubular atrophy and reduced numbers of functional nephrons, and diminished perfusion generating ischemia to those that remain. Chronic tissue hypoxia in CKD is clearly multifactorial, but is the etiology of the tubulointerstitial damage responsible for disease progression.[16]

Angiotensin II (AII), the primary functional component of the RAAS, is known to vasoconstrict efferent arterioles of the glomerulus.[32] The result is an increase in glomerular pressure

and filtration; in CKD, this amplifies the proteinuria. AII is also suspected of enhancing inflammation and fibrosis.[27,28,32] Angiotensin, renin, and aldosterone activate transforming growth factor-β, which is involved in both of these processes.[27,28] All of these factors participate in the progression of CKD.[32]

Nitric oxide (NO), a key component of vascular endothelial function, has been found to be deficient in CKD.[33] There are 3 subtypes of NO synthase, and all of them have roles in CKD pathology. Defects in the bioactivity of NO may contribute to alterations in renal angiogenesis, vascular permeability, thrombogenicity, and endothelium-dependent vasodilation. Several theories for the deficiency of NO have been proposed, although at this time researchers have been unable to determine if it occurs as a result of CKD or contributes to its progression.[33]

Hyperphosphatemia, hyperparathyroidism, and the lack of active vitamin D occur as renal function declines and recent animal and human research has identified a potential role for these factors in the further progression of CKD.[34] Previously felt to contribute minimally to disease progression, discovery that optimal management of blood pressure and proteinuria have not consistently slowed progression of CKD has stimulated renewed interest.

In CKD, the damaged nephrons are unable to function properly. The remaining nephrons compensate by enlarging and increasing their clearance capacity. Through this process, renal function remains relatively normal until 75% to 80% of the nephrons are damaged and nonfunctional. Although there may be no signs or symptoms at this point, the GFR has decreased.[12,13]

Stages of Chronic Kidney Disease

The progression of CKD is determined by staging systems. Two such systems are available: an older system reflecting degree of nephron loss as correlated with clinical presentation, and a newer one that chronicles progression through the decline in GFR (Tables 28-4 and 28-5). The recommendation is that diagnosis of CKD not be based on a specific pathology (e.g., diabetes mellitus), but rather on the presence of damage

---

TABLE 28-4

Stages of Chronic Kidney Disease According to Nephron Loss and Clinical Presentation

Stage	% Nephron Loss	Clinical Presentation
Decreased renal reserve	<75%	No signs or symptoms BUN and creatinine normal May not be diagnosed
Renal insufficiency	75%-90%	Polyuria, nocturia Slight elevation in BUN and creatinine May be controlled by diet and medication
End-stage renal disease	>90%	Azotemia/uremia Fluid and electrolyte abnormalities Osteodystrophy Anemia Dialysis or transplantation essential

---

TABLE 28-5

Stages of Chronic Kidney Disease According to GFR*

Stage	Description
Stage 1	Kidney damage with normal or increased GFR GFR >90 ml/min/1.73m^2
Stage 2	Mildly decreased GFR GFR 60-89 ml/min/1.73m^2
Stage 3	Moderately decreased GFR GFR 30-59 ml/min/1.73m^2
Stage 4	Severely decreased GFR GFR 15-29 ml/min/1.73m^2
Stage 5	End-stage kidney disease GFR <15 ml/min/1.73m^2 (or dialysis)

GFR, glomerular filtration rate

*National Kidney Foundation, Kidney Disease Outcomes Quality Initiative

to the kidney and the level of function according to GFR as shown in Table 28-5.[25] Screening for the complications of CKD is recommended to begin in Stage 3.[12]

In Stage 1 in the GFR-staging system shown in Table 28-5, patients' blood pressure and laboratory values are usually normal and they are asymptomatic, but they have some form of kidney damage such as a diagnosis of cystic kidney disease.[15] An initial reduction in GFR with or without documented kidney damage would be in Stage 2. This would include, for example, a diabetic patient with proteinuria or an older person with the predictable age-related diminishment of renal function. Again, patients may be asymptomatic without laboratory value changes, but hypertension frequently is present at this point and altered laboratory findings associated with other organ systems may be present. Beginning with Stage 3, patients are classified according to GFR, regardless of the existence of kidney damage. Although they may be otherwise asymptomatic in Stage 3, hypertension is nearly always noted. At Stage 4, diagnosis is made because manifestations are usually very apparent with the significant decline in renal function. By Stage 5, manifestations of end-stage renal disease are present and renal function is so impaired that dialysis is required.[15]

The staging system shown in Table 28-4 is useful because the terms *renal insufficiency* and *decreased renal reserve* are commonly used in clinical practice. Decreased renal reserve is not associated with signs or symptoms of renal failure, largely because the remaining nephrons accommodate the additional workload. Electrolyte and fluid balance are maintained within normal limits.[7] Although not abnormally elevated, creatinine levels are usually at the high end of the normal range—a common finding in the elderly population. Interventions for those at risk for CKD (see Box 28-3) should be initiated to help slow disease progression. At this point, kidney function is already impaired and significant deterioration is possible if the kidney is stressed. There may be small amounts of protein in the urine, so proteinuria screening is useful to identify patients at this early stage.[12] The stage of renal insufficiency is reached with further nephron damage. Although electrolyte levels remain within normal limits with the GFR decline, the metabolic wastes (creatinine and urea) are retained at levels proportional to nephron loss.[7] Impairment of the kidney's ability to concentrate the filtrate often results in increased urinary output (polyuria), often requiring the patient to get up at night to void (nocturia). End-stage renal disease develops when more than 90% of the kidneys' nephrons have been destroyed. At this point, the patient typically demonstrates the sequelae and complications of renal failure, seen as laboratory alterations and signs and symptoms associated with the inability of the kidneys to fulfill their multiple roles within the body. Without interventions, when the remaining nephrons number less than 5% to 10% of normal, death is inevitable.[7]

Complications of Chronic Kidney Disease

The consequences of CKD are affected by the intake of food and water and the degree to which renal function is impaired.[7] Some of the complications of CKD begin to appear when the GFR falls

below 60 ml/min/1.73m^2 (Stage 3 of the GFR-based classification).[12] Because of the breadth of roles the kidneys carry out in the body, the effects of their failure are seen in every body organ system.[7,12] Complications impact the gastrointestinal, neurologic, musculoskeletal, dermatologic, cardiovascular, and endocrine systems. Immune function, acid-base regulation, and the coagulation cascade are affected as well. In many cases, complications are interrelated, one contributing to or exacerbating the development of others. Laboratory alterations become significant as CKD progresses; typical values are shown in Table 28-2. Major complications of CKD are discussed below.

Hypertension and Cardiovascular Disease

If hypertension was not a precursor to CKD, it inevitably develops with decreasing renal function,[35] appearing in Stages 2 or 3.[15] The excess fluid volume and escalated atherosclerotic process, along with heightened RAAS activity and evidence of increased SNS activity are all involved in the development of hypertension in CKD.[35] Most people with CKD do not die from kidney failure, but rather from the results of cardiovascular disease, which is both a risk factor for and a complication of CKD.[12,21,33] The incidence of cardiovascular morbidity and mortality are markedly increased in CKD.[36,37] Cardiac complications are the basis for 24.5% of the hospitalizations—more than any other cause.[21] Although the risk of cardiovascular disease is greatest for those with end-stage disease, it has been found to be an issue at all stages of CKD.[23] Risk and mortality are both escalated proportionally to the decline in GFR.[12] Multiple factors have been identified that are conducive to this, including, but not limited to, dyslipidemias, anemia, electrolyte-induced dysrhythmias, hypertension, endothelial dysfunction (including inflammation, alterations in nitric oxide, oxidative stress), proteinuria, premature atherosclerosis, activity limitations, and volume overload.[15,23,36]

Uremic Syndrome

As renal function declines, retention of metabolic wastes increases, creating a toxic environment within the body. Uremia produces signs and symptoms in many body systems (see Table 28-3). Compared to the presentation in ARF, uremic syndrome in CKD is far more severe and its effects are more widespread even though the serum levels often must be much higher for manifestations to be apparent.

Metabolic Acidosis

Normally, the human body produces 50 to 80 millimoles more acids than bases during daily metabolism.[7] Metabolic acidosis occurs with the retention of acidic waste products of metabolism as part of uremia. It is also produced in association with hyperkalemia, when potassium ions in the blood are exchanged for intracellular hydrogen ions, lowering the pH of the blood (see Chapter 25). The kidneys lose their ability to secrete hydrogen ions or to produce bicarbonate, and with the limited capacity of the other buffers, pH can fall precipitously; coma develops and death will occur if the pH drops below 6.8.[7] Metabolic acidosis depresses cardiac as well as central nervous system function. The respiratory system attempts to compensate for metabolic acidosis by increasing the rate and depth of respirations.

Electrolyte Imbalances

The loss of renal mechanisms involved in electrolyte balance result in the retention of potassium, phosphorus, and magnesium in the blood. Each of these imbalances is associated with specific manifestations (see Chapter 24). Hyperkalemia is of special concern, as discussed with ARF, because it can be responsible for fatal cardiac dysrhythmias. The inability to eliminate phosphorus and the loss of the renal mechanisms involved in maintaining calcium balance results in the complication osteodystrophy, which is discussed next.

Renal Osteodystrophy

The disease of bone that develops in CKD due to alterations in endocrine function and mineral metabolism is termed *renal osteodystrophy*.[38] The inability of the kidney to excrete phosphorus in CKD results in elevated phosphorus levels in the blood. Since phosphorus and calcium maintain a reciprocal relationship in the body, as hyperphosphatemia develops in CKD, hypocalcemia likewise develops. Phosphorus begins to be retained in Stages 2 to 3 of CKD,[15,38] but is clearly evident by Stage 4.[15] The body's system of maintaining calcium balance is sophisticated, and involves the activation of parathyroid hormone (PTH) when the level is low. When this occurs because of CKD, the result is secondary hyperparathyroidism.[38] The most sensitive and earliest indicator of abnormal metabolism of bone is the elevated PTH.[15] The normal response to PTH release is the increase in serum calcium levels by: (1) increasing reabsorption by the kidney, (2) increasing absorption of dietary calcium, in the presence of vitamin D, which must be activated by the kidney, and (3) increasing resorption of bone.[7] Because of the renal damage in CKD, only the bone resorption mechanism is functional and the protein matrix may be markedly affected. Renal osteodystrophy presents as both high-turnover disease, where remodeling of bone is accelerated, and low-turnover disease, in which the new bone contains fewer cells.[38] Vascular and soft-tissue calcifications as well as osteoporosis are the end result of the prolonged elevation of PTH and altered bone and mineral metabolism.[15] The resulting bone pain, deformities, and fractures are significant long-term complications of CKD.[38] Renal osteodystrophy has been estimated to be present to some degree in 30% to 50% of patients not undergoing dialysis.[38] Additionally, abnormal PTH, calcium, and phosphorous levels are reported to have been identified as independent risk factors of cardiac-etiology mortality during dialysis.[23]

Malnutrition

Protein-energy malnutrition (PEM) is a common finding in advanced CKD[15]; by Stage 5, it affects 40% of the patients.[38] Decreased intake is due to the anorexia of uremic syndrome, changes in taste, the depression of chronic illness, as well as the dietary limitations imposed by disease. Additionally, there is a negative-nitrogen balance due to escalated protein catabolism and decreased protein synthesis. Medications and concomitant diseases such as diabetes may cause nausea, vomiting, and slowed gastric emptying. The best serum marker of PEM, albumin, may be invalid because of proteinuria, inflammation, or infection.[38] Malnutrition and inflammation are associated with atherosclerosis,[15] and malnutrition has a negative impact on CKD prognosis.[12]

Anemia

The development of anemia is an anticipated problem as CKD progresses.[23] It typically appears initially in stage 2.[21] The production of red blood cells by the bone marrow depends on numerous cofactors; perhaps the most significant of these is erythropoietin, which is produced by the kidneys.[7] Erythropoiesis, with all essential ingredients, requires about 5 days.[39] Lacking erythropoietin, fewer red blood cells are produced and anemia is a persistent problem. The problem is often further escalated by malnutrition, generating anemia due to nutritional deficits of iron, folate, and vitamin B_{12}. Chronic inflammation and elevations of PTH suppress bone marrow. At the same time, the uremia associated with CKD produces a toxic environment for red blood cells, reducing their normal life expectancy of 120 days. Blacks appear to have both a greater prevalence of anemia as well as more severe reductions in RBC counts and hemoglobin concentrations. By Stage 5 and the initiation of dialysis, approximately 66% of patients have hemoglobin levels <11 g/dl.[39] The cardiovascular compensatory efforts for the chronic anemia of CKD can lead to myocardial dilatation, hypertrophy, and remodeling.[23,39] The combination of worsening CKD, anemia, and heart failure is referred to as *cardiorenal anemia syndrome* and becomes a chain of escalating pathologies.[39]

KEY POINTS

- CKD is characterized by a gradual, irreversible loss of functional nephrons. Common causes are diabetes mellitus, recurrent pyelonephritis, glomerulonephritis, and polycystic kidney disease.
- Progression of CKD can be monitored by two staging systems: (1) percentage of nephron loss and (2) reduction in GFR. Although the correlation is not perfect, there is a relationship between these two systems in that GFR reduction occurs with nephron loss. Nephron loss of up to 75% is called the *stage of decreased renal reserve* and encompasses stages 1 and 2 of GFR diminishment. Laboratory values are normal, and the condition is usually asymptomatic. At the point where 75% to 90% of the nephrons have been destroyed, renal insufficiency is present, and patients have mild azotemia and may have polyuria and nocturia because of impaired urine concentration. The GFR reductions of stages 3 and 4 roughly correspond to this degree of loss. ESRD occurs when about 90% of the nephrons

are lost and is reflected by the marked reduction of GFR in stages 4 to 5. BUN and creatinine concentrations are markedly elevated, and manifestations of fluid and electrolyte abnormalities, renal osteodystrophy, and uremia are present.

- Complications of CKD include hypertension and increased cardiovascular risks, uremic syndrome, metabolic acidosis, electrolyte disturbances, renal osteodystrophy, malnutrition, and anemia.

CLINICAL MANAGEMENT

Clinical management of acute renal failure and chronic kidney disease requires a multidisciplinary approach. Collaboration among the nurse, physician, clinical pharmacist, and dietitian is essential to attain optimal patient outcomes.

Prevention

Prevention assumes a traditional perspective for acute renal failure: primary prevention of its development. With chronic kidney disease, although prevention of the myriad causes is certainly desirable, prevention also focuses on retarding the inevitable progression of the disease and reducing cardiovascular risk factors.

Acute Renal Failure

ARF is often entirely preventable.[3] Prevention is highly dependent on recognizing patients who are at risk for the development of ARF and establishing prophylactic interventions to decrease this risk.

Etiologies and risk factors for prerenal ARF should be identified, and whenever possible, treated swiftly.[9] Early consultation with a nephrologist is recommended. Hypotension due to hypovolemia should be addressed; medications that might be contributing (antihypertensives, opioids) should be decreased or terminated. Nutrition should be supported, and indwelling catheters and other invasive equipment should be removed as soon as possible to decrease the risk of infection. Infection should be monitored for and treated should it develop.[9] Maintaining adequate circulating volumes and supporting cardiac function, especially in those at risk for prerenal acute renal failure, are the primary foci for prevention.

Should prerenal oliguria develop, efforts should be initiated to enhance renal perfusion before ATN can occur. Two interventions that were previously staples of treatment of prerenal oliguria have been deemed to be harmful, or at the very least, likely to be ineffective.[40] Dopamine in the low-dosage range was previously believed to enhance renal perfusion; evidence is now indicating that this approach produces no difference from placebo therapy in the progression of ARF, the need for dialysis, or death. Again, compared to placebo therapy, loop diuretics made no difference in the recovery of renal function.[40] Aggressive management of conditions such as glomerulonephritis can prevent progression to intrarenal ARF.[3] Prevention of intrarenal ARF due to chemicals begins

with an awareness of the most likely agents; these are shown in Box 28-4. Whenever possible, their use should be limited and when used, serum levels may need to be monitored.[3] Single doses of aminoglycosides rather than multiple doses and liquid formulations of amphotericin B appear to be less nephrotoxic.[40] Of all the chemicals listed in Box 28-4, the most common culprit is radiocontrast media. Although more evidence is needed, the prophylactic administration of N-acetylcysteine (Mucomist) has been found to reduce kidney damage associated with the use of contrast media, especially when combined with maximizing hydration parenterally.[3,9,40] The use of low-osmolality contrast media has been found to reduce the development of nephrotoxicity, and nonionic iso-osmolar media appears even more efficacious, at least in those with diabetes.[9, 40]

Postrenal etiologies should be avoided whenever possible, but if they occur they should be rapidly identified and corrected.[3] Postrenal ARF is the least common and most readily identifiable; promptly addressing it will prevent the progression to ATN.

Numerous experimental interventions continue to be explored for their safety and efficacy in preventing acute renal failure.[3] Patients with a previous history of ARF and continuing impairment should be protected from sources of renal injury, including unnecessary surgery and anesthesia.[9]

Chronic Kidney Disease Progression

Effective therapeutic management of ATN increases the likelihood that it will not progress to CKD, but for the most part, prevention of this disease is directed at slowing progression to

---

BOX 28-4

Selected Chemicals Toxic to the Kidneys

- Acetaminophen
- Acyclovir (Zovirax)
- Allopurinol
- Aminoglycosides
- Amphotericin B (Fungizone)
- Angiotensin-converting enzyme inhibitors
- Certain cytotoxic chemotherapeutic agents
- Cocaine
- Cyclosporine (Sandimmune)
- Foscarnet (Foscavir)
- Heavy metals
- Hemoglobin; myoglobin
- Heroin
- Lithium
- Nonsteroidal anti-inflammatory drugs
- Pentamidine (Pentam 300 and others)
- Radiocontrast media*
- Uric acid
- Vasopressors (norepinephrine, high-dose dopamine)

Derived from: McKenry L, Tessier E, Hogan M: *Mosby's pharmacology in nursing*, ed 22, St. Louis, 2006, Mosby; Needham E: Management of acute renal failure, *Am Fam Physician* 72(9):1739-1746, 2005.
*Most common

end-stage renal disease. The results of several studies of patients diagnosed with chronic illness indicate that if their symptoms are not significant, they underestimate disease severity and may refuse therapy.[41] This means that patient education regarding CKD is essential. Since death is often due to cardiovascular pathologies, risk factors for these are also addressed.

The actual speed with which CKD progresses is primarily a factor of its origin, however it can differ significantly among those with the same causative disease.[12] By and large, glomerular diseases, polycystic disease, and both hypertensive and diabetic nephropathy progress more rapidly than do diseases affecting the tubular interstitium.[12] Interventions have varying degrees of evidence to support their implementation. The major evidence-based interventions are: (1) ACE inhibitors or A-II receptor blockers to reduce proteinuria,[12,17,20,30,42,43] (2) aggressive control of blood glucose levels in diabetic patients,[12,13,17,20] and (3) control of blood pressure levels in hypertensive patients.[12,13,17,20,43] Additional interventions with research support for their use consist of treatment of hyperlipidemia[12,13,20,36,37] and anemia,[12,13,16,20] maintaining nutritional status, and, in those with a GFR of <25 ml/min/1.73m^2, dietary protein of no more than 0.6 to 0.75 grams/kg of body weight.[12,13,26] Weight loss has been found to decrease proteinuria in obese patients.[24]

A number of other interventions are being studied for their role in slowing the progression of CKD. In many cases, data are limited, but given the pressing nature of the projected escalation in CKD, research has intensified. Some of these interventions include targeted immunosuppressive and immune-modulating drugs; gene therapy for hereditary disorders and pharmacogenomic approaches to treatment; new approaches to block RAAS components; antioxidant therapy; stem cell regeneration of renal parenchyma; glycosaminoglycan therapy; and smoking cessation.[17]

Evaluation for cardiovascular risk factors is also an important aspect of intervention, since the risk of morbidity and mortality rises proportionally with the decline of GFR.[12] All modifiable risks should be assessed, and interventions initiated as possible.

At a community level, screening for hypertension, diabetes, and chronic kidney disease are essential to stem the tide of these interrelated chronic diseases.[17,18] Underdiagnosis and treatment mediate the problem, and lack of awareness is the enemy of early diagnosis and treatment.

Therapeutic Interventions

At this time, recovery from ATN has not been accelerated by any individual or constellation of therapies.[3] Interventions are designed to support renal function and correct derangements while waiting for the kidneys to either recover or advance to CKD.[8] Efforts are made to slow progression of CKD (see previous discussion), but complications begin to be apparent by stage 4 of GFR reduction. At this stage, attention is directed to therapeutic interventions designed to minimize and treat complications of renal failure. An in-depth presentation of treatment is beyond the scope of this text; discussion is simply

---

BOX 28-5

Therapeutic Goals in Renal Failure

- Maintain volume status
- Prevention and treatment of acid-base and electrolyte disturbances
- Prevention and treatment of uremia
- Support nutritional needs
- Prevention and treatment of infection
- Prevention and treatment of anemia
- Improve quality of life
- Lower mortality and morbidity rates

---

an overview. Goals of therapeutic interventions for renal failure are summarized in Box 28-5.

Nutrition

Nutrition plays a large role in the treatment of CKD. Malnutrition is known to adversely affect CKD prognosis.[12] Advanced CKD produces gastrointestinal manifestations, anorexia, and changes in the sense of taste, which further complicate the necessary modifications in diet.[38] CKD increases insulin resistance and, combined with proteinuria and the nausea and anorexia, protein-energy malnutrition is a significant concern.[21] Caloric requirements are increased. Aspects of nutritional management of CKD include limiting dietary phosphorus, protein, sodium, and potassium; avoiding malnutrition; prevention of anemia; and countering disease and drug-induced constipation. Additionally, diet-related risk factors for cardiovascular disease must be considered. This can all seem overwhelming to patients, so involvement of a dietitian and thorough education considering concomitant conditions, personal likes and dislikes, eating habits, and financial resources is essential.

Hyperphosphatemia is addressed nutritionally, and later through drug management, as phosphorus is not removed by dialysis. Phosphorus intake should be limited to 800 to 1000 mg/day.[38] Since nearly all foods contain some phosphorous, the best place to begin with dietary reduction of phosphorus is by limiting dairy products to no more than 4 ounces of milk per day and using nondairy creamers. Taking processed meats out of the diet helps lower the intake of both phosphorus and sodium. Hypocalcemia is secondarily treated as the phosphorus levels are corrected, and directly approached pharmacologically and nutritionally.[38] Calcium intake is based on standard recommendations for age and gender, and should be less than 2000 mg/day.[15,38] Target ranges of both calcium and phosphorus are shown in Table 28-6.

Lists of foods high in sodium, potassium, and protein should be provided; patients can then be encouraged to identify their favorite foods and choose smaller portions or eat them less often.[38] Potassium levels are monitored by laboratory values, and adjustments are made accordingly. Sodium increases the retention of water, and should be limited to less than 2000 to 2400 mg/day.[15,38] Fluid intake restrictions fluctuate

TABLE 28-6

Target Ranges for Calcium and Phosphorus in CKD

Stage	Calcium	Phosphorus
3	8.4-9.5 mg/dl	2.7-4.6 mg/dl
4	8.4-9.5 mg/dl	2.7-4.6 mg/dl
5	8.4-9.5 mg/dl	3.5-5.5 mg/dl

Data from Legg V: Complications of chronic kidney disease: a close look at renal osteodystrophy, nutritional disturbances, and inflammation, *Am J Nurs* 105(6):40-49, 2005.

but should normally equal the volume of urine output plus 500 ml for insensible losses.[15] Protein intake varies, depending on protein losses and the individual limitations for each patient.[38] Patients undergoing dialysis are permitted higher protein intake.[14]

Maintaining higher hemoglobin levels has been found to be highly correlated with reduced mortality and hospitalizations, decreased left ventricular hypertrophy, and improved quality of life indicators in CKD.[14] Hemoglobin levels diagnostic of anemia are <11 g/dl for premenopausal women and prepubescent children with CKD, and <12 g/dl for postmenopausal women and adult males.[15] Adequate nutrition can defray the development of nutritional anemias, a common problem with significant dietary restrictions. Foods high in iron support the primary pharmacologic intervention for anemia due to inadequate erythropoietin formation and secretion by the kidney.

Pharmacology

When dietary measures to manage the calcium-phosphorous imbalance are inadequate, pharmacologic interventions are required.[38] Calcium and noncalcium phosphate binders decrease absorption of dietary phosphorous while supplemental vitamin D increases dietary calcium absorption. New calcimimetic agents have been found to suppress PTH secretion.[38]

Pharmacologic treatment of anemia in CKD is supported in numerous studies; energy levels, cardiac function, and work capacities are improved, disease progression is retarded, and mortality is decreased.[39,44] Synthetic erythropoietin (epotin alpha) is the primary intervention and is often initiated at stage 3 of CKD.[20,39]

Drug management for diabetes mellitus, hypertension, and hyperlipidemias are initiated or continued as needed in CKD.

Dialysis

The procedures, advantages, disadvantages, and expected outcomes of dialysis should begin to be discussed when the patient is in stage 3 of CKD.[13] When patients with CKD reach stage 5, dialysis is indicated.[45] The primary reason for the initiation of dialysis is the development of uremia.[14] Approximately two thirds of the total body urea content is removed by each dialysis treatment.[14] It may also be required if severe hyperkalemia is unresponsive to other interventions[3] or in cases of severe volume overload. If these conditions develop during the

oliguric stage of ATN, dialysis may be required temporarily. Dialysis supports all the treatment goals in Box 28-5.

Dialysis may be accomplished by hemodialysis, peritoneal dialysis, or continuous renal replacement therapy (CRRT). CRRT is limited to in-hospital acute renal failure patients. Most patients with end-stage renal disease (ESRD) go through hemodialysis treatments three times per week.[45] Hemodialysis was first carried out on humans in 1924; prior to that time, patients with ESRD simply died. In 1972, the national ESRD program was signed into law, giving all Americans the right to treatment; ESRD is the sole recipient of this status. Although a life-saving intervention, dialysis treatments have complications, some of which are life-threatening, and long-term morbidity remains quite high.[45] Dialysis remains the only therapeutic option for those with ESRD who are unable to obtain a transplant.

Transplantation

Kidney transplantation is an alternative to dialysis for patients with ESRD. As with other conditions in which transplantation is indicated, the primary limiting factor is the availability of organs. Kidneys are obtained from brain-dead and living donors. For most of those who choose it, transplantation allows the independence to return to normal activities of daily living and provides normal renal function. Even with the best possible tissue matching, antirejection drug therapy is required and the adverse effects of these medications may have a significant impact. Early transplantation has the lowest mortality and the best 5-year survival rate.[13]

KEY POINTS

- Prevention of ARF includes early identification of those at risk, maintenance of fluid volume status and cardiac output, avoiding whenever possible and monitoring nephrotoxic chemicals, and avoiding and aggressively treating infections. Prerenal and postrenal ARF are treated by addressing their specific etiologies. Intrarenal ARF (ATN) is treated with many of the same interventions used to support renal function in CKD.
- Slowing the progression of CKD is the focus of interventions until stages 4 to 5. Appropriate management of ATN, blood glucose control in diabetes, ACE inhibitors, or AII blockers to reduce proteinuria, and aggressive management of hypertension are the primary foci. Since cardiovascular disease is both a risk factor for CKD and accelerates progression, interventions are also included to retard it.
- Nutritional needs for patients in renal failure include increased calories as well as calcium and vitamin supplementation. Fluid, phosphorus, potassium, sodium, and protein intake are usually restricted, depending on the underlying pathologic process and stage of the disease.
- Drug therapy in CKD is used to control hypertension, anemia, and some of the electrolyte imbalances.

- Dialysis is used for some patients with ATN and patients with CKD in stages 4 or 5 in order to remove metabolic wastes and correct fluid and electrolyte abnormalities.
- Renal transplantation is a potential option for patients with ESRD. Kidney transplantation has been associated with a high degree of success.

SUMMARY

Renal failure can occur at any age. ARF has multiple causes that can be classified into one of three categories according to the physical location of the problem: prerenal, intrarenal, or postrenal. Each category has unique pathologic features and some variation in laboratory values. Intrarenal failure (ATN) is divided into three phases: oliguric, diuretic, and recovery. Interventions differ for each phase.

CKD is a progressive, irreversible process. It is characterized by stages of declining GFR producing increasing impairment in the ability of the kidney to maintain homeostasis. The clinical manifestations of CKD are determined by the degree of impairment of the kidneys' normal functions.

Key aspects of care include pharmacologic management of fluid overload, electrolyte abnormalities, and metabolic wastes; nutritional management; dialysis; and renal transplantation.

A clear understanding of the pathophysiology related to renal dysfunction is essential for any healthcare professional caring for patients in renal failure. The impact that renal failure has on all other body systems presents many challenges.

REFERENCES

1. Koeppen BM, Stanton BA: *Renal physiology,* ed 4, Philadelphia, 2007, Mosby.
2. Lameire N, Van Biesen W, Vanholder R: Acute renal failure, *The Lancet* 365:417-430, 2005.
3. Needham E: Management of acute renal failure, *Am Fam Physician* 72(9):1739-1746, 2005.
4. Gill N, Nally JV, Fatica RA: Renal failure secondary to acute tubular necrosis: Epidemiology, diagnosis, and management, *Chest* 128(4):2847-2863, 2005.
5. Ympa YP et al: Has mortality from acute renal failure decreased? A systematic review of the literature, *Am J Med* 118:827-832, 2005.
6. Goldenberg I, Matetzky S: Nephropathy induced by contrast media: pathogenesis, risk factors and preventive strategies, *Can Med Assoc J* 172(11):1461-1471, 2005.
7. Guyton AC, Hall JE: *Textbook of medical physiology,* ed 11, Philadelphia, 2006, Saunders.
8. Gammill HS, Jeyabalan A: Acute renal failure in pregnancy, *Crit Care Med* 33(10):S372-S384, 2005.
9. Abuelo JG: Normotensive ischemic acute renal failure, *N Engl J Med* 357:797-805, 2007.
10. McKenry L, Tessier E, Hogan M: *Mosby's pharmacology in nursing,* ed 22, St. Louis, 2006, Mosby.
11. Kuiper JW et al: Mechanical ventilation and acute renal failure, *Crit Care Med* 33(6):1408-1415, 2005.
12. Snyder S, Pendergraph B: Detection and evaluation of chronic kidney disease, *Am Fam Physician* 72(9):1723-1732, 2005.
13. Dinwiddle L, Burrows-Hudson S, Peacock E: Stage 4 chronic kidney disease: preserving kidney function and preparing patients for stage 5 kidney disease, *Am J Nurs* 106(9):40-51, 2006.
14. Meyer TW, Hostetter TH: Uremia, *N Engl J Med* 357:1316-1325, 2007.
15. McCarley PB, Burrows-Hudson S: Chronic kidney disease and cardiovascular disease—using the ANNA standards and practice guidelines to improve care, Part I: The epidemiology of chronic kidney disease: the risk factors and complications that contribute to cardiovascular disease, *Nephrol Nurs J* 33(6):666-674, 2006.
16. Nangaku M: Chronic hypoxia and tubulointerstitial injury: A final common pathway to end-stage renal failure, *J Am Soc Nephrol* 17:17-25, 2006.
17. Jaber BL, Madias NE: Progression of chronic kidney disease: can it be prevented or arrested? *Am J Med* 118:1323-1330, 2005.
18. Atkins RC: The epidemiology of chronic kidney disease, *Kidney Int* 67(Suppl 94):S14-S18, 2005.
19. Eikmans M et al: Genetic factors in progressive renal disease: the good ones, the bad ones and the ugly ducklings, *Nephrol Dial Transplant* 21(2):257-260, 2006.
20. Weiner DE: Causes and consequences of chronic kidney disease: implications for managed health care, *J Manage Care Pharm* 13(Suppl 3):S1-S9, 2007.
21. Burrows-Hudson S: Chronic kidney disease: An overview, *Am J Nurs* 105(2):40-49, 2005.
22. Chobanian AV et al: Seventh report of the joint national committee on prevention, detection, evaluation, and treatment of high blood pressure: the JNC 7 complete report, *Hypertension* 42:1206-1252, 2003.
23. McCarley PB, Salai PB: Cardiovascular disease in chronic kidney disease: recognizing and reducing the risk of a common CKD comorbidity, *Am J Nurs* 105(4):40-52, 2005.
24. Praga M, Morales E: Obesity, proteinuria and progression of renal failure, *Curr Opin Nephrol Hypertens* 15:481-486, 2006.
25. National Kidney Foundation, Kidney Disease Outcomes Quality Initiative, 2002. Retrieved October 30, 2007, from http://www.kidney.org/professionals/kdoqi/guidelines_ckd?p4_class_g1.htm.
26. Perico N et al: Pathophysiology of disease progression in proteinuric nephropathies, *Kidney Int* 67(Suppl 94):S79-S82, 2005.
27. Wolf G: Renal injury due to renin-angiotensin-aldosterone system activation of the transforming growth factor-β pathway, *Kidney Int* 70:1914-1919, 2006.
28. Harris RC, Neilson EG: Toward a unified theory of renal progression, *Annu Rev Med* 57:365-380, 2006.
29. Marín R et al: Systemic and glomerular hypertension and progression of chronic renal disease: The dilemma of nephrosclerosis, *Kidney Int* 68(Suppl 99):S52-S56, 2005.
30. Rodríguez-Iturbe B, Johnson RJ, Herrera-Acosta J: Tubulointerstitial damage and progression of renal failure, *Kidney Int* 68(Suppl 99):S82-S86, 2005.
31. Eardley KS, Cockwell P: Macrophages and progressive tubulo-interstitial disease, *Kidney Int* 68:437-455, 2005.
32. Remuzzi G et al: The role of renin-angiotensin-aldosterone system in the progression of chronic kidney disease, *Kidney Int* 68(Suppl 99):S57-S65, 2005.
33. Marin E, Sessa WC: Role of endothelial-derived nitric oxide in hypertension and renal disease, *Curr Opin Nephrol Hypertens* 16:105-110, 2007.
34. Ritz E, Gross ML, Dikow R: Role of calcium-phosphorous disorders in the progression of renal failure, *Kidney Int* 68(Suppl 99):S66-S70, 2005.
35. Phillips JK: Pathogenesis of hypertension in renal failure: Role of the sympathetic nervous system and renal afferents, *Clin Exp Pharmacol Physiol* 32(5-6):415-418, 2005.
36. Vaziri ND: Dyslipidemia of chronic renal failure: The nature, mechanisms, and potential consequences, *Am J Physiol Renal Physiol* 290:F262-F272, 2006.
37. Cases A, Coll E: Dyslipidemia and the progression of renal disease in chronic renal failure patients, *Kidney Int* 68(Suppl 99):S87-S93, 2005.
38. Legg V: Complications of chronic kidney disease: a close look at renal osteodystrophy, nutritional disturbances, and inflammation, *Am J Nurs* 105(6):40-49, 2005.

39. Dowling TC: Prevalence, etiology, and consequences of anemia and clinical and economic benefits of anemia correction in patients with chronic kidney disease: an overview, *Am J Health Syst Pharm* 64(13 Suppl 8):S3-S7, 2007.

40. Kellum J, LeBlanc M, Venkataraman V: Clinical evidence concise: acute renal failure, *Am Fam Physician* 76(3), 2007. Retrieved October 8, 2007, from http://www.aafp.org/afp/20070801/bmj/html

41. Thomas-Hawkins C, Zazworsky D: Self-management of chronic kidney disease: patients shoulder the responsibility for day-to-day management of chronic illness. How can nurses support their autonomy? *Am J Nurs* 105(10):40-48, 2005.

42. Epstein M: Aldosterone blockade: an emerging strategy for abrogating progressive renal disease, *Am J Med* 119:912-919, 2006.

43. Casas JP et al: Effect of inhibitors of the renin-angiotensin system and other antihypertensive drugs on renal outcomes: systematic review and meta-analysis, *Lancet* 366:2026-2033, 2005.

44. Spiegel DM: Anemia management in chronic kidney disease: what have we learned after 17 years? *Semin Dial* 19(4):269-272, 2006.

45. Rosner MH: Hemodialysis for the non-nephrologist, *South Med J* 98(8):785-791, 2005.

Disorders of the Lower Urinary Tract

Roberta J. Emerson

MEDIA RESOURCES

Additional Material for Study, Review, and Further Exploration

 CD Companion ■ Review Questions and Answers
■ Glossary (with audio pronunciations for selected terms)
■ Disease Profiles ■ Animations

 evolve **Website** at http://evolve.elsevier.com/Copstead/
■ Case Studies ■ Disease Profiles ■ WebLinks ■ Key Points Review

Online Course (Module 14)

KEY QUESTIONS

■ How do the pathophysiologic characteristics and management of stress, urge, mixed, overflow, and functional incontinence differ?

■ How are congenital abnormalities of the urinary collecting system detected and treated?

■ What are the risk factors and clinical manifestations for bladder cancer?

■ How do the manifestations of urethritis, cystitis, and painful bladder syndrome differ?

■ How do stones in the lower urinary tract present clinically?

The lower urinary tract encompasses several structures that together are responsible for the transport and elimination of urine from the body. These structures include the ureters, bladder, urethra, and associated urinary sphincters. The male prostate gland is anatomically located in this area, but is functionally involved in male reproduction; the prostate gland role and disorders are presented in Chapters 30 and 31, respectively. Ureters collect the urine formed in the kidneys from the renal pelvises and transport it to the bladder. The bladder is a hollow, muscular reservoir for urine that expands to store it and then contract to expel urine through the urethra. The process of micturition (voiding) is dependent on the coordinated activity of the nervous system, bladder contraction, and urethral sphincter relaxation. In addition to voiding dysfunction, disorders of the lower urinary tract can generally be classified as congenital, neoplastic, infective, inflammatory, or obstructive. These disorders are often interrelated. For instance, stasis of urine, which occurs with a variety of disorders, often leads to urinary tract infection (UTI). Infection of the kidney, pyelonephritis (see Chapter 27) and acute postrenal renal failure (see Chapter 28) can be caused by any number of pathologies affecting the lower urinary tract. Lower urinary tract disorders can result in significant health problems that have tremendous physical, psychosocial, and economic ramifications on patients and their families.[1,2]

LOWER URINARY TRACT

The role of the lower urinary tract is to transport urine formed by the kidneys and allow its appropriate removal from the body. The anatomy of the lower urinary tract is presented in Chapter 26. Urine movement from the kidneys to the bladder is due to the effect of gravity and is facilitated by peristaltic movement of the ureters. The bladder stores the urine and it is released through the urethra, ultimately by conscious decision. Anatomical integrity of the ureters and bladder, competent urethral sphincters, and an appropriately functioning nervous system are required for the lower urinary system to properly carry out its role.

Diagnostic Tests

Several of the procedures presented in Chapter 26 are used to diagnose urologic disorders discussed in this chapter. Other, more specialized diagnostic tests are often even more appropriate. A urinalysis is the simplest and cheapest test that can provide a wealth of information. For the lower urinary tract, it is primarily used in the diagnosis of infection. Although the abdominal radiograph known as a KUB (kidneys, ureters, and bladder) provides information regarding anatomy and may detect neoplasms or urinary stones, it is not the most frequently used procedure for this purpose. Ultrasonography, which is painless, does not involve radiation, and provides excellent visualization of the urinary system, is the most common initial screening study for infants and children with urinary problems. Fluoroscopic voiding cystourethrography or radionuclide voiding cystography may be required to yield more specific information than can be obtained by ultrasound.[3] Fluoroscopic voiding cystourethrography involves placing a catheter in the bladder and then filling it with sterile, iodinated, dilute contrast material. The catheter is then removed and the patient voids. Images of the bladder are taken prior to voiding to detect a ureterocele or tumor, and images taken during voiding can identify reflux or urethral abnormalities. Radionuclide voiding cystography also requires catheterization but involves the use of a small amount of radioactive material. A technetium 99m–labeled radiopharmaceutical is instilled in the bladder through the catheter, followed by sterile normal saline to fill the bladder. Once the catheter is removed, images are taken

with the bladder full and during voiding, but this procedure does not allow visualization of the urethra. The term *urodynamic testing* is used for procedures associated with diagnosing voiding dysfunction. There are multiple urodynamic tests and procedures and the choice of tests is based on clinical presentation and begins with the least invasive of the desired tests. The most common tests are cystometry (measurement of intrabladder pressure during filling); urethral pressure profilometry (measurement of intraluminal pressure along the length of the urethra); uroflowmetry (noninvasive method of measuring characteristics of urine flow); and pressure-flow micturition studies (invasive method of measuring characteristics of urine flow).[3] Electrophysiologic testing may also be done to determine pathologic processes underlying voiding dysfunction. Neurophysiologic tests provide information about the coordination between the bladder and the external sphincter. Neurophysiologic tests are much more involved and are completed only in very specialized laboratories.

Mechanics of Micturition

Micturition is often taken for granted by health care providers and patients, but is a complicated process. Understanding of the process begins with a review of the significant part the nervous system plays in the functioning of the structures of the lower urinary tract.

Nervous System Innervation of the Lower Urinary Tract

The central, autonomic, and peripheral nervous systems are all involved in urinary elimination. The brain stem coordinates relaxation of the internal sphincter and contraction of the bladder to enable urination, while the cerebral cortex primarily inhibits the process through conscious control of the external sphincter.[1] Any disease process affecting these areas can interfere with urination. This includes such pathologies as Parkinsonism, multiple sclerosis, traumatic brain injury, spinal cord injury, or stroke.

The smooth muscle of the bladder is innervated by both the sympathetic and parasympathetic branches of the autonomic nervous system (Figure 29-1). This innervation controls the detrusor muscle in the bladder wall and the bladder neck, ultimately controlling filling and emptying of the bladder. In other words, the bladder itself does not respond to voluntary control, but rather to neurologic reflexes. These nerves have both autonomic efferent motor and afferent sensory roles; efferent nerves control bladder smooth muscle, and afferent fibers transmit sensations of bladder stretch—distension and fullness—and pain. Injury or disease of the spinal cord in this region profoundly affects lower urinary tract function.

Sympathetic outflow of the autonomic nervous system to the bladder originates from the spinal cord region of L1-L2 and causes relaxation of the bladder allowing the storage of urine. Parasympathetic innervation of the urinary tract is supplied by the pelvic nerves, which exit the spinal cord at S2-S4. Their stimulation causes contraction of the detrusor muscle and relaxation of the internal sphincter (bladder

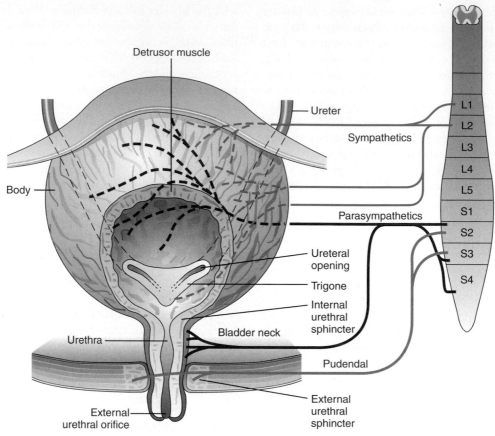

FIGURE 29-1 Bladder structure and innervation.

neck). Parasympathetic signals from the posterior urethra in response to stretch of the bladder musculature are primarily responsible for initiating bladder emptying.

The somatic nerve fibers of the peripheral nervous system control the voluntary skeletal muscle of the external bladder sphincter via the pudendal nerve. The peripheral nervous system is primarily responsible for muscle function at the pelvic floor.

Mechanism of Micturition

The softness, pliability, mucosal secretions, and submucosal cushioning of the urethra are responsible for the maintenance of a water-tight seal or "compression" of the urethra. The internal sphincter is located at the proximal portion of the urethra, where the convergence of the detrusor muscle fibers provides pressure to keep it closed. When the internal sphincter has normal tone, the bladder is prevented from emptying until the pressure in the body of the bladder rises above a specific threshold. The sequence of urination begins with the bladder filling with urine until a first sensation of fullness is felt. This causes the internal bladder pressure to trigger stretch receptors in the bladder wall. Activation of these receptors results in afferent communication to the nervous system to bring about contraction of the bladder destrusor muscle. The internal sphincter simultaneously relaxes, taking on a funnel shape.

The very noticeable urge to urinate causes an individual to consciously tighten the external sphincter. The external sphincter is located at the distal end of the urethra, surrounding it by a ring of skeletal muscle from the pelvic floor. This musculature provides the necessary tension needed to maintain continence at normal resting bladder pressures. The external sphincter allows voluntary emptying of the bladder or the prevention of urination. Usually, enough pressure to hold the urine in the bladder can be voluntarily generated until about 350-400 ml of urine has collected in the bladder. At this point an urgent sensation to void occurs and the resulting activation of the voiding centers in the brain (central nervous system) also helps inhibit the bladder from emptying. At the appropriate time, a coordinated nerve response allows the detrusor muscle to contract and the both urethral sphincters to relax, and voiding occurs. If an individual is able to coordinate urination at a suitable location and desired time, we consider the individual to be **continent.**

Normal adult bladder capacity is 300 to 500 ml, and the urge to void usually develops when 150 to 300 ml are present.[1] With an average fluid intake, this typically results in a voiding pattern of every four to five hours, with no need to awaken at night in order to void. With aging, bladder capacity declines to 200-350 ml; urination becomes more frequent (every three to four hours), and awakening at night to urinate is common. Under normal circumstances, the adult bladder contains less than 50 ml following voiding. This volume of postvoiding urine is called **residual urine.** Certain pathologies are associated with incomplete bladder emptying, and increased residual urine volumes.

KEY POINTS

- The lower urinary tract transports urine from the kidneys and facilitates its removal from the body. A variety of laboratory tests are used in the diagnosis of lower urinary tract disorders.
- Bladder innervation is supplied by sympathetic nerves that exit the spinal cord at L1 and L2 and allow relaxation and filling. Stimulation of parasympathetic nerves from S1-S4 results in bladder contraction and relaxation of the internal sphincter. The somatic pudendal nerve innervates the external bladder sphincter. The sympathetic system innervates blood vessels via the hypogastric plexus.
- Micturition requires central, autonomic, and peripheral nervous system functioning. It is a result of parasympathetic and voluntary motor control.

VOIDING DYSFUNCTION

Disorders of the lower urinary tract, such as infection, usually affect voiding secondarily. Voiding dysfunction can also be associated with pathologies affecting the central, autonomic, and peripheral nervous systems. However, voiding dysfunctions may also be associated with a wide variety of factors affecting control of micturition, including medications and access to toileting facilities. Voiding dysfunction encompasses several types of incontinence, and enuresis.

Incontinence. Issues of urinary continence in adults are 2 to 3 times more common among women than men until the age of 80 years.[1] The prevalence of urinary incontinence across women's lifetimes has been most recently estimated to range from a low of 8% to a high of 64.7%.[2,4] The significant variance in these data may be related to differences in the definition of incontinence between studies, actual differences among ethnic and social groups, and/or cultural constraints in reporting the problem. Surprisingly, prevalence in younger women from the age of 18 to 34 has been found to range from 10% to 18%. Prevalence of incontinence among women increases steadily so that by age 55 it reaches 30%.[2] The severity of the problem also escalates with age.[2] In 2000, the overall cost of incontinence in the United States was nearly $20 billion.[1] Itemization of these costs illustrates the complexity of the problem: 3% for diagnostic testing, 9% for routine care, 32% for treatments, and 56% for the indirect costs of nursing home admissions and loss of productivity.[1] However, incontinence is never normal under any circumstances and is not a normal part of aging.

Pathogenesis. Continence requires both physiologic and cognitive capabilities. Physiological requirements include an appropriately functional nervous system, and intact bladder and

BOX 29-1

Risk Factors for Incontinence

Risk Factors
Immobility
Impaired cognition
Medications (e.g., diuretics)
Morbid obesity
Smoking
Fecal impaction
Delirium
Environmental barriers to toileting
High-impact physical activities
Estrogen depletion
Low fluid intake
Pelvic muscle weakness
Childhood nocturnal enuresis
Pregnancy, vaginal delivery, or episiotomy

Pathologies
Urinary tract infection
Diabetes mellitus
Diabetes insipidus
Stroke
Multiple sclerosis
Parkinsonism
Spinal cord injury
Spinal cord defects

urethral function. Cognitively, individuals must have the ability to react to bladder urges and be motivated to be continent. Any disruption in these capabilities can result in an inability to attain or maintain continence. Risk factors associated with acute and chronic urinary incontinence are listed in Box 29-1.

Neurogenic bladder is a broad classification of voiding dysfunction in which the specific cause is a pathology that produces a disruption of nervous communication governing micturition. Patients with neurogenic bladder include those with central nervous system disorders (e.g., stroke, parkinsonism) and those with disorders affecting the autonomic innervation of the bladder (e.g., spinal cord injury, spinal cord anomalies such as meningocele). It results in an alteration in the ability to initiate voiding.

Urinary incontinence is not a part of normal aging, but it may be a result of factors such as disorders that are more common in the elderly or medications that induce urinary changes (e.g., diuretics). Age-related changes in the function or structure of the lower urinary tract, and the possible limitations in the mobility and independence of the elderly predispose them to incontinence.[1]

Acute incontinence has a sudden onset and is due to potentially reversible, more easily treatable conditions. Chronic urinary incontinence is usually classified by type, based on the specific characteristics of presentation.[1] These types are: urge, stress, mixed, overflow, and functional incontinence. The etiologies and interventions vary, so identification of the type of incontinence is clinically important.

Urge incontinence is the most common type among ambulatory older women[1] and is often seen in younger individuals as well.[2] It involves the sudden sensation of a need to urinate (urgency) and involuntary leakage of variable amounts of urine.[1,2] When associated with frequency and **nocturia** (a need to get up at night to void), it is termed *overactive bladder*.[1,2] In men, these symptoms frequently present with the enlargement of the prostate gland.[1] At times, urine may leak without any warning. This condition is most often due to an overactive destrusor muscle that suddenly contracts without the patient's desire for it to do so.[1,2] Causes of urge incontinence are numerous and require a diagnostic process of elimination. Identifiable causes include bladder infections that irritate the bladder lining, radiation therapy, and tumors or stones in the urinary tract. It is also possible that the cause is related to central nervous system damage to inhibitory pathways as would occur with stroke, dementia, parkinsonism, and multiple sclerosis. In cases in which a specific cause is not determined, urge incontinence is said to be *idiopathic*.[1,2]

Stress incontinence occurs when urine, typically in small amounts, is involuntarily lost with increases in intraabdominal pressure.[1] It is often precipitated by situations such as coughing, sneezing, laughing, or lifting heavy objects. Stress incontinence occurs in conjunction with weakening of the pelvic floor structures that then cause the bladder and urethra to be more mobile.[1,2] Childbearing predisposes some women to this type of incontinence.[1,2] One study reports that in women between 30 and 44 years of age with stress incontinence, 66% of the cases were ascribed to childbirth.[2] It is second to urge incontinence in frequency among elderly women, due to decreased estrogen and a history of vaginal deliveries.[1] It is also common among women who are younger or middle-aged.[2] Less often, stress incontinence can be due to an intrinsic sphincter deficiency secondary to a trauma or surgery to the proximal urethra, or by atrophy of the urethral tissues with aging.[1] Urethral atrophy with aging has been related to diminished estrogen availability.[1,4]

Mixed incontinence is a combination of both stress and urge incontinence.[1,2] It is common for these two types of incontinence to occur together, especially in older women. This often results in a greater volume of urine leakage, which markedly increases the disruption in activities of daily living.[1,2]

Overflow incontinence occurs when the bladder becomes so full that it leaks urine, or "overflows."[2] This can happen when an obstructed urethra prevents the bladder from emptying normally, such as with an enlarged prostate, urethral stricture, cystocele, or prolapsed uterus. Overflow incontinence can also happen in situations in which the bladder is too weak to contract and force the urine out such as in diabetes mellitus, or neurologic disorders such as multiple sclerosis or spinal cord injury that interfere with detrusor innervation (neurogenic bladder).[2]

Functional incontinence is related to physical or environmental limitations resulting in an inability to access a toilet in time.[2] The urinary system may work well, but inaccessible toilets, mobility disorders, cognitive dysfunction, or mental disabilities prevent normal toilet usage.[2] Healthcare workers can be critical in manipulating the environment to facilitate a person to successfully get to the toilet on time.[2]

Treatment. Management of incontinence begins with a review of reversible and contributing factors.[2] Patients should be assessed for reversible issues affecting the function of the lower urinary tract. These include potential drug-induced effects, UTIs or obstructions, fecal impaction, over-usage of alcohol or caffeine, and excess fluid intake. Impaired cognitive function may be due to chronic illness, depression, or delirium. All disorders associated with cognitive or neurologic function (e.g., stroke, parkinsonism) should be identified. Circumstances or conditions affecting mobility should also be acknowledged.[2]

Once reversible factors are addressed, treatment includes behavioral, pharmacologic, and surgical interventions, and depends on the cause of incontinence[1,2,4] (Table 29-1). Behavioral techniques include toileting assistance, bladder retraining, and pelvic muscle rehabilitation. Bladder retraining incorporates education, scheduled voiding with systematic delay of voiding to conform with the schedule, and positive

TABLE 29-1

Treatment Guidelines: Voiding Dysfunction

Condition	Treatment
Detrusor overactivity	Manage underlying condition (e.g., urethral obstruction, infection, bladder stones, bladder cancer, spinal cord tumors, spinal disk disease)
	Behavior modification
	Anticholinergics and/or musculotropic relaxants and/or tricyclic antidepressants (± intermittent catheterization)
	Electrical stimulation
	Biofeedback
	Neuromodulation
	Detrusor myectomy
	Augmentation enterocystoplasty (± intermittent catheterization)
	Continent urinary diversion
Low bladder compliance	Anticholinergics and/or musculotropic relaxants and/or tricyclic antidepressants (± intermittent catheterization)
	Neuromodulation
	Detrusor myectomy
	Augmentation enterocystoplasty (± intermittent catheterization)
	Continent urinary diversion
Sphincteric incontinence Intrinsic sphincter deficiency	Periurethral injections Pubovaginal sling Artificial urinary sphincter
Urethral hypermobility	Pelvic floor exercises (± biofeedback)
	Electrical stimulation
	Urethropexy or pubovaginal sling

reinforcement. Pelvic muscle rehabilitation may be as simple as the performance of exercises to strengthen pelvic muscles, or more complex to include techniques with vaginal weights, pelvic floor electrical stimulation, and biofeedback. Pelvic muscle rehabilitation is most effective with urge, stress, and mixed incontinence. Pharmacologic agents may be used to promote or inhibit physiologic activities associated with micturition, depending on the cause of incontinence. This may include anticholinergic agents, tricyclic agents, and vaginal or oral estrogen. The effectiveness of behavioral interventions is often increased by the addition of drug therapy. Surgical procedures for incontinence are variable, depending on the underlying anatomic or physiologic problems. Stress incontinence is the most amenable to surgical intervention. Surgical procedures to correct urge incontinence caused by detrusor overactivity are rare and are used as a last resort. Artificial sphincters are possible, but they only appear to resolve the problem 50% of the time and carry a 40% morbidity rate.[2]

Incontinence that is not resolved by behavioral, pharmacologic or surgical intervention occasionally may be managed by supportive approaches such as intermittent catheterization, indwelling catheterization, or incontinence undergarments.[2] Each of these devices creates the potential for further complications. UTIs are more likely with stasis of urine in the bladder and, in the case of catheterization, with continuous or intermittent introduction of a foreign object into the normally sterile bladder. Stasis of urine also increases the risk for bladder and renal calculi. Catheterization is never an appropriate solution solely for caregiver convenience. Management of incontinence with incontinence undergarments predisposes patients to skin breakdown.

Enuresis. Enuresis is the inappropriate wetting of clothes or bedding, and the term is generally used to refer to incontinence in children. Nocturnal enuresis is a common childhood condition and is defined as the involuntary urinary elimination at night by a child over the age of 5 years, without any congenital or acquired central nervous system disorder.[5,6] *Primary nocturnal enuresis* describes a child who has never achieved continence, whereas *secondary enuresis* refers to enuresis that develops after a period of at least 6 months of dryness.[6] In *monosymptomatic nocturnal enuresis*, the child has no urinary symptoms during the day and is continent at that time. *Polysymptomatic nocturnal enuresis* is diagnosed when the child has symptoms of urgency, frequency, or incontinence during the day in addition to nighttime enuresis. Secondary enuresis and polysymptomatic nocturnal enuresis are usually related to a UTI or to the introduction of stress or change in the child's life.[6]

Fifteen to twenty-five percent of 5-year-old children have *primary monosymptomatic nocturnal enuresis*.[6] It is more common among female children. About 15% of children over the age of 5 years continue to suffer from nighttime bed wetting[5]; it resolves at an annual rate of approximately 15%,[5,6] and by the age of 12 the prevalence is 4% to 8%.[6] This means that for the most part, enuresis is a result of maturational delay. Unfortunately, the problem continues for some

children and by adolescence, 1% to 3% are still wetting the bed at night.[6]

Etiology. *Primary monosymptomatic nocturnal enuresis* has several potential etiologic factors.[6] These generally fall into the categories of physiologic or genetic causes. Several of these may coexist. Previous beliefs that it was due to psychological or emotional disturbances have been disproven by research findings that show most affected children have no clinically significant problems with behavior and are found to be psychologically well adjusted.[6]

Physiologic factors include the inability to awaken in response to the urge to void, reduced bladder capacity, and nocturnal polyuria.[6] Nocturnal enuresis has been found to occur not only in the deepest stages of sleep, but in all stages. The issue then is that the child cannot wake up in response to the urge. Fifty percent of children who have been unresponsive to treatment have been found to have reduced bladder capacity, and some also had significant nocturnal instability of the detrusor muscle. This diminished capacity results in the need to urinate occurring prior to the bladder being full. The release of antidiuretic hormone (ADH/vasopressin) by the posterior pituitary gland normally increases at night, decreasing the volume of urine reaching the bladder. It has been hypothesized, and documented in at least one study, that children with nocturnal enuresis are less responsive to these changes. Since higher than normal levels of ADH were found in these children, a less sensitive feedback system or receptor defect has been suggested.[6]

The fact that parents and siblings of children with nocturnal enuresis also report a history of the problem has lead to the exploration of a genetic contribution.[6] The chance of a child having the condition is 77% if both parents had nocturnal enuresis. If one parent was affected, this risk drops to 43% to 44%. Genetic analysis has implicated at least three gene loci on chromosomes 12q, 13q, and 8q.[6]

Underlying diseases and anatomic abnormalities should also be eliminated as potential causes of nocturnal enuresis, as well as medications with diuretic or sedating effects.[5,6] Disorders such as diabetes mellitus, diabetes insipidus, chronic renal failure, UTI, neurologic disorders, and constipation are possible causes. Anatomic etiologies, such as ectopic ureter that empties outside the bladder in females, and posterior urethral valves or urethral stricture in males, must be ruled out, but these are rare causes of bedwetting.[5,6]

Diagnosis. Clinical workup for enuresis includes a thorough history of elimination patterns (which may necessitate having the parents keep a diary), urinalysis, and a physical examination to identify gross anatomic abnormalities.[6] If an infection is detected, renal and bladder sonograms and a voiding cystourethrogram should be obtained to rule out vesicoureteral reflux (backflow of urine from the bladder into the ureters toward the kidneys). In children who remain enuretic after many months of standard treatment, urodynamic testing to eliminate the possibility of neurologic causes may be warranted. Any effort to manage a child's enuresis prior to treating any underlying pathology is likely to be unsuccessful.[6]

Treatment. If both daytime and nighttime wetting are present, daytime wetting should be addressed first, to follow the normal maturational process of gaining continence.[5,6] Scheduled voiding is the initial approach to daytime enuresis. More complex multidimensional approaches involve urine retention and sphincter-control exercises, counseling, visualization, and hypnosis. Research has shown that biofeedback therapy may be useful in children when other approaches have failed.[5,6]

The decision to initiate treatment for nocturnal enuresis, after other etiologies have been eliminated, is based on the impact it is having on the child and family, and their readiness.[6] The approach is essentially behavioral therapy with or without pharmacotherapy.[6] "Dry bed training" refers to a comprehensive approach that includes enuresis alarms, waking routines, positive reinforcement, and bladder training, in a variety of combinations.[5] Nocturnal enuresis has been reported to have been successfully managed with bed wetting alarms in 62% to 78% of cases[6] although a meta-analysis found recidivism rates to be 50%.[5] Although there is insufficient evidence providing support for other behavioral interventions (fluid restrictions, nighttime awakenings, motivational interventions with "star charts" or tokens), they are harmless and anecdotal data provide some validation.[5] Pharmacotherapy to manage enuresis consists primarily of synthetic vasopressin (desmopressin acetate) and tricyclic antidepressants (e.g., imipramine).[5,6] Relapse rates with both of these drugs is quite high.[5,6] Anticholinergic therapy sometimes is used, in combination with vasopressin or alone, for children with reduced functional bladder capacity,[6] but is effective in less than 40% of cases. Pharmacologic treatment is not a cure; drug weaning is eventually necessary, and overall long-term effectiveness is poor.[6]

KEY POINTS

- Voiding dysfunction may be secondary to disorders of the lower urinary tract, due to pathologies affecting the central, autonomic, and peripheral nervous systems, or associated with a wide variety of factors affecting control of micturition, including medications and access to toileting facilities.
- Urge incontinence may be idiopathic, or due to bladder infections that irritate the bladder lining, radiation therapy, tumors or stones in the urinary tract, or central nervous system damage to inhibitory pathways (as would occur with stroke, dementia, parkinsonism, and multiple sclerosis).
- Weakening of pelvic muscles or intrinsic urethral sphincter deficiency results in stress incontinence.
- Mixed incontinence is a combination of both stress and urge incontinence.
- Obstruction of the urethra, or an underactive or inactive detrusor muscle causes overflow incontinence.
- Functional incontinence is related to physical or environmental limitations in reaching a toilet in time to void.
- *Neurogenic bladder* is a broad classification of voiding dysfunction in which the specific cause is a pathology that produces a disruption of nervous communication governing micturition.
- Treatment options for voiding dysfunction include behavioral, pharmaceutical, and surgical interventions.
- Enuresis is inappropriate wetting of clothing or bedding, with the term usually reserved for incontinence in children, particularly at night. The primary cause of enuresis is maturational delay.
- Treatment for enuresis is usually behavioral modification with or without pharmacologic intervention.

CONGENITAL DISORDERS

Vesicoureteral Reflux. Reflux of urine from the bladder to the ureter and renal pelvis, known as **vesicoureteral reflux (VUR),** is usually due to incompetence of the valvular mechanism at the ureter-bladder junction.

The incidence of vesicoureteral reflux in children without a UTI has been cited as 1% to 2%.[7] However, the incidence in infants and children with UTIs is much greater, between 30% to 40%. A genetic component is also present; in siblings of children in whom reflux had been diagnosed, the incidence is 27% to 51%. There is a 66% rate of VUR in the children of parents who have had a diagnosis of reflux. The specific mode of inheritance has not yet been identified; a major, dominantly inherited allele, multifactorial or polygenic traits, and an X-linked pattern have all been postulated.[7] Infants who have a family history of reflux should be routinely evaluated at as early an age as possible so that appropriate medical management may be initiated.[7,8]

Pathogenesis. Normally, the ureters enter the bladder at an oblique angle and then continue for 1 to 2 cm under the bladder mucosa before exiting inside the bladder cavity. As the bladder fills, pressure within it increases against the muscle wall and closes the ureteral passageway. In vesicoureteral reflux, closure of the ureteral passage is not successful, and the urine flows backward into the ureters, sometimes reaching the kidney.

Vesicoureteral reflux is classified as being of either a primary or secondary etiology. Congenital abnormalities at the ureterovesical junction are the cause of primary reflux.[9,10] These anomalies include situations in which the mucosal ureteral tunnel is short, which decreases the efficiency of the valvular mechanism, the orifice is more lateral, or the trigone area of the bladder is not well developed. Primary reflux is also associated with other abnormalities of the urinary system, among them ureteral duplication, ureterocele with duplication, ureteral ectopia, and paraurethral diverticula. Secondary reflux can occur from increased pressure within the bladder (neurogenic bladder, bladder outlet obstruction), inflammatory processes, or surgical procedures at or near the ureterovesical junction. The extent of reflux is graded from I to V (Figure 29-2).

Increased renal pelvis pressure and migration of bacteria from the bladder to the kidneys may result from reflux,

Calyx

Renal pelvis

Ureter

Malfunctioning valve

Functioning ureterovesicular valve

Bladder

Reflux into ureter only—no dilation

Urine

Grade I

Reflux into ureter, pelvis, and calyces with no dilation and normal calyceal fornices

Grade II

Mild dilation of ureter and mild dilation of renal pelvis

Grade III

Moderate dilation of ureter, pelvis, and calyces

Grade IV

Gross dilation of ureter, pelvis, and calyces

Grade V

FIGURE 29-2 International classification of vesicoureteral reflux. (From James SR, Ashwill JW: *Nursing care of children: principles and practice*, ed 3, Philadelphia, 2007, Saunders, p 576.)

producing pyelonephritis or renal scarring that may cause hypertension or renal insufficiency.[9] In the 1970s, in 50% of the cases of hypertension in children, VUR was documented as the specific etiology. At that time, up to 40% of the children treated at renal failure clinics had VUR. More recent data indicate that VUR is noted as the etiology of hypertension or renal insufficiency in only about 6% of the children. These differences may be due to changes in disease-coding procedures, and/or better diagnosis and treatment.[9]

Voiding dysfunction is also a possible result for children with VUR.[10] In a recent study of children with congenital VUR who were diagnosed before the age of 6 months, roughly 20% continued to have voiding dysfunction following the usual age of toilet training. These results were unaffected by the child's gender or severity of VUR.[10]

Diagnosis and Clinical Manifestations. Reflux may be discovered prenatally, during ultrasonography, when hydronephrosis is identified.[9] The other most common time of diagnosis is during the screening of children with a family history of VUR.[8] It may also be identified during evaluation for recurrent UTI, voiding dysfunction, renal insufficiency, or hypertension in children. Diagnostic tests such as voiding cystourethrography, intravenous pyelography, radionuclide renal scintigraphy, and computed tomography are performed to evaluate the status of the kidney and bladder system.

Treatment. In nearly 80% of cases, reflux resolves spontaneously as the child grows.[11] The factors predictive of spontaneous resolution are younger age at diagnosis, classification as grade I or II reflux, higher bladder capacity at the onset of reflux manifestations, and a history of prenatal hydronephrosis. This information is helpful in determining when and how to treat patients, given questions about safety and efficacy of long-term prophylactic antimicrobial therapy and surgical interventions.[11]

For those with VUR most likely to resolve spontaneously, observation and medical management when necessary are the initial therapeutic approaches.[11-12] During the period of observation, low-dose antibiotics specific for the most likely organisms are used to prevent infection by some practitioners. Others, because of the concern for the development of bacterial resistance, choose to obtain urinalysis screening periodically and initiate treatment only if a UTI is present. A recent study comparing the use of prophylactic antibiotics compared to monitoring and prompt treatment of UTIs in children with grades I and II VUR found no difference in outcomes.[12] Another study involving school-aged children with grades I to III VUR concluded that termination of the use of prophylactic antibiotics in selected school age children is safe practice.[13] The risk of significant upper UTI is low, and the development of new renal scars unlikely.[13]

Although open surgical intervention is still the standard treatment for high-grade VUR, minimally invasive endoscopic surgery is the surgical intervention of choice now for those with low and medium grade reflux.[14] In this approach, a bulking agent is inserted into the bladder wall below the ureteral orifice to create a prominent bulge that serves as a barrier to reflux. A variety of agents are being used, and cure rates of 44% to 90% after one injection and from 66% to 94% after subsequent injections have been reported.[12,14]

Obstruction of the Ureteropelvic Junction. Ureteropelvic junction obstruction (UPJO) is defined as a blockage (partial or complete) in urinary flow from the renal pelvis at the entry point of one or both ureters.[15] It is diagnosed more often in males, and more frequently presents unilaterally at the left ureter.[16] Bilateral UPJO has an incidence of 10% to 40% and is usually diagnosed in infants under the age of 6 months.[16] It may be either congenital or acquired; acquired UPJO may be due to such conditions as urinary tract stones, postoperative or inflammatory strictures, or neoplasms of the ureters.[15] An autosomal-dominant model of inheritance has been proposed but not verified.[16] An increased incidence in premature infants and twins has been noted, as well as an increased incidence of other urologic abnormalities in conjunction with UPJO.[16]

Pathogenesis. The exact etiology of UPJO remains unknown, but in the majority of cases, stenosis (narrowing) of the junction by either intrinsic or extrinsic factors is the cause of the obstruction. Excessive collagen in the muscle cells of the junction is a usual intrinsic source of UPJO, whereas compression from renal veins or arteries, "crossing vessels," is a possible external cause. Because uncrossing the vessels never solves the obstruction, it is likely that an intrinsic factor changes the structure of the renal pelvis producing these variations in the vasculature. The result of intrinsic and extrinsic UPJO is inefficient ureter drainage leading to progressive dilation of the renal pelvis and hydronephrosis. Eventually, structural damage to the renal parenchyma and kidney dysfunction will occur.

Diagnosis and Clinical Manifestations. The majority of UPJO diagnoses are made prenatally during maternal ultrasonography.[15,16] Neonates with hydronephrosis due to UPJO frequently have elevated serum creatinine levels and reduced urinary output, but it is not common for renal failure to be present in neonates with either unilateral or bilateral UPJO.[16] Other early signs and symptoms include a palpable flank mass in a newborn infant; abdominal, flank, or back pain; a UTI with fever; or hematuria without significant trauma. UPJO may also be asymptomatic and discovered incidentally on renal ultrasonography.

Treatment. Surgical intervention for UPJO has decreased since the late 1980s, in favor of more conservative approaches.[15] In the case of prenatally diagnosed UPJO, observation is considered most appropriate.[15,17] Conservative, observational management consists of frequent renal ultrasound to assess for hydronephrosis.

The intent of surgery is to relieve symptoms and/or maintain renal function, but for some asymptomatic cases, monitoring the patient has been found to be most appropriate.[15] The percentage of surgical interventions in children under 6 months of age has decreased from 34.2% in an assessment of 1988-1991 to 25.2% in a similar review encompassing 1997 to 2000.[17]

The timing of surgical intervention to correct UPJO is also controversial. Ultimately, it is a clinical decision based on the degree of obstruction, careful analysis of kidney function, and the overall health of the infant or child. Early surgical repair is usually warranted if function of the affected kidney decreases, in cases of bilateral obstruction, and in cases of congenital single kidney with obstruction.

Pyeloplasty is the surgical reconstruction of the UPJ, and it is a common pediatric surgery. It usually involves removal of the stenosed area of the junction and anastomosis of the ureter and renal pelvis. Endoscopic and laparoscopic techniques are being utilized widely in the United States.[17,18] An improvement in renal function is likely, although a small percentage of patients require a second surgical intervention due to the postoperative development of urine leakage or a return of the obstruction.[18] The use of a robotic endoscopic approach to surgery is increasingly popular in locations where it is available.[19]

Ureteral Ectopy. An ectopic ureter is a single ureter implanted in an abnormal location or a duplicate ureter. Alternative or duplicate sites of ureter implantation predispose the patient to infection and a potential reduction in renal function.

Pathogenesis. Ureters may implant anywhere along the route of migration of the mesonephric duct during fetal development. Ectopic ureters are significantly more common in females than in males.[20,21] In males, the ectopy is usually unilateral and is most frequently found implanted in the urethra, but the bladder neck, seminal vesicle, and vas deferens are also common sites. In females, ectopic ureters may be implanted in the urethra, vagina, cervix, ovarian tubes, or uterus.[20,21]

Diagnosis and Clinical Manifestations. An ectopic ureter is often found in conjunction with other genitourinary pathologies, including renal dysgenesis or agenesis, ectopic kidneys, abnormal ovaries or tubes, or abnormalities in the seminal vesicles.[20,21] The diagnosis of ureteral ectopy is frequently made during maternal ultrasonography. Hydronephrosis secondary to obstruction is the typical sonographic finding. Postnatally, the condition is diagnosed with intravenous urography, renal ultrasonography, and endoscopy in symptomatic individuals. The clinical manifestations of ureteral ectopy vary depending on the site of implantation, and identification may not be made until significantly later, often by decades.[20-23] In females the most common symptom is incontinence; other symptoms experienced by male and female patients are continence with dribbling, UTIs, obstruction, and pain.[20-22] Epididymitis may be the initial problem in males.

Treatment. Surgical alternatives vary according to the site of ureteral ectopy, the function of the affected kidney(s), and the presence of any other pathology.[20-23] In the case of a single ectopic ureter, when the opposing kidney is normal, nephroureterectomy is the recommended course of treatment. If the involved kidney has adequate function, the ureter may be reimplanted in a more physiologically acceptable site. Heminephrectomy and ureteropyelostomy are not uncommon. Laparoscopic nephrectomy and heminephrectomy are increasingly used because of the reduced mortality and better visualization of the surgical field with laparoscopic procedures.[20-23] Antenatal sonography may lead to earlier diagnosis and an increase in kidney-sparing surgery.

Ureterocele. A **ureterocele** is a congenital cystic dilatation of the distal end of the ureter (see Figure 29-2).

These cysts are called *intravesical* ureteroceles when they are entirely within the bladder itself.[24] Ureteroceles found in the neck of the bladder or in the urethra are *ectopic* or *extravesical* ureteroceles, and represent the majority of these anomalies.[25] Ectopic ureteroceles are the more common form in the pediatric population.

Etiology and Pathogenesis. Ureteroceles are most often identified prenatally or in infants and children; however, they may not be found until adulthood.[24] It is most likely that the etiology of ureteroceles is complex rather than unified. Most certainly there are multiple points in embryogenesis when ureterocele formation could occur, often with concomitant anomalies of the kidney(s). The microscopic structure of the muscle is abnormal, with smaller myocytes, decreased numbers of muscle bundles, and an absence of thick myofibrils. Ureteroceles occur more often in females than in males (6:1 ratio) and almost exclusively in Caucasians.

Ureteroceles may be classified as simple structures when they are not associated with duplicate collecting systems, but the majority present as duplicate systems with ectopic implantation. They are infrequently bilateral. When identified in adults, they are typically intravesical, simple, and unilateral.[24] The small orifice of the ureter poses an obstruction in the

collecting system and results in ureteral and renal calyx dilatation and often facilitates reflux and infection. If the ureterocele is large, obstruction of the bladder outlet may occur.[26]

Diagnosis and Clinical Manifestations. Ureteroceles are increasingly identified serendipitously during prenatal ultrasonography by the appearance of hydronephrosis and evidence of cystic dilatation.[26] After birth, confirmation with further assessment is necessary. UTIs are the most common manifestation in infants. In addition to the manifestations of UTI, patients with ureteroceles may present with either urinary retention or incontinence if the bladder outlet is obstructed, ureteral calculus, hematuria, urosepsis, or a general failure to thrive.

Anatomically, ureteroceles present with significant variability, requiring a thorough history, physical examination, and diagnostic testing. In addition to determining the precise presentation, diagnostic test results assist in determining the most appropriate surgical intervention.[24-27] Ultrasonography of the kidneys and bladder has the greatest sensitivity and is felt by many to be the only diagnostic assessment needed for ureterocele diagnosis.[26] The function of the urinary tract is also evaluated with voiding cystourethrograms, intravenous pyelograms, CT scans, MRI, and nuclear renal scans. These tests are most useful in guiding interventions, but are not necessary for ureterocele diagnosis. Prophylactic antibiotics are usually prescribed during diagnostic testing.

Treatment. Treatment goals for ureterocele include controlling infection, preserving urinary tract function, maintaining urinary continence, and removing obstruction.[25] Surgical interventions are necessary to accomplish these goals. Although a selected group of individuals may be managed without surgical intervention,[27] this is not generally a reasonable option and most require surgical manipulation.[24,25] The evolution of endoscopic equipment that is small enough even for neonates has increased the use of endoscopic surgery to accomplish the required procedures with less morbidity.[25,26] Endoscopic ureterocele decompression by incision or puncture is a frequent approach for intravesical ureteroceles in pediatric cases and may be also used for ectopic ureteroceles.[25] This incision or puncture may be appropriate for adults, but other techniques used include a combined percutaneous-transurethral approach.[24] Depending upon the anomalies found during diagnostic evaluation, the intervention may include transurethral incision of the defect, excision with reimplantation of the ureter, or partial nephrectomy and ureterectomy. In an acutely septic patient, a percutaneous nephrostomy to drain the upper collecting system may be needed.

KEY POINTS

- Congenital abnormalities of the bladder include misimplantation of ureters, strictures, an extra ureter, and ureterocele.
- These disorders cause problems by obstructing normal urine flow and predisposing to the retrograde flow of urine, urine stasis, and secondary infection; they are usually treated with surgical interventions.

NEOPLASMS

Primary cancers of the ureters or urethra are rare. Bladder cancer however, is quite common.

Bladder Cancer. It is predicted that there will be 68,810 new diagnoses of bladder cancer, with about 51,230 in men and 17,580 in women.[28] Lifetime risk is 1 in 85 for women and 1 in 27 for men; the risk for men is roughly 4 times that for women. Bladder cancer is the fourth most common cancer diagnosed in men in the United States (following prostate, lung, and colon cancers)[28,29] and the eighth most common in women.[29] Mortality rate for 2008 is estimated to be about 9,950 men and 4,150 women.[28] Although incidence is increasing, mortality is decreasing; there are more than ½ million bladder cancer survivors in the United States. Like most cancers, the risk of developing bladder cancer increases with age; approximately 90% of cases are in people over the age of 55. Incidence in whites is twice that in blacks, and the diagnosis in Hispanics is less frequent than blacks. Blacks, however, have more advanced stages of bladder cancer than whites at the time of diagnosis. At diagnosis, 74% of individuals have cancers that are limited to the bladder itself, while in 19% adjacent tissues are involved, and in 3% there are metastases to more distant sites.[28]

There are four general types of bladder cancer, differentiated by their histologic appearance.[28] Some of these bladder cancer histologies are also found in malignancies of the renal pelvis, ureters, and/or urethra. More than 90% of all cases of bladder cancer are *urothelial (transitional cell)* carcinomas originating in the transitional epithelium, or urothelium, which is the lining found throughout the urinary tract. *Squamous cell* carcinoma of the bladder represents only approximately 4% of the overall cases. This type of bladder cancer looks very similar to skin cancers under the microscope, and is quite invasive. One to two percent of bladder cancers are *adenocarcinomas*. These tumors, arising from glandular tissue, are also invasive in nature. *Small cell* bladder cancers account for less than 1% of all bladder cancers. These diverse types of malignancies may respond differently to the interventions for bladder cancer. A very rare malignancy called *rhabdomyosarcoma* is not usually included in discussions of bladder cancer. It may originate in the bladder but more frequently involves other organs and tissues. This cancer is uncommon in adults; it is more likely to occur in infants.[28] In 1998, the World Health Organization and International Society of Urological Pathology collaboratively created a system of evidence-based subtypes for urothelial bladder cancer that is more detailed.[28,29] These subtypes are based upon whether the tumors are invasive or noninvasive, and whether their configuration is flat or papillary. Subtypes are then combined (e.g., invasive papillary urothelial carcinoma) to allow for further characterizations of presentation.[28,29]

From diagnosis, through treatment to death, bladder cancer is the fifth most expensive cancer, with cost per annum greater than $3.4 billion.[30,31] These costs have increased since 2000, although most patients are being treated in outpatient settings.[31] In addition to the increase in diagnosed cases, this cost is primarily attributed to outpatient testing such as cystoscopies and CT scans.[31]

Etiology. Prevention of bladder cancer entails the avoidance of identified risk factors, and a diet high in fruits and vegetables.[28] One study, published in 2002, estimated that genetics contributed to 7% of bladder cancers, 12% to shared environmental effects, 4% to childhood environmental effects, and 77% to nonshared environmental effects,[32] but no more recent research is available. Bladder cancer risk usually is divided into environmental and inherited classifications, with environmental risk being the greatest and well supported by research.[28,29] Familial clustering of bladder cancer is documented in numerous case reports, but epidemiologic studies are limited.[29,32] One cause appears to be a mutation of the retinoblastoma gene responsible for an infantile cancer of the eye, which also results in an increased frequency of bladder cancer.[28,29,32]

Environmental risk factors for bladder cancer are shown in Box 29-2. Smoking is the greatest risk factor, although the association is not as strong as its association with lung cancers.[28,29] Smoking doubles the risk of bladder cancer. Carcinogenetic chemicals inhaled through cigarettes, cigars, or pipes enter the bloodstream and then are filtered and concentrated in the urinary tract. Up to 48% of deaths from bladder tumors in men and 28% in women are attributable to smoking. Occupational exposure to carcinogens and smoking may increase bladder cancer risk synergistically.[28,29] Specific occupations and chemical risks are listed in Box 29-2. Consumption of coffee, tea, or artificial sweeteners and the use of hair dyes and their association with bladder cancer have been studied extensively, with inconsistent results.[28,29] Chronic inflammation of the bladder by UTIs is associated with an increased risk of bladder cancer, especially the invasive squamous cell type. Other causes of inflammation, such as stones, have also been associated with the disease. Certain chemotherapy agents used in the treatment of other malignancies, and radiation therapy to the pelvis increase the risk of bladder cancer. Arsenic in drinking water and low fluid intake are both risk factors for bladder cancer.[28,29]

In children, the congenital anomaly of exstrophy of the bladder (bladder outside the abdominal cavity) may predispose to the development of bladder tumors, particularly adenocarcinomas.[28,29] Parasitic infections from schistosomiasis, especially prevalent in Egyptian males and in Africa, have been associated with squamous cell carcinoma as a result of urine-borne carcinogens formed during the infectious process and irritation by the parasitic ova.[28,29]

Pathogenesis. (See Chapter 7 for specific details of the pathogenesis of cancer). Bladder tumors occur most often at the trigone, the ureteral orifices, and the posterior and lateral walls of the bladder[29] (see Figure 29-1). Metastasis is through a direct route through the bladder wall to adjacent organs or through lymph nodes in the pelvis and abdomen. Once treated, tumors can recur at the original site, or an entirely new tumor may develop at another site. The sites of metastasis most

BOX 29-2

Environmental Risk Factors for Bladder Cancer

Smoking
Occupations
- Dye industry
- Rubber tire production
- Pesticide production
- Pharmaceuticals
- Leather dust
- Textiles
- Printing
- Painters
- Machinists
- Truck drivers (exposure to diesel fumes)

Arsenic in drinking water
Low fluid intake
Selected chemotherapeutic agents
Pelvic radiation therapy

commonly include the liver, lungs, bone, and adrenals. Other sites of metastasis are the heart, brain, and kidney.[29]

Clinical Manifestations. Hematuria is usually the initial symptom of bladder cancer.[28] However, in the early stages of bladder cancer, both gross and microscopic hematuria are often intermittent, and hematuria is associated with numerous urinary tract pathologies. Other common manifestations related to bladder cancer include frequency and urgency; dysuria is an uncommon finding. But again, all these symptoms are also seen with other conditions involving the urinary tract.[28] Because these signs and symptoms are so general, early diagnosis of bladder cancer requires a thorough workup by the health care provider.

Diagnosis. In most cases, diagnostic evaluation for bladder cancer is initiated because of the development of one or more of the above clinical manifestations. A thorough history may reveal risk factors for bladder cancer, or physical examination and diagnostic testing may indicate another etiology.

The most frequently used invasive test in the diagnosis of bladder cancer is a cystoscopy, with biopsy of any questionable tissue and washings of free cells for cytologic examination.[28,29,31,33] Fluorescent cystoscopy may be performed at the same time.[28] In this test, porphyrins are instilled into the bladder, where they are taken up by any cancer cells present. When a blue light is then shown through the cystoscope, malignant cells appear to glow due to the fluorescence of the porphyrins.[28] Blood and urine specimens will be tested for the presence of tumor markers.[28,30] The sensitivity and specificity of available tumor markers varies widely.[30] At this point, no tumor marker is sufficient for the diagnosis of bladder cancer, and they cannot definitively replace cystoscopy.[30] Additional imaging tests including intravenous pyelogram, retrograde pyelogram, chest x-ray, CT scan, MRI, bladder ultrasonography, and bone scans may be performed to assist with diagnosis and determine the presence of metastasis, which is part of the staging process.[28,29,33] The stage of the malignancy is an important contributor to treatment decisions, and also aids in the determination of prognosis.

Biopsied tissue and the examination of cells obtained during cystoscopy as well as those that might be found in the urine are key to the determination of the specific type and grade of the tumor. (See Chapter 7 for a thorough discussion of staging and grading). Examination of the urine for malignant cells (urinary cytology) is of the greatest value with urothelial tumors.[29] Examination of the biopsy also allows the determination of the depth to which the tumor has penetrated the bladder wall.[28,29] All of this information is used to guide the selection of the specific treatment approach.

Treatment. Treatment protocols are based on the tumor's features: the type of bladder cancer, and its grade and stage. The primary options are surgery, radiation therapy, chemotherapy, and immunotherapy.[28,29] Treatment selection is evidence-based, with available information continuously being updated. Surgery as the single treatment, or with other adjuvants, is the intervention for more than 90% of bladder cancers.[28,29] The specific approach to surgery varies with the stage. For noninvasive carcinoma in situ, endoscopic resection is usually performed. Transurethral resection (TUR) with appropriate cystoscopic and cytologic follow-up is the only treatment recommended for most superficial bladder cancers. For the 70% to 80% of patients with low-grade superficial cancers at the time of diagnosis, this is typically the first intervention. If the tumor is invasive, the area of the bladder where it is located is removed (partial cystectomy), and this is routinely followed by chemotherapy and radiation therapy. If necessary, surgeons may return to remove the entire bladder (**cystectomy**) should the patient not respond to the adjuvant interventions. In cases in which the tumor is large, or multiple bladder tumors are identified, a radical cystectomy is performed, where the bladder and surrounding nodes are removed; in men, the prostate gland is also removed, and in women the uterus, ovaries, fallopian tubes, and part of the vagina are also often removed. Under these circumstances, reconstructive surgery is necessary to provide for storage and elimination of urine.[28,29] There are numerous such procedures, and their discussion is beyond the scope of this text. Readers are referred to urologic surgical resources.

Radiation therapy may be provided prior to surgery to shrink the tumor, facilitating its eventual removal.[28,29] Or, it may be done following surgery in order to kill remaining malignant cells. In situations in which the cancer is advanced, palliative radiation therapy may reduce signs and symptoms such as obstruction, pain, and bleeding.[28,29]

Chemotherapy may also be given preoperatively, for the same reason as radiation therapy.[28,29] Or, as with radiation therapy, it is administered postoperatively to destroy cells left behind during surgery. In noninvasive or minimally invasive (stage I) bladder cancer, chemotherapy may be given by instillation into the bladder with a catheter (intravesical chemotherapy). When the cancer is more advanced, and cells have metastasized into neighboring lymph nodes or other tissues or organs, systemic chemotherapy is indicated. Immunotherapy may likewise be administered intravesically, depending on the individual tumor circumstances.[28,29]

The prognosis for noninvasive (stage 0/in situ) bladder cancer is excellent.[28,29,31] As the tumor invades deeper into the bladder wall, the survival rate begins to decline, and at 5 years following diagnosis, the mortality rate is 60% to 80%. Overall survival rates for persons with metastatic bladder cancer are poor. For patients with distant metastases, life expectancy averages 2 years. Ongoing research is being conducted on the efficacy of alternative chemotherapeutic agents. However, to date these drugs have not proved more efficacious than the standard treatments. Risk of recurrence of bladder cancer is high, even for superficial malignancies.[28,29,31]

KEY POINTS

- Bladder cancer is the fourth most common cancer diagnosed in men in the United States and the eighth most common in women.
- Risk of developing bladder cancer increases with age; smoking and occupational exposure to carcinogenic chemicals are thought to be the main predisposing factors.
- There are four general types of bladder cancer, differentiated by their histological appearance. More than 90% of bladder tumors originate from the transitional epithelium (urothelium) lining the urinary tract.
- Bladder cancer is primarily manifested as hematuria. Frequency and urgency may also be present. Dysuria is not common.
- The most frequently used invasive test in the diagnosis of bladder cancer is a cystoscopy, with biopsy of any questionable tissue and washings to free cells for cytologic examination.
- Treatment protocols are based on the tumor's features: the type of bladder cancer, and its grade and stage. The primary options are surgery, radiation therapy, chemotherapy, and immunotherapy.

INFLAMMATION AND INFECTION

Most inflammations of the lower urinary tract are due to infection. The normal defense mechanisms of the urinary tract are presented in detail in Chapter 27 with the discussion of pyelonephritis, infection of the kidney. Infections in the urinary tract are typically ascending in nature; they begin in the lower urinary tract and may progress to the kidney (upper urinary tract). By the time infection reaches the kidneys, the bladder and urethra are already infected. Involvement of the ureters does not seem to present with clinical manifestations.

Urethritis. Urethritis is an inflammation of the urethra. Inflammation of the urethra may lead to pain, burning, urinary incontinence, and, if it is due to an infectious organism, it may progress to infective cystitis. Urethritis can be caused from infection, external irritants or, in women, insufficient estrogen.

Infection of the urethra may be due to a wide variety of organisms.[34] Many patients are asymptomatic; if the cause is a sexually transmitted disease, they may not know they are infected until notified that their partner has an infection. Otherwise, the most common symptom is dysuria.[34-38] Dysuria is often the first indication, along with discharge, of many sexually transmitted diseases such as *Chlamydia trachomatis;* such infections are typically confined to the urethra.[34-38] There are many external irritants capable of producing urethritis: frequent catheterizations; repeated exposure to bubble baths; tight pants; perfumed soaps or powders; or poor personal hygiene. The urethra is an estrogen-dependent structure, and postmenopausal women are at increased risk for irritation and inflammation of the urethra. Good hygiene, adequate fluid intake, voiding after intercourse, avoiding irritants, and wearing cotton briefs that do not rub the urethral opening reduce the risk of developing urethritis. Additionally, postmenopausal women may benefit from a regular application of topical estrogen to the urethral opening. If due to a sexually transmitted organism, targeted pharmacologic therapy is indicated. Otherwise, urethritis due to infection is often not symptomatic until the organism progresses to the bladder, causing cystitis.

Cystitis. Cystitis, or inflammation of the bladder lining, may result from bacterial, fungal, or parasitic infections, chemical irritants, foreign bodies (e.g., stones), or trauma. By far the most common cause of cystitis—and the focus of this discussion—is bacterial infection.

Etiology and Pathogenesis. Normally, bacteria are cleared from the bladder by the flushing and dilutional effects of voiding. The high urea concentration and osmolarity, and low pH in urine act as natural barriers, killing invading bacteria in a normal bladder environment.

UTIs vary in prevalence by age, gender, race, and in males, circumcision status.[35] Risk factors are listed in detail in Box 29-3. In the pediatric population, uncircumcised male infants under 6 months of age and females less than 12 months of age have the highest prevalence.[35] Later in life, cystitis is more common in females than males.[35] UTIs annually affect 15% of adult women.[6] Recurrent infection will present in more than 25% of these.[36] A shorter urethra, as well as a colonization route from both the rectum and vagina to the urethra, is thought to facilitate the increased rate of infections in women.[36,38] They are common occurrences during pregnancy, and have been associated with an increased risk of fetal mortality, pyelonephritis, and premature delivery. Prostatic secretions, which are antibacterial, inhibit cystitis in men younger than 50 years. Use of spermicidal agents, with diaphragms or coated condoms, increases the risk of infection with *Escherichia coli* or *Staphylococcus saprophyticus.*[36] *Escherichia coli* is responsible for the majority of cases of bacterial cystitis, with additional possible culprits being *Staphylococcus saprophyticus, Klebsiella* species, *Proteus mirabilis, enterococci,* or β-*hemolytic streptococci.*[35-37] Fungal infections, mycoplasmas, and other anaerobic bacteria are occasionally responsible. Infections due to *Neisseria gonorrhoeae* or *Chlamydia trachomatis* are associated with sexually transmitted diseases but are typically limited to

BOX 29-3

Risk Factors for Cystitis

Factors Increasing Urinary Stasis
Intrinsic obstruction (stone, tumor of urinary tract, urethral stricture, BPH)
Extrinsic obstruction (tumor, fibrosis compressing urinary tract)
Urinary retention (including neurogenic bladder and low bladder wall compliance)
Renal Impairment

Foreign Bodies
Urinary tract calculi
Catheters (indwelling, external condom catheter, urethral stent, nephrostomy tube, intermittent catheterization)
Urinary tract instrumentation (cystoscopy, urodynamics)

Anatomic Factors
Congenital defects leading to obstruction or urinary stasis
Fistula (abnormal opening) exposing urinary stream to skin, vagina, or fecal stream
Shorter female urethra and colonization from normal vaginal flora
Obesity

Factors Compromising Immune Response
Aging
Human immunodeficiency virus infection
Diabetes mellitus

Functional Disorders
Constipation
Voiding dysfunction with detrusor sphincter dyssynergia

Other Factors
Pregnancy
Hypoestrogenic state
Multiple sex partners (women)
Use of spermicidal agents or contraceptive diaphragm (women)
Poor personal hygiene

From Lewis S et al: *Medical-surgical nursing: assessment and management of clinical problems,* ed 7, St. Louis: Mosby, 2007.

the urethra.[38] Additional risk factors include sexual activity, diabetes mellitus, poor personal hygiene, any type of bladder dysfunction causing urine stasis, and urinary catheterization and indwelling catheters. Catheter-associated UTIs are the most common nosocomial infection.[39]

Clinical Manifestations. In about 10% of individuals with bacteriuria, the infection is asymptomatic.[37] The majority of patients with cystitis experience an acute onset of frequency, urgency, dysuria, and pain, often in the suprapubic area. The urine may appear pink due to hematuria or cloudy due to the infectious organism. Common symptoms of cystitis in children include fever, irritability, poor feeding, vomiting, diarrhea, and ill appearance.[35,37] Children who are able to talk may also indicate dysuria, suprapubic pain, or incontinence, but even older children sometimes have difficulty localizing signs and symptoms.[35,37] Untreated cystitis may lead to renal damage secondary to progression of the infection to the upper urinary tract. Therefore, prompt intervention is essential.

Diagnosis and Treatment. Treatment algorithms for acute cystitis and recurrent cystitis are shown in Figures 29-3 and 29-4, respectively. Acute, uncomplicated UTI in women may be treated by telephone screening only, without being seen by a health care provider.[36] These women with no anatomical anomalies of the urinary tract, who have not recently had cystitis, and without symptoms suggestive of either vaginitis or cervicitis, may be treated empirically with a 3-day course of antibiotics.[36,38-40]

Men, children, and those women with recurrent infections, unresolved infections, atypical manifestations, or other problems identified above have complicated UTIs and require physical examination and diagnostic testing.[36-38] *Recurrent UTIs* are repeated infections within a short period after verified resolution of the earlier infection. Recurrent UTIs are fairly common in women but rare in healthy adult men. Recurrent infections in men should trigger a urologic examination that includes endoscopy. *Unresolved infections* are those in which bacteriuria remains after the initial treatment.[36,37]

Screening for UTI is often performed using a nitrite and leukocyte esterase dipstick.[36] Leukocyte esterase is indicative of **pyuria** (white blood cells in the urine), and most urinary pathogens reduce nitrates to nitrites. The sensitivity of dipstick urinalysis combined with visual appearance has been reported to be decreased in children; microscopic analysis is recommended.[35,36] A urine culture is unnecessary for most symptomatic patients with a positive dipstick. It is only recommended in situations in which the patient has manifestations suggesting pyelonephritis, fails to respond to empiric pharmacologic therapy, is pregnant, or has urinary calculi. A culture should be considered if the patient is immunosuppressed (because of the likelihood of atypical organisms) or has diabetes mellitus.[36] Under these circumstances, organisms are precisely identified and pharmacologic therapy is targeted.

Cystitis in younger men is managed with a 7- to 10-day course of antibiotics. In older men, a minimum of 14 and up to 28 days of antibiotic therapy is recommended. Unresolved infections are usually treated with targeted antimicrobials for 7 to 10 days. Urine culture and sensitivity are also necessary to ensure antibiotic effectiveness.[36] Some female patients are optimally treated with low-dose prophylactic antibiotics or an intermittent self-start antibiotic regimen in which the woman initiates antibiotic therapy after obtaining a midstream voided specimen.[36] In elderly women, topical estrogen can be effective to prevent recurring infection because bacteria colonize in the urethra due to de-estrogenization of the tissue due to menopause.[34,36] In some women, recurrent infections are related to sexual intercourse, and a postcoital prophylactic antibiotic program is an effective treatment option.[34,36,38,40] Persistent bacterial infections are nearly always due to an anatomic abnormality or pathology in the urinary tract. Such problems include calculi, prostatitis, foreign bodies, and duplicated or ectopic ureters.[36,40]

In children, administration of broad-spectrum antibiotics for 7 to 14 days is the treatment of choice.[35] The specific choice of therapy, including whether or not to start parenterally,

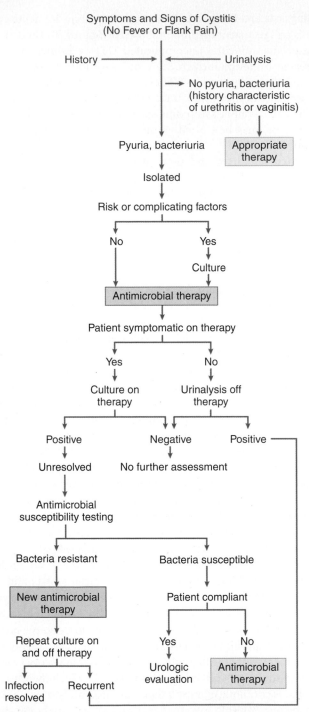

FIGURE 29-3 Management of acute cystitis. (From Walsh PC et al, editors: *Campbell's urology*, ed 4, Philadelphia, 2007, Saunders, p 255.)

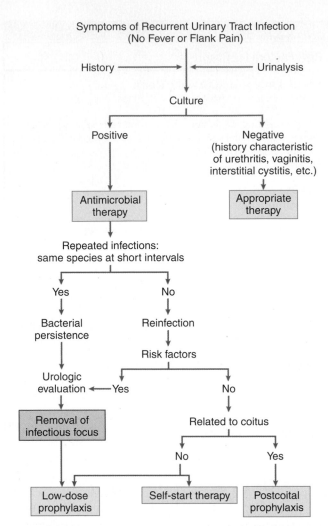

FIGURE 29-4 Management of recurrent UTI. (From Walsh PC et al, editors: *Campbell's urology*, ed 4, Philadelphia, 2007, Saunders, p 256.)

Pregnant women have the same prevalence of bacteriuria as nonpregnant women, but diagnosis and treatment are critical in pregnant women because of their greater propensity for pyelonephritis.[36,39] The increased likelihood of pyelonephritis is related to hydronephrosis and stasis of urine during pregnancy. Antibiotic therapy must be carefully chosen to avoid fetal harm.[36,39]

Bacteriuria significantly increases with age, so that 10% of men and at least 20% of women older than 65 years are affected.[36,37] Factors that predispose the elderly to cystitis include genitourinary abnormalities (e.g., calculi, benign prostatic hyperplasia, prostatitis), chronic illnesses (particularly diabetes mellitus and neurologic diseases), changes in urinary pH, decreased estrogen production in women, bowel incontinence, and greater prevalence of catheterization. A 7- to 10-day course of antibiotic treatment and close monitoring for adverse effects are recommended for symptomatic UTIs. Symptoms associated with bacteriuria in the elderly may include anxiety, confusion, lethargy, and anorexia as opposed to dysuria and fever. The diagnosis is often one of exclusion,

is contingent on many factors including age, illness severity, illness duration, and the ability to drink adequate fluids. However, children younger than 5 years should keep taking prophylactic doses of antibiotics until radiographic evaluation is completed. UTIs in children are often indicative of an underlying pathologic process (e.g., vesicoureteral reflux, ureteropelvic junction [UPJO] obstruction) and warrant prompt urologic evaluation.[35]

and urinalysis and culture are included in the diagnostic evaluation.

Interstitial Cystitis/Painful Bladder Syndrome.

Interstitial cystitis/painful bladder syndrome (IC/PBS) is a chronic condition consisting of bladder pain and a variety of other manifestations typically associated with other bladder pathologies.[41,42] However, these patients have no other identifiable pathology. Urgency, frequency, and nocturia are other common findings. The absence of a usable and consistent definition of the condition affects the determination of pathogenesis and delays diagnosis, resulting in the use of therapeutic and preventative interventions that are empiric. This condition can have a serious impact on quality of life, interfering with work, daily activities, sleep, family life, and sexual activities. Approximately one million Americans suffer from interstitial cystitis.[41,42]

The specific etiology is unclear, but theories suggest that injury occurs to the protective bladder lining due to activation of the inflammatory process.[41,42] Pain is usually present in several locations, but physical exam is often negative. In the majority of patients, the pain worsens with certain foods and/or drinks, and bladder filling, while urinary elimination results in a reduction of pain. The foods and drinks most often associated with pain are alcohol, citrus fruits, coffee, carbonated beverages, tea, chocolate, and tomatoes. Hydrodistention of the bladder and instillations of potassium chloride will often reproduce the pain. Biopsies and urodynamics often provide insufficient information to provide a diagnosis. Therefore, IC/PBS is diagnosed as a symptom-based syndrome, once other pathologies have been eliminated, and treatment is based on lifestyle modification and medications for symptom relief.[41,42]

KEY POINTS

- Urethritis is inflammation of the urethra. It is most often due to infection, either from the bladder or associated with a sexually transmitted disease. Sexually transmitted diseases are confined to the urethra; infections of other etiologies may ascend to the bladder before symptoms present. It may also be due to external factors such as frequent catheterizations or poor personal hygiene. Treatment depends on the cause.
- Cystitis is an inflammation of the bladder lining that may be due to infection, chemical irritants, stones, or trauma. Most cases have an infectious etiology and result from infection originating in the urethra.
- Factors predisposing to cystitis include: female gender, increased age, catheterization, diabetes mellitus, bladder dysfunction, poor personal hygiene, and any disorder causing urinary stasis. Manifestations include frequency, urgency, dysuria, possible suprapubic pain, and cloudy urine, although the infection may be asymptomatic. Most female patients are treated based only on this information. More complicated situations, and cystitis in men and children, may require urine culture, and/or further assessment.

- Symptoms of cystitis in older adults may be atypical and include lethargy, anorexia, confusion, and anxiety. Symptomatic cystitis in the elderly should be managed with close drug monitoring to avoid toxicity. Asymptomatic bacteriuria in the elderly should not be treated.
- Interstitial cystitis/painful bladder syndrome is a chronic condition consisting of bladder pain, and often urgency, frequency, and nocturia, when no other etiology can be identified. It is diagnosed based on this information. Treatment is based on the identification of contributory lifestyle factors, such as some foods and beverages. Avoidance of these factors is the primary intervention; medication may be added to manage ICS.

OBSTRUCTION

Obstruction of the lower urinary tract develops when a stone obstructs urine transport. Stones here produce some manifestations that are similar to those formed and lodged in the kidney.

Lower Urinary Tract Urolithiasis.

Stones, or calculi, usually form in the kidneys (*nephrolithiasis*). Nephrolithiasis is discussed in Chapter 27. The term **urolithiasis** is used for stones forming anywhere in the urinary tract, primarily in the kidney or ureters, as well as those that form or travel into the ureters, bladder, or urethra.[43] The manifestations of stones in the ureters and bladder vary somewhat from those when the stone is present in the kidneys, but the risk factors, stone composition, diagnostic tests, and treatment aspects are essentially the same. Refer to Chapter 27 for a detailed discussion of these topics. If diagnosis and treatment are not completed in a timely manner, the patient is at risk for the development of postrenal acute renal failure (Chapter 28).

Ureterolithiasis

Calculi in the ureters are usually those that were able to pass through the junction of the renal pelvis and ureters, as opposed to being formed there. In many cases, these stones are small, pass easily through the ureters, and cause no clinical manifestations. This intersection is a point where large kidney stones become wedged; manifestations then are those characteristic of nephrolithiasis.[43-45] Other stones enter the ureters and cause ureteral colic as they move. This is an acute, sharp, spasmodic pain, experienced in the flank area, possibly radiating into the umbilical region. Irritation of the ureters may result in hematuria. When the stone approaches the distal portion of the ureters, the pain may continue to be sharp in quality, but intermittent in nature. Or, instead of this presentation, the pain may increase, with radiation into the groin region, testicles, or labia. Additional manifestations, also seen with nephrolithiasis, include tachycardia, tachypnea, diaphoresis, nausea, and vomiting.[43]

Diagnostic approaches are the same as those used for nephrolithiasis, being sure to include this lower urinary tract region in scans. Therapeutic interventions for stones located in the ureters depend upon their size and shape, which governs their ability to reach the bladder.[43-47] For stones immobilized in the ureters, endoscopic lithotripsy is the preferred intervention in both adults and children.[43-47] Therapeutic and preventative interventions are otherwise the same as those presented in Chapter 27. These will affect stones formed anywhere in the urinary tract.

Bladder Urolithiasis

Formation of stones in the bladder is unusual; typically, if calculi are present in the bladder, they arrived there by migration from the kidney and ureters. If they do form in the bladder, it is most often secondary to urinary stasis. Regardless of the location of their formation, if they are present in the bladder, dysuria and frequency may be the only symptoms.[43] A stone in the bladder may irritate the urothelium (bladder lining) resulting in hematuria, and once the bladder neck or urethral orifice is reached, manifestations of obstruction may appear. Symptoms are immediately relieved when the stone leaves the bladder.[43] For the most part stones pass on, into the urethra, and exit the body. If stones originate in the bladder, they are nearly always composed of uric acid and are usually indicative of urinary retention and resulting stasis.

As with ureterolithiasis, diagnosis and interventions are similar to those for nephrolithiasis, again with concentration on the lower urinary tract. Relief of urinary obstruction and treatment of infection are the primary goals of treatment. Treatment of cystitis has been previously discussed. Cystitis together with bladder stones requires a thorough approach to treatment, with full diagnostic testing including culture and sensitivity, and close monitoring.[36] A urethral obstruction may be eliminated or converted to a partial obstruction by inserting a urinary catheter. Obstruction results in a risk for postrenal acute renal failure and requires prompt intervention. Endoscopic lithotripsy may be necessary.[43-47]

KEY POINTS

- Urolithiasis is most often due to stones traveling to the ureters, bladder, or urethra from the kidney. They may also originate in the bladder or ureters. Manifestations are associated with tissue irritation and obstruction.
- Manifestations of ureterolithiasis include ureteral colic, hematuria, tachycardia, tachypnea, diaphoresis, nausea, and vomiting. Individuals with stones that approach the bladder may continue to experience pain that continues to be sharp in quality, but intermittent in nature. Otherwise, the pain may increase and radiate into the groin region, testicles, or labia.
- Bladder urolithiasis is usually due to stones traveling from the ureters, but may form in the bladder, usually due to urinary stasis.
- Manifestations of bladder stones are often limited to dysuria and frequency; hematuria is possible. Obstructive signs and symptoms will present if stones obstruct the bladder neck or urethral orifice.

- Ureterolithiasis and bladder urolithiasis are similar to nephrolithiasis in terms of risk factors and stone characteristics. If infection is present, it is treated with appropriate antimicrobials, based on culture and sensitivity tests. Intervention for stones that do not pass spontaneously is endoscopic lithotripsy.

SUMMARY

Disorders involving the lower urinary tract are quite common. In adults, the most prevalent pathologic conditions are voiding dysfunction, malignancies, infections, and urinary stones. Incontinence as a result of bladder dysfunction affects millions of adults. The prevalence of incontinence increases with age and is more common in women than men. However, incontinence is not a result of the normal aging process, and patients should be urged to seek evaluation and treatment. Behavioral, pharmacologic, and surgical approaches may be used to manage voiding dysfunction. Interstitial cystitis/painful bladder syndrome is a chronic condition consisting of bladder pain and a variety of other manifestations typically associated with other bladder pathologies. However, these patients have no other identifiable pathology. Urgency, frequency, and nocturia are other common findings. Bladder cancer is the fourth most common type of cancer in men, and the eighth most common type in women. The primary clinical manifestation of bladder cancer is hematuria. Treatment is based on stage, grade, and type of cancer. Interventions include surgery, radiation, and chemotherapy.

Both childhood UTIs and enuresis should trigger more detailed urologic evaluation to rule out congenital disorders such as UPJO obstruction, ectopic ureters, ureterocele, and vesicoureteral reflux. Vesicoureteral reflux is the most prevalent congenital lower urinary tract disorder. It predisposes children to UTIs, which can result in kidney scarring and permanent renal impairment. Most cases of vesicoureteral reflux resolve spontaneously as the child ages. Before resolution, close medical management is necessary to prevent upper UTI and kidney damage.

Stones in the lower urinary tract usually arrive there after being formed in the kidney. Risk factors and treatment are much the same as those for nephrolithiasis, however manifestations of urolithiasis in the ureters or bladder differ.

REFERENCES

1. Gibbs CF, Johnson TM, Ouslander JG: Office management of geriatric urinary incontinence, *Am J Med* 120:211-220, 2007.
2. Sand PK, Appell R: Disruptive effects of overactive bladder and urge urinary incontinence in younger women, *Am J Med* 119:16S-23S, 2006.
3. Pagana KD, Pagana TJ: *Mosby's manual of diagnostic and laboratory tests*, ed 3, St. Louis, 2006, Mosby.
4. Palmer MH, Newman DK: Urinary incontinence and estrogen, *Am J Nurs* 107:35-37, 2007.
5. Lyon C, Schnall J: What is the best treatment for nocturnal enuresis in children? *J Fam Pract* 54:905-906, 909, 2005.

6. Berry AK: Helping children with nocturnal enuresis, *Am J Nurs* 106:56-63, 2006.

7. Pirker ME et al: Familial vesicoureteral reflux: influence of sex on prevalence and expression, *J Urol* 176:1776-1780, 2006.

8. MacNeily AE, Afshar K: Screening asymptomatic siblings for vesicoureteral reflux: sound science or religious rhetoric? *Can J Urol* 13:3309-3316, 2006.

9. Pohl HG et al: Vesicoureteral reflux and ureteroceles, *J Urol* 177:1659-1666, 2007.

10. Homayoon K et al: Voiding dysfunction: outcome in infants with congenital vesicoureteral reflux, *Urology* 66:1091-1094, 2005.

11. Knudson MJ et al: Predictive factors of early spontaneous resolution in children with primary vesicoureteral reflux, *J Urol* 178:1684-1688, 2007.

12. Faust WC, Pohl HG: Role of prophylaxis in vesicoureteral reflux, *Curr Opin Urol* 17:252-256, 2007.

13. Al-Sayyad AJ, Pike JG, Leonard MP: Can prophylactic antibiotics safely be discontinued in children with vesicoureteral reflux? *J Urol* 174:1587-1589, 2005.

14. Oberson C et al: Endoscopic and surgical treatment of vesicoureteral reflux in children, *Swiss Med Wkly* 137:471-475, 2007.

15. Lam JS, Breda A, Schulam PG: Ureteropelvic junction obstruction, *J Urol* 177:1652-1658, 2007.

16. Karnak I et al: Prenatally detected ureteropelvic junction obstruction: clinical features and associated urologic abnormalities, *Pediatr Surg Int* 24:395-402, 2008.

17. Nelson CP et al: Contemporary trends in surgical correction of pediatric ureteropelvic junction obstruction: data from the nationwide Inpatient sample, *J Urol* 173:232-236, 2005.

18. Sheu JC et al: Ureteropelvic junction obstruction in children: 10 years' experience in one institution, *Pediatr Surg Int* 22:519-523, 2006.

19. Casale P: Robotic pediatric urology, *Expert Rev Med Devices* 5:59-64, 2008.

20. Hernandez-Rey AE, Vitenson J, McGovern PG: Duplicated ectopic hydroureter presenting as a hydrosalpinx, with chronic pelvic pain and recurrent urinary infections, *Fertil Steril* 88:1677-1679, 2007.

21. Elzayat EA, Al-Mandil MS, Ethilali MM: Renal agenesis associated with ipsilateral ectopic ureters entering a large seminal vesicle cyst, *Can J Urol* 14:3463-3466, 2007.

22. Gordon M, Cervellione RM, Hennayake S: Constant urinary dribbling due to an ectopic ureter and delays in diagnosis, *Clin Pediatr* 46(6):544-546, 2007.

23. Funahashi Y et al: Radical prostatectomy for prostate carcinoma with ectopic ureters: a case report, *Nippon Hinyokika Gakkai Zasshi* 98:580-582, 2007.

24. Spatafora S, Pierfrancesco B, Leoni S: Combined percutaneous-transurethral incision for treatment of ureterocele in adults, *Urology* 68(6):1333-1335, 2006.

25. Kajbafzadeh A et al: Evolution of endoscopic management of ectopic ureterocele: a new approach, *J Urol* 177:1118-1123, 2007.

26. Nonmura K, Kakizaki H: Recent trends of genitourinary endoscopy in children, *Int J Urol* 12:607-614, 2005.

27. Han MY et al: Indications for non-operative management of ureteroceles, *J Urol* 174:1652-1655, 2005.

28. American Cancer Society: All about bladder cancer. Available at http://www.cancer.org/docroot/CRI/CRI_2x.asp?sitearea=LRN&dt=44. Accessed March 24, 2007.

29. Kirkali Z et al: Bladder cancer: epidemiology, staging and grading, and diagnosis, *Urology* 66:4-34, 2005.

30. Hong YM, Loughlin KR: Economic impact of tumor markers in bladder cancer surveillance, *Urology* 71:131-135, 2008.

31. Konety BR, Joyce GF, Wise M: Bladder and upper tract urothelial cancer, *J Urol* 177:1636-1645, 2007.

32. Czene K, Lichtenstein P, Hemminki K: Environmental and heritable causes of cancer among 9.6 million individuals in the Swedish Family-Cancer Database, *Int J Cancer* 99:260-266, 2002.

33. Legg JS: Bladder cancer imaging, *Radiol Technol* 79:333-346, 2008.

34. Dieterle S: Urogenital infections in reproductive medicine, *Andrologia* 40:117-119, 2008.

35. Shaikh N et al: Prevalence of urinary tract infection in childhood: a meta-analysis, *Pediatr Infect Dis J* 27(4):302-308, 2008.

36. Car J: Urinary tract infections in women: diagnosis and management in primary care, *BMJ* 332:94-97, 2006.

37. Mak RH, Kuo H: Pathogenesis of urinary tract infection: An update, *Curr Opin Pediatr* 18:148-152, 2006.

38. Sheffield JS, Cunningham FG: Urinary tract infection in women, *Obstetr Gynecol* 106:1085-1092, 2005.

39. Jacobsen SM et al: Complicated catheter-associated urinary tract infections due to *Escherichia coli* and *Proteus mirabilis*, *Clin Microbiol Rev* 21:26-59, 2008.

40. Katchman EA et al: Three-day vs longer duration of antibiotic treatment for cystitis in women: systematic review and meta-analysis, *Am J Med* 118:1196-1207, 2005.

41. Dell JR: Interstitial cystitis/painful bladder syndrome: appropriate diagnosis and management, *J Womens Health* 16:1181-1187, 2007.

42. Warren JW et al: Evidence-based criteria for pain of interstitial cystitis/painful bladder syndrome in women, *Urology* 71:444-448, 2008.

43. Colella et al: Urolithiasis/Nephrolithiasis: what's it all about? *Urol Nurs* 25:427-475, 2005.

44. Pietron PK, Karellas ME: Medical management of common urinary calculi, *Am Fam Physician* 74:86-94, 99–100, 2006.

45. Moe OW: Kidney stones: pathophysiology and medical management, *The Lancet* 367:333-344, 2006.

46. Galvin DJ, Perle MS: Upper urinary tract: the contemporary management of renal and ureteric calculi, *BJU Int* 98:1283-1288, 2006.

47. Ahmadnia H et al: Percutaneous treatment of bladder calculi in children: 5 years experience, *Urol J* 3:20-22, 2006.

Prostate and Breast Cancer

Sheila K. Smith

Other than some forms of skin cancer, prostate cancer is the most commonly occurring form of cancer in the U.S. and is the second leading cause of cancer deaths. In 2004 (the most recent year for which complete statistics are available) about 189,000 cases of prostate cancer were diagnosed, and 29,000 men died of the disease. Both incidence (the number of men who get the disease each year) and mortality rates are almost twice as high for African-American men as for Caucasian men, with lower rates among Hispanic, American Indian, and men of Asian descent. Deaths from prostate cancer have decreased significantly since the early 1990's due to improved screening and treatment. The incidence of prostate cancer has remained high, however, and more African American men die from prostate cancer than any other ethnic group.

The prostate gland is a small organ near the bottom of the male bladder. It is thought to protect the bladder from ascending bacteria, and it provides the transporting fluid for spermatozoa during ejaculation. About 70 years ago Dr. H. H. Young found that digital rectal examination, palpation of the two posterior lobes of the prostate through the rectal wall and Denonvilliers fascia, was a reliable way to examine the prostate for abnormalities. The posterior lobes, which contain most of the organ's glandular tissue, are the most likely place for a malignancy to develop. The American Cancer Society recommends that beginning at age 50 (40 for African-American men), all men who have a life expectancy of at least 10 years (5 years for African Americans) should have a digital rectal examination (DRE) and measurement of prostate-specific antigen (PSA) as part of their annual checkup. One study shows that most all malignant lesions will be detected if both forms of examination are used, but by itself, PSA is not an entirely reliable screening test. Risk factors are thought to include age, family history and ethnic heritage. Studies on preventive factors are looking at herbal supplements, the antioxidant lycopene, high levels of dietary fruits and vegetables, vitamin E, selenium, androgen levels, physical activity, and body weight/adiposity.

Once a malignancy is found, physicians decide treatment by considering the man's general health, age, life expectancy, and personal preferences for treatment. Prostate cancer is generally relatively slow growing. Because of this some research suggests that when prostate cancer is found in an otherwise healthy and active 75-year-old man, the disease should simply be tracked because surgery and irradiation could be more deadly than the growth of tumors in elderly men. For the growing numbers of men who would like to remain healthy and active well into their nineties, however, 75 may seem an arbitrarily young age at which to decide not to pursue treatment. For younger men with aggressively spreading disease there is little debate about the appropriateness of definitive treatment. Prostate cancer treatment, however, is also not without difficulties. Depending on the extent of surgical excision or radiation required, treatment can lead to impotence and urinary

Carcinoma of the prostate showing perineural invasion by malignant glands. (From Kumar V et al: Robbins and Cotran pathologic basis of disease, *ed 7, Philadelphia, 2005, Saunders.)*

Genital and Reproductive Function

incontinence. As compared to loss of life these may seem a small price to pay.

For women, breast cancer is the most common cancer except for some forms of skin cancer and is the leading cause of death between the ages of 40 and 55 years. Breast cancer is the second leading cause of cancer deaths among women. The American Cancer Society estimates that 1 woman in 8 will develop invasive breast cancer at some time in their life.

Research has revealed a number of factors that may contribute to the incidence of breast cancer. Women who smoke cigarettes are considered to be at higher risk because cigarette smoke is carcinogenic. Women exposed to ionizing radiation before the age of 40 are more likely to get breast cancer, and there is evidence that women who have not given birth or who first give birth when older than 30 years are at greater risk. Alcohol intake has also been implicated as a risk factor for breast cancer. Researchers suspect that high fat intake contributes to the likelihood of breast cancer, and epidemiologic studies show that obesity increases the risk in women after menopause. Exogenous estrogen (estrogen supplied as treatment for menopausal hormone replacement) has been found to contribute to the risk for breast cancer, especially when used for five years or longer.

The American Cancer Society recommends annual mammograms and annual clinical breast exams for women beginning at age 40 years. Women with a first degree relative (mother, sister) who developed breast cancer before age 40 should start their annual mammograms and clinical breast exams at least five years earlier than the diagnosis of the cancer in the primary relative. Women not yet 40 should have a clinical breast exam at least every 3 years. The American College of Obstetricians and Gynecologists takes an even stronger position and suggests that women 19 years and older consider annual clinical breast examinations. All women 19 and older should perform regular self breast examinations. It is the triad of mammogram, clinical breast exam, and self breast exam that has been found to be most effective in the early detection of breast cancer.

Men also develop breast cancer. While breast cancer in men is much less frequent than in women, the CDC reports 1,815 breast cancer diagnoses and 362 breast cancer deaths among men in 2004. For men as with women, early detection is the best protection and provides the best range of options for treatment.

For breast and prostate cancer, investigators are beginning to be able to advise us on ways to reduce our risk. Some of the circumstances—family history, for example—are beyond our control. Some measures can help, however: a healthy and active lifestyle, attention to lifetime quality nutrition with high levels of plant foods, limiting alcohol use, maintaining a healthy weight, avoiding exposures to chemical toxins, radiation, or unnecessary hormone treatment, and attention to early and ongoing screening activities, all are beginning to show evidence as effective approaches for minimizing the risk for breast and prostate malignancies.

30

Male Genital and Reproductive Function

Marvin Van Every • David Mikkelsen • Carolyn Spence Cagle

MEDIA RESOURCES

Additional Material for Study, Review, and Further Exploration

CD Companion ■ Review Questions and Answers
■ Glossary (with audio pronunciations for selected terms)
■ Disease Profiles ■ Animations

evolve **Website** at http://evolve.elsevier.com/Copstead/
■ Case Studies ■ Disease Profiles ■ WebLinks ■ Key Points Review

Online Course (Module 15)

KEY QUESTIONS

■ What is the role of the Sertoli cells in spermatogenesis?
■ What is the function of Leydig cells?
■ Which branch of the autonomic nervous system is responsible for penile erection? Ejaculation?
■ Which genitourinary structures develop embryologically from the wolffian ductal system in males?

■ How do the hypothalamic-pituitary gonadotropic hormones influence male reproductive function?
■ How do the processes of capacitation and acrosome reaction affect the fertilization process?

CHAPTER OUTLINE

This chapter provides a foundation for comprehending male genital and reproductive disorders, which are presented in Chapter 31. The anatomy and embryology of the male genitourinary tract—those organs involved in the processes of sexual reproduction and elimination of nitrogenous wastes—will be presented first. Because these organs are derived from common embryologic structures, the anatomy and embryology of the male genitalia and urinary system will be emphasized, and the differences in embryologic development between males and females will be considered when pertinent. The remainder of this chapter will deal with the physiologic processes of male reproduction.

ANATOMY

Upper Genitourinary Tract

The upper genitourinary tract consists of the kidneys and ureters. The kidneys receive their blood from the renal arteries, which arise directly from the aorta. They are usually solitary but will at times be duplicated. The ureteral blood supply is derived from multiple sources. The renal pelvis and upper part of the ureter receive blood from branches of the renal artery. The arterial blood supply of the middle ureter segment comes from the internal spermatic artery, and the lowermost ureter sections receive blood from the branches of the common iliac, internal iliac, and vesical arteries (Figure 30-1). The veins of the renal pelvis and ureter are usually paired with the arteries.

Lower Genitourinary Tract

Bladder

The bladder is a hollow muscular organ that serves as a reservoir for urine. The adult bladder normally has a capacity of 450 to 500 ml. When empty, the bladder lies behind the pubic symphysis and is mainly a pelvic organ. With overdistention or chronic urine retention, the abdomen may bulge, allowing easy palpation of the bladder in the suprapubic region.

The ureters enter the bladder posteroinferiorly. The ureteral orifices are situated on a crescent-shaped ridge and are approximately 2.5 cm apart. The triangular area demarcated by this interureteric ridge and bladder neck is called the *trigone* (Figure 30-2). As will be discussed later in the chapter, the **trigone** has a different embryologic origin from the rest of the bladder body, or fundus. The trigone is composed of mesoderm, and the fundus is composed of endoderm.

In males, the bladder lies anterior to the seminal vesicles, vasa deferentia, ureters, and rectum. The dome and part of the posterior bladder surfaces are covered by peritoneum and are thus in close proximity to the small bowel and the sigmoid colon. The neck of the bladder, which is the most inferior part, leads to the urethra. In males, the prostate lies between the bladder and the muscle layers of the pelvic floor that composes the urogenital diaphragm.

The arterial blood supply of the bladder comes from the superior, middle, and inferior vesical arteries, which originate from the anterior division of the hypogastric artery. Venous

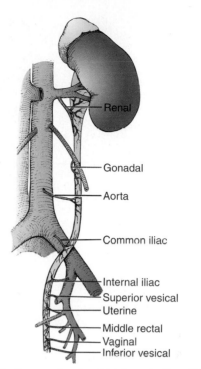

FIGURE 30-1 Sources of ureteral blood supply. (From Walsh PC et al, editors: *Campbell's urology*, ed 7, Philadelphia, 1998, Saunders, p 38.)

Labels: Renal, Gonadal, Aorta, Common iliac, Internal iliac, Superior vesical, Uterine, Middle rectal, Vaginal, Inferior vesical

drainage occurs by a rich plexus of veins that surround the bladder and ultimately drain into the hypogastric veins.

The bladder and urethra receive their nerve supply from both the sympathetic and parasympathetic divisions of the autonomic nervous system. The sympathetic fibers, originating mainly from the lower thoracic and upper lumbar segments (T11-T12 and L1-2), innervate the bladder and urethra as the hypogastric nerves. These sympathetic fibers are distributed more densely in the bladder base and proximal end of the urethra than in the bladder dome. The sympathetic nerves facilitate storage of urine. Studies have revealed differences in the bladder muscle receptors, with cholinergic receptors concentrated in the fundus and adrenergic receptors present in the trigone and proximal end of the urethra (Figure 30-3).

The parasympathetic nerve supply originates from the sacral segments (S2-S4), which proceed to form a plexus surrounding the bladder. In the male, a separate segment will reach the prostate and form the prostatic plexus. From this plexus, nerves emerge to innervate the erectile tissue of the male penis and the clitoris of the female (see Figure 30-3).

Branches of the bladder plexus penetrate the muscular coat of the bladder and become distributed throughout the detrusor. Parasympathetic muscle receptors are cholinergic in nature, and parasympathetic stimulation induces a detrusor contraction that causes bladder emptying.

Urethra

The male urethra, which extends from the bladder to the external opening (urethral meatus) at the tip of the penis, functions as a conduit for both the urinary and genital systems.

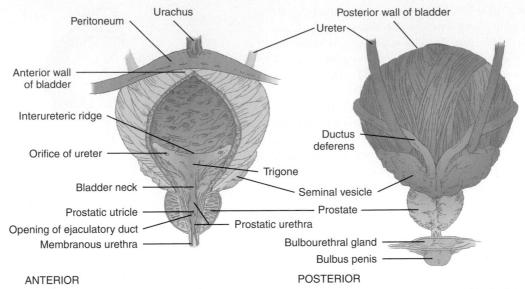

FIGURE 30-2 Anterior and posterior views of the prostate gland and related structures. The triangular area demarcated by the interureteric ridge and the bladder neck is the trigone. (From Black JM et al: *Medical-surgical nursing: clinical management for positive outcomes,* ed 6, Philadelphia, 2001, Saunders, p 940.)

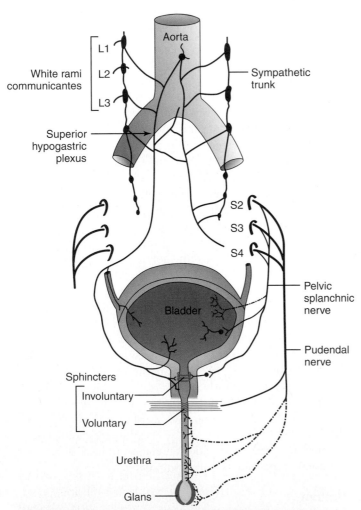

FIGURE 30-3 Diagram of nerve supply to bladder and urethra. (From Sauerland EK: *Grants dissector,* ed 10, Baltimore, 1991, Williams & Wilkins, p 66.)

It is commonly divided into three segments: the prostatic, the *membranous,* and the *penile* or *spongy urethra* (Figure 30-4).

Auxiliary Genital Glands

The auxiliary genital glands of the male consist of the *prostate,* the *seminal vesicles,* and the *bulbourethral glands.* These glands secrete products that contribute to the seminal fluid.

Prostate

The **prostate** lies below the bladder and has both a muscular and a glandular component. The normal prostate weighs about 20 g and measures about 3.5 cm transversely and about 2.5 cm in its vertical and anteroposterior dimensions. The prostate is conical and is anterior to the rectum. Its base is continuous with the bladder neck, and the inferior aspect of the prostate gland, or apex, lies adjacent to the urogenital diaphragm (Figure 30-5).

The prostate consists of a thin fibrous capsule with internally circular smooth muscle fibers and collagenous tissue that surround the urethra. Deep in this layer of connective and elastic tissue lies the prostatic stroma, which contains the prostatic epithelial glands. These glands drain into excretory ducts, which open chiefly on the floor of the urethra between the verumontanum and the vesical neck. The prostate is primarily a reproductive organ. It and the seminal vesicles produce the fluid that support the sperm. In fact, the sperm constitute a small amount of the semen with the vast majority of the seminal fluid coming from the prostate and seminal vesicles. A further function of the prostate gland is to act as a valve for the bladder.

The main blood supply of the prostate is derived from the inferior vesical artery, a branch of the hypogastric artery. Besides the prostate, this artery also supplies the distal portion of the ureter, the seminal vesicles, and part of the bladder.

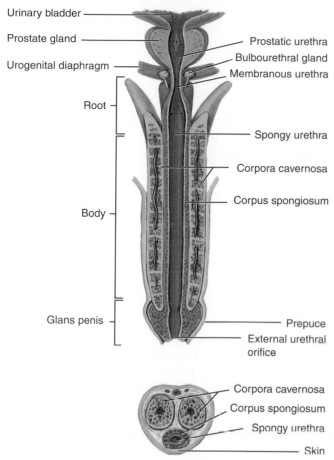

Urinary bladder

Prostate gland

Urogenital diaphragm

Prostatic urethra

Bulbourethral gland

Membranous urethra

Root

Spongy urethra

Corpora cavernosa

Corpus spongiosum

Body

Glans penis

Prepuce

External urethral orifice

Corpora cavernosa

Corpus spongiosum

Spongy urethra

Skin

FIGURE 30-4 Cross-sectional view of the penis emphasizing the membranous urethra, the urogenital diaphragm, the bulbourethral or Cowper gland, and the orifices of the bulbourethral glands. (From Applegate EJ: *The anatomy and physiology learning system: textbook,* ed 2, Philadelphia, 2000, Saunders, p 401.)

A complex plexus situated between the prostate and overlying tissue freely communicates with the inferior hypogastric veins and provides venous drainage to the prostate.

Seminal Vesicles

The **seminal vesicles** are paired organs that lie next to the prostate under the base of the bladder (see Figure 30-5). Their coiled pouches secrete a fluid important to the survival of spermatozoa.

Bulbourethral Glands

The **bulbourethral** or **Cowper glands** are located on each side of the membranous urethra within the urogenital diaphragm. They add a mucoid secretion to the semen.

External Genitalia

Scrotum

The **scrotum** (see Figure 30-5) is a pouchlike sac that lies below the penis and pubic symphysis. A septum of connective tissue divides the sac into two compartments. Each compartment contains a male gonad, or testis, with its associated

epididymis and the lower portion of the vas deferens protected by the spermatic cord and its coverings. The scrotum not only supports the testes but also, by relaxation and contraction of its muscular layer, helps regulate temperature of the testes.

The scrotal sac consists of several tissue layers. The scrotal skin overlies the dartos muscle layer, whose smooth muscle fibers are embedded in loose connective tissue. The dartos muscle functions to contract the scrotal pouch with cold and expand it with heat. Under the dartos layer are several fascial layers (see Figure 30-5) that are continuous with the muscular layers of the abdominal wall and make up the covering of the spermatic cord. The external spermatic fascia is continuous with the external oblique aponeurosis of the abdominal wall. A few slips of skeletal muscle derived from the internal oblique muscle layer make up the cremasteric muscle, which adds to the upper part of the cord. The internal spermatic fascia is a continuation of the transverse fascia of the abdominal wall, with the transversus abdominis muscle not contributing to the cord layers. Finally, the peritoneum provides the tunica vaginalis layers, which are actually cut off from the abdominal cavity by obliteration of the processus vaginalis.

The scrotum receives its blood supply from the external pudendal artery, a branch of the femoral artery. In addition, the scrotum receives blood from portions of the internal pudendal artery (a branch of the hypogastric artery), the cremasteric, and testicular arteries that transverse the spermatic cord.

Testes

The **testes** are the male reproductive organs responsible for sperm production. They average about 4 to 5 cm in length and 2 to 3 cm in thickness. The testes lie within the scrotum and are suspended by the spermatic cord. The testes are covered by a thick fascial layer called the tunica albuginea. This layer invaginates posteriorly to form the mediastinum testis. This fibrous mediastinum sends fibrous septa into each testis that separate it into many different lobules. Each lobule contains one to four seminiferous tubules that if stretched to full length would measure approximately 60 cm. Spermatozoa production occurs within the epithelial lining of the seminiferous tubules (Figure 30-6).

The seminiferous tubules have a basement membrane consisting of elastic and connective tissue that supports the seminiferous cells. The seminiferous cells are either **Sertoli cells** (supporting cells) or spermatogenic cells. Found between the seminiferous tubules and embedded in connective tissue, the interstitial **Leydig cells** produce and secrete testosterone, a hormone involved in the development of male sexual characteristics (Figure 30-7). The seminiferous tubules converge on the mediastinum testis. The tubules, which are connected by the straight efferent ducts, drain into the head of the epididymis.

The testicular blood supply is derived from the internal spermatics, which arise directly from the aorta below the renal arteries. They course inferiorly through the spermatic cord and anastomose with the cremasteric arteries and the arteries of the vas; these vessels also contribute to the blood supply.

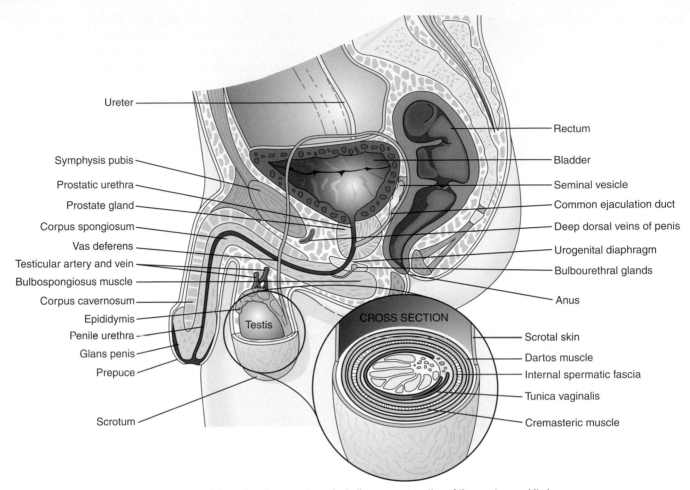

FIGURE 30-5 Male genitourinary anatomy, including a cross-section of the scrotum and its layers.

The blood from the testis returns through a plexus of veins in the spermatic cord (the pampiniform plexus) that forms the spermatic veins. The left internal spermatic vein enters the left renal vein, which subsequently enters the vena cava. The right internal spermatic vein enters the vena cava directly.

Epididymis and Ductus Deferens

The **epididymis** is a tightly coiled tube that lies along the top of and behind each testis. It is divided into the head, situated at the upper pole of the testes; the body, lying posterior to the testes; and the tail, which is attached to the inferior pole of the testes (see Figure 30-6). The body and the tail of the epididymis form one continuous tube that serves as a conduit for maturing spermatozoa. In the epididymis, sperm develop the ability to swim.

As the convoluted tube of the tail leaves its testicular attachments, it increases in diameter to become a thick, muscular tube called the **ductus deferens,** also called the **vas deferens.** Leaving the spermatic cord, the vas deferens follows an extraperitoneal course and passes caudally and laterally along the pelvic wall. As it passes medial to the distal end of the ureter, it bends caudally to reach the midline and lies on the posterior wall of the bladder just medial to the seminal vesicles.

It terminates in a dilated ampulla that courses underneath the base of the prostate. At this point the duct of the seminal vesicle joins with the duct of the ampulla, and the ejaculatory duct is formed. The ejaculatory ducts open in the prostatic urethra at the level of the verumontanum.

Penis

The **penis** is the male organ of copulation and urinary excretion. It is composed of three erectile bodies—two paired **corpora cavernosa,** which lie dorsally, and the *corpus spongiosum,* which contains the urethra (Figure 30-8). Grossly, the penis is divided into three segments. The root of the penis consists of the proximal ends of the corpora cavernosa, which attach to the pelvic bones, and the proximal end of the corpus spongiosum, which connects to the undersurface of the urogenital diaphragm. Together these attachments provide fixation and stability to the penis. The shaft of the penis consists of all three erectile bodies: the two cavernous bodies lying on the dorsum, and the corpus spongiosum, which occupies a depression on their ventral surface. Finally, the glans of the penis forms the distal segment of the corpus spongiosum.

The three erectile bodies have the capability to become engorged with blood and enlarge considerably with erection.

FIGURE 30-6 The anatomy of the testis and epididymis. Note the numerous compartments of the testis that are filled with seminiferous tubules gathering into the rete testis; they join to form a markedly convoluted tubule that becomes the epididymis, which is continuous with the vas deferens. The epididymis attaches to the dorsomedial aspect of the testis, and the vas deferens joins the other structures of the spermatic cord.

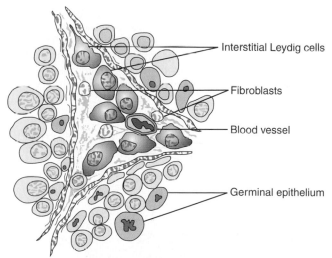

FIGURE 30-7 The interstitial Leydig cells, the cells that secrete testosterone, are located in the interstices between the seminiferous tubules. (From Guyton AC, Hall JE, editors: *Textbook of medical physiology*, ed 11, Philadelphia, 2006, Saunders, p 1003.)

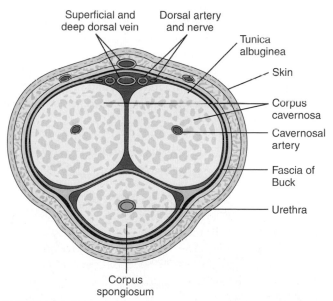

FIGURE 30-8 Transverse section through the penis. The paired upper structures are the corpora cavernosa. The single lower body surrounding the urethra is the corpus spongiosum.

Microscopically, these bodies have an internal spongelike network that consists of endothelium-lined spaces surrounded by smooth muscle.

Each corpus is enclosed in a fascial sheath, the tunica albuginea, and all are subsequently surrounded by a thick fibrous envelope known as the **fascia of Buck.** The overlying skin of the penis is remarkable for its thinness and looseness of connection with the fascial sheath of the penis. The skin of the penis is folded upon itself to form the **prepuce,** or **foreskin.** It is this penile skin overlying the glans that is removed with circumcision.

The arterial blood supply is primarily derived from the paired internal pudendal arteries, which are branches of the hypogastric arteries. Each internal pudendal artery branches several times in the penis. The deep or cavernous artery supplies the entire corpus cavernosum. The urethral artery supplies the corpus spongiosum, and the bulbar artery supplies the bulb of the corpus spongiosum. The dorsal artery continues along the dorsum of the penis and lies below the fascia of Buck and between two dorsal veins. It provides additional supply to the glans (Figure 30-9).

Venous drainage of the penis is through several channels. The cavernous veins drain the corpora cavernosa, and the circumflex veins join the deep dorsal vein of the penis to also drain the corpora. The superficial dorsal vein drains the glans and part of the distal portion of the corpora. Finally, a bulbar branch drains the bulbous urethra and proximal portion of the corpus spongiosum. Together these branches coalesce and pass through the urogenital diaphragm into the retropubic venous plexus of Santorini (see Figure 30-9).

The nerve supply of the penis is formed from both parasympathetic and sympathetic components. The parasympathetic fibers arise from S2-S4, and the sympathetic component is derived from the hypogastric plexus. Although the final neurotransmitters have not been completely defined, parasympathetic stimulation from the pudendal nerve results in relaxation of vascular resistance, which increases blood flow to the penis and creates an erection. The pudendal nerve also carries sensory fibers from the penis and enters the sacral spinal cord to contribute to penile erection.

Sympathetic nerve fibers may contribute to erectile capacity, but their role has not been proved conclusively. They do innervate the proximal involuntary sphincter of the bladder neck, where contraction prevents retrograde ejaculation of semen from the prostatic urethra into the bladder. They also innervate the muscles of the seminal vesicles and prostate, which when stimulated cause ejaculation of seminal fluid into the urethra.

KEY POINTS

- The upper genitourinary tract is composed of the kidneys and ureters. The lower genitourinary tract includes the bladder and urethra and the accessory male sexual organs.
- Ureters transport urine from the renal pelvis to the bladder. Ureters have several points of narrowing that predispose to obstruction: ureteropelvic junction, pelvic brim, and ureterovesical junction.
- The adult bladder has a normal capacity of 450 to 500 ml. With overdistention, the bladder may be palpable in the suprapubic region. The bladder is a muscular organ composed of several layers of muscle fibers. An important muscular landmark in the bladder is the trigone. Parasympathetic stimulation of the bladder results in bladder muscle contraction.
- The prostate is a key organ in the male genitourinary system with both reproductive and continence functions. It also causes many pathologic conditions as men age such as prostatitis, benign hyperplasia and cancer.
- The urethra extends from the bladder to the meatus at the end of the penis. In addition to transporting urine, the urethra has ducts that receive fluid from the prostate, seminal vesicles, and bulbourethral glands.
- The scrotal sac supports the testes and regulates their temperature. Testes contain several cell types important in sperm production and the development of secondary sex characteristics. Spermatogenic cells produce sperm in the testes. Sertoli cells serve to support and nurture spermatogenesis. Leydig cells produce and secrete testosterone.

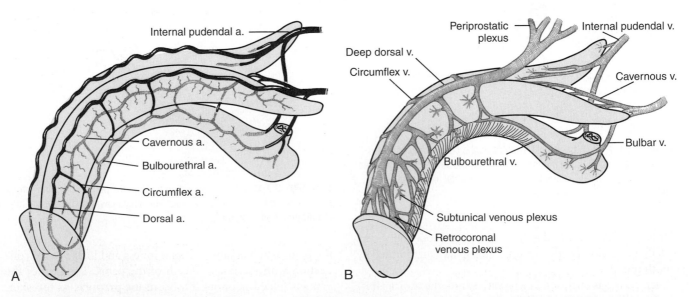

FIGURE 30-9 Penile arterial supply **(A)** and venous drainage **(B)**, longitudinal views. *a.,* Artery; *v.,* vein. (From Walsh PC et al, editors: *Campbell's urology,* ed 7, Philadelphia, 1998, Saunders, p 1160.)

- Situated in the testes, the epididymis serves as a collecting conduit for sperm. The epididymis is continuous with the ductus (vas) deferens. The vas travels along the pelvic wall and joins with the seminal vesicle duct at the prostate to form the ejaculatory duct. The ejaculatory ducts open into the urethra.
- Skin overlying the penis is very loose, which facilitates significant enlargement when the penis is engorged with blood during erection. Parasympathetic fibers forming the pudendal nerve are responsible for erection. Ejaculation is a function of the sympathetic nerve fibers.

EMBRYOLOGY

Developmental processes in the genital and urinary systems are intimately related. To facilitate understanding of this development, the two systems will be discussed in several subdivisions. The urinary system, which is composed of the nephric system and the vesicourethral unit, will be discussed first. The genital system, which is composed of the gonads, the genital ducts, and the external genitalia, will be discussed second.

Nephric System

The nephric system develops progressively through three distinct phases: the *pronephros, mesonephros,* and *metanephros.* The **pronephros** is the earliest state in humans but corresponds to the mature structure in primitive vertebrates. The pronephros consists of 6 to 10 pairs of tubules connected by a pronephric duct. It grows caudally to join the cloaca, a blind end of the hindgut. The pronephros is a temporary structure and, except for its duct, disappears by the fourth week of intrauterine life (Figure 30-10).

The **mesonephros** corresponds to the mature excretory organ of some amphibians. In humans it begins developing at about the fourth to fifth week of gestation.[1-4] The tubules of the mesonephros are more numerous and form a cuplike outgrowth into which capillaries push to form a primitive glomerulus. The tubules communicate with the mesonephric duct, which is derived from the preceding pronephric duct. The number of mesonephros tubules reaches a maximum by about 8 weeks of gestation and then degenerate.

The final stage of development, the **metanephros,** begins in the fourth week when the ureteral bud grows out of the mesonephric duct. The bud elongates in a dorsocranial direction, where it meets a mass of mesoderm, the nephrogenic blastema, and begins to differentiate into the ureter and renal collecting system.[1,4] The metanephros is derived from the nephrogenic blastema and eventually differentiates into the mature mammalian kidney.

Vesicourethral Unit

The blind end of the caudal hindgut forms the cloaca, which is separated from the outside by a thin membrane of tissue, the urogenital membrane. At about 4 weeks of gestation a septum grows downward and separates the cloaca into a posterior compartment, which will become the rectum, and an anterior compartment, which will form the urogenital sinus.

The urogenital sinus receives the mesonephric duct, which is progressively absorbed into this structure. The mesonephric duct distal to the ureteral bud is absorbed into the sinus, and its mesenchyme subsequently forms the bladder trigone. The ureter, which is derived from the ureteral bud, and the mesonephric duct, which differentiates into the vas deferens, merges into the sinus as well. In a complex pattern of development,

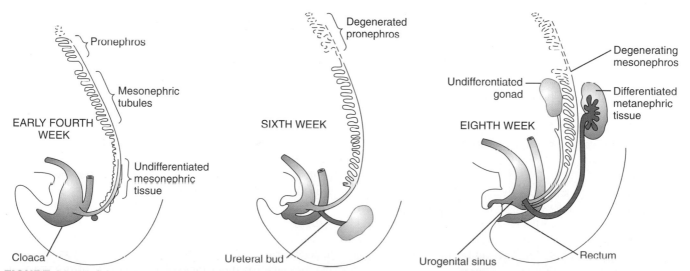

FIGURE 30-10 Schematic representation of the development of the nephric system. Only a few of the tubules of the pronephros are seen early in the fourth week, whereas the mesonephric tissue differentiates into mesonephric tubules that progressively join the mesonephric duct. The first sign of the ureteral bud from the mesonephric duct is shown. At 6 weeks, the pronephros has completely degenerated and the mesonephric tubules start to do so. The ureteral bud grows dorsocranially and has met the metanephrogenic cap. By the eighth week, cranial migration of the differentiating metanephros can be seen. The cranial end of the ureteric bud expands and starts to show multiple successive outgrowths. (From Tanagho FA, McAninch JW, editors: *Smith's general urology,* ed 13, East Norwalk, Conn, 1992, Appleton & Lange, p 18.)

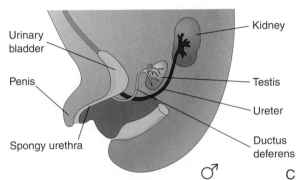

FIGURE 30-11 Diagrams showing division of the cloaca into the urogenital sinus and rectum; absorption of the mesonephric ducts; development of the urinary bladder, urethra, and urachus; and changes in location of the ureters. **A,** Lateral view of the caudal half of a 5-week embryo. The stages shown in **B** and **C** are reached by the 12th week. (From Moore KL, Persaud TVN, editors: *The developing human: clinically oriented embryology,* ed 8, Philadelphia, 2008, Saunders, p 258.)

the opening of the ureteral bud, which will eventually become the ureteral orifice, migrates upward and laterally. The opening of the mesonephric duct, which will become the ejaculatory duct, migrates downward and medially (Figure 30-11).

The urogenital sinus can be divided into two main segments. The ventral and pelvic portion, which receives the ureter, forms the bladder, part of the urethra in males, and the whole urethra in females. A phallic or urethral portion will receive the mesonephric ducts and in males will form a second part of the urethra. In females, this portion receives the müllerian ducts, which fuse distally to form the uterus and upper part of the vagina. The lower portion of the female urogenital sinus forms the lower part of the vagina and vaginal vestibule (Figure 30-12).

Gonads

The undifferentiated and primitive **gonads** are derived from the urogenital ridge, a dorsal region of thickening from which the primitive kidney also forms. The gonads serve as precursors to the testes in males and the ovaries in females. During the seventh week, an individual gonad begins to assume the characteristics of either a testis or an ovary.

In the presence of testis-determining factor, which is located on the Y chromosome, a gonad develops into a testis. The gland increases in size, and the cells of the epithelium grow centrally into the organ's mesenchyme. These ingrowths become radially arranged, form cords, and begin to converge

on the posterior aspect of the testis. The cords eventually differentiate into the seminiferous tubules, which produce spermatozoa. The testes descend behind the abdominal cavity in the retroperitoneal space and into the scrotum, usually by the eighth month of gestation.

In the absence of testis-determining factor, a gonad differentiates into an ovary, and a cortex forms from the germinal epithelium and ultimately gives rise to ovarian follicles containing ova. It descends only partially through the abdominal cavity and eventually lies adjacent to the fallopian tubes.

Genital Duct System

As the embryo develops, two different but related kinds of ducts form beside the undifferentiated gonads. The mesonephric, or **wolffian ducts,** as previously explained, develop as nephric ducts but will go on to form the male genital ducts. The **müllerian ducts** develop alongside the mesonephric ducts (paramesonephric) and are genital structures from the start.

Early in development, each of the two müllerian ducts arises lateral to the mesonephric ducts, either directly from the mesonephric ducts themselves or possibly from the adjacent epithelium of the primitive abdominal cavity. Both ducts grow caudally to enter the urogenital sinus.

If a gonad differentiates into a testis, the wolffian ducts subsequently develop into the male duct system consisting of the epididymis, vas deferens, seminal vesicles, and ejaculatory

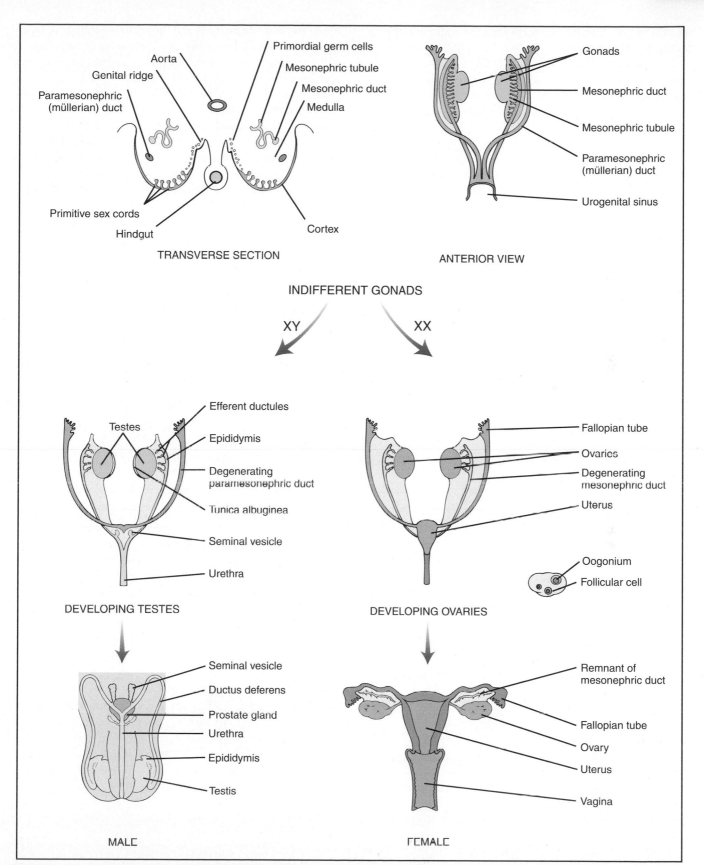

FIGURE 30-12 Transformation of the undifferentiated genital system into the definitive male and female systems. (From Nichols FH, Zwelling E: *Maternal-newborn nursing: theory and practice,* Philadelphia, 1997, Saunders, p 174.)

ducts. The müllerian ducts, except for a few rudimentary fragments, rapidly atrophy.

If, on the other hand, a gonad develops into an ovary, the müllerian ducts proceed to form the uterus, fallopian tubes, and upper part of the vagina. The mesonephric, or wolffian, ducts fail to develop further and remain rudimentary (see Figure 30-12).

External Genitalia

Development of the external genitalia begins at about 12 intrauterine weeks. Prior to this point, three small protuberances appear on the external aspect of the cloacal membrane. The genital tubercle is located anteriorly and the genital swellings are situated on either side of the membrane. In the seventh week, rupture of the urogenital membrane gives the urogenital sinus a separate opening on the undersurface of the genital tubercle.

In males, the genital or labioscrotal swellings migrate and fuse centrally to form the scrotum. The fused genital tubercles elongate. The elongated fused tubercles form a cylindric shape with a ventral groove communicating with the urogenital sinus. This groove subsequently becomes covered by folds of tissue and forms the penile urethra (Figure 30-13).

The female external genitalia closely resemble those of the male until about the eighth intrauterine week. At this

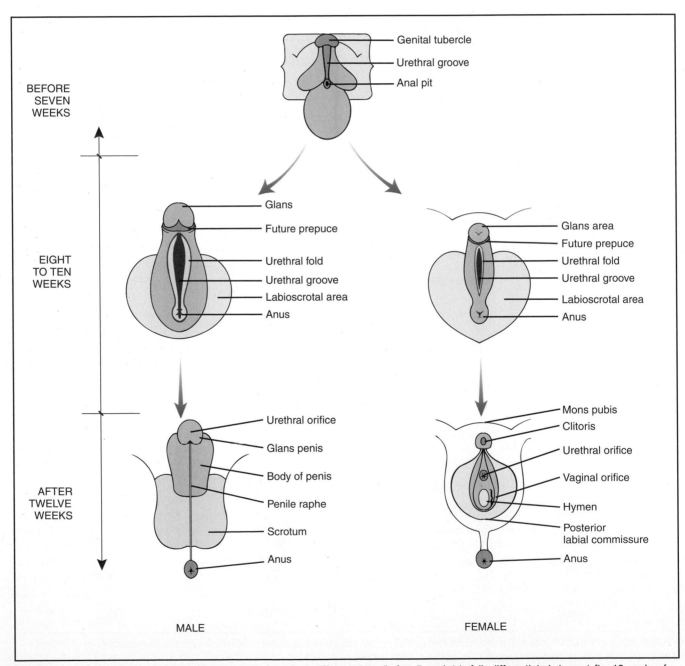

FIGURE 30-13 Development of the external genitalia from the indifferent stage (before 7 weeks) to fully differentiated stages (after 12 weeks of gestation). (From Nichols FH, Zwelling E: *Maternal-newborn nursing: theory and practice,* Philadelphia, 1997, Saunders, p 175.)

time the genital tubercle lags behind in growth and becomes the clitoris. The urogenital sinus shortens and widens somewhat to form the vaginal vestibule, and the genital swellings form the labia majora. The urethral folds become the labia minora.

KEY POINTS

- The fetal gonads can either become a testis or an ovary. The presence of the testis determining factor on the Y chromosome causes the testis to develop in the male fetus, while the absence of this factor allows the gonad to become an ovary in the female. Once the gonad has differentiated, it then is responsible for the cascade of events that lead to the formation of the female or male sexual organs and genitalia.
- During early embryonic development, the genital structures of males and females are similar. Two important ductal systems are the mesonephric (wolffian) ducts and the paramesonephric (müllerian) ducts. The mesonephric ducts develop to form the kidneys and the genital duct in males. In the presence of a testis, the wolffian ducts develop into the epididymis, vas deferens, seminal vesicles, and ejaculatory ducts. In the presence of an ovary, the müllerian ducts develop into the uterus, fallopian tubes, and upper part of the vagina, and the wolffian ducts fail to develop.
- Development of the external genitalia begins at about 12 weeks of gestation. In males the labioscrotal tissue fuses and elongates to form the scrotum and penis. In females, this tissue remains separated and forms the labia minora.

MALE REPRODUCTIVE PHYSIOLOGY

Hypothalamic-Pituitary-Testicular Axis

To fully understand male reproductive function, one must consider the endocrine function of the hypothalamic-pituitary-testicular axis. The components of this system function to maintain a constant level of the circulating hormones responsible for normal male sexual development and behavior, as well as the maturation of sperm necessary for fertility (Figure 30-14).

The hypothalamus is the integrating center for this hormonal axis. This organ coordinates neural messages from the central nervous system and humoral (blood-borne) messages from the testis to control the secretion of a small peptide hormone, gonadotropin-releasing hormone (GnRH). The pituitary stalk provides the route for GnRH to travel to the pituitary gland, which lies caudal to the hypothalamus. A system of veins, the pituitary portal system, traverses the pituitary stalk and maintains responsibility for transporting GnRH to the anterior portion of the pituitary gland.

In response to the secretion of GnRH, the pituitary synthesizes and releases two hormones, luteinizing hormone (LH)

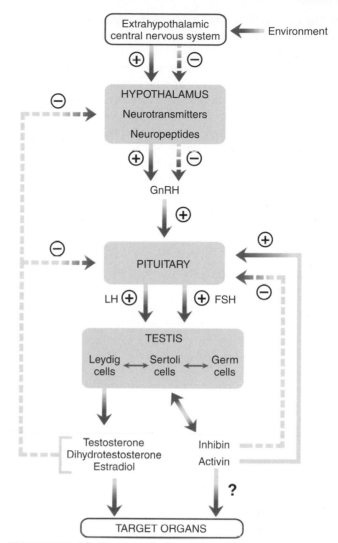

FIGURE 30-14 Diagram of the hypothalamic-pituitary-testicular axis. *GnRH,* Gonadotropin-releasing hormone; *LH,* luteinizing hormone; *FSH,* follicle-stimulating hormone. (Redrawn from Walsh PC et al, editors: *Campbell's urology,* ed 7, Philadelphia, 1998, Saunders, p 1240.)

and follicle-stimulating hormone (FSH). Although these hormones carry names related to their function in females, they are produced by both sexes through a feedback mechanism with GnRH for reproductive purposes.[5]

By binding to receptors on the surface of the testicular Leydig cells, LH mediates testosterone synthesis. Binding of LH produces an increase in the conversion of adenosine triphosphate to cyclic 3,5-adenosine monophosphate. This activity stimulates the production of other intracellular enzymes with subsequent increased synthesis of testosterone. Testosterone is then released into the bloodstream and adjacent seminiferous tubules.

Besides testosterone, other steroid hormones are synthesized, among them dihydrotestosterone, 17-hydroxyprogesterone, and estradiol. Dihydrotestosterone functions to differentiate and mature the male external genitalia and prostate.[6] In early puberty the production of androgen begins to increase, with normal adult plasma levels of testosterone and dihydrotestosterone being 300 to 1200 ng/dl and 30 to 60 ng/dl, respectively.

The function of FSH in male reproduction remains somewhat unclear. However, it appears that the production of sperm in the seminiferous tubules (spermatogenesis) requires the presence of high levels of both androgen and FSH.[7]

A feedback inhibition mechanism controls the secretion of both LH and FSH. Production of LH occurs in response to serum levels of testosterone and estradiol. The mechanism of the regulation of FSH is more hypothetical, but the existence of a nonsteroid factor called inhibin produced by Sertoli cells in response to FSH has been proposed.[8] In addition to inhibin, sex steroids also modulate FSH secretion through feedback inhibition on the pituitary.[7]

Spermatogenesis

To understand spermatogenesis, one must briefly consider the histology of the testis and its seminiferous tubules. As previously stated, Leydig cells occur in clusters in the interstitial tissue between the seminiferous tubules. These Leydig cells are responsible for the testicular production of testosterone.

The seminiferous tubules contain both germinal elements and supporting cells, which include the sustaining cells of the basement membrane and the Sertoli cells. The Sertoli cells rest on the basement membrane of the tubule and form a unique impermeable junction with each adjacent Sertoli cell. It is through this junction that the young germinal cells, or primary spermatocytes, migrate and pass from the basal compartment to the basement membrane and then to the central or adluminal compartment of the seminiferous tubule. The junction is also responsible for maintenance of the blood-testes barrier. This barrier ensures that the more mature spermatocytes and spermatids located in the adluminal compartment are behind the barrier and theoretically maintained in a constant intratubular environment to support the development of maturing sperm cells.[8]

The process of sperm production is called **spermatogenesis** and involves several phases (Figure 30-15). The proliferative phase involves division of the young germinal cells near the basement membrane (spermatogonia) either to replace their numbers or to produce daughter cells that will form spermatocytes. Next, a meiotic phase occurs in which spermatocytes undergo a reduction division. This division reduces

FIGURE 30-15 Process of meiosis in spermatogenesis.

the number of chromosomes to the monoploid number of 23 from the diploid number of 46. Finally, haploid spermatids undergo change to form mature **spermatozoa.**

As sperm cells mature and move from the basement membrane to the adluminal compartment, the Sertoli cells have an important nutritional role in the spermatogenic process. As the spermatid matures, it elongates and develops a tail, or **flagellum,** that attains a form similar to that of the mature spermatozoon. Mature spermatozoa are released into the tubular lumen and rapidly flow out to the rete testis and into the epididymis. Although each spermatogonium, one of the primitive male germ cells, requires about 70 days to develop into a mature sperm cell, or spermatozoon, within each tubule are spermatozoa in all stages of development. This characteristic allows new spermatozoa to be continuously produced across the male life span. The effects of aging on the male reproductive system are described in the Geriatric Considerations section.

Anatomy of Spermatozoa

The human spermatozoon is approximately 60 μm in length. The oval head contains a nucleus that is highly condensed and stabilized by cross-links between its molecules, which makes it very resistant to physical injury during its passage and storage in the epididymis. An outer membrane, the acrosome, contains the enzymes required for penetration of the female egg before fertilization.

The tail accounts for 90% of the length of the spermatozoon and is divided into a middle piece, principal piece, and end piece. The spermatozoon derives its motile ability from the motor apparatus of the tail, which is called the **axoneme.** The axoneme, which runs the length of the tail, is composed of a central pair of tubules surrounded by a ring of nine pairs of tubules (the 9 + 2 pattern). This ring of tubules is surrounded by a supporting structure of nine noncontractile dense fibers. Within the middle piece, a circular sheath of mitochondria[9] (Figure 30-16) surrounds these outer dense fibers.

The mitochondria contain the enzymes required for the production of adenosine triphosphate, the energy source for the cell. Within the axoneme are enzymes and structural proteins. These enzymes convert chemical energy from adenosine triphosphate to the mechanical energy of sperm cell movement to aid in fertilization of the egg.

Transport of Spermatozoa

Once mature spermatozoa are released from the Sertoli cells into the seminiferous tubules, they must pass through approximately 6 m of duct in the male reproductive tract before leaving the urethral meatus and being deposited in the vagina during sexual intercourse. From the seminiferous tubules, the spermatozoa are deposited into the rete testis, a collecting chamber for all the seminiferous tubules. From the rete testis, the sperm travel through the efferent ductules, 12 to 20 channels that pass into a single compact duct, the epididymis. The epididymis is a tightly convoluted duct that is divided into three regions: the caput (globus major), the corpus (body),

and the cauda epididymis (tail, or globus minor). Unfolded and stretched, the epididymis would measure 12 to 15 feet.

After leaving the epididymis, the sperm enter the ductus or vas deferens. Embryologically, this duct is derived from the mesonephric duct. It passes through the scrotum, traverses the inguinal canal into the pelvis, and then passes behind the bladder to enter the prostatic urethra at the ejaculatory ducts of the verumontanum. The terminal portion of the vas deferens is known as the **ampulla.** It is joined by the ducts of the seminal vesicle before entering the ejaculatory ducts.

As one passes in a proximal-to-distal direction from the efferent ducts to the vas deferens, the thickness of the muscle gradually increases. In the vas deferens, three interconnected smooth muscle layers form a thick muscular wall, with the ratio of wall thickness to lumen being the greatest in any human structure.[7] This thick muscular wall facilitates rapid sperm transport at the time of ejaculation.

Aside from serving as a conduit and storage depot for spermatozoa, the epididymis probably sustains maturational processes. Most studies have demonstrated that sperm taken directly from the testes are incapable of fertilizing eggs. It appears that the development of motility and increased fertility are acquired during transit through the epididymis.[7]

Because epididymal sperm are probably immotile, other mechanisms must be involved in their transport. Initially, spermatozoa are carried into the efferent ducts by fluid from the rete testis. Within the efferent ducts, motile cilia within the lumen function to reabsorb testicular fluid and help move spermatozoa into the epididymis. Within the epididymis, the spermatozoa are probably transported by rhythmic contraction of the smooth muscle cells.[7]

Ejaculation accelerates the passage of spermatozoa through the vas deferens and distal end of the epididymis. In young men, approximately 200 million sperm can be found in the

FIGURE 30-16 Anatomy of a mature sperm cell. (From Moore KL, Persaud TVN, editors: *The developing human: clinically oriented embryology,* ed 8, Philadelphia, 2008, Saunders, p 19.)

reservoir of the epididymis. About 50% are found in the cauda region. With ejaculation, sperm from the distal part of the epididymis and vas deferens are deposited into the prostatic urethra, where they account for less than 10% of the normal ejaculate.[10]

Erection, Emission, and Ejaculation

To penetrate the vagina and deposit sperm, the penis must be erect. The physiology of **erection** is a complicated interaction of vascular, neurologic, and hormonal factors. Although erection has classically been thought of as a parasympathetic function, it is more complex. Erection may be mediated by either local stimulation, which causes a reflexogenic erection through the sacral spinal cord, or psychological stimulation, which causes a psychogenic erection through cerebral centers. The presence of erections in patients with spinal cord injuries attests to the presence of reflex erections. Such patients have an intact sacral spinal cord and its reflex arc of afferent and efferent nerves below the site of spinal cord injury.

The penis receives sensory innervation from the pudendal sensory nerves entering the sacral spinal cord. The pudendal nerve is a mixed nerve that provides motor innervation to the pelvic floor musculature and penile sensory fibers. The efferent nerve to the erectile tissue is provided by sacral parasympathetic fibers. Although erection is possible in patients with spinal cord injuries, in intact men it is a much more controlled process influenced to a great extent by the cerebral cortex. Impulses may traverse the spinal cord from the cerebral cortex in the lateral columns and exit the spinal cord through sacral parasympathetic and possibly the thoracolumbar sympathetic nerves as well.[7]

During erection, the vascular spaces that make up the spongy vacuous tissues of the corpora cavernosa and corpus spongiosum fill with blood. The relaxation of smooth muscle tone in these structures that allows filling and subsequent penile erection is modulated by an undetermined neurotransmitter, most likely nitric oxide (NO). Research indicates that erectile function cannot be fully explained by parasympathetic or sympathetic mechanisms; this observation has led to consideration that nonadrenergic and noncholinergic neuromodulators may be involved in such function.[11] For example, penile injection of certain prostaglandins has been shown to induce smooth muscle relaxation and has been used to induce erections in some men experiencing erectile dysfunction.[12]

Ejaculation may be divided into two phases: *emission* and *ejaculation*. During **emission,** secretions from the periurethral glands, seminal vesicles, and prostate are deposited with sperm from the vasa deferentia and the cauda epididymis into the prostatic urethra. Control of emission is mediated primarily through the sympathetic nerves, which stimulate contraction of smooth muscle in these genital structures.

With **ejaculation,** the bladder neck or internal sphincter closes. This closure is also mediated through the sympathetic nervous system. Next, the external sphincter relaxes and the perineal and bulbourethral muscles surrounding the bulb of the corpus spongiosum contract and expel the ejaculate from the posterior urethra and through the urethral meatus.

The physiologic function of the secretory products of the accessory sex glands is uncertain. These secretions make up most of the seminal plasma, with the sperm and testicular fluid probably composing less than 10% of the final ejaculated semen volume. Although some investigators have demonstrated that sperm removed directly from the epididymis are capable of fertilization, these secretions most likely optimize conditions for sperm motility, survival, and transport in both the female and male reproductive tracts.

Capacitation

Capacitation of the spermatozoa refers to the multiple changes that activate the sperm and enhance their ability to participate in the final process of fertilization. Although sperm are anatomically complete and highly motile when ejaculated, the complex process of capacitation is necessary before the sperm are actually capable of fertilizing the egg. The capacitation process occurs over a period of 1 to 10 hours and occurs in sperm only after they have been introduced into the vagina of the female. Once the sperm are inside the female, the uterine and fallopian tube fluids wash away the various inhibitory factors that had suppressed sperm activity in the male genital ducts. During the time that the spermatozoa were in the fluid of the male genital ducts, they were continually exposed to many floating vesicles from the seminiferous tubules containing large amounts of cholesterol. This cholesterol, continually donated to the cellular membrane covering the sperm acrosome, toughens the outside membrane and prevents release of its enzymes. After ejaculation, the sperm that are deposited in the vagina swim away from the cholesterol vesicles upward into the uterine fluid, and they gradually lose much of their excess cholesterol during the next few hours. As the cholesterol is lost, the membrane at the head of the sperm becomes much weaker.

The membrane of the sperm head also becomes much more permeable to calcium ions. Large amounts of calcium enter the sperm to increase the powerful whiplike motion of the flagellum beyond its previously weak, undulating motion. In addition, the calcium ions probably also alter the intracellular membrane covering the leading edge of the acrosome, thus making it possible for the acrosome to release its enzymes very rapidly and easily as the sperm penetrates the granulosa cell mass surrounding the ovum. These enzymes are released even more rapidly and easily as the sperm attempts to penetrate the zona pellucida of the ovum itself.[13]

Acrosome Reaction

The head of a sperm is essentially a highly compact package of genetic chromatin material covered by a specialized **acrosome** and acrosomal (head) cap. Stored in the acrosome of the sperm are large quantities of hydrolytic (water-splitting) enzymes that are released during capacitation. The specialized acrosomal enzymes first break down cervical mucus to allow sperm to pass into the uterus and uterine tubes. If an ovum is present in the female reproductive tract when semen is introduced, continued release of acrosomal enzymes results in digestion of proteins in the structural elements of the outer covering of the egg. A high sperm count is essential for male fertility because the female ovum, once it is expelled from the ovarian follicle into the abdominal cavity and fallopian tube, contains multiple layers of granulosa cells. Before a sperm can fertilize the ovum, it must first pass through the granulosa cell layer, and then it must penetrate the thick covering of the ovum itself, the **zona pellucida.** It is believed that the acrosomal enzyme hyaluronidase plays an important role in opening pathways between the granulosa cells so that the sperm can reach the ovum.

On reaching the zona pellucida of the ovum, the anterior membrane of the sperm binds specifically with a receptor protein in the zona pellucida. Then the entire anterior membrane of the acrosome rapidly dissolves, and all the acrosomal enzymes are immediately released. Within minutes, these open a penetrating pathway for passage of the sperm head through the zona pellucida.

The head at first enters the perivitelline space lying beneath the zona pellucida but outside the membrane of the underlying oocyte. Within 30 minutes, the membranes of the sperm head and the oocyte fuse; the sperm genetic material enters the oocyte to cause fertilization, and the embryo begins to develop.

GERIATRIC CONSIDERATIONS

A decline in male fertility and reproductive organ function usually occurs with aging. However, the magnitude of functional decline of the male reproductive organs is variable. For example, some elderly men maintain their fertility into their 70s and 80s.

Male reproductive organ variability is due to organ-specific tissue changes. Active male germinal cells continue to produce spermatozoa (spermatogenesis), although the number of sperm produced declines proportionally over time. The testes become smaller as a result of increased connective tissue, fibrosis of the tubules, and decreased numbers of capillaries. The number of active seminiferous tubules declines with aging. The number of Leydig cells that produce testosterone decreases, leading to a decrease in testosterone with aging.

The arteries and veins in the penis become increasingly sclerotic. The penis itself becomes smaller, with an increase in fibroelastic tissue. Penile sensation is decreased. Sexually, the aging male has a longer refractory period after orgasm and decreased force of ejaculation.

KEY POINTS

- Normal male sexual development and spermatogenesis depend on the appropriate secretion of reproductive hormones. GnRH, secreted by the hypothalamus, induces the anterior pituitary gland to secrete LH and FSH. The bloodstream receives these hormones, which then travel to the testes where they bind to testicular cells.

- Leydig cells in the testes possess LH receptors and respond by increasing production of testosterone. Testosterone and related androgens are necessary for maturation of the male external genitalia. The function of FSH is less well understood, but it may be necessary for spermatogenesis.

- Spermatogenesis occurs when germinal cells within the seminiferous tubules undergo meiosis to form haploid (23 chromosomes) spermatids. Spermatids then develop into mature spermatozoa with the assistance of Sertoli cells. Sperm require 70 days to mature, and they are continuously produced and released into the epididymis.

- Sperm are well formed to perform their function in that they have a highly stabilized nucleus that is resistant to physical trauma, a mobile tail (axoneme) for swimming, and specialized enzymes to enhance penetration of the egg.

- Sperm traveling from their site of origin in the testes must travel through approximately 6 m of tubules before arriving at the penile meatus. This tubular system includes the seminiferous tubules in the testes, epididymis, vas deferens, and urethra. About 200 million sperm may be stored in the epididymal reservoir. Increased motility and fertility appear to be acquired by sperm as they pass through the epididymis. Sperm account for less than 10% of the ejaculate volume.

- The physiologic process of erection is a complex interplay of vascular, neurologic, and hormonal factors. The sacral parasympathetic nerves provide important innervation to the penis. Acetylcholine from parasympathetic nerves causes relaxation of penile smooth muscle with subsequent engorgement. Injected prostaglandins may also induce penile erections.

- The sympathetic nervous system mediates the process of ejaculation. Sympathetic actions include contraction of the internal sphincter to prevent retrograde ejaculation and relaxation of the external sphincter to allow emission.

- Sperm deposited in the vagina undergo further changes in a process known as capacitation. This process improves the chances of sperm successfully producing fertilization of an egg. Enzymes are released (acrosome reaction) to facilitate penetration of the ovum, a process that further increases the chances of successful fertilization.

SUMMARY

The male genitourinary tract may be divided into upper and lower tracts, with the upper tract composed of the kidneys and ureters and the lower tract composed of the bladder and urethra. Auxiliary genital glands that lie adjacent to or surround the urethra include the prostate, seminal vesicles, and bulbourethral glands. The external genitalia of the male consist of the scrotum, testes, epididymis, and penis.

Embryologic development of the male and female genital and urinary systems is closely related. The nephric system develops progressively through three distinct phases: the pronephros, mesonephros, and metanephros. The gonads are derived from the urogenital ridge, from which the primitive kidney also forms. Finally, the genital duct systems develop from two different but related ducts adjacent to the undifferentiated gonads, the müllerian ducts and the mesonephric, or wolffian, ducts.

Male reproductive function depends on an intact hypothalamic-pituitary-testicular endocrine axis. Spermatogenesis takes place in the seminiferous tubules. Spermatozoa mature in their transit through the male reproductive tract. Through erection, emission, and ejaculation, sperm enter the vagina. Through capacitation and the acrosome reaction, spermatozoa acquire the ability to fertilize ova residing in the female reproductive tract.

REFERENCES

1. Bullock N, Sibley G, Whitaker R: *Essential urology*, ed 2, Edinburgh, 1994, Churchill Livingstone, pp 1-2.
2. Zderic SA, Levin RM, Wein AJ: Voiding function and dysfunction. In Gillenwater JY et al, editors: *Adult and pediatric urology,* vol 2, ed 3, St Louis, 1996, Mosby, pp 1159-1219.
3. Redman JF: Anatomy of the genitourinary system. In Gillenwater JY et al, editors: *Adult and pediatric urology,* vol 1, ed 3, St Louis, 1996, Mosby, pp 3-61.
4. Kissane JM: Development and structure of the urogenital system. In Murphy WM, editor: *Urological pathology*, ed 2, Philadelphia, 1997, Saunders, pp 1-3.
5. Hoffman GE, Berghorn KA: Gonadotropin-releasing hormone neurons: their structure and function, *Semin Reprod Endocrinol* 15(1):5-17, 1997.
6. Grayhack JT, Kozlowski JM: Benign prostatic hyperplasia. In Gillenwater JY et al, editors: *Adult and pediatric urology,* vol 2, ed 3, St Louis, 1996, Mosby, pp 1501-1574.
7. Meacham RB, Lipschultz LI, Howards SS: Male infertility. In Gillenwater JY et al, editors: *Adult and pediatric urology,* vol 2, ed 3, St Louis, 1996, Mosby, pp 1747-1802.
8. Pyror JP: Male infertility. In Sant GR, editor: *Pathophysiologic principles of urology*, Oxford, 1994, Blackwell, pp 155-179.
9. Gondos B, Wong T-W: Non-neoplastic diseases of the testis and epididymis. In Murphy WM, editor: *Urological pathology*, ed 2, Philadelphia, 1997, Saunders, pp 277-341.
10. Pabst RZ: Investigations of the construction and function of the human ductus deferens, *Z Anat Entwicklungsgesch* 129(20):154-176, 1969.
11. Lerner SE, Melman A, Christ G: A review of an erectile dysfunction: new insights and more questions, *J Urol* 149(5):1246-1255, 1993.
12. O'Leary MP, Lue TF: Penile function. In Sant GR: *Pathophysiologic principles of urology*, Oxford, 1994, Blackwell, pp 181-207.
13. Guyton AC, Hall JE: Reproductive and hormonal functions of the male (and the pineal gland). In Guyton AC, Hall JE, editors: *Textbook of medical physiology*, ed 9, Philadelphia, 1996, Saunders, pp 1003-1016.

Alterations in Male Genital and Reproductive Function

chapter
31

Marvin Van Every • David Mikkelsen • Donna W. Bailey

MEDIA RESOURCES

Additional Material for Study, Review, and Further Exploration

CD Companion ■ Review Questions and Answers
■ Glossary (with audio pronunciations for selected terms)
■ Disease Profiles ■ Animations

evolve **Website** at http://evolve.elsevier.com/Copstead/
■ Case Studies ■ Disease Profiles ■ WebLinks ■ Key Points Review

Online Course (Module 15)

KEY QUESTIONS

■ What are the common causes of and clinical findings in priapism?
■ What are the common causes of primary and secondary impotence?
■ What are the usual clinical manifestations and significance of testicular cancer, testicular torsion, cryptorchidism, and hydrocele or spermatocele?

■ What clinical manifestations would lead to a suspicion of prostatitis, and how would confirmed prostatitis be treated?
■ How can benign prostatic hyperplasia be distinguished from prostate cancer?
■ What clinical manifestations are indicative of prostatic enlargement?

CHAPTER OUTLINE

The male genital system is susceptible to numerous congenital, acquired, and infectious conditions and, to a lesser extent, neoplasms. These disorders may interrupt the normal functions of urinary excretion and sexual function and fertility and directly affect the quality of life. This chapter will identify and explain the most common conditions that come to the attention of practitioners.

Disorders of the Penis and Male Urethra

CONGENITAL ANOMALIES

Micropenis. **Micropenis** is defined as a small, normally formed penis with a stretched length more than two standard deviations below the mean.[1] The normal range in newborns is 2.0 to 3.5 cm, so micropenis may be defined as a stretched length of less than 1.9 cm.[2]

Etiology and Pathogenesis. Penile development and growth are both testosterone dependent. Therefore, micropenis may result from defects in testosterone production or a deficiency that results in poor growth of the organs that are targets of this hormone.

Diagnoses and Treatment. Patients with micropenis must be evaluated for endocrine abnormalities. To check for these, one should measure serum levels of testosterone, luteinizing hormone, and follicle-stimulating hormone. Depending on what these measurements show, the problem may be determined to involve the hypothalamic-pituitary axis (Prader-Willi and Kallmann syndromes) or testicular disorders (Klinefelter syndrome).[3]

Treatment depends on providing testosterone, either intramuscularly or topically, to stimulate penile growth. Such treatment requires caution because growth may be altered by premature closure of the epiphyseal growth plates in the long bones. In rare cases, when micropenis fails to respond to testosterone, a female sex assignment is indicated.[3]

Urethral Valves. The vast majority of **urethral valves** are posterior in location and occur in the distal prostatic urethra. They are the most common cause of urinary obstruction in male newborns and infants. These valves are mucosal folds that resemble thin membranes and cause obstruction when the child attempts to void (Figure 31-1).

Etiology. Many theories have been given to explain how valves develop. It has been suggested that several different processes may occur to form different posterior valves. Most commonly, posterior valves may result from abnormal insertion and persistence of the distal wolffian ducts. Less frequently, a persistent urogenital membrane may result in valves and obstruction.[4]

Clinical Manifestations. Children with posterior valves may have variable degrees of obstruction. In the most severe cases, intrauterine renal failure may cause oligohydramnios (decreased amniotic fluid), pulmonary hypoplasia (incomplete lung development), and either stillbirth or extreme distress at the time of delivery. More frequently, inability to void is noted shortly after birth (normal voiding occurs within

48 hours after birth), or the infant has abdominal masses representing a thickened palpable bladder or hydronephrotic kidneys. Varying degrees of azotemia and renal failure occur with this scenario. Finally, urinary ascites (extravasated urine in the peritoneum) may result from a urinary leak that is usually difficult to localize. In an infant with abdominal distention, the diagnosis of urethral valves is confirmed by a plain abdominal radiograph showing the bowel "floating" in the center of the abdomen. Prenatal ultrasounds often suggest the diagnosis before birth so immediate evaluation and treatment can take place upon delivery.

Older infants with a urethral valve are less likely to have a palpable kidney or ascites. Rather, urinary infection, poor stream with straining to void, or occasionally hematuria may be present. Urethral valves in these older male infants may not produce much obstruction, thus making the diagnosis more difficult.[5]

Treatment. Management of posterior valves involves initial management of the metabolic abnormalities with appropriate fluid management and electrolyte replacement. In patients with a urinary tract infection, drainage of urine with a urethral or occasionally a suprapubic catheter is necessary. Finally, ablation of the valves with an endoscopic resectoscope should be performed. In infants, this step may be delayed and a cutaneous vesicostomy made to temporarily divert and drain the urine. This approach reduces the risk of traumatizing the infant's delicate urethra, which may create urethral stricture disease.

Rarely, urethral valves are located anteriorly in the penile urethra. Valves in this location are a very rare congenital anomaly and most likely represent urethral dilation or a diverticulum proximal to the valve.[6] Endoscopic resection will correct the problem.

Urethrorectal and Vesicourethral Fistulas

Etiology. **Urethrorectal** and **vesicourethral fistulas** are rare and almost always associated with an imperforate anus. Failure of the urorectal septum to develop completely leads to persistent communication between the rectum posteriorly and the urogenital tract anteriorly.

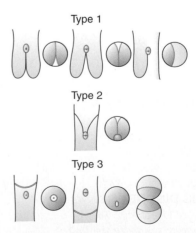

FIGURE 31-1 Posterior urethral valves. (Redrawn from Young HH, Frontz WA, Baldwin JC: Congenital obstruction of the posterior urethra, *J Urol* 3:289, 1919.)

Clinical Manifestations and Treatment. Children with a urethrorectal or vesicourethral fistula may pass fecal material and gas through the urethra. If the anus has formed normally with an external opening, urine may drain through the rectum. The diagnosis is made with cystoscopy and contrast-enhanced radiography to delineate a blind rectal pouch or communication. Surgery is needed to resect the fistula and open the imperforate anus.

Hypospadias. In hypospadias, the urethral meatus is located on the ventral undersurface of the penis or on the perineum (Figure 31-2). The condition may occur with varying degrees of severity. In the least severe cases, the meatus is located distally on the penis, either at the corona or on the undersurface of the glans. With increasing severity of the condition, the meatus assumes a more proximal location and is more often associated with chordee, or curvature of the penile shaft (Figure 31-3).

Etiology and Treatment. Hypospadias is the result of incomplete fusion of the urethral folds, so the meatus may be found anywhere along the phallus from the perineum to the glans. In the majority of cases hypospadias occurs distally, with about 85% of all cases involving the glans or corona.[7] Because incomplete fusion of urethral folds may indicate insufficient masculinization, it is recommended that the more severe penoscrotal and perineal openings be evaluated for conditions of intersex.[8]

FIGURE 31-2 Varying forms of hypospadias. **A,** Glandular hypospadias. **B,** Subcoronal hypospadias. Note the dorsal hood of foreskin. **C,** Penoscrotal hypospadias with chordee. **D,** Perineal hypospadias with chordee and partial penoscrotal transposition. **E,** Megameatal variant of hypospadias diagnosed following circumcision; note absence of hooded foreskin. (From Kliegman RM et al: *Nelson textbook of pediatrics,* ed 18, Philadelphia, 2007, Saunders, p. 2254.)

FIGURE 31-3 Epispadias **(A)** and hypospadias **(B)** showing possible locations of the urethral meatus. (From Black JM, Matassarin-Jacobs E: *Medical-surgical nursing: clinical management for continuity of care,* ed 6, Philadelphia, 2001, Saunders, p 971.)

Management of hypospadias involves surgical repair. Many procedures are available, with several repairs indicated for each type of hypospadias. The goal of surgery is a good overall cosmetic appearance that will allow the patient to stand and direct his urinary stream and will also allow normal sexual function.

Epispadias. In **epispadias,** the urethra opens on the dorsal aspect of the penis at a point proximal to the glans (see Figure 31-2). Although much less common than hypospadias, it can be considerably more disabling.

Etiology and Treatment. The embryogenesis of epispadias is related to another congenital condition, exstrophy of the bladder. In this condition, the abdominal wall fails to form below the level of the umbilicus. At birth, the back wall of the bladder is exposed to the external environment.[9] The development of epispadias is simply a mild degree of exstrophy, with a deficiency of abdominal wall formation present inferiorly. Most commonly, the defect extends proximally to involve the urinary sphincter and results in urinary incontinence. Less commonly, the urethral meatus is located more distally along the dorsum of the penis and is accompanied by urinary continence because the sphincter is not affected (see Figure 31-3).

Management of exstrophy and proximal epispadias with incontinence is difficult and involves staged surgical procedures to reconstruct a continent bladder neck and a functional urethra. The less common distal epispadias is usually managed with tubular reconstruction procedures similar to those used for repair of hypospadias.

ACQUIRED DISORDERS

Priapism. **Priapism** may be defined as a painful, persistent erection. The patient usually reports several hours of painful erection in which the corpora cavernosa are tense with congested blood. The corpus spongiosum and glans are characteristically soft and uninvolved.

Etiology and Treatment. The causes of priapism are multiple. Most cases are idiopathic, with the next most common cause being sickle cell disease. Other etiologic factors include anticoagulant therapy, diabetes mellitus, leukemia, and the use of certain antidepressant medications.[10] Recently, intracavernosal injection of vasoactive substances for the management of impotence has been noted to cause priapism. Although multiple causes exist, the common abnormality is probably an obstruction of venous drainage resulting in the buildup of viscous, poorly oxygenated blood in the corpora.[11] If the process is allowed to continue, fibrosis of the corpora cavernosa will eventually occur and may cause impotence.

Management of priapism may involve a combination of measures, depending on the cause and duration of the condition. Initial therapy for priapism secondary to sickle cell disease includes sedation and oxygen.[12] For the management of priapism secondary to other causes, initial measures may include aspiration of blood from the corpora, as well as injection of α-adrenergic agents.[13] If the priapism remains refractory to these initial measures, a surgical shunting procedure may be necessary in which a shunt is created between the erect corpora cavernosa and the detumesced corpus spongiosum.

Phimosis and Paraphimosis

Etiology, Clinical Manifestations, and Treatment. **Phimosis** occurs when the uncircumcised foreskin cannot be retracted over the glans of the penis (Figure 31-4, *A*). Phimosis is usually the result of chronic inflammation and infection from poor hygiene. Calculi and squamous cell carcinoma may occur, although it is usually the presence of erythema, tenderness of the phimotic foreskin, or a discharge that prompts the patient to seek medical attention.[14] Management involves treating the infection with antifungal agents or antibiotics, followed by circumcision.

Paraphimosis, on the other hand, occurs when a foreskin that has been retracted over the glans up onto the shaft of the penis cannot be replaced in its normal position (see

FIGURE 31-4 A, Phimosis. **B,** Paraphimosis.

Figure 31-4, *B*). In this condition, which is usually secondary to chronic inflammation under the foreskin, a constricting ring of skin forms around the base of the retracted glans. The constriction causes venous congestion of the glans, with further swelling and edema making the condition worse. Treatment entails reducing the paraphimotic foreskin back over the glans, which can usually be accomplished by compressing the glans to reduce the edema. Occasionally, a slit or formal circumcision is needed to manage the problem.

Peyronie Disease

Etiology and Treatment. Peyronie disease refers to the formation of palpable, fibrous plaque on the surface of the corpora cavernosa. This plaque subsequently causes curvature of the penis with painful, incomplete erections. No satisfactory treatment for this disease is available, although some cases may remit with time. Conservative therapies that have had limited success include the use of vitamin E or aminobenzoate potassium (Potaba). In addition, several operative procedures have been developed. These procedures involve excising the plaque and repairing the corporal defect with a graft.[15]

Urethral Strictures

Etiology. Urethral strictures are fibrotic narrowings of the urethra and are usually composed of scar tissue. Most acquired strictures are due to a prior infection such as gonorrhea or trauma. Traumatic causes can be both iatrogenic, such as large urethral catheters and instrumentation, and noniatrogenic, such as straddle injuries.

Clinical Manifestations and Treatment. A decreased urinary stream is the most common complaint. Other common complaints include urethral discharge, infection, and urine retention. Urethral strictures are usually diagnosed by cystoscopy or retrograde urethrography, which would demonstrate a narrowing of the urethra. Management of urethral strictures involves procedures to dilate, incise, or reconstruct the urethra, depending on the extent and duration of the stricture.

Erectile Dysfunction.

The physiologic process of penile erection is a complex interaction of the vascular, hormonal, and neurologic systems. **Impotence,** or the inability to attain an erection, may be primary or secondary. Primary impotence refers to the inability to attain an erection throughout life and is often related to deep-seated psychiatric problems of some duration. Occasionally, vascular trauma sustained during early childhood or adolescence may account for primary impotence.[16]

Etiology. Far more common than primary impotence is secondary impotence. An individual with secondary impotence is no longer able to achieve normal erections but did have normal erections in the past. The causes of secondary impotence are multiple and may be discovered by examining the patient's medical history. Common causes of secondary impotence are peripheral vascular disease, the use of certain medications, endocrine problems, trauma, iatrogenic causes, and psychological causes. To differentiate organic causes from psychogenic impotence, one relies on the history, physical, and basic laboratory testing such as serum glucose and testosterone. Penile tumescence testing can also be utilized to make this distinction.

Arterial insufficiency of the penis may occur from obstruction of the arterial supply. Several processes may account for this obstructive arteriosclerosis. Stenosis of the arteries secondary to atheromatous plaque may be the most common etiologic factor. Diabetes mellitus may not only result in occlusion of arterial vessels but may also cause a neuropathy of the pudendal nerve that might result in erectile dysfunction.[17] Most investigators have suggested that erectile dysfunction may result from excessive venous drainage from the penis. This occurs because the blood is not adequately trapped in the corpora.

The list of medications that may cause erectile dysfunction is long. Several antihypertensive agents, including propranolol, monoamine oxidase inhibitors, and thiazides, have been associated with varying degrees of impotence. Other medications linked to erectile dysfunction include phenothiazines, antihistamines, and some antidepressants.[18]

Endocrinopathy accounts for a small percentage of impotence cases.[19] Pituitary dysfunction resulting in decreased or no secretion of luteinizing hormone may result in decreased secretion of testosterone. Primary failure of the testes may also occur, resulting in decreased secretion of testosterone. Finally, excessive secretion of the hormone prolactin by the pituitary gland may result in low testosterone levels.

Trauma to the penis resulting in penile fractures and damage to penile erectile tissue may occasionally lead to partial or complete impotence. More common injuries include pelvic fractures with subsequent damage to the penile vascular and nervous supply. Iatrogenic trauma secondary to several commonly performed operations, including aortoiliac vascular surgery, and radical pelvic cancer operations may also result in impotence.

A newer concept in erectile dysfunction is the idea of vascular endothelial damage, which can be diffuse throughout the body. Some researchers believe impotence may be a precursor of CAD.

Finally, it must be remembered that successful sexual function depends not only on intact vascular, hormonal, and neurologic systems but also on intact psychological and social responses. Several psychological factors may be manifested as problems of low desire, erectile failure, or premature ejaculation. A discussion of the psychological contribution to impotence is beyond the scope of this book.

Treatment. Management of erectile dysfunction requires an initial evaluation to differentiate organic causes from psychogenic causes. Further evaluation to distinguish among the various organic causes may then be needed. Once a psychogenic cause has been ruled out, several therapeutic options exist. Surgical options include the insertion of an inflatable or semirigid prosthetic device into the corpora cavernosa. In the past few years, several investigators have discovered that intracavernous injection of various vasoactive substances can cause an erection. Several of these substances, including papaverine, phentolamine, and prostaglandin E_1, are commonly used and afford a nonsurgical treatment option.

Viagra, the first oral therapy for erectile dysfunction, is the citrate salt of sildenafil, a selective inhibitor of cyclic guanosine monophosphate (cGMP)–specific phosphodiesterase type 5 (PDE5). To understand its clinical pharmacology, a review of some of the physiologic mechanisms of erection follows. Briefly, erection of the penis involves release of nitric oxide in the corpus cavernosum during sexual stimulation. Nitric oxide then activates the enzyme guanylate cyclase, and the subsequently increased levels cGMP produce smooth muscle relaxation in the corpus cavernosum and allow inflow of blood. Sildenafil has no direct relaxant effect on isolated human corpus cavernosum, but it enhances the effect of nitric oxide by inhibiting PDE5, which is responsible for degradation of cGMP in the corpus cavernosum. When sexual stimulation causes local release of nitric oxide, inhibition of PDE5 by sildenafil causes increased levels of cGMP in the corpus cavernosum, smooth muscle relaxation, and inflow of blood to the corpus cavernosum, which results in erection. Sildenafil citrate at the recommended doses appears to have no effect in the absence of sexual stimulation and affords another nonsurgical treatment option. Two newer agents for erectile dysfunction are Levitra and Cialis. In any particular patient, one of the three available oral medications may work better than the others. None of these agents should be used in conjunction with nitrate medications.

Another nonsurgical alternative entails the use of a vacuum device to sustain an erection. Finally, in very specific cases of erectile dysfunction, surgical procedures may be done to revascularize the arterial supply of the penis or ligate the penile venous drainage.

INFECTIOUS DISORDERS

Sexually transmitted infections (STIs) are common in the male genital system. The following describes five of the most well-known infections. A more in-depth discussion of STIs is provided in Chapter 34.

Gonococcal Urethritis

Etiology and Clinical Manifestations. Gonococcal urethritis is associated with a gram-negative diplococcus, *Neisseria gonorrhoeae.* Most cases are acquired during sexual intercourse, with the incubation period lasting from 3 to 10 days. Gonorrhea classically produces a urethral discharge and a burning sensation during urination. The initial urethritis may resolve without treatment, but long-term complications may include urethral stricture, abscess, and fistula formation.

Diagnosis and Treatment. Management of this disease depends on the diagnosis, which is accomplished by identification of the gonococcus in stained smears or cultures from infected sites. Recommended treatment includes single-dose parenteral administration of ceftriaxone (125 mg IM), or azithromycin (1000 mg IM). Oral treatments include doxycycline or levofloxacin.

All persons with gonorrhea should receive appropriate follow-up care and evaluation and treatment for other sexually transmitted diseases. The potential presence of coexisting chlamydial infection is an important consideration.

Nongonococcal Urethritis

Etiology, Diagnosis, and Treatment. Nongonococcal urethritis has several specific causes. The organism most responsible is probably *Chlamydia trachomatis.* Chlamydia is an intracellular organism that usually causes a urethral discharge and dysuria. A second organism, *Ureaplasma urealyticum,* has also been implicated as a causative agent of nongonococcal urethritis. Urethral swabs can be used to culture the urethra and determine the causative organism. Treatment of nongonococcal urethritis involves oral antibiotics, either tetracycline or erythromycin, 500 mg four times daily for 7 days.[21] Parenteral treatment with azithromycin is also used.

Syphilis

Etiology and Diagnosis. Syphilis is caused by the organism *Treponema pallidum,* a spirochete that gains entrance to the body through the skin or mucous membranes. The initial site of involvement in males is usually the penis, where a characteristic painless, shallow ulcer (chancre) is formed. This primary chancre often becomes associated with enlarged inguinal lymph nodes.

The diagnosis of syphilis may be made by microscopic dark-field examination of serous drainage from the ulcer. In the absence of a dark-field microscope, the diagnosis may be made by either of two serologic tests, the rapid plasma reagin test or the Venereal Disease Research Laboratory (VDRL) test. Management of early or primary syphilis involves an intramuscular injection of benzathine penicillin G, 2.4 million units. For patients who are allergic to penicillin, tetracycline or erythromycin, 500 mg four times a day for 15 days is the treatment of choice.[22]

Genital Herpes

Etiology, Pathogenesis, Clinical Manifestations, and Treatment. Herpes simplex virus is a double-stranded DNA virus that may cause persistent or latent infections. Two subtypes are recognized. The majority of patients with genital herpes have type 2 virus, whereas type 1 infections usually involve the oral cavity. Vesicles grouped together on an erythematous base constitute the typical lesion seen in genital herpes. Symptoms of herpes usually arise several days after the sexual contact. They include local discomfort, neuralgic pain, and malaise.[23] Occasionally patients develop meningitis, encephalitis, or disseminated infections. Usually after 5 to 10 days the symptoms resolve, but the virus then travels up the nerves and settles into the basal ganglia of the spinal cord where it resides forever. Periodically it can spread back down the nerves and cause recurrent disease. Both forms of the virus (type 1 and type 2) can cause the disease.[23] To confirm the diagnosis, smears of the lesions to demonstrate intranuclear inclusions may be performed. In addition, viral cultures or tests to measure serum antibody to herpes simplex virus may also be obtained. Acyclovir and Valtrex have demonstrated efficacy in managing this disease. They work by preventing the formation of viral DNA chains by inhibiting viral DNA polymerase.

Genital Warts

Etiology, Clinical Manifestations, and Treatment. Genital warts, or **condylomata acuminata** (singular: condyloma acuminatum), are caused by various strains of papillomavirus. The disease may be transmitted when viral particles from lesions come in contact with another person during sexual intercourse. The relationship between genital warts and cervical carcinoma in women has received considerable attention.[24]

Male patients may have warts anywhere on the external genitalia, but commonly on the penile shaft or glans. Warts may also be found in the urethra, as well as around or within the anus. Treatment involves the topical application of podophyllin. The warts may also be removed with electrocautery or a carbon dioxide laser. A new vaccine for HPV should cut down on the prevalence of this virus.

NEOPLASTIC DISORDERS

Neoplasms of the Penis

Etiology. Although cancer of the penis is rare in the United States and accounts for fewer than 0.2% of cancer deaths, its prevalence fluctuates widely among various locations. The causes are poorly understood, but phimosis of the foreskin accompanied by chronic inflammation has been thought to be the primary etiologic factor. The incidence of penile cancer among circumcised men is extremely low.[25]

The majority of penile cancer cases are squamous cell carcinoma (97%). They usually occur on the glans or the inner surface of the foreskin. Metastasis occurs by lymphatic dissemination, with initial involvement of the palpable inguinal lymph nodes. Death from penile carcinoma is a result of uncontrolled lymphatic spread and subsequent necrosis of the overlying skin, debilitation, and sepsis.

Penile carcinoma is staged as follows[26]:

Stage I: The lesion is limited to the glans or foreskin.

Stage II: The tumor involves the shaft of the penis.

Stage III: The inguinal nodes are involved but the lesion is operable.

Stage IV: Disseminated disease.

The lesion of penile cancer is usually ulcerative and fungating in appearance and may be associated with pain, bleeding, and urethral discharge. Inguinal adenopathy is present in more than 50% of patients at the time of diagnosis, although frequently the adenopathy represents an inflammatory response secondary to the lesion rather than metastasis.

Treatment. Therapy for penile carcinoma depends on the stage of the lesion. Topical chemotherapy and radiation therapy may be considered for certain small superficial lesions. Larger distal penile lesions usually require partial penectomy, whereas proximal lesions may require total penectomy with creation of a perineal urethrostomy. Finally, removal of the involved inguinal lymph nodes by inguinal lymph-adenectomy may be performed in cases of suspected stage III disease. Systemic chemotherapy is also used to treat metastatic disease.

The prognosis of penile carcinoma depends on the stage of disease. The 5-year survival rate for men with tumors localized to the penis is 65% to 90%. With inguinal node involvement, 5-year survival rates drop to about 30% to 50%, and if distant metastases are present, the 5-year survival rate is virtually zero.[26]

KEY POINTS

- Congenital disorders of the penis may result from hormonal deficiencies or abnormalities in embryonic development. Micropenis, for example, is usually a result of testosterone deficiency. Urethral valves, fistulas, and malpositioning of the urinary meatus (hypospadias, epispadias) are related to abnormal embryonic development.

- Priapism is a persistent, painful erection, most commonly of unknown cause. Priapism may occur in conditions that cause obstruction of venous drainage, including sickle cell anemia, anticoagulant therapy, diabetes mellitus, and certain antidepressant medications.

- Phimosis and paraphimosis are disorders of the foreskin. Phimosis is associated with chronic inflammation and poor hygiene and results in a foreskin that cannot be retracted. Paraphimosis refers to a foreskin that remains retracted and cannot be returned to its normal position.

- Urethral strictures may be congenital or acquired. Most acquired strictures are secondary to gonorrheal infection or urethral trauma. Poor stream, bladder infections, and retained urine are common manifestations.

- Impotence is the inability to achieve a sustained erection. Causes of impotence are categorized as primary and secondary. Primary impotence is rare and usually related to adolescent vascular trauma or psychiatric problems. Secondary impotence may be due to a variety of factors, including vascular disease, medications, endocrine disorders, trauma, and psychological distress.

- A number of infections are sexually transmitted and affect the penis and urethra, including gonococcal urethritis, nongonococcal urethritis, syphilis, herpes, and genital warts. Gonococcal and nongonococcal urethritis and syphilis are effectively managed with antibiotics. Herpes and genital warts are associated with viruses and tend to be chronic, with intermittent recurrence.

- Penile neoplasms are rare, particularly in circumcised males. Phimosis and chronic inflammation may be important etiologic factors. Like other neoplasms, penile cancer has a better prognosis if managed before dissemination.

Disorders of the Scrotum and Testes

CONGENITAL DISORDERS

Cryptorchidism. **Cryptorchidism** means "hidden testis" and refers to any testis that occupies an extrascrotal position. The cryptorchid testis may be incompletely descended and as such be located intra-abdominally, within the inguinal canal, or just external to the canal but above the scrotum. Occasionally the testis may emerge from the external ring of the inguinal canal and be misdirected into an abnormal extrascrotal position. In this situation the testis may be called ectopic. An ectopic testis may be located in any of several locations but is most commonly found in a superficial inguinal pouch[27] (Figure 31-5).

The incidence of cryptorchidism is about 0.7% to 1.0% of male infants at 1 year of age. The cause of the condition is uncertain but may be related to an intrinsic testicular defect or a subtle hormonal deficiency.[27]

The incompletely descended, cryptorchid testis undergoes deleterious changes. The tubules become fibrotic, with a deficiency of spermatogenesis and subsequent infertility. More important is the increased incidence of testicular malignancy in cryptorchid testes.[28] Several studies have revealed an increased prevalence of testicular tumors in subjects with a history of cryptorchidism.

Treatment. Because of the increased risk of malignancy and infertility, treatment at an early age to bring the testis into a normal scrotal position is recommended. An operative procedure (*orchiopexy*) is usually required, although in certain situations descent may be stimulated by the administration of human chorionic gonadotropin, which is given in a series of intramuscular injections.[29]

ACQUIRED DISORDERS

Hydrocele

Etiology and Clinical Manifestations. A **hydrocele** consists of a fluid collection surrounding the testicle or spermatic cord and contained within the tunica or processus vaginalis (Figure 31-6). Scrotal swelling in infants or young boys may indicate a hydrocele. These congenital hydroceles exist because of communication between the abdominal cavity and scrotum through the processus vaginalis. The scrotum is characteristically small and soft in the morning but larger and tense at night as it fills with fluid from the abdominal cavity.

Hydroceles may also develop secondary to scrotal injury, radiation therapy, infection of the epididymis, or testicular neoplasms. More commonly, however, the cause is uncertain, with the hydrocele developing slowly over time and occurring in middle-aged or elderly men. These acquired hydroceles may vary in size and consistency from small and soft to large and tense. The fluid is usually clear and yellow.

Treatment. Because hydrocele is a benign condition, treatment is required only if the fluid collection becomes uncomfortable for the patient. Occasionally, a tense hydrocele might restrict circulation to the testicle. Management usually involves a surgical procedure to drain the fluid with either resection or plication of the hydrocele sac to prevent reaccumulation of the fluid. Aspiration of the hydrocele may be performed, although fluid often reaccumulates.

Spermatocele

Etiology and Treatment. **Spermatoceles** are painless, cystic masses containing sperm. Although they are usually small, they may be quite large and difficult to distinguish from a hydrocele. The cause of spermatoceles is uncertain; they may arise from the tiny tubules that connect the epididymis to the testis (vasa efferentia) or from the epididymis itself. Like hydroceles,

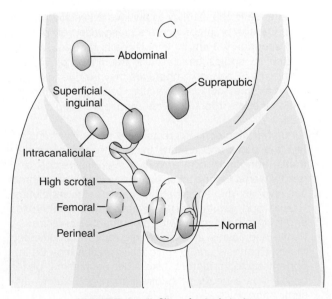

FIGURE 31-5 Sites of ectopic testes.

FIGURE 31-6 Hydrocele.

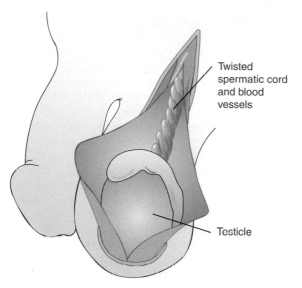

FIGURE 31-7 Testicular torsion.

spermatoceles need not be treated unless they become large enough to trouble the patient, in which case an operative procedure to excise the spermatocele may be performed.

Testicular Torsion. Torsion of the testicle is described as a twisting of the spermatic cord with subsequent compromise of the testicular vascular supply and testicular ischemia, followed by infarction (Figure 31-7). Although torsion may occur in the neonatal period, the majority of cases occur in prepubertal boys.

Clinical Manifestations. The diagnosis is suggested by the onset of severe pain in one testis, followed by swelling of the scrotum. Lower abdominal pain accompanied by nausea and vomiting may also occur. The condition may be differentiated from epididymitis (inflammation of the epididymis), which is also associated with scrotal swelling, by the presence of vascular echoes detected with a Doppler ultrasound stethoscope. A testis made ischemic by torsion will not echo sound, whereas the inflammation of epididymitis and its hypervascularity increase sound emission. Testicular nuclear scanning is the most definitive test, with torsion making the testis avascular.

Treatment. Management of torsion involves an operation to open the scrotum, untwist the testis, and "pex" (secure) it to the scrotal wall. Because the chance of torsion also involving the contralateral testis is increased, the contralateral testicle is "pexed" to the scrotal wall as well. If detorsion is accomplished within 12 hours of the event, the prognosis for testicular viability is usually good. If torsion has been present for more than 24 hours, viability of the testis is doubtful.

INFECTIOUS DISORDERS

Epididymitis

Etiology. Epididymitis, or inflammation of the testis, has several causes. It may occur as a result of trauma or the reflux of sterile urine up the vas deferens. However, the majority of cases are probably secondary to a bacterial cause, with both sexually transmitted organisms (*N. gonorrhoeae* and *C. trachomatis*) and non–sexually transmitted organisms (*Pseudomonas* and *Escherichia coli*) involved.

Clinical Manifestations and Treatment. With epididymitis the scrotum may be enlarged, reddened, and tender. The pain may radiate along the spermatic cord into the inguinal area. Fever may also occur, as may urethral discharge, cystitis, and cloudy urine. Laboratory testing usually reveals an elevated white blood cell (WBC) count, and urine culture may reveal the infecting organism.

Treatment for the condition involves bed rest, scrotal support, and administration of antibiotics. In advanced cases, incision and drainage with the intravenous administration of antibiotics may be needed to effectively manage a resulting scrotal abscess.

Fournier Gangrene

Etiology, Clinical Manifestations, and Treatment. Fournier gangrene is a severe but rare condition involving gangrenous necrosis of the scrotum. Symptoms are pain and swelling of the scrotum, fever and chills, and sepsis.[30] The diagnosis can often be made by history and physical examination. Additional tests such as ultrasound, computed tomography, or magnetic resonance imaging can also be helpful in diagnosis. Usually, an underlying disease such as diabetes, alcoholism, or another general debility predisposes the patient to such an aggressive infection. Extravasation of infected urine from urethral trauma, a perforated urethral diverticulum, or a non–urinary tract source such as a perirectal abscess may act as the source of infection. Treatment, which must be instituted swiftly, includes incision and drainage of fluctuant areas and debridement of necrotic tissue along with antibiotics. This often is a fatal disease unless it is managed quickly and aggressively.

NEOPLASTIC DISORDERS

Neoplasms of the Testis. Although testicular tumors are rare, with a prevalence of 3.7 cases per 100,000 population, their peak incidence is in late adolescence to early adulthood. These neoplasms therefore represent the most common solid tumors of men aged 20 to 34 years in the United States.[31] Testicular self-examination is an important tool for early detection because prompt treatment is associated with a higher success rate.

Etiology. Although the cause of testicular tumors is uncertain, a strong association is seen between cryptorchidism and the subsequent development of malignancy. Nevertheless, the majority of patients with testicular tumors have no history of cryptorchidism, which suggests that several unrecognized factors may be contributing to the pathogenesis.

Histologically, testicular tumors may be considered in two groups. In the first group are nongerminal neoplasms, including tumors that originate from either the Leydig cells or other stromal tissue cells of the testis. In the second group are germinal neoplasms, which are derived from the germinal cells of the testis. This group accounts for the vast majority (95%) of testicular tumors. Germinal neoplasms may be further subdivided into two groups: seminomas and nonseminomatous.

Treatment. Although germinal tumors may consist entirely of one histologic subtype, many contain elements of more than one subtype. Treatment and prognosis vary according to the subtype of germinal tumor. For example, seminoma in its early stages is exquisitely sensitive to and easily cured with radiation therapy. On the other hand, nonseminomatous germ cell tumors in the early stage are usually successfully managed with surgery. The prognosis is also variable. Pure choriocarcinomas are usually first seen at an advanced stage with distant metastases. Treatment is usually less effective for this aggressive lesion. However, the majority of germ cell tumors may be effectively managed even if lymph node metastases are present.

Except for choriocarcinomas, which disseminate by vascular means, testicular germ cell tumors usually metastasize through the lymphatic system. They usually disseminate in a stepwise manner, first involving the retroperitoneal lymph nodes lying adjacent to the great vessels. If unmanaged, the disease may progress to involve other lymph nodes and other organs such as the lungs.

Multiple staging systems have been devised to classify the extent of this disease. Most are a variation of the system proposed by Boden and Gibb in 1951.[31] One commonly used system is as follows:

Stage I: The tumor is confined to the testis.

Stage II: The tumor has spread to retroperitoneal lymph nodes.

Stage III: The tumor has spread to nodes above the diaphragm.

Stage IV: The tumor has spread to other organs.

Because the management of testicular tumors is complicated and somewhat controversial, a complete discussion is not possible here; however, several issues can be pointed out. After diagnosis of a testicular tumor, an operation to remove the testicle is performed. This procedure involves an inguinal incision with removal of the testis from the scrotum, followed by ligation and removal of the spermatic cord and testicle together. Histologic classification, additional staging studies, and other factors then determine further treatment. This treatment may involve close observation with frequent radiologic studies to determine new progression, surgery to remove the retroperitoneal lymph nodes (retroperitoneal lymphadenectomy), chemotherapy, or radiation therapy. Some situations may call for a combination of these measures.

KEY POINTS

- Cryptorchidism refers to a testis located in a position other than the scrotum. Often the testis has failed to descend completely and is located in the inguinal canal. Undescended testes are associated with infertility and an increased risk of testicular malignancy.
- A hydrocele is a collection of fluid in the testicle or spermatic cord, commonly associated with communication between the abdominal cavity and the scrotum (hernia). Hydroceles are benign and treated only if they become uncomfortable. A spermatocele is a cyst that contains sperm. Like hydroceles, they are benign and do not require treatment unless they cause discomfort.
- Testicular torsion refers to a twisting of the spermatic cord with subsequent testicular ischemia and infarction. Sudden onset of severe testicular pain is common. If the torsion is reduced within 12 hours, the testicle may be viable.
- Inflammation of the epididymis, called epididymitis, is most commonly associated with infectious agents. Manifestations include a swollen, tender, reddened scrotum with associated bladder infection and cloudy urine. Antibiotics are indicated. Aggressive infections of the scrotum may result in Fournier gangrene manifested by gangrenous necrosis of the scrotum.
- Although rare in the population, testicular cancer is the most common solid tumor in men aged 20 to 34 years. The great majority of testicular neoplasms originate in the germ cells. Most germ cell tumors can be effectively managed even after lymph node metastasis. Management includes surgical removal of the testis and spermatic cord, with irradiation and chemotherapy as indicated.

Disorders of the Prostate

Benign Prostatic Hyperplasia. **Benign prostatic hyperplasia,** also referred to as benign prostatic hypertrophy (BPH), is a very common disorder. An estimated 80% of men older than 60 years experience some degree of BPH. It is important to recognize that BPH and prostate cancer are not related entities, and no study has conclusively demonstrated that BPH predisposes to the development of prostate cancer.[32]

Etiology. Although the exact cause of BPH is unknown, the occurrence of the disease with aging suggests a relationship to changes in the aging male endocrine system. The process involves hyperplasia of the glands surrounding the prostatic urethra (Figure 31-8). As this tissue increases in size, it compresses the urethra and produces symptoms of bladder outlet obstruction.

Clinical Manifestations. Symptoms of obstruction may be minimal at first but may eventually progress to complete obstruction and urinary retention. A decrease in the force of the urinary stream, hesitancy or difficulty in initiating a urinary stream, and interruption of the stream may occur. Because the bladder may fail to empty completely, infection associated with residual urine may occur. Figure 31-9 illustrates possible complications of benign prostatic enlargement.

The diagnosis of BPH usually involves recognition of the characteristic symptoms. Rectal examination disclosing an enlarged prostate, urethral catheterization or bladder scanning to document a large postvoid urinary residual, and radiographic evidence of hypertrophy and obstruction on CT scan

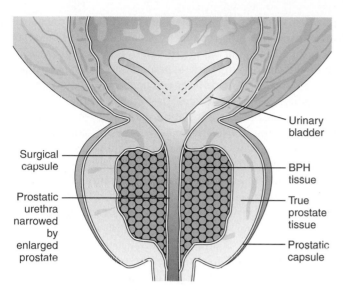

FIGURE 31-8 Gross appearance of hyperplastic prostatic tissue obstructing the prostatic urethra. *BPH,* Benign prostatic hypertrophy.

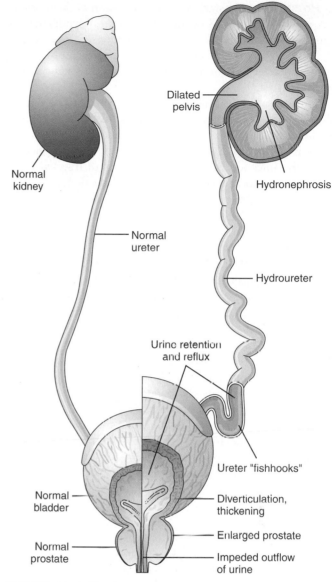

FIGURE 31-9 Sites for potential complications caused by benign prostatic enlargement *(right)* are compared with a normal kidney, ureter, bladder, and prostate *(left).*

or abdominal ultrasound are some of the measures that may be used to confirm the diagnosis. Urodynamics are sophisticated measures of urinary function that can help confirm the diagnosis.

Treatment. The treatment of BPH has changed markedly over the last several years. The first line of treatment is with medication such as alpha blockers or 5-alpha reductase inhibitors. The former treatment decreases the tension in the prostate by relaxing the muscle fibers in the gland. This reduces pressure in the bladder neck and urethra allowing easier flow. The latter treatment actually decreases the size of the gland by blocking the conversion of testosterone to dihydrotestosterone. This can shrink the gland by up to one-third and thereby reverse the years of growth that have caused impingement of the urethra.

The next forms of treatment are the minimally invasive treatments that are usually done in the office. These include microwave therapy, needle ablation, and some other forms of treatment to decrease the tissue squeezing the urethra closed. They are usually well tolerated but may not cause total relief of the obstruction, and the long-term results are variable.

The last form of treatment is surgery. The classic operation for BPH is called a transurethral resection of the prostate (TURP). This procedure uses a resectoscope that is passed through the penis and into the prostate. An electric wire is then used to resect chips of tissue from the interior of the gland to form an open channel for urination.

A newer alternative to the TURP is laser therapy. In this approach, a scope is passed via the urethra into the prostate, and the tissue is vaporized with a laser fiber to create an open channel.

In some patients with extremely large glands or other bladder pathology, an incision is made and an open simple prostatectomy can be performed to remove the adenoma (inner portion of the gland). This creates a large cavity and channel for the urine to pass through.

All of the treatments have various side effects and risks. Therefore, each patient has to have his treatment tailored to his specific situation.

GERIATRIC CONSIDERATIONS

BPH is a common disorder that affects about 80% of men older than 60 years. Although the exact cause is unknown, the occurrence of the disease with aging suggests a relationship to changes in the aging male endocrine system. Enlargement of the prostate gland and progressive compression of the urethra result in symptoms of obstruction.

Prostatitis. **Prostatitis,** or inflammation of the prostate, has several causes and encompasses several syndromes. A common classification of prostatitis proposed by Drach et al[32] in 1978 considers four types: acute bacterial prostatitis, chronic bacterial prostatitis, nonbacterial prostatitis, and prostatodynia.[34]

The causative organism in bacterial prostatitis is usually *E. coli,* with species of *Proteus, Klebsiella, Enterobacter, Pseudomonas, Serratia, Staphylococcus,* and *Enterococcus* occurring less commonly.[35] Possible routes of infection include ascending infection up the urethra, reflux of infected urine into the prostatic ducts, hematogenous infection, and invasion of rectal bacteria by direct extension or lymphogenous spread (Figure 31-10). Many cases of prostatitis result from periurethral infection associated with an indwelling urethral catheter.[36]

Clinical Manifestations, Diagnosis, and Treatment. Acute bacterial prostatitis is characterized by the onset of fever, chills, low back pain, and the voiding symptoms of frequency, urgency, and dysuria. Rectal examination usually reveals a tender, swollen prostate, and subsequent urinalysis may reveal WBCs and bacteria.

The diagnosis of bacterial prostatitis is usually suggested by the initial symptoms and signs. Microscopic inspection of the urine and expressed prostatic secretions may reveal WBCs and bacteria. A urine culture with sensitivity testing for the offending organism is recommended to direct therapy with an appropriate antibiotic. In the event of high fever and an elevated WBC count, intravenous antibiotics are recommended.

Chronic bacterial prostatitis may be associated with variable symptoms. Although some men with chronic bacterial prostatitis may report a history of acute bacterial prostatitis, many have no history of this problem. Most men complain of voiding symptoms with pain localized to various areas, including the perineum, back, suprapubic area, and occasionally, the testis. High-grade fever and chills are uncommon with this entity, as opposed to acute bacterial prostatitis.

In chronic bacterial prostatitis, pathogenic organisms may persist in prostatic tissues unaltered by the administration of several antibiotics. Because most antibiotics accumulate poorly in prostatic secretions, discontinuation of antibiotic use often results in reinfection and recurrence of symptoms. It is this occurrence of relapsing infections, often caused by the same organism, which is typical of chronic bacterial prostatitis. Several antibiotic agents, such as trimethoprim-sulfamethoxazole (Septra, Bactrim), when used for a prolonged period (4 to 6 weeks) have a better cure rate because of their capability to penetrate prostatic tissue.

Prostatitis may also occur secondary to nonbacterial inflammation. In fact, nonbacterial prostatitis probably accounts for the majority of cases of prostatitis. The symptoms of this entity are variable but usually include irritative voiding; symptoms of urgency, frequency, and nocturia; as well as occasional perineal and suprapubic pain. Although these symptoms are similar to those of bacterial prostatitis, patients have no history of positive urine cultures or urinary tract infections. Treatment may include a course of antibiotics, oral anti-inflammatory agents (e.g., ibuprofen), alpha blockers, prostatic massage, and occasionally, sitz baths. Symptoms are often intermittent, and patients should be reassured that the disease is not contagious and does not predispose to the development of cancer or other serious disease.

The final classification of prostatitis, **prostatodynia,** is typified by symptoms of prostatitis but no history of urinary tract infection and no evidence of inflammation in prostatic secretions. The cause of this entity is uncertain and may involve spasm of the pelvic floor musculature. Treatment may involve the use of α-adrenergic receptor–blocking agents and occasionally diazepam (Valium).[36]

Prostate Cancer. Other than skin cancers, prostate cancer is now recognized as the most prevalent form of cancer in men. About 200,000 cases are diagnosed annually in the United States, with approximately 35,000 deaths annually attributed to the disease. Prostate cancer ranks as the second leading cause of cancer death among men. Cancer of the prostate rarely occurs in men younger than 50 years, and its incidence increases with age. The majority (95%) of prostate cancers are adenocarcinomas with abnormal proliferation of prostatic glandular structures.[37]

Etiology. The precise cause of prostate cancer is undetermined, although genetic, hormonal, dietary, and viral factors have all been suggested. Varying degrees of aggressiveness of prostate cancer have been recognized, with different tumors expressing different malignant potential and ultimately carrying a different prognosis. Attempts to classify prostate cancer into separate groups of cancer have been made, with different tumors expressing different malignant potential and ultimately

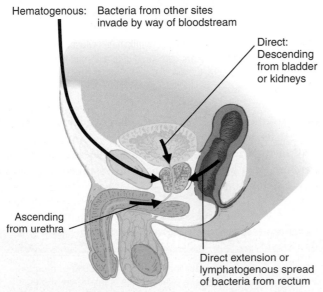

Hematogenous: Bacteria from other sites invade by way of bloodstream

Direct: Descending from bladder or kidneys

Ascending from urethra

Direct extension or lymphatogenous spread of bacteria from rectum

FIGURE 31-10 Postulated pathways of infection to the prostate gland. (From Black JM, Matassarin-Jacobs E: *Medical-surgical nursing: clinical management for continuity of care,* ed 6, Philadelphia, 2001, Saunders, p 963.)

carrying a different prognosis. Such attempts to classify prostate cancer into different groups consider the structure and internal architecture of tumor cells and their pattern of proliferation. For example, cells of the more aggressive or poorly differentiated prostate cancers have more indistinct cell borders, larger nuclei, and loss of acinar (gland) formation.

Prostate cancer is staged as follows:

Stage A: The tumor is microscopic and intracapsular.

Stage B: The tumor is palpable on rectal examination but confined to the prostate.

Stage C: The tumor has extended beyond the capsule of the prostate.

Stage D: The tumor has metastasized to distant organs.

Diagnosis. The diagnosis of prostate cancer may involve several clinical scenarios. The disease may be diagnosed after microscopic inspection of prostate tissue removed for the management of presumed BPH. Prostate cancer may also be detected on rectal examination in patients with or without voiding symptoms. Occasionally, patients have urinary retention or even azotemia and renal failure secondary to obstructive nephropathy. Much interest has focused on the search for effective measures to detect prostate cancer in its early and most easily manageable stages. Two new techniques, a blood test for serum prostate-specific antigen and transrectal ultrasonography, have generated considerable excitement within the field of urology. Several initial investigations have shown efficacy in the early detection of prostate cancer.

Once the diagnosis of prostate cancer is made, the lesion must be staged. Staging usually involves a bone scan to rule out bone metastases, chest radiography to rule out lung metastases, and occasionally abdominal and pelvic computed tomography to rule out abdominal lymphadenopathy.

Treatment. Management of prostate cancer depends on several factors, including the stage of the tumor, as well as the age and health of the patient. Debate exists over treatment for men with localized disease, with options ranging from aggressive therapy to "watchful waiting." Watchful waiting may be an option for older men with asymptomatic stage A prostate cancer. Younger men may be candidates for the more aggressive approach, which includes surgery to remove the prostate and surrounding tissue (radical prostatectomy), radiation therapy, or cryotherapy (freezing the gland). It is important to note that approximately 70% to 90% of men who undergo radical prostatectomy will experience impotence. Urinary incontinence may also occur. Given the effects of surgical intervention, it is important that patients have access to preoperative and postoperative counseling about issues arising from their diagnosis and the effect of various treatments and potential complications.

In addition to radical prostatectomy or radiation therapy, in some cases lymph nodes in the pelvis are also removed (pelvic lymph node dissection). Advanced lesions may respond to hormonal manipulation. Orchiectomy, oral administration of estrogens, or intramuscular injection of luteinizing hormone–releasing hormone agonists may reduce the patient's serum testosterone level. Many prostate cancers are androgen sensitive and may be temporarily controlled with androgen ablation. In more advanced cases that are no longer hormonally responsive, palliative measures such as spot radiation treatment of painful areas of bone metastasis and analgesics may be required.

GERIATRIC CONSIDERATIONS

Cancer of the prostate rarely occurs in men younger than 50 years, and its incidence increases with age. Symptoms vary depending on the stage of the disease. Men who are older and have stage A prostate cancer may be monitored closely without any treatment. Men with more advanced stage disease may be treated more aggressively.

KEY POINTS

- Symptoms of BPH include diminished force of the urinary stream, hesitancy, and poor bladder emptying. Transurethral resection of the obstructing prostatic tissue is the usual treatment.
- Inflammation of the prostate, or prostatitis, is characterized by low back pain, urinary frequency, urgency, and dysuria. Fever and chills may also be present with acute bacterial prostatitis. *E. coli* is the most commonly associated organism. Prostatitis may also occur in the absence of infection.
- Prostate cancer is usually detected as a lump or enlargement of the prostate gland. As with other cancers, early, accurate diagnosis is important for effective therapy. Surgical resection, radiation therapy, and hormone therapy (to reduce androgens) may be used. The choice of treatment depends on the grade and stage of the disease and the individual's age, general health, and life expectancy.

SUMMARY

Disorders of the penis and male urethra may be grouped into congenital and acquired anomalies, infections, and neoplasms. Common congenital anomalies include urethral valves and hypospadias. Common acquired disorders involve phimosis, urethral strictures, and impotence. Sexually transmitted diseases are some of the most common infections involving the penis and urethra; they include gonococcal urethritis, nongonococcal urethritis, syphilis, genital herpes, and genital warts. Neoplasms of the penis and urethra are relatively rare.

Congenital disorders of the scrotum and testes include cryptorchidism. This condition is one of the most common problems seen by pediatric urologists. Testicular torsion and Fournier gangrene are two of the more immediate urologic emergencies. Finally, neoplasms of the testes, although rare, may afflict younger men in the prime of life.

Disorders of the prostate account for a majority of the visits to a practicing urologist. Briefly, these disorders can be divided into problems of benign prostatic hyperplasia, prostatitis, and prostatic cancer. Prostate cancer is the most frequently diagnosed cancer in men, with more than 200,000 cases diagnosed and 35,000 deaths yearly.

REFERENCES

1. Underwood LE, Van Wyk JJ: Normal and aberrant growth. In Wilson JD, Foster DW, editors: *Williams textbook of endocrinology,* ed 9, Philadelphia, 1998, Saunders, pp 1117-1124.
2. Feldman KW, Smith DW: Fetal phallic growth and penile standards for newborn male infants, *J Pediatr* 86(3):395-398, 1975.
3. Kogan SJ, Williams DI: The micropenis syndrome: clinical observations and expectations for growth, *J Urol* 118(2):311-313, 1977.
4. Greenfield SP: Posterior urethral valves: new concepts. *J Urol* 157(3):996-997, 1997.
5. King LR: Posterior urethra. In Kelalis PP, King LR, editors: *Clinical pediatric urology,* ed 3, Philadelphia, 1992, Saunders.
6. Van Savage JG et al: An algorithm for the management of anterior urethral valves, *J Urol* 158(3 pt 2):1030-1032, 1997.
7. Zaontz MR, Packer MG: Abnormalities of the external genitalia, *Pediatr Clin North Am* 44(5):1267-1297, 1997.
8. Albers N et al: Etiologic classification of severe hypospadias: implications for prognosis and management, *J Pediatr* 131(3):344-346, 1997.
9. Beaudoin S, Simon L, Bargy F: Anatomical basis of a common embryological origin for epispadias and bladder or cloacal exstrophies, *Surg Radiol Anat* 19(1):11-16, 1997.
10. Mulhall JP, Honig SC: Priapism: etiology and management, *Acad Emerg Med* 3(8):810-816, 1996.
11. Powars DR, Johnson CS: Priapism, *Hematol Oncol Clin North Am* 10(6):1363-1372, 1996.
12. Fitzpatrick TJ: Spongiograms and cavernosograms: a study of their value in priapism, *J Urol* 109(5):843-846, 1973.
13. deHoll JD et al: Alternative approaches to the management of priapism, *Int J Impot Res* 10(1):11-14, 1998.
14. Golubovic Z et al: The conservative treatment of phimosis in boys, *Br J Urol* 78(5):786-788, 1996.
15. Licht MR, Lewis RW: Modified Nesbit procedure for the treatment of Peyronie's disease: a comparative outcome analysis, *J Urol* 158(2):460-463, 1997.
16. Bortolotti A et al: The epidemiology of erectile dysfunction and its risk factors, *Int J Androl* 20(6):323-334, 1997.
17. McMillan DE: Development of vascular complications in diabetes, *Vasc Med* 2(2):132-142, 1997.
18. Fabbri A, Aversa A, Isidori A: Erectile dysfunction: an overview, *Hum Reprod Update* 3(5):455-466, 1997.
19. Roy JB: Advances in the management of impotence, *J Okla State Med Assoc* 91(1):14-16, 1998.
20. Jones RB et al: Randomized trial of trovafloxacin and ofloxacin for single-dose therapy of gonorrhea. Trovafloxacin Gonorrhea Study Group, *Am J Med* 104(1):28-32, 1998.
21. Martin SJ et al: Levofloxacin and sparfloxacin: new quinolone antibiotics, *Ann Pharmacother* 32(3):320-336, 1998.
22. Centers for Disease Control and Prevention: 1998 guidelines for treatment of sexually transmitted diseases, *Morb Mortal Wkly Rep* 47(RR-1):1-111, 1998.
23. Patel R: Progress in meeting today's demands in genital herpes: an overview of current management, *J Infect Dis* 186:547-556, 2002.
24. Jablonska S, Majewski S: Human papillomavirus infection in women. Special aspects of infectious diseases in women, *Clin Dermatol* 15(1):67-79, 1997.
25. Micali G et al: Squamous cell carcinoma of the penis, *J Am Acad Dermatol* 35(3 pt 1):432-451, 1996.
26. Schellhammer PF, Grabstald H: Tumors of the penis. In Walsh PC et al, editors: *Campbell's urology,* ed 7, Philadelphia, 1997, Saunders.
27. Kogan SJ: Cryptorchidism. In Kelalis PP, King LR, editors: *Clinical pediatric urology,* ed 3, Philadelphia, 1992, Saunders.
28. Cortes D: Cryptorchidism: aspects of pathogenesis, histology and treatment, *Scand J Urol Nephrol Suppl* 196:1-54, 1998.
29. Gill B, Kogan S: Cryptorchidism. Current concepts, *Pediatr Clin North Am* 44(5):1211-1227, 1997.
30. Morpurgo E, Galandiuk S: Fournier's gangrene, *Surg Clin North Am* 82(6):1213-1224, 2002.
31. Morse MJ, Whitmore WF: Neoplasms of the testis. In Walsh PC et al, editors: *Campbell's urology,* ed 7, Philadelphia, 1997, Saunders.
32. Drach GW et al: Classification of benign diseases associated with prostatic pain: prostatitis or prostatodynia, *J Urol* 120(2):266, 1978.
33. Roehrborn CG et al: Guidelines for the diagnosis and treatment of benign prostatic hyperplasia: a comparative, international overview, *Urology* 58(5):642-650, 2001.
34. Nickel JC: Prostatitis: myths and realities, *Urology* 51(3):362-366, 1998.
35. Meares EM: Prostatitis and related disorders. In Walsh PC et al, editors: *Campbell's urology,* ed 7, Philadelphia, 1997, Saunders.
36. Walsh PC: Benign prostatic hyperplasia. In Walsh PC et al, editors: *Campbell's urology,* ed 7, Philadelphia, 1997, Saunders.
37. Catalona WJ: Carcinoma of the prostate. In Walsh PC et al, editors: *Campbell's urology,* ed 7, Philadelphia, 1997, Saunders.

Female Genital and Reproductive Function

Rosemary A. Jadack • Jane M. Georges

MEDIA RESOURCES

Additional Material for Study, Review, and Further Exploration

 CD Companion ■ Review Questions and Answers
■ Glossary (with audio pronunciations for selected terms)
■ Disease Profiles ■ Animations

evolve **Website** at http://evolve.elsevier.com/Copstead/
■ Case Studies ■ Disease Profiles ■ WebLinks ■ Key Points Review

 Online Course (Module 15)

KEY QUESTIONS

■ What are the major structures of the internal and external female reproductive tract?
■ What are the major hormonal events of the female reproductive cycle?
■ Which hormones are involved in breast development during pregnancy and lactation, and what are their specific functions?

■ What are the physiologic changes associated with pregnancy?
■ What gestational events occur in the fetus during each of the three trimesters of pregnancy?
■ What hormonal changes lead to menopause?
■ What physiologic changes and complications may result from menopausal hormone deficiencies?

CHAPTER OUTLINE

The female reproductive system is complex both in structure and in function. From birth to senescence, the organs of the female reproductive system function in concert with each other, with the brain, and with other endocrine organs. This integrated functioning constitutes some of the most intricate and elegant processes of the human body. This chapter presents an overview of these functions, beginning with the development of the female reproductive tract.

The major processes related to the reproductive tract throughout life, including the menstrual cycle, pregnancy, lactation, and menopause, are then described with an emphasis on recent research findings. Health care providers must also consider the developmental, cognitive, functional, social, and financial aspects of women's reproductive lives.[1,2] Because the functioning of the female reproductive system has an enormous impact on the life of the individual woman, increased importance has been placed on the active involvement of women in understanding their own health care needs. Health care professionals are encouraged to include women as collaborators in decisions about their reproductive health.[3,4]

REPRODUCTIVE STRUCTURES

Embryology

Until the sixth week of gestation, the gonads in both sexes are *bipotential*, which means that the gonads present in the embryo may become either testes or ovaries. Beginning about the seventh week, the so-called indifferent gonad begins to develop into either a male or a female derivative.[5] Recent research has demonstrated that SRY (sex-determining region of the Y chromosome) is the gene that influences the indifferent gonad to organize into a testis.[5] In a genetically female embryo, the gonad organizes into an ovary under the influence of one or more ovary-determining genes, which have not yet been well characterized. The cortex of the gonad accumulates nests of cells that differentiate into ovarian follicles, each containing a primary oocyte. The wolffian ducts, the primordial structures that are precursors to the male internal reproductive organs, begin to disappear, and the müllerian ducts, the structures that will develop into the female internal reproductive organs, become dominant.[6]

The external genitalia of both the male and female are identical until the eighth week of gestation. Like the gonads, the genitalia are bipotential until this time, with the capability of developing into organs of either sex. In a genetically male embryo, dihydrotestosterone, a metabolite of testosterone, binds to androgen receptors in the external genitalia and effects the differentiation of these structures into the male external genitalia. Without the influence of dihydrotestosterone, the bipotential external genitalia will spontaneously develop into female external genitalia.[5]

During the later period of fetal development, maternal hormones may have some influence on reproductive structures. Estrogens and progestins from the mother cause cervical enlargement, hypertrophy of the vaginal epithelium, and enlargement of the mammary gland of the female fetus.

These alterations may be present at birth but usually subside during the first 1 to 2 months.[7]

Organization of the Female Reproductive Organs

The internal organs of the female reproductive system include the ovaries, **oviducts** (fallopian tubes), uterus, cervix, and vagina (Figure 32-1). These organs are situated in the pelvic cavity and are supported and anchored in place by a series of ligaments (Figure 32-2).

Ovaries

The two ovaries, which are the female gonads, are located close to the lateral walls of the pelvic cavity. When the ovary is in its normal position, its long axis is nearly vertical with respect to the horizontal axis of the body. The size of the ovary varies with age and with the stage of the menstrual cycle. It is somewhat larger before than after pregnancy and further reduces in size with the aging process.[8]

The ovary is covered with a single layer of epithelium. Underneath the epithelium is a layer of dense fibrous connective tissue called the tunica albuginea. The tunica albuginea constitutes the outer portion of the cortex of the ovary. The remainder of the cortex consists of connective tissue called the *stroma*, which contains ova in various stages of maturation. The innermost part of the ovary, the medulla, consists of loose connective tissue that is richly supplied with blood and lymph vessels and nerve fibers.[9]

Before birth, hundreds of thousands of **oogonia** (cells that develop into ova) are present in the ovaries. Thus the entire lifetime supply of ova is established during embryonic development; no new oogonia arise after birth. Each oogonium is surrounded by a cluster of granulosa cells. The oogonium and its granulosa cells constitute a follicle. During prenatal development, the oogonia increase in size and become primary oocytes. By the time of full gestational development, the primary oocytes are in the prophase of the first meiotic division (Figure 32-3). During childhood and into adult life, the oocytes enter a nonactive phase. After puberty, a few of the oocytes develop in follicles each month in response to follicle-stimulating hormone (FSH) secreted by the anterior pituitary gland. The vast majority of follicles and their oocytes die by atresia. Generally, each month, only one mature follicle will develop to eject an oocyte through the wall of the ovary in the process of ovulation, which is described in more detail in the Menstrual Cycle section.

Oviducts

The two **oviducts,** also called the fallopian or uterine tubes, are each about 10 cm long and located in the upper margin of the broad ligament. Each oviduct runs laterally from the uterus to the uterine end of the ovary. The free end of the oviduct adjacent to the ovary is called the *infundibulum*. It is shaped like a funnel with long, fingerlike projections termed *fimbriae*. The ampulla, the longest part of the oviduct, has an inner lining consisting of ciliated mucous membrane

ANTERIOR VIEW OF ADNEXA

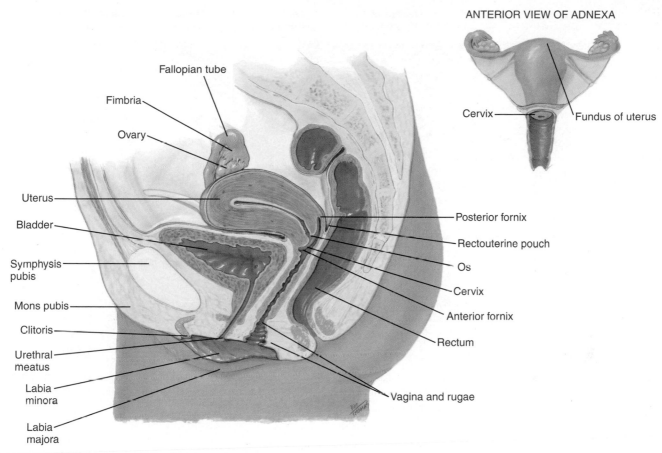

FIGURE 32-1 Cross-sectional view of the female reproductive system. (From Jarvis C: *Physical examination and health assessment,* ed 5, Philadelphia, 2008, Saunders, p 759.)

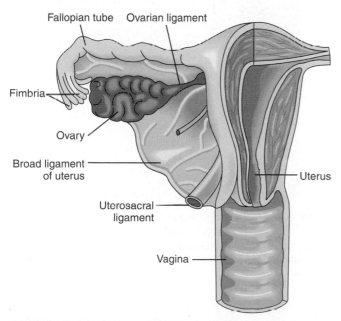

FIGURE 32-2 View of the female pelvis showing the ovarian and uterine ligaments.

arranged in longitudinal folds. Beneath this ciliated lining is a double layer of smooth muscle with a thick outer layer of peritoneal serosa. The oviduct has an active role in propelling the ovum toward the uterus; the current created by the beating cilia and the peristaltic contractions of the muscular wall are powerful forces that move ova along the oviduct. Once inside the oviduct, the ovum is moved through the ampulla to the isthmus (the short, narrow portion near the uterus) and finally through the intramural passageway to the uterus. Fertilization of the ovum occurs in the upper third of the oviduct, and the **zygote** (fertilized ovum) begins developing as it moves through the oviduct. If no fertilization occurs, the ovum undergoes degeneration in the oviduct.[9]

Uterus

The uterus varies in size, shape, location, and structure during various phases of a woman's life and reproductive status. In the nonpregnant state, the uterus is about 8 cm long, 4 cm wide in its upper part, and 2 cm thick. The rounded part of the uterus, which lies above and in front of the openings of the oviducts, is called the *fundus;* the main portion of the uterus is the *corpus,* or body. The lower, narrow portion of the uterus is the *cervix,* which extends downward to the opening within the vagina. The cervix contains a narrow canal that joins the

Follicular cells   Nucleus of primary oocyte   Zona pellucida   Theca interna   Cumulus oophorus

Antrum

filled with follicular fluid

A   B   C

FIGURE 32-3 Photomicrographs of sections from adult human ovaries. **A,** Ovarian cortex showing two primordial follicles containing primary oocytes that have completed the prophase of the first meiotic division. **B,** Growing follicle containing a primary oocyte. **C,** An almost mature follicle. (From Leeson CR et al: *Text/atlas of histology,* Philadelphia, 1988, Saunders.)

uterine cavity at the internal os and opens into the vagina at the external os.

The wall of the body and fundus of the uterus consists of three layers: endometrium, myometrium, and serosa (Figure 32-4). The outermost layer of the uterus, the serosa, consists of a single layer of mesothelial cells supported by a thin layer of loose connective tissue. The middle layer, the myometrium, consists of three layers of smooth muscle with the muscle fibers arranged in a different direction in each layer. The innermost lining of the uterus, the **endometrium,** consists of two layers: a thin deep layer called the *basilar layer* and a thick superficial layer referred to as the *functional layer.* During a woman's reproductive years, the endometrium displays a constant cyclic activity of alternate proliferation and sloughing of the functional layer in response to **estrogen** and **progesterone** secretion.[9] These changes will be discussed in more detail in the Menstrual Cycle section.

Vagina

The vagina is the sexual organ that enfolds the penis during sexual intercourse, serves as an exit for discarded endometrium, and forms the lower end of the birth canal. It is located anterior to the rectum and posterior to the urethra and urinary bladder. The vagina surrounds the cervix at one end and opens to the vestibule at its other end. The vagina is a highly elastic muscle that is capable of considerable distention. Two longitudinal ridges run along the anterior and posterior walls, with numerous transverse folds called *rugae.* The

FIGURE 32-4 The uterine wall consists of an epithelial lining *(E)* from which uterine glands *(G)* extend through the full thickness of the mucosa. Beneath the endometrium, a small portion of myometrium *(M)* is shown. (From Leeson CR et al: *Atlas of histology,* ed 2, Philadelphia, 1985, Saunders, p 261.)

vagina is lined by a mucous membrane of stratified squamous epithelium overlying a layer of connective tissue.[9] The vaginal wall is subject to thinning with aging; this and other age-related changes in the female sexual organs are described in the Menopause section.

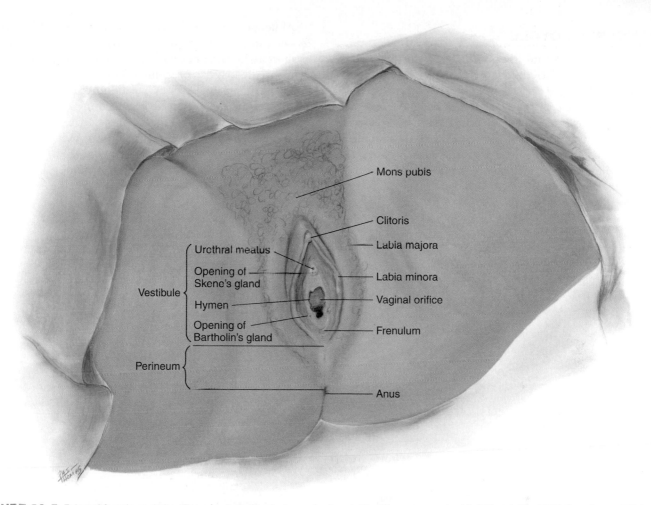

FIGURE 32-5 External female genitalia. (From Jarvis C: *Physical examination and health assessment,* ed 5, Philadelphia, 2008, Saunders, p 759.)

External Genitalia

The external female genital structures include the mons pubis, labia majora, labia minora, clitoris, and vestibule of the vagina (Figure 32-5). The mons pubis is a rounded elevation in front of the pubis symphysis. It consists primarily of an accumulation of fat. After puberty, the skin over it is covered by coarse hair. The labia majora, which are **homologous** (i.e., corresponding in structure) with the scrotum of the male, are folds of skin that run downward and backward from the mons pubis to the area behind the vaginal opening. After puberty, the labia majora become pigmented and covered with hair. The labia minora are two small folds of skin located between the labia majora on either side of the vaginal opening. The vestibule of the vagina is the cleft between the labia minora and contains the openings of the vagina, the urethra, and the ducts of the greater vestibular glands (also called *Bartholin glands*). These glands, along with the lesser vestibular or Skene glands, secrete mucus to provide lubrication during sexual intercourse.[8,9]

The clitoris is a body of erectile tissue that projects from the anterior end of the vulva at the anterior junction of the labia minora. It is about 2 cm long and 0.5 cm in diameter and is covered by a fold of tissue called the prepuce, which is formed by the merging of labial tissue. The glans of the clitoris is the rounded elevation on the free end of the body and is highly sensitive to stimulation. During sexual arousal, the erectile tissue of the clitoris becomes engorged with blood.[8,9]

KEY POINTS

- Organs of the female reproductive tract include the ovaries, oviducts, uterus, cervix, and vagina. Ovaries contain a lifetime supply of ova at birth. After puberty, a few of the ovarian follicles develop about every 28 days in response to secretion of FSH.
- The oviducts (fallopian tubes) actively propel the ovum toward the uterus by ciliary action and peristaltic contractions. The uterine lining undergoes a cyclic process of proliferation and then sloughing in response to estrogen and progesterone.
- External genitalia in the female include the mons pubis, labia majora, labia minora, clitoris, and vestibule of the vagina. The urinary meatus, vaginal opening, and vestibular gland ducts are located in the vaginal vestibule.

MENSTRUAL CYCLE

From **menarche** onward, the normal reproductive years of the female are characterized by rhythmic changes in hormonal secretion and corresponding changes in the sexual organs, which are called the *target organs* of the female hormones. This rhythmic pattern is called the **menstrual cycle.** Two significant results of the menstrual cycle are stimulation of the production of an ovum and preparation of the uterine endometrium for the implantation of a fertilized ovum at the appropriate phase of the cycle.[8]

Although considerable variation can be found in human females, an average menstrual cycle is 28 days long, with cycles as short as 20 days or as long as 45 days occurring in normal women. The first day of menstruation is considered the first day of the menstrual cycle. Ovulation occurs approximately 14 days before the next cycle begins; thus in a 28-day cycle, ovulation occurs on about day 14 of the cycle.

The release of hormones and accompanying response of the female sexual target organs are depicted in Figure 32-6. The principal female reproductive hormones are summarized in Table 32-1. As shown in Figure 32-6, the events of the

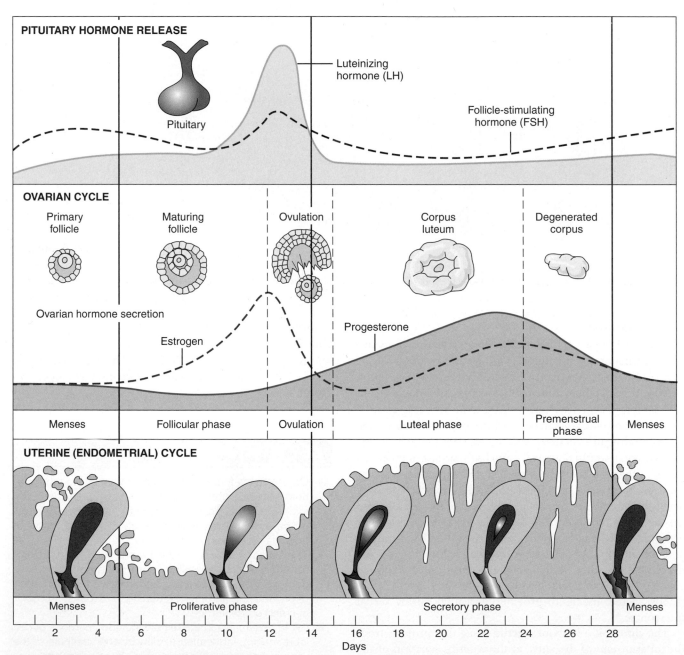

FIGURE 32-6 The menstrual cycle. The events that take place within the pituitary, ovary, and uterus are precisely synchronized. When fertilization does not occur, the cycle repeats itself about every 28 days.

TABLE 32-1

Principal Female Reproductive Hormones

Hormone	Target Organs	Significant Actions
Estrogen	Multiple sites throughout the body, including reproductive structures, bone, fat, and muscle tissues	Development of reproductive organs during puberty Development of secondary sex characteristics, including breast maturation, widening of the pelvis, and distribution of fat and muscle tissues in a distinctively female pattern Cyclic preparation of the endometrium for implantation of an ovum
Progesterone	Primarily uterus and breasts	Cyclic preparation and maintenance of the endometrium for implantation of an ovum Stimulation of development of breast lobes and alveoli
Follicle-stimulating hormone	Ovary	Stimulates ovarian follicle development; with luteinizing hormone, stimulates secretion of estrogen and ovulation
Luteinizing hormone	Ovary	Stimulates final development of the ovarian follicle, ovulation, and development of the corpus luteum

menstrual cycle require precise synchronization between the activities of the pituitary gland, ovary, and uterus. Beginning at the first day of the menstrual cycle, or the first day of menstruation, these events can be summarized as follows. The thickened functional layer of the endometrium of the uterus is gradually sloughed off, and about 35 ml of blood is lost. During this phase of the menstrual cycle, FSH is released by the pituitary gland and stimulates a group of follicles to develop in the ovary.

In the preovulatory phase, also called the proliferative phase, theca and granulosa cells in the developing follicles in the ovary secrete estrogen, which stimulates growth of the uterine endometrium once again. At about the midpoint of the cycle, an increase in estrogen secretion from the follicles occurs. This increase in estrogen is thought to render the anterior pituitary more responsive to luteinizing hormone–releasing hormone secreted by the hypothalamus.[10] The anterior pituitary gland then produces a burst of luteinizing hormone. FSH also increases about twofold at the same time, and these two hormones act synergistically to cause the extremely rapid swelling of the follicle that culminates in ovulation.[11] During the process of ovulation, the secondary oocyte is ejected through the wall of the ovary into the peritoneal cavity. The free end of the oviduct is strategically located so that the ovum enters its fimbriated end almost immediately.[9]

After ovulation, the postovulatory phase (also called the luteal phase) begins. During the luteal phase the site of the ruptured follicle becomes a **corpus luteum** (Latin for "yellow body"), which secretes estrogen and progesterone. These hormones stimulate continued thickening of the uterine endometrium. The cells of the corpus luteum become greatly enlarged and develop lipid, or fatty, areas that give the cells a distinctive yellow color. In a normal cycle, the corpus luteum grows to approximately 1.5 cm, with maximal development attained about 7 to 8 days after ovulation. If pregnancy does not occur, the corpus luteum begins to degenerate, and progesterone and estrogen levels in the blood fall markedly. Constriction of the spiral arteries located in the uterine wall occurs, and the portion

of the endometrium supplied by these arteries becomes ischemic. As the cells in the endometrium die, tissue is sloughed off and menstruation begins again. It is presently thought that prostaglandins liberated in the endometrium may have a role in stimulating the sloughing of endometrial tissue.[9,12]

If fertilization of the ovum occurs, the embryo arrives in the uterus on about the fourth day of development. Small glands in the endometrium stimulated by progesterone produce a nutritive fluid for the developing embryo. On approximately the seventh day after fertilization, the embryo implants itself in the thick endometrium of the uterus, and development of the **placenta** occurs. The placenta secretes the hormone human chorionic gonadotropin (hCG), which in turn signals the corpus luteum to continue to function. Subsequent events in pregnancy are described later in this chapter.

KEY POINTS

- The monthly reproductive cycle averages about 28 days. Beginning on the first day of menses, the important events of the cycle are as follows:
  1. The endometrial layer is sloughed off.
  2. The ovarian follicles are stimulated by pituitary FSH.
  3. Estrogen is secreted from the developing follicles.
  4. Proliferation of the endometrium occurs in response to estrogen.
  5. At the midpoint of the cycle, a burst of luteinizing hormone and a doubling of FSH secretion from the pituitary gland stimulate ovulation.
  6. The ruptured follicle changes into a corpus luteum and secretes estrogen and progesterone.
  7. In the absence of pregnancy, secretion of estrogen and progesterone drops rapidly and the endometrial lining sloughs off again to complete the cycle.
- With fertilization and implantation of the ovum, the developing placenta secretes hCG, which in turn stimulates the corpus luteum to continue to secrete estrogen and progesterone and thus prevent endometrial sloughing.

BREAST

The breast is an important accessory organ in sexual function and human reproduction. Although its primary physiologic function is **lactation** (production of milk) to nourish the human infant, the significance of the breast as a symbol of feminine sexuality in contemporary Western culture must also be recognized.

Structure of the Breast

The breasts are located anterior to the pectoralis major muscle and are separated from it by a layer of fat. The position of the breasts is maintained by fibrous bands called *Cooper ligaments,* which are easily stretched, especially if the breasts are large. Lymph drainage from the breasts is mainly toward the axillary lymph nodes, with some drainage toward the substernal and diaphragmatic lymph nodes.[13]

Each breast consists of 15 to 20 lobes of glandular epithelial tissue and a duct system embedded in interstitial tissue and fat. The secretory cells that constitute the glandular epithelium are arranged in grapelike clusters called *alveoli* (Figure 32-7). Ducts or openings from each alveolus unite to form a single duct from each lobe. These main ducts then enlarge slightly into ampullae immediately before opening onto the surface of the nipple. The nipple, located at the center of the adult female breast, is composed of bundles of smooth muscle fibers with erectile properties. The areola that surrounds the nipple has a diameter of 1.5 to 2.5 cm. The openings from the lactiferous ducts are arranged radially under the areola; thus 15 to 20 small openings are located on the surface of each nipple through which milk flows in a lactating female.[9]

Breast Development

The stages of development of the female breast are depicted in Figure 32-8. As shown in this figure, the breasts contain only rudimentary glands during childhood. At puberty, estrogen and progesterone, in the presence of growth hormone and prolactin, promote the development of glandular tissue and ducts and the deposition of fat characteristic of the adult female breast. Throughout the reproductive years, some women note swelling of the breast around the latter part of each menstrual cycle before the onset of menstruation. The water retention and subsequent swelling of breast tissue during this phase of the menstrual cycle are thought to be due to high levels of circulating progesterone stimulating the secretory cells of the breast.[13]

Lactation

During pregnancy, high concentrations of estrogen and progesterone produced by the corpus luteum and the placenta stimulate the development of glands and ducts in the breast.

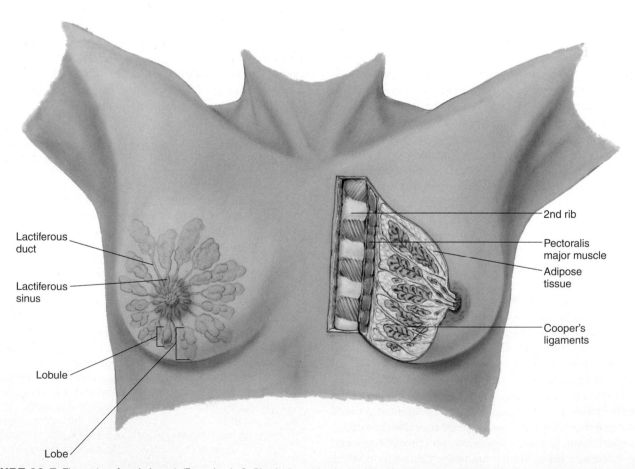

FIGURE 32-7 The mature female breast. (From Jarvis C: *Physical examination and health assessment,* ed 5, Philadelphia, 2008, Saunders, p 409.)

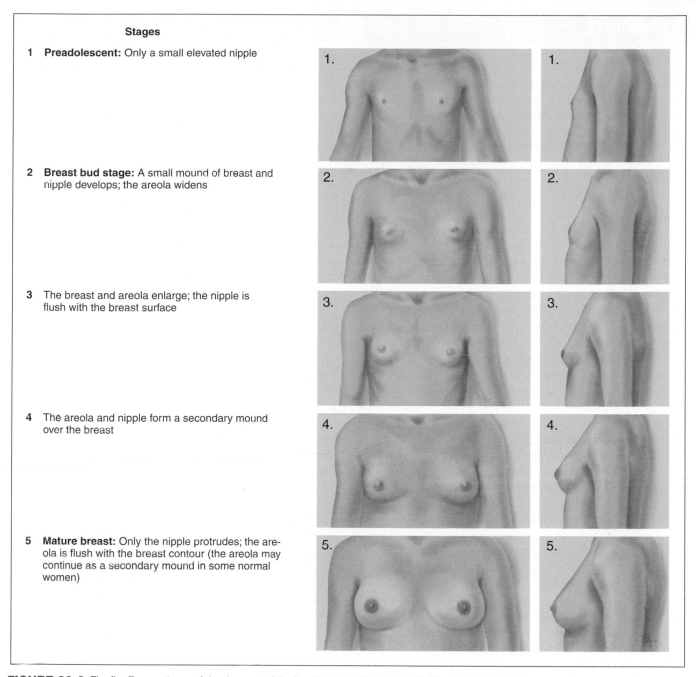

Stages

1 **Preadolescent:** Only a small elevated nipple

2 **Breast bud stage:** A small mound of breast and nipple develops; the areola widens

3 The breast and areola enlarge; the nipple is flush with the breast surface

4 The areola and nipple form a secondary mound over the breast

5 **Mature breast:** Only the nipple protrudes; the areola is flush with the breast contour (the areola may continue as a secondary mound in some normal women)

FIGURE 32-8 The five Tanner stages of development of the female breast. (From Jarvis C: *Physical examination and health assessment,* ed 5, Philadelphia, 2008, Saunders, p 411.)

During the first trimester of pregnancy, the ducts proliferate; in the second trimester, the ducts group together to form large lobules with new alveoli formation. In the third trimester, the existing alveoli dilate in preparation for lactation. Toward the end of pregnancy and until 1 to 3 days after childbirth, the mammary glands form colostrum, which contains protein and lactose but little fat. After birth of the infant, the hormone **prolactin** secreted by the mother's anterior pituitary gland stimulates milk production, and milk is produced by the third day after delivery. The initiation and maintenance of lactation are a complex neuroendocrine process involving sensory nerves in the nipples and breast tissue, the spinal cord and hypothalamus, and the pituitary gland. The suckling movements of the infant on the breast stimulate the release of prolactin from the anterior pituitary gland and **oxytocin** from the posterior pituitary gland. These hormones in turn stimulate lactation and ejection of milk from the alveoli into the ducts, where it is accessible to the infant. Oxytocin then promotes the actual release of milk, called the "milk ejection reflex."[9,14]

PREGNANCY

During the 9 months of human gestation, the single-celled zygote gives rise to an infant with a complex set of physiologic systems. The fertilized ovum contains the entire genetic complement—or encoded genetic instructions—to develop into a fully functioning term infant, given adequate nutrition and time. Three basic developmental processes—growth, **morphogenesis,** and cellular differentiation—are involved in this transformation.[7] Growth denotes the proliferation of new cells by mitosis, a necessary but not sufficient process for development. The arrangement of cells in a particular order is called *morphogenesis* and is essential to the elaboration of higher forms of life. In addition to growth and morphogenesis, cellular differentiation is needed for cells to specialize structurally and biochemically in a myriad of ways. This section describes the sequence of events in which growth, morphogenesis, and cellular differentiation function to transform a human zygote with encoded genetic information into a human infant. In addition, this section will describe the response of the mother's body to pregnancy. Information on genetic control of inheritance and genetic disorders is contained in Chapters 5 and 6, and the reader may wish to refer to these chapters for specific content in these areas.

Early Human Development

Fertilization of the ovum occurs in the oviduct. Within 24 hours after fertilization, the zygote begins a series of divisions by the process of mitosis; this process is referred to as *cleavage* (Figure 32-9). From a two-cell entity the zygote soon divides multiple times, and its cytoplasm begins to be partitioned into specific cells that will serve as the building blocks of the embryo. As more cleavage takes place, the embryo is transported through the oviduct to the uterus. This process takes about 4 days. The embryo receives nutrition during this time from secretions released by the epithelial cells lining the oviduct. After the embryo enters the uterus, the zona pellucida, the membrane surrounding the embryo, dissolves. At about day 4, the embryo arrives in the uterus and floats freely while receiving nutrition from secretions from the endometrial glands stimulated by progesterone.

At this point the cells of the embryo have arranged themselves into a hollow spherical structure called the *blastocyst* (Figure 32-10). The outer cells of the blastocyst, called the *trophoblast,* will ultimately become the protective and nutritive membranes (chorion and placenta) that surround the developing embryo. The inner cell mass, a small cluster of cells that projects into the cavity of the blastocyst, will develop into the structures of the embryo itself. If at this point the inner cell mass divides into two separate groups of cells, identical twins with an identical genetic complement will result. Fraternal twins develop when two ova are fertilized by two sperm cells and do not have an identical genetic complement.[7]

Implantation

On approximately day 7 after fertilization, the embryo attaches to the uterine lining and then implants itself in the endometrium. Enzymes secreted by the trophoblast erode a small portion of the uterine lining, and by day 10 of development the embryo has worked its way down into the endometrium completely. The opening in the uterine lining is closed, initially by a blood clot and then by regeneration of uterine epithelium; all subsequent development of the embryo takes place in the wall of the uterus.[9]

Fetal Membranes and Placenta

Fetal membranes protect the developing embryo or fetus and provide needed substrates for growth and development, particularly oxygen and nutrition. In addition, they serve the purpose of elimination of waste products of metabolism. All terrestrial vertebrates have four fetal membranes: amnion, yolk sac, chorion, and allantois.[9] In the developing human, the yolk sac is usually thought to be a vestigial structure, although it serves as an important temporary center for the formation of blood cells between the second and sixth weeks. The allantois is also considered vestigial, although its blood supply contributes to formation of the umbilical vessels.

The amnion begins to develop at a very early stage and eventually expands to surround the entire embryo. The space between the amnion and the embryo is called the **amniotic cavity**. It is filled with a clear amniotic fluid that keeps the embryo moist and provides a measure of protection against mechanical injury.

The **placenta** serves two basic functions. It is the organ of exchange between the developing fetus and the mother; it also provides nutrients to the fetus and removes wastes. It is also an endocrine organ and produces several hormones, most notably hCG. The placenta develops from both the chorion and maternal uterine tissue. After implantation, the chorion develops rapidly and forms highly vascularized villi as the embryonic circulation develops. The umbilical cord develops and connects the embryo with the placenta. Two umbilical arteries arise in the umbilical cord and connect with a rapidly proliferating network of capillaries in the villi. The umbilical vein, also located in the umbilical cord, carries blood from the villi back to the fetus.

The placenta eventually consists of the portion of the chorion in which villi develop, along with the uterine tissue between the villi that contains maternal capillaries and small

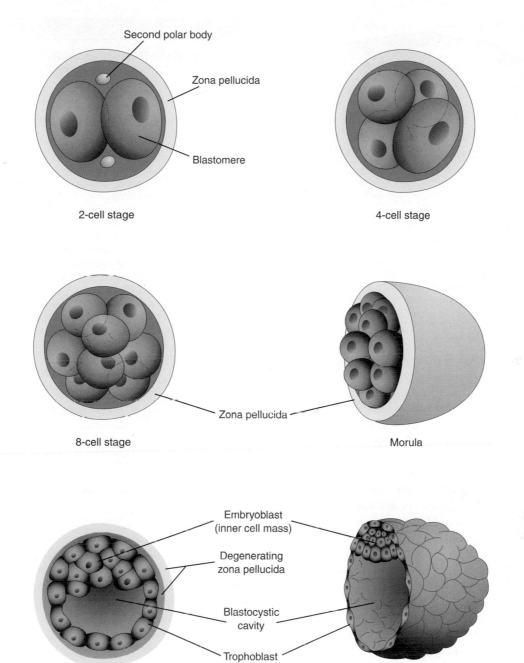

FIGURE 32-9 Early human development. Drawings illustrate cleavage of the zygote and formation of the blastocyst. (From Moore KL, Persaud TVN: *The developing human: clinically oriented embryology,* ed 8, Philadelphia, 2008, Saunders, p 36.)

pools of maternal blood. The placenta brings maternal blood adjacent to fetal blood, although the two circulatory systems are completely separate from each other. Thus oxygen and nutrient substrates pass from the maternal blood through the placental tissue and diffuse into the blood of the fetus, where these substances can be used for growth and development of various body tissues. Waste products of fetal metabolism from fetal blood then pass through the placenta into the maternal blood supply and are eventually transported to the maternal kidneys for disposal.[9]

The placenta, like the corpus luteum, secretes both estrogen and progesterone during pregnancy. These hormones serve a variety of purposes in pregnancy. Estrogen promotes enlargement of the uterus and growth of the ductal structure of the breast, as well as alters the elasticity of various pelvic ligaments and the symphysis pubis to allow passage of the infant through the pelvic structures during delivery. In addition to its role in providing early nutrition for the embryo, progesterone has the special effect of decreasing contractility of the gravid uterus, thus preventing spontaneous abortion.

FIGURE 32-10 Implantation of the early human embryo. (From Guyton AC, Hall JE: *Textbook of medical physiology,* ed 11, Philadelphia, 2006, Saunders, p 1029. Courtesy Arthur Hertig, MD.)

TABLE 32-2

Summary of Developmental Events in Human Fetal Life

Time from Fertilization	Key Events
36 hours	Embryo has achieved two-cell stage
4 days	Embryo reaches the uterus
7 days	Implantation of the embryo in the uterine wall
2.5 weeks	Differentiation of heart tissue
	Blood cell formation in the yolk sac and chorion
	Formation of the notochord and neural plate
3.5 weeks	Formation of the neural tube
	Heart tubes begin to beat
	Primordial eye and ear visible
	Respiratory system begins development
	Liver bud differentiates
	Blood vessels established
4 weeks	Formation of three primary brain vesicles
	Limb buds appear
2 months	Embryo capable of movement
	Cerebral cortex differentiating
	Gonad identifiable as testis or ovary
	Bones begin ossification and muscles are differentiating
	Major blood vessels in final positions
3 months	Fetus performs breathing and sucking movements
	Sex is clearly identifiable
5 months	Heartbeat is audible with a stethoscope
	Fetus moves freely through the amniotic cavity
6-9 months	Rapid growth with final differentiation of tissues and organs
266 days	Birth

In addition, progesterone may have a role in preparing the breasts for lactation, as described earlier in the Lactation section.

Of major importance in the role of the placenta as an endocrine gland is its production of hCG. From the time of implantation, the trophoblastic cells begin to secrete hCG, which sends a signal to the corpus luteum that a pregnancy has begun. The corpus luteum responds by increasing its size and its secretion of estrogen and progesterone, which then promote continued development of the endometrium and the placenta. In the absence of hCG, the corpus luteum would disintegrate, as it does in a nonfertilized menstrual cycle, and the endometrium would deteriorate and be sloughed off along with the embryo. Thus, hCG is an essential element in continuation of the pregnant state.[9]

Development of the Human Embryo and Fetus

From fertilization to the end of the eighth week, the developing organism is referred to as an *embryo;* from the ninth week until birth, the developing baby is referred to as a *fetus.* Development of the fetus proceeds in an orderly sequence of complex events. With recent developments in fetal physiology, it is possible to predict which structures will begin their development or function on a particular day of development after conception. Table 32-2 depicts some important developmental events from the time of fertilization to birth. Detailed information on the development of organ systems during fetal life is contained in the chapters in this book that focus on these organ systems; for example, Chapter 35 contains a description of the development of the gastrointestinal tract.

First Month

Rapid growth, morphogenesis, and cell differentiation occur early in development of the human embryo. By 2½ weeks of development, the notochord and neural plate are formed; these

structures eventually give rise to the central nervous system. In addition, the tissue that will form the heart has differentiated. By the end of the first month, an S-shaped heart beats about 60 times per minute, and the three primary vesicles of the brain have formed.

Second Month

Figure 32-11 shows an embryo in its seventh week. All of the organs continue to develop during the second month, and the embryo becomes capable of movement. The major blood vessels assume their final positions, and the heart assumes its final shape. The brain begins to transmit impulses to regulate function of the organ systems, and a few reflexes are now present. Although sex cannot be distinguished externally, either an ovary or testis has begun to form internally. At the end of the second month, the rudiments of all organs are present and the embryo is referred to as a *fetus.*[9]

Third Month

During the third month, the ears and eyes approach their final positions, and some of the bones become distinct. The fetus performs breathing movements consisting of moving amniotic fluid in and out of the lungs and can carry on sucking

Eyelid

Eye

Digital ray

Notch between digital
rays of hand

Liver prominence

Umbilical cord

Digital ray of foot plate

External acoustic meatus
(external ear canal)

Cervical flexure

Auricle of
external ear

Wrist

A

B

Actual size 16.0 mm

FIGURE 32-11 A and **B,** Human embryo in the seventh week of development. (In Moore KL: *The developing human: clinically oriented embryology,* ed 7, Philadelphia, 2003, Saunders, p 93. **A,** Courtesy Kazumasa Hoshino, MD, former Professor of Anatomy and Director of the Congenital Anomaly Center, Faculty of Medicine, Kyoto University, Japan. **B,** From Moore KL, Persaud TVN: *The developing human: clinically oriented embryology,* ed 8, Philadelphia, 2008, Saunders, p 88.)

movements. By the end of the third month, the fetus is almost 56 mm in length and weighs about 14 g (Figure 32-12).

Second Trimester

A *trimester* refers to a period of 3 months during pregnancy. During the second trimester, or months 4 to 6 of development, the fetus achieves independent mobility and can move freely through the amniotic cavity. The heartbeat of the fetus is now audible through a stethoscope and averages 150 beats per minute. By the fifth month of development, the fetus measures 250 mm (10 inches) in length, which is half its total length at birth.[7] Figure 32-13 shows a fetus in the second trimester at 17 weeks of development.

Third Trimester

By far the greatest growth of the fetus occurs during the third trimester. The weight of the fetus almost doubles during the last 2 months.[13] In addition, final differentiation of tissues and organs takes place. Survival of infants born prematurely during this time has increased markedly in the past few years because of an enhanced ability to sustain vital functions such as respiration and regulation of body temperature in neonatal intensive care settings.

Parturition

Parturition refers to the process by which the infant is born. Toward the end of pregnancy, the uterus becomes progressively more excitable until it begins strong rhythmic contractions that ultimately expel the infant.[11] At the present

time, the exact cause of the increased uterine activity remains unknown. However, two sets of effects have been suggested as contributing to the increased excitability of uterine musculature at this time: progressive hormonal changes and progressive mechanical changes.[13,15]

Hormonal Changes

During the latter part of pregnancy, large amounts of estrogen, which has a definite tendency to increase uterine contractility, are secreted. Concurrent with this enhanced estrogen release, the secretion of progesterone, which inhibits uterine contractility, remains constant or may decrease slightly. Thus it is hypothesized that the increased ratio of estrogen to progesterone secretion in the latter part of pregnancy may promote the increased contractility of the uterus.[13]

Oxytocin is a hormone secreted by the posterior pituitary gland that specifically causes uterine contraction and is thought to have a major role in promoting increased uterine contractility during parturition. The rate of oxytocin secretion is considerably increased at the time of labor (see the following discussion of mechanical changes), and the uterus displays increased responsiveness to a given dose of oxytocin at this time.[13,15]

Mechanical Changes

Stretching smooth muscle organs increases their contractility; in addition, intermittent stretching of smooth muscle can elicit contraction. Thus it is hypothesized that the stretch or irritation of the fetal head against the cervix begins a reflex

FIGURE 32-12 Photograph of the human fetus at 11 weeks of development. (From Moore KL, Persaud TVN: *The developing human: clinically oriented embryology,* ed 8, Philadelphia, 2008, Saunders, p 100. Courtesy Professor Jean Hay [Retired], Department of Anatomy, University of Manitoba, Winnipeg, Canada.)

action that causes the uterus to contract. As the cycle of stretching and contraction is repeated again and again, increased contractions result. In addition, stretching of the cervix causes the release of oxytocin from the posterior pituitary. Oxytocin then stimulates additional uterine contractions, thus initiating another feedback cycle of stretching and contraction.[13,16,17]

Response of the Mother's Body to Pregnancy

The presence of a developing fetus in the uterus creates an extra physiologic load for the pregnant woman, with resulting effects on her basal metabolism and specific organ systems. Normal physiologic responses to pregnancy are described here; complications of pregnancy are discussed in Chapter 33.

Metabolism During Pregnancy

As a result of increased secretion of many hormones, including thyroxine, adrenocortical hormones, and the sex hormones, the basal metabolic rate increases by about 15% during the latter half of pregnancy.[13] This increase in metabolism results in alterations in many organ systems, including the circulatory, respiratory, and urinary systems.

Changes in the Female Reproductive Organs

The hormones secreted during pregnancy, either by the placenta or the endocrine glands, directly promote alterations in body structures. In particular, the organs of the female reproductive tract increase markedly in size, with the uterus increasing from 30 to 1100 g and the breasts approximately doubling in size. Concurrently, the vagina enlarges with a widening of the vaginal introitus.

Changes in the Circulatory System

In the latter stages of pregnancy, about 625 ml of blood flows through the maternal circulation of the placenta each minute. This factor, along with a general increase in metabolism, causes an increase in maternal cardiac output to 30% to 40% above normal by the 27th week of pregnancy. However, for reasons not understood at the present time, cardiac output decreases to a little above normal during the last 8 weeks of pregnancy, although the high uterine blood flow continues.[13]

As shown in Figure 32-14, an increase in maternal blood volume occurs mainly during the latter half of pregnancy. This increase is mainly due to hormonal factors. Both aldosterone and estrogens, which are greatly increased in pregnancy, promote increased fluid retention by the kidneys. In addition, bone marrow increases its activity to produce an excess of red blood cells to accompany the excess vascular volume. At the time of parturition, the mother has an additional 1 to 2 extra liters of blood in her circulatory system.[13]

Changes in the Respiratory System

The increased basal metabolic rate and size of the pregnant woman result in an increase in oxygen utilization, with utilization of oxygen being 20% above normal at the time of birth. Concurrently, a commensurate amount of carbon dioxide is formed. In addition, the growing uterus is pressing upward against the abdominal organs, which in turn press against the diaphragm and cause a decrease in diaphragmatic excursion. The net result of these changes is an increase in minute ventilation of approximately 50% and a decrease in arterial P_{CO_2} to slightly below normal.[13]

Changes in the Urinary System

Because of an increased load of excretory products, the rate of urine formation in pregnancy is usually slightly increased. In addition, other alterations in urinary function occur. Renal tubule reabsorption of sodium, chloride, and water is increased as a result of increased production of steroidal hormones by the placenta and adrenal cortex. Concurrently, the glomerular filtration rate often increases by as much as 50%, a change that serves to increase the rate of water and electrolyte loss in the urine. These two events tend to balance each other out, with the result that only a moderate excess of water and salt accumulation occurs under normal circumstances.[11] However, in the condition of toxemia of pregnancy, excess water and salt accumulation may occur with life-threatening consequences.

FIGURE 32-13 A, Side view of human fetus at 17 weeks. **B,** Frontal view of 17-week fetus. (**A,** From Moore KL et al: *Color atlas of clinical embryology,* ed 2, Philadelphia, 2000, Saunders. **B,** Courtesy Dr. Robert Jordan, St. Georges University Medical School, Grenada.)

FIGURE 32-14 Effect of pregnancy on blood volume. (From Guyton AC, Hall JE: *Textbook of medical physiology,* ed 11, Philadelphia, 2006, Saunders, p 1035.)

Weight Gain and Nutrition During Pregnancy

The average weight gain during pregnancy is about 24 lb, with most of this gain occurring during the last two trimesters. Approximately 7 lb of this weight gain is the fetus; 4 lb of the increased weight is amniotic fluid, placenta, and fetal membranes; 2 lb represents an increase in uterine tissue; and another 2 lb of the weight gain is an increase in breast tissue. Thus an average 9-lb increase in weight occurs in the remainder of the woman's body. Approximately 6 lb of fluid may be excreted during the days following birth, after loss of the fluid-retaining hormones of the placenta.[13]

Appetite may be greatly increased during the latter part of pregnancy, in part because of fetal removal of food substrates from the mother's blood and partly because of hormonal factors. The developing fetus assumes priority in regard to many of the nutritional substrates of the mother's body fluids and will continue to grow even when maternal nutrition is inadequate. However, although fetal length may increase normally in the absence of adequate maternal nutrition, fetal weight will be considerably decreased, and abnormal bone formation and decreased size of many bodily organs of the fetus may result.[13]

If the intake of nutritional elements during pregnancy is inadequate, a number of deficiencies can be present in the mother. In particular, deficiencies of calcium, phosphates, iron, and vitamins may be present. As an example, approximately 375 mg of iron is needed by the fetus to form its blood, and an additional 600 mg is needed by the mother to form her own extra blood supply. Because the normal store of nonhemoglobin iron in the mother at the beginning of pregnancy is often about 100 mg and seldom above 700 mg, anemia will develop in a pregnant woman without sufficient iron intake in her food.[13] Important also is adequate folic acid intake, which has been shown to help prevent neural tube defects.[18]

MENOPAUSE

Although **menopause** is defined specifically as the last menstrual period in a woman's reproductive life, the term is often used to denote the entire period of years before and after this event in which the function of the ovaries is in transition. The terms *climacteric* and *perimenopause* are used in the health care literature to describe this transitional period. At about 45 to 52 years of age the supply of ovarian follicles declines, with the majority becoming atretic or degenerated. With the depletion of ovarian follicles, secretion of estrogen and progesterone by the ovaries declines, and the menstrual cycle becomes irregular. When too little estrogen is secreted to cause endometrial growth, menstrual periods stop permanently.[13]

The decline in ovarian hormone production that occurs in the perimenopausal period causes important physiologic changes in a woman's body. The decline in plasma estrogen levels may result in a number of distressing symptoms, although some women experience no symptoms during this time. Hot flushes, described by women as an unpleasant sensation of sudden warmth sweeping upward over the abdomen, chest, neck, and face, are experienced by nearly 75% of postmenopausal women. Although the precise cause of hot flushes is unknown, it is thought that decreased estrogen levels have an effect on the temperature-regulating center in the hypothalamus. Hot flushes are often accompanied by other symptoms of autonomic nervous system instability such as tachycardia, palpitations, and feelings of faintness. Other distressing symptoms, including pain and stiffness in the joints,

sleep pattern disturbances, and changes in gastrointestinal function, have been noted by women in the perimenopausal period. These symptoms are presently the focus of many nursing research projects examining the health of aging women. Although such psychological symptoms as increased nervousness have been reported in the medical literature as being related to hormonal imbalance in menopause, it has been established that psychological symptoms are not directly related to estrogen deficiency.[19] There is an increasing awareness of the importance of role of culture and other social factors in the understanding of how women view and experience menopause.[20]

With the decline in estrogen associated with perimenopause, many structural changes occur in various organs. These changes are summarized in Geriatric Considerations: Changes in the Female Reproductive System. The epidermis of the skin becomes thinner and less elastic throughout the entire body. The breasts may decrease in size; the labia may also lose their underlying fat and become thinner.[21] The vaginal epithelium may become thin and atrophied, with the result that sexual intercourse may be painful. The decline in estrogen also leads to osteoporosis and decreased bone density, particularly in white women, with resulting bone fractures. Exercise and supplemental calcium and vitamin D are recommended for postmenopausal women to prevent accelerated bone loss. At present, some authorities recommend estrogen therapy during the perimenopausal period to prevent and relieve symptoms such as hot flashes and vaginal atrophy. However, supplemental estrogen and progestin therapy has been associated with an increased risk of breast cancer and cardiovascular disease.[22,23] Newer treatments that have been developed for osteoporosis include bisphosphonates, calcitonin nasal spray, and raloxiphene.[24] Work continues on the development of selective estrogen receptor modulators that may retain some of the beneficial effects of estrogen while avoiding the bad effects.[25] Women in perimenopause may wish to discuss the risks and potential benefits of hormone replacement therapy and other menopausal therapies with their health care providers before making an informed decision about these medications.

GERIATRIC CONSIDERATIONS

Changes in the Female Reproductive System

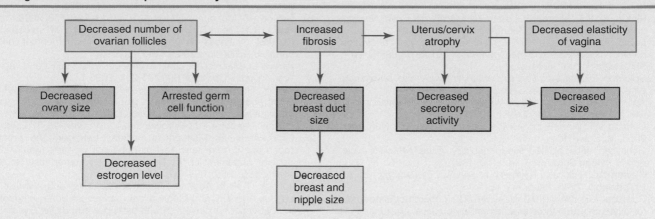

Female reproductive system function declines with organ-specific tissue changes. Active female germ cells decline over time with variable function before they are arrested in menopause. The ovaries become smaller and increasingly fibrotic and have fewer ovarian follicles.

The secretion of estrogen by the ovaries stops at menopause, resulting in a marked estrogen level decrease. The ovarian follicles become insensitive to gonadotropins (FSH and luteinizing hormone). However, the peripheral conversion of androgens to estrogen causes a small maintenance level of estrogen to persist at 10% to 30% of previous levels. The androgen-producing ovarian cells (hilar and thecal) continue to secrete testosterone in postmenopausal women.

The follicles, uterus, and cervix undergo atrophy with a decrease in size and secretory action. The vagina is reduced in size with a loss of elasticity and atrophy of the vaginal epithelium. The vascular supply to the vaginal walls decreases with reduced glycogen and mucopolysaccharide. The pH of Bartholin gland secretions is increased or alkaline due to the loss of estrogen.

The breasts decrease in size. Breast ducts become smaller and are replaced by fat tissue. Some fibrosis and calcification may occur within the ducts. The nipples are smaller with less nipple pigmentation. The aging female nipple may be normal or retracted.

SUMMARY

This chapter has described the major processes related to the human female reproductive tract, including the menstrual cycle, pregnancy, lactation, and menopause. In approaching this material, the reader must view the information presented within the current context of social change in which women are taking an active role in meeting their health care needs. In addition, recent research in the area of reproductive endocrinology has yielded a rapidly expanding understanding of the reproductive structures and their function.

The female reproductive structures are a complex set of organs with multiple, integrated functions. Careful review of the section on reproductive structures, including their embryologic development, will assist the reader in understanding the various alterations in these structures that occur throughout a woman's life. Although the hormonal and structural changes occurring in the female reproductive organs may at first seem overwhelmingly complex to the student, some basic concepts will help in organizing this material. First, the menstrual cycle has two significant results: production of an ovum and preparation of the uterus for implantation of the fertilized ovum. Second, the fertilized ovum contains the entire encoded genetic instructions

to produce a unique human individual. Third, pregnancy consists of three basic developmental processes—growth, morphogenesis, and cellular differentiation—to bring about this transformation, which will also result in multiple changes in the body of the mother. The breast, with its function of lactation, is also a component of the reproductive system and is subject to alterations throughout a woman's life span. Finally, menopause is not a discrete event but rather a process during which the supply of ovarian follicles declines. A review of these concepts will prepare the student for a better understanding of women's health concerns and provide a basis for approaching the next chapter, which considers alterations in reproductive functioning.

REFERENCES

1. Heavey EJ, Moysich KB, Hyland A et al: Differences in contraceptive choice among female adolescents at a state-funded family planning clinic, *J Midwifery Women's Health* 53(1):45-52, 2008.
2. Prunty MC, Sharpe L, Butow P et al: The motherhood choice: A decision aid for women with multiple sclerosis, *Patient Educ Couns* 71(1):108-115, 2008.
3. Wilmoth MC: The middle years: women, sexuality, and the self, *J Obstet Gynecol Neonatal Nurs* 25(7):615-621, 1996.
4. Albright MJ, Clinton HR: The perimenopause: a critical time in a woman's life, *Int J Fertil Menopausal Stud* 41(2):85-89, 1996.

5. Capel B: Sex in the 90s: SRY and the switch to the male pathway, *Annu Rev Physiol* 69:497-523, 1998.

6. Josso N: Embryology and control of fetal sex differentiation. In DeGroot LJ, Jameson JL, editors: *Endocrinology,* ed 5, Philadelphia, 2005, Saunders.

7. McKinney ES, Murray SS, Ashwill J: *Maternal-Child Nursing,* ed 2, Philadelphia, 2007, Saunders.

8. Lewis SL, Heitkemper MM, Dirksen SR et al: *Medical-surgical nursing: assessment and management of clinical problems,* ed 7, Philadelphia, 2007, Mosby.

9. Solomon EP: *Introduction to human anatomy and physiology,* ed 3, Philadelphia, 2008, Saunders.

10. Apter D: Development of the hypothalamic-pituitary-ovarian axis, *Ann N Y Acad Sci* 17(816):9-21, 1997.

11. Ganong WF: *Review of medical physiology,* ed 22, New York, 2005, McGraw-Hill.

12. Genazzani AR et al: Neuroendocrinology of the menstrual cycle, *Ann N Y Acad Sci* 17(816):143-150, 1997.

13. Guyton AC, Hall JE: *Textbook of medical physiology,* ed 11, Philadelphia, 2005, Saunders.

14. Cumbers MR, Chung ST, Wakerley JB: A neuromodulatory role for oxytocin within the supramammillary nucleus, *Neuropeptides* 41(4):217-226, 2007.

15. Blackburn ST: *Maternal, fetal, and neonatal physiology: a clinical perspective,* ed 3, Philadelphia, 2007, Saunders.

16. Fanchin R: Assessing uterine receptivity in 2001: ultrasonographic glances at the new millennium, *Ann N Y Acad Sci* 943:185-202, 2001.

17. Buhimschi CS, Buhimschi IA, Manilow AM et al: Uterine contractility in women whose fetus is delivered in the occipitoposterior position, *Am J Obstet Gynecol* 188(3):734-739, 2003.

18. Green NS: Folic acid supplementation and prevention of birth defects, *J Nutr* 132(8 Suppl):23565-23605, 2002.

19. Nelson HD: Menopause, *Lancet* 371(9614):760-770, 2008.

20. Hall L, Callister LC, Berry JA et al: Meanings of menopause: Cultural influences on perception and management of menopause, *J Holist Nurs* 25(2):106-118, 2008.

21. Farage M, Maibach H: Lifetime changes in the vulva and vagina, *Arch Gynecol Obstet* 273(4):195-202, 2006.

22. Writing Group for the Women's Health Initiative Investigators: Risks and benefits of estrogen plus progestin in healthy postmenopausal women: principal results from the Women's Health Initiative randomized controlled trial, *JAMA* 288:321-333, 2002.

23. North American Menopause Society: Estrogen and progestogen use in peri- and post-menopausal women: March 2007 position statement of the North American Menopause Society, *Menopause* 14(2):168-182, 2007.

24. Johnell O et al: Additive effects of raloxifene and alendronate on bone density and biochemical markers of bone remodeling in postmenopausal women with osteoporosis, *J Clin Endocrinol Metab* 87:985-992, 2002.

25. Riggs BL, Hartmann LC: Selective estrogen-receptor modulators: mechanisms of action and application to clinical practice, *N Engl J Med* 348:618-629, 2003.

Alterations in Female Genital and Reproductive Function

Rosemary A. Jadack • Jane M. Georges

MEDIA RESOURCES

Additional Material for Study, Review, and Further Exploration

CD Companion ■ Review Questions and Answers
■ Glossary (with audio pronunciations for selected terms)
■ Disease Profiles ■ Animations

evolve **Website** at http://evolve.elsevier.com/Copstead/
■ Case Studies ■ Disease Profiles ■ WebLinks ■ Key Points Review

 Online Course (Module 15)

KEY QUESTIONS

■ What are the differentiating factors of the common menstrual disorders?
■ What are the common etiologic factors leading to uterine prolapse, uterine retrodisplacement, cystocele, and rectocele?
■ How can the pain of endometriosis be differentiated from that of dysmenorrhea?
■ What is the rationale for routine Papanicolaou testing for cervical cancer?

■ What factors contribute to the high mortality rate of ovarian cancer?
■ What clinical findings would indicate the development of pregnancy-induced hypertension, placenta previa, and abruptio placentae in a pregnant woman?
■ How can benign and malignant breast lumps be clinically differentiated?

CHAPTER OUTLINE

The complex functioning of the female reproductive system described in Chapter 32 may be subject to alterations in structure and function throughout a woman's life that can have far-reaching effects on her health and well-being. This chapter is a survey of these alterations and describes the pathophysiologic basis of the most common disorders of the female reproductive system. In addition, current therapeutics for these alterations, including pharmacologic therapy, will be summarized. The information presented here is an introduction to these complex areas, and the reader may wish to consult in-depth gynecology and obstetrics texts for more detailed information.

Perhaps no other function of the human body is so closely linked to psychological, social, and spiritual concerns as reproductive function. Any alteration in reproductive status (or the perceived threat of such an alteration) may have profound effects on an individual. Clinicians caring for women experiencing alterations in functioning of the reproductive system should bear in mind the profundity of such alterations for the individual woman and must also maintain an awareness of the context in which women seek help for such problems. A clinical approach in which information is freely shared between caregiver and client and in which mutual decision making is an integral part of the therapeutic environment is a necessary component of care for women seeking help for reproductive concerns. Previous clinical approaches in which women's concerns were labeled as unimportant or merely psychogenic often resulted in anger, frustration with health care providers, and withdrawal from the health care delivery system. Women consumers of health care are now seeking active involvement in their own care, and clinicians who care for women experiencing the alterations described in this chapter need to approach women's health concerns with sensitivity and openness.

MENSTRUAL DISORDERS

Alterations in the normal functioning of the menstrual cycle include amenorrhea (no menses), abnormal uterine bleeding patterns, and dysmenorrhea (painful menstruation). Although many pathologic conditions can cause these alterations, an obvious cause is often not found.

Amenorrhea

Etiology and Pathogenesis. **Amenorrhea** is the absence or suppression of menstruation in a female age 16 years or older; it occurs if a woman misses three or more periods in a row.

Amenorrhea is normal before menarche (the first menstrual period at the time of puberty), after menopause, and during pregnancy and lactation.[1] At other times, it is considered pathologic and may result from a wide range of pathophysiologic causes (Figure 33-1). In the majority of cases, amenorrhea is due to an abnormal pattern of hormonal functioning that interrupts the normal sequence of events in which the endometrial tissue lining the uterus proliferates and then sloughs off. The endometrial tissue must be stimulated and regulated by the correct quantity and sequence of the female sex hormones estrogen and progesterone and the gonadotropic hormones follicle-stimulating hormone (FSH) and luteinizing hormone (LH). As described in Chapter 32, the menstrual cycle is dependent on the sequential changes in estrogen and progesterone levels. The initial rise in LH and FSH in the menstrual cycle occurs in response to a decline in estrogen and progesterone; estrogen levels then rise again in response to actions of the gonadotropic hormones, and the endometrium proliferates again in response to estrogen secretion. Thus events that prevent estrogen production, interfere with the normal fluctuations in estrogen levels, or block the action of estrogen on the endometrium will result in abnormal or absent menstrual flow.[2] Such events may include physical or emotional stress, which can interfere with normal production of the gonadotropic hormones and alter the pattern of estrogen functioning. In addition, ovarian, adrenal, or pituitary tumors may interfere with the normal production of female sex hormones or LH and FSH. Neoplasms of the ovaries or adrenal and pituitary glands may result in excess or deficient production of these hormones, with a consequent interruption in normal menstrual flow.

Treatment. Therapeutic strategies for amenorrhea are directed to correcting the cause of the interruption in hormonal functioning and may include the use of hormonal supplementation to reinstate a normal sequence of events in the menstrual cycle. If amenorrhea is the result of a neoplastic process, surgery may be indicated for tumor removal.

Abnormal Uterine Bleeding Patterns.
Irregular or excessive bleeding from the uterus is one of the most common alterations in the female reproductive system. Uterine bleeding that varies from a woman's normal pattern either in quantity or in frequency may occur at any age and for a variety of reasons.

Etiology, Clinical Manifestations, and Treatment. The most common alterations in uterine bleeding patterns and their

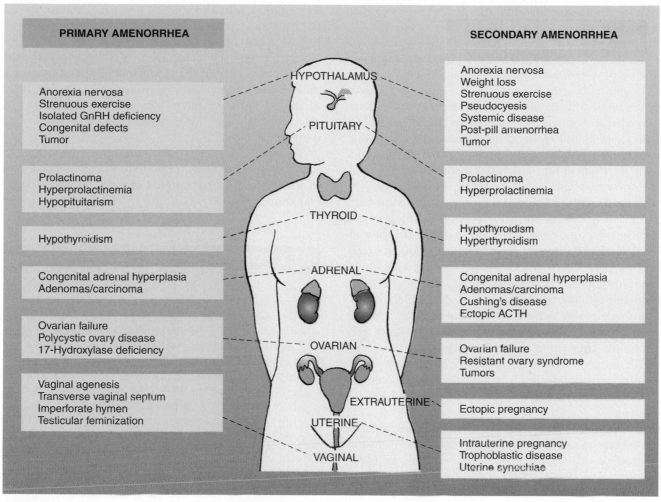

FIGURE 33-1 Causes of amenorrhea. GnRH, Gonadotropin-releasing hormone; ACTH, adrenocorticotropic hormone. (From Black JM, Hawks JH: *Medical-surgical nursing: clinical management for positive outcomes,* ed 8, Philadelphia, 2009, Saunders, p 915.)

causes are described here. **Metrorrhagia,** or bleeding between menstrual periods, usually results from slight physiologic bleeding from the endometrium during ovulation but may also result from other causes such as uterine malignancy, cervical erosions, and endometrial polyps or as a side effect of estrogen therapy.[1] **Hypomenorrhea,** or a deficient amount of menstrual flow, results from endocrine or systemic disorders that may interfere with proper functioning of the hormones in the menstrual cycle, or it may be due to partial obstruction of menstrual flow by the hymen or a narrowing of the cervical os. **Oligomenorrhea,** or infrequent menstruation, usually reflects failure to ovulate because of an endocrine or systemic disorder with accompanying inappropriate hormonal function. Similarly, **polymenorrhea,** an increased frequency of menstruation, may be associated with ovulation and may be caused by endocrine or systemic factors. **Menorrhagia,** an often debilitating increase in the amount or duration of menstrual bleeding, usually results from lesions of the female reproductive organs such as uterine leiomyomas, endometrial polyps, and adenomyosis. It is often managed

with surgery, oral contraceptives, and/or antiprostaglandins. More recently, a progestin-containing intrauterine device has shown promise in reducing menorrhagia, dysmenorrhea, and anemia.[3]

The term **dysfunctional uterine bleeding** is used to describe abnormal endometrial bleeding not associated with tumor, inflammation, pregnancy, trauma, or hormonal effects. Dysfunctional uterine bleeding is most common around the time of menarche and menopause and not as common in women prior to menopause.[4] In adolescents, dysfunctional uterine bleeding is most often due to immaturity in functioning of the pituitary and ovary, which have not yet properly orchestrated their activities.[5] Thus an imbalance may be present in the ratio of estrogen to progesterone. Absent or diminished levels of progesterone will result in a thick and extremely vascular endometrium that lacks structural support. As a result of this fragile structure, spontaneous and superficial hemorrhage occurs randomly throughout the endometrium. In addition, the blood vessels in the endometrium fail to constrict to limit the extent and duration of bleeding.[5] Uterine bleeding that is abnormal in both quantity and frequency can therefore occur in a noncyclic pattern.

In perimenopausal women, dysfunctional uterine bleeding may be the result of progressive degeneration and failure of the ovary to produce estrogen. As the number of ovarian follicles diminishes, the production of estrogen by the ovary becomes unpredictable, and the secretion of LH and FSH may also assume an unpredictable pattern. As in adolescents with dysfunctional uterine bleeding, diminished or absent production of progesterone may result in unopposed stimulation of the endometrium by estrogen, with subsequent unpredictable bleeding from a fragile endometrium.[4,5]

Dysmenorrhea. **Dysmenorrhea** is menstruation that is painful enough to limit normal activity or to cause a woman to seek health care. Dysmenorrhea is a widespread phenomenon that affects many women across the reproductive years, including girls of high school age through perimenopausal women. Although symptoms of dysmenorrhea tend to decrease with age, the traditional notion that childbirth permanently decreases symptoms is unfounded. In addition, the contention that women with dysmenorrhea tend to be neurotic has been refuted in well-designed psychiatric research studies.[5] Recent research into the physiologic process of uterine contractions has enhanced our understanding of the causes of dysmenorrhea and has thus resulted in better treatment.

Etiology and Clinical Manifestations. Dysmenorrhea is usually classified as primary (not related to any identifiable pathologic condition) or secondary (related to an underlying pathologic condition). The cramps that occur with primary dysmenorrhea are usually located in the suprapubic region and are sharp in quality. The pain may radiate to the inner aspect of the thighs and lower sacral area and may be accompanied by nausea, diarrhea, and headache.[2] Primary dysmenorrhea usually develops 1 or 2 years after menarche, when ovulatory cycles are established. Under the influence of progesterone, increased amounts of prostaglandins, potent hormone-like unsaturated fatty acids, are released from the endometrium. Prostaglandins have significant effects on smooth muscle and vasomotor tone; when released from the endometrium, prostaglandins promote uterine contractions and ischemia of the endometrial capillaries and thereby cause the cramping pain of dysmenorrhea.[5]

Secondary dysmenorrhea is characterized more often by dull pain that may increase with age. It is associated with pelvic disorders such as endometriosis, leiomyomas, or pelvic adhesions.[6]

Treatment. Recent therapeutic strategies for the management of primary dysmenorrhea have focused on the phenomenon of prostaglandin-induced enhanced uterine contractility. The use of prostaglandin synthetase inhibitors such as ibuprofen and naproxen, which inhibit the formation of prostaglandins, has been very effective in many women experiencing dysmenorrhea.[5] Other approaches that use steroid hormones, such as progestins or combined high-progestin/low-estrogen oral contraceptives, have also been advocated.

The rationale is that production of the high menstrual levels of prostaglandins needed to produce dysmenorrhea requires high levels of estrogen without progesterone in the proliferative phase of the menstrual cycle. Progestin administration therefore inhibits the production of prostaglandins and relieves the symptoms of dysmenorrhea.[5] However, the use of steroid hormones may involve significant risks, which the individual client must weigh against the benefits of such therapy.

Therapeutic strategies for secondary dysmenorrhea may involve diagnostic operative procedures such as laparoscopy, as well as medical and surgical therapy for the underlying condition.[3]

KEY POINTS

- Amenorrhea, the absence of menstruation, is most commonly due to hormonal disturbances. Stress and neoplasms (ovarian, adrenal, or pituitary tumors) may interfere with the normal patterns of hormone secretion. Treatment is aimed at the underlying cause of the hormonal imbalance.

- Irregular or excessive uterine bleeding is a common problem. Metrorrhagia is bleeding between periods, hypomenorrhea is reduced menstrual flow, oligomenorrhea is infrequent menstruation, polymenorrhea is an increased frequency of menstruation, and menorrhagia is prolonged and heavy bleeding during menstruation. These disorders may be associated with hormonal imbalances or primary lesions of the reproductive tract.

- Dysfunctional uterine bleeding is common at menarche and menopause and is due to irregular secretion of reproductive hormones. Other causes of abnormal bleeding, such as tumor, trauma, inflammation, and endocrine diseases, are ruled out before a diagnosis of dysfunctional uterine bleeding is made.

- Dysmenorrhea is painful menstruation, generally described as sharp suprapubic cramping severe enough to limit activity. Dysmenorrhea may be treated with prostaglandin inhibitors. Dysmenorrhea secondary to pelvic disorders (endometriosis, adhesions) generally has a dull quality and may increase with age.

ALTERATIONS IN UTERINE POSITION AND PELVIC SUPPORT

Alterations in uterine position and pelvic support may occur anytime during a woman's reproductive years. The major support for the uterus and upper part of the vagina is provided by the thickenings of the endopelvic fascia known as the *cardinal ligaments.* Although tearing of the cardinal ligaments during labor and delivery is rare, they can be stretched abnormally during a difficult or prolonged delivery and subsequently fail to support the pelvic organs adequately.[5] In addition, congenital defects in the muscles of the pelvic floor may promote

FIRST-DEGREE PROLAPSE   SECOND-DEGREE PROLAPSE   THIRD-DEGREE PROLAPSE

FIGURE 33-2 Degrees of uterine prolapse. (From Black JM, Hawks JH: *Medical-surgical nursing: clinical management for positive outcomes,* ed 8 Philadelphia, 2009, Saunders, p 930.)

alterations in position of the uterus and other pelvic structures. The two most common alterations in uterine position are **uterine prolapse** and **retrodisplacement** of the uterus. Other commonly occurring alterations resulting from a weakening of the vaginal and pelvic floor musculature are **cystocele** and **rectocele**.

Uterine Prolapse

Etiology. The axis of the uterus normally forms an acute angle with the axis of the vagina. This anatomic feature itself tends to prevent a prolapse, or sinking, of the uterus from its normal position. Descent of the uterus occurs when supporting structures, such as the uterosacral ligaments and the cardinal ligaments, relax and allow the relationship of the uterus to the vaginal axis to be altered. This relaxation permits the cervix to sag downward into the vagina. If the support of the vaginal wall is also compromised, the pressure of the abdominal organs on the uterus will gradually force it downward through the vagina into the introitus.[4] Uterine prolapse may occur at any age. In female infants and in women who have never given birth, congenital defects in the basic integrity of the pelvic supporting structures are usually responsible. Trauma to the ligaments during childbirth is the cause of uterine prolapse in women who have given birth, particularly if multiple deliveries have occurred. Uterine prolapse is classified as first-degree, second-degree, or third-degree according to the level to which the uterus has descended (Figure 33-2). In first-degree prolapse, the uterus is approximately halfway between the vaginal introitus and the level of the ischial spines. In second-degree prolapse, the end of the cervix has begun to protrude through the introitus. In third-degree or complete prolapse, the body of the uterus is outside the vaginal introitus. Figure 33-3 shows a third-degree, or complete, uterine prolapse.

Clinical Manifestations. The symptoms of uterine prolapse depend on the degree of severity of prolapse. The woman may become increasingly aware of a sensation of bearing down and discomfort in the vagina. If the prolapse has advanced to the second or third degree, she may note discomfort while walking or sitting and have difficulty urinating. In addition, as the end of the cervix begins to protrude outside the body, it may

FIGURE 33-3 Complete uterine prolapse. (From Parsons L, Sommers SC: *Gynecology,* ed 2, Philadelphia, 1978, Saunders, p 1443.)

be subject to trauma from friction and ulceration. Bleeding and ulceration of the cervix may be present.

Treatment. Uterine prolapse is one of the most common reasons for hysterectomy usually from the vaginal approach.[7] In patients who are at poor risk for surgery or who choose not to have a hysterectomy, a pessary, which is a small supportive device, is inserted to hold the uterus in place.[5]

Retrodisplacement of the Uterus.

The term **retrodisplacement** refers to situations in which the body of the uterus is displaced from its usual location overlying the bladder to a position in the posterior of the pelvis.[4] As shown in Figure 33-4, the uterus may be in one of five positions: anteverted, midposition, anteflexed, retroflexed, or retroverted.

Etiology and Clinical Manifestations. Retrodisplacement can be detected in 20% to 30% of all women.[8] It may be a normal variation and therefore be present throughout a woman's entire life, or it may develop after childbirth when the supporting structures are injured.

Anteverted

Midposition

Anteflexed

Retroflexed

Retroverted

FIGURE 33-4 The various positions of the uterus. Note that the classifications describe the position of the long axis of the uterus with respect to the long axis of the body. (From Jarvis C: *Physical examination and health assessment,* ed 5, Philadelphia, 2008, Saunders, p 777.)

In many women, no symptoms occur from uterine retrodisplacement. In some women, symptoms of pelvic pain or pressure, dysmenorrhea, and dyspareunia (painful intercourse) may be present. In addition, infertility has been associated with retrodisplacement.[5]

Treatment. If the woman has no symptoms, no treatment is indicated. The use of a pessary to support the uterus in a normal position may relieve the symptoms, but surgical correction is sometimes indicated when symptoms are severe.[5] Newer, less invasive, laparoscopic surgical procedures are also becoming increasingly popular.[8]

Cystocele

Etiology. A *cystocele* is a protrusion of a portion of the urinary bladder into the anterior of the vagina at a weakened part of the vaginal musculature (Figure 33-5, *A*). The defect in the vaginal wall is usually caused by injury during childbirth or surgery but may also result from the aging process or as an inherent weakness. Other predisposing factors include obesity and a history of lifting heavy objects. The pressure created by this protrusion causes the anterior vaginal wall to bulge in a downward direction.

Clinical Manifestations and Treatment. A wide range of symptoms may be present, depending on the degree of severity of the cystocele. A mild degree of protrusion of the bladder may result in no symptoms. In moderate to severe cases, a sensation of pressure is felt in the vagina, along with dysuria and back pain. Fullness at the vaginal opening may be observed, as may a soft, reducible mucosal mass bulging into the anterior of the vaginal introitus.

Surgical repair of the vagina is done to correct the cystocele and re-establish support of the anterior vaginal wall. The bladder is restored to a normal position by reinforcement of the weakened portion of the anterior vaginal wall.

Rectocele

Etiology. A *rectocele* (also called *proctocele*) is a protrusion of the anterior rectal wall into the posterior of the vagina at a weakened part of the vaginal musculature (see Figure 33-5, *B*). As for a cystocele, the defect in the vaginal wall is usually caused by injury during childbirth or surgery but may also occur with aging or as an inherent weakness. Other predisposing factors for a rectocele include multiparity, obesity, and postmenopausal status. The rectocele forms a bulging mass beneath the posterior vaginal mucosa and pushes downward into the lower vaginal canal. Gradually, the rectum may be torn from its fascial and muscular attachments to the pelvic wall. The levator ani muscles may also become stretched or torn.

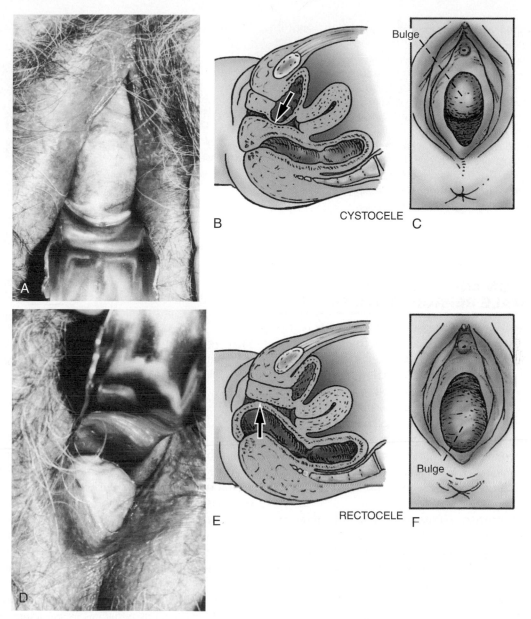

FIGURE 33-5 A-C, Cystocele. **B,** Note the bulging of the anterior vaginal wall. The urinary bladder is displaced downward. **C,** The cystocele pushes the anterior wall downward into the vagina. **D-F,** Rectocele. **E,** Note the bulging of the posterior vaginal wall. (**A** and **D,** From Huffman JW: *Gynecology and obstetrics,* Philadelphia, 1962, Saunders. **B, C, E,** and **F,** From Black JM, Hawks JH: *Medical-surgical nursing: clinical management for positive outcomes,* ed 8, Philadelphia, 2009, Saunders, p 930.)

Clinical Manifestations and Treatment. A wide range of symptoms may be present, depending on the degree of severity of the rectocele. The patient may report a history of difficulty in bowel evacuation and may have experienced chronic constipation with laxative and enema dependency. A feeling of pressure may also be reported, along with painful sexual intercourse. Physical examination reveals a mass bulging into the posterior of the vaginal introitus.[5]

Surgical repair of the vagina is done to correct the rectocele and re-establish support of the posterior vaginal wall. The rectum is restored to its normal location, and the levator ani muscles are brought together in proper position.

KEY POINTS

- Uterine prolapse occurs when supporting pelvic structures relax and the cervix sags downward into the vagina. Congenital defects, pregnancy, and childbirth are the usual contributing factors. Prolapse may be accompanied by a sensation of pelvic fullness and vaginal discomfort.
- Retrodisplacement of the uterus is common (20% to 30% of women) and may be congenital or due to pregnancy and childbirth. The body of the uterus is flexed or rotated into the posterior of the pelvis, which sometimes

leads to varied symptoms of pelvic pain or pressure, dysmenorrhea, and dyspareunia.

- A cystocele may result from weakness in the vaginal musculature that allows the urinary bladder to protrude into the anterior of the vagina. Contributing factors include childbirth, surgery, aging, obesity, and heavy lifting. Vaginal pressure, dysuria, and back pain may be present.
- A rectocele may result from weakness in the posterior vaginal musculature that allows the rectum to protrude into the vagina. Contributing factors are similar to those for cystocele. Symptoms include constipation, painful bowel evacuation, and painful intercourse.

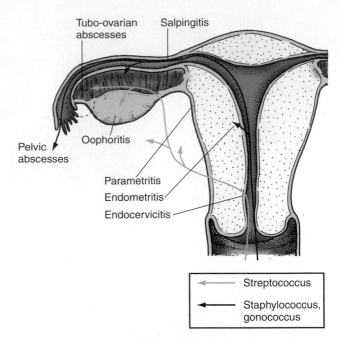

FIGURE 33-6 The spread of pelvic inflammatory disease. (From Ignatavicius DD, Workman ML: *Medical-surgical nursing,* ed 5, Philadelphia, 2006, Saunders, p 1896.)

INFLAMMATION AND INFECTION OF THE FEMALE REPRODUCTIVE TRACT

Inflammatory and infectious processes of the female reproductive tract may have effects that range from discomfort to life-threatening situations. Because the infectious agents responsible for inflammation and infection of the female genital tract may be sexually transmitted, some overlap in the discussion of these processes and sexually transmitted diseases is necessary. This chapter will describe the two principal inflammatory and infectious processes of the upper and lower female reproductive tract: pelvic inflammatory disease (PID) and vulvovaginitis. The reader may wish to refer to Chapter 34 for additional information on sexually transmitted infections.

Pelvic Inflammatory Disease. **Pelvic inflammatory disease** is any acute, subacute, recurrent, or chronic infection of the oviducts and ovaries with involvement of the adjacent reproductive organs (Figure 33-6). It includes inflammation of the cervix (cervicitis), uterus (endometritis), oviducts (salpingitis), and ovaries (oophoritis). When the connective tissue underlying these structures between the broad ligaments is also involved, the condition is called *parametritis*.[1]

Approximately 1 million women are treated for PID each year in the United States. In addition, significant reproductive health problems may occur as a result of PID. Twenty-five percent of all women who have had PID eventually experience one or more long-term health problems. Infertility is present in 20% of women who have had PID, and the incidence of ectopic pregnancy is increased six to ten times. Chronic pelvic pain, dyspareunia, pelvic adhesions, and chronic inflammation and abscesses of the oviducts and ovaries may all occur in women after PID.[5]

Etiology. Normally, cervical secretions provide protective and defensive functions for the reproductive organs. By providing a bacteriostatic barrier, cervical mucus prevents bacterial agents present in the cervix or vagina from ascending into the uterus. Therefore, conditions or surgical procedures that alter or destroy cervical mucus may impair this bacteriostatic mechanism. PID may follow the insertion of an intrauterine

device, pelvic surgery, abortion procedures, and infection during or after pregnancy. Bacteria may also enter the uterine cavity through the bloodstream or from drainage from other foci of infection such as a pelvic abscess, ruptured appendix, or diverticulitis of the sigmoid colon.[1]

PID can result from infection with aerobic and anaerobic organisms. *Neisseria gonorrhoeae* and *Chlamydia trachomatis* are the most common causative agents because they readily penetrate the bacteriostatic barrier of cervical mucus. However, a variety of bacterial organisms may contribute to the development of PID, including staphylococci, streptococci, diphtheroids, and coliforms such as *Pseudomonas* and *Escherichia coli*. These bacteria are commonly found in cervical mucus, and PID can result from infection by one or several of these bacteria. In addition, PID may occur after multiplication of bacteria in the endometrium that are normally nonpathogenic. During parturition, the traumatized endometrium favors the multiplication of bacteria.[1]

Clinical Manifestations. The associated signs and symptoms of PID vary with the affected part of the reproductive tract but generally include abdominal tenderness and tenderness or pain of the cervix or adnexa on palpation. In addition, the temperature may be elevated above 38° C and the white blood cell count elevated above 10,000/mm³. A pelvic abscess or inflammatory mass may be present on physical examination or ultrasound, and purulent vaginal discharge may be noted.[1,5]

Treatment. Early and aggressive use of antibiotic agents best suited for the causative organisms is essential in preventing the progression of PID. Various antibiotic regimens involving the use of multiple antimicrobial agents have been suggested by the Centers for Disease Control and Prevention for use in PID.[9] Inpatient hospitalization may be indicated for patients with rapidly progressing PID and those requiring surgical drainage of pelvic abscesses. Rupture of a pelvic abscess is a potentially life-threatening condition, and a total abdominal hysterectomy (removal of the uterus) with bilateral salpingo-oophorectomy (removal of both oviducts and ovaries) may be indicated in this situation.

Vulvovaginitis. Vulvovaginitis is an inflammation of the vulva (vulvitis) and vagina (vaginitis). Because the vulva and vagina are anatomically close to each other, inflammation of one location usually precipitates inflammation of the other. Vulvovaginitis may occur at any time during a girl's or woman's life and affects most females at some point in life.[1]

Etiology. Infection by *Candida albicans* (formerly called *Monilia*) accounts for approximately half of all reported cases of vulvovaginitis. (Infection by *Candida* is referred to as *candidiasis*.[5]) *C. albicans* is a fungus that requires glucose for growth; thus its growth may be promoted during the secretory phase of the menstrual cycle when glycogen levels increase in the vaginal environment. In addition, other conditions in which the glycogen content of the vagina is enhanced may favor candidiasis, such as diabetes, pregnancy, and the use of oral contraceptives. Other factors predisposing to the development of vulvovaginitis from *Candida* infection include the use of estrogen supplementation and antibiotics. Women using estrogen supplementation in the perimenopausal period may be at greater risk for candidal infection of the vagina inasmuch as the glycogen content of the vagina may increase with these therapies. The mechanism by which antibiotic use promotes candidiasis is presently unclear, but it is thought that destruction of the bacteria that normally exert the protective effect of consuming *Candida* results in overgrowth of the *Candida* population with subsequent infection.[1,5]

Other infectious agents that may result in vulvovaginitis include *Trichomonas vaginalis, Haemophilus vaginalis,* and *N. gonorrhoeae*. Viral agents that may cause vulvovaginitis include human papillomavirus (venereal warts, condylomata acuminata) or herpesvirus type 2. These organisms can be transmitted during sexual intercourse and are discussed in detail in Chapter 34.

In addition to infectious processes, vulvovaginitis may be promoted by conditions or agents that irritate the vulva and vagina. Chemical irritation or allergic reactions to detergents, feminine hygiene products, and toilet paper may be a causative factor. Trauma to the vulva or vagina or the atrophy of the vaginal wall that occurs postmenopausally may predispose to vulvovaginitis as well.[1]

Clinical Manifestations. Vulvovaginitis from candidiasis results in a thick, white discharge and red, edematous mucous membranes with white flecks adhering to the vaginal wall. Intense itching usually accompanies this discharge. The vaginal pH is usually normal (less than 4.5), and fungal organisms are often seen on microscopy. Vulvovaginitis from other infectious agents may involve a malodorous, purulent discharge. Irritation and subsequent inflammation of the vulva and vagina may be manifested by red, swollen labia, pain on urination and intercourse, and itching.

Treatment. Appropriate medical therapy for the causative organisms is usually instituted, including local antifungal preparations for vaginal candidiasis and local and systemic antibiotic therapy for vulvovaginitis caused by bacterial agents. Cool compresses and sitz baths provide relief of itching and burning of inflamed tissues. Avoidance of factors that promote irritation of the vulva, such as drying soaps, non-absorptive underwear, and tight clothing, is also of therapeutic benefit.[1]

Bartholinitis. Bartholinitis is an inflammation of the Bartholin glands, which are located on either side of the vaginal orifice and lubricate the vaginal introitus with a clear, viscous secretion. The location of Bartholin glands renders them susceptible to access by bacteria such as *N. gonorrhoeae, C. trachomatis,* and other organisms.

Clinical Manifestations and Treatment. Once bacteria are established, an abscess (also referred to as a *Bartholin cyst*) may form and cause tenderness and swelling at the site. Pus may be observed coming out of the duct orifice leading to the affected gland, and symptoms of fever and malaise are present in some individuals. Laboratory culture with proper diagnosis of the causative organism is performed, and appropriate antibiotic therapy is usually instituted. Surgical incision and drainage of the abscess may be necessary for effective management.

KEY POINTS

- PID refers to any infection of the oviducts, ovaries, and adjacent reproductive organs. It includes cervicitis, endometritis, salpingitis, and oophoritis. Manifestations and complications of PID include infertility, ectopic pregnancy, pelvic pain, dyspareunia, and abscesses.

- Intrauterine devices, abortion, and pelvic surgery predispose to PID. *N. gonorrhoeae* and *C. trachomatis* are the most common causative organisms, and treatment centers on aggressive antibiotic therapy.

- Inflammation of the vulva and vagina, or vulvovaginitis, is a common problem in women. Most cases are associated with fungal infection by *C. albicans* and are manifested as a white vaginal discharge and an irritated, itchy mucosa. Predisposing factors include chemical irritation from feminine hygiene products, trauma, allergic reactions, and antibiotic therapy that inhibits the growth of normal flora.

- Inflammation of the Bartholin glands, or bartholinitis, is typically a result of the entry and subsequent infection of the glands by *N. gonorrhoeae* or *C. trachomatis*. Tenderness, swelling, and pus may be present and signify the formation of an abscess within one of the Bartholin glands. Antibiotic therapy and surgical drainage are used to manage the abscess.

BENIGN GROWTHS AND ABERRANT TISSUE OF THE FEMALE REPRODUCTIVE TRACT

Benign growths and aberrant tissue in the female reproductive tract are not uncommon; for example, uterine leiomyomas develop in approximately 50% of all premenopausal women.[10] The presence of benign growths or aberrant tissue in the reproductive tract may cause no symptoms and go entirely unnoticed, or symptoms ranging from debilitating to life threatening may be present. The diagnosis of these growths or tissue may cause anxiety in the woman experiencing them; in spite of their benign classification, their presence can have devastating effects on the underlying reproductive structures.[11] This section focuses on three of the most common forms of benign growths and aberrant tissue in the female reproductive organs: uterine leiomyomas, ovarian cysts, and endometriosis.

Uterine Leiomyomas. Uterine **leiomyomas,** which are also called *myomas* or *fibroids,* are the most common form of uterine growths that appear in women. Their actual incidence is difficult to establish because many myomas are either too small or inaccessibly placed to be palpated. Uterine leiomyomas occur in approximately 50% of all premenopausal women and affect black women three times more often than white women. Age appears to be a factor in their development inasmuch as myomas are not found before the onset of puberty and rarely exhibit growth activity after menopause.

Etiology. Uterine leiomyomas make their appearance and exhibit growth activity during the reproductive years. Therefore, although the actual cause of myomas is presently unknown, it is thought that estrogen and human growth hormone may influence tumor formation by stimulating susceptible fibromuscular elements in the uterine wall. This theory is supported by the finding that tumor growth is enhanced by large doses of estrogen and the later stages of pregnancy, when human growth hormone and estrogen levels are high. In addition, uterine leiomyomas usually shrink or disappear after menopause, when estrogen levels decrease.[1]

Clinical Manifestations. Uterine leiomyomas can grow to a large size (Figure 33-7). Obviously, the presence of such a large mass within the uterus will cause symptoms of abdominal pain and pressure, but smaller myomas can result in such symptoms as well. Other symptoms associated with leiomyomas may include abnormal vaginal bleeding and discharge, depending on the location of the mass. If the myoma is sufficiently large to cause pressure on surrounding abdominal organs, backache, constipation, and urinary frequency or urgency may also be present.

Treatment. Treatment for uterine leiomyomas depends on such factors as the severity of symptoms, size and location of the leiomyoma, and the patient's age. Small myomas that cause no health problems are generally monitored carefully for growth patterns. Large or multiple masses that promote severe uterine bleeding or interfere with functioning of the gastrointestinal or urinary tract are surgically removed, and hysterectomy may be indicated.[1]

FIGURE 33-7 Uterine leiomyomas. (From Jarvis C: *Physical examination and health assessment,* ed 5, Philadelphia, 2008, Saunders, p 790.)

Ovarian Cysts. **Ovarian cysts** are sacs on an ovary that contain fluid or semisolid material. Ovarian cysts can develop at any time between puberty and menopause, including during pregnancy.

Etiology. The cause of the formation of ovarian cysts is presently unknown. They can arise in several locations in the ovaries:

1. Follicular cysts result when a maturing ovarian follicle fails to release an ovum; instead, the follicle continues to enlarge and produce estrogen.
2. Corpus luteum cysts occur when the corpus luteum fails to degenerate normally; the cyst continues to grow and produce progesterone.
3. Theca-lutein cysts are commonly bilateral and filled with clear, straw-colored fluid. Often their development is associated with hydatidiform mole, choriocarcinoma, or hormone therapy.[4]

Clinical Manifestations and Treatment. Normally, ovarian cysts produce no symptoms. They may be noted on periodic examination and may increase and decrease in size with the menstrual cycle. However, when an ovarian cyst ruptures, an ovarian vessel may tear, with variable amounts of intraperitoneal hemorrhage and abdominal pain. In persons with recurrent ovarian cysts, oral contraceptives may be recommended to prevent ovulation. Occasionally, immediate surgical intervention is indicated to control the hemorrhage and repair the site of rupture.[12]

Endometriosis. **Endometriosis** is the presence of endometrial tissue outside the lining of the uterine cavity. Because the only normal location for endometrial tissue is the endometrial lining of the uterus, the presence of this abnormal growth is associated with a variety of side effects ranging from mild symptoms to life-threatening consequences. These foci of abnormal endometrial tissue are called **endometriomas,** or endometrial implants, and usually occur within the pelvis. The most common sites of occurrence of endometriosis within the pelvis are the ovary, peritoneum of the cul-de-sac or pouch of Douglas, uterosacral ligaments, round ligament, oviduct, and the peritoneal surface of the uterus.[5] Less frequently, endometrial implants occur in other body sites such as the bladder or large intestine. Although endometriosis is a benign disease, it possesses certain characteristics of malignant disease, such as the ability to grow, infiltrate, and spread. Symptoms of endometriosis may have an abrupt onset or may develop over many years.

The actual incidence of endometriosis is unknown inasmuch as it exists in many women without any significant symptoms. Endometrial implants have been identified in at least 20% of women undergoing gynecologic surgery.[13] Active endometriosis usually occurs between 30 and 40 years of age, particularly in women who have never given birth. Endometriosis is rare in women younger than 20 years or after menopause. Although some authorities report a higher incidence of endometriosis in white women of higher socioeconomic levels,[3] these impressions may not be accurate given the tendency of this group to delay childbearing and to have enhanced access to health care. The infertility rate for women in whom endometriosis is diagnosed is about 30%.[14]

Etiology. At the present time, three major theories on the etiology of endometriosis have been proposed:

Transportation. Endometrial tissue flows backward through the oviducts during a normal menstrual period. After this retrograde flow, endometrial fragments implant on the ovary, peritoneal surfaces, and other areas.

Metaplasia. Inflammation or a hormonal change triggers metaplasia (conversion of one kind of tissue to a form that is not normal for that tissue). Thus, coelomic epithelium at certain sites converts to endometrial epithelium.

Induction. In this theory, a combination of transportation and metaplasia takes place, and regurgitated endometrium chemically induces mesenchyma to form endometrial epithelium. (At present, this theory is thought to be the most likely.[1])

Once the endometrial implants arise in their abnormal locations, they continue to be under hormonal influence, just as the endometrial lining of the uterus responds to hormonal influence. Thus they periodically proliferate and bleed in response to hormonal stimulation. In some instances they may rupture, usually immediately before or after a menstrual period. Endometriomas are filled with brown blood debris; when they rupture, their contents spill onto the sensitive pelvic peritoneum. This irritative discharge sets up a local chemical peritonitis, followed by the formation of fibrous tissue in the injured location. Dense tissue adhesions in the pelvis may result as the pelvic peritoneum undergoes repeated irritation by the cyclic activities of the endometrial implants.

Clinical Manifestations. The most prominent symptom of endometriosis is acquired dysmenorrhea, which produces pain in the lower part of the abdomen and in the vagina, posterior of the pelvis, and back. The pain usually begins 5 to 7 days before the peak of menses and lasts for 2 to 3 days. It differs from the pain of primary dysmenorrhea, which is more cramplike and concentrated in the abdominal midline. Pain may be extremely severe, although the degree of pain does not necessarily indicate the extent of disease. Dyspareunia and pain with defecation may also be present.[1,14] Significant changes in the pattern of menstrual flow may occur, with excessive bleeding that may progress to anemia and fatigue.

Treatment. Treatment varies according to the extent of disease. Many women with endometrial implants never experience symptoms and require no treatment; others experience a rapidly progressive set of severe symptoms requiring immediate intervention. Both medical and surgical treatment modalities may be used. Hormonal agents, including progestational steroids and antigonadotropic agents, may be used to produce a hormonal state similar to pregnancy or menopause. Because endometriosis responds to cyclic hormonal functioning, it is thought that the use of hormones to interrupt this cyclic pattern may result in atrophy of the endometrial implants. Surgical intervention includes removal or destruction of the endometriosis. If damage to the pelvic organs is widespread and the disease is progressing rapidly, total abdominal hysterectomy with removal of the oviducts and ovaries is performed.[15]

KEY POINTS

- Benign fibroid tumors, or leiomyomas, are the most common uterine tumor, affecting about 20% of women older than 35 years. Depending on their size, uterine leiomyomas may be characterized by abnormal vaginal bleeding, pelvic pain, constipation, and urinary frequency.

- Ovarian cysts are usually asymptomatic and may change in size with the menstrual cycle. Rupture of an ovarian cyst may result in severe abdominal pain and hemorrhage, which occasionally necessitates immediate surgical intervention.

- Endometriosis occurs when endometrial tissue grows in areas other than the uterine lining. Endometriosis may involve the ovary, peritoneum, oviduct, outer layer of the uterus, bladder, and intestine. Although considered benign, endometriosis tends to infiltrate and spread to adjacent tissues. Endometriosis may be initiated by reflux of the uterine lining through the oviducts into the abdominal cavity during menses.

- Ectopic endometrial tissues periodically proliferate and bleed in response to fluctuations of reproductive hormones. Dysmenorrhea, with pelvic, back, and lower abdominal pain, usually begins 5 to 7 days before the peak of menses and lasts for 2 to 3 days. The pain is more diffuse than that of primary dysmenorrhea. Treatment may include induction of a menopause-like state with hormone administration or the surgical excision of affected structures.

CANCER OF THE FEMALE GENITAL STRUCTURES

Malignant neoplasms occur in every part of the female reproductive system. This section describes the incidence and pathophysiologic aspects of the most common types of malignancies in female genital structures. For further information about the process of neoplasm development, the reader may wish to refer to Chapter 7 of this text.

Cancer of the Cervix

Etiology. Cancer of the uterine cervix is a neoplasm that can be detected in the early, curable stage by the Papanicolaou (Pap) test.[5] There are approximately one quarter of a million deaths worldwide per year from cervical cancer.[16] The main cause of cervical cancer appears to be certain human papillomavirus (HPV) types. Other factors include intercourse at a young age, multiple sexual partners, multiple pregnancies, and herpesvirus type 2 and other sexually transmitted infections.[1] Widespread screening with a yearly Pap test in women at risk has continued to decrease the mortality of cervical cancer. The American Cancer Society now recommends that after three consecutive negative Pap tests, women older than 30 years who are not at high risk can be tested every 2 to 3 years. Sexually active women younger than 21 years should also be tested within three years of first coitus. For women who have had a hysterectomy unrelated to cervical neoplasia, the Centers for Disease Control and Prevention no longer recommends Pap screening.[17] Low-risk women who have been screened regularly may also stop screening at age 70.

Clinical Manifestations. Preinvasive cervical cancer produces no symptoms, although the Pap test can detect changes in cells of the cervical epithelium, which may be present for 10 years before invasive cancer develops.[1,5] Early invasive cancer causes abnormal vaginal bleeding, persistent vaginal discharge, and pain and bleeding after intercourse.[1] When symptoms appear, the cancer has usually progressed beyond its early stages. Squamous cell carcinoma accounts for 95% of all invasive cervical cancers diagnosed, and adenocarcinomas account for most of the rest. Invasive carcinoma of the cervix spreads by direct extension to the vaginal wall, laterally into the parametrium toward the pelvic wall, and anteroposteriorly into the bladder and rectum. Metastasis to the pelvic lymph nodes is more common than spread to distant lymph nodes.[5]

Treatment. The treatment strategy depends on the clinical stage of the tumor at the time of diagnosis. Surgery—including cryotherapy, excision, and laser surgery for precancer and hysterectomy for invasive carcinoma—may be indicated. Chemotherapy and radiation therapy may be used in invasive disease. More than 55% of treated patients live 5 years or longer. Radical surgery, including *pelvic exenteration,* or removal of all the pelvic organs, can now be performed with limited morbidity. Treatment works best at early stages of cancer. The cure rate for stage I cervical cancer is 85% to 90%. The cure rate for stage IV cancer is only 5% to 10%.

Prevention. In 2006, the Food and Drug Administration (FDA) licensed the first vaccine developed to prevent cervical cancer and other diseases in females caused by certain types of human papillomavirus (HPV). The quadrivalent vaccine, Gardasil®, protects against four HPV types (6,11,16,18), which are responsible for 70% of cervical cancers and 90% of genital warts. The HPV vaccine is recommended for 11- to 12-year-old girls, but can be administered to girls as young as 9 years of age. The vaccine also is recommended for 13- to 26-year-old females who have not yet received or completed the vaccine series. Ideally, the vaccine should be administered before onset of sexual activity. However, females who are sexually active also may benefit from vaccination.[18,19]

Endometrial Cancer.
Cancer of the endometrial lining of the uterus is less common than cervical cancer in young women, but both types of cancer occur with equal frequency in postmenopausal women.[5] Related factors include infertility, late menopause (older than 55 years), obesity, diabetes, and hypertension. Unopposed estrogen therapy also increases the frequency.

Clinical Manifestations and Treatment. The most common initial symptom is bleeding between menstrual periods or postmenopausal bleeding. The diagnosis of endometrial cancer is based on histologic tissue examination. Treatment strategies for endometrial cancer include radiation therapy and total hysterectomy with possible removal of the ovaries and oviducts. The 5-year survival rate for patients in whom early endometrial cancer is diagnosed is approximately 85%.[20] The cure rate drops to 50% if the cancer has metastasized before diagnosis.

Ovarian Cancer.
Ovarian cancer has replaced cervical cancer as the leading cause of death from genital cancer. The peak incidence is between 60 and 80 years of age.[5] Because no symptoms are noted until late in the disease, the mortality rate is high, with only a 45% long-term survival rate.[20]

Clinical Manifestations and Treatment. When symptoms occur, they are related to intra-abdominal metastasis and include increasing abdominal girth, weight loss, abdominal pain, dysuria or urinary frequency, and constipation. Management of ovarian cancer includes removal of the uterus, ovaries, and oviducts. Radiation therapy and chemotherapy may be used in conjunction with surgery. Increasingly, prophylactic oophorectomy or salpingo-oophorectomy is being recommended in high-risk women.[21]

Vaginal Cancer.
Cancer of the vagina generally occurs in women in their early- to mid-fifties, although it has an increased incidence in young women whose mothers took diethylstilbestrol during pregnancy.[1] Because the vagina is a thin-walled structure with rich lymphatic drainage, vaginal cancer may metastasize to the bladder, rectum, vulva, pubic bone, and other surrounding structures.

Clinical Manifestations and Treatment. The primary signs and symptoms of vaginal cancer are vaginal spotting and discharge, pain, groin masses, and changes in urinary pattern.[5] Early-stage therapy is designed to treat the malignant area while preserving normal parts of the vagina. Radiation therapy or surgery varies based on the size, depth, and location of the tumor.[1] Preservation of a functional vagina is generally possible only in the early stages, although grafting from other body sites may be performed to avoid vaginal stenosis, particularly in younger women.[5]

Cancer of the Vulva

Clinical Manifestations and Treatment. Cancer of the vulva accounts for approximately 5% of all gynecologic malignancies. It can occur at any age, including infancy, but has a peak incidence in the mid-sixties. Factors that seem to predispose to the disease include sexually transmitted infections, chronic pruritus of the vulva with swelling and dryness, obesity, hypertension, diabetes, and never having been pregnant.[1]

Leukoplakic changes (the presence of whitish plaque-like or ulcerated lesions) in the vulva may precede the development of carcinoma. Once the carcinoma develops, vulvar masses may be present, with groin masses and abnormal urination and defecation later in the disease.[1] Management of vulvar cancer includes partial excision of the vulva to remove precancerous leukoplakic lesions and total vulvar excision for advanced disease.[5] Local relapse is common whether conservative or radical procedures are undertaken.[22]

KEY POINTS

- Cervical cancer may be detected by evaluation of cervical cells (Pap test). Early-stage cervical cancer may be asymptomatic. When they appear, symptoms include abnormal vaginal bleeding and discharge. Cervical cancer may spread to the vaginal wall, pelvis, bladder, rectum, and pelvic lymph nodes. The quadrivalent vaccine, Gardasil®, protects against four HPV types (6,11,16,18), which are responsible for 70% of cervical cancers and 90% of genital warts.
- Other cancers of the female reproductive tract include endometrial, ovarian, vaginal, and vulvar cancers. No routine screening tests are available for these cancers. Ovarian cancer has a high mortality rate because it is usually diagnosed after it has metastasized.

DISORDERS OF PREGNANCY

Pregnancy results in a number of physiologic alterations in the mother that are usually well tolerated, particularly if adequate prenatal care is available. However, pregnancy can result in a number of conditions that may be life threatening to the mother and the developing fetus. The most common pregnancy-related disorders are described here; in addition, for information concerning diabetes in pregnancy, the reader may wish to consult Chapter 41, which covers the topic of diabetes in depth.

Pregnancy-Induced Hypertension. Pregnancy-induced hypertension (PIH) is known by other names such as *toxemia* and *preeclampsia-eclampsia*. Hypertension complicates 0.5% to 10% of pregnancies in the United States and is one of the leading causes of pregnancy-related deaths.[23] PIH is characterized by a rapid rise in arterial blood pressure associated with the loss of large amounts of protein in the urine. Women at risk for the development of PIH include teenagers and women in their late thirties and early forties. In addition, the presence of multiple fetuses and the preexistence of hypertension, renal and cardiovascular disease, and diabetes may predispose to the development of PIH.[23]

Etiology, Clinical Manifestations, and Treatment. The exact causes of PIH are presently unknown, although poor nutrition and genetic and immunologic factors have been suggested. PIH is characterized by salt and water retention by the kidneys, weight gain, and edema. In addition, arterial spasm occurs in many parts of the body, most significantly in the kidneys, brain, and liver. Both renal flow and the glomerular filtration rate are decreased, a condition exactly opposite the normal changes in pregnancy. The renal effects are caused by thickening of the glomerular tufts, which contain a fibrinoid deposit in the basement membranes.[24]

The severity of symptoms of PIH is closely related to the retention of salt and water and the degree of the increase in arterial pressure. The increasing arterial pressure seems to promote a vicious cycle in which arterial spasm and other pathologic effects give rise to further increases in arterial pressure. Milder forms of the disease are managed with bed rest. Fetal well-being is periodically assessed, and the infant is delivered if conditions deteriorate or maturity is achieved.

In its severe form, PIH is characterized by extreme vascular spasticity throughout the body, clonic convulsions followed by coma, renal failure, liver malfunction, and extreme hypertension. Usually, this severe form occurs shortly before parturition. The mortality rate in women with severe PIH who are left untreated is high. However, the immediate use of rapidly acting vasodilating drugs, seizure prophylaxis, and rapid delivery have reduced the mortality rate from PIH to less than 1%.[24]

Hyperemesis Gravidarum. Hyperemesis gravidarum is a Latin term for excess of vomiting in pregnant women. Although transient nausea and vomiting occur in about half of women in the first trimester of pregnancy, in a few women these symptoms continue throughout the entire course of pregnancy. Intractable vomiting, or hyperemesis gravidarum, occurs in about 1 in 1,000 pregnancies, sometimes with life-threatening consequences.[24] Severe dehydration and electrolyte imbalance, hepatic and renal damage, encephalopathy, and ultimately death may ensue if the vomiting cannot be controlled.

Clinical Manifestations and Treatment. The causes of hyperemesis gravidarum are unknown, but it is thought that an abnormal response to the production of large amounts of human chorionic gonadotropin by the placenta may be implicated. Intravenous therapy to correct metabolic and nutritional abnormalities, antiemetic agents, and supportive care in a hospital environment may be needed to resolve the symptoms.

Placenta Previa and Abruptio Placentae

Etiology and Clinical Manifestations. **Placenta previa** is a condition in which the placenta is implanted abnormally over the internal cervical os. **Abruptio placentae** is premature separation of the placenta before delivery of the fetus. Placenta previa occurs in approximately 1 in 200 deliveries and is more common in women with multiple pregnancies and previous cesarean section; its cause is unknown. Placenta previa may occur in varying degrees of severity ranging from partial to entire coverage of the internal cervical os. Abruptio placentae, or premature separation of the placenta, occurs after 20 weeks of gestation in about 1% of deliveries. The detachment may be partial or complete and may cause overt or concealed hemorrhage.[5] Abruptio placentae can be caused by trauma, a short umbilical cord, occlusion of the inferior vena cava, PIH, or abnormal uterine anatomy.

Treatment. Therapeutic strategies for placenta previa and abruptio placentae include cesarean section for fetal distress or hemorrhage control. Medications designed to control preterm labor may also be administered.

Spontaneous Abortion. **Spontaneous abortion** is expulsion of the products of conception from the uterus before the period of fetal viability. It is usually called a *miscarriage* by laypersons, and it is differentiated from elective abortion. Although the precise incidence is unknown, it is estimated that 10% to 15% of pregnancies end in spontaneous abortion.

Etiology. Abnormal development accounts for a large percentage of aborted pregnancies. Some 61% of abortuses expelled in the first trimester demonstrate chromosomal abnormalities.[4] In addition, abnormal development may result from faulty implantation of the fertilized ovum or from an abnormality in the uterine environment. Maternal factors responsible for spontaneous abortion include both systemic and localized conditions. Infectious processes that may contribute to spontaneous abortion include cytomegalovirus, herpesvirus, and rubella infections. Abnormalities of the reproductive organs, immune disorders, endocrine malfunction, and physical and psychic trauma may all contribute to spontaneous abortion.[5]

Clinical Manifestations and Treatment. Associated signs and symptoms of spontaneous abortion include vaginal bleeding and abdominal cramps. The cramps may intensify as the cervix dilates for expulsion of the uterine contents. If the entire contents are expelled, the bleeding and cramps subside. However, if any contents remain, an incomplete abortion has occurred and intervention may be needed to control bleeding and to surgically remove the remaining uterine contents.

KEY POINTS

- PIH is characterized by a rapid rise in blood pressure and proteinuria. Renal blood flow and the glomerular filtration rate are reduced, and the kidneys retain salt and water. When severe, PIH may be associated with convulsions and coma. Antihypertensive therapy may be indicated.
- Excessive vomiting during pregnancy is termed *hyperemesis gravidarum*. Dehydration, electrolyte imbalance, hepatic and renal damage, and death may ensue.

- Placenta previa occurs when the placenta is implanted over the cervical os. Abruptio placentae is premature separation of the placenta. Both conditions may interrupt fetal oxygen supply and cause maternal hemorrhage. Cesarean section is indicated.
- It is estimated that 10% to 15% of pregnancies end in spontaneous abortion. Fetal abnormalities, faulty implantation, infections, and trauma increase the risk of spontaneous abortion.

Disorders of the Breast

The breast is considered an accessory organ of the female reproductive tract and is affected by many of the same factors that promote alterations in the other reproductive organs. Women's breast health has become a critical concern in the United States because the breast is the most common site of cancer in women between 25 and 75 years of age.[20] In addition, women are playing an increasingly important role in recognizing the symptoms of breast disease and are seeking earlier intervention with improved outcomes. It is essential that health care professionals continue to encourage this enhanced role and provide accurate information about breast health to their clients. This section includes information on specific breast disorders involving reactive-inflammatory breast disorders, benign breast disorders, and carcinoma of the breast. Before reading this information, the reader may wish to review the section on the structure and function of the breast in Chapter 32 of this text and the specific information on neoplasm development in Chapter 7.

REACTIVE-INFLAMMATORY BREAST DISORDERS

Breast disorders in which an inflammatory response occurs in reaction to irritation, injury, or infection include mammary duct ectasia, breast abscess, fat necrosis, and reactions to injections or implantation of foreign materials in the breast.

Mammary Duct Ectasia. Mammary duct ectasia is a chronic inflammatory process occurring in and around the terminal subareolar ducts of the breast (it is also referred to as *periductal mastitis*). It is more prevalent in older women, primarily postmenopausal women.[25] The Latin word **ectasia** means dilation, and in mammary duct ectasia the collecting ducts beneath the nipple and areola become dilated, thinned, and filled with secretions.

Pathogenesis. Over time, the ducts become distended with cellular debris, and the debris begins to have an irritating effect on the duct walls. The inflammatory response is initiated, and a zone of granulation tissue is created around a small cavity filled with thick yellowish or brownish material. This area will be palpable as a mass in the central area of the breast, beneath or near the areola. By the time the duct ectasia has grown into

FIGURE 33-8 Nipple retraction in the right breast as a result of mammary duct ectasia. (From Haagensen CD: *Diseases of the breast,* ed 3, Philadelphia, 1986, Saunders, p 359.)

a palpable mass, a reactive fibrosis will also have formed in the tissue around the mass. This fibrous thickening of the surrounding breast tissue causes dimpling and distortion of the breast and nipple inversion (Figure 33-8). However, a congenital inverted nipple is already present in some women with mammary duct ectasia, and it is thought that the presence of this nipple anomaly may in some way contribute to ductal wall irritation.[25]

Clinical Manifestations and Treatment. In addition to a palpable mass and dimpling or distortion of the breast or areola, women with mammary duct ectasia may have a persistent nipple discharge. These signs must be evaluated carefully because they may also be indicative of a malignant breast mass. A biopsy is usually performed to rule out the presence of a malignancy. After confirmation of the diagnosis of mammary ductal ectasia, surgical excision of the dilated subareolar ducts is performed.[25]

Breast Abscess. The majority of abscesses occurring in the breast are not associated with breast-feeding and are referred to as *nonlactational* breast abscesses (for a complete description of abscesses or mastitis related to lactation, the reader may wish to refer to an obstetric or maternity nursing text). Nonlactational breast abscesses are most often a recurring problem and usually affect persons with conditions that predispose to infections, such as diabetes, steroid therapy, or other skin lesions.

Etiology. Multiple factors may contribute to the formation of nonlactational breast abscesses. In some women, the presence of a congenital inverted nipple may predispose to abscess formation. Abscesses may also be part of the syndrome of mammary duct ectasia; in addition, women with the aforementioned pre-existing conditions that predispose to infections may be at increased risk for the development of an infectious process in the breast tissue. Unlike breast abscesses occurring during breast-feeding, in which *Staphylococcus aureus* is the most

common causative organism, nonlactational breast abscesses usually yield multiple organisms when cultured.

Clinical Manifestations and Treatment. Signs and symptoms of these abscesses include an area of tenderness, redness, and induration under the periareolar skin.[25] Unfortunately, nonlactational breast abscesses do not respond well to antibiotic therapy and often recur, and it is sometimes necessary to excise the major duct system beneath the areola to prevent further recurrence.[25]

Fat Necrosis. Necrosis refers to the death of a portion of tissue, and fat necrosis in the breast is the death of fat tissue after trauma or injury to the breast. The position of the breasts makes them vulnerable to trauma, particularly in larger women with pendulous breasts. This phenomenon is important for health care professionals to assess because fat necrosis may mimic or obscure carcinoma of the breast.

Clinical Manifestations and Diagnoses. Fat necrosis of the breast may have many of the same clinical signs as breast malignancy, including a painless mass in the breast that is firm, ill defined, and poorly mobile. Skin thickening and retraction may also be present. In addition, a mammogram may not provide a clear diagnosis.[16] Unfortunately, many women with pendulous breasts frequently sustain injuries to the breast and may be unable to recall any specific trauma; thus a diagnosis of fat necrosis may be difficult to make. If fat necrosis cannot be reliably distinguished from carcinoma based on clinical observation or mammography, excisional biopsy must be performed.[25]

Reactions to Foreign Material. Surgery to enlarge the female breast has become one of the most popular of all cosmetic surgical procedures in the past 25 years.[25] Since the early twentieth century, a variety of materials have been used for breast augmentation. Silicone implants, which consist of silicone gel encased in polyurethane or other materials, have been the most widely used devices for breast enlargement and have been implanted in more than 1 million women.[25] At present, controversy surrounds the use of silicone breast implants because some side effects, including irritation at the implantation area and other symptoms suggestive of an immune system response, have been reported. Currently, the recommendations surrounding silicone breast implants are conflicting. The use of silicone implants for routine cosmetic breast augmentation is specifically controlled in the United States, favoring implants filled with a saline solution. Health care professionals should be aware of the reported side effects of silicone breast implants inasmuch as a substantial segment of the female population in the United States and western Europe has undergone breast augmentation with these devices. In addition, persons with silicone implants who sustain blunt trauma to the chest are at risk for rupture of the implant, with subsequent leakage of the silicone gel into surrounding tissue. After chest trauma, the communication of information regarding the presence of silicone breast implants to other health care professionals is an important consideration in planning care and preventing further tissue exposure to silicone.

BENIGN BREAST DISORDERS

The term **benign breast disorders** encompasses a group of lesions affecting the breast. These disorders are usually divided into two categories: (1) fibrocystic breast disease and (2) specific benign neoplasms of the breast such as fibroadenomas, adenomas, and papillomas. It is important for health care professionals to understand the clinical significance of these benign disorders. Although these entities are "benign" in the sense of being differentiated from malignant breast neoplasms, clients experiencing them may be at risk for experiencing a psychological crisis and may need to be educated regarding their potential risk for breast malignancy.

Fibrocystic Breast Disease. Although the term **fibrocystic breast disease** is frequently used by health care professionals, it is important to understand that it is not a distinct disease entity.[25] Instead, it is a diagnosis classification that is applied to a condition in which the presence of palpable breast masses fluctuates with the menstrual cycle and may be associated with pain or tenderness. Laboratory examination of this breast tissue shows macroscopic and microscopic cysts, along with a variety of alterations in tissue structure such as fibrosis or overgrowth of stromal fibrous tissue. However, these alterations in breast tissue are present to some degree in all female breasts, which has led some authorities to question use of the term "disease" for such a widespread condition.[16] Until a more precise system for classifying this type of benign breast disorder is widely adopted, fibrocystic breast disease will probably continue to be used to describe this phenomenon of tender breast masses that occur on a cyclic basis.

Etiology and Clinical Manifestations. Hormonal imbalance in the reproductive years is thought to contribute to fibrocystic breast disease. Fibrocystic breast disease is more common in women aged 30 to 50 years. It is usually characterized by tenderness or pain in one or both breasts immediately before onset of the menstrual period. On palpation, the cysts tend to be firm, regular in shape, and mobile. They are located most often in the upper outer quadrant of the breasts, and their size may fluctuate throughout the menstrual cycle.[25]

Although it was previously thought that all women with fibrocystic breast disease were at increased risk for breast cancer, recent research has disproved this theory.[25] It is now known that only certain types of tissue changes may predispose a woman with fibrocystic breast disease to the development of breast malignancy. The vast majority of women with fibrocystic disease do not have these alterations in breast tissue and therefore are not at a substantially increased risk for breast cancer.[25]

Diagnoses and Treatment. Diagnostic studies can include ultrasound and needle aspiration of a cyst for histologic analysis (Figure 33-9). Danazol, a weak androgen, has shown efficacy in the treatment of fibrocystic breast disease. Oral contraceptives have also been recommended to control symptoms of fibrocystic breast disease. Other supportive measures include the application of local heat and use of a support bra. Nutritional therapies have shown success in some women,

FIGURE 33-9 Ultrasonic image of a cyst showing typical smooth margins, dark center, edge shadows, and a bright posterior wall. (From Donegan WL, Spratt JS: *Cancer of the breast,* ed 5, Philadelphia, 2002, Saunders, p 331.)

particularly avoidance of foods with methylxanthines such as tea, coffee, cola, and chocolate. It is thought that methylxanthines tend to stimulate cyclic adenosine monophosphate and thus increase metabolic activity in the breast.[25] A low-fat, high-carbohydrate diet has been shown to decrease breast swelling and tenderness.

Specific Benign Neoplasms. Specific benign neoplasms of the breast, such as fibroadenomas, adenomas, and papillomas, may occur at any time during a woman's life from childhood through old age. These neoplasms behave in a clinically "benign" fashion; that is, they do not invade the surrounding tissue or metastasize to other sites. They generally appear as freely movable, encapsulated masses that are sharply delineated from the surrounding breast tissue.[25] However, it is important to have any breast mass evaluated because biopsy and histologic examination may be needed to differentiate these benign neoplasms from breast carcinoma.

MALIGNANT DISORDER OF THE BREAST

Cancer of the Breast. Carcinoma of the breast remains the most common form of cancer in women between the ages of 25 and 75 years.[26] In the United States, it is the leading cause of death from all causes in women between the ages of 40 and 44 years. The incidence of breast carcinoma appears to be increasing in the United States, with an estimated 178,000 newly diagnosed cases per year.[26] Although the disease is more common in white women, its incidence in blacks and Asians is rising.[26] Breast cancer does occur in males but is 100 times less common.[26] Even though recent advances in early detection and treatment have afforded longer survival after diagnosis, invasive breast carcinoma remains an incurable disease that continues to take the lives of a large segment of the population.

Etiology. A substantial number of studies conducted in the past 20 years have begun to establish the risk factors and possible causes of breast cancer. Some factors that may place a woman at risk for breast cancer include hormonal influences, reproductive factors, dietary factors, family history, age, radiation exposure, and a history of cancer.[27] It should be noted that helping a client understand and interpret her personal breast cancer risk is a difficult task for a health care professional. The public media has given much attention to some of the risk factors for breast cancer but has not provided much context in which to interpret evaluations for individual risk factors.

Risk factors are characteristics related to the probability of a certain outcome—in this case, breast cancer. These risk factors may be either causally or correlatively associated with an outcome. For example, a factor may directly *cause* an outcome (as the smallpox virus causes smallpox) or may be *correlated* with an outcome (as not wearing a seat belt is correlated with an increased degree of injury in a motor vehicle accident). The distinction between causality and correlation is an important concept to impart to clients when discussing risk factors. A client may express concern, for example, that a certain risk factor will directly cause breast cancer to develop in her. The ability of a health care professional to describe and discuss risk factors in a knowledgeable way will greatly enhance the client's ability to make decisions regarding such issues as hormonal replacement therapy after menopause.

Hormonal Factors. Hormones are now thought to be a major factor in the development of breast cancer.[25] Length of exposure to the hormones secreted by the ovary (estrogen and progesterone) has been shown to affect the risk for breast cancer in the following way. If a woman has had an early (younger than 12 years) onset of menses and a late (older than 55 years) menopause, her risk is increased. Put another way, women with 40 or more years of menstrual activity have twice the breast cancer risk as women with fewer than 30 years of menstrual activity.[25] Postmenopausal hormone replacement therapy may increase the risk of breast cancer, and recent data show that the risk may be greater for women taking estrogen/progesterone combination therapies than for women taking estrogen only therapies.[28,29] For some women, the known benefits of these medications may outweigh effects on cancer risk. Future research is needed to clarify the way in which hormonal exposure may foster breast cancer development and the many interactive factors associated with taking hormonal medications.

Reproductive Factors. It has been observed in many research studies that giving birth at a young age (less than 18 years) is associated with a decreased risk of breast cancer and that giving birth for the first time at 35 years or older increases the risk.[25] In addition, parity (the number of children a woman has given birth to) has been associated with risk, with low parity increasing risk and high parity having a protective effect.[25] Breast-feeding is also associated with a decrease in breast cancer.[30]

Dietary Factors. It has been suggested that the amount of fat in the diet is a risk factor for breast cancer.[25] Researchers who favor this theory point to the relatively low rates of dietary fat ingestion in countries with low rates of breast cancer. Although the media has given a great deal of attention to this issue, scientific data have been inconclusive thus far.[25] Countries in which low-fat diets are widespread are typically nonindustrialized countries in which other factors, such as age at first delivery or parity, differ from those in westernized countries. No single dietary pattern or food has been shown to "cause" cancer, just as no specific food has been shown to prevent or cure it.

Family History. The role of heredity in contributing to breast cancer has long been recognized. Specific gene mutations such as *BRCA1* and *BRCA2* have been identified in high-risk families. Research studies have indicated that women with a mother or sister with breast cancer have an increased risk of developing breast cancer, even if specific gene mutations are not identified. Women with family risk factors and gene mutations need careful care and accurate information in order to make informed choices. Women with *BRCA1* and *BRCA2* are at risk for both breast and ovarian cancer and may benefit from prophylactic salpingo-oophorectomy to reduce their risk.[31] Another controversial option for some high-risk women is bilateral mastectomy. Finally, chemoprevention with selective estrogen receptor modulators (SERMs) may be an option for some high-risk women.[32] SERMs may not be recommended in low- to average-risk women because they have their own adverse effects such as thromboembolic events and endometrial cancer.

Age. Breast cancer is extremely rare in young women. The incidence of breast cancer begins to increase by 25 to 30 years of age and continues to increase with advancing age.[25]

Other Factors. Other factors, such as radiation exposure and a history of cancer, have been shown to be risk factors for the development of breast cancer.[25] Several potential factors have been suggested, such as exposure to low-frequency electric or magnetic fields and a virus transmitted through lactation. More research is required to establish the role of these potential factors.[32]

Clinical Manifestations. Most breast cancers are discovered by the woman herself. She usually finds a single lump that is painless, hard, and poorly movable. Therefore, self breast examination is an important health promotion skill. Mammography is also an important clinical tool, and according to current screening guidelines, most women should have yearly mammograms beginning at age 40.[26] Improvements in technology, such as digital mammography, have greatly increased the ability to identify breast cancers.

Half of malignant tumors occur in the upper outer quadrant of the breast.[25] Other signs of advanced tumor development include dimpling of the skin (Figure 33-10), nipple retraction, changes in breast contour, and bloody discharge from the nipple. Breast cancer is diagnosed by a number of techniques that use films (mammography, xerography) (Figures 33-11 and 33-12), computerized technologies (digital mammography), and by thermography, a technique in which "hot spots" indicate increased metabolic activity. A person of any age with a suspected breast mass should undergo mammography and biopsy.

FIGURE 33-10 Skin dimpling caused by an underlying malignant tumor. (From Donegan WL, Spratt JS: *Cancer of the breast,* ed 5, Philadelphia, 2002, Saunders, p 321.)

FIGURE 33-12 Mammographic image of a typical cancer. (From Donegan WL, Spratt JS: *Cancer of the breast,* ed 5, Philadelphia, 2002, Saunders, p 328.)

Central ray

Divergent ray

FIGURE 33-11 Placement of the breast for mammography, along with the direction of the x-rays.

FIGURE 33-13 Ultrasound scan of a carcinoma. Note the ragged appearance of this invasive, malignant lesion. (From Donegan WL, Spratt JS: *Cancer of the breast,* ed 5, Philadelphia, 2002, Saunders, p 332.)

Most breast carcinomas arise in the epithelium of the glandular ducts of the breast. The lesion(s) have infiltrating edges that begin to invade normal breast tissue (Figure 33-13). After this invasion, malignant cells begin to scatter or disseminate into the lymph system of the axilla (Figure 33-14). The breast is in close proximity to the large system of axillary lymph nodes, which makes easy dissemination of malignant cells possible. The major way by which breast carcinoma causes morbidity and death is through the dissemination of malignant cells to other body sites, most commonly lung, liver, and bone.[25] **Metastasis** (or spread of carcinoma) to these other body sites signifies a poorer prognosis. The prognosis is vastly better for persons with no evidence of spread of malignant cells to the regional lymph nodes. The 5-year survival rate is 98% when no lymph node involvement is found at surgery but averages 83% when lymph node involvement is present.[26] For women with distant spread (metastases), the rate drops to 26%. The more positive lymph nodes (nodes with malignant cells) that are found at surgery, the less favorable the prognosis.

Treatment. Treatment for breast cancer includes surgery, chemotherapy, radiation therapy, and supportive measures. Surgical therapy is a controversial area, and various options are available. Breast conserving therapy, which includes removal of only the lesion is called a **lumpectomy.** Lumpectomy or lumpectomy in conjunction with either chemotherapy and/or radiation is becoming increasingly preferred. Removal of only the breast is a simple **mastectomy.** Other surgical interventions include a **modified radical mastectomy,** in which the breast is removed and a portion of the axillary lymphatic system is dissected, and a **radical mastectomy,** in which the

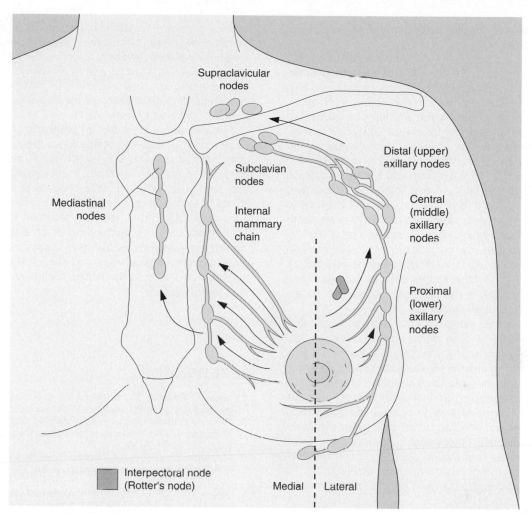

FIGURE 33-14 Lymphatic spread of breast cancer. In general, lateral lesions in the breast metastasize to axillary and supraclavicular nodes, whereas medial tumors tend to metastasize to the internal mammary and mediastinal lymph nodes, as well as the supraclavicular nodes. (From Skarin AT, editor: *Atlas of diagnostic oncology,* ed 3, St Louis, 2003, Mosby, p 260.)

breast, lymphatic drainage, and underlying pectoral muscles are removed.[25]

Chemotherapy entailing a variety of hormonal and antineoplastic agents is also used. Malignant cells appear to have cytoplasmic hormone receptors that bind to hormone molecules and promote cellular division and growth. Selective estrogen receptor modulators (SERMS), estrogen antagonists, are the most common agents used. Popular examples of SERMs include tamoxifen and raloxifene. Antineoplastic agents are given to control the spread of malignant cells.[25]

Radiation therapy may be used as an adjunct to the aforementioned therapy and to control pain by shrinking large tumor masses. Other supportive measures in advanced disease include operations to reduce the bulk of tumors.[25]

Continuum of Care. Breast cancer is characterized by a wide variation in clinical course. Many patients who undergo therapy for breast carcinoma are able to achieve a satisfying quality of life. Educational and support programs for breast cancer patients and their families, both preoperatively and postoperatively, have been an important means of providing emotional support. Programs for continuing care after mastectomy have helped patients and families face the adaptive challenges of living with breast cancer. Follow-up care includes early detection of recurrent disease, with an emphasis on breast self-examination, yearly mammography, and regular examination by health care professionals.

KEY POINTS

- Chronic inflammation of the subareolar ducts may result in mammary duct ectasia. Fibrous thickening results in a palpable central mass, breast distortion and dimpling, and nipple inversion. Persistent nipple discharge may occur. These signs are similar to those of malignancy and are carefully evaluated by biopsy. Surgical excision may be performed.
- Breast abscesses in nonlactating women are commonly associated with chronic infection, diabetes, and steroid

therapy. These abscesses respond poorly to antibiotics and tend to recur.

- Fibrocystic breast disease is a condition in which palpable breast masses are present and fluctuate with the menstrual cycle. Breast cysts are firm, mobile, and tender, and are usually located in the upper outer quadrant. There is no evidence that women with fibrocystic breasts are at higher risk for breast cancer. A low-fat, high-carbohydrate diet; danazol; heat therapy; and avoidance of methylxanthines may be recommended.

- Breast cancer is the most common cancer in women between 25 and 75 years of age. Malignant tumors tend to be painless, hard, and fixed in place, in contrast to benign breast tumors, which are mobile and encapsulated. Risk factors for breast cancer include a high-fat diet, a first-degree relative with breast cancer, increasing age, radiation exposure, and a previous malignancy. In addition, reproductive factors such as the age at first pregnancy and the number of pregnancies may be associated with altered cancer risk.

- Breast cancer may spread to the regional lymphatics and disseminate to other sites. Localized breast cancer, without lymph node involvement, has a 98% 5-year survival rate. The survival rate falls to 85% when lymph nodes are cancerous and to 26% when there are distant metastases. Depending on the extent of tumor spread, surgery may be performed to remove the tumor only (lumpectomy), the affected breast only (simple mastectomy), the affected breast and involved lymph nodes (modified radical mastectomy), or the breast, lymphatics, and underlying muscle (radical mastectomy). In addition, radiation therapy and chemotherapy may be initiated.

SUMMARY

This chapter has described the most prevalent women's reproductive health problems at the present time. Any alteration in reproductive status may have profound implications for the individual; thus the reader should review this material carefully to acquire the ability to distinguish the differences and similarities in these alterations.

Commonly occurring alterations in reproductive health for women may have serious consequences and require immediate intervention. Menstrual disorders may have multiple manifestations, and such disorders as amenorrhea and abnormal uterine bleeding may occur at any time throughout a woman's life. Alterations in uterine position and pelvic support, including uterine prolapse, retrodisplacement of the uterus, cystocele, and rectocele, may result in severe symptoms and require surgical correction. Inflammation and infection of the female reproductive tract, including PID and vulvovaginitis, may have far-reaching effects for the individual experiencing them.

The reader should pay particular attention to the section on benign growths and aberrant tissue of the female reproductive tract given the widespread nature and potentially serious consequences of these lesions. A thorough understanding of uterine leiomyomas, ovarian cysts, and endometriosis includes the ability to define these syndromes as described in this book, as well as an ability to explain them to clients. In addition, the reader is urged to review the material regarding the efficacy of the Pap smear in detecting cervical cancer at an early stage.

The section on disorders of pregnancy highlighted the most important aspects of this topic; the reader will probably wish to use this information as a basis for a more in-depth study of this area in a specialized course in maternal-child nursing. Finally, because of the widespread threat to women's health posed by disorders of the breast, the reader should pay particular attention to the final section. Specifically, the reader must be able to compare and contrast the differences between benign breast disorders and carcinoma of the breast and discuss the meaning and importance of various risk factors for breast carcinoma in a knowledgeable way.

REFERENCES

1. Hacker NF, Moore JG, Gambone JC: *Essentials of obstetrics and gynecology,* ed 4, Philadelphia, 2004, Saunders.
2. Practice Committee of the American Society for Reproductive Medicine: Current evaluation of amenorrhea, *Fertil Steril* 87(5 Suppl):S148-S155, 2006.
3. Hubasher D, Grimes DA: Noncontraceptive health benefits of intrauterine devices: a systematic review, *Obstet Gynecol Surv* 57:120-128, 2002.
4. Albers JR, Hull SK, Wesley MA: Abnormal uterine bleeding, *Am Fam Physician* 69(8):1915-1926, 2004.
5. Curtis MG, Overholt S, Hopkins MP: *Glass's office gynecology,* ed 6, Baltimore, 2005, Williams & Wilkins.
6. Diamond MP, Freeman ML: Clinical implications of postsurgical adhesions, *Hum Reprod Update* 7:567-576, 2001.
7. Keshavarz H et al: Hysterectomy surveillance—United States, 1994-1999, *MMWR Morb Mortal Wkly Rep* 51(ss-5):1-8, 2002.
8. Yen CF, Wang CJ, Lin SL et al: Combined laparoscopic uterosacral and round ligament procedures for treatment of symptomatic uterine retroversion and mild uterine decensus, *J Am Assoc Gynecolog Laparosc* 9(3):359-366, 2002.
9. Centers for Disease Control and Prevention: Sexually Transmitted Diseases Treatment Guidelines, *MMWR Morb Mortal Wkly Rep* 55(RR-11), 2006.
10. Day Baird D et al: High cumulative incidence of uterine leiomyomas in black and white women: ultrasonic evidence, *Am J Obstet Gynecol* 188(1):100-107, 2003.
11. Kimura I et al: Ovarian torsion: CT and MR imaging appearances, *Radiology* 190(2):337-341, 1994.
12. Knudsen UB et al: Management of ovarian cysts, *Acta Obstet Gynecol Scand* 83(11):1012-1021, 2004.
13. Mahmood TA, Templeton A: Prevalence and genesis of endometriosis, *Hum Reprod* 6(4):544-549, 1991.
14. Farquhar C: Endometriosis, *BMJ* 334(7587):249-253, 2007.
15. Winkel CA, Scialli AR: Medical and surgical therapies for pain associated with endometriosis, *J Women's Health Gend Based Med* 10(2):137-162, 2001.
16. Parkin DM, Bray FI, Devesa SS: Cancer burden in the year 2000: the global picture, *Eur J Cancer* 37(Suppl 8):S4-S66, 2001.
17. Saraiya M et al: Observations from the CDC. An assessment of Pap smears and hysterectomies among women in the United States, *J Women's Health Gend Based Med* 11:103-109, 2002.
18. Koutsky LA et al: A controlled trial of a human papillomavirus type 16 vaccine, *N Engl J Med* 347:1645-1651, 2002.

19. Markowitz LE et al: Quadrivalent human papilloma virus vaccine: Recommendations of the advisory committee on immunization practices, *MMWR Morb Mortal Wkly Rep* 56(RR02):1-24, 2007.

20. American Cancer Society: *Cancer Facts and Figures*, Atlanta, 2006, American Cancer Society.

21. Rebbeck TR et al: Prophylactic oophorectomy in carriers of BRCA1 or BRCA2 mutations, *N Engl J Med* 346:1616-1622, 2002.

22. Rouzier R et al: Local relapse in patients treated for squamous cell vulvar carcinoma: incidence and prognostic value, *Obstet Gynecol* 100:1159-1167, 2002.

23. Chang J et al: Pregnancy-related mortality surveillance. United States, 1991-1999, *MMWR Morb Mortal Wkly Rep* 52(SS02):1-8, 2003.

24. American College of Obstetricians and Gynecologists: *Diagnosis and management of preeclampsia and eclampsia,* ACOG Practice Bulletin No 33, Washington, DC, 2002, The College.

25. Harris JR et al: *Diseases of the breast*, ed 3, Philadelphia, 2004, Lippincott Williams & Wilkens.

26. American Cancer Society: *Cancer Facts and Figures,* Atlanta, 2007, American Cancer Society.

27. Haile RW et al: A case-control study of reproductive variables, alcohol, and smoking in premenopausal bilateral breast cancer, *Breast Cancer Res Treat* 37(1):49-56, 1996.

28. Stefanick ML, Anderson GL, Margolis KL: Effects of conjugated equine estrogens on breast cancer and mammography screening in postmenopausal women with hysterectomy, *JAMA* 295:1647–1657.

29. Writing Group for the Women's Health Initiative Investigators: Risks and benefits of estrogen plus progestin in healthy postmenopausal women: principal results from the Women's Health Initiative randomized controlled trial, *JAMA* 288:321-333, 2002.

30. Collaborative Group on Hormonal Factors in Breast Cancer: Breast cancer and breastfeeding: collaborative reanalysis of individual data from 47 epidemiological studies in 30 countries, including 50,302 women with breast cancer and 96,973 women without the disease, *Lancet* 360:187-195, 2002.

31. Kauff ND et al: Risk-reducing salpingo-oophorectomy in women with a BRCA1 or BRCA2 mutation, *N Engl Med* 346:1609-1615, 2002.

32. U.S. Preventative Services Task Force: Chemoprevention of breast cancer: recommendations and rationale, *Ann Intern Med* 137:56-58, 2002.

Sexually Transmitted Infections

Rosemary A. Jadack • Jane M. Georges

KEY QUESTIONS

▪ What are the characteristic clinical manifestations and lesions of gonorrhea and chlamydial infection?

▪ How do the pathologic changes and clinical manifestations of syphilis differ during the incubation, primary, secondary, and tertiary phases?

▪ How do the lesions of herpes simplex, syphilis, and lymphogranuloma venereum differ?

▪ Which sexually transmitted diseases remain localized, and which have systemic consequences?

▪ What are the causative organisms and characteristic lesions of the following localized sexually transmitted diseases: chancroid, granuloma inguinale, molluscum contagiosum, and condylomata acuminate (genital warts)?

CHAPTER OUTLINE

An epidemic of sexually transmitted infections (STIs) currently exists in the United States.[1,2] About one million gonococcal infections are reported each year to the Public Health Service, and it is estimated that 3 million to 4 million chlamydial infections occur each year.[1,3] The true incidence of these infections is likely to be significantly higher inasmuch as many sexually transmitted infections go unreported. The cost of STIs, in both economic and personal terms, is extremely high. It is estimated that the annual total cost associated with managing acute pelvic inflammatory disease associated with STIs in women amounts to more than $3 billion.[1] In addition, the personal costs to the individual experiencing an STI may include pain, disfigurement, psychosocial difficulties, and reproductive problems. It has been estimated that about 15 million persons acquire a new STI each year in the United States.[3] Because of the epidemic status of these diseases and the enormous costs associated with them, it is imperative that health care providers become sufficiently knowledgeable to assess their patients' STI status and educate them about STIs in an accurate and compassionate manner.

The term **sexually transmitted infections** refers to a large group of disease syndromes that can be transmitted sexually, regardless of whether the disease has manifestations in genital structures.[1] In older texts, STIs are referred to as *sexually transmitted diseases* (STDs) and *venereal diseases*. Although STIs are more prevalent in the 15- to 25-year-old age group, they can occur at any age. These diseases are sometimes contracted by nonsexual transmission, as when a newborn infant contracts an STI from an infected mother during passage through the birth canal.[1]

A list of sexually transmitted organisms grouped according to type of pathogen is found in Box 34-1. As the box shows, the list of pathogens that can be transmitted sexually is quite extensive, and the diseases that these pathogens can produce are equally extensive. Many pathogens produce multiple diseases, and many diseases may be caused by more than one pathogen. A useful approach to learning the complex pathophysiologic processes of STIs is to group STIs according to the disease manifestations that the patient is most likely to exhibit

when first seen by the health care provider. These categories of STIs and the disease manifestations associated with them are listed in Table 34-1. This chapter describes each of these categories and the pathophysiologic processes associated with each relevant STI.

Some diseases listed in Table 34-1 are discussed elsewhere in this volume but have been included here for completeness. In particular, the reader may wish to refer to Chapter 33 for more detailed information on pelvic inflammatory disease and vulvovaginitis. Also, certain systemic infections are potentially transmitted by sexual contact. Cytomegalovirus infection, hepatitis A and B, and human immunodeficiency virus (HIV) have the potential for sexual transmission. These diseases are covered in detail in Units III and X, along with more in-depth information concerning infectious processes and immune responses. Before studying this chapter, the reader may wish to refer to Chapters 8 and 9 for a review of basic terminology such as *incubation period* and *period of communicability*. Health care providers caring for persons at risk for STIs should be aware of the potential for acquisition of systemic diseases by sexual contact and include assessment of these diseases as part of their overall clinical evaluation.

URETHRITIS, CERVICITIS, SALPINGITIS, AND PELVIC INFLAMMATORY DISEASE

Three types of STI are manifested by *urethritis* (inflammation of the urethra), *cervicitis* (inflammation of the uterine cervix), and/or *salpingitis* (inflammation of the oviduct or fallopian

---

BOX 34-1

Sexually Transmitted Organisms

Bacterial Pathogens
Calymmatobacterium granulomatis
Chlamydia trachomatis
Gardnerella vaginalis
Haemophilus ducreyi
Mycoplasma hominis
Neisseria gonorrhoeae
Shigella
Group B streptococci
Ureaplasma urealyticum
Treponema pallidum

Fungal Pathogens
Candida albicans
Candida glabrata

Viral Pathogens
Human immunodeficiency virus
Cytomegalovirus
Herpes simplex virus
Hepatitis virus
Human papillomavirus
Molluscum contagiosum virus

Protozoan Pathogens
Entamoeba histolytica
Giardia lamblia
Trichomonas vaginalis

TABLE 34-1

Sexually Transmitted Infections Categorized According to Disease Manifestations

Disease Manifestations	Disease
Urethritis, cervicitis, and salpingitis	Gonorrhea
	Nongonococcal urethritis
	Pelvic inflammatory disease
Ulcerative lesions with systemic involvement	Syphilis
	Lymphogranuloma venereum
	Herpes simplex virus
Ulcerative lesions only	Chancroid
	Granuloma inguinale (donovanosis)
Nonulcerative lesions	*Molluscum contagiosum*
	Genital warts (*Condylomata acuminata*)
Vulvovaginitis	Trichomoniasis
	Candidiasis
	Gardnerella vaginalis vaginitis
Systemic infections	Cytomegalovirus
	Hepatitis
	AIDS
Enteric infections	Giardiasis
	Campylobacter enteritis
	Shigellosis
	Amebic dysentery

tube). **Gonorrhea** is an inflammation of epithelial tissue by the organism *Neisseria gonorrhoeae*. In men, nongonococcal urethritis refers to urethritis resulting from a pathogen other than the gonococcus, which is usually *Chlamydia trachomatis*. In women, mucopurulent cervicitis refers to an inflammation of the cervix, which is usually caused by either *Chlamydia trachomatis* or *Neisseria gonorrhoeae*. *Pelvic inflammatory disease,* which was described in Chapter 33, is usually the result of acute salpingitis caused by gonococcal or chlamydial infection that has extended into nearby pelvic tissue.[1,3]

Gonococcal Infection.
Gonorrhea is associated with gram-negative diplococcus, *Neisseria gonorrhoeae*.

Etiology and Clinical Manifestations. In gonorrhea, disease transmission occurs through contact with exudates from the mucous membranes of infected persons, usually by direct contact. The gonococcus then attaches to and penetrates columnar epithelium and produces a patchy inflammatory response in the submucosa with a polymorphonuclear exudate.[1] Although usually asymptomatic in women, gonorrhea may produce purulent vaginal discharge, dysuria, and abnormal vaginal bleeding. The most commonly affected areas in women are the cervix, the urethra, the Skene and Bartholin glands, and the anus. Among females, adolescents (age 15 to 19 years) and young adults (age 20 to 24 years) now have the highest rates of gonorrhea.[3] In men, symptoms of urethritis, including dysuria and a purulent urethral discharge accompanied by redness and swelling at the site of infection, usually occur after a 3- to 6-day incubation period. Among males, young adults (age 20 to 24 years) have the highest rates of gonorrhea.[3] In both sexes, infection and inflammation of the pharynx, conjunctivae, and anus may be present. Direct extension of the infection with gonococci occurs by way of the lymphatic system. In the female, extension may spread unilaterally or bilaterally to the oviducts, with subsequent salpingitis. In the male, direct extension of the infection most frequently occurs to the epididymis.[1,3]

Once gonococcal infection has spread to other areas, localized infection occurs and may cause the formation of cysts and abscesses. Purulent exudate containing the organism causes damage to tissue, and fibrous tissue replaces inflamed tissue. This hardened, fibrous tissue may result in scarring and narrowing of the urethra, epididymis, or oviducts. In women, partial or complete closure of the oviducts results in sterility. Infection of the oviducts may also result in pelvic inflammatory disease if exudate is released into the peritoneal cavity.[1,4,5] As described in Chapter 33, pelvic inflammatory disease may be an acute or chronic condition causing widespread damage to the pelvic organs in the female.

Nongonococcal Infection

Etiology. Nongonococcal urethritis and cervicitis are often caused by strains of *C. trachomatis* that act on columnar epithelium in a manner similar to that noted for the gonococcus. The symptoms of infection with *Chlamydia* are generally less severe than those of gonorrhea. As with gonorrhea, the infection may spread by extension to the oviducts, and pelvic inflammatory disease may eventually result. Upper reproductive tract infection, whether symptomatic or subclinical, is an important cause of infertility and ectopic pregnancy.[6] Transmission of *Chlamydia* during birth may result in **ophthalmia neonatorum,** or infection of the eyes in the newborn.[1,2]

Treatment. Resistance of *N. gonorrhoeae* to antimicrobial agents continues to spread and intensify. Newer antimicrobial agents such as ceftriaxone, cefixime, spectinomycin, and cephalosporin are now being used to manage uncomplicated gonococcal infections. In 2007, the Centers for Disease Control and Prevention no longer recommended fluoroquinolones for treatment of gonococcal infections due to fluoroquinolone resistance in *N. gonorrhoeae*.[7,8] Unless chlamydial infection is ruled out, dual therapy for gonococcal and chlamydial infection consisting of azithromycin or doxycycline added to one of the above agents is recommended.[7] Pelvic inflammatory disease is also generally managed with two agents to cover potential chlamydial and gonorrheal infection. A number of organizations now recommend *Chlamydia* (as well as gonorrhea) screening for sexually active adolescents and women through age 25 who have no symptoms in order to reduce the sequelae of infection.[9]

> ### KEY POINTS
>
> - Urethritis, cervicitis, salpingitis, and pelvic inflammatory disease are commonly due to gonorrhea or chlamydial infection. Transmission is usually by direct contact with infected mucous membranes. The symptoms of chlamydial infection are similar but usually less severe than those of gonorrhea.
> - Gonorrhea may produce purulent discharge, dysuria, and abnormal vaginal bleeding. Cysts and abscesses may form in localized areas of infection, followed by scarring and fibrosis. Inflammation of the pharynx, conjunctivae, and anus may be present. Antibiotic therapy is indicated.

DISEASES WITH SYSTEMIC INVOLVEMENT

Several STIs cause a distinctive ulcerative lesion and disseminate throughout the body to affect multiple organ systems. Most prominent of this type of STI are syphilis, herpesvirus infections, and lymphogranuloma venereum.

Syphilis.
Syphilis is a systemic infection of the vascular system consisting of five distinct stages: incubation, primary and secondary stages, latency, and late syphilis.[1] Syphilis is communicable by persons with primary, secondary, or early latent syphilis.[1] The incidence of syphilis has varied in the United States since reporting began in 1941. The rate of primary and secondary syphilis decreased during the 1990s to its lowest levels since 1941. However, overall rates increased again between 2001 and 2006, primarily among men who have sex with men (MSM) and men and women who engage in high-risk sexual behavior.[3] An estimated 5.7 cases of primary and secondary syphilis per 100,000 population occur annually.[3]

Etiology. Syphilis is caused by *Treponema pallidum*, an anaerobic spirochete. Syphilis is acquired when *T. pallidum* penetrates intact mucous membrane or abraded skin during sexual contact. (The process of transmission of congenital syphilis is described later.) Some of the *T. pallidum* pathogens remain at the original invasion site, whereas others migrate to regional lymph nodes within hours. During this incubation phase, *T. pallidum* is disseminated throughout the body and can invade and multiply in any organ system.[1]

Pathogenesis. During all stages of syphilis, invasion of tissue by *T. pallidum* results in pathologic changes in the vascular system. The inflammatory response in endothelial tissue causes the infiltration of lymphocytes and plasma cells, with subsequent endothelial swelling. The terminal arterioles and small arteries may become obliterated and no longer functional. Finally, long-term inflammation of vascular tissue results in the formation of hardened, fibrous thickening in the blood vessels and eventually tissue necrosis.[2]

After the initial incubation period of 10 to 90 days, the primary phase begins with the formation of a **chancre,** a painless, ulcerative lesion that arises at the original spirochete portal of entry (Figure 34-1). The chancre may go unnoticed in a female if it occurs on the cervix or in the vagina; in fact, most cases of syphilis in women go undiagnosed until recognized by positive testing of the blood in the latent phase. In males, the chancre may form on the genitalia; in both sexes, chancres may erupt on the anus, fingers, lips, tongue, nipples, tonsils, or eyelids.[1]

Untreated chancres will resolve spontaneously within 3 to 6 weeks and are followed by the secondary stage of syphilis, which is characterized by a low-grade fever, malaise, sore throat, headache, lymphadenopathy, and mucosal or cutaneous rash (Figure 34-2). This secondary stage occurs as

T. pallidum is spread throughout the bloodstream and lymphatic system. The secondary stage is also self-limiting and is followed by a latent phase in which no symptoms are present. During the latent stage, the affected person will test positive for syphilis on serologic assays and may still experience infectious mucocutaneous lesions during the early latent stage. Thus, the early latent stage is considered contagious. The latent stage is of variable length and may last more than 40 years.[2] In approximately two thirds of patients, the infection remains asymptomatic and never causes a recurrence of symptoms. If syphilis remains untreated, then late syphilis—the final, destructive phase of the disease—will eventually develop in approximately one third of affected people.[1] The manifestations of late syphilis depend on the area of arterial lesions and the extent of circulatory insufficiency.[2] Body systems particularly at risk are the cardiovascular and central nervous systems. Damage to the cardiovascular system may include aortic necrosis and subsequent aortic insufficiency; damage to the central nervous system may be progressively widespread, with degeneration of the cortical neurons and, eventually, paresis, blindness, and mental deterioration.[1]

Transmission of *T. pallidum* from the mother to the fetus may occur transplacentally at any point during pregnancy, but an inflammatory response to the pathogen does not develop in the fetus until around the 15th week of gestation. Therefore, treatment of infected women before the 15th week may prevent damage to the fetus. Infection with syphilis before birth may result in physical deformities and developmental disabilities in the infant. Infants born to untreated or inadequately treated mothers will have active infection and must be treated.[1] A presumptive diagnosis of syphilis is generally based on a positive result of a serologic screening test, such as the Venereal Disease Research Laboratory (VDRL) or

FIGURE 34-1 Typical syphilitic chancre, a painless, ulcerative lesion that arises at the original spirochete portal of entry. (From Morse SA et al: *Atlas of sexually transmitted diseases and AIDS,* ed 3, St Louis, 2003, Mosby, p 28.)

FIGURE 34-2 Typical generalized skin rash of secondary syphilis. (From Morse SA et al: *Atlas of sexually transmitted diseases and AIDS,* ed 3, St Louis, 2003, Mosby, p 29.)

rapid plasmid reagin (RPR) test, followed by a positive result of a treponemal serologic test.[2] Dark-field examination of tissue and exudates or direct fluorescent antibody tests may also be useful.

Treatment. Benzathine penicillin is the first choice for the management of syphilis. If the affected person is allergic to penicillin, tetracycline or doxycycline is given. Treatment is administered to all individuals with positive evidence of syphilis on laboratory testing and to people who have had sexual contact with infected individuals.[1] Response to antibiotic treatment is monitored by repeating laboratory testing for evidence of syphilis at regular intervals up to 24 months after therapy.[7] Management during pregnancy is complex, but it focuses on maternal cure and prevention of congenital syphilis.[10]

Lymphogranuloma Venereum. **Lymphogranuloma venereum (LGV)** is a highly contagious systemic infection caused by a number of closely related strains of *Chlamydia*. The disease occurs more commonly in the tropics but has been reported rarely in the United States.[11] LGV develops more often in males than in females and has a higher incidence among sexually active young adults.

Etiology and Pathogenesis. Like syphilis, LGV has stages of development in which an initial lesion forms and systemic disease occurs after dissemination via the lymphatic system. Three stages occur in LGV: (1) a primary lesion; (2) regional inflammation of the lymphatic system (also called *lymphadenitis*); and (3) late complications resulting from progression of the lymphadenitis.[1]

After invasion of the mucosa by *Chlamydia* during sexual contact, a painless lesion appears on the genitalia after a 1- to 3-week incubation period. The lesion may range from a slight erosion to a small papule and often goes undetected (Figure 34-3). This lesion heals spontaneously in a few days. During this period, the pathogens are disseminated to regional lymph nodes, primarily the inguinal lymph nodes.

About 2 weeks after appearance of the primary lesion, the inguinal lymph nodes begin to swell, and the systemic

FIGURE 34-3 Lymphogranuloma venereum is characterized by a small, transient genital ulcer with swollen, extremely painful inguinal lymph nodes. (From Lewis SM et al: *Medical surgical nursing,* ed 6, St Louis, 2004, Mosby, p 1392.)

symptoms of fever and malaise develop. The nodal swelling is a manifestation of inflammation of the lymphatic system in which lesions filled with polymorphonuclear leukocytes are forming in the lymph nodes. Spread of the inflammation throughout adjacent lymph nodes causes multiple nodes to become matted together and form a large abscess. These abscesses are said to be regional because they develop in one or more areas along the lymphatic system. If a person with LGV remains untreated, the abscesses rupture through the skin and other body cavities to create chronic fistulas. Thus, as the regional lymphadenitis progresses, complications such as perianal and rectovaginal fistulas develop, along with strictures of the rectum. Other complications include extreme swelling of the genitalia; this occurs because the normal lymph drainage of this area is impeded.[7] The diagnosis is usually made by serologic testing (antibody titers).

Treatment. Doxycycline is the recommended antibiotic with erythromycin being the alternative. Surgical treatment may include aspiration of lymph nodes as needed; rectal strictures and fistulas may require surgical correction.[7]

Herpesvirus Infections. **Herpesviruses** are an important group of viral agents that produce infection in humans. Two types of herpes simplex virus (HSV)—type 1 and type 2—may be sexually transmitted and are discussed in this section. HSV type 1 is most often associated with herpetic infections above the waist, typically in the oral cavity and on the lips, but also in the eyes or on the epidermis. HSV type 1 can be transmitted sexually, and it is present in saliva, stool, and urine. The vesicles resulting from type 1 infection in the oral cavity are commonly referred to as *cold sores* or *chancres* and often affect children younger than 5 years.[1] HSV type 2 is implicated in most genital, anal, and perianal herpes and is sometimes referred to as *genital herpes* for this reason. Type 2 HSV can also result in oral lesions after sexual contact. Serologic studies indicate that one in five individuals in the United States have been infected with type 2 HSV.[12] Although type 2 is primarily transmitted through sexual contact, pregnant mothers can transmit the infection to newborns during vaginal delivery.[1]

Etiology. HSV types 1 and 2 have certain characteristics in common. Both produce an initial infection that is self-limiting. The lesions produced by this infection heal, but HSV continues to be present in the body. Recurrence of the lesions, usually in the area of the initial infection, may take place as the virus is reactivated. Recurrence of either type may be triggered by an infectious disease, emotional stress, or immunosuppression.[2] The exact mechanism for reactivation of the virus is presently unknown, but it is thought that ganglion neurons may contain latent forms of the virus and then receive a trigger to stimulate replication of the virus under certain conditions.[1]

Clinical Manifestations. Genital infection with HSV type 2 is manifested by the appearance of fluid-filled vesicles after a 3- to 7-day incubation period. In the female, the cervix is usually the primary infection site, although the labia, perianal skin, vulva, or vagina may also be involved (Figure 34-4). In the male, the

FIGURE 34-4 Primary genital herpes in the female showing herpetic vesicles and tender ulcerations. (From Morse SA et al: *Atlas of sexually transmitted diseases and AIDS,* ed 3, St Louis, 2003, Mosby, 2003, p 247.)

vesicles are located on the glans penis, foreskin, or penile shaft (Figure 34-5). Extragenital lesions may appear on the mouth or anus. In both males and females, the vesicles, which are usually painless at first, may rupture and develop into extensive shallow, painful ulcers. The virus may enter the lymphatic system and create localized lesions there; thus, the inguinal lymph nodes may be edematous and tender. Rarely, the virus spreads to visceral organs and can produce areas of necrosis in the liver, adrenal glands, lungs, and central nervous system.[2] In newborns and people with weak immune defenses (particularly people with acquired immunodeficiency syndrome), HSV type 2 may result in severe damage to these organ systems, with high related mortality.[1] Most HIV-infected individuals are HSV-2 seropositive, and perirectal involvement is common.[12,13]

HSV type 1 infections may appear as single or multiple fluid-filled, tender vesicles in the oral cavity or on the lips. Usually, the appearance of the lesions is preceded by 1 or 2 days of paresthesia before the chancre or "cold sore" erupts. These lesions will generally crust and heal within 3 to 10 days. HSV infections are usually diagnosed by cell culture.[2] Exudate from early lesions gives the most positive results.

Treatment. Normally, HSV type 1 lesions are self-limiting and respond to measures that promote good oral hygiene. HSV type 2 genital lesions are usually self-limiting but may be extremely painful. The use of antiviral agents such as acyclovir, famciclovir, and valacyclovir has been shown to accelerate healing time and reduce the duration and severity of symptoms in initial episodes of HSV type 2 infection.[7,14] Long-term or episodic suppression may also be used to reduce the number or severity of recurrent episodes.[7] Consistent use of condoms reduces transmission from men to women.[15,16] If HSV type 2 lesions are active in a pregnant mother at term, a cesarean section may be recommended to reduce the risk of transmission to the newborn.[5]

KEY POINTS

- Syphilis is caused by an anaerobic spirochete that is transmitted sexually but disseminates throughout the body during incubation. Manifestations of early syphilis include chancre formation at the portal of entry, which spontaneously resolves in 3 to 6 weeks if untreated. General malaise, fever, sore throat, and rash may then occur, followed by an asymptomatic latent phase. The latent phase may last more than 40 years. Late syphilis is characterized by central nervous system degeneration, blindness, and paresis.
- LGV is a highly contagious systemic infection caused by strains of *Chlamydia*. An initial painless genital lesion appears after 1 to 3 weeks of incubation. The infection spreads to regional lymph nodes and is accompanied by fever and malaise. Infected lymph nodes become abscessed and may rupture through the skin and body cavities, causing fistula formation.
- HSV types 1 and 2 are implicated in cases of genital herpes. Herpes lesions are fluid-filled vesicles that appear 3 to 7 days after infection. The virus may enter the lymphatics and cause inguinal lymph node tenderness. Although the lesions may disappear, the virus remains in the body, thus predisposing to recurrence. Herpes may be transmitted from mother to newborn during birthing.

DISEASES WITH LOCALIZED LESIONS

Ulcerative Lesions

Two types of STIs result in the formation of ulcerative lesions but do not progress to systemic involvement. **Chancroid** (also called soft chancre) and **granuloma inguinale** are both manifested by ulcerative lesions, although their pathophysiologic courses differ.

FIGURE 34-5 Recurrent genital herpes in the male showing herpetic ulcerations **(A)** and ulcers with grayish exudate **(B)**. (From Morse SA et al: *Atlas of sexually transmitted diseases and AIDS,* ed 3, St Louis, 2003, Mosby, p 248.)

Chancroid

Etiology. Chancroid is an ulcerative, infectious disease of the genital tract caused by the sexually transmitted anaerobic bacillus *Haemophilus ducreyi.* Chancroid was relatively rare in the United States until the past decade. Since 1981, small epidemic outbreaks of chancroid have been reported in the United States. In terms of outbreaks in Western countries, there is an approximately 10:1 male-to-female ratio.[1] Chancroid is a cofactor for human immunodeficiency virus infection.

Pathogenesis and Clinical Manifestations. *Haemophilus ducreyi* initially invades the genital skin or mucous membranes at sites traumatized by sexual contact. The patient generally has one or more painful genital ulcers, unlike the chancre in syphilis, which is generally solitary and painless. Fresh lesions may occur from autoinoculation (self-infection). The ulcerated lesions may enlarge, continue to erode

(Figure 34-6), and produce destruction of surrounding tissue. In addition, inguinal lymph nodes may become tender and painful as the infection is disseminated to this region. If the infection goes untreated, the enlarged lymph gland (called a *bubo*) may rupture, draining pus and leaving a large inguinal ulcer. The infection is communicable until the lesions heal, which may be a period of weeks.[1] Scarring may occur in advanced cases. Diagnosis is usually made by culture for *H. ducreyi.*

Treatment. Anti-infective agents recommended for management of chancroid include azithromycin, erythromycin, ceftriaxone, and ciprofloxacin.[7] Large ulcers may not heal for more than 2 weeks. As with all STIs, sexual partners should be treated simultaneously and re-exposure avoided until therapy is completed. Aspiration of enlarged inguinal lymph nodes may also be indicated.[1]

FIGURE 34-6 The eroded, purulent ulcer of chancroid. (From Morse SA et al: *Atlas of sexually transmitted diseases and AIDS*, ed 3, St Louis, 2003, Mosby, p 56.)

Granuloma Inguinale

Etiology. *Calymmatobacterium granulomatis* is the causative agent of granuloma inguinale. This intracellular bacterium is also referred to as a *Donovan body* and the disease as *donovanosis*. Granuloma inguinale is rare in the United States, with the highest incidence in homosexual males.[1,2]

Pathogenesis and Clinical Manifestations. Transmission of granuloma inguinale is not clearly understood. It is generally thought to be an STI, but the disease is also seen in adults who are not sexually active and in young children, possibly as a result of autoinoculation. The causative bacterium is found in the rectum of nondiseased persons, which suggests that the organism may be part of the normal gastrointestinal flora in some persons.[2] The communicability of the disease is relatively low, and it is generally believed that repeated exposure is necessary.[1]

The incubation period is variable and ranges from a few days to months. The initial sign of the disease may be a painless papule or nodule that subsequently ulcerates into an enlarging, granulomatous, red velvety ulcer. The raised mass of granulation tissue may look more like a tumor than an ulcer. The lesions are highly vascular and bleed easily with minor contact. Single or multiple lesions may coalesce, or lesions may spread to nearby tissue.[2] Secondary infection of the ulcers and expanding tissue necrosis in lesions may lead to erosion of the genitals. In addition, the formation of scar tissue on genital structures during the healing process may produce urethral occlusion.[2] Lymph node involvement is minimal, and inguinal swelling is usually due to the presence of subcutaneous granulomas.[1] Diagnosis is by identification of the dark-staining Donovan bodies on biopsy or tissue crush preparations.

Treatment. Doxycycline is given for at least 3 weeks or until all lesions are healed.[7] Alternative agents include trimethoprim-sulfamethoxazole, ciprofloxacin, erythromycin, and azithromycin.[7] Long-term follow-up should be provided because this disease may recur.[1]

Nonulcerative Lesions

Molluscum contagiosum and infections caused by human papilloma virus (HPV) (also called genital warts) are two prevalent types of STIs that produce nonulcerative lesions. Both are caused by viral agents that invade superficial layers of the epidermis during sexual contact.

Molluscum Contagiosum

Etiology. Molluscum contagiosum is a viral skin disease caused by a member of the poxvirus family.[2] (The term *poxvirus* refers to a viral agent that causes an eruption, or "pox," on the skin.) The manifestations are much milder than those of smallpox or chickenpox. Two forms of the disease exist. One affects children and is transmitted by skin-to-skin contact and indirect contact; the other affects young adults and is transmitted during sexual contact.[1]

Pathogenesis and Clinical Manifestations. After invasion of the epidermis by the virus, pink to white lesions with an exudative core appear on the genitalia. The lesions are multiple, are slow to develop, and remain stable for long periods. The disease is usually asymptomatic, tends to be self-limiting, and lasts on average 2 years.[1,2]

Treatment. The goal of treatment is primarily to prevent spread of the infection for cosmetic reasons. The lesions can be removed by minor surgery or frozen with liquid nitrogen. Sexual contacts of affected persons should be examined to prevent further spread.[1]

Human Papillomavirus Infections

Etiology. Human Papillomavirus (HPV) infections cause epithelial lesions of the anogenital region.[1] Also called *genital warts* or *Condylomata Acuminata*, HPV is predominantly transmitted sexually in young adults, with the highest prevalence in the 16- to 25-year-old age group.[3] The risk of contracting the disease by sexual contact with an infected person is high; lesions will develop in up to two thirds of the sexual contacts of affected persons. Nonsexual transmission has also been documented, and lesions have been found in infants.[1] The period of communicability is unknown but is thought to last as long as the lesions persist, and perhaps even after they are clinically removed.[1]

Pathogenesis and Clinical Manifestations. After invasion of the epidermis by HPV, an incubation period of 1 to 20 months (usually about 4 months) precedes the appearance of lesions. It is thought that the virus infects single epithelial cells and stimulates the cells to divide and proliferate into the wartlike lesions. The lesions are single or multiple, soft pink to brown, and usually elongated. They often occur in cauliflower-like clusters (Figure 34-7). The lesions are generally asymptomatic but may be pruritic (itchy), painful, or friable (bleed easily). In females, HPV may be found in the vagina and cervix, as well as in the anogenital area.[1] In males, they may occur in the anterior urethra and anogenital area.

Treatment. External genital warts may be treated with patient applied podofilox or imiquimod topical preparations.[7] Providers can administer cryotherapy, podophyllin, trichloroacetic acid, bichloroacetic acid, or surgery.[7] Patient-applied preparations are also available, and include podofilox (0.5%) and imiquimod (5%) cream. Alternative regimens include intralesional interferon and laser surgery. Malignant transformation to invasive carcinoma has been observed with some types of genital warts. Persistent infections of HPV types 6, 11, 16, and 18 are thought to be responsible for 70% of cervical cancers and 90% of genital warts. Therefore, it is generally agreed that affected persons should be treated or monitored carefully.[9] Because HPV has been associated with cervical cancer, there has been an increasing use of human papillomavirus testing in evaluating abnormal Papanicolaou smears.[1]

In 2006, the Food and Drug Administration (FDA) licensed the first vaccine developed to prevent cervical cancer

FIGURE 34-7 Human papillomavirus of the vulva. (From Morse SA et al: Atlas of sexually transmitted diseases and AIDS, ed 3, st. Louis, 2003, Mosby, p. 268.)

and other diseases in females caused by certain types of human papillomavirus (HPV) (see Chapter 33). The HPV vaccine is recommended for 11- to 12-year-old girls, but can be administered to girls as young as 9 years of age. The vaccine also is recommended for 13- to 26-year-old females who have not yet received or completed the vaccine series. Ideally, the vaccine should be administered before onset of sexual activity. However, females who are sexually active also may benefit from vaccination.[17,18]

KEY POINTS

- Chancroid is caused by infection with an anaerobic bacillus. Initially the lesion is a small erythematous papule, and after 2 to 3 days the painful lesion ulcerates. Lesions resemble those of syphilis; however, the lesions of syphilis are painless.
- Granuloma inguinale is caused by an intracellular bacterium. The initial papule is painless and subsequently ulcerates into a growing granulomatous ulcer resembling a tumor.
- Molluscum contagiosum is associated with infection by a poxvirus. Genital lesions are pink to white with an exudative core. The disease is usually asymptomatic and self-limiting.
- Condylomata acuminata, or genital warts, are associated with infection by human papillomavirus. Warts are pink to brown and painless and may occur in clusters. Persistent human papillomavirus infection is an important risk factor for cervical cancer.

ENTERIC INFECTIONS

Until recently, information regarding the transmission of enteric infections of the gastrointestinal tract through sexual contact was limited. Recent research in this area has increased the knowledge base of health care providers, and the term **gay bowel syndrome** has been coined to describe the transmission and subsequent infection with enteric pathogens through sexual contact. It must be stressed that despite the specific reference to homosexual males by the term *gay*, such disorders are *not* limited to the homosexual community. Enteric pathogens may be transmitted sexually among any individuals who engage in direct or indirect fecal-oral contact. Enteric organisms that may be transmitted through sexual contact include *Giardia, Campylobacter, Shigella,* and the agents causing amebic dysentery.[4]

The pathophysiologic process of enteric infections of the gastrointestinal tract is described in Chapter 36, and the reader may wish to refer to this material. In general, persons who have acquired enteric infections by sexual contact will have variable manifestations. Some individuals may experience no symptoms, whereas others will have marked symptoms of enteritis or proctitis. All individuals who engage in oral-anal sexual practices should be monitored for the presence of enteric

infections with laboratory studies and diagnostic examinations. Education for persons at risk for sexually transmitted enteric infections includes an emphasis on protective hygienic practices. Infected persons should avoid all sexual contact until all partners are examined and treated if necessary. After completion of appropriate therapy for enteric infections, affected individuals should be retested for assessment of therapeutic effectiveness.[5]

SUMMARY

Because of the epidemic nature of STIs, it is essential for readers preparing for careers in the health sciences to have a complete grasp of the material in this chapter. The STIs considered in the chapter are grouped according to the disease manifestations that the patient is most likely to exhibit. Gonorrhea, most chlamydial infections, and pelvic inflammatory disease are manifested by urethritis, cervicitis, or salpingitis. A second group of STIs cause ulcerative lesions with systemic involvement. Syphilis, herpes, and LGV all cause a distinctive ulcerative lesion and may disseminate throughout the body to affect multiple organ systems.

In reviewing the material on STIs related to ulcerative and nonulcerative lesions, the reader should compare and contrast the appearance of these lesions and consider the differing pathophysiologic characteristics of each type. Finally, the reader should consider how he or she would incorporate this material into an overall assessment process. Nurses and other health care providers caring for persons at risk for STIs should be aware of the potential for acquisition of these diseases as well. The overall goal in learning the material in this chapter is to be able to assess and educate clients with STIs in a comfortable and accurate manner.

REFERENCES

1. Holmes KK et al, editors: *Sexually transmitted diseases,* ed 4, New York, 2007, McGraw-Hill.
2. Borchardt KA, Noble MA, editors: *Sexually transmitted diseases: epidemiology, pathology, diagnosis, and treatment,* Boca Raton, Fla, 1997, CRC Press.
3. Centers for Disease Control and Prevention: *Sexually transmitted disease surveillance,* Atlanta, 2007, U.S. Department of Health and Human Services.
4. Horner PJ et al: Gonorrhoea: signs, symptoms, and serogroups, *Int J STD AIDS* 3(6):430-433, 1992.
5. Hacker NF et al, editors: *Essentials of obstetrics and gynecology,* Philadelphia, 2004, Saunders.
6. Jossens MO, Schacter J, Sweet RL: Risk factors associated with pelvic inflammatory disease of differing microbial etiologies, *Obstet Gynecol* 83(6):989-997, 1994.
7. Centers for Disease Control and Prevention: Sexually transmitted diseases treatment guidelines, 2006, *MMWR Morb Mortal Wkly Rep* 55(No. RR-11):1-93, 2006.
8. Centers for Disease Control and Prevention: Update to CDC's *Sexually Transmitted Diseases Treatment Guidelines, 2006:* Fluoroquinolones no longer recommended for treatment of gonococcal infections, *MMWR Morb Mortal Wkly Rep* 56(14):332-336, 2007.
9. U.S. Preventive Services Task Force: Screening for chlamydial infection: recommendations and rationale, *Am J Prev Med* 20(3S):90-94, 2001.

10. Wendel GD et al: Treatment of syphilis in pregnancy and prevention of congenital syphilis, *Clin Infect Dis* 35(Suppl 2):S200-S209, 2002.
11. Centers for Disease Control and Prevention: Lymphogranuloma venereum among men who have sex with men: Netherlands, 2003-2004, *MMWR Morb Mortal Wkly Rep* 53(42):985-988, 2004.
12. Fleming DT et al: Herpes simplex virus type 2 in the United States, 1976 to 1994, *N Engl J Med* 337:1105-1111, 1997.
13. Schacker T et al: Frequency of symptomatic and asymptomatic herpes simplex type 2 reactivations among human immunodeficiency virus-infected men, *J Infect Dis* 178:1616-1622, 1998.
14. Mostad MB et al: Cervical shedding of herpes simplex virus in human immunodeficiency virus–infected women: effects of hormonal contraception, pregnancy, and vitamin A deficiency, *J Infect Dis* 181:58-63, 2000.
15. Corey L: Challenges in genital herpes simplex virus management, *J Infect Dis* 186(Suppl 1):S29-S33, 2002.
16. Wald A et al: Effect of condoms on reducing the transmission of herpes simplex virus type-2 from men to women, *JAMA* 285:3100-3106, 2001.
17. Koutsky LA et al: A controlled trial of a human papillomavirus type 16 vaccine, *N Engl J Med* 347:1645-1651, 2002.
18. Markowitz LE et al: Quadrivalent human papilloma virus vaccine: Recommendations of the advisory committee on immunization practices, *MMWR Morb Mortal Wkly Rep* 56(RR02):1-24, 2007.

PART 6

Alterations in Metabolism and Nutrition

Frontiers of Research

Advances in Treatment of Gastrointestinal Disorders

Sheila K. Smith • Michael J. Kirkhorn

When the gastrointestinal (GI) system is working properly, we are happy not to have to think about it. When it shows signs of stress or disease, we think about it only reluctantly. It seems so complicated—its coilings, its odd junctures, its paradoxical purposes—in nourishing the body and disposing of wastes, processes sustaining life in two invaluable but seemingly contradictory ways. It is vitally important that the GI system work properly in both of its essential functions. The standard textbook listing of GI disorders is unappetizing: gastritis, peptic ulcer disease, pancreatitis, bowel obstruction, Crohn disease, irritable bowel syndrome, GI bleeding, colitis, and cancer. Most of us have had at least an episodic experience with the unpleasantness, serious inconvenience, and discomfort of a GI disorder. Thinking about living with such symptoms on an everyday basis, sometimes at a life-threatening level of severity, can help us appreciate the significance and disruptive impact of serious GI disease. Life-threatening fluid and electrolyte imbalances, pH disorders, altered nutritional and immune status, significant anemias, bleeding disorders, and massive infection can all result from disordered GI functioning.

Research on a variety of fronts is leading to greater knowledge about some of the more significant GI disorders. As with other medical conditions, a paradigm shift is occurring in the understanding of many causes of GI disease. Disorders of the GI tract are increasingly understood to involve interplay between personal lifestyle, nutrition, genetic constitution, and environmental factors. The role of *Helicobacter pylori* in the development of peptic ulcer disease and gastric cancer is an important example of this interplay. *H. pylori* is a factor in nearly all cases of ulcer formation in patients who are not taking nonsteroidal anti-inflammatory agents. However, a large proportion of the population has *H. pylori* as a component of their normal flora, and these individuals never develop peptic ulcer disease or cancer. Perhaps psychoneuroendocrine or psychoimmune factors (i.e., stress) will be shown to affect host resistance or the clinical expression of gastric cancer and peptic ulcer, as has occurred with other diseases.

Another example of a significant host-environment relationship is seen with *Clostridium difficile (C. difficile)* and the development of antibiotic-related colitis. *C. difficile* is a spore-forming bacterium that can cause extensive inflammatory damage to the intestinal mucosa, leading to pain, diarrhea, dehydration, and septicemia. Many people carry *C. difficile* as a resident organism; others may become exposed to it as health care workers. The majority of cases, however, develop as nosocomial infections secondary to an antibiotic-related decrease in GI organisms, the decreased immunity of illness processes, and concomitant exposure to and overgrowth of *C. difficile* bacteria. *C difficile* colitis can take weeks to months to resolve, requiring its own unpleasant and sometimes ineffective antibiotic regimen. Adding *C. difficile* colitis to an already ill person's list of diagnostic conditions does not help to cultivate a sense of trust and confidence in the health care system.

Colorectal cancer, the most common GI malignancy, is common in the United States and is a major source

Helicobacter pylori *gastritis. Numerous darkly stained* Helicobacter *organisms along the luminal surface of the gastric epithelial cells with no tissue invasion by bacteria. (From Kumar V et al: Robbins basic pathology, ed 7, Philadelphia, 2003, Saunders.)*

Gastrointestinal Function

of concern throughout the world. Colorectal cancer accounts for about 11% of all cancers in both men and women, as well as about 11% of cancer-related deaths. Each year more than 150,000 new cases occur in the United States, and more than 55,000 persons die from the disease. Physicians are encouraged by their ability to cure colon cancer if malignant polyps are detected early. Researchers have also identified noncancerous lesions that are responsible for the later development of some colon cancers. They provide early warning, often appearing years before the cancer itself. Early colonoscopy screening, beginning at age 50, helps detect the hyperplastic polyps that precede cancer. During colonoscopy, the polyps are removed to reduce the possibility of colon cancer. Only 6% of colon cancers are inherited; for those individuals it is especially important to begin colonoscopy screening early, as malignant changes can emerge as early as young adulthood. Genetic studies also promise an effective screening test.

The liver is another target of intense interest. The liver provides major metabolic, protein/nutrient synthesis, filtration, and elimination functions. Failed liver physiology leads to severe illness and death. A British researcher reports that about 60% of patients suffering from severe, acute alcoholic hepatitis die during the first 6 weeks after hospitalization. Alcoholic hepatitis is frequently found in patients in whom cirrhosis eventually develops, a potentially fatal disease in which the functioning cells of the liver are replaced with fibrotic tissue that impedes hepatic blood flow and cell function. The most common cause of non-alcoholic liver disease is chronic hepatitis C. The Centers for Disease Control and Prevention estimate that there are 38,000 new cases of acute hepatitis C in the United States annually. Very few of these are diagnosed. In studies, approximately 15% to 25% of patients with acute hepatitis C virus cleared the infection spontaneously. Up to 85%, however, develop chronic infection, and a high percentage of them develop cirrhosis or liver cancer.

Clinicians are encouraged by their improved ability to diagnose, treat, and manage a variety of liver diseases. Among these improvements are new developments in liver transplantation, including the possibility of grafting transplanted tissue onto the diseased liver to allow it to recover. Viral suppression in hepatitis C treatment has improved to allow preservation of hepatic function for many, many years when combined with appropriate lifestyle health behaviors.

In industrialized nations where advanced technology is available, new imaging strategies are aiding in the diagnosis of GI diseases. Computed tomography can be used to diagnose pancreatitis, Crohn disease, fatty infiltration of the liver, or metastases in cases of cancer. Innovations have also led to far less painful recovery for surgical patients. Each year, more than 500,000 Americans undergo surgical treatment of gallbladder disease—a formerly excruciatingly painful condition. Laparoscopic cholecystectomy affords a minimally invasive surgical approach and is an appropriate choice for many patients. Rather than making a single large incision, surgeons remove the gallbladder and stones through four small abdominal incisions. Usually the patient is able to go home in a day or two, at a significant cost savings.

Gastrointestinal Function

Jeffrey S. Sartin

MEDIA RESOURCES

Additional Material for Study, Review, and Further Exploration

 CD Companion ▪ Review Questions and Answers
▪ Glossary (with audio pronunciations for selected terms)
▪ Disease Profiles ▪ Animations

ⓔvolve **Website** at http://evolve.elsevier.com/Copstead/
▪ Case Studies ▪ Disease Profiles ▪ WebLinks ▪ Key Points Review

 Online Course (Module 16)

KEY QUESTIONS

- What are the major structures of the gastrointestinal tract and their corresponding functions?
- How does the autonomic nervous system influence gastrointestinal motility?
- How do segmental and propulsive movements influence the digestive and absorptive functions of the small intestine?
- What are the major secretions of each of the following secretory cells and glands: salivary, gastric, intestinal epithelium, pancreas, and gallbladder?

- How and where are complex carbohydrates, proteins, and lipids digested and absorbed?
- How and where are water and electrolytes absorbed?
- What alterations in gastrointestinal function occur in association with very young or very old age?

CHAPTER OUTLINE

The gastrointestinal (GI) system consists of the GI tract and the related solid organs of digestion. Beginning with the mouth and pharynx, the GI tract includes the esophagus, stomach, and small and large intestines (Figure 35-1). These components can be thought of as a continuous tube about 7 m in length running from the mouth to the anus. Other parts of the GI system that are located outside the GI tract include the salivary glands, the pancreas, and the biliary system (liver, gallbladder, and bile ducts).

The function of the GI system is to provide nutrients for the body. The process of ingesting nutrients, propelling them through the GI tract, and transforming them into a form capable of absorption into the body's internal milieu constitutes a remarkable interface of the human organism with the external environment. The general functions of the GI tract in providing nutrients for the body can be divided into (1) GI motility, including propulsive and mixing movements; (2) secretion of digestive juices; (3) digestion of nutrients; and (4) absorption of nutrients.[1,2] This chapter describes each of these functions in detail and provides an overview of the structure and organization of the GI tract and its growth and alteration across the life span.

STRUCTURE AND ORGANIZATION OF THE GASTROINTESTINAL TRACT

Embryology

As early as the fourth week of gestation, the GI system begins to form from the primitive gut structures of the foregut, midgut, and hindgut.[3] The foregut gives rise to the pharynx, esophagus, stomach, the duodenum proximal to the opening of the common bile duct, the hepatobiliary system, and the pancreas. The trachea and esophagus share a common developmental origin, and incomplete partitioning of these structures may lead to **tracheoesophageal fistula,** a developmental anomaly characterized by an abnormal connection between the trachea and esophagus, often accompanied by **esophageal atresia,** a condition in which the esophagus is closed off in a blind pouch. These disorders occur in about 1 in 4000 live births, with about one-third of the infants affected by this anomaly born prematurely. These disorders are two of the most serious surgical emergencies in newborns and require immediate diagnosis and surgical correction.[4] The current prognosis for

such infants is very good, with about 90% survival beyond the neonatal period.

The midgut gives rise to the small intestine (below the opening of the common bile duct), the cecum, the appendix, the ascending colon, and the proximal portion of the transverse colon. Failure of normal partitioning between the foregut and midgut can lead to **intestinal atresia,** a condition in which the lumen of the small intestine is obliterated. This anomaly is one of the most common causes of intestinal obstruction in the newborn and necessitates prompt surgical correction.[4] Failure of the midgut to develop or rotate properly with respect to the umbilical cord can result in **omphalocele,** a congenital herniation of viscera into the base of the umbilical cord.

The hindgut gives rise to the distal part of the transverse colon, the descending and sigmoid colon, the rectum, and the superior portion of the anal canal. Congenital malformations resulting from inappropriate development of the anorectal portion of the GI tract include colonic or anal agenesis, a condition in which the rectal pouch ends blindly above the surface of the perineum. This condition has been rarely reported with congenital varicella syndrome.[5] Other developmental anomalies of this portion of the GI tract include anal stenosis, in which the anal aperture is small, and anal membrane atresia, in which the anal membrane covers the aperture and creates an obstruction.

After its initial embryologic development, the GI tract continues to grow in length and diameter until somatic growth ends after puberty. The degree of growth and development of the GI tract during childhood appears to depend on the same general factors as growth of the rest of the body. Such general factors as nutritional adequacy, insulin, growth hormone, thyroid hormone, cortisol, androgens, and estrogens may play a role in its development, as well as such specific factors as the direct effect of ingested nutrients, GI hormones, and secretions.[6]

Functional Anatomy

Each part of the GI tract is uniquely adapted for a specific function in the process of providing nutrients for the body—a process that continues from birth to death. Each major component of the GI tract is described as a basis for understanding the overall structure and innervation of the GI tract.

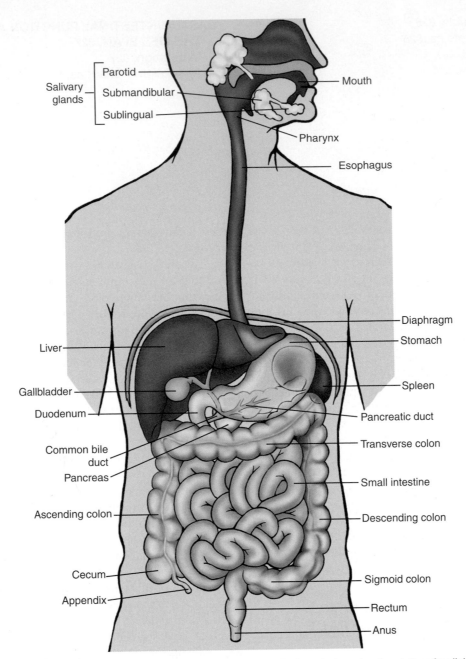

FIGURE 35-1 The gastrointestinal system. (From Monahan FD, Neighbors M: *Medical surgical nursing: foundations for clinical practice,* ed 2, Philadelphia, 1998, Saunders, p 950.)

Oral Cavity and Pharynx

The mouth, or oral cavity, is the usual point of entry for nutrients and is the site of the initial breakdown of nutrient substances into a form usable by the body. Food is pushed toward the side of the mouth by the tongue to facilitate chewing and grinding on the surfaces of the molar and premolar teeth. As the food is manipulated and broken down, it is moistened by saliva secreted by three major pairs of salivary glands: the parotid, submandibular, and sublingual glands (Figure 35-2). Saliva serves three major functions: (1) by its moistening action, saliva allows the tongue to convert a mouthful of food

into a bolus, or semisolid mass, that can be swallowed easily; (2) by its moistening action, saliva changes dry foods into a solute form and allows for taste perception by the papillae on the surface of the tongue, which are sensitive to chemical differences among food molecules; and (3) the digestive enzyme contained in saliva, **salivary amylase** (also called *ptyalin*), initiates carbohydrate digestion by effecting the breakdown of polysaccharides (also called *starch*) into the simpler molecular structures of dextrin and maltose.[7,8] Important changes in oral structure and function that occur during aging are detailed in Geriatric Considerations: Changes in the Mouth.

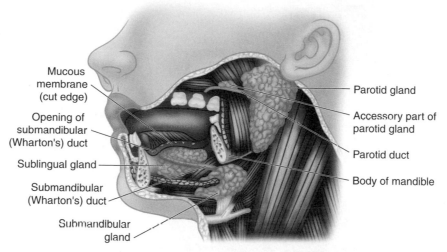

FIGURE 35-2 Oral cavity. Structures of the mouth and location of the salivary glands. (From O'Toole M, editor: *Miller-Keane encyclopedia and dictionary of medicine, nursing, and allied health,* ed 7, Philadelphia, 2003, Saunders.)

GERIATRIC CONSIDERATIONS

Changes in the Mouth

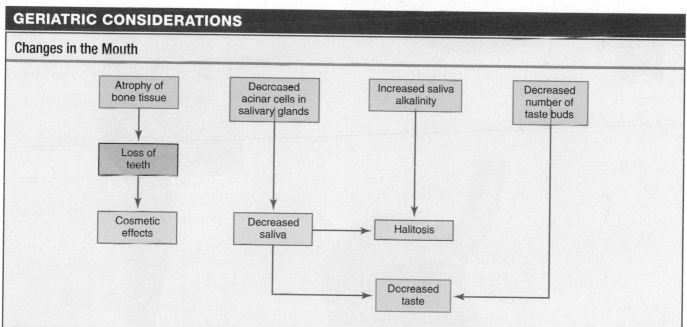

Elderly people experience a decline in taste. This decline is due to both an increase in the sensation threshold for all four tastes and a decrease in the number of papilla. For example, children have more than 200 taste buds, whereas the elderly have fewer than 100. Of the four basic tastes, the elderly experience a particular decrease in salt and sugar tastes.

The elderly also experience a decrease in the number of acinar cells in the salivary glands, leading to a reduction in the amount and secretory rate of saliva. The saliva becomes more alkaline as well.

The decrease in the amount of saliva and the increased alkalinity contribute to halitosis (bad breath).

Loss of teeth in the elderly is due to atrophy of gum and bone tissue as well as actual tooth wear and tear. The enamel of the teeth may wear away, exposing dentin. As a result of secondary dentin deposition with aging, the size of the pulp chamber is decreased and the pulp is limited to the root cavity only. There is controversy as to whether the loss of gingival epithelial tissue is pathologic or a normal part of aging.

The pharynx, or throat, is about 12 cm long and serves as the entryway for both the respiratory and the GI systems. The oropharynx is the portion of the pharynx posterior to the mouth and is separated from the nasopharynx, the portion of the pharynx posterior to the nose, by the soft palate. The laryngopharynx is the portion of the pharynx that opens into the larynx and the esophagus. During swallowing, the soft palate is pulled upward to close off the nasopharynx. The bolus of food being swallowed is propelled by reflex movements of muscles in the pharynx through the laryngopharynx and into the esophagus. Simultaneously, the opening to the larynx is closed by the epiglottis. This coordinated set of actions prevents food substances and liquids from inadvertently entering the respiratory system, a potentially life-threatening occurrence referred to as *aspiration.*

FIGURE 35-3 Physiologic anatomy of the stomach. *HCL,* Hydrochloric acid. (From Herlihy B: *The human body in health and illness,* ed 3, Philadelphia, 2007, Saunders, p 402.)

Esophagus

The esophagus is a muscular tube approximately 25 cm in length. Passage of food through the esophagus is greatly facilitated by mucus secreted by cells in the epithelial lining. Extremely rough or fibrous foods may potentially penetrate the mucous lining of the esophagus and cause damage. The stratified squamous epithelium lining the esophagus is constantly renewed by cells moving to the surface from below, thus providing a means of renewal for such damage. The esophagus propels nutrients to the stomach by means of strong muscular contractions (a capability that may be affected by aging). **Presbyesophagus,** or an abnormal esophageal motility pattern occurring with advanced age, is described in detail in the Age-Related Changes section. When the body is in an upright position, gravity assists in the downward movement of food to the stomach. However, the muscular contractions of the esophagus are extremely strong and are sufficient to transport nutrients to the stomach even in the absence of gravity, just as persons living (and eating) in the weightless conditions of space have demonstrated.[1,3]

At the lower end of the esophagus, about 2 to 5 cm above its juncture with the stomach, the circular muscle of the esophagus functions as a sphincter; this region is referred to as the **lower esophageal sphincter (LES).** Although anatomically this sphincter is no different from the remainder of the esophagus, it remains tonically constricted, in contrast to the mid- and upper portions of the esophagus, which are completely relaxed under normal conditions.[2] Thus the LES serves to prevent the highly acidic gastric contents from moving in a retrograde motion back into the esophagus. Under certain conditions the LES does not function properly, and reflux of gastric contents into the esophagus may occur. The resulting subjective sensation of irritation and spasms of the distal portion of the esophagus is often referred to as *heartburn* or *dyspepsia.*

Stomach

The stomach (Figure 35-3) is essentially an elastic food reservoir and is the site of the start of the digestive process. Under normal circumstances, its capacity is 1000 to 1500 ml, although a capacity of as much as 6000 ml is possible.[2] The portion of the stomach immediately below the LES is called the *cardia.* The fundus is the part of the stomach that continues lateral to and above the cardia; the body of the stomach extends from the cardia to the antrum, which stretches from the angulus to the pylorus. The antrum differs markedly from the rest of the stomach in function and is distinguished by the absence of rugae, the folds present in the mucous membrane of the other areas of the stomach. The **pylorus** is a muscular sphincter between the stomach and duodenum that serves to control gastric emptying and limit the reflux of bile from the small intestine.

The stomach is lined with simple columnar epithelium containing millions of gastric glands that extend down to the mucosa. A typical gastric gland is shown in Figure 35-4. As shown in this illustration, gastric glands are lined by several types of specialized cells. Chief cells produce pepsinogen, the

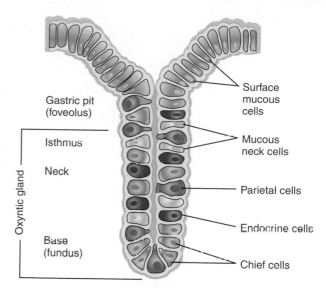

FIGURE 35-4 Gastric mucosa and gastric glands.

inactive form of the enzyme pepsin; parietal cells produce hydrochloric acid and also a substance called intrinsic factor that is needed for adequate intestinal absorption of vitamin B_{12}.[9] Mucous cells produce an alkaline mucus that serves to shield the stomach wall and neutralize the acidity in the immediate area of the lining. A layer of mucus more than 1 mm thick continuously bathes the free surfaces of the gastric epithelial lining. In addition to these cells, gastrin cells are located in the antral epithelium and have surface microvilli that monitor intragastric pH. The role of these cells and the substances they secrete in the digestion of nutrients are described in detail in the Secretory Function section.

Small Intestine

The small intestine of an adult is approximately 5 to 6 m long (the longest portion of the GI tract). The first 22 cm of the small intestine is called the *duodenum;* the *jejunum* constitutes the next 2 m, and the *ileum* forms the remainder. The entire inner wall of the small intestine is marked by circular folds of a mucous membrane called the *plicae circulares;* these permanent ridges do not stretch out when the intestine is distended.

On microscopic examination, the lining of the small intestine contains millions of fingerlike projections called **intestinal villi** (Figure 35-5). Like the circular folds just described, these villi serve to increase the surface area of the intestine for digestion and absorption of nutrients. Each villus has its own microscopic projections called *microvilli,* which in turn are covered by a fuzzy coat (called the **brush border** because of its brushlike appearance when viewed with an electron microscope) containing many digestive enzymes. The combined effect of the circular folds, villi, and microvilli is to increase the surface area of the small intestine by about 600 times, thereby creating a remarkably efficient milieu for nutrient digestion and absorption. Figure 35-6 shows a microscopic section of the small intestine.

FIGURE 35-5 The intestinal wall showing the layers of muscle, mucosal villi, and the brush border microvilli. Villi contain blood capillaries and a lacteal (lymph capillary). Villi and microvilli significantly increase the surface area available for absorption. (From Thibodeau GA, Patton KT: *Anatomy and physiology,* ed 6, St Louis, 2007, Mosby, p 938.)

Between the villi are situated the intestinal glands, or crypts of Lieberkühn. The intestinal glands secrete about 2 L of fluid daily into the lumen of the intestine, but most of the fluid is quickly reabsorbed by the villi. Goblet cells throughout the intestinal mucosa secrete large amounts of mucus. In addition, specialized mucous glands located in the first few centimeters of the duodenum, called *Brunner glands,* release the thick coating of mucus needed in that area to protect the mucosa from the potentially damaging effects of acidic gastric juice that may enter through the pylorus.

Although the details of the process of digestion and absorption of nutrients in the intestinal mucosa will be covered in greater detail in subsequent sections, a unique and salient feature of the villus epithelial cells is described here. Villus epithelial cells have both digestive and absorptive functions, apparently dependent on their current stage of maturation.

The rapidly dividing cells at the base of the intestinal glands are responsible for secretion, but as they migrate to the villus, they mature into absorptive cells and are eventually pushed out of the villus tip. Turnover of cells in the small intestine occurs in 48 to 72 hours, one of the fastest cell turnover rates in the body. Therefore, conditions such as malnutrition or substances that interfere with cell replication or protein synthesis, such as chemotherapeutic agents, may adversely affect intestinal function.

The **ileocecal valve,** a sphincter between the small and large intestines, is normally closed so that the contents of the large intestine cannot move in a retrograde fashion back into the small intestine. In response to a peristaltic contraction bringing intestinal contents toward it, the ileocecal valve opens.

Large Intestine

The large intestine (Figure 35-7) is so termed because of its 6.5-cm diameter, which is greater than the diameter of the small intestine. The large intestine is a 1.5-m-long muscular tube that forms a frame around the small intestine. The vermiform appendix, which is attached to the cecum, is a worm-shaped blind tube containing specialized lymphatic structures. It is generally considered a vestigial structure that probably serves a role as an incubator and warehouse for commensal bacteria.[10] Inflammation of the appendix, or appendicitis, is a potentially life-threatening occurrence that can lead to peritonitis if not diagnosed and managed promptly.

FIGURE 35-6 Microscopic section of the small intestine. (From Kumar V et al: *Robbins basic pathology,* ed 7, Philadelphia, 2003, Saunders, p 803.)

FIGURE 35-7 Divisions of the large intestine. (From Thibodeau GA, Patton KT: *Anatomy and physiology,* ed 6, St Louis, 2007, Mosby, p 941.)

FIGURE 35-8 Normal colon histology showing a flat mucosal surface and abundant vertically oriented crypts. (From Kumar V et al: *Robbins basic pathology,* ed 7, Philadelphia, 2003, Saunders, p 803.)

Stomach: Reservoir for food, mixing, and initial digestion of proteins (by the enzyme pepsin); secretion of hydrochloric acid, intrinsic factor, and gastrin. The pyloric sphincter prevents reflux of intestinal contents.

Small intestine: Digestion and absorption of nearly all nutrients in the duodenum and jejunum; absorption of bile salts in the terminal ileum. The brush border contains numerous digestive enzymes. The enzymes secretin and cholecystokinin are secreted by intestinal mucosa.

Pancreas and gallbladder: The pancreas delivers digestive enzymes and bicarbonate to the duodenum. The gallbladder delivers bile salts to the duodenum.

Large intestine: Reabsorption of water and storage of feces. Feces are delivered to the rectum for defecation.

The portion of the large intestine from the cecum to the rectum is known as the *colon.* The ascending colon extends from the cecum straight up to the lower border of the liver; the transverse colon then extends across the abdomen, anterior to the small intestine. The descending colon then turns downward on the left side of the abdomen, finally becoming the S-shaped sigmoid colon, which empties into the rectum. The rectum has its outlet at the anus, the opening for elimination of feces (see Figure 35-7).

The mucosa of the large intestine has no villi and does not produce digestive enzymes (Figure 35-8). The epithelial surface of the colon consists of absorptive cells that predominantly absorb water and electrolytes.[11] Mucus-producing goblet cells line the glandular crypts present in the surface epithelium. Endocrine cells are also present, but the function of hormones in the large intestine is presently not well understood. The turnover time of cells in the colonic mucosa is 3 to 8 days, comparatively longer than that of cells in the small intestine.

KEY POINTS

- Tracheoesophageal fistula, esophageal and duodenal atresia, and anal agenesis are congenital disorders that occur with abnormal development of the GI tract. These disorders are usually manifested as obstructions.
- The major structures and corresponding functions of the GI tract can be summarized as follows:
  Mouth and salivary glands: Mastication, moistening, and the beginning of starch digestion (by the enzyme salivary amylase) of foodstuff.
  Pharynx: Transport of food to the esophagus and protection of the airway from aspiration of food particles.
  Esophagus: Movement of food to the stomach by peristaltic waves. The LES prevents reflux of stomach contents.

GASTROINTESTINAL MOTILITY

The way in which nutrients and their eventual waste products are propelled through the GI tract is a complex and fascinating process involving an exquisitely timed set of autoregulatory actions and responses. A summary of the characteristics of the intestinal wall, innervation of the gut, and hormonal control of GI motility is presented as a basis for a description of the means by which nutrients move through the GI tract.

Characteristics of the Intestinal Wall

A typical cross-section of the intestinal wall is depicted in Figure 35-9. From the outer surface inward are five main layers: the serosa, a longitudinal muscle layer, a circular muscle layer, the submucosa, and the mucosa. A small layer, the muscularis mucosa, is located between the mucosa and submucosa. The muscular movements of the GI tract are performed mostly by the different layers of the smooth muscle, which extends from the distal end of the esophagus through most of the large intestine. However, skeletal muscle has a key role in motility at both ends of the GI tract; motility from the mouth through the proximal portion of the esophagus at the upper end and through the external sphincter of the anus at the lower end is mediated by the action of skeletal muscle.[2,12]

The general characteristics of smooth muscle are covered in Chapter 5. Specific characteristics of smooth muscle in the gut that render its function possible include the close proximity of these smooth muscle fibers to each other. In most areas of the GI tract, smooth muscle fibers are extremely close; about 12% of their membrane surfaces are actually fused with the membranes of other adjacent muscle fibers to form a *nexus,* or junction. This close proximity of smooth muscle fibers in the GI tract allows intracellular current to travel very easily from one muscle fiber to another. Action potentials originating in one smooth muscle fiber in the GI tract are generally propagated from fiber to fiber; therefore, the GI tract acts as

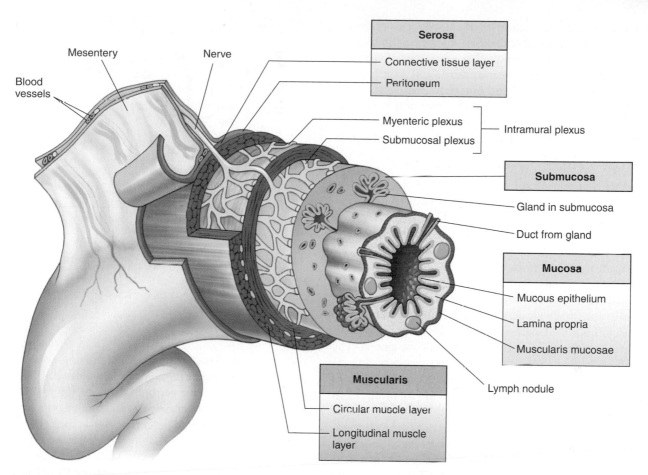

FIGURE 35-9 Cross-section of a typical segment of the intestinal wall showing the four principal layers and associated structures: mucosa, submucosa, muscularis, and serosa. Although different areas of the GI tract specialize in function, the anatomy of the wall is similar in structure. (From Thibodeau GA, Patton KT: *Anatomy and physiology,* ed 6, St Louis, 2007, Mosby, p 927.)

a **functional syncytium,** where separate cells have the ability to function in a unified manner.[1]

Neural Control

Movement of nutrients through the GI tract is controlled by the central nervous system through its autonomic division and is modulated by numerous hormonal interactions.[2,3,9,13] In addition, the GI system has an intrinsic nervous system of its own that controls most GI functions.[14] The **intrinsic nervous system** is composed of two layers: (1) the myenteric, or Auerbach, plexus, which lies between the longitudinal and circular muscular layers; and (2) the submucosal, or Meissner, plexus, which lies in the submucosa. The myenteric plexus is largely responsible for control of GI movements; the submucosal plexus serves to control secretion and is also involved in many sensory functions, with information being received from the gut epithelium and stretch receptors in the intestinal wall. The entire intrinsic nervous system, including both the myenteric plexus and the submucosal plexus, is responsible for many reflexes that occur locally in the GI tract, such as those causing the localized secretion of digestive juices by the submucosal glands or an increase in gut smooth muscle activity.

In general, when the myenteric plexus is stimulated, activity in the GI tract increases. This stimulation results in four principal effects: (1) tonic contraction of the intestinal wall increases; (2) rhythmic contractions increase in intensity; (3) rhythmic contractions increase in rate; and (4) the velocity of conduction of excitatory waves along the intestinal wall increases. As part of the parasympathetic nervous system, these excitatory fibers of the myenteric plexus are primarily cholinergic (i.e., secrete acetylcholine), in addition to one or more other excitatory transmitter substances. However, some myenteric plexus fibers have an inhibitory effect and may secrete purine-based transmitter substances such as adenosine triphosphate.[15]

Input from the sympathetic and parasympathetic nervous systems can strongly affect the activity of the intrinsic nervous system. In general, sympathetic stimulation decreases the activity of the intrinsic nervous system whereas parasympathetic stimulation increases its activity.

Parasympathetic Innervation
The parasympathetic supply to the GI tract is divided into cranial and sacral divisions. Cranial parasympathetic stimulation is transmitted almost entirely by the vagus nerves, which

provide extensive innervation to the esophagus, stomach, pancreas, and the first half of the large intestine (with little innervation of the small intestine). The sacral parasympathetic division originates in the second, third, and fourth sacral segments of the spinal cord and innervates the distal half of the large intestine. The sigmoid, rectal, and anal regions of the large intestine are especially well supplied with parasympathetic fibers; these fibers have a key role in the defecation reflex.

Sympathetic Innervation

The sympathetic fibers that innervate the GI tract have their origin in the spinal cord between T8 and L3. After exiting the cord, the preganglionic fibers enter the sympathetic chains and then pass through these chains to various ganglia located adjacent to the GI tract, such as the celiac ganglion and the mesenteric ganglia. From these locations, postganglionic fibers radiate out to all parts of the gut. These sympathetics supply essentially all parts of the GI tract, in contrast to the concentration of parasympathetic innervation at locations close to the entry and exit points of the gut.[2,15] The sympathetic nerve endings in the GI tract secrete norepinephrine, which promotes the inhibitory effect of the sympathetic nervous system on the GI tract in the following ways: Norepinephrine acts directly on smooth muscle in the GI tract to inhibit activity; in addition, norepinephrine has an inhibitory effect on the neurons of the intrinsic nervous system of the GI tract. Strong stimulation of the sympathetic nervous system can effectively shut down motility in the gut and can block the movement of nutrients through the GI tract. Gastrointestinal sympathetic activity can also initiate vomiting through a complex sequence of events mediated by various neurotransmitters.[3,16]

Afferent Nerve Fibers

The GI tract is richly supplied with afferent nerve fibers arising from the gut that transmit important information about the status of the GI tract. Afferent fibers that have their cell bodies in the submucosal plexus and terminate in the myenteric plexus transmit signals in response to irritation of the gut mucosa, excessive distention, or the presence of specific chemical substances. These signals can result in excitation or, in some circumstances, inhibition of intestinal motility or secretion. Other afferent fibers with cell bodies in the dorsal root ganglia of the spinal cord or cranial nerve ganglia can transmit signals to higher levels of the central nervous system by traveling along sympathetic or parasympathetic pathways. For example, the vagus nerves contain many afferent fibers that transmit signals to the medulla; this information is then used to initiate and modulate vagal signals that control many important functions of the GI tract.

Electrical Activity of Gastrointestinal Smooth Muscle

Electrical activity is almost constantly present in the smooth muscle layers of the GI tract. Two basic types of electrical wave activity have been identified in the gut: slow waves

FIGURE 35-10 Membrane potentials in intestinal smooth muscle. (From Guyton AC, Hall JE: *Textbook of medical physiology*, ed 11, Philadelphia, 2006, Saunders, p 772.)

and spikes (the latter named for the spiking appearance of these sudden increases in membrane potential).[1,2] These two types of electrical wave patterns are shown in Figure 35-10. **Slow-wave electrical activity** represents an ongoing basic oscillation in membrane potential that occurs in the smooth muscle of the GI tract, especially in the muscle in the longitudinal layer. Normally, between 3 and 12 slow waves occur per minute, ranging from −40 to −50 millivolts in amplitude. Slow waves can be any degree of intensity and are not the "all-or-nothing" type of action potential seen in other smooth muscle fibers in the body. In contrast to these nearly continuous slow waves, spikes occur under certain circumstances. When the muscle layer in the GI tract is stimulated by being stretched or by the effects of acetylcholine or parasympathetic excitation, the intracellular resting membrane potential of the muscle fibers becomes relatively more positive. The entire potential level of the slow waves is raised—an effect called *depolarization*.[1,17,18] As shown in Figure 35-10, when the depolarization rises above a certain level (around −40 mV), sudden increases in the membrane potential, or spikes, start to appear on the peaks of the slow waves. If the resting potential rises further, spikes appear more frequently. With very strong stimulation, the spikes generally disappear because the membrane now remains entirely depolarized. Figure 35-10 also illustrates the response of smooth muscle fibers to stimulation by norepinephrine or sympathetic excitation. In this situation, the resting membrane potential is decreased, or hyperpolarized, and electrical activity is almost abolished.

Hormonal Control

The following section on secretory function of the GI tract describes in detail the role of hormones in controlling GI secretion. It is important to note that many of these same hormones are involved in controlling motility in different portions of the GI tract. Gastrin, which is secreted by specialized endocrine cells (G cells) of the stomach mucosa in response to food entry, increases stomach motility and is the primary mediator of gastric acid secretion. In addition, it promotes increased constriction of the LES, which serves to prevent reflux of stomach contents into the esophagus. Gastrin may also have a small effect in increasing motility of the small intestine and gallbladder.[2,3,19]

Cholecystokinin, which is secreted mainly by I cells of the jejunum in response to the entry of fatty substances, has an extremely strong effect in increasing contractility of the gallbladder. This stimulation of gallbladder activity results in an outpouring into the small intestine of bile, which plays an important role in promoting fat digestion and absorption. Cholecystokinin also stimulates pancreatic secretion, helps regulate gastric emptying and bowel motility, and induces satiety.[3]

Secretin, which is produced by the mucosa of the duodenum in response to the entry of acidic gastric juice from the stomach, stimulates pancreatic fluid and bicarbonate secretion, with the effect of neutralizing the acidity of intestinal contents. It also has a mild inhibitory effect on motility in most of the GI tract.[2,3.]

Other important gastrointestinal polypeptide hormones include vasoactive intestinal polypeptide (VIP), glucagon, glucose-dependent insulinotropic polypeptide (GIP—formerly called *gastric inhibitory polypeptide*), somatostatin, motilin, leptin, and ghrelin.[3] Somatostatin analogues have been used therapeutically to treat some forms of diarrhea and to reduce fluid output from pancreatic fistulae.[20] Ghrelin is a peptide that increases appetite, stimulates growth hormone secretion, and produces weight gain. It has been the focus of intense research recently as a mediator for obesity, with the potential for a therapeutic anti-obesity drug that would block ghrelin's effects on the body.[21,22]

Movement in the Gastrointestinal Tract

Contraction of Gastrointestinal Smooth Muscle

In general, most contraction in the GI tract occurs in response to **spike potentials;** slow waves without superimposed spikes ordinarily do not give rise to contraction. Spike potentials occurring in GI smooth muscle are analogous to action potentials in cardiac muscle and are responsible for the membrane changes that initiate contraction. As calcium enters the cell membrane and passes to the interior of the smooth muscle, it initiates a reaction between actin and myosin,[1] a process described in detail in Chapter 17.

The electrical activity occurring in the smooth muscle of the gut gives rise to tonic contractions and rhythmic contractions, both of which occur in most types of smooth muscle. Tonic contraction is continuous, instigated by pacemaker cells that are believed to reside at the interface between the longitudinal and circular muscle layers.[23] The intensity of tonic contraction may vary with the frequency of spike potentials. In turn, the intensity of tonic contraction in a specific segment of the gut will determine the amount of pressure in that segment. The degree of tonic contraction in the sphincters of the GI tract determines the amount of resistance to the movement of intestinal contents along the tract. Thus the degree of contraction exerted by the pyloric, ileocecal, and anal sphincters serves to regulate the movement of nutrients through the GI tract.

The degree of rhythmic contraction varies in different parts of the GI tract. These differing rhythmic frequencies are dependent on the rate of slow-wave activity in a particular segment and may occur at rates of 3 to 12 times per minute. These slow wave–dependent contractions are responsible for the mixing and peristaltic propulsive movements present in the GI tract.

Two types of muscular activity are involved in the digestive and absorptive functions of the GI tract: mixing movements and propulsive movements. In different portions of the GI tract these movements may serve different functions to achieve proper digestion and absorption of nutrients. For example, mixing movements in the stomach and small intestine promote digestion by mixing the digestive juices with the food that enters from above. In the small intestine and proximal segment of the large intestine, mixing movements facilitate absorption by bringing newly arrived intestinal contents into contact with absorbing surfaces. In the case of propulsion, the rate at which nutrients are propelled through the GI tract depends on the function of the different organs of the tract. For example, the passageway for nutrients from the mouth through the pharynx and esophagus is simply a conduit; essentially no digestive or absorptive function occurs here. Thus the transit of nutrients through these regions is quite rapid. In contrast, transit from the stomach and through the small and large intestines is quite slow. This slow rate of passage allows for completion of the digestive and absorptive processes that occur in these portions of the GI tract.

Although the characteristics of mixing and propulsive movements differ in various parts of the GI tract and will be described separately in the next section, a description of the general characteristics of these movements is presented here.

Propulsive Movements

The basic propulsive movement of the GI tract is called *peristalsis* (Figure 35-11). Nutrients are propelled by the slow advancement of a circular constriction that squeezes the materials in front of the constricted area forward. Peristalsis is an inherent property of any smooth muscle tube that, like the intestine, is a functional syncytium. However, effective intestinal peristalsis requires the presence of an intact myenteric nerve plexus. The usual stimulus for peristalsis is distention of the intestinal walls. The entry and subsequent stretching of the intestinal wall by a bolus of food will have the effect of stimulating the gut wall 2 to 3 cm above this point, and a circular constriction will then occur and propel the food with a peristaltic movement. Although peristalsis can move in both directions in the gut (either toward the mouth or toward the anus), it normally moves toward the anus. The exact cause of

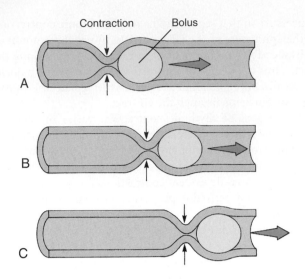

FIGURE 35-11 Peristalsis is a progressive type of movement, propelling material from point to point along the GI tract. **A,** A ring of contraction occurs where the GI wall is stretched, pushing the bolus forward. **B,** The moving bolus triggers a ring of contraction in the next region, which pushes the bolus even farther along. **C,** The ring of contraction moves like a wave along the GI tract, pushing the bolus forward. (From Thibodeau GA, Patton KT: *Anatomy and physiology,* ed 6, St Louis, 2007, Mosby, p 965.)

this generally anal direction of peristalsis is still being debated by physiologists; it is thought that the myenteric plexus may be organized in such a way that preferential transmission of signals downward occurs simultaneously with relaxation of the portion of the intestine below the distended stimulus point. This posited ability of the GI tract to propel nutrients downward while relaxing an adjacent lower portion to receive these nutrients is sometimes referred to as the "law of the gut."[1,2]

Mixing Movements

Mixing movements that serve to keep the intestinal contents thoroughly mixed on a constant basis are caused by either peristaltic contractions or local constrictive contractions of small segments of the gut wall. These movements may vary according to the specific function of each portion of the GI tract (see the Secretory Function section).

Movement of Nutrients

The path taken by foods ingested into the GI tract as these nutrients travel down the tract and are digested and absorbed and their waste products eventually excreted will be traced beginning with the mouth. Although this process is described here as a linear sequence, it is important to note that several steps may occur simultaneously. The individual steps involved in nutrient ingestion constitute a synergistic process, and an inability to perform one phase of the process will ultimately have a profound effect on the entire GI tract. In addition, individuals manifest a great deal of variability in such aspects of digestive function as tolerance of certain nutrients

and defecation patterns. Such variations may represent age-related differences or conditioned responses to environmental cues.

Chewing

The entry of solid food into the mouth results in the action of chewing, an important first step in the process of nutrient digestion. The process of moving the food around in the mouth and mixing it with saliva results in stimulation of the taste buds and olfactory epithelia; this sensory input greatly increases the subjective enjoyment of eating. As the food is mixed with saliva, it becomes softened and formed into a mass of appropriate size (bolus) that can be swallowed. The action of the molars and premolars in crushing more rigid forms of foods serves to prepare rough substances for transport down the esophagus. Although the act of chewing is under voluntary control, it is also partly reflexive in nature. The entry of food into the mouth has been shown to stimulate chewing in animals in the absence of full cerebral function. The movements of the skeletal muscles responsible for chewing are coordinated by impulses traveling through cranial nerves V, VII, IX, X, XI, and XII. Interruption of the proper transmission of impulses through these nerve tracts places an individual at risk for decreased voluntary control of the chewing function, with a resultant risk of aspiration.

Swallowing

Swallowing is the transport of material from the mouth to the stomach. The process of swallowing has been divided into three stages that describe the regions through which the bolus of nutrients passes on its way to the stomach: (1) the oral stage, (2) the pharyngeal stage, and (3) the esophageal stage.[2,3,9]

During the oral stage, the bolus is passed from the mouth to the pharynx through the space called the *fauces*. The bolus, either solid or liquid, is rolled toward the back of the tongue, and the front of the tongue is then pushed up against the hard palate. Respiration is inhibited briefly in this phase, as the pharyngeal muscles constrict to force the bolus of food into the pharynx. In the pharyngeal stage the bolus is passed through the pharynx into the esophagus, a process taking about one-fifth of a second. Continued contraction of the pharyngeal muscles and the position of the tongue prevent reentry of the bolus into the oral cavity. The soft palate is pulled upward to close off the nasopharynx; simultaneously, food is prevented from entering the larynx by elevation of the larynx and approximation of the vocal cords, both of which actions serve to close the glottis. As these openings are closed off, the pharyngeal constrictors contract and force the bolus of food into the esophagus. Respiration is now resumed, and pressure in the pharynx rises as a result of the muscular activities that have occurred.

The muscular characteristics of the esophagus are of particular importance in effecting the third, or esophageal, stage of swallowing. The upper one-third of the esophagus consists of skeletal muscle, whereas the lower two-thirds is composed of predominantly smooth muscle. In the normal resting stage, the upper part of the esophagus is closed by the tonic contraction of a band of skeletal muscle that serves as the pharyngoesophageal sphincter. The pressure exerted by the pharyngoesophageal sphincter in this region is normally about 20 to 40 cm H_2O above atmospheric pressure; this zone of high pressure keeps air from entering the esophagus during inspiration. Almost immediately after initiation of a swallow, the sphincter relaxes and pressure in the region drops to atmospheric pressure, thus allowing the bolus to be forced into the esophagus by the pressure generated in the pharynx. Pressure in the pharyngoesophageal junction region then rises as a result of contraction of skeletal muscle in this area, thus preventing reflux of food from the esophagus back to the pharynx. Pressure in this region then gradually subsides to a resting level as muscular relaxation occurs.

If the bolus being swallowed is a liquid, it is propelled through the esophagus by the initial force of swallowing and travels by gravity to the stomach in about 1 second. If the bolus is a semisolid mass, it is propelled down the esophagus by means of a peristaltic wave. This esophageal peristalsis is caused by a contraction of circular muscle that forces the bolus ahead of it toward the stomach, with a transit time of about 4 to 6 seconds.

Although no well-differentiated muscular structure is located in the area where the esophagus joins the stomach, the region approximately 2 to 5 cm above the juncture with the stomach is referred to as the LES and is described in the Esophagus section. Almost immediately after initiation of a swallow, pressure at the LES drops and remains low during the time that a peristaltic wave is passing down through the lower end of the esophagus. Once the bolus has passed through the lower esophageal region and pressure in the lower portion of the esophagus has fallen to a resting level, the pressure in the LES rises and remains elevated for about 10 seconds before falling to a resting level once again.[2]

Neural Control of Swallowing. Figure 35-12 illustrates the neural pathways involved in the swallowing mechanism. Swallowing receptors in the posterior of the mouth and throat transmit impulses in response to a stimulus to the mucous membranes in the mouth, such as the presence of a moderate amount of fluid. These impulses travel mainly through the trigeminal nerve into the reticular substance of the medulla oblongata, where the swallowing center is located. Once this center has been activated, the sequence of muscular reactions described earlier occurs automatically and usually cannot be voluntarily stopped. The swallowing center then sends impulses over a number of efferent nerves to the numerous skeletal and smooth muscles involved in the swallowing process to allow the complete act of swallowing to occur in the appropriate sequence. The glossopharyngeal and hypoglossal nerves are primarily concerned with the oral and pharyngeal stages, whereas the vagus nerve is important in activating the esophageal stage.

The gag reflex is an important protective mechanism that aborts the normal swallowing response and helps eliminate potentially harmful ingestions. The afferent limb of the reflex

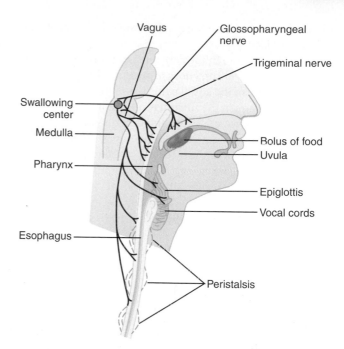

FIGURE 35-12 Neural pathways of the swallowing mechanism. (From Guyton AC, Hall JE: *Textbook of medical physiology,* ed 11, Philadelphia, 2006, Saunders, p 782.)

is controlled by the glossopharyngeal nerve (cranial nerve IX), and the efferent limb is by the vagus nerve (cranial nerve X). Disorders of the gag reflex such as stroke or neuropathy can lead to life-threatening obstruction or aspiration.

Motor Functions of the Stomach

The motor functions of the stomach include the storage of ingested nutrients for variable lengths of time and the discharge of gastric contents into the small intestine at an appropriate rate for optimal digestion and absorption. The stomach also aids in the digestive process by its mixing movements, which convert large pieces of food to a finer, liquid consistency.

Gastric Filling and Storage. On entering the stomach from the esophagus, newly arrived food forms concentric circles in the body and fundus of the stomach, with the newest food lying closest to the esophagus and older food lying closer to the stomach wall. The smooth muscle in the fundus and body of the stomach can adapt to the volume of contents so that relatively large contents can be introduced with little increase in intragastric pressure. The fundus and body of the stomach maintain a consistent pressure at all times. This tonic contraction continually presses on the food mass and aids in its delivery to the pyloric antrum.

Peristaltic contractions occur in the stomach once every 20 seconds. These rippling peristaltic waves begin in the corpus and move at a velocity of about 1 to 2 cm/sec. When they reach the more thickly walled pyloric antrum, they become much more vigorous and also increase in speed. These strong peristaltic contractions in the pyloric antrum are largely responsible for mixing ingested nutrients with gastric secretions. As ingested food is churned and mixed to a greater degree of fluidity, the mixture takes on a milky white sludge appearance and is then called **chyme.**

Emptying. As pressure in the antrum rises momentarily as the result of peristaltic contraction, a pressure differential exists between pressure in the antral pylorus and the duodenal bulb. The higher pressure in the antrum is sufficient to overcome resistance of the pyloric sphincter, and the contents of the stomach are then propelled into the duodenum. Concurrently, the degree of constriction of the pyloric sphincter may increase or decrease, depending on several factors discussed in the next section. Because this process is dependent on the muscular activity of the antrum as well as pyloric muscle tone, gastric emptying is largely regulated by mechanisms that affect each of these regions.

Regulation of Gastric Emptying. Factors that may affect the rate at which the stomach empties include the degree of distention of the gastric wall and release of the hormone **gastrin** in response to certain types of food in the stomach. Both of these factors increase the rate of gastric emptying by increasing the force of antral contractions while simultaneously inhibiting pyloric constriction. Distention of the gastric wall results in stimulation of mechanoreceptors in the stomach with subsequent activation of reflexes over the vagus and the intrinsic nerve plexuses. These neural influences, along with contractile activity (which is a direct response to the stretch of gastric muscle), constitute a major mechanism in providing the stimulus for gastric emptying. Gastric emptying time can vary depending upon the food ingested (e.g., whether solid or liquid) and generally ranges from 1 to several hours.[3]

Gastrin is a hormone released from the antral mucosa in response to stretching of the gastric wall, as well as the presence of certain foods, particularly meat. The role of gastrin in promoting the secretion of highly acidic gastric juices will be discussed later. With respect to stomach emptying, gastrin has a key role by enhancing peristalsis while at the same time relaxing the pylorus.[24]

In addition to these influences, many of the mechanisms that affect gastric emptying are initiated in the duodenum. Reflex nervous signals are transmitted from the duodenum back to the stomach in response to intraluminal stimuli; these signals probably have a key role in controlling both peristaltic activity and the degree of pyloric constriction. Stimulation of the duodenum in a variety of ways has the effect of slowing gastric emptying; both the chemical and physical properties of chyme entering the duodenum may affect the rate of gastric emptying. A variety of both duodenal cells and receptors, including osmoreceptors, mechanoreceptors, and chemoreceptors, respond to intraluminal stimuli to produce hormonal and reflex inhibition of gastric motor activity and enhancement of pyloric tone. The presence in the duodenum of chyme containing the breakdown products of proteins, and to a lesser extent fats, may impede gastric emptying. Also, the presence of highly acidic or highly hypertonic or hypotonic chyme in the duodenum may inhibit the rate of gastric emptying. The degree of distention of the duodenum, as well as the presence of any degree of irritation of the duodenum, may serve to impede stomach emptying. These inhibitory mechanisms have a protective function and are effective in preventing the intestinal mucosa from overloading its digestive and absorptive abilities and potentially being damaged by chemical or mechanical sources.

Although regulation of gastric emptying is largely dependent on factors in the stomach and duodenum, gastric motility may be stimulated or inhibited reflexively from a variety of regions of the body. For example, stomach emptying is inhibited when the ileum is full and when the anus is mechanically distended. Stimulation of visceral and somatic pain receptors may result in inhibition of gastric motility. Various strong emotions such as anger, fear, and anxiety may produce changes in motility of the stomach, but whether these states tend to predispose an individual to inhibition or excitation of gastric motility is not always predictable.[3,25]

Vomiting. Vomiting is rapid emptying of the contents of the stomach through the esophagus and into the mouth. The major force for vomiting is supplied by the skeletal muscle of the diaphragm and abdomen, rather than by contraction of the muscles of the stomach wall. Vomiting is the result of an extremely complex set of neural events coordinated by the nucleus tractus solitarius (NTS), a center located in the medulla. Afferent impulses from receptors in various regions of the body, including the sensory nerve endings of the pharynx, abdominal viscera, and the labyrinths, arrive at this center to initiate the vomiting reflex. This reflex causes closure of the glottis and trachea, relaxation of the gastroesophageal sphincter, and contraction of the diaphragm and the abdominal muscles, which forcibly expels the contents of the stomach.

Motility of the Small Intestine

After intact food entering the mouth has been liquefied and partially digested in the stomach, it enters the small intestine, where the major part of digestion and absorption occurs. As in other parts of the GI tract, movements of the small intestine can be described as propulsive and mixing movements, which in the small intestine generally occur simultaneously.

Propulsion. Chyme is propelled through the small intestine by peristaltic waves that move at a rate of 0.5 to 2 cm/sec, with a faster rate at the proximal part of the intestine and a slower rate in the terminal portion. Approximately 3 to 5 hours is normally needed for the passage of chyme from the pyloric sphincter to the ileocecal valve, but this period may vary in some disease states. Peristaltic activity in the small intestine is greatly increased after the ingestion of a meal. The increase in contractile activity in the stomach caused by distention of the stomach wall is conducted principally through the myenteric plexus down along the wall of the small intestine. This so-called gastroenteric reflex serves to increase the activity of the small intestine, with an enhancement of both intestinal motility and secretion.

The usual stimulus for peristalsis in the small intestine is distention of the intestinal walls; stretch receptors in the gut wall are sensitive to circumferential stretch and initiate a local myenteric reflex in response to this stimulation. The resulting

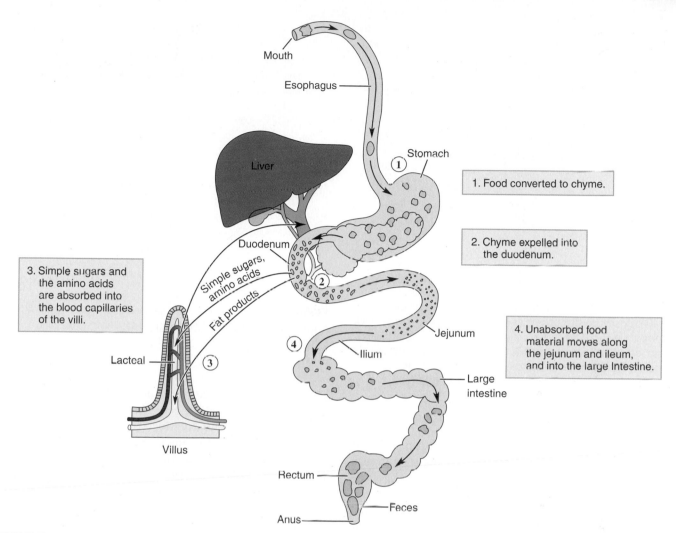

FIGURE 35-13 Chyme and the process of absorption of nutrients. (Modified from Herlihy B: *The human body in health and illness,* ed 3, Philadelphia, 2007, Saunders, p 416.)

contraction of longitudinal muscle, followed by the contraction of circular muscle, spreads downward in a peristaltic motion.

The peristaltic waves in the small intestine not only propel chyme downward toward the ileocecal valve but also spread out the chyme along the intestinal mucosa, thus facilitating the process of absorption of nutrients (Figure 35-13). As additional chyme enters the small intestine, this spreading process intensifies as peristalsis increases. When chyme reaches the ileocecal valve, it is sometimes stationary for several hours until the individual eats another meal and a new gastroenteric reflex intensifies the peristaltic process and propels the remaining chyme through the ileocecal valve.

Certain disease states, particularly those that involve intense irritation of the intestinal mucosa, may result in a peristaltic rush, a powerful peristaltic wave that travels long distances in the small intestine in a short period. The peristaltic rush clears the contents of the small intestine into the colon, thus relieving the small intestine of either irritating substances or excessive distention.[2,9]

Mixing. In addition to propulsive peristaltic movements, a set of movements characterized as **segmentation contractions** also occur in the small intestine. The primary effect of these contractions is progressive mixing of solid chyme particles with secretions of the small intestine. As their name implies, segmentation contractions involve contraction of the small intestine in regularly spaced segments that have the appearance of sausages (Figure 35-14). As one set of segmentation contractions is completed, a new set begins, with contractile points located at different locations along the small intestine. Segmentation contractions occur at a rate of 7 to 12 times per minute and effectively chop and mix the chyme, as well as assist in propelling the chyme toward the ileocecal valve (see Figure 35-14).

Control of Motility. The electrical and mechanical activities of the small intestine are closely associated. Slow waves, as described previously in this chapter, occur at the membranes of the longitudinal smooth muscle, with frequencies of 11 to 12 per minute in the duodenum decreasing to 7 to 9 per minute in the terminal ileum. Slow waves do not directly produce

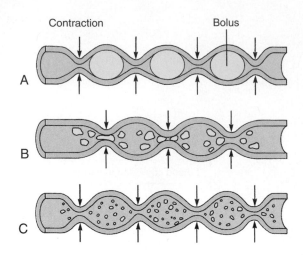

FIGURE 35-14 Segmentation. Segmentation is a back-and-forth action that breaks apart chunks of food and mixes in digestive juices. **A,** Ringlike regions of contraction occur at intervals along the GI tract. **B,** Previously contracted regions relax and adjacent regions now contract, effectively "chopping" the contents of each segment into smaller chunks. **C,** Locations of the contracted regions continue to alternate back and forth, chopping and mixing the contents of the GI lumen. (From Thibodeau GA, Patton KT: *Anatomy and physiology,* ed 6, St Louis, 2007, Mosby, p 967.)

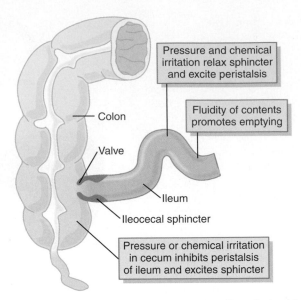

FIGURE 35-15 Emptying of the ileocecal valve. (From Guyton AC, Hall JE: *Textbook of medical physiology,* ed 11, Philadelphia, 2006, Saunders, p 788.)

muscular contractions in the small intestine but provide the conditions under which contractions can occur. Although slow waves determine the velocity and direction of peristalsis, other factors determine whether action potentials and thus contraction will occur. Local mechanical and chemical stimulation by chyme is probably largely responsible for the initiation and continuance of contraction in the small intestine. Thus when the intestinal tract becomes overly distended or when the mucosa becomes irritated, myenteric reflexes enhance the electrical activity of the gut and spike potentials are superimposed on the slow waves. These spike potentials then spread through both longitudinal and circular muscle, and contraction results.

Intestinal motility may also be influenced by stimulation from sources extrinsic to the colon. Stimulation of the vagus nerve generally causes increased intestinal motility, with sympathetic stimulation resulting in inhibition. Intestinal motility can be altered reflexively by stimulation of many sensory areas. For example, trauma to organs outside the GI tract, such as irritation of the peritoneum or urinary tract, may cause intestinal inhibition. A condition called *paralytic ileus,* in which intestinal motility is inhibited as the result of reflex inhibition, may occur as a response to intra-abdominal infection or surgery in this area.[3,26]

Much current research is focused on the involvement of gastrointestinal hormones in the regulation of GI tract motility.[2,3,25] Cholecystokinin, a hormone released from the mucosa of the jejunum in response to fatty substances in chyme, has been shown to block the increased gastric motility caused by gastrin. Another hormone, secretin, which is released mainly

from the duodenal mucosa in response to gastric acid entering the duodenum, has the general effect of decreasing GI motility. A hormone called *GIP,* which is released from the upper portion of the small intestine in response to fat in chyme, as well as to carbohydrates, is known to inhibit gastric motility under some conditions. These hormones will be described in more detail in the Secretory Function section.

Ileocecal Sphincter

Chyme from the small intestine is eventually propelled downward to the terminal ileum immediately proximal to the cecum, where the last 2 to 3 cm of the muscular coat is thicker than that in the rest of the ileum. This region, called the *ileocecal sphincter,* has a resting high pressure (about 20 cm H_2O above atmospheric pressure) and is normally closed. Distention of the distal ileum lowers the pressure in the ileocecal sphincter. Thus when intestinal contents are present in the terminal ileum at sufficient quantity and are ready to be propelled into the cecum, the sphincter reflexively relaxes and the intestinal contents are pushed into the cecum by the propulsive movements of the distal small intestine. Conversely, distention of the cecum after it is filled with contents passing through the ileocecal valve results in increased pressure in the sphincter, which prevents reflux flow back into the ileum (Figure 35-15).

Motility of the Colon

The movements of the colon are effective in promoting the two major functions of the colon: (1) absorption of water and electrolytes from chyme and (2) storage of the fecal mass until it can be expelled from the body by defecation.

Colonic Movements. For most of the time, the large intestine in humans is inactive. However, the presence of material in the proximal end of the colon results in a type of mixing movement in the haustra (the outpouchings in the colon wall), termed **haustral churning,** that is similar to the segmenting movements in the small intestine. This movement is the major type of motility in the large intestine. Haustral churning exposes the contents of the large intestine to the mucosa, thus promoting the absorption of water. Normally, about 500 ml of chyme enters the proximal part of the colon each day. Out of this total volume, 400 ml—mostly water and electrolytes—is reabsorbed before defecation takes place, with an average volume of 100 ml of feces remaining for eventual disposal from the body.[1,26]

At infrequent intervals of about three to four times a day, a strong peristaltic movement termed a *mass movement* occurs and propels the fecal material long distances. These strong contractions may reach a peak of 100 cm H_2O pressure in the segment undergoing the contraction. Fecal material may be transported all the way from the ascending colon to the descending colon by a mass movement. Feces are then stored in the distal end of the colon until defecation takes place.

Defecation. Under normal conditions, it takes about 18 hours for intestinal contents to reach the distal end of the colon after leaving the small intestine. Fecal material is stored in the distal part of the colon for varying lengths of time; defecation may take place 24 hours or longer after the ingestion of food. Ordinarily the rectum is empty, but fecal material is occasionally shifted into it after one of the mass movements, and the resulting distention of the rectum initiates the urge to defecate. The act of defecation is a combination of voluntary and involuntary movements. Contraction of the distal end of the colon and relaxation of the internal anal sphincter, which are regions composed of smooth muscle, are involuntary movements. Relaxation of the external anal sphincter, which consists of striated muscle, is a voluntary movement. Other voluntary movements that may assist in the act of defecation are contraction of the abdominal muscles and forcible expiration with closure of the glottis (the Valsalva maneuver, often referred to as "bearing down").

Regulation of Colonic Motility. Movements in the proximal portion of the colon are largely initiated by distention in the colonic walls, which stimulates contractile activity by triggering short reflexes through the intrinsic nerve plexuses. Although the proximal part of the colon receives extrinsic innervation via the vagus nerve, it functions in a relatively autonomous manner in the absence of extrinsic motor innervation and is thus a somewhat self-regulating structure. Extrinsic nerves may occasionally modify proximal colonic activity, however; for example, entry of food into the stomach or duodenum may result in a mass contraction in the proximal end of the colon. Sometimes termed the gastrocolic or duodenocolic reflexes, these strong mass movements are most evident after the first intake of nutrients in the morning and are often followed by a strong need to defecate.

In contrast, the distal part of the colon is somewhat more dependent on its extrinsic nerve supply, so movements in this region, including the act of defecation, may be entirely abolished after injury to these nerves. However, weak movements return eventually, and defecation can still occur without voluntary control after the initial response to injury has passed.[3]

SECRETORY FUNCTION

Secretion of Gastrointestinal Juices

The many glands associated with the GI tract generally produce enzymes that participate in the digestive process to break down the major nutrient components of carbohydrates, fats, and proteins. The somewhat archaic term *juices* is still used to describe the fluids secreted in the GI tract, which contain a complex mixture of salts and protein enzymes. Thus the glands located in the stomach are said to produce gastric juice and the glands of the intestinal wall produce intestinal juice. Secretion of these digestive juices is stimulated by various factors, including mechanical and chemical stimulation by chyme, parasympathetic stimulation (in certain regions of the GI tract), and various hormones.

Gastrointestinal Hormones

Table 35-1 lists the major hormones of the GI tract and their sources, target organs, major actions, and factors that stimulate release. These hormones are released from the GI mucosa in response to distention or the presence of certain nutrient substances. They are then absorbed into the blood and carried to glands in target tissues (i.e., tissues on which they exert their effects), where they stimulate secretion. Chemically, GI hormones are polypeptides or polypeptide derivatives. Receptors for the peptide hormones are widely distributed throughout the body, including in the brain and central nervous system, and much current research is focused on the varied effects of these complex chemicals.[27,28]

In addition to their effects on motility, as mentioned above, gastrin, secretin, cholecystokinin, and GIP have critical roles in mediating secretion of gastrointestinal juices. Gastrin is secreted by the stomach mucosa and stimulates the exocrine (secretory) cells of the gastric glands to produce their specific products, including hydrochloric acid. Research over the last 2 decades has shown that gastrin exerts its primary effect on enterochrommafin-like cells (ECL cells), provoking them to release histamine.[29] Histamine, an amine with multiple roles in human physiologic processes, including an ability to constrict bronchial smooth muscle, diffuses readily into nearby parietal cells to induce acid release (Figure 35-16). The development of specific medications that block the action of histamine (H_2 antagonists) led to the first effective treatment for peptic ulcers, by reducing gastric acid secretion.

Secretin was one of the first of the many hormones of the body to be discovered. The most potent stimulus for secretin release is hydrochloric acid, and the presence of acidic chyme in the duodenum promotes its release into the blood from the duodenal mucosa. It is carried to the pancreas, where it stimulates the secretion of a large volume of alkaline juice rich in sodium bicarbonate. In the duodenum, sodium bicarbonate then neutralizes the HCl of the chyme, thus protecting the duodenal mucosa from potential damage and creating a slightly alkaline medium that is optimal for chemical digestion by pancreatic intestinal enzymes. Although the liver produces bile continuously, secretin is effective in increasing the rate of bile secretion. Hormonal regulation is the most important mechanism governing the activity of the pancreas, and cholecystokinin has a key role in stimulating the release of large amounts of digestive enzymes from the pancreas. Cholecystokinin also stimulates the gallbladder to release the bile it stores. GIP acts to slow stomach emptying by decreasing gastric motor activity.[1,24]

Stimulation of the parasympathetic nerves to certain regions of the GI tract will also increase the rates of glandular secretion. Those glands in the upper portion of the GI tract that are innervated by the vagus and other cranial parasympathetic nerves (particularly the salivary, esophageal, and gastric glands, the pancreas, and some duodenal glands) are especially

TABLE 35-1

Major Hormones of the Gastrointestinal Tract

Hormone	Source	Target Organ	Major Actions	Stimulated By
Gastrin	Stomach (mucosa)	Stomach (gastric glands)	Stimulates gastric glands to secrete specific substances	Distention of the stomach by food; other specific substances (e.g., partially digested proteins, caffeine)
Secretin	Duodenum (mucosa)	Pancreas	Stimulates release of the alkaline component of pancreatic juice	Acidic chyme acting on the duodenal mucosa
		Liver	Increases bile secretion rate	
Cholecystokinin	Duodenum (mucosa)	Pancreas	Stimulates release of digestive enzymes	Presence of fatty acids and partially digested proteins in the duodenum
		Gallbladder	Stimulates gallbladder contraction and emptying	
Glucose-dependent insulinotropic polypeptide (gastric inhibitory peptide)	Duodenum (mucosa)	Stomach	Reduces motor activity of the stomach; slows rate of gastric emptying	Presence of fat or carbohydrate in the duodenum

FIGURE 35-16 Schematic diagram of the complex regulation of acid (H^+) secretion from parietal cells in the gastric pits. Gastrin stimulates enterochrommafin-like cells (ECL), which in turn release histamine onto H_2 receptors on the parietal cell. Gastrin also stimulates acid secretion directly as does acetylcholine. *PSNS,* Parasympathetic nervous system; *ACh,* acetylcholine.

subject to parasympathetic stimulation. Glands in the distal portion of the large intestine are also affected by parasympathetic stimulation because this region is innervated by the pelvic parasympathetic nerves. In the small intestine, the major stimulus for intestinal secretion is local and mechanical stimulation of the intestinal wall, which initiates the excitation of local myenteric reflexes and subsequent release of secretions.

DIGESTION AND ABSORPTION

Substances contained in foods that are important to maintenance of the body include carbohydrates, fats (also called *lipids*) proteins, vitamins, inorganic salts, and water. Many of the nutrient constituents that make up intact food substances are structurally complex and cannot be easily absorbed from the GI tract in their original forms. During the process of digestion, digestive juices and the enzymes contained in these secretions convert these complex organic molecules to smaller molecules (Figure 35-17). These simpler compounds are then capable of absorption, or transfer across the wall of the small intestine into the blood and lymph, which in turn transport them to the cells. This complex task of digestion and absorption of nutrients is the primary task of the GI tract, and an inability to perform this function would be life-threatening. This section describes the mechanisms of digestion of the three major groups of nutrients—carbohydrates, lipids, and proteins—and then considers the absorption of these substances.

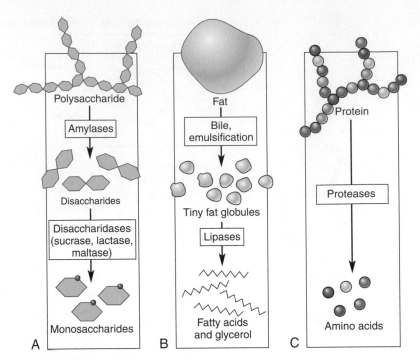

FIGURE 35-17 Chemical digestion. **A,** Amylases and disaccharidases break carbohydrates down into monosaccharides. **B,** Lipases break fats down to fatty acids and glycerol. The large fat globule must first be emulsified by bile. **C,** Proteases and peptidases break proteins down into amino acids. (From Herlihy B: *The human body in health and illness,* ed 3, Philadelphia, 2007, Saunders, p 415.)

TABLE 35-2

Summary of Carbohydrate, Protein, and Lipid Digestion

Location of Digestive Process	Source of Digestive Enzyme or Substance	Basic Digestive Process
Carbohydrates		
Mouth, stomach	Salivary glands (salivary amylase)	Polysaccharides → salivary amylase maltose + dextrin
Small intestine lumen	Pancreas (pancreatic amylase)	Undigested polysaccharides/dextrins → pancreatic amylase → maltose
Brush borders	Intestine (maltase, sucrase, lactase)	Maltose → maltase → glucose + glucose
		Sucrose → sucrase → glucose + fructose
		Lactose → lactase → glucose + galactose
Lipids		
Small intestine	Liver	Lipid particle → bile salts → emulsified fat (triglycerides)
	Pancreas	Triglyceride → lipase → fatty acids + glycerol
Proteins		
Stomach	Stomach (gastric glands)	Protein → pepsin polypeptides
Small intestine lumen	Pancreas	Polypeptides → trypsin, chymotrysin → tripeptides + dipeptides → carboxypeptidase → free amino acids
Brush borders (and within cytoplasm of epithelial cells)	Small intestine	Tripeptides and dipeptides → peptidase → free amino acids

---

Digestion of Carbohydrates

In terms of calories, carbohydrates account for approximately half of the American diet. The major digestible carbohydrate in food is the polysaccharide plant starch, a large molecule composed of straight and branched chains of glucose. A summary of carbohydrate digestion is presented in Table 35-2.

Digestion of starch begins in the mouth as the enzyme salivary amylase breaks down polysaccharides to the much smaller disaccharide molecules maltose and dextrin. In the stomach, this action of salivary amylase continues until the enzyme is eventually inactivated by the acidic gastric juice. In the duodenum, the pancreatic enzyme amylase completes the task of splitting any remaining undigested polysaccharides and dextrins to small maltose units. Then maltase, an enzyme located in the brush border of the epithelial cells lining the duodenum, hydrolyzes each maltose molecule to two molecules of glucose. Other carbohydrates that are present in the diet in smaller quantities are the disaccharides sucrose, which is table sugar (glucose-fructose), and lactose, which is milk sugar (glucose-galactose). These two carbohydrates remain chemically unaltered until they reach the duodenum. There the enzyme sucrase in the brush border converts the sucrose to the monosaccharides glucose and fructose. Lactose is acted on by lactase, which splits it into the monosaccharides glucose and galactose.[6,30]

Glucose, the major product of carbohydrate digestion, accounts for about 80% of the monosaccharides obtained from food, whereas fructose and galactose account for the other 20%. Humans do not secrete an enzyme capable of digesting cellulose, a plant polysaccharide found in the cell walls of plants and present in large amounts in fibrous vegetables. Although cellulose consists of glucose molecules, it contains molecular linkages different from those of starch. Thus much of this complex carbohydrate passes through the digestive tract without being digested and is excreted in the feces.

Digestion of Lipids

Lipids in the diet are mostly in the form of triglycerides but also include phospholipids, cholesterol, and fat-soluble vitamins A, D, E, and K. Digestion of lipids occurs in the small intestine, where fats are emulsified by the action of bile; neither salivary nor gastric enzymes appear to have any effect on triglycerides. As the lipid particles enter the duodenum from the stomach, bile exerts a detergent action on them in which the surface tension of the particles is decreased. This decrease in surface tension promotes breakup of the particles into smaller particles as they are pushed around by the mixing movements of the small intestine. The emulsification process is an entirely mechanical action inasmuch as bile contains no enzymes and thus performs no chemical digestion.

Eventually, the detergent action of bile salts reduces the particles of fat to tiny droplets so that their surface area is greatly increased. This enhancement of surface area allows for maximal exposure to pancreatic lipase, an enzyme, which (along with intestinal lipase, to a lesser extent) hydrolyzes the triglycerides to free fatty acids and glycerol. Some monoglycerides (glycerol with one fatty acid still attached) may remain; in fact, some fat may escape digestion entirely or be reduced only to diglycerides (glycerol with two fatty acids attached).[31] A summary of triglyceride digestion is presented in Table 35-2.

Cholesterol, a steroid type of lipid, is ingested in the form of cholesterol esters, which cannot be directly absorbed. An esterase in pancreatic juice degrades cholesterol esters to cholesterol and fatty acid, which then undergo absorption.

Digestion of Proteins

Proteins are composed of molecular subunits called *amino acids* that are linked together by peptide bonds. Protein that undergoes digestion in the small intestine includes both protein from food and protein from desquamated cells and the many enzymes of the GI tract. This protein of endogenous origin constitutes a sizable portion of the total protein subjected to digestion and absorption.[32]

Protein digestion involves breakage of the peptide bonds by hydrolysis and release of free amino acids. It begins in the stomach with the action of the enzyme pepsin, which is secreted by the gastric glands. By its action on peptide bonds, pepsin reduces most protein to intermediate-sized polypeptides. Pepsin is also capable of breaking down collagen, a protein component of intercellular connective tissue, thus rendering cellular proteins more accessible to enzymatic action in the GI tract. In the duodenum, the trypsin and chymotrypsin contained in pancreatic juice reduce the polypeptides to small peptides (tripeptides and dipeptides). Carboxypeptidase, which has its source in the pancreas, and peptidases in the brush borders of the intestinal epithelial cells split some of these peptides into free amino acids. Free amino acids, in addition to dipeptides and tripeptides, are absorbed into the intestinal epithelial cells. Within the cytoplasm of epithelial cells the small peptides are then hydrolyzed by various peptidases into free amino acids before their passage into the circulation. Numerous proteolytic enzymes are involved in protein digestion, and each enzyme acts on a slightly different type of peptide linkage. Protein digestion is summarized in Table 35-2.

Absorption

Intestinal absorption is the movement of water and dissolved materials, such as the products of nutrient digestion, vitamins, and inorganic salts, from the inside of the small intestine through the semipermeable intestinal membrane and into the blood and lymph. A major feature of the intestinal absorptive surface is the villus, the small fingerlike projection lined with epithelial cells that was described earlier in this chapter. Within each villus is a network of capillaries that branch from a miniscule artery and empty into a miniscule vein. A central lymph vessel called a *lacteal* is also located in the villus. In the process of absorption, nutrient molecules pass through the single layer of epithelial cells lining the villus and through the single layer of cells forming the wall of the capillary or lacteal. A number of transport systems specific to certain nutrient components function in the intestinal epithelium to promote this process of absorption.[4]

Operation of the intestinal transport systems is dependent on adenosine triphosphate (ATP) production by the epithelial cells. These systems are capable of moving the products of nutrient digestion and inorganic salts from the intestinal lumen into the blood against electrochemical gradients (active transport). In addition to active transport, some molecules may move across the intestinal epithelium by passive means when a difference in concentration on the two sides of the epithelium exists. The rate of molecular transfer based on diffusion gradients is dependent not only on the magnitude of the difference in concentration, but also on the size of the molecules and the lipid solubility of the substances involved.

Almost all substances capable of intestinal absorption disappear from the lumen of the small intestine by the time that the intestinal contents reach the mid-jejunum. The ileum is not involved in absorption to any significant degree, as the proximal regions of the small intestine have usually done the work of absorption before the intestinal contents reach the ileal region. Nevertheless, the distal end of the small intestine has the capability of absorption and may do so in situations in which absorption has not taken place in the proximal part of the small intestine. Thus about 50% of the small intestine can be surgically removed without compromising absorptive ability. However, it is important to note that vitamin B_{12} and bile salts are absorbed specifically in the terminal ileum and that surgical removal of this portion of the small intestine will result in impaired absorption of these substances.[6] Intrinsic factor produced by the parietal cells of the gastric antrum is also required for B_{12} absorption; intrinsic factor deficiency leads to a condition known as *pernicious anemia*.[3]

The intestinal contents arriving at the terminal ileum contain no digestible carbohydrate, very little fat, and only 15% to 17% nitrogen-containing substances. Most of the contents of the terminal ileum consist of bacteria, desquamated epithelial cells, digestive secretions, and the residue of foods that are undigested and therefore unabsorbed, such as the cellulose walls of fibrous plants and connective tissue from animal sources.

Carbohydrates

Carbohydrates are absorbed in the form of monosaccharides. Polysaccharides and disaccharides lack the capacity for absorption; apparently the intestinal epithelium is impermeable to carbohydrates of such high molecular weight, and no transport systems exist for these types of carbohydrate molecules. The monosaccharides glucose and galactose are absorbed by an active, energy-requiring process in which a carrier molecule located on the luminal border of epithelial cells transports glucose and galactose across the border. It is theorized that the same carrier molecule that ferries glucose and galactose also carries sodium and that the carrier affinity for sugar is greatest when sodium is bound to the carrier. In contrast to the other monosaccharides, the monosaccharide fructose is absorbed passively by means of a diffusion gradient.[6]

Lipids

Absorption of lipids occurs by a highly complex, unique process. As fatty acids and monoglycerides are freed during digestion, they become dissolved in bile salt micelles, which are colloidal particles composed of many molecules. Within the micelles, the products of lipid digestion are now soluble and can be absorbed far more efficiently. The bile salt micelles transport the lipid products to the epithelial brush borders, where the monoglycerides or fatty acids, which are highly soluble in the lipid cell membrane, diffuse into the epithelial cells and leave the micelle behind. The micelle is now emptied of its cargo and can pick up more fatty acids and monoglycerides and transport them to the cell membrane.

Bile salts, which are required for micelle formation, are absorbed mostly in the terminal ileum and then recycled in the liver. In the absence of bile, the amount of lipid absorbed in this manner is reduced by more than 25%. In this situation, the absorption of fat-soluble vitamins (vitamins A, D, E, and K) is compromised. Several cholestatic conditions, such as primary biliary cirrhosis and primary sclerosing cholangitis, may be associated with deficiencies of fat-soluble vitamins.[33-35]

Monoglycerides may be further degraded into glycerol and fatty acids by the enzyme lipase within the epithelial cell. Short-chain fatty acids (those with fewer than 12 carbon atoms) can be absorbed directly into the blood at this point. Long-chain fatty acids and glycerol, however, are reassembled into triglycerides by the endoplasmic reticulum. These newly synthesized triglycerides are aggregated into droplets that become progressively larger during passage through the cell. These lipid droplets are stabilized by enclosure with absorbed cholesterol and phospholipids and encased by a protein coat. The final product, called a *chylomicron*, passes out of the cell and into the lacteal of the villus. From the lacteal, chylomicrons pass through a series of lymph vessels that eventually drain into the general circulation.

Proteins

Amino acids are transported across the epithelial membrane by means of an active transport carrier system in much the same way as monosaccharides are. It is currently thought that different carrier systems exist to carry the different chemical classes of amino acids (i.e., neutral, basic, dicarboxylic, and imino acids). As is the case for the transport of sugars, brush border membrane carriers are involved in the transfer of amino acids across the intestinal epithelial cell; these carriers require energy and are coupled to the transport of sodium. After being transported to the epithelial cells of the villi, amino acids diffuse through the base of the cell and into the blood. Both amino acids and monosaccharides are transported directly to the liver by the hepatic portal vein.

Water and Electrolytes

Water and inorganic ions, which are in the GI tract as a result of ingestion and secretion, are absorbed mainly from the small intestine and, to a lesser extent, from the colon. The process of absorption of water and ions is the same in both the small and large intestine: sodium is actively transported to the blood, and water follows passively in response to the osmotic gradient created by the removal of sodium from the intraluminal fluid. About 8000 ml of water is absorbed every day by the small intestine and about 300 to 400 ml by the colon. Frequently, diarrhea is the result of failure of the small intestine to absorb water appropriately. If large quantities of water are allowed to enter the colon from the small intestine because of some malfunction of the small intestine's absorptive ability, the colonic absorptive mechanism may be overwhelmed, and diarrhea is the result (Figure 35-18).

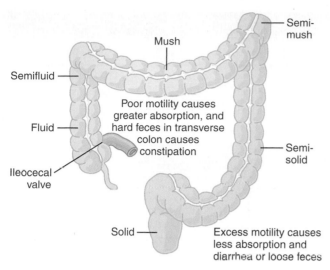

FIGURE 35-18 Absorptive function of the large intestine. (From Guyton AC, Hall JE: *Textbook of medical physiology,* ed 11, Philadelphia, Saunders, 2006, p 788.)

KEY POINTS

- Digestion, the process of converting large molecules to simpler forms, is accomplished by mechanical and enzymatic processes. Digestion is a necessary prelude to absorption because only simple molecules can cross the intestinal epithelia.

- Digestion of complex carbohydrates is initiated in the mouth, where salivary amylase begins to cleave large molecules into disaccharides. Pancreatic amylase continues this process in the small intestine. Disaccharides (maltose, sucrose, lactose) are cleaved into monosaccharides (glucose, fructose, galactose) by brush border enzymes (maltase, sucrase, lactase) on the intestinal epithelia. Glucose and galactose are absorbed across the intestinal epithelia by a sodium-dependent cotransporter. Fructose is absorbed passively by facilitated diffusion. Monosaccharides then travel via the bloodstream to the liver.

- Lipid digestion begins in the small intestine, where bile salts from the gallbladder mix and emulsify the fatty substances. Emulsification mechanically separates the lipids into small drops that are more accessible to enzymatic digestion. Pancreatic lipase and brush border lipases digest the fats into free fatty acids and glycerol, which remain associated with the bile salts and form micelles. Cholesterol is digested by pancreatic esterase. Fatty acids are transported to the intestinal epithelia by micelles. Free fatty acids diffuse out of the micelle and into the epithelial cell passively. Epithelial cells synthesize large protein-lipid complexes (chylomicrons) that enter the lymphatic system.

- Protein digestion begins in the stomach, where HCl from parietal cells activates pepsinogen to pepsin. Pepsin cleaves proteins into smaller polypeptides. Pepsin is neutralized in the duodenum, and pancreatic trypsin, chymotrypsin, and carboxypeptidase take over protein

digestion. Brush border peptidases split tripeptides and dipeptides into single amino acids. Amino acid transport into intestinal epithelial cells is mediated by a sodium-dependent cotransport system similar to monosaccharide transport. Small peptides may also undergo endocytosis and be cleaved into amino acids within the epithelial cells.

- Amino acids pass into the bloodstream and travel to the liver.

- Absorption of water occurs passively by osmosis. An osmotic gradient for water absorption is created as electrolytes are absorbed.

GASTROINTESTINAL FUNCTION ACROSS THE LIFE SPAN

Maturation

During the first months of life, the newborn's GI tract undergoes many maturational changes. In the first 3 to 4 months of life, sucking reflexes are present, and extrusion reflexes protect against the ingestion of solids that the immature GI tract is still unable to digest. The pressure in the LES remains low during this time, and "spitting up" of gastric contents is common because intragastric pressure often exceeds LES pressure. Gastric motility is not well coordinated for the first 3 to 4 months, so antral mixing is inadequate for the digestion of solid foods. At about 12 weeks of age, intestinal peristalsis similar to that in adults begins to develop, but it is one-third slower. This slower transit in infants may serve to improve nutrient digestion and absorption by increasing the exposure of nutrients to the intestinal mucosa. The motor function of the large intestine appears to be fully developed at birth. During the first 2 years of life, the secretory and absorptive functions of the intestine mature and begin a pattern of functioning that continues into senescence.[6,11]

Age-Related Changes

Changes in GI function in older adults occur simultaneously with other age-related changes such as a decrease in lean body mass and impaired homeostasis of multiple body systems. Within the GI tract, a variety of changes occur that may place an aging individual at risk for health problems related to GI functioning and nutrition. Important elements of this process are summarized in Geriatric Considerations: Changes in the Gastrointestinal System.

Loss of dentition and reduced taste and smell acuity may promote a decreased interest in food intake as chewing becomes difficult and the sensory enjoyment associated with food becomes impaired. A condition called **presbyesophagus,** in which esophageal motility is slowed or disorganized, may develop in older adults. Presbyesophagus may be manifested as difficulty in swallowing and may cause discomfort as food passes through the esophagus. The incidence of hiatal hernia, where part of the stomach moves into the chest cavity through an enlarged diaphragmatic opening, is also increased in the

GERIATRIC CONSIDERATIONS

Changes in the Gastrointestinal System

As a person ages, gastrointestinal muscle strength and movement decrease, leading to reduced peristalsis and decreased gastrointestinal motility throughout the system.

In the esophagus, the elderly person experiences greater numbers of muscle movements that do not propel the contents onward. These nonperistaltic waves are common in the lower esophagus. The phenomenon of presbyesophagus—in which the esophageal sphincter fails to relax and the lower esophagus becomes dilated—may not necessarily be normal to the elderly.

In the stomach, decreased numbers of parietal and chief cells result in diminished acid (HCl) and pepsin secretion. This leads to increased pH and a more alkaline secretion. The protective alkaline viscous mucus in the stomach is also decreased. The loss of smooth muscle in the stomach can delay emptying time, which increases and prolongs the exposure of gastric epithelial cells to the gastric contents.

The small intestinal smooth muscle, Peyer patches, and lymphatic follicles are decreased. Normal intestinal absorption in the elderly is not well understood and may be influenced by a number of factors, including bowel motility, epithelial membranes, vascular perfusion, and gastrointestinal membrane transport. However, absorption of lipids, amino acids, glucose, calcium, and iron is known to be decreased. Normal changes in the large intestine have been difficult to determine. As a result of smooth muscle changes, anal sphincter tone decreases.

---

aging population, affecting 69% of persons over 70 years. The transit time for intestinal contents to pass through the GI tract is increased in older persons; this factor, coupled with a decreased perception of the sensory stimuli that produce the urge to defecate, may promote constipation in the aging population. Conversely, a confused or neurologically impaired older individual may experience fecal incontinence because the sensation and tone of the rectum diminish with aging.[6,36]

KEY POINTS

- Infants may experience GI dysfunction because of immaturity of the GI tract. Motility is not well coordinated until 3 to 4 months of age, making digestion of solids difficult in infancy. Pressure in the LES is low, which leads to "spitting up" and gastric distention. Maturation of the GI tract is complete by about 2 years of age.
- Elderly individuals may experience GI dysfunction for a number of reasons. Poor dentition, loss of taste and smell acuity, and reduced esophageal motility may lead to poor intake of nutrients. Hiatal hernia and constipation are common in the elderly.

SUMMARY

This chapter describes the structure of the human GI system and the process by which it provides nutrients for the body. A thorough understanding of the structure of the GI tract, GI motility, secretion of digestive juices, digestion of nutrients, and absorption of nutrients is needed as a basis for understanding other principles of health and disease.

GI motility is a complex process involving a set of carefully timed autoregulatory action responses (Figure 35-19). You may wish to trace the path and destiny of the apple you ate for lunch as an example of this process. As you track the movement of nutrients through the GI tract, consider the ways in which secretion of digestive juices occurs in response to the ingestion of your apple, which contains a great deal of carbohydrate (fructose), small amounts of protein, and minimal lipid. Consider also how digestion and absorption of these nutrients are occurring. What part of the apple will you use, for example, for energy to study this text? What part of the apple will your body "throw away," and how will this be accomplished? Finally, will your GI tract respond the same way to eating an apple when you are 85 years old? A careful review of the elegant and nearly

Mouth
Breaks up food particles
Assists in producing
spoken language

Salivary glands
Saliva moistens and
lubricates food
Amylase digests
polysaccharides

Pharynx
Swallows

Esophagus
Transports food

Liver
Breaks down and builds up
many biological molecules
Stores vitamins and iron
Destroys old blood cells
Destroys poisons
Bile aids in digestion

Stomach
Stores and churns food
Pepsin digests protein
HCl activates enzymes, breaks
up food, kills germs
Mucus protects stomach wall
Limited absorption

Gallbladder
Stores and concentrates bile

Pancreas
Hormones regulate blood glucose levels
Bicarbonates neutralize stomach acid
Trypsin and chymotrypsin digest proteins
Amylase digests polysaccharides
Lipase digests lipids

Small intestine
Completes digestion
Mucus protects gut wall
Absorbs nutrients, most water
Peptidase digests proteins
Sucrases digest sugars
Amylase digests polysaccharides

Large intestine
Reabsorbs some water
and ions
Forms and stores feces

Anus
Opening for elimination
of feces

Rectum
Stores and expels feces

FIGURE 35-19 Summary of digestive function. (From Thibodeau GA, Patton KT: *Anatomy and physiology,* ed 5, St Louis, 2007, Mosby, p 985.)

automatic function of the human GI tract will prepare you to care for individuals experiencing interruptions in proper nutrient digestion and absorption.

REFERENCES

1. Guyton AC, Hall JE: *Textbook of medical physiology,* ed 11, Philadelphia, 2006, Saunders.
2. Johnson LR: *Gastrointestinal physiology,* ed 7, Philadelphia, 2006, Mosby.
3. Sleisenger MH, Feldman M, Friedman LS: *Sleisenger and Fordtran's gastrointestinal and liver disease: pathophysiology, diagnosis, management,* ed 8, Philadelphia, 2006, Saunders.
4. Yazbeck S: Gastrointestinal emergencies of the neonate. In Roy CC, Silverman A, Alagille D, editors: *Pediatric clinical gastroenterology,* ed 4, St Louis, 1995, Mosby.
5. Sauve RS, Leung AK: Congenital varicella syndrome with colonic atresias, *Clin Pediatr* 42(5):451-453, 2003.
6. Shils ME: *Modern nutrition in health and disease,* ed 10, Philadelphia, 2006, Lippincott Williams & Wilkins.
7. Pedersen AM et al: Saliva and gastrointestinal functions of taste, mastication, swallowing and digestion, *Oral Dis* 8(3):117-129, 2002.
8. Herrera JL, Lyons MF 2nd, Johnson LF: Saliva: its role in health and disease, *J Clin Gastroenterol* 10(5):569-578, 1988.
9. Yamada T et al: *Textbook of gastroenterology,* ed 4, Philadelphia, 2003, Lippincott Williams & Wilkins.
10. Randal Bollinger R, Barbas AS, Bush EL et al: Biofilms in the large bowel suggest an apparent function of the human vermiform appendix, *J Theor Biol* Sep 7; [Epub ahead of print 2007].
11. Gebruers EM, Hall WJ: Role of the gastrointestinal tract in the regulation of hydration in man, *Dig Dis* 10(2):112-120, 1992.
12. Current concepts in research of gastrointestinal motility: international symposium, Aarhus, Denmark, July 18-20, 1991, *Dig Dis* 9(6):321-443, 1991.
13. Thomson AB et al: Small bowel review: normal physiology part 2, *Dig Dis Sci* 46(12):2588-2607, 2001.
14. Burns AJ, Thapar N: Advances in ontogeny of the enteric nervous system, *Neurogastroenterol Motil* 18(10):876-887, 2006.
15. McIntyre AS, Thompson DG: Review article: adrenergic control of motor and secretory function in the gastrointestinal tract, *Aliment Pharmacol Ther* 6(2):125-142, 1992.
16. Hornby PJ: Central neurocircuitry associated with emesis, *Am J Med* 111(Suppl 8A):106S-112S, 2001.

17. Huizinga JD: Action potentials in gastrointestinal smooth muscle, *Can J Physiol Pharmacol* 69(8):1133-1142, 1991.

18. Sanders KM: Ionic mechanisms of electrical rhythmicity in gastrointestinal smooth muscles, *Annu Rev Physiol* 54:439-453, 1992.

19. Thulin L, Johansson C: Gastrointestinal hormones, *Acta Chir Scand Suppl* 482:69-72, 1978.

20. de Herder WW, Lamberts SW: Somatostatin and somatostatin analogues: diagnostic and therapeutic uses, *Curr Opin Oncol* 14(1):53-57, 2002.

21. Nonogaki K: Ghrelin and feedback systems, *Vitam Horm* 77:149-170, 2007.

22. Wiedmer P, Nogueiras R, Broglio F et al: Ghrelin, obesity and diabetes, *Nat Clin Pract Endocrinol Metab* 3(10):705-712, 2007.

23. Publicover NG, Sanders KM: Myogenic regulation of propagation in gastric smooth muscle, *Am J Physiol* 248:G512-G520, 1985.

24. Jenkins AP et al: Effects of bolus doses of fat on small intestinal structure and on release of gastrin, cholecystokinin, peptide tyrosine-tyrosine, and enteroglucagon, *Gut* 33(2):218-223, 1992.

25. Surrenti C, Maggi CA: Sensory nerves in the gastrointestinal tract: changing concepts and perspectives, *Ital J Gastroenterol* 23(2):94-99, 1991.

26. Karaus M, Wienbeck M: Colonic motility in humans: a growing understanding, *Baillieres Clin Gastroenterol* 5(2):453-478, 1991.

27. Berna MJ, Jensen RT: Role of CCK/gastrin receptors in gastrointestinal/metabolic diseases and results of human studies using gastrin/CCK receptor agonists/antagonists in these diseases, *Curr Top Med Chem* 7(12):1211-1231, 2007.

28. Rehfeld JF, Friis-Hansen L, Goetze JP et al: The biology of cholecystokinin and gastrin peptides, *Curr Top Med Chem* 7(12):1154-1165, 2007.

29. Barocelli E, Ballabeni V: Histamine in the control of gastric acid secretion: a topic review, *Pharmacol Res* 47(4):299-304, 2003.

30. Marks V et al: Gut hormones in glucose homeostasis, *Proc Nutr Soc* 50(3):545-552, 1991.

31. Titus E, Ahearn GA: Vertebrate gastrointestinal fermentation: transport mechanisms for volatile fatty acids, *Am J Physiol* 262(4):R547-R553, 1992.

32. Dockray GJ, Forster ER, Louis SM: Peptides and their receptors on afferent neurons to the upper gastrointestinal tract, *Adv Exp Med Biol* 298:53-62, 1991.

33. Hofmann AF: Cholestatic liver disease: pathophysiology and therapeutic options, *Liver* 22(Suppl 2):14-19, 2002.

34. Sokol RJ: Fat-soluble vitamins and their importance in patients with cholestatic liver diseases, *Gastroenterol Clin North Am* 23(4):673-705, 1994.

35. Jorgensen RA, Lindor KD, Sartin JS et al: Serum lipid and fat-soluble vitamin levels in primary sclerosing cholangitis, *J Clin Gastro* 20(3):215-219, 1995.

36. Orr WC, Chen CL: Aging and neural control of the GI tract, IV: clinical and physiological aspects of gastrointestinal motility and aging, *Am J Physiol Gastrointest Liver Physiol* 283(6):G1226-G1231, 2002.

Gastrointestinal Disorders

Jeffrey S. Sartin

MEDIA RESOURCES

Additional Material for Study, Review, and Further Exploration

 CD Companion ▪ Review Questions and Answers
▪ Glossary (with audio pronunciations for selected terms)
▪ Disease Profiles ▪ Animations

evolve **Website** at http://evolve.elsevier.com/Copstead/
▪ Case Studies ▪ Disease Profiles ▪ WebLinks ▪ Key Points Review

 Online Course (Module 16)

KEY QUESTIONS

▪ What are the common causes of the following general manifestations of gastrointestinal disorders: pain, nausea, vomiting, diarrhea, and constipation?
▪ What are the predisposing factors and characteristic manifestations common to inflammatory disorders of the gastrointestinal tract?

▪ What are the common causes of and clinical findings in functional and mechanical bowel obstructions?
▪ What are the common causes of and clinical findings in malabsorption?
▪ What warning signs may indicate cancer of the gastrointestinal tract?

CHAPTER OUTLINE

Alterations in function of the gastrointestinal (GI) tract may have far-reaching consequences in an individual's life. The ability to take in nutrients, convert them to usable forms for body functions, and dispose of their waste products goes beyond physiologic function and is intimately associated with social and psychological functioning. A person with an alteration in GI function may experience great emotional distress and be unable to participate fully in social activities, which in American society are largely centered on food consumption. Certain symptoms that may accompany GI disorders, such as chronic diarrhea and abdominal pain, may severely limit an individual's ability to maintain employment. It has been estimated that 200,000 people miss work daily because of GI-related problems.[1] In addition, GI diseases account for more hospital admissions in the United States than any other category of disease. Because many chronic GI conditions begin in midlife and continue into old age, their prevalence will likely increase as the U.S. population continues to age.

This chapter describes the pathophysiologic process of the most common disorders of the GI tract and summarizes current treatment for these conditions. Because knowledge about many GI disorders is expanding rapidly, some current research on selected GI conditions is described. Finally, because of the intimate relationship between GI function and the integrity and well-being of the person, a discussion of the psychological and emotional aspects of GI disorders across the life span is included.

MANIFESTATIONS OF GASTROINTESTINAL TRACT DISORDERS

As a basis for discussing individual types of GI disorders, a description of some common manifestations of these disorders and their pathophysiologic mechanisms is presented. Common manifestations include dysphagia, esophageal and abdominal pain, intestinal gas, vomiting, and alterations in bowel patterns.

Dysphagia

Dysphagia is a subjective difficulty in swallowing (Figure 36-1). It may include the inability to initiate swallowing or the sensation that the swallowed solids or liquids "stick" in the esophagus. In certain disorders, **odynophagia,** or pain with swallowing, may accompany dysphagia. The physiologic mechanism of normal swallowing is described in Chapter 35; the reader may wish to refer to this information.

Categories

The pathophysiologic basis for dysphagia usually falls into three major categories: (1) problems in delivery of the bolus of food or fluid into the esophagus as a result of neuromuscular incoordination; (2) problems in transport of the bolus down the body of the esophagus as a result of altered esophageal peristaltic activity; and (3) problems in bolus entry into the stomach as a result of lower esophageal sphincter (LES) dysfunction or obstructing lesions.[2]

In the first category of dysphagia, individuals have a decreased ability to accomplish the initial steps of swallowing in an orderly sequence. The normal sequence of pharyngeal contraction, closure of the epiglottis, upper esophageal sphincter relaxation, and initiation of peristalsis by contraction of the striated muscle in the upper portion of the esophagus is altered, or certain steps in the sequence may be absent. Persons experiencing this type of dysphagia may cough and expel the ingested food or fluids through their mouth and nose or aspirate when they attempt to swallow. These symptoms are usually worse with liquids than with solids in this type of swallowing dysfunction.

The second type of dysphagia may be the result of any disorder, structural or neuromuscular, in which the peristaltic activity of the body of the esophagus is altered. The presence of: (1) esophageal **diverticula,** or outpouchings of one or more layers of the esophageal wall, (2) **achalasia,** a disorder of esophageal smooth muscle function, or (3) structural disorders such as neoplasms or strictures may interfere with proper peristaltic activity in the esophagus.[3,4] This alteration in peristalsis may

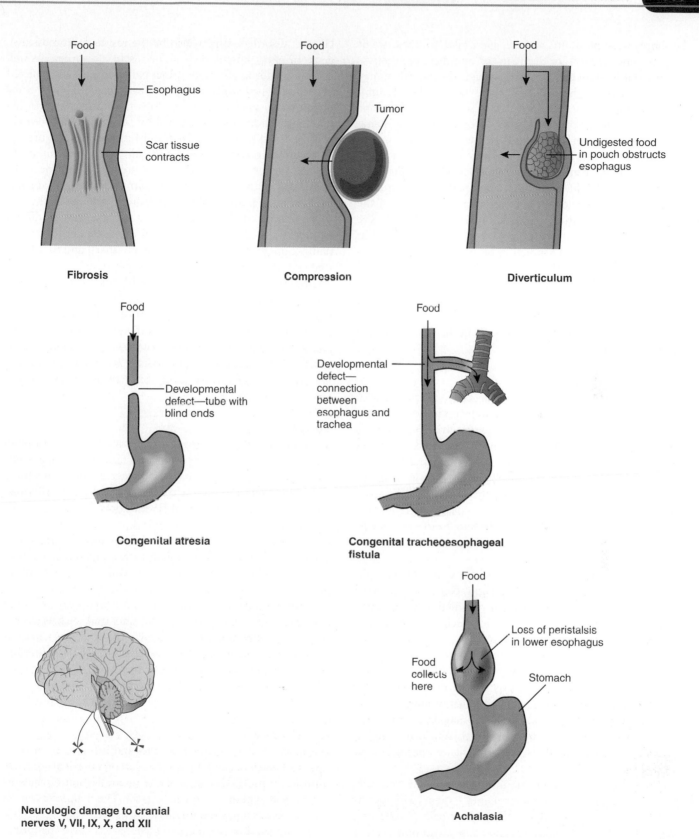

FIGURE 36-1   Causes of dysphagia. (From Gould BE: *Pathophysiology for the health professions,* ed 2, Philadelphia, 2002, Saunders, p 382.)

be simply weak peristaltic activity, aperistalsis (the absence of all peristaltic activity), or disorganized and therefore ineffective peristalsis. With this type of dysphagia the individual may have the sensation that food is "stuck" behind the sternum. Initially, dysphagia may be noted with solid foods; if the underlying pathologic process fosters a worsening of peristaltic ability, the passage of liquids may also become impaired.

The third category of dysphagia, which results from problems of bolus entry into the stomach, is secondary to any condition in which the LES functions improperly or is obstructed by a lesion. Tumors of the mediastinum, lower part of the esophagus, and gastroesophageal junction may invade the myenteric plexus or produce an obstruction at the LES, thus interrupting normal LES function by neural invasion or direct obstruction. In addition, motor disorders resulting from neuromuscular diseases or chronic lower esophageal inflammation from the reflux of acidic gastric contents may limit the ability of the LES to function properly. This type of dysphagia may be manifested as tightness or pain in the substernal area during the swallowing process.

Esophageal Pain

Two types of pain occur in the esophagus: (1) heartburn (also called **pyrosis**) and (2) pain located in the middle of the chest, which may mimic the pain of angina pectoris. Heartburn is caused by the reflux of gastric contents into the esophagus and is a substernal burning sensation that may radiate to the neck or throat. Two probable mechanisms contribute to the development of heartburn.[2] First, the highly acidic gastric contents may be a noxious stimulant to sensory afferent nerve endings in the esophageal mucosa. Second, heartburn may be produced by a spasm of the esophageal muscle brought on by acid stimulation.

Chest pain other than heartburn may be the result of esophageal distention or powerful esophageal contractions. These stimuli may arise from esophageal obstruction or a condition called *diffuse esophageal spasm,* in which high-amplitude, simultaneous contractions in the smooth muscle portion of the esophagus may be randomly interspersed with normal-appearing peristalsis.[1]

This type of esophageal pain is similar to that of angina pectoris, particularly in its pattern of radiation into the neck, shoulder, arm, and jaw. Odynophagia may accompany diffuse esophageal spasm and be indistinguishable from esophageal chest pain except that it is brought on specifically by swallowing.

Herpetic or candidal infections of the esophagus generally occur in immunocompromised patients. Patients with esophagitis may experience a dull, aching chest pain. Swallowing may worsen the pain sensation and cause symptoms such as heartburn or chest pain.

Abdominal Pain

Pain in the abdominal region may be the first sign of a disorder of the GI tract and is often an important impetus for seeking medical care. Although abdominal pain may result from GI tract disorders, it may also be the result of reproductive, genitourinary, musculoskeletal, or vascular disorders, as well as toxins or drug use. Abdominal pain is usually categorized into three types, which may manifest separately or in combination: (1) visceral pain develops from stretching or distending an abdominal organ or from inflammation. The pain is diffuse and poorly localized and has a gnawing, burning, or cramping quality; (2) somatic pain arises from injury to the abdominal wall, the parietal peritoneum, the root of the mesentery, or the diaphragm. In contrast to visceral pain, it is sharper, more intense, and generally well localized to the area of irritation; and (3) referred pain is felt at a location distant from the source of the pain but in the same dermatome or neurosegment. Referred pain is usually sharp and well localized and may be felt in the skin or deeper tissues.

Abdominal pain may be acute with instantaneous onset, such as pain due to a perforated ulcer or a ruptured internal organ. A more gradual development of abdominal pain may accompany such chronic states as diverticulitis or ulcerative colitis (UC). Abdominal pain seldom occurs as a solitary manifestation of GI disorders but is usually accompanied by other manifestations such as vomiting or alteration in bowel patterns to a variable degree.

Vomiting

Vomiting is the forceful expulsion of gastric contents through the mouth. Usually accompanied by a feeling of nausea, vomiting results from a coordinated sequence of abdominal muscle contractions and reverse esophageal peristalsis. Although vomiting is a common sign of GI disorders, it may also occur with metabolic, endocrine, labyrinthine, and cardiac disorders, as well as with infection and fluid and electrolyte imbalances. It is also associated with such nonpathologic causes as pharmacologic agents, surgery, and the first trimester of pregnancy.

Vomiting associated with GI disorders may be the result of alterations in the integrity of the GI tract wall, such as gastroenteritis, or alterations in the motility of the GI tract, such as intestinal obstruction. The characteristics of the vomitus and the presence of blood or fecal matter may suggest the nature of the GI disorder and the level of the GI tract at which the disorder is located.

Intestinal Gas

Gas normally occurs in the GI tract and is the result of swallowed air, bacterial and digestive action on intestinal contents, diffusion from the blood, and the neutralization of acids by bicarbonate within the upper GI tract. The manifestations of excess intestinal gas may include excessive belching, distention of the abdomen, and excessive flatus. These manifestations may occur singly or in combination and may stem from a variety of causes. Belching is a normal phenomenon caused by the eructation of swallowed air but may also be the result of a motility disorder or gastric outlet obstruction. Abdominal distention may be due to failure to adequately digest some particular nutrient such as the sugar lactose. In the absence of adequate lactase (the digestive enzyme that breaks down lactose into glucose and galactose in the intestine), lactose undergoes bacterial fermentation, which results in gas production in the intestinal lumen. In some individuals, abdominal distention from excess gas may result from a defect in intestinal motility in which the intestinal contents are not propelled in a regular fashion, rather than from the production of too much gas. Excessive flatus may have causes similar to those of abdominal distention. Usually it is the result of increased amounts of gas produced by the action of bacteria on nutritional substrates that are particularly gas-producing, such as certain vegetables and legumes. Some individuals are particularly sensitive to the flatulent effects of beans, for instance.

Alterations in Bowel Patterns

Both constipation and diarrhea are difficult to define with precision, as a wide variation in bowel pattern can be found in different individuals. In addition, cultural and family socialization may play a role in the way in which an individual perceives bowel patterns. Alterations in bowel patterns may be the result of a change in GI tract motility or may be a component of a functional GI disorder such as irritable bowel syndrome (IBS).

Constipation

Constipation may be defined as small, infrequent, or difficult bowel movements.[3,5] Authorities have agreed on a norm of fewer than three stools per week as a guideline for defining constipation.[1] Dietary factors, particularly a diet low in fiber, have been shown to contribute to constipation. The presence of cellulose, the carbohydrate component of dietary fiber that is indigestible in the human intestine, may be effective in promoting regular peristaltic movement in the GI tract by forming bulk within the intestinal lumen to stimulate propulsion. In addition, because exercise stimulates intestinal peristalsis, a lack of exercise has been implicated in the development of constipation. In elderly persons the slowed rate of peristalsis that occurs with the aging process, coupled with a decreased level of physical activity, may promote chronic constipation. These factors may eventually contribute to the development of fecal impaction, a condition in which a firm, immovable mass of stool becomes stationary in the lower GI tract. Constipation may also be the result of pathologic conditions, including processes that alter the motility of the GI tract such as intestinal obstruction or processes that alter the integrity of the GI tract wall such as diverticulitis.

Diarrhea

Diarrhea is defined as an increase in the frequency and fluidity of bowel movements and is often a primary sign of GI tract disorders. While stool weight in excess of 200 g/24 h is one easily obtainable, objective definition of diarrhea,[4] most persons consider increased liquidity as the primary determinant.[6] Diarrhea may be present as an acute or chronic manifestation. Acute diarrhea may be the result of an acute infection, emotional stress, or leakage of stool around impacted feces.

Chronic diarrhea is usually defined as symptoms greater than 4 weeks and may be the result of a chronic GI tract infection (often associated with immune system compromise), alterations in the motility or integrity of the GI tract, malabsorption, or certain endocrine disorders.[7] Diarrhea that occurs on an episodic basis may be related to a food allergy or may be due to the ingestion of irritants to the GI tract or caffeine. Diarrhea in children frequently results from infection, although malabsorption, anatomic defects, and allergy may also be causative factors.[8]

Pathophysiologic Mechanisms. Four major pathophysiologic mechanisms have been identified in the development of diarrhea: (1) In osmotic diarrhea, increased amounts of poorly absorbable, osmotically active solutes such as a carbohydrate or magnesium sulfate cause sodium and water influx into the bowel lumen, resulting in diarrhea; (2) in secretory diarrhea, a pathophysiologic event such as the presence of a bacterial toxin causes enhanced secretion of chloride ion and water in the small intestine by simultaneously stimulating active secretion and inhibiting resorption. Diarrhea of 1 L or more per day may result from this inappropriate secretion of fluid across the intestinal mucosa.[3] Causes of secretory diarrhea include enterotoxins produced by such organisms as *Vibrio cholerae* and *Staphylococcus aureus*; (3) exudative diarrhea is the result of exudation of mucus, blood, and protein from sites of active inflammation into the bowel lumen. This creates an increased osmotic load and a subsequent shift of water across the epithelium. In addition, if a large surface area of the bowel has an alteration in its integrity, intestinal absorption will be severely impaired, further compounding the diarrhea produced. Diarrhea associated with Crohn disease and UC may be the result of this exudative process,[3,7] and (4) diarrhea related to motility disturbances is a result of the decreased contact time of chyme with the absorptive surfaces of the intestinal lumen. If inadequate absorption takes place in the small intestine, large amounts of fluid will be delivered to the colon and may overwhelm the absorptive capability of the colon and cause diarrhea. In addition, if the fatty acids and bile salts present in chyme have not been adequately absorbed in the small intestine, they may induce a secretory diarrhea once they reach the colon, further compounding the process of diarrhea formation. Diarrhea associated with the postgastrectomy dumping syndrome and IBS are examples of this type of diarrhea.[5,7]

KEY POINTS

- Dysphagia is the perception of difficulty in swallowing. Dysphagia caused by neuromuscular disorders may be accompanied by coughing and aspiration, particularly with liquid ingestion. Altered esophageal peristalsis is associated with the sensation that food has become "stuck" behind the sternum. LES dysfunction may be manifested as substernal pain.

- Pain is a common symptom of GI disorders. A heartburn type of pain is associated with esophageal reflux. Chest pain similar to anginal pain may result from esophageal distention and obstruction. Abdominal pain may be visceral (diffuse, poorly localized), somatic (sharp, well localized), or referred (at a distance from the source but in the same dermatome).
- Nausea and vomiting are manifestations of many GI and other disorders. Alterations in bowel motility or integrity are causative factors. Excess gas may result from altered motility or lack of digestive enzymes. Gas is generated by swallowed air and bacterial action on nutritional substrates.
- Constipation is defined as small, infrequent (less than three per week), or difficult bowel movements. Lack of exercise, lack of dietary fiber, slowed peristalsis, and pathologic conditions that alter motility (e.g., obstruction) may produce constipation.
- Diarrhea is defined as an increased frequency and fluidity of bowel movements. Acute infection, stress, fecal impaction, malabsorption, and ingestion of bowel irritants may produce diarrhea. Osmotic diarrhea is due to increased amounts of poorly absorbed solutes in the intestine. Secretory diarrhea is usually due to toxins that stimulate intestinal fluid secretion and impair absorption. Exudative diarrhea (mucus, blood, protein) results from inflammatory processes. A decreased transit time in the small intestine results in diarrhea because the absorptive capacity of the large intestine is exceeded.

Disorders of the Mouth and Esophagus

The mouth and the esophagus are the portals of entry for nutrients into the GI tract. An impairment in the proper functioning of these structures may have a profound effect on the ability of the individual to ingest adequate nutrients and begin the initial steps of the digestive process. Although disorders of the mouth and esophagus may not be acute, life-threatening emergencies, they may have severe long-term consequences for the well-being of the individual experiencing them.

ORAL INFECTIONS

Stomatitis

Etiology. Stomatitis is defined as an inflammation of the oral mucosa that may extend to the buccal mucosa, lips, and palate. Among its causes are pathogenic organisms, including bacteria and viruses; mechanical trauma; exposure to such irritants as alcohol, tobacco, and other chemical substances; certain medications, particularly chemotherapeutic agents; radiation therapy; and nutritional deficiencies, especially vitamin deficiencies. Stomatitis is a common manifestation of human immunodeficiency syndrome.[9] Stomatitis may also be idiopathic; that is, with no identifiable cause.[10]

Acute Herpetic Stomatitis

Etiology and Clinical Manifestations. One of the most commonly encountered types of stomatitis is acute herpetic stomatitis, also called *herpetic gingivostomatitis* or *cold sores*. It is caused by infection with herpes simplex virus, which has an affinity for the skin and nervous system. This type of stomatitis is commonly acquired by children between the ages of 1 and 3 years, although it may occur at any age. In primary infection, a brief period of prodromal tingling and itching may be present along with fever and pharyngitis. Vesicles may erupt on any part of the oral mucosa, particularly the tongue, gums, and cheeks. Vesicles form on an erythematous base, eventually rupture, and leave a painful ulcer. Once herpes simplex virus is acquired, it remains latent in the dorsal ganglia of the spinal cord and may be reactivated by physical or emotional stressors.

Treatment. The pharmacologic therapy used for stomatitis depends on its cause. The antiviral drugs acyclovir, famciclovir, and valacyclovir have been approved for treating acute herpetic stomatitis. Unfortunately, in a large number of cases stomatitis is idiopathic or not amenable to specific therapy (e.g., stomatitis due to chemotherapy). In all types of stomatitis, measures designed to provide adequate oral hygiene and increase comfort in the oral cavity will be helpful in preventing decreased nutritional intake during the period of inflammation and assist in promoting the healing process. Topical mucosal barriers and corticosteroids may be of some benefit, e.g., triamcinolone (Kenalog) in Orabase,[9] while pentoxyphylline, colchicines, and thalidomide have been used for recalcitrant cases.[11]

ESOPHAGEAL DISORDERS

Gastroesophageal Reflux. Gastroesophageal reflux disease (GERD) is the backflow of gastric contents into the esophagus through the LES. GERD may or may not produce symptoms.

Pathogenesis. The production of GERD is a multifactorial process. Any condition or agent that alters the closure strength and efficacy of the LES or increases intraabdominal pressure may predispose an individual to GERD. For example, the closure strength of the LES may be adversely affected by the intake of fatty foods, caffeine, and ethanol; cigarette smoking; sleep position; or obesity. In addition, pharmacologic agents such as progesterone-containing medications (e.g., birth control pills), narcotics, benzodiazepines, calcium-channel blockers, and theophylline may decrease the pressure of the LES. Pregnancy increases the risk of reflux both by increasing intraabdominal pressure and through hormonal mechanisms. Certain anatomic features, especially hiatal hernia, have been associated with GERD. The extent and severity of damage to the esophagus from GERD reflect the frequency and duration of exposure to refluxed material, as well as the volume and acidity of the gastric juices being refluxed.[3,4,12,13] The role of *Helicobacter pylori*, a cause of gastric and duodenal ulceration, in GERD is poorly understood and controversial.[14]

Clinical Manifestations. The most common manifestations of GERD are heartburn, regurgitation, chest pain, and dysphagia. These symptoms are related to **reflux esophagitis,** which is esophageal inflammation caused by the highly acidic refluxed material. Complications of persistent GERD include esophageal strictures, Barrett esophagus (see Complications section), and pulmonary symptoms—cough, asthma and laryngitis—due to reflux into the breathing passages.

Treatment. Appropriate therapy is directed to increasing LES pressure, enhancing esophageal clearance, improving gastric emptying, and suppressing gastric acidity. Dietary and behavioral changes, such as avoiding tobacco and aggravating food and drink, are indicated for all patients, while over-the-counter antacids and histamine (H_2)-blocking medications may be effective for occasional GERD. Proton pump inhibitors (PPI) are the mainstays of treatment for chronic GERD and have proven very successful in halting and even reversing the changes of chronic GERD.[15] If reflux esophagitis has progressed in severity, tissue damage, including ulceration, fibrotic scarring, and strictures, may be present in the distal third of the esophagus. Upper GI endoscopy is indicated for patients with ongoing symptoms, and some patients with stricture may require endoscopic dilatation. Surgical intervention, such as thoracoscopic Nissan fundoplication, may be helpful for intractable GERD.[16]

Complication. **Barrett esophagus** is a complication of chronic GERD and represents columnar tissue replacing the normal squamous epithelium of the distal esophagus. It carries a significant risk for esophageal cancer, and patients with Barrett esophagus should undergo regular endoscopic screening for cancer, along with pharmacologic control of their reflux.[17]

Hiatal Hernia. A **hiatal hernia** is a defect in the diaphragm that allows a portion of the stomach to pass through the diaphragmatic opening into the thorax. Two types of hiatal hernia are commonly recognized: (1) a sliding hernia, in which both a portion of the stomach and the gastroesophageal junction slip up into the thorax so that the gastroesophageal junction is above the diaphragmatic opening, and (2) a paraesophageal hernia, in which a part of the greater curvature of the stomach rolls through the diaphragmatic defect (Figure 36-2). "Mixed" hiatal hernias with features of both of these types may also occur. Sliding hernias are three to ten times more common than paraesophageal and mixed hernias combined. The incidence of hiatal hernia increases with age, and this form of hernia occurs more often in women than in men.

Etiology. Although the cause of the anatomic deformity leading to hiatal hernia is not well understood, certain conditions seem to predispose to loosening of the muscular band around the esophageal and diaphragmatic junction. Conditions in which intraabdominal pressure increases, such as ascites, pregnancy, obesity, and chronic straining or coughing, have been associated with the development of hiatal hernia.

Clinical Manifestations and Treatment. Individuals with hiatal hernia are predisposed to GERD and may experience symptoms such as heartburn, chest pain, and dysphagia. Ulcerations can develop along the mucosal surface of the stomach as it slides through the diaphragmatic opening, so-called Cameron ulcers. This is a rare cause of chronic upper GI blood loss.[18] Hiatal hernia can be a potentially life-threatening situation if a large portion of the stomach becomes caught above the diaphragm and is incarcerated, although this is extremely rare. Medical therapy for hiatal hernia is exactly the same as that for GERD, detailed above. Indications for surgery would be acute incarceration or intractable reflux.

Mallory-Weiss Syndrome

Etiology. **Mallory-Weiss syndrome** is bleeding caused by a tear in the mucosa or submucosa of the cardia or lower portion of the esophagus. The tear is usually longitudinal and is primarily caused by forceful or prolonged vomiting in which the upper esophageal sphincter fails to relax during the vomiting process. Approximately 75% of individuals with Mallory-Weiss syndrome are men with a history of excessive ingestion of alcohol or salicylates.[2] Other factors and conditions that may contribute to the development of esophageal tearing in Mallory-Weiss syndrome are coughing, straining during bowel movements, trauma, hiatal hernia, esophagitis, and gastritis.

Clinical Manifestations and Treatment. Manifestations of Mallory-Weiss syndrome include vomiting of blood and passing of large amounts of blood rectally after an episode of forceful vomiting. Epigastric or back pain may also be present.

Diaphragm · Esophagus · Hiatus · Stomach — Normal stomach

Part of fundus above diaphragm — Sliding hiatal hernia

Sac and peritoneum in mediastinum — Paraesophageal hernia

FIGURE 36-2 Types of hiatal hernia. (From Gould BE: *Pathophysiology for the health professions,* ed 2, Philadelphia, 2002, Saunders, p 383.)

Bleeding may range in severity from mild to massive. It is often profuse when the tear is near the cardia of the stomach and may proceed to fatal shock in this circumstance. Identification is made by endoscopic examination during an episode of acute upper GI bleeding. The majority of patients require at least one blood transfusion, but in most cases bleeding stops spontaneously.[19] Control of active bleeding may be achieved through endoscopic multipolar electric coagulation or similar techniques, epinephrine injection, or through interventional radiologic procedures (vasopressin infusion, Gelfoam embolization, etc.).[7,20] In selected cases, surgical intervention may be necessary.

Esophageal Varices. Esophageal varices represent a complication of portal hypertension, which in Western society is generally the result of cirrhosis due to alcoholism or viral hepatitis. In developing tropical countries, chronic infection with *Schistosoma* species is a major cause of portal hypertension. Varices will affect more than half of cirrhotic patients, and approximately 30% of them experience an episode of variceal hemorrhage within 2 years of the diagnosis of varices.[21] The diagnosis and management of varices is discussed in detail in Chapter 38.

KEY POINTS

- Stomatitis is inflammation of the oral mucosa. It may result from pathogenic organisms, trauma, chemical irritants, chemotherapy, radiation therapy, or nutritional deficiencies.
- Common esophageal disorders are GERD with esophagitis, hiatal hernia, and bleeding. Reflux esophagitis is manifested as heartburn, chest pain, and dysphagia and may be precipitated by gastric overdistention or poor LES tone. Fatty foods, cigarettes, morphine, theophylline, and progesterone may inhibit LES tone.
- Hiatal hernias may be sliding or rolling (paraesophageal). Conditions that increase intraabdominal pressure predispose to the development of hiatal hernia. Esophageal reflux often accompanies hiatal hernia, and the manifestations are similar: heartburn, chest pain, dysphagia.
- Bleeding from the esophagus may pose a life-threatening situation. Mallory-Weiss syndrome is bleeding caused by tears in the lower end of the esophagus or upper part of the stomach. Alcohol and salicylate ingestion appear to be factors. Esophageal bleeding may also be precipitated by coughing, straining, or esophagitis. Rupture of esophageal varices is a dreaded complication of cirrhosis with portal hypertension and carries a high mortality rate.

Alterations in Integrity of the Gastrointestinal Tract Wall

Alterations in the integrity of the GI tract may occur at any location along the 30 feet or so of its length resulting from an infection, inflammatory process, or weakness of the intestinal wall.

Such alterations may present as an acute, life-threatening situation or as a chronic, disabling condition. When the integrity of the GI tract wall is compromised, the ability to perform digestive and absorptive functions may also be compromised because the surface area or motility (or both) are altered.

INFLAMMATION OF THE STOMACH AND INTESTINES

Gastritis

Etiology. **Gastritis** is defined as an inflammation of the stomach lining. Acute inflammation of the stomach lining may occur after the ingestion of alcohol, aspirin, or irritating substances, as well as due to viral, bacterial, or autoimmune illnesses. (Some experts prefer use of the term *gastropathy* for toxic gastric inflammation, and *gastritis* for inflammation due to infection or autoimmune disorders.)[22] In Western countries, overuse of nonsteroidal antiinflammatory drugs (NSAIDs) and overindulgence in alcohol and tobacco are preeminent causes of acute gastritis.

Pathogenesis. Chronic gastritis is currently the focus of extensive research. The factors promoting chronic gastritis have always been poorly understood. However, in 1983, identification of the bacterium *Helicobacter pylori* proved to be a landmark event.[23] Since that time, *H. pylori* has generated worldwide attention for its role in the promotion of chronic gastritis, peptic ulcer disease (PUD), and gastric carcinoma. Circumstantial evidence suggests that the mode of transmission of *H. pylori* is primarily person to person.[24] Some studies suggest a fecal-oral route, with the possibility of a reservoir in water sources.

It is now known that *H. pylori* causes chronic, superficial gastritis in virtually all infected persons.[3] Once established in the gastric mucosa, *H. pylori* sets up a destructive pattern of persistent inflammation. This persistent inflammation may resolve spontaneously, with clearance of the organism over time, leading to a decreased prevalence of *H. pylori* infection among older individuals. Consequences of *H. pylori* gastritis include peptic ulcer disease (PUD) (discussed below), atrophic gastritis, gastric adenocarcinoma, and mucosa-associated lymphoid tissue (MALT) lymphoma. The diagnosis and management of *H. pylori* infection will be discussed below.

Clinical Manifestations. While gastritis may be asymptomatic, manifestations of acute gastritis include anorexia, nausea, vomiting, and postprandial discomfort. Occasionally, **hematemesis** may occur in response to damage to the gastric epithelial mucosa. These manifestations usually disappear when the causative agent is removed, and the gastric epithelium undergoes a process of renewal after sloughing off the layer of damaged cells.

Gastroenteritis

Etiology. **Gastroenteritis** refers to inflammation of the stomach and small intestine, and may occur on an acute or chronic basis. Chronic gastroenteritis is usually the result of another GI disorder, such as UC, and is discussed in a later section. Acute gastroenteritis is the result of direct infection of the GI tract lining by a pathogenic organism such as Norwalk virus; or by the ingestion of preformed bacterial toxins (e.g., *Staphylococcus aureus, Bacillus cereus*); or by the ingestion of bacteria that produce toxins *(Clostridium perfringens)*. Acute gastroenteritis may also be caused by an imbalance in the normal bacterial flora of the GI tract precipitated by the introduction of an unusual bacterial strain, as may occur during travel.

Clinical Manifestations and Treatment. Acute gastroenteritis in adults is usually a self-limiting, nonfatal disease with manifestations of diarrhea, abdominal discomfort and pain, nausea, and vomiting. An elevated temperature and malaise may also be present. The manifestations vary according to the type of causative pathologic organism and the region of the GI tract affected. Many pathogenic organisms induce a severe secretory type of diarrhea (see the earlier discussion on the pathophysiologic mechanism of secretory diarrhea). In children and the elderly, fluid losses from diarrhea and vomiting can have serious consequences and may be life-threatening, particularly in underdeveloped countries. Supportive treatment designed to provide fluid and electrolyte replacement may thus be required for many patients experiencing severe acute gastroenteritis.

Peptic Ulcer Disease. The term **peptic ulcer disease** refers to disorders of the upper GI tract caused by the action of acid and pepsin. These disorders may include injury to the mucosa of the esophagus, stomach, or duodenum and may range from a slight mucosal injury to severe ulceration (Figures 36-3 and 36-4). Peptic ulcer disease seems to be the result of an increase in factors that tend to injure the mucosa relative to factors that tend to protect it. Factors such as the gastric mucosal barrier and the ability of the mucosa to renew

epithelium serve to protect it against injury. On the other hand, the presence of acid, which potentiates the actions of pepsin and other injurious substances such as aspirin and NSAIDs, will promote injury to the mucosa.

Previously, PUD was attributed to stress and an irritative diet, and treatment revolved around removing any hint of spice in diet and lifestyle. In recent years, however, research has suggested that the organism *H. pylori* is a major precipitant of PUD, along with NSAIDs. A brief review of the current understanding of the pathogenesis of PUD is presented as a basis for further discussion of the manifestations and management of PUD.

Etiology and Pathogenesis. Most peptic ulcers arise in the stomach and duodenum. Although the precise mechanisms of ulcer formation remain incompletely understood, the process involves the interplay of mucosal defense mechanisms, pepsin, and acid.[3] In the stomach, it is thought that a breakdown in the normally protective epithelial lining occurs (Figure 36-5). In the formation of a gastric peptic ulcer, the barrier of the epithelial layer and the slightly alkaline layer of mucus may be interrupted by the chronic presence of such injurious substances as aspirin, NSAIDs, alcohol, and bile acids, which may be regurgitated from the duodenum. These substances apparently strip away the surface mucus and cause degeneration of the epithelial cell membranes, with diffusion of acid into the gastric epithelial wall.

Inappropriate excess secretion of acid is a major factor in the development of PUD in the duodenum (Figure 36-6). Studies have documented that the basal activity of the vagus nerve is increased in persons with PUD of the duodenum, particularly during a fasting state and at night. This stimulates the pyloric antrum cells to release gastrin, which travels via the bloodstream and acts on the gastric parietal cells to release hydrochloric acid (HCl). The result is an inappropriately high level of HCl in the duodenum.

H. pylori has a key role in promoting both gastric and duodenal ulcer formation (Figure 36-7). It has been reported that up to 75% of persons with duodenal ulcers and 60% of

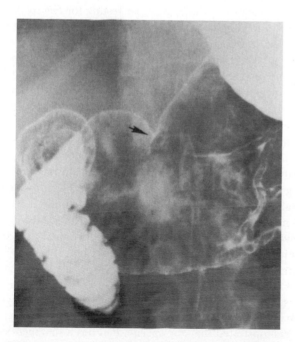

FIGURE 36-3 Radiograph of an ulcer in the lesser curvature of the stomach *(arrow)*. (From Laufer I: *Double contrast gastrointestinal radiology with endoscopic correlation,* Philadelphia, 1979, Saunders.)

FIGURE 36-4 Photograph of an ulcer. (From Sleisenger MH, Fordtran JS, editors: *Gastrointestinal disease,* ed 5, Philadelphia, 1993, Saunders.)

FIGURE 36-5 Lesions caused by peptic ulcer disease. (From Phipps WJ et al: *Medical-surgical nursing: health and illness perspectives,* ed 7, St Louis, 2003, Mosby, p 1027.)

FIGURE 36-6 Duodenal bulbar ulcer. (From Sleisenger MH, Fordtran JS, editors: *Gastrointestinal disease,* ed 5, Philadelphia, 1993, Saunders.)

persons with gastric ulcers have *H. pylori* infection.[3] *H. pylori* thrives in acidic conditions; thus, infection with *H. pylori* renders a person with PUD subject to a slow rate of ulcer healing and a high rate of recurrence, and clearance of *H. pylori* promotes ulcer healing.[25] Although the precise mechanisms of the development of PUD remain complex and poorly understood, *H. pylori* virulence is associated with several factors, including the presence of unique, lengthy DNA sequences known as *pathogenicity islands*, particularly the *cytotoxin-associated gene A* (CagA).[26]

Other cofactors in the development of PUD have been investigated. Stress has long been considered a key factor in PUD. Glucocorticoids released in response to stress may have a role in the promotion of excess acid production or the destruction of gastric mucosal defenses. Smoking is an important risk factor, as identified by epidemiologic studies showing that PUD is twice as likely to develop in smokers as in nonsmokers.[27] In addition, smoking is related to poor ulcer healing and high rates of ulcer recurrence. Heredity is thought to have a role in the development of PUD. Certain patterns of gastrin release and pepsin secretion have been identified as genetic traits in families with an increased incidence of PUD.[16] Somewhat surprisingly, there is little evidence of a pathogenic role for alcohol, spicy foods, and caffeine.[3]

Clinical Manifestations and Diagnoses. Manifestations of PUD include epigastric burning pain that is usually relieved by the intake of food (especially dairy products) or antacids. The pain of gastric ulcers typically occurs on an empty stomach but may present soon after a meal. Duodenal ulcer pain classically occurs 2 to 3 hours after a meal and is relieved by further food ingestion. Other manifestations that may occur in individuals with PUD include nausea, abdominal upset, and chest discomfort. A significant proportion of ulcers are asymptomatic, and life-threatening complications, such as GI bleeding, may occur in patients with no warning. The symptoms of PUD are not specific enough to allow for a diagnosis, and malignant conditions can mimic benign PUD.

Diagnosis can be accomplished by upper GI barium contrast radiography or by endoscopy. The finding of a duodenal ulcer indicates a high probability of *H. pylori* and a low probability of malignancy, and the condition can be managed on this basis. All gastric ulcers should be visualized with endoscopy and biopsied to rule out malignancy and confirm the presence of *H. pylori*.[3] Whether testing for *Helicobacter* is necessary for uncomplicated duodenal ulcers, given the very high pretest probability, is somewhat controversial. Most authorities do recommend testing for this organism in the case of gastric ulcers. Testing modalities include noninvasive tests such as the urease breath test and serology, and endoscopic tests such as the tissue urease test, histology, and bacterial culture.[28]

Treatment. The major treatment objectives for PUD are to encourage healing of the injured mucosa by reducing gastric acidity and to prevent recurrence. Proton pump inhibitors are generally given to block acid secretion. Agents such as sucralfate form a protective coating over the injured mucosa and may be useful under some circumstances. Eradication of *H. pylori* infection with antibiotics has led to a marked reduction in the recurrence rate of PUD to less than 10%.[26,29,30]

In addition to these pharmacologic strategies, such measures as smoking cessation, avoidance of aspirin and NSAIDs, and stress reduction are all part of a comprehensive program to manage PUD. At the present time, no conclusive research has demonstrated that any specific diet has a therapeutic effect. Susceptible people are generally advised to avoid foods that seem to exacerbate symptoms, including caffeinated beverages and alcohol.

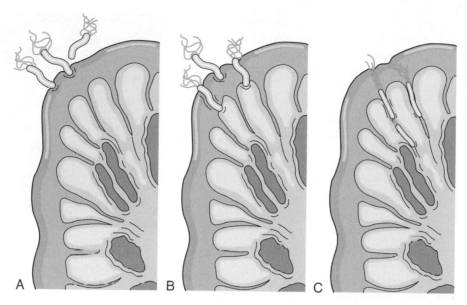

FIGURE 36-7 Penetration of the mucosal layer by *Helicobacter pylori*. **A,** After penetration, *H. pylori* forms clusters near membranes of surface epithelial cells. **B,** Some attach to the cell membrane. **C,** Others lodge between the epithelial cells.

INFLAMMATORY BOWEL DISEASE

The term **inflammatory bowel disease (IBD)** refers to the two separate disease entities of UC and Crohn disease. IBD is generally a life-altering chronic illness with serious consequences for people and their families who must cope with it. Both UC and Crohn disease have their onset most commonly in childhood and young adulthood, with obviously profound implications. This section describes the pathophysiologic aspects of UC and Crohn disease; a later section in this chapter discusses the psychosocial aspects of IBD.

Ulcerative Colitis. Ulcerative colitis (Figure 36-8) is an inflammatory disease of the mucosa of the rectum and colon. Approximately one-fifth of patients have total colitis, one-third have subtotal disease extending beyond the sigmoid, and one-half have disease limited to the rectum and rectosigmoid.[3] The changes are usually most severe in the rectum and extend for a variable extent around the colon, although there are several exceptions to this general rule. IBD is typically characterized by exacerbations and remissions. Its causes are poorly understood, but recent research has focused on genetic, environmental, and immunologic factors.[31] The immunologic basis for the disease is supported by the fact that UC frequently accompanies other autoimmune conditions such as thyroid disease and pernicious anemia. The incidence in North America is about 15 per 100,000.

Etiology and Clinical Manifestations. Ulcerative colitis begins as an inflammation at the base of the crypts of Lieberkühn. Damage to the crypt epithelium results, with eventual invasion of leukocytes and the formation of abscesses in the crypts. When multiple abscesses form in close proximity and begin to coalesce, large areas of ulcerations develop in the epithelium. Concurrent with this destructive process are attempts at repair of damaged tissue, along with the development of fragile and

FIGURE 36-8 Ulcerative colitis. (From Sleisenger MH, Fordtran JS, editors: *Gastrointestinal disease,* ed 5, Philadelphia, 1993, Saunders.)

highly vascularized granulation tissue. The manifestations of UC are the result of these processes and include abdominal pain, diarrhea, and rectal bleeding. Bleeding occurs as a result of mucosal destruction and ulceration, as well as damage to newly developed granulation tissue. Diarrhea is a result of the mucosal destruction in the colon, which leads to a decreased ability of the bowel to absorb water and sodium and thus to an increased volume of fluid in the intestinal contents.

The progression of UC may be highly variable. In some individuals it may have very mild manifestations; in others it may rapidly progress to a life-threatening disorder. Five percent to 10% of persons with UC have only one attack, with no further recurrence. However, 65% to 75% of those with UC experience an intermittent series of exacerbations and remissions. Rarely, patients with UC will manifest toxic megacolon, a life-threatening condition in which the colon becomes massively enlarged. This condition generally requires urgent colectomy. A number of conditions in other organ systems complicate UC, the most devastating of which is the relentlessly progressive liver condition primary sclerosing cholangitis, which occurs in 3% of UC patients.[3]

An additional concern is increased risk for the development of colon cancer in persons who have had UC for more than 7 to 10 years. Authorities recommend monitoring these individuals carefully with regular endoscopy and biopsy. The presence of high-grade dysplasia should prompt consideration of prophylactic complete colectomy. Recent surgical advances, such as the ileoanal pouch, have allowed colectomy patients to avoid colostomy and have close to normal bowel function.

Treatment. Management of UC is complex and ever evolving. Corticosteroids have long been the mainstay of treatment of acute exacerbations, but side effects limit their long-term use. Patients with signs of systemic toxicity, especially those with impending or full-blown toxic megacolon, should receive broad-spectrum antibiotics. Important categories of disease-modifying agents include the salicylate analogs, and immunomodulating agents such as azathioprine and mercaptopurine. Intravenous followed by oral cyclosporine is a relatively new treatment for steroid-refractory UC that may help patients avoid colectomy.[32] Infliximab (Remicade) is another option for refractory UC whose exact role has yet to be determined.[33]

Crohn Disease. **Crohn disease,** also called *regional enteritis and granulomatous colitis,* is an inflammation of the GI tract that extends through all layers of the intestinal wall (Figure 36-9). It most commonly affects the proximal portion of the colon and, less often, the terminal ileum. It may affect multiple portions of the colon, with intervening normal areas left in between the affected regions. The manifestations of Crohn disease differ in some respects from those of UC, although some overlap may occur and distinction may be difficult. In Crohn disease, abdominal pain is often constant and is usually in the right lower quadrant of the abdomen. A palpable abdominal mass may be present in the right lower quadrant, reflecting significant ileocecal involvement. The stool may be bloody, although not usually to the extent as with UC. The cause of Crohn disease is unknown at the present time. There are fascinating parallels with UC as well as unexpected distinctions. For instance, smoking has been shown to protect against UC but to increase the risk of Crohn disease.[34] The incidence in North America is approximately 5 per 100,000, and up to 5% of people with Crohn disease have one or more affected relatives.

Etiology and Pathogenesis. Certain features of the pathogenesis of Crohn disease differ from those of UC. Crohn disease appears to be the result of a process in which the lymphoid and lymphatic structures of the GI tract become blocked. Subsequent engorgement and inflammation of surrounding tissue leads to the development of deep linear ulcers in the bowel wall. Eventually, all layers of the GI tract wall may become involved, and the portion of intestine that is affected may become thickened by fibrous scar tissue. Deep fissures

FIGURE 36-9 Crohn disease. (From Sleisenger MH, Fordtran JS, editors: *Gastrointestinal disease,* ed 5, Philadelphia, 1993, Saunders.)

may develop into fistulas, which may extend into adjacent tissue of other organs such as the bladder wall or even the skin.[2]

Clinical Manifestations. The manifestations of Crohn disease are the result of the pathologic changes described above, as the bowel becomes incapable of adequately absorbing the intestinal contents. Complications such as perianal fissures, fistulae, and abscesses are common in Crohn disease and may be the symptoms that lead individuals to seek health care. The onset and course of Crohn disease may vary a great deal; unlike UC, the symptoms present during a period of Crohn exacerbation may be subtle but persistent. At the present time, it is unclear whether a significantly increased incidence of intestinal cancer occurs in persons with Crohn disease. However, when Crohn disease involves the large bowel, the risk of colorectal cancer appears to be similar to that of UC of similar extent.[35] Toxic megacolon and primary sclerosing cholangitis also occur with Crohn disease but are much less frequent than in patients with UC.

Treatment. Because the etiology of Crohn disease is unknown, therapeutic strategies are focused on alleviating and reducing inflammation. Therapeutic drug categories are similar to those for UC. The antibiotic metronidazole is particularly useful for colonic Crohn disease. New types of treatments include the anti–tumor necrosis factor agent infliximab, which has shown particular success, as well as other investigational anticytokine treatments.[31] Despite these advances, there is no cure for this challenging condition.

ENTEROCOLITIS

Antibiotic-Associated Colitis (Pseudomembranous Colitis)

Etiology. **Antibiotic-associated colitis** (AAC), also known as **pseudomembranous colitis,** is an acute inflammation and necrosis of the large intestine caused primarily by *Clostridium difficile,* usually affecting the mucosa but sometimes extending to other layers.[36] Exposure to antibiotics is the major factor predisposing to the development of this disorder, and patients with cancer or who have undergone abdominal surgery are at particular risk. The disease is mediated by bacterial toxins, leading to mucosal necrosis and the characteristic pseudomembrane composed of leukocytes, mucus, fibrin, and inflammatory cells.

Clinical Manifestations and Treatment. Resulting manifestations include diarrhea (often bloody), abdominal pain, fever, and rarely, colonic perforation. AAC is a major cause of fever among hospitalized patients receiving antibiotics. Treatment involves stopping the offending antibiotic, if possible, treating ischemia and other contributing conditions, and using antibiotics such as oral metronidazole or vancomycin. Recurrences are relatively common and may necessitate retreatment.

Necrotizing Enterocolitis

Etiology. **Necrotizing enterocolitis** (NEC) is a disorder occurring most often in premature infants (less than 34 weeks gestation) and infants with low birth weight (less than 5 lb or 2.25 kg). This disorder is characterized by diffuse or patchy intestinal necrosis accompanied by sepsis.

Clinical Manifestations and Treatment. Early manifestations include a distended abdomen and stomach. The major complication of NEC is intestinal perforation, which may necessitate surgery. Various theories regarding the etiologic progression of NEC include perinatal oxygen deficit with insufficient blood flow to the viscera, and the use of hypertonic feeding formulas in newborn infants. Over 90% of infants with NEC have a history of milk feeding as well. A special form of necrotizing enterocolitis, called *typhlitis,* may afflict adult cancer patients with neutropenia and carries a grave prognosis. Management of neonatal and adult forms of NEC includes careful supportive care, including fluid management and broad-spectrum antibiotics. Early surgical consultation is essential for this syndrome, and surgery is necessary for patients with evidence of significant ischemia or perforation.

Appendicitis

Etiology. The most common cause of emergency surgery on the abdomen, **appendicitis** is an inflammation of the vermiform appendix. The classic hypothesis suggests that obstruction of the appendiceal lumen, usually by a fecalith or, less commonly, lymphoid hyperplasia or parasitic worms, causes most cases of appendiceal inflammation. In an unknown number of cases appendiceal inflammation may be self-limited and may remit (e.g., with relief of the obstruction). If left unchecked, inflammation generally leads to necrosis of the appendix, with subsequent abscess formation and life-threatening peritonitis. Rarely appendicitis may occur in a subacute or stuttering fashion over several days or weeks.

Clinical Manifestations and Treatment. Appendicitis is twice as common before age 45 years as after, and affects men somewhat more often than women. This peak incidence is between ages 10 and 19 years. The earliest manifestation of appendicitis is generalized periumbilical pain accompanied by nausea and, occasionally, diarrhea. The pain is often described as "migrating" or localizing to the lower right abdomen (**McBurney's point**) due to distention of the serosa from inflammatory edema, at which time fever usually manifests. Experienced

FIGURE 36-10 Colonic diverticula are evident as small outpouchings of colonic mucosa through the muscular tunicas *(arrow).* (From Sleisenger MH, Fordtran JS, editors: *Gastrointestinal disease,* ed 5, Philadelphia, 1993, Saunders.)

surgeons generally operate in suspicious cases. Less typical cases should be assessed with computed tomography (CT), or ultrasound, if the patient is a child or pregnant women or if CT is not readily available. Such an approach yields a relatively low false-positive surgical rate of around 5%.[3] Surgical removal of the appendix, either through an open procedure or laparoscopically, is the treatment of choice for appendicitis. Administration of antibiotics with replacement of fluid and electrolytes may be necessary. Localized abscesses secondary to perforation may be managed with percutaneous tube drainage and antibiotics alone, if there are no signs of diffuse peritonitis.[37]

Diverticular Disease

Etiology. The term diverticular disease generally refers to **diverticulosis**, or the presence of diverticula in the colon. Diverticula are acquired herniations of the mucosa and submucosa through the muscular coat of the colon (Figure 36-10) that probably result from a combination of structural and functional factors. In particular, areas of weakness in the bowel wall, especially where blood vessels enter, are subject to damage from high intraluminal pressures. Colonic diverticulosis is very common in Western countries and is associated with a diet low in fiber; this lack of fiber presumably fails to provide enough bulk to dampen pressure variations in the intestine. The prevalence of diverticulosis increases with age; about 30% of the general population at 60 years of age and about 80% at 80 years will have diverticula in the colon.[1] Most persons experience no manifestations of diverticulosis, and by itself diverticulosis is not considered a pathologic condition. However, when diverticula become inflamed, the condition is referred to as **diverticulitis** (see Box 36-1 for the terminology of diverticulosis).

Clinical Manifestations and Treatment. Inflammation of diverticula can lead to serious consequences such as the development of abscesses in the bowel wall, peritonitis, and intestinal obstruction. Manifestations of diverticulitis include acute lower abdominal pain (usually left lower quadrant in location), fever, and leukocytosis. Constipation is common, but one-quarter of patients may have diarrhea. During an acute episode of diverticulitis, the administration of broad-spectrum antibiotics is indicated, and on occasion percutaneous or surgical drainage of an abscess may be necessary. Recurrence of diverticulitis is common. Long-term complications include colonic strictures and fistulae, which may necessitate surgery.

KEY POINTS

- Alterations in intestinal wall integrity are generally a result of infection, inflammation, or weakness of the muscular layers. General symptoms include pain, bleeding, and diarrhea.
- Gastritis may be acute or chronic. Acute gastritis is generally precipitated by the ingestion of irritating substances, including alcohol and aspirin. Chronic gastritis may lead to atrophy of the gastric mucosa and the subsequent decreased production of HCl and intrinsic factor. Acute gastroenteritis is usually due to the ingestion of pathogenic organisms or preformed bacterial toxins and is characterized by self-limited vomiting, diarrhea, and abdominal pain.
- PUD may affect the esophagus, stomach, and duodenum. Gastric ulcers are thought to be due to breakdown of the protective mucus layer that normally prevents the diffusion of acids into gastric epithelia. Duodenal ulcers are caused by excessive acid secretion that is mediated by increased vagal activity. The organism *H. pylori* has been implicated in the pathogenesis of both gastric and duodenal ulcers. PUD is characterized by epigastric pain that is relieved by food or antacids. Perforation and bleeding are the major complications of PUD. Management of PUD is aimed at minimizing acid secretion and eradicating *H. pylori*.
- Ulcerative colitis and Crohn disease are chronic inflammatory disorders of the bowel. Ulcerative colitis (inflammation and ulceration of the colon and rectal mucosa) is manifested as bloody diarrhea and abdominal pain. There is an increased risk for colon cancer in persons who have had ulcerative colitis for more than 7 to 10 years. Crohn disease generally affects the proximal portion of the colon or the terminal ileum. Involvement of all layers of the intestinal wall predisposes to fistula

formation and malabsorption. Crohn disease may result from blockage and subsequent inflammation of lymphatic vessels. Chronic abdominal pain and diarrhea are common. Management of ulcerative colitis and Crohn disease is aimed at reducing inflammation.
- Acute inflammation of the intestinal wall may manifest as pseudomembranous enterocolitis or necrotizing enterocolitis. Abdominal pain, diarrhea, fever, and sepsis may result. The use of broad-spectrum antibiotics has been implicated in the etiologic development of pseudomembranous enterocolitis. Necrotizing enterocolitis, which occurs most often in infants, is thought to be due to bowel ischemia.
- Appendicitis is characterized by right lower quadrant pain, nausea and vomiting, and systemic signs of inflammation. Surgical removal of the appendix is necessary. Untreated appendicitis may result in rupture of the appendix and subsequent peritonitis; localized abscesses may be managed with tube drainage and antibiotics alone.
- Diverticula of the colon are very common in Western society because of a low intake of dietary fiber. Low-bulk stools result in the development of high intraluminal pressure, which predisposes to diverticula formation. Diverticulosis is generally asymptomatic. Inflammation of the diverticula, or diverticulitis, is manifested as fever and lower abdominal pain. Antibiotics and surgery may be required for management of complicated diverticulitis.

Alterations in Motility of the Gastrointestinal Tract

Disorders of the GI tract that alter its regular propulsive ability may have a negative effect on nutrient absorption. In the case of increased motility, the transit time of substances passing through the GI tract may be too fast to allow for adequate absorption. Conversely, a blockage or constriction of the GI tract may result in slowed or absent motility, which also prevents normal ingestion and processing of nutrient substances. As with alterations in the integrity of the GI tract wall, these alterations in GI motility may be acute or chronic, with many implications for the lifestyle of the patient.

MOTILITY DISORDERS

Irritable Bowel Syndrome. Irritable bowel syndrome is a complex entity that remains incompletely understood despite decades of intensive research. A clear definition of this syndrome has not been agreed on by all authorities; nevertheless, certain defining characteristics have been established. Typically, IBS is the presence of alternating diarrhea and constipation accompanied by abdominal cramping pain in the absence of any identifiable pathologic process in the GI tract.[3] (Other terms that have been used for this syndrome include *spastic colitis* and *irritable colon syndrome*.) Many authorities point out that the quantity of symptoms is not as important as their effect on the normal lifestyle of an individual. Persons with IBS may miss work, curtail their social life, and avoid sexual intercourse. This is an extremely common disorder affecting up to 20% of the U.S. population.[7] It is important to differentiate IBS, in which no pathologic process of the GI tract has been identified, from *inflammatory bowel disease,* in which a specific pathologic process is identifiable.

Etiology and Pathogenesis. The etiologic factors and pathogenesis of IBS are presently obscure. Most evidence seems to show that IBS is primarily a disorder of bowel motility. Some studies have demonstrated that the myoelectric activity of the colon of persons with IBS is altered. In particular, the slow wave activity of the colon, which usually occurs at a rate of three to six times per minute, is markedly increased in IBS.[1,3] Moreover, the sensory response to distension and stimulation seems to be heightened. Whether these findings are the result of genetic factors or such environmental factors as episodic infection, psychological stressors, or dietary patterns remains unknown.

Clinical Manifestations and Treatment. The manifestations of IBS may vary greatly, with some persons experiencing only diarrhea or constipation and others experiencing an alternating pattern of both. In addition to cramping abdominal pain, manifestations such as nausea and mucus in the stool may also be present. The severity of manifestations range from barely noticeable to incapacitating. Current therapy focuses on the use of antidiarrheal agents and antispasmodic medications as appropriate. No study has shown a clearly demonstrable benefit for a particular agent.[38] The 5-hydroxytryptamine (serotonin) 3 receptor antagonist alosetron has shown favorable results for the diarrhea-predominant form of IBS, while the 5-HT 4 receptor agonist tegaserod has been useful for patients with constipation as the main manifestation. However, both of these products have been associated with significant side effects, necessitating the Food and Drug Administration (FDA) to restrict their use. Ingestion of a diet with increased amounts of fiber has proved useful in many cases and is thought to promote a more normal pattern of myoelectric activity by providing a regular propulsive stimulus in the gut.[30] Perhaps more than with most GI disorders, patients with IBS may benefit from support groups, internet-based resources, and alternative therapies.

Intestinal Obstruction. Intestinal obstruction is partial or complete blockage of the intestinal lumen of the small or large bowel. Mechanical obstructions are caused by blockage of the intestine by adhesions, hernia, tumor, inflammation, and stricture (as in Crohn disease), impacted feces, volvulus, or intussusception. (Volvulus and intussusception are covered in more detail in the following sections.) Functional obstruction or ileus refers to the loss of propulsive ability by the bowel and may occur after abdominal surgery or in association with hypokalemia, peritonitis, severe trauma, spinal fractures, ureteral distention, and the administration of medications such as narcotics. Ogilvie syndrome is a rare severe motility problem characterized by recurrent bouts of ileus.

Etiology and Pathogenesis. The most common location for gastrointestinal obstruction is the small bowel (90% of cases). The most frequent contributing factors are previous abdominal surgery with adhesions and congenital abnormalities of the bowel. Metastatic carcinoma, particularly cancer of the intestinal tract or female reproductive organs, is an important cause of obstruction and should be considered in patients with obstruction who have never had abdominal surgery. The severity and types of symptoms initially accompanying an intestinal obstruction vary with its cause and location.

With obstruction of the bowel lumen, fluid and gas begin to accumulate proximal to the obstructed location. The distention produced by trapped fluid and gas causes water and electrolytes to be secreted into the obstructed lumen of the small bowel. Distention also results in the impedance of venous return, and the bowel wall becomes edematous. The absorptive ability of the bowel wall is compromised, and fluid and gas continue to accumulate as additional water and electrolytes are secreted into the lumen. The pressure on the bowel wall exerted by the excess fluid and gas may result in leakage of fluid through the wall into the peritoneum, as well as necrosis of the bowel wall.

In addition to the process just described, other complications may be present with blockage of the intestinal lumen. Impairment of bowel circulation leads to ischemia, a process referred to as *strangulation.* Bacteria may translocate across the bowel wall into the bloodstream to produce fever and other signs of sepsis. As blood escapes from the engorged veins, significant loss of blood and plasma from the affected segment may result in the rapid development of shock. In addition, the strangulated segment may become gangrenous, with resulting peritonitis, or become perforated, with the leakage of highly toxic bacterial material into the peritoneal cavity.[3] If left untreated, a person with an intestinal obstruction of the small bowel has a high risk of death from shock and vascular collapse.

Clinical Manifestations and Treatment. The manifestations of an intestinal obstruction depend on its site and duration. Obstructions in the upper jejunal area usually result in vomiting, dehydration, and electrolyte depletion. In obstruction of the distal portion of the small bowel or ileus, constipation may be an early manifestation, with massive accumulation of fluid in the lumen occurring later. Dehydration may progress to hypovolemic shock if the obstruction is left untreated. In obstructions of the colon, massive gas distention may be present. The fluid and electrolyte losses associated with colonic obstruction may not be as severe as those seen in obstruction of the small bowel. Blockage of the colon by a tumor is the most common cause of colonic obstruction, and perforation of the bowel wall adjacent to the tumor may occur in association with an obstruction.

Therapeutic strategies for intestinal obstruction include surgical intervention to correct or remove the source of a mechanical obstruction. Supportive therapy, including decompression of the bowel with specialized tubes or endoscopy, and fluid and electrolyte replacement therapy may be needed during an acute obstructive episode.

Volvulus. **Volvulus** is twisting of the bowel on itself, causing intestinal obstruction and blood vessel compression (Figure 36-11). The two most common sites for the development of volvulus are the cecum and the sigmoid colon.[3] A volvulus may be the result of an anomaly of rotation, an ingested foreign body, or an adhesion; however, the cause cannot always be determined. Volvulus tends to occur in elderly individuals with coexistent medical conditions. With the sudden tight twisting of the bowel on its mesentery, blood flow to the bowel is impeded. Gangrene, necrosis, and perforation may develop, resulting in a life-threatening situation. If both ends of a bowel segment are twisted, a closed-loop obstruction results, with the manifestations described earlier for intestinal obstruction. Treatment varies according to the severity and location of the volvulus and includes the therapeutic approaches described for intestinal obstruction.[3,7]

Intussusception. **Intussusception** is a telescoping or invagination of a portion of the bowel into an adjacent distal portion (Figure 36-12). It is most common in infants and occurs three times more often in males than in females.[3] In most cases involving infants, the actual cause is unknown, although intussusception has been linked to viral infections[39] and the use of some forms of rotarvirus vaccine. In older children, it may be associated with alterations in intestinal motility or a condition called Meckel diverticulum, in which a congenital abnormality consisting of a blind tube is present in the distal end of the ileum. In adults, intussusception usually results from the presence of benign or malignant tumors.

As a bowel segment undergoes intussusception, peristalsis acts to pull more bowel along with it. The resulting area of tightened, invaginated bowel becomes edematous; venous engorgement with hemorrhage may occur. Intestinal obstruction of the bowel may develop, with eventual gangrene, shock, and perforation of the bowel if surgical treatment is delayed.[7]

Megacolon. **Megacolon** can be congenital or acquired at any age. Perhaps the most common cause in Western countries is prolonged constipation/obstipation, usually chronic in nature. This is particularly common in younger children who are dealing with the psychological aspects of toilet training and bowel control. Although most of these children are psychologically normal, a small number of children with **encopresis** have experienced sexual abuse, and its presence should be considered.[40] Significant voiding issues also plague the other end of the age spectrum, and constipation/obstipation in the elderly may lead to megacolon, particularly when the sufferer has relied on regular enemas or laxatives for many years.

Hirschprung disease (see below) is characterized by the congenital absence of autonomic smooth muscle ganglia. The aganglionic bowel segment contracts but without the reciprocal relaxation needed to propel the intestinal contents forward. Stasis of stool and dilation of the proximal end of the colon result in megacolon, or massive dilation of the colon. **Chagas disease** caused by *Trypanosoma cruzii* is a common cause of acquired colon neuronal dysfunction and megacolon in Central and South America but is rarely seen in the United States. As discussed earlier in the chapter, antibiotic-associated colitis may result in acute megacolon, which is a surgical emergency. Finally, the idiopathic syndrome of intestinal pseudo-obstruction (**Ogilvie syndrome**) may rarely result in megacolon.

Hirschsprung Disease. **Hirschsprung disease** is a congenital disorder of the large intestine in which the autonomic nerve ganglia in the smooth muscle are absent or markedly reduced. In 90% of individuals with Hirschsprung disease, the aganglionic segment is in the rectosigmoid area, but occasionally the entire colon may be affected.[3] Hirschsprung disease occurs in approximately 1 in 5000 live births and is occasionally familial.[41] It is more common in males than in females, with a ratio of 3.8:1.[3] The disease often coexists with other anomalies, particularly Down syndrome. Although Hirschsprung disease is most commonly identified in infants and children, it may be present in adults as a long-standing undiagnosed condition.

FIGURE 36-11 Volvulus. Intestine twists at least 180 degrees, causing obstruction and ischemia. (From Black JM et al: *Medical-surgical nursing: clinical management for positive outcomes,* ed 8, Philadelphia, 2008, Saunders, p 714.)

FIGURE 36-12 Intussusception. A portion of bowel telescopes into adjacent (usually distal) bowel. (From Black JM et al: *Medical-surgical nursing: clinical management for positive outcomes,* ed 8, Philadelphia, 2008, Saunders, p 714.)

In infants, Hirschsprung disease may have severe, life-threatening effects. Fecal stagnation may result in enterocolitis with bacterial overgrowth, profuse diarrhea, hypovolemic shock, and intestinal perforation. Interventions such as colonic lavage may be performed to empty the bowel until the infant is stable enough to withstand surgical intervention, which is the definitive treatment.

KEY POINTS

- IBS is manifested by bouts of alternating diarrhea and constipation in the absence of an identifiable GI pathologic process. The cause is unclear; however, the slow wave activity of the bowel is markedly increased. A high-fiber diet and antidiarrheal agents may be recommended.
- Intestinal obstructions may be mechanical or functional. Mechanical obstructions are due to adhesions, hernia, tumors, impacted feces, volvulus (twisting), or intussusception (telescoping). Mechanical obstructions are characterized by increased bowel sounds initially, accompanied by abdominal pain, nausea, and vomiting. Functional obstructions are due to conditions that inhibit peristalsis, such as narcotics, anesthesia, surgical manipulation, peritonitis, hypokalemia, and spinal cord injuries. Functional obstructions are characterized by the absence of bowel sounds. Uncorrected obstruction may lead to intestinal wall edema, ischemia, and necrosis. Bowel gangrene, sepsis, and shock can result. Surgical intervention or decompression with an intestinal tube is often required.
- Hirschsprung disease is a familial, congenital disorder of the large intestine in which the autonomic ganglia are reduced or absent. Stasis of stool and megacolon may occur in the abnormally innervated section of bowel. Megacolon can also be acquired as an adult.

Malabsorption

Malabsorption refers to failure of the GI tract to absorb or normally digest one or more dietary constituents.[1] It is typically manifested as diarrhea, with the passage of inappropriately processed intestinal contents resulting in impaired fluid absorption. A variety of pathologic processes produce malabsorption syndromes, including intestinal enzyme abnormalities (e.g., lactase deficiency), infection (e.g., AIDS enteritis), and radiation enteritis, among others. The types of malabsorption syndromes discussed here result from a mucosal disorder of the small bowel or from the surgical removal of portions of the stomach or small bowel.

MUCOSAL DISORDERS

Myriad disorders affect the mucosa of the small intestine. Because the small intestine is the principal site of digestion and absorption of nutrients, a defect in this area has the potential for causing malabsorption of fat, protein, carbohydrate, vitamins, and minerals. Crohn disease, described earlier, may result in damage to the mucosa of the distal portion of the ileum, which is the site of vitamin B_{12} and bile acid absorption. Other important mucosal disorders of the small intestine are celiac disease and tropical sprue.

Celiac Disease

Etiology. **Celiac disease** (also called celiac sprue) is characterized by intolerance of gluten, a protein in wheat and wheat products. Current research suggests that celiac sprue is an immune disorder triggered by exposure to gliadin (a specific wheat gluten) in genetically predisposed persons.[3,42] Environmental, genetic, and immune factors play pivotal roles in determining the nature of symptoms. The main pathologic finding is villus atrophy, with a decrease in the activity and amount of surface epithelial enzymes. The resulting malabsorption of ingested nutrients may promote malnutrition and severe debilitation.

Celiac disease affects twice as many females as males and may have a familial inheritance pattern. The incidence in the general population is 1 in 3000, and those affected are primarily of northwestern European ancestry. The onset of celiac disease may present in infancy, when gluten-containing products are first introduced into the diet, but is more common in the fourth and fifth decades.[43]

Diagnosis and Treatment. In the past the diagnosis of celiac disease relied on intestinal biopsy showing the typical pathologic manifestations. New blood tests assay for anti–tissue transglutaminase antibody (anti-ttG) and the more specific immunoglobulin A (IgA) endomysial antibody (EMA) have a high degree of sensitivity and specificity, although in general biopsy is still recommended for confirmation. Effective treatment includes the elimination of all gluten from the diet, which results in significant improvement in the intestinal mucosa, and the administration of supplemental iron, folate, and in specific cases B_{12} and fat-soluble vitamins (A, D, E, K). Refractory cases may be treated with oral corticosteroids or other immunomodulating agents.[3] Importantly, while the overall risk for malignancy is no higher than the general population, the incidence of certain types of intestinal malignancy, especially lymphoma, is modestly increased among sprue patients.[44]

Tropical Sprue

Etiology. **Tropical sprue or enteropathy** is a malabsorptive syndrome of unknown cause prevalent in equatorial countries. In tropical sprue, the mucosa of the small intestine atrophies, with resulting malabsorption, malnutrition, and B_{12} and folic acid deficiency. Although this entity often seems to occur in epidemics, no single organism has been implicated in its development. Its incidence is high in persons living in or visiting tropical climates, and it appears to affect adults more often than children.[5] While environmental factors seem preeminent, a genetic component may be present in some cases.

Clinical Manifestations and Treatment. The atrophy of the small intestinal mucosa may have severe effects. Massive malabsorption may result from failure of the mucosa to produce the enzymes needed for digestion. Manifestations include severe diarrhea with blood-tinged stools, abdominal distention, and steatorrhea (the presence of excess fat in the stool). In the Caribbean, tropical sprue is strongly linked to the presence of enterotoxin-producing coliforms and responds well to broad-spectrum antibiotics.[3] The response of patients from other areas (e.g., India) to treatment is less predictable than that of patients with Caribbean sprue. Treatment includes antidiarrheal medication and prolonged antimicrobial therapy as well as replacement of deficient vitamins, particularly folic acid.

MALABSORPTION DISORDERS AFTER SURGICAL INTERVENTION

Surgical procedures in which a portion of the stomach or small bowel is removed may result in loss of the ability to absorb nutrients properly, either through a loss of appropriate motility patterns or through a loss of the surface area of the small

bowel needed for adequate absorption. Two types of disorders of malabsorption may occur after surgical intervention on the stomach or small bowel: dumping syndrome and short-bowel syndrome.

Dumping Syndrome

Etiology. Dumping syndrome is a term used to describe the literal dumping of stomach contents into the proximal portion of the small intestine because of impaired gastric emptying (Figure 36-13). This loss of normal, gradual pyloric emptying may occur after removal of all or part of the stomach (gastrectomy), a procedure performed commonly for PUD in previous years, but more recently primarily for control of obesity.

Pathogenesis, and Clinical Manifestations. With the normal reservoir function of the stomach now impaired, a large volume of hyperosmolar food is dumped rapidly into the small intestine, with consequences that may be severe. The hyperosmolar

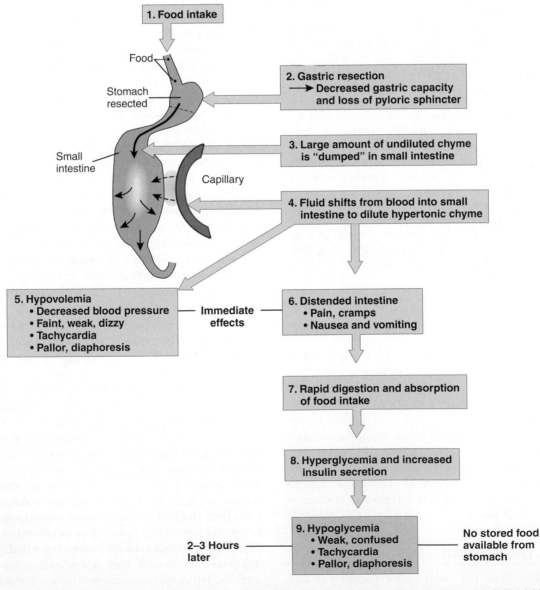

FIGURE 36-13 Dumping syndrome (postgastrectomy). (From Gould BE: *Pathophysiology for the health professions,* ed 2, Philadelphia, 2002, Saunders, p 390.)

contents of the small intestine draw water into the lumen and stimulate bowel motility, with manifestations of diarrhea and abdominal pain. In addition, the rapid absorption of a large amount of glucose and a subsequent rise in blood glucose levels promotes an excessive rise in plasma insulin. The elevated insulin level then causes a rapid fall in blood glucose levels 1 to 3 hours after a meal. This sudden reversal is referred to as "rebound hypoglycemia."[3]

Treatment. Persons who have undergone a gastrectomy procedure will require specific instruction regarding eating small meals six to eight times a day rather than three large meals. Restriction of carbohydrate intake may be needed to limit glucose absorption. Medications to reduce bowel motility have been helpful in promoting a more normal pattern of bowel function in this population.

Short-Bowel Syndrome

Etiology. **Short-bowel syndrome** refers to the severe diarrhea and significant malabsorption that develop after the surgical removal of large portions of the small intestine.

Pathogenesis and Clinical Manifestations. The severity of the manifestations depends on the amount and location of the bowel resected. In particular, removal of the distal two-thirds of the ileum and the ileocecal valve may result in severe malabsorption. Because the ileocecal valve serves to regulate the transit time of intestinal contents, its removal may promote a transit time that is too rapid for adequate absorption of nutrients. In addition, loss of large portions of the small intestine will result in a diminished ability to absorb water, electrolytes, protein, fat, carbohydrates, vitamins, and trace elements.

Treatment. The small intestine displays an amazing ability to adapt after bowel resection. The remaining villi may enlarge and lengthen, thus increasing the absorptive surface area of the bowel. The presence of orally ingested nutrients is needed for this adaptive process to occur, and a gradual increase in oral intake after bowel resection may promote gradual improvement in absorptive ability. Intravenous nutritional support may be required temporarily or indefinitely following surgical foreshortening of the gut.

KEY POINTS

- Malabsorption occurs when the small bowel fails to absorb one or more dietary components. Diarrhea and abdominal discomfort are the usual manifestations. Malabsorption may occur because of mucosal dysfunction (Crohn disease, celiac disease, tropical sprue), enzyme deficiencies, or surgical alterations that affect transit time and absorptive surface area.
- Celiac disease appears to be caused by a familial intolerance of gluten-containing foods. Ingestion of gluten leads to inflammation and atrophy of the intestinal villi. A reduced surface area and decreased brush border enzymes impair nutrient absorption.
- Dumping syndrome occurs with loss of pyloric sphincter regulation, generally after gastric surgery for ulcers

or cancer. Rapid dumping of chyme into the duodenum causes an osmotic shift of water into the lumen, and diarrhea. Glucose absorption may be rapid and lead to overshoot of insulin secretion and rebound hypoglycemia.
- Short-bowel syndrome follows surgical procedures involving removal of large sections of the small intestine. Rapid transit time and reduced surface area for absorption lead to diarrhea and malabsorption.

Neoplasms of the Gastrointestinal Tract

Neoplasms may develop in every region of the GI tract. They vary in their severity and in their ability to disrupt normal GI functioning. The most common neoplastic processes of the GI tract are summarized here; the reader may wish to refer to the chapter on neoplasms as a background for understanding these specific types of neoplasms occurring in the GI tract.

ESOPHAGEAL, GASTRIC, AND SMALL INTESTINAL CANCERS

Esophageal Cancer

Etiology. Esophageal cancer accounts for 1% to 2% of all cancers and affects men three times more often than women.[1] It usually develops in men older than 60 years, with a 1-year survival rate of less than 20%.[45] Although the cause of esophageal cancer is presently unknown, several predisposing factors have been identified, including genetic predisposition, dietary habits (especially ingestion of foods high in nitrosamine content), environmental exposures, and chronic irritation of the esophagus from heavy smoking and alcohol use. Chronic severe reflux, especially that associated with **achalasia,** is a prominent risk factor as well.

Most esophageal tumors are squamous cell carcinomas; fewer than 10% are adenocarcinomas. The incidence of adenocarcinoma of the gastroesophageal junction is increasing and seems to reflect an increased prevalence of **Barrett esophagus** (discussed earlier in the chapter). Interestingly, infection with *H. pylori* seems to protect against development of this form of esophageal cancer.[3,46]

Pathogenesis and Treatment. Tumors of the esophagus are usually infiltrating, and the disease may spread extensively to surrounding organs by way of the esophageal lymphatics at an early stage. Invasion of surrounding structures may lead to the formation of esophagobronchial or esophagopleural fistulas, with subsequent pneumonia or abscess. The tumor may partially constrict the lumen of the esophagus, and surgery, radiation therapy, or other measures may be considered to maintain a patent esophagus. Endoscopic procedures of benefit include stent placement and ablation of the tumor through heat probe and laser techniques. If the individual survives the initial extension of the tumor, the liver and lungs are the usual sites of distant metastasis.[45] Regardless of the cell type, the prognosis is extremely poor.

Gastric Carcinoma. Gastric carcinoma is common throughout the world; however, certain population groups appear to be at higher risk than others.[1,45] In Japan, the prevalence of gastric adenocarcinoma is about 10 times the prevalence in the United States. The incidence is higher in men older than 30 years than in other age and sex groups. The overall 5-year survival rate is approximately 10%, although the prognosis depends on the stage of the disease at the time of diagnosis.[45] Early stage gastric cancer has not penetrated the major muscle layer of the stomach wall and is associated with a more favorable survival rate than seen in more advanced disease.

Etiology. Research into the etiologic development of gastric cancer is a rapidly expanding area. A recent consensus Committee of the World Health Organization concluded that sufficient evidence has amassed that *H. pylori* has a role in promoting gastric cancer, with a twofold increased risk compared with that in uninfected individuals.[3] In particular, the development of multifocal atrophic gastritis induced by persistent *H. pylori* infection is a critical step in the development of gastric cancer.[14] Epstein-Barr virus is another viral oncogene that has been identified as contributing to the global burden of gastric cancer.[47] Other risk factors are similar to those for esophageal cancer, with the exception that alcohol is not a significant contributor to gastric carcinoma.[3] Aspirin use seems to be protective against stomach cancer.[48] Small numbers of gastric neoplasms may have different histologic characteristics, including lymphoma and carcinoid tumors, and have distinct clinical courses.

Clinical Manifestations and Treatment. Unfortunately, early gastric cancer typically has no manifestations and is rarely identified in countries that do not have a widespread screening program. Gastric carcinoma extends rapidly to the regional lymph nodes and surrounding organs by way of the lymphatic system, the blood stream, and direct extension through the wall of the stomach. Advanced gastric cancer (Figure 36-14) has penetrated the muscle layer of the stomach and produces manifestations such as anorexia, weight loss, and GI bleeding.

Surgical resection of the tumor with appropriate surrounding margins of tissue remains the only effective treatment for this cancer.

Small Intestinal Neoplasms. Neoplasms of the small intestine may be benign or malignant. Fairly unusual, they account for fewer than 5% of GI tumors.[1] Tumors of the small intestine (usually adenocarcinomas) occur most often in persons older than 50 years. Carcinoid tumors, lymphoma, and sarcoma represent less common forms of intestinal tumors. Depending on the extent and type of tumor, partial or complete obstruction of the small bowel may occur.

Clinical Manifestations and Treatment. If the tumor is located near the ampulla of Vater, the common bile duct may become obstructed, with resulting biliary stasis and jaundice. Bleeding and ulceration of small intestinal tumors are common manifestations. Treatment may include surgical intervention to remove the tumor and the affected portion of the small intestine, as well as chemotherapy for lymphomas and carcinoid tumors.

FIGURE 36-14 Ulcerating gastric cancer. (From Sleisenger MH, Fordtran JS, editors: *Gastrointestinal disease*, ed 5, Philadelphia, 1993, Saunders.)

COLONIC POLYPS AND COLON CANCER

Cancer of the colon and rectum is identified in more than 130,000 men and women in the United States each year, with the incidence equally distributed between men and women.[3] It is second only to lung cancer as a cause of cancer deaths. It is well accepted that adenomatous colonic polyps are the major precursor in the development of colon cancer.[3,45]

Colon Polyps. The term **polyp** refers to any protrusion into the lumen of the GI tract. Polyps may be benign or malignant, although most clinicians use the term *polyp* to refer to a benign or not-yet-malignant lesion. Polyps can have several forms; a *sessile polyp* is a raised protuberance with a broad base, while a *pedunculated polyp* is attached to the bowel wall by a stalk that is narrower than the body of the polyp. Benign adenomatous polyps of the colon predispose to malignant adenocarcinoma of the colon through dysplasia and neoplastic degeneration. In fact, some adenomatous polyps may already contain a focus of carcinoma (carcinoma in situ). Many people with polyps have no manifestations, although polyps may cause occult or gross bleeding and abdominal pain due to obstruction. Treatment will vary according to the size and type of polyp and its location in the colon. Biopsy and subsequent removal of polyps may be performed during sigmoidoscopy or colonoscopy. Figure 36-15 shows various colonic polyps. Several benign colon polyps, including the common hyperplastic variety, may be found on endoscopic biopsy and carry no cancer risk.

Colon Cancer

Etiology and Risk Factors. Although no specific cause of colon cancer has been identified, a number of risk factors have been identified. The risk of colon cancer increases with advancing age. After age 40 the annual incidence of colon cancer accelerates, doubling every decade until age 80.[1] Dietary factors also seem to increase the risk; a high-fat, low-fiber diet has been proposed as an associated factor. Certain bowel conditions may predispose an individual to colon cancer, including adenomatous polyps, UC, and Crohn disease of the colon

FIGURE 36-16 Barium enema demonstrating extensive mucosal destruction from a primary lymphoma of the right colon *(arrowhead).* (From Sleisenger MH, Fordtran JS, editors: *Gastrointestinal disease,* ed 5, Philadelphia, 1993, Saunders, p 1484.)

FIGURE 36-15 Photographs of colonic polyps. (Courtesy LE Copstead.)

(see previous discussions). A hereditary predisposition may also be present; the probability of colorectal cancer in a person who has a first-degree relative with the disease is greater than 15%, compared with a 5% risk in the general population.[1]

An important familial condition to consider is a hereditary polyposis syndrome, which presents in one of several discreet forms, the most notable of which are familial adenomatous polyposis and Gardner syndrome. More common are the so-called hereditary nonpolyposis colorectal cancer syndromes. Clues to a familial syndrome include at least three close relatives with colorectal cancer, colorectal cancer involving at least two generations, and one or more cases of colorectal cancer occurring before age 50 years.[3] Colon cancer screening guidelines have recently been updated; for the individual at average risk, annual fecal occult blood testing plus flexible sigmoidoscopy every 5 years, or colonoscopy every 10 years, is recommended.[49] Persons with an increased risk for colon cancer based on family history should undergo more aggressive colon cancer screening.

Clinical Manifestations. The manifestations of colon cancer depend on the anatomic location and function of the bowel segment containing the tumor. On the right side of the colon, the site of water and electrolyte absorption, tumor growth tends to extend along the bowel rather than surround the lumen (Figure 36-16). Although no signs of obstruction are present, black, tarry stools, which signify bleeding into the intestinal lumen, are a significant finding. On the left side of the colon, a tumor may cause manifestations of obstruction in the early stages of its growth. Feelings of intermittent abdominal cramping and fullness may be present, and "ribbon" or pencil-shaped stools may occur. Typically, the individual may note that the passage of stool or flatus relieves the abdominal pain. As tumor growth progresses, blood or mucus may be present in the stool. When the tumor is located in the rectum, early manifestations may include a change in bowel habits, often beginning with an urgent need to defecate upon awakening in the morning or alternating constipation and diarrhea. Later in the progression of tumor growth, a sensation of rectal fullness and a dull ache may be felt in the rectum or sacral region.

Treatment. The treatment and prognosis for colon cancer depend on several factors, including the extent of tumor invasion through the colon wall, cell type and degree of dysplasia, tumor genetics, and the presence or absence of local or distant tumor metastases.[3,50] The 5-year survival rate is directly related to the extent of tissue invasion. The traditional Dukes classification scheme (Table 36-1) has been modified and expanded over the last several decades; currently the tumor-node-metastasis (TNM) classification is accepted as the standard scheme. The most effective treatment is surgery to remove the malignant tumor and adjacent tissue and lymph nodes that may contain cancer cells. The surgical formation of a **colostomy,** or an artificial opening of the colon on the abdominal wall, may be performed after removal of the affected bowel segment. Chemotherapy and radiation therapy are used as supportive measures in addition to surgical intervention. Chemotherapy in particular has advanced rapidly over the last two decades and has significantly improved the prognosis for moderately advanced (i.e., with nodal metastases) colon cancer.[50,51]

TABLE 36-1

Modified Dukes Classification for Colorectal Cancer

Dukes Category	Definition	5-Yr Survival (%) After Treatment
A	Cancer limited to the mucosa or submucosa	90
B1	Cancer penetrates into but not through the muscularis propria	80
B2	Cancer penetrates through the muscularis	70
C1	Same as B1, plus lymph node metastases	50
C2	Same as B2, plus lymph node metastases	50
D	Distant metastases are present	<30

KEY POINTS

- Warning signs for cancer of the GI tract include black, tarry, bloody, or pencil-shaped stool and a change in bowel habits. Risk factors for GI cancer include a low-fiber, high-fat diet, polyps, and chronic irritation or inflammation.
- The prognosis for GI cancer is related to the extent of spread in the body. Surgical removal of tumors followed by chemotherapy, radiation therapy, or both is the usual treatment. Early detection is associated with a better prognosis.

Psychosocial Aspects of Gastrointestinal Disorders

STRESS OF LIFESTYLE CHANGES

GI disorders may have profound effects on the psychosocial functioning of the affected individual. Moreover, these disorders may place great stress on the family attempting to cope with the demands of that person's illness. Nutrition and bowel elimination are behaviors that are dependent on cultural norms; changes in these basic areas of human activity brought about by a GI disorder may have a variety of meanings to different individuals. A teenager affected by a chronic GI disorder such as Crohn disease may be unable to participate in social eating activities and thus may feel isolated from peers. IBS in a young adult who is beginning the most productive

years of life may curtail the ability to function fully in the roles of spouse, parent, and wage earner. Finally, the onset of GI disorders, particularly a neoplastic process, in a middle-aged or older individual may not only limit that person's ability to perform activities of daily living but may also bring about an increased awareness of aging and mortality.

In the past, much of the health care literature, including nursing texts, tended to stereotype individuals with chronic disorders of the GI tract as having behavioral disorders. Aberrant psychological characteristics, it was thought, were somehow associated with or even responsible for certain diseases of the GI tract, such as Crohn disease and UC. It is now recognized that the pathogenic process is almost never the result of primarily psychological causes, although some chronic diseases of the GI tract may be aggravated by emotional factors.[1,3] The stress of coping with a chronic, disabling illness may result in psychological trauma; in addition, any type of illness represents a threat to the integrity of the person. Individuals experiencing a chronic GI disorder may exhibit the psychological effects of such threats and will benefit from a sensitive approach to meeting their needs.

SUMMARY

This chapter has described the major alterations in the GI tract that may occur across the human life span. Because of the strong links between cultural and psychological functioning and activities associated with the GI tract, an in-depth understanding of these alterations is essential for health care professionals.

Disorders of the GI tract may have many manifestations, including dysphagia, pain, vomiting, gas, and alterations in bowel elimination patterns. Disorders may occur in any portion of the GI tract, from the mouth to the anus, and may be the result of alterations in the integrity of the GI tract wall (as in UC) or alterations in motility (as in IBS). Disorders of malabsorption, such as celiac disease, may seriously limit the individual's ability to utilize dietary nutrients and are therefore potentially life threatening. Patients who have undergone surgery on the GI tract may also be at risk for malabsorption. Neoplasms of the GI tract are prevalent in the U.S. population, and the reader will want to review the associated risk factors for these neoplasms very carefully. Finally, readers who are preparing for a career in health care should carefully consider the information provided on the psychosocial aspects of GI disorders and identify ways to provide optimal care for patients with these disorders.

REFERENCES

1. Avunduk C: *Manual of gastroenterology,* ed 4, Philadelphia, 2008, Lippincott Williams & Wilkins.
2. Gitnick G: *Current gastroenterology,* vol. 14, St Louis, 1994, Mosby.
3. Sleisenger MH, Feldman M, Friedman LS: *Sleisenger and Fordtran's gastrointestinal and liver disease: pathophysiology, diagnosis, management,* ed 8, Philadelphia, 2006, Saunders.
4. Yamada T et al: *Textbook of gastroenterology,* ed 4, Philadelphia, 2003, Lippincott Williams & Wilkins.
5. Haubrich WS, Schaffner F, Berk JE: *Bockus gastroenterology,* ed 5, Philadelphia, 1995, Saunders.
6. Wenzl HH, Fine KD, Schiller LR et al: Determinants of decreased fecal consistency in patients with diarrhea, *Gastroenterology* 108(6):1729-1738, 1995.
7. Barrett KE: Mechanisms of inflammatory diarrhea, *Gastroenterology* 103(2):710-711, 1992.
8. Kneepkens CM, Hoekstra JH: Chronic nonspecific diarrhea of childhood: pathophysiology and management, *Pediatr Clin North Am* 43(2):375-390, 1996.
9. Scully C, Gorsky M, Lozada-Nur F: The diagnosis and management of recurrent aphthous stomatitis: a consensus approach, *J Am Dent Assoc* 134(2):200-207, 2003.
10. Perry HO: Idiopathic gingivostomatitis, *Dermatol Clin* 5(4):719-722, 1987.
11. Bruce A, Rogers RS: New and old therapeutics for oral ulcerations, *Arch Dermatol* 143(4):519-523, 2007.
12. Hillemeier AC: Gastroesophageal reflux: diagnostic and therapeutic approaches, *Pediatr Clin North Am* 43(1):197-212, 1996.
13. Weinberg DS, Kadish SL: The diagnosis and management of gastroesophageal reflux disease, *Med Clin North Am* 80(2):411-429, 1996.
14. Vakil N: Gastroesophageal reflux disease and *Helicobacter pylori* infection, *Rev Gastroenterol Disord* 3(1):1-7, 2003.
15. Coron E, Hatlebakk JG, Galmiche JP: Medical therapy of gastroesophageal reflux disease, *Curr Opin Gastroenterol* 23(4):434-439, 2007.
16. Liu JY et al: Determining an appropriate threshold for referral to surgery for gastroesophageal reflux disease, *Surgery* 133(1):5-12, 2003.
17. Spechler SJ: Barrett's esophagus and esophageal adenocarcinoma: pathogenesis, diagnosis, and therapy, *Med Clin North Am* 86(6):1423-1445, vii, 2002.
18. Weston AP: Hiatal hernia with cameron ulcers and erosions, *Gastrointest Endosc Clin N Am* 6(4):671-679, 1996.
19. Bharucha AE, Gostout CJ, Balm RK: Clinical and endoscopic risk factors in the Mallory-Weiss syndrome, *Am J Gastroenterol* 92(5):805-808, 1997.
20. Morales P, Baum AE: Therapeutic alternatives for the Mallory-Weiss tear, *Curr Treat Options Gastroenterol* 6(1):75-83, 2003.
21. Navarro VJ, Garcia-Tsao G: Variceal hemorrhage, *Crit Care Clin* 11(2):391-414, 1995.
22. Carpenter HA, Talley NJ: Gastroscopy is incomplete without biopsy: Clinical relevance of distinguishing gastropathy from gastritis, *Gastroenterology* 108(3):917-924, 1995.
23. Marshall B: Unidentified curved bacilli on gastric epithelium in active chronic gastritis, *Lancet* 1:1273-1274, 1983 (letter).
24. Malaty HM et al: Transmission of *Helicobacter pylori* infection: studies in families of healthy individuals, *Scand J Gastroenterol* 26:927-932, 1991.
25. Walsh JH, Peterson WL: The treatment of *Helicobacter pylori* infection in the management of peptic ulcer disease, *N Engl J Med* 333:984-991, 1995.
26. Atherton JC: CagA, the cag pathogenicity island and *Helicobacter pylori* virulence, *Gut* 44:307-308, 1999.
27. Kurata JH, Nogawa AN: Meta-analysis of risk factors for peptic ulcers: nonsteroidal anti-inflammatory drugs, *Helicobacter pylori,* and smoking, *J Clin Gastroenterol* 24:2-17, 1997.
28. Bickston SJ, Peura DA: Diagnostic tests for *Helicobacter pylori* infection. In Rose BD, editor: *UpToDate.* Available at www.utdol.com. Accessed December 5, 2007.
29. Suerbaum S, Michetti P: Medical progress: *Helicobacter pylori* infection, *N Engl J Med* 347:1175-1186, 2002.
30. Shiotani A, Graham DY: Pathogenesis and therapy of gastric and duodenal ulcer disease, *Med Clin North Am* 86(6):1447-1466, 2002.
31. Podolsky DK: Medical progress: inflammatory bowel disease, *N Engl J Med* 347:417-429, 2002.
32. Cohen RD, Stein R, Hanauer SB: Intravenous cyclosporin in ulcerative colitis: a five-year experience, *Am J Gastroenterol* 94(6):1587-1592, 1999.
33. Rutgeerts P et al: Infliximab for induction and maintenance therapy for ulcerative colitis, *N Engl J Med* 353(23):2462-2476, 2005.
34. Cosnes J et al: Smoking cessation and the course of Crohn's disease: an intervention study, *Gastroenterology* 120:1093-1099, 2001.
35. Lewis JD, Deren JJ, Lichtenstein GR: Cancer risk in patients with inflammatory bowel disease, *Gastroenterol Clin North Am* 28(2):459-477, 1999.
36. Hurley BW, Nguyen CC: The spectrum of pseudomembranous enterocolitis and antibiotic-associated diarrhea, *Arch Intern Med* 162(19):2177-2184, 2002.
37. Oliak D et al: Initial nonoperative management for periappendiceal abscess, *Dis Colon Rectum* 44(7):936-941, 2001.
38. Klein KB: Controlled treatment trials in the irritable bowel syndrome: a critique, *Gastroenterology* 95(1):232-241, 1988.
39. Buettcher M, Baer G, Bonhoeffer J et al: Three-year surveillance of intussusception in children in Switzerland, *Pediatrics* 120(3):473-480, 2007.
40. Loening-Baucke V: Encopresis, *Curr Opin Pediatr* 14(5):570-575, 2002.
41. Parisi MA, Kapur RP: Genetics of Hirschsprung disease, *Curr Opin Pediatr* 12(6):610-617, 2000.
42. Schuppan D: Current concepts of celiac disease pathogenesis, *Gastroenterology* 119(1):234-242, 2000.
43. Kagnoff MF: Celiac disease: a gastrointestinal disease with environmental, genetic, and immunologic components, *Gastroenterol Clin North Am* 21(2):405-425, 1992.
44. Askling J, Linet M, Gridley G et al: Cancer incidence in a population-based cohort of individuals hospitalized with celiac disease or dermatitis herpetiformis, *Gastroenterology* 123(5):1428-1435, 2002.
45. Daly JM et al: *Gastrointestinal oncology,* Philadelphia, 2001, Lippincott Williams & Wilkins.
46. Chow WH et al: An inverse relation between cagA+ strains of *Helicobacter pylori* infection and risk of esophageal and gastric cardia adenocarcinoma, *Cancer Res* 58:589-590, 1998.
47. Takada K: Epstein-Barr virus and gastric carcinoma, *Mol Pathol* 53(5):255-261, 2000.
48. Thun MJ et al: Aspirin use and risk of fatal cancer, *Cancer Res* 53(6):1322-1327, 1993.
49. Trowbridge B: Colorectal cancer screening, *Surg Clin North Am* 82(5):943-945, 2002.
50. Skibber JM, Minsky BD, Hoff PM: Cancer of the colon. In DeVita DT, Hellman S, Rosenberg SA, editors: *Cancer: principles and practice of oncology,* Philadelphia, 2001, Lippincott Williams & Wilkins.
51. National Comprehensive Cancer Network (NCCN): Clinical Practice Guidelines in Oncology. Available at www.nccn.org/professionals/physician_gls/PDF/colon.pdf. Accessed December 10, 2007.

chapter 37

Alterations in Function of the Gallbladder and Exocrine Pancreas

Jeffrey S. Sartin

MEDIA RESOURCES

Additional Material for Study, Review, and Further Exploration

CD Companion ▪ Review Questions and Answers
 ▪ Glossary (with audio pronunciations for selected terms)
 ▪ Disease Profiles ▪ Animations

evolve **Website** at http://evolve.elsevier.com/Copstead/
 ▪ Case Studies ▪ Disease Profiles ▪ WebLinks ▪ Key Points Review

 Online Course (Module 16)

KEY QUESTIONS

- How is bile produced, stored, and secreted?
- How is pancreatic enzyme secretion regulated?
- What factors predispose to formation of cholesterol gallstones?
- What is the relationship between cholecystitis and cholelithiasis?
- What clinical and laboratory findings are indicative of acute pancreatitis?

- What serious complications may result from acute pancreatitis?
- How do the etiologic factors, clinical presentation, and management of chronic pancreatitis differ from those of acute pancreatitis?

CHAPTER OUTLINE

tones have been discovered in the gallbladders of Egyptian and Chinese mummies, suggesting that gallbladder disease has been present in humans for thousands of years. More than 700,000 operations to remove the gallbladder (cholecystectomy) are performed annually in the United States, and the incidence of new gallstones is 1 million to 2 million cases per year.[1,2] The incidence of acute pancreatitis varies according to geographic area but has been reported to range from 5 to 24 per 100,000 population in the United States and Europe.[3] Many health care professionals will encounter diseases of the pancreaticobiliary system frequently and need an in-depth understanding of the mechanisms that promote them. (As cancer of the pancreas and biliary system is relatively rare, it will not be discussed in detail.) This chapter describes the pathophysiology of diseases of the gallbladder, the biliary tree, and the exocrine pancreas, and summarizes current treatments.

Structure and Function of the Pancreaticobiliary System

The pancreaticobiliary system is composed of the gallbladder and cystic duct; the intrahepatic, hepatic, and common bile ducts; and the endocrine and exocrine pancreas. The extrahepatic biliary tree and the gallbladder form a controlled system for delivering **bile** to the intestinal tract. (For additional background, refer to Chapter 35, which describes the physiology of digestion in the gastrointestinal lumen.)

The **gallbladder** is a distensible sack of about 30 to 50 ml capacity that connects via the cystic duct with the common hepatic duct to form the common bile duct. The common bile duct, which is about 3 inches long, runs behind the duodenum to terminate at the ampulla of Vater, a complex structure that also forms the terminating point of the main pancreatic duct. The pancreatic duct runs proximally in the pancreas and branches off dorsally to drain the tail of the pancreas. Thus, the ampulla of Vater forms the major aqueduct through which important digestive secretions enter the intestinal tract (Figure 37-1).

EMBRYOLOGY OF THE PANCREATICOBILIARY SYSTEM

In about the third or fourth week of gestation, the hepatic diverticulum forms from the primitive foregut.[4,5] It is composed of specialized progenitor liver cells that will eventually form the entire liver, biliary tree, and ventral pancreas. The dorsal pancreas forms from a separate outcropping of cells lying on the opposite side of the primitive foregut.

At 5 weeks, three buds can be seen in the hepatic diverticulum. The cranial bud contains specialized liver cells (hepatoblasts), which will form the liver. The liver sinusoids develop and feed into the developing bile canaliculi, which drain into intralobular ductules and then into interlobular ducts. The caudal bud develops into the gallbladder, which joins the

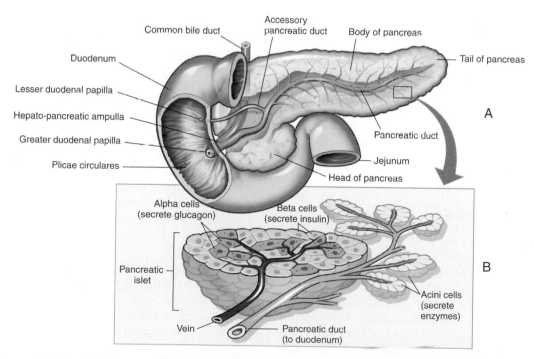

FIGURE 37-1 A, The pancreaticobiliary system showing the anatomic placement of the gallbladder and pancreas, the junction of the common bile duct and the pancreatic duct in the ampulla, and the ampulla of Vater. **B,** Exocrine acinar cells are arranged around pancreatic ducts and secrete enzymes and bicarbonate into the pancreatic juice that enters the duodenum, whereas endocrine cells of the pancreatic islets secrete hormones into the interstitial space where they diffuse into capillaries and enter the bloodstream. (From Thibodeau GA, Patton KT: *Anatomy and physiology,* ed 6, St Louis, 2007, Mosby, p 949.)

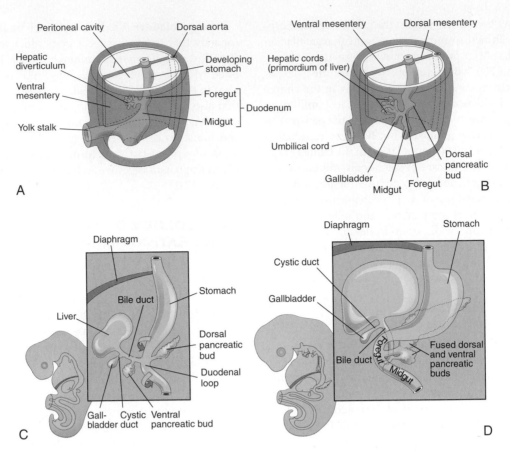

FIGURE 37-2 Stages in the embryonic development of the liver, pancreas, and duodenum at 4 weeks **(A)**, 5 weeks **(B and C)**, and 6 weeks **(D)**. (From Moore KL, Persaud TVN: *The developing human: clinically oriented embryology,* ed 8, Philadelphia, 2008, Saunders, p 218.)

common hepatic duct via the developing cystic duct to form the common bile duct. The gallbladder and the hepatic ducts are initially hollow, but they fill in with development and become solid cords. With further differentiation, they hollow out once again to become the tubes and reservoir for bile flow. During the second trimester, the fetus produces bile, which gives coloring to the fetal meconium. Finally, the basal bud transforms into the ventral pancreas (Figure 37-2).[4,5]

PHYSIOLOGY OF BILE

Normal **bile** is composed primarily of water, electrolytes, and organic solutes. It has a low protein content, containing mainly bile acids, pigment, cholesterol, and phospholipids.[1] Bile acids consist mostly of primary bile salts (cholic and chenodeoxycholic acid) and secondary bile salts (deoxycholic, ursodeoxycholic, and lithocholic acids). Bile is formed in the liver and then modified and stored in the gallbladder and bile ducts prior to secretion into the intestinal tract. The major functions of bile are to aid in the digestion of lipids in the diet and to transport waste products (particularly bilirubin), immunoglobulins (IgA), toxins, and cholesterol into the intestine for eventual disposal or reabsorption. After secretion into the bile canaliculi, bile flows through the canals of

Hering, ductules, interlobular ducts, septal ducts, and right and left lobar ducts, and into the common bile duct (see Figure 37-1).[6]

The principal function of the gallbladder is the concentration and storage of bile. During the fasting state, the muscular sphincter at the ampulla of Vater is contracted, promoting flow of bile into the gallbladder. Only about half of the bile is stored during this time; the rest flows into the duodenum. At the same time that bile is flowing into the gallbladder, absorption is also occurring so that within 4 hours up to 90% of water in bile can be removed, leaving a very concentrated mixture of sodium, bile salts, and other electrolytes.[6]

With the first morning meal, a hormonally and neurally regulated contraction of the gallbladder occurs, releasing the concentrated bile into the duodenum. Bile acids eventually will be absorbed again in the terminal ileum and travel by the portal circulation to be secreted again into the bile. (Bile acids are reabsorbed on average two or three times.) A small amount of the bile acid pool (less than 5%) enters the colon, where primary bile salts undergo bacterial transformation into secondary bile salts (Figure 37-3).[7]

After secretion into the bile, bile salts have dual properties, being **hydrophilic** (soluble in water) at one end and

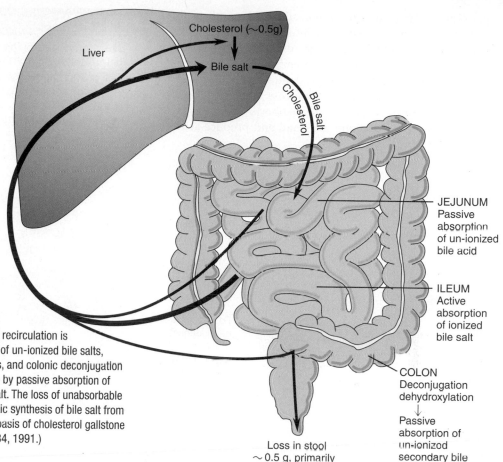

FIGURE 37-3 Enterohepatic bile salt recirculation is maintained by passive jejunal absorption of un-ionized bile salts, active ileal absorption of ionized bile salts, and colonic deconjugation and dehydroxylation of bile salts followed by passive absorption of lipid-soluble un-ionized secondary bile salt. The loss of unabsorbable bile salt is balanced by the de novo hepatic synthesis of bile salt from cholesterol. (From Cooper AD: Metabolic basis of cholesterol gallstone disease, *Gastroenterol Clin North Am* 20:34, 1991.)

FIGURE 37-4 Bile acid–lecithin–cholesterol mixed micelle. Polar ends of bile acid and lecithin are oriented outward, whereas hydrophobic, nonpolar portions make up the interior. Cholesterol is solubilized within the hydrophobic, nonpolar center. (From Saunders KD et al: Pathogenesis of gallstones, *Surg Clin North Am* 70:1197-1216, 1990.)

hydrophobic (insoluble in water) at the other. Thus, these molecules tend to aggregate into clusters called *micelles*, which surround lipids such as cholesterol and allow them to go into solution (Figure 37-4). Micelles are not good stabilizers of cholesterol alone, but another molecule, lecithin, also secreted in large amounts in the bile, is readily incorporated in the core of the micelle to greatly enhance the solubility of cholesterol. In this way, bile keeps cholesterol partly solubilized. Precipitation of cholesterol from bile occurs at high concentrations, predisposing to formation of gallstones.[7]

FUNCTIONAL ANATOMY OF THE PANCREAS

The pancreas is really two organs in one: it functions as both an endocrine and an exocrine organ. On the one hand, hormones such as insulin, glucagon, and somatostatin are produced and secreted into the vascular system (characteristic of an endocrine organ). On the other hand, every 24 hours the pancreas secretes more than 1 liter of digestive juice into the digestive tract (characteristic of an exocrine organ).[6]

Embryologically, the pancreas is composed of two fused organs: a dorsal and a ventral pancreas (Figure 37-5). Microscopically, the pancreas is somewhat lobular and arranged into exocrine glands. The pancreatic juices are secreted into the glandular acini, which eventually drain into the main pancreatic duct and then enter the intestinal tract. The juices themselves are composed of both active digestive enzymes (e.g., amylase, lipase) and precursor or proenzymes (e.g., trypsinogen). Their release during a meal is controlled by hormones secreted from the small intestinal mucosa: **cholecystokinin** (CCK) and **secretin**. When this regulation is deranged, enzymes may be released within the gland and produce **acute pancreatitis.**

KEY POINTS

- Bile is produced by hepatocytes in the liver and stored in the gallbladder. The main components of bile are bile acids, pigment, cholesterol, and phospholipids. Bile salts are important for digestion and absorption of fats from the small bowel. Bile is an important route for excretion of waste products, particularly bilirubin.

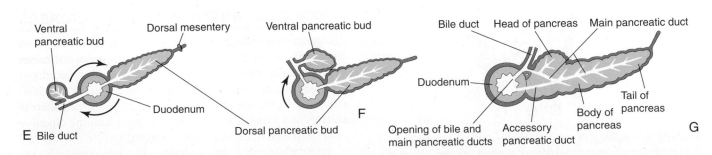

FIGURE 37-5 Stages in the embryonic development of the pancreas from the fifth to eighth week **(A-D)**, and a diagram of the progressive development of the bile duct and main pancreatic duct **(E-G)**. (From Moore KL, Persaud TVN: *The developing human: clinically oriented embryology*, ed 8, Philadelphia, 2008, Saunders, p 223.)

The gallbladder receives bile from the liver, concentrates bile by absorbing water, and then contracts to expel stored bile into the common bile duct, which terminates in the duodenum.

■ The pancreas is both an endocrine organ (secreting insulin, glucagon, and somatostatin into the bloodstream) and an exocrine gland (secreting digestive juice into the duodenum). Some pancreatic enzymes are secreted in active form (amylase, lipase), whereas others are proenzymes that are activated in the duodenum (trypsinogen). Release of pancreatic enzymes is stimulated by cholecystokinin and secretin.

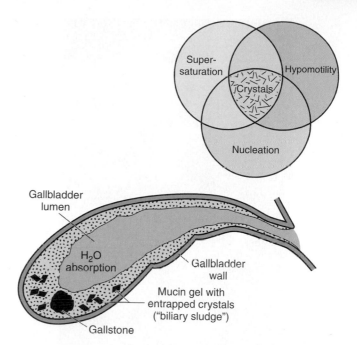

FIGURE 37-6 The three principal phases responsible for the formation of cholesterol gallstones illustrated with a Venn diagram. (From Feldman M et al: *Sleisenger and Fordtran's gastrointestinal and liver disease: pathophysiology, diagnosis, management,* ed 7, Philadelphia, 2002, Saunders, p 1069.)

Disorders of the Gallbladder

PATHOPHYSIOLOGY OF CHOLESTEROL GALLSTONE FORMATION

The majority of gallstones among patients in the United States are cholesterol stones.[1] In general, the formation of cholesterol stones in the gallbladder (**cholelithiasis**) can be broken down into three phases: (1) supersaturation of bile with cholesterol; (2) nucleation of crystals; and (3) hypomotility allowing stone growth (Figure 37-6).

As described previously, cholesterol eventually precipitates from supersaturated bile. If conditions are right for the formation of cholesterol gallstones, nucleation occurs in which the cholesterol crystals aggregate together. Continued growth of the crystals then becomes a balance between cholesterol growth–promoting factors and factors that tend to cause stone dissolution. A significant factor that promotes the continued growth of stones is hypomotility or stasis of bile within the gallbladder. **Stasis** in this context means a condition of inactivity or staying. Patients with high spinal cord injuries, patients receiving total parenteral nutrition, and persons who undergo prolonged fasting or rapid weight loss have impaired emptying and are at particular risk for development of cholesterol gallstones. Other risk factors for cholelithiasis include pregnancy, oral contraceptives, obesity, diabetes mellitus, and octreotide therapy (analogue of somatostatin).[1]

About 25% of gallstones in Western countries are due to pigment stones, which contain a mixture of pigment polymers and calcium salts. "Black" pigment stones are most common and are associated with cirrhosis and hemolysis, or they may be idiopathic. "Brown" pigment stones differ in their composition and are much more common in developing countries, where they are associated with biliary parasitosis and bacterial colonization and infection.[1]

CHOLELITHIASIS AND CHOLECYSTITIS

Currently, about 20 million people in the United States have gallstones (cholelithiasis). The incidence of gallstones is related to age, sex, and a variety of medical factors. Gallstones are twice as common in women as in men. Native Americans, particularly the Pima Indians of North America, are markedly susceptible to gallstones, and American Caucasians somewhat less so. European Caucasians are intermediate in prevalence, and persons of Asian descent are at the lowest risk. Obesity correlates with the development of gallstones, but so does rapid weight loss in an obese individual. However, the presence of gallstones does not necessarily mean that an individual will have any symptoms. In many individuals, gallstones are completely asymptomatic and require no treatment.[8] Cholelithiasis in children is usually associated with an underlying systemic disease such as cystic fibrosis or sickle cell disease. It is often symptomatic and requires treatment by gallbladder removal.

The term **cholecystitis** refers to inflammation of the gallbladder wall. The continued presence of gallstones in the gallbladder ultimately promotes inflammatory changes in the gallbladder wall, with fibrosis and thickening.[9] Cholecystitis is classified as acute or chronic, according to its clinical manifestations. The clinical manifestations of each are described, followed by diagnostic and treatment methods.

Chronic Cholelithiasis
Clinical Manifestations. The chief complication of chronic cholelithiasis is biliary colic, a persistent epigastric or right upper abdominal pain. Often the pain radiates to the back and is accompanied by nausea, vomiting, sweating, and flatus. A typical episode lasts several hours. Biliary colic is typically caused by intermittent obstruction of the cystic duct by a gallstone

FIGURE 37-7 Chronic cholecystitis demonstrated by a thickened gallbladder wall and luminal cholesterol gallstones. (From Cotran RS et al: *Robbins pathologic basis of disease*, ed 6, Philadelphia, 1999, Saunders, p 897.)

(Figure 37-7), although some authorities point to spasm of the sphincter of Oddi as etiologic.

Symptoms may be precipitated by a meal, but they often occur spontaneously and may occur at night. The pain often increases steadily for 15 minutes and persists for an hour or more, then slowly decreases. Attacks may recur on a frequent or infrequent schedule. Patients often describe additional symptoms, including fatty food intolerance, belching, flatus, bloating, and epigastric burning.[8]

Diagnosis and Treatment. The diagnosis of chronic cholelithiasis depends on imaging studies, particularly ultrasonography, and is essentially the same as that described for acute cholecystitis.

In cases of chronic cholelithiasis with no or very few recurrent symptoms, "watchful waiting" may be considered.[8,9] However, patients with significant recurrences of biliary colic are candidates for one of the three current modes of treatment for cholecystitis: cholecystectomy (surgical removal of the gallbladder), chemical dissolution of gallstones, or lithotripsy (mechanical breaking up of gallstones within the gallbladder). These will be discussed in more detail in the Acute Cholecystitis section.

Acute Cholecystitis

Clinical Manifestations. Acute cholecystitis is defined as acute inflammation of the gallbladder wall. It is characterized by severe right upper abdominal pain that may radiate to the back. Abdominal tenderness and fever are often present. The pathogenesis of acute cholecystitis is not well understood. Cholelithiasis is present in about 90% of patients. Obstruction of the cystic duct is present in almost all cases, suggesting that stasis of bile in the gallbladder is important in the pathogenesis of the disease. Bacterial infection may also be present in acute cholecystitis, although it is not thought to be the direct cause of the inflammatory process. Laboratory evaluation may reveal leukocytosis, mild elevations of the bilirubin and serum transaminases, and, elevated amylase levels.[9,10]

If left untreated, the inflammatory process will escalate, and gangrene of the gallbladder wall with rupture may occur. This may lead to peritonitis and septic shock, a localized abscess, or a **cholecystoenteric fistula** (fistula between the gallbladder and gastrointestinal tract).

Acalculous cholecystitis is an important subgroup of acute cholecystitis. As the name implies, it occurs in patients without pre-existing gallstones. It tends to occur in the setting of major surgery, critical illness, trauma, or burn-related injury. Patients tend to be predominantly male and older than 50 years, and total parenteral nutrition (TPN) is a common cofactor. It carries a somewhat more serious implication than stone-associated cholecystitis, in part because of the associated medical conditions. In fact, gangrene of the gallbladder wall and perforation, **emphysematous cholecystitis,** and **empyema** all develop more rapidly than in calculous cholecystitis.[1]

Diagnosis. Evaluation for possible cholecystitis includes an appropriate history and physical examination, laboratory studies, and an imaging study designed to evaluate the gallbladder and biliary tree. Ultrasound of the abdomen is the procedure of choice early in the diagnostic evaluation. Typically, the ultrasound scan reveals the presence of stones, occasionally in the cystic duct, as well as thickening of the gallbladder wall and distention of the lumen. It may also point to another diagnosis of right upper quadrant pain, such as a liver neoplasm or hydronephrosis of the kidney. The sensitivity and specificity of ultrasound for stones larger than 2 mm in diameter approach 95%.[10] Sensitivity rates for acalculous cholecystitis are somewhat lower.[11]

However, the presence of cholelithiasis and a thickened gallbladder wall are not definitive evidence of cholecystitis, and other diagnostic tests are used on occasion. Hepatobiliary scintigraphy (or cholescintigraphy) by hydroxyiminodiacetic acid (HIDA) scanning provides a good functional assessment of gallbladder excretion, which is markedly impaired with cholecystitis. Computed tomography (CT), magnetic resonance cholangiography (MRCA), and endoscopic retrograde cholangiopancreatography (ERCP) are useful for selected cases. The latter carries a risk of perforation and pancreatitis, and so is reserved for cases requiring intervention (stent placement, biopsy, or special contrast studies).

Treatment. Treatment for cholecystitis depends on the severity of symptoms and the patient's clinical status. Acute cholecystitis may necessitate intervention, but surgeons generally prefer to allow a "hot" gallbladder to "cool down" before performing surgery, particularly if the patient is considered a high surgical risk. The benefit of antibiotics for uncomplicated cholecystitis remains unclear, but broad-spectrum antibiotics are generally administered in the setting of acute cholecystitis. Percutaneous catheter drainage or endoscopic drainage with stent placement may be performed to relieve obstruction, particularly if infection is involved. If the patient's condition precludes surgery, these may be the main treatments, and drains can be left in place indefinitely. Advanced acute cholecystitis complicated by empyema, gangrene, or emphysematous change is a surgical emergency.

Laparoscopic cholecystectomy was first performed in 1987 and has benefited from rapid development of video **laparoscopy** instrumentation. Laparoscopic cholecystectomy is now the treatment of choice for symptomatic gallstones. The procedure is usually performed with four small incisions through which instruments are inserted. The gallbladder is freed either by electrosurgical or laser excision and is then withdrawn through one of the small incisions. Advantages of the laparoscopic technique include minimal scarring, less postoperative pain than after laparotomy, shortened hospital stays, and a rapid return to daily activities.[12]

Open cholecystectomy was first performed in the nineteenth century and remains an extremely safe operation with low morbidity and mortality. However, the length of the incision and accompanying postoperative pain render many patients extremely immobile after the procedure. Altered anatomy or scarring from previous surgery or the presence of common bile duct stones may necessitate a traditional cholecystectomy. A laparoscopic procedure may be converted to an open one intraoperatively if necessary (e.g., upon finding a malignant tumor in the vicinity of the gallbladder). Complications of cholecystectomy (either laparoscopic or open) can include infection, inadvertent transection of the common bile duct, and the rare but debilitating syndrome of recurrent sclerosing cholangitis.

Some patients, such as elderly or debilitated persons, may be poor surgical risks and cannot undergo the stress of surgery.[13] Nonoperative methods to manage gallstones, such as **chemodissolution** with a variety of bile acids or organic solvents and **lithotripsy,** have been tried as alternatives to surgery. Chemodissolution is the use of chemical substances, such as bile acids or organic solvents, to dissolve gallstones. Such agents as chenodeoxycholic acid (CDCA), a secondary bile salt, are administered orally. However, this approach has several major drawbacks, including diarrhea in about 50% of patients and a low overall efficacy. Extracorporeal shock wave lithotripsy (ESWL), which involves the breaking up of gallstones using shock waves, is another nonsurgical approach. The objective is to fragment stones into pieces small enough to be passed through the cystic duct, or small enough to allow dissolving agents to work. ESWL is safe and relatively effective, under proper circumstances. The disadvantages include strict selection criteria (e.g., stones less than 2 cm in diameter), resulting in a low percentage of eligible patients. The gallbladder also is left in place, allowing for possible recurrence of

gallstones and necessitating the concurrent use of dissolving agents such as CDCA to prevent new stone formation.

For the most part, in the near future the management of gallstone disease is likely to remain surgical, with traditional or laparoscopic cholecystectomy being the major forms of intervention.

Chronic Cholecystitis

Clinical Manifestations. Chronic cholecystitis is defined as chronic inflammation of the gallbladder wall due to persistent low-grade irritation from gallstones or to recurrent attacks of acute cholecystitis. Diabetes mellitus and obesity are important predisposing factors. Although many patients suffer from intermittent biliary colic or have symptomatic acute attacks, a surprising number of patients experience no symptoms. Chronic cholecystitis may lead to many of the complications described above for acute cholecystitis, including biliary sepsis, as well as a specific type of scarring known as a calcified or *porcelain* gallbladder, which is associated with a higher risk of cancer.[1]

KEY POINTS

- Lecithin is an important component of bile that helps keep cholesterol from precipitating into crystals. Crystals of cholesterol may initiate gallstone formation. The relative concentrations of cholesterol, lecithin, and bile acids appear to determine the likelihood of cholesterol gallstone formation. Bile hypomotility or stasis contributes to growth of cholesterol stones.
- Gallstones occur more frequently in women than in men. Ethnicity, obesity, and rapid weight loss are predisposing factors. Gallstones may be asymptomatic or associated with symptomatic cholecystitis. Colicky pain due to intermittent obstruction of the cystic duct by a stone is the chief complaint. Symptoms of chronic cholecystitis include epigastric or right upper quadrant pain radiating to the back, nausea, vomiting, sweating, fat intolerance, bloating, and flatus.
- Acute cholecystitis is acute inflammation of the gallbladder associated with abdominal pain, leukocytosis, and fever. Cholelithiasis is present in about 90% of patients; obstruction of the cystic duct is present in nearly all patients.
- Treatment for cholecystitis includes surgical removal of the gallbladder (cholecystectomy), chemodissolution, ESWL (lithotripsy) for stones, antibiotics if indicated, and management of pain. Cholecystectomy is the mainstay of therapy.

Disorders of the Pancreas

PANCREATITIS

Acute Pancreatitis

Etiology and Pathogenesis. Acute **pancreatitis** is an inflammatory process involving the pancreas that may range from mild and inconveniencing to severe and life-threatening. After an

BOX 37-1

Conditions Predisposing to Acute Pancreatitis

Gallstones
Biliary sludge and microlithiasis
Other causes of mechanical ampullary obstruction
Alcohol
Hypertriglyceridemia
Hypercalcemia
Drugs
Infections and toxins
Trauma
Pancreas divisum
Vascular disease
Pregnancy
Post-ERCP
Postoperative pancreatitis
Hereditary pancreatitis
Structural abnormalities
- Duodenum/ampullary region
- Bile duct
- Sphincter of Oddi dysfunction
- Main pancreatic duct

From Feldman M et al: *Sleisenger and Fordtran's gastrointestinal and liver disease: pathophysiology, diagnosis, management,* ed 7, Philadelphia, 2002, Saunders, p 914.

ERCP, Endoscopic retrograde cholangiopancreatography.

attack, the exocrine and endocrine functions of the pancreas may remain impaired for a variable period. Pancreatitis affects between 1 and 5 per 10,000 individuals in the United States annually. Predisposing factors for pancreatitis have been well known for more than 100 years (Box 37-1); in the United States the most common causes are biliary tract disease, hypertriglyceridemia, and ethanol-associated pancreatitis.[1] Although the exact mechanisms leading to pancreatitis are not fully understood, three possible pathways are known (Figure 37-8). The most prominent factor is obstruction of the pancreatic duct by a stone or other cause (usually unknown), with release of digestive enzymes within the parenchyma, followed by enzyme activation and then autodigestion of the pancreas.[14] Edema leading to vascular insufficiency and ischemic injury is a contributing factor. Other possible mechanisms include acinar cell injury from alcohol or drugs, trauma, or viral infection; and defective intracellular transport of proenzymes within acinar cells.

Up to 66% of first cases of pancreatitis are associated with alcoholism.[15] While there is clearly an association of alcohol with pancreatitis, the causal mechanism has not been determined. Transient increases in pancreatic exocrine secretion, contraction of the sphincter of Oddi, and direct toxic effects on acinar cells have all been postulated from experimental studies.[9] Many authorities now think that most cases of alcoholic pancreatitis are sudden exacerbations of chronic pancreatitis, presenting as apparent de novo acute pancreatitis.[14] According to this view, chronic alcohol ingestion causes secretion of protein-rich pancreatic fluid, leading to deposition of inspissated protein plugs and obstruction of small pancreatic ducts, followed by the train of events described above. However, other pathologic studies show no evidence of chronic pancreatitis in up to 40% of acute alcoholic pancreatitis patients.[16]

Clinical Manifestations. The presentation of acute pancreatitis usually begins with steady, boring pain in the epigastrium or left upper quadrant, which gradually increases in intensity. It often radiates or penetrates through to the back and is accompanied by nausea and vomiting. Tenderness on palpation may be exquisite. Bowel sounds are reduced but not absent. Abdominal distention may be present. Fever is common but is usually low grade initially. In more severe pancreatitis, this clinical picture is accompanied by signs of circulatory instability, respiratory insufficiency, and, occasionally, shock.[17]

Diagnosis. The laboratory evaluation of acute pancreatitis begins with measurements of serum pancreatic enzymes. Serum lipase and amylase levels rise more or less in tandem during the first 12 hours and remain elevated for several days. Lipase is more specific and persists longer, and therefore has become the preferred test for most clinicians. Serum aminotransferases (aspartate aminotransferase, alanine aminotransferase) may also be elevated. Marked elevation of the alkaline phosphatase and bilirubin levels suggest the possibility of biliary disease or obstruction, particularly by gallstones. Associated laboratory findings include leukocytosis, hyperlipidemia (which may be marked), and hypocalcemia.[1,9]

The diagnosis of acute pancreatitis is based on the signs and symptoms, laboratory data, and imaging studies of the pancreas and surrounding organs. Radiographs of the abdomen may reveal an ileus pattern or the "sentinel loop" (a distended loop of small bowel in the area of the pancreas). Ultrasound can provide a bedside technique to visualize the pancreas, gallbladder, common bile duct, and other abdominal structures, but is limited by poor image resolution due to bowel gas. Computed tomography (CT) of the abdomen is the gold standard for evaluation of the pancreas and allows depiction of the pancreas in remarkable detail, including edema and abscess or cyst formation as well as the degree of peripancreatic involvement. The differential diagnosis of acute pancreatitis includes perforated peptic ulcer, acute cholecystitis, mesenteric vascular disease, and a variety of other illnesses (some associated with elevated amylase levels) (Box 37-2), most of which may be differentiated on the basis of CT and other radiographic tests.

Grading systems allow prediction of the clinical course of acute pancreatitis. Ranson's criteria are a widely used benchmark for prognostic assessment, and are particularly useful with modifications based on CT scoring.[18] Early monitoring in the intensive care unit is indicated for patients with a high number of risk factors. One particularly important finding on contrast CT is the presence of significant pancreatic necrosis. Acute necrotizing pancreatitis carries a high risk for progression to infected pancreatic necrosis, a devastating complication with a high morbidity and mortality.

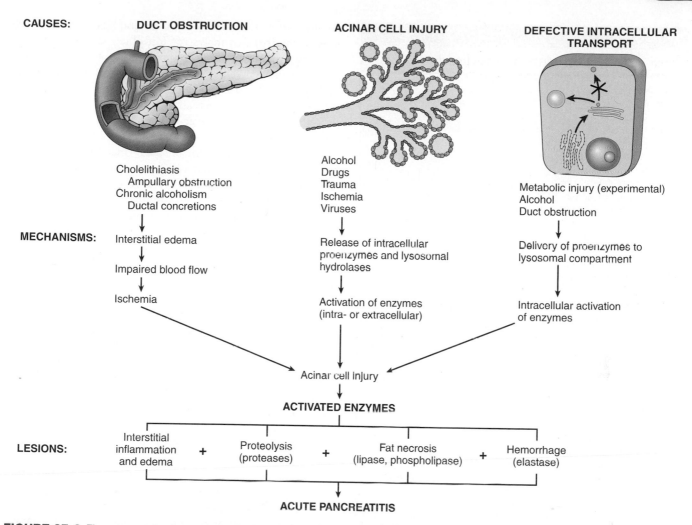

FIGURE 37-8 Three proposed pathways in the pathogenesis of acute pancreatitis. Obstruction of the duct, extrinsic injury and intrinsic metabolic mechanisms lead to injury of pancreatic cells. Injured cells release activated pancreatic enzymes that cause autodigestion and inflammation of the pancreas. (From Kumar V et al: *Robbins basic pathology,* ed 8, Philadelphia, 2007, Saunders, p 678.)

Treatment. Conservative management is indicated for mild to moderate cases of acute pancreatitis. In general, withholding oral feedings, providing nasogastric suction for significant adynamic ileus, and providing careful volume replacement with IV fluids are indicated. Analgesics are administered parenterally. All narcotics should be used carefully because of the potential of sphincter of Oddi dysfunction, although recent studies show that no single agent is contraindicated.[19] This treatment is often sufficient when carried out for 3 to 7 days, after which the acute episode subsides and oral intake may gradually be resumed.

Severe pancreatitis, particularly in the setting of acute necrotizing pancreatitis, may result in multisystem organ dysfunction, requiring aggressive support in the intensive care unit setting. Nutritional deficits develop rapidly with extensive catabolism (tissue breakdown) and lack of caloric intake; total parenteral nutrition is usually indicated with pancreatitis of more than a few days duration or if complications arise.[7] Additional supportive measures include calcium administration to reverse severe hypocalcemia, correction of magnesium deficiency, and control of hyperglycemia. Causes of death from severe pancreatitis include respiratory failure (usually associated with adult respiratory distress syndrome), acute renal failure, and acute intraabdominal sepsis. Mechanical ventilation and hemodialysis may be required in complicated cases.

Bacterial infection is a critical determinant of poor outcome in acute necrotizing pancreatitis. Some authorities advocate broad-spectrum antibiotics (e.g., carbapenems) directed to common pathogens such as *Escherichia* and *Klebsiella* species for all patients with acute necrotizing pancreatitis, although definitive studies are lacking.[1] In the patient with fever and signs of sepsis, empiric antibiotics should be administered, and any significant fluid collections found on CT scan should be aspirated for culture and sensitivity.

Abscess or hemorrhage may complicate pancreatitis with or without significant pancreatic necrosis and may necessitate surgical intervention. Open laparotomy with debridement of devitalized tissue (necrosectomy) and major pancreatic resection (pancreatectomy) are the main surgical options.[20] Drains are typically left in place postoperatively, and repeated

BOX 37-2

Causes of Increased Serum Amylase Activity

Pancreatic diseases
- Acute pancreatitis
- Complications of pancreatitis
- Acute exacerbation of chronic pancreatitis
- Pancreatic tumors, cysts

Other serious intraabdominal diseases
- Acute cholecystitis
- Common bile duct obstruction
- Perforation of esophagus, stomach, small bowel, or colon
- Intestinal ischemia or infarction
- Intestinal obstruction
- Acute appendicitis
- Acute gynecologic conditions such as ruptured ectopic pregnancy and acute salpingitis

Diseases of salivary glands
- Mumps
- Effects of alcohol

Tumors
- Ovarian cysts
- Papillary cystadenocarcinoma of ovary
- Carcinoma of lung

Renal insufficiency
Macroamylasemia
Miscellaneous
- Morphine
- Endoscopy
- Sphincter of Oddi stenosis or spasm
- Anorexia nervosa
- Head trauma with intracranial bleeding
- Diabetic ketoacidosis
- Human immunodeficiency virus

From Feldman M et al: *Sleisenger and Fordtran's gastrointestinal and liver disease: pathophysiology, diagnosis, management,* ed 7, Philadelphia, 2002, Saunders, p 914.

debridement may be needed to remove infective debris and necrotic tissue.

Localized complications of acute pancreatitis may result in prolonged morbidity for the patient. The most common localized complication is pancreatic **pseudocyst.** This is a collection of fluid within or adjacent to the pancreas that often has a direct communication to the pancreatic duct. It is called a *pseudocyst* because, unlike a true cyst, it contains no epithelial lining. A pseudocyst can develop rather acutely or more subacutely, as the patient recuperates from the acute illness. The presentation often includes fever, tachycardia, and an abdominal mass and tenderness. Complications of pseudocysts include infection (usually termed an *infected pseudocyst,* as opposed to the pancreatic abscess described above), spontaneous rupture, or hemorrhage. Management of pseudocyst includes endoscopic or surgical drainage of the cyst, either externally or internally, usually into the stomach or bowel.[1,20]

Pancreatic ascites may occur and may represent a persistent leak in the main pancreatic duct. It is usually painless and often massive. The fluid may find its way into unusual places, including the pleural space and mediastinum.[21] Pancreatic ascites may be detected by ultrasonography or CT, and diagnosis is confirmed by analysis of fluid obtained by aspiration, in particular the amylase level. Management is often conservative, with prolonged parenteral nutrition. Improvement may occur following the endoscopic placement of a stent (a thin-walled tube) into the main pancreatic duct.

Other complications of acute pancreatitis include common bile duct obstruction, portal or splenic vein thrombosis, peptic ulcer disease, and chronic fistula formation.

Endoscopic treatment may be carried out for gallstone pancreatitis in selected cases. Indications for *urgent* ERCP with ampullotomy (incision of the ampulla) include biliary sepsis, recalcitrant severe pancreatitis, and jaundice.[1] In milder cases, traditional conservative therapy followed by elective ERCP is acceptable. The risks of ERCP include exacerbation of pancreatitis, and so the need for this procedure must be carefully considered.

Chronic Pancreatitis

Etiology and Pathogenesis. Chronic pancreatitis is defined histologically as the presence of chronic inflammatory lesions in the pancreas, and in practice is the persistence of symptoms secondary to pancreatic dysfunction over weeks and months. Destruction of exocrine parenchyma and fibrosis precedes the destruction of endocrine parenchyma. After a variable time, most patients with chronic pancreatitis develop calcifications that become visible on radiologic films of the abdomen or CT. Chronic pancreatitis is most often associated with alcohol consumption, although a small percentage of cases are idiopathic, hereditary, or associated with hyperparathyroidism (hypercalcemia), trauma, or various other factors.[1,14]

The association of alcohol ingestion with chronic pancreatitis is profound. Autopsy studies have shown that the changes of chronic pancreatitis are present in 45% of alcoholics, even those without symptoms, and that this rate is 40 to 50 times higher than that in nondrinkers.[1,9] Exactly how alcohol causes chronic pancreatitis is not known (see the previous discussion of alcohol and acute pancreatitis). One recent theory suggests that the initial factors include an increase in the protein concentration in pancreatic juice coupled with reduction in a specific "pancreatic stone protein" that inhibits the formation of pancreatic protein plugs.[22] This biochemical situation allows the formation of protein plugs that can later calcify, in addition to causing obstruction to the flow of pancreatic juice. A key element seems to be necrosis, followed by fibrosis, perhaps analogous to cirrhosis of the liver. Ischemic and antioxidant damage may occur as well. Another facet of alcohol-associated pancreatitis is its tendency to progress after alcohol consumption is stopped.

Clinical Manifestations. The presentation of chronic pancreatitis may consist of bouts of acute pancreatitis with progressive signs of persistent pancreatic dysfunction after the acute attack subsides. Alternatively, an insidious onset of pain in the epigastrium that radiates to the back may be the first symptom. About 10% to 15% of patients will not present with pain but rather with the sequelae of chronic pancreatitis, including diabetes mellitus, malabsorption, and weight loss.[23] The mortality is 3% to 4% per year. Interestingly, the incidence of pancreatic carcinoma does not appear to be substantially increased in patients with chronic pancreatitis.

The pain of chronic pancreatitis is often the major form of debility. Nerve fibers from the pancreas pass to the celiac plexus and then to spinal sympathetic ganglia. The events that actually trigger the pain are not well understood. There may be a relation to ductal pressures or possibly to ischemia in the pancreas. The pain is often accompanied by nausea and is steady and boring in nature. The pain is usually located in the upper abdomen, particularly in the epigastrium, and radiates to the back in more than half of cases. In alcoholic pancreatitis, continued drinking affords temporary anesthesia but may foster recurrences of pain. Cessation of drinking may allow for a better long-term prognosis. After about 5 years of continual pain, many patients note a decrease in the symptoms (i.e., the pain "burns out").

Endocrine and exocrine pancreatic insufficiency lead to diabetes mellitus, malabsorption, and weight loss. Diabetes mellitus arises from progressive loss of endocrine cells in the pancreatic islets and usually requires exogenous insulin administration; diabetic ketoacidosis is an unusual finding. Weight loss may be aggravated by poor intake as a result of pancreatic pain. Malabsorption of fat does not occur until pancreatic enzyme output drops to 10% of normal. Along with the malabsorption of fat, the absorption of fat-soluble vitamins (A, D, E, and K) may be impaired, leading to coagulopathy and night vision problems.

Further complications of chronic pancreatitis are similar to those of acute pancreatitis and include pseudocyst, pancreatic ascites, and obstruction of the common bile duct. Obstruction of the bile duct may lead to elevated values on liver function tests and the need to intervene either surgically or endoscopically. Alkaline phosphatase and bilirubin levels may become markedly elevated if obstruction is severe. Unusual complications include thrombosis of the portal and splenic veins. This may lead to gastrointestinal hemorrhage from gastric varices.[17] Peptic ulcer disease is also increased in patients with chronic pancreatitis, although a definite causal relationship has not been established.

Diagnosis. The diagnosis of chronic pancreatitis is usually suggested by the clinical history, physical examination findings, and routine blood chemical analyses. Biochemical studies of pancreatic function may be helpful. Confirmation of the diagnosis is aided by plain radiographs showing calcifications in the area of the pancreas. Abdominal ultrasound, CT, or magnetic resonance cholangiopancreatography (MRCP) are usually performed with reasonable sensitivities and specificities. ERCP is reserved for suspicious cases that cannot be confirmed by other techniques, or for cases in which biopsy or cytologic examination are necessary to rule out malignancy.[1] It shows the pancreatic duct to range from almost normal in early cases, to markedly dilated or beaded—the "chain of lakes" appearance (Figure 37-9). A common finding is truncation of the secondary branches of the pancreatic duct.

Treatment. The treatment for chronic pancreatitis is directed toward pain control, exocrine and endocrine insufficiency, and

FIGURE 37-9 Endoscopic retrograde cholangiopancreatogram in a patient with chronic pancreatitis shows marked narrowing and irregularity of the main pancreatic duct body and tail (arrows). (From Feldman M et al: *Sleisenger and Fordtran's gastrointestinal and liver disease: pathophysiology, diagnosis, management,* ed 6, Philadelphia, 1998, Saunders, p 952.)

management of complications. By far the most challenging is the management of pain. Absolute abstention from alcohol is paramount to prevent worsening of symptoms. For almost 40 years, analgesics and surgical intervention have been the mainstay of pain control, and celiac plexus block is helpful for some patients. With the advent of ERCP, less drastic forms of intervention are now possible. Pancreatic sphincterotomy is indicated for the management of single or multiple stones. Endoscopic drains may be placed for pseudocysts of the pancreas if they are adjacent to the stomach or duodenum. Obstruction of the common bile duct can be managed with endoscopically placed biliary stents. Strictures of the main pancreatic duct can be managed with indwelling pancreatic stents.[24]

If endoscopic management fails or is not appropriate in a given patient, surgery may be indicated. Various procedures, such as the pylorus-preserving Whipple procedure (pancreaticoduodenectomy), may be used, generally with favorable results regarding relief of pain. Complete and distal pancreatic resections are rarely used for this condition. As with management of acute pancreatitis, the judgment of the surgeon is paramount to prevent the catastrophic complications that can result from surgery on the pancreas.

Pancreatic enzyme replacement has become a standard therapy for chronic pancreatitis, both for its effects on steatorrhea and for the management of chronic pain.[1] As proteases (e.g., trypsin, chymotrypsin, and elastase) exert a controlling influence on pancreatic secretion, feedback regulation should result in relief of pain following oral administration of pancreatic enzymes. Unfortunately, only 20% to 30% of patients with the typical alcohol-induced type of disease respond to such therapy. Responses seem to be higher in patients with small-duct disease. Acid suppression with an H_2-blocker or proton-pump inhibitor is indicated to reduce inactivation of the enzymes from gastric acid. Research has also been undertaken on octreotide, a synthetic long-acting analog of somatostatin that has been shown to inhibit CCK release and both basal and neural-stimulated pancreatic secretion.[1] Octreotide is being used increasingly for abdominal pain unresponsive to pancreatic enzyme replacement.[25]

Management of exocrine insufficiency can usually be accomplished with low-fat diets and pancreatic enzyme supplementation. Likewise, endocrine insufficiency in the form of diabetes mellitus is managed with diet and either oral hypoglycemic agents or insulin.[7]

duct may be performed. Pancreatic enzyme therapy may be helpful in reducing pain by providing negative feedback, which reduces pancreatic secretion.

SUMMARY

The pancreaticobiliary system is central to the digestion of food because it provides necessary digestive enzymes and lipid-emulsifying agents that allow the intestine to absorb nutrients. This chapter has considered alterations in the function of the gallbladder and exocrine pancreas. A major disease of the pancreaticobiliary system is the formation of cholesterol gallstones, which can lead to acute and chronic cholecystitis and acute and chronic pancreatitis. New forms of surgical and nonsurgical interventions for the management of gallstone disease have become available in the past few years, with conventional open surgery remaining a useful option. These interventions, as well as interventions for acute and chronic pancreatitis, are currently the focus of much clinical research.

KEY POINTS

- Acute pancreatitis is commonly associated with biliary tract disease and excessive ethanol ingestion. Activation of pancreatic proenzymes to active forms within the pancreas leads to autodigestion and inflammation of the gland. The manifestations of acute pancreatitis may be mild or severe and include a steady, boring pain in the epigastrium or left upper quadrant, nausea, vomiting, a tender abdomen, reduced bowel sounds, and fever. In severe cases, circulatory shock may occur. Elevated serum amylase and lipase levels are indicative of pancreatitis.
- Management of acute pancreatitis is aimed at reducing pancreatic secretion. Because chyme entering the duodenum is the primary stimulus for pancreatic secretion, food is withheld and nasogastric suctioning may be instituted. Complications of acute pancreatitis include hyperglycemia, nutritional deficit, and pancreatic hemorrhage, infection, abscess formation, or necrosis. Antibiotics, fluid management, total parenteral nutrition, and insulin may be indicated to manage complications.
- Chronic pancreatitis is closely associated with alcohol use. Acute pancreatitis due to biliary obstruction rarely progresses to chronic pancreatitis. Chronic pancreatitis results in progressive destruction of endocrine and exocrine function. Manifestations of chronic pancreatitis are more insidious than those of acute pancreatitis. Epigastric pain, diabetes mellitus, malabsorption, and weight loss may be the presenting problems.
- The complications of chronic pancreatitis are similar to those of acute pancreatitis. Therapy is directed to pain control, amelioration of endocrine and exocrine deficiency, and monitoring for and management of complications. Surgery to correct obstruction of the pancreatic

REFERENCES

1. Yamada T et al: *Textbook of gastroenterology*, ed 4, Philadelphia, 2003, Lippincott Williams & Wilkins.
2. Avunduk C: *Manual of gastroenterology*, ed 3, Philadelphia, 2002, Lippincott Williams & Wilkins.
3. Go VLW, Everhart JE: Pancreatitis. In Everhart JE, editor: *Digestive diseases in the United States: epidemiology and impact.* NIH Publication No. 94-1447, Washington, DC, 1994, U.S. Department of Health and Human Services.
4. Moore KL, Persaud TVN, Torchia MG: *The developing human: clinically oriented embryology*, Philadelphia, 2008, Saunders.
5. Moore KL, Persaud TVN, Shiota K: *Color atlas of clinical embryology*, ed 2, Philadelphia, 2000, Saunders.
6. Guyton AC, Hall JE: *Textbook of medical physiology*, ed 11, Philadelphia, 2006, Saunders.
7. Shils ME: *Modern nutrition in health and disease*, ed 10, Philadelphia, 2006, Lippincott Williams & Wilkins.
8. Goroll AH, Mulley AG: *Primary care medicine*, ed 3, Philadelphia, 2000, Lippincott Williams & Wilkins.
9. Feldman M, Friedman LS, Sleisenger MH: *Sleisenger and Fordtran's gastrointestinal and liver disease: pathophysiology, diagnosis, management*, ed 7, Philadelphia, 2002, Saunders.
10. Shea JA et al: Revised estimates of diagnostic test sensitivity and specificity in suspected biliary tract disease, *Arch Intern Med* 154(22):2573-2581, 1994.
11. Mirvis SE et al: The diagnosis of acute acalculous cholecystitis: a comparison of sonography, scintigraphy, and CT, *AJR Am J Roentgenol* 147(6):1171-1175, 1986.
12. Orlando R, Russell JC: Managing gallbladder disease in a cost-effective manner, *Surg Clin North Am* 76:117-128, 1996.
13. Behrman SW et al: Laparoscopic cholecystectomy in the geriatric population, *Am Surg* 62:386-390, 1996.
14. Cotran RS, Kumar V, Collins T: *Robbins pathologic basis of disease*, ed 6, Philadelphia, 1999, Saunders.
15. Laoser C, Faolsch UR: A concept of treatment in acute pancreatitis: results of controlled trials and future developments, *Hepatogastroenterology* 40:569-573, 1993.
16. Renner IG, Savage WE, Pantoja JL et al: Death due to acute pancreatitis: a retrospective analysis of 405 autopsy cases, *Dig Dis Sci* 30(10):1005-1018, 1985.

17. Clochesy JM et al: *Critical care nursing,* Philadelphia, 1996, Saunders.

18. Chatzicostas C et al: Computed tomography severity index is superior to Ranson criteria and Apache II and III scoring systems in predicting acute pancreatitis outcome, *J Clin Gastroenterol* 36(3):253-260, 2003.

19. Thompson DR: Narcotic analgesic effects on the sphincter of Oddi: a review of the data and therapeutic implications in treating pancreatitis, *Am J Gastroenterol* 96(4):1266-1272, 2001.

20. Townsend CM et al: *Sabiston textbook of surgery: the biological basis of modern surgical practice,* ed 15, Philadelphia, 2001, Saunders.

21. Maringhini A, Ciambra M, Patti R: Ascites, pleural, and pericardial effusions in acute pancreatitis, *Dig Dis Sci* 41:848-852, 1996.

22. Yamedera K, Moriyama T, Makino I: Identification of immunoreactive pancreatic stone protein in pancreatic stone, pancreatic tissue and pancreatic juice, *Pancreas* 5(3):255-260, 1990.

23. Haubrich WS, Schaffner F, Bork JE: *Bockus gastroenterology,* ed 5, Philadelphia, 1995, Saunders.

24. Treacy PJ, Worthley CS: Pancreatic stents in the management of chronic pancreatitis, *Aust N Z J Surg* 66:210-213, 1996.

25. Singh VV, Toskes PP: Medical therapy for chronic pancreatitis pain, *Curr Gastroenterol Rep* 5(2):110-116, 2003.

chapter

38

Liver Diseases

Jeffrey S. Sartin

MEDIA RESOURCES

Additional Material for Study, Review, and Further Exploration

CD Companion ▪ Review Questions and Answers
▪ Glossary (with audio pronunciations for selected terms)
▪ Disease Profiles ▪ Animations

  Website at http://evolve.elsevier.com/Copstead/
▪ Case Studies ▪ Disease Profiles ▪ WebLinks ▪ Key Points Review

Online Course (Module 16)

KEY QUESTIONS

▪ What role does the liver play in nutrient metabolism, bile synthesis, storage of vitamins and minerals, urea synthesis, clotting factor synthesis, and detoxification?
▪ Which manifestations of liver disease are due to hepatocellular failure, and which are due to portal hypertension?
▪ How do the different types of viral hepatitis vary with regard to mode of transmission and severity of symptoms?

▪ What clinical and laboratory findings would lead to a diagnosis of liver cirrhosis?
▪ What treatment modalities are available to patients with end-stage liver failure?

CHAPTER OUTLINE

The liver is a vital but vulnerable organ. Its role in digestion of fats, storage of sugars, blood detoxification, and protein production makes it indispensable; in contrast to the kidney and heart, there are no "artificial livers." Nevertheless, the liver is susceptible to a wide variety of metabolic, circulatory, toxic, microbial, and neoplastic insults. In some instances the disease is primary to the liver, as in viral hepatitis and hepatocellular carcinoma (HCC). More often the hepatic involvement is secondary, a consequence of some of the more common diseases of humans, such as cardiac decompensation, metastatic cancer, alcoholism, and infections. This chapter will focus on primary diseases of the liver.

STRUCTURE AND FUNCTION OF THE LIVER

The liver, the largest parenchymal organ of the body, averages 1500 g. It is located in the right upper quadrant of the abdomen, beneath the diaphragm, and is anatomically divided into a right and left lobe and then further subdivided according to the pattern of its blood supply and biliary drainage. It is covered by a connective tissue capsule, the Glisson capsule, which in turn is covered by visceral peritoneum, reflections of which form the various suspensory hepatic ligaments. These structures demarcate the bare area of the liver directly in contact with the diaphragm (Figure 38-1).[1-3]

The liver has a dual blood supply. Arterial inflow from the aorta via the celiac trunk and hepatic artery provides 25% of the organ's blood supply. The remainder comes from the portal vein, which drains the capillary bed of the alimentary canal and pancreas (Figure 38-2). This oxygen-depleted venous blood is rich in substances absorbed and secreted by the gut. These afferent blood vessels then branch throughout the liver in association with the bile ducts and form the portal triads (consisting of the portal veins, hepatic arteries, and bile ducts). Eventually, blood from both the hepatic artery and the portal vein drains into the hepatic sinusoids, which surround sheets of liver cells, or hepatic plates (Figure 38-3). The sinusoids are lined by endothelial cells and Kupffer cells (a type of phagocytic macrophage). This blood drains into the central veins, which finally coalesce into the hepatic vein and empty into the inferior vena cava. Any obstruction to the flow of blood may result in a rise in portal venous pressure proximal to the level of blockage. This condition is called **portal hypertension** and is a central pathophysiologic event in many liver diseases. The liver also has a rich and complex lymphatic drainage system.

The liver is one of the most metabolically active organs in the body and functions simultaneously as a digestive organ, an endocrine organ, a hematologic organ, and an excretory organ (Box 38-1). All of these functions are elegantly interwoven with such redundancy that more than 80% of the liver may be destroyed before life is threatened.

General Manifestations of Liver Disease

Whether primary or secondary, all hepatic derangements tend to cause similar signs and symptoms that are directly attributable to loss of hepatocellular function or disruption of blood flow through the liver. Because of the liver's considerable reserve, however, manifestations appear only when the injury is significant and diffuse or so strategically located that it obstructs biliary outflow.

Hepatocellular Failure

Hepatocellular failure results in a number of typical manifestations, including jaundice, muscle wasting, ascites, excessive bleeding, deficiencies of important blood proteins and vitamins, glucose imbalance, and impaired hormone production (Table 38-1). At its most basic the liver is a sophisticated biochemical factory, and these conditions all derive from problems with processing the essential molecules of the body. Inadequate protein metabolism leads to decreased production of clotting factors and hypoalbuminemia. Decreased serum albumin in turn leads to generalized edema as a result of low serum oncotic pressure. Abnormal storage and release of glucose in the form of glycogen may result in bouts of either hyperglycemia or hypoglycemia. Reduced production of bile salts by the liver impairs absorption of the fat-soluble vitamins A, D, E, and K from the gastrointestinal (GI) tract. Lack of vitamin D may lead to osteomalacia (impaired bone

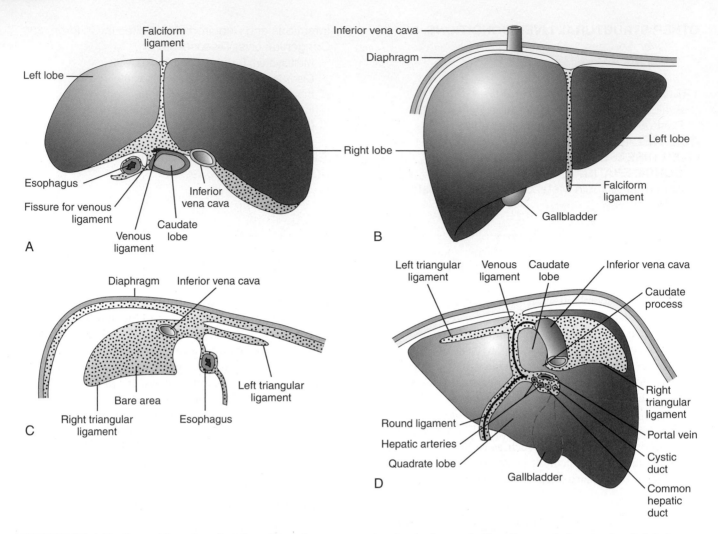

FIGURE 38-1 The liver and its peritoneal relations. *Stippled* areas represent surfaces not covered with peritoneum. **A,** Superior view. **B,** Anterior view. **C,** The diaphragm, viewed from in front, showing the position of the bare area of the liver. **D,** Visceral surface of the liver, viewed from behind. (Redrawn from Gardner E et al: *Anatomy: a regional study of human structure,* ed 3, Philadelphia, 1969, Saunders, p 414.)

homeostasis); lack of vitamin K contributes to poor blood clotting factor production. Altered lipoprotein processing leads to dyslipidemias, particularly hypertriglyceridemia.

Hepatocellular failure is associated with impaired processing of endogenous steroid hormones and the by-products of protein metabolism, as well as decreased clearance of exogenous drugs and toxins. Impaired metabolism of estrogen leads to feminization in men (gynecomastia, impotence, testicular atrophy, female hair distribution), irregular menses in women, palmar erythema, and spider telangiectasia. Impaired conversion of ammonia to urea may lead to hepatic encephalopathy, which will be discussed later in this chapter.

Jaundice

Etiology and Pathogenesis. Jaundice, the green-yellow staining of tissues by bilirubin, results from impaired bilirubin metabolism and is one of the most characteristic signs of liver disease. A study of the mechanisms of bilirubin metabolism is essential to an understanding of liver disease and may serve as a paradigm for other hepatic processes (Figure 38-4).[4-6]

As red blood cells age or are damaged by disease, they lyse and release oxygen-carrying hemoglobin molecules. These are taken up by the reticuloendothelial system, which separates heme from globin, and through the action of heme oxygenase opens the heme ring to release the central iron atom. This process yields biliverdin, which in turn is converted by the enzyme bilirubin reductase to bilirubin. (A small percentage of bilirubin is derived from the premature destruction of immature cells in the bone marrow and spleen and from heme proteins such as myoglobin and the cytochromes in the liver.) Bilirubin is released into the plasma and transported to the liver tightly bound to the plasma protein albumin. The free unconjugated bilirubin is lipid soluble and can be displaced from albumin by fatty acids and certain organic anions (e.g., sulfonamides, salicylates). The neonate is particularly sensitive to free unconjugated bilirubin, which can diffuse into the brain and cause a type of encephalopathy known as **kernicterus** (see the Liver Diseases and Pediatric Considerations section).

FIGURE 38-2 Schematic diagram of the portal circulation. Blood from the aorta supplies the alimentary canal. Venous blood from the intestine reaches the sinusoids of the liver by way of the portal vein. Venous blood from the liver reaches the inferior vena cava by way of the hepatic veins.

FIGURE 38-3 Liver lobule.

BOX 38-1

Summary of Normal Liver Function

The Liver as a Digestive Organ
Bile salt secretion for fat digestion
Processing and storage of fats, carbohydrates, and proteins
    absorbed by the intestines
Processing and storage of vitamins and minerals

The Liver as an Endocrine Organ
Metabolism of glucocorticoids, mineralocorticoids, and sex
    hormones
Regulation of carbohydrate, fat, and protein metabolism

The Liver as a Hematologic Organ
Temporary storage of blood
Removal of bilirubin from bloodstream
Hematopoiesis in certain disease states
Synthesis of blood clotting factors

The Liver as an Excretory Organ
Excretion of bile pigment
Excretion of cholesterol via bile
Urea synthesis
Detoxification of drugs and other foreign substances

TABLE 38-1

Pathophysiology Underlying the Symptoms and Signs of Liver Disease

Symptoms/Signs	Pathophysiologic Mechanism
Weakness, fatigue, anorexia, weight loss, muscle wasting	Failure of multiple metabolic functions
Fever	Liver inflammation, decreased reticuloendothelial function with increased risk of infection
Bruising, increased bleeding	Thrombocytopenia secondary to splenic enlargement, decreased synthesis of clotting factors I, II, V, VII, VIII, IX, and X
Palmar erythema, cutaneous spider telangiectases, irregular menses, gynecomastia, impotence, female body hair distribution in men, testicular atrophy	Altered metabolism of sex hormones, chronic debilitation
Hepatic encephalopathy	Abnormal protein metabolism
Fetor hepaticus	Decreased detoxification
Pruritus	Decreased bile salt excretion
Cyanosis	Arteriovenous shunts in lungs, liver
Jaundice	Biliary obstruction, decreased bilirubin synthesis, decreased bilirubin excretion
Hyperdynamic circulation, wide pulse pressure, tachycardia	Generalized vasodilation (? Hormonally mediated)
Ascites, peripheral edema	Portal hypertension, sodium and water retention, low serum albumin secondary to decreased hepatic synthesis
Splenomegaly	Portal hypertension
Hepatomegaly	Cirrhosis (liver may be small), hepatitis, vascular congestion, bile duct obstruction, infection, benign infiltrative disease (e.g., fatty liver, amyloidosis, hemochromatosis), malignant infiltrative disease (e.g., metastatic cancer, lymphoma, large space-occupying lesions such as neoplasm, abscess)
Varices (esophageal, gastric, rectal, ectopic) or abnormal abdominal vascular pattern (caput medusae, umbilical bruit)	Portal hypertension with collateral blood flow around hepatic blockage
Osteomalacia, hypocalcemia, night blindness, coagulopathy	Fat-soluble vitamin malabsorption and loss of fat-soluble vitamin reserves A, D, and K; loss of vitamin K metabolism (a cofactor for I, II, VII, VIII, IX, and X)
Anemia	Multifactorial: blood loss, chronic disease, vitamin B_{12} deficiency, splenic sequestration
Leukopenia	Hypersplenism secondary to portal hypertension
Hypoglycemia	Altered glycogenolysis, gluconeogenesis
Hyperglycemia	Portosystemic shunting with delayed hepatic uptake of absorbed glucose
Hypercholesterolemia	Obstructive jaundice with decreased cholesterol excretion

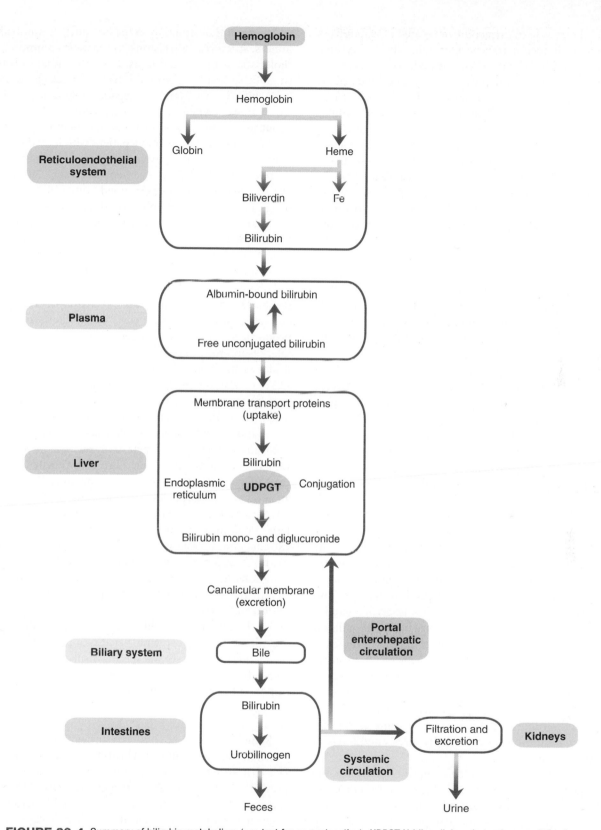

FIGURE 38-4 Summary of bilirubin metabolism (see text for an explanation). *UDPGT,* Uridine diphosphate glucuronyltransferase.

Liver cells are able to extract unconjugated bilirubin from the plasma with special transport proteins. In the cytosol, bilirubin is quickly bound, or conjugated, to water-soluble derivatives of glucuronic acid by action of the enzyme uridine diphosphate glucuronosyltransferase (UDPGT) located in the endoplasmic reticulum. This process yields water-soluble bilirubin monoglucuronide and diglucuronide, which is then actively excreted into microscopic bile ducts (canaliculi). Bilirubin is then transported through the biliary system as a component of bile to the small intestine. Because it cannot be absorbed in the small intestine, it passes to the colon where bacterial β-glucuronidase enzymes break it down to urobilinogen. A small fraction of urobilinogen is absorbed from the colon and re-excreted by the kidneys and the liver. In the presence of liver disease, the hepatic fraction decreases and the urinary fraction increases, thus accounting for the rise in urinary urobilinogen seen with liver dysfunction. With complete obstruction to bile flow or with intestinal obstruction above the colonic level, urinary urobilinogen falls to zero, as no bilirubin reaches the colon. (The function of bile salts and the other components of bile flow are discussed in Chapter 37.)

Therefore, jaundice may result from dysfunction anywhere along this complex pathway. Classically, it is divided into prehepatic, hepatic, and posthepatic or cholestatic, but much overlap occurs.

Prehepatic. The most common causes of prehepatic jaundice are hemolysis and ineffective erythropoiesis. The resorption of large hematomas in patients with mild liver disease is a frequent and harmless cause of mild jaundice due to unconjugated hyperbilirubinemia.

Hepatic. Dysfunction of each of the hepatic steps in bilirubin metabolism may cause jaundice. In the neonate, immature UDPGT levels may result in physiologic jaundice of the newborn. Various genetic disorders of UDPGT synthesis are characterized by high levels of unconjugated bilirubin in the blood. Mutant UDPGT enzymes can produce the common and benign Gilbert syndrome, in which low levels of unconjugated hyperbilirubinemia may be increased by fasting or illness (e.g., viral gastroenteritis). Other UDPGT mutations cause the Crigler-Najjar type 1 and 2 syndromes with severe neonatal unconjugated hyperbilirubinemia (see the Liver Diseases and Pediatric Considerations section). Most of the liver diseases to be discussed later, such as viral hepatitis, alcoholic liver disease, and autoimmune hepatitis, result in jaundice because dysfunction within the liver cell results in elevated levels of conjugated bilirubin.

Posthepatic. At the level of canalicular bilirubin transport, the rare inherited Dubin-Johnson and Rotor syndromes cause conjugated hyperbilirubinemia. Both conditions have an excellent prognosis. At the canalicular posthepatocytic level, many drugs such as the phenothiazines and the sex hormones may cause jaundice.[7] In susceptible women, the high sex hormone levels of normal pregnancy can cause benign cholestasis of pregnancy.[8] This condition is also associated with defective transport of bile salts and is characterized by jaundice and intense pruritus.

Mechanical obstruction to the bile ducts from obstructing tumors, strictures, or gallstones is the most common cause of cholestatic jaundice. Some experts differentiate obstructive jaundice caused by a gross mechanical blockage to bile flow in the biliary tract from intrahepatic cholestatic jaundice, the latter implying a defect at the microscopic level.

Evaluation. Evaluation of a jaundiced patient may be used as a model for investigation of any patient with liver disease. After a complete history and physical examination are obtained and routine laboratory data reviewed (see Table 38-1), specific liver-related tests may be performed (Table 38-2). The underlying cause, such as alcoholic liver disease, a drug reaction, or metastatic or primary malignancy, is often suggested by the history and physical examination. Physical stigmata of chronic liver disease include telangiectasia, ascites, palmar erythema, gynecomastia, testicular atrophy, hair loss (in men), and central obesity with peripheral muscle wasting.

Diagnostic Tests. Biochemical tests usually fall into one of several categories. A significant elevation in transaminases out of proportion to the other liver enzymes indicates a hepatocellular disorder (i.e., hepatitis). Alcoholic and other toxic hepatitides virtually always show the aspartate aminotransferase (AST) markedly elevated in comparison with the alanine aminotransferase (ALT), whereas in viral hepatitis the reverse is usually true. Predominant elevations of alkaline phosphatase (ALP) indicate intrahepatic cholestasis and are often due to an infiltrative process (e.g., metastatic carcinoma, sarcoidosis). Elevated bilirubin can be either direct (conjugated) or indirect (unconjugated). Although an overwhelming liver process in an adult will produce elevations of both, as a practical matter unconjugated hyperbilirubinemia points to significant hemolysis. Predominant conjugated bilirubin elevation points to extrahepatic cholestasis due to biliary obstruction. It is noteworthy that jaundice in patients with cirrhosis often shows elevations in all parameters, reflecting the widespread liver dysfunction and obstruction of the bile canals and small vessels due to scarring.

Evaluation of hepatocellular and cholestatic disorders may include evaluation for viral hepatitis (Table 38-3), various biochemical assays (see the specific disorders discussed later), or needle biopsy of the liver. Needle biopsies may be carried out "blind" or may be directed by ultrasound or computed tomography (CT), allowing examination of a specific target such as a mass lesion.

Radiologic imaging with ultrasonography is often helpful for significant liver disease. This is particularly true given the fact that structural liver abnormalities such as tumors may present with any of the above enzyme patterns or with a mixed picture. CT provides more information and has a special role in evaluating the content of iron in the liver in cases of suspected hemochromatosis. Specific visualization of the bile ducts may necessitate percutaneous transhepatic cholangiography or endoscopic retrograde cholangiopancreatography (ERCP; see Chapter 37), though magnetic resonance cholangiopancreatography (MRCP) has rapidly gained acceptance as a noninvasive way of evaluating the liver and biliary tree in great detail.

TABLE 38-2

Common Laboratory Tests in Liver Disease

Test	Normal Range	Significance
AST/SGOT	5-40 U/ml	Elevated levels indicate hepatocellular inflammation or necrosis
ALT/SGPT	5-35 U/ml	AST much greater than ALT in alcoholic liver disease
		AST less specific; may be of skeletal muscle, myocardial, kidney, or liver origin
		ALT more specific for liver disease
Alkaline phosphatase	35-150 U/ml	Elevated in cholestasis, infiltrative liver disease (cancer, granulomas, etc.)
		May be of bone origin
γ-Glutamyl	10-48 U/ml	Elevated in cholestasis and hepatocellular disease transpeptidase
		Used to confirm that elevated alkaline phosphatase is of hepatic origin
		Disproportionately elevated in alcoholic liver disease
		May be induced by many drugs (e.g., phenobarbital)
5'-Nucleotidase	2-11 U/ml	Elevated in cholestasis
		Very specific to the liver
Total bilirubin	<1.0 mg/dl	Elevated levels diagnose jaundice
Indirect bilirubin	<0.8 mg/dl	Elevated in hemolysis, Gilbert disease
Prothrombin time	11.5-14 sec	Prolongation suggests decreased hepatic synthetic function
Serum albumin	3.5-5.5 g/dl	Decreased level suggests decreased hepatic synthesis
Serum globulin	2.5-3.5 g/dl	Elevated in autoimmune hepatitis
Urine bilirubin	0	Increased with elevation of serum conjugated (direct) bilirubin, zero in unconjugated (indirect) hyperbilirubinemia
Urinary urobilinogen	0-4 mg/24 hr; spot test ± on urine dipstick	Zero in complete biliary or proximal bowel obstruction
		Increase may suggest liver disease
		Nonspecifically insensitive
		Primary utility because its presence on urine dipsticks allows simple office/bedside testing or screening with one-time urinalysis

Portal Hypertension

Manifestations of liver disease not attributed to hepatocellular failure are mainly due to impaired blood flow through the liver as a result of increased resistance from fibrosis and degeneration of liver tissue. Sluggish blood flow through the liver results in increased pressure in the portal circulation (**portal hypertension**) (Figure 38-5). In this condition, venous drainage of much of the GI tract is congested. Symptoms are surprisingly few early in the course, but as abnormal vascular patterns progress anorexia may result. The end results of elevated venous pressure are varices, particularly esophageal, but also gastric and hemorrhoidal. A pathognomic feature of advanced liver disease is superficial periumbilical varices, known as *caput medusae*, or *the head of Medusa*. Portal hypertension may present as an accumulation of peritoneal fluid, or **ascites**. A serious consequence of portal hypertension is uncontrolled bleeding from esophageal varices, which are prone to rupture.

Gastroesophageal Varices

Etiology. Esophageal varices result mainly from portal hypertension, which in Western society is generally the result of alcoholic or posthepatitis cirrhosis. In developing tropical countries, chronic infection with *Schistosoma* species is a major cause of portal hypertension. Recently, it has been recognized that vasoactive hormones, as well as increased splanchnic blood flow and increased vascular resistance in the liver, have a prominent role in the formation of variceal esophageal veins.[1] Gastric varices may occur in connection with or independently from esophageal varices.

Pathogenesis. Gastroesophageal varices are merely one of a number of collateral venous pathways that dilate in response to elevated portal pressure in an attempt to transport blood from the splanchnic bed around the cirrhotic liver and back to the heart. Other common pathways include spontaneous splenorenal shunts, a variety of deep and usually entirely asymptomatic portosystemic shunts; dilated veins in the small intestine, colon, and rectum are also not uncommon.[1] Unfortunately, part of the very complex venous network that surrounds the proximal part of the stomach and esophagus lies just beneath the mucosa, rendering it especially liable to rupture when portal pressures reach a critical level. Rupture results in massive, often life-threatening upper GI bleeding (Figure 38-6).

Clinical Features. Varices will affect more than half of cirrhotic patients, and approximately 30% of them experience an episode of variceal hemorrhage within 2 years of the diagnosis of varices.[1] Variceal size is the main determinant of risk for bleeding, which is often catastrophic and is one of the main causes of death (20% to 33%) in persons with long-standing cirrhosis. The mortality after an episode of significant variceal bleeding is as high as 50%. The diagnosis is made mainly endoscopically, but varices may be seen on upper GI barium examinations as well, and occasionally on CT scans of the abdomen.

Bleeding from gastroesophageal varices is one of the most dreaded complications of portal hypertension. The initial symptoms and signs are those of major upper GI hemorrhage and include hematemesis, melena, and rapid intestinal transit

TABLE 38-3

Immunologic Markers in Viral Hepatitis

Marker	Description
Hepatitis A	
Anti-HAV IgM	Acute infection with HAV, but may persist for months
Anti-HAV IgG	Past infection with HAV
	Implies immunity to the virus
Hepatitis B	
Hepatitis B surface antigen (HBsAg)	Surface protein coat of HBV
	Implies active infection
	Detectable 2-6 wk after infection
	Remains present as long as infection is active
Hepatitis B surface antibody IgM (HBsAb)	Antibody to surface protein of HBV
	Detectable shortly after or with clearance of HBsAg
	Implies resolution of infection and immunity to HBV
Hepatitis B core antibody IgM (HBcAb IgM)	Antibody to inner core protein of HBV
	Detectable 3-5 wk after infection
	Implies recent infection
Hepatitis B core antibody IgG (HBcAb IgG)	As for HBcAb IgM, but implies past infection
Hepatitis e antigen (HBeAg)	Soluble fraction of HBV
	Detectable 2-6 wk after infection
	Implies ongoing infection with high infectivity
	May resolve independently of HBsAg
Hepatitis B e antibody (HBeAb)	Antibody to soluble fraction of HBV
	Detectable when HBeAg clears
	Implies decreased infectivity
HBV DNA polymerase activity	Same significance as HBV DNA
Hepatitis C	
Anti-HCV	Antibody to HCV antigens
	May not be detectable early in infection
	Does not indicate immunity to the virus
	Rapidly evolving area; many commercially available assays of different sensitivity and specificity
	Many false-positive and false-negative results
HCV RNA by PCR	Assay for level of viremia
	Correlates positively with activity of infection
	Clears with resolution of infection
	Technically difficult; available through reference laboratories
Hepatitis D (Delta)	
Hepatitis delta antigen (HDAg)	Assay for 35-nm RNA virus
	Detectable 2-10 wk after infection
	Implies early infection
Anti-HDV	Implies past or chronic infection
	Does not indicate immunity to the virus
Hepatitis E	
HEV RNA by PCR	Detects presence of virus
HEV antibody IgG and IgM	Not well standardized
Hepatitis G	
HGV by PCR	Measures level of viremia

PCR, Polymerase chain reaction.

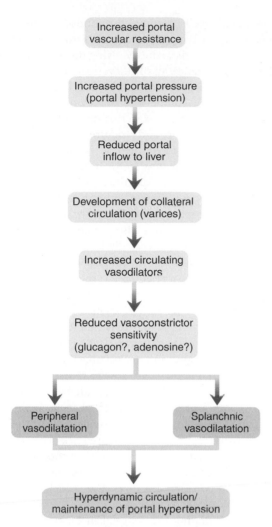

FIGURE 38-5 Pathophysiologic process of portal hypertension. (Redrawn from MacMathuna P: The pathogenesis of variceal rupture, *Gastrointest Endosc Clin North Am* 2[1]:1-8, 1992.)

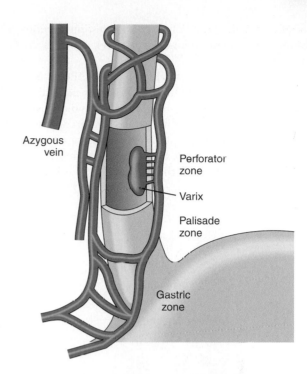

FIGURE 38-6 Gastroesophageal venous anatomy. (Redrawn from MacMathuna P: The pathogenesis of variceal rupture, *Gastrointest Endosc Clin North Am* 2[1]:1-8, 1992.)

and vigorous bleeding, even bright red rectal bleeding. These characteristics may be associated with profound anemia and symptoms and signs of shock. In most cases, concomitant evidence of chronic liver disease and portal hypertension is seen. There are two distinct phases of the variceal hemorrhage process: one, coincident with and shortly after the bleeding; and two, a period of 6 to 8 weeks following the initial bleed, where there is a high risk of rebleeding. The greatest risk of rebleeding occurs in the first 72 hours.

Treatment. Initial treatment is directed at fluid resuscitation, correcting the coagulopathy, and stopping further bleeding. Large-bore intravenous lines are placed, and fluid resuscitation is carried out with normal saline. Blood components and clotting factors are replaced as needed. Any coagulopathy may necessitate administration of parenteral vitamin K, fresh frozen plasma, and platelet infusions if profound thrombocytopenia is present. Recombinant Factor VIIa has been shown in numerous small studies to be helpful in reversing the coagulopathy associated with advanced liver disease and may be considered for patients whose prothrombin time (PT) fails to normalize with the above measures.[9]

Primary acute pharmacologic management rests on drugs that can effectively lower portal pressure by dilating alternative collateral pathways, reducing splanchnic blood flow, or both. Traditionally, in the United States the agent of choice has been vasopressin, an analog of antidiuretic hormone, administered by continuous intravenous infusion. Although effective in controlling variceal bleeding, its use may be associated with angina pectoris, severe abdominal cramping, and, with long-term infusion, hyponatremia. These side effects often limit both the dose administered and the duration of therapy. Nitroglycerin is very effective in lowering portal pressure, counteracts some of these side effects, and is generally given concomitantly with vasopressin by the intravenous route.[3]

In recent years, octreotide acetate, a synthetic analog of the naturally occurring hormone somatostatin, has been effectively used as a replacement for vasopressin.[10] It is administered as an initial intravenous bolus followed by continuous infusion, which may be administered for as long as 3 to 5 days. In the doses used, the drug is remarkably free of side effects and more effective than vasopressin. However, it should be noted that no drug treatment has shown a mortality benefit for this condition.

Metoclopramide and β-blockers have been used as ancillary treatments in the past and may be considered for selected patients. Intravenous H_2 blockers or proton pump inhibitors are also often administered. The use of prophylactic antibiotics is controversial but is recommended by the American

Association for the Study of Liver Diseases; intravenous ceftriaxone or an oral quinolone for a 1-week course is the preferred regimen.[11]

Emergency esophagogastroduodenoscopy (EGD) is crucial in determining the site of bleeding, as well as excluding other causes of upper GI bleeding. In addition to its diagnostic role, EGD actively addresses bleeding varices. **Endoscopic sclerosis** of esophageal varices is accomplished by passing a flexible needle through the gastroscope and injecting various sclerosant solutions into and around the bleeding varix (Figure 38-7).

FIGURE 38-7 Endoscopic sclerosis of varices.

Such treatment results in initial thrombosis of the vein with hemostasis. Repeated injections cause fibrosis and obliteration of the varix and fibrosis of the overlying mucosa. This process can effectively obliterate all of the varices at risk of bleeding. Unfortunately, this treatment may be associated with a variety of acute and chronic complications, including drug reactions to the sclerosing solutions, exacerbation of bleeding, perforation, ulceration, infection, and stricture formation.[5]

An alternative treatment method is endoscopic ligation of esophageal varices (Figure 38-8). In this technique, a special apparatus is preloaded onto the gastroscope so that the endoscopist can suction a varix into a special chamber at the end of the gastroscope and then ligate the varix with a small rubber band. This technique also results in immediate loss of flow in the varix and eventually leads to thrombosis and fibrosis. The area ligated simply sloughs off over the next week or so without significant residual ulceration or scarring. This method requires fewer sessions than endoscopic sclerosis to completely obliterate the varices, seems to be associated with a lower complication rate, and may be more effective in the management of bleeding gastric varices.[6] However, it is technically more challenging and not suitable for all patients.[12]

Endoscopic techniques have shown a mortality benefit relative to drugs alone but fail to control acute bleeding in 10% to 20% of patients. Unfortunately, both of these methods may result in an increase in venous pressure proximal to the area treated, perhaps resulting in an increased risk of bleeding from congestive gastroenteropathy (a diffuse venous congestion that may result in both chronic and acute severe blood loss).

Balloon tamponade of varices was widely used before the availability of endoscopic treatment. A variety of tubes are available, including the Sengstaken-Blakemore tube, the Minnesota tube, and the Linton-Nachlas tube.[13] All consist of a gastric balloon that is passed by mouth or transnasally,

| Site of bleeding identified | Contact made between ligator and varix | Suction applied to draw varix into ligator lumen | O ring released around neck of varix | Hemostasis achieved |

FIGURE 38-8 Endoscopic band ligation of varices.

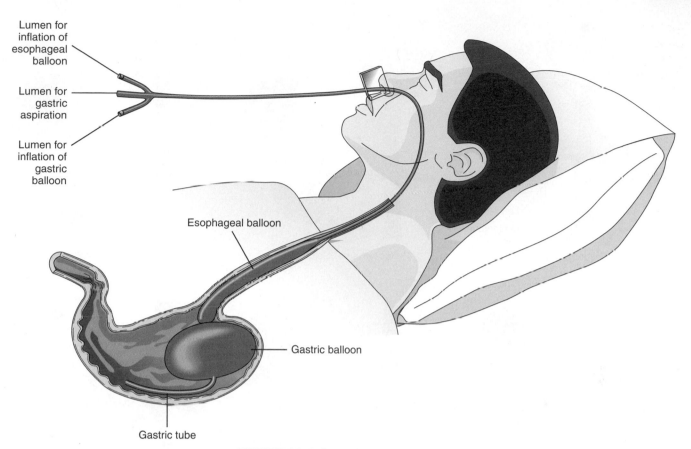

Lumen for
inflation of
esophageal
balloon

Lumen for
gastric
aspiration

Lumen for
inflation of
gastric
balloon

Esophageal balloon

Gastric balloon

Gastric tube

FIGURE 38-9 Sengstaken-Blakemore tube.

inflated to volumes specific to each tube, and held in gentle traction against the gastric varices in the fundus, thus resulting in compression hemostasis and occlusion of blood flow from the fundus of the stomach up into the esophageal varices (Figure 38-9). In addition, some tubes have an esophageal balloon that may be inflated to specific pressures against the esophageal varices directly. Suction of oropharyngeal and gastric secretions is accomplished with integral or separate drainage tubes. Aspiration of stomach contents, migration of the tube with airway compression, pressure necrosis of the esophagus and stomach, balloon rupture, and rebleeding after the maximal inflation period of 24 hours all limit the usefulness of balloon tamponade to a temporizing role.

Chronic pharmacologic management of portal hypertension is frequently successful with nonselective β-blockers such as propranolol or nadolol. The drug is carefully titrated to reduce the initial resting heart rate by 25%. These drugs may be used prophylactically in patients with known portal hypertension and are often prescribed following endoscopic therapy as part of a combined approach to variceal bleeding prevention. It should be noted that studies have not yet shown a consistent survival benefit for this intervention, however. In addition to β-blockers, oral long-acting nitrates such as isosorbide mononitrate act synergistically with β-blockers to reduce portal pressure and have been studied for prevention of variceal hemorrhage.[14,15] Side effects limit use of nitrates as

primary prophylaxis, but these agents could be considered for secondary prophylaxis in patients who fail β-blockers alone.

If the aforementioned measures are ineffective, a number of surgical and radiologic procedures are possible. Although rarely used in the United States, esophageal transection and reanastomosis with ligation of other collateral channels has been used in other countries.[1] Surgery to reduce portal pressure is very effective in decreasing the rate of rebleeding, but it may not alter overall survival. A variety of surgical techniques are used, all of which create an alternative connection between the splanchnic and systemic circulation. These techniques include portacaval, mesocaval, splenorenal, and distal splenorenal shunts (Figure 38-10). A discussion of the specific indications and technical aspects of these shunts is beyond the scope of this text, but each has certain specific indications, advantages, and disadvantages.[16]

In recent years a radiographic procedure called transjugular intrahepatic portosystemic shunting (TIPS) has been developed that combines angiographic and ultrasonographic techniques.[1] The hepatic vein is cannulated by the transjugular route. A needle is then passed into a main portal vein branch. Catheters are passed over this guidewire along with balloon dilation of the tract so created. This step is then followed by placement of an expandable metallic stent, thus creating a portosystemic shunt (portal vein to hepatic vein) within the liver itself. This procedure is technically very demanding and

Normal (without anastomosis)

Portal vein
Splenic vein
Inferior vena cava
Left renal vein
Mesenteric vein

Portacaval side-to-side shunt

Portacaval end-to-side shunt

Cavomesenteric shunt

Central splenorenal shunt

Distal splenorenal shunt

FIGURE 38-10 Portosystemic shunt operations.

may be complicated by hemorrhage, infection, stent migration, stent stenosis, and occlusion, both acute and chronic. In addition, hepatic encephalopathy and congestive heart failure may result. The primary use of this modality is as a bridge to allow stabilization of patients who are candidates for liver transplantation.[17]

Treatment of esophageal varices is often unsatisfactory. Ideally, the underlying condition for varices (i.e., portal hypertension) should be reversed. The only consistently effective way to accomplish this goal is by liver transplantation (see the Transplantation section), which is limited in its application to a select group of patients.

Portal Systemic Encephalopathy
Hepatic Encephalopathy

Pathogenesis. Hepatic encephalopathy is a complex neuropsychiatric syndrome characterized by symptoms ranging from mild confusion and lethargy to stupor and coma. Some patients exhibit dementia, psychotic symptoms, spastic myelopathy, and cerebellar or extrapyramidal signs. The classic physical finding is asterixis, or "liver flap," a spastic jerking of the hands held in forced extension. Hepatic encephalopathy is associated with fulminant hepatic failure or severe chronic liver disease, conditions in which liver function is severely depressed and blood is shunted around the liver. The arterial ammonia level correlates positively with the level of encephalopathy in most patients, consistent with its central role in the pathogenesis of hepatic encephalopathy as one of the primary causes of neuronal dysfunction. The exact cause is unclear, and other contributing factors such as elevated mercaptan levels, enhanced activation of certain neurotransmitter receptors (including gamma-amino butyric acid and benzodiazepine receptors), and elevated levels of aromatic amino acids (false neurotransmitters) remain under investigation.[1,18]

Clinical Manifestations. Hepatic encephalopathy is usually precipitated by certain well-defined clinical developments, including hypokalemia, hyponatremia, alkalosis, hypoxia, hypercarbia, infection, use of sedatives, GI hemorrhage, protein meal gorging, renal failure, and constipation. In some patients, progressive liver failure leads to chronic encephalopathy without other exacerbating factors.

Hepatic encephalopathy is graded 1 to 4:

Grade 1: Confusion, subtle behavioral changes, no flap
Grade 2: Drowsy, clear behavioral changes, flap present

Grade 3: Stuporous but can follow commands, marked confusion, slurred speech, flap present

Grade 4: Coma, no flap

Treatment. The first step in treatment of hepatic encephalopathy consists of correcting any identifiable precipitating factors, such as gastrointestinal bleeding. Restriction of dietary protein to 60 g or less daily is indicated for patients with chronic encephalopathy, along with enhanced elimination of the toxic nitrogenous substances produced by intestinal digestion (see below). Critically ill patients should receive peripheral or central glucose infusions along with vitamins, especially thiamine. As the patient's ammonia levels drop, protein may be reintroduced into the diet. The initial amount of 20 g/day is increased by 10 or 20 g/day every few days to an ultimate 0.75 to 1.0 g of protein per kilogram of body weight daily.[19] Observation for worsening encephalopathy is crucial at this time. When protein is restricted, it is essential to provide at least 400 g of carbohydrate daily. Vegetable protein may be better tolerated than animal protein. High dietary fiber intake may help by decreasing constipation. If dietary measures fail, oral defined-formula feedings containing essential amino acids and enriched with branched-chain amino acids may be indicated.

Osmotic diuretics or antibiotics are used to enhance elimination of nitrogenous wastes. Lactulose is the standard osmotic cathartic and may be given orally or by enema. (Standard precautions must be taken before any cathartic is administered, including ruling out bowel obstruction and monitoring electrolytes, particularly in patients with renal insufficiency.) Some evidence suggests that a lactulose-related change in pH also inhibits ammonia production by the gut flora, possibly by selecting for bacterial populations that are less ammoniagenic. No serious adverse reactions have been reported with lactulose therapy, although flatulence and abdominal cramping may occur. The dosage should be individually titrated so that two soft, acidic stools are passed daily.

Oral antibiotics have been used for many years to suppress the intestinal flora that break down dietary protein and release ammonia. Amoxicillin and rifamixin are currently used for this purpose. Bacterial overgrowth is one of the complications that limit the long-term use of antibiotics; therefore, this treatment is reserved for persons who cannot tolerate lactulose. Neomycin, the first antibiotic widely used in hepatic encephalopathy, is no longer recommended because of side effects.[1]

Cerebral Edema

Pathogenesis. Swelling of the brain (cerebral edema) often develops in patients with grade 3 or 4 hepatic encephalopathy and results in an increase in intracranial pressure. Both vascular and toxic mechanisms have been implicated as etiologic factors. With increasing intracranial pressure, blood perfusion of the brain is decreased (cerebral perfusion pressure = carotid artery pressure − intracranial pressure) with resulting cerebral hypoxia. Cerebral edema is a major cause of death in patients with acute hepatic failure.[20,21]

Clinical Manifestations. Clinically, cerebral edema is suggested by deepening coma, systolic hypertension, and extensor rigidity (decerebrate posture), followed by pupillary dilation and, if brainstem herniation occurs, respiratory arrest. Some highly specialized referral centers monitor patients with advanced hepatic encephalopathy by extradural pressure monitors to permit early detection. Unfortunately, complications of extradural monitors occur up to 20% of the time and include infection and intracranial bleeding.[1,22]

Treatment. Cerebral edema is managed primarily by the intravenous infusion of mannitol, which by increasing serum osmolarity draws water from the brain and thus reduces the swelling. Patients should be kept in the semi-Fowler position (head and trunk elevated 30 degrees). The barbiturate sodium pentothal is used as a second-line agent for patients with recalcitrant intracranial hypertension and those who cannot tolerate the fluid volume component of mannitol therapy (e.g., those in heart or kidney failure). Moderate hypothermia with the use of cooling blankets has looked promising in preliminary trials as well.[23] Aggressive treatment allows patient survival in 60% of cases, until liver failure resolves or liver transplantation can be accomplished.

Conditions of Advanced Liver Disease
Ascites

Etiology, Pathogenesis, and Clinical Manifestations. Ascites, or the pathologic accumulation of fluid in the peritoneal cavity, can occur in patients with advanced liver disease complicated by portal hypertension and hypoalbuminemia (Figure 38-11). Abdominal distention results from an inappropriate osmotic gradient across the pleura, with the intraabdominal accumulation of sodium, water, and protein.[1,24] Other causes of ascites are malignancy, infection, pancreatitis, hypothyroidism, vasculitis, nephrosis, cardiac failure, constrictive pericarditis, Budd-Chiari syndrome, and portal vein thrombosis. The specific chemical and cellular composition of the ascites varies with its cause.

Abdominal paracentesis should be performed in all patients with new ascites and in those with known ascites who have experienced significant worsening of their condition.[1] The fluid should be examined for total protein, albumin, and cell count. Optional tests include culture for bacteria, fungi and mycobacteria; cytology; amylase; glucose; and lactate dehydrogenase. A small amount of ascites may not require specific therapy. However, with increasing volumes, abdominal discomfort, abdominal or umbilical herniation, respiratory embarrassment, or infection may occur.

Treatment. Dietary sodium should be restricted to 88 mEq (2.0 mg) per day in patients with ascites. In motivated patients, this is perhaps the most helpful intervention that can be undertaken. Bed rest is useful, although strict bed rest can result in decubitus ulcers, deconditioning, and other problems. Diuretics are necessary for the majority of patients. The aldosterone antagonist spironolactone works in the distal nephron as a weak diuretic that also inhibits potassium secretion, thus sparing serum potassium. A delay of 2 to 3 days may occur before the full effect of the drug is seen, and the dosage should not be increased more frequently. Many authorities

FIGURE 38-11 Pathophysiologic process of ascites. (Redrawn from Dudley FJ: Pathophysiology of ascites formation, *Gastroenterol Clin North Am* 21:215-235, 1992.)

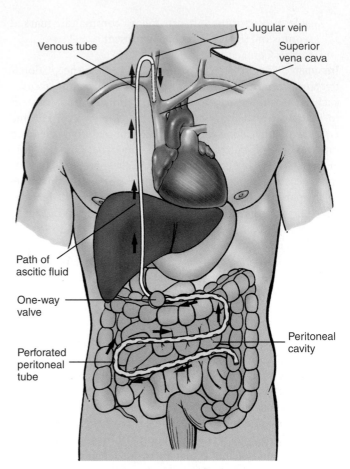

FIGURE 38-12 LeVeen shunt. Arrows show direction of flow of ascitic fluid out of the peritoneal cavity, through the shunt, into the superior vena cava. (From Monahan FD, Neighbors M: *Medical-surgical nursing: foundations for clinical practice*, ed 2, Philadelphia, 1998, Saunders, p 1146.)

suggest adding a loop diuretic such as furosemide from the beginning and increasing the dose at a ratio of 4:10 with spironolactone.[1] It is helpful to monitor both urinary sodium and potassium levels periodically. When the urinary sodium level exceeds the urinary potassium level, spironolactone is exerting its maximal effect. Serum potassium levels must be carefully controlled.

The goal is the loss of approximately 0.5 kg of body weight daily, although in patients with peripheral edema, slightly more rapid weight loss is tolerable. More rapid losses may result in diuretic-induced renal impairment, intravascular volume depletion and severe electrolyte abnormalities, and hepatic encephalopathy. Diuresis should be continued until the ascites is barely detectable. Free water restriction is prescribed if hyponatremia is present or develops during treatment, although compliance with a strict regimen is unlikely.

In patients who do not respond to both diuretic therapy and sodium restriction, the use of 25% albumin infusions may help initiate diuresis. However, the effect of this treatment is often short lived and not without a risk of overexpansion of the intravascular volume, with congestive heart failure,

pulmonary edema, and precipitation of variceal hemorrhage all possible.[25] Alternatively, large volumes of ascitic fluid can be removed from the peritoneal space through paracentesis. This "large-volume therapeutic paracentesis" is a very rapid and effective treatment that can be safely instituted if the intravascular volume is maintained by appropriate measures.[25] Diuretic and dietary treatment should be continued, but in severe cases, large-volume paracentesis may be repeated as needed.

Shunting procedures such as the LeVeen (Figure 38-12) and Denver shunts have been used. These one-way valves connect the peritoneal space with the venous system, usually at the jugular vein. These shunting procedures, although useful, carry significant risks and are best reserved for a small subset of ascites patients who have refractory ascites and are not candidates for liver transplantation.[26] The use of Transjugular Intrahepatic Portosystemic Stenting (TIPS) has largely replaced traditional surgical procedures for treatment of refractory ascites (see discussion above). Diuretic-resistant ascites is also an indication for liver transplantation in the patient who meets other criteria.

FIGURE 38-13 Pathophysiologic process of spontaneous bacterial peritonitis. (Redrawn from Garcia-Tsao G: Spontaneous bacterial peritonitis, *Gastroenterol Clin North Am* 21:257-275, 1992.)

Spontaneous Bacterial Peritonitis

Pathogenesis and Clinical Manifestations. Patients with cirrhosis and ascites suffer from a variety of defects in host defense that predispose to infection in the peritoneal cavity. This observation is especially true in patients who have ascites with a low protein concentration. These defects include diminished opsonic activity of the ascitic fluid, diminished reticuloendothelial function, and transmigration of gut bacteria across the intestinal wall and into the ascites (so-called monomicrobial non-neutrocytic bacterascites).[1,27] Chronic alcoholics demonstrate abnormal white blood cell function as well (Figure 38-13).

Typically, patients with spontaneous bacterial peritonitis (SBP) have a single infecting organism of gut origin in the fluid. This pattern is in marked distinction to patients with secondary infection of the ascites, as may occur after traumatic gut perforation, for instance, in which a polymicrobial infection is typical. The onset of spontaneous bacterial peritonitis may be subtle, with only mild abdominal discomfort or general clinical deterioration, including worsening hepatic encephalopathy, renal failure, or a nonspecific "septic" picture. Significant fever may be lacking. The most important diagnostic study is abdominal paracentesis. An ascitic polymorphonuclear leukocyte count greater than 250/cm³ suggests the diagnosis, although it should be noted that a low count does not rule out the diagnosis, and bacterial culture remains the gold standard.

Treatment. Antimicrobial therapy should be initiated promptly in suspected cases of spontaneous bacterial peritonitis pending culture results. Third-generation cephalosporins and quinolone antibiotics are effective empirical therapy. Use of long-term oral antibiotics for prophylaxis in at-risk patients with cirrhosis is controversial but may be considered for selected patients. Use of a narrow-spectrum agent such as sulfamethoxazole-trimethoprim therapy is preferable to agents of the quinolone class.[28] Overall, the occurrence of spontaneous bacterial peritonitis is a poor prognostic sign, as it is typically associated with end-stage liver disease.

Hepatorenal Syndrome

Etiology and Pathogenesis. Patients with liver failure may experience acute kidney failure with rising serum creatinine levels and oliguria. The kidney itself is normal, but intrarenal blood flow is seriously disturbed. This disturbance in blood flow appears to be due to an imbalance between vasoconstricting and vasodilating mechanisms related to the liver disease.[1,29] The course is usually acute and progressive, but chronic cases are occasionally seen. Differentiation from reversible causes of renal failure is essential. Hepatorenal syndrome may be precipitated by overly vigorous diuretic therapy or paracentesis, severe diarrhea, nonsteroidal antiinflammatory drugs, variceal bleeding, and sepsis.

Prognosis and Treatment. The prognosis depends on the severity of the liver disease and is generally poor.[30] Treatment is primarily preventive and supportive; hemodialysis should be considered only as a bridge to definitive therapy. Fortunately, liver transplantation generally results in return of normal renal function, providing no undue delay has occurred.

- The liver is a vital, multifunctional organ located in the right upper quadrant beneath the diaphragm. Blood is supplied to the liver by the hepatic artery and the portal vein. The portal vein drains the capillaries of the alimentary canal and pancreas. Arterial and portal blood flows into the hepatic sinusoids, which have direct contact with hepatic cells.
- The functions of the liver are multiple and include metabolism of fats, proteins, and glucose; synthesis and secretion of bile salts; storage of vitamins and minerals; metabolism and detoxification of endogenous and exogenous substances; and urea synthesis.
- Manifestations of liver disease are attributable to hepatocellular failure and portal hypertension. Jaundice, decreased clotting factors, hypoalbuminemia, decreased vitamins D and K, and feminization are attributed to hepatocellular failure. Portal hypertension may result in GI congestion with the development of esophageal or gastric varices, hemorrhoids, splenomegaly, and ascites. Bleeding from varices is often massive and life threatening; various pharmacologic, endoscopic, and surgical treatments are now available.
- Symptoms of hepatic encephalopathy range from confusion and lethargy to coma. A spastic flapping tremor of the hands, called asterixis, is a classic finding. The severity of the encephalopathy correlates positively with serum ammonia levels. Encephalopathy may be precipitated by conditions that increase protein metabolism, such as GI hemorrhage and increased protein consumption, and by conditions that further impair hepatocyte function. Treatment may include protein restriction, antibiotics to reduce ammonia production by intestinal organisms, and lactulose to enhance ammonia excretion in the stool. Cerebral edema is a common cause of death in patients in deep hepatic coma.
- Ascites is a pathologic accumulation of fluid in the peritoneal cavity. It occurs commonly in liver disease because of the increased fluid transudation that occurs with portal hypertension and hypoalbuminemia. In severe ascites, treatment may be instituted to ameliorate pain and respiratory difficulty. Sodium restriction, diuretics, and intermittent paracentesis are commonly prescribed. Surgical shunting procedures that allow accumulated peritoneal fluid to flow back into the circulation through a one-way valve may be effective.
- Spontaneous bacterial peritonitis is infection of ascites by a single organism unrelated to bowel perforation or surgical procedures. Antibiotic therapy alone is usually curative.
- Hepatorenal syndrome is a type of functional renal failure caused by severe liver disease. The prognosis is poor and is contingent on the outcome of the liver disease.

Disorders of the Liver

HEPATITIS

Acute Viral Hepatitis

Hepatitis is inflammation of the liver parenchyma. Acute hepatitis may be caused by many viruses, among them cytomegalovirus and Epstein-Barr virus. However, the term *viral hepatitis* is usually applied to illnesses caused by hepatitis A, hepatitis B, and hepatitis C viruses (Table 38-4). A fourth virus, known as the *delta agent*, is a defective RNA virus that

TABLE 38-4

Comparison of Hepatitis Viruses

Virus	Hepatitis A	Hepatitis B	Hepatitis C	Hepatitis D	Hepatitis E
Type of virus	ssRNA	Partially dsDNA	ssRNA	Circular defective ssRNA	ssRNA
Viral family	Hepatovirus; related to picornavirus	Hepadnavirus	Flaviridae	Subviral particle in Deltaviridae family	Calicivirus
Route of transmission	Fecal-oral (contaminated food or water)	Parenteral, sexual contact, perinatal	Parenteral; intranasal cocaine use is a risk factor	Parenteral	Fecal-oral
Mean incubation period	2-4 weeks	1-4 months	7-8 weeks	Same as HBV	4-5 weeks
Frequency of chronic liver disease	Never	10%	~80%	5% (coinfection); ≤70% for superinfection	Never
Diagnosis	Detection of serum IgM antibodies	Detection of HBsAg or antibody to HBcAg	PCR for HCV RNA; 3rd-generation ELISA for antibody detection	Detection of IgM and IgG antibodies; HDV RNA serum; HDAg in liver	PCR for HEV RNA; detection of serum IgM and IgG antibodies

dsDNA, double-stranded DNA; *ELISA,* enzyme-linked immunosorbent assay; *HBcAg,* hepatitis B core antigen; *HBsAg,* hepatitis B surface antigen; *HBV,* hepatitis B virus; *HCV,* hepatitis C virus; *HDAg,* hepatitis D antigen; *HDV,* hepatitis D virus; *HEV,* hepatitis E virus; *PCR,* polymerase chain reaction; *ssRNA,* single stranded RNA.

From Washington K: Inflammatory and infectious diseases of the liver. In Kumar V et al: *Robbins basic pathology,* ed 8, Philadelphia, 2007, Saunders, p 640.

requires the helper function of hepatitis B virus and so occurs only as a coinfection with that agent. Hepatitis E virus is a recently described agent common mainly in developing countries.

Despite variation in the symptoms, signs, and epidemiologic progression of these diseases, it is often clinically impossible to differentiate them in a given patient without appropriate serologic tests (Figure 38-14) (see Table 38-2).

Hepatitis A

Pathogenesis and Clinical Manifestations. Hepatitis A virus (HAV) is an RNA virus that is usually spread by the fecal-oral route. The infection has a 2- to 7-week incubation period (see Figure 38-14). The illness may be asymptomatic or mildly symptomatic without jaundice (anicteric); the latter occurs especially in children, with the patient exhibiting nonspecific GI symptoms. The majority of adults develop hepatitis with

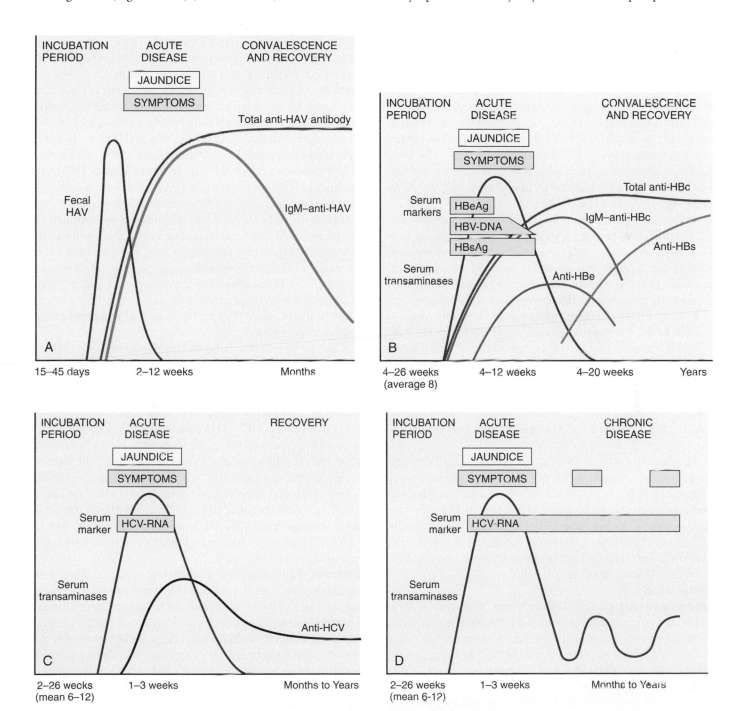

FIGURE 38-14 Comparison of clinical course and serologic tests in viral hepatitis. **A,** Hepatitis A only occurs in an acute form. **B,** The acute phase of Hepatitis B—a small number of patients may not clear the virus during this stage and become chronic carriers. **C,** Acute hepatitis C is often not diagnosed because the symptoms tend to be mild. **D,** Most patients with hepatitis C infection are unable to clear the virus and develop chronic hepatitis C. (From Kumar V et al: *Robbins basic pathology, ed 8,* Philadelphia, 2007, Saunders, pp 641, 642, 644.)

jaundice. The prodromal symptoms of icteric hepatitis consist of malaise, anorexia, nausea, low-grade fever, and right upper quadrant pain. This is followed by jaundice lasting 2 weeks on average. The clinical course is generally self-limited, although fulminant and fatal attacks occur rarely, particularly in patients with preexisting chronic active hepatitis B or C infection. Two uncommon prolonged syndromes are recognized: prolonged cholestasis and relapsing hepatitis.[1]

Diagnosis, Treatment, and Prevention. HAV infection is diagnosed through serologic testing. Presence of anti-HAV immune globulin G (IgG) indicates previous infection, and presence of immune globulin M (IgM) indicates acute infection. The test is highly reliable within several weeks of exposure.

Treatment does not change the course of acute HAV infection. Supportive management includes rest and a nutritious diet. Alcohol, acetaminophen, and other potential hepatotoxins should be avoided. HAV is a common infection control concern, particularly in the community setting.[31] The usual fecal-oral precautions, such as careful hand washing, segregation, and cleaning of laundry and personal items, should be undertaken by patients and contacts.

Active immunization is indicated for risk groups (e.g., foreign travelers, persons with chronic active hepatitis B or C, persons in institutions) using an inactivated whole-virus vaccine that is highly immunogenic and effective in preventing acute hepatitis A.[32] An intramuscular dose is followed by a booster 6 to 12 months later, providing lifelong immunity in at least 98% of recipients.[33] The vaccine is ideally administered at least 2 weeks pre-exposure (e.g., before travel to a developing country) but can also be administered in the setting of a community outbreak. It is effective even among persons with advanced chronic liver disease. Hepatitis A vaccination was added to the routine childhood vaccination schedule by the Advisory Committee on Immunization Practices (ACIP) of the Centers for Disease Control and Prevention (CDC) in 2006.

Patients exposed to HAV who are anti–HAV antibody negative should receive passive immunization with pooled human immune globulin, in addition to active vaccination. An intramuscular dose should be given within 2 weeks of exposure. Passive immunity lasts 4 to 6 months and does not diminish vaccine effectiveness. However, subclinical infections may develop in some exposed patients, whereas other patients have a clinically evident but attenuated illness.

Hepatitis B

Pathogenesis and Clinical Manifestations. Hepatitis B virus (HBV) is a partially double-stranded DNA virus that is highly prevalent worldwide. Probably 300 million persons, or 5% of the world population, have chronic HBV infection. Chronic infection in the United States affects approximately 1 to 1.25 million people, most of them immigrants from endemic countries. In contrast to HAV, HBV is spread by parenteral contact with infected blood or blood products, including contaminated needles, and by sexual contact. Perinatal infection is a major route in endemic (mainly developing) countries. Other risk factors for HBV infection include working in a health care

setting (3% of cases in the United States), transfusions and dialysis (1% each), acupuncture, tattooing, extended overseas travel, and residence in an institution.[1]

HBV has an incubation period of 2 to 6 months. The prodrome of HBV infection is often longer and more insidious than that of HAV infection and may involve a variety of immune complex–related phenomena, including urticaria and other rashes, arthralgia and arthritis, angioedema, serum sickness, and glomerulonephritis. Severity of illness ranges from no symptoms to moderate illness to fulminant hepatitis (1% of cases). The jaundice phase for most HBV infections is similar in degree and duration to that of HAV infections, although serious extrahepatic illness occurs more frequently.

Diagnosis. The serologic diagnosis is somewhat complicated (see Figure 38-14). A typical screening panel for HBV infection includes surface antigen (HBsAg), surface antibody (HbsAb), core antigen (HBcAg), and core antibody (HBcAb). In brief, with acute infection HBV core antigen (HBcAg) appears first, followed by seroconversion to core antibody (HBcAb). Presence of HBV surface antigen (HBsAg) shows up early and may persist, indicating *active infection*; development of surface antibody (HBsAb) points to resolution and immunity. (It should be noted that conversion from surface antigen to surface antibody positivity can take as long as 1 year after acute infection, so treatment should not be considered right after infection.) In chronic infection, hepatitis B e antigen (HBeAg) is associated with viral replication and infectivity, whereas hepatitis B e antibody (HBeAb) indicates minimal replication and infective potential.

Chronic infection is indicated by HBsAg positivity. There are two important features of chronic infection: ongoing liver inflammation and active viral replication. Liver damage may be deduced from persistently elevated liver enzymes and confirmed by liver biopsy. Viral replication can be measured by molecular testing (HBV DNA by hybridization) and is associated with a positive HBeAg. Persons who have a detectable virus and are HBeAg positive can readily transmit the virus to their contacts, and should be counseled regarding appropriate sexual and blood exposure precautions (including no blood donation). Patients with chronic HBV and cirrhosis are at risk for development of HCC, and periodic screening (e.g., at 6 to 12 month intervals) with ultrasound and α-fetoprotein determinations is recommended.

Treatment. Fulminant hepatitis is a life-threatening illness with high mortality. Care for patients with acute hepatitis is largely supportive, and those with fulminant hepatitis may require aggressive treatment for coagulopathy, encephalopathy, cerebral edema, and other manifestations. Liver transplantation is the only definitive treatment for progressive liver failure in acute hepatitis. Most nonfulminant HBV infections resolve spontaneously, although about 5% of acute hepatitis cases progress to chronic infection. Management of acute HBV infection is similar to that of HAV infection in terms of supportive care.

Management of chronic HBV infection has advanced dramatically over the last decade.[34,35] Endpoints are defined as elimination of hepatitis B DNA from the blood and conversion from E antigen positivity to E antibody positivity. Currently available therapies are interferon-α, lamivudine, adefovir, entacavir, and telbivudine. Interferon-α was the first effective treatment available and may be given daily or weekly (in the pegylated form) for 24 to 48 weeks with a response rate of about 33%. A significant proportion of patients experience a flare-up of acute hepatitis, and therefore this treatment cannot be used for patients with advanced liver disease (e.g., cirrhosis) or significant comorbidities. Lamivudine, adefovir, entavavir, and telbivudine are oral nucleoside analogs that are generally given for several years. Lamivudine has the advantage of being significantly cheaper than the other options, but increasing drug resistance limits its role as primary therapy. Entecavir is the treatment of choice for most patients, with a response rate of about 67% and E antibody seroconversion rate of 21%. It can be used in patients with cirrhosis as well. The drawback is the cost, as the treatment is extremely expensive ($20 to $25 per day). Telbivudine has a higher durable response rate, but it cannot be used for lamivudine-resistant strains of HBV. Adefovir has significant nephrotoxicity, and its use is reserved for patients with resistant strains.

Patients with chronic active hepatitis B infection are at risk for fulminant hepatitis with a superimposed hepatitis A infection and should be vaccinated against hepatitis A using the killed, two-dose vaccine. They are also at risk for fulminant hepatitis or more rapid progression of liver disease if they contract hepatitis D virus (see Hepatitis D section), so they should avoid risk factors for this virus such as injecting drug use and unprotected sex.

Prevention. HBV vaccine is a recombinant vaccine that is highly immunogenic with no material of human origin. (Thus, there is no risk of transmission of other agents such as HIV.) Adults are vaccinated intramuscularly with three doses of HBV vaccine given at 0, 1, and 6 months. Simultaneous administration of hepatitis B immune globulin (HBIG) and other vaccines has no effect on efficacy. After the full course, the antibody response rate is 95% for normal hosts.[1] The response rate is slightly lower in obese individuals, smokers, and men, and significantly lower in patients with cirrhosis or chronic renal failure, organ transplant recipients, children with celiac disease, and immunosuppressed patients. The effect of vaccination is considered long-lasting, and booster shots are not required. Post-vaccination testing is not recommended but could be considered for certain high-risk groups (e.g., sexual partners of chronic carriers).

Universal immunization is indicated for neonates in this country and has been suggested for individuals of any age, but especially for the following high-risk groups: sexually active individuals with multiple sex partners, male homosexuals, users of illicit drugs, household contacts of HBV carriers, hemodialysis patients, residents of institutions, health care workers, patients needing frequent transfusions, and those planning to reside in high-risk areas (e.g., the Far East and sub-Saharan Africa).[37] If exposed to HBV, a susceptible person should receive one dose of HBIG and HBV vaccine as soon as possible

after exposure and then complete the vaccination program. The issue of how to deal with persistent nonresponders, especially health care workers, is unsettled, but most authorities recommend a full three-shot course according to the usual schedule.[36]

The administration of immune globulin containing high levels of hepatitis B surface antibody (HBIG) affords effective post-inoculation prophylaxis if given within 7 days of exposure. The indications for HBIG are as follows: (1) neonates born to HBsAg-positive mothers; (2) prophylaxis after needlestick or sexual exposure in nonimmune persons; and (3) after liver transplantation in patients who are HBsAg positive prior to transplantation.[1,37] The usual dose is 0.05 to 0.07 ml/kg given intramuscularly, with the same dose repeated 25 to 30 days later. (See reference for dosing recommendations for perinatal vaccination.[37]) The immune status of the recipient may be determined before treatment to avoid unnecessary administration. HBV vaccine should be given concomitantly with HBIG in most cases.

Hepatitis C

Pathogenesis and Clinical Manifestations. Hepatitis C virus (HCV; previously categorized as non-A, non-B hepatitis virus) is a single-stranded RNA virus that belongs to the Flavivirus family. Our knowledge of HCV is evolving rapidly but has lagged behind that of HAV and HBV for two important reasons: lack of a suitable cell line for replication in the laboratory and an extremely high mutation rate. Worldwide about 3% of the population is chronically infected, with a somewhat lower rate in the United States. The mode of transmission of HCV closely resembles that of HBV, although sexual and perinatal transmission are much less likely. The main pool of infected individuals in the United States acquired HCV through intravenous drug use or blood transfusions prior to availability of the screening test in 1990. HCV remains an important occupational risk for health care workers, with the risk after a single needlestick being about 3%, as opposed to 30% for HBV or 0.3% for HIV. A significant number of seropositive persons have no known risk factors for HCV.

Acute HCV infection is usually asymptomatic. Clinical illness, when it occurs, is usually mild, with transaminase levels rarely exceeding 1000 IU/L. Only 15% of acute infections resolve, with the remainder progressing to chronic active infection (see Figure 38-14). The course is erratic, with wide fluctuations on liver enzymes (primarily ALT). A number of extrahepatic manifestations occur, the most prominent of which are a medium-vessel vasculitis (polyarteritis nodosa), essential mixed cryoglobulinemia, and membranoproliferative glomerulonephritis.[1] Chronic infection seems to progress to significant liver disease about 20% of the time, although there are no reliable noninvasive ways to predict who will progress. HCV infection is currently one of the most common causes of end-stage liver disease with cirrhosis in the United States. If untreated, as with hepatitis B, chronic active HCV infection with cirrhosis predisposes to HCC. Of the three recognized serotypes, Type 1 is most common in the United States but has a lower response rate to treatment.

Treatment. Management of acute HCV infection is the same as for other acute viral strains (i.e., supportive and expectant unless complications or subacute hepatic failure develop). Treatment of acute HCV infection with antiviral agents is not currently recommended, and immune globulin is not helpful in preventing infection in the acute exposure setting. Between 20% and 40% of acute seropositive patients will convert to seronegativity and an undetectable viral load during the first 6 months after infection, so early treatment is not recommended. Chronic infections should be assessed by a viral load and viral genotype, and a liver biopsy to stage disease activity should be considered for those with a Type 1 virus.[1]

The current standard of treatment for chronic HCV infection is pegylated interferon-α, given intramuscularly once weekly, and ribavirin orally twice daily.[1,38] The response rate overall is about 60%; for the more common Type 1 infection (85% of cases) it is 45%, and for the less common types 2 and 3 it is 85%. Side effects are significant and include cytopenias, malaise, and flulike symptoms, as well as induction or aggravation of depression and anxiety. In fact, in many patients the latter side effects are severe and have resulted in suicides. About 5% to 10% of recipients drop out of treatment because of side effects. The expense is considerable—from $8,000 to $15,000 per year—and insurance coverage in the past has been inconsistent. Treatment for Type 1 virus lasts 48 weeks, and for other types 24 weeks. New treatments for HCV infection are currently a burgeoning area of research.

Patients with chronic active hepatitis C infection should be vaccinated against hepatitis A and B and counseled regarding blood-borne precautions. As the issue of sexual transmission is unsettled, the Centers for Disease Control and Prevention does not currently recommend barrier methods for patients with long-term sexual partners because of the apparent low risk of infection.

Hepatitis D (Delta)

Pathogenesis and Clinical Manifestations. Hepatitis D virus (HDV) is an incomplete viral organism that requires the presence of HBV for replication. It may occur coincident with or subsequent to initial infection with hepatitis B. The disease is primarily transmitted by parenteral routes and by intimate personal contact, like hepatitis B.[1] In the United States and northern Europe, HDV infection is most prevalent in persons exposed to blood and blood products (e.g., drug addicts and hemophiliacs). HDV infection tends to accelerate the progress of liver disease associated with HBV infection. In fact, fulminant hepatitis may result from HDV infection superimposed on chronic HBV infection. As HDV is a deficient virus, its persistence is determined by the duration of the HBV infection. Diagnosis is by anti-HDV IgM and IgG enzyme-linked immunosorbent assays (ELISA).

Treatment and Control. HDV infection is controlled through the same measures used to prevent transmission of other hepatitis viruses: safe sexual practices, screening of blood products, avoidance of intravenous drug use, and vaccination of susceptible persons with the HBV vaccine. There is no specific vaccine or treatment for HDV.

Hepatitis E

Pathogenesis and Clinical Manifestations. Hepatitis E virus (HEV) is one of the most common causes of acute hepatitis in developing countries. Cases in developed countries are usually related to recent travel. HEV is an RNA virus spread via the fecal-oral route, especially through contaminated water. Parenteral transmission may occur.

The incubation period is 2 to 9 weeks. The prodrome and icteric illnesses are similar to those of HAV infection but usually last only 2 weeks. It is assumed that many subclinical cases occur, but in the absence of widely available serologic testing, subclinical infection is difficult to determine. Fulminant hepatic failure may occur, especially in pregnant woman (see the Liver Diseases and Pediatric Considerations section).

Treatment. Treatment is supportive. Because no vaccine is available, the only prophylaxis is avoidance of undercooked foods, careful hand washing, and drinking of safe water and beverages (i.e., canned, bottled, or purified through the usual means).

Chronic Hepatitis

Chronic hepatitis encompasses a group of diseases characterized by inflammation of the liver that lasts 6 months or longer. The most prominent of these conditions is chronic active viral hepatitis, but chronic hepatitis may be due to toxic, autoimmune, or metabolic causes as well.

Chronic Persistent Hepatitis

Chronic persistent hepatitis, often called *triaditis* or *transaminitis,* is an archaic term for a chronic, low-grade liver inflammation of any cause. The inflammation is confined to the portal triads without destruction of normal liver structures, but serum transaminase levels are elevated. The condition may be asymptomatic or may be associated with mild, nonspecific symptoms. Progressive liver disease does not usually develop, and no drug treatment is indicated. The illness has an excellent prognosis. However, other more serious liver diseases may pass through a phase that is histologically indistinguishable from chronic persistent hepatitis and may progress (e.g., chronic viral hepatitis).

Current classification schemes emphasize: (1) etiologic factor, (2) histologic grade, and (3) stage in terms of fibrosis. Therefore, chronic persistent hepatitis would generally correspond to a liver condition with mild disease activity and minimal or no fibrosis by biopsy.

Chronic Active Hepatitis

Pathogenesis and Clinical Manifestations. On the other hand, **chronic active hepatitis** is a progressive, destructive inflammatory disease that extends beyond the portal triad to the hepatic lobule (piecemeal necrosis). In current nomenclature, grade and stage span the spectrum from mild to severe. The disease could spontaneously arrest with any degree of fibrosis or could progress to macronodular or micronodular cirrhosis. Symptoms typical of acute hepatitis are often seen. Eventually chronic active hepatitis often culminates in cirrhosis and end-stage liver disease.

Four main subgroups of patients with chronic active hepatitis are identified. First, as discussed above, a minority of newly infected HBV patients but a majority of those with HCV will go on to have chronic active hepatitis. The second subgroup (mainly young women) manifest autoimmune hepatitis and exhibit a variety of immunologic markers, including antinuclear antibodies and anti-smooth muscle antibodies. In addition, these patients frequently suffer from a second autoimmune disease such as Hashimoto thyroiditis. In the third subgroup are patients with chronic hepatitis induced by therapeutic agents such as minocycline or nitrofurantoin. In the fourth subgroup are patients with a metabolic liver disorder such as Wilson disease or hemochromatosis. A small number of patients have neither a suggestive history nor any detectable markers that would place them in any of the four main groups; advanced liver disease in this group is usually termed **cryptogenic cirrhosis.**

Diagnosis. The diagnosis of chronic hepatitis is made on the basis of the clinical setting and abnormal liver enzymes. Serologic studies are indicated to screen for viral hepatitis and autoimmune hepatitis. Serum iron and ferritin studies are performed to diagnose hemochromatosis, and a serum ceruloplasmin is used to screen for Wilson disease. A liver biopsy may be performed to confirm the diagnosis and to exclude specific causes. Biopsy also allows for grading and staging, as discussed earlier in the chapter.

Autoimmune hepatitis is characterized by the presence of several autoantibodies as well as a polyclonal hypergammaglobulinemia. Antinuclear antibody (ANA) is generally positive at a high level. Anti-smooth muscle antibodies (ASMA) are less sensitive than ANA but highly specific for autoimmune hepatitis. The finding of highly positive autoimmune markers in the presence of significant hepatitis, in the absence of other tests indicative of viral or metabolic liver disease, is pathognomonic for this condition. There is some overlap between conditions, however, and in questionable cases a liver biopsy is indicated.

Management of Autoimmune Hepatitis. Corticosteroids and immunosuppressive drugs have been used since the early 1960s for the management of autoimmune chronic active hepatitis. Their use is based on the assumption that immunologic mechanisms either cause or maintain ongoing hepatic inflammation. Corticosteroids alone or in combination clearly lower mortality in chronic active hepatitis, most noticeably in symptomatic patients and those with very severe pathologic lesions demonstrated on liver biopsy. Current guidelines recommend prednisone with azathioprine until a remission is induced (usually within 18 to 24 months, as indicated by significant improvement in liver function test results).[39] Subsequently, steroids can be tapered off over 6 weeks or so, with azathioprine tapered off more slowly; 65% to 80% of patients will respond to this initial regimen. Cyclosporine is another treatment option for nonresponders. Treatment with corticosteroids is generally accompanied by well-known complications: arterial hypertension and fluid retention, hypokalemia, glucose intolerance, mental status changes, cataracts, thinning of skin and bones, suppression of the adrenal gland, avascular necrosis of the joints, rounding of the face (moon facies), loss of muscle mass, and central adiposity, as well as increased risk for certain infections. Suddenly stopping long-term treatment with corticosteroids may result in acute adrenal insufficiency with hypotension and shock.

Management of drug-induced chronic active hepatitis involves stopping the offending drug. Specific antidotes or treatments are available for some of these conditions.[1] Specific treatments for Wilson disease and hemochromatosis are discussed later in the chapter.

KEY POINTS

- Acute viral hepatitis is generally classified as hepatitis A, B, C, D (delta), and E infection. Modes of transmission and severity of symptoms differ among types.
- HAV infection is also known as enteric hepatitis because it is generally transmitted by ingestion of contaminated substances. Symptoms are flulike and tend to be less severe than those of HBV infection. Early treatment with γ-globulin and vaccination after exposure may be effective in preventing disease.
- HBV infection is also known as serum hepatitis because its usual route of transmission is through infected blood. The incubation period is longer, and the severity of symptoms (particularly jaundice) is greater than in HAV infection. Hepatitis B immune globulin (HBIG) is effective after inoculation if given within 7 days of exposure. HBV vaccine is recommended as part of the childhood vaccination regimen and for high-risk individuals, and after exposure. Treatment is with intramuscular interferon-α for 4 months, or with oral lamivudine for 1 to 2 years.
- HCV, also known as non-A, non-B hepatitis virus, resembles HBV in its routes of transmission. Chronic HCV infection develops in 85% of cases and is usually asymptomatic until advanced liver disease intervenes. Immune globulin does not protect against HCV infection. Treatment is with intramuscular pegylated interferon and oral ribavirin for 6 to 12 months.
- HDV coinfects with HBV and requires the presence of HBV to be active. Infection appears to accelerate and worsen HBV infection symptoms. Prevention of HBV infection also prevents HDV infection.
- HEV is a common virus in the developing world that causes an illness similar to HAV infection but has a high mortality rate in pregnant women.
- Chronic hepatitis is characterized by persistent inflammation of the liver lasting 6 months or more. Autoimmune disease, viral hepatitis (B and C), toxins, and metabolic diseases may result in chronic hepatitis. Chronic active hepatitis may progress to cirrhosis. Corticosteroids (prednisone) and immunosuppressants (azathioprine) are common therapeutics for autoimmune hepatitis.

CIRRHOSIS

Cirrhosis represents the irreversible end stage of many different hepatic injuries, including severe acute hepatitis, chronic hepatitis, the metal storage diseases, alcoholism, and toxic hepatitis. It is characterized by diffuse hepatic fibrosis surrounding nodules of liver tissue and results in permanent alteration in hepatic blood flow and liver function. The pathophysiology of cirrhosis and complications have been reviewed earlier in this chapter. We will discuss briefly the sequelae of chronic biliary disease and alcoholic liver disease.

Biliary Cirrhosis

Etiology and Pathogenesis. **Biliary cirrhosis** represents the end result of continuous, ongoing inflammation of the bile ducts, which may be due to macroscopic or microscopic biliary obstruction. Persistent biliary obstruction results in inflammation and scarring of the liver, with obliteration of the bile ductules. The end result is diffuse and widespread fibrosis with regenerative nodule formation (islands of healthy liver tissue within a background of fibrosis), and the consequences of portal hypertension described above. The prototypical form of microscopic biliary disease is **primary biliary cirrhosis** (PBC), an autoimmune condition often associated with systemic lupus erythematosus and other autoimmune illnesses. It is usually associated with positive tests for ANA and anti-mitochondrial antibodies (AMA).

Examples of large-duct obstruction include gallstone disease, chronic biliary fluke infestation, and primary sclerosing cholangitis (PSC). The biliary flukes endemic in Asia, *Opisthorchis* and *Clonorchis* species, are acquired by eating raw fish that carry larval cyst forms.[40] *Fasciola hepatica* is found in all sheep-producing and cattle-producing areas of the world and infects humans as accidental hosts; it is acquired by eating fecally contaminated watercress and other aquatic plants that harbor the immature cysts. Immigrants from infected areas may be at risk for these chronic infestations.

Diagnosis and Treatment. The diagnosis of PBC depends upon appropriate serologic results and liver biopsy. Ursodeoxycholic acid (ursodiol, UDCA) is the only approved treatment for PBC and may delay development of end-stage liver disease. Methotrexate and colchicine are other therapies whose efficacy has yet to be elucidated in studies. Supportive care is similar to that for other conditions with impaired bile metabolism, including supplementation with fat-soluble vitamins. In spite of these measures, most patients will eventually go on to require liver transplantation for prolonged survival.

The diagnosis of biliary flukes in immigrants and (less commonly) foreign travelers can usually be made by serial stool examinations for parasitic ova, and serologic testing is often helpful. Treatment with antiparasitic agents (praziquantel, mebendazole or albendazole) will eliminate the live worms but will not necessarily prevent recurrent episodes of cholangitis and other consequences.

Primary Sclerosing Cholangitis

Etiology and Pathogenesis. Primary sclerosing cholangitis (PSC) is an autoimmune condition generally seen in patients with ulcerative colitis; 80% of PSC patients have coexistent ulcerative colitis, whereas 3% to 5% of ulcerative colitis patients develop PSC.[1] It is characterized by recurrent episodes of cholangitis, with progressive biliary scarring and obstruction. Secondary forms of sclerosing cholangitis, such as that

following bile duct injury during surgery, behave in a similar fashion.

Diagnosis and Treatment. Diagnosis is primarily by means of endoscopic retrograde cholangiopancreatography showing the typical beaded and atrophic appearance of the biliary tree; liver biopsy is often performed for staging reasons. Medical and endoscopic treatments are merely palliative, and the only effective recourse is liver transplantation.[41] The end result of recurrent cholangitis of any cause is cirrhosis, and such patients are predisposed to cholangiocarcinoma.

Alcoholic Liver Disease

Alcoholic liver disease is manifested by fatty liver, hepatitis, and cirrhosis. One or more of these manifestations may be found in alcoholic patients.

Alcoholic Fatty Liver

Etiology. **Alcoholic fatty liver** *(alcoholic steatohepatitis)* is an accumulation of fat in the liver cells. It is caused by more fat being delivered to the hepatocyte than it can normally metabolize or by a defect in fat metabolism within the cell.

Diagnosis and Treatment. Steatohepatitis is not exclusively alcohol related. Indeed, diabetes mellitus, obesity, protein malnutrition, total parenteral nutrition, drugs, and many other factors may result in a similar pathologic process. It is usually mild and asymptomatic, and is often diagnosed incidentally on ultrasound or CT examination or by liver biopsy for another reason. Liver enzymes are often mildly abnormal, generally serum transaminases. Hypertriglyceridemia is commonly found and at times may be dramatically elevated (e.g., greater than 1000 mg/dl). Occasionally, there is significant liver enlargement, abdominal discomfort, and even portal hypertension. Treatment involves stopping alcohol intake and providing appropriate nutrition. Nonalcoholic steatohepatitis (NASH) may be managed with weight reduction, control of diabetes and hyperlipidemia, or other treatment directed at the underlying cause. Although the exact risk is unclear, it has been estimated that between 3% and 15% of persons with untreated NASH will go on to progressive liver fibrosis and cirrhosis.[42]

Alcoholic Hepatitis

Pathogenesis and Clinical Manifestations. **Alcoholic hepatitis** is an active inflammation of the centrilobular region of the liver. The liver cells show pathologic changes of hepatocyte necrosis with neutrophilic infiltration and intracellular inclusions known as Mallory bodies. This form of liver disease often occurs in chronic alcoholics who "go on a bender" and binge on quantities much greater than their usual intake. Clinically the illness ranges from mild to very severe, with the worst cases characterized by hepatomegaly, fever, signs of acute liver failure, and encephalopathy. Hepatitis may be complicated by acute alcohol withdrawal and delirium tremens. Mortality rates as high as 33% are seen with this condition.[1]

Diagnosis and Treatment. The diagnosis is supported by the history, if the patient is reliable. The finding of a serum AST (SGOT) markedly higher than ALT (SGPT) strongly suggests a toxic etiology, rather than acute viral hepatitis. Viral serologies, serum acetaminophen levels, and tests for certain metabolic disorders (e.g., serum ceruloplasmin for Wilson disease) may help sort out diagnostic dilemmas.

As one of the pathogenetic factors in alcoholic hepatitis is malnutrition and vitamin deficiencies, special attention should be given to nutrition. Thiamine 100 mg daily and a multivitamin should be administered routinely, and B[12] and folate levels should be measured and replenished as necessary. Patients with an elevated prothrombin time or INR should receive subcutaneous vitamin K. Corticosteroid therapy with prednisolone is recommended for seriously ill patients, especially those with declining liver function and coma.[39, 44]

TOXIC LIVER DISORDERS

Metal Storage Diseases

Hereditary Hemochromatosis

Pathogenesis and Diagnosis. Hereditary hemochromatosis (HH) is one of the most common autosomal recessive disorders in the world. In European populations, approximately 1 in 10 persons is a heterozygous carrier, and 0.3% are homozygous persons with disease.[45] Studies in the United States show a prevalence of HH homozygosity of 0.44 percent for Caucasians, 0.027 percent for Hispanics, and 0.014 percent for African Americans.[46] The prevalence among Asians is extremely low. However, despite the high prevalence of the gene, the number of persons with clinical hemochromatosis is considerably smaller—less than 1% of homozygotes. This is due to incomplete penetrance of the gene and environmental factors.

The disease is caused by the activity of a mutant gene called *HFE,* which allows excessive and uncontrolled iron absorption by the GI tract. The usual *HFE* mutation has been identified as C282Y, but other mutations can occur and act in a similar way. A small number of patients with HH are heterozygotes for *HFE;* disease in this population may result from as-yet-unidentified mutations or other factors. The result of these mutations is iron deposition in numerous organs; in advanced disease, the body may contain 20 g or more of iron, mainly in the liver, pancreas, and heart. Because of menstruation and perhaps endocrinologic factors, hemochromatosis is much less common in women than in men (ratio of 1:5 to 1:10).[45]

The liver is usually the first organ to show evidence of involvement, with hepatomegaly and elevated liver enzymes. Specific manifestations in organ systems other than the liver include diabetes mellitus, hyperpigmentation, polyarthritis, hypogonadism, and heart failure. (In previous times the condition was often known as "bronze diabetes" because of the association of diabetes and bronze discoloration of the skin.) In advanced disease fibrosis and macronodular cirrhosis of the liver develop insidiously and represent the major cause of death. Splenomegaly is common, although portal hypertension and its complications (see discussion above) occur less frequently than with other forms of liver disease. HCC develops in about 30% of persons with hemochromatosis, exclusively in the setting of cirrhosis.[45] Therefore, early diagnosis and treatment are critical.

Clinical Manifestations and Diagnosis. The diagnosis is suggested by clinical features and family history. Plasma iron and transferrin saturation are increased, and serum ferritin is dramatically elevated, often to several thousand micrograms per liter (normal 10 to 200). The diagnosis of hereditary hemochromatosis is confirmed by genetic analysis for the *HFE* gene. In selected cases liver biopsy may be performed, demonstrating iron deposition in periportal hepatocytes.[1] The diagnosis of hereditary hemochromatosis should prompt investigation of other family members for carriage and expression of the *HFE* gene.

It should be noted that a second large category of iron overload syndromes exists, that of *secondary* hemochromatosis. This may occur with chronic hereditary dyserythropoietic states (e.g., sideroblastic anemia and thalassemia), in alcoholic patients with liver disease, and in patients with excessive iron ingestion over a period of many years. Hemochromatosis related to anemias is generally the result of repeated blood transfusions and iron intake. Of mainly historical interest is an interesting condition called *Bantu siderosis,* which occurred among South African tribesmen who imbibed beer fermented in iron pots. All of these secondary forms of hemosiderosis are not associated with the *HFE* gene.

Treatment. The mainstay of treatment for hemochromatosis is repeated phlebotomy. The typical protocol is weekly phlebotomy of 500 ml (1 unit) of whole blood until the hematocrit drops below 37%, at which time maintenance phlebotomy of 1 unit is carried out every 2 to 3 months. Patients who do not tolerate phlebotomy may be treated with subcutaneous or intramuscular deferoxamine, a drug that chelates iron and facilitates its renal excretion. Deferoxamine is much less efficient than phlebotomy and requires adequate renal function. If identified early, hereditary and acquired hemochromatosis carries an excellent prognosis in terms of preventing heart failure and liver disease. Diabetes may still develop, however, and iron removal does not change hypogonadism or arthritis. Liver transplantation is available for patients with irreversible cirrhosis whose heart involvement does not preclude surgery.

Wilson Disease (Hepatolenticular Degeneration)

Etiology. Wilson disease, or hepatolenticular degeneration, is a rare autosomal recessive disorder in which excessive amounts of copper accumulate in the liver and other organs. As with hereditary hemochromatosis, it has now been linked to a specific abnormal protein, ATP7B, which results in retention of copper in the liver as well as impaired incorporation of copper into ceruloplasmin. Most patients are compound heterozygotes with more than one of several mutations involving the *ATP7B* gene. The condition may present at any time before age 30, generally with either significant hepatic dysfunction or neuropsychiatric illness. Patients with a neuropsychiatric presentation virtually always have occult compensated cirrhosis at the time of diagnosis.

Clinical Manifestations. Hepatic disease is more common in children than adults and begins as hepatomegaly, fatty infiltration of the liver, and elevated liver enzymes. Great variability in liver disease is seen, and Wilson disease may manifest as acute hepatitis progressing to fulminant hepatic failure, a condition very similar to autoimmune hepatitis with numerous extrahepatic symptoms, or insidious development of macronodular cirrhosis with portal hypertension. Neurologic involvement presents as a movement disorder or rigid dystonia, or occasionally as primarily psychiatric symptoms. Other manifestations include renal tubular acidosis with a Fanconi-like syndrome, cardiomyopathy, hypogonadism, metabolic bone disease (i.e., vitamin D–resistant rickets), and arthritis.

Diagnosis. Clinical signs and symptoms suggest the diagnosis, in particular the finding on slit-lamp examination of the brownish Kayser-Fleischer rings at the margin of the cornea. However, lack of Kayser-Fleischer rings does not exclude the diagnosis. Unlike hereditary hemochromatosis, genetic analysis is not the primary diagnostic pathway; it should be reserved for those with proven metabolic abnormalities because of variability in the genetic mutations that cause copper overload syndromes. The combination of low serum ceruloplasmin and elevated 24-hour urinary copper excretion is highly suggestive of Wilson disease.[1] Results of 24-hour urinary copper excretion after penicillamine administration provide additional diagnostic proof in ambiguous cases. The liver biopsy technique for copper determination is technically demanding and is not routinely performed. As with hereditary hemochromatosis, genetic screening of close relatives should be carried out.

Treatment. Treatment involves dietary modification and copper removal therapy. Patients should try to eliminate copper-rich foods from their diet, including organ meats, shellfish, nuts, chocolate, and mushrooms.[1,19] (Vegetarians require specific dietary counseling.) Dietary measures include testing home water sources and filtering water with a high copper content. Oral chelation therapy is the mainstay of treatment for Wilson disease, and the currently preferred agent is trientine. Alternative agents include penicillamine and zinc. Patients receiving this treatment early in the course of the disease will show marked improvement and protection against liver and neurologic disease.[1] Even patients with advanced Wilson disease may expect some functional recovery. Treatment is lifelong, and noncompliance leads to definite progression.

Side effects are less common with trientine than with the older therapy, penicillamine. A mild anemia and gastritis may occur with this medication, also a transient worsening of neurologic symptoms. Finally, ammonium tetrathiomolybdate is occasionally used for severe neurologic Wilson disease because, unlike penicillamine, it is not associated with early transient neurologic deterioration.[47] As with hemochromatosis, liver transplantation has a limited but useful role.

Toxic Metabolic Agents
Acetaminophen Poisoning

Etiology. Many drugs and toxins cause liver damage. Unfortunately, treatment is often limited to withdrawal of the offending agent and administration of supportive care. Standard measures, including gastric lavage, induced emesis, and activated charcoal, are used in cases of acute ingestive poisoning. Specific antidotes are few, although heavy metal intoxication may be managed with chelating drugs. Acetaminophen overdose is an important exception that bears further discussion.

Pathogenesis and Clinical Manifestations. Acetaminophen (paracetamol, in Britain and Europe) is a widely used, nonprescription analgesic and antipyretic that is frequently implicated in suicide attempts and accidental poisonings. In fact, a multicenter study recently showed that acetaminophen overdose was responsible for 39% of cases of acute hepatic failure in the United States.[48] Oral acetaminophen is rapidly absorbed and metabolized (Figure 38-15). A toxic metabolite, N-acetyl-p-benzoquinone imine, is formed and rapidly detoxified by reaction with glutathione. However, acute ingestion of at least 140 mg of acetaminophen per kilogram of body weight may expose the liver to high levels of the toxic metabolite with resultant hepatic necrosis. Importantly, repeated ingestion of smaller amounts may cause harm in children, the elderly, patients with pre-existing liver disease, persons abusing alcohol, and persons on other possibly hepatotoxic drugs. Significant liver damage is rare if serum acetaminophen levels are less than 150 and 37 g/ml, respectively, 4 and 12 hours after ingestion. Given the many variables affecting acetaminophen toxicity,

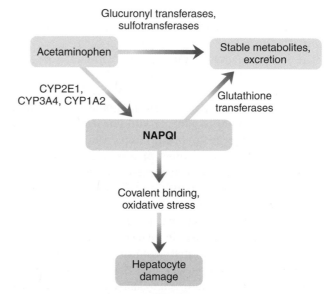

FIGURE 38-15 Mechanism of acetaminophen toxicity. The majority of an administered dose of acetaminophen is conjugated with sulfate or glucuronic acid to form stable metabolites that are promptly excreted in urine. Under most circumstances, only a minority of the total acetaminophen dose undergoes bioactivation to the reactive intermediate N-acetyl-p-benzoquinone imine (NAPQI). This species is capable of binding to intracellular proteins and mediating cell injury or death. The liver enzymes capable of bioactivating acetaminophen to NAPQI are CYP2E1, CYP3A4, and CYP1A2. Accumulation of NAPQI in the liver does not generally occur because the liver has sufficient ability to detoxify this metabolite through glutathione conjugation. (Redrawn from Fontana RJ, Watkins PB: Genetic predisposition to drug-induced liver disease, *Gastroenterol Clin North Am* 24:811-823, 1995.)

it is imperative for clinicians evaluating a suspected case to refer to a published nomogram and obtain periodic drug levels of acetaminophen.[49] (Screening for ingestion of other drugs, such as tricyclic antidepressants, should also be done.)

Within several hours of ingestion, the patient generally experiences nausea, vomiting, and diarrhea. After these symptoms, there is often a temporary "window" period, in which the patient feels well and may wish to withdraw from medical care. Within 24 to 48 hours, signs of hepatic injury occur, including abnormal liver enzyme levels. If untreated, progressive liver failure with jaundice, encephalopathy, hypoglycemia, coagulopathy, and even death may occur, generally within the first week. Patients surviving one week generally experience complete recovery of normal liver function without sequelae.

Treatment. Initial treatment, as for any poisoning, involves decontamination with induced emesis or lavage and activated charcoal (which will not interfere with use of acetylcysteine). The proper use of acetylcysteine for patients with clearly toxic levels can effectively prevent hepatic necrosis and its fatal consequences if started in a timely fashion.[50] Acetylcysteine, a mucolytic solution often used in patients with bronchial diseases, stimulates liver production of reduced glutathione, which can then keep up with blood levels of toxic metabolites.[49] Acetylcysteine is nontoxic but may cause rash and frequently induces vomiting because of its foul odor and taste.

OTHER STRUCTURAL LIVER CONDITIONS

Liver Abscess

Pathogenesis, Clinical Manifestations, and Diagnosis. Pyogenic liver abscess is a very common condition worldwide. In the United States it represents most commonly a complication of ascending cholangitis with or without gallstones, "upstream" seeding from a distal intestinal infection (e.g., appendicitis, through the portal vein), or hematogenous seeding from an endovascular infection.

Liver abscess should be considered in any patient with fever and right upper abdominal pain. Nausea and vomiting are common, and jaundice from biliary obstruction may rarely be present. Frequently, tender hepatosplenomegaly and sometimes a palpable mass are noted. Typical signs of pyogenic infection are usually present, including leukocytosis, an elevated erythrocyte sedimentation rate, and elevated liver enzymes, usually in a "mixed" pattern. As the primary diagnostic considerations include acute cholecystitis and cholangitis, imaging of the liver with ultrasonography or CT is usually carried out. Ultrasound-guided or CT-guided thin-needle aspiration of abscesses is recommended to provide the necessary material for Gram stain and cultures; blood cultures should also be obtained.

Pyogenic liver abscess from abdominal sources generally contains enteric aerobic and anaerobic gram-negative bacteria. *Escherichia coli*, *Klebsiella* species, and *Bacteroides fragilis* are particularly important. Abscesses of hematogenous origin are more heterogeneous. *Streptococcus viridans* and related streptococcal species are commonly seen. *Staphylococcus aureus* is seen in the setting of endocarditis or widespread bacteremia.

Other uncommon causes of cystic liver abnormalities should be considered, in particular hydatid liver cysts secondary to *Echinococcus* species and amebic liver abscess. These conditions are virtually always seen among persons who have lived in developing countries for many years. Their appearance on ultrasound and CT is usually characteristic, and serologies are available to assist with diagnosis. (Aspiration of echinococcal cysts is contraindicated because of the possibility of anaphylactic shock due to leakage of immunogenic cyst material.) Fungal and mycobacterial infections of the liver are usually granulomatous and diffuse, but in certain settings, such as in neutropenic patients, localized infection with an organism such as *Aspergillus* may be seen.

Treatment. Large (2.0 cm) solitary or multiple liver abscesses require drainage, formerly a surgical procedure. However, at present CT-guided and ultrasound-guided percutaneous drainage tubes are the standard of care and may be placed with minimal morbidity and discomfort. These should be kept in place until drainage has essentially resolved.

Antibiotic coverage should be directed at likely organisms. A third-generation cephalosporin such as ceftriaxone can be used alone or in combination with metronidazole, if anaerobic bacteria are likely. A β-lactam with β-lactamase inhibitor (e.g., ampicillin/sulbactam) is an excellent choice, but it must be given four times daily. Ertapenem is a new, once-daily carbapenem with broad aerobic and anaerobic coverage and is a good choice for outpatient administration. As 3 to 4 weeks of antibiotic administration is generally required, the latter part of the treatment course could be given orally, using an oral quinolone such as levofloxacin with or without oral metronidazole. Therapy should be adjusted depending on culture results.

Trauma

Etiology and Clinical Manifestations. The liver is the most common solid organ to be injured by penetrating abdominal trauma (such as gunshot wounds, stab wounds, or rib fractures) and the second most commonly injured organ in blunt trauma. Damage or injury to the liver should be suspected when any upper abdominal or lower chest trauma is sustained. The liver is frequently injured by steering wheels in vehicular accidents. Common injuries to the liver include simple lacerations, multiple lacerations, avulsions, and crush injuries.

The gravity of liver wounds arises from the fact that the liver is a highly vascular organ receiving approximately 29% of the body's cardiac output. When hepatic trauma occurs, blood loss can be massive. The patient generally exhibits the typical signs of hemorrhagic shock: hypotension, tachycardia, tachypnea, pallor, diaphoresis, and confusion. Hemoglobin/hematocrit may be normal early on but eventually will reflect significant blood loss. Clinical manifestations include right upper quadrant pain with abdominal tenderness, distention, guarding, and rigidity. Abdominal pain exaggerated by deep breathing and referred to the shoulder may indicate diaphragmatic irritation.

Treatment. Treatment entails the administration of fresh whole blood or packed red blood cells and fresh frozen plasma, as well as massive fluid infusion to maintain adequate intravascular volume and hematocrit.[51] Most patients require surgical management, although some may be treated angiographically or expectantly with medical support. Postoperatively, a patient with hepatic trauma is usually admitted to a critical care unit and monitored for persistent bleeding. The complete blood cell count and coagulation parameters must be closely monitored for trends in changes.

Malignancy

Etiology. Malignancy in the liver usually develops as a metastatic process. Because of the vascularity and lymphatic drainage of the liver, the organ is a common site for metastasis from primary cancers of the esophagus, stomach, colon, rectum, breast, and lung—among many other possibilities.

Primary hepatic malignancy (cancer originating within the liver) is rare in the United States. However, in other parts of the world such as Africa, it is one of the most common sites of malignancy because of a high prevalence of chronic hepatitis B virus infection. Primary liver tumors include HCCs (discussed in the next section), cholangiocarcinoma, and angiosarcoma. Hepatoblastoma is the most common malignant tumor in children. Lymphoma, especially T-cell lymphoma, may occasionally arise primarily in the liver. Benign liver tumors are much less common, with the exception of cavernous hemangioma.

Clinical Manifestations and Diagnosis. The most common form of primary hepatic malignancy is **hepatocellular carcinoma** (HCC), often referred to as *hepatoma*. HCC is an uncommon malignancy of middle-aged persons, more frequent in men than in women. The incidence may be increasing in the United States as a result of increasing HBV and HCV prevalence; it is always preceded in these situations by cirrhosis. Signs and symptoms of HCC include hepatomegaly, abdominal pain, weight loss, nausea, and, in advanced cases, jaundice and ascites. HCC has an extraordinary number of paraneoplastic syndromes, including hypercalcemia, erythrocytosis, hypoglycemia, thyrotoxicosis, and hypertrophic osteoarthropathy (finger clubbing).[1]

Space-occupying masses of the liver may first be suggested by abnormal liver-related enzymes, especially alkaline phosphatase. α-Fetoprotein is often dramatically elevated in cases of HCC, although some false-positive results can occur. Definitive diagnosis requires imaging of the liver with ultrasonography, CT, or magnetic resonance imaging, although on occasion the tumor may be diffuse and not diagnostic. These studies also allow guided needle biopsy of the liver lesion.

Treatment. The only treatment for HCC is hepatic resection. Unfortunately, because of advanced diffuse liver disease or multifocal tumors, such treatment is not usually possible. Partial resection is preferred, but complete hepatectomy followed by liver transplantation is a radical option for tumor localized to the liver. Other treatments include systemic chemotherapy and chemotherapy directed selectively to the liver via portal vein or hepatic artery cannulation.[52] Other novel palliative treatments include hepatic artery ligation, direct percutaneous injection of alcohol into hepatic tumors, cryotherapy, and other thermal techniques.

TRANSPLANTATION

Patients with end-stage liver disease that has not responded to conventional medical or surgical intervention are potential candidates for **liver transplantation** (Boxes 38-2, 38-3, and 38-4). In adults, diseases currently managed by orthotopic (in-place) liver transplantation (OLT) include end-stage cirrhosis from chronic active hepatitis, alcoholic liver disease, primary biliary cirrhosis, and primary sclerosing cholangitis; and hepatic metabolic diseases such as hemochromatosis and Wilson disease.[1,53] Liver transplantation is rarely performed for patients with malignant neoplasms, although there is clearly a subset of patients with HCC who are candidates for this procedure.[54] The major indication for pediatric OLT is biliary atresia following a failed Kasai procedure (portoenterostomy) or delayed recognition of the diagnosis. Other major pediatric indications include α1-antitrypsin deficiency and other metabolic disorders. Currently about 5000 liver transplantations are performed yearly, although the waiting list contains about three times that number.

BOX 38-2

Conditions Treated with Liver Transplantation

Cirrhosis Secondary To
Viral hepatitis
Alcoholic hepatitis
Autoimmune hepatitis
Cryptogenic source (no cause determinable)

Metabolic Liver Diseases
Wilson disease
α1-Antitrypsin deficiency
Hemochromatosis, neonatal
Glycogen storage disease
Tyrosinemia
Byler disease
Crigler-Najjar syndrome
Miscellaneous others

Cholestatic Liver Diseases
Primary biliary cirrhosis
Sclerosing cholangitis
Biliary atresia
Miscellaneous others

Acute Liver Failure
Drug reactions
Toxins (e.g., mushroom poisoning)
Viral hepatitis
Acute Budd-Chiari syndrome, other ischemic insult

BOX 38-3

Indications for Liver Transplantation

Acute Liver Disease
Fulminant liver failure with progressive encephalopathy
Prothrombin time >10 seconds above control
Bilirubin <15 mg/dl and rising

Chronic Liver Disease
Bilirubin >15 mg/dl
Intractable hepatic encephalopathy
Intractable ascites
Serum albumin <2.5 mg/dl
Prothrombin time ≥20 sec
Hepatorenal syndrome

BOX 38-4

Contraindications to Liver Transplantation

Absolute Contraindications
End-stage cardiopulmonary disease
Metastatic cancer
Active sepsis
Acquired immunodeficiency syndrome
Psychiatric illness preventing compliance with treatment

Relative Contraindications (Vary Greatly Among Transplant Centers)
Renal failure
Hepatitis B infection
Liver cancer
Portal vein thrombosis
Active alcoholism

Evaluation of the Transplantation Patient

Potential transplantation patients undergo extensive physiologic and psychological evaluation by physicians, nurses, psychologists, and social workers to identify potential contraindications to the procedure. Conditions that would normally preclude OLT include uncontrolled bacterial sepsis, failure of other major organ systems, extrahepatic malignancy, and more. Additional identified risk factors include portal vein thrombosis, previous portosystemic shunt operations, current alcohol or drug addiction, a poor psychosocial support system, and psychological instability. Many of these conditions are relative contraindications that diminish the chance of a successful outcome, but they do not always preclude transplantation. One group whose numbers are growing is patients with HIV and end-stage liver disease, and this group is increasingly being considered for OLT.[55]

Patients with viral hepatitis are particularly susceptible to recurrence in the transplanted organ and must be managed with care. Recent data show that patients transplanted for HBV who are treated indefinitely with high-dose HBIG have low recurrence rates, with acceptable survival and quality of life.[56] In contrast to HBV, it has not been possible to develop an effective regimen to prevent recurrent HCV infection.[57] A promising approach is pre-emptive antiviral therapy started shortly after OLT but before histologic recurrence is established; in particular, the use of long-acting pegylated interferons is currently the focus of ongoing clinical trials.[58]

After the patient has been identified as a candidate and a donor organ has been procured, the actual surgical procedure can take 8 to 22 hours to complete. The procedure involves five anastomoses between recipient and donor organs, including the following vascular anastomosis sites: suprahepatic inferior vena cava, infrahepatic vena cava, portal vein, hepatic artery, and biliary tract. The biliary anastomosis site varies, depending on the patient's extrahepatic biliary tract.

Posttransplantation Management

A cornerstone of posttransplantation management is immunosuppression to prevent rejection of the transplant graft. The rejection response after liver transplantation most often occurs between postoperative days 4 and 10. Clinical manifestations of acute rejection include tachycardia, fever, right upper quadrant or flank pain, diminished bile flow through the T tube drain or a change in bile color, and increasing jaundice. Laboratory findings include elevated serum bilirubin, transaminase, and alkaline phosphatase levels and increased prothrombin time. Following the successful use of cyclosporine, a number of immunosuppressive drugs have appeared and provide several choices for improving outcome. Immunosuppressives may be broadly categorized into three groups: initial immunosuppression, maintenance immunosuppression, and management of acute cellular rejection.[1] Prednisone is the primary posttransplantation immunosuppressive and is steadily tapered off in favor of maintenance drugs. The calcineurin inhibitors cyclosporine and tacrolimus are begun during induction and represent the mainstays of maintenance therapy. In many centers, tacrolimus has supplanted cyclosporine as the preferred immunosuppressive. Adjunctive maintenance agents include either mycophenolate mofetil or the older drug azathioprine. Acute rejection is generally managed with high-dose corticosteroids. Patients who fail to respond to steroids can be treated with infusion of one of several agents, including muromonab (OKT3), mycophenolate mofetil (MMF), or an interleukin-2 receptor blocker (e.g., basiliximab).

Side effects limit the usefulness of all these drugs and are a main source of morbidity and mortality among transplant recipients. The main nonimmunologic side effects of cyclosporine and tacrolimus are hypertension and renal insufficiency. Blood levels must be carefully monitored. Side effects of mycophenolate mofetil and azathioprine include bone marrow suppression with cytopenias. Problems with the acute antirejection infusions include hypersensitivity and cytokine reactions, and a heightened risk of opportunistic infection, especially cytomegalovirus, immediately after use. Among the many side effects of prednisone are hypertension and hyperglycemia. The main consequence of all these treatments is immune suppression and increased risk for infection.

Early infections are generally due to issues involving surgical technique and pre-existing infection (e.g., cholangitis) and have declined significantly in recent years.[1] They usually represent nosocomially acquired pathogens. Infections in the middle period from 1 to 6 months often represent viral infection or reactivation. Trimethoprim-sulfamethoxazole (TMP-SMX) is usually prescribed for prophylaxis against bacterial infection and *Pneumocystis carinii (jiroveci)* for the first year. Of particular concern and the focus of several prophylactic strategies is cytomegalovirus. Cytomegalovirus occurs at a high rate among seronegative recipients who receive a liver from a seropositive recipient, and reactivation rates are significant as well. In the middle and late periods fungal infection is important, especially *Aspergillus* species, and lymphoproliferative disorder due to Epstein-Barr virus is seen. OLT recipients should be instructed to avoid exposure to environmental or food-borne mold, which could increase their risk for fungal infection. Another important preventive strategy is appropriate vaccination, particularly annual influenza shots. (Live virus vaccinations, such as varicella, yellow fever, etc., should be avoided.)

Critical issues in the posttransplantation period include the following: hypertension, renal dysfunction, hyperlipidemia and cardiovascular disease, obesity, osteoporosis, and increased risk for cancer. Psychological issues are especially prominent, and caregivers and family should be alert for signs of depression and anxiety. Many of the antirejection medications exacerbate these symptoms. With careful follow-up, OLT recipients can live productive lives for many years after transplantation. Chronic rejection, often in the setting of progressive ductopenia, and recurrence of primary pretransplantation liver disease tend to cause graft failure with time. Actuarial survival at 5 years is approximately 88% for persons with cholestatic liver disease, 78% for patients with noncholestatic liver disease who are HCV negative, and 70% for persons with HCV.[59]

Age-Related Liver Disorders

LIVER DISEASES AND PEDIATRIC CONSIDERATIONS

Liver disease in infants and children not only encompasses pediatric variations of adult liver diseases but also includes conditions unique to that age group. Many of these conditions present at birth or shortly thereafter, although several may appear in later life.

Abnormal Bilirubin Metabolism in the Neonatal Period

Physiologic jaundice of the newborn is a harmless condition lasting no longer than 2 weeks after delivery. (Bilirubin metabolism in the neonatal period has already been discussed; see above section on jaundice.) Immature bilirubin conjugation and transport mechanisms are the primary causes, along with increased gut absorption of bilirubin. Hyperbilirubinemia is not considered physiologic or normal if the bilirubin is greater than 5 mg/dl on the first postpartum day, 10 mg/dl on the second, or 13 mg/dl at any time.[60] It should be noted that breast-fed babies have a higher incidence of hyperbilirubinemia than do bottle-fed babies because the β-glucuronidase in breast milk results in increased unconjugated bilirubin in the gut, which can be absorbed. If significant hyperbilirubinemia occurs, breast-feeding can be stopped.

Pathologic bilirubin levels should lead to an immediate evaluation to exclude congenital hemolytic disorders, Crigler-Najjar syndrome, hypothyroidism, congenital pyloric stenosis, sepsis, resorbing hematomas, and other conditions associated with an elevated serum bilirubin level.

Kernicterus refers to brain injury as a result of hyperbilirubinemia. It is a serious complication of the neonatal period, generally occurring in the setting of premature birth, neonatal jaundice, and especially hemolytic disease of the newborn.[61] In brief, the immature blood-brain barrier allows free unconjugated bilirubin to enter the brain, leading to encephalopathy. The term *kernicterus* refers to yellowish staining of permanently damaged brain tissue, primarily in the basal ganglia and thalamus. Despite decades of research, the exact pathophysiologic mechanisms by which elevated bilirubin causes brain damage have not been elucidated. Unfortunately, most infants die of this condition, and survivors often suffer from cerebral palsy, movement disorders, and mental retardation. Drugs that displace bilirubin from albumin seriously worsen the condition.

If recognized early, treatment with exchange transfusions, phenobarbital (to increase the levels of UDPGT; see previous discussion), and phototherapy ("bili-lights") may prevent these catastrophic consequences.[62] Phototherapy with light in the 450-nm-wavelength band is used to treat unconjugated hyperbilirubinemia in infants. Light at this wavelength converts unconjugated lipid-soluble bilirubin into water-soluble photoisomers that can be excreted by the kidneys, thus lowering the bilirubin level.

Infectious and Acquired Hepatidites in Children

Acute hepatitis A virus infection is often mild or asymptomatic in children. The prevalence of childhood infection correlates inversely with the quality of sanitation and hygiene. Treatment is supportive, and prevention guidelines parallel those for adults. Universal childhood vaccination is recommended in the United States and in many countries around the world.

Globally, **hepatitis B virus infection** is a common childhood disease, with vertical transmission from an HBsAg-positive mother to the infant being the most common mechanism of spread. Infected blood products and drugs are modes of infection in less developed areas. Features suggesting immune complex disease such as arthritis, fever, papular acrodermatitis (a rash not seen in adults), renal disease, and hematologic complications are more common in children. The incidence of chronic infection is also much higher after neonatal or childhood infection, which has grave long-term consequences because of the late sequelae of cirrhosis and HCC.

Passive immunization with HBIG should be given within 12 hours of birth to children of HBsAg-positive mothers. Active immunization with HBV vaccine should be given as a series of intramuscular injections at birth and at 1 and 6 months of age. Identical prophylaxis should be given to children of high-risk mothers even if not screened for HBsAg and to children otherwise exposed to HBV. In 1991, the Public Health Service recommended universal childhood HBV vaccination.[36] Strategies include infant vaccination, possibly with a booster dose in young adulthood, or adolescent vaccination.

Unlike HBV, **hepatitis C virus** is less commonly spread vertically, and effective screening of blood products has greatly reduced the risk of childhood infection. **Hepatitis delta virus** may be spread by the intrafamily route as a coinfector with hepatitis B.

Acute **hepatitis E virus** is especially virulent in adolescents and young adults, with a high mortality rate in pregnant women. In endemic regions, it is the most common cause of childhood hepatitis and is indirectly a cause of infant mortality.

Many systemic viruses may cause biochemical or clinical hepatitis in the pediatric population, including Epstein-Barr virus, cytomegalovirus, herpesvirus, and adenovirus. Neonatal hepatitis is part of the so-called TORCH syndrome and may be caused by a variety of congenital infections, including cytomegalovirus, herpesvirus, varicella, *Toxoplasma*, and syphilis. Encephalitis and retinitis may accompany these conditions, with lifelong sequelae. The finding of an enlarged liver and elevated transaminases in the newborn should necessitate a search for congenital infection.

Reye syndrome is primarily a disease of children, although adult cases are reported. The syndrome usually occurs shortly after a viral illness such as influenza or chickenpox, and begins with nausea and vomiting rapidly progressing to coma. The exact pathophysiologic mechanism is unknown, but significant mitochondrial dysfunction of hepatocytes occurs.[63] Reye syndrome is characterized by fatty infiltration of the liver with severe hepatic dysfunction, including encephalopathy, coagulopathy, and elevated levels of hepatocellular enzymes. Mortality may be as high as 40%. A strong association with aspirin use during the preceding viral illness has been noted, but other drugs may be causative as well.[63] (Because of the risk of Reye syndrome, aspirin is contraindicated for childhood viral illnesses.) Treatment of Reye syndrome is supportive, and if the child survives, recovery is complete. As with other toxic hepatitides, liver transplantation is reserved for irreversible disease.

Congenital Liver Disease

Many heritable diseases of the liver occur in childhood. These may be broadly characterized as enzyme deficiencies affecting multiple organ systems including the liver (e.g., α_1-antitrypsin deficiency), disorders of bilirubin metabolism (e.g., Crigler-Najjar syndrome), inborn errors affecting other metabolic pathways, intrahepatic ductopenic conditions, and extrahepatic ductopenia (biliary atresia).

Multisystem Enzyme Deficiencies

α_1-**Antitrypsin deficiency** is an autosomal recessive condition that commonly affects children and young adults, although it may not become obvious until later in life. α_1-Antitrypsin is an enzyme inhibitor found in many tissues that prevents normal enzymes, such as elastase and collagenase, from causing damage to those tissues. Production of this enzyme is genetically controlled by a gene that has many allelic variations (gene types). Although numerous abnormal alleles have been identified, the most common pathologic form, which causes both liver and lung disease, is the protease inhibitor Z variant *PiZZ*, which produces α_1-ATZ protein.[1] This defective α_1-antitrypsin protein accumulates in the liver and produces the diagnostic granules seen microscopically, although the exact mechanism of liver damage is unclear. A characteristic centrilobular emphysema, pancreatic insufficiency, and cirrhosis may occur. Treatment by liver transplantation is often precluded by these other problems. Gene therapy for α_1-antitrypsin deficiency is an area of active investigation.[1]

Cystic fibrosis is an autosomal recessive condition primarily known as a cause of lung disease in children. However, this relatively common genetic disease may also cause pancreatic insufficiency, intestinal obstruction, gallstone disease, neonatal giant cell hepatitis, bile duct obstruction, and biliary cirrhosis. Treatment is directed at complications.[64] Ursodeoxycholic acid improves the biochemical indices of liver injury; however, conclusive evidence that the drug halts the progression to cirrhosis is lacking. Gene therapy for the pulmonary disease is in the experimental phase.

Wilson disease and **hemochromatosis** are single-gene-mutation illnesses with significant liver involvement and have been discussed earlier in the chapter.

Disorders of Bilirubin Metabolism

Inherited defects in bile acid metabolism can manifest as impaired synthesis or transport. The first group includes **cerebrotendinous xanthomatosis,** a steroid hydroxylase deficiency that leads to premature atherosclerosis and encephalopathy. However, manifestations do not generally include liver disease. Children treated with chenodeoxycholic acid have shown marked improvement. Peroxisomes are responsible for β oxidation in the final steps of bile acid synthesis, and numerous hereditary peroxisomopathies have been described. The most well known of these conditions is X-linked adrenal leukodystrophy, which is manifested by progressive neurologic dysfunction and adrenal insufficiency. Treatments for this and related conditions remain generally ineffective, but investigational therapies have been frequently tried.[65] X-linked adrenal leukodystrophy was recently the subject of a major movie focusing on the experimental "Lorenzo's oil."[66]

Disorders of bile acid transport include **Gilbert syndrome,** a very common (about 10% of the Caucasian population in the United States), entirely benign, autosomal dominant condition that results in mild unconjugated (indirect) hyperbilirubinemia. It is caused by decreased bilirubin glucuronidation.

Awareness of this disorder is important to avoid inappropriate evaluation of these patients.

Crigler-Najjar syndrome is a rare autosomal recessive disorder marked by significant unconjugated hyperbilirubinemia.[67] In type I Crigler-Najjar syndrome, the near-total absence of bilirubin conjugation results in high levels of unconjugated bilirubin crossing the immature blood-brain barrier. This condition presents shortly after birth, and neonates usually die of kernicterus or suffer irreversible neurologic damage. Liver transplantation following phototherapy and plasma exchange transfusion has been lifesaving in rare instances. In type II Crigler-Najjar syndrome, some conjugating capability exists and is enhanced by the administration of phenobarbital. These patients rarely experience bilirubin encephalopathy and can lead normal lives. Treatment consists of phototherapy, phenobarbital, and potentially liver transplantation. Gene therapy is an active area or research for Crigler-Najjar syndrome.

Progressive familial intrahepatic cholestasis (PFIC) is a rare autosomal recessive disorder involving severe jaundice, pruritus, and malabsorption due to a defect in bile salt excretion. PFIC type I, or **Byler syndrome,** is caused by a single-gene mutation and traces back to an Amish kindred descended from Jacob Byler. Other genetic defects cause different types of PFIC with similar manifestations. Medical therapy with ursodeoxycholic acid is helpful in some children, and biliary diversion procedures have given symptomatic relief to some patients by decreasing the bile acid pool.[1] In the past the disease was uniformly fatal, but liver transplantation has been shown to normalize bile acid synthesis and growth in selected patients.[68]

Other rare disorders of bile salt transport exist and are generally fatal in infancy. These chronic cholestatic diseases, such as North American Indian childhood cirrhosis and cholestasis-lymphedema syndrome (Aagenaes syndrome), are undergoing investigation at the molecular genetic level and are generally linked to single-gene mutations.

Inborn Errors of Metabolism

A very broad range of enzyme abnormalities resulting from single-gene mutations, generally autosomally recessive, may show up in children. These result in abnormal processing of lipids, glycogen, amino acids and proteins, lipopolysaccharides, and other substances. The pathologic process generally results from excessive accumulation of precursor substances in target organs, such as the brain and spinal cord. The liver is often the primary site of processing and may be the target of toxic accumulation as well. The latter may result in signs of liver disease, including hepatomegaly, liver enzyme elevation, and jaundice. Inborn errors that show up in the neonatal period are usually fatal unless immediate treatment is undertaken. Inborn errors presenting in infancy and later years may be amenable to specific therapies. Liver or bone marrow transplantation[69] may be effective for some of these conditions, and many of them are foci of intense research regarding gene therapy. The diagnosis of any inborn error of metabolism should

prompt a thorough investigation of family history and appropriate genetic counseling and testing of family members.

As noted above, given the heterogeneity and rarity of these conditions, they will not be discussed further in this chapter, and the interested reader is referred to a standard text on the subject.[70]

Intrahepatic Cholestatic Conditions

Intrahepatic cholestasis may be defined as cholestatic liver disease in which the pathologic process is confined to the liver (i.e., the extrahepatic biliary system is normal).[71] One cause of this condition is neonatal hepatitis, which can be idiopathic, viral, or secondary to an inborn error of metabolism. (Viral hepatitis and inborn errors were discussed earlier in the chapter.) The second category of these illnesses includes conditions in which the number of bile ducts is decreased and inadequate to accommodate normal bile metabolism and transport.

Alagille syndrome, or arteriohepatic dysplasia, is the most common form of inherited intrahepatic cholestasis. This autosomal dominant condition has incomplete penetrance and expressivity, and is associated with typical bony and cardiovascular malformations, as well as a paucity of intrahepatic bile ducts. The disease generally progresses slowly; pruritus, hypercholesterolemia, xanthomas, and neurologic complications due to vitamin E deficiency may occur if untreated. Patients may be maintained on ursodeoxycholic acid until liver transplantation, which is the current treatment of choice.[72]

Several other conditions manifest a paucity of intrahepatic bile ducts. Some of these arise from defective bile transport mechanisms and are discussed in the Inborn Errors of Metabolism section.

Extrahepatic Cholestatic Conditions (Biliary Atresia)

Extrahepatic ductopenia is often referred to as **biliary atresia.** Biliary atresia or, as some authors prefer, *progressive obliterative cholangiopathy,* can be either congenital or acquired. The latter occurs in the setting of certain autoimmune illnesses and is one of the principle forms of chronic rejection of a transplanted liver allograft. Biliary atresia is a rather common birth defect, occurring in 1/10,000 to 1/15,000 live births (and is therefore much more common than intrahepatic cholestatic conditions).[1] Distinguishing between this disorder and idiopathic neonatal hepatitis can be challenging, but the liver biopsy findings are usually characteristic. Infants and children with biliary atresia have progressive cholestasis with all the usual concomitant features: pruritus, malabsorption with growth retardation, fat-soluble vitamin deficiencies, hyperlipidemia, and eventually cirrhosis with portal hypertension. Some children have recurrent episodes of bacterial cholangitis as well. A cholangiogram should be obtained to assess the possibility of a correctable obstruction. The Kasai procedure is often performed to create a hepatoportoenteric connection, which may allow adequate bile drainage. This procedure is not usually curative but ideally does "buy time" until the child can achieve growth and undergo liver transplantation.

KEY POINTS

- Cirrhosis is the irreversible end stage of many different hepatic injuries. The liver is fibrotic, scarred, and nodular. Symptoms of cirrhosis are due to hepatocellular failure and portal hypertension.
- Biliary cirrhosis is associated with chronic bile duct obstruction with resultant backup of bile in the liver. Gallstones and extrahepatic and intrahepatic bile duct inflammation are common causes.
- Alcoholic cirrhosis is associated with chronic alcohol ingestion, which may precipitate fatty liver, hepatitis, and, finally, cirrhosis.
- The liver is subject to damage because of its role in storing and detoxifying potentially injurious substances. Metal storage diseases are genetic disorders in which excessive minerals are absorbed and subsequently deposited in the liver. Hemochromatosis is characterized by excessive iron absorption and is manifested by elevated serum ferritin and iron levels. Phlebotomy is the usual treatment. Wilson disease is due to excessive accumulation of copper in the liver and other organs. Copper chelators are effective in preventing liver damage.
- Acetaminophen is converted to a toxic metabolite in the liver that is normally rapidly detoxified by liver enzymes. In acetaminophen overdose, the detoxification reaction may be overwhelmed and liver necrosis results. Treatment is with acetylcysteine.
- Liver abscesses are suspected in patients with fever, nausea, vomiting, and right upper quadrant pain. Ascending biliary infection, abdominal infections transported by the portal vein, and direct extension of infection from neighboring structures are usual sources of infection. Antibiotics and drainage are commonly prescribed.
- The liver commonly sustains injury during penetrating and blunt trauma to the abdomen. Because the liver is highly vascular, trauma may produce extreme blood loss and hemorrhagic shock. Liver trauma is manifested by abdominal tenderness, distention, guarding, and rigidity.
- In the United States, cancer of the liver is usually metastatic and rarely primary. Tumors of the esophagus, stomach, colon, rectum, breast, and lung commonly seed in the liver. HCC is more common in other parts of the world but its incidence is increasing in the United States, with HBV and HCV as important contributing factors.

LIVER DISEASES AND GERIATRIC CONSIDERATIONS

Liver size and blood flow decrease with aging, but this observation has little functional significance. Drugs whose metabolism is primarily related to hepatic blood flow and drugs processed by the mixed-function oxidase system (cytochromes) may have a prolonged serum half-life requiring careful monitoring and dose adjustment. Routine blood test results of liver-related enzymes are not changed by aging.

In the United States, HCC is usually the result of years of injury from alcohol or chronic viral hepatitis and is therefore more often seen in older people. The prognosis is unfortunately dismal (see discussion earlier in the chapter).

Ischemic hepatitis is usually associated with underlying cardiovascular disease and episodes of hypotension, as during surgery or sepsis, and is more common in older patients. Typically, serum transaminases rise rapidly and the prothrombin time is prolonged. Recovery may be rapid, but the prognosis depends on the severity of the underlying disorder. Ischemic hepatitis alone is rarely a cause of death in such patients. Right-sided heart failure may result in passive hepatic congestion with ascites and (rarely) liver failure. In developing countries, constrictive pericarditis and uncorrected valvular heart disease due to rheumatic fever are still significant causes of intractable ascites and should be considered in the differential diagnosis.

Metabolic liver diseases rarely present in the geriatric population. **Hemochromatosis** in women often occurs after menopause and may present as new-onset diabetes mellitus, heart failure, arthritis, cirrhosis, or HCC. Typically, **autoimmune liver diseases** are seen in young to middle-aged people. However, autoimmune chronic active hepatitis may be a cause of "cryptogenic" cirrhosis in older women. **Primary biliary cirrhosis** is uncommon in later life. **Primary sclerosing cholangitis (PSC)** may afflict older persons with long-standing ulcerative colitis, even those who had colectomies many years, even decades, earlier.

Because **alcohol abuse** generally starts early in life, older patients bear the cumulative injury of years of exposure and are likely to show signs of advanced liver disease. Treatment is the same as in younger patients, but attention must be given to the older patients' social circumstances and intercurrent medical problems. Symptoms and signs of alcohol intoxication and hepatic encephalopathy may be confused with senile dementia and made worse by concomitant drug use (e.g., minor tranquilizers, opiates).

The diagnosis of **acute viral hepatitis** may be more difficult in older people because of nonspecific symptoms in mild cases and decreased clinical suspicion. Acute HAV infection is less common as a result of the higher incidence of immunity, but it may be more severe with higher mortality rates in the elderly. The end results of HBV and HCV infection often become evident in elderly persons, and in the United States the increased prevalence of persons living with these viruses will mean more elderly patients with liver disease in coming decades.

Older patients with chronic HBV and HCV infection may be treated with the standard treatments, but comorbid medical problems, intolerance to the side effects of treatment, and advanced liver disease may preclude treatment in many persons. The indications for **liver transplantation** do not change with advancing years, and no arbitrary age limits have been set on transplantation. However, there may be subtle barriers in effect, and the allocation of organs remains a highly controversial issue. Each patient must be evaluated individually regarding the propriety of transplantation and the likelihood of success.

SUMMARY

Disorders of the liver are diverse and complex. Because the liver is vital to most life processes, even mild disorders can cause life-threatening alterations. Health care professionals need a good understanding of hepatobiliary anatomy and physiology to appreciate the effects of these disorders on patients.

Many liver disorders are the consequence of lifestyle choices such as alcoholism and drug abuse. Health care professionals are in a position to explain the risks of detrimental lifestyles and their relationship to liver diseases so as to prevent occurrence of these diseases.

Medical treatment entails the use of drugs from many different classes. Because the liver is central to the metabolism of many of these drugs, their use requires special attention. Before any drug is given to a patient with liver disease, it is essential to become completely familiar with it by consulting a good pharmacology text or drug information source.

REFERENCES

1. Sleisenger MH, Feldman M, Friedman LS: *Sleisenger and Fordtran's gastrointestinal and liver disease: pathophysiology, diagnosis, management*, ed 8, Philadelphia, 2006, Elsevier Saunders.
2. Moore KL, Persaud TVN, Torchia MG: *The developing human: clinically oriented embryology*, Philadelphia, 2008, Saunders.
3. Moore KL, Persaud TVN, Shiota K: *Color atlas of clinical embryology*, Philadelphia, 2000, Saunders.
4. Guyton AC, Hall JE: *Textbook of medical physiology*, ed 11, Philadelphia, 2006, Elsevier Saunders.
5. Johnson LR: *Gastrointestinal physiology*, ed 7, Philadelphia, 2006, Mosby.
6. Kamisako T et al: Recent advances in bilirubin metabolism research: the molecular mechanism of hepatocyte bilirubin transport and its clinical relevance, *J Gastroenterol* 35(9):659-664, 2000.
7. Gurakar A et al: Androgenic/anabolic steroid–induced intrahepatic cholestasis: a review with four additional case reports, *J Okla State Med Assoc* 87:399-404, 1994.
8. Davies MH et al: The adverse influence of pregnancy upon sulphation: a clue to the pathogenesis of intrahepatic cholestasis of pregnancy, *J Hepatol* 21:1127-1134, 1994.
9. Bosch J et al: Recombinant factor VIIa for upper gastrointestinal bleeding in patients with cirrhosis: a randomized, double-blind trial, *Gastroenterology* 127(4):1123-1130, 2004.
10. Imperiale TF, Teran JC, McCullough AJ: A meta-analysis of somatostatin versus vasopressin in the management of acute esophageal variceal hemorrhage, *Gastroenterology* 109(4):1289-1294, 1995.
11. Garcia-Tsao G et al: Prevention and management of gastroesophageal varices and variceal hemorrhage in cirrhosis, *Hepatology* 46:922, 2007.
12. Laine L, Cook D: Endoscopic ligation compared with sclerotherapy for treatment of esophageal variceal bleeding: a meta-analysis, *Ann Intern Med* 123(4):280-287, 1995.
13. D'Amico G, Pagliaro L, Bosch J: The treatment of portal hypertension: a meta-analytic review, *Hepatology* 22(1):332-354, 1995.
14. Gournay J et al: Isosorbide mononitrate and propranolol compared with propranolol alone for the prevention of variceal rebleeding, *Hepatology* 31(6):1239-1245, 2000.
15. Bosch J, Garcia-Pagan JC: Prevention of variceal rebleeding, *Lancet* 361(9361):952-954, 2003.
16. Rikkers LF, Sorrell WT, Gongliang J: Which portosystemic shunt is best? *Gastroenterol Clin North Am* 21:179-196, 1992.
17. Escorsell A et al: TIPS versus drug therapy in preventing variceal rebleeding in advanced cirrhosis: a randomized controlled trial, *Hepatology* 35(2):385-392, 2002.
18. Butterworth RF: The astrocytic ("peripheral-type") benzodiazepine receptor: role in the pathogenesis of portal-systemic encephalopathy, *Neurochem Int* 36(4-5):411-416, 2000.
19. Shils ME, Olson JA: *Modern nutrition in health and disease*, ed 8, Philadelphia, 1994, Lea & Febiger.
20. Crippin JS, Gross JB Sr, Lindor KD: Increased intracranial pressure and hepatic encephalopathy in chronic liver disease, *Am J Gastroenterol* 87:879-882, 1992.
21. Blei AT, Larsen FS: Pathophysiology of cerebral edema in fulminant hepatic failure, *J Hepatol* 31(4):771-776, 1999.
22. Blei AT et al: Complications of intracranial pressure monitoring in fulminant hepatic failure, *Lancet* 341:157-158, 1993.
23. Jalan R et al: Moderate hypothermia prevents cerebral hyperemia and increase in intracranial pressure in patients undergoing liver transplantation for acute liver failure, *Transplantation* 75:2034, 2003.
24. Schrier RW, Gurevich AK, Cadnapaphornchai MA: Pathogenesis and management of sodium and water retention in cardiac failure and cirrhosis, *Semin Nephrol* 21(2):157-172, 2001.
25. Runyon BA: Management of adult patients with ascites caused by cirrhosis, *Hepatology* 27(1):264-272, 1998.
26. Stanley MM et al: Peritoneovenous shunting as compared with medical treatment in patients with alcoholic cirrhosis and massive ascites: Veterans Administration Cooperative Study on Treatment of Alcoholic Cirrhosis with Ascites, *N Engl J Med* 321(24):1632-1638, 1989.
27. Runyon BA et al: A rodent model of cirrhosis, ascites, and bacterial peritonitis, *Gastroenterology* 100(2):189-193, 1991.
28. Singh N et al: Trimethoprim-sulfamethoxazole for the prevention of spontaneous bacterial peritonitis in cirrhosis: a randomized trial, *Ann Intern Med* 122(8):595-598, 1995.
29. Watt K, Uhanova J, Minuk GY: Hepatorenal syndrome: diagnostic accuracy, clinical features, and outcome in a tertiary care center, *Am J Gastroenterol* 97(8):2046-2050, 2002.
30. Arroyo V, Guevara M, Gines P: Hepatorenal syndrome in cirrhosis: pathogenesis and treatment, *Gastroenterology* 122(6):1658-1676, 2002.
31. Alexander IM: Viral hepatitis: primary care diagnosis and management, *Nurse Pract* 23(10):13-26, 1998.
32. General recommendations on immunization: recommendations of the Advisory Committee on Immunization Practices (ACIP) and the American Academy of Family Physicians (AAFP), *MMWR Morb Mortal Wkly Rep* 51(RR02):1-36, 2002.
33. Braconier JH, Wennerholm S, Norrby SR: Comparative immunogenicity and tolerance of Vaqta and Havrix, *Vaccine* 17(17):2181-2184, 1999.
34. Marcellin P: Advances in therapy for chronic hepatitis B, *Semin Liver Dis* 22(Suppl 1):33-36, 2002.
35. Wai CT, Lok AS: Treatment of hepatitis B, *J Gastroenterol* 37(10):771-778, 2002.
36. Hepatitis B virus: A comprehensive strategy for eliminating transmission in the United States through universal childhood vaccination: recommendations of the Immunization Practices Advisory Committee (ACIP), *MMWR Morb Mortal Wkly Rep* 40(RR13):1-19, 1991.
37. Updated U.S. Public Health Service guidelines for the management of occupational exposures to HBV, HCV, and HIV and recommendations for postexposure prophylaxis, *MMWR Morb Mortal Wkly Rep* 50(RR11):1-42, 2001.
38. McHutchison JG, Fried MW: Current therapy for hepatitis C: pegylated interferon and ribavirin, *Clin Liver Dis* 7(1):149-161, 2003.
39. Czaja AJ, Freese DK: Diagnosis and treatment of autoimmune hepatitis: American Association for the Study of Liver Disease recommendations, *Hepatology* 36(2):479-497, 2002.
40. Gorbach SL, Bartlett JG, Blacklow NR: *Infectious diseases*, ed 3, Philadelphia, 2004, Lippincott Williams & Wilkins.
41. Lee YM, Kaplan MM: Management of primary sclerosing cholangitis, *Am J Gastroenterol* 97(3):528-534, 2002.
42. Angulo P, Keach JC, Batts KP et al: Independent predictors of liver fibrosis in patients with nonalcoholic steatohepatitis, *Hepatology* 30(6):1356-1362, 1999.

43. Crosse KI, Anania FA: Alcoholic hepatitis, *Curr Treat Options Gastroenterol* 5(6):417-423, 2002.

44. O'Shea RS, McCullough AJ: Treatment of alcoholic hepatitis, *Clin Liver Dis* 9(1):103-134, 2005.

45. Braunwald E et al: *Harrison's principles of internal medicine*, ed 15, New York, 2001, McGraw-Hill.

46. Adams PC et al: Hemochromatosis and iron-overload screening in a racially diverse population, *N Engl J Med* 352(17):1769-1778, 2005.

47. Brewer GJ et al: Treatment of Wilson disease with ammonium tetrathiomolybdate, III: Initial therapy in a total of 55 neurologically affected patients and follow-up with zinc therapy, *Arch Neurol* 60(3):379-385, 2003.

48. Ostapowicz G et al: Results of a prospective study of acute liver failure at 17 tertiary care centers in the United States, *Ann Intern Med* 137(12):947-954, 2002.

49. Ahya SN et al: *The Washington manual of medical therapeutics*, ed 30, Philadelphia, 2001, Lippincott Williams & Wilkins.

50. Makin AJ, Wendow J, Williams R: A 7-year experience of severe acetaminophen-induced hepatotoxicity (1987-1993), *Gastroenterology* 109:1907-1916, 1995.

51. Clochesy JM et al: *Critical care nursing*, Philadelphia, 1996, Saunders.

52. Ravoet C, Bleiberg H, Gerard B: Non-surgical treatment of hepatocarcinoma, *J Surg Oncol* (Suppl)13:104-111, 1993.

53. Keeffe EB: Liver transplantation: current status and novel approaches to liver replacement, *Gastroenterology* 120(3):749-762, 2001.

54. Yu AS, Keeffe EB: Management of hepatocellular carcinoma, *Rev Gastroenterol Disord* 3(1):8-24, 2003.

55. Boyd AE et al: Liver transplantation and HIV: a case series of 7 patients, *Conf Retroviruses Opportunistic Infect* 8(Feb 4-8):217 (abstract 578), 2001.

56. Shouval D, Samuel D: Hepatitis B immune globulin to prevent hepatitis B virus graft reinfection following liver transplantation: a concise review, *Hepatology* 32:1189-1195, 2000.

57. Sheiner P: The efficacy of prophylactic interferon alfa-2b in preventing recurrent hepatitis C after liver transplantation, *Hepatology* 28:831-838, 1999.

58. Samuel D et al: Interferon-alpha 2b plus ribavirin in patients with chronic hepatitis C after liver transplantation: a randomized study, *Gastroenterology* 124(3):642-650, 2003.

59. Wiesner RH et al: Recent advances in liver transplantation, *Mayo Clin Proc* 78(2):197-210, 2003.

60. Sherlock S, Dooley J: The liver in infancy and childhood. In: *Diseases of the liver and biliary system,* ed 10, Oxford, 1997, Blackwell.

61. Hansen TW: Mechanisms of bilirubin toxicity: clinical implications, *Clin Perinatol* 29(4):765-778, 2002.

62. Bratlid D: Criteria for treatment of neonatal jaundice, *J Perinatol* 21(Suppl)1:S88-S92, 2001; discussion, S104-S107.

63. Casteels-Van Daele M et al: Reye syndrome revisited: a descriptive term covering a group of heterogeneous disorders, *Eur J Pediatr* 159(9):641-648, 2000.

64. Sokol RJ, Durie PR: Recommendation for management of liver and biliary tract disease in cystic fibrosis, *J Pediatr Gastroenterol Nutr* 28:S1-S13, 1999.

65. McGuinness MC, Wei H, Smith KD: Therapeutic developments in peroxisome biogenesis disorders, *Expert Opin Investig Drugs* 9(9):1985-1992, 2000.

66. Suzuki Y et al: The clinical course of childhood and adolescent adrenoleukodystrophy before and after Lorenzo's oil, *Brain Dev* 23(1):30-33, 2001.

67. Ishak KG: Inherited metabolic diseases of the liver, *Clin Liver Dis* 6(2):455-479, 2002.

68. Ismail H et al: Treatment of progressive familial intrahepatic cholestasis: liver transplantation or partial external biliary diversion, *Pediatr Transplant* 3(3):219-224, 1999.

69. Yeager AM: Allogeneic hematopoietic cell transplantation for inborn metabolic diseases, *Ann Hematol* 81(Suppl 2):S16-S19, 2002.

70. Behrman RE, Kliegman RM, Jenson HD: *Nelson textbook of pediatrics*, ed 16, Philadelphia, 2000, Saunders.

71. Bezerra JA, Balistreri WF: Cholestatic syndromes of infancy and childhood, *Semin Gastrointest Dis* 12(2):54-65, 2001.

72. Balistreri WF: Intrahepatic cholestasis, *J Pediatr Gastroenterol Nutr* 35(Suppl 1):S17-S23, 2002.

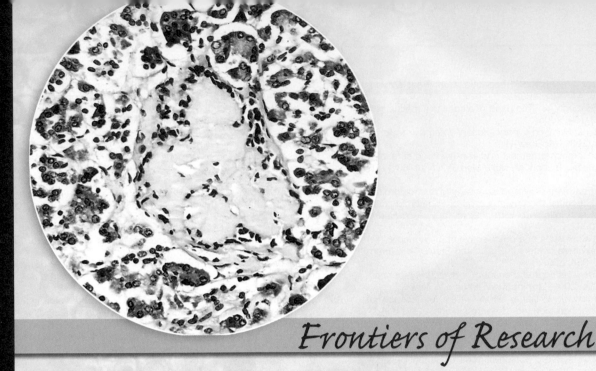

Diabetes Mellitus

Sheila K. Smith

Diabetes mellitus refers to a group of clinical syndromes characterized by abnormal carbohydrate, fat, and protein metabolism resulting in excessive levels of glucose in the blood. High blood glucose (hyperglycemia) is caused by defects in pancreatic insulin secretion, insulin sensitivity at the cellular level, or both. Insulin is a hormone produced by the beta (β) cells of the pancreas. Under conditions of normal physiology, insulin lowers blood glucose by acting as a protein transporter of glucose from the bloodstream into the tissue cells, where it can be used as an important source of energy. Similarly, insulin promotes the uptake of free fatty acids into adipose tissue, and the uptake of amino acids for the synthesis of proteins. Thus insulin acts as a "storage" hormone. Under the influence of insulin, glucose is stored by the liver and muscle cells as glycogen; fat tissue is deposited; and muscle tissue is built. Normally a low level of insulin is released continuously, 24 hours per day. This is known as the *basal* supply of insulin. In addition, the rise in plasma glucose that occurs with eating a meal triggers the pancreas to release a postmeal (postprandial) insulin "bolus," thereby assisting the body to make use of the ingested energy source.

When insulin is lacking or if the tissue cells have become resistant to insulin, glucose cannot be absorbed from the bloodstream. Several forms of impaired glucose metabolism have been identified. These are categorized as: (1) Diabetes type 1; (2) pre-diabetes; (3) diabetes type 2; (4) metabolic syndrome; and (5) gestational diabetes. In all cases, glucose utilization is diminished, fat metabolism is increased, and the breakdown of proteins is increased. The clinical picture is one of abnormally elevated blood glucose levels frequently accompanied by high plasma lipid levels and muscle atrophy from the breakdown of protein tissues.

Diabetes mellitus type 1 (DM1), previously referred to as *childhood-onset diabetes,* results from complete loss of insulin production. Patients with DM1 experience rapid, permanent autoimmune destruction of pancreatic β cells. A genetic predisposition for DM1 has been identified, but it

seems that an environmental "trigger" may be necessary as well. Viral infections seem to be one mechanism for stimulating the immune system to attack the pancreas. Because destruction of the β cells occurs rapidly with DM1, the onset of symptoms is similarly rapid. With new onset, DM1 patients are acutely and often seriously ill. They experience the classic signs of diabetes: abnormal thirst, increased fluid consumption, frequent urination, and weight loss from the metabolism of fats and proteins for energy. Excess glucose that has not moved into cells is passed through the kidneys, causing the polyuria, polydipsia, and glycosuria ascribed to diabetes mellitus. In addition, because fats have been used to supply energy, these patients frequently present in ketoacidosis which can be life-threatening. Therapy for DM1 patients requires immediate insulin replacement, both in basal and bolus forms. To date, no effective therapy has been discerned that can prevent the development of DM1 in susceptible individuals.

Pre-diabetes refers to the earliest clinical form of diabetes mellitus type 2 (DM2). In pre-diabetes, an insulin resistance has developed causing the start of higher-than-normal blood sugars. There is a decreased ability of the cells to take up glucose, but not yet enough to be diagnosed as full diabetes. This condition is also known as *impaired glucose tolerance.* Many of these individuals will go on to develop DM2, though aggressive exercise, weight loss, dietary control, and medication therapy have been found to prevent or delay its onset.

DM2, previously referred to as *adult-onset diabetes,* has a more heterogeneous clinical course than DM1. Patients with DM2 still have insulin production by the pancreatic β cells, but insulin resistance at the tissue cell level causes blood glucose levels to rise. Blood sugars can be elevated both in the fasting state and in the postprandial state. Defects in DM2 include pancreatic insulin production, cellular insulin resistance, and excessive hepatic release of stored glucose (gluconeogenesis). Significant lifestyle modifications and often several medications are required for the management of DM2. Over time,

Amyloidosis of a pancreatic islet in type 2 diabetes. (From Kumar V et al: Robbins and Cotran pathologic basis of disease, ed 7, Philadelphia, 2005, Saunders, p 1200.)

Endocrine Function, Metabolism, and Nutrition

the function of the pancreatic β cells declines further, eventually resulting in the need for insulin therapy. Development of DM2 appears to be both genetic and environmental: nearly 100% of identical twins will develop the disorder, even if raised apart. Recently, however, the world has seen a near epidemic of DM2, especially with the development of more and more sedentary lifestyles, driving instead of walking, fewer forms of physical work, more processed foods, and especially with the use of highly processed corn sweeteners.

Regardless of the type of diabetes mellitus causing hyperglycemia, prolonged excessive blood glucose eventually leads to devastating multisystem damage. Microvascular complications predominantly affect the retina, glomerulus, and peripheral nervous system, resulting in impaired vision, renal failure, and loss of tactile sensation, respectively. Macrovascular complications include accelerated atherosclerosis in the coronary arteries, the systemic arteries, and the central nervous system. It is not surprising, then, to find that in the developed world, diabetes mellitus is the leading cause of blindness and renal failure leading to hemodialysis. Diabetes mellitus is the leading cause of lower extremity amputation in Europe and North America. Diabetes mellitus and its associated cholesterol abnormalities are major comorbid conditions contributing to the epidemic of atherosclerosis afflicting the world population. Diabetes is now regarded as a cardiovascular disease equivalent in terms of risk for myocardial infarction, stroke, and peripheral vascular disease. In other words, diabetes is our newest form of heart disease. The constellation of diabetes, overweight, hypertension, a pro-inflammatory state, and dyslipidemia is the condition known as *metabolic syndrome.*

Clinical research into diabetes therapy offeres insights into prevention of microvascular and macrovascular complications. There remains controversy as to whether maintaining near-normal blood glucose control is sufficient to prevent complications. In the 1993 Diabetes Control and Complication Trial (DCCT), 1,440 subjects with DM1 were randomly selected to receive either "conventional therapy" with 1 to 2 injections of intermediate and short-acting insulin daily, or "intensive treatment" with an insulin infusion pump or insulin injections at least 3 times daily. Subjects treated with intensive therapy experienced more hypoglycemia but noted a 76% decrease in the incidence of retinopathy over conventionally treated subjects. Intensive-therapy subjects with mild retinopathy on enrollment noted a 54% reduction in disease progression over their conventionally-treated counterparts. Early diabetic nephropathy, causing abnormal renal leaking of small amounts of protein (microalbuminuria), was reduced by 39% in the intensive-therapy group. Finally, diabetic neuropathy was reduced by 60% in the intensive-therapy group during the 10 years of intervention. The results of the DCCT indicate that the goal of therapy for all patients with DM1 should be reduction of blood glucose to values as near normal as possible without causing frequent hypoglycemia.

By comparison, newer and surprising findings from the recent Action to Control Cardiovascular Risk in Diabetes (ACCORD) trial that involved more than 10,000 patients studied for three and a half years with treatment and follow-up, revealed that intensifying glycemic control *harmed patients* with DM 2. This multicenter clinical study, sponsored by the National Heart, Lung, and Blood Institute, was designed to evaluate whether tight control of blood sugar in DM 2 would "reduce the rate of cardiovascular events" in high risk patients.[1] The news has shocked clinicians worldwide, since diabetes educators have been advocating tight glycemic control for most patients with DM 2 based on DCCT and two additional international studies (Kumamoto Study, 1995; and United Kingdom Prospective Diabetes Study, 1998). At a 2008 conference of the American Diabetes Association's Annual Scientific Sessions, findings of ACCORD underscore that intensifying therapy to achieve glycemic control may create additional risk for death in patients who are middle aged or older and are at high risk for cardiovascular disease. Special consideration may now be essential for high-risk patients with multiple risk factors and heart disease. The controversy continues, and in the words of William Cefalu, MD, who writes in a recent *New England Journal of Medicine* ". . . a targeted glycosylated hemoglobin level of approximately 7% may be appropriate in this high-risk population, especially when the use of aggressive pharmacologic therapy is under consideration."[2]

[1]Gerstein HC et al: *Effects of intensive glucose lowering in type 2 diabetes* N Engl J Med *358(24):2545-2559, 2008.*
[2]Cefalu WT: *Glycemic targets and cardiovascular disease.* N Engl J Med *358(24):2633-2635, 2008.*

Endocrine Physiology and Mechanisms of Hypothalamic-Pituitary Regulation

Jacquelyn L. Banasik

MEDIA RESOURCES

Additional Material for Study, Review, and Further Exploration

CD Companion ■ Review Questions and Answers
■ Glossary (with audio pronunciations for selected terms)
■ Disease Profiles ■ Animations

ⓔvolve **Website** at http://evolve.elsevier.com/Copstead/
■ Case Studies ■ Disease Profiles ■ WebLinks ■ Key Points Review

Online Course (Module 17)

KEY QUESTIONS

■ How does the lipid or water solubility of hormones affect their transport in the circulation?
■ What are the general mechanisms of action of lipid-soluble and water-soluble hormones on target cells?
■ How do target cells regulate their responsiveness to endocrine hormones?
■ How do feedback mechanisms control the secretion of hormones?

■ What are the anterior and posterior pituitary hormones, their target tissues, and their negative-feedback mechanisms?
■ How are thyroid and steroid hormones synthesized?
■ What are the normal actions on target cells of antidiuretic hormone, growth hormone, thyroid hormone, and steroid hormones?

CHAPTER OUTLINE

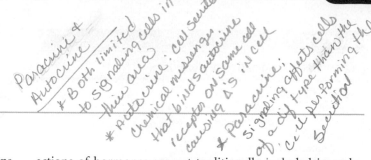

The endocrine system is composed of cells and organs that are specialized to synthesize and secrete hormones into the bloodstream to act at distant target cells. The nervous and endocrine systems are closely integrated, and many of their actions are coordinated at the level of the hypothalamus. Endocrine systems are particularly suited for regulating complex functions that involve numerous tissues and organs such as growth, metabolism, fluid balance, responses to stress, and reproduction.[1] It is now appreciated that all cells in an organism are involved in cell-to-cell communication, not just the specialized endocrine cells, therefore the term *classical* endocrine systems is sometimes used to designate specialized endocrine glands. This chapter describes general principles of endocrine communication systems and explores the details of hypothalamic-pituitary regulation of antidiuretic hormone, oxytocin, growth hormone, prolactin, gonadotropins, thyroid hormone, and corticosteroid hormones. Disorders of these systems are discussed in Chapters 40 and 41. Reproductive function and disorders can be found in Unit IX.

HORMONE STRUCTURE AND ACTION

A **hormone** may be defined as a blood-borne chemical messenger (ligand) that has an effect on target cells anatomically distant from the secreting cell (Figure 39-1). Chemical messengers may also act in a **paracrine** or **autocrine** fashion; the hormone molecule is secreted by one cell and affects adjacent cells, or the original secreting cell. Paracrine and autocrine

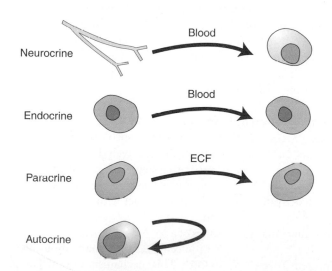

FIGURE 39-1 Terminology and comparison of cell-to-cell signaling pathways. *ECF,* Extracellular fluid.

actions of hormones are not traditionally included in endocrine system physiology; however, the same signaling molecules can have autocrine, paracrine, and hormonal actions.[2] As an example, estrogen acts locally within the ovary potentiating maturation of ova but is required systemically for outward female sexual differentiation. Secretion of hormones into the bloodstream by neurons may be termed **neurocrine** signaling.

Chemical Structure of Hormone Classes

Hormones may be classified according to chemical structure as peptides, tyrosine-derived catecholamines and thyroid hormones, and steroids. (Box 39-1). The great majority of endocrine hormones are peptides (small proteins) and are water soluble and easily transported through the circulation to target cells.[2] The catecholamines (dopamine, epinephrine, and norepinephrine) are also water soluble. Water-soluble hormones usually travel free in solution in the plasma, although some are partially protein-bound. Water-soluble hormones are unable to cross the plasma membrane to enter cells and therefore must exert their actions by binding to receptors located on the surface of target cell membranes.[1]

Thyroid and steroid hormones are lipid-soluble molecules and dissolve poorly in blood. Thyroid hormones (T_3 and T_4) are derived from tyrosine amino acids to which iodine has been attached. The steroid hormones are derived from cholesterol. Thyroid and steroid hormones require transport proteins (globulin) to convey them through the circulation. In some cases these transport proteins are specialized to carry a certain hormone (thyroxine-binding globulin, cortisol-binding globulin), but hormones can also be carried by "nonspecific proteins," such as albumin.[1] The transport proteins are manufactured by the liver. At the target cell, the hormone detaches from the transport protein and diffuses through the lipid-containing cell membrane to activate intracellular receptors in the cytoplasm or nucleus.[1]

Mechanisms of Hormone Action

Hormones with Cell Membrane Receptors

Hormones exert their actions by binding to target cell receptor proteins. The target cell receptors for water-soluble hormones have a hormone-binding site located on the external portion of a specific cell-surface receptor. Once hormone-receptor binding takes place, a change in the conformation of the receptor protein conveys a signal to the interior of the cell. Some receptors generate second messengers, such as cyclic adenosine monophosphate (cAMP) within the cell, while others become activated enzymes. The intracellular activities occurring after hormone-receptor binding may include changes

BOX 39-1

Chemical Classification of Hormones

Water-Soluble
Peptides
Adrenocorticotropic hormone
Angiotensin II
Atrial natriuretic hormone
Antidiuretic hormone (vasopressin)
Calcitonin
Cholecystokinin
Follicle-stimulating hormone
Growth hormone
Glucagon
Hypothalamic-releasing hormones
Insulin
Insulin-like growth factor-1
Luteinizing hormone
Oxytocin
Parathyroid hormone
Prolactin
Secretin
Thyroid-stimulating hormone
Tyrosine-Derived Amines
Dopamine
Epinephrine
Norepinephrine

Lipid-Soluble
Tyrosine-Derived Thyroid Hormones
Triiodothyronine
Thyroxine
Steroids
Aldosterone
Cortisol
Corticosterone
Estrogen
Progesterone
Testosterone
Vitamin D

[handwritten: Phosphorlation means: Attaching phosphates to target proteins to ∆ their activity.]

in cell membrane permeability; activation or inactivation of enzymes; cellular maintenance, growth, and differentiation; protein synthesis; and genetic expression via RNA and DNA synthesis in the cell nucleus.[2] A more detailed explanation of receptor mechanisms can be found in Chapter 3.

G-Protein-Linked Receptors. Hormones can be described as "first messengers"; the hormone carries a message from the secreting cell to the target cell. A **second messenger** is generated within the cell in response to the first message. The term *second messenger* is usually applied to the products generated by a class of receptors called G-protein linked. These receptors undergo a conformational change upon binding to a hormone that allows them to interact with a class of proteins, called G-proteins, located on the inner side of the cell membrane (Figure 39-2). G-proteins have three subunits and when activated by the receptor, one of these subunits (alpha) binds to a GTP molecule and then dissociates from the other subunits (beta-gamma).[3] The activated alpha subunit is able to move along the inner membrane and interact with target enzymes,

inducing them to produce the second messenger. There are several different forms of G-proteins that have different target enzymes and produce different sets of second messengers (see Chapter 3). The most important of these for endocrine systems are the G_s and the G_q subtypes. Hormones that bind to receptors that are linked to G_s increase the production of cAMP within the cell. The usual downstream target of cAMP is an enzyme called Protein kinase A. Kinases are enzymes that attach phosphates (phosphorylation) to target proteins to change their activity. Enzymes within the cell called phosphorylases work to remove the attached phosphates. Phosphorylation-dephosphorylation is a common strategy for controlling enzyme activity in cells. Activation of Protein kinase A causes varied cellular effects depending on the cell type. Important examples of hormones that are linked to increased cAMP production through activation of the G_s pathway include adrenocorticotropic hormone (ACTH), thyroid-stimulating hormone (TSH), follicle-stimulating hormone (FSH), luteinizing hormone (LH), epinephrine (beta receptors), parathyroid hormone, antidiuretic hormone (ADH), and glucagon.[1]

The G_q pathway is linked to production of two second messengers, diacylglycerol (DAG) and inositol trisphosphate (IP_3). Norepinephrine and epinephrine can activate the G_q pathway by binding to alpha-1 receptors on target cells. The DAG and IP_3 work together to increase the activity of protein kinase C, which then phosphorylates downstream target proteins to change cell behavior.

Protein Kinase Receptors. A second class of surface receptors important in endocrine signaling is the protein kinase receptor family. These receptors either become activated kinases themselves or are associated with cytoplasmic kinases on their inner domain (Figure 39-3). Both types of receptors phosphorylate their target proteins upon binding of the hormone to an external binding site. An important example of a receptor kinase is the insulin receptor that phosphorylates tyrosine amino acids in its targets and activates several different intracellular signaling cascades (Chapter 41). Growth hormone and prolactin receptors are associated with Janus kinase (JAK) on the cytoplasmic side and become activated when the hormone binds to the outside of the receptor causing a conformational change that pulls two JAK enzymes closer together.[1] The JAK enzymes become activated and phosphorylate their target proteins initiating a signaling cascade.

Amplification of Hormone Activity

The process of intracellular activation by secondary signals occurs via a cascade effect. Progressively larger numbers of chemical reactions occur at each step, so that activation of one receptor at the cell surface can activate numerous G-proteins.[3] Each activated G-protein may interact with 100 or more targets enzymes, such as adenylate cyclase. Each activated enzyme produces many molecules of a second messenger (cAMP), and each second messenger molecule activates many molecules of protein kinase, and so forth. This mechanism of signal *amplification* explains why minute amounts of circulating hormone cause significant and rapid cellular and systemic effects.

[handwritten: Amplification means it the effects keep building so small amt Hormone can have big effect.]

[handwritten notes: intrinsic = structure belonging solely to a part; Extrinsic = coming from outside]

FIGURE 39-2 Mechanism of G-protein–linked receptor signaling in endocrine cells. Activation of the receptor by a hormone on the outside of the cell changes the conformation of the receptor and activates its target G-proteins. Common G-proteins in endocrine systems are Gs (which activates adenylyl cyclase to produce cAMP) and G_q (which activates phospholipase C to produce DAG and IP_3).

FIGURE 39-3 Some endocrine receptors have intrinsic kinase activity, while others have kinases associated with their inner domain. In either case, hormone binding to the outer part of the hormone triggers a conformational change in the receptor that initiates kinase activities. Kinases phosphorylate target proteins and alter their activity.

[handwritten note: Thyroid + steroid diffuse easily because they are lipid soluble]

Hormones with Intracellular Receptors

Thyroid and steroid hormones diffuse easily through the lipid bilayer of cell membranes. Receptors for these hormones are located in the cytoplasm or, more frequently, the nucleus of the target cell (Figure 39-4). Binding of the hormone causes a change in affinity of the receptor for binding sites on DNA in the cell nucleus.[4] Gene expression is changed by binding of the hormone-receptor complex to specific DNA binding sites. The events that result from the interaction between nuclear

DNA and the receptor include messenger RNA transcription, processing, and translation into specific proteins (see Chapter 5 for a review of protein synthesis). In general, the onset of action of lipid-soluble hormones is slow compared with that of the water-soluble hormones described above and there is no amplification cascade. Changes in DNA transcription and protein synthesis occur over hours to days.

FIGURE 39-4 Lipid-soluble hormones diffuse through the plasma membrane and bind to intracellular receptors. The hormone-receptor complexes are DNA-regulatory proteins that regulate messenger RNA transcription, processing, and translation into proteins.

phosphorylation of target proteins, which changes their activity and initiates intracellular signaling cascades.

■ Steroid and thyroid hormones are lipid-soluble and carried in the circulation by transport proteins. They can diffuse through lipid bilayers, and their receptors are in the cytoplasm or nucleus. Intracellular hormone-receptor complexes bind to specific targets on nuclear DNA and alter gene expression.

HORMONE REGULATION

Hormone Synthesis, Secretion, and Metabolism

Hormone synthesis and secretion may take place in several different cell types, but one site is generally considered to be the primary endocrine tissue and is responsive to feedback about the need for the hormone or its effects. For example, endothelial cells throughout the vascular system produce small amounts of angiotensin II (AII); however, the primary endocrine control is through the renin-angiotensin-aldosterone cascade in which specialized cells in the kidney trigger AII production in response to changes in extracellular volume and pressure.

Most endocrine hormones are polypeptides manufactured on the rough endoplasmic reticulum and stored in vesicles within the cells. A review of protein synthesis can be found in Chapter 5. The initial forms of the polypeptide hormones are usually larger molecules called *prohormones* or *pre-prohormones*. These must be cleaved by specific enzymes to release the active form of the hormone.[1,2] Sometimes this cleavage occurs after the hormone is packaged into vesicles and the fragments are released into the bloodstream along with the hormone. In some cases, such as with insulin secretion, this is clinically useful as a marker of hormone synthesis.

Insulin and its C-peptide fragment are produced in a 1:1 ratio and the concentration of C-peptide, which is more stable in the circulation, can be used as a measure of insulin production.

Because they are water-soluble, peptide hormones can be contained within the lipid bilayer of the vesicles and stored until a trigger results in exocytosis of the hormone into the extracellular space. Catecholamines are also water-soluble and stored in vesicles until they are released by exocytosis. However, they are formed by enzymes within the cytoplasm that begin with tyrosine and through a series of steps convert it first to dopamine; depending on the cell type, dopamine may be the final hormone or it can be converted to norepinephrine and then to epinephrine.

Steroid and thyroid hormones cannot be stored within vesicles because they are lipid-soluble and would simply diffuse out of the cell. The strategy for synthesis and storage is much different for each of these hormones. When a steroid hormone is needed, increased production of the hormone closely precedes hormone release into the circulation.[2,5] Steroid hormones are formed on demand from cholesterol that is either stored in the cell or retrieved from the circulating lipoproteins. The stimuli that trigger steroid secretion induce the enzymes in the pathway to synthesize the necessary hormones from cholesterol. Once formed, steroid hormones can simply diffuse through the plasma membrane and into the circulation. The strategy for trapping thyroid hormones within the thyroid gland until they are needed is quite different. Hormone synthesis precedes secretion by weeks or months. Triiodothyronine (T_3) and thyroxine (T_4) are synthesized in the thyroid follicle, bound to a protein called *thyroglobulin*.[6] Thyroglobulin is a large water-soluble protein that is trapped within the thyroid follicle. Secretion occurs via cleavage of the thyroid hormone from thyroglobulin in response to systemic needs determined by the hypothalamus and the pituitary gland. Free T_3 and T_4 are lipid-soluble and diffuse from the thyroid cells. Thyroid and steroid synthesis and release are detailed later in this chapter.

Factors Affecting Hormone Secretion

Secretion of endocrine hormones is dependent on the interplay of many factors. Most of the hormones controlled by the anterior pituitary gland are secreted in cyclic patterns. These cycles are regulated by the hypothalamus and may occur in response to feeding-fasting cycles, light-dark cycles, sleep-wake cycles, or in a 24-hour (circadian) period. Cycles also occur over longer periods (e.g., the 28-day menstrual cycle) or over years (e.g., the hormones that control reproductive differentiation and maturity).[1] Acute systemic needs or stressors can partially override cyclic patterns and modify hormone secretion. An example of this is activation of the stress response that alters the normal circadian pattern of cortisol secretion. Knowledge of the cyclical nature of hormone release is important when comparing measured serum concentrations to normal ranges and when attempting to provide hormone replacement therapy that mimics the normal physiologic pattern.

Feedback Control of Secretion

The most common mechanism regulating hormone production and secretion is *negative feedback* control in which some aspect of the secreted hormone is sensed and regulates further secretion.[4] An example of negative feedback is the interaction between the hypothalamic-pituitary system and the respective hormone-releasing glands controlled by this system. For example, thyrotropin-releasing hormone (TRH) is secreted by the hypothalamus when the central nervous system senses an inadequate supply of thyroid hormones in the circulation. TRH stimulates the synthesis and release of thyroid-stimulating hormone (TSH) from specific cells in the anterior pituitary gland; TSH then stimulates the synthesis and release of the thyroid hormones T_3 and T_4 from the thyroid follicle. The resulting increase in plasma thyroid hormone concentration exerts an inhibitory effect, or negative feedback, on the release of TSH by the anterior pituitary gland and TRH from the hypothalamus.[7,8] The negative feedback loop is a mechanism for maintaining hormone activity within a normal range or *set point* of normal activity. The set point is genetically determined and influenced by age, gender, circadian cycles, and current internal and environmental conditions. The regulatory influences are multiple and complex, but often there is a particular variable that is influenced by the hormone's activity and provides most of the feedback regulation. These feedback systems are detailed for the hormones of the pituitary system in later sections of this chapter. Knowledge of feedback controls is helpful when evaluating patients for endocrine diseases (see Chapter 40).

Hormone Metabolism and Excretion

The plasma concentration of a hormone depends not only on the rate of synthesis and release of the hormone but also on how rapidly the hormone is metabolized and excreted. Like other compounds, hormones are frequently degraded and excreted by the liver and kidneys. Water-soluble hormones may be excreted in the urinary filtrate. Lipid-soluble hormones, which are bound to plasma proteins and stored in adipose tissue, are less readily metabolized and remain in the circulation for a more prolonged period.[2] In addition to metabolism by the kidneys and liver, hormones are often degraded by the target cell after binding to receptors. *Half-life* is a term used to describe the duration of hormone activity in the circulation and may be expressed in minutes, hours, or days.[9] The half-life is the time for a hormone to reach one-half of its original concentration in the blood and is influenced by the rate of uptake by cells, degradation, and excretion.

Pharmacologic Hormone Concentrations

It is important to differentiate between physiologic and pharmacologic hormone activity. Physiologic hormone concentrations are extremely low in most cases, and pharmacologic levels of hormones are usually several-fold greater than would normally be secreted by endocrine tissues. Pharmacologic levels occur as a consequence of either pathologic processes or the administration of large doses of hormones. The tissue response to pharmacologic hormone concentrations may be significantly different from those caused by physiologic levels of hormones.[2]

Regulation of Receptor Responses

Tissue response to circulating hormone is only partially determined by the amount of hormone present in the circulation. Although virtually all body tissues are exposed to circulating hormones, specific hormones elicit a response only from certain cells and tissues. The ability of a cell to respond to a particular hormone depends on the presence of specific receptors for that hormone on or in the cell. Target cells are able to regulate their responsiveness to hormones by altering the receptor number, affinity, and efficiency of coupling to intracellular responses.[3]

Receptor Specificity and Affinity

The concept of *receptor specificity* is important for understanding the targeted responses of the endocrine system. Specificity refers to the molecular "fit" of a hormone within a receptor binding pocket. Specificity cannot easily be separated from the concept of *affinity*. Affinity describes the degree of "tightness" of the hormone-receptor bond, or the inclination of the hormone to remain bound to the receptor. Specificity and affinity determine whether a cell with a receptor will respond to a hormonal stimulus and the hormone concentration at which the receptor effectively can bind the hormone. The potency of the hormone, or the amount of hormone required to elicit a cellular response, is dependent in part on the affinity of the receptor for a particular hormone. The higher the affinity of the receptor for a hormone, the lesser the amount of hormone needed to produce a response.[3,9] Therefore, hormones that circulate in very minute amounts may have a large effect on cellular activity because of the tightness of the hormone-receptor bond.

"Cross-specificity" between hormones of similar structure may occur. For example, prolactin and growth hormone both can bind to the prolactin receptor, but with differing affinities. Under normal circumstances, the plasma concentration of growth hormone is not adequate to bind a significant number of prolactin receptors. However, in the condition called *acromegaly*, in which excessive concentrations of growth hormone lead to massive bone and tissue overgrowth, milk may be secreted from the mammary glands secondary to growth hormone stimulation of prolactin receptors.[10]

Receptor Down-Regulation and Up-Regulation

A factor determining the degree of response to a circulating hormone is the number of cell receptors available for hormone binding. When cells are exposed to high concentrations of hormone for a prolonged period, a common result is that the cell decreases the number of receptors. This phenomenon is known as *down-regulation*. An example of down-regulation occurs with insulin receptors in obese individuals. An increase in the plasma insulin level commonly occurs in obese individuals. This increased concentration of insulin does not result in an increase in cellular activities in most cells because the number of insulin receptors is down-regulated in response to the high plasma insulin concentration.[3] Down-regulation probably serves a protective function: the cells are protected against excessive activity despite pathologic processes that cause excessive hormone levels. *Up-regulation*, or an increase in the number of receptors in response to chronically low hormone concentrations, may also occur. Up-regulation would make the cell more sensitive to the hormone, and hormone-dependent cellular activity could occur at normal or nearly normal levels despite a lower than normal hormone concentration.[3]

Another mechanism for altering hormone responsiveness is through regulation of the coupling mechanism between receptor activation and its intracellular responses.[3] For example, the cytoplasmic domain of a receptor can be phosphorylated or otherwise altered so that it cannot effectively interact with its target G-protein. Additionally, the enzymes such as phosphorylases that remove phosphates from proteins, and phosphodiesterases that degrade cyclic nucleotides can be up-regulated or downregulated to turn off the cellular responses more or less quickly. Many of these regulatory mechanisms are not fully understood.

Permissiveness

One effect that hormones may have on target cells is to increase the number of receptors for other hormones, thus enhancing the effect of the second hormone. This phenomenon is known as *permissiveness*. For example, one effect of thyroid hormone on adipose cells is to increase the number of receptors for epinephrine. When the adipose tissue is subsequently exposed to epinephrine, a greater release of fatty acids (used in providing energy for cellular processes) takes place than would occur in the absence of thyroid hormone.[2] Permissiveness also allows cellular events to occur in sequence. One effect of estrogen, secreted early in the menstrual cycle, is to increase the number of uterine receptors for progesterone. The uterus is therefore sensitive to progesterone when it is present during the last part of the menstrual cycle, and normal proliferative changes take place.[11]

Hormone Agonists and Antagonists

To produce a cellular effect, a hormone must bind to the receptor and initiate a series of events that lead to a change in cellular activity. A chemical may bind to a receptor without initiating the typical intracellular changes; this chemical is described as a hormone **antagonist** or **blocking agent**.[9] **Agonists,** on the other hand, bind hormone receptors and cause the same intracellular events that would occur with hormone-receptor binding. A large number of pharmacologic agents have agonist or antagonist effects on receptors for hormones. For example, hormone antagonists that compete with epinephrine and norepinephrine for receptor sites are frequently used to block the cardiac stimulatory properties of these hormones and thus decrease cardiac workload. Conversely, agonist medications that mimic hormone activity are frequently given as hormone replacement therapy in deficiency syndromes.

KEY POINTS

- Hormone concentration in the bloodstream depends on the rate of secretion and degradation by the liver, kidneys, and target tissues. Lipid-soluble hormones are less readily metabolized than peptides and usually have a longer half-life.
- The secretion of most hormones is regulated by negative-feedback mechanisms. Target gland hormones feed back to inhibit secretion of the initial hormone and keep the response within a normal range or set point.
- Only target cells producing the specific receptor for a hormone will respond to a particular hormone. High-affinity receptors enable hormone-binding at very low physiologic concentrations of hormone.
- The number of hormone receptors on a cell's surface may adapt to changes in cell environment. Down-regulation refers to a decrease in the number of receptors in response to excessive hormone. Up-regulation refers to an increase in receptor number in response to low hormone concentration. Receptors may also be uncoupled from their intracellular signaling cascades.
- Permissiveness: Receptor number and responsiveness may be enhanced by the presence of other hormones.
- Chemicals other than the usual hormone may be able to bind to the hormone's receptors. Chemicals that bind receptors and block activity are antagonists; those that bind receptors and activate them are agonists.

HYPOTHALAMIC-PITUITARY ENDOCRINE SYSTEM

The pituitary gland is located beneath the hypothalamus in the sella turcica, a pocket of bone at the base of the skull (Figure 39-5).[12] In adults, the pituitary gland is composed of distinct anterior and posterior lobes. The pituitary gland is connected to the hypothalamus by the pituitary stalk, which contains a portal system that transports capillary blood from the hypothalamus to the capillaries of the anterior pituitary gland. Neurons whose cell bodies lie within the hypothalamus send their axons down the pituitary stalk and terminate in the posterior pituitary gland. Synthesis and secretion of the various pituitary hormones are controlled, directly or indirectly, by the hypothalamus. Release of posterior pituitary hormones occurs when action potentials generated in the hypothalamic neurons travel down the axons of the pituitary stalk and trigger exocytosis of hormone from the nerve terminals in the posterior pituitary gland. The hypothalamus regulates endocrine function of the anterior pituitary gland by secreting releasing hormones and inhibiting hormones that are carried to anterior pituitary endocrine cells by the pituitary portal system.

The pituitary gland is also called the *hypophysis,* and the anterior and posterior lobes are sometimes referred to as the *adenohypophysis* and the *neurohypophysis,* respectively. The posterior pituitary gland secretes two important peptide

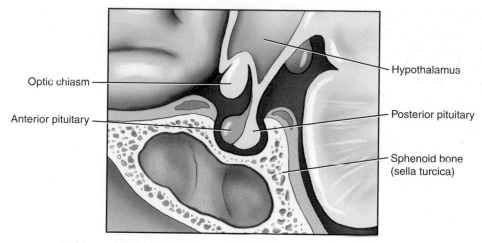

FIGURE 39-5 Anatomic relationship of the hypothalamus and pituitary gland.

TABLE 39-1

Endocrine Cell Types of Adenohypophysis

Cell Type	Corticotrope	Thyrotrope	Gonadotrope	Somatotrope	Lactotrope
Primary hypothalamic regulation	Corticotropin-releasing hormone (CRH) (41-aa peptide) (stimulatory)	Thyrotropin-releasing hormone (TRH) (tripeptide) (stimulatory)	Gonadotropin-releasing hormone (GnRH) (decapeptide) (stimulatory)	Growth hormone–releasing hormone (GHRH) (44-aa peptide) (stimulatory) and somatostatin (tetradecapeptide) inhibitory	Dopamine (catecholamine) inhibitory and prolactin-releasing factor (stimulatory)
Tropic hormone secreted	Adrenocorticotropic hormone (ACTH) (39-aa peptide)	Thyroid-stimulating hormone (TSH) (glycoprotein hormone)	Follicle-stimulating hormone and luteinizing hormone (FSH and LH) (glycoprotein hormone)	Growth hormone (GH) (ca. 22-kDa protein)	Prolactin (ca. 23-kDa protein)
Receptor	MC2R (G_s-linked GPCR)	TSH receptor (G_s-linked GPCR)	FSH and LH receptors (G_s-linked GPCRs)	GH receptor (JAK/STAT-linked cytokine receptor)	PRL receptor (JAK/STAT- linked cytokine receptor)
Target endocrine gland	Zona fasciculata and zona reticularis of the adrenal cortex	Thyroid epithelium	Ovary (theca and granulosa*) and testis (Leydig, Sertoli)	Liver (but also direct actions, especially in terms of metabolic effects)	No endocrine target organ; not part of an endocrine axis
Peripheral hormone involved in negative feedback	Cortisol	Triiodothyronine (T_3)	Estrogen†, progesterone, testosterone, inhibin‡	IGF-I	None

*Both follicular and luteinized thecal and granulose cells.
†Estrogen can also have a postive feedback in women.
‡Inhibin selectivity inhibits FSH release from the gonadotrope.
IGF-I, Insulin-like growth factor -1.
From Porterfield SP, White BA: *Endocrine physiology,* ed 3, Philadelphia, 2007, Mosby, p 118.

hormones: antidiuretic hormone (vasopressin) and oxytocin. The anterior lobe of the pituitary gland has five endocrine cell types that secrete 6 different peptide hormones: (1) somatotropes, which secrete growth hormone (GH); (2) gonadotropes, which secrete gonadotropins (luteinizing hormone [LH], follicle-stimulating hormone [FSH]); (3) thyrotropes, which secrete thyroid-stimulating hormone (TSH, thyrotropin); (4) corticotropes, which secrete adrenocorticotropic hormone (ACTH); and finally (5) lactotropes, which secrete prolactin (PRL).[10] The hormones produced by the anterior pituitary gland have direct actions on other endocrine tissues and the liver (Table 39-1).

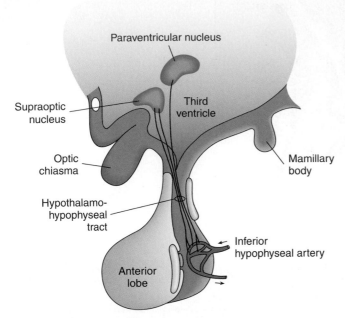

FIGURE 39-6 Axons from the paraventricular and supraoptic nuclei in the hypothalamus project down the pituitary stalk, and the axon terminals lie within the posterior pituitary gland. Oxytocin and antidiuretic hormone are produced in the hypothalamic neuron cell bodies and then transported to the axon terminals, where they are released into the bloodstream in response to action potentials. (From Porterfield SP, White BA: *Endocrine physiology,* ed 3, Philadelphia, 2007, Mosby, p 110).

FIGURE 39-7 Antidiuretic hormone (ADH) acts on renal tubule Gs-protein–linked receptors to trigger movement of water channels (aquaporins) to the apical cell membrane. The aquaporins increase membrane permeability to water, allowing it to be absorbed through the process of osmosis. ADH thus decreases the osmolality of the extracellular fluids and creates a more concentrated urine. *ATP,* Adenosine triphosphate; *cAMP,* cyclic adenosine monophosphate.

Hormones of the Posterior Pituitary Gland

The posterior pituitary gland consists of nerve axons whose neuronal cell bodies originate in the supraoptic and paraventricular nuclei of the hypothalamus (Figure 39-6). Posterior pituitary hormones, oxytocin and antidiuretic hormone, are produced in the neurons of the hypothalamus and, packaged in vesicles, travel along the length of the nerve axons to the posterior pituitary gland. Release of antidiuretic hormone or oxytocin occurs as a result of depolarization of the appropriate hypothalamic neurons and conduction of action potentials to the nerve terminals in the posterior pituitary gland.[10] Antidiuretic hormone is released in response to altered serum osmolality and hypotension and causes water retention by increasing water reabsorption by the renal collecting duct.[10] Oxytocin is released during sexual activity, childbirth, and breast-feeding and causes uterine and milk duct contractions.[10]

Antidiuretic Hormone

Antidiuretic hormone is a 9–amino acid peptide that differs by two amino acids from oxytocin, another 9–amino acid peptide. The circulating half-life of ADH is about 15 to 20 minutes, and it is destroyed by proteolysis in the kidney and liver.[10] The most important regulator of ADH release is the osmolality of plasma, which is detected by specialized neurons called *osmoreceptors* that are found in the hypothalamus. The osmoreceptors have a set point that influences the stimulation and suppression of ADH. When body fluids become too concentrated, ADH is released, leading to increased reabsorption of water in the kidneys. ADH secretion is also stimulated by the baroreceptors in response to hypovolemia and low arterial blood pressure.

The primary targets for ADH are vasopressin 2 (V2) receptors on the basolateral membrane of distal renal tubule cells. ADH causes pores, called *aquaporins,* to move from the cytoplasm to the cell membranes of apical tubular epithelial cells (Figure 39-7). These pores allow free diffusion of water from the tubular fluid into the cell. Water then flows out the basolateral membrane and into the interstitium. The enhanced reabsorption conserves water in the body, creates a concentrated urine, and reduces serum osmolality (see Chapter 26).

Oxytocin

Oxytocin is structurally similar to ADH, and there is some overlap in biologic activity. Oxytocin can inhibit diuresis. Oxytocin has a half-life of 3 to 5 minutes. Oxytocin is known for its actions on breast and uterus, but other actions are likely because it is produced in males as well as females. Sexual intercourse can stimulate oxytocin release in men and women. Its role in men is not understood, but in women it is proposed to affect sperm motility through uterine contractions. Oxytocin also stimulates uterine contractions during labor. It is not

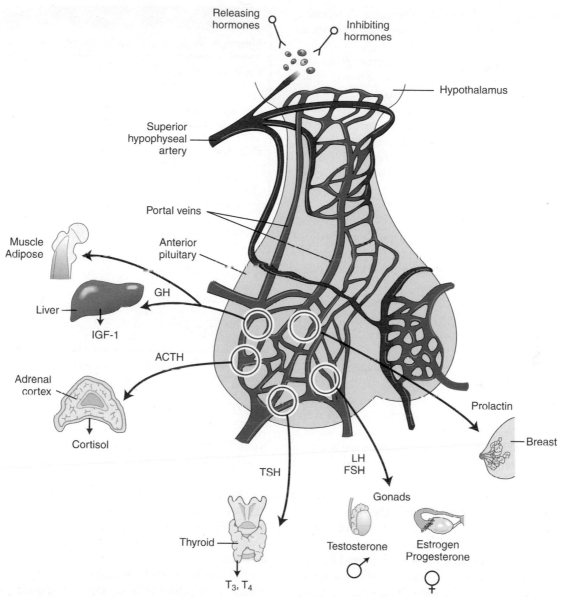

FIGURE 39-8 Relationship of the hypothalamic releasing and inhibiting hormones, anterior pituitary hormones, and target gland hormones. *GH*, growth hormone; *FSH*, follicle-stimulating hormone; *LH*, luteinizing hormone; *TSH*, thyroid-stimulating hormone; *ACTH*, adrenocorticotropic hormone; IGF-1, insulin-like growth factor-1.

thought to initiate labor, but once labor has begun, stretching of the cervix increases oxytocin release, which increases the intensity of uterine contractions.[10] This is an example of a positive feedback loop in which stretching of the cervix induces oxytocin release, resulting in more forceful uterine contraction and further stretching of the cervix.

Oxytocin release is triggered by stimulation of the nipple and areola which have sensory receptors that send neuronal signals to the hypothalamic nuclei. Oxytocin then binds to myoepithelial cells surrounding the milk ducts causing them to contract and eject milk during breast feeding. This reflex can be triggered centrally without breast stimulation as a conditioned response to the sight or sound of an infant.

Hormones of the Hypothalamus and Anterior Pituitary Gland

The hypothalamic-pituitary endocrine system is a three-tiered axis that includes hypothalamic releasing and inhibiting hormones, anterior pituitary hormones, and target organ hormones (Figure 39-8). Releasing and inhibiting factors are secreted into a capillary bed that is contained within the hypothalamus by hypothalamic neurons having short axons. Hypothalamic hormones diffuse into the capillary network, travel down the portal vein, and then diffuse from the anterior pituitary capillary network into the tissue where they bind receptors on pituitary cells.[12] All of the hypothalamic releasing and inhibiting factors are peptides, with the exception of dopamine, and all are water-soluble. Therefore all releasing and inhibiting factors interact with cell surface receptors on the target pituitary cells.

The three-tiered hypothalamic-pituitary-target system provides an opportunity for fine modulation of hormone action on target tissues. The hypothalamic and pituitary hormones exemplify the complexity of endocrine interactions. In addition to feedback from target organ hormones, the hypothalamus processes numerous neuronal signals into an integrated response by the anterior pituitary gland. Each of the major anterior pituitary hormones is briefly described below.

Growth Hormone

Pituitary GH secretion is controlled by hypothalamic release of growth hormone–releasing hormone (GHRH) and growth hormone–inhibiting hormone (somatostatin). GHRH binds to receptors on pituitary somatotropes and stimulates release of GH, whereas somatostatin inhibits GH release. Under normal physiologic conditions, the anterior pituitary gland secretes small pulsatile amounts of GH each day. Sleep studies indicate a circadian pattern to GH secretion, with secretion being greatest during deep, slow-wave sleep (stage 3 or 4). GH secretion is greatest during adolescence and decreases in the elderly.[10]

GH is a 191–amino acid protein that is similar in structure to prolactin. A major target for GH is the liver, where it affects liver metabolism and also induces the production of another endocrine hormone called *insulin-like growth factor-1* (IGF-1). Previously, IGF-1 was called *somatomedin*. IGF-1 is an anabolic hormone that increases the growth of bone and cartilage tissues of the body. GH is not the only stimulus for the production of IGF-1, nor is the liver the only source. Insulin is an important co-stimulator of IGF-1 along with GH.[10] GH also has direct effects on some cells and binds to receptors on muscle and adipose tissue, increasing muscle mass and decreasing fat mass by inducing lipolysis. It affects metabolic processes by increasing the rate of protein synthesis, decreasing protein catabolism, slowing carbohydrate utilization, and increasing mobilization of fats and the use of fats for energy (Box 39-2).[4] Insufficient GH is exhibited as short stature in children, whereas excesses may lead to increased height in children and excessive growth of nonadipose tissues in adults (see Chapter 40).

Feedback regulation of GH release is complex and is affected by several hormones including estrogen, testosterone, and thyroid hormone, which stimulate GH release. Perhaps the most important negative feedback is through IGF-1. Hypoglycemia and a rise in amino acids in the blood stimulate the release of GH as does starvation and exercise.

Prolactin

The lactotropes that secrete prolactin are the second most numerous cell type in the anterior pituitary gland, after the somatotropes (which are the most numerous). Prolactin is a 199–amino acid protein that acts directly on numerous cell

---

BOX 39-2

Metabolic Actions of Growth Hormone

Carbohydrates
Increases blood glucose
Decreases peripheral insulin sensitivity
Increases hepatic output of glucose
Administration results in increased serum insulin levels

Proteins
Increases tissue amino acid uptake
Increases incorporation into proteins
Decreases urea production
Produces positive nitrogen balance

Lipids
Is lipolytic
Can be ketogenic after long-term administration, particularly if insulin is deficient

Insulin-Like Growth Factor
Stimulates IGF production
Stimulates growth
Is mitogenic

From Porterfield SP, White BA: *Endocrine physiology,* ed 3, Philadelphia, 2007, Mosby, p 117.

---

types.[10] Prolactin is best known for its trophic effects on breast tissue development and lactation and its ability to suppress reproductive function in both men and women. Prolactin exerts its inhibitory effects on fertility through suppression of hypothalamic gonadotropin-releasing hormone. Numerous other functions for prolactin have been proposed, and it has been noted that it increases during sexual orgasm, stress, and exercise.

Prolactin secretion is normally under tonic (constant) inhibition by prolactin-inhibiting factor. The prolactin-inhibiting factor is dopamine produced in the hypothalamus. Drugs that block dopamine receptors can release prolactin from its normal inhibition, resulting in abnormal breast development in males (gynecomastia) or inappropriate milk secretion in females (galactorrhea). During pregnancy, the number of pituitary lactotropes increases under the influence of placental estrogen. Estrogen and nipple stimulation increase prolactin synthesis and release from the anterior pituitary gland.

Gonadotropins

The gonadotropins, FSH and LH, are produced together within the gonadotropes in the anterior pituitary gland, however they are segregated into different packaging vesicles and are not necessarily released in equal amounts.[10] FSH and LH are proteins and bind to their specific respective receptors on target cells in the ovary or testes. In general, FSH and LH stimulate testosterone production in men (see Chapter 30) and estrogen and progesterone production in women.[11] These relationships are complex in women and change over the menstrual cycle (see Chapter 32). Release of FSH and LH is stimulated by hypothalamic gonadotropin-releasing hormone in a pulsatile fashion, and inhibited by negative feedback from sex steroids (except for the midcycle positive-feedback LH surge induced by estrogen at the time of ovulation in women).

Thyroid Stimulating Hormone

Thyrotropes release TSH in response to hypothalamic thyrotropin releasing hormone (TRH). TSH is a glycoprotein that binds to TSH receptors on follicle cells of the thyroid gland. TRH is released according to a diurnal (daily circadian) rhythm with its lowest period in the evening. Stress, starvation, and infection reduce the secretion of TRH. Negative feedback regulation of TRH and TSH is achieved primarily by the concentration of circulating T_3. TSH regulates all aspects of thyroid function, including growth of the gland, hormone synthesis, and hormone secretion.[8,10] The details of thyroid hormone synthesis and action on target tissues are described later in this chapter.

Adrenocorticotropic Hormone

ACTH is produced by corticotropes in the anterior pituitary gland in response to hypothalamic corticotropin-releasing hormone (CRH). ACTH is a 39–amino acid peptide that is derived from cleavage of a large preprohormone called pro-opiomelanocortin (POMC). Although POMC has the protein sequences for melanocyte-stimulating hormone and endorphin in its structure, human corticotropes express only the enzyme for cleaving ACTH as the sole hormone from this preprohormone.[5,10] ACTH circulates unbound in the circulation and has a half-life of about 10 minutes. It binds to Gs-coupled receptors on cells in the adrenal cortex and stimulates the production of cortisol and adrenal androgens. ACTH also has trophic effects on the adrenal cortex and supports the structure and synthetic enzymes of the gland. Withdrawal of ACTH results in adrenal cortical atrophy. ACTH in high concentration stimulates darkening of the skin by stimulating melanocyte receptors on skin cells. Normally keratinocytes in the skin produce melanocyte-stimulating hormone (MSH) in response to ultraviolet light, which can bind to MSH receptors on neighboring skin melanocytes in a paracrine fashion. ACTH can cross-react with melanocyte MSH receptors, and in high concentrations ACTH can produce abnormal skin pigmentation.

CRH and ACTH secretion demonstrate a significant diurnal pattern, with a peak upon wakening in the morning and a valley in the evening (Figure 39-9) Negative feedback regulation of ACTH is accomplished by the actions of cortisol, which suppress CRH and ACTH release. Regulation of the hypothalamic-pituitary-adrenal (HPA) axis is complex and is affected by acute and chronic stress (see Chapter 2). The adrenal cortex produces three types of steroid hormones: glucocorticoids, mineralocorticoids, and androgens. The details of adrenocortical steroid hormone synthesis and action on target tissues are described later in this chapter.

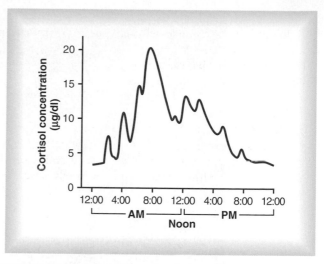

FIGURE 39-9 Typical pattern of cortisol secretion showing a diurnal (circadian) rhythm, with highest secretion occurring in the morning upon awakening and lowest levels in the late evening. (From Guyton AC, Hall JE: *Textbook of medical physiology*, ed 11, Philadelphia, 2006, Saunders, p 956.)

KEY POINTS

- Oxytocin and antidiuretic hormone (vasopressin) are synthesized in hypothalamic neurons that send axons to the posterior pituitary gland. Oxytocin is released during childbirth and suckling. Antidiuretic hormone is released in response to increased serum osmolality and decreased blood pressure.
- Major hormones of the anterior pituitary gland are GH, TSH, prolactin, ACTH, and gonadotropins (FSH, LH). The release of anterior pituitary hormones is regulated by releasing and inhibiting hormones secreted into pituitary portal blood by the hypothalamus. Many factors influence the secretion of releasing and inhibiting hormones, including circadian rhythms, hormone release from target cells, stress, and pain.

THYROID HORMONES

Thyroid Hormone Synthesis and Secretion

The thyroid gland, a two-lobed gland, lies in the neck region on either side of and anterior to the trachea. It secretes the thyroid hormones thyroxine (T_4) and triiodothyronine (T_3).[12] The thyroid gland is composed of microscopic follicles made up of a single layer of epithelial cells forming a ball, with their apical surface toward a pocket in the middle filled with colloid and their basal surfaces facing the interstitial fluid and capillary system (Figure 39-10). Follicular cells perform all the functions required to make and secrete thyroid hormones.[7,8] They trap dietary iodine and transport it into the colloid, synthesize thyroglobulin protein, and transport it into the colloid along with the enzyme thyroid peroxidase. Thyroid peroxidase acts on thyroglobulin to produce thyroid

FIGURE 39-10 Histology of thyroid follicle demonstrating single layer of epithelial follicular cells (FC) surrounding a core of colloid (C). The parafollicular cells (P) produce another hormone called *calcitonin,* which is involved in calcium regulation. (From Porterfield SP, White BA: *Endocrine physiology,* ed 3, Philadelphia, 2007, Mosby, p 142).

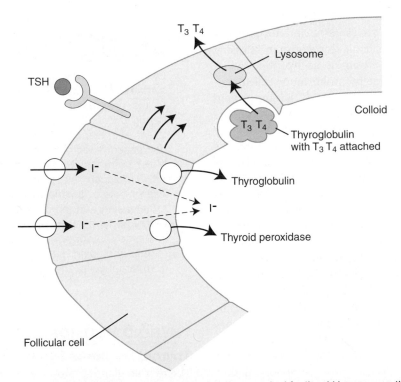

FIGURE 39-11 The follicular cells in the thyroid gland perform all of the functions required for thyroid hormone synthesis. Iodide is transported from the circulation into the inner core along with the protein thyroglobulin, which is synthesized within the cells. Follicles also produce a thyroid peroxidase enzyme and secrete it on the apical surface next to the colloid. Thyroid peroxidase activates and attaches iodides to tyrosine amino acids in the thyroglobulin. Two iodotyrosines are then coupled together, but remain attached to thyroglobulin. Simulation by TSH initiates a cascade that induces the follicle cell to endocytose some of the colloid, followed by combining it with a lysosome that cleaves the T_3 and T_4 from the thyroglobulin. T_3 and T_4 can then diffuse from the cell into the circulation.

hormones (Figure 39-11). First it oxidizes iodide and couples it to tyrosine amino acids in thyroglobulin. Some tyrosines receive two iodides (diiodotyrosine, DIT) and others have only one (monoiodotyrosine, MIT). Two iodotyrosines are then attached together by thyroid peroxidase to form T_4 (two DIT) or T_3 (one DIT and one MIT). Approximately 90% of the thyroid hormone is in the form of T_4, and 10% is in the form of T_3. The thyroid hormones remain attached to thyroglobulin, a storage protein, which accumulates in the thyroid follicles. By remaining attached to thyroglobulin, the lipid-soluble

Thyroxine (T_4)

Triiodothyronine (T_3)

FIGURE 39-12 The structure of thyroxin (T_4) and triiodothyronine (T_3).

T_3 and T_4 are trapped within the water-soluble colloid. When stimulated by TSH, the follicular cells endocytose a portion of the colloid containing thyroglobulin with its attached thyroid hormones. The endocytic vesicle combines with a lysosome, and the thyroid hormones are cleaved from thyroglobulin. Released T_4 and T_3 are lipid-soluble and diffuse from the follicle and into the circulation (Figure 39-12).

Thyroid Action on Target Cells

Thyroid hormones are carried in the circulation bound to thyroid-binding proteins. Ninety percent of the circulating thyroid hormone is T_4, and 10% is T_3. A small percentage of thyroid hormone (less than 1%) is dissolved in the plasma as free hormone and is able to cross directly into the target cell. Once in the cell, T_3 is able to bind to its receptor and exert its actions. T_4 is acted upon by cellular enzymes that cleave one of the iodine molecules to form either the active T_3 or a mirror image of T_3 called *reverse T_3*. This stereoisomer of T_3 has no known biologic activity. The ratio of production of T_3 and reverse T_3 is normally about 1:1, but is influenced by altered metabolic states such as starvation.[8] Most of the actions of thyroid hormone on target cells are mediated through alterations in gene transcription. The nuclear thyroid receptor has much higher affinity for T_3 than T_4 and primarily binds T_3 to form a complex that binds to specific DNA sequences and alters gene activity. Many of these genes influence the metabolic rate of the cell. The general physiologic effects of thyroid hormones are shown in Table 39-2. Excesses and deficits of thyroid hormone are exhibited by alterations in growth, development, and metabolic rate (see Chapter 40).

Inactive because it won't fit in the receptor (handwritten note in margin)

KEY POINTS

- Follicular cells in the thyroid gland perform all the functions required to make and secrete thyroid hormones. They trap dietary iodine and transport it into the colloid, synthesize thyroglobulin protein, and transport it into the colloid along with the enzyme thyroid peroxidase.
- Thyroid peroxidase oxidizes iodide and couples it to tyrosine amino acids in thyroglobulin. Two iodotyrosines are then attached together to form T_4 (two DIT) or T_3 (one DIT and one MIT). Approximately 90% of the thyroid hormone is in the form of T_4, and 10% is in the form of T_3.

- When stimulated by TSH, the follicular cells endocytose a portion of the colloid. The endocytic vesicle combines with a lysosome, and the lipid-soluble T_4 and T_3 are released and diffuse from the follicle and into the circulation.
- Actions of thyroid hormone on target cells are mediated through alterations in gene transcription. The nuclear thyroid receptor binds T_3 to form a complex that binds to specific DNA sequences and alters gene activity.
- Thyroid hormone increases metabolic rate and is essential for normal growth and development.

STEROID HORMONES

Steroid Hormone Synthesis and Secretion

The adrenal glands are located atop the kidneys and are composed of an inner medulla and an outer cortex. The adrenal medulla secretes epinephrine and norepinephrine in response to sympathetic nervous system stimulation and is discussed in Chapter 40. The hormones produced by the adrenal cortex are called **steroids** and include (1) glucocorticoids (cortisol), (2) mineralocorticoids (aldosterone), and (3) sex steroids (androgens).[11] The synthesis and secretion of these hormones, especially cortisol, are considered essential for life, regulating the body's response to normal and abnormal levels of physiologic and psychological stress. The activities of these three hormones can be remembered as regulating the "three S's": sugar, salt, and sex.

The adrenal cortex has distinct zones that differ in histologic appearance, regulation, and enzymes for steroid synthesis (Figure 39-13). The outer *zona glomerulosa* produces the mineralocorticoid, aldosterone, in response to stimulation by AII. The middle *zona fasciculata* produces the glucocorticoid, cortisol, in response to stimulation of ACTH from the pituitary gland.[5] The inner *zona reticularis* is adjacent to the adrenal medulla and produces the androgen, DHEA. All of these hormones are synthesized from cholesterol, and some of the cholesterol-derived precursors feed enzymatic pathways in all three zones (Figure 39-14) This is an important concept because it explains why an enzyme deficiency in one pathway (e.g., cortisol synthesis) may lead to an overproduction in another pathway (e.g. DHEA) as precursors are shunted. This is what happens in a disorder called *congenital adrenal hyperplasia* (see Chapter 40).

TABLE 39-2

Physiologic Actions of Thyroid Hormones

	HYPOTHYROID	EUTHYROID	HYPERTHYROID
Metabolic rate	Decreased BMR	—	Increased BMR
Proteins	↓ Synthesis, ↓ degradation, ↓ turnover (% BW as protein will ↓)	Protein anabolic	↑ Synthesis, ↑ degradation, ↑ turnover (catabolic if insufficient dietary protein)
Lipids	↓ Synthesis, ↓ degradation, ↓ turnover (% BW as lipid increases), ↓ serum cholesterol	↑ Beta oxidation, ↑ lipolysis, ↑ lipogenesis	↑ Synthesis, ↑ degradation, ↑ turnover (% of BW as lipid decreases), ↓ serum cholesterol
Glucose	Normal	Normal	Normal serum glucose; abnormal glucose tolerance test
Glycogen	↓ Synthesis, ↓ degradation, ↓ turnover, glycogen accumulates	—	↑ Synthesis, ↑ degradation, ↑ turnover; glycogen is depleted
Actions with SNS	—	—	Excess mimics effects of ↑ β-adrenergic stimulation; can ↑ number and affinity of β-receptors and ↑ adenylyl cyclase sensitivity
Direct cardiovascular actions	↓ Amplitude of ECG waves	↑ HR, ↑ CO, ↑ contractility, ↑ pulse pressure, ↑ actin, and myosin	↑ Amplitude of ECG waves

BMR, basal metabolic rate; *BW,* body weight; *CO,* cardiac output; *ECG,* electrocardiogram; *HR,* heart rate; *SNS,* sympathetic nervous system.
From Porterfield SP, White BA: *Endocrine physiology,* ed 3, Philadelphia, 2007, Mosby, p 155.

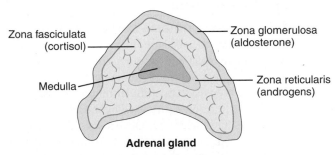

Adrenal gland

FIGURE 39-13 The adrenal gland is composed of the adrenal medulla at the innermost core, surrounded by the cortex. The adrenal cortex is composed of three anatomically and physiologically distinct layers, the zona glomerulosa, the zona fasciculata, and the zona reticularis. Each zone produces a different adrenocortical hormone.

As previously noted, steroid hormones are lipid-soluble and diffuse from the adrenocortical cells as they are synthesized, so they are made on demand and not stored in the cells. The stimulus for both cortisol and androgen synthesis and secretion is ACTH, whereas aldosterone synthesis and secretion is under control of AII (Figure 39-15). The activity of aldosterone synthase, the enzyme that performs the last 3 steps to produce aldosterone, is stimulated by AII binding to its Gq receptors on adrenocortical cells in the zona glomerulosa.[5]

Steroid Action on Target Cells

Steroid hormones travel in the circulation bound to proteins, including corticosteroid-binding globulin (transcortin) and albumin. Cortisol and androgens bind tightly with their binding proteins, but aldosterone does not and has a shorter half-life in the circulation. Steroids diffuse through their target cell membranes and bind with their respective cytoplasmic receptors. The hormone-receptor complex rapidly translocates into the nucleus where it binds to specific DNA sequences to alter responsive genes.

Glucocorticoids, principally cortisol, are named for their primary effect on glucose metabolism. Cortisol affects nearly every tissue in the body and exhibits a broad range of effects (Box 39-3). Glucocorticoids oppose the effects of insulin and raise blood sugar. This is accomplished by decreasing glucose uptake by many body cells (decreased glycogenesis), and increasing glucose synthesis in the liver from glycogen and amino acid and glycerol substrates in protein and fat stores (glycogenolysis, gluconeogenesis). Glucocorticoids also contribute to protein catabolism by releasing muscle stores of proteins, providing amino acids for glucose production in the liver. Glucocorticoids promote lipolysis and increased blood cholesterol. Glucocorticoids protect against the damaging physiologic effects of stress (see Chapter 2) and regulate the inflammatory and immune responses.[13]

Mineralocorticoids, principally aldosterone, function to maintain normal salt and water balance by promoting sodium retention and potassium excretion at the distal renal tubules. Aldosterone production is regulated primarily by the renin-angiotensin system associated with the juxtaglomerular cells of the kidney in response to a reduction in renal perfusion, and by a high serum potassium level (see Chapter 26).

[Handwritten annotations:]
Produced in Response to Renin-Angiotensin syst Kidney
Produced in response
* Cortisol is Produced in Response to Stimulation of ACTH in Ant Pit

FIGURE 39-14 Adrenal cortex steroid hormone synthesis. Steroid hormones are synthesized from cholesterol and have some common precursors. *DHEA*, dehydroepiandrosterone.

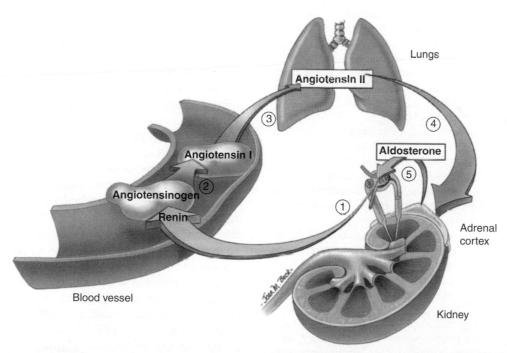

FIGURE 39-15 Renin-angiotensin mechanism for regulating aldosterone secretion. *(1)* When the incoming blood pressure in the kidneys drops below a certain level, the juxtaglomerular apparatus secretes **renin** into the blood. *(2)* Renin, an enzyme, causes angiotensinogen (a normal constituent of blood) to be converted to angiotensin I. *(3)* Angiotensin I circulates to the lungs, where converting enzymes in the capillaries split the molecule, forming angiotensin II. *(4)* Angiotensin II circulates to the adrenal cortex, where it stimulates the secretion of aldosterone. *(5)* Aldosterone causes increased reabsorption of sodium, which causes increased water retention. As water is retained, the volume of blood increases. The increased volume of blood creates higher blood pressure, which then causes the renin secretion to stop. (From Thibodeau GA, Patton K: *Anatomy and physiology,* ed 6, St Louis, 2007, Mosby, p 621.)

BOX 39-3

Biologic Actions of Cortisol

Metabolic
    Hyperglycemic
    Glycogenic
    Gluconeogenic
    Lipolytic
    Protein catabolic
Insulin antagonist in muscle and adipose tissue
Inhibits bone formation, stimulates bone resorption
Necessary for vascular response to catecholamines
Anti-inflammatory
Suppresses immune system
Inhibits antidiuretic hormone secretion and action
Stimulates gastric acid secretion
Necessary for integrity and function of gastrointestinal tract
Stimulates red blood cell production
Alters mood and behavior
Permissive for calorigenic, lipolytic effects of catecholamine

From Porterfield SP, White BA: *Endocrine physiology,* ed 3, Philadelphia, 2007, Mosby, p 175.

KEY POINTS

- The hormones produced by the adrenal cortex are called **steroids** and include (1) glucocorticoids (cortisol), (2) mineralocorticoids (aldosterone), and (3) sex steroids (androgens).
- The adrenal cortex has distinct zones. The outer *zona glomerulosa* produces aldosterone, in response to stimulation by AII. The middle *zona fasciculata* produces cortisol in response to stimulation of ACTH from the pituitary gland. The inner *zona reticularis* is adjacent to the adrenal medulla and produces androgens.
- Steroids diffuse through their target cell membranes and bind with their respective cytoplasmic receptors. The hormone-receptor complex rapidly translocates into the nucleus where it binds to specific DNA sequences to alter responsive genes.
- Cortisol affects nearly every tissue in the body and exhibits a broad range of effects on metabolism including increasing plasma glucose, regulating immune and inflammatory reactions, and inhibiting bone and collagen synthesis. Cortisol is a vital hormone in the response to acute stress.
- Aldosterone secretion increases in response to low blood pressure and reduced perfusion of the kidney, which stimulate the renin-angiotensin-aldosterone cascade. Aldosterone increases sodium and water reabsorption in the distal tubule of the kidney and promotes the excretion of potassium in the urine.

CATEGORIES OF ENDOCRINE DISEASE

Endocrine pathologic processes can be divided into three general categories: disorders of hyposecretion, hypersecretion, and target cell hyporesponsiveness. These are discussed in relation to specific endocrine diseases in Chapter 40.

Hyposecretion

Primary hyposecretion occurs when an endocrine gland, such as the thyroid or adrenal cortex, releases an inadequate amount of hormone to meet physiologic needs. Secondary hyposecretion occurs when secretion of a tropic hormone such as TSH or ACTH is inadequate to cause the target gland to secrete adequate amounts of hormone. The diagnosis of hormone deficiency is complex inasmuch as knowledge of tropic and releasing hormone levels, as well as the deficient hormone level, is necessary. For example, in a *primary* thyroid hormone deficiency, serum thyroid hormone would be low but TSH levels would be high because the anterior pituitary gland would not be receiving negative feedback from thyroid hormone. However, in *secondary* thyroid hormone deficiency, thyroid hormone and TSH concentrations both would be abnormally low.

Hypersecretion

Hypersecretion disorders can also be either primary or secondary.[14] When a diseased endocrine gland secretes an abnormally high amount of its hormone, the tropic pituitary hormone will be at an unusually low plasma level because of excessive negative feedback. Alternatively, if hypersecretion is secondary to elevated tropic hormone levels, the plasma concentration of both hormones will be elevated. For example, in Cushing disease, the pituitary gland becomes hyperactive and oversecretes ACTH, which induces the adrenal cortex to produce too much cortisol (causing symptoms of cortisol excess). Excessive plasma hormone levels can also occur from hormone secretion by an ectopic source, as sometimes occurs with malignancies.

Hyporesponsiveness

Hyporesponsiveness (hormone resistance) of the target tissues will cause the same set of clinical symptoms as hyposecretion. The usual reason for hyporesponsiveness is lack of or a deficiency in cellular receptors, although postreceptor mechanisms such as second-messenger dysfunction can also cause decreased cellular response. If the target cell does not have appropriate receptors for a hormone, the clinical symptoms will be the same as if inadequate hormone levels were reaching the target cells. However, plasma concentrations of hormone would be expected to be normal or high because of the lack of negative feedback to hormone-secreting organs. Nephrogenic diabetes insipidus is an example of kidney tubule resistance to the effect of ADH because of defective receptors on the tubular cells.[14] Some forms of diabetes mellitus also are characterized by tissue resistance to the effects of insulin (see Chapter 41).

KEY POINTS

- Endocrine disorders occur because of hyposecretion, hypersecretion, or lack of responsiveness by target cells. Hyporesponsiveness is clinically similar to hyposecretion and usually results from a lack of functional receptors.

■ Endocrine disorders may be due to abnormal tropic signals from the pituitary gland (secondary disorder) or to dysfunction of target glands (primary disorder).

SUMMARY

The endocrine system, together with the nervous system, is responsible for coordination of cellular activity between many body systems and organs. Hormone secretion occurs in response to a variety of stimuli, including psychological or physiologic stress, electrolyte and metabolite levels, and normal circadian cycles. Increases or decreases in the quantity of a particular circulating hormone tend to regulate levels of that hormone through negative feedback mechanisms. The cellular responses to hormones are complex and controlled by many other factors in addition to the circulating hormone levels.

REFERENCES

1. Porterfield SP, White BA: Introduction to the endocrine system. In Porterfield SP, White BA, editors: *Endocrine physiology,* ed 3, Philadelphia, 2007, Mosby, pp 1-24.
2. Chin WW: Molecular and cellular biology. In Lavin N, editor: *Manual of endocrinology and metabolism,* ed 3, Philadelphia, 2002, Lippincott Williams & Wilkins, pp 44-49.
3. Alberts B et al: Mechanisms of cell communication. In Alberts B et al, editors: *Molecular biology of the cell,* ed 5, New York, 2008, Garland Science, pp 879-964.
4. Guyton AC, Hall JE: Introduction to endocrinology. In Guyton AC, Hall JE, editors: *Textbook of medical physiology,* ed 11, Philadelphia, 2006, Saunders, pp 905-917.
5. Porterfield SP, White BA: The adrenal gland. In Porterfield SP, White BA, editors: *Endocrine physiology,* ed 3, Philadelphia, 2007, Mosby, pp 163-196.
6. Costanzo LS: Endocrine physiology. In Costanzo LS, editor: *Physiology,* ed 3, Philadelphia, 2006, Saunders, pp 377-440.
7. Guyton AC, Hall JE: Thyroid metabolic hormones. In Guyton AC, Hall JE, editors: *Textbook of medical physiology,* ed 11, Philadelphia, 2006, Saunders, pp 931-943.
8. Porterfield SP, White BA: The thyroid gland. In Porterfield SP, White BA, editors: *Endocrine physiology,* ed 3, Philadelphia, 2007, Mosby, pp 141-162.
9. Brunton L: Pharmacokinetics and pharmacodynamics: the dynamics of drug absorption, distribution, action, and elimination. In Brunton L et al, editors: *Goodman and Gilman's manual of pharmacology and therapeutics,* ed 11, New York, 2007, McGraw-Hill, pp 1-40.
10. Porterfield SP, White BA: The hypothalamus-pituitary complex. In Porterfield SP, White BA, editors: *Endocrine physiology,* ed 3, Philadelphia, 2007, Mosby, pp 107-140.
11. Costanzo LS: Reproductive physiology. In Costanzo LS, editor: *Physiology,* ed 3, Philadelphia, 2006, Saunders, pp 441-462.
12. Thibodeau GA, Patton KT: Endocrine systems. In Thibodeau GA, Patton KT, editors: *Anatomy and physiology,* ed 6, Philadelphia, 2007, Mosby, pp 593-644.
13. Guyton AC, Hall JE: Adrenocortical hormones. In Guyton AC, Hall JE, editors: *Textbook of medical physiology,* ed 11, Philadelphia, 2006, Saunders, pp 944-960.
14. Ball SG: Vasopressin and disorders of water balance: the physiology and pathophysiology of vasopressin, *Ann Clin Biochem* 44(Pt 5):417-431, 2007.

chapter

40

Disorders of Endocrine Function

Jacquelyn L. Banasik

MEDIA RESOURCES

Additional Material for Study, Review, and Further Exploration

  CD Companion ■ Review Questions and Answers
   ■ Glossary (with audio pronunciations for selected terms)
   ■ Disease Profiles ■ Animations

evolve **Website** at http://evolve.elsevier.com/Copstead/
   ■ Case Studies ■ Disease Profiles ■ WebLinks ■ Key Points Review

 ■ **Online Course (Module 17)**

KEY QUESTIONS

■ How can primary and secondary endocrine disorders be differentiated?

■ What etiologic factors would lead to clinical manifestations of hormone excess or deficiency?

■ What are the etiologic factors, clinical findings, and management of growth hormone excess and deficiency?

■ What are the etiologic factors, clinical findings, and management of thyroid hormone excess and deficiency?

■ What are the etiologic factors, clinical findings, and management of adrenocortical hormone excess and deficiency?

■ What are the etiologic factors, clinical findings, and management of adrenal medullary hormone excess?

■ What are the etiologic factors, clinical findings, and management of parathyroid excess and deficiency?

■ What are the etiologic factors, clinical findings, and management of antidiuretic hormone (ADH) excess and deficiency?

CHAPTER OUTLINE

Together with the nervous system, the endocrine system (the glands and the hormones they secrete) regulates body processes involving growth, maturation, metabolic functions, fluid balance, responses to stress, and reproduction.[1,2] This regulation is carried out through the actions of the hormones produced and secreted by the endocrine cells. **Hormones** are chemical messengers that travel through the bloodstream to exert physiologic effects on specific target cells and tissues. In the healthy state, hormones are released by endocrine glands when their action is needed and inhibited when their effect is attained.

Endocrine disease is marked by either hyperfunction (excessively high blood concentrations of a hormone, or conditions that mimic high hormone levels) or hypofunction (depressed levels, or conditions that mimic low hormone levels). Some endocrine disorders have such striking characteristics that recognition is obvious. Other symptoms of endocrine disease may be nonspecific and more difficult to detect. Observing and interviewing skills are important because, with the exception of the thyroid and testicles, the endocrine glands cannot be directly examined. Laboratory diagnostic tests are especially important in assessing the endocrine system.

This chapter describes alterations in the anterior pituitary regulatory system, growth hormone, thyroid hormone, and adrenal hormones; as well as parathyroid hormone disorders and posterior pituitary disorders of antidiuretic hormone (vasopressin) secretion. Disorders of prolactin and the gonadotropins (follicle-stimulating hormone, and luteinizing hormone) are discussed in Unit IX. Disorders of insulin secretion are discussed in Chapter 41.

BASIC CONCEPTS OF ENDOCRINE DISORDERS

Etiology of Endocrine Disorders

Dysfunction, either hyposecretion or hypersecretion, may originate in the hypothalamus/pituitary, the hormone-producing gland, or the target tissue (Figure 40-1). The etiology of endocrine disorders may be congenital, infectious, autoimmune, neoplastic, idiopathic, or iatrogenic. The onset of the disorders can be slow and insidious or abrupt and life threatening. The age at onset may range from birth to old age.

Abnormal hormone production occasionally results from an inborn genetic defect. Such defects may cause excessive production of hormone precursors due to an enzymatic block in the synthetic pathway, and enzyme deficiencies that impair hormone synthesis. An important example is congenital adrenal hyperplasia in which infants develop enlarged adrenal glands, but have a deficiency of cortisol production. If genetic defects do not cause a complete block of synthesis, increased pituitary stimulus may compensate by causing glandular hyperplasia, resulting in near normal hormone levels.

Autoimmune disorders commonly cause endocrine dysfunction, particularly in women. The pathogenesis of autoimmunity is incompletely understood, but involves both a genetic predisposition and an environmental trigger (see Chapter 10).

Antibodies are produced against certain antigens on self tissue cells, resulting either in hyperfunction of the endocrine gland (e.g. hyperthyroidism of Graves disease) or in immune destruction of the gland, eventually leading to hypofunction (e.g. adrenal insufficiency of Addison disease).

Hormones may be produced by abnormal tissue sites. Such *ectopic* hormone production is usually associated with a malignant tumor. Although different tumors can produce hormones, some cell types are more commonly associated with specific tumors. For example, some lung tumors produce antidiuretic hormone, leading to water intoxication and hyponatremia. Endocrine disorders can also be classified as functional disorders caused by nonendocrine disease such as chronic renal failure, liver disease, or heart failure.

In some cases endocrine disease occurs when the target tissue fails to respond to a hormone. The presence of normal or elevated hormone levels without normal hormonal action indicates hormone resistance. This problem is also illustrated by diminished or absent response to the administration of exogenous hormones. The mechanisms of hormone resistance may be genetic or acquired and may include defects at receptor sites, antibody reaction to hormone receptors, and defective postreceptor hormone action.

Finally, some endocrine disorders may be induced by medical treatments, such as therapy for a nonendocrine disorder. These iatrogenic disorders can also be caused by chemotherapy, radiation therapy, or surgical removal of glands. Commonly, a treatment for endocrine hyperfunction involves removal or destruction of glandular tissue with resultant chronic hypofunction. Chronic hormone replacement therapy may then be needed.

Classification of Endocrine Disorders

Endocrine disorders involving control by the anterior pituitary gland commonly are classified as **primary** (intrinsic malfunction of the hormone-producing target gland) or **secondary** (malfunction of the hypothalamus/pituitary cells that control the hormone-producing target gland). The clinical presentation of an endocrine disorder of primary or secondary etiology is similar, however diagnosing the source of the problem may be important in determining the best treatment. Measurement of serum concentrations of pituitary and target gland hormones allows differentiation between primary and secondary endocrine etiologies.

Clinically useful measures are available for thyroid, cortisol, and gonadal hormones. Laboratory diagnosis is based on an understanding of the feedback loop communication between the hypothalamic pituitary system and the target gland. When the *primary* gland fails, inadequate hormone is produced, low levels of hormone are present in the circulation, but blood levels of the corresponding trophic pituitary hormone levels become very elevated (Figure 40-2). For example, in primary hypothyroidism, the thyroid fails to secrete and serum levels of thyroxine (T_4) become lower. TSH levels rise as the pituitary gland attempts to stimulate the malfunctioning thyroid. In contrast, in secondary hypothyroidism, the pituitary gland

FIGURE 40-1 Examples of endocrine disorders and their pathogenesis. *SIADH,* Syndrome of inappropriate antidiuretic hormone secretion.

fails to release TSH, secondarily reducing thyroid gland production, so both thyroxine and TSH levels are abnormally low in the circulation. It is important to recall that the hormones released by the target gland are the ones that produce clinical signs and symptoms and that they are the starting point for interpretation of laboratory test results, followed by interpretation of the pituitary hormone results.

KEY POINTS

- Endocrine disorders occur because of hypersecretion, hyposecretion, or nonresponsiveness by target cells.
- *Hypersecretion* is usually due to secreting tumors, autoimmune disease, or excessive stimulation of the gland by trophic signals.

- *Hyposecretion* may be due to failure or congenital absence of glandular tissue, autoimmune destruction, surgical removal of the gland, or lack of normal trophic signals.
- *Hyporesponsiveness* is clinically similar to hyposecretion and is due to hormone receptor dysfunction. This phenomenon is called *tissue resistance.*
- Endocrine disorders involving the hypothalamic-pituitary system are often classified as primary or secondary.
- Primary endocrine disorders result from intrinsic defects within the hormone-secreting gland.
- Secondary disorders result from abnormal pituitary secretion of trophic signals. Manifestations of an endocrine disorder are due to abnormal target gland function and are therefore similar whether the etiologic classification is primary or secondary.

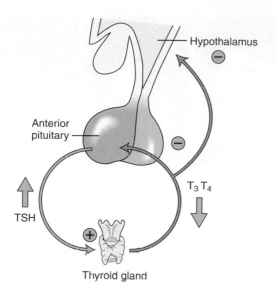

FIGURE 40-2 Diagnosing endocrine disorders as primary or secondary is based on the hypothalamic-pituitary and target tissue feedback loops. In this example, the low T_3 and T_4 are indicative of hypothyroidism. The elevated TSH indicates that the pituitary gland is responding appropriately and is not the source of the hypothyroidism. A diagnosis of primary hypothyroidism would be made based on these laboratory results.

TABLE 40-1

Signs and Symptoms of Growth Hormone Imbalance

Growth Hormone Excess	Growth Hormone Deficiency
Children	
Increased linear growth and tall stature	Delayed growth
	Fine features
	Short stature, proportionate
Adults	
Soft-tissue hyperplasia	May be associated with
Increased bone density	hyposecretion of other
Large hands, feet	pituitary hormones
Coarse facial features	
Thick, leathery skin	
Weight gain	
Glucose intolerance	

GROWTH HORMONE DISORDERS

Growth hormone is produced in the anterior pituitary gland under the influence of hypothalamic releasing (growth hormone releasing hormone) and inhibiting (somatostatin) factors. Its primary target organ is the liver, but GH also has direct effects on several tissue types. In general GH increases lean body mass, reduces fat mass, and induces the liver to release glucose under conditions of hypoglycemia. Please refer to Chapter 39 for details of GH synthesis, regulation, and activity. The major signs and symptoms of GH imbalance are summarized in Table 40-1.

Growth Hormone Deficiency

Etiology and Pathogenesis. Deficiencies in GH secretion can be classified into several major categories: (1) decreased GH secretion, (2) defective GH action (structurally abnormal GH or defective GH receptor), and (3) defective IGF-1 (somatomedin) generation.

Growth hormone deficiency is most clinically relevant in children. A birth history of prolonged labor or breech delivery is common, but GH deficiency may also be present in children who are born with midline craniocerebral defects, most likely due to congenital malformations or as sequelae of a chromosomal anomaly. Deficiencies in GH and other pituitary hormones should be considered in any child with nystagmus, retinal abnormalities, and other mid line or midfacial abnormalities, such as cleft lip or palate. The association between GH deficiency and other midline abnormalities appear to occur because the pituitary gland is developing during the same stage of fetal life as the other midline structures.

Classic Growth Hormone Deficiency

Children with GH deficiency have a variety of presentations, depending on the cause of the deficiency, the age at onset, and the severity of the disorder. The basis for this defect may be failure of the hypothalamus to stimulate pituitary GH secretion or failure of the pituitary to produce GH.

The most common tumors to influence hypothalamic-pituitary function are midline brain tumors. These include gliomas of the optic nerve and craniopharyngiomas. Craniopharyngiomas arise from cells at the junction of the anterior and posterior pituitary gland, are believed to be present at birth, and are slow growing. Craniopharyngiomas may grow to a large size without producing typical signs of increased intracranial pressure (vomiting, headache, oculomotor abnormalities). In older children, delayed growth may be the first symptom of a craniopharyngioma. Radiation therapy for brain tumors or leukemia may cause damage to hypothalamic and pituitary function. Traumatic insult to the skull or sella turcica may damage the pituitary gland, interrupting vascular connections and hypothalamic stimulation.

Clinical Manifestations. GH-deficient infants usually have normal birth length and weight. They may manifest hypoglycemia because GH and cortisol are necessary to maintain the euglycemic state. Hypoglycemia may present after fasting, which could be as brief as 3 hours in an infant. Recurrent episodes of hypoglycemia may lead to seizures and permanent cerebral damage. Boys developing GH deficiency in utero may have micropenis and undescended testicles.

GH-deficient children fall below the third percentile of growth in comparison with their peers. Dental eruption is delayed, and the development and setting of the permanent teeth are irregular. The hair is thin, and the nail growth is poor. Older children have greater fat mass and decreased muscle mass, with delayed bone formation. Delayed puberty is common if other anterior pituitary hormones are also affected.[3]

Children's growth should be evaluated annually. If growth velocity is abnormal, an endocrinologic evaluation and physiologic tests to stimulate GH release can be planned. Many pharmacologic agents are available that stimulate GH secretion in children, including insulin, arginine, levodopa, and clonidine. Children's neurosecretory GH patterns can be studied by obtaining timed serum GH samples during a normal nighttime sleep cycle.

Treatment. Hormonal replacement therapy for GH-deficient children has been available for several decades. The most obvious effect of GH replacement is stimulation of linear growth in children whose bones have not fused. With treatment, children experience an increase in growth velocity as well as depletion of the excess fat stores noted in GH-deficient children. GH injections are given subcutaneously 3 to 7 days a week.[4] The greatest response occurs during the first year of treatment.

Adults

Acquired GH deficiency in adults has only recently been recognized and treatment approved by the Food and Drug Administration.[5] Adults may become GH deficient after resection of pituitary tumors or after traumatic head injuries, but these patients are usually evaluated for deficiency of pituitary hormones other than GH. There is controversy regarding the manifestations of GH deficiency acquired in adulthood. There appears to be increased mortality due to cardiovascular causes when adults do not receive GH replacement following pituitary damage. GH-deficient adults have diminished lean body mass, hypercholesterolemia, and decreased bone density.[6] Research seems to indicate that individualized therapy for GH-deficient adults is beneficial in these circumstances.[7]

Growth Hormone Excess

Etiology and Pathogenesis. GH excess is nearly always due to uncontrolled production of the hormone by a benign somatotropic tumor in the pituitary gland. GH stimulates the liver to produce IGF-1, and these two hormones act in concert to cause upregulated growth of soft and bony tissues. Because GH secretion varies significantly over the course of the day, the serum level of IGF-1, which is more stable, may be measured as an indicator of GH secretion. If the tumor presents in childhood before the skeletal epiphyses are closed, rapid growth results in *pituitary giantism*. These children experience markedly accelerated growth velocity and quickly exceed the 95th percentile on pediatric growth charts. When the disorder is allowed to progress untreated, some of these children may grow to 8 feet or more in height and usually suffer an early cardiovascular death related to cardiomegaly and heart failure.

In adults, GH excess is called *acromegaly* and may be clinically subtle. Acromegaly occurs with equal frequency in men and women during the fourth and fifth decades of life. After the skeletal epiphyses close, bony growth occurs at the short bones, such as the hands and feet.

Clinical Manifestations of Acromegaly. Patients usually notice increased ring and shoe size, which progressively advances over several years. Enlargement of the frontal sinus causes a prominent brow, and growth of the mandible results in

FIGURE 40-3 Progressive development of facial features of acromegaly. (From Lewis SM et al: *Medical-surgical nursing,* ed 6, St Louis, 2004, Mosby, p 1304.)

progressive underbite *(prognathism)* (Figure 40-3). Soft tissues also slowly hypertrophy, causing coarsening of facial features and skin tags. Internal organs increase in size, resulting in goiter (thyroid enlargement) and cardiomegaly. Other manifestations include deepening of the voice secondary to vocal cord thickening and enlargement of the tongue, resulting in sleep apnea. Colonic polyps become more common, with the potential for malignant degeneration. It is estimated that the average patient with acromegaly has an active tumor for 7 or more years before seeking evaluation. Most often the changes are attributed by the patient and his or her family as "just growing older." Abnormalities in bone and soft-tissue growth are mostly irreversible. Patients may develop symptoms of increased intracranial pressure if the pituitary tumor enlarges significantly, including headache and visual disturbances. Some patients may develop glucose intolerance or hyperglycemia, and GH has been called a *diabetogenic* hormone for this reason.

Treatment. Effective therapy for acromegaly involves surgically removing the tumor while counteracting the effects of excess GH.[8] Octreotide, a synthetic form of somatostatin, suppresses production of GH. Surgery is usually performed using a transsphenoidal approach, but often the tumor is too large to completely resect. Radiation may be used postoperatively in these cases.[9]

KEY POINTS

- Hyposecretion of GH results in decreased linear growth in children. In some cases decreased linear growth occurs despite normal GH levels, and abnormalities of IGF-1 generation or responsiveness are suspected.
- GH deficiency may be idiopathic or related to tumors, radiation, or trauma. The diagnosis is confirmed by a finding of decreased GH levels in the blood and deficient GH release in response to hypoglycemia or other stimulants.

- Excessive GH production is usually due to pituitary adenoma. Excess GH during childhood results in increased linear growth and giantism. Excess GH secretion after closure of bone epiphyses results in increased bulk and acromegaly.
- Features of acromegaly include a protruding jaw, increased bone density, increased growth of soft tissues (e.g., nose, ears), and large hands and feet. Excessive GH secretion causes persistent hyperglycemia and increased insulin production in some individuals.
- Serum IGF-1 measurement is used to assess for acromegaly. High IGF-1 and an elevated GH level that is not suppressed by administration of oral glucose aids in the diagnosis. Treatment entails surgical removal or pharmacologic palliation of the pituitary tumor.

THYROID HORMONE DISORDERS

Secretion of the thyroid hormones, triiodothyronine (T_3) and thyroxine (T_4) is under control of thyroid-stimulating hormone (TSH) secretion from the anterior pituitary gland. Thyroid hormones are important for normal growth and development of tissues throughout the body and an important regulator of metabolism. The thyroid hormones, T_3 and T_4, are lipid-soluble and are able to cross the cell membranes of cells by simple diffusion. The details of thyroid hormone synthesis, regulation, and activity are described in Chapter 39.

Hypothyroidism

Etiology and Pathogenesis. **Hypothyroidism** may be congenital in origin or acquired later in life. The majority of cases of hypothyroidism are primary, due to intrinsic dysfunction of the thyroid gland. Congenital hypothyroidism (*cretinism*) may result from a variety of causes. Thyroid dysgenesis (lack of thyroid gland development) accounts for most congenital hypothyroidism. Abnormal TSH receptors and defective synthesis of thyroid hormone are other mechanisms causing congenital hypothyroidism.[10]

Lymphocytic thyroiditis (Hashimoto thyroiditis, or autoimmune thyroiditis) is the most common cause of acquired hypothyroidism. Lymphocytic thyroiditis is characterized by an enlarged thyroid gland (Figure 40-4) caused by lymphocytic infiltration. Thyroid hormone production decreases, stimulating the release of TSH from the pituitary gland, indicating a hypoactive thyroid gland. Hypothyroidism and its clinical symptoms progress as the gland becomes fibrotic.

Other causes of acquired hypothyroidism include irradiation of the thyroid gland, surgical removal of thyroid tissue, and iodine deficiency.[11] Iodine is essential for the formation of T_4 and T_3. Lack of iodine prevents production of both T_4 and T_3 but does not stop the formation of thyroglobulin. As a result, insufficient hormone is available to inhibit production of TSH by the anterior pituitary gland. This imbalance allows the pituitary gland to secrete excessively large quantities of TSH. The TSH then causes the thyroid cells to secrete tremendous amounts of thyroglobulin (colloid) into the follicles, and the gland grows larger and larger, producing a **goiter** (see Figure 40-4). An enlarged thyroid (goiter) is not always associated with hypothyroidism and can be present in euthyroid and hyperthyroid states.

Some foods contain "goitrogenic" substances that interfere with thyroid hormone synthesis. Such goitrogenic substances occur in some varieties of turnips and cabbage, but the clinical

FIGURE 40-4 An enlarged thyroid gland (goiter) can be present in hypothyroid, hyperthyroid, and euthyroid states. Note enlargement at the base of the neck. (From Wilson JD, Foster DW, editors: *Williams textbook of endocrinology*, ed 8, Philadelphia, 1992, Saunders, p 425.)

significance of these goitrogens is considered to be minimal. The drug lithium inhibits thyroid hormone synthesis and secretion and causes hypothyroidism in up to 20% of patients treated for bipolar disease.[12]

Secondary hypothyroidism is caused by defects in TSH production. Individuals who have been exposed to severe head trauma, cranial neoplasms, brain infections, cranial irradiation, and neurosurgery can be left with secondary hypothyroidism.[11]

Clinical Manifestations. Routine screening of newborns has resulted in early treatment of most infants with congenital hypothyroidism. Few clinical manifestations are present at birth. In untreated infants, symptoms appear in the first months of life and include a dull appearance; a thick, protuberant tongue; and thick lips (leading to feeding difficulties). Other signs include prolonged neonatal jaundice, poor muscle tone, bradycardia, mottled extremities, umbilical hernia, and a hoarse cry. Thyroid hormone is essential for normal central nervous system development; mental retardation will occur unless thyroid replacement is started early in infancy. Older children who acquire hypothyroidism have essentially the same clinical manifestations as adults. In addition, growth retardation, delayed bone development, and delayed or precocious puberty may occur.[12]

In general, individuals with hypothyroidism have decreased basal metabolic rates as the basis for many of their signs and symptoms. Patients report subjective feelings of weakness, lethargy, cold intolerance, and decreased appetite. Bradycardia, narrowed pulse pressure, and mild to moderate weight gain may occur. Elevated serum cholesterol and triglycerides are common as is an increased incidence of atherosclerosis. The thyroid gland may become enlarged (goitrous), the skin may be cool and dry, and constipation may be present. Depression and difficulties with concentration and memory occur. Women with acquired hypothyroidism may experience menstrual irregularities, with increased flow and clotting.[12] Table 40-2 summarizes the general signs and symptoms of thyroid imbalance.

Myxedema occurs in severe or prolonged thyroid deficiency. The term *myxedema* is in reference to the generalized, non-pitting edema that patients with long-term hypothyroidism tend to demonstrate. The edematous-looking skin is from the accumulation of glycosaminoglycans (mucopolysaccharides) in the interstitial spaces, which then retain fluid. Thyroid hormone normally prevents the accumulation of glycosaminoglycans within subcutaneous tissues. Individuals with hypothyroid-induced myxedema usually present in an altered mental state, with alterations in thermoregulation and a history of a precipitating event such as sepsis, trauma, or the use of certain medications.[10] Without medical intervention, patients may lapse into so-called myxedema coma, a medical emergency with upward of 60% mortality. Figure 40-5 shows the typical features of patients with myxedema.

TABLE 40-2

Typical Signs and Symptoms of Thyroid Imbalance

Hyperthyroidism	Hypothyroidism
Sleeplessness, nervousness	Lethargy
Muscle weakness, fatigue	Weakness
Susceptibility to infection	
Skin texture warm, silky, damp	Dry, pale, cool, coarse skin
Heat intolerance	Cold intolerance
Increased appetite with weight loss	Weight gain
Increased gastric motility	Constipation
Tachycardia, narrow pulse pressure, palpitations, angina	Bradycardia, wide pulse pressure
Dyspnea	Dyspnea, chest pain
Enlarged thyroid, may be diffuse or nodular	Thyroid may be diffusely enlarged (goiter) or may not be palpable
Hair silky, nail loose or detached from nail bed	Hair coarse
Hyperreflexia	Sluggish return of reflexes; mental impairment: slowed cognitive ability, poor memory, forgetfulness, depressed affect; deafness (in one-third of population)
Eye symptoms: burning, tearing, diplopia, lid lag, prominent eyes (exophthalmia with Graves disease), stare, eyelid tremors when closed	Facial edema (especially periorbital); thinned lateral aspect of eyebrows
Absence of forehead wrinkling on upward gaze	
Decreased or absent menses	Heavy, prolonged menses; infertility; decreased libido

FIGURE 40-5 Typical facial puffiness and dull expression of patients with myxedema. (From Seidel HM et al: *Mosby's guide to physical examination,* ed 5, St Louis, 2003, Mosby. Courtesy Paul W. Ladenson, MD, The Johns Hopkins University and Hospital, Baltimore, Md.)

In individuals with typical presentations of hypothyroidism, the diagnosis can be confirmed by measuring serum thyroid hormone levels. Since the most common cause of hypothyroidism is thyroid failure (primary hypothyroidism), nearly all patients will have elevated TSH levels because of the lack of negative feedback exerted by T_3 and T_4.[11] Serum TSH is a sensitive indicator of thyroid hypoactivity, and a rise in TSH often is detectable long before many symptoms develop. A decline in T_4 and T_3 levels may not occur until later in the course of disease. In the rare case of hypothalamic-pituitary dysfunction, both serum TSH and serum T_4 will be inappropriately low (Table 40-3).

Treatment. The goal of treatment is to return the individual with congenital or acquired hypothyroidism and thyroiditis to a euthyroid state. When serum thyroid levels are replaced too quickly, patients may experience insomnia, anxiety, and mood lability. Once treatment has begun, those individuals with a goiter usually experience a regression in glandular enlargement.[13]

Oral levothyroxine is used to replace or supplement hormone production from an underactive thyroid. Patients notice an increase in exercise tolerance, decreased fatigue, and improved mentation with therapy. Resolution of symptoms occurs gradually over weeks. Rarely, adrenal insufficiency may coexist with hypothyroidism, and patients may develop symptoms of nausea and vomiting as their thyroid disorder is treated (see the section on adrenocortical insufficiency). Intravenous levothyroxine may be used in myxedema coma. As the goal of therapy is reached and patients return to a "euthyroid" state, the serum TSH level should return to the normal range. Overtreatment with thyroid hormone can be detected by a serum TSH that is below the normal range. Overtreatment should be avoided in part because it contributes to osteoporosis.

Hyperthyroidism

Etiology and Pathogenesis. Mechanisms that can produce hyperthyroidism and thyrotoxicosis include thyroid follicular cell hyperfunction with increased synthesis and secretion of T_4 and T_3 (e.g., Graves disease), thyroid follicular cell destruction with release of preformed T_4 and T_3 (e.g., Hashimoto thyroiditis), and ingestion of excessive thyroid hormone or iodide preparations. The increased serum levels of thyroid hormones increase the metabolic rate (see Table 40-3).

TABLE **40-3**			
Thyroid Hormone Levels in Various States			
State	**Serum T_4 (µg/dl), Range**	**Serum T_3 (ng/dl), Range**	**Serum TSH (µU/ml), Range**
Euthyroid	4.5-11.5	60-180	0.5-4.5
Infants (<2 wk)	8.0-15.0	—	0.5-4.5
Children (prepubertal)	6.5-11.5	80-220	0.5-4.5
Hyperthyroid	>11.5	—	<0.15
Hypothyroid	<1.0-5.0	—	>10

Hyperfunction of thyroid follicular cells can be either autonomous (primary) or mediated through stimulation of TSH receptors by substances such as TSH (secondary) or TSH receptor antibodies (autoimmune). The basic abnormalities underlying ideopathic hyperfunction are unknown. Primary hyperfunction can be caused by adenomas and, rarely, thyroid carcinoma. Inflammation of thyroid follicular cells, with release of preformed thyroid hormone, can be associated with viral or autoimmune processes. Examples are the toxic thyroiditis of Hashimoto disease and subacute thyroiditis. Acute or chronic ingestion of thyroid hormone preparations can produce excess levels of thyroid hormones. Excessive intake of iodides may also result in thyrotoxicosis. Iodine is not usually ingested in toxic amounts, but some medications (such as amiodarone) have a high iodine content.

The most common etiology of hyperthyroidism is from autoantibodies that bind and stimulate TSH receptors on the thyroid gland.[10] This stimulation leads to a diffuse toxic goiter and a type of primary hyperthyroidism called **Graves disease.**[12] The etiology of Graves disease is unknown, but it has been associated with certain genetic markers (e.g., *HLA B8, HLA DR3*) and is more common in women than men. There is an increased incidence during the second and third decades of life. In response to the high circulating T_3 and T_4 levels that are stimulated by autoantibodies, the pituitary gland stops producing TSH, and serum TSH falls to very low levels.

Clinical Manifestations. Symptoms of hyperthyroidism include changes in behavior, insomnia, restlessness, tremor, irritability, palpitations, heat intolerance, diaphoresis, and an inability to concentrate that interferes with work performance (see Table 40-2). Increased basal metabolic rate may result in weight loss, although appetite and dietary intake increase. In women, amenorrhea or scant menses is a frequent finding.[12]

Individuals with Graves disease usually present with thyromegaly (diffusely enlarged thyroid), thyrotoxicosis, and, often, **exophthalmos** (enlargement of retro-orbital muscles causing protrusion of the eyes) (Figure 40-6). Spasm and retraction of the eyelids leads to widening of the palpebral fissure, resulting in exposed sclera. Lid lag develops, and severe, progressive exophthalmos may occur. Eye complaints may include vision changes and photophobia. The exophthalmos of Graves disease is not from elevated thyroid hormones and is thought to develop as a result of autoimmune antibody injury to ocular structures. Fibroblasts and fat cells behind the eye become infiltrated with immune cells, followed by release of inflammatory cytokines, swelling, and accumulation of glycosaminoglycans. Reduction of circulating thyroid hormone levels often does not prevent progression of the exophthalmos.

Undetectable TSH levels are the best indicator of primary hyperthyroidism. Serum T_4 and T_3 levels are elevated. A 24-hour radioactive iodine uptake study can confirm the diagnosis of Graves disease when the scan shows diffuse homogeneous uptake of tracer and can exclude the presence of thyroid neoplasms.

FIGURE 40-6 Patients with the usual ophthalmopathy found in Graves disease. **A,** Patient with periorbital swelling, exophthalmos, and chemosis (edema). **B,** Woman with widening of the palpebral fissures owing to lid retraction and proptosis. (From Larsen PR, Ingbar SH: The thyroid gland. In Wilson JD, Foster DW, editors: *Williams textbook of endocrinology,* ed 8, Philadelphia, 1992, Saunders, p 426.)

Thyroid storm is a form of life-threatening thyrotoxicosis that occurs when excessive amounts of thyroid hormones are acutely released into the circulation. This may occur under conditions of psychological or physiologic stress or with physical manipulation of the gland during diagnostic or surgical procedures. Thyroid storm presents with the clinical features of elevated temperatures, significant tachycardia, cardiac arrhythmias, and congestive heart failure. Extreme restlessness, agitation, and psychosis may occur. The patient may also experience vomiting, nausea, and diarrhea; jaundice may develop due to hepatic dysfunction.[14] Prompt treatment of thyroid storm is required (see the Treatment section that follows).

Treatment. Depending on the degree of symptoms, hyperthyroidism may be treated with medications, such as β-blockers to quickly block symptoms; drugs to inhibit thyroid hormone production, or radioactive iodine to destroy part of the thyroid gland. Surgical removal of the thyroid gland usually is reserved for hyperthyroidism associated with tumors and may result in hypoparathyroidism due to inadvertent resection of one or more parathyroids. In the rare case of hyperthyroidism secondary to pituitary adenoma, surgical or laser destruction of the anterior pituitary gland may be undertaken.

Antithyroid drugs called thionamides (propylthiouracil, methimazole) block the activities of the enzyme thyroid peroxidase and inhibit thyroid hormone production by follicular cells. These drugs do not prevent release of hormone, and because the typical thyroid gland contains a 2- to 3-month supply of already-made hormone, the onset of symptom reduction is slow. Thionamides produce a gradual reduction in the basal metabolic rate and the disappearance of symptoms (decreased size of the gland). Patients with Graves disease may receive these medications for months to years, depending on their response to the drugs and patient preferences. Relapse frequently occurs once medications are stopped.

Radioactive iodine treatment to ablate the gland, thereby curtailing its ability to produce excess thyroid hormones, is now the treatment of choice for Graves disease. Hypothyroidism occurs following radioactive iodine therapy in 50% to 80% of patients, so patients should be prepared for the likelihood of lifelong thyroid replacement therapy.

Because thyroid storm is a life-threatening form of thyrotoxicosis, aggressive management to achieve metabolic balance is mandated. Measures are taken to block the production and actions of thyroid hormone. Antithyroid drugs, such as propylthiouracil, are given followed by iodine administration to further inhibit release of T_3 and T_4 after an effective blockade of new hormone synthesis has been initiated. β-Blockers used for their antiadrenergic effects also inhibit the peripheral conversion of T_4 to T_3. Careful monitoring of individuals receiving treatment for thyroid storm must be provided. Antipyretic therapy (cooling blankets, ice packs, acetaminophen) may be started to achieve peripheral cooling. Fluid replacement is provided and the cardiovascular status monitored during stabilization of the individual's condition. The addition of glucocorticoids to the pharmacologic regimen improves survival. Thyroid storm is fatal if untreated. With treatment, the mortality is between 20% and 30%; therefore, aggressive, multifocused preventive measures must be implemented early in individuals who present with thyroid storm.[14]

KEY POINTS

- Thyroid hormone (T_3, T_4) is produced in follicular cells of the thyroid gland. The synthesis and secretion of thyroid hormone are stimulated by TSH from the pituitary gland. Thyroid hormone is an important stimulator of growth and cellular metabolism.
- Hypothyroidism may be primary (due to congenital agenesis, autoimmune destruction, irradiation, trauma, surgical removal of the gland, or iodine deficiency) or secondary to pituitary hyposecretion of TSH.
- TSH level is helpful in differentiating between primary (high TSH) and secondary (low TSH) causes of

hypothyroidism. Low serum T_3 and T_4 levels confirm the diagnosis of hypothyroidism.

- Manifestations of hypothyroidism are attributable to a generalized decrease in metabolism. Untreated congenital hypothyroidism results in profound mental and physical retardation (cretinism).

- Manifestations of hypothyroidism include nonpitting edema (myxedema), slowed mentation, weight gain, dry skin, constipation, decreased heart rate, decreased pulse pressure, lethargy, and loss of the outer third of the eyebrow. Severe hypothyroidism may lead to myxedema coma, characterized by bradycardia, hypothermia, hypotension, and decreased level of consciousness. Treatment centers on hormone replacement therapy.

- Hyperthyroidism may be primary (Graves disease, autoimmune, tumor related, inflammatory) or secondary to pituitary hypersecretion of TSH. The blood level of TSH is helpful in differentiating primary (low TSH) from secondary (high TSH) hyperthyroidism. High levels of T_3 and T_4 confirm the diagnosis of hyperthyroidism.

- The manifestations of hyperthyroidism result from a generalized increase in metabolism. Hyperactivity, irritability, insomnia, weight loss, increased appetite, heat intolerance, diarrhea, and palpitations are common. Most individuals have a detectably enlarged thyroid gland. Exophthalmos is immune-mediated and occurs with Graves disease.

- Thyroid storm may be precipitated by stress or manipulation of the gland. It is characterized by tachycardia, hypertension, high temperature, and cardiac dysrhythmias. Treatment includes β-blockers to control cardiovascular symptoms, antithyroid drugs to reduce thyroid production, radioactive iodine to ablate the gland, and surgical removal of tumors.

ADRENOCORTICAL HORMONE DISORDERS

The adrenal cortex synthesizes three different classes of steroid hormones including glucocorticoids, mineralocorticoids, and androgens. Cortisol is the primary glucocorticoid, and its concentration in the circulation provides negative feedback regulation of the hypothalamus and pituitary gland to suppress adrenocorticotropic hormone (ACTH) release. Aldosterone secretion is not regulated by the hypothalamic-pituitary system and is instead regulated by the presence of angiotensin II in the circulation. **Androgenic** hormone secretion by the adrenal cortex plays a relatively minor role in the development and maintenance of secondary sex characteristics, except in children with adrenogenital syndromes, which produce virilization in the female and precocious sexual development in the male. Physiologically, adrenal androgens are the main source of androgens in the female. As with mineralocorticoids, there is no known feedback mechanism to suppress ACTH production associated with adrenal sex hormone plasma levels. The details of adrenocortical hormone synthesis, regulation, and activity are discussed in Chapter 39.

Adrenocortical Insufficiency

Etiology and Pathogenesis. Hyposecretion of adrenocortical hormones can result from disease of the adrenal cortex (primary adrenocortical insufficiency, **Addison disease**), from the inadequate secretion of ACTH from the anterior pituitary gland (secondary adrenal insufficiency), or from a lack of CRH secretion from the hypothalamus due to hypothalamic malfunction or injury (tertiary adrenal insufficiency). Although hyposecretion of all the adrenocortical hormones may occur, the most severe clinical manifestations of adrenocortical insufficiency occur because of inadequate levels of circulating cortisol.

The syndrome of **congenital adrenal hyperplasia,** a rare cause of adrenal insufficiency in pediatric populations, is due to specific enzymatic defects in the biosynthesis of cortisol by the adrenal glands. Severe and life-threatening symptoms of adrenal insufficiency occur because of lack of circulating cortisol. The lack of negative feedback results in overproduction of ACTH, leading to hyperplasia of the adrenal glands and excessive androgen secretion.[15,16] Congenital adrenal hyperplasia is discussed at the end of the section on adrenal insufficiency.

Primary adrenal insufficiency (Addison disease) is caused by destruction of the adrenal gland through idiopathic or autoimmune mechanisms, tuberculosis, trauma or hemorrhage of the adrenals (often associated with anticoagulant therapy), fungal disease (e.g., histoplasmosis), and neoplasia. Because of the high functional reserve, symptoms of adrenal insufficiency may or may not be recognized until 90% of the cortical tissue has been rendered nonfunctional.

Secondary adrenal insufficiency (hypothalamic-pituitary dysfunction) is usually iatrogenic in origin because of the large numbers of patients receiving corticosteroid therapy for chronic illnesses. Prolonged exposure to pharmacologic doses of exogenous corticosteroids suppresses ACTH and CRH stimulation of the adrenal gland through negative feedback. If corticosteroid administration is suddenly halted, or if the individual experiences a sudden stress-induced increase in need for cortisol, the adrenal gland will be unable to respond by increasing cortisol secretion. Acute and severe manifestations of adrenal insufficiency ensue. Secondary adrenal insufficiency can also occur because of damage to the anterior pituitary gland or hypothalamus by tumors, infection, radiation, postpartum necrosis, trauma, or surgery.[15]

Addisonian crisis or acute adrenal insufficiency represents a true medical emergency caused by inadequate levels of glucocorticoids and mineralocorticoids in the circulation. This may occur as the result of a slowly developing and unrecognized ACTH or cortisol deficiency in which secretion is adequate for the normal demands of life but inadequate for increased stress or trauma. Individuals who are taking corticosteroids on an ongoing basis may also develop acute life-threatening adrenal insufficiency if the corticosteroid is suddenly withdrawn.

Clinical Manifestations. The clinical manifestations of adrenal insufficiency (Table 40-4) occur because of inadequate levels of circulating cortisol and aldosterone (Figure 40-7). Diminished

TABLE 40-4

Signs and Symptoms of Adrenocortical Hormone Imbalance

Cushing Syndrome	Adrenocortical Insufficiency
Truncal obesity	Weakness
Moon face	Hypotension
Buffalo hump	Hypoglycemia
Hirsutism	Hyperpigmentation (Addison disease)
Muscle wasting	
Striae	Hyperkalemia
Petechiae	Weight loss
Glucose intolerance	
Hypertension	
Hypokalemia	

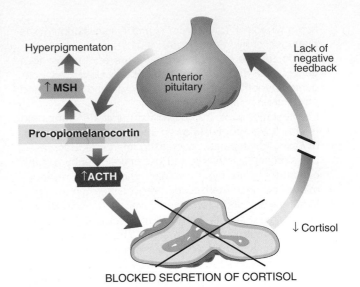

FIGURE 40-7 Primary adrenocortical insufficiency (decreased cortisol production) leads to hypersecretion of melanocyte-stimulating hormone (MSH) and adrenocorticotropin hormone (ACTH) because of lack of negative feedback. MSH and ACTH are derived from the same precursor molecule, pro-opiomelanocortin. Even though ACTH levels are high, the adrenal gland is unable to produce adequate levels of cortisol.

vascular tone, reduced cardiac output, and inadequate circulating blood volume all contribute to potentially lethal vascular collapse. Clinical manifestations may appear gradually, especially if adrenal destruction is slow and incremental, such as in autoimmune adrenal insufficiency. Symptoms are more dramatic if adrenal destruction is sudden (hemorrhage) or if a stressor, such as trauma, causes sudden decompensation in a patient with chronic adrenal insufficiency.

Early signs of primary adrenal insufficiency include anorexia, weight loss, weakness, malaise, apathy, electrolyte imbalances, and hyperpigmentation of the skin caused by unsuppressed ACTH production (Figure 40-8). Salt craving may be present as a result of sodium deficit. If the condition is unrecognized or left untreated, gastrointestinal symptoms can develop, including nausea, vomiting, diarrhea, and dehydration. The patient may be hypotensive or tachycardic. The sudden onset of nausea, vomiting, anorexia, and hypotension suggests acute adrenal insufficiency, which is a medical emergency.[16]

Diagnosis. The diagnosis of acute adrenal insufficiency is made on clinical grounds, taking into account the patient's medical history (use of steroids, trauma, anticoagulation), physical examination, and biochemical findings. Decreased plasma cortisol levels assist in the diagnosis; however, since acute decompensation progresses to death so rapidly, levels are often drawn and therapy is initiated presumptively. Resolution of symptoms may be remarkably rapid with therapy.

In cases of chronic adrenal insufficiency, an ACTH provocation test can be given. Cosyntropin, synthetic ACTH, is given IV, and serum samples of cortisol are measured 30 and 60 minutes after administration. Serum cortisol levels should increase following this stimulus if the adrenal cortex is functioning normally. A failure to produce cortisol indicates a primary adrenal insufficiency. Abdominal CT or MRI can be performed to determine the size of the adrenal glands. Small adrenal glands occur with autoimmune destruction, whereas tuberculous glands are large and calcified, and hemorrhagic glands are large and smooth.

Treatment. The treatment for adrenal insufficiency entails replacing the absent or deficient hormones usually produced by the adrenal cortex in a manner that mimics natural production as closely as possible. About 2/3 of the daily dosage may be given in the morning and 1/3 in the evening to more closely mimic physiologic adrenal cortical function. In the case of adrenal crisis, intravenous glucocorticoids can be administered intermittently until the symptoms (hypotension, hypoglycemia) resolve; the dose is then titrated downward. In addition, volume replacement is needed to replace the increased urine output associated with renal sodium excretion.[17]

Stress situations increase the dose requirements for individuals on chronic replacement therapy. Acute illness (increased temperature causes an increase in metabolic rate), injury (e.g., trauma, surgery, burns), and psychological episodes that affect an individual's ability to function normally (death of a significant relative) may double or triple the needed daily corticosteroid dose. If illness or injury restricts the patient's ability to tolerate oral intake, replacement must be given parenterally.[16]

Congenital Adrenal Hyperplasia. Congenital adrenal hyperplasia is also called *adrenogenital syndrome* and occurs when an enzyme needed for cortisol production is lacking because of a gene defect. Because circulating cortisol levels are inadequate to provide negative feedback to the anterior pituitary gland, ACTH secretion is elevated. This leads to adrenal hypertrophy and overproduction of steroid precursors in the gland, which are shunted into the production of androgens. In the newborn, classic congenital adrenal hyperplasia is

FIGURE 40-8 Altered pigmentation in adrenocortical insufficiency. **A,** Increased pigmentation across the bridge of the nose. **B,** Generalized hyperpigmentation with vitiligo. (From Bondy PK, Rosenberg LE: *Metabolic control and disease,* ed 8, Philadelphia, 1980, Saunders, p 1462.)

a life-threatening condition because of inadequate circulating cortisol.

Infants are frequently diagnosed at birth because of the effects of excessive androgens on the genitals of the newborn. Virilization of a female fetus's genitalia occurs. The female infant may be born with an enlarged clitoris and fused labia, resembling a scrotal sac (Figure 40-9). Male infants with congenital adrenal hyperplasia may have an enlarged penis and hyperpigmented scrotum, but the examiner may not recognize these subtle signs.

Depending on the enzymes affected, androgen overproduction may occur at any time from birth to early adult life. If it occurs in an adult female, she may develop such virile characteristics as a beard, a much deeper voice, baldness, masculine distribution of pubic hair, growth of the clitoris to resemble a penis, and deposition of proteins in the skin and muscles to yield typical masculine characteristics.

In adult men, the virilizing characteristics of adrenogenital syndrome are less obvious because male virilizing characteristics are normally associated with testosterone secreted by the testes. Therefore, the diagnosis is difficult to make.[18] In the prepubertal male, adrenogenital syndrome usually causes precocious puberty.

In all cases, treatment with glucocorticoids is necessary to avoid the complications associated with adrenal insufficiency as previously described. In addition, exogenous glucocorticoid therapy suppresses pituitary secretion of ACTH, allowing the adrenal cortex to atrophy and the overproduction of adrenal androgens to cease.

Hypercortisolism

Etiology and Pathogenesis. Hyperfunction of the adrenal cortex results in conditions characterized by **hypercortisolism.** Primary adrenocortical hyperfunction is caused by disease of

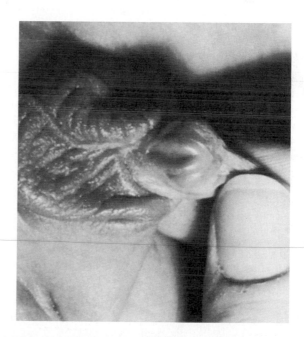

FIGURE 40-9 Female infant with congenital adrenal hyperplasia demonstrating virilization of the genitalia. Note the enlarged clitoris and the fused labia, which resemble a scrotal sac. (From Hurwitz LS: Nursing implications of selected endocrine disorders, *Nursing Clin North Am* 15:528, 1980.)

the adrenal cortex (adrenal adenoma). Secondary disease is caused by hyperfunction of the anterior pituitary ACTH-secreting cells, and tertiary disease is caused by hypothalamic dysfunction or injury. The term **Cushing syndrome** is used to describe the clinical features of hypercortisolism, regardless of cause. **Cushing disease** is the diagnosis reserved for pituitary-dependent conditions.[15]

In pediatric and adult populations, hypercortisolism is frequently caused by the excessive production of pituitary ACTH by microadenomas or adenomas. Ectopic ACTH production by nonpituitary tumors can also stimulate the adrenal glands. In the United States, exogenous steroids used in the management of various diseases, such as asthma and connective tissue diseases, is the most common cause of Cushing syndrome.[17]

Clinical Manifestations. An individual with excess circulating glucocorticoids typically develops a round face with prominent, flushed cheeks, often referred to as "moon facies" (see Table 40-4). There is a noticeable weight gain with increasing total body fat, especially in the abdomen. A cervical fat pad, capillary friability, and thinning of the skin with the formation of purple striae and ecchymoses over the abdomen, arms, and thighs develop. Muscle mass decreases and muscle weakness develops. Cortisol increases tissue resistance to the effects of insulin and may contribute to glucose intolerance or hyperglycemia. Figure 40-10 shows the common clinical manifestations of Cushing syndrome.

Hypertension may develop as a consequence of the salt-retaining activity of cortisol and of the increased blood volume.

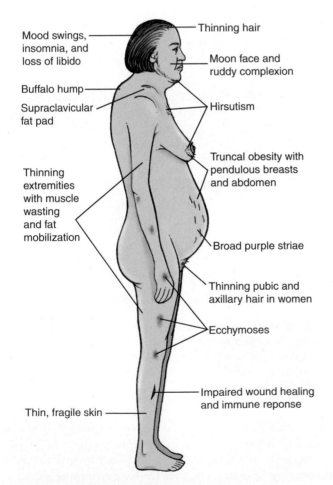

Mood swings, insomnia, and loss of libido

Thinning hair

Buffalo hump

Moon face and ruddy complexion

Supraclavicular fat pad

Hirsutism

Thinning extremities with muscle wasting and fat mobilization

Truncal obesity with pendulous breasts and abdomen

Broad purple striae

Thinning pubic and axillary hair in women

Ecchymoses

Impaired wound healing and immune reponse

Thin, fragile skin

FIGURE 40-10 Common clinical manifestations of Cushing syndrome. (From Monahan FD, Neighbors M: *Medical-surgical nursing: foundations for clinical practice,* ed 2, Philadelphia, 1998, Saunders, p 1286.)

An associated reduction of serum potassium is commonly found because of the excessive exchange of sodium for potassium in the renal tubules. With chronic Cushing syndrome, demineralization of the bones (osteoporosis) and resulting fractures may occur. The cortisol excess may be accompanied by increased androgen production (excessive hair production, acne, menstrual irregularities).

Emotional changes include depression, emotional lability, anxiety, and irritability. Rarely, euphoria is noted. Decreases in short-term memory, concentration, and attention span may be present.

The diagnosis of adrenocortical excess depends on reliable, accurate laboratory measurements. A serum ACTH level may be helpful in differentiating between primary (low ACTH) and secondary (high ACTH) hypercortisolism. Urinary free cortisol levels will be elevated in all forms. A 24-hour urine collection is typically done to exclude inappropriate diagnoses due to diurnal variations in cortisol production. If the ACTH is elevated or normal and the 24-hour urinary free cortisol is found to be elevated, a dexamethasone suppression test may be used to differentiate between pituitary causes and ectopic causes of excessive ACTH production. Most pituitary adenomas (Cushing disease) demonstrate a relative resistance to feedback inhibition by cortisol. When a more potent glucocorticoid is given (dexamethasone) the pituitary gland responds by reducing ACTH production. Sometimes Cushing syndrome is a result of ectopic production of ACTH by cancer cells. In this case, the suppression test will fail to reduce ACTH production because the cancer cells do not respond to feedback control. A negative suppression test will necessitate a diagnostic evaluation to find the ectopic cancer source.

Treatment. The choice of treatment for Cushing syndrome is based on its etiology. Patients who have Cushing syndrome as a result of exogenous glucocorticoid therapy should have doses reduced if possible. Care must be taken to taper doses slowly to avoid acute adrenal insufficiency. For pituitary disease (Cushing disease), transsphenoidal hypophysectomy or laser ablation may be done. Figure 40-11 shows a woman before and after treatment for Cushing syndrome.

Unilateral adrenalectomy is used if the cause of the hypercortisolism is an adrenal tumor. Bilateral removal of the adrenal glands is rarely necessary because most tumors are unilateral. Lifelong steroid replacement is usually necessary following this surgery. Radiation therapy may be an option if surgery is contraindicated.[15]

Chemotherapeutic agents that block cortisol production can also be utilized either alone or in conjunction with surgery and radiation. When any of these therapies is used, the patient should be assessed for adrenal insufficiency.

Hyperaldosteronism. Excessive aldosterone production may be from primary hyperaldosteronism (Conn syndrome) or secondary to conditions associated with poor kidney perfusion. Conn syndrome usually occurs as a result of aldosterone-secreting tumors. Aldosterone is not under pituitary control and in this case, "secondary" refers to disease processes or conditions that stimulate the renin-angiotensin-aldosterone

FIGURE 40-11 A woman with Cushing syndrome before **(A** and **C)** and after **(B)** removal of an adrenal adenoma. (From Wyngaarden JB et al: *Cecil textbook of medicine,* ed 19, Philadelphia, 1992, Saunders, p 1285.)

cascade. These include heart failure, reduced kidney perfusion, and liver cirrhosis.

Aldosterone facilitates salt and water retention by the kidney. Because aldosterone acts on the distal renal tubule to promote sodium exchange for the potassium lost in the urine, individuals with hyperaldosteronism usually have decreased potassium levels. The drug spironolactone is an aldosterone antagonist and therefore is useful in the medical management of aldosterone excess. Spironolactone increases sodium excretion and potassium retention. Sodium restriction and potassium replacement may also be necessary.[15]

- The adrenal cortex produces three classes of steroid hormones: (1) glucocorticoids, (2) mineralocorticoids, and (3) sex steroids. Glucocorticoid synthesis is regulated by the pituitary secretion of ACTH. Mineralocorticoid synthesis is regulated by the renin-angiotensin system. The glucocorticoid cortisol provides the primary negative-feedback mechanism to inhibit ACTH release.

- Adrenocortical insufficiency may be primary (Addison disease), in which case it is characterized by high ACTH levels in the blood and hyperpigmentation of skin related to excessive pituitary secretion, or it may be secondary, in which case it is characterized by low ACTH levels.

- Primary adrenal insufficiency may follow autoimmune destruction of, surgical removal of, or trauma to the gland. Exogenous administration of steroids suppresses ACTH, resulting in adrenocortical atrophy. Sudden withdrawal of exogenous steroids may result in adrenal insufficiency.

- Inherited defects in biosynthetic enzymes necessary for cortisol production may affect one or more of the steroid hormone synthesis pathways. Cortisol deficiency results in pituitary release of ACTH, stimulating the adrenal gland to enlarge (congenital adrenal hyperplasia). Excess androgens may be synthesized, leading to masculinization of females and precocious puberty in males.

- Manifestations of primary adrenocortical insufficiency include weight loss, salt wasting, volume depletion, low blood pressure, hypoglycemia, and hyperkalemia. Stress may lead to severe symptoms (Addisonian crisis), including circulatory collapse (hypotension). Treatment includes hormone replacement therapy. Dosages are generally increased during periods of stress (e.g., surgery).

- Excess cortisol production due to pituitary hyperstimulation of the adrenal cortex is termed *Cushing disease.* Hypercortisolism of any other cause is termed *Cushing syndrome.* ACTH excess may be due to pituitary adenoma or exogenous production by nonpituitary tumors. Cushing syndrome is commonly due to administration of exogenous steroids.

- Clinical manifestations of Cushing disease and Cushing syndrome include moon facies, cervical fat pad, central obesity, thin extremities, weight gain, thin skin, striae, hypertension, and hyperglycemia. Plasma cortisol levels and the urinary excretion of cortisol metabolites are increased. Surgical removal of ACTH-producing tumors or removal of the adrenal gland is the usual treatment.
- Primary hyperaldosteronism (Conn syndrome) is usually due to adrenal tumor. Aldosterone enhances sodium and water reabsorption and potassium excretion from the kidney, leading to hypervolemia, hypertension, and hypokalemia.

ADRENAL MEDULLA

Pheochromocytoma

Etiology and Pathogenesis. The adrenal medulla secretes two important catecholamine hormones in response to stimulation by the sympathetic nervous system. Epinephrine, or adrenaline, accounts for about 80% of the adrenal medulla's secretion; norepinephrine accounts for the other 20%. Norepinephrine is also the neurotransmitter produced by the postganglionic sympathetic fibers. Sympathetic effectors such as the heart, smooth muscle, and glands have receptors for norepinephrine. Both epinephrine and norepinephrine can bind to the receptors of sympathetic effectors to prolong and enhance the effects of sympathetic stimulation.

Pheochromocytoma is a tumor of chromaffin tissue that results in the excessive production and release of catecholamines. It is usually benign, but in about 10% of cases the tumor exhibits malignant behavior. It is usually found in the adrenal medulla, but it may also arise in other sites where there is chromaffin tissue, such as the sympathetic ganglia. Like adrenal medullary cells, the tumor cells of a pheochromocytoma produce and secrete the catecholamines epinephrine and norepinephrine in response to sympathetic stimulation. Excessive release of these catecholamines results in severe hypertension.[19] The hypertension in individuals with pheochromocytoma is influenced by the level of sympathetic nervous system stimulation, the circulating catecholamine levels, and the cardiovascular response to these changes.

Clinical Manifestations. The most common problem experienced by an individual with a pheochromocytoma is intermittent or persistent hypertension. Bouts of the classic triad of headache, tachycardia, and diaphoresis strongly suggest the diagnosis of pheochromocytoma. Sporadic hypertensive episodes may occur with stress, excitement, physical activity, ingestion of certain drugs, and the smoking of tobacco products. Other symptoms may include tremor, nervousness, emotional lability, pallor, fatigue, generalized gastrointestinal complaints, and orthostatic hypotension. Signs of a hypermetabolic state may be present, such as fever, weight loss, polyuria, and polydipsia.[20]

Because most pheochromocytomas are located on the adrenal glands, abdominal CT or MRI are commonly employed diagnostic tools. Uncontrolled hypertension can lead to end-organ damage and stroke, so prompt diagnosis and aggressive therapy are necessary.[21]

Treatment. The usual treatment for this condition is surgical removal of the tumor. Before surgery, sympathetic blocking medications are prescribed to manage blood pressure and relieve symptoms.

If surgery is contraindicated, treatment with drugs to block catecholamine production is possible. However, surgery is the only curative therapy. If both adrenal glands are surgically removed, lifetime treatment for adrenocorticoid insufficiency is necessary. After a period of stabilization, the sympathetic nervous system is able to compensate for the loss of adrenal medullary function and no replacement is necessary. Because there is an increased risk of recurrence of the tumor in later years, annual follow-up is recommended.[21]

KEY POINTS

- The adrenal medulla releases catecholamines into the bloodstream when stimulated by the sympathetic nervous system. Catecholamines increase heart rate, blood pressure, and glucose release from the liver.
- A pheochromocytoma is a catecholamine-secreting tumor that is usually located in the adrenal medulla. Excessive catecholamine release from the tumor causes intermittent or persistent hypertension, headache, tachycardia, tremor, and irritability. Most tumors are benign, and surgical removal relieves the disorder. Adrenergic blocking agents may be used to manage the hypertension until surgical treatment is accomplished.

PARATHYROID GLAND DISORDERS

Regulation and Actions of Parathyroid Hormone

The parathyroid glands are small glands located at the upper and lower poles of the thyroid. There are usually four parathyroid glands, although there are reports of fewer or more than four being found during surgery. The parathyroid glands detect serum calcium concentration and help maintain constant levels through the regulation of calcium absorption and resorption from bone (Figure 40-12). The absorption of calcium from intestine and renal tubules is dependent on vitamin D and is impaired in conditions such as renal failure, in which active vitamin D is deficient (see Chapter 28).

Serum calcium levels provide the feedback necessary to regulate parathyroid hormone (PTH) secretion. A decrease in serum calcium causes a release of PTH. An elevated serum calcium level leads to suppression of PTH secretion. Parathyroid hormone (PTH) is not under control of the hypothalamic-pituitary

↓ Serum calcium level

↑ PTH secretion

| PTH promotes calcium and phosphate resorption from bone | PTH promotes calcium reabsorption and phosphate excretion from the renal tubule | PTH promotes calcium absorption from the GI tract |

↑ Serum calcium level

↓ PTH secretion

FIGURE 40-12 Parathyroid hormone *(PTH)* increases serum calcium level through its effects on bone, renal tubules, and intestine. *GI,* Gastrointestinal.

system. Parathyroid hormone acts on bones, intestine, and renal tubules to increase serum calcium levels. In the bone, PTH increases osteoclastic activity, resulting in the release of calcium from bone into extracellular fluid. Renal calcium reabsorption increases under the effect of PTH, thus decreasing urinary calcium excretion.

Calcitonin, produced by thyroid parafollicular cells, also influences the processing of calcium by bone cells. Calcitonin controls the calcium content of the blood by increasing bone formation by osteoblasts and inhibiting bone breakdown by osteoclasts. Although the role of calcitonin in calcium homeostasis is not entirely clear, calcitonin tends to decrease blood calcium levels and promote conservation of hard bone matrix.

The clinical manifestations of parathyroid hormone dysfunction are those of hypercalcemia and hypocalcemia and related changes in neuromuscular excitability. A discussion of serum calcium regulation and disorders can be found in Chapter 24.

Hyperparathyroidism

Etiology and Pathogenesis. The causes of primary hyperparathyroidism remain unclear. Despite an elevated serum calcium level, PTH continues to be secreted. Some forms of hyperparathyroidism can have a genetic origin. Hyperparathyroidism from a single parathyroid adenoma occurs in 80% of surgically proven cases. Hyperplasia of the parathyroid is found in the remainder of the cases.

In hyperparathyroidism, bone resorption and formation rates are increased. Serum calcium levels do not rise uncontrollably; indeed, excessive parathyroid gland secretion rarely causes hypercalcemic crisis. Malignant tumors elsewhere in the body can also release PTH and are a more frequent cause of extreme hypercalcemia and hypercalcemic crisis.[22]

A hyperparathyroid state during pregnancy leads to perinatal and neonatal complications. The newborn's PTH production will be suppressed by maternal hypercalcemia, and neonatal hypocalcemia and tetany can develop. This presentation in a newborn may be the first indication of the need for investigative studies in the mother if the disorder was asymptomatic during pregnancy.[23] In chronic renal failure, hyperparathyroidism may result from reduced production of active vitamin D (which impairs calcium absorption) and from impaired glomerular filtration (which limits excretion of phosphate in the urine). Some drugs, such as lithium and thiazides, may increase serum calcium levels, leading to a misdiagnosis of hyperparathyroidism.

Clinical Manifestations. The presentation of hyperparathyroidism is related to the level of hypercalcemia and the hyperparathyroid state. Hyperparathyroidism may present as asymptomatic hypercalcemia. Individuals are prone to kidney stones and to bone demineralization (osteoporosis). Severe hypercalcemia causes a wide variety of effects, dominated by polyuria and dehydration. Anorexia, nausea, vomiting, and constipation may develop. Various cardiac problems can arise including bradycardia, heart block, and cardiac arrest.

Often, asymptomatic cases of hyperparathyroidism are found on screening serum chemistry laboratory reports that note mild elevations in serum calcium levels. In primary hyperparathyroidism (not secondary to renal disease), serum calcium levels are elevated and serum phosphorus levels are low to low-normal. Urinary excretion of calcium and phosphate is elevated, as are serum PTH levels.

Treatment. Surgical removal of the abnormal parathyroid gland is the treatment of choice. Individuals with asymptomatic hyperparathyroidism may defer or refuse surgery. In such cases, medical management may work for a time. Medical management includes hydration (to prevent kidney stone formation) and ambulation to maintain bone density.

For hypercalcemic crisis, rapid volume expansion with normal saline reverses dehydration. Volume replacement also results in improved glomerular filtration rate and increased calcium excretion. Diuretics may be used to increase calcium excretion by the kidney.

Hypoparathyroidism

Etiology and Pathogenesis. Hypoparathyroidism most frequently occurs as a consequence of parathyroid or thyroid surgery or surgery in the area of these glands. The resulting iatrogenic hypoparathyroidism may be temporary or permanent. In some cases it may take years to develop.

Hypoparathyroidism can occur following the removal of one hyperfunctioning parathyroid gland. The hyperfunctioning gland suppresses the function of the other parathyroid glands, creating a temporary state of deficiency. Permanent hypoparathyroidism rarely follows initial surgery. Permanent hypoparathyroidism may develop following thyroidectomy because of damage to parathyroid gland blood supply, post-surgical swelling, or fibrosis.[22]

Congenital lack of parathyroid tissue and idiopathic hypoparathyroidism are causes of hypoparathyroidism in infants and children. Autoimmune processes may also target and damage the parathyroid gland.

Clinical Manifestations. Clinical manifestations of hypoparathyroidism occur as a result of low serum calcium levels. The manifestations of acute hypocalcemia include circumoral numbness, paresthesias of the distal extremities, muscle cramps, fatigue, hyperirritability, anxiety, depression, nonspecific electroencephalographic changes, increases in intracranial pressure, and prolongation of corrected Q-T intervals on the electrocardiogram. Severe manifestations of hypocalcemia include carpopedal spasm, laryngospasm, and seizures. The clinical signs of hypocalcemia include neuromuscular irritability associated with tetany. Tetany is indicated by the Chvostek sign (ipsilateral contraction of the facial muscles that is elicited by tapping the facial nerve anterior to the ear) or Trousseau sign (carpal spasm produced by pressure ischemia of the nerves in the upper arm during inflation of a blood pressure cuff for 3 to 5 minutes above the systolic blood pressure).

The serum calcium level is low (5 to 7 mg/dl), and the phosphorus level is high (7 to 12 mg/dl). Levels of antibodies to the parathyroid gland are high if an autoimmune mechanism is operant.

Treatment. Emergency treatment with IV calcium is needed if an individual presents in acute hypocalcemic crisis (tetany, laryngospasm, and convulsions). Calcitriol, an activated form of vitamin D, should also be given in the emergent phase. Long-term treatment includes oral calcium supplement and vitamin D.[22] Serum calcium levels should be maintained in the low-normal range in an attempt to avoid hypercalciuria, which may contribute to stone formation.

glands. Adequate hydration may help prevent the formation of kidney stones.

- Hypoparathyroidism may be idiopathic, autoimmune, or secondary to surgical removal of the parathyroid gland. The manifestations result from low serum calcium levels, which increase neuromuscular excitability. Paresthesias, cramps, spasms, tetany, and seizures may result. Elicitation of Chvostek and Trousseau signs indicates neuromuscular hyperexcitability. Treatment entails calcium (and vitamin D) supplementation rather than PTH replacement.

ANTIDIURETIC HORMONE DISORDERS

ADH (vasopressin) is secreted from the posterior pituitary gland in response to changes in blood osmolality. The details of ADH synthesis, regulation, and activity are described in Chapter 39. Concepts related to physiologic effects on renal water handling can be found in Chapter 26; Chapter 24 includes details of body fluid regulation and osmolality.

Diabetes Insipidus

Etiology and Pathogenesis. **Diabetes insipidus** is a disorder of insufficient ADH activity characterized by excessive loss of water in the urine. ADH acts directly on the renal collecting ducts and distal tubules, increasing membrane permeability to and reabsorption of water. Damage to the ADH-producing cells in the hypothalamus can occur with closed head trauma, intracranial tumors, and neurosurgery.[24] Some pharmacologic agents can lead to abnormalities in ADH secretion (Table 40-5). For example, the diuresis that follows alcohol ingestion occurs because of decreased ADH secretion.[25]

Diabetes insipidus (DI) is a term meaning *a large diuresis of inappropriately dilute urine.* In adults with DI, 30% of cases are idiopathic, 20% are caused by the surgical treatment of brain tumors, 16% result from nonsurgical brain trauma, 25% are secondary to brain tumors, and 9% follow

---

KEY POINTS

- PTH is an important regulator of serum calcium levels. Low serum levels of ionized calcium are a potent stimulus for PTH release. PTH increases calcium absorption from the GI tract in concert with Vitamin D, the resorption of calcium and phosphate from bones, and the reabsorption of calcium from the urine filtrate. PTH also increases the excretion of phosphate by the kidney. Disorders of PTH secretion are manifested as alterations in serum Ca^{2+} levels.

- Hyperparathyroidism may be idiopathic or may be due to a parathyroid adenoma. Its manifestations result from high serum calcium levels and bone demineralization. High serum calcium levels decrease neuromuscular excitability. Treatment entails removing the abnormal

---

TABLE 40-5	
Agents That Cause Alterations in Antidiuretic Hormone Secretion	
Agents That Enhance Release	**Agents That Suppress Release**
Vincristine	Phenytoin
Cyclophosphamide	Alcohol
Prostaglandin E_2	α-Adrenergic agents
β-Adrenergic agents	
Histamine	
Hypercapnia	
Morphine and narcotic analogs	
Nicotine	
Clofibrate	
Carbamazepine	
Barbiturates	
Hypoxia	

a hypophysectomy.[26] ADH deficiency may be accompanied by other hypothalamic-pituitary hormone deficiencies. Damage to the posterior pituitary gland may cause temporary or permanent deficiency of ADH. With insufficient amounts of ADH, urine cannot be concentrated and free water is lost, causing hyperosmolality and hypernatremia. This is called *central DI* because the ability to produce and release ADH from the pituitary gland is lost. *Nephrogenic DI* occurs when the kidney is unable to respond to ADH because of chronic renal disease, serum electrolyte abnormalities, or drugs (e.g., lithium). The clinical presentation of both forms of DI is similar, and measurement of serum ADH may be helpful in determining the etiology.

Clinical Manifestations and Diagnosis. The development of **polyuria** (excessive urination) and **polydipsia** (excessive drinking) is the hallmark of DI. The patient may void as much as 15 L of urine daily. Specific gravity of the urine will be greatly decreased. If the thirst center of the hypothalamus is functional, the patient will consume up to 15 L of water to maintain osmolar balance. Symptoms persist at night (nocturia), interrupting normal sleep patterns. Usual patterns of behavior and work habits can be affected by the need to frequently drink and urinate. If the thirst center has been damaged, DI becomes a life-threatening illness because increased water losses from the kidneys (due to the absence of ADH) are not counteracted by increased thirst and fluid intake.

DI results in hypernatremia (water deficit) from loss of water without concurrent loss of sodium. Hypernatremia is associated with serum sodium concentrations in excess of 145 mEq/L and indicates a body water deficit relative to sodium. Signs and symptoms are those of dehydration (water deficit) and include thirst, dry mucous membranes, poor skin turgor, decreased saliva and sweat production, disorientation, lethargy, and seizures.[25] The early neurologic symptoms are thought to be due to shrinkage and dehydration of neuronal cells, which are more sensitive to osmolality changes than other cell types.

Most sudden, critical presentations are straightforward, with documented hypotonic polyuria, hypernatremia, and hypertonicity indicating a defect in secretion of ADH. Individuals presenting with the sudden onset of polyuria and polydipsia should undergo laboratory studies, including tests for glucose, urine and serum electrolytes, serum creatinine, and blood urea nitrogen (BUN) levels. The results of these tests should exclude diabetes mellitus and kidney disease as the basis for the presenting complaints. A comparison of serum and urine osmolality is needed, as is a urine specific gravity measurement. Dilute urine in the presence of water deficit and hypernatremia along with abnormally low serum ADH levels are diagnostic of central DI.

A water deprivation test may be used to confirm the diagnosis. Water intake is restricted, and the urine osmolality is measured hourly. When a plateau in urine osmolality is reached, vasopressin is injected subcutaneously. With central DI, urine osmolality increases following vasopressin

administration. Polyuria and polydipsia also resolve. In the case of nephrogenic DI, little or no response to vasopressin occurs.

Treatment. Daily replacement of ADH is needed for the management of DI. DDAVP (1-deamino-8-D-arginine vasopressin), a synthetic analog of ADH, can be given by nasal insufflation.[24] One dose lasts between 8 and 24 hours. Free access to fluids is necessary, and home testing of urine specific gravity may be useful for some individuals to allow them to adjust their dose of DDAVP independently. Careful education and follow-up of these individuals are needed.

Syndrome of Inappropriate Antidiuretic Hormone Secretion

Etiology and Pathogenesis. Inappropriate secretion of excessive amounts of ADH is referred to as *syndrome of inappropriate antidiuretic hormone* secretion (SIADH). The excessive ADH is from ectopic production and has been noted in association with several types of tumors, the most common of which are primary lung malignancies. Nonmalignant lung disorders are also capable of ADH synthesis, or stimulation of central ADH production, especially pulmonary tuberculosis. Drug-induced ADH secretion occurs with the administration of a number of medications, including (but not limited to) chlorpropamide, carbamazepine, morphine, and barbiturates.

SIADH results in hyponatremia when free water is inappropriately conserved and "dilutes" the serum to a sodium concentration below the normal range (<135 mEq/L). In hyponatremia there is an excess of water relative to solute. Cells swell, and the effects of cellular swelling on neurons can be profound. Adrenal insufficiency and hypothyroidism may also cause increased ADH secretion, and hyponatremia. Both of these hormonal deficiencies must be excluded before SIADH is diagnosed.

Clinical Manifestations. Clinical manifestations are due to the hypotonicity of body fluids.[26] SIADH is characterized by hyponatremia. Urine osmolality is inappropriately high because of increased water reabsorption in the renal tubules and collecting ducts. Serum osmolality is low because of dilution by the reabsorbed water (Figure 40-13). The symptoms of SIADH include weakness, muscle cramps, nausea and vomiting, postural blood pressure changes, poor skin turgor, fatigue, anorexia, and lethargy. In very severe cases, confusion, hemiparesis (motor weakness on one side of the body), seizures, and coma may occur. Laboratory findings include low serum sodium, hematocrit, and BUN levels as a result of expansion of the extracellular fluid volume.

Treatment. Free water restriction is implemented for individuals with SIADH. Water restriction should result in a slow, steady rise in serum sodium levels and osmolality. If severe symptoms develop, intravenous (IV) administration of saline, combined with diuretic therapy, may cause loss of free water. Hyponatremia should be corrected slowly to avoid rapid changes in brain cell volume. If hyponatremia is persistent, drugs such as lithium may be used to block the effects of ADH.

FIGURE 40-13 The syndrome of inappropriate antidiuretic hormone secretion leads to hyponatremia by two mechanisms: (1) dilution of plasma and (2) increased excretion of sodium by the kidneys. Sodium excretion is increased because of the expanded plasma volume, which enhances sodium filtration and reduces sodium reabsorption. *ADH,* Antidiuretic hormone.

deprivation, which is promptly corrected with administration of vasopressin.

- DI is treated with ADH hormone replacement therapy (DDAVP) and fluid therapy.
- SIADH is associated with pulmonary tumors, central nervous system disease, and certain drugs. Excess ADH stimulates the renal tubules to reabsorb water despite decreased blood osmolality.
- Clinical manifestations of hyponatremia are associated with cellular swelling and neurologic dysfunction (e.g., confusion, coma). Water restriction and diuretics may be administered to manage hyponatremia. Detection and management of the underlying cause are paramount.

SUMMARY

Endocrine disorders present as hyperfunction or hypofunction of hormone actions. An understanding of the usual actions of hormones is useful in predicting the signs and symptoms that will be apparent with excesses and deficits. Several important hormone systems are controlled by the hypothalamic-pituitary system and disorders may occur from intrinsic defects in the target gland (primary) or abnormalities in pituitary secretion of trophic hormones (secondary). Diagnosis relies on laboratory evaluation of pituitary gland and target gland hormone levels because the signs and symptoms are similar regardless of primary or secondary etiology. The etiologies of endocrine disorders are similar regardless of the particular gland involved and include tumors, autoimmune disorders, and destruction, suppression, removal, or failure to develop, Treatment strategies are also limited and for hyperfunction include surgical removal, ablation, or drugs to block synthesis. Replacement therapy is available for most endocrine deficiency disorders and is tailored to mimic normal secretion inasmuch as possible.

KEY POINTS

- ADH secretion is primarily regulated by osmoreceptors in the hypothalamus that respond to changes in extracellular osmolality. An increase in osmolality stimulates secretion of ADH. Renal distal and collecting tubules respond to ADH by becoming more permeable to water. In the presence of ADH, water is reabsorbed from the urine filtrate, resulting in a concentrated urine.
- Central DI is due to lack of production of ADH by the hypothalamus or release by the posterior pituitary gland. Central DI may be idiopathic or related to brain surgery, trauma, or tumor.
- Nephrogenic DI is caused by lack of renal collecting tubule responsiveness to ADH. Nephrogenic DI may be caused by receptor abnormalities, renal disease, medications, or electrolyte imbalance.
- Most commonly, DI causes polydipsia accompanied by thirst, polyuria, and increased serum sodium and osmolality. Increased osmolality may cause cellular shrinkage with neurologic signs and symptoms. The diagnosis is confirmed when dilute urine is formed during water

REFERENCES

1. Porterfield SP, White BA: The hypothalamus-pituitary complex. In Porterfield SP, White BA, editors: *Endocrine physiology,* ed 3, Philadelphia, 2007, Mosby, pp 107-140.
2. Costanzo LS: Endocrine physiology. In Costanzo LS, editor: *Physiology,* ed 3, Philadelphia, 2006, Saunders, pp 377-440.
3. Hintz RL: The pituitary gland and growth failure. In Lavin N, editor: *Manual of endocrinology and metabolism,* ed 3, Philadelphia, 2002, Lippincott Williams & Wilkins.
4. Attanasio AF, Shalet SM: Growth hormone and the transition from puberty into adulthood, *Endocrinol Metab Clin North Am* 36(1):187-201, 2007.
5. Biller BM: Concepts in the diagnosis of adult growth hormone deficiency, *Horm Res* 68(Suppl 5):59-65, 2007.
6. Colao A et al: Effect of growth hormone (GH) and/or testosterone on the prostate in GH-deficient adult patients, *J Clin Endocrinol Metab* 88:88-94, 2003.
7. Murray RD, Shalet SM: Adult growth hormone replacement: lessons learned and future direction, *J Clin Endocrinol Metab* 87:4427-4428, 2002.

8. Melmed S et al: For the Acromegaly Treatment Consensus Workshop participants: guidelines for acromegaly management, *J Clin Endocrinol Metab* 87:4054-4058, 2002.

9. Lipscombe L, Asa SL, Ezzat S: Management of lesions of the pituitary stalk and hypothalamus, *Endocrinologist* 13:38-51, 2003.

10. Hershman JM: Hypothyroidism and hyperthyroidism. In Lavin N, editor: *Manual of endocrinology and metabolism*, ed 3, Philadelphia, 2002, Lippincott Williams & Wilkins.

11. Gudmundsdottir A, Schlecte JA: Central hypothyroidism, *Endocrinologist* 12:218-223, 2002.

12. Porterfield SP, White BA: The thyroid gland. In Porterfield SP, White BA, editors: *Endocrine physiology*, ed 3, Philadelphia, 2007, Mosby, pp 141-162.

13. Nieuwlaat WA, Hermus AR, Huysmans DA: Nontoxic, nodular goiter: new management paradigms, *Endocrinologist* 13:31-37, 2003.

14. Nayak B, Burman K: Thyrotoxicosis and thyroid storm, *Endocrinol Metab Clin North Am* 35(4):663-686, 2006.

15. Porterfield SP, White BA: The adrenal gland. In Porterfield SP, White BA, editors: *Endocrine physiology,* ed 3, Philadelphia, 2007, Mosby, pp 163-196.

16. Cooper MS, Stewart PM: Corticosteroid insufficiency in acutely ill patients, *N Engl J Med* 348:727-734, 2003.

17. Stern N, Tuck ML: The adrenal cortex and mineralocorticoid hypertension. In Lavin N, editor: *Manual of endocrinology and metabolism*, ed 3, Philadelphia, 2002, Lippincott Williams & Wilkins.

18. Azziz R: Polycystic ovary syndrome, insulin resistance, and molecular defects of insulin signaling, *J Clin Endocrinol Metab* 87:4085-4087, 2002.

19. Yu J, Pacak K: Management of malignant pheochromocytoma, *Endocrinologist* 12:291-299, 2002.

20. Landberg L, Young JB: Catecholamines and the adrenal medulla. In Wilson JD, Foster DW, editors: *Williams textbook of endocrinology*, ed 9, Philadelphia, 1998, Saunders.

21. Karagiannis A, Mikhailidis DP, Athyros VG et al: Pheochromocytoma: an update on genetics and management, *Endocr Relat Cancer* 14(4):935-956, 2007.

22. Brickman AS: Disorders of calcitropic hormones in adults. In Lavin N, editor: *Manual of endocrinology and metabolism*, ed 3, Philadelphia, 2002, Lippincott Williams & Wilkins.

23. Recker BF: Pregnancy at risk: metabolic and renal alterations. In Dickason EJ, Silverman BL, Schult MO, editors: *Maternal-infant nursing care*, ed 2, St Louis, 1994, Mosby.

24. Ball SG: Vasopressin and disorders of water balance: the physiology and pathophysiology of vasopressin, *Ann Clin Biochem* 44(Pt 5):417-431, 2007.

25. Loh JA, Verbalis JG: Diabetes insipidus as a complication after pituitary surgery, *Nat Clin Pract Endocrinol Metab* 3(6):489-494, 2007.

26. Moses AM et al: Central diabetes insipidus due to cytomegalovirus infection of the hypothalamus in a patient with acquired immunodeficiency syndrome: a clinical, pathological and immunohistochemical case study, *J Clin Endocrinol Metab* 88:51-54, 2003.

chapter

41

Diabetes Mellitus

Lorrie J. Dawson

MEDIA RESOURCES

Additional Material for Study, Review, and Further Exploration

CD Companion ■ Review Questions and Answers
■ Glossary (with audio pronunciations for selected terms)
■ Disease Profiles ■ Animations

ⓔvolve **Website** at http://evolve.elsevier.com/Copstead/
■ Case Studies ■ Disease Profiles ■ WebLinks ■ Key Points Review

Online Course (Module 17)

KEY QUESTIONS

■ Which hormones are involved in regulation of serum glucose, and under what physiologic conditions would each be secreted?
■ What are the differentiating characteristics of type 1 and type 2 diabetes?
■ How do the pathophysiologic processes differ among the various types of diabetes?

■ What clinical findings are associated with hyperglycemia, and how do they differ from those of hypoglycemia?
■ How is diabetes mellitus diagnosed, monitored, and managed?
■ What are the acute and chronic complications of diabetes mellitus?

CHAPTER OUTLINE

The public health impact of diabetes mellitus is enormous. In the United States, nearly 21 million persons (7% of the population) have diabetes mellitus, although it is estimated that only 70% are aware of their diagnosis. Should this trend continue unabated, worldwide the number of persons with diabetes will rise to 366 million by 2015.[1] The annual cost of diabetes to the U.S. medical care system was estimated to be $176 billion in 2007, with half of the total cost attributed to inpatient diabetes care.[2] Diabetes mellitus is the sixth leading cause of death and a major cause of disability in the United States. It increases the risk for heart disease, end-stage renal disease, blindness, amputation, and complications of pregnancy. The disease disproportionately affects non-Caucasian and elderly individuals.[3]

REGULATION OF GLUCOSE METABOLISM

Because diabetes mellitus affects the utilization of all energy nutrients, it is helpful to review energy nutrient metabolism to understand the disease process of diabetes mellitus. The energy requirements of humans are predominantly met by glucose and fats. Produced from endogenous glycogen stores in the muscles and liver or manufactured from such substrates as amino acids and lactate, glucose is supplied to the bloodstream from the gastrointestinal tract and liver. Glucose is typically present in greater quantities in extracellular fluid than within cells.[3]

The plasma membranes of cells are variously permeable to glucose, and the diffusion of glucose into some cells is controlled by glucose transporters (GLUT 1-4) specific to each tissue. The glucose transporters of endothelial cells of the brain and erythrocytes (GLUT 1) do not require activation with the hormone insulin. Heart, adipose, and skeletal muscle cells possess insulin receptors on the cell membrane that bind to insulin and activate glucose transporters (GLUT 4), increasing glucose-transport threefold immediately.[4] Activated glucose transporters translocate to the cell membrane and facilitate the diffusion of glucose. Insulin may have additional, as yet undefined, roles in glucose uptake.[5]

Hormonal Regulation

Protein and fat metabolism are regulated by the anabolic effects of insulin. Insulin is synthesized in the pancreas by the β cells of the islets of Langerhans. The islets are groups of cells dispersed throughout the pancreas. Within the islets can be found β cells that produce insulin in the form of proinsulin, α cells that produce glucagon, δ cells that produce somatostatin, and F cells that produce pancreatic polypeptide. Proinsulin is produced and packaged into granules. Enzymes within the granules cleave proinsulin into insulin and C-peptide, with some remaining proinsulin. Granules release their contents into the bloodstream by exocytosis. Insulin appears to increase the uptake and decrease the release of amino acids by skeletal muscle, thus inducing protein synthesis and preventing muscle breakdown. The amount of stored fats in the form of triglyceride is potentiated by the action of insulin in preventing fat breakdown and inducing lipid formation. Insulin also appears to have a role in growth by stimulating the secretion of IGF-1 (somatomedin).[5]

Normal glucose metabolism is usually described in reference to the fed and fasting (or absorptive and postabsorptive) states. The fed state occurs after ingestion of a meal and is characterized by utilization and storage of ingested energy nutrients. The fasting state is characterized by utilization of stored nutrients for the energy needs of the body.[5]

In the fed state, glucose from ingested food provides the primary energy source (Figure 41-1). The post-meal rise in blood glucose and the presence of certain gastrointestinal hormones stimulate the production of insulin. Initial stimulation produces a brief rise in insulin secretion, termed the *first phase*. The continued presence of increased glucose produces the second phase of insulin secretion, a state characterized by insulin synthesis. Amylin is a peptide hormone produced by pancreatic β cells and co-secreted with insulin. Amylin acts upon the area postrema (AP) in the brain to inhibit gastric emptying, suppress glucagon release, and induce satiety.[6]

The ingestion of nutrients stimulates the release of glucose-dependent insulinotropic polypeptide (GIP) and glucagon-like peptide 1 (GLP-1) from cells in the gut. Both hormones stimulate production of insulin in the presence of glucose, promote proliferation of β cells, and inhibit apoptosis. The presence of these hormones and their effect on blood glucose is known as the *incretin* effect, as they are not secreted with parenteral nutrition. In addition, GLP-1 delays gastric emptying, inhibits glucagon production, and increases satiety.[7]

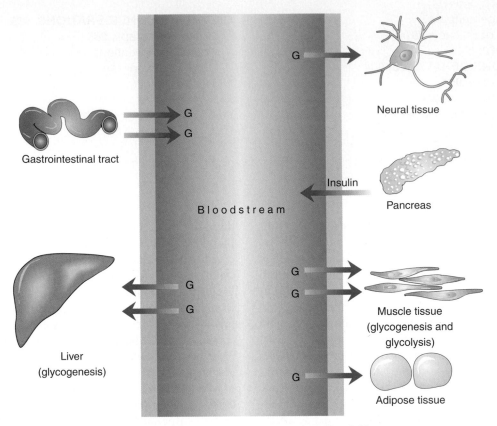

FIGURE 41-1 Energy metabolism in the fed state. *G*, Glucose.

The presence of insulin stimulates the diffusion of glucose into adipose and muscle tissue and inhibits the production of glucose by the liver. After diffusion into the cell, glucose may be oxidized for the energy needs of the cell, a process termed *glycolysis.* Most ingested glucose is utilized in *glycogenesis* (production of glycogen in the muscle and the liver).

In the fasting state, glucose is produced by glycogenolysis (breakdown of stored glycogen) in the liver and muscles and by gluconeogenesis (production of glucose from amino acids and other substrates) in the liver (Figure 41-2). Insulin levels, no longer stimulated by an influx of ingested glucose, fall to a basal level. The catabolic effects of the absence of insulin are evident in the stimulation of glycogenolysis and are accompanied by a rise in glucagon levels. If insulin is the hormone that dominates the fed state, glucagon dominates the fasting state. Glucagon-stimulated glycogenolysis and gluconeogenesis are responsible for up to 75% of glucose production in the fasting state. The primary source of energy to muscle tissue in the fasting state is free fatty acids produced by lipolysis (breakdown of fat from adipose tissue). Lipolysis is stimulated by the fall in plasma insulin.[8]

Other hormones referred to as *counterregulatory hormones* have a role in glucose metabolism in the fasting state. Corticosteroids stimulate gluconeogenesis and counteract the hypoglycemic action of insulin. Growth hormone increases peripheral insulin resistance and prevents insulin from suppressing hepatic glucose production. Catecholamines augment glucose production by prompting hepatic glycogenolysis and gluconeogenesis.[8]

Exercise

Increasing activity requires increased fuel for muscle tissue. At the onset of exercise, insulin levels drop and glucagon and catecholamine levels initially rise and increase the production of free fatty acids, the primary energy source of resting muscle (Figure 41-3). Falling insulin levels and increased glucagon levels stimulate glycogenolysis. Under the influence of catecholamines, muscle tissue shifts from using primarily fatty acids for fuel to using stored glycogen. The relative absence of insulin and increased production of glucagon also stimulate hepatic glycogenolysis. Glucose released by the liver increasingly meets the energy needs of muscle tissue as exercise continues. After 10 to 40 minutes of exercise, blood glucose use by muscle tissue increases 7 to 20 times. The interactions of hormones thus produce the mixture of glucose and free fatty acids used by muscle tissue during exercise.[8]

Muscle tissue is affected not only by the influence of hormones but also by exercise itself. The postreceptor activities of glucose transporters are enhanced by muscular contraction. The resulting increase in insulin sensitivity can last as long as 16 hours. Thus in normal metabolism, increased insulin sensitivity allows normal blood glucose values in the presence of lower levels of circulating insulin.

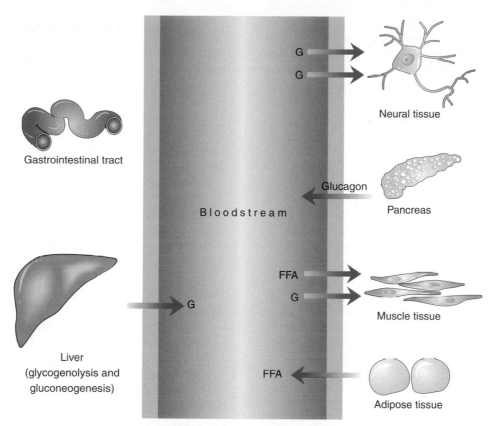

FIGURE 41-2 Energy metabolism in the fasting state. *G,* Glucose; *FFA,* free fatty acids.

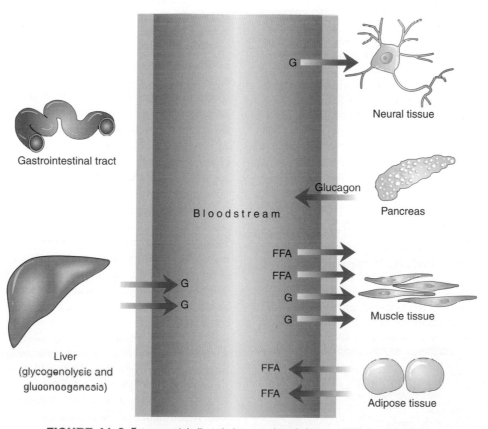

FIGURE 41-3 Energy metabolism during exercise. *G,* Glucose, *FFA,* free fatty acids.

Stress

During stress such as injury, illness, and pain, stress hormones, including corticosteroids and catecholamines, interact to ensure continuous supplies of glucose. Corticosteroids increase the production of glucose in the liver and elevate the production of glucagon. Glucocorticoids also decrease the utilization of glucose by muscle tissue by diminishing the effect of insulin on glucose transporters and by generating a decline in the number of insulin receptors and their function.

Catecholamines increase serum glucagon levels, increase glucose production by the liver, and decrease the use of glucose by muscle and fat tissue. The production of fatty acids that is triggered by the action of catecholamines further inhibits glucose uptake in the periphery. The series of events produced by traumatic stress is referred to as *stress hyperglycemia*.

Psychological stress can produce metabolic changes comparable with those of physical stress. Deterioration in metabolic control has been noted in stressed diabetic subjects. However, the response is by no means universal. An actual decrease in blood glucose levels has frequently been observed during acute stress, perhaps reflecting differing individual responses to psychological stress (e.g., disordered eating).[8]

KEY POINTS

- Plasma membrane permeability to glucose is determined by the type and density of glucose transport proteins in the membrane. In some tissues, particularly muscle and fat, the density of glucose transporters is regulated by insulin. Insulin binding to receptors on the cell surface results in translocation of glucose transporters to the cell surface. Glucose enters the cell passively by facilitated diffusion. Neurons and erythrocytes have glucose transporters that do not require insulin.

- The metabolic effects of insulin include enhancing protein synthesis and inhibiting gluconeogenesis, enhancing fat deposition and inhibiting lipolysis, and stimulating cellular growth by enhancing somatomedin secretion. Insulin is synthesized in pancreatic β cells as proinsulin. Proinsulin is stored in granules, where it is cleaved into insulin and C-peptide. A postprandial rise in glucose and other substrates stimulates the release of insulin into the bloodstream. During fasting, when blood glucose levels fall, the decrease in insulin and the increase in glucagon secretion lead to lipolysis, glycogenolysis, and gluconeogenesis.

- Exercise has complex effects on glucose metabolism. The decrease in insulin production and the increase in glucagon and catecholamines lead to elevated blood glucose levels. However, exercising muscle has increased insulin sensitivity, which facilitates glucose uptake for as long as 16 hours after exercise.

- A number of hormones released during stress increase blood glucose levels and oppose the effects of insulin. Catecholamines, glucocorticoids, and glucagon may precipitate stress hyperglycemia.

GLUCOSE INTOLERANCE DISORDERS

Classification of Glucose Intolerance Disorders

Diabetes mellitus is not a single disease entity; as many as 30 different disorders may be called diabetes. Criteria for diagnosing the different conditions, all associated with glucose intolerance, were established by the Expert Committee on the Diagnosis and Classification of Diabetes Mellitus in 1997, and most recently updated in 2008.[9]

Classifications include four clinical classes and two pre-diabetes classes (Box 41-1). The four clinical classes are type 1 diabetes mellitus, type 2 diabetes mellitus, other specific types of diabetes mellitus, and gestational diabetes mellitus. Pre-diabetes classes are impaired glucose tolerance and impaired fasting glucose tolerance.

Diabetes Mellitus

Guidelines for the diagnosis of diabetes mellitus have been developed by the Expert Committee for the Classification of Diabetes Mellitus (Box 41-2).[9] The diagnostic criteria were revised in 1997 to more accurately reflect the degree of hyperglycemia associated with the onset of diabetic complications. The same diagnostic criteria apply in type 1, type 2, and other specific types of diabetes mellitus, and some of the same pathophysiologic processes are present in these disorders. The diagnostic criteria for impaired fasting glucose (IFG) was revised in 2003, and in 2008 IFG and impaired glucose tolerance (IGT) were classified as pre-diabetes.[9] The pathophysiologic and etiologic mechanisms of type 1 and type 2 diabetes mellitus are different, with resulting differences in sequelae.

Type 1 Diabetes Mellitus. Type 1 diabetes mellitus is, by definition, characterized by destruction of the β cells of the pancreas. Type 1 diabetes can occur at any age but is most commonly diagnosed in individuals between the ages of 5 and 20 years. Type 1 diabetes affects about 5% to 10% of individuals with diabetes mellitus in the United States. The incidence is 1 in every 400 to 600 children and adolescents. Caucasian populations are more susceptible to type 1 diabetes mellitus than are African-American, Hispanic, Asian, or Native American populations. Little difference is noted in the incidence of type 1 diabetes mellitus under the age of 15. However, more men than women are affected in the population.[10]

Etiology. The two forms of type 1 diabetes mellitus are immune-mediated and idiopathic. Immune-mediated type 1 diabetes is the result of an autoimmune attack on the β cells of the pancreas. A strong association with the presence of a gene or genes in the major histocompatibility complex on chromosome 6 has been observed. Genes in the major histocompatibility complex (MHC) are responsible for the creation of cell surface proteins (human leukocyte antigens, or HLAs) that interact with lymphocytes to stimulate or suppress antibody production. The DR3 and DR4 MHC genes are associated with the development of type 1 diabetes mellitus.[11]

Environment and heredity are factors in the development of immune-mediated type 1 diabetes mellitus.[8] The incidence

---

BOX 41-1

Classifications of Glucose Metabolism Disorders

Type 1 Diabetes Mellitus
  Immune mediated
  Idiopathic

Type 2 Diabetes Mellitus

Other Specific Types of Diabetes
Genetic Defects of β-Cell Function
Chromosome 12, *HNF1A* (formerly *MODY3*)
Chromosome 7, glucokinase (formerly *MODY2*)
Chromosome 20, *HNF4A* (formerly *MODY1*)
Chromosome 13, insulin promoter factor-1 (IPF-1, MODY4)
Chromosome 17, HNF-1β (MODY5)
Chromosome 2, *Neuro*D1 (MODY6)
Mitochondrial DNA
Others
Genetic Defects in Insulin Action
Type A insulin resistance
Leprechaunism
Rabson-Mendenhall syndrome
Lipoatrophic diabetes
Others
Diseases of the Exocrine Pancreas
Pancreatitis
Trauma pancreatectomy
Neoplasia
Cystic fibrosis
Hemochromatosis
Fibrocalculous pancreatopathy
Others
Endocrinopathies
Acromegaly
Cushing syndrome
Glucagonoma
Pheochromocytoma
Hyperthyroidism
Somatostatinoma
Aldosteronoma
Others

Drug or Chemical Induced
Pyriminil (Vacor)
Pentamidine
Nicotinic acid
Glucocorticoids
Thyroid hormone
Diazoxide
β-Adrenergic agonists
Thiazides
Phenytoin (Dilantin)
Interferon-α
Others
Infections
Congenital rubella
Cytomegalovirus
Others
Uncommon Forms of Immune-Mediated Diabetes
Stiff-man syndrome
Anti-insulin receptor antibodies
Others
Other Genetic Syndromes Sometimes Associated with Diabetes
Down syndrome
Klinefelter syndrome
Turner syndrome
Friedreich ataxia
Huntington chorea
Laurence-Moon-Beidl syndrome
Myotonic dystrophy
Porphyria
Prader-Willi syndrome
Others

Gestational Diabetes Mellitus

Pre-Diabetes Mellitus
Impaired glucose tolerance
Impaired fasting glucose tolerance

Data from American Diabetes Association: Diagnosis and Classification of Diabetes Mellitus, *Diabetes Care* 31(S1):S55-S60, 2008.

---

of immune-mediated diabetes in identical twins when one twin is affected is 25% to 50%. Viral infection or exposure to a toxic agent may be the responsible environmental influence.

Antibodies against glutamic acid decarboxylase 65 (GAD65), insulinoma-antigen 2(IA-2), or insulin frequently appear early in the onset of immune-mediated diabetes. Antibodies may be present for as long as 9 years before diagnosis. The order of appearance of antibodies is not necessarily obvious; however, the presence of multiple antibodies is highly predictive of type 1 diabetes.[11] The presence of hyperglycemia indicates that autoimmune destruction of β cells has reached the point at which insulin secretion is inadequate.

Recognition of the autoimmune component in the pathogenesis of immune-mediated type 1 diabetes has led to varying attempts to prevent the disease. Immunosuppressive agents such as cyclosporine and azathioprine have been effective in some human studies. Oral delivery of insulin from animal species to reduce the reaction to islet cell antibodies has been proposed as a preventive measure, as has nicotinamide.[11]

The etiologic progression of idiopathic type 1 diabetes mellitus is not known. Idiopathic diabetes is associated with β-cell destruction without autoimmune markers or HLA association.

Pathogenesis and Clinical Manifestations. Type 1 diabetes mellitus is characterized by an absolute insulin deficiency, and thus glucose cannot enter muscle and adipose tissue (Figure 41-4). Production of glucose by the liver is no longer opposed by insulin. Overproduction of glucagon by pancreatic α cells stimulates glycogenolysis and gluconeogenesis. Plasma blood glucose levels rise. When the maximal tubular absorptive capacity of the kidney is exceeded, glucose is lost in the urine, and the resulting glycosuria and osmotic fluid loss eventually lead to profound hypovolemia. Tissues dependent on insulin for glucose transport do not have glucose available as a substrate. Neural tissue in the brain responds to this emergency by promoting eating behavior. The thirst, (polydipsia), increased urination (polyuria), and hunger (polyphagia) resulting from the aforementioned processes are the classic symptoms of diabetes.[8]

Continued insulin deficiency and other hormonal influences (increased levels of catecholamines, cortisol, glucagon, and growth hormone, in part caused by hypovolemia, physical stress, or insulin deficiency itself) lead to lipolysis in body tissues. As the catabolic process continues, metabolism of fats stored in adipose tissue leads to the production of fatty acids. The resulting fatty acids undergo transformation to keto acids in the liver. Hepatic gluconeogenesis in response to tissue glucose deprivation is also responsible for the increased production of keto acids. Under normal circumstances, keto acids can be used by neural and muscle tissue in energy metabolism. When the normal pathway is saturated, the pH falls (6.8 to 7.3) and ketone bodies are present in the urine, thus sharply increasing osmotic fluid loss. Metabolic acidosis ensues as the bicarbonate concentration decreases, and diabetic ketoacidosis results. In response to the metabolic acidosis, extracellular

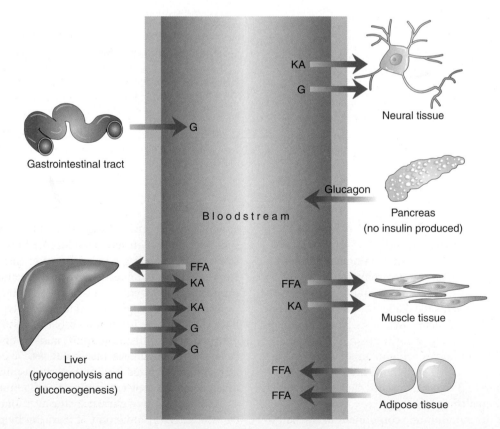

FIGURE 41-4 Pathophysiology of energy metabolism in diabetes mellitus type 1. *G,* Glucose; *FFA,* free fatty acids; *KA,* keto acids.

hydrogen ions are exchanged for intracellular potassium ions. Serum potassium levels rise (transient hyperkalemia) and excess potassium is excreted into the urine, eventually leading to a net potassium loss. Losses of sodium, magnesium, and phosphorus also occur as total body water decreases. Serum levels of the ions may be normal or elevated owing to hypovolemia. Hypovolemia also accounts for an increased hematocrit, hemoglobin (Hb), protein, white blood cell count, creatinine, and serum osmolality (Table 41-1). Lactic acidosis, or an excessive amount of lactate, a product of glucose metabolism, can also be present because of hypovolemia and possibly reduced uptake of lactate by the liver as a result of acidosis. Hypovolemia and muscle catabolism are responsible for the significant weight loss present in persons with ketoacidosis and often at diagnosis of type 1 diabetes. Hypovolemic shock can lead to death if the patient is not promptly treated.[8]

Respiratory compensation for the metabolic acidosis in the form of deep, labored respirations that are "fruity" in odor (Kussmaul respirations) results in lowered Pco_2 values (compensatory respiratory alkalosis). Ketoacidosis may be the initial symptom of a new diagnosis of type 1 diabetes. Other factors that may precipitate ketoacidosis are intercurrent illness and inadequate treatment. The need for hospitalization for diabetic ketoacidosis is greatest for individuals <45 years of age, (39.7 per 1000 individuals with diabetes).[8]

Type 2 Diabetes Mellitus

Etiology. Individuals with type 2 diabetes mellitus are resistant to the action of insulin on peripheral tissues. Type 2 diabetes mellitus affects 90% to 95% of individuals with diabetes in the United States. Non-Caucasian and elderly populations are disproportionately affected. The prevalence of diabetes is 8.7% in the non-Hispanic white population, 13.3% in non-Hispanic blacks, and 9.5% in Hispanic/Latino-Americans. The prevalence of diabetes in Native American populations ranges from 8.1% to 27.6%. Overall, close to 21% of American individuals older than 60 years have diabetes mellitus. One of every 6 overweight adolescents age 12 to 19 has type 2 diabetes,

about 2 million in all. The prevalence of diabetes mellitus is 10.9% among men age 20 or older and 8.8% in women of the same age.[3]

Risk factors include aging and a sedentary lifestyle, but the most powerful predictor is obesity. Excessive abdominal (visceral) fat introduces a greater threat of diabetes mellitus (and cardiovascular disease) than does lower body obesity. The initial symptoms of polydipsia, polyuria, polyphagia, and weight loss may be subtle or absent in type 2 diabetic patients.[3]

Epidemiologic studies indicate a strong genetic component, but no specific Human Leukocyte Antigen (HLA) type has been identified. Studies indicate that the prevalence of type 2 diabetes mellitus in identical twins when one twin is affected is close to 100%.[12]

Pathogenesis and Clinical Manifestations. Type 2 diabetes is characterized by a relative lack of insulin. The processes instrumental in producing the relative lack of insulin are insulin resistance and β-cell dysfunction (Figure 41-5).[3,12]

The insulin resistance of type 2 diabetes mellitus is defined as a requirement for more insulin for the same biological action, along with lowered glucose utilization at all levels of insulin concentration. A decreased number of insulin receptors and such postreceptor defects as decreased action of glucose transporters are associated with insulin resistance. Impaired glycogen synthesis may also be a factor in the development of type 2 diabetes.[13] Impaired production of insulin by the pancreatic β cells that intensifies as the disease progresses is also present in type 2 diabetes mellitus. Individuals with type 2 diabetes mellitus ultimately have an absent first-phase insulin response and a diminished second-phase response.

Basal insulin secretion may be higher than normal in type 2 diabetes. Glucagon secretion is increased absolutely or relatively (relative to insulin levels). The incretin effect, stimulation of insulin secretion by GLP-1 and GIP, is diminished in type 2 diabetes.[7,12] Individuals with type 2 diabetes may be predominantly insulin resistant or predominantly insulin deficient.

Type 2 diabetes mellitus is a progressive disease characterized by the development of insulin resistance, at first compensated for by increased insulin production and hyperinsulinemia. Decompensation occurs as the impaired β cells are unable to produce sufficient insulin to overcome insulin resistance. Insulin levels, however, remain elevated above normal until later in progression of the disease. Relatively decreased insulin levels, continued insulin resistance, and hyperglucagonemia result in the hyperglycemia of diabetes. Hyperglycemia itself may then increase insulin resistance and further diminish insulin secretion. The latter process has been termed *glucose toxicity*.[12]

The relative lack of insulin seen in individuals with type 2 diabetes mellitus leads to similar but not identical sequelae as the absolute lack of insulin of type 1 diabetes mellitus. The initial symptoms of polyuria, polydipsia, and polyphagia may be present, possibly in a more subtle form. Ketoacidosis is an uncommon occurrence in type 2 diabetes. The presence of endogenous insulin in type 2 diabetes suppresses the lipolysis that leads to the production of ketone bodies and

---

TABLE 41-1

Diabetic Ketoacidosis and Nonketotic Hyperglycemic Hyperosmolar Coma

Parameter	Diabetic Ketoacidosis	Nonketotic Hyperglycemic Hyperosmolar Coma
Glucose	>300 mg/dl	>600 mg/dl
Urine ketones	Moderate to high	None
pH	6.8-7.3	Normal
Na+, K+	Low, normal, or high	Low, normal, or high
Hct, Hb, protein, WBC, Cr, BUN, serum osmolality	High	High

BUN, Blood urea nitrogen; *Cr,* creatinine; *Hb,* hemoglobin; *Hct,* hematocrit; *WBC,* white blood cell count.

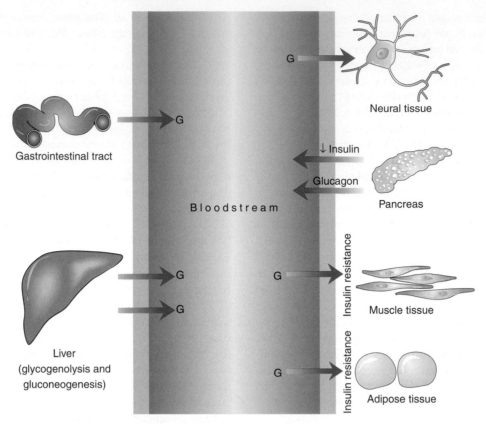

FIGURE 41-5 Pathophysiology of energy metabolism in diabetes mellitus type 2. *G,* Glucose.

subsequently ketoacidosis in type 1 diabetes mellitus. More common in type 2 diabetes mellitus, especially in older individuals, is nonketotic hyperglycemic hyperosmolar coma, characterized by severe hyperglycemia with no or slight ketosis and striking dehydration. Nonketotic hyperglycemic hyperosmolar coma is more likely to occur in institutionalized patients, especially patients unable to recognize or respond appropriately to thirst. Diabetic ketoacidosis and nonketotic hyperosmolar coma can be life-threatening events, especially in the elderly. Seventy percent of all cases of nonketotic hyperglycemic hyperosmolar coma occur in individuals older than 64 years. The mortality rate is approximately 11%.[14]

Other Specific Types of Diabetes

- Genetic defects of β cells: The genetic defects of β cells follow an autosomal dominant pattern of inheritance and are characterized by a defect in the production of insulin. Affected individuals are identified before they reach 25 years of age, respond to oral sulfonylureas, and are nonketotic. The disorder is also referred to as "mature-onset diabetes of the young" (MODY).
- Genetic defects in insulin action: The disorders listed in Box 41-1 result in relatively rare, genetically determined defects of the insulin receptor.
- Diseases of the exocrine pancreas: Diseases of the pancreas can affect the insulin-producing capability of the organ (see Box 41-1).

- Endocrinopathies: Excessive production of insulin antagonists (e.g., cortisol, growth hormone, glucagon, epinephrine) affects glucose metabolism (see Box 41-1).
- Drug- or chemical-induced diabetes: Many chemicals can affect the ability of the pancreas to produce insulin (see Box 41-1).
- Infections: Destruction of the β cells of the pancreas has been linked to various infectious agents (see Box 41-1).
- Uncommon forms of immune-mediated diabetes.
- Certain autoimmune disorders are linked to glucose intolerance (see Box 41-1).
- Other genetic syndromes sometimes associated with diabetes: Certain genetic syndromes are linked to glucose intolerance (see Box 41-1).

Gestational Diabetes Mellitus. Gestational diabetes mellitus (GDM) is by definition a disorder of glucose intolerance of variable severity with onset or first recognition during pregnancy. Approximately 4% (may range from 1% to 14% depending on population) of pregnancies are affected by gestational diabetes. GDM represents 90% of all pregnancies complicated by diabetes.[9]

Etiology. In its pathophysiologic characteristics, gestational diabetes mellitus closely resembles type 2 diabetes mellitus. As in type 2 diabetes, tissue insulin resistance is present during normal pregnancy. Insulin resistance in normal pregnancy is most likely precipitated by the presence of placental hormones: human chorionic somatomammotropin, estrogen, and cortisol. The weight gain of pregnancy is also responsible for an increase in insulin resistance. During pregnancy, women require two to three times as much insulin as they do in the nonpregnant state. Women with gestational diabetes are unable to produce sufficient insulin to meet their needs during pregnancy.[9]

Risk factors for gestational diabetes mellitus include severe obesity, history of gestational diabetes, previous offspring weighing more than 9 lb at birth, presence of glycosuria, or a strong family history of type 2 diabetes. High-risk individuals should be screened as soon as possible after confirmation of pregnancy. Because insulin needs rise sharply in the 24th to 28th weeks of pregnancy, it is recommended that all pregnant women older than 25 years be screened for gestational diabetes during the 24th to 28th weeks with either 50 or 100 grams of oral glucose. Younger pregnant women who are obese, have a first-degree relative with diabetes, are members of an ethnic/racial group with a high prevalence of diabetes (e.g., African-American, Hispanic, Asian, Native American), have a history of abnormal glucose tolerance, or have a history of poor obstetrical outcome should also be screened. If the venous plasma glucose concentration is 140 mg/dl or greater with 50 g of glucose, an oral glucose tolerance test is performed using 100 g load (Table 41-2).[15] Untreated gestational diabetes can result in metabolic abnormalities and stillbirth. However, the most common complications of gestational diabetes are macrosomia and neonatal hypoglycemia. Macrosomia (birth weight greater than 4,000 g or >90% for gestational age) is a result of increased glucose, free fatty acids, and amino acids delivered to the fetus. Neonatal hypoglycemia is due to increased production of insulin by the fetal pancreas in response to the chronic stimulation of hyperglycemia while in utero.[16,17]

Treatment. Management of gestational diabetes mellitus includes dietary counseling, exercise, and blood glucose and urine ketone monitoring. If hyperglycemia persists, insulin therapy should be initiated. Only glyburide does not cross the placenta to cause fetal hypoglycemia; this sulfonylurea may be used in gestational diabetes mellitus.[15,16]

Glucose tolerance will return to normal after parturition in 97% of women with gestational diabetes mellitus. Women with gestational diabetes mellitus have a markedly increased risk for the development of type 2 diabetes mellitus or an impairment in glucose tolerance later in life, especially within the first 5 years postpartum.[17] In subsequent pregnancies, recurrence varies between 30% and 84% in women with a history of gestational diabetes mellitus.[18]

Pre-Diabetes

Impaired Glucose Tolerance and Impaired Fasting Glucose Tolerance

Guidelines for diagnosing the categories of impaired glucose tolerance (IGT) and impaired fasting glucose tolerance (IFG) are listed in Box 41-2. Impaired glucose tolerance and IFG are intermediate stages between normal glucose metabolism and the onset of diabetes. They represent risk factors for the development of diabetes and are also risk factors for the onset of cardiovascular disease. The latter association is not fully understood.

Screening for Diabetes

Because of the high prevalence of undiagnosed type 2 diabetes mellitus, current recommendations are to screen all adults over the age of 45 for diabetes at least every 3 years. There is some controversy regarding screening individuals with asymptomatic disease. Individuals with risk factors should be screened at more frequent intervals (Box 41-3).[15] No diagnostic criteria use Hb_{A1c} as yet because of a lack of standardization of methods of measurement.

BOX 41-3
Screening for Diabetes

Testing should be considered in all adults over age 30 who are overweight (BMI ≥ 25 kg/m²*) and have additional risk factors:

Physical inactivity
 First-degree relative with diabetes
 Members of a high-risk ethnic population (e.g., African American, Latino, Native American, Asian American, and Pacific Islander)
 Women who delivered a baby weighing >9 lb or were diagnosed with GDM
 Hypertension (≥140/90 mm Hg) or on therapy for hypertension
 HDL cholesterol level <35 mg/dl and/or a triglyceride level >250 mg/dl
 Women with polycystic ovarian syndrome
IGT or IFG on previous testing
Other clinical conditions associated with insulin resistance (e.g., severe obesity and acanthosis nigricans)
History of CVD
In the absence of the above criteria, testing for pre-diabetes and diabetes should begin at age 45 years.
If results are normal, testing should be repeated at least at 3-year intervals, with consideration of more frequent testing depending on initial results and risk status.

Data from American Diabetes Association: Standards of Medical Care in Diabetes, *Diabetes Care* 31(S1):S12-S54, 2008.

HDL, High-density lipoprotein; *IGT*, impaired glucose tolerance; *IFG*, impaired fasting glucose tolerance.

TABLE 41-2		
Diagnosis of GDM with a 100-g or 75-g glucose load		
	100-g glucose load	**75-g glucose load**
Fasting	95 mg/dl	95 mg/dl
1-hour	180 mg/dl	180 mg/dl
2-hour	155 mg/dl	155 mg/dl
3-hour	140 mg/dl	**

Two or more blood glucose determinations must be equal to or greater than these values to establish the diagnosis. The test should be done in the morning after an overnight fast of between 8 and 14 hours and after at least 3 days of unrestricted diet (150 g carbohydrate per day) and unlimited physical activity. The subject should remain seated and should not smoke throughout the test.

Data from American Diabetes Association: Diagnosis and Classification of Diabetes Mellitus, *Diabetes Care* 31(S1):S55-S60, 2008.

Screening for gestational diabetes is discussed in the Gestational Diabetes Mellitus section. It is not recommended that routine screening for type 1 diabetes mellitus be performed. No agreement has been reached on the blood level of immune markers that represents a risk for type 1 diabetes or on treatment after identification of the presence of such markers.[15]

KEY POINTS

- Diabetes mellitus is an endocrine disorder diagnosed by the presence of chronic hyperglycemia. Diabetes is diagnosed if any of the following conditions occurs on more than one occasion: a random sampling of blood glucose above 200 mg/dl with classic signs and symptoms, a fasting blood glucose level of greater than 126 mg/dl, or a blood glucose concentration greater than 200 mg/dl 2 hours after a 75-g oral glucose load.

- The classification of diabetes mellitus includes two broad categories: (1) actual glucose intolerance and (2) the risk of glucose intolerance. Disorders of actual glucose intolerance include type 1, type 2, other specific types, and gestational diabetes. Pre-diabetes categories include individuals with impaired glucose tolerance and those with impaired fasting glucose tolerance. Individuals at risk for glucose intolerance include those with a history of glucose intolerance and those with a positive family history, obesity, or other risk factors.

- Persons with type 1 diabetes have an absolute insulin deficiency caused by pancreatic β-cell failure. Immune-mediated type 1 diabetes is associated with a specific HLA genetic makeup and may be autoimmune. Idiopathic type 1 diabetes is not an autoimmune process. Type 1 diabetes may affect people of any age. Classic manifestations include polyuria, polydipsia, polyphagia, and weight loss. Persons with type 1 diabetes are more prone to the development of ketoacidosis because of lipolysis associated with absolute insulin deficiency.

- Persons with type 2 diabetes have a relative insulin deficiency caused by decreased tissue sensitivity and decreased responsiveness to insulin. A decreased number of insulin receptors or abnormal translocation of glucose transporters is suspected. As the disease progresses, pancreatic insulin production may become impaired. Obesity, female sex, family history, older age, and lack of exercise are risk factors. Individuals with type 2 diabetes are prone to the development of nonketotic hyperglycemic hyperosmolar coma.

- Gestational diabetes is a disorder of glucose intolerance that is diagnosed during pregnancy. Placental hormones and weight gain are contributing factors. High infant birth weight and neonatal hypoglycemia are common complications. Gestational diabetes is a risk factor for the later development of type 2 diabetes.

- Ketoacidosis occurs primarily in type 1 diabetes mellitus as a result of increased lipolysis and conversion to ketone bodies. Excessive ketones result in metabolic acidosis, which is recognized by a fall in pH and bicarbonate levels. Ketoacidosis may occur in patients with type 2 diabetes mellitus under severe stress, such as concomitant sepsis, stroke, or myocardial infarction. Acidosis-induced hyperkalemia and compensatory hyperventilation (Kussmaul respirations) resulting in reduced arterial carbon dioxide are associated findings.

- Hyperosmolar coma is more common in type 2 diabetes because endogenous insulin suppresses ketone formation and thus prevents ketoacidosis. Hyperglycemia may go untreated for a time and result in persistent glycosuria with osmotic diuresis. Dehydration may be manifested as high osmolality and hemoconcentration of erythrocytes, proteins, and creatinine.

CLINICAL MANIFESTATIONS AND COMPLICATIONS

Acute Hyperglycemia

Etiology. Acute hyperglycemia is most commonly caused by alterations in nutrition, inactivity, inadequate use of antidiabetic medications, or any combination of these factors. Persistent fasting hyperglycemia can occasionally be attributed to the dawn phenomenon, which is a rise in blood glucose concentration in the early morning hours attributed to increased growth hormone, cortisol, glucagon and epinephrine release.[8,12]

Complications. A primary concern of individuals with diabetes and their health care providers is avoiding the acute and chronic complications of diabetes. Acute complications of diabetes include the signs and symptoms of hyperglycemia—polydipsia, polyphagia, and polyuria—and concomitant metabolic and fluid problems. Prolonged insulinopenia can result in ketoacidosis and nonketotic hyperglycemic coma with the accompanying more severe electrolyte and fluid derangements.[15]

Acute complications of diabetes also include infections, most commonly of the skin, urinary tract, and vagina. Infections that particularly affect elderly diabetic patients include malignant otitis externa, necrotizing fasciitis, and persistent candidal infections. Tuberculosis infection and reactivation can be a particular problem in diabetic residents of extended care facilities.[15]

Nausea, fatigue, and a generally decreased sense of wellbeing frequently accompany hyperglycemia. Blurred vision is a common short-term problem of acute hyperglycemia. These symptoms can be quite distressing and uncomfortable. Acute complications are directly linked to hyperglycemia and recede as euglycemia is approached.[15]

Chronic Hyperglycemia

Chronic complications associated with diabetes are extensive and are generally placed into two categories: vascular and neuropathic. The vascular complications are further subdivided into macrovascular and microvascular components. Microvascular complications affect the capillaries, and macrovascular complications involve damage to large vessels.[15]

Vascular Complications

Macrovascular Complications

Macrovascular complications of diabetes mellitus are defined as damage to the large blood vessels providing circulation to the brain, heart, and extremities. These complications include cardiovascular disease and stroke (38.1% of all individuals with diabetes mellitus over the age of 35), as well as peripheral vascular disease. The presence of heart and blood vessel disease is increased twofold to fourfold in individuals with diabetes and is responsible for more than half of all deaths.[3] Ischemic cerebrovascular accidents (strokes) are more prevalent in individuals with diabetes and are associated with poorer outcomes. Cerebrovascular accidents are responsible for almost 1% of hospitalizations of individuals with diabetes mellitus.[3]

Diabetes is an independent risk factor for coronary artery disease. However, several important risk factors for coronary artery disease—dyslipidemia, hypertension, and impaired fibrinolysis—are present in uncontrolled diabetes and decrease with improved blood glucose control. The latter risk factor may be linked to the presence of the compensatory hyperinsulinemia of type 2 diabetes mellitus.[12,15] Reduction of insulin resistance by such hygienic measures as caloric restriction and exercise, and possibly by pharmacologic means, may be of principal importance in reducing the incidence of macrovascular complications. Conventional measures of risk reduction, including measures to control dyslipidemia and hypertension, continue to be considered essential. Improved glycemic control is thought to affect the microvasculature rather than the macrovascular complications.

Microvascular Complications

The microvascular complications of diabetes, retinopathy and nephropathy, are thought to result from abnormal thickening of the basement membrane in capillaries. Capillary basement membrane thickening has been shown to increase with the length of time after diagnosis and with persistent hyperglycemia.[15]

Hyperglycemia has been shown to disrupt platelet function and growth of the basement membrane. The presence of proteins altered by high glucose levels (advanced glycosylation end products) is also believed to play a part in the pathogenesis of microvascular complications. Thickening of capillary basement membranes has been shown to decrease with improved glycemic control.[19] Other risk factors for microvascular disease include hypertension and smoking.

Retinopathy is evident in less than 10% of those diagnosed with diabetes for less than 5 years. However, greater than 50% of patients diagnosed with diabetes for more than 20 years are found to be suffering with some degree of retinopathy. Because of the prevalence of long-standing undiagnosed diabetes mellitus, as many as 21% of individuals with newly diagnosed type 2 diabetes are affected by retinopathy.[12]

Retinopathy is the primary cause of new cases of blindness in adults in the United States. The incidence of diabetic retinopathy appears to correlate with the duration of diabetes. Retinopathy is a progressive disease involving three stages: background retinopathy, preproliferative retinopathy, and proliferative retinopathy. Background retinopathy is characterized by microaneurysms and small hemorrhages in the retinal capillaries. Background retinopathy usually does not affect visual acuity. Preproliferative and proliferative retinopathy involves further damage to retinal capillaries, with the latter condition characterized by capillary neovascularization. The small new capillaries are particularly prone to hemorrhage. Proliferative retinopathy is managed with laser photocoagulation.[8,12,20,21]

Nephropathy affects 20% to 40% of individuals with type 1 diabetes. Fewer individuals with type 2 progress to end-stage renal disease.[19] Diabetic nephropathy accounts for 40% of cases of end-stage renal disease. Ethnic origin is a risk factor in the development of diabetic nephropathy, with African-American, Hispanics, and Native American diabetic individuals experiencing an increased rate of end-stage renal disease as compared with Caucasians.[19, 21] The characteristic lesion of diabetic nephropathy is glomerulosclerosis, or thickening and hardening of the basement membrane of capillaries in the glomeruli. Filtration, an essential component of kidney function, occurs in the glomerulus. The first stage of diabetic nephropathy is an increase in the glomerular flow rate, or the rate of blood flow through the glomerulus. This increased flow rate leads to hyperfiltration in the glomerulus, or a rise in the rate at which blood is filtered. The mechanisms leading to the increase in glomerular flow rate are unclear but are evidently related to poor glycemic control. As hyperfiltration progresses, the glomeruli become damaged. The resulting glomerulosclerosis leads to blockage and leaking of the capillaries. Protein is characteristically seen in the urine, at first in small amounts (microalbuminuria) and then grossly. As diabetic nephropathy advances, the glomerular filtration rate drops and renal failure ensues. Hypertension is an important contributing factor to diabetic nephropathy. Management of hypertension with medications that inhibit angiotensin-converting enzyme has been shown to reduce the rate of renal failure, end-stage renal disease, and mortality.[20]

Neuropathic Complications

Diabetic neuropathy produces symptoms in 60% to 70% of individuals with diabetes and is responsible for 6.8 per 1,000 diabetic population hospitalizations. Neuropathic complications are divided into autonomic dysfunction and sensory dysfunction. Autonomic complications include gastrointestinal disturbances, bladder dysfunction, tachycardia, postural hypotension, and sexual dysfunction. Approximately 35% to 50% of men with diabetes experience erectile dysfunction. Sensory disturbances include carpal tunnel syndrome and paresthesias or lack of sensation in the feet. Neuropathy is largely responsible for the increased risk of serious foot problems in individuals with diabetes. The rate of lower extremity amputation in individuals with diabetes is 15 to 40 times higher than in nondiabetic individuals. More than 60% of all nontraumatic amputations in the United States are performed on individuals with diabetes.[21-23]

Diabetes in humans and experimentally induced diabetes in animals are associated with decreased levels of myoinositol in peripheral nerves. Myoinositol is a cell membrane component normally found in abundance in nerve tissue. Several theoretical explanations have been proposed for the myoinositol link to neuropathy. Glucose appears to compete with myoinositol in transport into the cell. Degradation of glucose to sorbitol and fructose (the polyol pathway) occurs in the nerves in the presence of hyperglycemia and insulinopenia. Increased activity of the polyol pathway also appears to be linked to reduced myoinositol in the peripheral nerves. Focal ischemic lesions of the nerves may also have a role in diabetic neuropathy. Pathologic findings include degeneration or loss of nerve fibers resulting in decreased nerve function.[8]

Glycemic control has been shown to improve nerve function in animals and in humans and to decrease perceived pain. In addition to hyperglycemia, hypertriglyceridemia, obesity, smoking, and hypertension are modifiable vascular risk factors for the development of neuropathy.[21] Other risk factors associated with neuropathy include male sex, white race, older age, and possibly height >175.5 cm.[22] In addition, the elderly, non-Hispanic blacks, and Mexican Americans are disproportionately affected.[23] Strong evidence linking prolonged hyperglycemia to neuropathy and the microvascular complications of diabetes was provided by the Diabetes Control and Complications Trial, a 9-year multicenter prospective study designed to examine the effect of intensive insulin therapy on the development of retinopathy. Renal and neurologic indices were also examined. Subjects in this trial were individuals with type 1 diabetes and no or mild retinopathy at baseline.[24] The experimental group was intensively treated with three or more insulin injections daily or with insulin delivered by a pump. The incidence of initial retinopathy was reduced by 76%, and progression of existing retinopathy was reduced by 54% in the experimental group. Indices of beginning nephropathy such as microalbuminuria and albuminuria were reduced in the experimental group by 39% and 54%, respectively. Symptomatic neuropathy was reduced by 60% in the experimental group. Dilemmas presented by the Diabetes Control and Complications Trial include the presence of a significant increase in severe hypoglycemia in the experimental group and some question about the validity of extrapolating all results to individuals with type 2 diabetes. A large study on the effect of lowering blood glucose in type 2 diabetes has also yielded data on decreased morbidity and mortality with improved glycemic control (United Kingdom Prospective Diabetes Study).[25]

Complications in Pregnancy

Pregnancy in women with type 1 diabetes has been complicated by an increased risk for perinatal infant mortality and congenital anomalies. Metabolic control during pregnancy reduces the risk of perinatal mortality to a rate approximating that of the general population. An increased rate of congenital malformations continues to attend pregnancies in women with type 1 diabetes. Because the affected organs develop early in the first trimester, excellent glycemic control before conception is recommended.[15] Untreated maternal hyperglycemia can result in increased rates of macrosomia, shoulder dystocia, and preeclampsia as well as death, fractures, and nerve palsies.[26, 27]

KEY POINTS

■ The acute complications of hyperglycemia are hyperosmolar coma, ketoacidosis, and infection. Hyperglycemia may be associated with nausea, fatigue, and blurred vision.

■ The chronic complications of hyperglycemia are primarily caused by vascular and neuropathic dysfunction. Individuals with diabetes are prone to vascular complications, including coronary artery disease, stroke, and peripheral vascular disease. These complications are related to dyslipidemia, hypertension, and impaired fibrinolysis. Retinopathy and nephropathy are thought to be due to hyperglycemia-induced thickening of retinal and glomerular basement membranes. Neuropathy is manifested as pain and loss of sensation. Excessive glucose is thought to interfere with myoinositol in neurons.

TREATMENT AND EDUCATION

The usual treatment goals in diabetes are achieving metabolic control of blood glucose levels and preventing acute and chronic complications. The American Diabetes Association recommends as goals a preprandial blood glucose level between 70 and 130 mg/dl and a postprandial blood glucose level less than 180 mg/dl for adults with diabetes.[15] A glycemic control algorithm to guide treatment is presented in Figure 41-6. The goals of treatment are accomplished by diet, exercise, medication, and such hygiene practices as daily foot care and smoking cessation. Each treatment involves lifestyle changes that are difficult to accomplish initially and challenging to maintain. Treatment must be individualized to the type of diabetes and the individual patient.[28]

Nutrition

Nutrition has often been called the cornerstone of diabetes therapy. Ideas about the optimal dietary prescription have been far from constant throughout recorded history. From wheat, fruit, and beer in ancient Egypt through blood pudding and rancid meats in 19th century France to more recent investigations of fiber and fat, nutritional controversies are far from over.

In a position statement, the American Diabetes Association has listed four recommendations for nutritional therapy in patients with diabetes (Box 41-4).[28] Accomplishing the goals can involve changes in composition of the diet, meal patterns and timing, and caloric consumption. All the energy nutrients—carbohydrates, fats, and protein—have an essential role in optimal nutrition. Obesity and eating disorders such as bulimia have an important impact on nutritional status.

Goals
A1C ≤ 6.0%[1]
Fasting SMBG ≤ 100 mg/dL
2-hr PP SMBG ≤ 140 mg/dL
*Avoid hypoglycemia; i.e., glucose
<60 mg/dL or <70 mg/dL if
IHD/CAD*

Initial Intervention[2]
1. Diabetes education *and*
2. SMBG *and*
3. Medical nutrition, weight
   control, exercise[3] *and*
4. Dual therapy or consider
   monotherapy if A1C < 6.5%

Options for Dual/Combination Therapy[4]

Metformin[5]	+ TZD
Metformin or TZD	+ DPP-4 or SU*[6] or Meglitinide
Metformin + TZD or SU*	+ Exenatide or DPP-4 or AGI
Metformin + TZD, AGI or SU*	+ Insulin

*SU is not recommended if A1C < 6.5%

Goals not met after 3 months

Add additional oral agent or exenatide[7] if A1C
less than 1% above goal
Otherwise add insulin as third agent

Goals achieved

Continue therapy
A1C every 3-6 months

Abbreviations

A1C	=	Glycosylated hemoglobin
AGI	=	Alpha-glucosidase inhibitors
CAD	=	Coronary artery disease
DPP-4	=	Dipeptidyl peptidase-4 inhibitor
IHD	=	Ischemic heart disease
PP	=	Postprandial
SMBG	=	Self-monitored blood glucose
SU	=	Sulfonylurea

Goals not met after 3 months

Add insulin
Consider referral to endocrinologist

[1] Goals must be individualized. A1C ≤ 6% is the goal if possible *without significant hypoglycemia*. Less stringent treatment goals may be appropriate for patients with a history of severe hypoglycemia, patients with limited life expectancies, very young children and individuals with comorbid conditions. A1C is referenced to a non-diabetic range of 4-6% using DCCT-based assay. ADA Clinical Practice Recommendations. *Diabetes Care* 2007;30(suppl 1):S9-S10.

[2] If initial presentation is hyperglycemia PLUS weight loss, use insulin, with or without oral agents, as the initial intervention. Other agents may be introduced as glycemic control improves.

[3] These interventions should be maintained life-long.

[4] Consider stopping/reducing dose of SU as a component of therapy due to risk of hypogycemia as A1C approaches goal.

[5] Metformin is the only FDA-approved oral antidiabetic agent in children (≥ age 10); other agents may be used at the discretion of the clinician.

[6] If a SU is selected, low dose glipizide ER or glimepiride are recommended because they have a lower incidence of hypoglycemia than glyburide.

[7] DPP-4 inhibitor should not be used in combination with exenatide.

FIGURE 41-6 Algorithm to achieve glycemic control for type 2 diabetes mellitus in children and adults. *A1c,* glycosylated hemoglobin; *ER,* extended release; *PP,* postprandial; *SMBG,* self-monitoring of blood glucose; *SU,* sulfonylurea *TZD,* thiazolidinedione; *UKPDS,* United Kingdom Prospective Diabetes Study; (Reprinted with permission from the Texas Diabetes Council)

BOX 41-4

American Diabetes Association Recommendations for Nutritional Therapy

Achieve and maintain
- Blood glucose levels in the normal range or as close to normal as is safely possible
- A lipid and lipoprotein profile that reduces the risk for vascular disease
- Blood pressure levels in the normal range or as close to normal as is safely possible

To prevent, or at least slow, the rate of development of the chronic complications of diabetes by modifying nutrient intake and lifestyle

To address individual nutrition needs, taking into account personal and cultural preferences and willingness to change

To maintain the pleasure of eating by only limiting food choices when indicated by scientific evidence

Data from American Diabetes Association: Nutrition Recommendations and Interventions for Diabetes, *Diabetes Care* 31(S1):S61-S78, 2008.

Protein

Protein is used in the repair and growth of tissues. Proteins are composed of amino acids and contain 4 calories per gram. The addition of protein to a meal will stimulate the secretion of insulin without increasing plasma blood glucose. Protein consumption should not be used to treat or prevent nighttime hypoglycemia. Growth, development, and maintenance, as well as glycemic control, are considered to occur optimally at the recommended daily allowance of 0.8 grams protein per kilogram of body weight. Most Americans exceed this guideline. High-protein diets are not recommended for weight loss.[15,28]

Chronic high-protein intake is linked to heightened glomerular flow rates and renal hypertrophy. It is thought that continued renal hyperfunction can lead to nephropathy in diabetic patients. There is conflicting evidence concerning benefits of restricting dietary protein. Studies indicate that it may be beneficial in improving renal function in type 1 diabetes; however not in type 2 diabetes. Current recommendations are 0.8 g per kg and any protein restriction diets should be planned by a registered dietitian.[15,28]

Present recommendations also call for not exceeding the recommended daily allowance for protein (10% to 35% of calories) except in cases of increased need, as in gestation, childhood, and adolescence.

Fat

Fats are composed of fatty acids and other substances. Fats contain 9 cal/g. Dietary fats are classified as saturated, monounsaturated, and unsaturated based on their molecular structure. Dietary saturated fat and dietary cholesterol may contribute to hypercholesterolemia. Elevated serum cholesterol levels have been identified as an important risk factor for cardiovascular disease. Hypertriglyceridemia, or an elevated level of fatty acids in the bloodstream, is linked to hyperglycemia and is an independent risk factor for cardiovascular disease in diabetes.

Fat metabolism is dependent on the appropriate presence of insulin. Untreated diabetes is associated with hypertriglyceridemia, elevated levels of very-low–density lipoprotein, and lowered high-density lipoprotein levels. Although effective treatment reduces the incidence of dyslipidemia, the risk of cardiovascular disease may not be affected.[15,28] The ideal diet for control of serum lipids continues to be a source of controversy. A diet high in carbohydrates and low in all sources of fat has been shown to reduce total and low-density lipoprotein cholesterol but contribute to hypertriglyceridemia, reduced high-density lipoprotein cholesterol, and a deterioration in glycemic control.[18] A diet high in monounsaturated fat has been shown to lower serum triglycerides and very low–density lipoprotein cholesterol, raise high-density lipoprotein cholesterol, and promote euglycemia in patients with diabetes.[15,28]

Current recommendations include limiting saturated fat to less than 7% of total intake, minimizing trans fat consumption, and enjoying two or more servings of fish per week that provide n-3 polyunsaturated fatty acids. It is recommended that not more than 200 mg of cholesterol be consumed daily.[28]

Carbohydrates

Carbohydrates are categorized as monosaccharides (simple sugars) and polysaccharides (complex carbohydrates or starches). Carbohydrates contain 4 cal/g. For many years the American Diabetes Association recommended restriction of carbohydrate, especially sucrose. The atherogenic potential of the resulting high-fat diet became a cause of concern.

Current recommendations are for an individualized diet that includes carbohydrates from fruits, vegetables, whole grains, legumes, and low-fat milk. Carbohydrate intake can be monitored by carbohydrate counting, exchanges, or experienced estimation. Glycemic load and index may be of additional benefit. Sucrose-containing foods can be included in moderation and should be substituted for other carbohydrate-containing foods or covered appropriately with insulin or oral hypoglycemics. The use of artificial sweeteners and sugar alcohols are condoned at levels established by the FDA.[15,28]

Alcohol

Alcohol contains 7 cal/g. Moderate alcohol intake does not appear to have a deleterious effect on glycemic control. Alcohol intake increases the risk of sulfonylurea- or insulin-induced hypoglycemia because of the ability of alcohol to suppress gluconeogenesis. For this reason, alcohol intake should always be accompanied by food intake with these agents. Intake of alcohol should be limited to 1 drink per day (or less) for women and 2 or less per day for men. It is recommended that alcohol be avoided in the presence of poor glycemic control, pancreatic or liver disease, severe triglyceridemia, advanced neuropathy, pregnancy, and alcoholism.[28]

Obesity and Eating Disorders

Obesity is the strongest risk factor for type 2 diabetes, in addition to being a risk factor for cardiovascular disease in women. Obesity is defined as a body mass index (BMI) of greater than 30 kg/m². BMI is calculated by dividing body weight in kilograms by the square of the height in meters. Increased risk for health problems occurs at a body mass index of equal to or greater than 25.2 kg/m². A body mass index of 18.5 to 24.9 kg/m² is considered normal. Weight management is a chronic and difficult problem for many individuals. No single strategy has been shown to be effective for all individuals. Current recommendations for management of obesity include the use of a nutritionally complete diet, a program of maintenance, and exercise.[28] Consult Chapter 42 for additional nutritional risk factors related to obesity.

Eating disorders such as bulimia and anorexia may be more common in women with type 1 diabetes. Inducing weight loss by reducing insulin has also been noted. In order for clinicians to be aware of eating disorders in their patients, careful assessment is necessary.

Exercise

Exercise, one of the oldest treatments for diabetes, was prescribed in India in 500 BC. Exercise can have a role in both type 1 and type 2 diabetes in terms of lowering blood glucose levels and promoting health maintenance. Exercise lowers such cardiovascular risk factors as high blood pressure and dyslipidemia, increases work capacity, reduces stress, prevents bone loss, and improves reaction time. Exercise may also be beneficial in weight reduction.[29]

The effects of exercise on fuel utilization and insulin sensitivity are comparable to exercise-induced changes in normal metabolism. As glucose production increases and plasma insulin levels drop, the reduction in tissue insulin resistance can result in a net fall in blood glucose. Exercise has the potential to decrease insulin requirements in type 1 diabetes, decrease and possibly eliminate the need for pharmacologic agents in type 2 diabetes, and reduce the risk for heart disease in all persons with diabetes. It has been shown to prevent the onset of type 2 diabetes in persons who are genetically at risk.[29]

Although the benefits of exercise are numerous, there are associated risks. Individuals with type 1 diabetes are at risk for hypoglycemia and ketoacidosis. Exercise in individuals with type 2 diabetes can be associated with hypoglycemia, cardiac dysfunction, orthopedic injury, and worsening of some complications.

When insulin or an oral hypoglycemic agent is used in the management of diabetes, the usual fuel metabolism of exercise is disturbed. Inappropriately high insulin levels result in decreased hepatic glucose production and increased tissue insulin sensitivity. The latter processes can lead to hypoglycemia. Replacement of expended glycogen and continued insulin sensitivity can result in hypoglycemia as long as 24 hours after activity.[29]

When insulin levels are inappropriately low, hepatic glucose production is increased and tissue insulin sensitivity is decreased. The production of free fatty acids increases, probably because of the influence of exercise-stimulated production of catecholamines. Hyperglycemia and ketosis may be a result of exercise under insulinopenic conditions. Safeguards must be built into exercise programs to prevent hypoglycemia, ketoacidosis, injury, cardiac compromise, and exacerbation of diabetic complications.

The exercise prescription is as essential in diabetes management as the medication or nutrition prescription. To achieve maximal metabolic and cardiovascular benefit, exercise must be performed for 20 to 45 minutes at least 3 days a week and must incorporate aerobic activity at 50% to 70% $\dot{V}O_{2max}$ (maximal aerobic capacity), which approximates 65% to 80% of the maximal heart rate. The maximal heart rate is often estimated as 220 minus age (in years). However, even rather small increases in activity have been associated with improved metabolic profile. Patients with autonomic neuropathy should be taught a method of judging exercise intensity by perceived exertion. The Centers for Disease Control and Prevention recommend an exercise program of moderate intensity for at least 30 minutes, 5 or more days per week or vigorous-intensity for 20 minutes, 3 or more days per week.[29]

Before an exercise program is begun, a physical examination should rule out the presence of such limiting diabetic complications as retinopathy and neuropathic foot ulcers or malformations. Routine screening for cardiovascular problems in diabetic patients is no longer recommended. Clinicians should use judgment in this area and encourage high-risk patients to start with low-intensity exercise for short periods to start. To avoid orthopedic injury, the exercise session should be preceded by a warm-up period involving mild activity or stretching. Exercise should be initiated at a low intensity and duration and gradually increased. Patients must be counseled to wear appropriate clothing and footwear and to carefully inspect their feet after the exercise session.

Individuals using insulin or insulin secretagogues are encouraged to eat 15 gm of carbohydrates if blood glucose levels are <100 mg/dl, or to reduce the dose of injected insulin when exercise is anticipated. A consistent exercise program can facilitate such adjustments. Patients should be encouraged to have rapidly acting carbohydrate available should it become needed. Exercise should be avoided if ketosis is present, as it can indicate an acute shortage of insulin. Exercise under the

latter conditions can lead to increased hyperglycemia. Exercise when blood glucose values are greater than 250 mg/dl is safe if ketosis is not present.[28,29]

Pharmacologic Agents
Oral Antidiabetic Agents

Along with diet and exercise as initial treatment of type 2 diabetes, metformin is recommended at the time of diagnosis. When initial treatment fails, either insulin, sulfonylureas, or thiazolidinediones can be added to achieve the recommended A1C of less than 7%. Current guidelines call for timely implementation and titration of oral agents as well as insulin to achieve euglycemia.[30] Sulfonylurea drugs have been used in the management of type 2 diabetes for more than 40 years. These drugs have been joined by other agents with different mechanisms of action. Table 41-3 includes a list of common antidiabetic agents.

Sulfonylureas exert their hypoglycemic effect by inducing insulin release by β cells, augmenting the action of insulin in glucose disposal, diminishing insulin clearance by the liver, and reducing hepatic glucose production. Because sulfonylureas are ineffective in the management of type 1 diabetes, stimulation of β cells is known to be a crucial factor in the action of these oral agents. Enhanced insulin secretion appears to be a short-term effect, possibly caused by a reduction in insulin requirements as a result of the other hypoglycemic activities of sulfonylurea agents.[30]

The so-called *first-generation agents* (those formulated earliest) are tolbutamide, chlorpropamide, and tolazamide. Second-generation agents include glyburide, glipizide, and glimepiride. Use of first-generation agents is not recommended unless patients have a well-established history of previous use with good results. Second-generation agents are more

TABLE 41-3

Oral Antidiabetic Agents

Oral Antidiabetic Agent	Onset (hours)	Duration (hours)	Comment
Tolbutamide	0.3	8-12	Useful in renal disease
Chlorpropamide	1	24-70	Antidiuretic action
Acetohexamide	1	12-24	Uricosuric agent Contraindicated in renal disease
Tolazamide	3-4	14	Useful in renal disease
Glyburide	1	24	No disulfiram effect
Glipizide	1	Up to 24	No disulfiram effect
Glimepiride	1	24	Extrapancreatic action
Metformin	1-2	24	Diarrhea, slight risk of lactic acidosis
Acarbose	1	14-24	Decreases intestinal absorption of carbohydrate

potent than first-generation agents, possibly because of increased capacity to bind to the plasma membrane of the β cell. In addition, they are more predictable, have fewer side effects, and represent more convenient dosing. Glyburide appears to characteristically increase basal secretion of insulin and glipizide to heighten postprandial insulin production. Glipizide is preferred with renal impairment. Glimepiride appears to selectively exert extrapancreatic hypoglycemic effects.[15]

The side effects of sulfonylureas include hypoglycemia, nausea, dizziness, headache, allergic reactions, flushing with alcohol use (disulfiram effect), and other rarer blood disorders. Sulfonylureas that are metabolized to inactive compounds by the liver are considered safer for use in renal disease. Duration of action is another safety issue. After insulin, sulfonylureas are the major cause of severe hypoglycemia caused by a drug. The longer acting sulfonylureas chlorpropamide and glyburide are responsible for the majority of cases of severe hypoglycemia and fatal hypoglycemic coma.

Metformin, classified as a biguanide, suppresses hepatic gluconeogenesis and enhances glucose uptake by peripheral tissues without causing hypoglycemia. Metformin has been used alone and in combination with a sulfonylurea drug and sitagliptin. Metformin is associated with improvement in dyslipidemia and weight loss. Side effects include nausea and diarrhea. A rare side effect, lactic acidosis, is one-tenth as likely to occur with metformin as with the related phenformin.[31] Because of the possibility of lactic acidosis, metformin is contraindicated in individuals with liver or renal disease. Metformin should be discontinued for 48 hours after procedures using contrast dyes.

Acarbose and miglitol, α-glucosidase inhibitors, diminish postprandial hyperglycemia by delaying carbohydrate absorption. They can be used alone and in combination with sulfonylurea drugs, metformin, or insulin. Side effects include symptoms related to decreased gastrointestinal absorption (e.g., flatulence and diarrhea). They do not cause hypoglycemia but can complicate management of hypoglycemia if used in combination with a sulfonylurea. Sulfonylurea-induced hypoglycemia cannot be managed with sucrose when acarbose is being used because of drug-induced delayed sucrose absorption.[15,30]

Rosiglitazone and piaglitazone, two thiazolidinedione drugs, increase tissue sensitivity to insulin and inhibit hepatic gluconeogenesis. Thiazolidinediones are thought to decrease insulin resistance, increase glucose uptake, and redistribute fat. In addition, they are thought to preserve β-cell function, decrease vascular inflammation, and minimally decrease hepatic glucose production. Thiazolidinediones were initially approved for use only in individuals with type 2 diabetes mellitus who require the use of insulin. Because thiazolidinediones do not increase pancreatic production of insulin, they cannot by themselves cause hypoglycemia. However, the improvement in insulin sensitivity can result in hypoglycemia in individuals treated with another hypoglycemic drug. Troglitazone, the first marketed thiazolidinedione, caused hepatic failure and was withdrawn from use. Evidence of rare liver damage with

thiazolidinediones has led to the recommendation that liver enzymes be checked regularly. Controversy regarding risk of myocardial infarction (rosiglitazone) and congestive heart failure (rosiglitazone and pioglitazone) has led to black box warning for the drugs. They are still recommended as additional therapy, however caution is advised.[30]

After an initial trial of metformin, diet, and exercise, insulin, sulfonylureas, or thiazolidinediones may be chosen as another pharmacologic agent for type 2 diabetes. If treatment goals are not met, additional oral agents may be prescribed. When prescribed along with an appropriate meal plan, oral antidiabetic agents can be very effective in the management of type 2 diabetes mellitus. Primary failure of the drug is considered to have occurred when initiation of oral agent therapy does not result in a significant decline in blood glucose levels. Primary failure can be due to misdiagnosis of type 1 diabetes mellitus or inadequate adherence to the diet and exercise regimen. Secondary failure, or hyperglycemia after an effective initial response to the drug, is often due to dietary nonadherence but may also be due to the progressive β-cell dysfunction of type 2 diabetes mellitus.[15,30]

Incretins and Amylins

The newest oral agent for management of diabetes is sitagliptin, a DPP-4 inhibitor that inhibits the enzymatic breakdown of the incretin hormones, GLP-1 and GIP. It has minimal side effects and can be used alone or in conjunction with metformin, thiazolidinediones, sulfonylureas, or sulfonylurea + metformin.[32]

Exenatide is a GLP-1 mimetic that delays gastric emptying, inhibits release of glucagon, and increases satiety. It is an injectable medication with the common side effects of nausea and hypoglycemia. Exenatide can be used alone or in combination with sulfonylureas, metformin, or thiazolidinediones. It is not currently indicated for use with insulin, therefore is not appropriate for use among individuals with type 1 diabetes.[32]

Pramlinitide is an amylin-mimetic and can be used in conjunction with insulin for the management of glycemia. It may not be mixed with insulin and should be injected separately. Insulin requirements are usually decreased by 50% with pramlinitide; in addition, minimum carbohydrate and caloric intake are required for its use. It is contraindicated in patients with hypoglycemia unawareness or gastroparesis. Both incretin and amylin mimetics have been effective in weight loss and lowering A1C when used in conjunction with metformin or a sulfonylurea (both) or insulin (pramlinitide only).[32]

Insulin

Insulin therapy is required in 100% of persons with type 1 diabetes mellitus and 35% with type 2 diabetes mellitus.[8] Persons with type 1 diabetes mellitus require replacement of the deficient hormone in as physiologic a manner as possible. The role of insulin in type 2 diabetes mellitus is more complex.[12,15]

Because type 2 diabetes mellitus is a progressive disease, many if not most individuals will need insulin at some time, either because of increasing insulin resistance or because of β-cell dysfunction. Glucose toxicity, a phenomenon in which insulin resistance and decreased production of insulin are worsened by hyperglycemia, may respond to insulin therapy. Insulin may be necessary in type 2 diabetes intermittently during times of physiologic stress that increase insulin requirements (e.g., intercurrent illness, surgery, inactivity, weight gain). However, with resolution of the stress, the individual may be able to discontinue insulin use.[12,15]

Types of insulin are classified into four groups according to their duration of action: rapid acting, short acting, intermediate acting, and long acting (Table 41-4). The most commonly used insulins in the rapid-acting category are aspart, glulisine, and lispro. Regular insulin is considered short acting. Intermediate-acting agents include NPH and lente. Glargine and determir are in the long-acting category.[15] An oral inhaled insulin preparation was briefly on the market for use as a mealtime insulin; however it was not well-received and was subsequently discontinued.

Patterns of insulin use vary with the type of diabetes and the degree of desired metabolic control. For patients with type 1 diabetes mellitus, a minimum of 2 or more daily injections of a mixture of rapid-acting and long-acting insulins has been used to control postprandial and fasting hyperglycemia. A popular regimen includes use of long-acting Lantus with preprandial injections of a rapid-acting insulin.[15]

Intensive insulin schedules are an attempt to mimic normal insulin secretion closely and are considered important for optimal control. One such schedule calls for the use of rapid-acting insulin before meals and long-acting insulin at bedtime. Other schedules use long-acting insulin twice daily: at breakfast and before dinner, or at breakfast and at bedtime. In the latter schedule, the long-acting insulin stands in for basal insulin secretion. Insulin doses can be adjusted by the use of an algorithm based on capillary blood glucose monitoring, estimation of the carbohydrate content of the next meal, or both. Patients can work with a certified diabetes educator to determine their insulin sensitivity factor (how much insulin is required to lower blood glucose) and insulin-to-carbohydrate ratio (how much insulin is needed per x grams of carbohydrate).[15, 28]

Continuous subcutaneous insulin infusion (CSII) by means of an insulin pump has been used to approximate nondiabetic insulin secretion in situations in which intensive insulin therapy has not been effective. CSII technology supplies a constant infusion of regular or more commonly, a rapid-acting insulin to mimic basal insulin and delivers a premeal bolus dose programmed by the user. Improvement in glycemic control has been noted with CSII. Complications associated with CSII therapy (infected infusion sites, ketoacidosis, and hypoglycemic coma) have resulted in a 34.5% rate of discontinuation of pump use.[33]

Other insulin delivery devices include jet injectors and insulin pens. Jet injectors, mechanisms that deliver a spray of insulin under the skin, increase the rate of insulin absorption. Insulin pens include the insulin, measuring device, and needle in one pen-sized instrument. Delivery of inhaled insulin is under study.

Pancreas transplantation has been performed in individuals with diabetes since 1966 and has shown consistent improvement in patient outcomes. Pancreas transplantation restores normal metabolism but must be accompanied by lifelong treatment with immunosuppressive agents.

In the management of type 2 diabetes, insulin is initiated early in the course of the disease to achieve and maintain glycemic control. It can be used concurrently with other antidiabetic agents. Intensity of the regimen is based on the needs of the patient. Long-acting insulin or rapid-acting insulin only can be used to improve fasting or postprandial glycemia, respectively, depending upon the patients needs. Normally fasting glucose is targeted first; if A1C goals are not met, prandial insulin is initiated. Mixed formulations are beneficial, and require only 1 to 2 injections per day, in type 2 diabetes as well.[8,15,34]

The action of insulin is affected by many elements, including climate, alteration in blood flow, tobacco use, and the injection site. Insulin is absorbed most rapidly from the abdomen, less rapidly from the arm, and most slowly from the legs and buttocks. Insulin is absorbed more rapidly from areas that are exercised or massaged after injection.[8,15]

Hypoglycemia Complications. Hypoglycemia is the most common complication of hypoglycemic therapy and the most hazardous. The incidence of hypoglycemia has been estimated at 20% in individuals treated with sulfonylureas, 35% in individuals with type 2 diabetes treated with insulin, and 100% in individuals with type 1 diabetes mellitus. Severe hypoglycemia occurs in as many as 44% of insulin-treated individuals. Hypoglycemia may cause or be a factor in 2% to 4% of deaths in individuals with type 1 diabetes mellitus.[34] Neural tissue depends on a constant supply of glucose for normal function. When insufficient food intake, unplanned activity, or an inappropriate insulin or sulfonylurea dose lowers the blood glucose concentration excessively, counterregulatory mechanisms are activated to ensure a continued supply of glucose to the brain. The production of glucagon, catecholamines, corticosteroids, and growth hormone is increased. The latter hormones increase glucose production by mechanisms outlined earlier in this chapter.

Symptoms of hypoglycemia produced by counterregulatory mechanisms include pallor, tremor, diaphoresis, palpitation, and anxiety. Neuroglycopenic symptoms noted in hypoglycemia are hunger, visual disturbance, weakness, paresthesias, confusion, agitation, coma, and death. In long-standing diabetes, neuropathy can alter the counterregulatory mechanisms. Hypoglycemic unawareness, in which the diabetic patient does not experience counterregulatory symptoms, can be the result.[15]

Alcohol interferes with counterregulatory processes by suppressing gluconeogenesis. Alcohol intake has resulted in fatal hypoglycemic coma even in the absence of other hypoglycemic drugs. The combination of alcohol and insulin or sulfonylurea drugs can be particularly dangerous.

TABLE 41-4

Insulin and Other Injectable Antihyperglycemic Medications*

Drug Class	Action	Brand Name	Generic Name	Appearance	Rx or OTC	Drug Type
Insulin	Rapid	Humalog	Insulin Lispro	Clear	Rx	Insulin Analog
		NovoLog	Insulin Aspart	Clear	Rx	Insulin Analog
		Apidra	Insulin Glulisine	Clear	Rx	Insulin Analog
		Exubera	Inhaled Dry Powder Insulin	Powder	Rx	Regular Insulin; Inhaled
	Short	Humulin R Novolin R	Regular Insulin; Injectable	Clear	OTC	Regular Insulin; Injected
	Intermediate	Humulin N Novolin N	Isophane Insulin	Cloudy	OTC	Isophane Insulin
	Long	Levemir	Insulin Detemir	Clear	Rx	Long-Acting Insulin Analog
		Lantus	Insulin Glargine	Clear	Rx	Long-Acting Insulin Complex
	Combination Products	Humulin 70/30 Novolin 70/30	70% Isophane/ 30% Regular	Cloudy	OTC	NPH and Regular Combination
		NovoLog 70/30	70% Aspart Protamine/30% Aspart	Cloudy	Rx	NPH-like and Rapid Acting Combination
		Humalog Mix 75/25	75% Lispro protamine/25% Lispro	Cloudy	Rx	NPH-like and Rapid Acting Combination
		Humulin 50/50	50% Isophane/ 50% Regular	Cloudy	OTC	NPH and Regular Combination
Non-Insulin Injectables						
Incretin Mimetic	Adjunct Therapy	Byetta	Exenatide		Rx	GLP-1 Analog
Amylin Analog		Symlin	Pramlintide		Rx	Amylin Analog

*Data from Dipiro JT et al: *Pharmacotherapy: a pathophysiologic approach,* McGraw-Hill, 2008, pp 1216-1217.

Other Complications of Insulin Therapy. Another typical complication of insulin therapy is lipodystrophy. Lipoatrophy has been linked to the use of insulin from animal sources and is manifested as hollows in the surface of the skin caused by the destruction of subcutaneous adipose tissue. Lipohypertrophy is characterized by an increase in subcutaneous tissue because of insulin-stimulated growth of adipose tissue at the injection sites. Avoiding repeated injections at the same site is recommended to prevent lipodystrophy.[34]

An acute complication of insulin use can be insulin edema, or a localized or generalized accumulation of fluid. Weight gain can accompany initiation of insulin therapy, especially when glycemic control is improved. A third complicating factor in insulin therapy is insulin resistance. Insulin resistance is exacerbated by obesity and can necessitate the use of large insulin doses. An appropriate diet and exercise program is as important to insulin-treated individuals as it is to other patients with diabetes.[28,29,34]

Stress Management

Living with diabetes can be stressful. The tasks of blood glucose monitoring, medication administration, meal planning, and preventive care to avoid complications can be demanding. Fearing the onset of complications and their impact in addition to living with complications are parts of the psychological impact of diabetes. Depression is more likely to be diagnosed in individuals with diabetes and is correlated with deterioration of glycemic control.[35] Stress management can have an important role in diabetes care by improving quality

Onset (In Hours Unless Noted)	Peak (Hours)	Duration (Hours)	Compatible Mixed With	Storage/ Expiration	Typical Dosing/Comments
15-30 min	1-2	3-4	NPH	Refrigerate/28 days at room temp	15 minutes prior to meal or immediately after meals
15-30 min	1-2	3-5	NPH	Refrigerate/28 days at room temp	5-10 minutes before meal
15-30 min	1-2	3-4	NPH	Refrigerate/28 days at room temp	15 minutes before or within 20 minutes after meal
10-30 min	1-2	6	None	Room temp/discard after 90 days of opening foil	Within 10 minutes prior to meal
0.5-1	2-3	3-6	NPH	Refrigerate/28 days at room temp	30 minutes prior to meal
2-4	4-6	8-12	Insulin Analogs/ Injectable Regular Insulin	Refrigerate/28 days at room temp	One, two, or three times daily
2	6-9	14-24	None	Refrigerate/42 days at room temp	Once or twice daily
4-5	Peakless	22-24	None	Refrigerate/28 days at room temp	Once daily, at the same time each day *Some patients may need to split the dose twice daily
30 min	1.5-16	24	None	Refrigerate/28 days at room temp	30 minutes prior to meal
15 min	1-4	24	None	Refrigerate/28 days at room temp	15 minutes prior to meal
15 min	1-6.5	24	None	Refrigerate/28 days at room temp	15 minutes prior to meal
30 min	2-5.5	24	None	Refrigerate/28 days at room temp	30 minutes prior to meal
	2	10	None	Refrigerate/30 days after opening	Within 60 minutes prior to morning and evening meals *When initiating, taking close to meals may minimize side effects
	20 min	3	None	Refrigerate/28 days at room temp or refrigerated	Immediately prior to each major meal (≥ 250 kcal or 30g of carbohydrate)

of life and reducing the possible impact of stress on glycemic control.

Assessment of Efficacy

Several measures are used by clinicians to determine the adequacy of glycemic control. One indirect but very useful indication of blood glucose levels is the level of glycosylated hemoglobin. Hemoglobin becomes glycosylated when glucose is nonenzymatically attached to one of its terminal amino acids. Four glycosylated hemoglobin products are formed: HbA_{1a1}, HbA_{1a2}, HbA_{1b}, and HbA_{1c}. The latter is produced in the largest quantity and is used in most assays.[15]

Because erythrocytes are freely permeable to glucose, the quantities of glycosylated hemoglobin formed are proportional to the quantity of glucose in the blood plasma. Glycosylated hemoglobin values will reflect mean blood glucose levels for the life of the average erythrocyte (100 to 120 days). Highly significant correlations have been found between HbA_{1c} levels and mean blood glucose.[34] The presence of abnormal hemoglobins or hemolytic anemia can skew results. The normal value for HbA_{1c} varies with the laboratory technique but is usually less than 7%. Results of the A1C-Derived Average Glucose (ADAG) Trial will be published in 2008 and will provide an average glucose number that correlates with an A1C rather than reporting a percentage; this should increase a patients' understanding of their overall glycemic control.[15]

HbA_{1c} values are used clinically to estimate long-term control and to set and evaluate therapeutic goals. Values of less than 7% or as close to normal as possible without adverse effects are considered desirable. Depending upon individual circumstances and life expectancy, less stringent goals may be appropriate. HbA$_{1c}$ values cannot be used for day-to-day management of therapy.[15]

Assessment of glycemia on a daily basis was attempted in the past by the use of testing for glycosuria. However, the blood glucose level at which glucose is measurable in the urine, the glycemic threshold, varies from individual to individual, is usually unacceptably high, and cannot be used to establish the presence of hypoglycemia.

Venous blood can be drawn in a clinic or office and analyzed for glucose content. Office laboratory evaluation is inconvenient and expensive. The advent of capillary blood glucose monitoring in the late 1970s provided a solution to the problem of short-term evaluation of glycemic control. Individuals with diabetes and health professionals can use a drop of capillary blood applied to a glucose oxidase reagent strip to measure the blood glucose level. The treated strips are generally read in 5 to 45 seconds. Test strips are read visually or by a meter. Some test strips can be read both ways.[15]

The First and Second Consensus Development Conference on Self-Monitoring of Blood Glucose, convened by the American Diabetes Association and other involved agencies, formulated several goals for the use of capillary blood glucose monitoring. The goals included use of capillary blood glucose monitoring to achieve and maintain a specific level of glycemic control, prevent and manage hypoglycemia, avoid severe hypoglycemia, adjust care in response to changes in lifestyle in individuals requiring pharmacologic therapy, and determine the need for initiating insulin therapy in women with gestational diabetes mellitus.[36]

Capillary blood glucose monitoring has been shown to be an accurate reflection of venous blood glucose when performed by health professionals and by individuals with diabetes. However, unacceptable variation has been found in some studies. Hematocrit, altitude, temperature, humidity, hypotension, hypoxia, and hypertriglyceridemia can affect results. Accuracy can be affected by such performance errors as underloading or overloading the strip, incorrect placement of the sample, and improper sample handling. Training improves performance.[36]

Diabetic individuals using capillary blood glucose monitoring have frequently reported enthusiasm and increased insight into the relationship between blood glucose and such factors as diet, exercise, and stress or have reported increased feelings of well-being. Capillary blood glucose monitoring has been associated with improved glycemic control. Monitoring of capillary blood glucose levels is simply a feedback mechanism that provides immediate information on the effects of a change in therapy.[36]

Hazards are associated with the use of capillary blood glucose monitoring. Institutional use of capillary blood glucose monitoring involves potential handling of blood, with the concomitant risk of transmission of such blood-borne diseases as hepatitis B and human immunodeficiency virus infection. The American Association of Diabetes Educators has published guidelines for the safe use of capillary blood glucose monitoring in institutional and home settings. Patient use of capillary blood glucose monitoring has also been associated with such hazards as hand infection and improper disposal of used medical waste. Hand washing and use of a fresh lancet for every test have been recommended to prevent finger infection. Proper disposal of lancets and insulin syringes to avoid injury to household members and waste disposal personnel is essential and mandated by law in many municipalities.[37]

In the replacement of testing for glycosuria with capillary blood glucose monitoring, testing for ketonuria should not be neglected. The presence of ketones in the urine can be an indication of diabetic ketoacidosis and may be harmful to a developing fetus in diabetes complicated by pregnancy. All individuals with diabetes should be tested for ketonuria when blood glucose values are greater than 300 mg/dl, during intercurrent illness, during pregnancy, and in the presence of symptoms of diabetic ketoacidosis (nausea, vomiting, abdominal pain).[38]

Education

Individuals with diabetes must meet physical and financial challenges and uncertainty about the future. They must also learn a variety of skills, some relatively easy to master, others more demanding. Persons with diabetes must learn to perform biological tests and interpret results correctly, measure and administer medication (often injectable medication), manage the side effects of medications, plan meals, design an exercise program, perform foot inspection and care, and accomplish other difficult tasks. Many of these tasks would require a license if performed on another person.

Few other chronic diseases make so many demands on patients. For this reason, diabetes education is considered an essential component of diabetes treatment. Participation in a diabetes education program has been shown to increase patient knowledge about diabetes and improve performance of self-care procedures and psychological outlook. Benefit has been shown in such biochemical indices as blood glucose, HbA$_{1c}$, and serum lipids. Hospitalization rates have been decreased by 19% to 87%, and the rate of diabetic ketoacidosis decreased by 86% after educational intervention. A reduction in the incidence of foot lesions, amputation, and congenital malformations has been demonstrated and has led to health care cost savings. The efficacy of education programs is increased when behavior change approaches are emphasized.[39]

Many individuals with diabetes lack essential skills for performing diabetes self-care. Less than half of all individuals with diabetes have attended a diabetes education program. It is the position of the American Diabetes Association that diabetes education is a critical constituent of diabetes care and should be a benefit included in third-party reimbursement.[39]

BOX 41-5

National Standards Established by the American Diabetes Association

Structures

Standard 1

The Diabetes Self Management Education (DSME) entity will have documentation of its organizational structure, mission statement, and goals and will recognize and support quality DSME as an integral component of diabetes care.

Standard 2

The DSME entity shall appoint an advisory group to promote quality. This group shall include representatives from the health professions, people with diabetes, the community, and other stakeholders.

Standard 3

The DSME entity will determine the diabetes educational needs of the target population(s) and identify resources necessary to meet these needs.

Standard 4

A coordinator will be designated to oversee the planning, implementation, and evaluation of diabetes self-management education. The coordinator will have academic or experiential preparation in chronic disease care and education and in program management.

Processes

Standard 5

DSME will be provided by one or more instructors. The instructors will have recent educational and experiential preparation in education and diabetes management or will be a certified diabetes educator. The instructor(s) will obtain regular continuing education in the field of diabetes management and education. At least one of the instructors will be a registered nurse, dietitian, or pharmacist. A mechanism must be in place to ensure that the participant's needs are met if those needs are outside the instructors' scope of practice and expertise.

Standard 6

Written curriculum reflecting current evidence and practice guidelines, with criteria for evaluating outcomes, will serve as the framework for the DSME entity. Assessed needs of the individual with pre-diabetes and diabetes will determine which of the content areas listed below are to be provided:

Standard 7

An individual assessment and education plan will be developed collaboratively by the participant and instructor(s) to direct the selection of appropriate educational interventions and self-management support strategies. This assessment and education plan and the intervention and outcomes will be documented in the education record.

Standard 8

A personalized follow-up plan for ongoing self management support will be developed collaboratively by the participant and instructor(s). The patient's outcomes and goals and the plan for ongoing self management support will be communicated to the referring provider.

Outcomes

Standard 9

The DSME entity will measure attainment of patient-defined goals and patient outcomes at regular intervals using appropriate measurement techniques to evaluate the effectiveness of the educational intervention.

Standard 10

The DSME entity will measure the effectiveness of the education process and determine opportunities for improvement using a written continuous quality improvement plan that describes and documents a systematic review of the entitles' process and outcome data.

Data from: Funnell MM, Brown TL, Childs BP et al: National Standards for Diabetes Self-Management Education, *Diabetes Care* 31:S97-S104, 2008.

Individuals with diabetes are a diverse group with wide variations in age, ethnic background, disease duration, education, and intellectual abilities. For this reason, diabetes education must be tailored to the individual's needs. Individuals with newly diagnosed diabetes will need education in such survival skills as medication administration and the management of hypoglycemia. More comprehensive education is best provided after the initial disturbance of the diagnosis has receded. Individuals with low literacy skills will benefit from educational materials designed for their special needs. The education of elderly individuals must take sensory deficits into consideration. The short attention spans of children necessitate special guidelines for educating the young.[15]

To ensure quality in diabetes education programs, national standards have been established by the American Diabetes Association. The standards define key content areas and provide guidelines for assessment, setting of objectives, follow-up, and other areas (Box 41-5). Diabetes education programs that can demonstrate adherence to the national standards are officially recognized by the American Diabetes Association.[15]

KEY POINTS

- The mainstays of diabetic treatment are diet, exercise, and drug therapy. Education is an integral part of treatment, enabling individuals with diabetes to follow the diabetic regimen and avoid complications. The efficacy of therapy can be assessed by monitoring blood glucose and HbA_{1c} levels. Blood glucose monitoring is useful for assessing short-term efficacy. HbA_{1c} is a better measure of the long-term efficacy of therapy. A mean blood glucose level less than 170 mg/dl (HbA_{1c} level of 7% or less) is desirable.

- The recommended diabetic diet includes 15% to 35% of calories from protein sources; carbohydrates obtained from fruits, vegetables, whole grains, legumes, and low-fat milk; and limiting saturated fat to <7% and total cholesterol to <200 mg, as well as minimizing trans fat intake. High-protein intake may hasten the development of nephropathy. For individuals with type 2 diabetes, a diet geared toward weight loss may be beneficial. Even modest weight loss usually improves glycemic control.

- Exercise has several benefits for an individual with diabetes. Insulin requirements may be reduced, weight loss facilitated, and the risk of cardiovascular complications decreased. Exercise may precipitate hypoglycemia, so insulin injections or dietary intake may have to be adjusted. Oral antidiabetic agents may be successfully used in type 2 diabetes. The sulfonylureas exert their effects primarily by stimulating the release of endogenous insulin. They also reduce insulin degradation and suppress the release of glucose from the liver. Metformin suppresses hepatic gluconeogenesis and enhances glucose uptake by peripheral tissue; thiazolidinediones enhance glucose uptake by peripheral tissue; and acarbose delays absorption of ingested carbohydrate.
- Insulin replacement therapy is required in patients with type 1 and in about one-third of patients with type 2 diabetes mellitus. Insulin is classified according to its onset, peak, and duration of action. A combination of insulins may be given to produce optimal control. A long-acting insulin (glargine or detemir) and a rapid-acting insulin (aspart, lispro, glulisine) are commonly used to mimic basal and prandial insulin, respectively.
- Hypoglycemia is the most common complication of pharmacologic therapy. Symptoms are mediated primarily by activation of the sympathetic nervous system stress response. Secretion of catecholamines, glucagon, corticosteroids, and growth hormone rises in an attempt to increase blood glucose levels. Pallor, tremor, diaphoresis, weakness, and decreased consciousness are the usual manifestations of hypoglycemia.

PEDIATRIC CONSIDERATIONS

Diabetes has been diagnosed in approximately 176,500 children and adolescents younger than 20 years. One in every 400 to 600 children and adolescents has type 1 diabetes. Eighteen new cases per population of 100,000 are diagnosed yearly. The overwhelming majority have type 1 diabetes, with an approximately 5% prevalence of genetic defects in the β cell.[1,3,8]

Type 1 diabetes is characterized by destruction of the β cells of the pancreas with resulting insulinopenia. Type 1 diabetes in children is often manifested acutely as diabetic ketoacidosis when insulin secretion falls below insulin needs. A condition termed the "honeymoon period" can occur if the diagnosis occurs during a time of increased insulin needs, such as during a viral illness. When the illness is resolved, insulin needs can fall below residual insulin production and normoglycemia results without the use of exogenous insulin. The honeymoon period rarely lasts more than 1 year and is usually shorter.[8,9]

Goals of Therapy

Goals of therapy for children include achieving normal growth and development, avoiding acute and chronic complications of diabetes, addressing psychosocial issues, and educating children regarding self-care.[15]

Acute Complications

Whenever children with type 1 diabetes mellitus experience hyperglycemia, the resulting glycosuria can precipitate dehydration. The threat of dehydration is especially severe during episodes of diabetic ketoacidosis. Supplemental fluids and insulin may be necessary during these times.[15]

Diabetic ketoacidosis can occur when insulin administration is inadequate for needs. Diabetic ketoacidosis frequently accompanies the diagnosis of type 1 diabetes mellitus. Avoiding diabetic ketoacidosis involves knowledge of appropriate care during times of increased insulin need, such as during intercurrent illness. To ensure early detection of incipient diabetic ketoacidosis, children and adolescents should be tested for ketonuria when the blood glucose concentration is greater than 240 mg/dl and during intercurrent illness.[8,15]

Hypoglycemia can be difficult to detect in very young children. Caregivers should be alert for behavioral changes such as lethargy, pallor, and sleep disturbances.

Chronic Complications

Chronic complications of diabetes are rarely manifested during adolescence. Screening for neuropathy and nephropathy and determinations of serum lipid levels should occur on a regular basis. Adolescent girls must be counseled on the importance of excellent metabolic control before initiation of pregnancy.[15,26]

Treatment

Insulin requirements are approximately 1.0 units per kg per day. An intensive regimen of at least 3 injections per day is recommended to prevent chronic complications. The administration of very small doses of insulin in infants and children may necessitate the use of a dilutent.[8,15]

Insulin needs increase during times of physiologic stress, such as during intercurrent illness or puberty. Children who are inadequately treated with insulin will not grow or mature normally.

Children are usually able to begin administering insulin and performing capillary blood glucose monitoring with supervision when they are of school age. The age may vary with different children. When administering insulin, the abdomen is the least preferred site because of insufficient abdominal subcutaneous fat.

Diabetic teaching of such self-management skills as insulin injection, capillary blood glucose monitoring, and recognition and treatment of hypoglycemia should include all caregivers. Baby sitters and teachers will need information on prevention, recognition, and management of hypoglycemia. All educational materials used with children should be age appropriate.[15,40]

Children must be provided with a caloric intake adequate to meet needs for energy expenditure, growth, and maturation. Calorie intake is usually calculated as 1,000 cal/day plus 100 added calories for each year until age 11 years. From age 11 to age 18 years, an additional 100 calories is added for girls and an additional 200 calories for boys. Growth should be plotted at each medical appointment to assess adequate nutrition and adequate insulinization. After the age of 2 years, recommended dietary guidelines for percentage of fat, carbohydrate, and protein are the same as for adults.[15,28]

Exercise is encouraged, with careful attention to adequate nutritional intake. Insulin doses may need to be adjusted to plan for unusual levels of activity, such as during long-distance bike riding or hiking.[29]

Following a regimen designed to prevent acute and chronic complications of diabetes is difficult under the best of conditions. The goals of treatment are best accomplished when meals, medication, exercise, and blood glucose monitoring are consistent. Achieving consistency while also achieving developmental goals of separation and independence is very difficult. Peer pressure during adolescence can lead to poor adherence to therapeutic regimens. Concern regarding weight can lead to omission of insulin injections or other forms of eating disorders.[35]

The child and family need support and counseling to develop effective strategies for achieving desired goals. Disturbed family functioning can have an impact on children and adolescents with diabetes and can lead to an increased frequency of hospitalization for diabetic ketoacidosis.[35]

Genetic defects of the β cell are usually diagnosed in individuals younger than 25 years. These individuals are not likely to become ketotic. Management is identical to that of type 2 diabetes in young adults.

KEY POINTS

- Children and adolescents with diabetes overwhelmingly have type 1 diabetes mellitus (5% have genetic defects of the β cell). In type 1 diabetes, insulin is required at diagnosis or shortly thereafter.
- Goals of therapy for children include achieving normal growth and development, avoiding acute and chronic complications of diabetes, addressing psychosocial issues, and educating children regarding self-care.
- Acute complications of diabetes in children and adolescents include hyperglycemia leading to dehydration, possible diabetic ketoacidosis, and hypoglycemia. Hypoglycemia may manifest differently in children than in adults.
- Chronic complications in children and adolescents are rare. Screening for complications should nevertheless be initiated. Adolescent girls should be counseled on issues regarding diabetes and pregnancy.
- Insulin needs will vary according to growth stages, exercise, and intercurrent illness. Regular capillary blood glucose monitoring is crucial for determining the efficacy of treatment. The age at which children will perform insulin measurement and administration and capillary blood glucose monitoring independently will vary. Nutritional needs are calculated at 1,000 cal/day, with 100 added calories per year until age 11 and an additional 100 calories for girls and an additional 200 calories for boys until age 18.

- Education in self-care activities should be appropriate for age and include other family members. Support for the person with diabetes and the family is important. Counseling may be helpful in some circumstances.

GERIATRIC CONSIDERATIONS

The prevalence of type 2 diabetes mellitus increases with age. Adults older than 60 years constitute nearly 50% of the diabetic population of the United States. The prevalence of diabetes in the elderly is almost 21% for individuals age 60 or older and more than doubles that of younger adults age 40 to 59 years old.[1]

The increase in risk for type 2 diabetes in older adults is multifactorial. Aging often involves increased adiposity and a decrease in lean body mass and activity levels. The latter factors contribute to insulin resistance. Insulin secretion also diminishes with age. The risk of diabetes in the elderly is likewise increased by surgery, illness, and the use of such medications as steroids and diuretics.[1]

Diabetes in the elderly can be difficult to diagnose because of fluctuating blood glucose values in response to food intake and activity and because of inconsistent or absent symptoms of hyperglycemia. Chronic complications of diabetes such as neuropathy and retinopathy are frequently present at diagnosis and indicate glucose intolerance of long duration.[15]

Goals of Therapy

Goals of treatment for the elderly include prevention of acute complications, prevention and management of chronic complications, attention to psychosocial issues, and education regarding self-care.[15,41,42]

Acute Complications

Uncontrolled hyperglycemia in the elderly may be asymptomatic or may produce such classic symptoms as polyuria and fatigue. Polydipsia is less common because of decreased thirst perception. Hyperglycemia can result in increased perception of pain and slowing of intellectual processes. The risk of infection is greater when blood glucose values are over 200 mg/dl. Such infectious disease processes as malignant otitis externa and reactivation of chronic tuberculosis are linked to hyperglycemia. Elderly individuals with diabetes are two times as likely to be hospitalized for kidney infections as individuals without diabetes.[15,24,34]

Chronic hyperglycemia can cause mild to moderate dehydration in the elderly that can be exacerbated by age-related changes in kidney function and water conservation. The resulting electrolyte imbalances can increase the risk of falls.

Elderly people with type 2 diabetes mellitus are not prone to ketosis, but they are at risk for nonketotic hyperglycemic hyperosmolar coma. Particular risk factors include impaired thirst recognition, polypharmacy, dementia, and intercurrent illness. Profound dehydration can occur and lead to a significant mortality rate for this complication (10% to 50%).[34]

Older individuals with type 2 diabetes mellitus must be instructed in care during intercurrent illness and advised to perform capillary blood glucose monitoring on a regular basis to avoid undetected hyperglycemia.[40]

Hypoglycemia can occur when an elderly individual with diabetes is treated with a sulfonylurea or insulin. Hyperglycemia can occur atypically with symptoms of lethargy or focal neurologic dysfunction. Elderly individuals may have age-related decreases in counterregulatory function or an inability to report hypoglycemic symptoms. Glycemic targets for these individuals may be higher. The risk of injury during a hypoglycemic episode warrants careful observation of blood glucose values and regular evaluation of treatment of all elderly individuals with diabetes.[15]

Chronic Complications

The increased prevalence of heart and blood vessel disease, kidney disease, eye disease, and foot disease in patients with diabetes overlaps with the increased prevalence of these conditions in the general elderly population. Diabetes increases the incidence and severity of these diseases.

Aging-related changes can present a particular problem in the performance of diabetic foot care. Orthopedic deformity, loss of protective subcutaneous fat, and atherosclerotic changes are all common problems of the elderly. Inspection of the feet and nail care can be compromised by changes in visual acuity and joint function. Assistance with foot care is often necessary to minimize the risk of diabetic complications involving the feet.[15,19,40]

Treatment

Oral antidiabetic agents must be chosen carefully to avoid age-related adverse effects. Oral agents with a shorter duration of action are preferable. Elderly individuals with diabetes should be evaluated for changes in renal and hepatic function. Oral agents metabolized in an impaired system should be avoided. Metformin is not appropriate for individuals with decreased liver and renal function because of the increased risk of lactic acidosis.[15]

Insulin is safe to use with caution in the elderly. Thin elderly individuals can be highly sensitive to insulin and may require very small amounts to control hyperglycemia. Some elderly individuals are quite sensitive to regular insulin. Daily or twice-daily dosing of a long-acting insulin may be preferable.

Age- or illness-related changes in vision, manual dexterity, and cognition can diminish the ability to measure and administer insulin. Magnification devices and the use of prefilled syringes can be of assistance.

Exercise is of benefit to individuals of all ages. Exercise plans must often be modified to account for orthopedic or other mobility problems. Armchair exercise can be an excellent way for elderly individuals to stay active.[29]

Appropriate food intake can help control hyperglycemia and reduce the risk of chronic complications in the elderly, as in all individuals with diabetes. The quality and quantity of nutrients must be assessed carefully in the elderly. Elderly individuals may be obese, malnourished, or both. Increasing the nutritional value of a meal plan that is low in calories because of choice or a desire to lose weight is an important and difficult goal. Dental and other oral disease or dysfunction can have an impact on nutritional intake.[28]

Education of the elderly in diabetic self-care practices can be challenged by age-related changes in vision, hearing, and cognition. Simple, clearly written educational materials and less complex therapeutic regimens can be of assistance. Caretakers and family members should be included in education sessions if possible. Family or other assistance can ensure safe performance of diabetic self-care activities while maintaining as much independence as possible.[15]

KEY POINTS

- The increased prevalence of type 2 diabetes mellitus in the elderly is multifactorial and due to increased adiposity, decreased lean body mass, decreased activity levels, decreased insulin secretion, the hyperglycemic effect of certain medications, intercurrent illness, and surgery. Varying blood glucose values can lead to difficulty in diagnosis.

- Goals of treatment for the elderly include prevention of acute complications, prevention and management of chronic complications, attention to psychosocial issues, and education regarding self-care.

- Acute complications of diabetes in the elderly include hyperglycemia, often asymptomatic, which can lead to dehydration, increased risk of infection, and nonketotic hyperglycemic hyperosmolar coma. Hypoglycemia can occur atypically and may lead to injury.

- Heart and blood vessel disease, foot problems, visual disabilities, and kidney disease have a significant presence in the aging population in general, as well as being chronic complications of diabetes. Avoiding foot problems can be particularly challenging given the frequent presence of orthopedic deformity and other common aging-related changes, as well as the decreased ability to perform appropriate foot care.

- Oral antidiabetic agents should be carefully chosen with consideration of renal and hepatic function. Short-acting agents are preferable. When insulin treatment is necessary, visual or orthopedic and other changes may hinder measurement of insulin. Adaptive devices can be helpful. Exercise should be encouraged and may have to be modified for people with limited mobility or other limiting factors. Meal planning for elderly individuals should emphasize appropriate amounts of foods with high nutritional value.

- Simple, clearly written educational material can be helpful for individuals with visual or cognitive impairments. Caretakers or family members should be included in education sessions if necessary.

SUMMARY

Diabetes mellitus, the most common endocrine disorder, affects millions of Americans.[1] Diabetes is characterized and diagnosed by chronic hyperglycemia, the result of a relative or absolute deficiency of insulin; however, the metabolism of all energy nutrients is altered. Of the four clinical classes of diabetes, the most common are type 2 and type 1 diabetes. Type 2 diabetes is characterized by insulin resistance and a reduction in insulin production leading to a relative insulin deficiency.[12] Type 1 diabetes is the result of destruction of the insulin-producing β cells of the pancreas because of an autoimmune or idiopathic process.[8]

Sequelae of insulin deficiency include the acute and chronic complications of diabetes. Acute complications include diabetic ketoacidosis in type 1 and nonketotic hyperglycemic hyperosmolar coma in type 2 diabetes. Chronic complications include cardiovascular disease, retinopathy, nephropathy, and neuropathy.

The goals of treatment are glycemic control and prevention of complications. Treatment is individualized and encompasses an individualized diet, regular exercise, and appropriate use of medications such as oral antidiabetic agents; incretin and amylin mimetics; and insulin. The efficacy of treatment and the presence of complications of therapy are evaluated by capillary blood glucose monitoring. Patient education is an essential component in teaching skills associated with treatment.[15]

Special considerations attend the treatment and education of individuals with diabetes in the pediatric and geriatric age groups. Children and adolescents require careful monitoring to adjust insulin levels for variations in maturation, exercise, and intercurrent illness. The elderly may have chronic complications of diabetes or other impairments of mobility, vision, or cognition that affect treatment.[15]

Educational materials must be appropriate for age in children and be accessible for elderly individuals with visual or cognitive impairments.[15,40]

REFERENCES

1. Wild S, Roglic G, Green A et al: Global prevalence of diabetes: estimates for the year 2000 and projections for the year 2030, *Diabetes Care* 27:1047-1053, 2004.
2. American Diabetes Association: Economic Costs of Diabetes in the U.S. in 2007, *Diabetes Care* 31:1-20, 2008.
3. National Institute of Diabetes and Digestive and Kidney Diseases. National diabetes statistics fact sheet: general information and national estimates on diabetes in the United States, 2005, Bethesda, MD: U.S. Department of Health and Human Services, National Institutes of Health, 2005.
4. Scheepers A, Joost HG, Schurmann A: The glucose transporter families SGLT and GLUT: Molecular basis of normal and aberrant function, *J Parenter Enteral Nutr* 28:364-372, 2004.
5. Spiegel A, Carter-Su C, Taylor SI et al: Mechanism of action of hormones that act at the cell surface. In Wilson RH et al, editors: *Williams textbook of endocrinology*, ed 11, Philadelphia, 2008, Saunders.
6. Hartter E, Svoboda T, Ludvik B et al: Basal and stimulated plasma levels of pancreatic amylin indicate its co-secretion with insulin in humans, *Diabetologia* 34:52-54, 1991.
7. Drucker DJ: The biology of incretin hormones, *Cell Metab* 3:153-165, 2006.
8. Eisenbaeth GS, Polonsky KS, Buse JB: Diabetes mellitus. In Wilson RH et al, editors: *Williams textbook of endocrinology*, ed 11, Philadelphia, 2008, Saunders.
9. American Diabetes Association: Diagnosis and Classification of Diabetes Mellitus, *Diabetes Care* 31:S55-S60, 2008.
10. Gale EAM, Gillispie KM: Diabetes and Gender, *Diabetologia* 44:3-15, 2001.
11. Pihoker C, Gilliam LK, Hampe CS et al: Autoantibodies in diabetes, *Diabetes* 54:S52-S61, 2005.
12. Buse JB, Polonsky KS, Purant CF: Type 2 Diabetes mellitus. In Wilson RH et al, editors: *Williams textbook of endocrinology*, ed 11, 2008, Saunders.
13. Nikoulina SE, Ciaraldi TP, Carter L et al: Impaired muscle glycogen synthase in type 2 diabetes is associated with diminished phosphatidylinositol 3-kinase activation, *J Clin Endocrinol Metab* 86:4307-4314, 2001.
14. Kitabchi AE, Umpierrez GE, Murphy MB et al: Hyperglycemic Crisis in Adult Patients with Diabetes, *Diabetes Care* 29:2739-2748, 2006.
15. American Diabetes Association: Standards of medical care in diabetes—2008, *Diabetes Care* 31:S12-S54, 2008.
16. Coustand DR: Pharmacological Management of Gestational Diabetes: an overview, *Diabetes Care* 30(S2):S206-S208, 2007.
17. Kim C, Newton KM, Knopp RH: Gestational diabetes and the incidence of type 2 diabetes—a systematic review, *Diabetes Care* 25:1862-1868, 2002.
18. Kim C, Berger DK, Chamany S: Recurrence of gestational diabetes mellitus: a system review, *Diabetes Care* 30:1314-1319, 2007.
19. American Diabetes Association: Nephropathy in diabetes, *Diabetes Care* 27:S79-S83, 2004.
20. Vijan S, Hayward RA: Treatment of hypertension in type 2 diabetes mellitus: blood pressure goals, choice of agents, and setting priorities in diabetic care, *Ann Intern Med* 138:593-602, 2003.
21. Tesfaye S, Chaturvedi N, Eaton SE et al: Vascular risk factors and diabetic neuropathy, *N Engl J Med* 352:341-350, 2005.
22. Cheng YJ, Gregg EW, Kahn HS et al: Peripheral insensate neuropathy—a tall problem for U.S. adults? *Am J Epidemiol* 164:873-880, 2006.
23. Gregg EW, Sorlie P, Paulose-Ram R et al: Prevalence of lower-extremity disease in the U.S. adult population ≥40 years of age with and without diabetes, *Diabetes Care* 27:1591-1597, 2004.
24. American Diabetes Association: Implications of the diabetes control and complications trial, *Diabetes Care* 26:25-27, 2003.
25. American Diabetes Association: Implications of the United Kingdom Prospective Diabetes Study, *Diabetes Care* 26:28-32, 2003.
26. Kwik M, Seeho SKM, Smith C et al: Outcomes of pregnancies affected by impaired glucose tolerance, *Diabetes Res Clin Pract* 77:263-268, 2007.
27. Crowther CA, Hiller JE, Moss JR et al: Effect of treatment of gestational diabetes mellitus on pregnancy outcomes, *N Engl J Med* 352:2477-2486, 2005.
28. American Diabetes Association: Nutrition recommendations and interventions for diabetes. A position statement of the American diabetes association, *Diabetes Care* 31:S61-S78, 2008.
29. American Diabetes Association: Physical activity/exercise and diabetes mellitus, *Diabetes Care* 26:73-77, 2003.
30. Nathan DM, Bus JB, Davidson MB et al: Management of hyperglycemia in type 2 diabetes: a consensus algorithm for the initiation and adjustment of therapy. Update regarding thiazolidinediones: a consensus statement from the American Diabetes Association and the European Association for the study of diabetes, *Diabetes Care* 31:173-175, 2008.
31. Bloomgarden ZT: Metformin, *Diabetes Care* 18:1078-1080, 1995.
32. Jones MC: Therapies for diabetes: pramlinitide and exenatide, *Am Fam Physician* 75:1831-1835, 2007.
33. Weissberg-Benchall J, Antisdel-Lomaglio J, Seehadri R: Insulin pump therapy: a meta-analysis, *Diabetes Care* 26:1079-1087, 2003.
34. Cryer PE: *Hypoglycemia: pathophysiology, diagnosis and treatment*, New York, Oxford University Press, 1997

35. Laing SP, Swerdlow AJ, Slater SD et al: The British Diabetic Association Cohort Study. II. Cause-specific mortality in patients with insulin-treated diabetes mellitus, *Diabetes Med* 16:466-471, 1999.

36. Jacobson AM: The psychological care of patients with insulin-dependent diabetes mellitus, *N Engl J Med* 334:1249-1253, 1996.

37. American Diabetes Association: Tests of glycemia in diabetes, *Diabetes Care* 26:106-108, 2003.

38. American Association of Diabetes Educators: Infection control guidelines for patient education as a means of preventing blood-borne disease transmission during diabetes self-care procedures, *Diabetes Educ* 17:321-325, 1991.

39. Goldstein DE, Little RR, Lorenz RA et al: Tests of glycemia in diabetes, *Diabetes Care* 27:1761-1773, 2004.

40. American Diabetes Association: Third-party reimbursement of diabetes care, self-management education, and supplies, *Diabetes Care* 19(Suppl 1):S96-S97, 2008.

41. American Diabetes Association: National standards for diabetes self-management education, *Diabetes Care* 31:S97-S104, 2008.

42. U.S. Department of Health and Human Services: Healthy People 2010, Washington DC: Government Printing Office, 2000.

Alterations in Metabolism and Nutrition

Daniel J. Guerra

MEDIA RESOURCES

Additional Material for Study, Review, and Further Exploration

 CD Companion ■ Review Questions and Answers
■ Glossary (with audio pronunciations for selected terms)
■ Disease Profiles ■ Animations

evolve **Website** at http://evolve.elsevier.com/Copstead/
■ Case Studies ■ Disease Profiles ■ WebLinks ■ Key Points Review

KEY QUESTIONS

■ How does acute physiologic stress affect body metabolism?
■ What information about nutritional status can be gained from each of the following biochemical tests: serum albumin, transferrin, prealbumin, red blood cell and white blood cell counts, blood urea nitrogen, serum creatinine, and urinary nitrogen excretion?

■ What anthropometric measurements are used to assess nutritional status?
■ What information gained from a nutritional assessment would indicate potential or actual nutritional problems?
■ How do insulin, glucagon, catecholamines, thyroid hormone, cortisol, and growth hormone affect the metabolism of fats, sugars, and proteins?

CHAPTER OUTLINE

Each moment, millions of biochemical reactions occur within the body to generate or dissipate energy to meet physiologic needs. The process, known as **metabolism,** uses energy to sustain the body's vital functions.[1] Metabolism converts biochemical reactions to energy by synthesizing and breaking down molecules. These interrelated and dynamic reactions meet the unique requirements of each independent cellular activity.[2] Adequate nutrition is needed for growth and metabolism, organ function, tissue repair, and response to infection.

Many hospitalized patients experience a significant degree of physiologic stress and multiple organ dysfunction, both of which increase specific and general nutritional needs. Treatment modalities, altered intake, and restricted mobility may also require nutritional adjustment. In many cases, these problems can be averted if nutritional assessment and therapy are started early. This chapter reviews normal nutrient metabolism and nutritional assessment and progresses to a comprehensive discussion of nutritional and metabolic alterations.

METABOLIC PROCESSES

Metabolism is the sum of all the physical and chemical processes by which living organized substance is produced and maintained (anabolism), and also the transformation by which energy is made available for the uses of the organism (catabolism). Metabolism may be dissected along interconnecting pathways, which fall into three discrete programs:

1. **Intermediary metabolism** can be defined as that biochemical process involved with the interconversions of small organic molecules in living cells through evolutionarily adapted pathways, which are under multiple layers of regulation.
2. **Primary metabolism** includes metabolic pathways and the machinery of DNA replication, recombination, transcription, RNA processing, translation, and protein processing.
3. **Secondary metabolism** refers to the synthesis, accumulation and degradation of molecules that are not specifically essential for normal cell processes.

Intermediary metabolism is the key to cell biology: it provides energy and the molecular structures including lipids, proteins, nucleic acids, and carbohydrates essential to cellular architecture including cytoskeleton, membrane systems, and organelle formation. These "intermediates" are also used in anti-metabolite responses, signal transduction, and energy storage, and in mineral and water balance in the cell.

The key to metabolism is the control or regulation of the concentration of metabolites in given cell types such that the cell is always poised to deal with nutritional and communicative requirements. Cells must be receptive to membrane-associated signaling such that transfer of lipids, or glucose or amino acids or a suite of signaling molecules can be recruited and secreted by the activated cell, At the same time, the cell must be in an energetically favorable state; this requires both

production and utilization of energy, usually in the form of ATP, although many nucleotides take part in this energy transfer (e.g., cAMP, GTP, NAD(P)H, FAD etc).

The positioning or constancy of the cell at any particular time may be referred to as the steady state. It is in dynamic non-equilibrium.

The reactions leading to the assimilation of organic molecules either auto or heterotrophic are organized into metabolic pathways. A pathway can be considered a sequential vectorial transfer of substrate to product where the individual catalytic events are carried out by specific enzymatic reactions.

- Enzymes in a pathway can be organized in clusters sometimes via simple compartmentalization and sometimes via more specific protein/protein interactions such as multi-subunit and polyprotein complexes. Intermediates in a pathway are vectorially transferred to the next enzyme active site; even though this process may be nothing more than simple diffusion. The rate of the reactions are such that flux through the pathway is guaranteed and intermediates do not simply diffuse away from the catalysis.
- Soluble and discrete enzymes likely carry out glycolysis within the cytosol. When this pathway design is utilized, it may be enhanced catalytically by compartmentalization, as the TCA cycle is sequestered in the mitochondrial matrix. Another pathway that is utilized in eukaryotic cells is that found in plant FAS. Here, the proteins are aggregated but not covalently attached. They can be separated as individual catalysts but are believed to exist as protein aggregates in the stroma of the chloroplast. FAS I as found in mammals and yeast is a multi-protein or polyprotein covalently linking all of the component proteins in a highly efficient multienzyme complex. Another form of order is that found in the oxidative phosphorylation reactions of the inner mitochondrial membrane leading from the utilization of NADH and the subsequent electrochemical proton pumping coupling to ATP synthesis. These are membrane-bound complexes.

Pathways are functionally separated and regulated.

- *Catabolism and degradative metabolism.* Dietary foods are combusted or oxidized finally to CO_2 and H_2O. The electrons from these reactions are largely driven to molecular oxygen, and the production of ATP is coupled to this reduction of oxygen (see Chapter 3). Some of the electrons driven off during the oxidation of carbon are used to make NADPH that in turn provides reducing power for biosynthesis. Glycolysis and the TCA cycle are the major metabolic routes, as well as fatty acid beta-oxidation, amino acid catabolism to ketogenic (TCA) or glucogenic products, purine degradation to uric acid, and pyrimidine degradation to beta alanine, NH_3 and CO_2. Along these degradation pathways intermediates for biosynthesis are formed and used (e.g., oxidative pentose phosphate pathway, flavin nucleotides).
- *Biosynthesis or anabolism.* This metabolism involves several unique biosynthetic routes each coupled to the energy state of the cell and the specific cell type, age, and degree

of stimulation/signaling. NADPH is the preferred bioreductant in biosynthesis. ATP is also usually required to overcome thermodynamic unfavorability of biosynthetic reactions. Thioester intermediates are also commonly used in biosynthesis. During biosynthesis, substrates are replenished from the catabolite pools, as are NADPH and ATP. Examples of biosynthetic pathways include gluconeogenesis, fatty acid synthesis, amino acid and nucleotide biosynthesis, and protein synthesis. DNA replication and transcription are anabolic pathways as are processing of proteins including important covalent modifications like acylation, prenylation, glycosylation, and glypiation.

Anabolism and Catabolism

Anabolism refers to the constructive phase of metabolism and involves the synthesis of organic molecules by cells. More complex or larger molecules are built from simple ones, and in the process energy is consumed. Anabolism occurs continuously along with catabolism, but is more prominent during times of rest, healing, pregnancy, lactation, and growth. Hormonal secretions such as insulin and sex hormones may also trigger anabolism. Obesity, with the accumulation of adipose tissue via net synthesis of lipids such as triacylglycerol, is a form of anabolism.[3] Conversely, **catabolism** is the degradative phase of metabolism. Complex molecules are broken down into simpler substances, often with the concurrent release or production of energy. During times of disease, stress, fever, or starvation or during the release of certain hormones such as thyroid hormone and cortisol, catabolism dominates the body's metabolic processes. The resultant tissue wasting may lead to cellular injury or death if excessive catabolism is left unregulated.[4] Anabolism and catabolism occur simultaneously and together create the dynamic, homeostatic balance of substance and energy known as metabolism.

The metabolic process requires nutrients in the form of carbohydrates, fats, and proteins. Each of these three nutrients is altered or broken down into simpler substances. Lipids may be directly sequestered into adipose cells after limited lipolysis and synthesis into lipoproteins for transport. Enzymes and coenzymes mediate the metabolism of glucose, fatty acids, amino acids, and nucleic acids. In this fashion, the body's continual cellular energy requirements are met.[4] Energy produced by metabolic processes is used to create the energy currency of the body known as **adenosine** triphosphate (ATP; See Chapter 3).[4]

Cells use energy to perform essential physiological and biochemical processes. **Energy** can be measured in kilocalories; 1 kcal represents the amount of energy required to raise the temperature of 1 kg of water from 15° C to 16° C. During catabolism of fuel molecules, approximately 40% of the available energy ultimately is converted to ATP or NADPH (nicotinamide adenine dinucleotide phosphate, reduced form), with the remaining 60% producing heat.[2] The energy released as heat is important for maintaining body temperature.

Metabolic Rate

Several factors determine the body's energy requirements or metabolic needs, including the basal metabolic rate (BMR), growth, stress, activity level, and the energy necessary for digestion.[4]

The **basal metabolic rate** refers to the rate of energy consumption by resting tissue. It is a measurement of the energy used in maintenance of the body at rest after a 12-hour fast.[4] It represents the energy used in maintaining basic body processes such as respiration, cellular metabolism, circulation, glandular activity, and the maintenance of body temperature.[4] The body's BMR is determined by calculating oxygen use during a specific period. The normal range for BMR is generally between 0.8 and 1.43 kcal/min.[4] Several factors that affect an individual's BMR are described in Table 42-1. Body stature and size affect BMR by the amount of heat lost from the body surface. BMR also is an important determinant of total daily energy expenditure (TEE).[5] Age is also an important determinant of BMR. A growing child's BMR is significantly higher than an adult's, primarily because of an increased rate of cellular activity, surface-to-volume ratio, and the generation of new tissue.[4] Conversely, as one ages, the BMR gradually declines by about 2% per decade. Body composition, determined by the amount of fat and lean tissue, also affects BMR. Muscle tissue requires more oxygen than adipose tissue, which explains why athletes have an approximately 5% higher BMR than nonathletes.[2] One contribution to this observation among athletes is the enhanced beta-oxidation of fatty acids in this group.[6] Women typically have a metabolic rate 5% to 10% less than that of men, probably because of differences in body mass. Women also tend to have more adipose tissue than men, and fat is less metabolically active than muscle.[3] Pregnancy increases the BMR by about 20% to 28%, or 300 kcal/day, as a consequence of increased uterine and mammary gland size, fetal development, and additional cardiopulmonary workload.[4] Other factors affecting BMR include nutritional status, muscle tone, sleep, fever, environmental temperature, and stress.[2]

Almost any alteration in the body's normal homeostatic state will alter its energy requirements and BMR. Many diseases are known to dramatically increase the body's energy requirements; including chronic obstructive and restrictive

TABLE 42-1

Examples of Factors Affecting Basal Metabolic Rate

Increasing Metabolism	Decreasing Metabolism
Childhood growth	Aging process
Exercise	End-stage illness
Sympathetic stimulation	Starvation
Shivering	Sleep
Fever	Tropical climates
Thyroid hormone	Calorie restricted diets
Muscle tissue	Reduced muscle-mass
Pregnancy	
Stress	
Male sex hormone	

pulmonary disease, hyperthermia, burns, cancer, diabetes, and Graves disease (hyperthyroidism).

> **KEY POINTS**
>
> - Anabolism refers to energy-requiring processes involving synthesis of biomolecules. Catabolism refers to energy-producing processes during which biomolecules are broken down into simpler forms. Metabolism refers to the dynamic state of simultaneously occurring anabolism and catabolism.
> - The BMR is the rate of energy utilization when the body is at rest. Examples of factors affecting the BMR include body size and composition, age, nutritional status, muscle mass, fever, stress, and pregnancy.

NUTRIENT METABOLISM

Metabolism in general is controlled by both the nervous system and the endocrine system. Four major hormones involved in substrate metabolism are insulin, glucagon, catecholamines, and cortisol. The effects of these four hormones on carbohydrate, fat, and protein metabolism are summarized in Tables 42-2 to 42-4. Both the nervous system and the endocrine system directly affect metabolism by release of the catecholamines epinephrine and norepinephrine, which during times of stress inhibit insulin secretion. The pancreatic hormones insulin and glucagon have a crucial role in the metabolic processes that govern the body's energy requirements. These hormones function antithetically, with insulin lowering blood glucose levels and glucagon ultimately increasing blood glucose levels.[2] Growth hormone affects metabolism by decreasing cellular uptake and use of glucose. High levels of growth hormone tend to decrease affinity for insulin at the receptor site such that even increased secretion of insulin by the pancreas has diminutive effects on blood glucose levels. Glucocorticoid hormones, primarily cortisol, stimulate gluconeogenesis by the liver. Blood glucose levels six to ten times normal may occur with significant cortisol secretion. Left uncorrected, diabetes mellitus may develop (see Chapter 41).[3]

Carbohydrates

Carbohydrates are the main energy source for the body. Approximately 45% to 65% of the recommended diet should consist of carbohydrates.[7] Dietary carbohydrates are starches or sugars. Carbohydrates are classified into the three categories of **monosaccharides** (simple sugars), **oligosaccharides** (2 to 10 joined monosaccharide units), and **polysaccharides** (10 to 10,000 monosaccharide units). They range from very simple sugars consisting of three to seven carbons to incredibly complex polymers made up of repeating units of thousands of monosaccharides.[4]

Dietary monosaccharides are the six-carbon sugars of glucose, mannose, fructose, and galactose. Glucose, the most physiologically important of the group, is the form of sugar normally found in the bloodstream. Glucose is derived from the catabolism of more complex carbohydrates during the process of digestion. Fructose and galactose are also eventually converted to glucose by the liver, although fructose can directly enter metabolism via phosphorylation.[8] Once in the bloodstream, glucose is either oxidized to provide cellular energy, metabolized to fatty acids, or stored in the liver and muscles as glycogen. Blood sugar levels then reflect the difference between the amount of glucose released into the bloodstream by the liver and the amount of glucose taken up by the cells for energy.[3]

Intracellular Glucose Metabolism

Once in the cell, glucose undergoes various biochemical transformations including a form of anaerobic oxidation called glycolysis (See Chapter 3). Glycolysis is the metabolic

TABLE 42-3

Hormonal Actions on Fat Metabolism

Hormone	Actions
Insulin	Increases fatty acid uptake by fat cells
	Promotes glucose uptake by fat cells
Glucagon	Promotes lipolysis in fat cells
Catecholamines	Increases fat mobilization
	Increase serum free fatty acid levels
Cortisol	Increases fat cell membrane permeability

TABLE 42-2

Hormonal Actions on Carbohydrate Metabolism

Hormone	Actions
Insulin	Stimulates glucose uptake by cells
	Stimulates glycolysis
	Inhibits gluconeogenesis
Glucagon	Stimulates glycogen breakdown
	Increases gluconeogenesis
Catecholamines	Maintain blood glucose level during stress
	Diminish glucose uptake by cells
	Increase glycogen breakdown
Cortisol	Stimulates gluconeogenesis
	Diminishes glucose uptake by cells

TABLE 42-4

Hormonal Actions on Protein Metabolism

Hormone	Actions
Insulin	Actively transports amino acids into cells
	Accelerates cellular protein synthesis
Glucagon	Stimulates protein breakdown into amino acids
	Increases amino acid transport into hepatic cells
Cortisol	Increases protein catabolism

sequence that converts glucose to pyruvate and, depending on several variables including oxygen availability and energy needs, eventually yields the end products of carbon dioxide and water.[4] Catabolism of glucose may occur anaerobically along the Embden-Meyerhof (glycolysis) pathway, which is a 10-step process altering the chemical composition of glucose to pyruvic acid and results in a net gain of two ATP molecules for each molecule of glucose that enters the pathway. Pyruvic acid has two important roles in the catabolic process of carbohydrates. It provides the body with acetyl coenzyme A, which is required for conversion to fatty acids or to energy, and it is the initial step for the second stage of carbohydrate metabolism, the tricarboxylic acid (TCA) cycle (also called the *citric acid cycle* or the *Krebs cycle*) and oxidative phosphorylation. The TCA cycle occurs in the mitochondrial matrix. Oxidative phosphorylation (see Chapter 3) produces a total of about 30 molecules of ATP for each molecule of glucose. Although other pathways exist, the interrelated glycolytic, TCA cycle, and respiratory chain enzymes can produce nearly all of the energy required for cellular functioning.[4] Figure 42-1 illustrates the metabolism of carbohydrate, fat, and protein through the anaerobic glycolytic pathway and the TCA cycle. The TCA cycle and the respiratory chain require molecular oxygen (aerobic) to function.

Depending on needs, glucose is catabolized for the production of energy, synthesized into lipid, stored as polymers of glycogen, or re-synthesized. **Gluconeogenesis** refers to the process by which glucose is formed from noncarbohydrate sources, including amino acids supplied by muscle tissue and glycerol supplied from fat breakdown.[7] The glucose made through this mechanism may either be stored in the liver as glycogen or released into the bloodstream. During periods of fasting, gluconeogenesis and glycogenolysis provide the necessary glucose to meet the metabolic requirements of the brain and other glucose-dependent tissues.[3]

Hormonal Control of Glucose Metabolism

Many hormones affect glucose levels by altering carbohydrate metabolism. The only hormone known to lower blood glucose levels is insulin. Hormones that tend to raise blood glucose levels include glucagon, growth hormone, glucocorticoid hormones, epinephrine and norepinephrine, and thyroid hormone. Table 42-2 describes the major hormonal effects on glucose metabolism.

Insulin, a peptide hormone formed from its precursor proinsulin and synthesized by β cells in the pancreas, is secreted in response to increased blood glucose levels. Minutes after ingestion of a meal, insulin levels in the blood rise significantly, peak in 30 minutes, and level off in about 3 hours. Between meals, when blood glucose levels tend to drop, insulin levels also remain low. At that time, glucose and amino acid stores are used for cellular energy requirements.[3]

Insulin directly affects glucose metabolism by promoting glucose uptake by the liver, which then favors the synthesis

FIGURE 42-1 Metabolic integration of carbohydrate, fat, and protein metabolism. Anaerobic pathway: glycolysis moves with downward arrows, gluconeogenesis moves with upward arrows. *CoA,* Coenzyme A. (From Mahan LK, Arlin MT: *Krause's food, nutrition and diet therapy,* ed 8, Philadelphia, 1992, Saunders, p 345.)

of glycogen. Glucose formation (**gluconeogenesis**) and the breakdown of glycogen to form glucose (**glycogenolysis**) are inhibited by insulin. The active transport of glucose across cellular membranes into muscle and adipose tissue is facilitated by insulin and has a direct lowering effect on blood glucose levels.[9] Individuals with diabetes mellitus have either insulin hyposecretion or cellular hyporesponsiveness to insulin as a consequence of receptor down-regulation. Obese and elderly persons are especially at risk for insulin receptor down-regulation with resultant diabetes. Diabetes mellitus is discussed in Chapter 41.

Glucagon is a peptide hormone secreted by α cells in the pancreas and also by some cells lining the gastrointestinal tract. Acting in a fashion opposite that of insulin, glucagon increases blood glucose levels.[10] As blood glucose levels begin to drop, plasma glucagon levels begin to rise. The two primary effects of glucagon, then, are to promote the breakdown of liver glycogen with subsequent release of glucose into the bloodstream and to promote liver gluconeogenesis. These actions tend to bring serum glucose levels back to normal. Conversely, as glucose levels rise, glucagon secretion is diminished and serum glucose levels drop toward normal. The diametric actions of insulin and glucagon partially explain why increased glucagon secretion may also have a role in the elevated blood glucose levels seen in people with diabetes mellitus.[2]

Catecholamines, epinephrine and norepinephrine, are derived from the amino acid tyrosine and serve a role in carbohydrate metabolism to maintain blood glucose levels during times of stress. As the stress response occurs, catecholamines stimulate the conversion of glycogen to glucose in the muscles and liver. Although muscles, unlike the liver, cannot release glucose into the general circulation, mobilization of muscle glycogen frees up unused blood glucose for other tissues such as the brain and the peripheral nervous system. The second primary action of epinephrine during the stress response is to stimulate glucagon secretion and prevent insulin release from the pancreas, thereby preventing glucose movement into muscle cells. Epinephrine also promotes glycogenolysis by the liver and muscles and reduces glucose uptake by muscle tissue. The role of catecholamines in glucose metabolism is very similar to that of glucagon and opposite that of insulin.[2]

Cortisol is derived from cholesterol and is the primary **glucocorticoid** hormone secreted from the adrenal cortex. Cortisol is an insulin antagonist and helps to maintain serum glucose levels. During fasting, cortisol permissively enables other hormonal changes to occur, such as decreased insulin production and increased glucagon and epinephrine secretion. The end result is promotion of gluconeogenesis and lipolysis. If cortisol deficiency occurs simultaneously with fasting, hypoglycemic reactions significant enough to alter brain functioning can occur. A recent study indicated that cortisol deficiency may be a significant cause of morbidity and mortality in critically ill surgical patients, who frequently are poorly nourished.[11]

Growth hormone has a role in carbohydrate metabolism, although it is minor in comparison with its role in growth regulation and protein anabolism; however, it can have a significant impact on glucose regulation under certain circumstances. Growth hormone's effects parallel those of cortisol: growth hormone increases gluconeogenesis in the liver and inhibits glucose uptake by muscle cells.[2] Growth hormone disinhibits gene expression in the liver in favor of transcription of **phosphoenolpyruvate (PEP)** carboxykinase, a key enzyme in hepatic gluconeogenesis.[12] Elevated serum growth hormone levels tend to increase blood glucose levels. As a result, the insulin-secreting β cells in the pancreas are stimulated. If this process is not corrected, the β cells will eventually be exhausted. It is for this reason that diabetes mellitus eventually develops in individuals with excessive growth hormone, as in acromegaly.[3]

Thyroid hormone tends to raise blood glucose levels. In carbohydrate metabolism, the primary mode of action is to increase glucose absorption from the intestines and stimulate the release of epinephrine. Thyroid hormone also promotes the rate of insulin destruction. Ultimately, thyroid hormone causes an increase in cellular oxygen consumption and the basal metabolic rate of tissues.

Fats

Fats, the most concentrated form of energy, are derived de novo and from animal fats and vegetable oils. Fats supply 9 kcal of energy per gram, as compared with 4 kcal from glucose and 4 kcal from protein. Fats are 98% **triacylglycerol (TAG)**. Like carbohydrates, fats are made up of carbon, hydrogen, and oxygen. The bulk of each TAG molecule consists of fatty acids containing 4 to 30 carbon atoms. Fats are frequently categorized as **saturated** or **unsaturated.** Figure 42-2 shows the chemical composition of some common saturated and unsaturated fatty acids. The degree of hydrogen **saturation** refers to the number of double bonds between the carbon atoms in

---

18-Carbon Fatty Acids

Stearic acid	$CH_3(CH_2)_{16}COOH$ (C18:0) (saturated)
Oleic acid	$CH_3(CH_2)_7CH{=}CH(CH_2)_7COOH$ (C18:1Δ9) (monounsaturated)
Linoleic acid	$CH_3(CH_2)_4CH{=}CHCH_2CH{=}CH(CH_7)COOH$ (C18:2Δ9,12) (polyunsaturated)

FIGURE 42-2 Chemical composition of some fatty acids.

the chain. If a fatty acid chain contains all the hydrogen atoms possible with no double bonds, it is called a **saturated fatty acid.** Those fatty acids with one double bond are typed as **monounsaturated,** and those with several double bonds are called **polyunsaturated.**[4]

Fats in the form of TAG supply approximately two thirds of the cell's total energy requirements. Whereas the human body is able to economically store approximately 140,000 kcal of usable fats in adipose tissue, it can store only 24,000 kcal of protein and a mere 800 kcal of carbohydrate in an adult male.[10] Carbohydrates and amino acids not immediately used by the tissues are converted to fat and stored, along with ingested fat, as adipose tissue. Fat deposits are extremely important in the economical use of metabolites. If intake exceeds expenditure, obesity results. During times of fasting, the body quickly reverts to the breakdown and use of fats as its energy source.[11] All tissues in the body, with the exception of brain cells, can metabolize and use fats as an energy source as effectively as glucose.[10]

Almost all fats are absorbed into the lymph system from the intestinal mucosa. They are then converted to a chylomicron consisting of 80% triglyceride, 9% cholesterol, 7% phospholipid, and 4% lipoprotein coat.[13] Chylomicrons empty into the venous blood at the thoracic duct and are carried to the liver for metabolism or assimilated into adipose tissue. Once in the liver, TAG is generally hydrolyzed into glycerol and fatty acids in a process known as **lipolysis.** When released, the fatty acids, bound to albumin, are quickly assimilated into tissue. Oxidation in tissue begins when acetyl coenzyme A binds to the end of a fatty acid. Progressing through a series of reactions known as β oxidation, the fatty acid chain is shortened by two carbon atoms until all the carbon atoms have been transferred to coenzyme A. Acetyl coenzyme A then enters the TCA cycle and oxidative phosphorylation, with each 2-carbon segment producing 2 molecules of carbon dioxide and 12 molecules of ATP. During prolonged fasting, acetyl-CoA is converted into ketone bodies that can traverse the blood-brain barrier and provide energy to the brain (see below). The average fatty acid contains approximately 18 carbon molecules, with 146 ATP molecules being produced during catabolism.[2] Unlike fatty acids, glycerol (the other component of triglycerides) can only be metabolized by a few tissues. Glycerol is generally carried to the liver, where it is either oxidized for energy or used to generate new triglycerides.

Within the liver, fatty acids are generally transformed to acetyl coenzyme A, which is further processed into one of three compounds collectively known as **ketone bodies.** Once released into the bloodstream, ketones have a critical role as an energy source for tissues able to oxidize them in the Krebs cycle. During the fasting state, tissues use ketones as a primary energy source, with glucose reserved for brain metabolism. If the fasting state continues, many areas of the brain begin to use ketone bodies as an energy source. As the brain begins to use ketones, less protein is broken down to provide glucose. For this reason, the body is able to withstand periods of fasting with minimal protein breakdown and tissue disruption.[2]

The liver is the major organ responsible for lipid metabolism and regulation of serum lipid levels. The four primary functions of the hepatic system in regard to lipid metabolism are: (1) synthesis of triglycerides from carbohydrates and protein, (2) synthesis of phospholipids and cholesterol from TAG, (3) desaturation of fatty acids, and (4) utilization of TAG as an energy source.[4] Liver disease can significantly alter any of these processes and cause serious metabolic disturbances. A fatty liver is characterized by fat deposits in the liver cells caused either by ingestion of hepatotoxic substances such as alcohol or halocarbons or by diets significantly low in protein for a prolonged period (see Chapter 38). Infections managed with protein synthesis–inhibiting antibiotics such as tetracycline, and malignancies may also lead to increased fat deposits within the liver by adversely affecting the hepatic cells or biliary tract. Increased mobilization of fatty acids from adipose tissue to the liver occurs in certain conditions, such as diabetes mellitus, starvation, and obesity, where lipogenesis exceeds the ability of the liver to export the fat as lipoproteins.[14] Metabolic studies of critically ill patients indicate that fatty acid breakdown occurs at a much higher rate than patient caloric needs require. This excess lipolysis may cause fatty liver.[15]

Hormonal Control of Lipid Metabolism

Because carbohydrates and lipids may both be metabolized along the anaerobic glycolytic pathway, hormones that affect carbohydrate metabolism also affect lipid metabolism. Table 42-3 describes the hormones considered to have the greatest effect on lipid metabolism. These hormones include insulin, thyroid hormone, glucocorticoids, mineralocorticoids, growth hormone, epinephrine, and norepinephrine. Insulin prevents fat utilization by indirectly causing fatty acids to be taken up by adipose tissue and by decreasing the activity of hormone-sensitive lipase, which promotes the movement of fat out of adipose tissue. Glucocorticoids increase fat cell membrane permeability, whereas mineralocorticoids increase the activity of hormone-sensitive lipase. Epinephrine and norepinephrine increase fat mobilization by stimulating the activity of hormone-sensitive lipase, thus increasing the serum free fatty acid level. Growth hormone increases fatty acid mobilization and use by tissues as an energy source.[4]

Proteins

Proteins are composed of nitrogen, carbon, hydrogen, oxygen, and, occasionally, sulfur. When hydrolyzed, they yield amino acids. Twenty-two amino acids have been identified in protein, 8 of which are essential—meaning that they must be supplied through the diet.[13] These include phenylalanine, valine, threonine, tryptophan, isoleucine, methionine, leucine, and lysine. The distinction between essential and non-essential amino acids is somewhat unclear, as some amino acids can be produced from others. Several amino acids are considered to be conditionally essential and must be supplied by the diet under conditions of reduced ability to synthesize them in the body. For example, tyrosine can be synthesized from phenylalanine, but when a patient is on a phenylalanine-restricted diet, then tyrosine can't be synthesized and must be provided in the diet. Muscle tissue, bones, teeth, skin, and hair are made up primarily of protein. To function properly, most body processes require an adequate supply of proteins, many of which must be obtained through a balanced diet. Children, because of their rapid growth, require more protein per kilogram of body weight than adults do. In addition, when compared with adults, children also need a larger percentage of their dietary intake of protein to contain essential amino acids.

Once ingested, proteins are broken down into amino acids or peptides and are absorbed through the intestinal lumen. They are then carried to the liver through the portal vein. The liver regulates protein metabolism through enzymatic breakdown of amino acids; formation of nonessential amino acids from simple precursors; and detoxification of ammonia, urea, uric acid, and other catabolic end products. Proteins are rapidly metabolized by the liver, which enables a quick response to changing metabolic demands. Amino acids supplied in excess of metabolic requirements are degraded to by-products such as urea, uric acid, or creatinine, and the remaining carbon molecules are converted to carbohydrate and fat or oxidized for energy.[16] Of particular importance is the conversion of amino acids to keto acids, which are carbohydrate-like in structure and created by removal of the amino group during deamination. These keto acids may then enter the TCA cycle, where they provide energy for liver metabolism, or they may be converted to fatty acids by the liver.

Protein metabolism can be measured in terms of **nitrogen balance.** If nitrogen intake approximates output, an equal nitrogen balance exists. If dietary intake of proteins exceeds output, a **positive nitrogen balance** occurs. Protein anabolism exceeds catabolism during periods of rapid growth, pregnancy, and the formation of new tissue. Experimentally, positive nitrogen balance has been induced in malnourished patients through the administration of growth hormone.[17] A **negative nitrogen balance** occurs when protein breakdown exceeds daily protein intake and synthesis. If the daily caloric intake is insufficient, the body catabolizes dietary and tissue protein for energy, as is the case after severe burns and during fever, illness, or stress.[2]

Hormonal Control of Protein Metabolism

Anabolic and catabolic protein metabolism is controlled by various hormones. Table 42-4 lists the major hormonal effects on protein metabolism. Hormones that also promote protein synthesis include growth hormone, especially during growth spurts; testosterone in specific reproductive organs during puberty; and thyroid hormone indirectly, by increasing the metabolic rate. Insulin also promotes the active transport of amino acids across cell membranes and accelerates protein synthesis within the cell. Insulin, in concert with growth hormone, is required for normal growth and development of children and adolescents. Glucagon, whose actions diametrically oppose those of insulin, promotes gluconeogenesis by stimulating the breakdown of protein into amino acids and increasing their transport into hepatic cells. Glucagon also enables the conversion of amino acids into glucose precursors.

KEY POINTS

- Metabolism of carbohydrate, fat, and protein supplies energy to support the cell's energy-requiring processes and provides building blocks for the synthesis of cellular biomolecules. The primary hormonal regulators of nutrient metabolism are insulin, glucagon, catecholamines, cortisol, thyroid hormone, and growth hormone.
- Insulin is secreted from pancreatic β cells in response to elevated serum glucose levels. Binding of insulin to receptors on target cells (muscle, adipose tissue) facilitates the transport of glucose into cells and reduces blood glucose levels. Insulin inhibits lipolysis and gluconeogenesis.
- Glucagon is secreted from pancreatic α cells in response to low blood glucose levels. Glucagon promotes glycogenolysis and gluconeogenesis (from protein and glycerol) by the liver, thereby increasing blood glucose levels.
- Catecholamines increase glycogenolysis and gluconeogenesis by the liver, thereby increasing blood glucose levels. Catecholamines also stimulate lipolysis in adipose cells by enhancing the action of hormone-sensitive lipase. Glucagon secretion is enhanced and insulin secretion is inhibited by catecholamines.
- Cortisol enhances the actions of glucagon and catecholamines and promotes glycogenolysis, gluconeogenesis, and lipolysis, thus raising blood levels of glucose and fatty acids.
- Thyroid hormone tends to raise blood glucose levels. In carbohydrate metabolism, the primary mode of action is to increase glucose absorption from the intestines and stimulate the release of epinephrine. Thyroid hormone also enhances the rate of insulin destruction. Ultimately, thyroid hormone causes an increase in cellular oxygen consumption and the general metabolic rate of tissues.
- Growth hormone increases blood glucose by inhibiting uptake by muscle cells and by stimulating gluconeogenesis in the liver. Growth hormone enhances the cellular uptake of amino acids and stimulates protein synthesis.
- The main sources of cellular energy are glucose and fatty acids. Glucose is the primary energy source for the brain, although the brain can use ketones. Ketones are produced from fatty acids by the liver, particularly under conditions of decreased carbohydrate intake or fasting.

AGING AND METABOLIC FUNCTION

Without doubt, the aging process has an effect on normal metabolism. It is sometimes difficult, however, to distinguish the effects of aging from the effects of chronic illness, drug therapy, or obesity.

There seems to be little difference in the ability of healthy people, young or old, to metabolize glucose and little difference in insulin secretion by the β cells in the pancreas. What does appear to occur with the aging process is a change in tissue sensitivity to insulin. Although many possible causes

Geriatric Variations Associated with Aging and Metabolic Function

- With aging comes a change in tissue sensitivity to insulin because of an alteration in the molecular make-up of insulin. Elderly persons have higher levels of circulating serum proinsulin than younger adults do. The aging process may also alter insulin receptor sites and thereby render insulin less effective.
- The aging process may affect lipid metabolism as proportionate body fat increases. Although caloric intake generally decreases, a concurrent loss of lean body mass and decline in energy expenditure begin with adulthood.
- A decline in the resting metabolic rate also occurs with aging. This change is related to several factors, such as reduced lean body mass, reduced lipogenic enzyme response to glucose, and decreased catecholamine secretion after a meal.

for this phenomenon have been proposed, such as reduced carbohydrate intake, decreased muscle mass, and lowered activity levels, the reason appears to lie in an alteration in the molecular makeup of insulin. The elderly have higher levels of circulating serum proinsulin than younger adults do. It is also believed that the aging process alters insulin receptor sites and thus renders insulin less effective (insulin resistance).[18]

The aging process may also affect lipid metabolism as proportionate body fat increases. Although caloric intake generally decreases, a concurrent loss of lean body mass and a decline in energy expenditure begin with adulthood. A decline in the resting metabolic rate also occurs with the aging process. This change is related to several factors, such as reduced lean body mass, reduced lipogenic enzyme response to glucose, and decreased catecholamine secretion after a meal. Although cross-sectional studies demonstrate that cholesterol and triglyceride serum levels tend to rise with age, evidence is increasing that this change may be due more to obesity than to the aging process itself. As a risk factor, hyperlipidemia poses less threat for coronary artery disease and atherosclerosis with the aging process.[18]

A decrease in the quantity of skeletal muscle normally occurs with aging. Although this decrease in muscle is associated with factors such as physical inactivity and a decrease in the number of neurons to muscle cells, endocrine factors also influence the loss of muscle mass. The decreased growth hormone secretion noted in elderly individuals leads to decreased protein synthesis.[18]

Box 42-1 summarizes some of the effects that the aging process has on normal metabolism.

KEY POINTS

- Aging is associated with a change in tissue sensitivity to insulin and altered insulin receptor sites, factors hypothesized to render insulin less effective.
- As proportionate body fat increases with aging, lipid metabolism may be affected.
- The resting metabolic rate slows with aging.

NUTRITIONAL ALTERATIONS OF PHYSIOLOGIC STRESS

Metabolic Response

The response of the body to starvation is different from the response to physiologic stress.[19] Starvation is a gradual process in which the metabolic rate decreases and carbohydrate reserves are exhausted. As insulin levels dwindle, free fatty acids are released for energy use. Despite the available free fatty acids, protein is used for energy by means of gluconeogenesis because the body's tissues prefer glucose as an energy source. This is in part because of the requirement for molecular O_2 to carry out fatty acid β-oxidation. This preference creates a negative nitrogen balance. As starvation continues, overall energy needs are reduced and the tissues that usually require glucose for function adapt by using ketones for energy. Then lipolysis provides the source of needed energy, and the use of protein as an energy source decreases. This change is an adaptive response through which the body strives to conserve lean body mass. Overall, the result is minimal depletion of the body's protein. Decreased serum glucose and urinary nitrogen excretion, along with elevation in ketones and free fatty acids, characterizes starvation. Fasting (voluntary starving) alone is not associated with a high mortality unless it is prolonged, as it is in anorexia nervosa. Figure 42-3 provides a summary of the physiologic effect of starvation.

With physiologic stress, conservation of lean body mass does not occur. The metabolic rate increases rather than decreases, and a high sustained rate of catabolism (breakdown of protein to meet energy needs) results. Protein is used as an energy source by gluconeogenesis through release of muscle stores of protein-derived amino acids. This adaptation quickly results in a negative nitrogen balance. Cell mass is redistributed in response to the stressor, with an increase in the production of acute phase proteins. The degree of hypermetabolism, hypercatabolism, and negative nitrogen balance associated with a physiologic stress depends on the type, duration, and severity of the stressor present.

Phases of Catabolic Response

Typically, the catabolic response to stress occurs in two phases: the immediate phase, lasting 5 to 8 days, and the subsequent adaptive phase. The physiologic effects of each phase are summarized in Figures 42-4 and 42-5.

The immediate phase of **catabolism** is characterized by increased sympathetic nervous system stimulation with release of glucagon, glucocorticoids, and catecholamines. The resultant decreased production and circulation of insulin cause a pseudodiabetic state. Hyperglycemia develops from decreased circulating insulin and decreased utilization of glucose by muscle and other tissues (insulin resistance).

An energy deficit is created, and alternative mechanisms of glucose production are needed. The oxidation of branched-chain amino acids occurs for two reasons: to meet energy requirements and for the amino acids to provide the liver a substrate for the synthesis of acute phase proteins

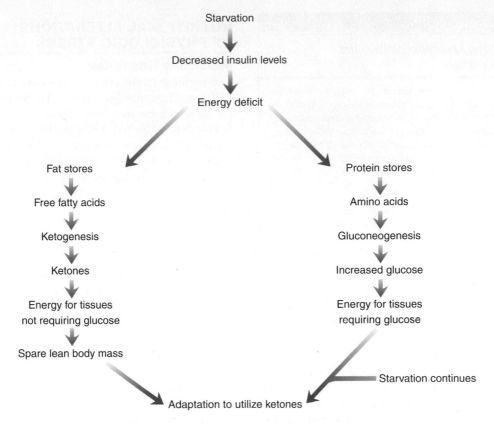

FIGURE 42-3 Catabolic response to starvation.

FIGURE 42-4 Immediate catabolic response to stress. *SNS*, Sympathetic nervous system.

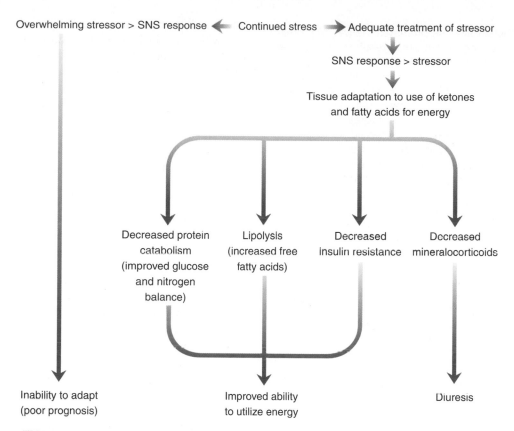

FIGURE 42-5 Adaptive phase of the catabolic response to stress. *SNS,* Sympathetic nervous system.

(immunoglobulins, lymphocytes, and leukocytes). As the amino acids are mobilized to meet energy needs, alanine is formed (ammonia plus pyruvate) and stimulates gluconeogenesis. Sodium and water are retained secondary to an increase in aldosterone, which results in potassium loss. The mineralocorticoid aldosterone is released as a result of stimulation of the sympathetic nervous system. During this phase, fat is not well used as an energy source because some level of insulin is present and has an antilipolytic action.

The nutritional result of the immediate phase of stress on the body is hyperglycemia, negative nitrogen balance, and retention of fluid and sodium. This protective mechanism uses skeletal muscle to meet energy requirements and protects the rest of the body's tissue from breaking down during periods of high-energy need. An overall loss of nitrogen and other electrolytes, including magnesium, phosphorus, and zinc, takes place.

The adaptive phase occurs if the sympathetic nervous system response can selectively keep up with the stressors present. Hypermetabolism, a condition caused by excessive trauma, helps keep the system active, thus providing essential energy needs and new protein synthesis during severe stress.[20] If the stressors overwhelm the body's response system, the effect on prognosis will be negative. In the adaptive phase, the body begins to use ketones and fatty acids (lipolysis) for energy and conserve proteins. As the sympathetic nervous system response lessens, insulin resistance decreases and glucose utilization

improves. Return of aldosterone levels to normal results in diuresis. The overall result is an improvement in negative nitrogen balance as the serum glucose level improves. This phase is similar to the response of the body during starvation, when fat is used to meet energy requirements. Chronic conditions such as diabetes, liver disease, or renal disease restrict the body's ability to move into the adaptive phase during physiologic stress. Chronic system failure or inadequate support of the current disease process complicates the course of recovery. Nutritional support is used more efficiently by the body's tissue during the adaptive phase than during the immediate phase. It is in this phase that nutrition can have a vital role in recovery. The combination of starvation and a physiologic stress increases the risk for morbidity and mortality. When poor nutritional status coincides with physiologic stress, the body's response is weakened. The ability to mobilize the immune response also decreases with impaired cell-mediated immunity, humoral immunity, and alteration of the tissue barriers to infection.

KEY POINTS

■ Acute physiologic stress results in activation of the sympathetic nervous system. The immediate phase is characterized by a high metabolic rate, sustained catabolism, hyperglycemia, and salt and water retention.

The sympathetic response promotes the use of protein stores for gluconeogenesis, which results in a negative nitrogen balance. Fat stores are poorly utilized.

- After 5 to 7 days of acute physiologic stress, the body may enter an adaptive phase that more closely resembles the normal response to starvation. Ketones and fatty acids from the lipolysis of fat stores are used for energy, and body proteins are conserved. Glucose utilization improves and hyperglycemia resolves. Aldosterone secretion diminishes and edema resolves. During the adaptive phase, nutrients supplied to the body are used more efficiently than during the immediate phase.

- Physiologic stress increases energy and protein requirements. An increase in needed calories of 20% to 50% above baseline is typical. Because glucose is poorly utilized during the immediate phase, carbohydrate intake is controlled to avoid exacerbation of hyperglycemia and excessive carbon dioxide production. Protein should supply about 16% of the total energy needs. Fats are given to fill the remaining caloric requirements. Vitamin and mineral replacement may also be required.

EFFECTS OF MALNUTRITION

Cardiovascular System

The cardiovascular system may be injured by malnutrition. Deficiencies in thiamine and selenium can cause primary cardiomyopathy.[21] Protein-energy malnutrition as seen in an acutely ill patient can result in visceral protein loss and decreases in myocardial function.[22] A decrease in heart size and atrophy of cardiac muscle could result in decreased cardiac output. The increase in extracellular fluid commonly associated with physiologic stress could further compromise cardiac output. In compensation, the cardiac muscle fibers lengthen in response to increased workload. This compensation, together with a decreased oxygen demand secondary to decreased intake, curtails the development of cardiac failure. However, if the cardiac muscle is diseased, malnutrition will contribute to uncompensated heart failure.

Even though the body compensates to prevent heart failure in a malnourished patient, heart failure is common even in a healthy heart when starvation is corrected by refeeding. Refeeding increases the metabolism of the stressed state, and cardiac output is increased to meet oxygen demands. This added stress could lead to heart failure. In addition, providing a high-carbohydrate diet (RQ = 1) during the refeeding period would increase carbon dioxide production and result in increased work of breathing, which places further demand on the heart. It is necessary to provide some of the energy needs with fat to decrease the carbon dioxide production, particularly for patients with concurrent respiratory failure. The patient must resume feeding with caution and be carefully monitored for signs and symptoms of cardiac failure. In addition, rapid weight loss secondary to malnutrition has been associated with ventricular dysfunction and dysrhythmias, so cardiac monitoring is an essential component in the care of such patients.

Cardiac cachexia associated with chronic congestive heart failure promotes malnutrition. The mechanisms involved in cardiac cachexia are shown in Figure 42-6. A vicious cycle exists, with congestive heart failure causing malnutrition, and malnutrition further contributing to the congestive heart failure.

FIGURE 42-6 Cyclic effect of malnutrition on chronic congestive heart failure. *GI,* Gastrointestinal.

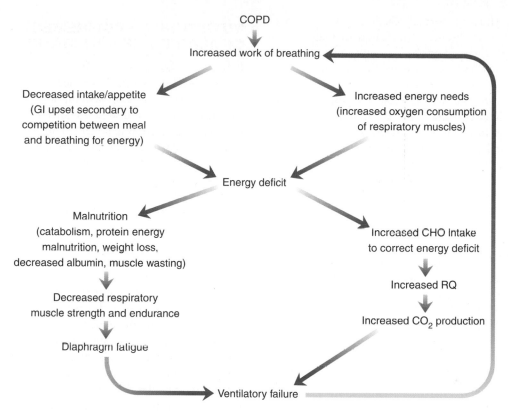

FIGURE 42-7 The increased work of breathing with chronic obstructive pulmonary disease *(COPD)*. *CHO,* Carbohydrate; *RQ,* respiratory quotient; *GI,* gastrointestinal.

Respiratory System

Malnutrition affects the functioning of the lungs. It decreases the structure of the lung parenchyma because the use of protein for energy reduces protein synthesis. This structural alteration can cause increased lung compliance and result in increased work of breathing.[23] Respiratory muscle function is decreased as a result of visceral protein loss, and both endurance and contractility are affected.

Malnourished patients often suffer from decreased vital capacity and respiratory muscle strength. If vital capacity and muscle strength fall below 50% of predicted norms, respiratory failure is probable owing to retention of carbon dioxide. Malnutrition also decreases the immune response in the lung. Surfactant stability is decreased, contributing to decreased lung compliance and microatelectasis. The result of an alteration in immune function and structural changes is an increase in respiratory infections. Infections develop easily and are not controlled by the protein-deficient immune system. The consequences of energy deficit in chronic obstructive pulmonary disease are summarized in Figure 42-7. When a patient has respiratory distress and must work harder to breathe, the caloric requirement for breathing alone can increase to 10 times normal levels. Inadequate intake and increased utilization further contribute to the effects of malnutrition on the respiratory system.

TABLE 42-5

Effects of Deficiency of Selected Nutrients on Immunity

Deficient Nutrient	Immune System Change
Vitamin C	Decreased mobility of neutrophils
Vitamin A	Lymphoid tissue atrophy
Vitamin B group	Lymphoid tissue atrophy
Amino acids	Decreased immunoglobulins, interferons, and acute phase proteins
Fatty acids	Impaired lymphocyte function
Iron	Decreased bacterial activity of phagocytes
Zinc	Lymphoid tissue atrophy
Selenium	Decreased antibody production

Immune System

Increased rates of infection in malnourished patients secondary to depression of the immune system and defense mechanisms are caused by nutrient deficiency. Changes in the immune system vary according to the type of nutrient lacking (Table 42-5). For example, lack of protein can impair the immune response from lack of amino acids necessary for immunoglobulin and interleukin synthesis.[24] As previously mentioned, cellular immunity (delayed cutaneous hypersensitivity), which is needed for reaction to an antigen in skin testing, is often depressed in undernourished patients. In addition, the total lymphocyte count decreases. Thus the normal reaction that occurs with antigen stimulation is absent or decreased in malnutrition secondary to both decreased synthesis of immune system cells and a decrease in antibody response to stimulation (humoral immunity).

Malnutrition also causes a decrease in lymphoid tissue mass, a decrease in circulating T and B lymphocytes, depression of phagocytic function, and a decrease in complement activity. The overall result is a decrease in resistance and an increased infection rate. In the critical care setting, the high number of invasive procedures and indwelling lines increases the potential for infection and complicates the patient's recovery.

KEY POINTS

- The cardiovascular, respiratory, and immune systems are particularly susceptible to the effects of malnutrition.
- Cardiac atrophy and reduced cardiac output may be associated with heart failure, particularly during refeeding, which increases the myocardial workload.
- Respiratory muscle atrophy and fatigue and deficient surfactant production impair effective respiration.
- Immune system depression is associated with an increased risk of infection.

NUTRITIONAL REQUIREMENTS OF ALTERED HEALTH STATES

Infection, Sepsis, and Fever

A complex interaction exists between the development of infection, the immune system, and nutritional intake.[25] Malnutrition contributes to the infectious process by directly depressing the immune system. This depression impairs the patient's defense mechanism and opens a path for infection to develop unchecked. Infection then potentiates malnutrition through inhibition of nutrient assimilation and stimulation of metabolic rate (fever).

Fever is a common symptom accompanying infection. Fever increases metabolic needs by 7% for each 1° F increase (13% for each 1° C increase). Energy requirements can increase by 40% when a high fever (above 104° F) is present. The metabolic response to fever is both anabolic and catabolic, which greatly increases nutrient requirements.

It is known that peptide mediators stimulated by macrophages initiate the metabolic alterations associated with infection. The mediator-stimulated response is summarized in Figure 42-8. This process is complex, with the need for protein synthesis requiring the availability of amino acids.[26] Although catabolism may be detrimental in some aspects, it is also a protective mechanism that provides needed substrates for activation of the immune response to infection. Nutritional

FIGURE 42-8 Mediator-stimulated response.

support is often aimed at decreasing catabolism, but it is also important to provide substrate (amino acids) for the protective mechanisms that catabolism supports.

Infection is a stressor that increases energy expenditure as a result of fever, increased immune cell demand, and catabolism. The body's metabolic response to the infection is to increase available glucose. Often the demand is too great for the body to manage; for example, sepsis can increase energy expenditure 20% to 60% above basal energy requirements. Nutritional support is needed to supply additional energy and the necessary substrates so that body stores are not excessively depleted.

Surgery

Adequate nutrition before and after surgery promotes wound healing, prevents infection, and decreases complications and mortality. A patient should be in the best nutritional condition possible before surgery.[27] A common cause of protein energy malnutrition in postoperative patients is starvation. The combination of poor presurgical nutrition and postoperative starvation may increase complications after surgery, such as separation of the layers of the surgical wound. Obesity, malnutrition, and dehydration are among the causes of this serious postoperative problem.

Nutritional needs in the postoperative period depend on the extent and type of surgery, as well as the presurgical nutritional status. The postoperative energy requirement can increase from 10% to 35% above BMR. Frequently, postoperative oral intake is delayed in critically ill patients well beyond the return of bowel function. This combination of increased need with decreased intake can have a major impact on wound healing. The functions of various nutrients in wound healing have long been established and are listed in Table 42-6. In addition, nitrogen loss through wounds can be large and create a greater need for increased protein intake. Protein intake sufficient to replace losses and promote anabolism will be required, together with nonprotein calories for energy requirements. As with every patient, individual assessment and determination of exact needs are required.

Trauma

The general catabolic response to stress is also seen in trauma patients.[28] Energy expenditure is increased by 15% to 30%. Increased carbohydrate intake will be needed, but patients must be observed for complications of high carbohydrate intake, such as glucose intolerance. Nitrogen loss secondary to catabolism and to cellular damage can be high. Circulating hormones in the immediate phase have an anti-insulin effect that decreases glucose utilization; therefore, gluconeogenesis is increased to meet energy needs. As with other stress states, the catabolism of protein provides a source of amino acids for acute phase protein synthesis by the liver (see Chapter 9). Because trauma is a sudden stress, catabolism is much greater than anabolism because the body has not had enough time to replenish the proteins lost. This dominance of catabolism results in excessive negative nitrogen balance and significant loss of skeletal muscle, which is a problem in post-trauma rehabilitation.

With other forms of physiologic stress, fatty acids cannot be used as a source of energy. In trauma patients, however, it is thought that fatty acids can be used because of extremely high levels of catecholamines, which mobilize fat through the stimulation of lipases. In addition, if glycogen stores are intact, an initial source of glucose and free fatty acids is available. Glucose utilization is maintained in trauma patients, so glucose is an effective source of energy during the immediate phase. These differences in the nutritional effect of physiologic stress on trauma patients stem from both the suddenness of the stress and the state of health of such patients before admission.

Burns

A burn is an extreme physiologic stressor that results in significant hypermetabolism.[29] In addition, the destruction of skin increases energy expenditure through evaporative heat loss. The energy needs of a burn patient increase 50% to 100% from the basal metabolic requirement. Because of individual variations such as preburn nutritional status, other physiologic stresses present, activity level, stage of burn, and age,

TABLE 42-6	
Role of Nutrients in Wound Healing	
Nutrient	**Role in Wound Healing**
Proteins (amino acids and albumin)	Maintain osmotic pressure to decrease edema; maintain cell-mediated immune responses; cellular proliferation, including neurovascular components, lymphocytes, and fibroblasts
Carbohydrates (glucose)	Meet energy requirements of cells involved in the healing process and prevention of infection
Fats (essential fatty acids)	Components of cellular membranes; building blocks for eicosanoids such as prostaglandins, which regulate cellular function
Vitamins	Roles in cellular function, including capillary function and formation, enzyme cofactors, immune cell function, clotting mechanism, calcium and phosphorus metabolism, collagen synthesis
Minerals	Roles in cellular function, including oxygen transport, immune cell function, collagen synthesis, cellular proliferation

indirect calorimetry is the best method for determination of individual needs.

As with other stressors, negative nitrogen balance is increased by catabolism and by the use of amino acids to form stress proteins. In addition, burn wounds directly contribute to protein loss because soluble proteins leak from the wound and proteolysis is activated. Fatty acids are also increased in response to the release of stress hormones and breakdown of lipoproteins. The effective utilization of this available energy source in the immediate post-burn phase may be impaired.

Cancer

The nutritional effects of cancer can be severe and result in what is commonly termed **cancer cachexia**.[30] Cachexia is associated with the end stage of cancer but can also develop earlier. The cause of cachexia is inadequate nutritional intake relative to energy requirements and increased anaerobic glycolysis. It results in significant weight loss, muscle weakness, and anorexia. A major cause of cachexia is anorexia associated with the malignancy and with the treatment. Sensory changes such as changes in smell or taste may be associated with cancer treatment and malnutrition. These changes can contribute significantly to the anorexia experienced during cancer treatment. Thus cancer patients often enter the critical care environment with mild to severe malnutrition.

Beyond the anorexia and sensory changes, abnormalities of intermediate metabolism in cancer promote tissue loss. The normal response to decreased intake is a decreased resting metabolic rate. Abnormalities in substrate metabolism in cancer patients increase total energy expenditure and raise the resting metabolic rate. The tumor also requires energy for growth, often using anaerobic metabolism (because tumor cells may not have sufficient capillary supply), which increases lactic acid production and promotes an increase in gluconeogenesis. The metabolism of vitamins, minerals, and enzymes is also thought to be altered. Because both nutrient intake and substrate metabolism are altered, nutritional support is difficult to achieve and frequently ineffective in reversing the existing cachexia.

Immobility

The main nutritional effect of immobility is loss of calcium from nonstressed bone, a process that can elevate serum calcium and phosphorus levels. This demineralization is best managed with weight-bearing as early as possible rather than calcium supplementation. Calcium supplementation during immobility may increase the risk of developing renal calculi. A physical therapist should be consulted early to assist in prevention of demineralization. Because negative calcium balance can increase in a catabolic state, serum calcium levels must be monitored and abnormalities treated.

A second effect of immobilization is nitrogen loss as tissue mass is decreased from disuse atrophy. This loss can total 2 to 3 g/kg per day and require up to 10 to 15 g of protein to replenish the daily loss, which further emphasizes the need for early physical therapy and aggressive range-of-motion exercises.

KEY POINTS

- Infection is associated with fever and an increased metabolic rate. For each 1° F increase in body temperature, metabolic needs increase 7%. The synthesis of acute phase proteins and immune factors requires sufficient amino acid substrates.
- A major nutritional problem in postoperative patients is starvation. In addition, nitrogen loss through wounds may be significant.
- Major trauma is associated with a 15% to 30% increase in energy expenditure. Glucose utilization is maintained. Trauma victims are usually in good nutritional health before admission.
- Major burns are extreme physiologic stressors that result in an increase in energy expenditure of 50% to 100% above baseline. Protein loss from burned areas is high.
- Cancer cachexia is a result of several factors, including anorexia, poor intake, and preferential nutrient utilization by tumor cells.
- Immobility is associated with muscle atrophy and bone demineralization.

SUMMARY

Metabolism is a dynamic and continuous process affecting every organ and physiologic process in the human system. The building phase of anabolic metabolism occurs concurrently with the energy-consuming and tearing-down phase of catabolic metabolism. Phases of metabolism either release or require energy in the form of ATP. The rate at which metabolism occurs in the resting human system is referred to as the basal metabolic rate, and the process releases both heat and energy. The metabolic fate of carbohydrate, protein, and fat depends on cellular needs and systemic regulatory functions. The endocrine system greatly affects metabolism. Only one hormone, insulin, is known to lower serum glucose levels by decreasing liver glucose production and promoting the transfer of glucose into cells. Although each works in a unique manner, growth hormone, cortisol, epinephrine, thyroid hormone, and glucagon all work in concert to maintain or raise blood glucose levels.

Physiologic stress is accompanied by changes in metabolism that alter nutrient utilization and increase nutrient requirements. The degree to which these changes occur varies with the type and severity of the particular stress. If the patient is not provided with adequate nutrition when one or more stressors are present, the hypermetabolism, hypercatabolism, and negative nitrogen balance associated with the physiologic stress will have detrimental effects on recovery.

Health care professionals must be aware of the impact of stressors on the nutritional status of the body, as well as the impact of nutrition on the well-being of body systems. If this point is well understood, appropriate interventions can be taken to prevent some of the complications that can develop when nutritional support is inadequate.

Most well-nourished patients can tolerate a short period of inadequate intake (about 5 days) without untoward effects. However, critically ill patients require early nutritional support because of the magnitude and intensity of the stressors. Identification of the various risk factors and the nutritional needs of patients is an essential part of nursing care for critically ill patients. Overfeeding of patients should also be avoided because specific complications can develop with inappropriate nutritional support. Nurses must also understand nutritional interventions so that decisions regarding nutritional support for the patient can be based on specific nutritional assessments and knowledge of individual needs.

REFERENCES

1. Keesey RE: Physiological regulation of body weight and the issue of obesity, *Med Clin North Am* 73(1):15-27, 1989.
2. Widmaier EP, Raff H, Strang KT: *Vander, Sherman & Luciano's human physiology: the mechanisms of body function*, ed 9, New York, 2004, McGraw-Hill.
3. Mahan LK, Escott-Stump S: *Krause's food and nutrition therapy*, ed 12, St Louis, 2008, Saunders.
4. Guyton AC, Hall JE: *Textbook of medical physiology*, ed 11, Philadelphia, 2006, Saunders.
5. Froehle AW, Shoeninger MJ: Intraspecies variation in BMR does not affect estimates of early hominin total daily energy expenditure, *Am J Phys Anthropol* 131(4):552-559, 2006.
6. Sjodin AM et al: The influence of physical activity on BMR, *Med Sci Sports Exerc* 28(1):85-91, 1996.
7. U.S. Department of Health and Human Services: The Report of the Dietary Guidelines Advisory Committee on Dietary Guidelines for Americans, 2005, http://www.health.gov/DietaryGuidelines/dga2005/default.htm.
8. Jijakli H et al: Anomeric specificity of the stimulatory effect of D-glucose on D-fructose phosphorylation by human liver glucokinase, *J Biol Chem* 278(7):4531-4535, 2003.
9. Ignatavicius DD, Workman ML: *Medical-surgical nursing: critical thinking for collaborative care*, ed 5, Philadelphia, 2006, Elsevier Saunders.
10. Bray GA: Nutrient balance and obesity: an approach to control of food intake in humans, *Med Clin North Am* 73(1):29-45, 1989.
11. Tepperman J, Tepperman HM: *Metabolic and endocrine physiology*, ed 5, Chicago, 1987, Year Book Medical Publishers.
12. Wang GL et al: Growth hormone corrects proliferation and transcription of phosphoenolpyruvate carboxykinase in livers of old mice via elimination of CCAAT/enhancer binding protein alpha-Brm complex, *J Biol Chem* 282(2):1468-1478, 2007.
13. Kumpf V, Chessman K: Enteral nutrition. In DiPiro JT, Talbert RL, Yee GC et al, editors: *Pharmacotherapy: a pathophysiologic approach*, ed 7, New York, 2008, McGraw-Hill, pp 2399-2415.
14. Griffin JE, Ojeda SR: *Textbook of endocrine physiology*, ed 3, Oxford, 1996, Oxford University Press.
15. Klein S et al: Lipolytic response to metabolic stress in critically ill patients, *Crit Care Med* 19(6):776-779, 1991.
16. Goldman L, Ausiello D: *Cecil textbook of medicine*, ed 23, Philadelphia, 2008, Elsevier Saunders.
17. Ziegler TR et al: Metabolic effects of recombinant human growth hormone in patients receiving parenteral nutrition, *Ann Surg* 208(1):6-16, 1988.
18. MacLennan WJ, Peden NR: *Metabolic and endocrine problems in the elderly*, London, 1989, Springer-Verlag.
19. Kinney J, Weissman C: Forms of malnutrition in stressed and unstressed patients, *Clin Chest Med* 7(1):19-28, 1986.
20. Cartwright MM: The metabolic response to stress: a case of complex nutrition support management, *Crit Care Nurs Clin North Am* 16(4):467-487, 2004.
21. Van Heerebeek L et al: Myocardial structure and function differ in systolic and diastolic heart failure, *Circulation* 113:1966-1973, 2006.
22. Webb JG, Kiess MC, Chan-Yan CC: Malnutrition and the heart, *Can Med Assoc J* 135(7):753-758, 1986.
23. Openbrier D, Covey M: Ineffective breathing pattern related to malnutrition, *Nurs Clin North Am* 22(1):225-247, 1987.
24. Beisel W: Role of nutrition in immune system diseases, *Compr Ther* 13(1):13-19, 1987.
25. Keusch G, Farthing M: Nutrition and infection, *Annu Rev Nutr* 6:131-154, 1986.
26. Pomposelli J: Role of biochemical mediators in clinical nutrition and surgical metabolism, *J Parenter Enteral Nutr* 12(2):212-218, 1988.
27. Bellanton R: Preoperative parenteral nutrition in the high risk surgical patient, *J Parenter Enteral Nutr* 12(2):115-121, 1988.
28. Anderson B: The metabolic needs of head trauma victims, *J Neurosci Nurs* 19(4):211-215, 1987.
29. Lang CE: *Nutritional support in critical care*, Gaithersburg, MD, 1987, Aspen.
30. Kern K, Norton J: Cancer cachexia, *J Parenter Enteral Nutr* 12(3):286-298, 1988.

PART 7

Alterations in Neural Control and Integration

Frontiers of Research

Pain and Its Control

Sheila K. Smith • Timothy A. Harbst • Michael J. Kirkhorn

Through the sensation of pain, the brain monitors the body's organs and sounds the alarm when something goes wrong. Responding to complicated signaling processes, the brain and neurotransmitters are also able to provide relief from pain.

Pain is a pervasive human condition. One estimate suggests that nearly one third of the U.S. population has some form of chronic pain not associated with malignancy. Cancer offers its own peculiar challenges because it often causes sharp and lasting pain. As cancer advances in the body, pain becomes more severe. Cancer patients are not the only ones who suffer pain that is difficult or impossible to endure without assistance. Burn patients nearly always experience severe pain; more than half of a sample of medical-surgical patients said that they experienced "excruciating" pain; arthritis, osteoporosis, and other rheumatology pain can be extremely debilitating.

The study of naturally occurring chemicals for pain control and their receptors in the central nervous system dates back to the early 1970s. In 1973, researchers at Johns Hopkins University, New York University, and Uppsala University reported that brain cells had receptors that might accommodate opiates like morphine. Naturally-occurring opiate-like chemicals called *enkephalins* were already known to exist and were able to decrease pain by inhibiting muscle contractions. Based on this knowledge, researchers hypothesized that the newly discovered brain receptors must also interact with endogenous opiates. Within a few years, researchers isolated enkephalins and endorphins in the brain, suggesting that pain might be controlled through natural processes without resorting to potentially addictive opiates. Kosterlitz also learned that there are different kinds of opiate receptors: some that relieve pain and others that can cause addiction.

Researchers study pain not only to relieve it but also because it is a useful diagnostic tool. The body senses danger in its external as well as internal environment with a network of pain receptors—free nerve endings—in the skin and in certain internal tissues. When they are stimulated, pain impulses move along two separate paths from the dorsal spinal roots into the spinal cord to various destinations in the brain. When the signals reach their destinations, the outcome is clear: we hurt, we know how much, and except in the case of "referred pain," we know precisely where and when the pain occurs. However, the brain's response is more than an alarm: the brain controls pain as well.

Pain control resides in the central and peripheral nervous systems' analgesia systems—complex networks capable of controlling the input of pain signals to the nervous system by releasing neurotransmitters, blocking pain signals at their entry point to the spinal cord and by blocking other reflexes triggered by pain signals. The analgesia system and other areas of the brain have opiate receptors, which also dull pain. Researchers do not entirely understand the brain's intricate opiate system, but it is clear that activation of the analgesia system either by nervous signals entering the periaqueductal gray area of the brainstem or by the administration of morphine-like drugs suppresses many pain signals.

The study of pain management is relatively new. One model looks at four phases of pain perception and

Astrocytes. Glia cells found throughout the central nervous system in both gray and white matter. (From Kumar V et al: Robins and Cotran pathologic basis of disease, ed 7, Philadelphia, 2005, Saunders, p 1350. Courtesy Dr. J. Corbo, Brigham and Women's Hospital, Boston.)

Neural Function

the physiologic or chemical mediators involved. The goal is to interrupt the generation and transmission of the pain action potential at a level, or combination of levels, appropriate to the specific pain physiology, perception, and response. The four phases are identified as *transduction,* which occurs at the periphery with the pain stimulus; *transmission,* occurring as the action potential is transmitted to the spinal cord and up to higher brain centers; *pain perception,* an activity of the brain, bringing the pain sensation to conscious awareness; and *pain modulation,* experienced as modification of the pain sensation over time.

For example, transduction begins at the periphery with exposure to a sufficient quantity of noxious stimuli. This might be mechanical injury, thermal injury, or a noxious chemical. Chemical mediators are released in response to the injury—prostaglandins, bradykinins, serotonins, substance P, and histamines. These mediators facilitate the generation of an electronic action potential. Appropriate pain management for this level of the nociceptive or sensory process is targeted at interrupting the generation of an action potential. Analgesics accomplish this by decreasing the influx of sodium into the neuron (e.g., anticonvulsants work in this way), or by interfering with the production of chemical mediators (e.g., prostaglandins, substance P; NSAIDs, capsaicin, and corticosteroids operate in this way). The pain of herpes zoster or shingles is a condition for which pain management would be appropriately targeted at the periphery.

Transmission, occurring when nociceptive fibers transmit pain sensations to the spinal cord and on up to higher brain centers, is facilitated by the neurotransmitters ATP, glutamate, and substance P. Ascending spinothalamic tracts transmit the pain impulse to the thalamus. Treatment of pain impulses at this level includes antagonists such as methadone or ketamine that can inhibit the binding of excitatory amino acids within the spinal cord. TENS units (transcutaneous electrostimulation) is a mechanical approach used to compete with pain stimuli at the spinal cord level.

Pain perception, occurring within the brain, involves the reticular system for the autonomic response, the limbic system for the emotional and behavioral response, and the somatosensory cortex for cognitively localizing and characterizing the pain. At this level of pain physiology, cognitive-behavioral strategies can be used to direct attention away from the pain sensation. Approaches such as distraction, relaxation, imagery, biofeedback, and cognitive restructuring have proven to be very helpful adjuncts in the relief of pain.

Finally, modulation occurs as the pain impulse is processed and sent back down the spinal cord. Endogenous opioids are released, as well as serotonin, norepinephrine, GABA, and neurotensin. These neurotransmitters inhibit the transmission of the pain impulse and produce central and local analgesia. Treatments targeted at this level include the use of tricyclic antidepressants and anticonvulsants. Chronic pain conditions are neuropathic and should be treated at all appropriate levels.

Unfortunately, pain management continues to be hindered both by lack of a good working knowledge of pain pathology and by misconceptions about patients with pain. The patient's report of pain is the single most reliable indicator of pain, but we need to know what kind of pain in order to target the correct treatment. Is the pain due to a transient and spontaneously resolving phenomenon (a pin prick, a muscle strain)? Is the pain the symptom of other tissue pathology (a wound, arthritis, osteoporosis, pancreatitis)? Or is the pain due to chronic conditions signaling nerve pathology or central processing defects (sciatica, fibromyalgia, migraine headaches, diabetic neuropathy)? Are there co-existing conditions that intensify the pain? A correct diagnosis is needed to correctly manage chronic pain, as well as accurate identification of complicating conditions and triage for psychosocial needs and supports.

chapter

43

Structure and Function of the Nervous System

Jacquelyn L. Banasik

MEDIA RESOURCES

Additional Material for Study, Review, and Further Exploration

CD Companion ■ Review Questions and Answers
■ Glossary (with audio pronunciations for selected terms)
■ Disease Profiles ■ Animations

ⓔvolve **Website** at http://evolve.elsevier.com/Copstead/
■ Case Studies ■ Disease Profiles ■ WebLinks ■ Key Points Review

 Online Course (Module 18)

KEY QUESTIONS

■ How do the central nervous system (CNS), peripheral nervous system, and autonomic nervous system interrelate?
■ How is the CNS protected and supported?
■ What structures are located in each of the four principal areas of the brain: cerebrum, diencephalon, cerebellum, and brainstem?
■ What neurologic functions have been mapped to particular locations in the brain?
■ How do the properties of neuronal action potentials and neuronal communication through synapses relate to the functions of the nervous system?

■ How is the somatotopic organization of sensory receptors and muscles maintained in the CNS?
■ How is voluntary muscle activity initiated and executed?
■ How do the properties of the mind, including, thought, memory, learning, consciousness, and sleep, relate to the physiologic substance of the nervous system?

CHAPTER OUTLINE

The nervous system is a complex network of neurons and supportive cells that enables rapid communication between sensory receptors, central processing neurons, and functional responses. Much has been discovered about the mechanisms of sensory input and motor output, but the physiologic bases of thought, consciousness, emotion, and learning remain elusive. The idea that the mind is within the biological realm has only recently been generally accepted, although the effects of mind-altering drugs on emotions, appetite, sleep, thought, and sensory perception have long been recognized. Research continues to reveal the great complexity of neurologic function. A bewildering array of neurotransmitter signaling molecules and an even greater number of neurotransmitter receptors have been identified. Recently, the long-held notion that neurons cannot regenerate in the mature brain has been disproved, and neuronal stem cells have been identified in certain areas. Each discovery brings us closer to understanding neural physiologic processes and gives hope for finding effective therapies for the devastating diseases that affect them. This chapter provides an overview of neural structure and function and is the basis for understanding the neurologic disorders in the chapters that follow.

Structural Organization

The nervous system is traditionally divided into three principal anatomic units: the central nervous system (CNS), the peripheral nervous system (PNS), and the autonomic nervous system (ANS). These systems are not anatomically or functionally distinct, and they work together as an integrated whole. Therefore, when function, rather than anatomy, is the topic of concern, the nervous system is more conveniently divided into the sensory, motor, and higher brain functions. This chapter begins with a review of the major anatomic features of the nervous system, then addresses neurologic function at the cellular and synaptic level, and concludes with a summary of sensory, motor, and cognitive functions.

CENTRAL NERVOUS SYSTEM

The CNS includes the brain and spinal cord. Its primary functions are receiving and processing sensory information and creating appropriate responses to be relayed to muscles and glands. It is the site of emotion, memory, cognition, and learning. The CNS is bathed in cerebrospinal fluid (CSF) and shielded from the periphery by the blood-brain barrier. The CNS interacts with the neurons of the PNS through synapses in the spinal cord and cranial nerve **ganglia.** The cranial and spinal nerves constitute the PNS.

Support and Protection of the Central Nervous System

Nervous tissue has the consistency of gelatin, so measures to support and protect its fragile structure are necessary. In addition, the CNS must be shielded from circulating substances that would interfere with neurotransmission. These protective functions are provided by the skull and vertebral column, meninges, cerebrospinal fluid (CSF), and blood-brain barriers. The bony structures of the skull and vertebral column encase the brain and cord and protect them from external trauma, whereas the CSF and meninges provide buoyancy and shock-absorbing capacity.

The meninges are composed of three layers that serve to suspend and maintain the shape and position of the nervous tissue during head and body movements. The brain is suspended within layers of meninges that are fixed to the skull. In this manner, the brain turns with the movement of the skull. The CSF circulates within the subarachnoid space, giving buoyancy to the brain and making an average 1500-g brain mass resistant to distortion, which could occur from gravity alone were it not for the buoyancy effect.[1] The three meningeal layers are the *dura mater, arachnoid,* and *pia mater* (Figure 43-1).

The dura mater, the outermost meningeal layer, is a thick, tough, collagenous membrane. It is composed of two layers, one contiguous with the periosteum of the skull and the other, which is adherent to the first, covering the surface of the brain. The tough dura protects the soft tissue of the brain. Support and stability are also provided by dural septa that invaginate into the cranial cavity. The falx cerebri is a thin wall of dura that folds down the cortical midline, separating the two hemispheres (see Figure 43-1). The tentorium cerebelli is a septum that separates the cerebellum and brainstem from the rest of the cerebrum. The dural septa fix the brain in place by their tentlike structure and limit its movement within the skull. Venous sinuses that collect venous blood from cerebral veins are located between the two layers of the dura at the base of the septum.

FIGURE 43-1 Principle membranes of the cranial meninges. Cerebrospinal fluid flows in the subarachnoid space and is reabsorbed by arachnoid villi within the dural sinuses.

Beneath and continuous with the dura is the arachnoid layer. The spaces between the dura and the skull and between the dura mater and the arachnoid are potential spaces. Only in the presence of pathologic processes, notably epidural and subdural hemorrhages, do these spaces become evident (see Chapter 44). Unlike the dura mater, the arachnoid is a thin, delicate membrane. It is semitransparent and weblike in appearance, hence its name. From the arachnoid layer come strands of collagenous connective tissue called *trabeculae* that extend down to the pia mater, forming a subarachnoid space. The CSF flows in this space.

The pia mater, the third meningeal layer, is also very thin. However, unlike the other meningeal layers, the pia is attached to the brain and closely follows its contours over every **sulcus** and into every **gyrus**. Consequently, the subarachnoid space between the arachnoid and the pia mater is not evenly distributed. The arachnoid meshes with the pia via the trabeculae in such a subtle manner that it is often difficult to differentiate one from the other. Consequently, the two layers together are often referred to as the *leptomeninges*.

The meninges that cover and provide protection to the spinal cord are similar to those of the brain, with a few variations (Figure 43-2). The spinal dura, for example, has no periosteal layer, so it is a single rather than a double layer. It is continuous with the foramen magnum at the base of the skull and is separated from the spinal vertebral periosteum by an epidural space. Thus, in the spinal cord, the epidural space is a true space, unlike its counterpart in the cranium, which is only a potential space. Within this space lie fatty connective tissue and a vertebral venous plexus.

The spinal arachnoid, much like that covering the cerebrum, is closely adherent to the spinal dura. Between the arachnoid layer and the pial lining is the CSF-filled subarachnoid space. The spinal meninges end at approximately the second sacral vertebra. However, the spinal cord ends between the first and second lumbar vertebrae (L1 to L2). This results in a large subarachnoid cistern, called the *lumbar cistern*, which is a favored place to obtain CSF samples (see Figure 43-2). The spinal pia is much tougher and thicker than the cerebral pia. Projecting along the length of each side is the dentate

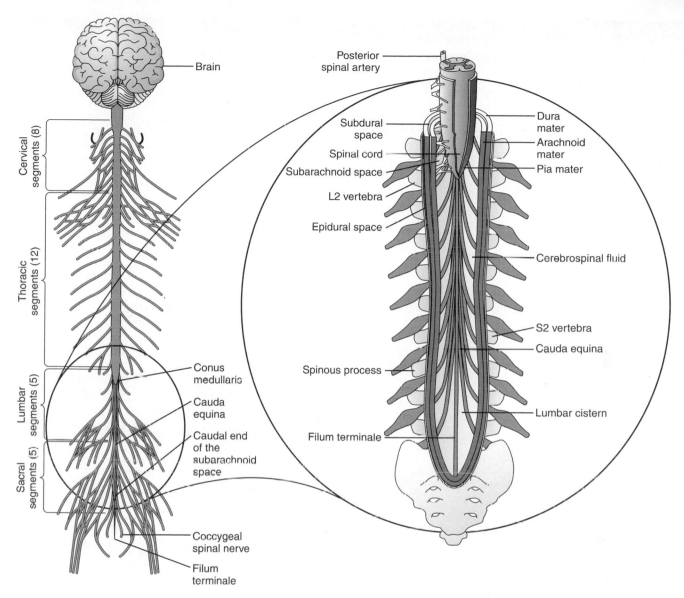

FIGURE 43-2 The spinal cord, spinal nerves, and meninges. Spinal meninges are similar to cranial membranes. Spinal meninges end at S2, creating a CSF-filled cistern below the spinal cord. The cauda equina (horse tail) is formed by the lumbar and sacral nerves, which protrude from the end of the spinal cord.

ligament, which anchors the spinal cord to the arachnoid and through it to the dura. Another pial projection connects the tail of the spinal cord (the cauda equina) at level L1 to L2 to the **caudal** end of the spinal dural sheath, where it is tethered to the end of the vertebral column. This projection is called the *filum terminale*.

The majority of CSF is produced by the choroid plexus, located in the lateral and third ventricles of the brain, at a rate of approximately 500 ml/day.[2] The composition of normal CSF is compared to plasma in Table 43-1. CSF is absorbed at about the same rate at which it is produced, so that only 150 to 175 ml is in circulation at any time.[2] The large C-shaped lateral ventricles occupy the center of each hemisphere. They communicate with the third ventricle in the diencephalon by way of the intraventricular foramen. The third ventricle is linked

to the fourth ventricle by way of the cerebral aqueduct, which lies between the pons and the medulla (Figure 43-3). The CSF flows from the fourth ventricle through the median or lateral aperture and into the subarachnoid space. It flows around the spinal cord and up over the cerebral hemispheres to the arachnoid villi, where it is absorbed into the venous system.

CSF is absorbed by the arachnoid villi, which are small tufts of the arachnoid that invaginate into the dural sinus, especially along the superior sagittal sinus. These tufts bring CSF into close approximation with venous blood. CSF flows into the venous system through one-way valves as a consequence of bulk flow or pressure gradient differences. Although the CSF flows readily into the venous sinus, flow in the opposite direction cannot occur[2]; that is, the fluid in the venous sinus cannot flow into the subarachnoid space. This mechanism is part

TABLE 43-1

Composition of Cerebrospinal Fluid Compared to Plasma and Selected Cerebrospinal Fluid Abnormalities

Substance	Normal CSF	Abnormal CSF	Plasma
Na$^+$ (mEq/L)	148	—	136-145
K$^+$ (mEq/L)	2.9	—	3.5-5.0
Cl$^-$ (mEq/L)	120-130	—	100-106
Glucose (mg/dl)	50-75	↓ Infection	70-100
Protein (mg/dl)	15-45	↑ Inflammation	6800
PH	7.3	—	7.4
Red blood cells (high-power field)	None	↑ Trauma, subarachnoid hemorrhage	—
White blood cells (high-power field)	<5	↑ Infection (e.g., meningitis)	—
Pressure (mm H$_2$O)	70-180	↑ Mass lesions	—

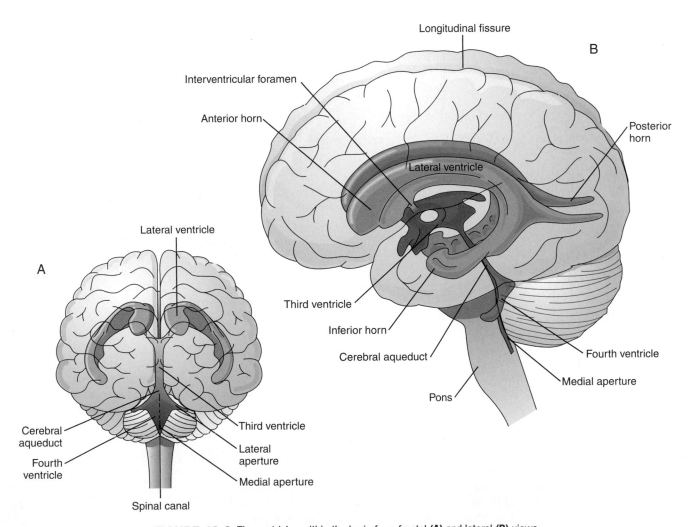

FIGURE 43-3 The ventricles within the brain from frontal **(A)** and lateral **(B)** views.

of a system of barriers between the extracellular space in the nervous system and the rest of the body.

The rate of production of CSF is independent of blood pressure or intraventricular pressure.[2] Thus, CSF will continue to be produced even when its path of circulation or absorption is blocked. If this occurs, the amount of CSF increases, as

does the size of the ventricles. This pathologic process is called *hydrocephalus.* Although hydrocephalus is usually caused by blockage of CSF pathways, it can also be caused by overproduction and malabsorption of CSF (see Chapter 45).

Blood supply to the brain is provided by two pairs of arteries; the anterior circulation is supplied by the internal

FIGURE 43-4 Blood supply to the brain. **A,** The internal carotid and vertebral arteries supply blood to the anterior and posterior aspects of the brain. **B,** At the base of the brain, the internal carotid and vertebral arteries join to form the circle of Willis. **C,** Major venous drainage from the brain.

carotid arteries, and the posterior circulation is supplied by the vertebral arteries (Figure 43-4). The cerebral circulation is discussed in detail in Chapter 44 as it relates to stroke. The internal carotid arteries have three principal branches: the anterior and middle cerebral arteries and the posterior communicating arteries. The vertebral arteries enter the skull at the foramen magnum and join at the level of the pons to form the basilar arteries. The ring of vessels that unites the anterior and posterior circulation at the base of the brain is known as the

circle of Willis (see Figure 43-4, B). The cerebral veins drain into large vascular channels called sinuses that are formed by folds in the dura. From the sinuses, venous blood returns to the heart by way of the jugular veins (see Figure 43-4, C).

The extracellular fluid that bathes the neurons is carefully shielded from elements in the CSF and blood by cellular barriers. Specialized tight junctions between the cells that line the CSF spaces and between the endothelial cells of brain capillaries prevent leakage of molecules through the spaces between the cells (Figure 43-5). Therefore, substances must move through the plasma membranes of these barrier cells to access the CNS. Lipid-soluble molecules move through more easily than water-soluble ones. Thus, the flow of ions, nutrients, drugs, proteins, and other charged or polar substances is highly restricted.[2] The blood-brain barrier is a crucial structure for protecting the brain, but it may also restrict access of beneficial molecules, such as antibiotics and cancer drugs, making treatment more difficult.

The integrity of the blood-brain barrier is maintained in part by CNS cells called *astrocytes.* These specialized **glial** cells have foot processes that contact the brain capillaries and are thought to help regulate transport across the capillary endothelium[3] (see Figure 43-5). The blood-brain barrier is less effective in infancy and can also be compromised by ischemia and chemical injury in adults.

A similar barrier exists between the circulating CSF and the interstitial fluid of the CNS, the CSF-brain barrier. The ependymal cells that line the ventricles are tightly joined and regulate the movement of water-soluble elements between the CSF and neurons. In addition, these cells serve the important function of removing unwanted substances from the CNS and secreting them into the CSF for eventual removal by the venous system.

Some areas of the brain have the need to sample the contents of the blood or CSF more directly to make regulatory adjustments in respiratory, autonomic, or endocrine functions, and these areas therefore have more permeable barriers. These areas include the hypothalamus, pituitary, and other circumventricular organs (around the ventricles).

The Brain

Various schemes have been used to subdivide the structures of the brain using embryologic, evolutionary, and anatomic frameworks (Table 43-2). In this section, an anatomic framework is used that includes the cerebrum, diencephalon, cerebellum, and brainstem (Figure 43-6).

Cerebrum

The cerebrum is divided into left and right hemispheres by the longitudinal fissure and is the largest part of the brain. The cerebral cortex is the outermost layer of the cerebrum and is composed of gray matter arranged in six histologically distinct layers[4] (Figure 43-7). Each layer makes connections with other parts of the brain. The cortex is characterized by its convoluted exterior having ridges (gyri), grooves (sulci), and deeper depressions (fissures). The sulci and fissures are used as landmarks to divide the cerebral cortex into lobes. The central sulcus separates the frontal and parietal lobes, the lateral sulcus separates the temporal lobe from the parietal and frontal lobes, and the parieto-occipital line defines the occipital lobe (Figure 43-8).

Some anatomic locations are particularly associated with certain brain functions. These functions have been characterized through lesion studies in which an area of brain is damaged and then the functional losses studied, and by mapping procedures during which the cerebral cortex is stimulated and responses are recorded. Functional specialization of brain loci

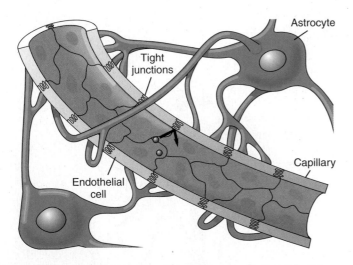

FIGURE 43-5 Tight junctions between brain capillary endothelial cells prevent polar and charged molecules from passing between cells. Astrocytes have foot processes on the capillary that help to maintain integrity of the blood-brain barrier.

TABLE 43-2

Subdivisions of the Brain Using Embryologic, Evolutionary, and Anatomic Frameworks

	Framework		
Structure	**Embryologic**	**Evolutionary**	**Anatomic**
Cerebral hemisphere	Telencephalon	Forebrain (includes diencephalon)	Cerebrum
Thalamus	Diencephalon	—	Diencephalon hypothalamus
Midbrain	Mesencephalon	Midbrain	—
Cerebellum	Metencephalon (includes pons)	Cerebellum	Cerebellum
Medulla	Myelencephalon	Hindbrain	Brainstem (includes midbrain, pons)

FIGURE 43-6 The four principal anatomic areas of the brain. The star at the top shows orientation of the brain: *A*, anterior; *P*, posterior; *S*, superior; *I*, inferior. (From Thibodeau GA, Patton KT: *Anatomy and physiology*, ed 6, St Louis, 2007, Mosby, p 483.)

FIGURE 43-7 The cortex of the brain is histologically divided into six layers that differ in their connections to other parts of the nervous system. (From Ransom and Clark [after Brodmann]: *Anatomy of the nervous system*, Philadelphia, 1959, Saunders.)

are listed in Table 43-3. A partial map of Brodmann areas is shown in Figure 43-9. Although the concept of functional anatomic areas is clinically useful, one should realize that even though an area may be critical for a particular function, it is not wholly responsible for that function, and many brain areas may be involved. A certain degree of reassignment of brain function from one area to another can occur, allowing the brain to adapt to loss of normal neural function.

Functional areas of the cortex that can be mapped to specific sensory receptors or muscles are called *primary* areas. Primary areas are surrounded by secondary areas that provide greater character to sensations and greater complexity to movements. In addition to primary and secondary cortical areas, there are large areas of association cortex that add interpretive and learned responses. The organization of primary and secondary cortex is best characterized for the somatosensory cortex and motor cortex (which are discussed later in the Somatosensory Cortex and the Central Control of Motor Function sections, respectively).

Cortical areas involved in visual perception are located in the occipital lobe. Brodmann area 17 is the primary visual cortex, and areas 18 and 19 are the secondary visual cortex. Interpretive association areas for vision are found in the adjacent temporal and parietal lobes. The primary auditory cortex

FIGURE 43-8 The four principal lobes of the cerebral cortex. (From Thibodeau GA, Patton KT: *Anatomy and physiology,* ed 6, St Louis, 2007, Mosby, p 490.)

TABLE **43-3**	
Functional Areas of Brain Specialization	
Area	**Specialized Function**
Occipital lobe	Visual cortex and association areas
Parietal lobe	Somatosensory cortex and association areas
Temporal lobe	Hearing and equilibrium, emotion, and memory
Frontal lobe	Motor cortex and association areas; prefrontal cortex involved in complex thought, ethical behavior, and morality
Limbic structures	Emotions, short-term memory, olfaction
Basal ganglia	Initiation and planning of learned motor activities
Broca and Wernicke areas	Interpretation and expression of language

is located on the superior temporal lobe, whereas vestibular information projects to the inferior temporal lobe.

Language expression and interpretation have been mapped to areas in the temporal lobe, particularly the Wernicke area (Brodmann areas 39, 40, and 22). One hemisphere, usually the left, is dominant for language. Lesions in this area lead to difficulty recognizing written words (alexia) and spoken language (receptive aphasia). Another area closely associated with speech is the Broca area (Brodmann area 44) in the frontal lobe. Damage to this region interferes with the ability to use language (expressive aphasia). In most cases, receptive and expressive aphasia occur together (see Chapter 44).

The frontal lobe is usually credited with control over emotional responses, ethical behavior, and morality. It is also the site of initiative and motivation. Patients with lesions of the frontal lobe may fail to conform to societal behavioral norms.

Another small cortical lobe, the central lobe or insula, lies deep in the lateral cerebral fissure under the junction of the frontal, parietal, and temporal lobes. Little is known about its specific functions, although it is thought to regulate visceral and intestinal functions.

The limbic lobe and **limbic system** are the parts of the cerebrum most closely associated with memory and emotion. The limbic lobe is a ring of cortex on the medial surface of each hemisphere containing the cingulate gyrus, isthmus, and parahippocampal gyrus (Figure 43-10). Olfaction (the perception of smell) occurs within the limbic cortex. The limbic system is a group of structures that encircle the brainstem.

FIGURE 43-9 A partial Brodmann map of the cerebral cortex. Note the locations of Broca and Wernicke areas, which are important in the expression and understanding of language. (From Thibodeau GA, Patton KT: *Anatomy and physiology,* ed 6, St Louis, 2007, Mosby, p 495.)

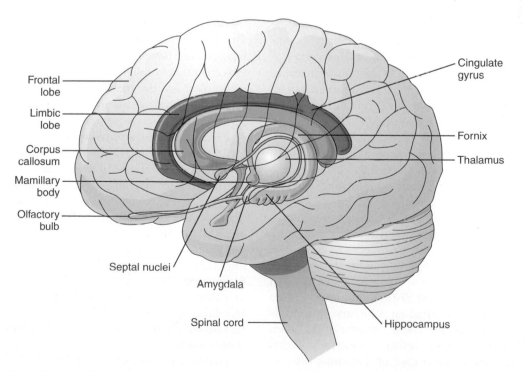

FIGURE 43-10 The limbic system is composed of a group of structures deep in the brain that are important In memory and emotion These structures include the limbic lobe, amygdala, fornix, hippocampus, olfactory cortex, and portions of the thalamus.

FIGURE 43-11 The basal ganglia include the caudate nucleus, putamen, globus pallidus, subthalamic nuclei, and substantia nigra.

Some of these lie within the anatomic division of the cerebrum, whereas others are within the diencephalon and upper brainstem. In addition to the limbic lobe, the limbic system includes the amygdala, fornix, hippocampus, and portions of the thalamus (see Figure 43-10). Lesions of the limbic system, particularly the hippocampus, cause impairment of short-term memory.

The **basal ganglia** are large masses of gray matter that lie deep within the cerebral hemispheres. They are intimately involved in the initiation, coordination, and execution of movement.[5,6] The basal ganglia include the caudate nucleus, putamen, globus pallidus, subthalamus, and substantia nigra (Figure 43-11). The caudate nucleus and putamen together are called the *striatum*. The five basal ganglia structures occur in pairs, with each cerebral hemisphere containing a set.

The basal ganglia are connected by complex neural circuits that incorporate sensory information about the current muscle conditions, cortical input about desired motor activities, and cerebellar signals about timing and coordination. The basal ganglia then relay motor signals to the thalamus, which projects to areas of the motor cortex. Finally, the program of desired muscle activity is conveyed to the primary motor cortex, which activates neurons projecting to muscle groups. Much of what is known about the function of basal ganglia has been learned from studying Parkinson disease. Parkinson disease is characterized by difficulty initiating voluntary movements (akinesia), stiff muscles (rigidity), and a tremor of the hands when idle (rest tremor). Improvement in symptoms occurs when the patient is given a precursor of dopamine (DA, levodopa), which can cross the blood-brain barrier. Drugs that block acetylcholine are also effective. Studies of these patients

revealed degeneration of DA-secreting neurons that project from the substantia nigra to the striatum. As these neurons slowly degenerate over many years, the amount of DA secreted decreases, downstream GABA pathways become dysregulated, and the relative activity of acetylcholine-secreting neurons in the basal ganglia is increased.[7] We do not know what causes Parkinson disease, but a number of drugs (those that block DA) are known to produce a similar clinical syndrome (see Chapter 45).

In addition to the gray matter of the cerebral cortex and the basal ganglia, the cerebrum contains thick layers of white matter that consist of myelinated axons. Some of these axons connect the two cerebral hemispheres (commissural fibers), some connect one area of cortex to another within the same hemisphere (association fibers), and others connect the cortex with lower brain centers, including the thalamus, basal ganglia, brainstem, and spinal cord (projection fibers). The corpus callosum and the anterior commissure connect the two hemispheres. The corpus callosum is a massive bundle of fibers crossing the brain just above the lateral ventricles and is the principal means of communication between the hemispheres.

In summary, the cerebrum is the largest brain structure, garnering about 70% of the neurons and supporting cells of the brain to accomplish its diverse and complex functions. Each of the 100 billion neurons in the brain may make hundreds of synaptic connections with other neurons, providing an incomprehensible number of potential interactions. Discovering the ways in which the substance of the cerebrum relates to the workings of the mind is truly one of the great remaining mysteries of science.

Diencephalon

The diencephalon lies deep in the brain, forming a connecting structure between the upper brainstem (midbrain) and the cerebral hemispheres. The principal structures of the diencephalon are the thalamus, hypothalamus, pineal gland, epithalamus, and ventral thalamus (Figure 43-12). The third ventricle also traverses the diencephalon.

The thalamus is the principal receiving site and relay center for impulses traveling to the cerebral cortex from the spinal cord, cerebellum, and basal ganglia. In addition to processing and relaying sensory information, the thalamus is integrally involved in executing motor activities through its projections to the motor cortex. The thalamus also is involved in propagating the constant background electrical activity of the brain, which can be detected by electroencephalography. Large groups of neurons sending impulses between the thalamus and cortex are responsible for the typical waveforms noted on the electroencephalogram during sleep, rest, and wakeful activities. Connections between the brainstem reticular activating system and thalamus are necessary to maintain consciousness.

Thalamic connections, including the limbic and association cortex, are integral to the expression of those qualities considered to be human: emotion, language, creativity, and

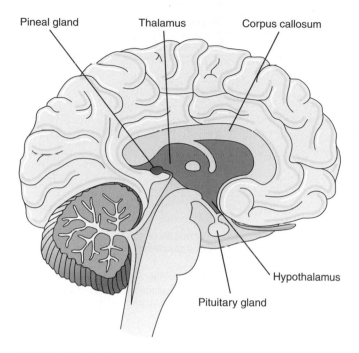

FIGURE 43-12 The diencephalon includes the thalamus, hypothalamus, pineal gland, and hypothalamic extension to the pituitary gland.

complex thought. Indeed, the thalamus is much more than a relay station; it is a complex integrative center that makes possible the functioning of higher brain centers.[8]

The hypothalamus is located just beneath the thalamus on the floor of the diencephalon. The inferior aspect of the hypothalamus extends downward to form the pituitary gland (hypophysis). The posterior pituitary gland is an extension of the neuronal tissue of the hypothalamus, whereas the anterior pituitary gland is derived from glandular tissue (Figure 43-13). Hormones secreted by the pituitary gland enter the systemic circulation and influence target cells at a distance. Neurons in the hypothalamus regulate the secretion of anterior pituitary hormones by releasing and inhibiting hormones (see Chapter 39 for a discussion of the endocrine system).

The hypothalamus is also an important regulatory center for the ANS and for basic functions, such as sleep, body temperature, appetite, and sex drive. Input from sensors of blood pressure, osmolarity, blood oxygen, carbon dioxide and pH, and temperature is received and integrated into appropriate regulatory responses. Perhaps more than any other structure, the hypothalamus is responsible for homeostasis of life-sustaining functions, including cardiovascular, respiratory, metabolic, fluid and electrolyte, and stress responses.

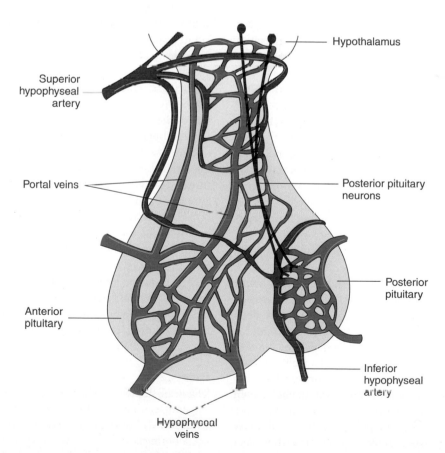

FIGURE 43-13 Anatomy of the hypothalamus and pituitary gland. Note that the posterior pituitary gland is connected to the hypothalamus by neuronal axons, whereas the anterior pituitary gland receives signals by way of a portal vein system. The portal veins drain blood from the capillaries of the hypothalamus and take it to the capillaries of the anterior pituitary gland.

The epithalamus contains the pineal gland, thought to be important in regulating circadian rhythms in response to light-dark cycles. The ventral thalamus contains the basal ganglia structure called the *subthalamic nucleus.*

Cerebellum

The cerebellum is located in the posterior fossa behind the pons. It is separated from the cerebrum by the tentorium cerebelli. The main roles of the cerebellum are to coordinate and smooth movements and to maintain posture and balance. The cerebellum compares the desired motor program with the moment-to-moment execution of the movement and makes instantaneous adjustments to improve the match.[9] The cerebellum receives information from proprioceptors in muscles and joints and from the vestibular apparatus in the inner ear about the position of the head in space. Some of the fastest-conducting neurons in the nervous system are involved in relaying sensory information to the cerebellum.

The cerebellar cortex is folded much as the cerebral cortex is folded, in a way that significantly increases surface area. Its tightly folded shape gives it a banded appearance. The cortical ridges on the surface of the cerebellum are called *folia.* The white matter beneath is called the *medullary* center and is made up of fibers running to and from the cerebellar cortex.

The cerebellum is divided anatomically, first by the posterolateral fissure, which separates the flocculonodular lobe (the region immediately inferior to the middle cerebellar peduncles) from the main body, the corpus cerebelli (Figure 43-14). Another prominent landmark is the primary fissure, which subdivides the corpus cerebelli into the anterior and posterior lobes. The midline body is called the *vermis,* and it is straddled on either side by the cerebellar hemispheres. The portion of the hemisphere that is adjacent to the vermis is called the *paravermal zone.*

The prominent tracts that attach the cerebellum to the brainstem are called the *inferior, middle,* and *superior* cerebellar peduncles. The inferior cerebellar peduncle is composed primarily of afferent fibers coming from the spinal cord and the brainstem. The middle peduncle contains afferent fibers from the contralateral pontine **nuclei.** The superior cerebellar peduncle is composed of major efferent pathways leaving the cerebellum.

Deep within the medullary center in each cerebellar hemisphere are the cerebellar nuclei. These include the dentate nuclei, the interposed nuclei, and the fastigial nuclei. The deep cerebellar nuclei are the final pathway of cerebellar output.

The lateral hemispheres form the biggest part of the cerebellum. Their major neural activity involves a feedback loop in which input from several areas of the cerebral cortex is received by the cerebellar hemispheres and dentate nuclei, then sent back to the motor and premotor cortex. This circuit is believed to influence the planning and programming of voluntary movements, especially learned, skilled movements (those that become more rapid, precise, and automatic with practice).

The major input to the paravermal region, also called the intermediate cortex, consists of somatotopically arranged

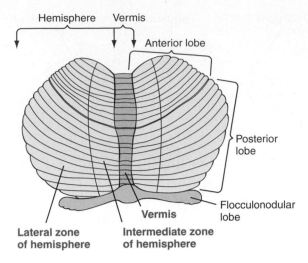

FIGURE 43-14 Lobes of the cerebellum from the posteroinferior view. (Adapted from Guyton AC, Hall JE, editors: *Textbook of medical physiology,* ed 11, Philadelphia, 2006, Saunders, p 699.)

projections from the motor cortex and spinal cord. The primary output from this region is through the interposed nucleus to the red nucleus and also back to the motor cortex by way of the thalamus. The intermediate cerebellum therefore can influence spinal cord and motor neurons through the corticospinal tract and the rubrospinal tract, where it is involved in interpreting and responding to the position and velocity of the moving body.

The vermis receives input and contains representation of the trunk as conveyed by the spinocerebellar tracts. It sends output to the vestibular nuclei and the reticular formation by way of the fastigial nucleus and through direct projections to the vestibular nuclei. The vestibulospinal and reticulospinal tracts in turn influence spinal motor neurons. This area of the cerebellum, then, is most involved with regulation of posture and stereotyped movements that are programmed in the brainstem and spinal cord.

The flocculonodular lobe receives most of its transmissions by way of the inferior cerebellar peduncle from the vestibular nerve and nuclei. Because of this primary source of input, this lobe is often referred to as the vestibulocerebellum. Its role is to maintain equilibrium and mediate the eye movements needed for visual tracking.

Lesions of the cerebellum result in ataxia (impaired balance), intention tremor, past pointing (failure of finger-to-nose test), and dysdiadochokinesia (failure of rapid movements).

Brainstem

The brainstem is a stalk of neural tissue that lies between the upper spinal cord and the diencephalon. It has three parts; from top to bottom these are the midbrain, pons, and medulla oblongata. The brainstem is critical for transmission of impulses between the brain and spinal cord. Vital centers for regulating respiratory and cardiovascular function are located in the medulla and pons. In addition, the reticular activating

TABLE 43-4

Cranial Nerves

Cranial Nerve	Origin	Function
I (Olfactory)	Nasal mucous membrane	Olfaction
II (Optic)	Retina	Vision
III (Oculomotor)	Midbrain	Movement of eyeball, eyelid, constriction of pupil
IV (Trochlear)	Lower midbrain	Lateral eye movements
V (Trigeminal)		
Ophthalmic	Forehead, eyes	Sensation from forehead, eye, scalp
Maxillary	Upper jaw, lip	Sensation from cheek, upper lip
Mandibular	Lower jaw area	Sensation from chin and lower jaw, motor chewing
VI (Abducens)	Lower pons	Lateral eye movements
VII (Facial)	Pons	Taste from anterior tongue, control of muscles of face
VIII (Vestibulocochlear)	Cochlea	Hearing
	Inner ear	Equilibrium
IX (Glossopharyngeal)	Medulla	Taste from posterior tongue, secretion of saliva, swallowing
X (Vagus)	Medulla	Monitors oxygen, carbon dioxide, and pH levels in the blood; senses blood pressure; inhibits cardiac action and extensive gastrointestinal activities
XI (Spinal accessory)	Medulla and cervical cord	Voice production, movement of head and shoulders
XII (Hypoglossal)	Medulla	Movements of tongue during speech and swallowing

neurons that maintain consciousness and alertness traverse the brainstem to reach the thalamus. Ten of the 12 pairs of cranial nerves originate from nuclei in the brainstem; only cranial nerves I (olfactory) and II (optic) originate elsewhere (diencephalon).

The midbrain or mesencephalon contains the cerebral peduncles, consisting of motor tracts to the spinal cord; the superior and inferior colliculi, which control head and eye movements; and the red nucleus, part of a major motor tract. Cranial nerve III (oculomotor) emerges from the midbrain and is prone to compression when pressure in one of the cerebral hemispheres is elevated. Increased intracranial pressure (e.g., from tumor, ischemia, edema, bleeding) is commonly manifested by dysfunction of cranial nerve III resulting in abnormal pupil size and poor reactivity to light (see Chapter 44). Cranial nerve IV (trochlear) also emerges at the level of the midbrain.

The pons (Latin for *bridge*) connects the midbrain above to the medulla below. The dorsal pons consists of reticular formation fibers, ascending sensory tracts, and descending motor tracts. Two respiratory centers (pneumotaxic and apneustic) located in the dorsal pons work in coordination with the principal respiratory centers in the medulla. The ventral pons contains the relay nuclei (pontine nuclei) for fibers projecting from the cortex to the cerebellum. The major pathway of voluntary motor control, the corticospinal tract, also passes through the ventral pons on its way from the motor cortex to the spinal cord.

The medulla oblongata makes up the lower third of the brainstem and is continuous with the spinal cord. Nuclei within the reticular formation of the medulla form the vital centers that regulate cardiac, vascular, and respiratory function. The medulla also contains centers that coordinate swallowing, vomiting, coughing, and sneezing. The medulla is the site of decussation (crossing over) of the major sensory (dorsal column) and motor (corticospinal) tracts such that innervation of one side of the body is connected to the opposite (contralateral) cerebral hemisphere. The corticospinal tract neurons decussate within ridges on the ventral surface of the medulla called *medullary pyramids*. Motor tracts that do not cross over within the pyramids (e.g., tectospinal, vestibulospinal) are sometimes referred to as extrapyramidal tracts; disorders associated with function of these tracts (balance, posture, gait) may be called *extrapyramidal disorders* (e.g., Parkinson disease). Although the anatomic correlation is not quite accurate, use of the term persists in a clinical context.

All of the remaining cranial nerves (VI, VII, VIII, IX, X, XI, and XII) originate in the medulla. The cranial nerves themselves are part of the PNS and are discussed in that section. The name, origin, and function of the 12 cranial nerves are included in Table 43-4.

The Spinal Cord

The spinal cord conveys nervous impulses between the brain and 31 pairs of spinal nerves that innervate sensory organs and muscle cells of the body. The spinal cord mediates spinal reflexes involved in maintenance of posture, protective responses to pain, urination, and muscle tone. A great deal of integration and processing occurs in the gray matter of the spinal cord, whereas the white matter contains bundles of myelinated axons forming tracts that run up and down the cord. Tracts in the spinal cord are **somatotopically** organized such that the innervation of a particular body region is connected to a specific region in the cerebral cortex.

Transverse process

Spinal nerves

Intervertebral disk

Vertebra

Intervertebral foramen

Spinal cord

FIGURE 43-15 The spinal cord travels down the center of the vertebral column. A foramen at the intersection of two vertebrae forms an exit point for the spinal nerves.

The typical adult spinal cord is about 18 inches long, extending from the base of the skull (foramen magnum) to the first or second lumbar vertebra (L1 to L2).[10] The vertebral column extends for several more inches, providing a reservoir for CSF and exit points for the lumbar and sacral spinal nerves. The vertebral column is formed by interlocking sections of bone separated and cushioned by intervertebral disks. At the lateral aspect of the intersection of two vertebrae is an opening (intervertebral foramen) that provides a passageway for spinal nerves to exit the cord. The spinal cord travels in a small lumen (1 cm) in the center of the vertebral column and is itself only slightly larger than the diameter of a pencil[10] (Figure 43-15).

On cross-section the spinal cord has a butterfly pattern of gray matter surrounded by white matter (Figure 43-16). Three bumps on the butterfly wings are called *horns*: the ventral horn (motor neurons), the dorsal horn (sensory neurons), and the lateral horn (sympathetic neurons). The horns consist of neuron cell bodies, synapses, and small unmyelinated interneurons. The white matter is divided into columns that contain tracts of nerve fibers traveling to and from the brain. These are the posterior (dorsal) columns, anterior columns, and lateral columns. Some of the neurons in the columns convey signals from one level of the cord to another and are important in reflex and postural adjustments. The principal ascending sensory tracts include the dorsal column–lemniscal

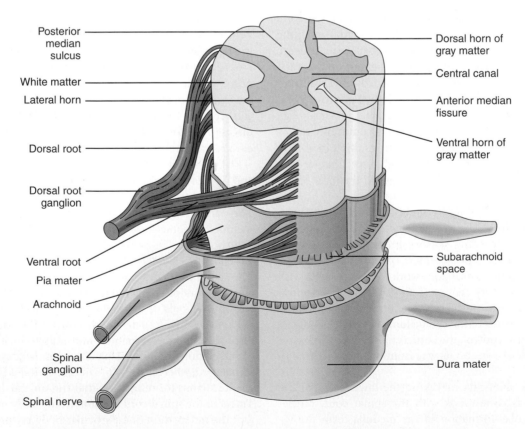

Posterior median sulcus

White matter

Lateral horn

Dorsal root

Dorsal root ganglion

Ventral root

Pia mater

Arachnoid

Spinal ganglion

Spinal nerve

Dorsal horn of gray matter

Central canal

Anterior median fissure

Ventral horn of gray matter

Subarachnoid space

Dura mater

FIGURE 43-16 The spinal cord in cross-section, showing the butterfly pattern of white and gray matter.

FIGURE 43-17 The main ascending *(left)* and descending *(right)* tracts of the spinal cord.

and the anterolateral (spinothalamic) tracts, which send **afferent** signals to the brain. The principal descending motor tracts include the corticospinal, rubrospinal, reticulospinal, and vestibulospinal tracts. These tracts are located in specific regions of the cord (Figure 43-17). Sensory and motor pathways are discussed in later sections of this chapter.

Spinal nerves divide into two sections as they make contact with the spinal cord: the ventral and dorsal roots (Figure 43-18). Ventral roots contain motor neurons that originate in the anterior horn and travel in the spinal nerve to skeletal muscles. Dorsal roots carry sensory information from somatic receptors to neurons in the posterior horn. The cell bodies of sensory afferents collect together in the dorsal root ganglion. Autonomic nerves also travel in the spinal cord and exit and enter the cord by way of the ventral and dorsal roots.

The points at which sensory neurons enter the cord and at which motor neurons exit represents the separation of the CNS and PNS.

PERIPHERAL NERVOUS SYSTEM

The PNS consists of the 31 pairs of spinal nerves and the 12 pairs of cranial nerves. These nerves are myelinated with Schwann cells, which differ somewhat from the oligodendrocytes that form the myelin sheaths of CNS neurons. By convention, groups of cell bodies are called *ganglia* in the PNS

and *nuclei* in the CNS. A major exception to this naming rule is the basal ganglia of the CNS. The PNS is not protected by CSF, meninges, or bony coverings as is the CNS; however, a sheath of connective tissue covers the nerves and provides support.

The PNS serves both afferent sensory functions and efferent motor functions of the somatic and autonomic systems. Cranial nerves III, VII, IX, and X and spinal nerves S2 and S3 contain parasympathetic neurons, and spinal nerves T1 to L2 contain sympathetic neurons.[11]

Cranial Nerves

As previously noted, all of the cranial nerves originate in the brainstem except cranial nerves I and II, which originate in the diencephalon[12] (Figure 43-19). Cranial nerve I is strictly sensory, transmitting olfactory signals from the 10 million to 20 million olfactory neurons in the nasal cavities to the olfactory bulbs. The olfactory bulb neurons then project to the olfactory cortex. Cranial nerve II is also sensory, conveying visual information from the retina to the brain. The optic nerve is unusual in that it is an extension of the CNS, myelinated by oligodendrocytes rather than Schwann cells. The neurons from the medial retina decussate in the optic chiasm, whereas the lateral retina neurons do not. Thus, the right visual field projects to the left hemisphere and the left visual field projects to the right hemisphere. Damage to one hemisphere, as occurs

FIGURE 43-18 Spinal nerves split to form dorsal and ventral roots as they emerge from the spinal cord. Ventral roots carry motor efferent neurons, whereas dorsal roots carry sensory afferent neurons.

in stroke, often interrupts visual signals from the corresponding sides of each retina—a condition known as homonymous hemianopsia (see Chapters 44 and 46).

Cranial nerves III, IV, and VI innervate motor structures in the eyes. Cranial nerve III mediates pupil constriction. The trigeminal nerve (cranial nerve V) is so named because it has three branches, which provide sensory innervation of the forehead and eyes (ophthalmic branch); upper lip, teeth, and palate (maxillary branch); and lower jaw (mandibular branch). The mandibular branch is both sensory and motor. Cranial nerve VII is also mixed sensory and motor, detecting taste in the anterior two thirds of the tongue and innervating muscles of facial expression. Cranial nerve VII also contains autonomic fibers that innervate salivary and lacrimal (tear) glands.

Cranial nerve VIII has two important sensory functions: transmitting auditory information from the cochlea and vestibular information from inner ear structures. The vestibular neurons of cranial nerve VIII interact with the neurons of cranial nerves III and VI to reflexively control eye movements during head rotation such that a visual image can remain fixed on the retina. This reflex, the oculovestibular reflex, is commonly assessed in the unconscious patient to evaluate brainstem function (see Chapter 44).

Cranial nerve IX innervates tongue and pharyngeal muscles, conveying taste from the posterior tongue and controlling pharyngeal motion during swallowing. Cranial nerve IX also has autonomic functions and transmits sensory information from the carotid baroreceptors and carotid bodies to the brainstem. Cranial nerve X, the vagus nerve, contains parasympathetic afferent and efferent fibers that innervate many visceral structures, including the heart, lungs, and gastrointestinal (GI) tract from pharynx to anus. Sensory information from aortic baroreceptors and aortic bodies is conveyed to the brainstem by the vagus nerve.

Cranial nerve XI innervates muscles of the larynx, neck, and shoulders and mediates voice production and neck and head movements. Cranial nerve XII innervates tongue muscles and controls their action during speech and swallowing.

Spinal Nerves

The 31 pairs of spinal nerves are named after the vertebral segments from which they emerge. There are 8 cervical, 12 thoracic, 5 lumbar, 5 sacral, and 1 coccygeal pair of spinal nerves. The first cervical nerve exits above C1, whereas the others all exit below the vertebral segment; thus there is one more pair of cervical spinal nerves (8) than there are cervical vertebrae (7).

Except for spinal nerves T2 to T12, the spinal nerves travel a distance from the cord and then merge into a large group called a *plexus.*[12] In the plexus, nerve fibers are recombined into different groups and emerge as peripheral nerves (Figure 43-20). There are five plexuses: (1) the cervical plexus (C1 to C4), (2) the brachial plexus (C5 to C8, T1), (3) the lumbar plexus (L1 to L4), (4) the sacral plexus (L4 to L5, S1 to S3), and (5) the coccygeal plexus (S4 to S5, coccygeal) (Table 43-5). Because of this recombination of nerve fibers in the plexus,

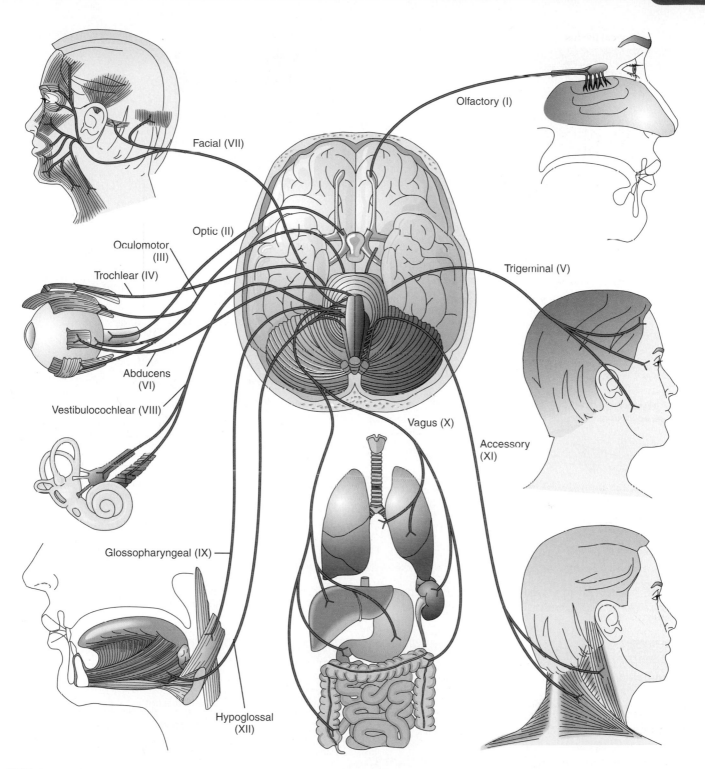

FIGURE 43-19 View of the inferior aspect of the brain showing the origin and distribution of the 12 cranial nerves. Only one of each pair is shown.

the spinal nerves and peripheral nerves have different somatic distributions. The segment of the body innervated by a spinal nerve is called a *dermatome*, whereas the peripheral nerve innervates a peripheral nerve field. Knowledge of dermatomes and peripheral nerve distribution can help the clinician differentiate between radiculopathy from spinal nerve compression

(dermatomal sensory changes) and peripheral neuropathy. (Dermatomal and peripheral nerve maps are located in Chapter 47.)

The intercostal nerves (T2 to T12) do not form plexuses; they travel in a course parallel to the ribs to innervate intercostal muscles and skin on the trunk and abdomen.

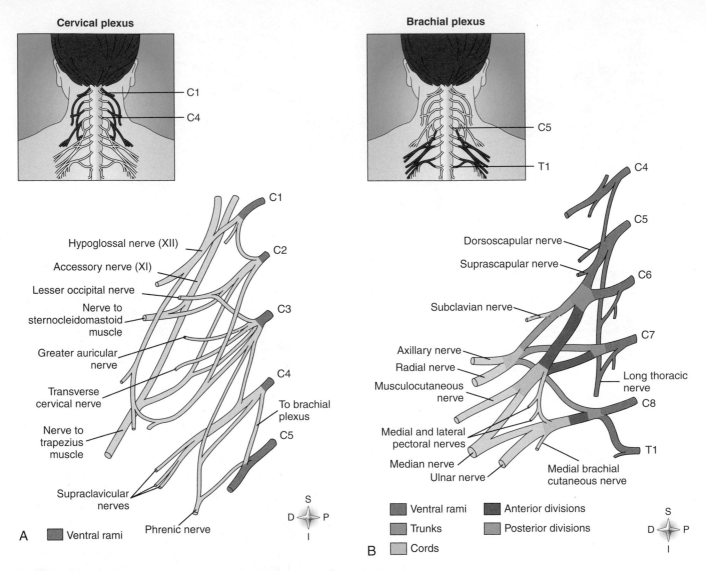

FIGURE 43-20 Examples of neuronal organization at the plexi showing reassortment of spinal nerves into peripheral nerves. **A,** Cervical plexus. **B,** Brachial plexus. (From Thibodeau GA, Patton KT: *Anatomy and physiology,* ed 6, St Louis, 2007, Mosby, pp 520-521.)

TABLE 43-5			
Spinal Nerve Plexuses			
Plexus	**Spinal Nerves**	**Peripheral Nerves**	**Distribution**
Cervical	C1-C4	Phrenic	Diaphragm
		Cutaneous	Neck
		Ansa cervicalis	Hyoid bone
Brachial	C5-C8, T1	Axillary	Upper arm
		Ulnar	Forearm, wrist, 5th digit
		Median	2nd-4th digits
		Radial	Thumb
		Musculocutaneous	Upper arm
Lumbar	L1-L4	Femoral (saphenous)	Hip, knee (lower leg)
		Obturator	Inner thigh
Sacral	L4-L5, S1-S3	Superior gluteal	Gluteus medius, minimus
		Inferior gluteal	Gluteus maximus
		Sciatic (tibial, peroneal)	Thigh, leg, foot
		Pudendal	Perineum
Coccygeal	S4-S5, coccygeal	Coccygeal fibers	Skin on coccyx

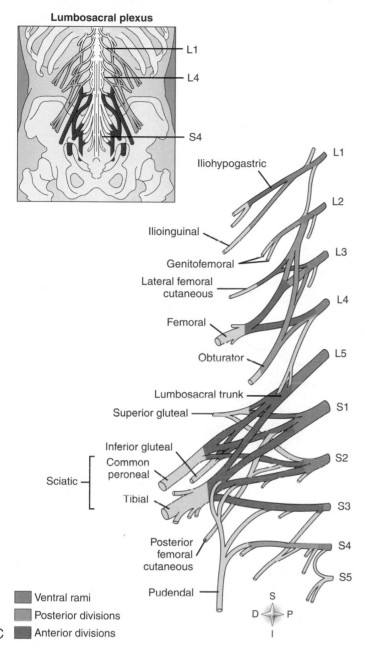

Lumbosacral plexus

L1
L4
S4

Iliohypogastric — L1

L2

Ilioinguinal

Genitofemoral — L3

Lateral femoral
cutaneous

L4

Femoral

Obturator — L5

Lumbosacral trunk

Superior gluteal — S1

Inferior gluteal

Common
peroneal — S2

Sciatic

Tibial

S3

Posterior
femoral
cutaneous — S4

S5

Pudendal

Ventral rami
Posterior divisions
Anterior divisions

C

FIGURE 43-20—cont'd C, Lumbosacral plexus (because of
their overlap the lumbar and sacral plexi are often considered together
as in this example).

AUTONOMIC NERVOUS SYSTEM

The ANS is composed of neurons in the CNS and PNS that
mediate automatic or involuntary functions. The ANS has
both sensory afferents and motor efferents that primarily
innervate visceral organs and blood vessels. As previously described, the hypothalamus and brainstem contain neurons responsible for integrating autonomic sensory information and
creating appropriate homeostatic responses. This response is
communicated to the effector organs by parasympathetic nervous system (PSNS) efferents located in cranial nerves III, VII,

IX, and X, and spinal nerves S2 to S3 and by sympathetic nervous system (SNS) neurons in spinal nerves T1 to L2.[11]

The distribution of parasympathetic nerves is shown in
Figure 43-21. Note the extensive role that cranial nerve X (vagus) has in cardiovascular, respiratory, and GI function. The
distribution of sympathetic nerves is shown in Figure 43-22.
Note that after leaving the spinal cord, sympathetic neurons
converge on a chain of ganglia that runs parallel to both sides of
the spinal cord. Some sympathetic neurons synapse on secondary neurons in the ganglia, and others travel to other plexuses or
ganglia before synapsing (see Figure 43-22). The neurons that
emerge from the spinal cord are called *preganglionic neurons,*
whereas the neurons traveling to the target cell are called *postganglionic neurons.* This terminology is also used for the PSNS
system; however the parasympathetic preganglionic neurons
are long, traveling all the way to the target organ, and they do
not terminate in ganglia.[11] The postganglionic neurons are short
and are located within the target organ (see Figure 43-21).

The neurotransmitter secreted by preganglionic neurons is
acetylcholine for both the SNS and PSNS. The postganglionic
neurotransmitters differ (Figure 43-23). The SNS secretes
norepinephrine (NE) in most cases, although sweat glands
and skeletal muscle vessels are innervated by acetylcholine
secreting SNS neurons. The PSNS secretes acetylcholine as
the postganglionic neurotransmitter. Acetylcholine is also the
neurotransmitter of the motor neurons that innervate skeletal muscle; however, the target cell receptors differ. Skeletal
muscle contains nicotinic acetylcholine receptors, whereas
autonomic organs contain muscarinic acetylcholine receptors
(see Figure 43-23).

The effect of the SNS and PSNS on target organs is nearly
always antagonistic. If one contracts smooth muscle, the other relaxes it; if one stimulates glandular secretion, the other
inhibits it; if one speeds up a process, the other slows it down.
The effects of SNS and PSNS stimulation on major target organs are shown in Table 43-6.

A specialized extension of the SNS is found in the adrenal
gland. The adrenal medulla receives preganglionic neurons
from SNS neurons emerging from the spinal cord, which stimulate the gland to secrete epinephrine (and smaller amounts of
NE) into the bloodstream. These hormones have effects similar to those of direct SNS stimulation.

The manner in which target cells respond to SNS stimulation depends on the types of receptors they possess. Several
subtypes of receptors bind and respond to NE and epineph-
rine; these include α_1, α_2, β_1, β_2, β_3, and several DA receptors
(see Table 43-6). (The details of autonomic regulation of car-
diac, genitourinary, and GI function can be found in Chapters
17, 29, and 35, respectively.)

The coordination of SNS and PSNS activity within a target organ is accomplished by centers in the brainstem and
hypothalamus with input from sensory neurons and cortical
neurons. Most of these systems work on a negative-feedback
principle to achieve homeostasis. Negative feedback requires
accurate sensory input about the conditions being regulated.
Much of this feedback is provided by the vagus nerves, which

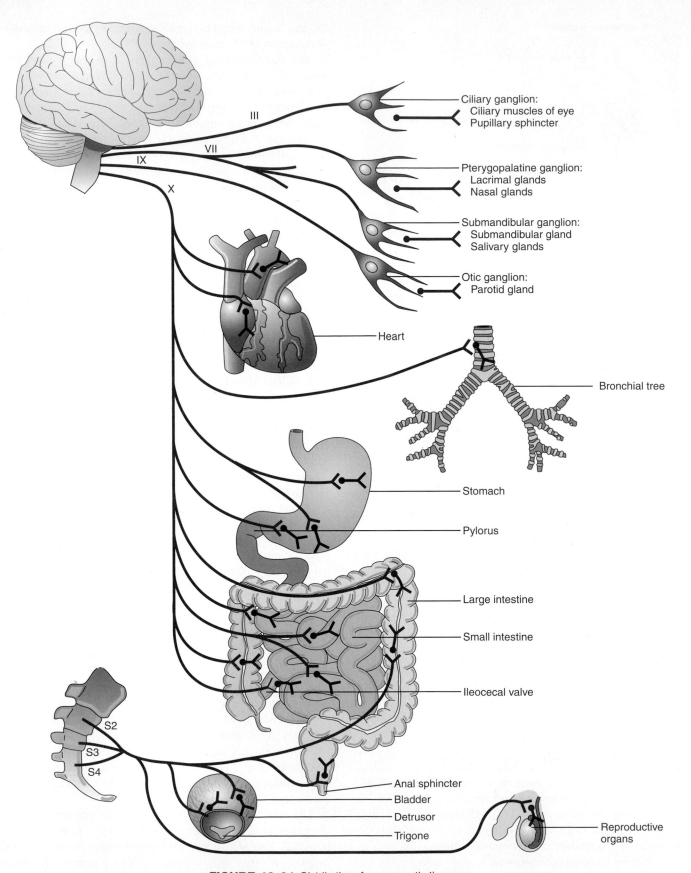

FIGURE 43-21 Distribution of parasympathetic nerves.

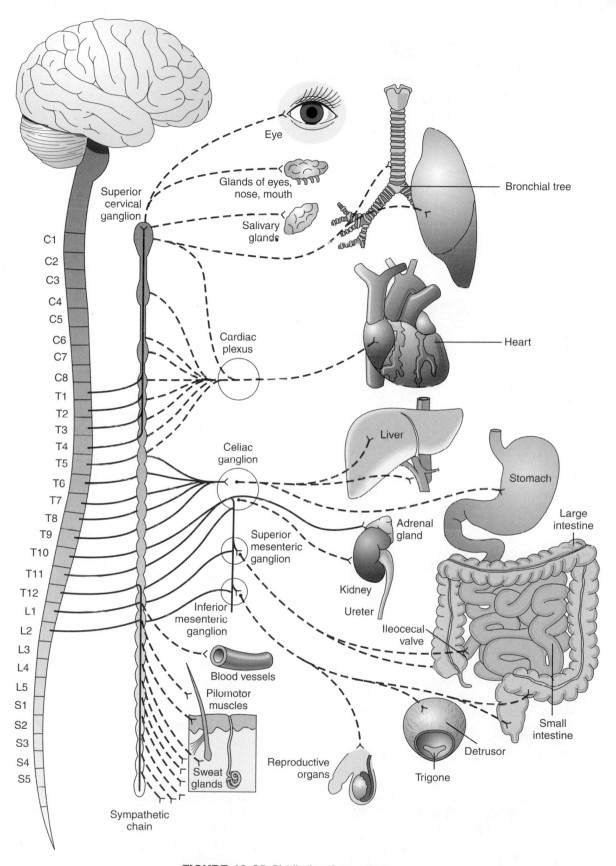

FIGURE 43-22 Distribution of sympathetic nerves.

FIGURE 43-23 Comparison of preganglionic and postganglionic neurotransmitters in the sympathetic and parasympathetic systems. Acetylcholine *(ACh)* is the neurotransmitter of the motor neuron, but its receptor differs from that of the parasympathetic terminations. *NE,* Norepinephrine; *N,* nicotinic receptors; *M,* muscarinic receptors.

obtain extensive sensory information from receptors in the GI tract and aorta. This sensory input is processed in lower brain centers and does not reach the level of perception.

KEY POINTS

- The nervous system can be divided into three principal systems: (1) the central nervous system (CNS), consisting of the brain and spinal cord; (2) the peripheral nervous system (PNS), consisting of 31 pairs of spinal nerves and 12 pairs of cranial nerves; and (3) the autonomic nervous system (ANS), consisting of the sympathetic and parasympathetic branches.
- Meninges affix the brain to the skull so that the brain is suspended and supported. Meninges have three layers: (1) The dura mater is the tough outer layer attached to the periosteum of the skull. (2) The arachnoid is a delicate weblike membrane spanning the space between the dura mater and the pia mater. (3) The pia mater covers the contours of the brain surface. The spinal cord has a similar arrangement of meningeal coverings.
- Cerebrospinal fluid (CSF) is produced in the brain ventricles and circulates in the subarachnoid spaces, providing cushioning and nutritive functions.
- The brain is protected by specialized tight junctions between the cells of the capillary endothelium (blood-brain barrier) and between the ependymal cells that line the ventricles (CSF-brain barrier).

- The brain can be anatomically divided into four principal structures: (1) the cerebrum (cerebral cortex, basal ganglia, limbic cortex, and corpus callosum); (2) the diencephalon (thalamus and hypothalamus); (3) the cerebellum; and (4) the brainstem (midbrain, pons, and medulla).
- Certain cortical areas are closely associated with specific functions: the frontal lobe contains the motor cortex and is involved in complex thought, motivation, and morality; the temporal lobe contains the auditory and vestibular centers and parts of the language center; the occipital lobe contains the visual cortex; the parietal lobe contains the somatosensory cortex; the limbic area is involved in memory and emotion.
- Basal ganglia are located deep within the cerebral hemispheres and are important in the control of skeletal muscles. Parkinson disease is an important example of basal ganglia dysfunction characterized by akinesia, rigidity, and rest tremor.
- The thalamus is a centrally located structure that processes and relays most of the signals traveling to and from the cortex and lower centers. Connections between the thalamus and the brainstem and cortex are needed to maintain consciousness and allow higher brain functions.
- The hypothalamus and brainstem are important structures regulating the ANS. The sympathetic nerves originate in spinal cord segments T1 to L2. The parasympathetic nerves emerge from the sacral segments and also travel in cranial nerves III, VII, IX, and X.

TABLE 43-6					

Effects of the Autonomic Nervous System on Organ System Function

| Organ | Sympathetic | | | Parasympathetic | |
	Action	Receptor	Action	Receptor
Heart				
SA node, heart rate	↑	β_1	↓	M
AV nodal conduction	↑	β_1	↓	M
Contractility	↑	β_1	↓ (atria only)	M
Vascular Smooth Muscle				
Skin; splanchnic	Constricts	α_1		
Skeletal muscle	Dilates	β_2		
Skeletal muscle	Constricts	α_1		
Endothelium			Releases EDRF	M
Bronchioles	Dilates	β_2	Constricts	M
Gastrointestinal Tract				
Smooth muscle, walls	Relaxes	α_2, β_2	Contracts	M
Smooth muscle, sphincters	Contracts	α_1	Relaxes	M
Saliva secretion	↑	β_1	↑	M
Gastric acid secretion			↑	M
Pancreatic secretion			↑	M
Bladder				
Wall, detrusor muscle	Relaxes	β_2	Contracts	M
Sphincter	Contracts	α_1	Relaxes	M
Male genitalia	Ejaculation	α	Erection	M
Eye				
Radial muscle, iris	Dilates pupil (mydriasis)	α_1		
Circular sphincter muscle, iris			Constricts pupil (miosis)	M
Ciliary muscle	Dilates (far vision)	β	Contracts (near vision)	M
Skin				
Sweat glands, thermoregulatory	↑	M*		
Sweat glands, stress	↑	α		
Pilomotor muscle (goose bumps)	Contracts	α		
Lacrimal glands			Secretion	M
Liver	Gluconeogenesis; glycogenolysis	α, β_2		
Adipose tissue	Lipolysis	β_1		
Kidney	Renin secretion	β_1		

From Constanzo LS: *Physiology,* ed 3, Philadelphia, 2006, Saunders, p 54.
AV, Atrioventricular; *EDRF,* endothelial-derived relaxing factor; *M,* muscarinic receptor; *SA,* sinoatrial.
*Sympathetic cholinergic neurons.

Neuronal Structure and Function

The ways in which the nervous system achieves its rapid communication function can be understood by examining the structure and behavior of neurons and neuronal synapses.

NEURONS AND SUPPORTIVE CELLS

The nervous system is composed of two principal cell types: neurons, which generate and transmit nerve impulses, and glial cells, which provide supportive functions to neurons but do not transmit impulses. There are approximately 10 glial cells per neuron and about 100 billion neurons in the CNS.[13]

Neurons

A neuron has three basic components: (1) the cell body containing cellular organelles, (2) the dendrites that receive signals and conduct them to the cell body, and (3) the axon that generates and conducts action potentials. Neurons can be categorized according to their structure or by the neurotransmitters they secrete. Neurons come in three basic configurations based on the location of the cell body and the relative length and number of dendrites and axons[13] (Figure 43-24).

Multipolar neurons have a large number of dendrites extending from the cell body and one axon. Most neurons are of

FIGURE 43-24 The three basic types of neurons: multipolar, bipolar, and unipolar.

FIGURE 43-25 The four types of neuroglial cells: astrocytes, microglia, ependymal cells, and oligodendrocytes.

FIGURE 43-26 Oligodendrocytes wrap around nerve axons to form a myelin sheath. The nodes of Ranvier are the small spaces between the oligodendrocytes. *CF, C*-fiber (unmyelinated). (From Kessel RG, Kardon RH: *Tissues and organs: a text-atlas of scanning electron microscopy,* San Francisco, 1979, Freeman, p 80.)

this type. Bipolar neurons have only one dendrite and one axon extending from the cell body. These neurons are prevalent in the retina, cochlea, and olfactory structures but are rare elsewhere. Unipolar neurons have a single process protruding from the cell body, which splits to form a dendrite and axon. This arrangement makes the cell body appear to be off-center. Unipolar neurons are prevalent in the somatosensory nerves in which the cell bodies are grouped in the dorsal root ganglia. The dendrites extend to the sensory receptors and the axons enter the spinal cord.

Neurons also can be grouped as excitatory or inhibitory based on the nature of the neurotransmitter they secrete. Each neuron secretes one principal neurotransmitter, which is excitatory if it depolarizes the target neuron or inhibitory if it results in hyperpolarization.

Glia

Glial cells in the nervous system (neuroglia) serve a number of supportive functions, but they are not capable of generating action potentials. Four types of neuroglia are recognized: oligodendrocytes, astrocytes, microglia, and ependymal cells (Figure 43-25). The Schwann cells of the PNS are similar to oligodendrocytes. Both of these cell types form the myelin sheath that wraps around nerve axons to insulate and speed

the rate of action potential conduction (Figure 43-26). Myelin gives the white matter its color.

Astrocytes serve many functions in the CNS. Some astrocytes have foot processes that contact the brain capillaries and help maintain integrity of the blood-brain barrier. Astrocytes regulate ionic balance of the interstitial fluid and may influence the transfer of nutrients from capillaries to neurons. Astrocytes also participate in nervous system signaling and have been shown to release molecules such as D-serine, which binds to neuron receptors and modulates neurotransmission.[14]

Microglia are derived from the monocyte-macrophage cell type and provide phagocytic functions within the CNS.[15] Ependymal cells line the ventricles and central canal of the spinal cord, producing CSF and maintaining the CSF-brain barrier.

Terminally differentiated neurons are not capable of cell division and cannot replace themselves if they die. However, certain areas of the brain, particularly the hippocampus and ventricles, are populated by neural stem cells. These cells are capable of cell division to produce two daughter cells, one of which retains stem cell characteristics while the other may differentiate into a neuron or glial cell (Figure 43-27). Specific signals are thought to guide the new cell as it migrates to the brain tissue and begins differentiation. Approximately half of the newborn cells will not find a suitable place and undergo apoptosis (programmed cell death).[16] The discovery that neural stem cells provide a reservoir for producing new neurons has numerous implications for treating neurodegenerative disorders such as Alzheimer disease, Parkinson disease, as well as brain damage after stroke and trauma. However, the methods for stimulating proliferation and coaching the neurons to migrate to the right places to make the correct synaptic connections have not been elucidated.

The term *neural plasticity* is used to describe the potential for the brain to change its structure and function. Traditionally, neural plasticity was thought to be a result of recruitment of formed neurons into new functional networks. With the discovery of neural stem cells, plasticity in some regions of the brain is likely to include the addition of new neurons as well as reassignment of the participants in the neuronal circuits. Neural plasticity is used to advantage to train different brain areas to assume new functions. For example, when a person suffers a stroke causing destruction of neurons in the motor cortex, it is possible to train nearby cortical neurons to take over some of the lost motor functions. Persistent attempts to use the muscles in an affected area may recruit cortical neurons into the neuronal circuit and improve motor strength and co-ordination over time. Neural plasticity is a fundamental process that endows the brain with the potential for memory and learning. Within certain boundaries, it appears that greater exposure to a particular stimulus prompts the brain to dedicate more neurons to that stimulus (and a lack of stimulation allows the brain to reassign neurons to a different function). And so the old adage "use it or lose it" appears to hold true for the brain. However, with significant effort, it is possible to reclaim at least some of what was lost.

Neural
stem cells

Newborn
neural
precursor

Neural
stem
cell

Neurons

Glial cell

Apoptosis

FIGURE 43-27 Schematic drawing of neural stem cell proliferation. Stem cells can differentiate into glial cells or neurons under the right conditions, but half fail to find a home and undergo apoptosis (programmed cell death).

NEURONAL COMMUNICATION

Neurons communicate through the release of neurotransmitters into the synapses adjacent to target neurons. Postsynaptic neurons have receptors for these neurotransmitters and respond by changing the flow of ions through channels in the cell membrane.

Sufficient depolarization of the membrane results in the generation of action potentials, which transmit signals quickly from one end of the axon to the other. Action potentials reaching the axon terminal open voltage-gated Ca^{2+} channels and stimulate the release of neurotransmitter into the next synapse. Not all neurotransmitters are excitatory; some are inhibitory and suppress the formation of action potentials in the postsynaptic neuron. Most neurons have many contacts, some inhibitory and some excitatory, such that the response of the postsynaptic neuron is a summation of all the input.

Membrane Potentials

A detailed discussion of membrane potentials can be found in Chapter 3, and the major points are reviewed here. All cells of the body contain slightly more negatively charged molecules than positively charged ones. These negative ions are trapped intracellularly because they cannot pass through the plasma membrane. Positive ions are attracted to the cell membrane by the negatively charged cellular ions. Because the cell membrane is permeable at rest to K^+ ions, but not to Ca^{2+} or Na^+ ions, potassium accumulates in the cell to neutralize the intracellular anions. The unequal distribution of K^+ across the cell membrane creates a concentration gradient, pulling K^+ back out of the cell. At equilibrium, the electrical gradient pulling K^+ into the cell and the chemical gradient pulling it out are balanced. This equilibrium point leaves a few extra negatively charged ions inside the cell with no positive ion to neutralize them. The negative ions line up on the inside of the cell membrane to interact with positive ions on the other side (Na^+, K^+, Ca^{2+}). This separation of charge across the membrane at rest creates a membrane potential that can be measured and is about −65 to −90 mV.[17] The membrane potential changes when the concentration of K^+ changes and when the permeability of the membrane to other ions changes.

Excitable cell types, like nerve and muscle, have ion channels in their cell membranes that open and close in response to fluctuations in membrane voltage. The most important voltage-gated ion channels in nerves are the fast Na^+ channels and the K^+ channels. Fast sodium channels allow Na^+ influx during the upstroke of the action potential, whereas potassium channels allow K^+ to leave the cell and help repolarize the membrane (see Chapter 3).

An action potential is initiated when neurotransmitters bind to receptors on the dendrite and cell body and allow cations, especially Na^+, to leak in. These channels are not voltage-gated channels; they are ligand-gated channels that open in response to a neurotransmitter binding to their receptor domain. If sufficient Na^+ leaks into the cell to raise the membrane potential to threshold, the fast voltage-gated Na^+

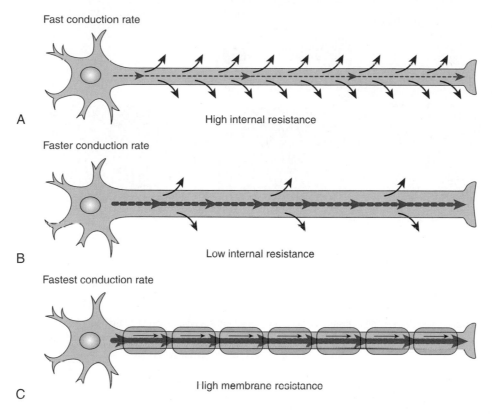

Fast conduction rate

A

High internal resistance

Faster conduction rate

B

Low internal resistance

Fastest conduction rate

C

High membrane resistance

FIGURE 43-28 The rate of action potential conduction down an axon depends on the relative degree of internal resistance to current flow. When the diameter is small **(A)**, there is higher internal resistance and slower conduction than in large-diameter neurons. A larger diameter **(B)** reduces internal resistance and speeds up the rate of conduction. Myelination **(C)** produces the fastest rate of conduction by increasing membrane resistance and decreasing internal resistance.

channels open and an action potential results. Opening of fast Na^+ channels in one section of the membrane allows Na^+ to flow in and bring the next section to threshold, thus opening the fast Na^+ channels in that section. This pattern repeats over and over again down the length of the axon. Threshold represents the amount of membrane depolarization required to cause fast Na^+ channels to flip into their open conformation (see Chapter 3). The axon hillock, the point at which the axon emerges from the cell body, is the usual site of action potential initiation because it has a high density of fast Na^+ channels and, therefore, a lower threshold.

Voltage-gated K^+ channels assist with repolarization because K^+ is allowed to flow out of the cell. During an action potential, the electrical gradient holding K^+ in the cell temporarily disappears as the membrane voltage moves toward zero. Potassium flows out of the cell passively down its concentration gradient. The Na^+-K^+ pumps work continuously to remove Na^+ from the cell interior and bring K^+ back in. The majority of a nerve cell's energy expenditure is used to power the Na^+-K^+ pumps.

The speed at which an action potential travels is determined by axonal diameter and myelination. Larger and myelinated neurons conduct impulses more quickly (Figure 43-28). In myelinated neurons, action potentials are generated only at the nodes of Ranvier, allowing the impulse to hop quickly

from node to node down the axon. This is called *saltatory conduction.*

Synaptic Transmission

The great majority of synapses responsible for signal transmission in the CNS function by using neurotransmitters. A neurotransmitter is released from the synaptic terminal of one neuron, proceeds across the synaptic cleft, and acts on the receptor proteins in the membrane of the second neuron to excite, inhibit, or modify its activity. The response at the postsynaptic membrane depends on the type of ion channel that is opened or closed when the neurotransmitter binds to the receptor. The neurotransmitter is therefore a chemical messenger that stimulates a response that is built into the postsynaptic cell. Once neurotransmitters are released into the synaptic cleft, their potential to activate the postsynaptic receptors is limited by deactivation processes. Neurotransmitters are either actively transported back into the axon terminals for reuse or destroyed by enzyme activity.

An *excitatory postsynaptic potential* (EPSP) results when a neurotransmitter has a depolarizing effect on the postsynaptic membrane. The EPSP may be too small to bring the axon hillock to threshold, and EPSPs from several presynaptic neurons may be required to generate an action potential. Thus postsynaptic potentials are not all-or-none phenomena, as are

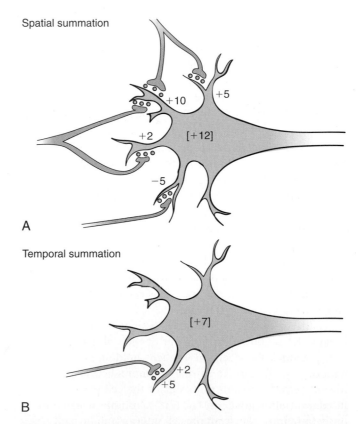

FIGURE 43-29 Neurotransmitter *(NT)* receptor classes. **A,** Ionotropic receptors are channel proteins that open when a neurotransmitter binds to them. **B,** Metabotropic receptors activate intracellular signaling cascades that generate second messengers in the cell when the neurotransmitter binds.

action potentials. Neurotransmitters that produce EPSPs do so by opening channels in the membrane that allow Na^+ influx. In some cases, the receptor itself is a channel *(ionotropic receptor)*; in others, the receptor is linked to the channel through a second messenger cascade *(metabotropic receptor)* (Figure 43-29). In general, the ionotropic receptors are concerned with producing changes in membrane potential, whereas the metabotropic receptors influence complex cytoplasmic signaling cascades that affect synthesis, metabolism, gene expression, and ion channels. The ion channels regulated by metabotropic receptors may participate in action potential generation, but receptor activation also exerts more long-lasting effects on cell structure and behavior.

Some neurotransmitters inhibit depolarization and may produce hyperpolarization of the postsynaptic membrane by opening Cl^- or K^+ channels. Chloride ions leaking into the cell or potassium ions leaking out of the cell serve to short-circuit the effect of sodium ion influx, thus making it more difficult to reach threshold. This effect is called an *inhibitory postsynaptic potential* (IPSP). Neurotransmitters that result in IPSPs include γ-aminobutyric acid (GABA) and glycine.

Most synapses in the CNS have many presynaptic neurons, some producing EPSP and some producing IPSP. The membrane potential of the postsynaptic membrane is an algebraic sum of all the IPSP and EPSP occurring at any one moment in time. This is called *summation* and is the basis of neuronal processing and integration (Figure 43-30). The term *spatial summation* is applied when multiple presynaptic neurons release their neurotransmitters onto one postsynaptic neuron at the same time. The IPSPs and EPSPs sum algebraically to produce the overall postsynaptic potential. *Temporal summation* occurs when one presynaptic neuron fires in rapid succession so that it releases more neurotransmitter onto the postsynaptic

FIGURE 43-30 Summation. **A,** Spatial summation occurs when two or more presynaptic neurons release neurotransmitter onto one postsynaptic cell at the same time. The various excitatory postsynaptic potentials and inhibitory postsynaptic potentials add algebraically to determine the overall postsynaptic potential (PSP) reaching the axon hillock. **B,** Temporal summation occurs when one presynaptic neuron fires in rapid succession such that a previous PSP has not fully dissipated before the next PSP is added to it.

cell before the postsynaptic neuron has completely recovered from a previous dose.

Neurotransmitters

Neurotransmitters are grouped according to their chemical structure into six principal categories[17] (Box 43-1). *Acetylcholine* is the sole neurotransmitter in its class and is prevalent in numerous areas in the CNS. It is the neurotransmitter in autonomic ganglia, postganglionic parasympathetic synapses, and neuromuscular junctions. There are two major types of acetylcholine receptors; the nicotinic receptors (N) are of the ionotropic variety and the muscarinic receptors (M) are metabotropic (Table 43-7). When acetylcholine is released into the synapse, it is quickly degraded by acetylcholinesterase to limit the duration of action (Figure 43-31). Choline is actively taken back up into the presynaptic membrane for resynthesis. Acetylcholine receptors located on the presynaptic membrane provide a negative feedback loop, whereby the presynaptic neuron monitors the amount of acetylcholine in the synapse. Acetylcholinesterase inhibitor drugs are used for diseases, such as Alzheimer disease and myasthenia gravis, in which there is a deficiency of acetylcholine in the synapse and for reversing the effect of neuromuscular blocking drugs.

The *amines* include DA, NE, epinephrine, serotonin (5-hydroxytryptamine, 5HT), and histamine. Amines are particularly involved in the limbic system, hypothalamus, and basal ganglia. NE is the neurotransmitter released at SNS post-ganglionic nerve endings. DA, NE, and serotonin are important in regulating thought processes and mood. Antipsychotic and mood-altering drugs change the activity of one or more of these amines in the brain (see Chapters 48 and 49). DA-secreting neurons project to the striatum (basal ganglia), pituitary gland, limbic system, and frontal cortex (Figure 43-32, *A*). DA can be degraded by enzymes in the extracellular fluid (catechol-*O*-methyltransferase, COMT) or by enzymes in the presynaptic nerve (monoamine oxidase, MAO). The primary means of clearing DA from the synapse is by active reuptake into the presynaptic membrane (see Figure 43-32, *B*). There are at least five DA receptor subtypes all of which are metabotropic and linked to the production of second messengers (see Table 43-7). Abnormality of DA metabolism is apparent in various diseases, including Parkinson disease and schizophrenia.

Some neurons have an enzyme for the hydroxylation of DA to form NE. The NE-secreting neurons originate in the brainstem (locus coeruleus) and project widely throughout the brain including the cerebral cortex, cerebellum, limbic structures, brainstem, and spinal cord (see Figure 43-32, *C*). Most of the NE released into the synapse is cleared by active reuptake into the presynaptic neuron, where it can be repackaged for release or broken down by MAO. A number of receptor subtypes can bind NE in the synapse, and all are of the metabotropic variety

---

BOX 43-1

Six Major Classes of Neurotransmitters

Acetylcholine

Amines
Dopamine
Norepinephrine
Epinephrine
Serotonin
Histamine

Amino Acids
Excitatory
Glutamate
Aspartate
Inhibitory
Glycine
γ-Aminobutyric acid

Polypeptides
Substance P, other tachykinins
Vasopressin
Oxytocin
Corticotropin-releasing hormone
Thyrotropin-releasing hormone
Growth hormone–releasing hormone
Somatostatin
Gonadotropin-releasing hormone
Endothelins

Enkephalins
β-Endorphin, other derivatives of pro-opiomelanocortin
Cholecystokinin
Vasoactive intestinal polypeptide
Neurotensin
Gastrin-releasing peptide
Gastrin
Glucagon
Motilin
Secretin
Calcitonin gene–related peptide α
Neuropeptide Y
Activins
Inhibins
Angiotensin II
Galanin
Atrial natriuretic peptide
Brain natriuretic peptide

Purines
Adenosine
Adenosine triphosphate

Gases
Nitric oxide
Carbon monoxide

TABLE 43-7

Mechanism of Action of Selected Nonpeptide Neurotransmitters

Transmitter	Receptor	Second Messenger	Net Channel Effects
Acetylcholine	Nicotinic	—	↑ Na^+, other small ions
	M_1	↑ IP_3, DAG	↑ Ca^{2+}
	M_2 (cardiac)	↓ cAMP	↑ K^+
	M_3	↓ cAMP	
	M_4 (glandular)	↑ IP_3, DAG	
	M_5	↑ IP_3, DAG	
Dopamine	D_1, D_5	↑ cAMP	
	D_2	↓ cAMP	↑ K^+, ↓ Ca^{2+}
	D_3, D_4	↓ cAMP	
Norepinephrine	$\alpha_{1A}, \alpha_{1B}, \alpha_{1D}$	↑ IP_3, DAG	↓ K^+
	$\alpha_{2A}, \alpha_{2B}, \alpha_{2C}$	↓ cAMP	↑ K^+, ↓ Ca^{2+}
	β_1	↑ cAMP	
	β_2	↑ cAMP	
	β_3	↑ cAMP	
5HT*	$5HT_{1A}$	↓ cAMP	↑ K^+
	$5HT_{1B}$	↓ cAMP	
	$5HT_{1D}$	↓ cAMP	↓ K^+
	$5HT_{2A}$	↑ IP_3, DAG	↓ K^+
	$5HT_{2C}$	↑ IP_3, DAG	
	$5HT_3$	—	↑ Na^+
	$5HT_4$	↑ cAMP	
Adenosine	A_1	↓ cAMP	
	A_2	↑ cAMP	
Glutamate	Metabotropic†		
	Ionotropic		
	AMPA, Kainate	—	↑ Na^+
	NMDA	—	↑ Na^+, Ca^{2+}
GABA	$GABA_A$	—	↑ Cl^-
	$GABA_B$	↑ IP_3, DAG	↑ K^+, ↓ Ca^{2+}

From Ganong WF: *Review of medical physiology*, ed 21, New York, 2003, Lange/McGraw-Hill, p 99.
AMPA, α-Amino-3-hydroxy-5-methyl-4-isoxazolepropionate; *cAMP*, cyclic adenosine monophosphate; *DAG*, diacylglycerol; *GABA*, γ-aminobutyric acid; *5HT*, serotonin; *IP₃*, inositol triphosphate; *NMDA*, N-methyl-ᴅ-aspartate.
*$5HT_{1E}$, $5HT_{1F}$, $5HT_{2B}$, $5HT_{5A}$, $5HT_{5B}$, $5HT_6$, and $5HT_7$ receptors also cloned.
†Eleven subtypes identified; all decrease cAMP or increase IP_3 and DAG, except one, which increases cAMP.

and linked to second-messenger cascades (see Table 43-7). The receptor subtype α_2 is commonly located on the presynaptic membrane where it provides a negative-feedback loop for the presynaptic cell to monitor the amount of NE in the synapse (see Figure 43-32, *D*). Stimulation of the presynaptic α_2 receptor by NE or by α_2-agonist drugs reduces the amount of NE released into the synapse by the neuron.

Serotonin is another amine that affects numerous areas of the brain in a pattern similar to that of NE (see Figure 43-32, *E*). Numerous serotonin receptor subtypes have been identified, including one ionotropic ($5HT_3$) and several metabotropic (see Table 43-7). Like NE and DA, serotonin is cleared from the synapse by an active reuptake carrier on the presynaptic membrane (see Figure 43-32, *F*). It is also subject to degradation by MAO in the presynaptic cell. Like other NT, serotonin can bind to presynaptic receptors that regulate its release. Numerous drugs have been developed to manage disorders associated with serotonin pathways, including depression, anxiety, and migraine headache. The class of medications known as selective serotonin reuptake inhibitors

blocks the reuptake carrier for serotonin. The tricyclic antidepressants also block reuptake of serotonin, but they are less specific than the selective serotonin reuptake inhibitors and also affect reuptake of other amines.

The category of *amino acids* can be subdivided into excitatory and inhibitory mechanisms of action. Glutamate and aspartate are the principal excitatory amino acids. Glutamate neurons are widely distributed throughout the brain, and it is considered to be the primary excitatory neurotransmitter. Glutamate is involved in memory and has been implicated as a neurotoxin when released in excessive amounts (Chapter 44). Glutamate is removed from the synapse by active reuptake transporters on the presynaptic membrane. When energy stores are low because of interrupted blood supply or hypoxia, the transporters do not function effectively and glutamate remains in the synapse where it can behave as a neurotoxin. Most glutamate receptors are ionotropic; the metabotropic types are poorly understood. The α-amino-3-hydroxy-5-methyl-4-isoxazolepropionate (AMPA) receptors are classic ligand-gated sodium channels that depolarize the

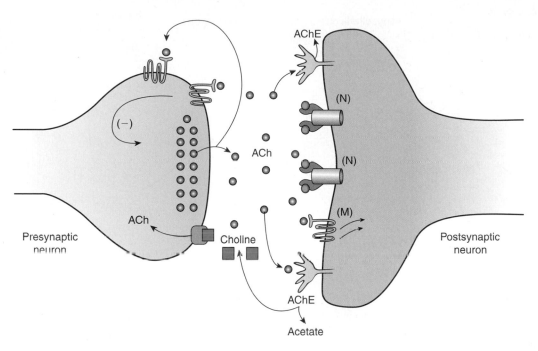

FIGURE 43-31 The acetylcholine synapse. Acetylcholine *(ACh)* released into the synapse binds to nicotinic *(N)* or muscarinic *(M)* receptors on the postsynaptic membrane. ACh also can bind to presynaptic receptors that are linked to a decrease in ACh release (negative feedback). Acetylcholinesterase *(AChE)* quickly degrades the ACh into acetate and choline. Choline is actively taken back into the presynaptic neuron for resynthesis.

postsynaptic membrane. The *N*-methyl-D-aspartate (NMDA) receptors are interesting because they will not open unless the binding of glutamate is paired with a cotransmitter (such as glycine or D-serine) and concurrent depolarization of the membrane.[14] The NMDA receptor is a ligand-gated calcium ion channel, but it is blocked by a magnesium ion when the postsynaptic membrane is polarized (Figure 43-33). It only opens in response to glutamate binding if a depolarization is produced at the same time by another neurotransmitter-receptor interaction. The depolarization releases the blocking magnesium ion from the channel, so that when glutamate binds, the channel opens to allow calcium influx. It is also unusual to use calcium ions to produce membrane depolarization as it can function to trigger signaling cascades within the cell. The NMDA receptor is thought to be responsible for long-term changes in the synapse that may relate to long-term memory. Drugs that interfere with NMDA receptors block memory; those that activate these receptors produce hallucinations and nightmares.

Glycine and GABA are inhibitory amino acids and are located throughout the spinal cord and brain. A large number of synapses (30%) are inhibitory in nature, and GABA is the principal neurotransmitter in these synapses. GABA is formed by decarboxylation (removal of CO_2) of glutamate, which transforms it from an excitatory amino acid to an inhibitory one. The GABA receptors are of two types: $GABA_A$ is a classic ligand-gated chloride channel that produces an IPSP when activated. The $GABA_B$ receptor is a metabotropic receptor that also produces an IPSP and is linked to cytoplasmic signaling cascades within the cell. Barbiturates and benzodiazepines are thought to exert their depressive effects by increasing GABA activity.

A long list of neurotransmitters is found in the *neuropeptide* category (see Table 43-7). Neuropeptides may function as the primary neurotransmitter in the synapse, but more often they are released together with another neurotransmitter. Amines and neuropeptides are commonly released together into synapses.[17] The neuropeptides have long-lasting effects on the postsynaptic cell, mediating changes in receptor number or structure and altering the responses of intracellular signaling pathways. Well-known neuropeptides include substance P, endorphins, and enkephalins, which are involved in the transmission and perception of pain. Neuropeptides are synthesized in the neuronal cell body and not in the nerve terminal like other neurotransmitters. The amount produced depends on the degree of gene activity that produces messenger RNA to direct the synthesis of the neuropeptide. Once synthesized and packaged into vesicles, the neuropeptides must be actively transported along the axon to the nerve terminal. All neuropeptide receptors are linked to second messenger cascades. Neuropeptides are released in very small quantity in comparison to other neurotransmitters, and reuptake mechanisms are not required to turn off their activity. The neuropeptide with its bound receptor may be internalized into the postsynaptic cell, where the receptor is degraded or recycled to the synaptic membrane.

Purines, including adenosine triphosphate (ATP) and adenosine, function as neurotransmitters in various brain regions. Adenosine is thought to be continuously released by most neurons and modulates neurotransmission by blocking neurotransmitter release. Adenosine may be important in

A Dopamine

B Dopamine

C Norepinephrine

D Norepinephrine

E Serotonin

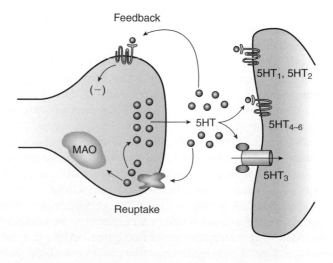

F Serotonin

FIGURE 43-32 Amine synapses. **A,** Dopamine *(DA)* distribution in the brain. **B,** The DA synapse. **C,** Norepinephrine *(NE)* distribution in the brain. **D,** The NE synapse. **E,** Serotonin *(5HT)* distribution in the brain. **F,** The 5HT synapse. *COMT,* Catechol-*O*-methyltransferase; *MAO,* monoamine oxidase.

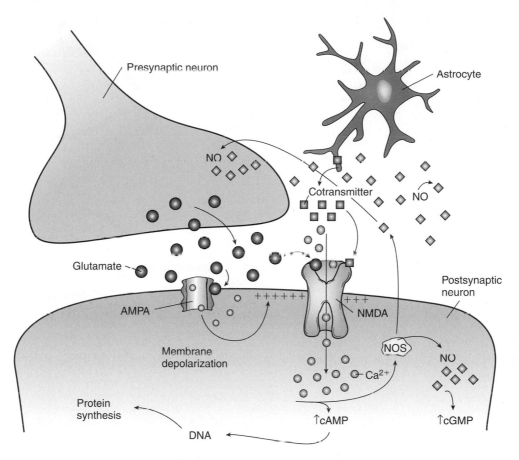

FIGURE 43-33 The glutamate synapse. Glutamate signaling is complex, having several receptor subtypes and costimulating molecules. The *N*-methyl-D-aspartate *(NMDA)* receptor is of special interest because it requires binding of glutamate and a cotransmitter (glycine or D-serine). In addition, the NMDA ion channel is blocked by Mg^{2+} and cannot open unless the postsynaptic membrane is already depolarized. Glutamate binding to its a-amino-3-hydroxy-5-methyl-4-Isoxazolepropionate *(AMPA)* receptors can provide this depolarization by allowing sodium influx. When the NMDA channel opens, it allows calcium ions to flow in, triggering intracellular signaling cascades that produce nitric oxide *(NO)*. Nitric oxide is a gas that can diffuse throughout the synapse. NMDA receptor activation has been linked to long-term changes in synaptic efficiency. *NOS,* nitric oxide synthase.

preventing seizure activity. The role of ATP as a neurotransmitter continues to be elucidated. There are at least two ATP receptor subtypes, one metabotropic and one an ionotropic-type cation channel. Little is known about either type.

Nitric oxide (NO) is a gas that can diffuse through cell membranes and therefore does not require a synaptic receptor for its activity. NO has several different potential targets within cells. For example, NO can bind and stimulate guanylyl cyclase, an enzyme that produces cyclic guanosine monophosphate (cGMP), a second messenger in the cell, or it can alter the activity of ion pumps, metabolic enzymes, and DNA transcription factors.[17] Unlike other neurotransmitters that are produced and released by presynaptic neurons, NO can be synthesized in the postsynaptic neuron and diffuse locally to affect presynaptic neurons. The functions of NO are not completely known, but it is thought to be important in memory and pain perception. One trigger known to stimulate NO is activation of the previously described NMDA receptor. The calcium ions that flow in through the open NMDA receptor cause activation of an enzyme called nitric oxide synthase (NOS), which produces NO. NO may be the messenger that alerts the presynaptic membrane that the paired stimuli required to open the NMDA receptor were received.[18]

Neuronal Circuits

Patterns of neuronal synaptic connections are called *neuronal circuits.* Activity in particular groups of neurons in one or more circuits is the basis of nervous system function: thoughts, memories, sensations, movements, and learning.

Divergence is a term used to describe neuronal circuits in which one presynaptic neuron makes contact with more than one postsynaptic neuron (Figure 43-34). Divergence is a strategy used to send sensory input to a large number of receiving neurons. *Convergence* occurs when many presynaptic neurons synapse with one postsynaptic neuron (see Figure 43-34). This arrangement is typical in the motor pathways, in which sensory, reflex, and voluntary inputs must be integrated into a response by the motor neurons that innervate skeletal muscle. Convergence is a mechanism of processing and integration of input.

The efficiency of circuits can be altered by changes in synaptic function. Synaptic transmission can be facilitated or

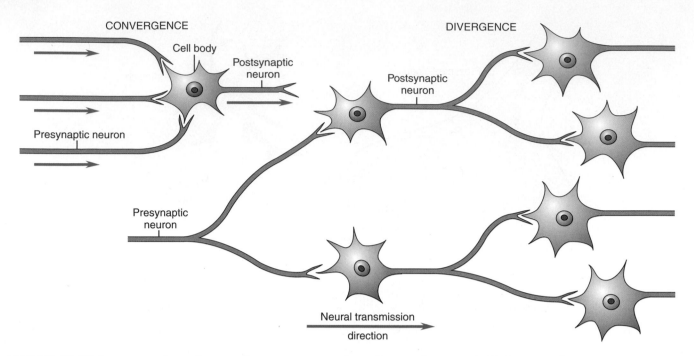

FIGURE 43-34 Convergence of several presynaptic neurons on one postsynaptic neuron is compared with divergence of one presynaptic neuron to several postsynaptic neurons.

inhibited in various ways. Alteration in the ease of synaptic transmission is the basis of memory and is discussed in more detail in the Consciousness, Memory, and Sleep section at the end of this chapter.

NEURAL DEVELOPMENT, AGING, AND INJURY

Development

The nervous system starts to take shape during the third week of embryonic development. At this time, three primary tissues of the embryo are distinguishable: the ectoderm, endoderm, and mesoderm. A thickened plate of ectoderm, running longitudinally on the dorsal surface of the embryo (neural plate), gives rise to the CNS and PNS. By the end of the third week, the neural plate folds to form a neural tube. Openings at either end of the neural tube are called *neuropores*. The neural tube is the precursor of the future brain and spinal cord.

Fusion of cells and formation of the neural tube starts in the cervical region of the future spinal cord and then progresses rapidly in a **rostral** direction toward the future brain. Failure of the neural tube to close properly is a cause of congenital malformation of the nervous system. Anencephaly (absent brain) results from failure of the rostral portion to close, whereas failure of the caudal portion results in myelomeningocele. In this defect, the spinal cord and meninges are displaced into a sac on the back (see Chapter 45). A reduction in neural tube defects has been achieved through prenatal maternal supplementation with folic acid.[19]

At the end of the fourth week of gestation, three primary vesicles are evident at the rostral end of the neural tube: the prosencephalon, or forebrain; the mesencephalon, or midbrain; and the rhombencephalon, or hindbrain.[20] The mature brain develops from these three primary structures. The prosencephalon divides to form the cerebral hemispheres and diencephalon; the mesencephalon forms the upper part of the brainstem (midbrain); and the rhombencephalon divides to form the cerebellum and lower brainstem (pons and medulla).

Neurons grow and divide at an incredible rate during embryologic development and make primitive synaptic connections according to a basic architecture that is genetically programmed. The number of neurons and synapses ultimately dedicated to particular functions is determined in large part by their use. For example, if no visual sensory input is relayed to the primary visual cortex (as occurs with congenital cataracts), the cortical neurons will be reassigned to other functions. Similarly, a person born without arms will lack representation of these structures in the primary somatosensory cortex. In contrast, greater stimulation appears to increase the number of neurons dedicated to a particular function. Critical periods in the early neonatal period have been identified when neuronal assignment to specific functions is determined.[21] In recent years it has been recognized that a significant degree of neural plasticity exists throughout life; however, it is much less than that during early childhood. The brain continues to increase in size until puberty and remains stable until middle age.

Aging

A gradual loss of neurons in later adulthood does not result in significant alteration in brain function during the usual life span. However, the older one gets, the greater the neurologic

GERIATRIC CONSIDERATIONS

Changes in the Nervous System

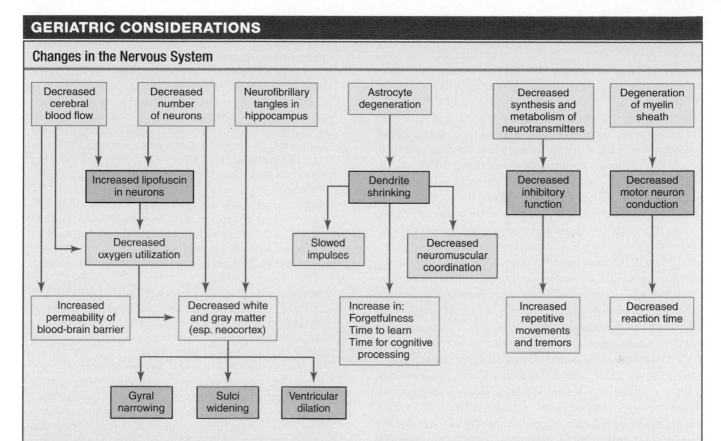

With aging, brain atrophy and a decrease in brain weight occur. This is evidenced by a decrease in white matter and gray matter up to 0.5% per year, with gyral narrowing, sulci widening, and ventricular dilation. There is a gradual atrophy and loss of neurons in the brain and spinal cord over time; but neuron loss is not uniform within the brain. Most of the neuron loss is in the neocortex (20%), Purkinje cells of the cerebellum, substantia nigra, and locus coeruleus. Some parts of the brain, such as the vestibular nucleus, have no neuron loss. Blood supply to the brain is decreased owing to the decreased metabolic demands and brain atrophy. There is also increased permeability of the blood-brain barrier.

Intracellularly there is an increase in lipofuscin, which hampers cellular oxygen use, crowds intracellular organelles, and reduces the number of mitochondria. There are also neurofibrillary tangles in the hippocampus and neuritic plaques that are found only in the elderly.

Nerve fibers in the brain decrease in number and show signs of splitting or fragmentation. The cortex, subcortex, and cerebellar astrocytes degenerate. Nerve axons develop swellings near their ends

called neuroaxonal dystrophy. The relevance of these swellings is unknown. Dendrites shrink decreasing the number of messages received from other cells and synaptic linkages. This causes slowing of impulses and decreases neuromuscular coordination. These changes result in decreased short-term memory, reduced speed of learning, prolonged new information processing, increased reaction time, diminished abstract reasoning, and impaired perception.

Changes in the secretion and metabolism of neurotransmitters also impact the aging brain. There is a decrease in norepinephrine and dopamine secretion with an increase in monoamine oxidase. The reduction of dopamine leads to decreased inhibitory motor functions.

In the spinal cord, posterior root fibers and sympathetic nerve fibers of the autonomic nervous system decline in number. Peripherally, there is degeneration of the motor nerve fibers and myelin sheath. Motor neuron axons remain intact. Decreasing motor neuron conduction velocity and prolonged muscle action potentials lead to decreased reaction times. Reflexes may be decreased or absent. There is an increased risk of falls.

---

impairment. Excessive neuronal degeneration in adulthood is called Alzheimer disease or senile dementia, and is distinguished from the normal changes of aging. The effects of aging on nervous system function are summarized in Geriatric Considerations: Changes in the Nervous System.

Injury

Mature neurons are terminally differentiated cells that are unable to undergo mitosis. Injury to neurons usually results in neuronal cell death and loss of function; however, some

regrowth is possible in peripheral nerves if the injury is not severe. Stem cells in the brain are capable of producing new, immature neurons; however, the likelihood that they will find and repair a site of injury and make appropriate synaptic connections is uncertain.

Injury to axons of neurons in the PNS results in degeneration of the distal segment (**wallerian degeneration**).[19] Within a few days to a week, the axons break into irregular fragments, and after 3 weeks they disappear completely. In the axonal segment proximal to the injury, a small section also degenerates.

If the nerve is myelinated, degeneration usually extends back to the next one or two nodes of Ranvier. As axons and myelin sheaths degrade, Schwann cells of the injured nerve swell and divide. Over the next 2 to 3 weeks, continuous columns of short Schwann cells mark the course of the lost axons. If there is little separation between the ends of a divided nerve, the proliferating Schwann cells bridge the gap. If the divided ends are further apart, the proliferating Schwann cells form bulbous swellings at the end of the nerves and the surviving axons form fine fibrils, which extend into the surrounding Schwann cells at random. Those fibrils that find a column of Schwann cells in the distal part of the nerve grow down the column. There is often good functional return to the nerve secondary to this process. If continuity is not restored, the distal end gradually becomes replaced by collagenous scar tissue.

Damaged axons in the CNS show a pattern of degeneration that is similar to that of peripheral neurons. Damaged axons become irregular and beaded, break up, and disappear, but the process is significantly slower. Methods using stains for β-amyloid precursor protein to identify axonal injury in the CNS have revealed that axonal injury is a common event even in mild concussion.[22] Axonal damage impairs axonal streaming and causes a buildup of β-amyloid precursor protein proximal to the injury. This buildup is taken as evidence of axonal injury. Contrary to previously held notions, a significant degree of axonal repair appears to occur in CNS neurons when the injury is not too severe.[22] If neurons that were the principal source of stimulation to some other group of neurons are damaged and die, that other group of neurons may also degenerate because of the loss of trophic (growth and survival) signals. Researchers continue to discover new nerve growth and survival factors. Eventually they may find ways to minimize neuronal degeneration after injury and encourage repair or replacement.

KEY POINTS

- The fundamental unit of the nervous system is the neuron. Neurons have three basic parts: cell body, dendrites, and axon. The dendrites receive signals and transmit them to the cell body. The axon generates and conducts action potentials. Conduction of action potentials is faster in large and myelinated axons.
- Neuronal communication through chemical synapses can be summarized as follows: Stimulation from other neurons occurs primarily at the dendrite and cell body. Action potentials are initiated at the axon hillock and conducted down the axon to the axon terminal, where neurotransmitter is stored. Depolarization of the terminal opens voltage-gated calcium channels. Calcium influx mediates exocytosis of neurotransmitter into the interneuronal synapse. Neurotransmitter binds and activates specific receptors on the postsynaptic cell, changing its ion conductance. With sufficient depolarization of the postsynaptic cell, an action potential is generated.

- There are six categories of neurotransmitters based on their chemical structure: acetylcholine, amines, amino acids, neuropeptides, purines, and gases.
- Excitatory neurotransmitters create excitatory postsynaptic potentials (EPSPs) in the postsynaptic neuron due to opening of channels that allow Na^+ or Ca^{2+} influx. Inhibitory neurotransmitters create inhibitory postsynaptic potentials (IPSPs) in the postsynaptic neuron due to opening of channels that allow Cl^- influx or K^+ efflux. The summation of EPSPs and IPSPs at the axon hillock determines whether an action potential will be initiated.
- Neuroglial cells are supportive cells in the CNS. Oligodendroglial cells form insulating myelin sheaths, astroglial cells moderate extracellular fluid composition, microglial cells are derived from circulating monocytes and destroy foreign materials, and ependymal cells form CSF.
- Development of the nervous system follows a basic architecture that is genetically programmed. However, the brain is quite plastic, especially during infancy, and alters the assignment of neurons to certain functions based on the degree of stimulation.
- Neurons in the CNS that are severely injured generally do not regenerate. Peripheral neurons may regenerate if the Schwann cells provide a pathway for growth. Neural stem cells in the ventricles and hippocampus of the brain can proliferate to produce either glial or neuronal cells depending on specific cues, most of which have yet to be elucidated.

Sensory Function

The discussion of sensory function in this chapter is restricted to the somatosensory system. The special senses of hearing, vision, taste, and olfaction are discussed in Chapter 46. Neural pathways related to pain transmission are discussed in detail in Chapter 47.

Transmission of sensory signals begins with activation of specialized dendritic processes, called *sensory receptors,* at the ends of sensory afferents that project to the spinal cord (or brainstem in the case of some cranial nerves). Secondary neurons in the cord are activated and carry the signals up the cord to the brain. The thalamus is the principal receiving site for somatosensory signals, which are then relayed to various brain areas, including the somatosensory cortex in the parietal lobe.

An important principle of sensory transmission is that somatotopic organization is maintained from receptor to somatosensory cortex. This property allows for precise localization of the origin of sensory signals. The somatosensory system conveys a number of different sensory modalities, including fine touch, vibration sense, pressure, temperature, itch, crude touch, and pain. In general, different modalities are sensed by different types of sensory receptors.

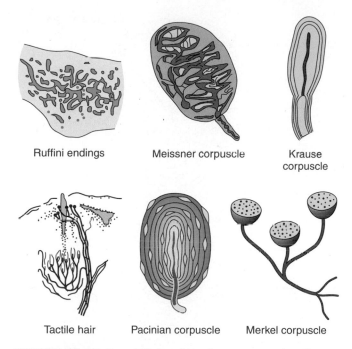

FIGURE 43-35 Common types of somatosensory receptors. Sensory receptors are specialized to respond to particular types of stimuli.

FIGURE 43-36 Relationship between stimulus intensity and action potential generation. As the stimulus increases, the receptor potential is greater, and action potentials are generated at a faster rate. (From Guyton AC, Hall JE, editors: *Textbook of medical physiology,* ed 11, Philadelphia, 2006, Saunders, p 574.)

SENSORY RECEPTORS

Sensory receptors are specialized terminations of the dendrites of primary sensory neurons. The receptor may be a free nerve ending or may have various connective tissue elaborations that affect its responsiveness (Figure 43-35). All types of receptors respond to stimuli by altering their membrane permeability to ions, thus creating a change in the membrane voltage. These receptor potentials are similar to the EPSPs generated in postsynaptic neurons, except that the stimulus is not a neurotransmitter. Different receptor types respond to different kinds of stimuli: mechanical stretch, changes in temperature, or the binding of chemicals. When a stimulus depolarizes the receptor sufficiently, voltage-gated fast Na^+ channels in the membrane open and an action potential is generated. The rate of action potential generation by the receptor depends on the intensity of the stimulus (Figure 43-36).

Some receptors are rapidly adapting and generate action potentials only when a change in the stimulus intensity occurs. The pacinian corpuscle is a classic example of a rapidly adapting receptor that is well suited to transmitting the sense of vibration. Tonic receptors adapt slowly and are good for conveying information about stimulus intensity over time. Free nerve endings, such as pain receptors, are usually tonic receptors.

Impulses generated by receptors are transmitted to the dorsal root of the spinal nerve. Depending on the sensory modality, the nerve impulses may travel up the **ipsilateral** side of the cord or may cross the spinal cord to travel up the **contralateral** side. In general, the well-localized sensations of touch, pressure, and vibration travel up the ipsilateral side of the cord, whereas the sensations of pain, itch, and temperature usually cross over and travel to the brain on the contralateral side. Regardless of pathway taken, somatosensory signals eventually converge on the somatosensory cortex in the hemisphere opposite from the location of the primary receptor.

SENSORY PATHWAYS

Two major tracts, the dorsal column–medial lemniscal tracts and the anterolateral tracts, carry information from the spinal segments to the brain[23] (Figure 43-37). The dorsal column–medial lemniscal tract carries fine touch, vibration sense, and proprioception and remains ipsilateral until the level of the medulla. As the fibers progress upward, they gradually move toward the midline, so that those corresponding to the lower extremities occupy the medial white column and those representing the arm are more lateral. From the nuclei in the medulla, neurons of the dorsal column pathway cross to the opposite side and travel up the brainstem, where they form the medial lemniscus, and then on to the thalamus. In the thalamus, fibers synapse with tertiary neurons, which in turn pass upward in a great band of fibers known as the *internal capsule,* and then travel on to the primary sensory cortex.

The anterolateral tract (previously called the *spinothalamic tract*) carries impulses for sensations of pain, itch, and temperature from small myelinated (Aδ) and unmyelinated (C-fiber) neurons. These neurons ascend one or more spinal segments before entering the posterior horn and synapsing with their secondary neuron. A few secondary fibers ascend ipsilaterally in the Lissauer fasciculus all the way to the thalamus. However, the majority of fibers cross the midline and ascend as the anterolateral tract. Fibers from the lower extremities and trunk are pushed laterally as they ascend in the spinal cord by the addition of fibers from the upper extremities and upper body, which enter medially.

FIGURE 43-37 Comparison of the two major ascending somatosensory tracts. *Left,* Dorsal column–medial lemniscal tract. *Right,* Anterolateral tract. Note that the dorsal column tracts do not cross the midline until the level of the medulla, whereas the anterolateral tracts cross at the spinal cord level.

On their way to the thalamus, these fibers give off collaterals to the reticular formation of the brainstem and the periaqueductal gray matter in the midbrain, where it is believed that one of their functions is pain inhibition (see Chapter 47). Secondary fibers of the anterolateral tract terminate in several thalamic regions. Tertiary neurons project from the thalamus to the somatosensory cortex. Thus, although the sensations of fine touch and pain are separated in the cord, they reunite in the somatosensory cortex that lies in the cerebral hemisphere opposite the site of sensory receptor origin.

SOMATOSENSORY CORTEX

The primary somatosensory cortex is organized in columns of gray matter that correspond to specific body locations. All modalities of sensation are grouped together in adjacent sections. The somatotopic representation of the body along a strip of cortex creates a distorted picture of the human body, called a homunculus map[23] (Figure 43-38). Body areas with a greater density of receptors garner a larger part of the homunculus map. The homunculus map was created by stimulating

discrete areas of the cortex in awake subjects and recording the sensations that they reported. The *perception* of sensation from the body occurs at the level of the somatosensory cortex.

KEY POINTS

- The body is somatotopically represented in the spinal cord and cerebral cortex. Stimulation of points in the primary somatosensory cortex results in discrete sensations in the contralateral side of the body.
- Projections to the somatosensory cortex begin in sensory receptors throughout the body. Receptors send axons to the spinal cord through the dorsal root. Stimulation of receptors by mechanical deformation, temperature, or chemicals alters membrane permeability, resulting in receptor potentials. The intensity of the stimulus is reflected in the rate of action potentials generated.
- Sensations of touch and proprioception (dorsal column–medial lemniscal tract) project up to the medulla on the ipsilateral side, then cross over and project to the thalamus.

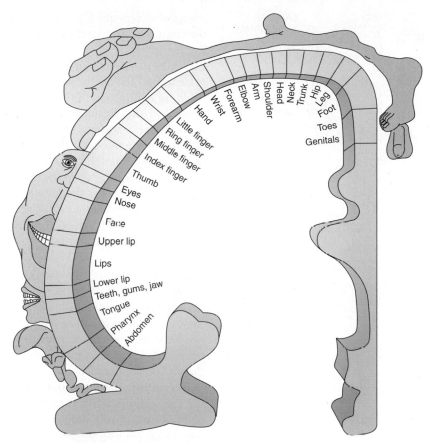

FIGURE 43-38 Topographic organization of the body on the somatosensory cortex, forming a homunculus map.

- Sensations of pain, temperature, and itch (anterolateral tract) usually cross the cord near the level of entry and travel to the brain on the contralateral side.
- Sensory information from both tracts is transmitted from the thalamus to the same areas of the somatosensory cortex by way of the internal capsule.

Motor Function

The execution of voluntary movement requires interaction among basal ganglia, cerebellum, and several regions of the cortex. The final program of voluntary muscle activity is transmitted from the primary motor cortex down the spinal cord by way of the corticospinal tract. As previously noted, the corticospinal tract decussates in the medullary pyramids and travels down the spinal cord to control muscles on the contralateral side of the body (Figure 43-39). The corticospinal tract primarily controls distal muscles of the arms, wrists, fingers, lower legs, feet, and toes. These are the muscles capable of fine-motor control. Another group of motor tracts innervate large proximal muscle groups and axial muscles that control posture and balance. These tracts include the vestibulospinal, reticulospinal, and tectospinal tracts. Motor tracts descending from the brain synapse on the cell bodies of motor neurons that lie in the anterior horn of the spinal cord and project to skeletal muscles.

MOTOR NEURONS

Motor neurons travel from the anterior horn of the spinal cord through the ventral root and within the spinal and peripheral nerves to finally innervate target muscles. Alpha motor neurons release acetylcholine into neuromuscular junctions, depolarizing skeletal muscle cells and contracting all the fibers in the *motor unit*. A motor unit consists of a single motor neuron and all of the muscle fibers under its control. Some motor units are large, containing hundreds of muscle cells, whereas others may contain only one muscle cell per motor neuron. Smaller motor units produce finer gradations of muscle control.

A single action potential in the α motor neuron is sufficient to release enough neurotransmitter to contract the motor unit. Therefore, the point of control of muscle contraction is at the cell body of the α motor neuron that lies within the anterior horn. A typical motor neuron receives hundreds of synaptic inputs, which summate to control the generation of action potentials. Some presynaptic inputs are from corticospinal neurons; others are sensory inputs from primary sensory afferents and spinal cord interneurons.

Gamma motor neurons are small fibers that innervate structures within the body of the muscles, called *muscle spindles*. Muscle spindles are specialized sensory receptors that sense the length or stretch within the muscle and relay the information to the spinal cord. The γ motor neurons

FIGURE 43-39 The corticospinal tract showing decussation at the level of the medulla.

contract muscle fibers within the muscle spindle and regulate the spindle sensitivity. Excessive γ motor neuron activity occurs in some types of brain coma, making the spindles hypersensitive and the muscles stiff and resistant to stretch (see discussions of decerebrate and decorticate rigidity in Chapter 44).

SPINAL REFLEXES

A great deal of motor coordination is exerted in the spinal cord through complex reflex pathways. These pathways allow upper motor neurons from the brain to initiate preprogrammed movements, rather than having to excite and inhibit each and every lower motor neuron individually. For example, experiments in lower animals have demonstrated that pressure on the pads of the feet initiates complex walking movements even when the brain is no longer functional.

Spinal reflexes allow sensory information from pain receptors, proprioceptors, and muscle spindles to alter muscle

contraction very quickly, even before the information reaches the brain. The stretch reflex and withdrawal reflex are illustrative examples.

The stretch reflex can be demonstrated by tapping the patellar tendon (below the knee) with a rubber hammer, which results in contraction of the quadriceps muscle and elevation of the lower leg. Evaluation of deep tendon reflexes is helpful in localizing a motor abnormality to the PNS or CNS. The deep tendon reflex tests the reflex arc between the sensory muscle spindles and the α motor neurons. Tapping the tendon produces a quick stretch in the muscle fibers of the quadriceps muscle and stimulates the muscle spindles. The muscle spindle sends action potentials along neurons (group Ia) that enter the dorsal horn of the spinal cord and then synapse directly on α motor neurons in the anterior horn that activate the muscle in which the spindles lie (Figure 43-40). Other branches of the group Ia neurons make connections with antagonistic muscle groups and inhibit their contraction. The stretch reflex makes only one synapse (monosynaptic) and produces a very quick response in the muscle. The physiologic function of the muscle spindle stretch reflex is to provide feedback to α and γ motor neurons to adjust the strength of muscle contraction to match the load on the muscle.

The withdrawal reflex is an important protective mechanism that allows reflexive withdrawal of a body part from a physical threat while simultaneously making postural adjustments to avoid loss of balance. The withdrawal reflex is polysynaptic, making connections with interneurons in the cord to affect muscles on both sides of the body. A simplified model of the withdrawal reflex is shown in Figure 43-41. Note that a painful stimulus to one extremity results in activation of flexor muscles and inhibition of extensor muscles on the ipsilateral side. This allows quick withdrawal of the extremity from the source of injury. Connections with muscle groups on the opposite side of the cord stimulate extensors and inhibit flexors to stabilize posture.

CENTRAL CONTROL OF MOTOR FUNCTION

Corticospinal tract neurons originate in the primary motor cortex, which is arranged in a similar manner to the somatosensory cortex. The motor homunculus map (Figure 43-42) shows that muscles of the face, lips, tongue, and hands occupy most of the cortical neurons. These areas have small motor units and produce fine-motor control. Activation of corticospinal neurons from the primary motor cortex is the last CNS step in executing a voluntary motor command. A great deal of neural activity occurs before the primary motor cortex is activated.

First, a motivation to move is needed to spur an individual to action. Little is known about motivation; however, signals from the limbic system are thought to be important. Circuits between the basal ganglia and association areas of the cerebral cortex plan the intended movement. Somewhat different circuits are involved in new situations, such as first learning to type, than are involved in the execution of learned, but

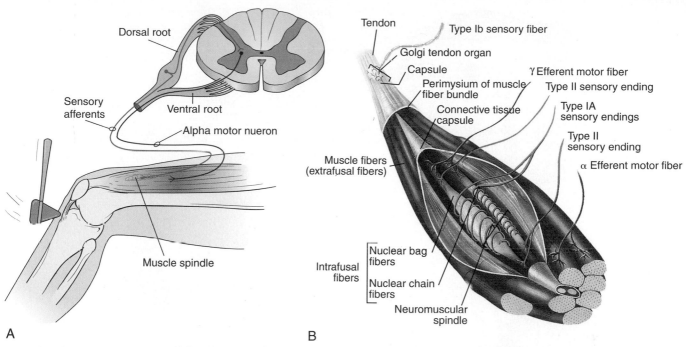

FIGURE 43-40 Diagram of the stretch reflex in which activation of the muscle spindle stimulates contraction of the stretched muscle. **A,** Stretch of the muscle sends action potentials to the cord, which make a monosynaptic connection to motor neurons from the same muscle fibers. **B,** Detailed view of the muscle spindle apparatus showing Type 1 and Type 2 sensory fibers that are large, myelinated and rapidly conducting neurons that detect stretch. The γ motor neurons contract the spindle to keep it taut and sensitive to further stretch, while the α motor neurons contract the muscle fibers. Also shown in this figure is another stretch receptor located at the juncture between the muscle and the tendon called the *Golgi tendon organ*. Muscle shortening during contraction stimulates the Golgi tendon organ, causing it to send signals to the cord that inhibit muscle contraction. This is thought to protect the muscle from excessive contraction that could tear it from its tendon insertion points on the bone. (**B** from Thibodeau GA, Patton KT: *Anatomy and physiology,* ed 6, St Louis, 2007, Mosby, p 559.)

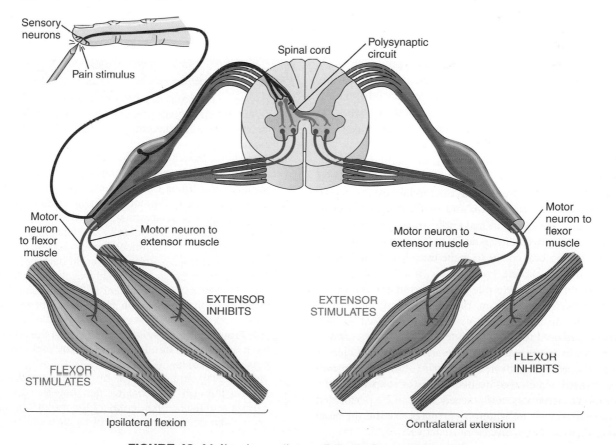

FIGURE 43-41 Neural connections mediating the flexor-withdrawal reflex.

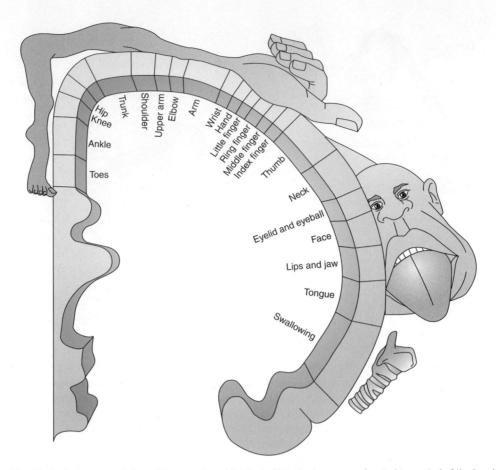

FIGURE 43-42 Cortical representation of the muscles of the body. Note the large area devoted to control of the hands and face.

subconscious, patterns of movement (e.g., typing 100 words per minute).[5] An important part of the planning process involves the somatosensory cortex, which provides information about the spatial coordinates of all body parts in relation to the physical surroundings (e.g., placement of the fingers on the keyboard).

The cerebellum serves to adjust the timing and intensity of movements to improve the similarity between the intended and actual movements. Neurons in the cerebellum learn with practice. Visual, proprioceptive, and vestibular information are used by the cerebellum to make adjustments in the execution phase of the movement. In addition, the cerebellum functions with the cerebral cortex to make muscle adjustments in advance of the movement. For example, if a person is asked to lift what appears to be a pile of bricks, but the bricks are made of lightweight Styrofoam, the unsuspecting subject will throw the pile up into the air. Visual cues and past learned experiences are used to gauge the intensity of muscle contraction. The brain learns quickly, however, and if the subject is asked to repeat the maneuver, the intensity of muscle contraction will exactly match that needed to lift the load smoothly. Once a motor activity is well-learned and can be performed "automatically," the cerebellum participates less and the basal ganglia and cortical neurons are most active.[5]

KEY POINTS

- The body is somatotopically represented in the motor cortex. Stimulation of points in the primary motor cortex results in discrete movements in the contralateral side of the body.
- Projections from the motor cortex (corticospinal tract) travel by way of the internal capsule, cross over at the medulla, and travel down the contralateral spinal cord to synapse on α motor neurons in the anterior horn. The α motor neurons innervate skeletal muscle.
- Extrapyramidal tracts (tectospinal, vestibulospinal, reticulospinal) from subcortical nuclei innervate antigravity muscles and are primarily involved in balance, posture, and movement of large proximal muscle groups.
- A great deal of motor activity is preprogrammed into neuronal connections in the spinal cord. These connections produce reflexive alterations in muscle contraction in response to sensory information about the tension on the muscle or the need to move a body part away from a painful stimulus.
- The planning and execution of movements is accomplished through neuronal circuits between the basal ganglia and association areas of the motor cortex. The cerebellum contributes primarily to the learning phase

of motor skill by making instantaneous adjustments in muscle force and timing to improve the match between the intended and the actual movement.

Consciousness, Memory, and Sleep

That the cerebral cortex is integral to the elaboration of complex thought, learning, memory, and so-called higher brain functions is well supported by lesion studies, yet little is known about the ways in which these higher functions are accomplished. Each thought involves neuronal circuits in portions of the cerebral cortex, thalamus, limbic system, and reticular formation of the brainstem. A thought or memory is not stored in any one place; rather it is the outcome of a pattern or circuit of neuronal activation.[24] Neurons in the limbic system, especially the amygdala, are thought to determine the general emotional value of the thought as being pleasant, painful, or neutral, whereas neurons in the cerebral cortex add the specific details, including remembered sensations and visual and auditory images. Consciousness and memory are prerequisites to thinking.

CONSCIOUSNESS AND MEMORY

Consciousness can be defined as awareness of the surroundings and of one's own thoughts and sensations. The neural correlates of consciousness are not known; however, continuous activation of neuronal circuits between the thalamus and cortex and thalamus and brainstem are believed to be necessary.[25] Consciousness is assessed by the expression of motor behaviors, such as speech, response to questions, and body movements. However, behavioral responses are not necessarily an outcome of consciousness. A person completely paralyzed with neuromuscular blocking agents is still conscious even though all outward behaviors are suppressed. It is difficult to know the level of brain activity in an individual who cannot move. Brain waves are frequently measured in an attempt to assess brain activity, and a correlation with consciousness is assumed. Alpha waves are thought to reflect search and retrieval functions and θ waves are associated with memory encoding tasks. Groups of neurons firing synchronously produce the regular oscillations of brain waves that seem to underlie consciousness. Much remains to be discovered before the phenomenon of consciousness and its counterpart, unconsciousness, are understood.

To think and learn, one must be able to remember past events and link them to current circumstances. Memory is a synaptic phenomenon in which neurons in the memory trace or circuit alter the efficiency of synaptic transmission. Greater stimulation of neurons in the memory circuit results in longer-lasting effects. Once the memory trace is established, it can be reactivated by the thinking mind to reproduce the memory. Reactivation by the mind is called *retrieval* and may be enhanced by rehearsal or strategies to link the memory trace with associated circuits that are already established.

Experiences that have important consequences, such as pain or pleasure, are usually enhanced and stored as memory traces, whereas experiences of little consequence may be suppressed. The value of a memory is determined primarily by the limbic system, which helps the brain learn to ignore information of little consequence (which can be construed as a form of negative memory, or remembering to ignore). This is an important function, as it prevents preoccupation and overload of brain circuits with useless stimuli.

Some memories last for a short time, and others persist for a lifetime. The mechanisms for different types of memory are mostly unknown; however, it is believed that short-term alteration of *presynaptic* neurons in the memory trace is responsible for short-term memory, whereas long-term memory requires more permanent changes in the *postsynaptic* neurons.[24] A certain time period is required for memories to be consolidated into long-term memory. An interruption of the consolidation phase, by head trauma, for example, results in loss of memory for events occurring just prior to the injury.

Some examples of presynaptic modulation are shown in Figure 43-43. The interaction between the presynaptic and postsynaptic neurons is modified by activity of the modulating neuron. For example, the modulating neuron could send a signal from the limbic system to indicate that the incoming signal was important. The modulating neuron would then enhance neurotransmitter release from the presynaptic neuron to facilitate transmission to the postsynaptic cell. Presynaptic inhibition could suppress synaptic transmission by preventing or reducing the amount of neurotransmitter released from the presynaptic neuron.

Longer-term memory is thought to occur because of long-term changes in synaptic efficiency. In some cases memory may incorporate new neurons into the memory circuit. The hippocampus is an important limbic structure that must be intact for memory to be consolidated. It is also a site of neural stem cell proliferation, leading some to conclude that memory involves the growth of new neurons.[16] Changes in synaptic efficiency could include alterations in receptor number or structure and changes in the components of second-messenger cascades. Protein synthesis in the involved neurons is necessary to consolidate long-term changes in synaptic efficiency.[24] Memories are thought to be stored in the brain in association with memories of similar qualities that share some of the same neuronal circuits. Information is added to the memory circuit that is already in place. This makes it easier to learn information that is connected to previously learned material. Learning something completely new, such as a foreign language, requires a great deal of rehearsal.

SLEEP

Sleep is a state of decreased arousal from which a person is easily awakened. Different levels of brain activity from wakefulness to deep sleep are characterized by different electroencephalographic waveforms. Brain waves become progressively slower and more synchronized with deeper levels of sleep.

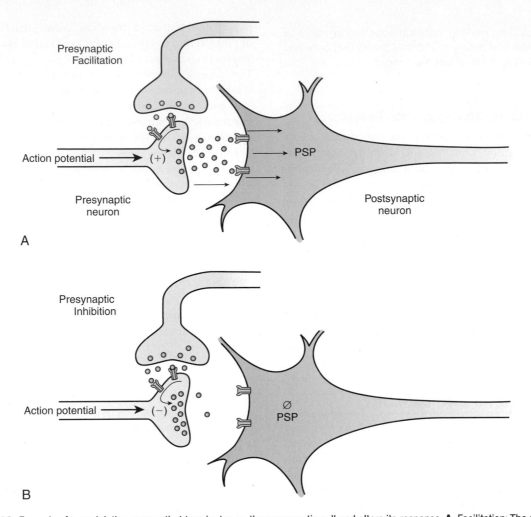

A

B

FIGURE 43-43 Example of a modulating neuron that terminates on the presynaptic cell and alters its response. **A,** Facilitation: The presynaptic neuron releases more neurotransmitter into the synapse when an action potential arrives. **B,** Inhibition: The presynaptic neuron releases less neurotransmitter into the synapse with each action potential. *PSP,* Postsynaptic potential.

These waveforms are called α, β, θ, and δ waves (Figure 43-44). The α and β waves are found in awake individuals. Alpha waves predominate during a relaxed state with the eyes closed; β waves occur during visual stimulation and with active problem solving. Beta waves are also apparent during a stage of sleep called *rapid eye movement* (REM) sleep. Both θ and δ waves occur during deep sleep.

Most sleep is of the restful, slow-wave type of deep sleep. Interspersed at about 90-minute intervals are episodes of REM sleep, which last 5 to 30 minutes. REM sleep is characterized by irregular breathing and heartbeat, rapid eye movements, depressed muscle tone, and active dreaming.[26] The number and length of REM episodes usually increases over the course of the night. Individuals who have been awake for a prolonged period spend more time in deep sleep at the beginning of sleep and begin to have more REM sleep as the brain becomes more rested.[26] Dreams occur in both types of sleep but are more likely to be remembered when they occur during REM sleep.

The mechanisms of the sleep-wake cycle and the reason the brain needs to sleep are not well understood. Experiments

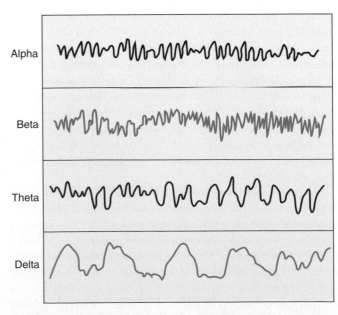

FIGURE 43-44 Brain waves are categorized according to frequency and synchrony as α, β, θ, and δ.

in animals have demonstrated that sleep is an active process initiated by sleep-inducing substances within the brain. CSF removed from sleep-deprived animals promptly produces sleep when injected into another animal. Production of sleep-inducing substances within the brain occurs during wakefulness; they gradually accumulate, producing a desire to sleep. A period of sleep is thought to inhibit production of sleep-inducing chemicals, and they are cleared from the CNS.

The physiologic significance of sleep to neural functioning is unknown, although the behavioral consequences of sleep deprivation are well characterized. Prolonged sleep deprivation produces hallucinations, disordered thought processes, and personality changes. It has been noted that the smaller the animal and the higher the metabolic rate, the greater the sleep requirement. Non-REM sleep is associated with lowering of metabolism and body temperature and may provide an opportunity to avoid or repair metabolism-induced brain damage.[26] REM sleep is associated with an active brain; however, certain types of neurons—those that secrete amines—are turned off during REM sleep. The younger and more immature brain spends more time in REM sleep, and some have speculated that the brain is laying down circuits for genetically programmed or instinctive neural pathways.[26] Less time is spent in REM sleep with aging.

through the secretion of neurotransmitters into synapses between neurons. Neurotransmitters bind to specific receptors to exert their effects on the membrane potential of the target cell.

Activation of groups of neurons in a particular circuit is the basis for neuronal processing of information, thoughts, and memories and for learning. Although certain brain locations have been associated with particular functions, most brain activities require participation by neurons in widespread locations. The ability of the nervous system to learn and adapt is remarkable in the early childhood period, and a significant degree of neural plasticity is maintained throughout life. However, damage to large numbers of neurons in a particular location usually results in significant disability because mature neurons cannot regenerate and neural stem cells may not survive or establish appropriate connections.

KEY POINTS

- Thoughts and memories are not stored in a particular location in the brain; rather, they are the outcome of activation of neurons in a neuronal circuit.
- Memories are stored by altering the synaptic efficiency of neurons in the memory trace. Short-term memory is thought to result from presynaptic mechanisms, whereas long-term memory is consolidated by more permanent changes in the postsynaptic neurons.
- Sleep is characterized as REM sleep (β waves) and deep sleep (θ and δ waves). Most sleep is of the deep-sleep variety, interspersed with periods of REM activity at about 90-minute intervals. Sleep is an active process produced by sleep-inducing chemicals in the brain. The nature of these chemicals and the reason that the brain requires sleep remain unknown.

SUMMARY

The nervous system is a complex network of neurons and supporting cells that provides the body with a rapid means of communication. The anatomy of the nervous system has been extensively studied, but the functional mechanisms of thought, memory, emotion, and sleep are poorly understood. The nervous system can be partially understood by examining the function of individual neurons and their synaptic connections. Neural communication occurs primarily

REFERENCES

1. Nolte J: *The human brain: an introduction to its functional anatomy*, ed 6, St Louis, 2008, Mosby.
2. Guyton AC, Hall JE: Cerebral blood flow, cerebrospinal fluid, and brain metabolism. In Guyton AC, Hall JE, editors: *Textbook of medical physiology*, ed 11, Philadelphia, 2006, Saunders, pp 761-770.
3. Abbott NJ, Rönnbäck L, Hansson E: Astrocyte-endothelial interactions at the blood-brain barrier, *Nat Rev Neurosci* (1):41-53, 2006.
4. Guyton AC, Hall JE: Somatic sensations: I. General organization, the tactile and position senses. In Guyton AC, Hall JE, editors: *Textbook of medical physiology*, ed 11, Philadelphia, 2006, Saunders, pp 585-597.
5. Doyon J, Penhune V, Ungerleider LG: Distinct contribution of the cortico-striatal and cortico-cerebellar systems to motor skill learning, *Neuropsychologia* 41:252-262, 2003.
6. Costa RM: Plastic corticostriatal circuits for action learning: what's dopamine got to do with it? *Ann N Y Acad Sci* 1104:172-191, 2007.
7. Nelson MV, Berchou RC, LeWitt PA: Parkinson's disease. In Dipiro J et al, editors: *Pharmacotherapy: a pathophysiologic approach*, ed 6, New York, 2005, McGraw-Hill, pp 1075-1088.
8. Sherman SM: The thalamus is more than just a relay, *Curr Opin Neurobiol* 17(4):417-422, 2007.
9. Salman MS: The cerebellum: it's about time! But timing is not everything—new insights into the role of the cerebellum in timing motor and cognitive tasks, *J Child Neurol* 17(1):1-9, 2002.
10. Thibodeau GA, Patton KT: Central nervous system. In Thibodeau GA, Patton KT: *Anatomy and physiology*, ed 6, St Louis, 2007, Mosby, pp 471-514.
11. Guyton AC, Hall JE: The autonomic nervous system and the adrenal medulla. In Guyton AC, Hall JE, editors: *Textbook of medical physiology*, ed 11, Philadelphia, 2006, Saunders, pp 748-760.
12. Thibodeau GA, Patton KT: Peripheral nervous system. In Thibodeau GA, Patton KT, editors: *Anatomy and physiology*, ed 6, St Louis, 2007, Mosby, pp 515-552.
13. Thibodeau GA, Patton KT: Nervous system cells. In Thibodeau GA, Patton KT. *Anatomy and physiology*, ed 6, St Louis, 2007, Mosby, pp 431-470.
14. Scolari MJ, Acosta GB: D-serine: a new word in the glutamatergic neuro-glial language, *Amino Acids* 33(4):563-574, 2007.
15. Chan WY, Kohsaka S, Rezaie P: The origin and cell lineage of microglia: new concepts, *Brain Res Rev* 53(2):344-354, 2007.
16. Zhao C, Deng W, Gage FH: Mechanisms and functional implications of adult neurogenesis, *Cell* 132(4):645-660, 2008.

17. Guyton AC, Hall JE: Organization of the nervous system, basic functions of synapses, "transmitter substances." In Guyton AC, Hall JE, editors: *Textbook of medical physiology*, ed 11, Philadelphia, 2006, Saunders, pp 555-571.

18. Feil R, Kleppisch T: NO/cGMP-dependent modulation of synaptic transmission, *Handb Exp Pharmacol* 184:529-560, 2008.

19. Frosch MP: The nervous system. In Kumar V et al, editors: *Robbins basic pathology*, ed 8, Philadelphia, 2007, Saunders, pp 859-902.

20. Chugani HT: A critical period of brain development: studies of cerebral glucose utilization with PET, *Prev Med* 27:184-188, 1998.

21. Hensch TK: Critical period plasticity in local cortical circuits, *Nat Rev Neurosci* 6(11):877-888, 2005.

22. Medana IM, Esiri MM: Axonal damage: a key predictor of outcome in human CNS diseases, *Brain* 126:515-530, 2003.

23. Castanzo L: Neurophysiology. In Castanzo L: *Physiology*, ed 3, St Louis, 2006, Saunders, pp 65-110.

24. Richter-Levin G, Akirav I: Emotional tagging of memory formation—in the search for neural mechanisms, *Brain Res Rev* 43:247-256, 2003.

25. Tononi G, Koch C: The neural correlates of consciousness: an update. *Ann N Y Acad Sci* 1124:239-261, 2008.

26. Siegel JM: Why we sleep, *Sci Am* 289(5):92-97, 2003.

Acute Disorders of Brain Function

Angela R. Starkweather • Jacquelyn L. Banasik

MEDIA RESOURCES

Additional Material for Study, Review, and Further Exploration

CD Companion ■ Review Questions and Answers
■ Glossary (with audio pronunciations for selected terms)
■ Disease Profiles ■ Animations

evolve Website at http://evolve.elsevier.com/Copstead/
■ Case Studies ■ Disease Profiles ■ WebLinks ■ Key Points Review

Online Course (Module 18)

KEY QUESTIONS

■ What are the proposed mechanisms and potential consequences of secondary brain injury?

■ What brain components determine intracranial pressure, and under what conditions might each contribute to elevated intracranial pressure?

■ How are level of consciousness and cranial nerve reflexes used to assess changes in neurologic status in the brain-injured patient?

■ What are the common manifestations of types of traumatic brain injury (focal, polar, diffuse) and hemorrhage (epidural, subdural, subarachnoid)?

■ How do the three most common causes of stroke (thrombi, emboli, and hemorrhage) differ with regard to risk factors, prevention strategies, and acute management?

■ How do the clinical manifestations of ischemic stroke vary depending on the location of cerebral artery obstruction?

■ What are the common long-term sequelae of stroke, and how are they managed?

■ What is the cause and usual presentation of cerebral aneurysm and arteriovenous malformation?

■ How do meningitis and encephalitis differ with regard to usual infective organisms, cerebrospinal fluid analysis findings, clinical manifestations, and treatment?

CHAPTER OUTLINE

Disorders of brain function can result from a wide variety of pathophysiologic processes. The focus of this chapter is on primary causes of acute brain injury including brain trauma, cerebrovascular disease, brain hemorrhage, and central nervous system (CNS) infections. These conditions are considered to be acute because they generally have a sudden onset and progress rapidly. Thus, early detection and prompt management are necessary to prevent death and minimize morbidity. However, the majority of patients who survive acute injury to brain structures will be left with some degree of permanent neurologic damage and chronic dysfunction. The designation of acute and chronic disorders is, therefore, somewhat arbitrary. The chronic aspects of neurologic diseases, including seizure disorders and dementias, are discussed in Chapter 45. Acute neurologic dysfunction often is a complication of diseases primarily affecting other systems. Hypoglycemia, renal failure, liver failure, human immunodeficiency virus infection, drug overdoses, fluid imbalances, and many others may cause acute brain dysfunction. Accurate determination of the source of acute alterations in brain function is an important step in developing an appropriate treatment plan. However, there are many common elements in the pathogenesis of acute brain injuries, regardless of etiologic factors. These cellular aspects are presented as a foundation for understanding the specific disorders that follow.

MECHANISMS OF BRAIN INJURY

The mechanisms of brain injury are varied, complex, and incompletely understood. Mechanical trauma, ischemia, cellular energy failure, reperfusion injury, excitotoxins, edema, vascular failure, and injury-induced apoptosis (programmed cell death) are all factors thought to be operative in most kinds of acute brain injury. These mechanisms are often separated into two categories: primary injury and secondary injury. The primary injury is that which occurs immediately at the onset of brain injury. This definition implies that there is little that can be done to reverse the process once it has occurred. For example, in the case of head trauma, some tissues will be irreversibly damaged at the time of impact owing to mechanical forces. This damage represents the primary injury. Similarly, with the sudden cessation of blood flow to an area of brain tissue, as occurs in stroke, an area of irreversible ischemia in cells may develop quickly, and this constitutes the primary injury. Brain tissue necrosis occurs rapidly as cells lose membrane integrity, rupture, and release their intracellular contents into the extracellular space. Cytotoxic edema quickly follows, which can cause deleterious effects to surrounding brain tissue.

Secondary injury refers to the development of further neurologic damage subsequent to the primary injury, and this may progress over days or weeks. Delayed cell death may involve necrosis from further acute injury or may be a delayed consequence of the primary injury. Cells that die slowly after injury are said to undergo apoptosis or programmed cell death. Apoptosis requires energy and protein synthesis, and the cells shrink and die in a tidy fashion without releasing their internal contents. Necrosis follows severe ischemic injury, whereas apoptosis is associated with moderate injury. A critical factor in determining the neuronal cell fate after injury is the degree of adenosine triphosphate (ATP) depletion. If ATP levels fall profoundly, increased membrane permeability and necrosis ensue. If the ATP level is partially maintained for a period of time after the injury, apoptosis is the likely consequence. Mild reductions in ATP are associated with reversible injury and cellular recovery.[1] ATP reduction is a consequence of ischemia and hypoxia, which accompany many types of acute brain injury including trauma and stroke.

Mechanisms of secondary injury are the subject of much interest because of the potential to effectively intervene to limit brain damage. Unfortunately, effective means of preventing secondary damage have remained elusive, leading to high rates of mortality and morbidity. The effort to elucidate mechanisms of secondary injury and develop effective treatments would seem worthwhile because the degree of primary injury is thought to be small in most cases.[2] Thus, the high rates of mortality and morbidity may be attributed in large part to mechanisms of secondary injury.

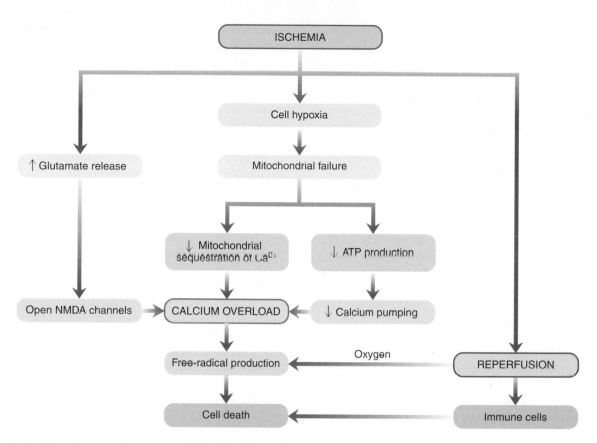

FIGURE 44-1 Sequence of neuronal cell injury following acute ischemia. Calcium overload is a key event in producing cellular damage.

Ischemia and Hypoxia

Ischemia occurs when the delivery of oxygenated blood is below the level needed to meet metabolic demands of the brain tissue. Ischemia is a contributing factor in most forms of acute brain injury, either as the primary insult (e.g., stroke) or as part of the secondary response to injury (e.g., vasospasm, vascular compression, or abnormal autoregulation). Hypoxia is a deficiency of oxygen at the cellular level, which may occur as a result of decreased blood flow (ischemia) or decreased blood oxygenation (hypoxemia). In practice, ischemia and hypoxia usually occur together and are considered together in this discussion. Ischemia results in immediate neurologic dysfunction because of the inability of neurons to generate the ATP needed for energy-requiring processes. In addition, ischemia sets the stage for secondary injury by oxygen free radicals, excitatory amino acids, and inflammatory cells.

Cellular Energy Failure

Neuronal tissue is highly sensitive to oxygen deprivation because it has great ATP requirements and limited capacity for anaerobic metabolism during ischemia. The normal brain receives about 15% of the total cardiac output and garners 20% of the body's oxygen consumption (750 ml/min), despite contributing only 2% of the body weight.[3] Neurons are dependent on glucose for production of ATP; however, they store little in the form of glycogen. Thus, when oxygen supply is decreased, not only is oxidative phosphorylation impaired, but the low

supply of stored glucose restricts anaerobic production of ATP as well. Brain cells tolerate loss of ATP for several minutes; about 5 to 10 minutes of complete occlusion is necessary for irreversible brain damage in humans. Complete occlusion of blood flow is rare but even a partial occlusion, if allowed to continue for a sufficient amount of time, may produce irreversible brain damage. Once blood flow to cerebral neurons diminishes, two mechanisms can independently lead to brain cell death; anaerobic metabolism and the deterioration of ion gradients.

A general sequence of events following acute brain ischemia has been proposed (Figure 44-1).[4,5] The critical event is mitochondrial dysfunction owing to lack of cellular oxygen.[5] Recall that oxygen is required to accept electrons from the mitochondrial electron transport chain. In the absence of oxygen, the transport proteins and cytochromes remain reduced and unable to accept any more electrons from the Krebs cycle (tricarboxylic acid cycle). Anaerobic glycotic pathways are initiated in the affected region to compensate for the loss of oxygen and to provide a source of energy. Glycolysis may continue for a short time, producing pyruvate, which is converted to lactate. However, this conversion releases H^+ and contributes to cellular acidosis, a damaging by-product of glycolysis. Toxicity of hydrogen ions leads to loss of neuronal integrity.

Inadequate energy supply leads to deterioration of ion gradients. Most of the ATP used by neurons is for maintenance of ion gradients across the plasma membrane. The sodium-potassium (Na^+-K^+) pump consumes three fourths of the ATP in a typical neuron.[6] Anoxic depolarization causes potassium to leave the cell and sodium, chloride and calcium ions to enter. Energy also is required to maintain calcium balance and regulate neurotransmitter synthesis and reuptake. Not surprisingly, energy failure results in neuronal dysfunction, injury, and, if severe or prolonged, necrotic cell death. Ischemia also is the probable inciting factor for apoptosis (see Chapter 4).

The mitochondria are also important regulators of calcium ion concentration in the cell. The mitochondrial membrane contains calcium transporters that sequester calcium ions within the mitochondria when cytoplasmic calcium levels are elevated. Mitochondrial energy failure impairs the ability of mitochondria to perform this sequestering function. Thus, the mitochondria become severely overloaded with calcium, which activates enzymes (phospholipases) that damage mitochondrial membrane structures. Ischemic cells are prone to calcium overload because pumps that move calcium out of the cell are energy dependent. Calcium ions have a large electrochemical gradient for diffusion into the neuron and tend to accumulate intracellularly.

Unfortunately, the activity of many intracellular enzymes is regulated by intracellular calcium. Calcium overload is thought to be a critical factor leading to activation of enzyme cascades, which disrupt function and cause irreversible damage to cell membranes (lipid peroxidation). One might speculate that measures to inhibit calcium entry into damaged cells would be of therapeutic benefit. One way to reduce calcium influx is by administration of calcium channel–blocking agents. These drugs block voltage-gated calcium channels. Unfortunately, clinical trials with calcium channel–blocking agents have failed to show benefit.[7] Other avenues for inhibiting calcium overload are being investigated, including those that block the effect of glutamate receptors described below.

Excitatory Amino Acids

Calcium may gain entry into cells by portals other than voltage-gated channels. Glutamate is an excitatory amino acid neurotransmitter thought to be important in learning and memory. Overstimulation of neurons by glutamate is associated with cell injury, leading to its designation as an *excitotoxin*. Glutamate binds two kinds of receptors that are linked to the opening of ion channels in the plasma membrane of neurons. *N*-Methyl-D-aspartate (NMDA) receptors have received the most attention, but α-amino-3-hydroxy-5-methyl-isoxazolepropionic acid (AMPA) channels are also thought to contribute to the neurotoxic effects of glutamate. Activation of AMPA receptors results in opening of Na^+ channels in the membrane, which leads to depolarization. Depolarization then affects the NMDA channels by removing a Mg^{2+} ion that usually blocks the NMDA channel (Figure 44-2). Subsequent binding of glutamate to the NMDA receptor opens it and allows Ca^{2+} to enter the cell accompanied by inflow of water, which results in cytotoxic edema, a rapid swelling of neurons.

As previously described, calcium overload mediates a cascade of events leading to cell injury.

The amount of glutamate in the synapses is usually tightly regulated by release and reuptake controls. In the presence of neuronal injury, excessive glutamate may be released because of impaired membrane integrity. With concomitant ischemia, reuptake mechanisms fail to remove excess glutamate from the synapse because they are energy-dependent processes. Excess glutamate stimulates nearby neurons, which then take up large amounts of injurious calcium ions. Small neurons in the cerebral cortex and hippocampus are particularly prone to glutamate excitotoxicity, and selective damage in these areas may occur. In addition to the calcium overload mechanism of injury, NMDA receptor activation stimulates nitric oxide (NO) production in neurons. NO is a neurotransmitter, but in excess it may increase the production of reactive nitrogen species (RNS), which function as free radicals to damage cellular components. The potential neuroprotective effects of controlling glutamate release or activity has been investigated. Studies with NMDA receptor–blocking agents have indicated benefit in some patients; however, conscious patients have experienced neuropsychiatric side effects, including hallucinations.[7] Further research is needed to evaluate the role of glutamate-blocking agents in acute brain injury.

Reperfusion Injury

Reestablishing perfusion to an area of prior ischemia is a matter of great urgency if neuronal tissue is to be salvaged. The longer and more severe the period of ischemia, the greater the extent of necrosis. However, previously ischemic cells face new dangers with the return of blood flow. In particular, the return of oxygen brings the potential for oxygen free radical formation, and the flow of blood allows inflammatory cells to invade the area. The secondary injury that occurs after re-establishing blood flow has been termed *reperfusion injury* and has been studied extensively in cardiac tissues. The mechanisms in the brain appear to be similar. During the period of ischemia, brain cells accumulate substrates for oxidative phosphorylation, including the free radical–forming metabolites of adenosine monophosphate (AMP), xanthine, and hypoxanthine. When oxygen re-enters the cell, erratic transfer of electrons to oxygen can produce a number of reactive oxygen products that behave as free radicals, damaging cell structures. These include hydroxyl radicals (OH·), superoxide (O_2^-), and peroxide (H_2O_2). Cell membranes may undergo lipid peroxidation in response to free radical damage, with subsequent formation of arachidonic acid. The arachidonic acid cascade yields more oxygen free radicals as well as mediators of inflammation.[1]

The role of immune mechanisms in reperfusion injury of brain tissue is only partially understood. Previously, the CNS was thought to be relatively shielded from immune cells because of the low permeability of the blood-brain barrier (BBB). However, the BBB is believed to be compromised with ischemia because the capillary endothelial cells are injured. Inflammatory cytokines, including interleukin-1 (IL-1), interleukin-6 (IL-6), and tumor necrosis factor (TNF), increase in the brain during

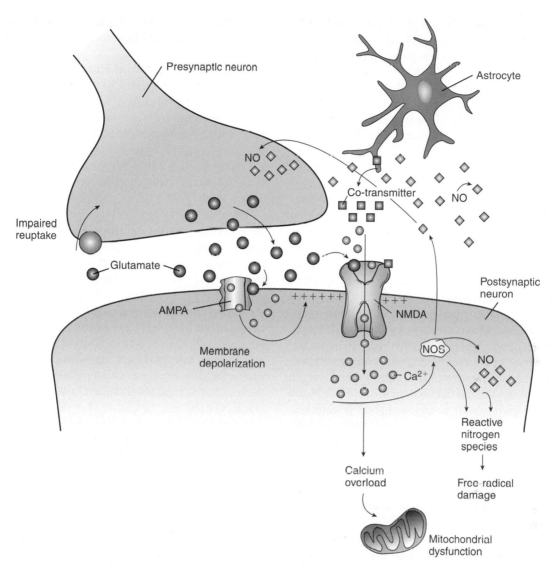

FIGURE 44-2 Mechanism of glutamate-mediated calcium influx. Impaired removal of glutamate from the synapse by energy-requiring reuptake mechanisms on the presynaptic membrane contributes to excessive glutamate in the synapse. Glutamate binds to the N-methyl-D-aspartate *(NMDA)* channel, causing it to open and allow calcium influx. A previous depolarization is necessary to remove the Mg^{2+} that normally blocks the channel. Excessive calcium entry impairs mitochondrial function and triggers nitric oxide production. Excessive nitric oxide can increase cell damage through free radical production. *AMPA,* α-Amino-3-hydroxy-5-methyl-4-isoxazolepropionate; *NO,* nitric oxide; *NOS,* Nitric oxide synthase.

ischemic injury and are thought to attract neutrophils to the area and contribute to brain inflammation.[8] The importance of neutrophil recruitment to secondary injury remains controversial, but it may contribute further free radical generation and vascular obstruction by aggregated neutrophils. Trauma and inflammation also promote platelet aggregation in cerebral vessels with subsequent reduction in perfusion and worsening of ischemia.

Abnormal Autoregulation

Under normal conditions, blood flow through brain tissue is controlled primarily by autoregulation. Cerebral vessels respond to metabolic factors including pH, carbon dioxide, and oxygen levels. Cerebral blood flow is closely matched to metabolic needs despite wide fluctuations in perfusion

pressure. Blood flow is maintained at a fairly constant rate over a range of mean arterial pressure (MAP) from about 50 to 150 mm Hg.[6] Above and below these levels, autoregulation fails. Hypotension predisposes to ischemia, whereas severe hypertension may lead to vascular damage and brain edema.

Appropriate autoregulation is necessary to provide a steady supply of oxygen and nutrients to brain cells and to remove metabolic wastes. Cerebral vessels dilate when mean arterial blood pressure falls or when brain metabolism increases. Anything that interferes with the ability of the vessels to dilate can lead to ischemia. Thrombi, emboli, vasospasm, neutrophil aggregation, and tissue edema may inhibit vasodilating autoregulatory mechanisms. Alternatively, vascular injury may impair vasoconstricting mechanisms and allow hyperperfusion and edema formation. Depending on the cause, autoregulation may be impaired locally, as in an area of thrombosis, or globally, as in generalized cerebral edema.

Autoregulation is influenced by the partial pressures of carbon dioxide ($Paco_2$) and oxygen (Pao_2) in the arterial blood. The response to a change in $Paco_2$ is very brisk: as $Paco_2$ levels fall, cerebral vessels constrict, and as $Paco_2$ levels rise, the cerebral vessels dilate. A rise in $Paco_2$ can increase cerebral blood flow significantly. The response to changes in Pao_2 is much less dramatic.

The autoregulatory response to $Paco_2$ remains robust, except in severely brain-injured patients, and can cause detrimental increases in cerebral blood flow when respiratory compromise leads to hypercapnia. Excessive cerebral blood volume can exacerbate cerebral edema. Conversely, hyperventilation to produce low $Paco_2$ results in prompt vasoconstriction and, often, a reduction in intracranial pressure (ICP). Hyperventilation had been used for many years as standard therapy in the treatment of patients with increased ICP. However, prolonged hyperventilation does more harm than good because it critically reduces cerebral blood flow to responsive vessels and triggers tissue ischemia in these areas.

Loss of matching between oxygen supply and demand occurs when autoregulatory mechanisms fail. Cerebral oxygen demand is correlated with the degree of neuronal activity and may vary widely from region to region. Excessive catecholamine or excitatory amino acids can significantly increase cerebral metabolism. In the context of impaired blood flow, these neurotransmitters may contribute to ischemia by increasing cerebral oxygen demand. Likewise, seizure activity greatly increases neuronal metabolism and can precipitate ischemia.[9] Efforts to reduce release of excitatory neurotransmitters through hypothermia, rest, and pain control may be beneficial. Pharmacologic suppression of brain seizures is imperative in the patient with cerebral ischemia. Drug-induced coma, with agents such as barbiturates, has been advocated to reduce brain metabolism.[10]

Hypothermia is a strategy for reducing brain metabolism and protecting the brain from ischemic injury. A number of animal and human studies suggest that cerebral injury can be delayed, and possibly avoided, by cooling the brain.[6] Possible mechanisms include inhibition of glutamate release, inhibition of IL-1 release, reduced cerebral metabolic rate, and suppression of inflammation. The effects of hypothermia on patient outcomes and the optimal degree of hypothermia remain controversial. Moderate degrees of cooling (28° C to 32° C) are associated with platelet dysfunction and coagulopathy.[6] Shivering negates the usefulness of hypothermia by increasing oxygen demand, and must be suppressed, usually by pharmacologic means. Further research is ongoing to determine the therapeutic window for effectiveness, appropriate duration, and safe rewarming protocols.[6]

Two related concepts important to the discussion of autoregulation are cerebral edema and increased ICP. Swelling and space-occupying lesions (mass lesions), such as tumors or hematomas, may increase the pressure within the cranium such that blood supply is compromised. Measures to reduce

cerebral edema, remove mass lesions, and prevent elevations of ICP help to maintain functional autoregulation.

Increased Intracranial Pressure

ICP is the pressure exerted by the contents of the cranium, and it normally ranges from 0 to 15 mm Hg.[11] Elevated ICP may occur in most types of acute brain injury and is associated with impaired neurologic function due to compression of brain structures. In all but very young children, the skull is a rigid, closed system with a set volume and a finite ability to accommodate changes in volume before elevations in ICP occur.

The volume of the cranium is made up of three components: brain tissue, cerebrospinal fluid (CSF), and blood. A relationship known as the Monro-Kellie hypothesis describes the compensatory responses to a change in volume in any of the three components.[12] A slight increase in one component can be offset by a reduction in the volume of the other two. An increase in brain volume, as might occur with cerebral edema, can be offset by a reduction in the CSF space and the space occupied by the cerebral vasculature. The ability to accommodate changes in volume without significant increases in pressure is called *compliance*. Intracranial compliance is limited because of the rigid skull; although small increases in intracranial volume may be absorbed, moderate changes result in significant increases in ICP (Figure 44-3).

Each of the cranial components has a varying capability to compensate for the others. Cerebral blood vessels can reduce their volume through vasoconstriction. The CSF compartment

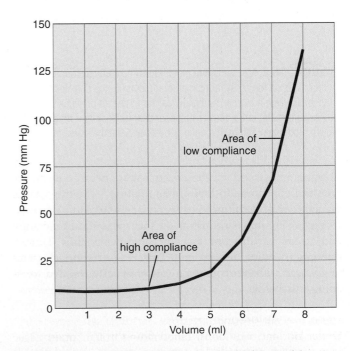

FIGURE 44-3 A volume-pressure curve showing intracranial compliance. Small increases in volume have little effect on pressure, but larger increases exceed the ability to compensate, and pressure rises dramatically.

Common Causes of Increased Intracranial Pressure

Increased Brain Tissue Volume
Tumor
Hemorrhage
Infection
Cytotoxic edema
Vasogenic edema
Ischemia and necrosis

Increased Cerebrospinal Fluid Volume
Obstructive hydrocephalus
Nonobstructive hydrocephalus
Pseudotumor cerebri

Increased Blood Volume
Increased right atrial pressure
Dural sinus thrombosis
High arterial Pa_{CO_2}
Acidosis

FIGURE 44-4 Generalized brain edema with increased intracranial pressure. The convolutions of the brain surface (gyri) are flattened, and the space between them is reduced. (From Kumar V, Cotran R, Robbins S: *Robbins basic pathology,* ed 8, Philadelphia, 2007, Saunders, p 861.)

is capable of significant reduction in volume by shunting CSF to the spinal cord or into the venous system via the arachnoid villi. The brain parenchyma has little ability to reduce its volume to compensate for CSF or blood volume expansion. In young children, an increase in ICP may manifest as an increase in head circumference. This occurs because the cranial bones have not yet fused, and the skull can expand to accommodate the increased intracranial volume.

In the healthy brain, transient changes in ICP are common and well tolerated. Sneezing, coughing, straining, and head-dependent positions all cause elevated ICP, but they are without consequence because ICP quickly returns to normal. In the brain-injured person, however, transient elevations in ICP can be very dangerous and poorly tolerated.

Etiology. The most common causes of increased ICP include stroke, trauma, and tumors, but many other primary and secondary disorders can cause significant elevations in ICP (Box 44-1). These disorders have common features in that they all affect the volume of CSF, blood, or brain tissue. An increase in brain tissue volume commonly occurs from conditions that cause cerebral edema. Edema of brain tissues is due to accumulation of fluid in interstitial or intracellular spaces.

Interstitial edema is usually secondary to increased capillary pressure, damage to the capillary endothelium from a chemical injury, or sudden increase in vascular pressure beyond autoregulatory limits. This type of edema has been termed *vasogenic,* and it results in extravasation of electrolytes, proteins, and fluid into the intercellular space. Vasogenic edema is a consequence of stroke, ischemia, and severe hypertension, and may occur surrounding brain tumors. The edema is often localized to a particular brain region where the BBB has been disrupted. Thus the swelling may be unilateral, occurring in one brain hemisphere or the other. Unilateral swelling often is poorly tolerated because midbrain structures

are compressed, and can lead to shifting of cerebral tissue or brain herniation.

Intracellular edema, called *cytotoxic edema,* occurs when ischemic tissue swells because of cellular energy failure. A lack of ATP allows Na^+ to accumulate in the cell, creating an osmotic force to draw in water. Cytotoxic edema predominates in cases of global ischemia. Global ischemia occurs when oxygenation of the whole brain is impaired, as would occur with cardiac arrest or severe hypoxemia. Generalized brain edema flattens the gyri and reduces the spaces between them (Figure 44-4).

In many cases of acute brain injury, vasogenic and cytotoxic edema occur together. Cerebral edema, when severe, can start a cyclic process that promotes further edema of increasing severity and contributes to increased ICP. As edema fluid collects, it compresses local vessels, preventing adequate blood and oxygen from reaching the cells. This results in ischemia, which in turn triggers vasodilation and increased capillary pressure, further fluid leakage into the injured tissue, and increased edema. Vasogenic edema tends to be a delayed process in terms of the secondary effects of brain injury, progressively worsening during the first several days after injury. Clearance of brain edema occurs primarily by absorption into the CSF system.[3]

In addition to edema, a number of space-occupying processes, such as tumors, hematomas, and abscesses, can increase intracranial volume and contribute to elevated ICP. These mass lesions are often unilateral and may result in severe compression of vital brain structures.[13] Attempts by the brain to accommodate the expanding mass result in typical findings on computed tomography (CT) scans (Figure 44-5). The ventricles are reduced in size, and midline structures are displaced.

Excessive accumulation of CSF (hydrocephalus) is another important cause of increased ICP. Elevated CSF volume causes

FIGURE 44-5 Right subacute subdural hematoma on weighted CT scan. Note the shift in midline structures. (From Grossman RI, Yousem DM: *Neuroradiology,* ed 2, St Louis, 2003, Mosby, p 249.)

FIGURE 44-6 Normal-pressure hydrocephalus. (From Grossman RI, Yousem DM: *Neuroradiology,* ed 2, St Louis, 2003, Mosby, p 377.)

the ventricles to enlarge and press on cerebral brain structures (Figure 44-6). Hydrocephalus may be a primary disorder or may develop due to obstruction proximal to the arachnoid granulations (obstructive; non-communicating hydrocephalus) or at the level of the arachnoid granulations (communicating; non-obstructive hydrocephalus). Obstructive hydrocephalus commonly occurs when a lesion blocks the flow of CSF out of the ventricle, whereas non-obstructive hydrocephalus is common following subarachnoid hemorrhage as residual blood clogs the arachnoid villi and prevents the CSF from being reabsorbed.

Increased intravascular cerebral blood volume is unlikely to be a primary cause of high ICP, but it may contribute to pressure elevations initiated by ischemia or trauma. High $Paco_2$ or loss of autoregulatory controls can lead to vasodilation and increased cerebral blood volume.

Manifestations. Manifestations of elevated ICP include headache, vomiting, and altered level of consciousness (drowsiness). The patient may complain of blurry vision, and evaluation of the fundi may reveal edema of the optic disk (papilledema). As ICP rises to higher levels, the level of consciousness decreases, and pupil responsiveness to light becomes impaired. Eventually the patient will exhibit altered respiratory patterns and will become unresponsive to stimulation and unable to move, verbalize, or open the eyes. Prolonged elevations of ICP are thought to damage brain structures by compressing the blood supply and causing ischemia.

Patients exhibiting manifestations of elevated ICP, or those with significant risk for elevated ICP, may be monitored with a pressure device inserted into the brain parenchyma through an opening in the skull (burr hole). The pressure device is connected to an electrical transducer, and the ICP waveforms can be monitored continuously (Figure 44-7). In general, a high ICP is associated with poor outcome. Different ICP waveforms are thought to carry different prognoses. The normal ICP waveform is characterized by three pressure peaks called P1, P2, and P3. These waves are reflections of changes in ICP associated with each arterial pulsation. Normally P1 is higher than P2, and P2 is higher than P3 (see Figure 44-7). As ICP begins to increase, the pattern of waves remains normal, but the peak and mean pressures are higher. Further increases in ICP are characterized by a P2 wave that exceeds P1 and a dampening of the individual waveforms (plateau waves).[14]

Plateau waves reflect severe pathologic increases in ICP due to changes in cerebral volume. Plateau waves can reach 50 to 100 mm Hg. After the plateau period the ICP slowly decreases, but it usually remains elevated above baseline. These waves reflect a potentially life-threatening situation, and if the pathologic process is not stopped, a cycle of increased ICP followed by vasodilation to maintain constant blood flow through swollen tissues continues, which in turn further increases ICP. An extreme increase in ICP can precipitate an intense reaction by the sympathetic nervous system as it attempts to maintain cerebral perfusion through the compressed blood vessels. This has been termed an *ischemic response* or *Cushing reflex*. The systolic blood pressure can jump to values exceeding 200 mm Hg, accompanied by bradycardia and a widening pulse pressure. The Cushing reflex generally is viewed as a "last ditch" effort by the brain to re-establish cerebral perfusion.[12]

FIGURE 44-7 Intracranial pressure *(ICP)* monitoring can be used to continuously measure ICP. The ICP tracing shows normal, elevated, and plateau waves. At high ICP the P2 peak is higher than the P1 peak, and the peaks become less distinct and plateau.

Brain Compression and Herniation

A dreaded complication of elevated ICP is brain compression and herniation. Compression of midbrain and brainstem structures is associated with rapid neurologic demise unless corrected quickly. Important midline structures include the reticular activating system (RAS), which is necessary for maintaining consciousness, and vital regulatory centers for cardiovascular and respiratory control. Radiologic examination by CT scan or other means (e.g., magnetic resonance imaging [MRI]) is useful in evaluating the patient with increased ICP who exhibits a change in neurologic status. CT scans may show midline shifts and herniations when ICP is sufficiently elevated.

Herniation refers to the protrusion of brain tissue through an opening in the supporting dura of the brain.[15] Several types of brain herniation have been described according to their anatomic locations. The brain parenchyma is divided into compartments by the supporting structure of the dura. The dura folds into the space between the cerebral hemispheres to form the falx cerebri and folds in from the lateral aspects to form the tentorium, which separates the cerebellum from the cerebral hemispheres (Figure 44-8). The most

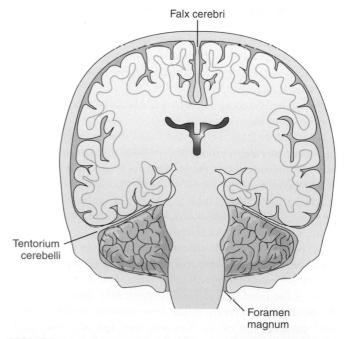

FIGURE 44-8 Schematic drawing of the normal brain compartments showing the dural folds that form the falx cerebri and the tentorium.

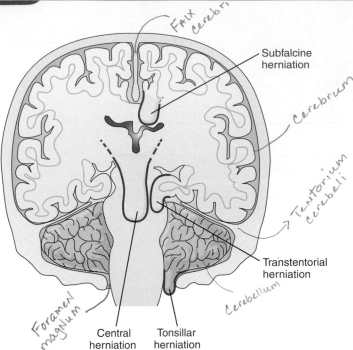

FIGURE 44-9 Herniations occur when brain tissue is pushed through openings beside the dural folds or the foramen magnum.

FIGURE 44-10 CT scan of acute hemorrhage with mass effect and subfalcine herniation and shift of the lateral ventricle. (From Grossman RI, Yousem DM: *Neuroradiology,* ed 2, St Louis, 2003, Mosby, p. 263.)

common herniations occur through openings in these structures (Figure 44-9).

There is a small space between the tip of the falx cerebri and the corpus callosum through which the neurologic lobe of the cerebral cortex can herniate (Figure 44-10). This is called a *subfalcine* or *neurologic hernia.* Subfalcine herniation occurs when a lesion in one hemisphere is large enough to cause a lateral shift across the midline of the intracranial cavity, forcing the neurologic gyrus under the falx cerebri. This results in distortion and compression of the internal cerebral vein. Subfalcine herniation can be asymptomatic and generally carries a better prognosis than other types of brain herniation. The greatest danger results from compression of blood vessels, particularly the ipsilateral anterior cerebral artery, which can cause further cerebral ischemia and edema and contribute to the ICP elevation.

The tentorium is a rigid dural fold that separates the cerebellum and cerebral hemispheres. Midbrain structures pass between the infoldings of the dura in a structure called the *incisura.* With transtentorial herniations, a part of the brain protrudes through this space. Tentorial herniations are of two types: (1) bilateral herniations, which cause central transtentorial herniation, and (2) lateral herniations, in which one hemisphere compresses midbrain structures to the side and herniates through the tentorial opening (see Figure 44-9).

Central tentorial herniation results from expanding lesions in the frontal, parietal, and occipital lobes that force a downward displacement of the hemispheres and basal nuclei with compression of the diencephalon and adjoining midbrain. Transtentorial herniation can occur rapidly or slowly, depending on the type of lesion. The speed with which the

process is recognized is a critical factor in patient survival. Slowly dilating or odd-shaped pupils is an ominous sign that indicates compression of the third cranial nerve and midbrain. Transtentorial herniations are associated with significant intracranial hypertension and may initiate vascular compression and CSF obstruction, which then contribute to the existing problem of ischemia and hypertension.

Uncal herniation is a type of tentorial herniation that typically occurs with expanding lesions in the temporal lobe. As the lobe shifts, the basal edge of the uncus and the hippocampal gyrus bulge over the edge of the incisura (see Figure 44-9). In the process, the third cranial nerve and the posterior cerebral artery are compressed. The pupil on the same side (ipsilateral) as the lesion often becomes dilated and unresponsive to light (fixed). Flattening of the midbrain interferes with the ascending RAS and depresses the level of consciousness. The ipsilateral cerebral peduncle is also compressed, resulting in contralateral motor dysfunction. Compression of the contralateral cerebral peduncle is also common, leading to the confusing symptom of ipsilateral motor dysfunction.

Tonsillar herniation is less common than the other herniation syndromes and involves the shift of the cerebellar tonsils through the foramen magnum and compression of the medulla and upper cervical cord (see Figure 44-9). This typically occurs in patients with cerebellar lesions. Because of the proximity of the cerebellum to the brainstem, tonsillar herniation evolves very rapidly and can result in death in a matter of minutes. Signs usually include precipitous changes in blood pressure and heart rate, small pupils, disturbances in conjugate gaze, ataxic breathing, and quadriparesis.

Management

Management of increased ICP is often based on the results of CT or MRI. Processes amenable to surgical intervention can be detected and treated. Removal of excess CSF, tumors, abscesses, and hematomas can dramatically improve ICP. Nonsurgical processes such as cerebral edema, intracerebral bleeding, and infections are managed medically.

Traditionally, ICP measurements and determinations of cerebral perfusion pressure (CPP) have been used to guide therapy. A CPP of greater than 60 mm Hg is generally thought to be sufficient to ensure adequate blood flow and to prevent ischemia. CPP is calculated by subtracting the ICP from the MAP. Thus, as ICP increases, a higher MAP is required to maintain CPP. More recently, the value of assessing more direct measures of cerebral oxygenation has been recognized. Measures of oxygen utilization by the brain are thought to provide a better assessment of brain ischemia. The oxygen level of jugular venous blood can be intermittently or continuously monitored and compared with arterial oxygen levels. An increasing difference between arterial and venous oxygen (A-VDO_2) is thought to indicate inadequate delivery of blood to the brain.

With these new assessment tools, it became obvious that measures to reduce ICP were not always associated with improvement in brain oxygenation, and in some cases they were detrimental. Controversy regarding the appropriate treatment of increased ICP continues, and the focus of management has shifted from ICP control to management of cerebral oxygenation. The roles of previously established therapies such as hyperventilation, brain dehydration with diuretics, head-up and neutral body positions, and administration of corticosteroids have been called into question. Previously discarded therapies, such as hypothermia, hypertonic saline infusion, and drug-induced comas, are being reintroduced. Despite these controversies in medical management, the value of careful observation and assessment of neurologic function are unquestioned. Many times subtle changes in neurologic function are detectable early in the process of evolving brain injury. Several tools have been developed to help standardize neurologic examination and are discussed in the following section.

KEY POINTS

- Primary brain injury occurs as a direct result of the initial insult. Secondary injury refers to progressive damage resulting from the body's physiologic response to the initial insult.
- Ischemia is an important mechanism of brain injury that occurs when the blood supply is inadequate to meet metabolic needs. A lack of oxygen results in mitochondrial failure, ATP depletion, and accumulation of intracellular calcium ions.
- Excessive release of excitatory amino acids, like glutamate, is thought to contribute to calcium overload during acute brain injury. Calcium overload is a critical

event leading to cell dysfunction, membrane damage, and cell necrosis.

- Reperfusion injury occurs when blood flow is reintroduced to previously ischemic but viable cells. Free radicals are generated, which damage cell structures. Inflammatory cells are recruited to the area and may increase edema, block vessels, and contribute to free radical production.
- Autoregulation of cerebral blood flow achieves appropriate flow to meet metabolic needs despite changes in blood pressure and metabolism. Autoregulation is effective over a range of MAP from 50 to 150 mm Hg. Hypoxia and high $Paco_2$ result in dilation of cerebral vessels. Hyperventilation with low $Paco_2$ results in cerebral vasoconstriction.
- Pressure in the cranium is a product of the volume of brain tissue, blood, and CSF. Increases in any one component are partially offset by reductions in the others to maintain ICP.
- Brain swelling is a common cause of increased ICP. Edema may result from changes in vascular competency that lead to transudation of fluid into intercellular spaces (vasogenic), or from cellular swelling (cytotoxic) owing to a deficiency in cellular ATP.
- Normal ICP ranges from 0 to 15 mm Hg. Transient increases are well tolerated, but chronically increased ICP results in compression of vessels and brain tissue, leading to cellular ischemia and brain damage. High ICP may precipitate herniation of brain tissue through dural compartments.

MANIFESTATIONS OF BRAIN INJURY

Depending on the severity and location of brain injury, a wide variety of clinical manifestations may occur. Patients may present with symptoms ranging from minor headache and visual disturbances to complete loss of consciousness. Patients with significant acute injuries require frequent neurologic assessments to detect changes that may evolve rapidly. Level of consciousness, cranial nerve reflexes, and brain hemodynamics provide important clues to neurologic status.

Level of Consciousness

A change in level of consciousness is one of the most sensitive indicators of altered brain function. Efforts have been made to standardize the terms used to describe level of consciousness (Table 44-1). In practice, however, it is best to use a full description due to lack of consistency in interpretation of the terms. Consciousness is a state of alertness and attentiveness to one's environment and situation. A fully conscious individual is awake, alert, and oriented to time, person, place, and current circumstances. Consciousness is thought to be dependent on activity in the RAS neurons, which project to the thalamus, and in tracts between the thalamus and cortex.[16] Although consciousness may be suddenly and completely lost, the decline is usually progressive. Cortical neurons are most

TABLE 44-1

Terms Used to Describe Altered Level of Consciousness

Term	Description
Confused	Unable to think clearly or engage in effective problem solving; orientation to time, place, person impaired; easily aroused by verbal stimuli
Delirious	Restless and disoriented, may have hallucinations; easily aroused, but may have difficulty with attention
Lethargic	Uninterested in surroundings or events; sluggish in thought and motor activities; does not engage spontaneously in activities
Obtunded	Falls asleep unless stimulated; arousable with voice or touch, but quickly returns to sleep
Stuporous	In a deep state of sleep; vigorous stimulation is required to arouse, and a wakeful state is not maintained
Comatose	Unable to be aroused, even with vigorous painful stimuli; motor responses, such as withdrawal or posturing, may occur

BOX 44-2

Glasgow Coma Scale

Eye Opening
4. Spontaneously (eyes open, does not imply awareness)
3. To speech (any speech, not necessarily a command)
2. To pain
1. Never

Verbal Response
5. Oriented (to time, person, place)
4. Confused speech (disoriented)
3. Inappropriate (swearing, yelling)
2. Incomprehensible sounds (moaning, groaning)
1. None

Motor Response
6. Obeys commands
5. Localizes pain (deliberate or purposeful movement)
4. Withdrawal (moves away from stimulus)
3. Abnormal flexion (decortication)
2. Extension (decerebration)
1. None (flaccidity)

sensitive, and cognitive and memory functions are impaired early, leading to confusion.

Delirium, a primary disorder of attention, is characterized by an acute onset of severe confusion, motor signs, slurred speech, altered consciousness, and hallucinations. As RAS function is compromised, the patient becomes difficult to arouse and requires increasingly noxious stimuli to produce verbal or motor responses. Eventually complete loss of consciousness may occur, a condition called *coma*. The **Glasgow Coma Scale** can be used to assess levels of consciousness with greater reliability among different observers (Box 44-2). Sudden or progressive changes in level of consciousness should prompt a thorough neurologic examination to determine the cause and best course of therapy.

Glasgow Coma Scale

The Glasgow Coma Scale (GCS) is a standardized tool developed for the purpose of assessing the level of consciousness in acutely brain-injured patients. It can also be used to evaluate patients with an altered level of consciousness as a result of other neurologic insults such as hemorrhage or craniotomy. Numeric scores are given to arousal-directed responses of eye opening, verbal utterances, and motor reactions. The best response is scored, bilateral responses are recorded for motor reactions, and consistent application of a painful stimulus is required for accuracy. When used correctly, the GCS has a high degree of interrater reliability.

The eye opening response is a simple measure of alertness. Normally, the eyes open spontaneously in response to verbal stimuli. If the eyes do not open in response to verbal stimuli, noxious stimuli, such as compression of the nail beds, may be applied. It is important to be consistent and vigorous enough

to achieve the best response from the patient. In patients with acute space-occupying lesions, eye opening is usually depressed in conjunction with impaired response to pain and motor function. Spontaneous eye opening in the acute phase is an encouraging sign, as it implies that the arousal mechanism in the brainstem is intact.

The verbal response on the GCS reflects orientation. A full score in this category indicates that the patient is alert and fully oriented: the patient knows his or her name, current location, and the time of day. In the next level down the patient is awake and can pay attention to a certain degree, but is confused as to who he or she is and does not know the time or the location. If attention is poor and the verbal responses consist of yelling and swearing, it is scored as an inappropriate response. Incomprehensible verbalizations are unintelligible sounds or mumbling. Absence of verbalization is given a score of 1. As in the eye opening category, noxious stimuli are applied to achieve the best verbal response from the patient.

Motor response is a powerful predictor of outcome. Motor response is scored as the best level of response the patient is able to perform. Each extremity is evaluated to avoid misinterpretation secondary to muscle paralysis. At the highest level, the patient can obey a command to move. At the next level down, the patient does not obey commands, but when a painful stimulus is applied, the patient moves in a purposeful manner to avoid the stimulus; the patient is able to localize the source of pain. As status deteriorates, the patient withdraws only the extremity from the painful stimulus. This is not considered a purposeful response. Further deterioration results in abnormal posturing movements. *Decorticate* posturing is characterized by an abnormal flexor

Decorticate posture

Decerebrate posture

FIGURE 44-11 Abnormal motor activity with coma. Decorticate posturing is indicated by flexed wrist and arm and extended legs and feet. Decerebrate posturing is indicated by arm and leg extension.

response of the arms and wrists. The legs and feet extend and internally rotate (Figure 44-11). The level below decorticate posturing is called *decerebrate* or *abnormal extension*. The arms extend with external rotation of the wrists. The legs and feet extend and rotate internally (see Figure 44-11). The lowest level of motor response is no response to painful stimuli (i.e., flaccidity in all four limbs). It is important to emphasize that all limbs must be tested separately, as motor responses may be preserved on one side only, and levels of involvement may vary from side to side. Higher initial scores tend to predict better recovery. On the GCS, the level of coma occurs on a continuum from mild (>12), to moderate (9 to 12), to severe (<8). The lowest total score of 3 indicates likely fatal damage, especially if both pupils fail to respond to light and oculovestibular responses are absent; however, the severity and prognosis are predicted more accurately by also considering diagnostic imaging and other factors.[17]

Cranial Nerve Reflexes

The GCS score alone is not sufficient to accurately determine the status of the patient with an acute insult to the brain. Assessment of the integrity of brainstem function is also important and is indicated by various brainstem reflexes including the pupil light reflex, oculovestibular reflex, and corneal reflex.

Pupil Reflex

Pupillary assessment provides important information about the function of the brainstem and cranial nerves II and III. The normal pupillary response to light results from an intact afferent cranial nerve II (optic) detecting the light and stimulating the intact efferent cranial nerve III (oculomotor) to constrict the pupils. The response of the pupil to light, in terms of both its shape and the speed of reaction, is a function of cranial nerve III.

The pupillary response is recorded by noting pupil size in millimeters, shape, and reactivity to light. Careful monitoring of the pupillary response to light during the acute phase is critical, as a failing response may be the first indication of brain compression from increasing ICP. Mild dilation of a pupil with sluggish or absent light response is ominous. This phenomenon results from pressure on the oculomotor nerve (cranial nerve III) by lateral displacement of midbrain structures. An oval pupil may be an early indicator of dangerously poor compliance and transtentorial herniation. The oval pupil represents a transitional pupil that can return to normal responsiveness if ICP is controlled.

Other pupillary responses indicate damage to the optic nerve. The afferent pupillary defect is a paradoxical response that is detected with the swinging-light test. As the examiner swings a light from the normal eye to the abnormal eye, the abnormal pupil responds by dilating instead of constricting. This occurs because the light signals transmitted to the Edinger-Westphal nucleus in the midbrain through the injured optic nerve are insufficient to maintain constriction brought on by stimulation of the normal eye.

Bilaterally small pupils suggest a destructive lesion in the pons or the presence of certain drugs. Bilaterally fixed and dilated pupils suggest inadequate cerebral perfusion. This could be related to hypotension or increased ICP. If perfusion is not interrupted for too long, a normal pupillary response returns with adequate flow.

Eye movements are important indicators of brainstem function. Cranial nerves III, IV, and VI are responsible for normal eye movements. Abnormalities of eye movement are useful in localizing the site of brain dysfunction. Abnormal eye movements seen in the brain-injured patient can include nystagmus, dysconjugate eye movements, and ocular palsies. **Nystagmus** is a persistent rhythmic or jerky movement in one or both eyes. **Dysconjugate movements** occur when the eyes do not move together in the same direction. Ocular palsies occur when one or more cranial nerves are dysfunctional such that motor paralysis of the eye muscles impairs movements in one or more directions.

Oculovestibular Reflex

The oculovestibular reflex normally detects head movements (via receptors in the semicircular canals) and causes appropriate adjustments of eye position such that an object can remain fixed on the retina even though the head is moving. An impaired oculovestibular reflex implies brainstem dysfunction. Two tests can be performed to evaluate this reflex in the unconscious patient: the doll's-eyes test and the cold calorics test.

The oculocephalic or doll's-eyes test is performed only in patients in whom a lateral spine radiograph has been obtained to rule out spinal injury. The test is performed by holding open the patient's eyelids and rotating the head from one side to the other (Figure 44-12). If the brainstem is intact, the eyes will turn in a direction opposite to the direction of head rotation. If the eyes do not move in conjugate fashion or are asymmetrical, the response is abnormal and brainstem function is impaired. If the eyes remain fixed at the midline and do not move, the response is said to be absent. An absent response indicates severe brainstem impairment.

The oculovestibular response or cold calorics is a similar test of brainstem function using cold water instillation into the ear. Cold against the tympanic membrane causes action potentials from the vestibular apparatus to change and simulates the neuronal response to head rotation. If the brainstem is intact, the normal response will be a tonic deviation of both eyes toward the side that is irrigated. Dysconjugate or asymmetrical eye movement is abnormal. If there is no eye movement, the response is absent. Testing of the oculovestibular response is one of the essential examinations performed in patients thought to be brain dead. Patients with depression of brain function due to metabolic abnormalities usually retain an intact oculovestibular response. Certain drugs, such as

Normal response

Absent response

FIGURE 44-12 Doll's eyes response is indicated by an absent (abnormal) response to the oculocephalic head turning test and indicates brainstem damage. In the normal response, the eyes turn in a direction opposite to head rotation. In the absent response, the eyes stay midline and do not turn when the head is rotated.

barbiturates and high doses of phenytoin, can severely depress the oculovestibular response. In the absence of drug effect, an absent response to cold calorics is a poor prognostic sign indicating minimal chance of brain recovery.

Corneal Reflex

A simple test of cranial nerve function is the corneal reflex. A wisp of cotton is touched to the cornea of the eye to elicit a blink response. Absence of blink is another indicator of severely impaired brain function.

Brain Hemodynamics and Metabolism

Monitoring of hemodynamic and metabolic parameters commonly is done in the patient with acute brain injury. Hypotension is poorly tolerated and must be promptly detected and managed to prevent further ischemia. Blood pressure can be monitored continuously by an indwelling arterial catheter. In general, the MAP should not fall below about 70 mm Hg. However, this may be too low in patients with chronic hypertension or elevated ICP. In patients with ICP monitors, CPP should not fall below 60 mm Hg:

$$CPP = MAP - ICP$$

Elevated temperature increases the metabolic rate of neuronal tissue and is poorly tolerated. Measures to keep body temperature at 37° C or lower are usually employed, and in some cases hypothermia may be purposefully induced to reduce brain metabolism. The adequacy of brain perfusion in meeting metabolic demands of the brain can be estimated by the arteriovenous oxygen difference (A-VDO_2). An arterial oxygen level (PaO_2) and a jugular vein oxygen level (PjvO_2) are obtained simultaneously and used to calculate the A-VDO_2:

$$A - V_{DO_2} = PaO_2 - PjvO_2$$

Alternatively, oxygen saturation can be used to derive similar information. Monitoring devices can be applied for continuous measurement of arterial (SaO_2) and venous saturation (SjvO_2). The A-V difference can then be calculated and expressed as a percentage:

$$(SaO_2 - SjvO_2) \div SaO_2 \times 100$$

This value reflects the degree of cerebral extraction of oxygen. An increase in the cerebral oxygen extraction is thought to reflect an inadequate rate of cerebral blood flow. It has been suggested that the percent extraction should not exceed a critical value of 40% and the SjvO_2 should remain greater than 50%.[18] Measures such as less aggressive hyperventilation, volume replacement, and blood pressure support may help return the extraction ratio back toward normal. Treating potential sources of increased brain metabolism, such as fever, seizures, agitation, and pain, can be helpful in restoring the balance between cerebral oxygen demand and supply.

KEY POINTS

- A change in level of consciousness often is an early indicator of compromised neurologic status. Normal consciousness is apparent as alertness and orientation to time, person, place, and situation.
- The Glasgow Coma Scale is used to assess level of coma by scoring alertness (eye opening response), orientation (verbal response), and motor control (movements). The highest score is given to demonstration of spontaneous eye opening, full orientation, and obeying of motor commands.
- Pupillary responses indicate the function of the brainstem and cranial nerves II and III. Changes in size, shape, and reactivity of the pupil may be an early indicator of impending brain herniation. Eye movements controlled by cranial nerves III, IV, and VI may be impaired with increased ICP. Nystagmus, dysconjugate gaze, and ocular palsies may be evident.
- An absent doll's-eyes response when the subject's head is turned and an abnormal response to activation of the oculovestibular reflex upon installation of cold water in the ear are very poor prognostic signs.
- Hemodynamic and metabolic assessments are helpful in maintaining adequate balance between cerebral oxygen supply and demand. Measures to restore the balance should be taken if cerebral oxygen extraction exceeds 40%.

Traumatic Brain Injury

Traumatic brain injury (TBI) refers to injuries of brain tissues sustained as a consequence of trauma. The term is sometimes used interchangeably with head injury; however, injuries to the cranium do not always result in brain injury. Confusion in terms has led to difficulty in determining actual rates of traumatic brain injury, but there is no doubt that it is a major public health concern.

EPIDEMIOLOGY

It is estimated that 7 million to 10 million new cases of head injury occur each year in the United States[19] and that as many as 85% of these go unreported.[20] Among the 1.5 million cases diagnosed annually, about 50,000 result in death. In the United States, an estimated 5.3 million individuals are living with permanent TBI-related disability.[6] Falls, sports injuries, and transportation-related trauma are important causes of TBI. The great majority of traumatic brain injuries in the United States are sustained in automobile accidents, whereas other forms of transportation are more significant contributors in other countries. The worldwide incidence of TBI may approach 500 million annually.[20]

Certain age, gender, and ethnic groups are at higher risk for sustaining TBI. In the United States, 15- to 24-year-olds are at highest risk. Males are twice as likely as females to sustain TBI and are more than three times more likely to die from their injuries. African Americans have a slightly higher risk than white and Hispanic Americans. Individuals at the lowest socioeconomic levels have the highest per capita rates of brain injury.[20]

It is difficult to quantify the social, medical, and economic impact of TBI. The cost of acute hospital care for a moderately to severely brain-injured patient is substantial, and the long-term care, rehabilitation, and loss of productivity for survivors add significantly to the cost. One in five patients who are hospitalized for TBI and survive will have a substantial long-term disability.

Prevention of TBI is an important initiative for public health. Because most TBI is associated with automobile accidents, efforts to prevent driving while under the influence of alcohol and other drugs, driver education, seatbelt use laws, and safer roads and automobiles may be most helpful. Helmet use by motorcyclists significantly reduces crash mortality. It is interesting to note that public concern does not seem to reflect the magnitude of the problem, and TBI is likely to continue to have a major impact on the health care system for years to come.

Early rescue from the trauma scene and immediate emergency management are important in the effort to reduce morbidity and mortality after TBI. Half of TBI fatalities occur within 10 minutes of the traumatic event.[20] Victims who survive until hospitalization require expert monitoring and intervention.

BOX 44-3

Traumatic Coma Data Bank Classification of Computed Tomography Imaging

Diffuse Injury I
No visible intracranial pathology seen on CT scan

Diffuse Injury II
Cisterns are present with a shift 0 to 5 mm and/or lesion densities present
No high- or mixed-density lesion greater than 25 ml
May include bone fragments and foreign bodies

Diffuse Injury III (with Swelling)
Cisterns compressed or absent
Shift 0 to 5 mm
No high- or mixed-density lesion greater than 25 ml

Diffuse Injury IV (with Shift)
Shift greater than 5 mm
No high- or mixed-density lesion greater than 25 ml

Evacuated Mass Lesion
Any lesion surgically evacuated

Nonevacuated Mass Lesion
High- or mixed-density lesion greater than 25 ml, not surgically evacuated

TYPES OF TRAUMATIC BRAIN INJURY

TBI is often characterized according to severity, location of injury, and mechanism of injury. There are different prognoses and management strategies for the different types of TBI.

Severity of TBI usually is based on the patient's GCS score on admission to the hospital or the lowest score in the first 48 hours postadmission. A GCS score of 8 or less is defined as a severe injury; moderate injury is defined by a GCS score of 9 to 12; mild injury is associated with a GCS score greater than 12. Injury severity can also be estimated by the degree of brain injury detected on CT examination. The Traumatic Coma Data Bank criteria (Box 44-3) determines the degree of diffuse injury noted on CT scan to predict injury severity.

In general, an increased severity score is thought to be associated with a poorer prognosis; however, the predictive value of these tools is not very high. Some authors have suggested that the duration of postinjury amnesia is a useful predictor of outcome,[20] but this measure often cannot be made early in the course of treatment and may not be timely enough to be helpful.

Injury severity and outcome are somewhat dependent on the physiologic state of the brain prior to the trauma. Physical factors such as bone thickness, dural stability, brain atrophy, drug effects, previous brain damage, pre-existing dementia, and cerebral atherosclerosis have an impact on the outcome of TBI. There is so much individual variation in brain response to injury that making a prognosis statement is often guesswork. After 48 to 72 hours following the injury, a better estimate of outcome is possible because the degree of secondary injury will be manifest.

PRIMARY INJURY

Primary injury is the result of the initial trauma on neural tissue. Primary injuries are commonly described as *focal, polar,* or *diffuse.* Although such injuries rarely occur in pure form, they are discussed separately for the sake of simplicity.

Focal injuries (coup) are those that are localized to the site of impact to the skull. The extent of the damage is quite variable. They may be superficial or extend deep into the brain matter. Local injury to the brain can result in specific neurologic symptoms, depending on the site. An injury over the motor cortex may result in contralateral weakness of the face and arm, whereas an injury to the frontal lobe can lead to **apraxia,** impulsive behavior, and poor judgment. However, localized hemorrhages or significant edema may act as space-occupying lesions and result in increased ICP, brain shifting, and herniation. In such cases, symptoms may include a decreased level of consciousness, cranial nerve dysfunction, and contralateral muscle weakness.

Polar injuries (coup contracoup) occur as a consequence of the brain shifting within the skull and meninges during the course of an acceleration-deceleration movement resulting in local injury at two opposite poles of the brain. This is commonly the case in motor vehicle accidents in which the head, traveling at the same high speed as the motor vehicle, is abruptly stopped by an obstacle such as the windshield. As a result, the frontal and temporal poles are crushed against the anterior and middle cranial fossae, damaging the tips and inferior surface of the temporal and frontal lobes. Damage may cause bruising or bleeding and, in combination with edema, may result in significant intracerebral mass lesions. Most forces to the head have a lateral rotational component; thus, one side of the brain typically is more severely injured than the other. Patients with polar injuries may or may not need significant acute care, depending on the severity of the injury. Polar injuries can, however, be a significant factor in the extent of subsequent cognitive impairment, affecting rehabilitation and long-term recovery.

Diffuse injuries occur when movement of the brain within the cranial cavity causes widespread neuronal damage. The brain is often subject to shifting and rotational forces during injury. The combined force causes stretching and shearing of the axonal white matter, known as *diffuse axonal injury.* Patients with severe diffuse axonal injury frequently are comatose from the time of injury. Coma is a consequence of axonal damage in the cerebral cortex or reticular activating center in the brainstem and can be prolonged. Recovery may be limited to a severely disabled or vegetative state. In addition to falls and motor vehicle accidents, diffuse injury is an unfortunate consequence of vigorous shaking, particularly of babies and the elderly, who have greater mobility of the brain within the skull.

BOX 44-4

Grades of Concussion

Grade 1
Transient confusion (inattentiveness, inability to maintain a coherent stream of thought and carry out goal-directed movements)
No loss of consciousness
Concussion symptoms or mental status abnormalities on examination resolve in less than 15 minutes

Grade 2
Transient confusion
No loss of consciousness
Concussion symptoms or mental status abnormalities (including amnesia) on examination last more than 15 minutes

Grade 3
Any loss of consciousness
- Brief (seconds)
- Prolonged (minutes)

BOX 44-5

Management Recommendations for Concussion

Grade 1
Remove from contest
Examine immediately and at 5-minute intervals for the development of mental status abnormalities or postconcussive symptoms at rest and with exertion
May return to contest if mental status abnormalities or postconcussive symptoms clear within 15 minutes

Grade 2
Remove from contest and disallow return that day
Examine on-site frequently for signs of evolving intracranial pathologic process
A trained person should re-examine the athlete the following day
A physician should perform a neurologic examination to clear the athlete for return to play after one full asymptomatic week at rest and with exertion

Grade 3
Transport the athlete from the field to the nearest emergency department by ambulance if still unconscious or if worrisome signs are detected (with cervical spine immobilization, if indicated)
Perform a thorough neurologic evaluation emergently, including appropriate neuroimaging procedures when indicated
Admit to hospital if any signs of pathologic process are detected or if the mental status of the athlete remains abnormal

In addition to categorizing primary injuries according to location as focal, polar, or diffuse, they can be differentiated by the mechanism of injury: concussion, contusion, and intracranial hematoma. *Concussion* is the term applied when head injury produces an alteration in consciousness, but no evidence of brain damage is found on physical or radiologic examination. Concussion is a common consequence of sports-related head trauma. Concussion is graded according to severity (Box 44-4), and management differs depending on the grade of concussion (Box 44-5).[21] *Contusion* is said to be present when CT or MRI reveals an area of brain tissue damage (necrosis, laceration, bruising). An intracranial hematoma is a localized collection of blood within the cranium resulting from vascular damage.

Intracranial Hematomas

Three types of hematoma can occur after traumatic head injury: epidural (extradural), subdural, and subarachnoid (Figure 44-13). Hematomas may expand slowly or rapidly, progressively compressing brain structures and increasing ICP. The types of hematoma differ in their clinical presentation and significance. Recognition and prompt management of intracranial hematomas can significantly improve outcome in the patient with TBI.

Epidural Hematoma

Epidural hematomas are collections of blood in the epidural space, which lies between the inner surface of the skull and the dura mater (extradural). Vessels that travel within the dura are susceptible to injury in conjunction with skull fractures. Fracture of the temporal bone commonly disrupts the middle meningeal artery, resulting in an acute epidural hemorrhage. Because the source of bleeding in most epidural hematomas is arterial, the hematoma can expand rapidly, causing acute

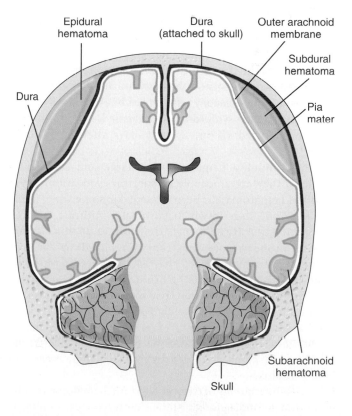

FIGURE 44-13 Locations of epidural, subdural, and subarachnoid hematomas.

deterioration of neurologic function. Often, the severity of the primary injury is minor, and the patient may suffer only a brief period of disturbed consciousness followed by a period of normal cognition (lucid interval). Then consciousness rapidly deteriorates as the epidural hematoma expands and compresses brain structures.

Rapid evaluation by CT is recommended to detect the hematoma, and surgical intervention to remove the hematoma is necessary in most cases. Patients with promptly managed epidural hematomas usually have an excellent prognosis because the associated primary injury is minimal.

Subdural Hematoma

Subdural hematomas form in the space between the dura and the outer arachnoid membrane (see Figure 44-5). The vessels traversing this area are called *bridging veins*. Bridging veins drain venous blood from the surface of the brain, crossing the arachnoid and subdural spaces before emptying into the venous sinuses. Venous sinuses are relatively fixed to the dura and are immobile, whereas the brain, which floats in the CSF, is quite mobile. With a sudden change in head velocity, as occurs with falls and vehicular accidents, the brain moves, the venous sinuses remain stationary, and the bridging veins between the two are stretched and sheared apart.

Because venous blood is under low pressure in the head, the rate of hematoma formation is usually slower than that of an epidural bleed. When subdural bleeds do produce an acute deterioration in neurologic status, the severity of the primary injury is likely to be high. Acute subdural hematomas produce symptoms within 24 hours of injury and have a worse prognosis than epidural or subacute subdural bleeds.

Subacute subdural hematomas can present a diagnostic challenge because the symptoms may be so delayed that the patient does not associate them with a head injury event. Venous bleeding is usually self-limited but may slowly progress and produce symptoms of increased ICP (headache, vomiting, blurred vision) 2 to 10 days after the primary event.

When subdural hematomas are large and sufficiently localized, they are amenable to surgical evacuation. If the subdural hematoma has been present for some time, it enters a chronic stage in which fibroblasts infiltrate the area and granulation tissue forms. Hematomas at this chronic stage are prone to rebleeding from thin-walled capillaries in the new granulation tissue. The risk of rebleeding is highest in the first few months.[3] Chronic subdural hematomas are a common finding at autopsy of elderly individuals. In addition to the increased incidence of falls, the elderly usually have some degree of cerebral atrophy, which makes the brain more mobile within the skull. In the elderly, the likelihood of damage to bridging veins is high even with minor trauma.

The manifestations of chronic subdural hematoma may be subtle and go undiagnosed. In the elderly, changes in mentation may be erroneously attributed to dementia. Chronic subdural hematomas are detectable by CT and MRI, and if they are symptomatic they may be managed by surgical removal of the clot and surrounding reactive tissue.

Subarachnoid Hemorrhage

The space between the outer arachnoid membrane and the pia mater is the subarachnoid space. The pia mater is tightly bound to the surface of the brain. The subarachnoid space is filled with CSF. Traumatic subarachnoid bleeding is due to rupture of the bridging veins that pass through the space, in a manner similar to subdural bleeding. Although trauma is an important cause of subarachnoid hemorrhage, it is more commonly associated with rupture of cerebral aneurysms or arteriovenous malformations (AVMs). In that case, bleeding is arterial in origin.

Blood in the CSF manifests with meningeal irritation and a bloody spinal tap. Blood in the subarachnoid space can spread throughout the CSF spaces and may not organize into a confined hematoma. Blood in the CSF produces severe headache in the conscious person and predisposes to secondary vasospasm and ischemia. It also predisposes to clogging of ventricular drainage, which leads to hydrocephalus. Further discussion of manifestations and management of subarachnoid hemorrhage is included in the Cerebral Aneurysm section.

SECONDARY INJURY

Mechanisms of secondary injury are initiated by TBI, resulting in ischemia, increased ICP, and altered vascular regulation. Most of the research on secondary mechanisms of injury has been conducted in the TBI model. Often the damage done by secondary mechanisms far exceeds that of the primary trauma.

In contrast to other types of brain injury, patients with TBI must be carefully evaluated for skull fractures, epidural and subdural hematomas, and injuries to other body systems. Concomitant trauma may complicate the brain injury. For example, uncontrolled hemorrhage can lead to hypovolemia and hypotension, which contributes to brain ischemia. Injuries to the chest can compromise ventilation and produce hypoxemia and hypercarbia, which contribute to cerebral dilation and increased ICP. Attention to other life-threatening injuries may extend the time until radiologic examination of the head can be accomplished, thus delaying surgical management of lesions.

Once the TBI patient's condition is stabilized, many other sources of secondary injury still loom. Brain swelling from both cytotoxic and vasogenic edema may increase for 48 to 72 hours after injury. Ruptured vessels may rebleed or spasm, and CSF drainage can become clogged. Open skull fractures predispose to CNS infections, as do ICP monitors, burr holes, and surgical incisions. Seizures and fever may develop, significantly increasing the brain's metabolic rate and further contributing to brain ischemia. Inflammation and free radical damage continue to cause injury to cells even after ischemia has resolved. Monitoring and managing a patient's course through the myriad perils of secondary injury requires expert knowledge and skill.

TREATMENT

After cardiopulmonary stabilization, the first priority in the TBI patient is radiologic screening of the brain for surgically correctable lesions. Hematomas, depressed skull fractures, and bleeding vessels require prompt surgical intervention. Surgical decompression by craniectomy, ICP monitors, and CSF drainage devices also may be done during surgery. Further therapy is individualized, seeking to maintain ICP, cerebral blood flow, and cerebral oxygen utilization within optimal ranges. Treatment recommendations are controversial, but in patients with acceptable cerebral blood flow, maintenance of normal body temperature or mild hypothermia, normal $Paco_2$, normal serum glucose level, and normal intravascular volume is suggested.[17] Acutely elevated ICP can be managed with administration of mannitol (osmotic diuretic), sedation, hypothermia, and mild hyperventilation. Repeat radiologic examination is indicated to determine if a new surgical lesion has developed. If it has not and the patient continues to exhibit high ICP, more aggressive measures may be attempted, including diuretics, hypertonic saline, moderate hyperventilation, and barbiturate coma; however the outcome is likely to be poor.

Patients with open head injuries may be treated with prophylactic antibiotics to prevent CNS infection. Sometimes fractures at the base of the skull are not visible on the routine CT scan but allow drainage of CSF into the nasal sinuses. Head-injured patients who have drainage of clear fluid from the ears or nose should be evaluated for basilar skull fracture. CSF drainage fluid can be differentiated from normal nasal mucus because it has a high glucose content and tends to separate into layers (halo) on tissue paper. Other findings with basilar skull fracture are bilateral periorbital hematomas (black eyes, "raccoon sign") and bruising under the ear (Battle's sign). The presence of basilar skull fracture increases the risk of CNS infection.

Although morbidity and mortality after acute TBI remain high, significant advances in prehospital, hospital, and rehabilitative care continue to occur. The care received during the first hour of injury can dramatically affect outcome. Efforts to improve prehospital management are likely to have the greatest impact on patient outcomes.

KEY POINTS

- Most head injuries are incurred in motor vehicle accidents, falls, and sports accidents. Young males aged 15 to 24 years are the most common victims. The seriousness of head injury can be classified according to Glasgow Coma Scale scores as mild (>12), moderate (9 to 12), or severe (<8).
- Injury that is directly due to the initial impact is called *primary injury*. Primary injuries are classified as focal, polar, or diffuse. Focal injuries are localized to the site of skull impact. Polar injuries are due to acceleration-deceleration movement of the brain within the skull, resulting in double injury. Diffuse injury is due to movement of the brain within the skull, resulting in widespread axonal injury.
- Disruption of the vasculature can result in intracranial hemorrhage. Epidural hematomas are associated with skull fracture and progress rapidly because they are arterial in origin. Subdural hematomas are associated with shearing of bridging veins and may develop slowly. Traumatic subarachnoid hemorrhage is also due to trauma to bridging veins.
- Secondary injury is a consequence of the body's response to the primary injury. Mechanisms are similar to those described for nontraumatic brain injury. In addition, concomitant injuries and cardiopulmonary impairment may contribute.
- The management of head injury is directed primarily to detecting and managing surgical lesions and reducing brain damage from secondary injury. Normovolemia, normothermia (or mild hypothermia), normal glucose level, and normal Pao_2 and $Paco_2$ values are recommended for most patients. In those with high ICP, diuretics, hyperventilation, and drug-induced coma may be tried. Open head injuries constitute a risk for CNS infections, and prophylactic antibiotics may be used.

Cerebrovascular Disease and Stroke

Cerebrovascular diseases cause abnormalities of cerebral perfusion including transient ischemic attacks (TIA), ischemic stroke, and hemorrhagic stroke. *Stroke* is a term applied to cerebrovascular events that result in a localized area of brain infarction and was previously termed *cerebrovascular accident* (CVA). The term *brain attack* has been popularized to educate the public about the importance of seeking care early, as is recommended for heart attack.

The symptoms of stroke usually are sudden in onset and may include the following: (1) numbness or weakness of the face, arm, or leg, especially affecting only one side of the body; (2) confusion, trouble in speaking or in understanding others; (3) visual disturbances in one or both eyes; (4) dizziness, loss of balance, and difficulty with walking; and (5) severe headache. Persons experiencing any of these symptoms, even temporarily, should seek medical care immediately.

EPIDEMIOLOGY

More than 700,000 new and recurrent strokes occur each year in the United States, making stroke the third leading cause of death.[22] The majority of these victims survive, with most requiring long-term care and rehabilitation. Currently, there are about 5 million stroke survivors living in the United States. Stroke is the leading cause of serious disability. Among long-term survivors (>6 months), 50% have **hemiparesis,** 30% cannot walk, 26% are unable to independently perform activities of daily living, 19% are aphasic, 35% are clinically depressed, and 26% are institutionalized in a nursing home.[22] Females account for 61% of all stroke fatalities. Seventy-eight percent of stroke victims are older than 65 years. Stroke death rates are significantly higher for black males and females than for their white counterparts.

Risk factors for stroke are similar to those for other atherosclerotic vascular diseases and include hypertension, diabetes, hyperlipidemia, cigarette smoking, advancing age, and family history. A previous stroke significantly increases the risk for suffering a subsequent stroke. Cardiac disease complicated by atrial fibrillation is an important risk factor for embolic types of strokes. Strokes can be categorized according to cause as ischemic and hemorrhagic strokes. Ischemic strokes are by far the most common (88%) and include thrombotic and embolic types.[22]

ISCHEMIC STROKE

Ischemic strokes result from sudden occlusion of a cerebral artery secondary to thrombus formation or embolization. Thrombotic and embolic strokes are grouped together because the clinical presentation and treatment are similar. However, etiologic risk factors and preventive measures are different and are discussed separately.

Thrombotic strokes are associated with atherosclerosis and hypercoagulable states. Risk reduction strategies for thrombotic stroke are those aimed at reducing atherosclerosis and platelet aggregation. Significant atherosclerotic plaques in the carotid arteries are sometimes evident as carotid bruits. Assessment for the presence of carotid bruits in all individuals older than 50 years may help identify persons at risk so that prevention strategies can be initiated early.

Emboli usually are from a cardiac source, although disruptions in carotid artery plaques may lead to downstream embolization. Cardiac sources include thrombi formed in the cardiac chambers (mural thrombi) and thrombi or vegetations on valve leaflets. Because atrial fibrillation allows stagnation of blood in the left atrium, it is associated with a high risk of mural thrombi, which can dislodge and travel to the cerebral circulation. Patients with chronic atrial fibrillation commonly receive anticoagulant medications to prevent this occurrence.

Sudden blockage of a cerebral artery by a thrombus or embolus produces acute ischemia in the territory served by the artery. Insufficient blood flow to brain tissue results in oxygen deprivation and rapid cerebral deterioration. Neurologic deficits become evident after just 1 minute of insufficient oxygen. If the ischemia continues for several minutes, irreversible cellular damage can occur. With further progression, the local area becomes infarcted and necrotic. Surrounding the infarct is a much larger area of ischemic but viable cells, called the **penumbra.** The penumbra receives some partial or collateral flow and may recover if the ischemia is mild or perfusion is restored in a timely manner. Salvaging the penumbra is the aim of early thrombolytic therapy; however, treatment must be instituted within 3 hours of stroke onset to be maximally effective.

In some cases, the obstructing clot is efficiently lysed by the endogenous fibrinolytic system before permanent tissue damage occurs. If the associated neurologic deficits completely resolve, the episode is called a *transient ischemic attack* (TIA). The neurologic symptoms of a TIA typically last only minutes, but they may last as long as 24 hours. Symptoms resolve completely without evidence of neurologic dysfunction. TIAs are important warning signs of thrombotic disease and carry a significant risk for subsequent stroke. The occurrence of one or more TIA episodes increases the risk of stroke by about ten-fold.[23]

Patients who present with TIAs should undergo evaluation to determine the origin of their symptoms. Unless contraindicated, these patients are started on daily aspirin therapy to prevent thrombus formation. Carotid endarterectomy or angioplasty may prevent stroke in a subset of patients experiencing TIAs who have carotid artery plaques occluding more than 70% of the arterial lumen.[24]

Manifestations of ischemic stroke are related to the cerebral vasculature involved (Figure 44-14) and the area of brain tissue the vessel supplies. The middle cerebral artery is most commonly occluded, resulting in damage to the lateral hemisphere. Contralateral **hemiplegia,** hemisensory loss, and contralateral visual field blindness are usual. If the dominant hemisphere is affected, global aphasia will occur. Occlusion of smaller branches of the middle cerebral artery produce more limited neurologic findings. Occlusions of the other cerebral arteries have different neurologic manifestations depending on the brain area they normally perfuse (Table 44-2).

Occlusion of the small penetrating arterioles can produce small lesions called *lacunar infarcts.* The basal ganglia, pons, cerebellum, and internal capsule are common sites of lacunar infarcts. These lesions are sometimes not observable on CT scan. The prognosis for recovery from a lacunar infarct is usually good, and neurologic manifestations are more circumscribed, often affecting purely motor or sensory functions.

HEMORRHAGIC STROKE

Intracerebral hemorrhage is a hemorrhage within the brain parenchyma and usually occurs in the context of severe and often long-standing hypertension. It carries a 38% mortality, with death usually occurring within minutes to hours.[22] In contrast, subarachnoid hemorrhage occurs under the arachnoid membrane and above the pia mater. Two common structural abnormalities that can cause subarachnoid hemorrhage (cerebral aneurysms and arteriovenous malformations) are discussed in the Cerebral Aneurysm and Arteriovenous section. Most intracerebral hemorrhagic strokes occur in the basal ganglia or thalamus (see Figure 44-10). If the hemorrhage is large, it may significantly increase ICP, which can lead to herniation and death. The prognosis for hemorrhagic stroke depends on the patient's age, the location and size of the hemorrhage, and how rapidly the hemorrhage produces brain distortion and shift. The degree of secondary injury and associated morbidity and mortality is significantly higher for hemorrhagic stroke than for ischemic stroke.

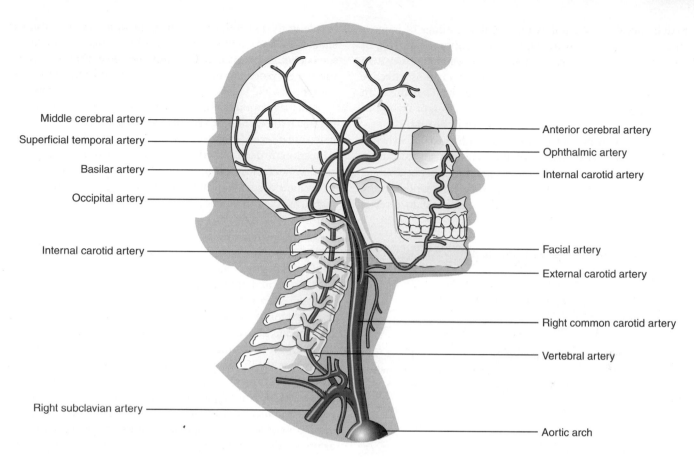

FIGURE 44-14 Cerebral vasculature showing fields of perfusion.

TABLE 44-2

Manifestations of Ischemic Stroke According to Location of Arterial Blockage

Cerebral Artery	Territory of Perfusion	Clinical Manifestations
Anterior cerebral	Medial aspect of frontal lobes	Contralateral hemiparesis; contralateral sensory loss; impaired cognition and decision making, aphasia (left-sided stroke); incontinence
Middle cerebral	Most of lateral cerebral hemisphere, internal capsule, and basal ganglia	Contralateral hemiplegia; contralateral sensory loss; aphasia (left-sided stroke); homonymous hemianopsia; altered consciousness; neglect syndrome
Posterior cerebral	Occipital lobe and medial aspect of temporal lobe	Visual defects including homonymous central blindness and color blindness; memory impairment
Basilar and vertebral	Thalamus	Sensory loss, mild hemiparesis
	Cerebellum and brainstem	Disturbances of gait, speech, swallowing, and vision

---

TREATMENT

Initially, after the patient's airway, respiratory, and cardiovascular function are assured, an assessment of stroke severity and associated neurologic deficits is made. An initial CT scan is used to determine the type of stroke and treatment, as treatment pathways differ between ischemic and hemorrhagic stroke. Patients who have experienced a hemorrhagic stroke secondary to hypertensive disease often have extremely high blood pressure. Bringing their blood pressure into normotensive ranges could result in ischemia. In these circumstances it is best to keep the patient mildly hypertensive with the goal of normalizing the blood pressure once the patient is medically stable.[7,10] Patients who have experienced a hemorrhagic stroke are at risk for increased intracranial pressure and are assessed and treated much as patients with a traumatic head injury. Thus, the remaining discussion will focus on treatment of ischemic stroke.

The goals of therapy for acute ischemic stroke are to minimize infarct size and preserve neurologic function. Aspirin may be administered following negative findings of hemorrhagic stroke on CT scan. The administration of 325 mg of aspirin immediately affects platelet aggregation and may help inhibit thrombus size. Thrombolytic therapy is most effective in limiting infarct size if it is initiated early. The American Heart Association guidelines for administration of thrombolytic therapy in ischemic stroke are shown in Box 44-6.

It is critical to prevent further cerebral hypoxia or ischemia after ischemic stroke. Thus, volume depletion, hemoconcentration, hypotension, and arterial obstruction must be avoided. As with the hemorrhagic stroke patient, careful blood pressure management is critical. Overhydration can result in cerebral

---

BOX 44-6

American Heart Association Guidelines for Administration of Thrombolytic Therapy in Ischemic Stroke

Intravenous recombinant tissue plasminogen activator (0.9 mg/kg) with 10% administered as a bolus followed by a 1-hour infusion is recommended for ischemic strokes presenting within 3 hours of symptom onset.

Inclusion Criteria (All Yes Boxes Must Be Checked Before Treatment)
Yes
☐ Age 18 years or older
☐ Clinical diagnosis of ischemic stroke causing a measurable neurologic deficit
☐ Time of symptom onset well established to be less than 180 minutes before treatment would begin

Exclusion Criteria (All No Boxes Must Be Checked Before Treatment)
No
☐ Evidence of intracranial hemorrhage on noncontrast head CT scan
☐ Only minor or rapidly improving stroke symptoms
☐ High clinical suspicion of subarachnoid hemorrhage even with normal CT scan
☐ Active internal bleeding (e.g., gastrointestinal/genitourinary bleeding within 21 days)
☐ Known bleeding diathesis, including but not limited to platelet count less than 100,000/mm³
☐ Patient has received heparin within 48 hours and had an elevated aPTT
☐ Recent use of anticoagulant (e.g., warfarin) and elevated PT (more than 15 seconds)/INR
☐ Intracranial surgery, serious head trauma, or previous stroke within 3 months
☐ Major surgery or serious trauma within 14 days
☐ Recent arterial puncture at noncompressible site
☐ Lumbar puncture within 7 days
☐ History of intracranial hemorrhage, arteriovenous malformation, or aneurysm
☐ Witnessed seizure at stroke onset
☐ Recent acute myocardial infarction
☐ Systolic blood pressure greater than 185 mm Hg, or diastolic blood pressure greater than 110 mm Hg at time of treatment

aPTT, Activated partial thromboplastin time; *CT,* computed tomography; *INR,* international normalized ratio; *PT,* prothrombin time.

---

edema in the ischemic area of the brain and raise ICP. Patients should have their ability to swallow evaluated *before* they take any food or liquids orally. Injury to cranial nerves V, VII, IX, X, or XII can place a patient at risk for respiratory aspiration and further compromise the individual's health and potential for recovery.

Anticoagulation therapy may be used in ischemic stroke, especially if the event is progressive. A stroke is termed *progressive* if an initial focal deficit worsened or fluctuated before hospital admission or deteriorated on serial examinations after admission. Patients who receive thrombolytic therapy should not receive anticoagulation therapy because the risk of bleeding is high. Throughout the course of therapy, it is essential to monitor clotting parameters and recognize the potential for hemorrhage into the ischemic area. Even in the absence of thrombolytic or anticoagulant therapy, a significant number of ischemic strokes convert to hemorrhagic lesions. A sudden change in neurologic function should prompt re-evaluation by CT. Numerous clinical studies on antioxidants, glutamate blockers, and calcium channel blockers have failed to show benefit, and early fibrinolytic therapy remains the cornerstone of treatment.[7]

Management of the stroke patient also must include efforts to prevent stroke recurrence. Evaluation and management of risk factors is an essential part of prevention. The survivor of a stroke is at high risk for a subsequent stroke if precipitating factors are still present. Patients who have experienced thrombotic strokes are also at significant risk for other vascular events, such as myocardial infarctions. Secondary prevention varies according to the cause of the stroke. For hemorrhagic strokes, careful monitoring and control of blood pressure is essential. For ischemic strokes of embolic origin, efforts are made to identify and remove the source of emboli. Usually the source is the heart, and therapy includes control of dysrhythmias, anticoagulation therapy, and antiplatelet drugs such as aspirin. The most common cause of embolic stroke is atrial fibrillation. Conversion of this dysrhythmia to normal sinus rhythm can sometimes be accomplished with antiarrhythmic agents or electrical cardioversion. Measures to improve left ventricular function may help to reduce atrial pressure and correct atrial fibrillation. Patients with long-standing atrial fibrillation require anticoagulation therapy. When abnormal valves are suspected to be the source of emboli, evaluation for surgical replacement may be indicated.

Secondary prevention for thrombotic stroke includes lifestyle modifications to address modifiable risk factors, including smoking cessation and lowering of serum lipid levels. In addition, the long-term daily use of aspirin or other antiplatelet agents (e.g., clopidogrel bisulfate) has been recommended. Some patients may benefit from surgical removal of carotid artery plaque by endarterectomy or angioplasty. Placement of rigid tubes, called *stents,* in the area of plaque removal may be helpful in preventing reocclusion.

STROKE SEQUELAE

Recovery after stroke depends on the size and location of the cerebral infarct, comorbid conditions, and rehabilitative efforts. Stroke rehabilitation begins during the acute hospitalization phase and continues after the patient has returned to the community. Many patients have residual or permanent deficits, in motor, sensory, language, and cognitive functions that necessitate intensive strategies to maximize the likelihood of return to a productive life.

Motor and Sensory Deficits

Motor impairment from a stroke is initially characterized by flaccidity, which is a decrease in or absence of muscle tone in the affected extremities. Most commonly, motor paralysis is contralateral to the side of the brain in which the stroke occurs. Thus a stroke on the right side of the brain results in left-sided body paralysis, whereas left brain strokes result in right-sided body paralysis. Footdrop, outward rotation of the leg, and dependent edema are common features in the lower extremity. In the upper extremity, the arm may separate from the shoulder if not supported. Muscles in the affected limbs tend to atrophy from lack of tone and use. Many of the complications can be limited with therapeutic interventions, including frequent range-of-motion exercises, elevation of edematous limbs, use of elastic stockings, and maintenance of body alignment.

Starting at about 6 weeks after the stroke, recovery of motor function is evident by the onset of spasticity. Spasticity is the resistance of muscle groups to passive stretch with an increase in tone. Increased flexor tone is usually seen in the upper extremities and increased extensor tone in the lower extremities. Passive or active range-of-motion exercises and positioning are critical to maintenance of function, as uncontrolled spasticity can result in contractures of the limbs, including adduction of the shoulder, pronation of the forearm, and finger flexion. In the lower extremity, the patient may have problems with hip and knee extension. If spasticity in a paretic extremity is not evident within 3 months, motor function is not likely to return to the affected limb.

Sensory impairment occurs in the same locations as the motor paralysis. A lack of sensory information from the paralyzed side contributes to the phenomenon of *neglect* (also called *hemiattention*). The patient seems not to realize that the affected body parts belong to him. Loss of the visual field on the paralyzed side also contributes to neglect. Contralateral field blindness is called *homonymous hemianopsia* because the same side of the retina in each eye is blinded (Figure 44-15). Patients with neglect may crush, burn, or otherwise injure the

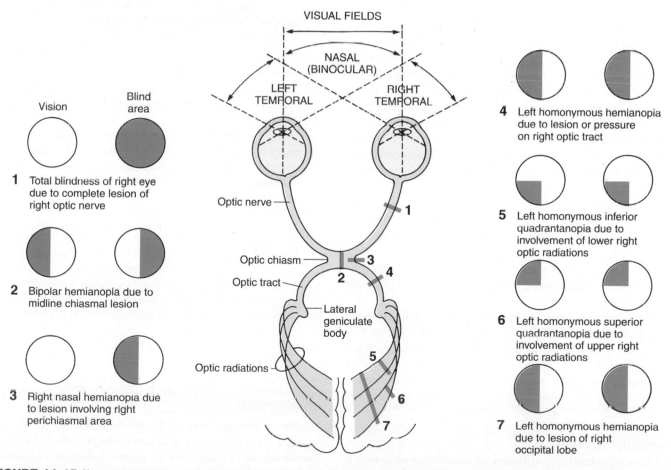

FIGURE 44-15 Homonymous hemianopsia. A right-sided brain stroke may cause lesions that disturb visual fibers and result in blindness in the left visual field. The optic pathway from the other side remains intact. (From Black JM, Hawks JH: *Medical-surgical nursing: clinical management for positive outcomes,* ed 8, Philadelphia, 2008, Saunders, p 1850.)

neglected body parts without realizing it. Poor hygiene of affected extremities may be apparent. Neuropsychological studies have shown that objects in the field of neglect are usually ignored. When asked to draw the numbers on the face of a clock, all 12 are drawn on one side. Self-portraits may be conspicuous for the distortion or omission of structures on the neglected side. Neglect is associated with a high risk for falls and other injuries.

Language Deficits

Aphasia is an integrative language disorder that occurs with brain damage to the dominant cerebral hemisphere (usually left) and involves all language modalities. Characteristics of aphasia include a reduced vocabulary, reduced verbal attention span, and reduced ability to use learned linguistic rules. Aphasia is associated with lesions in the primary language centers (Broca and/or Wernicke areas) as well as in adjacent cortical areas. Aphasia is categorized according to the location of the lesion and the linguistic deficit. The following is a brief description of those categories.

Broca aphasia, also known as verbal motor or expressive aphasia, results from a lesion in the third frontal convolution of the left hemisphere in most persons. Patients speak with poorly articulated and sparse vocabulary and in the simplest grammatical constructions.

Wernicke aphasia, also known as sensory, acoustic, or receptive aphasia, is characterized by impaired auditory comprehension and speech that is fluent but empty of content. This form of aphasia is caused by lesions in the posterior portion of the first temporal gyrus of the left hemisphere. Speech is frequently circumlocutory or tangential and contains paraphasic errors and jargon. Word finding and naming difficulties are a prominent feature of this disorder. Patients with Wernicke aphasia are unable to monitor their own language production and cannot comprehend or monitor the language production of others.

Anomic aphasia results from lesions in the parietotemporal area in proximity to the angular gyrus. This is a fluent aphasia with intact grammatical structure. Patients have greater word-finding difficulties than those with Wernicke aphasia but do not make paraphasic errors and have intact comprehension. However, their speech is typically constructed of simple words.

Conduction or central aphasia is associated with increased paraphasic errors and a reduced ability to repeat words. It is associated with a lesion in the arcuate fasciculus in the left hemisphere. Patients are well aware that they are making language errors. However, the more they struggle to find the correct words, the more likely they are to repeat paraphasic errors.

Cognitive Deficits

Patients experience impairments of cognition owing to diffuse cortical or subcortical injuries that affect the ability to be alert, to concentrate or attend to stimuli, to remember, and to reason. Cognitive impairment varies according to the area of brain affected and the severity of the injury. Injuries that disturb an individual's ability to maintain an alert status are the most severe. Increasing cognitive skill is necessary for the function of memory and the ability to learn and associate, to discriminate, to separate, and to categorize various stimuli. The highest levels of cognitive function include analysis, synthesis, and reasoning abilities.

Cognitive impairment is commonly evidenced as language deficit, impaired spatial relationship skills, short-term memory impairment, and poor judgment. Patients who do not retain the ability to learn are unlikely to benefit from rehabilitative services.

KEY POINTS

- Stroke is the sudden onset of neurologic dysfunction due to cerebrovascular disease. The most common cause of stroke is thrombosis, followed by embolization and intracranial hemorrhage.
- Thrombi form at atherosclerotic plaques, causing sudden occlusion of an already narrowed vessel. If the clot is quickly lysed, the deficits may completely disappear, a phenomenon associated with a TIA. Emboli are usually a consequence of clots from within the heart chambers due to disease or dysrhythmia. Hemorrhagic stroke is usually associated with uncontrolled hypertension.
- Stroke symptoms depend on the area of brain affected, which in turn depends on the vessel occluded: internal carotid, anterior cerebral, middle cerebral, or posterior cerebral artery. Common manifestations include contralateral motor and sensory loss, aphasia, and contralateral visual field loss.
- Treatment is aimed at limiting the size of the brain infarction, supporting bodily functions, and initiating aggressive rehabilitation strategies. Acute therapy with thrombolytic agents may limit infarct size in patients with ischemic stroke.
- Stroke is associated with long-term deficits in motor, sensory, language, and cognitive abilities. Initially, affected muscles are flaccid, with spasticity occurring after about 6 weeks. Prevention of contractures is a major concern. Aphasia may be described as expressive or receptive. Most individuals with aphasia have impaired integrative ability involving all language modalities. Concentration, memory, and reasoning may be impaired.

Cerebral Aneurysm and Arteriovenous Malformation

Structural abnormalities of the cerebral arteries predispose to intracerebral bleeding and hemorrhagic stroke. Cerebral aneurysms and AVMs are the two most common causes of subarachnoid hemorrhage. Early recognition and surgical management of these conditions are necessary to prevent significant mortality and morbidity associated with rupture.

Cerebral Aneurysm

Etiology. An aneurysm is a lesion of an artery that results in dilation and ballooning of a segment of the vessel. Aneurysm rupture occurs in about 15,000 Americans each year, or 6 per 1,000,000.[25] The prevalence is higher in women than in men, and rupture most often occurs between the ages of 30 and 60 years. Intracerebral aneurysms are found in about 6% of the general population, and more than half remain unruptured and undiagnosed.[25] Thus, other factors are likely to be important in precipitating aneurysm rupture. High blood pressure, acute alcohol intoxication, and recreational drug use (especially cocaine) have been implicated. The annual risk of rupture in persons with aneurysms is 1% to 2%. Larger aneurysms and those located in the posterior circulation are more prone to rupture.[25]

Approximately 15% of patients with ruptured cerebral aneurysms die before they receive medical attention. Of those who do receive hospital care, 25% to 50% die during the acute phase.[26]

Pathogenesis and Manifestations. Although the exact pathogenesis is not understood, saccular aneurysms are believed to result from congenital defects of the medial layer of the artery. This structural weakness permits gradual ballooning at the site as a consequence of arterial pressure effects over years. A common location for saccular aneurysms is the arterial bifurcations, where turbulent blood flow might have a greater impact on a weakened vessel wall. Ninety-five percent of cerebral aneurysms are located in the circle of Willis. Ten percent to 20% of affected individuals have more than one aneurysm.

Saccular aneurysms (berry aneurysms) are round and are the most common (Figure 44-16). The aneurysmal sac is composed of thickened intima and adventitia, the media layer having abruptly ended at the sac edge (Figure 44-17). Rupture of the aneurysm generally occurs from the dome of the sac or at the edge of the atheromatous plaque.

Warning leaks may occur before an aneurysm ruptures and often produce severe headache, which is typically described by the patient as "the worst headache I have ever had," and if recognized and treated as such, can significantly improve related morbidity and mortality.[26] Patients may also complain of photophobia (visual sensitivity to light), nausea/vomiting, and stiff neck. A stiff and painful neck results from meningismus caused by the irritating properties of blood in the CSF. After rupture, the onset of symptoms is very rapid. Sudden injection of blood into the subarachnoid space raises ICP and distorts intracranial structures. Secondary cerebral vasospasm, a pathologic narrowing of the major vessels around the area of rupture, typically occurs from day 4 to day 14. This process significantly reduces cerebral blood flow and results in increased cerebral ischemia and possibly infarction. Vasospasm is due to the presence of blood in the CSF. The next most serious consequence of the initial rupture is rebleeding. The risk for rebleeding is highest in the first 14 days. Patients are also at risk for developing hydrocephalus from clogging and obstruction of CSF flow through the ventricular system.

Diagnostic procedures for detecting ruptured aneurysm include CT or MRI to confirm a subarachnoid hemorrhage. If the scan is negative but suspicion of subarachnoid hemorrhage is high, a lumbar puncture for CSF analysis can be done. Blood in the CSF is indicative of subarachnoid hemorrhage. A cerebral angiogram is obtained to demonstrate the location of aneurysms in preparation for surgical management.

Treatment. The primary treatments for aneurysms are surgical stabilization by clipping or placement of endovascular coils for embolization. Prognosis is favorable if the aneurysm is detected and managed before significant rupture occurs. In most cases, the aneurysm is not diagnosed until after subarachnoid or intracerebral hemorrhage has occurred, and mortality is higher. Early surgery in stable patients with subarachnoid hemorrhage

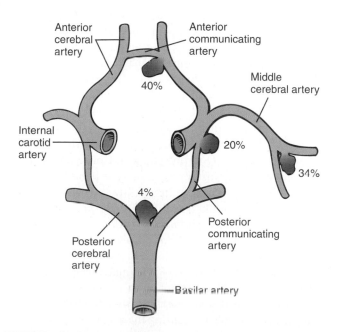

FIGURE 44-16 Saccular (berry) aneurysms are most commonly found in the circle of Willis, particularly at arterial bifurcations. (From Kumar V et al: *Robbins basic pathology,* ed 8, Philadelphia, 2007, Saunders, p 867.)

FIGURE 44-17 Gross view of a massive saccular aneurysm in the circle of Willis. (From Kumar V et al: *Robbins basic pathology,* ed 8, Philadelphia, 2007, Saunders, p 867.)

is associated with a lower overall mortality. Aneurysm clipping is accomplished by placement of a permanent vascular clip at the neck of the aneurysm. Coil devices may be inserted under radiographic guidance to thrombose or sclerose the area. The 1-year mortality rate of aneurysm clipping or coil placement in unruptured aneurysm is 10% to 12%.[25]

In patients experiencing subarachnoid hemorrhage as a consequence of ruptured aneurysm, the complications of cerebral vasospasm and hydrocephalus must be monitored and managed. Vasospasm can be managed by keeping blood volume and blood pressure at normal to high levels. Calcium channel blockers may be used to reduce vasospasm. In addition to hemodynamic monitoring, careful and frequent neurologic assessments are essential to monitor stability and indicate the first signs of deterioration so that rapid intervention can be undertaken.

Arteriovenous Malformation

Etiology. AVMs are the second most common cause of spontaneous subarachnoid hemorrhage, but can also cause intracerebral hemorrhage. The majority of AVMs are diagnosed in patients between 20 and 40 years.[27] Ninety percent of AVMs are found in the cerebral hemispheres and only about 10% in the posterior fossa. AVMs are vascular lesions thought to be congenital; however, they are rarely diagnosed in the pediatric population.[27]

The risk of clinically recognizable hemorrhage from an AVM is 2% to 3% per year.[27] The risk of rebleeding within the first year after an initial hemorrhage is 6%. The mortality associated with AVM rupture is 10% to 15%—much lower than with aneurysm rupture.[26]

Pathogenesis and Manifestations. In the normal vascular system, the capillaries are situated between the arterioles and the venules. In an AVM, the capillary system fails to develop appropriately, and arterial blood is shunted directly into the venous system. Exposure of the high-capacitance venous system to the high pressure of the arteries causes the vessels to progressively enlarge, as do the arteries and veins that feed and drain the lesion. Eventually the AVM becomes a congested mass of enlarged vessels.

Because of their abnormal structure and the high vascular pressure, AVMs are vulnerable to hemorrhage. Hemorrhage is the initial manifestation in 50% of cases of AVM; 25% are manifested by seizures and the rest by varying degrees of vascular steal syndrome. The abnormal shunting of blood into the AVM, called *vascular steal syndrome,* causes progressive neurologic dysfunction as a result of ischemia in normal tissue.

Treatment. Once the AVM and vascular bed is evaluated, it may be surgically removed. Alternatively, gamma knife or stereotactic radiosurgery can be used to deliver precisely aligned beams of gamma radiation to shrink the abnormal vascular tissue. For deep or very large AVMs, other approaches (e.g., irradiation and glue embolization) may be used.[27] Supportive therapy for AVMs that rupture and cause subarachnoid hemorrhage is similar to that described for ruptured cerebral aneurysms.

Central Nervous System Infections

Infections of the CNS include meningitis, encephalitis, and abscesses. A frequent consequence of bacterial infections is obstructive hydrocephalus, as the bacteria, white blood cells, and cellular debris block CSF reabsorption in the arachnoid villi.

Organisms gain access to the CNS by various portals of entry. These include the bloodstream, by direct extension from a primary site (e.g., sinuses), by extension along peripheral and cranial nerves, and through maternal-fetal exchange. Factors contributing to infections include such conditions as immunocompromise, debilitation, poor nutrition, radiation therapy, steroid therapy, and contact with vectors. Meningitis and cerebral abscess are most commonly associated with bacterial infections, whereas encephalitis is usually viral.

Meningitis. Meningitis is the most common sequela to microbial invasion of the CNS. Most frequently, meningitis is bacterial in origin, but it can also be viral or fungal. Persons with acquired immunodeficiency syndrome (AIDS) have an increased susceptibility to infection and have an increased prevalence of meningitis of viral, fungal, or parasitic origin.

Etiology. The bacteria most frequently involved in causing meningitis in adults are *Streptococcus pneumoniae* and *Neisseria meningitidis*.[28] *Haemophilus influenzae* type B (HIB) is a causative agent in children; however, the incidence has fallen dramatically since the introduction of the HIB vaccines.[28] The bacteria that cause meningitis usually reach the CNS by way of the bloodstream or by extension from cranial structures, such as the paranasal sinuses or ears. Some of the organisms responsible for causing meningitis may be normal inhabitants of the nasopharynx. Pathogens can also gain access to the CNS through breaks in the barrier system, as occur with penetrating head wounds or skull fractures or following neurosurgery in which the dura is penetrated. The overall mortality rate for meningitis is approximately 10% for *N. meningitidis* and 26% for *S. pneumoniae* infection.[28]

Pathogenesis and Clinical Manifestations. Bacterial meningitis is a pyogenic infection that invades the **leptomeninges** and the subarachnoid space. Because of its involvement in the subarachnoid space, the infection travels readily around the brain and spinal cord. The accumulation of inflammatory exudate frequently results in obstructive hydrocephalus and exudative invasion into the sheaths of the blood vessels and spinal and cranial nerves.

The combination of headache, fever, stiff neck (meningismus), and signs of cerebral dysfunction (confusion, delirium) is the classic presentation of meningitis. Deterioration in level of consciousness is progressive and often rapid. Patients who deteriorate rapidly often demonstrate dramatic tachypnea. About one third of patients experience seizures. Cranial nerve involvement is also common and is most often seen as ocular palsies, facial weakness and/or deafness, and vertigo.

The diagnosis of meningitis is usually made by lumbar puncture. Typical CSF findings are shown in Table 44-3. Gram stain of the CSF will reveal the causative organism in most patients. In addition to the causative organism, classic CSF findings include white blood cell counts between 1000 and 10,000/mm³ with a predominance of neutrophils. The CSF glucose level is reduced and often extremely low, and patients with bacterial or fungal meningitis have increased protein levels.

Treatment. Recovery from bacterial meningitis depends largely on how quickly effective treatment is started. Treatment includes general supportive care, intravenous antibacterial drug therapy targeting the specific pathogen, and management of any complications. Complications from meningitis can include visual impairment, optic neuritis, deafness, headache, seizures, personality changes, motor weakness, hydrocephalus, endocarditis, and pneumonia. Much of the damage to CNS structures is not a direct result of the pathogen; rather, it is the immune response that is injurious. Antibiotic therapy, with

resultant bacterial cell wall lysis, can increase the immune-mediated injury. This has led some investigators to recommend the use of corticosteroids during the antibiotic treatment phase. A significant reduction in mortality was achieved in some studies in adults receiving dexamethasone beginning with the initiation of antibiotics.[28]

Prevention strategies include public education promoting prompt and appropriate management of sinusitis, mastoiditis, ear infections, and pneumonia. Strict aseptic techniques for all procedures involving a break in the CNS barrier system may help prevent nosocomial CNS infections. Vaccination against *N. meningitidis* provides short-term protection (a few years) and may be useful prior to situations in which exposure is more likely, such as during the college years.

Encephalitis

Etiology. Encephalitis, an inflammation of the brain, can be caused by the same infectious agents as meningitis, although viruses are most often the pathogen. There are no well-established diagnostic criteria for acute encephalitis, and the manifestations mimic other brain injuries. The diagnosis of acute viral encephalitis is often a diagnosis of exclusion.

The most common types of viral encephalitis in the United States include West Nile virus, western equine encephalitis, and herpes simplex encephalitis. In 2002, the largest encephalitis outbreak in U.S. history, with more than 3800 cases and 225 deaths, was attributed to the West Nile virus.[29] West Nile is transmitted by infected mosquitoes (*Culex* species) during summer months in the United States. Previously, West Nile virus was confined to more tropical areas and considered to be fairly benign. Its usual hosts are birds, and it may affect horses and humans. Dogs and cats do not appear to be affected.[30]

Western equine encephalitis is transmitted by the mosquito *Culex tarsalis*, which breeds in sunlit grassy marshes, ground pools, and streams. Birds are the preferred host, and humans are not usually infected unless the population of *C. tarsalis* far outnumbers the bird host population. In the eastern United States, western equine encephalitis is carried by the mosquito vector *Culiseta melanura* and rarely infects humans. Western equine encephalitis is primarily a disease of the summer months, typically May to September. It most often infects the very young and those older than 50 years.

Herpes simplex encephalitis is an important cause of sporadic and often fatal (70%) encephalitis in the United States. It results from spread of the herpes simplex virus type 1 to the CNS. This can occur as a primary or secondary infection or as a reactivation of latent virus. There is no seasonal incidence of this disease.

Pathogenesis and Manifestations. The incubation period for West Nile ranges from 3 to 14 days, and symptoms usually last 3 to 6 days. Most infections are mild and asymptomatic. Twenty percent of infected individuals develop a febrile illness with headache, malaise, muscle pain, or rash. Approximately 1 in 150 infections results in severe neurologic disease, most commonly encephalitis, but some cases of meningitis have been reported. Advanced age is a significant risk factor for developing a more severe infection. The manifestations of

TABLE 44-3

Typical Cerebrospinal Fluid Findings in Bacterial Meningitis

CSF Variable	Typical Findings	Normal
White blood cell count	1000-5000 cells/mm³ (up to 10,000) (high)	<5
Neutrophils	≥90% (high)	60%-80%
Protein	80-500 mg/dl (high)	30 mg/dl
Glucose	≤40 mg/dl (low)	50-80 mg/dl
Gram stain	Positive (60%-90% of cases)	Negative
Culture	Positive (70%-85% of cases)	Negative
CSF opening pressure	>20 cm H₂O (high)	<15 cm H₂O

CSF, Cerebrospinal fluid.

severe infection include fever, muscle weakness or flaccid paralysis, headache, and changes in mental status.[30]

The incubation period for western equine encephalitis is 5 to 15 days. Onset of symptoms is typically rapid, and symptoms include general malaise, mild headache, and, often, nausea and vomiting. A moderately elevated temperature develops and the headache usually becomes severe. Lethargy and irritability are often present after a few days. In an uncomplicated infection, symptoms persist for about 10 days and then gradually subside. In severe cases, lethargy progresses to stupor alternating with extreme restlessness. In fatal cases, the progression of disease is rapid, culminating in coma and death.

The manifestations of herpes simplex encephalitis are variable. The patient may initially complain of flulike symptoms. Subsequent lethargy, confusion, and delirium are common and may evolve into coma. Some patients may experience a much more rapid course with acute necrotizing encephalitis and widespread destruction of white matter and extensive brain edema. Herpes simplex encephalitis is typically associated with a profound memory impairment and changes in personality.

The diagnosis of encephalitis is usually made from the history, clinical findings, and lumbar puncture in which there is a normal or mildly elevated white blood cell count, a small increase in protein, and a normal glucose. Viral serology may detect the virus in a minority of cases. Some viral infections can be diagnosed by detecting antibodies in serum or cerebrospinal fluid. Since IgM does not cross the BBB, an elevated IgM antiviral antibody titer in CSF is highly suggestive of CNS infection by the virus. In many cases of acute encephalitis, no causative organisms can be identified. A brain biopsy may be the only means to confirm the diagnosis.

Treatment. In general, the management of encephalitis is supportive and symptomatic. As with all severe illnesses, respiratory and cardiovascular support is imperative. Patients with encephalitis must be carefully hydrated as they frequently show signs and symptoms of excessive antidiuretic hormone secretion and water retention. Those with moderate to severe disease require careful and ongoing neurologic assessment. Seizures are a common complication in encephalitis secondary to hypoxia, tissue destruction, toxic encephalopathy, inflammatory vasculitis, and hyponatremia. All patients with moderate to severe illness should be monitored for intracranial hypertension. Although there is no definitive drug treatment, steroids may be given to control edema, anticonvulsants to prevent seizures, analgesics for headache, and antipyretics for hyperthermia. Patients in whom herpes simplex encephalitis has been diagnosed should be treated with antiviral medications such as acyclovir. Intravenous immunoglobulin, interferon-α, and ribavirin have been tried in some forms of viral encephalitis, but their efficacy is not yet proven.[29]

Brain Abscess

Etiology. A brain abscess is a localized collection of pus within the brain parenchyma. **Pyogenic** (pus-producing) pathogens reach the brain by a number of routes, including: (1) penetrating wounds, (2) direct extension or retrograde thrombophlebitis of an infected neighboring structure (e.g., mastoiditis, sinusitis), or (3) blood-borne dissemination from a distant infected site (e.g., lungs). Most brain abscesses are bacterial. The most common infective organisms are streptococci, staphylococci, and anaerobes.[31]

Pathogenesis and Manifestations. Brain abscess presents as a space-occupying lesion in the brain. Most patients experience symptoms 1 to 4 weeks after the initial infection. The abscess has a focal infected core in which the central portion contains an abundance of neutrophils and tissue debris (pus). The peripheral portion of the abscess is made up of inflammatory granulation tissue. Around the abscess is perifocal edema with proliferation of surviving astrocytes. In the chronic phase, the core of the abscess is liquefied and the peripheral portion forms a collagenous capsule that in turn is surrounded by fibrous gliosis. A CT scan typically shows an outer ring surrounding a low-density core (Figure 44-18).

Treatment. Management of a brain abscess depends on its location and accessibility, and usually involves drainage or excision. A critical feature in management is the administration of intravenous antibiotics, which is required for several weeks. Recently, the treatment of patients with brain abscess has become increasingly challenging because of the increase in unusual bacterial, fungal, and parasitic infections, particularly in immunosuppressed patients. Postinfection care must address residual neurologic deficits of cognitive, motor, or sensory function.

FIGURE 44-18 CT scan of a cerebral abscess showing typical ring with decreased core density and an edematous area surrounding the abscess. (From Grossman RI, Yousem DM: *Neuroradiology,* ed 2, St Louis, 2003, Mosby, p 285.)

KEY POINTS

- Meningitis is usually a consequence of bacterial infection in the CNS. Infection may be introduced through the bloodstream or by invasion from infected sinuses or ears. Fever, stiff neck, and headache are common. Seizures may occur. The diagnosis is based on an elevated CSF white blood cell count and the presence of bacteria in the CSF.

- Obstructive hydrocephalus is a serious complication of meningitis that leads to increased ICP. Antibiotics are used for treatment.

- Encephalitis is inflammation of the brain that is most commonly due to viral infection. Common causes of viral encephalitis in the United States include West Nile virus, western equine encephalitis, and herpes simplex virus. Management is based on symptoms and may include steroids, anticonvulsants, analgesics, and antipyretics. Antiviral agents (e.g., acyclovir) are helpful in the treatment of herpes simplex encephalitis. Other antiviral agents are under investigation.

- Brain abscesses are usually due to pus-forming bacteria. Abscesses may be asymptomatic at first, later showing manifestations of a progressive space-occupying lesion. Drainage or excision and antibiotics are indicated.

SUMMARY

Acute disorders of brain function are characterized by rapidly progressing neurologic deficits and life-threatening complications. The cellular pathophysiologic process is similar for most types of brain injury and includes mechanisms of ischemia, cellular calcium overload, and free radical and immune-mediated damage. The development of increased ICP with compression of vital brain structures is a potential complication of all types of brain injury.

Efforts to minimize brain damage are focused on recognizing and managing secondary brain damage. Careful monitoring and management of body temperature, blood pressure, volume status, and respiratory function are essential. Efforts to reduce brain ischemia are important because it is thought to be a critical factor in acute brain injury.

The acute brain injury disorders presented in this chapter, including TBI, stroke, vascular rupture, and CNS infections, are all largely preventable. Efforts at prevention are paramount because often the outcome of acute brain injury is poor.

REFERENCES

1. Guyton AC, Hall JE, editors: *Textbook of medical physiology*, ed 11, Philadelphia, 2005, Saunders, pp 52-64.
2. Centers for Disease Control and Prevention: *Heads up for physicians about mild traumatic brain injury (MTBI)*, Bethesda, Md, 2007, Department of Health and Human Services.
3. Bramlett HM, Dietrich WD: Progressive damage after brain and spinal cord injury: pathomechanisms and treatment strategies, *Progress Brain Res* 161:125-141, 2007.
4. MacDonald JF, Xiong ZG, Jackson MF: Paradox of Ca^{2+} signaling, cell death and stroke, *Trends Neurosci* 29:75-81, 2006.
5. Annunziato L, Cataldi M, Pignataro G et al: Glutamate-independent calcium toxicity: introduction, *Stroke* 38:661-664, 2007.
6. Schouten JW: Neuroprotection in traumatic brain injury: a complex struggle against the biology of nature, *Curr Opin Crit Care* 13:134-142, 2007.
7. Merenda A, Bullock, R: Clinical treatments for mitochondrial dysfunctions after brain injury, *Curr Opin Crit Care* 12:90-96, 2006.
8. Ferrer I: Apoptosis: future targets for neuroprotective strategies, *Cerebrovas Dis* 21:9-20, 2006.
9. Werner, C, Engelhard, K: Pathophysiology of traumatic brain injury, *Brit J Anaesth* 99:4-9, 2007.
10. Marklund N, Bakshi A, Castelbuono DJ et al: Evaluation of pharmacological treatment strategies in traumatic brain injury, *Curr Pharm Des* 12:1645-1680, 2006.
11. Broderick J, Connolly S, Feldmann E et al: Guidelines for the management of spontaneous intracerebral hemorrhage in adults, *Stroke* 38:2001-2023, 2007.
12. Cushing H: *Studies in intracranial physiology and surgery*, London, 1926, Oxford University Press, pp 19-23.
13. Smith M: Intensive care management of patients with subarachnoid haemorrhage, *Curr Opin Anaesth* 20:400-407, 2007.
14. American Association of Neuroscience Nurses: *Guide to the care of the patient with intracranial pressure monitoring*, Glenview, Ill, 2005, American Association of Neuroscience Nurses.
15. Barker E: *Neuroscience nursing: A spectrum of care*, ed 3, New York, 2007, Mosby, pp 515-520.
16. Kielan K: Mind time: the temporal factor in consciousness, *J Psychophys* 19:232-233, 2005.
17. Brain Trauma Foundation: Guidelines for the management of severe traumatic brain injury, ed 3, *J Neurotrauma* 24, S1-S106, 2007.
18. Vespa P: Brain tissue oxygen monitoring: a measure of supply and demand, *Crit Care Med* 34:1850-1852, 2006.
19. Pickelsimer EE, Selassie AW, Sample, PL et al: Unmet service needs of persons with traumatic brain injury, *J Head Trauma Rehab* 22:1-13, 2007.
20. Parikh S, Koch M, Narayan RK: Traumatic brain injury, *Internat Anesth Clin* 45:119-135, 2007.
21. Greenberg MS: *Handbook of neurosurgery*, ed 6, New York, 2006, Thieme Medical Publishers.
22. American Heart Association: *Heart disease and stroke statistics—2007 update*, Dallas, 2007, American Heart Association.
23. American Heart Association: Stroke symptoms—warning signs. Available at http://www.american heart.org.
24. American Heart Association/American Stroke Association: Guidelines for prevention of stroke in patients with ischemic stroke or transient ischemic attack, *Stroke* 37:577-617, 2006.
25. Molyneux AJ, Kerr RS, Yu LM et al: International subarachnoid aneurysm trial (ISAT) of neurosurgical clipping versus endovascular coiling in 2143 patients with ruptured intracranial aneurysms: a randomised comparison of effects on survival, dependency, seizures, rebleeding, subgroups, and aneurysm occlusion, *Lancet* 366:809-817, 2005.
26. Stevens RD, Nyquist PA: The systemic implications of aneurysmal subarachnoid hemorrhage, *J Neurol Scien* 261:143-156, 2007.
27. Friedlander RM: Arteriovenous malformations of the brain, *New Engl J Med* 356:2704-2712, 2007.
28. Nelson RP: Bacterial meningitis and inflammation, *Curr Opin Neurol* 19:369-373, 2006.
29. DeBiasi RL, Tyler KL: Viral meningitis and encephalitis, *Continuum: Life Learn Neurol* 12:58-94, 2006.
30. Murray K, Baraniuk S, Resnick M et al: Risk factors for encephalitis and death from West Nile virus infection, *Epidem Infect* 134:1325-1332, 2006.
31. Shakeri M, Vahedi P: Cerebral echinococcosis in the children and young adults, *Neurosurg Quart* 17:241-244, 2007.

Chronic Disorders of Neurologic Function

Joni D. Nelsen-Marsh

◀ MEDIA RESOURCES

Additional Material for Study, Review, and Further Exploration

CD Companion ■ Review Questions and Answers
■ Glossary (with audio pronunciations for selected terms)
■ Disease Profiles ■ Animations

 Website at http://evolve.elsevier.com/Copstead/
■ Case Studies ■ Disease Profiles ■ WebLinks ■ Key Points Review

 Online Course (Module 18)

◀ KEY QUESTIONS

■ How are the various types of seizures recognized, classified, and treated?
■ How is Alzheimer dementia diagnosed and managed?
■ What are the similarities between Alzheimer and vascular dementia?
■ What are the proposed neurotransmitter alterations in Parkinson disease, and how are drugs used to restore balance?
■ What are the similarities and differences between multiple sclerosis and amyotrophic lateral sclerosis?
■ How are congenital disorders, such as cerebral palsy, hydrocephalus, and spina bifida, manifested in the newborn?

■ How does the level of spinal cord injury relate to expected functional losses and clinical manifestations?
■ What is the role of immune mechanisms in Guillain-Barré syndrome amyotrophic lateral sclerosis and multiple sclerosis?
■ What are the causes of facial paralysis in Bell palsy, and how is this condition different from other chronic disorders of neurologic function?

◀ CHAPTER OUTLINE

atients experiencing neurologic dysfunction from chronic disease states present a challenge to health care professionals, who must strive to maximize the patient's function and quality of life. This chapter focuses on common chronic disabilities of neurologic function including those primarily affecting the brain such as seizures, dementia, Parkinson disease, cerebral palsy, and hydrocephalus. Disorders of the spinal cord include multiple sclerosis (MS), spina bifida, and spinal cord injury. Guillain-Barré syndrome and Bell palsy are examples of disorders affecting the peripheral nervous system.

BRAIN AND CEREBELLAR DISORDERS

Seizure Disorder. **Seizures** are a transient neurologic event of paroxysmal abnormal or excessive cortical electrical discharges that are manifested by disturbances of skeletal motor function, sensation, autonomic visceral function, behavior, or consciousness. Symptoms are not constant, and the length of time between seizure episodes is extremely variable. A seizure may only occur once in a person's lifetime. Epilepsy or seizure disorder refers to recurrent seizures. Seizures are a component of many diseases. Epilepsy affects 2.7 million Americans. About 10% of Americans will experience a seizure during their lifetime.[1]

Etiology. Seizures have many causes, and under the right circumstances anyone can experience one. A seizure disorder can be acquired as a consequence of cerebral injury or other pathologic process, including structural lesions such as tumors, blood clots, or infection. Other causes include metabolic and nutritional disorders such as electrolyte and water imbalance, hypoxia, acidosis, pyridoxine deficiency, acute withdrawal from alcohol, therapeutic medication overdose or medication adverse effect, and exposure to toxins such as heavy metals or street drugs. If seizures develop as a result of a structural change such as head injury or stroke, the onset is not predictable. In some cases, seizures may not develop for months or years after the structural change has occurred. In some cases, no explanation for the seizure disorder can be found. These individuals are classified as having **idiopathic** seizures.

A seizure event is often triggered by specific stimuli, usually unique for each individual. Physical inducements include specific sensory stimuli such as flashing lights, loud noises, and rhythmic music. Fever, physical exhaustion, inadequate nutrition, menses, hyperventilation, injury, and drugs can also prompt seizure activity. Psychosocial factors include family and environmental stress, shock, and emotional stress.

Pathogenesis. Seizures are due to an alteration in membrane potential that makes certain neurons abnormally hyperactive and hypersensitive to changes in their environment. These physiologically abnormal neurons form an **epileptogenic focus,** i.e., an area of the brain from which the seizure emanates. The epileptogenic focus functions autonomously, emitting excessively large numbers of paroxysmal electrical discharges. Nerve cells in this area can recruit neurons in adjacent areas as well as synaptically related neurons in distant areas of the brain, greatly increasing the number of neurons involved in the seizure activity. Recruitment can also incorporate neurons in the opposite hemisphere. Clinical symptoms become evident when a sufficient number of neurons have been excited. Seizures are classified according to clinical symptoms and the electroencephalographic features. Clinical manifestations depend on the area of the brain involved, the area of origin, and the areas to which the seizure spreads.

Clinical Manifestations. Seizures may be classified as partial, in which only part of the brain surface is affected (also known as focal seizures), or generalized, in which the whole brain surface is affected during the seizure (Box 45-1).

Generalized Seizures. Episodes in which the entire brain is involved from the onset of the seizure are referred to as **generalized seizures.** Involvement of the thalamus and reticular activating system results in loss of consciousness. Metabolic or toxin induced seizures tend to be generalized. This category includes the following: absence (petite mal), atypical absence, myoclonic, atonic (drop attack), or tonic-clonic (grand mal) seizures.

Absence or petite mal seizures usually occur only in children and are sometimes identified in children manifesting poor academic performance. They are very brief (2 to 10 seconds), and episodes are characterized by staring spells that last only seconds. Onset and termination of attacks are abrupt. During the spell, the individual is unaware of the surrounding environment and is usually motionless; however, it is not unusual for the person to continue walking or performing a routine motor task. If the seizure activity occurs during conversation, the individual may pause or miss a few words. Absence seizures almost always occur during childhood and resolve by age 20 years, although another seizure type may occur later in life.[2]

Atypical absence seizures have accompanying myoclonic jerks and automatisms (such as lip smacking or repetitive

---

BOX 45-1

Classifications of Seizures

Generalized Seizures: The Entire Brain Surface Is Affected During the Seizure

Absence (petit mal)
Atypical absence
Myoclonic
Atonic (drop attack)
Clonic
Tonic
Generalized tonic-clonic (grand mal)

Partial Seizures: Part of the Brain Surface Is Affected During the Seizure

Simple partial: There is no impairment of consciousness during the seizure.
Complex partial: There is impairment of consciousness during the seizure.
With secondary generalization: Onset begins as simple partial, and then progresses to impairment of consciousness.

semi-purposeful movements) with the staring spell. The electroencephalographic patterns are unique to each syndrome. Myoclonic seizures are extremely brief and are characterized by a single jerk or multiple jerks of one or more muscle groups. Atonic seizures or drop attacks are characterized by a sudden and complete loss of muscle tone. Falls and injuries are common with this type of seizure activity. Myoclonic episodes may also be associated with atonic seizures. Tonic-clonic seizures involve stiffening and repetitive jerking of muscle groups.

Tonic-clonic or grand mal seizures are characterized by a sudden loss of consciousness followed by muscle rigidity (tonic phase). The individual falls, and initial motor signs include opening of the mouth and eyes, extension of the legs, and adduction of the arms. There may be tongue biting or a high-pitched cry as the whole musculature is in spasm and air is forced out of the lungs through closed vocal cords. Respiration is arrested, and cyanosis may occur. Bowel and bladder incontinence frequently occurs. The tonic phase may last 10 to 15 seconds and is followed by clonic activity. There is often violent but rhythmic muscular contractions. During this phase the eyes roll, the face grimaces, and the pulse accelerates. Salivation increases and the patient may become diaphoretic. The clonic phase usually lasts 1 to 2 minutes with a gradual decline in the amplitude of the clonic jerks. The individual remains apneic until the end of the clonic phase that is marked by a deep inspiration.

During the terminal or postictal phase, the individual may regain consciousness or drift into a deep coma-like state. Disorientation and confusion are common. If allowed, the individual may sleep for several hours. Other findings include headache, drowsiness, nausea, muscle soreness, no memory of the seizure event, and retrograde amnesia. During the seizure, the person is at risk for injury from the initial fall as well as from the muscle contractions of the clonic phase.

A potentially life-threatening situation known as **status epilepticus** occurs in some seizure disorders. Status epilepticus is a continuing series of seizures without a period of recovery between seizure episodes. It can occur with all types of seizures but is of largest concern in tonic-clonic seizures. Irreversible brain damage and possible death from hypoxia, cardiac arrhythmias, or lactic acidosis can occur if the airway is not maintained and seizure activity is not halted. Whether non-convulsive status epilepticus causes neuronal damage is still a matter of debate; studies have shown that the increased metabolic activity of the brain that occurs during status epilepticus may cause ischemic brain damage, especially in elderly patients.[3]

Partial Seizures. Partial seizures are those in which activity is restricted to one brain hemisphere. They are further divided into three categories: simple partial, complex partial, and partial seizures that are secondarily generalized.

In simple partial seizures, the individual does not have a change in level of consciousness. The symptoms may be motor, sensory, autonomic, or any combination of the three. Motor symptoms may be limited to one part of the body. Sensory seizures may result in tingling or numbness that spreads or "marches" to different parts of the limb or body

(depending on the location of the seizure activity in the brain) or may involve the special senses, producing auditory (buzzing sounds), olfactory, or visual manifestations (flashing lights). Autonomic symptoms may include pupillary (pupil dilation), skin (diaphoresis, flushing), or respiratory changes.

Complex partial seizures have many different combinations of cognitive, affective, and psychomotor symptoms. Either loss or alteration of consciousness may occur when the seizure begins. After the attack, the individual may feel drowsy or confused. At the onset of impairment of consciousness, the individual often displays automatisms. Aggressive behavior may be displayed as well, especially if bystanders attempt to restrain the individual. Complex partial seizures often last several minutes and may be followed by a postictal state.

Partial seizures that are secondarily generalized are the third subtype of partial seizures. This category comprises seizures that begin as simple partial seizures then progress to involve both brain hemispheres. Once generalized, these seizures are clinically similar to primary generalized seizures.

Aura/Prodrome. Some people may have a subjective sense of an impending seizure. This **prodromal period** may be characterized by any one of several phenomena such as a type of myoclonic jerking, headache, lethargy, mood alterations, palpitations, or epigastric sensations, which may precede the actual seizure by several hours. In about half of cases there is some type of movement or odd sensory experience (visual, auditory, olfactory, or gustatory) that occurs seconds before consciousness is lost and that is remembered by the individual after recovery from the seizure. This experience is known as an *aura.* Although the individual may interpret the aura as an indication that a seizure is about to occur, in fact it is the beginning of the seizure episode. Auras can be significant, as they may be a clue to the location of the epileptogenic focus.

Diagnosis and Treatment. The diagnosis and management of seizure disorders is based on patient history, physical and neurologic examination results, and electroencephalographic studies. Electroencephalograms (EEGs) may be normal between seizures, so activation techniques (sleep deprivation, hyperventilation) may be used to elicit the pathologic mechanism. Laboratory studies are frequently used to investigate possible metabolic abnormalities as well as therapeutic serum levels in those already using anticonvulsant drugs. Lumbar puncture may be utilized when there is a suspicion of a CNS infection.[4] Initial studies ruling out structural causes may include computed tomography (CT) or magnetic resonance imaging (MRI).

Treatment of an individual experiencing a seizure is concentrated on maintaining an airway and protecting the individual from injury. Recording the course of the seizure episode is useful for identifying the location of the epileptogenic focus and for noting any change in the patient's seizure pattern. This data is useful in treatment planning. The information recorded should include the time of onset and duration of the seizure, precipitating factors, presence of a prodrome or aura, sequence of seizure activity, autonomic signs, level of consciousness, and postictal state.

Long-term treatment depends on the cause of the seizure disorder. In seizures resulting from a metabolic abnormality, infection, or tumor, the precipitating source is removed. If the seizures are due to irreversible or unidentifiable factors, anticonvulsant medications specific to the type of seizure are the best management. The decision to treat after one seizure is controversial when an identifiable cause has not been found.[4] The objective of therapy is to achieve seizure control with a minimum of side effects. Medication is continued until there have been no seizures for at least 3 years and is then gradually withdrawn.[2] If seizures continue despite treatment at a maximal dose of a single medication, a second agent is added and the dosage is increased depending on patient tolerance. The first drug is then gradually withdrawn. Anticonvulsant medication is a form of control, not a cure.

Treatment also includes patient education in the avoidance of activating factors (e.g., stress, loud noise, alcohol). Patients should be advised to avoid situations that could be dangerous or life threatening if seizures should reoccur (e.g., driving or swimming). State laws vary widely on when patients with seizure disorder are allowed to drive again.[4] Compliance to the treatment plan is sometimes difficult due to side effects of pharmacologic interventions. However, most patients are able to achieve optimal seizure control and lead active and productive lives. For some patients with seizure disorder uncontrolled by medications, surgical excision of the seizure focus may be an option. Vagal nerve stimulation for adults and adolescents with partial-onset seizures may provide an alternative approach to treatment.

KEY POINTS

- Seizure disorder is characterized by recurrent episodes of abnormal electrical impulses in the brain. Some individuals appear to have a lower-than-normal threshold for seizure activity. Seizure activity may occur in anyone, given the right conditions. Head injury, meningitis, brain tumors, and metabolic disorders (electrolyte imbalance, fever, acidosis) may predispose an individual to having seizures.
- Initiation of seizure activity may occur in a particular brain area (the epileptogenic focus). Nearby and distant neurons may then be recruited into the seizure. When sufficient neurons are involved, the seizure becomes clinically evident as involuntary movement or unusual sensations.
- Seizures are classified as partial or generalized. Partial seizures involve a part of the brain; generalized seizures involve the entire brain at the onset. Partial seizures are further classified as simple, in which consciousness is retained, and complex, in which consciousness is impaired. Seizures may begin as partial and then generalize to affect the entire brain. Generalized seizures include absence, myoclonic, atonic, and tonic-clonic types. Consciousness is always impaired in generalized seizures.

- Status epilepticus is a serious condition in which seizures occur continuously, resulting in intense brain metabolism. Ischemic brain damage may result. Management of a seizure in progress is aimed at maintaining the individual's airway and protecting the person from trauma. Close attention is given to the quality and progression of seizure activity. Anticonvulsant medications are used to suppress seizure activity.

Dementia. **Dementia** is not a specific disease but rather a syndrome associated with many pathologic processes. It is characterized by progressive deterioration and continuing decline of memory and other cognitive changes. Personality and behavior changes accompany the cognitive deterioration. Judgment, abstract thinking and complex task performance are all affected. The onset of dementia may be insidious, and the affected individual may initially appear uninterested or lacking initiative. Many demented patients have **agnosia** or lack of insight into their cognitive deficiencies.

Approximately 10% of adults 65 years of age or older and 50% of those older than 95 have some form of dementia.[5] In 2007, there were more than 5 million individuals in the United States living with Alzheimer disease, and it is estimated that someone in America develops Alzheimer disease every 7 seconds.[6] Alzheimer disease accounts for 50% to 60% of all dementias, while vascular dementia is common in 15% to 20% of demented individuals.[5]

Etiology. Multiple causes/types of dementia exist, and a full discussion of each is beyond the scope of this chapter. Some examples of dementia-causing illness include alcoholism, intracranial tumor, normal-pressure hydrocephalus, Parkinson disease, Lewy body disease, Huntington disease, multiple sclerosis, Pick disease, Creutzfeldt-Jakob disease, and bovine spongiform encephalopathy (mad cow disease). Unfortunately these also can occur in combination causing severe disease. Because Alzheimer- and vascular-type dementias are the first and second most common causes of dementia, they will be discussed in detail. The subsequent discussion of treatment of individuals with dementia will be more general because the care issues are similar regardless of type of dementia.

It is important to consider all potential causes of cognitive change when dealing with patients with mental status change. Both delirium and depression in the elderly can cause signs and symptoms that resemble those of dementia. Delirium is a global mental dysfunction that includes disturbed consciousness, decreased awareness of the environment, inability to maintain attention, disrupted sleep-wake cycles, drowsiness, restlessness, emotional lability, incoherence, and hallucinations.[2] Symptoms of delirium tend to have an abrupt onset and may fluctuate often, becoming worse at night. Delirium can result from numerous causes such as medication/polypharmacy, metabolic abnormalities, nutritional deficiencies, and infection, among others. Delirium may occur more frequently in individuals with an underlying dementing illness.

Pathogenesis. The hallmark pathophysiologic changes associated with Alzheimer disease include intracellular neurofibrillary tangles and extracellular amyloid (senile) plaques (Figure 45-1). Due to these changes, diffuse neuronal damage and brain atrophy occurs.[7] The brain of a patient with Alzheimer disease often weighs less that 1,000 grams at autopsy compared to normal weight of 1380 grams. The temporoparietal and anterior frontal regions of the brain are chiefly affected exhibiting enlarged sulci, ventricles, and atrophic gyri (Figure 45-2). Neurofibrillary tangles are composed of helical filaments formed from hyperphosphorylated protein tau, also known as neural thread protein.[8] In the central nervous system, neural thread proteins bind and help stabilize microtubules (the cell's internal support structure or skeleton). Inflammatory changes, lipid abnormalities, and aging are among the processes thought to be responsible for activating the phosphorylating enzymes altering the structure of the tau proteins.[9] Neurofibrillary tangles are well correlated with dementia, but are not specific just to Alzheimer disease and are found in other neurodegenerative disease processes.[8] The second, but most specific change in the brain of patients with Alzheimer disease is the deposition of extracellular amyloid plaques.

It is not known whether amyloid plaques cause Alzheimer disease or result from it. The number of senile plaques seems to correlate with the severity of disease. In plaques, β-amyloid is a protein fragment snipped from a larger protein— **amyloid precursor protein (APP)**—during metabolism. APP is a member of a large family of proteins that are associated with cell membranes. During metabolism, APP becomes embedded in the membrane of the nerve cell, partly inside and partly outside the cell. While APP is embedded in the cell membrane, proteases cleave APP apart. β-Amyloid is produced only when the cleavage happens at the wrong place in APP.

After β-amyloid is formed, it is not known how it moves through or around the nerve cells. In the final stages of its

Plaque surrounding amyloid deposit   Neurons filled with neurofibrillary tangles

FIGURE 45-1 Amyloid plaques and neurofibrillary tangles. (Courtesy James King-Holmes and Science Photo Library.)

FIGURE 45-2 Axial (horizontal) CT scan section through the temporal lobes. **A,** Normal. **B,** Alzheimer disease. (Courtesy James King-Holmes and Science Photo Library.)

journey, it joins with other β-amyloid filaments and fragments of dead and dying neurons to form the dense, insoluble plaques that are a hallmark of Alzheimer disease in brain tissue. Inflammatory processes including acute phase response, complement activation, and accumulation of activated microglia and astrocytes accompany the amyloid deposition and neurofibrillary tangle formation.[9,10] The accumulation of β-amyloid also causes oxidation of lipids, activation of apoptotic genes, disruption of cell membranes, and excitotoxicity from the neurotransmitter glutamate.[7,9] Recent Alzheimer research is suggesting that the formation of neurofibrillary tangles and amyloid plaques are the body's compensatory mechanism to protect neurons from oxidative stress, but eventually result in axonal cell damage and death.[7,9]

Much interest exists in the neurotransmitter systems in relation to Alzheimer disease. Damage in Alzheimer disease involves changes in three mechanisms: nerve cell communication, metabolism, and repair. Several studies have found abnormalities in the cholinergic system, including reduced activity of choline acetyltransferase (the enzyme necessary for acetylcholine synthesis) and decreased acetylcholine synthesis (Figure 45-3). Some researchers believe that β-amyloid may be responsible for lower choline levels in nerve cells and decreased acetylcholine levels. The degeneration of cells in the nucleus basalis, a band of gray matter in the ventral portion of the medulla oblongata, has also been linked to diminished levels of acetylcholine in the cerebral cortex, a finding that provides further evidence for the significant role of the cholinergic system in Alzheimer disease.[11,12]

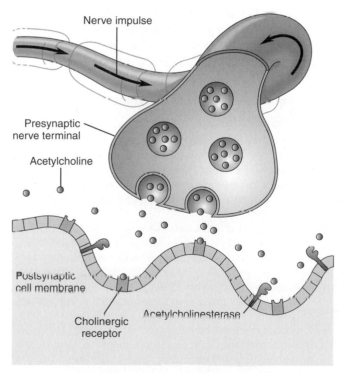

FIGURE 45-3 The cholinergic synapse.

Labels on figure:
Nerve impulse
Presynaptic nerve terminal
Acetylcholine
Postsynaptic cell membrane
Cholinergic receptor
Acetylcholinesterase

Vascular dementia results from single cerebrovascular insults such as cerebral infarction, from multiple lacunar infarcts or from microvascular pathology. Microvascular insults may not show any localizing clinical symptoms and may be found incidentally on brain imaging. However, the presence of these also does not automatically mean a diagnosis of vascular dementia.[13] Symptoms of vascular dementia are identical to Alzheimer dementia. Most research/reports present vascular dementia and Alzheimer dementia as entirely separate entities; however there is increasing evidence that particularly in elderly patients the brain lesions associated with both often coexist. There is emerging evidence that the cascade of events leading to the development of Alzheimer disease plaques and tangles may be due to ischemic insults of cerebrovascular disease.[14,15]

The primary risk factors for the development of Alzheimer disease include age and family history. Epidemiologic studies show that individuals who have an affected first-degree relative with Alzheimer disease have a fourfold greater risk of developing the disease. The risk is greater if there are individuals in more than one generation with the disease.[16] Three main genes have been identified and are thought to be responsible for autosomal dominant familial Alzheimer disease. Presenilin I, Presenilin II, and APP are believed to increase Amyloid beta protein.[16] These genes are rare, accounting for only 5% of Alzheimer disease cases, usually the early onset variant.[13,14] The major gene associated with late onset Alzheimer disease is apolipoprotein e 4 (APOe4). By age 85, those who are homozygous for the APOe4 allele have a 50% to 90% chance of developing Alzheimer disease. Those who are heterozygous have a 45% chance of developing the disease. Carrying the APOe4 gene has also been associated with increased risk of atherosclerosis and cerebrovascular disease, strengthening the link between Alzheimer disease and vascular dementia.[13,14] Lifestyle has also been linked to the risk of Alzheimer disease. Head trauma, diabetes, and depression have been linked to an increased incidence of the disease as well as marital status, urban living, and inactive mental and physical lifestyle.[13] Risk factors for vascular dementia include those for stroke, hypertension, and diabetes.[13,14] Clearly both vascular dementia and Alzheimer disease include a complex interplay of genetic, environmental and lifestyle factors.

Clinical Manifestations. Regardless of when patients first present with dementia, it is likely that brain disease has been present for quite some time. Most patients experience a gradual onset with a chronic progressive decline in cognitive functioning. There is memory loss, especially in short-term memory, whereas long-term memory may be preserved. Thinking ability declines, and there is a decreasing ability to function at work and in social settings. Anxiety and agitation are common. As the disease progresses, individuals have increasing difficulty with judgment, problem solving, and communication. Assistance may be necessary for completing activities of daily living (ADLs). Difficulty with eating and swallowing, and weight loss are common. Loss of bladder and bowel control and eventual complete loss of the ability to ambulate occurs in the late stages. Accidents and infection are common causes of death.[10]

Diagnosis and Treatment. The initial evaluation of a patient thought to have dementia of any type begins with a complete history and physical examination. This should address the patient's overall general health and any coexisting medical conditions. All manageable causes for dementia or delirium should be ruled out. It is recommended that the evaluation should include a complete blood cell count, chemistry panel, thyroid function, vitamin B_{12} levels, and syphilis serology. Other testing such as Lyme serology, HIV, urinalysis with culture/sensitivity, heavy metal assays, sedimentation rate, and other vitamin levels may be warranted in certain patient situations.[5] Other evaluations such as a chest x-ray and lumbar puncture may also be helpful.[2,5,8] Neuroimaging may include CT and MRI/MRA, which may identify vascular disease, normal pressure hydrocephalus, tumors, abscesses, or subdural hematoma.[5] PET (positron emission tomography) scans are not routinely recommended at this point, but show promise in identifying Alzheimer disease when combined with a history of genetic risk.[5,8] Mental status examinations, the clock drawing test, and tests of functional status are recommended.[5] A current list of the patient's medications, including over-the-counter medications, must also be reviewed. Medications with anticholinergic actions/side effects are a common cause of changes in cognitive functioning in the elderly.

Early diagnosis and intervention is key in the management of dementia. The financial and legal ramifications of dementia can be devastating to patients and their families and caregivers. If the diagnosis is made before the onset of severe cognitive disability, the patient can be involved in decisions regarding long-term care, power of attorney, and living will issues. Early diagnosis is also vital to initiating therapy as early as possible.

Currently, two classes of drugs are approved by the Food and Drug Administration for the treatment of Alzheimer disease. The first class is the acetylcholinesterase inhibitors: tacrine (Cognex), donepezil (Aricept), rivastigmine (Exelon), and galantamine (Reminyl). These agents are indicated for use in patients with mild to moderate Alzheimer disease. Although not a cure, the acetylcholinesterase inhibitors have been shown to stabilize cognitive function and slow progression of the illness.[12,17] Acetylcholinesterase inhibitors have also been shown to improve cognitive functioning in patients with vascular dementia.[14]

The second class of drugs used in the treatment of Alzheimer disease is known as the N-methyl-D-aspartate (NMDA) receptor antagonists. Currently only one drug in this class is available in the United States. Memantine (Namenda) is indicated for the treatment of moderate to severe Alzheimer-type dementia. This drug blocks stimulation by the neuroexcitatory transmitter glutamate. Again, this medication is not a cure, but slows progression of the disease.[8] Studies using combination therapy of acetylcholinesterase inhibitors and NMDA antagonists are showing modest improvement in cognitive functioning.[17] Studies using NMDA antagonists for vascular dementia have not shown conclusive benefit.[13]

Many other medications, although not approved for use in treating Alzheimer disease, are used to manage the symptoms, such as depression, sleep disturbance, agitation, and psychosis. These medications include antidepressants, anxiolytics, antipsychotics, and mood stabilizers.[18]

A variety of alternative medications have been used in the management of Alzheimer disease, including estrogen, gingko biloba, antioxidants such as vitamin E, and nonsteroidal anti-inflammatory drugs (NSAIDs). The data regarding estrogen therapy shows no benefit in slowing disease progression or improving cognitive functioning and may increase risk for CVA and vascular dementia.[17] Early observational research is showing reduced occurrence of Alzheimer disease in patients using NSAIDs and aspirin. However, randomized controlled trials using prednisone in Alzheimer patients failed to show any improvement in symptoms.[12] Studies also do not conclusively support the use of gingko biloba, and concerns of adverse affects have been reported.[12,17] Research is currently underway exploring the role of oxidative stress and homocysteine levels and Alzheimer disease. Use of antioxidants, vitamin B, and folate may prove useful in the prevention of the disease. Early research on the use of 3-hydroxy-3-methylglutaryl coenzyme A (HMG-CoA) reductase inhibitors, the lipid-lowering medications also known as the *statins,* is showing promise in reducing the risk of the developing Alzheimer disease and vascular dementia, especially those with APOe4 genetic changes.[14]

Other treatments for dementia include optimal management of other coexisting illnesses, interventions aimed at wellness, nutritional management, and protection from injury. In early stages of the disease, most patients are cared for at home, often by family members. It is important that the home environment be safe and that there be measures in place to control wandering. Consistent routines and familiar surroundings allow the patient to feel more comfortable and experience less confusion. As the disease progresses, the individual with dementia may have to be placed in an alternative living situation such as a nursing home or assisted-living program. Caring for the caregivers of patients with dementia is important.

KEY POINTS

- Dementia refers to progressive degeneration of cognitive function due to organic causes. In many instances the cause is unknown. There are limited definitive treatments for dementia, none of which are a cure. It is important to first rule out manageable causes of mental impairment.
- The dementia of Alzheimer disease is characterized by degeneration of neurons in temporal and frontal lobes, brain atrophy, amyloid plaques, and neurofibrillary tangles. The synthesis of brain acetylcholine is deficient. The cause of Alzheimer disease remains unknown, although genetic factors and environmental triggers are suspected.
- The behavioral problems of individuals with Alzheimer disease progresses from forgetfulness to total inability for self-care. Depression and psychosis may be significant.

Parkinson Disease. Parkinson disease is a disorder of mobility that affects 1.5 million Americans. It is estimated that 60,000 new cases are diagnosed each year. While it usually develops after age 65, 15% of those diagnosed are under age 50.[2,19]

Etiology. Parkinson disease may be idiopathic or acquired. Idiopathic Parkinson disease is that in which no demonstrable cause is identified. Common causes of acquired **parkinsonism** include infection, intoxication, and trauma.[2] Typically, parkinsonism due to drug toxicity evolves rapidly, unlike the slow insidious onset of the idiopathic disease. Side effects of drugs of the phenothiazine class (e.g., chlorpromazine, prochlorperazine, and thioridazine) and butyrophenone class (e.g., haloperidol) may manifest in a parkinsonian syndrome at toxic levels. Discontinuing the medication generally results in improvement in the symptoms. However, the additional use of the anticholinergic antiparkinsonian drugs may aid in more rapid recovery. The rest of this discussion of Parkinson disease refers to the most common idiopathic type.

Pathogenesis. Parkinson disease results from degeneration of the pigmented dopaminergic neurons found in the substantia nigra (Figure 45-4) and, to a lesser extent, neurons elsewhere in the brain. Eosinophilic cytoplasmic inclusions known as Lewy bodies may be found in the surviving neurons. Incidentally, Lewy bodies are found along with amyloid plaques at autopsy in the brains of some patients with a severe form of dementia. This suggests a possible link with Alzheimer disease. The exact cause of this degeneration is unknown, but oxidative stress, genetics, and environmental toxins have been implicated.[20]

A number of genes have been identified as having a role in the development of Parkinson disease. In particular, identification of a mutation in the α-synuclein gene has become the focus of much interest. Although mutations of the gene are a rare cause of Parkinson disease, α-synuclein is abundant in neurons, specifically in presynaptic terminals, and is a major component of Lewy bodies.[20] Another gene identified in the development of Parkinson disease is *parkin*. This gene is thought to have a role in protein degradation and clearance. Mutations in this gene may be associated with abnormal protein accumulations within the neuron.[20] Although genes have received much attention in Parkinson disease research, environmental factors have also been studied. High caffeine intake has been found to have an inverse relationship to the risk of developing the disorder.[21] Long-term exposure to the pesticide rotenone and the herbicide paraquat have been linked to increasing risk for Parkinson disease.[22] Whatever the cause of the degeneration of the dopaminergic cells, 75% to 80% of the neurons have died before any symptoms of the disease become apparent.

Clinical Manifestations and Treatment. Because of the insidious onset, earlier evidence of Parkinson disease may be discovered in a thorough health history. Frequently, the very early signs of the disorder (loss of flexibility, aching, and fatigue) are overlooked by the patient or are attributed to the aging process. Initially, symptoms are usually worse on one side of the body and then progress to involve both sides. Tremor is often the first symptom recognized that prompts patients to seek treatment. The tremor is generally at rest, unilateral affecting distal extremities. Hand tremors may be described as pill-rolling movements. Attempts to passively move the extremities are met with cogwheel rigidity. As Parkinson disease progresses, the tremor will often become bilateral/more generalized. Additional early signs of the disease include bradykinesia, rigidity, hypokinesia, loss of facial expression, and infrequent eye blinking (Figure 45-5). Again, these symptoms may be overlooked by patients but are usually apparent to observant family members.

As the disease progresses, additional functional changes are noted. The patient's handwriting may become small (micrographia) and cramped, with evidence of tremor. Speech may become low in volume, monotonous, and dysarthric. There may be a mumbling quality to the speech. The effects of bradykinesia are evident in the patient's swallowing function, ability to initiate activity, and mobility. Swallowing becomes delayed so much so that the individual may drool, and patients are at risk for aspiration. The effect of the disease on the ability to initiate activity is evident when the individual rises from a chair or begins to walk from a standing-still position. However, many people with Parkinson disease are able to act quickly in times of emergency, such as fire. This phenomenon is known as paradoxical kinesia.

Additional difficulties in mobility are evident from the lack of spontaneous position changes while the individual is sitting in one position, from the decreased or absent arm swing while the individual is walking, and from the shuffling gait. Impairment of postural reflexes presents particular safety problems for the individual with Parkinson disease in

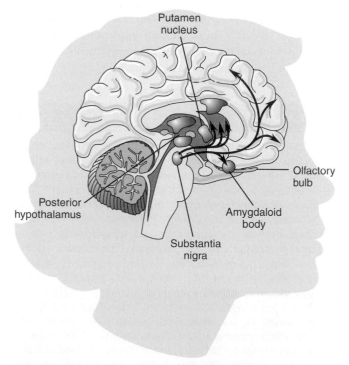

FIGURE 45-4 Dopaminergic neurons and their pathways in the human brain.

Tremor

Masklike face

Arms flexed
at elbows
and wrists

Tremor

Stooped
posture

Rigidity

Hips and
knees
slightly
flexed

Short,
shuffling
steps

FIGURE 45-5 Clinical manifestations of Parkinson disease. (From Monahan FD, Neighbors M: *Phipp's Medical-surgical nursing: health and illness perspectives,* ed 8, Philadelphia, 2007, Saunders, p 1446.)

maintaining balance, as evidenced by propulsive or retropulsive gaits. Involvement of the autonomic nervous system may result in orthostatic hypotension, which adds yet another risk to the individual's health. Because of these various impairments, falls are a common problem. Depression is present in many patients with Parkinson disease. Daytime sleepiness is also common as well as sleep disturbances and restless leg syndrome.[21] Dementia is prevalent in patients with Parkinson disease.

There is no known cure for Parkinson disease. Treatments are aimed at slowing the progression of the disease and managing symptoms. The mainstay of Parkinson therapy has been aimed at increasing the level of dopamine in the CNS. Dopamine precursors such as levodopa are one approach to increasing dopamine levels. Dopamine itself cannot be used because it does not cross the blood-brain barrier efficiently. Outside the CNS, levodopa is metabolized to dopamine and

then to adrenaline and noradrenaline, which cause nausea and hypotension. To minimize these side effects, levodopa is combined with carbidopa. This agent blocks the conversion of levodopa to dopamine in the periphery, allowing it to cross the blood-brain barrier.[23] Long-term use of levodopa has been associated with "on-off" phenomena (in which the action of the drug suddenly stops, leaving the patient with sudden onset of symptoms) or abnormal movements called *dyskinesias.* Other medications aimed at increasing the level of dopamine in the CNS include dopamine agonists (pramipexole, ropinirole); medications to slow the metabolism of dopamine (monoamine oxidase inhibitors such as selegiline, catechol-O-methyltransferase inhibitors); and others, such as amantadine, which has been shown to be helpful with akinesia and dyskinesia).[23,24] Anticholinergic medications may help with tremor, rigidity, or drooling.

Surgical options for the management of Parkinson disease have received much recent attention. Deep brain stimulation involves the surgical implantation of a high frequency thalamic electrical stimulator that interrupts the tremor-causing nerve impulses and can decrease the need for Parkinson medication.[23,24] Tissue transplantation of adrenal tissue or fetal brain tissue in an attempt to increase the level of dopamine in the CNS is very controversial and has not been consistently shown to improve the symptoms of Parkinson disease.[2]

Ablative surgical techniques of thalamotomy and pallidotomy create small lesions in the thalamus or pallidum; this can improve rigidity, tremor, and bradykinesia.[2,23] Symptoms are better controlled with medication following the surgery. These surgical techniques are considered for patients who have been unresponsive to the medical treatments or who are unable to tolerate the side effects. These surgical techniques have high morbidity associated with them and are rarely used. Early antioxidant research shows modest improvement in symptoms in patients taking coenzyme Q_{10} supplements.[24] Genetic research on Parkinson disease continues.

KEY POINTS

- Parkinson disease may be idiopathic or a consequence of the use of certain drugs. Dopamine deficiency in the basal ganglia (substantia nigra, caudate, and putamen) is associated with symptoms of motor impairment. Difficulty initiating and controlling movements results in akinesia, tremor, and rigidity. Tremor occurs at rest, and hand tremors may be described as pill-rolling movements. Attempts to passively move the extremities are met with cogwheel rigidity. There is a general lack of movement, loss of facial expression, drooling, propulsive gait, and absent arm swing.

- Treatment is aimed at restoring brain dopamine levels or activity by administration of dopamine precursors, dopamine agonists, monoamine oxidase inhibitors, and anticholinergics. Antidepressant therapy may also help alleviate depression, and surgical procedures may be helpful for motor symptoms.

Cerebral Palsy

Etiology and Pathogenesis. Cerebral palsy refers to a diverse group of crippling syndromes that appears during childhood and involves permanent, nonprogressive damage to the developing brain. Such damage occurs during fetal development; before, during, or shortly after birth; or during early infancy. Damage occurs in the upper motor neurons that control voluntary and involuntary muscle movement. The symptoms of this damage remain for life. Cerebral palsy is classified on the basis of neurologic signs and symptoms, with the major types involving spasticity, ataxia, dyskinesia, or a combination. Cerebral palsy is one of the most common crippling disorders of childhood, with an incidence of between 2 and 2.5 of 1,000 births in the United States.[25] Etiologic factors include prenatal infections or diseases of the mother; mechanical trauma to the head before, during, or after birth; nerve-damaging poisons; or reduced oxygen supply to the brain. Neonatal hypoglycemia, **kernicterus,** prematurity, and low birth weight are also risk factors. Often the cause is multifactorial, and in 70% to 80% of cases a single cause cannot be identified.[25,26]

Clinical Manifestations. Spastic cerebral palsy manifests with hypertonia, prolonged primitive reflexes, exaggerated deep-tendon reflexes, clonus, rigidity of the extremities, scoliosis, and contractures. This type of cerebral palsy is the most common and accounts for greater than 70% of cases.[26] Spastic paralysis often affects one entire side of the body (hemiplegia), both legs (paraplegia), both legs and one arm (triplegia), or all four extremities (quadriplegia). A "scissors" gait and toe walking are common. Dyskinetic/athetoid cerebral palsy manifests with extreme difficulty in purposeful movement and fine-motor coordination. Movements are slow, jerky, uncontrolled, and abrupt, resulting from injury to the **basal ganglia** or **extrapyramidal tracts.** The uncontrolled movements may increase during times of stress and disappear during sleep. This is the second most common form of cerebral palsy and accounts for approximately 10% to 20% of cases.[25,27] Ataxic cerebral palsy is associated with gait disturbances and instability. The infant with this type of cerebral palsy may have hypotonia at birth, but stiffness of the trunk muscles develops by late infancy. Persistence of truncal stiffness affects the child's gait and ability to maintain equilibrium. Pure ataxic cerebral palsy is rare. This palsy denotes maldevelopment of the cerebrum or its pathways, which if severe may be associated with significant cognitive impairment.[10] More typically, a child will have a mixed disorder with clinical manifestations of each of the types.

Children with cerebral palsy often have neurologic complications such as seizures (35% to 50%), intellectual difficulties ranging from mild to severe (50% to 75%), and visual problems (50%).[25] Other associated clinical manifestations include hearing impairment, communication disorders, respiratory problems, bowel and bladder problems, and orthopedic disabilities.

Treatment. There is no cure for cerebral palsy, and the goal of management is to increase functionality. Treatment varies according to the nature and extent of brain damage. Due to problems with muscle spasticity and contracture, muscle relaxation is a large part of therapy. Muscle relaxant medications are common. Several studies have also supported the use of *botulinum toxin* (Botox) to reduce pain and increase joint range of motion.[28] Anticonvulsant drugs are necessary when seizures are among the symptoms of the disorder. Orthopedic surgery, casts, braces, and traction may be useful to correct some types of associated disability. A comprehensive rehabilitation program including early muscle training and special exercises may help the child with cerebral palsy lead a more productive life.

KEY POINTS

- Cerebral palsy refers to a diverse group of crippling syndromes that appear during childhood and involve permanent, nonprogressive damage to motor control areas of the brain.
- Cerebral palsy may be classified on the basis of neurologic signs and symptoms, with the major types involving spasticity, ataxia, dyskinesia, or a mix of one or more of the three.
- Etiologic factors include prenatal infections or diseases of the mother; mechanical trauma to the head before, during, or after birth; exposure to nerve-damaging poisons; or reduced oxygen supply to the brain.
- Treatment varies according to the nature and extent of brain damage. Muscle relaxants, anticonvulsant drugs, orthopedic surgery, casts, braces, and traction are among the therapies used.

Hydrocephalus

Etiology. Hydrocephalus is a condition caused by abnormal accumulation of cerebrospinal fluid (CSF) in the cerebral ventricular system. Figure 45-6 illustrates the normal flow of CSF. Hydrocephalus is generally associated with a congenital defect, usually a neural tube defect. Viral infections or other neurotoxic agents acquired during pregnancy have been implicated with the congenital forms. It also occurs occasionally in adults and elderly persons as a consequence of mass lesions, trauma, hemorrhage, or infections such as meningitis. There are three types of hydrocephalus: (1) normal-pressure hydrocephalus; (2) obstructive hydrocephalus; and (3) communicating hydrocephalus.

Normal-pressure hydrocephalus is a condition in which CSF volume increases without change in intracranial pressure because brain tissue has been lost. The cause of normal pressure hydrocephalus remains unknown, but it is thought to be from an abnormality of the normal absorption of CSF. Ventricles become distended, compressing brain tissue and the cerebral vessels. There is no net change in intracranial pressure. Patients with this form of hydrocephalus demonstrate a triad of symptoms: gait instability, urinary incontinence, and dementia.[29] If the problem is identified quickly, symptoms may improve/resolve with appropriate treatment.

Superior
sagittal sinus

Choroid plexus   Dura mater   Interventricular
of third ventricle   foramen

Subarachnoid
space

Arachnoid
villi

Cerebral
aqueduct

Choroid plexus
of fourth ventricle

Central canal
of spinal cord

Foramen of
Magendie

FIGURE 45-6 The ventricular system of the brain and the distribution of the cerebrospinal fluid (CSF). CSF is formed in the ventricles, passes to the subarachnoid space outside the brain and spinal cord, and moves through small valvelike structures into the large veins of the head.

In obstructive hydrocephalus, there is an obstruction at some point in either the intraventricular or extraventricular pathways of the ventricular system. The cause of obstructive hydrocephalus usually is a congenital abnormality, such as stenosis of the foramina of the fourth ventricle or spina bifida cystica. Other etiologic factors include intraventricular hemorrhage, which is a common complication in premature infants.[10]

Communicating hydrocephalus (sometimes referred to as *acquired communicating hydrocephalus*) is identified by an abnormality in the capacity to absorb fluid from the subarachnoid space. There is no obstruction to the flow of fluid between the ventricles. Infections, trauma, and tumors have been identified as etiologic factors.[10]

Pathogenesis and Clinical Manifestations. Usually the obstructive type of hydrocephalus is caused by a block in the aqueduct of Sylvius, resulting from premature closure before birth in affected babies or from a brain tumor at any age (Figure 45-7). As fluid is formed by the choroid plexus in the two lateral and the third ventricles, the volumes of these three ventricles increase greatly. This flattens the brain into a thin shell against the skull. In neonates, the increased pressure also causes the whole head to swell because the skull bones have not fused.

The communicating type of hydrocephalus is usually caused by blockage of fluid flow in the **subarachnoid space**

Ischemia and
necrosis of
brain tissue

Dilated lateral
ventricles

Third ventricle

Flow of CSF
blocked here

FIGURE 45-7 Hydrocephalus. *CSF,* Cerebrospinal fluid. (From Gould BE: *Pathophysiology for the health professions,* ed 2, Philadelphia, 2002, Saunders, p 490.)

around the basal regions of the brain or blockage of the **arachnoid villi** themselves. Fluid therefore collects both inside the ventricles and on the outside of the brain. If it occurs in infants when the skull is still pliable and can be stretched, the head swells tremendously.

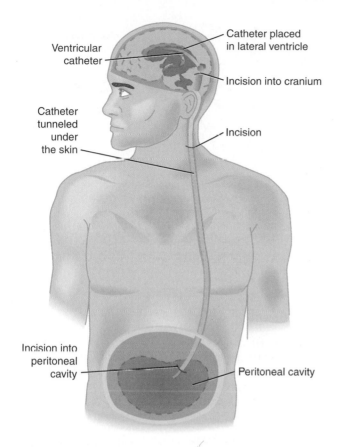

FIGURE 45-8 Ventriculoperitoneal shunt placed for chronic hydrocephalus. (From Black JM et al: *Medical-surgical nursing: clinical management for positive outcomes,* ed 8, Philadelphia, 2008, Saunders, p 1933.)

FIGURE 45-9 The cerebrum and the cerebellum work together to control muscles. Impulses from the cerebrum travel simultaneously to skeletal muscle and to the cerebellum. The cerebellum compares the intended movement with the actual movement and sends impulses to both the cerebrum and the muscle tissue, coordinating and smoothing muscle activity. (From Thibodeau GA, Patton KT: *Anatomy and physiology,* ed 4, St Louis, 2003, Mosby, p 388.)

Treatment. Medical treatment has been used with only limited success in controlling the secretion of CSF and relieving hydrocephalus. The most effective treatment is surgical correction employing a shunting technique. The basic components of the shunt are a ventricular catheter, a valve, and a distal catheter. Multiple perforations along the ventricular catheter permit the drainage of fluid from the ventricle. The valve is constructed so that fluid will flow in one direction only, and some valves have a pumping chamber to facilitate drainage. The distal catheter may be positioned at any of a number of sites, the most common being the peritoneal cavity (ventriculoperitoneal shunt) (Figure 45-8). The shunt thus extends all the way from one of the ventricles to the peritoneal cavity where the fluid can then be absorbed and excreted. Another surgical approach is endoscopic third ventriculostomy. This involves making a hole in the third ventricle to allow free flow of CSF into the basal cisterns for reabsorption. This surgery is used for obstructive hydrocephalus.[30] It should be emphasized that the correlation between degree of hydrocephalus and impaired cognitive function often results from additional complications, such as severe congenital malformations, acute or chronic infections, or progressive brain tumors.

KEY POINTS

- Hydrocephalus is a condition characterized by abnormal accumulation of CSF in the cerebral ventricular system.
- There are three types of hydrocephalus: normal-pressure hydrocephalus, due to an increased volume of CSF without change in CSF pressure; obstructive hydrocephalus, due to an obstruction to the flow of CSF; and communicating hydrocephalus, in which absorption of CSF is abnormal.
- The most effective treatment for hydrocephalus is surgical correction employing a shunt.

Cerebellar Disorders. The cerebellum performs three general functions in the control of skeletal muscles: (1) together with activity of the cerebral cortex, it coordinates the activities of muscle groups to produce skilled movement; (2) it functions below the level of consciousness to maintain posture and make movements smooth, steady, efficient, and coordinated; and (3) it controls skeletal muscles to maintain balance (see Chapter 43). Figure 45-9 illustrates the cerebrum and cerebellum working together to coordinate muscle movement.

Impulses from the motor control areas of the cerebrum travel down the corticospinal tract and through peripheral nerves to skeletal muscle tissue. Simultaneously, the impulses go to the cerebellum. The cerebellum compares the motor commands of the cerebrum to information coming from receptors in the muscle. In effect, the cerebellum compares the intended movement to the actual movement. Impulses then travel from the cerebellum to both the cerebrum and the muscle tissue to adjust or coordinate the movements to produce the intended action.[10]

Etiology and Clinical Manifestations. Cerebellar disorders may have myriad causes. Abscess, hemorrhage, tumors, trauma, viral infection, and chronic alcoholism have been implicated. Identification and eradication of the causal agent determines treatment and prognosis. The clinical manifestations of cerebellar disorders primarily include **ataxia** (muscle incoordination), hypotonia, intention tremors, and disturbances of gait and balance.[10] Disturbances of gait and balance vary, depending on the muscle groups involved. The walk, for instance, is often characterized by staggering or lurching and by a clumsy manner of raising the foot too high and bringing it down with a clap. Loss of cerebellar function does not result in paralysis.[10]

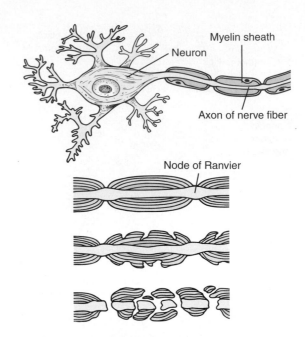

FIGURE 45-10 Changes in the nerve sheath, as seen in multiple sclerosis. Myelin is made by the oligodendrocyte and coats nerves, facilitating nervous impulse. In patients with multiple sclerosis, the myelin degenerates in patches, causing nerve transmission to become erratic. (From Black JM et al: *Medical-surgical nursing: clinical management for positive outcomes,* ed 8, Philadelphia, 2008, Saunders, p 1909.)

KEY POINTS

- The cerebellum is responsible for coordinated control of muscle action, excitation and inhibition of postural reflexes, and maintenance of balance.
- Etiologic factors in cerebellar disorders may include the following: abscess, hemorrhage, tumors, trauma, viral infection, or chronic alcoholism.
- Clinical manifestations of cerebellar disorders primarily include ataxia, hypotonia, intention tremors, and disturbances of gait and balance.

SPINAL CORD AND PERIPHERAL NERVE DISORDERS

Multiple Sclerosis

Etiology. **Multiple sclerosis** is a chronic demyelinating disease of the CNS that causes significant disability in young adults. It is thought to be an autoimmune disorder that results in inflammation and scarring (sclerosis) of the myelin sheaths covering nerves. It is estimated that 400,000 Americans have MS. The age of onset ranges from 20 to 50 years, and is two to three times more common in women than in men. Epidemiologic studies show that MS occurs at a higher rate among individuals from Caucasian northern European descent and those who live in northern latitudes (above the 37th parallel). Several studies indicate that those who were born and spent the early years of life (first 15 years) in northern areas carry an increased risk of MS even if they migrate south at some time later in their lives.[31]

MS is an unpredictable disease with a wide variety of clinical presentations. Symptoms can vary from day to day, and the disease may cause only mild disability with occasional exacerbations. In some individuals, however, MS may cause extreme progressive disability. Despite great advances in research, the exact cause of MS is unknown. Genetics may have a role. Nontwin first-degree relatives have a 10% to 40% higher chance of developing MS.[31]

Pathogenesis. In MS, the **demyelination** of nerves can occur anywhere in the CNS. There does not seem to be any predictable pattern in the timing or location of the lesions. However, structures most frequently affected are the optic nerves; the oculomotor nerves; and the corticospinal, cerebellar, and posterior column systems. Figure 45-10 illustrates demyelination. Myelin facilitates nerve conduction; the inflammation and scarring that occurs with MS slows or interrupts the conduction of nerve impulses. The triggering event for this process is not understood. It is theorized that an exposure to a viral infection or environmental toxin initiates the autoimmune attack in a genetically predisposed individual. Both humoral and cellular immune factors have been implicated in demyelination. Antibodies to specific myelin proteins have been found in both the serum and CSF of MS patients. T-cell lymphocyte–mediated damage to the myelin has also been implicated in causing the autoimmune damage and sustaining inflammation.[32]

Clinical Manifestations and Treatment. Symptoms of MS vary widely and depend upon the location of damage to the myelin.

TABLE 45-1

Multiple Sclerosis Symptoms

Area of Dysfunction	Symptoms
Cranial nerve dysfunction	Blurred central vision; faded colors; blind spots (optic neuritis)
	Diplopia
	Dysphagia
	Facial weakness, numbness, pain
Motor dysfunction	Weakness
	Paralysis
	Spasticity
	Abnormal gait
Sensory dysfunction	Paresthesias
	Lhermitte sign (electric shock–like sensation radiating down spine into extremities)
	Decreased proprioception
	Decreased temperature perception
Cerebellar dysfunction	Dysarthria
	Tremor
	Incoordination
	Ataxia
	Vertigo
Bowel and bladder dysfunction	Fecal urgency, constipation, incontinence
	Urinary frequency, urgency, hesitancy, nocturia, retention, incontinence
Cognitive dysfunction	Decreased short-term memory
	Difficulty learning new information
	Word-finding trouble
	Short attention span
	Decreased concentration
	Mood alterations (depression, euphoria)
Sexual dysfunction	Women: decreased libido, decreased orgasmic ability, decreased genital sensation
	Men: erectile, orgasmic, and ejaculatory dysfunction
Fatigue	Overwhelming weakness not overcome with increased physical effort

Adapted from Inglese M: Multiple sclerosis, new insights and trends, *Am J Neuroradiol* 27:954-957, 2006; Calabresi PA: Diagnosis and management of multiple sclerosis, *Am Fam Physician* 70(10):1935-1944, 2004.

TABLE 45-2

Clinical Course of Multiple Sclerosis

Course	Characteristics
Relapsing-remitting Most common form; approximately 85% of MS patients have this form	Clearly defined exacerbations (relapses) with acute decline in neurologic function; followed by periods of partial/complete recovery and remissions; remissions may last months to years
Primary-progressive Relatively rare; approximately 10% of MS patients have this form	Slow but almost continuous decline in neurologic function; plateaus or temporary minor improvements may occur; relapses/remissions not present; severe disability develops early
Secondary-progressive Prior to use of disease-modifying drugs; approximately 50% of relapsing-remitting patients develop this form	Begins as relapsing-remitting; followed by steady decline in neurologic function with or without occasional relapses, remissions, or plateaus
Progressive-relapsing Relatively rare; approximately 5% of patients have this form	Progressive from the outset, but with clear exacerbations with or without recovery

Adapted from McPhee SJ, Papadakis MA editors: *Current medical diagnosis and treatment*, ed 46, New York, 2007, McGraw-Hill; Inglese M: Multiple sclerosis: new insights and trends, *Am J Neuroradiol* 27:954-957, 2006; National MS Society: What is MS? Available at: http://www.nationalmssociety.org.

They include impaired visual acuity or blurred vision, diplopia, weakness, numbness, tingling, extreme fatigue, imbalance, movement disorders, spasticity, coordination difficulties and gait disturbance, bladder and/or bowel difficulties, vertigo, pain, and paresthesia. Neurobehavioral symptoms may include depression, emotional lability, sexual dysfunction, as well as memory and cognitive impairment (Table 45-1). In later stages of the disease, spastic paralysis of the limbs may be present due to upper motor neuron damage. Symptoms may be exacerbated by heat, infection, trauma, and stress. Relapses are also common in the postpartum period following pregnancy.[2] There are four main categories to classify the clinical course of MS (Table 45-2).

There is no conclusive test for MS. The diagnosis is based on clinical characteristics, imaging, and laboratory evidence. Clinical characteristics include objective abnormalities of CNS function in two parts of the CNS and a temporal sequence of at least two attacks that were remitting or relapsing in nature or followed a slow stepwise progression. Advances in neuroimaging techniques have become quite useful in the diagnosis of MS. MRI of the brain and spinal cord may show presence of demyelination (plaques). CNS lesions that are disseminated in time and space (occur in different parts of the CNS at least 3 months apart) with no better explanation is one diagnostic criteria for MS.[33] Evoked potential recording of nerve stimulation in the visual and other nerve pathways may be helpful. Laboratory tests may show mild lymphocytosis and elevated serum protein, especially following an acute relapse. Elevated immunoglobulin G (IgG) in the CSF with the presence of discrete bands of IgG (oligoclonal bands) may also be present.[2,34]

There is no cure for MS. Treatment centers not only on managing the symptoms of the disease but also at minimizing the damage inflicted by the autoimmune attack on myelin. Corticosteroids such as prednisone are used to reduce edema and the inflammatory response in acute exacerbations. Recovery may be hastened by the use of these agents; however, the extent of recovery is unchanged.[2] Five drugs are currently approved by the FDA as disease-modifying agents for use in treating MS. Four are administered by injection: beta-interferon-1a (Avonex, Rebif), interferon-1b (Betaseron) and glatiramer acetate (Copaxone). These medications reduce the number of attacks in relapsing-remitting MS. A fifth medication, mitoxantrone (Novantrone) is an antineoplastic medication that has been shown to be most helpful in decreasing symptoms of progressive relapsing MS. Natalizumab (Tysabri) is a monoclonal antibody that has been shown to decrease the movement of myelin damaging auto-antibodies across the blood-brain barrier, but has been removed from general use by the FDA due to concern of adverse effects. It is being used in limited, well-controlled trials.[2,33,34,35]

Management of symptoms frequently requires participation from multiple disciplines, including medicine, nursing, speech pathology, neuropsychiatry, social services, and vocational services. Treatment with an array of medications such as antispasmodics, anticholinergics, antidepressants, and antimicrobials helps to manage symptoms. Treatment also includes avoidance of complications such as urinary tract infections, constipation/impactions, respiratory infections, and pressure sores.

Research in MS continues to examine the immune system role. Viruses such as the Epstein-Barr virus have been implicated.[32] Low levels of vitamin D have also been implicated as an associated risk factor, as this is a common finding in people living in higher latitudes.[35] The lipid-lowering medications HMG-CoA inhibitors, otherwise known as statins, have been shown to decrease the number and size of plaques in patients with MS. These agents have some action against the immune cells responsible for demyelination.[2]

KEY POINTS

- MS is a demyelinating disease of the CNS that primarily affects young adults. The risk of contracting MS is greater for persons living above the 37th parallel. The cause of MS is unknown, but immunologic abnormalities and environmental factors are suspected.
- Demyelination can occur throughout the CNS but most frequently affects the optic and oculomotor nerves and spinal nerve tracts.
- In most cases symptoms are slowly progressive, and the disease is marked by exacerbations and remissions.
- Symptoms include double vision, weakness, poor coordination, and sensory deficits. Bowel and bladder control may be lost. Memory impairment is common.
- Management is symptomatic. Short-term steroid therapy may be helpful during acute exacerbations, and immune-modifying drugs may slow the progression of symptoms.

Spina Bifida

Etiology and Pathogenesis. Spina bifida is a developmental anomaly characterized by defective closure of the bony encasement of the spinal cord (neural tube) through which the spinal cord and meninges may or may not protrude. If the anomaly is not visible, the condition is called *spina bifida occulta*. If there is an external protrusion of the saclike structure, the condition is called *spina bifida cystica* and is further classified according to the extent of neural involvement (e.g., meningocele, meningomyelocele, or myelomeningocele) (Figure 45-11).

Both environmental factors and genetics appear to be a factor in the etiologic development of neural tube defects.[10] These include alcohol, vitamin excess (vitamin A) or vitamin deficiency (folate), congenital rubella, anticonvulsant drugs, and chromosomal abnormalities.[36] Substituting another anticonvulsant drug may be recommended for pregnant women or for those considering pregnancy. Supplementation of folic acid prior to conception and during pregnancy also appears to decrease the prevalence of neural tube defects.[10,36]

Clinical Manifestations. In spina bifida occulta, the posterior vertebral laminae have failed to fuse. The defect is extremely common and occurs to some degree in 5% of the population.[36] The vast majority of these vertebral defects are located in the lumbosacral regions, most commonly in the fifth lumbar vertebra and the first sacral vertebra, and may be detected prenatally through ultrasound and α-fetoprotein testing.

Spina bifida occulta may be manifested by changes in the skin and body hair: either very coarse or silky hair along the spine; a midline dimple with or without a sinus tract; a cutaneous port-wine angioma; and/or a subcutaneous mass typically representing a lipoma or dermoid cyst.[36] Spina bifida occulta usually causes no serious neurologic problems. Common lumbosacral defects can cause gait disturbances, positional deformities of the feet, or bladder/bowel dysfunction. These symptoms become evident in childhood during periods of rapid growth.

In the **meningocele** form of spina bifida cystica, a saclike cyst filled with CSF protrudes through the spinal defect but does not involve the spinal cord. Meningoceles occur with equal frequency in the cervical, thoracic, and lumbar areas. A **myelomeningocele** or **meningomyelocele** deformity contains meninges, CSF, and a portion of the spinal cord that protrudes from the vertebral defect in a cystlike sac. These defects most often occur in the lumbar or lumbosacral region of the spine, as these are the last areas of the neural tube to close during fetal development. These defects may be detected in prenatal ultrasound and with α-fetoprotein testing.[10] The bony prominences of the unfused neural arches are palpable at the lateral borders of the defect. The sac includes a transparent membranous covering that may have neural tissue attached to its inner surface. This membrane may be intact at birth or leak CSF, thereby increasing the risk of infection and neural damage. These infants are delivered via caesarean section to decrease the trauma to the exposed neural tissue, and surgical closure is attempted soon after delivery.[36] They often suffer from permanent neurologic damage resulting in motor weakness or paralysis and sensory deficit below the level of the

FIGURE 45-11 Photographs of infants with spina bifida cystica. **A,** Spina bifida with meningomyelocele in the lumbar region. **B,** Spina bifida with myeloschisis in the lumbar region. Note that the nerve involvement has affected the lower limbs. (Courtesy Dr. Dwight Parkinson, Department of Surgery and Department of Human Anatomy and Cell Science, University of Manitoba, Winnipeg, Manitoba, Canada. In Moore KL, Persaud TVN: *The developing human: clinically oriented embryology,* ed 8, Philadelphia, 2008, Saunders.)

spinal defect; bowel and bladder dysfunction; scoliosis; hydrocephalus; and seizures. Often the problems worsen as the child grows and the cord ascends within the vertebral canal, pulling primary scar tissue and thereby tethering the cord.[10]

Treatment. Treatment for this common disorder is based on the severity of the defect and neurologic dysfunction. The use of folic acid during the period prior to conception has been shown to significantly decrease the risk of having a child with a neural tube defect. It is recommended that all women of childbearing age take 0.4 mg of folic acid daily for prevention. In fact, in the United States common foods are being supplemented with folic acid to decrease the incidence of this deformity.

KEY POINTS

- Spina bifida is a developmental anomaly characterized by defective closure of the bony encasement of the spinal cord (neural tube) through which the spinal cord and meninges may or may not protrude.
- If the anomaly is not visible, the condition is called *spina bifida occulta*. If there is an external protrusion of the saclike structure, the condition is called *spina bifida cystica,* and is further classified according to extent of neural involvement (e.g., meningocele, myelomeningocele).
- The natural history of myelomeningocele supports an early and aggressive operative approach before significant clinical deterioration begins. A cesarean section before rupture of amniotic membranes and onset of labor may decrease the degree of paralysis.
- Folic acid supplementation taken before conception and during pregnancy appears to decrease the prevalence of neural tube defects.

Amyotrophic Lateral Sclerosis

Etiology and Pathogenesis. Amyotrophic lateral sclerosis (ALS) is a progressive degenerative disease affecting both the upper and lower motor neurons characterized by muscle wasting and atrophy of the hands, arms, and legs. There are pathologic changes in the spinal cord that include degeneration of the lateral columns where the corticospinal tracts are located. ALS is also known as Lou Gehrig disease after the famed "Iron Man" of the New York Yankees who died from the disease. ALS affects an estimated 30,000 Americans at any given time. It most commonly strikes between the ages of 40 and 60 with a higher incidence in men than women. The majority of ALS cases occur at random; however, 5% to 10% of cases are familial.[37] There is also a higher incidence of the disease in military veterans, especially those of the first Persian Gulf War.[38] Although ALS is classified as a single disease entity, emerging evidence suggests that it is a clinical syndrome with several possible causes. It appears that sporadic cases of ALS are multifactorial and related to several environmental factors and a genetic predisposition. Smoking is the only probable risk factor identified at this point. Several unproven risk factors have been considered. These include lead or agricultural chemical exposure, physical prowess, and intake of the dietary supplement glutamate.[39]

Genetic research has determined at least four different genetic mutations that are involved in ALS. One in particular involves a gene responsible for coding a free-radical–scavenging enzyme superoxide dismutase 1 (SOD1). SOD1 is the basis for much ALS research, and there seems to be multiple intracellular enzymatic pathways affected causing premature programmed cell death, or **apoptosis** (see Chapter 4) of the neurons. Like Alzheimer and Parkinson diseases, ALS has been linked with oxidative stress and cellular damage. Neurons are highly susceptible to damage from oxygen-free radicals and the activation of immune cells that propagate further cellular injury. High levels of the neurotransmitter glutamate have also been found in the CSF of ALS patients and are thought to be associated with the neuronal degeneration.[10] Other factors that may be involved in the pathogenesis include protein aggregation, mitochondrial dysfunction in motor neurons, and defective axonal transport.[39]

Clinical Manifestations and Treatment. Most patients with ALS demonstrate muscle weakness and atrophy. The earliest symptoms may be muscle twitching, cramping, and stiffness. Often the hands or upper extremities are affected first. The weakness is progressive and eventually affects the muscles that control speech, swallowing, and breathing. Finding hyperreflexia in a weak atrophied extremity is highly suggestive of ALS. Most individuals die from respiratory failure within 3 to 5 years from the onset of symptoms.[39] Despite the marked physical disability, most patients maintain their sensory and cognitive functions.

ALS is a diagnosis of exclusion, based on the patient's clinical signs and symptoms. Electromyography (EMG), nerve conduction studies, MRI, and serum laboratory testing may be used to rule out other causes of weakness, such as MS, brain and spinal tumors, human immunodeficiency virus, and Lyme disease.

The only FDA-approved treatment for ALS is riluzole (Rilutek), a glutamate inhibitor. This medication is not a cure, but its use can prolong life for several months and may delay the need for mechanical ventilation.[11] Patients with ALS benefit from a multidisciplinary approach to care to prevent complications from immobility as well as to address both physical and psychological needs. Clinical trials are currently underway evaluating the use of NMDA receptor antagonist memantine (Namenda). Other drugs that are also being evaluated are the antibiotic cephtriaxone, Coenzyme Q10, Tamoxifen, and thalidomide.

KEY POINTS

- ALS is a progressive disease affecting both the upper and lower motor neurons. The cause of ALS remains unknown. Weakness and wasting of the upper extremities usually occur, followed by impaired speech, swallowing, and respiration.
- ALS usually strikes between the ages of 40 and 60, and it is more common in men than in women. The mean survival time is about 3 years from the time of diagnosis.
- Clinical manifestations include weakness, atrophy, cramps, stiffness, and irregular twitching of muscle fibers.
- Diagnosis is based on clinical signs and symptoms, EMG, nerve conduction studies, MRI, and serum laboratory testing.
- Riluzole (Rilutek) is a glutamate inhibitor, which may be helpful in management of ALS.

Spinal Cord Injury. Spinal cord injuries are among the most devastating and costly problems faced by patients and their families. Marked changes in lifestyle are required for survivors. Medical advances in the emergent management of spinal cord injuries and their associated complications have been responsible for increasing survival rates. Continuing research is focused on minimizing the incidence of injury and the mortality/morbidity of spinal cord injury.

Etiology. Spinal cord injury is primarily a problem of the young. Males are three to four times more likely to have suffered a spinal cord injury, and these injuries are most common on the weekends and during the summer months. Motor vehicle crashes contribute the highest number of spinal cord injuries, followed by violence (primarily gunshot wounds), followed by falls and recreational accidents.[40] Alcohol and risk-taking behavior are often involved. Other causes of spinal cord injuries include birth injuries, herniated intravertebral disk, or bone spurs related to degenerative changes of aging and osteoporosis. Injuries to the spinal cord are classified by level, degree (complete or incomplete), and mechanism of injury (Box 45-2).

BOX 45-2

American Spinal Injury Association Impairment Scale

- **A** = Complete: No motor or sensory function is preserved in the sacral segments S4 to S5.
- **B** = Incomplete: Sensory function (but not motor function) is preserved below the neurologic level and includes the sacral segments S4 to S5.
- **C** = Incomplete: Motor function is preserved below the neurologic level, and more than half of key muscles below the neurologic level have a muscle grade less than 3.
- **D** = Incomplete: Motor function is preserved below the neurologic level, and at least half of key muscles below the neurologic level have a muscle grade of 3 or more.
- **E** = Normal: Motor and sensory function are normal.

From American Spinal Injury Association: http://www.asia-spinalinjury.org/publications/2006_Classif_worksheet.pdf.

A Flexion

B Hyperextension

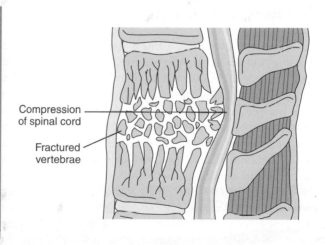

C Compression

FIGURE 45-12 Mechanisms of spinal cord injury. Many situations may produce these consequences. This figure shows examples only. **A,** Flexion injury of the cervical spine ruptures the posterior ligaments. **B,** Hyperextension injury of the cervical spine ruptures the anterior ligaments. **C,** Compression fractures crush the vertebrae and force bony fragments into the spinal canal.

Pathogenesis. Spinal cord injury results from compression (tumor, hematoma, or bony encroachment) and from blunt trauma causing contusion or penetration/transection of neural tissue. The major mechanisms of injury are hyperflexion, hyperextension, and compression (Figure 45-12). Flexion injury with tearing of the posterior ligaments and dislocation is the most unstable injury and is often associated with severe neurologic deficits. Hyperextension injury is the most common. Aside from the primary injury to the spinal cord, damage also results from secondary injury. Secondary events result in edema, ischemia, excitotoxicity, and inflammation, causing increased cell death, disruption of the blood-brain barrier, cavitation, and demyelination, which are detrimental to functional recovery. Not all of these processes are well-understood, but substantial damage occurs due to these events. In animal models, neutrophils appear at the primary injury site within 2 to 4 hours.[41] Oxidative and proteolytic enzymes produced by the neutrophils sterilize the damaged area and prepare it for "repair." However, these neutrophils can cause further damage. Macrophages also infiltrate the area and contribute to further damage by releasing pro-inflammatory cytokines, reactive oxygen species, nitric oxide, and proteases. T-lymphocytes, which are responsible for cell-mediated immunity, have also been identified in the site of injury. Whether T-lymphocytes cause secondary injury or help with healing is still a matter of debate. Animal studies have yet to determine the role of complement in this destructive inflammatory cascade.[42]

The systemic hemodynamic changes that occur after spinal cord injury are a major factor in the resulting damage to the spinal cord. Due to the injury to the spinal cord, autoregulation is lost resulting in a profound drop in systemic blood pressure. This adds to the ischemia of the tissue. In addition, spinal cord injuries are often accompanied by trauma to other organ tissue causing hypoxia, hypotension, hyperthermia/hypothermia, and hypoglycemia or hyperglycemia.

Clinical Manifestations. Immediately following injury to the spinal cord, there is complete loss of function below the level of injury. This may occur even in incomplete injuries to the spinal cord, causing the injury to appear more severe than it actually is. This phenomenon, known as **spinal shock,** can last from a few hours to a few weeks. Symptoms below the level of injury include flaccid paralysis of all skeletal muscles; loss of all spinal reflexes; loss of pain, proprioception, and other sensations; bowel and bladder dysfunction with paralytic ileus; and loss of thermoregulation. A return of spinal reflexes indicates the end of spinal shock. As reflex function returns, spastic paraplegia or quadriplegia develops with hyperreflexia and extensor plantar responses, but a flaccid atrophic (lower motor neuron) paralysis may be found depending on the segments of the cord affected. The bladder and bowel may regain some reflex function.[2]

In patients with cervical or upper thoracic cord injury, **neurogenic shock** is a life-threatening complication. Neurogenic shock is a form of distributive shock caused by the loss of brainstem and higher center control of the sympathetic nervous system. The loss of sympathetic outflow results in hypotension caused by peripheral vasodilation. Bradycardia occurs (secondary to the overriding parasympathetic influence), and there is a loss of the cardiac accelerator reflex. The loss of impulses from the temperature regulatory center in the brain prevents the ability to sweat below the level of injury.

A chronic, ongoing complication of spinal cord injuries occurring at or above the T6 vertebra is **autonomic dysreflexia.** This is a potentially life-threatening complication that may occur any time after spinal shock has resolved. It is characterized by a sudden episode of hypertension, headache, bradycardia, upper-body flushing and lower body vasoconstriction, piloerection (goose bumps), and sweating. The usual stimulus initiating autonomic dysreflexia is activation of visceral or cutaneous pain receptors below the level of injury. A full bladder or constipation is a common cause.

Stimulation of afferent pain receptors causes activation of sympathetic efferents in the cord and reflex vasoconstriction. Sustained activation of sympathetic neurons below the level of cord injury increases blood pressure significantly. The hypertension initiates the baroreceptor response. Baroreceptors mediate inhibition of heart rate and vasodilation of vessels above the level of injury. This is responsible for the upper body flushing. Descending signals from the brain cannot pass the cord injury, so inhibition of sympathetic neurons below the level of injury does not occur. Blood pressure may be dangerously high, and this may precipitate intracranial hemorrhage.[43]

Treatment. Management of spinal cord injuries includes appropriate stabilization of spinal vertebra components to prevent further trauma to the spinal cord. This may be accomplished surgically with internal fixation; or with external fixation and bracing.[44] During neurogenic shock, patients require intensive care to maintain oxygenation and blood pressure. The use of high-dose methylprednisolone initiated within the first 8 hours after injury and continued for 24 hours may preserve some function by decreasing the secondary injury to the spinal cord.[2,44] The benefit of this medication is modest at best, but it offers some hope of improving function. Ongoing assessment is critical. Methodical neurologic evaluations are important in determining improvement or deterioration in function. Treatment for autonomic dysreflexia includes removing or alleviating the painful stimulus, and in certain situations the use of adrenergic receptor–blocking medications to manage the hypertensive crisis.

Individuals suffering from spinal cord injuries have chronic and ongoing problems with spasticity and contracture related to upper motor neuron damage. They are also at high risk for respiratory and urinary tract infection, skin pressure sores, septicemia, and fecal impaction. Much of the care of patients with spinal cord injuries is aimed at preventing these complications and maximizing function. The rehabilitation phase for these patients is lengthy with emphasis on independence and self-care. Ongoing care of patients with spinal cord injuries is multidisciplinary and should also address the psychosocial impact of this life-changing event. Levels of injury and expected functional ability are summarized in Table 45-3.

KEY POINTS

- Spinal cord injury is usually traumatic, a result of motor vehicle accidents, falls, penetrating wounds, or sports injuries. The cord may be compressed, transected, or contused. Further injury may result from hemorrhage, swelling, and ischemia after injury.

TABLE 45-3

Levels of Injury and Expected Functional Ability for Patients with Spinal Cord Injury

Level	Normal Activity	Functional Expectation
C4	Head control Mouth control Shoulder/scapular movement Diaphragm movement	Can use adaptive devices (i.e., mouth stick) for phone, reading, computer Total dependence for transfers/ADLs Pulmonary toileting concerns; skin care issues
C5	Shoulder flexion Elbow flexion Increased scapular motion	Can use adaptive devices for self-feeding; can move wheelchair short distances (electric wheelchair preferred); can perform ADLs and bed mobility with assistance; needs pulmonary toileting assistance
C6	Good elbow flexion Wrist extension Shoulder rotation and abduction	Independent with grooming/feeding with adaptive devices; weak hand grasp; can roll over in bed; can drive with car adaptations; can transfer with assistance; can self-propel wheelchair
C7	Elbow extension Strong wrist extension Good shoulder movement	Can transfer to wheelchair independently; can perform most ADLs independently; excellent bed mobility
T1	Normal hand strength Normal upper body strength	Bed and wheelchair independent; can perform self-catheterization
T10	Normal strength/motion above umbilicus	May stand for exercise with braces; still wheelchair dependent for ambulation
L2-L5	Some leg and thigh movement	Can ambulate indoors with braces/canes
Sacral segments	Mild weakness in lower extremities	Can ambulate with braces/canes; still significant bowel/bladder dysfunction

ADLs, Activities of daily living.

- Spinal shock occurs immediately following injury and is characterized by temporary loss of reflexes below the level of injury. Muscles are flaccid, and skeletal and autonomic reflexes are lost. The end of spinal shock is noted when reflexes return and flaccidity is replaced by spasticity.
- Neurogenic shock may occur after spinal cord injury due to peripheral vasodilation. Hypotension and circulatory collapse may occur. High spinal cord injuries may also affect respiratory muscles, leading to ventilatory failure.
- Autonomic dysreflexia is an acute reflexive response to sympathetic activation below the level of injury. Visceral stimulation (full bladder or bowel) and activation of pain receptors below the injury are common initiating stimuli. Manifestations include hypertension, bradycardia, flushing above the level of injury, and clammy skin below the level of injury. Prompt removal of the offending stimulus is indicated.

Guillain-Barré Syndrome

Etiology and Pathogenesis. Guillain-Barré syndrome, also known as *acute idiopathic polyneuropathy* or *polyradiculo neuropathy,* is an inflammatory demyelinating disease of the peripheral nervous system or a lower motor neuron disorder. Between 0.6 and 1.9 cases per 100,000 individuals occur annually, with an increasing incidence in the aging population. It is one of the most common causes of non-traumatic paralysis in the Western world. There is a slight male preponderance.[10]

The cause of Guillain Barré syndrome is not well understood, but it sometimes follows an infection, inoculation, or surgical procedure 1 to 8 weeks prior to the onset of signs and symptoms. *Campylobacter jejuni* enteritis has been associated with the syndrome.[2] The basis for Guillain-Barré syndrome is probably immunologic, but the exact mechanism is unknown. There is segmental demyelination, and most evidence suggests that this damage is T-cell and B-cell mediated. Aggregates of lymphocytes are found at the sites of demyelination. This process slows or stops nerve conduction. Primarily motor neurons are affected, but sensory nerves may also be involved.[45]

Clinical Manifestations and Treatment. Patients with Guillain-Barré syndrome have progressive ascending weakness or paralysis. It usually begins in the legs, spreading often to the arms and face. The respiratory muscles may also be affected. The severity and extent of neurologic deficit may vary greatly between patients. Most patients reach the peak of disability in 10 to 14 days. Sensory nerves may also be affected, but to a lesser extent than motor neurons. Patients may experience paresthesia or dysesthesia; neuropathic pain may also be present. During this time, patients may demonstrate loss of autonomic regulation, with consequent changes in blood pressure and heart rhythm, and may require intensive care for ventilatory and circulatory support.

Diagnosis of Guillain-Barré syndrome is made through patient history, physical examination, and nerve conduction studies. The CSF characteristically contains high protein concentrations. Other laboratory studies and imaging are used to rule out other causes for neurologic dysfunction.

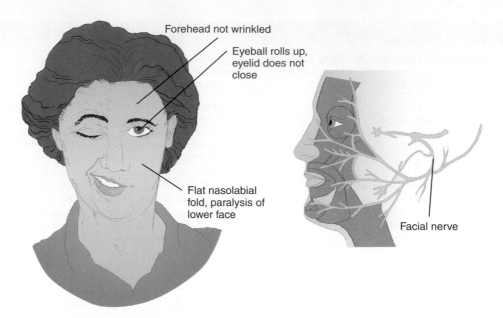

Forehead not wrinkled

Eyeball rolls up, eyelid does not close

Flat nasolabial fold, paralysis of lower face

Facial nerve

FIGURE 45-13 Bell palsy. Location of the branches of the facial nerve (cranial nerve VII) corresponds to the areas of peripheral facial paralysis. (From Black JM et al: *Medical-surgical nursing: clinical management for positive outcomes,* ed 8, Philadelphia, 2008, Saunders, p 1886.)

The majority of patients experience spontaneous recovery; however, 10% to 20% of patients may be left with a mild disability. Severe fatigue persists in 80% of patients and is unrelated to age, duration, or severity of illness.[46] Gradually, neurologic function returns, often in a descending pattern with upper extremities recovering earlier than lower extremities. Treatment within 14 days of onset of symptoms with plasmapheresis, especially in those with severe or rapidly progressing symptoms, has been shown to have some value. Intravenous immunoglobulin is also helpful.[2,45] Nursing care of these patients is aimed at preventing complications of immobility.

KEY POINTS

- Guillain-Barré syndrome is characterized by muscle weakness that begins in the lower extremities and spreads to the proximal spinal neurons.
- The cause is unknown; however, a postinfectious immunologic mechanism is suspected.
- Treatment is supportive, and spontaneous recovery usually occurs.

Bell Palsy

Etiology and Pathogenesis. Bell palsy is an acute idiopathic paresis or paralysis of the facial nerve involving an inflammatory reaction at or near the stylomastoid foramen or in the bony facial canal with probable compression, ischemia, and demyelination occurring.[2,47] The incidence peaks in the 40s.[47] There is mounting evidence that Bell palsy is caused by a viral infection. Antibodies to the herpes simplex and herpes zoster virus have been found in patients with Bell palsy.

Clinical Manifestations and Treatment. Symptoms of Bell palsy develop rapidly over 24 to 48 hours. Physical examination shows unilateral facial weakness with facial droop and diminished eye blink, **hyperacusis,** and decreased lacrimation (Figure 45-13). Patients may complain of a heavy sensation in their face as well as a decreased sense of taste, but sensation of the face is generally intact. Posterior auricular pain may be present. In the diagnosis of Bell palsy, other causes of facial paralysis, such as bacterial infection (otitis media), tumor, trauma, and cerebrovascular accident (stroke), must be ruled out. MRI, CT, and EMG can be helpful in certain situations. Laboratory testing is of limited value.

Management of Bell palsy is controversial. Most patients recover facial nerve function spontaneously within approximately 3 weeks. However, approximately 15% of patients are left with some level of residual disability.[47] Patients with the poorest prognosis for complete recovery are individuals older than 60 years, those with diabetes, and those who have had symptoms lasting longer than 3 months.[47] Prevention of corneal damage due to the inability of the eye to close is vital. Lubricating drops, ointments, and nighttime eye patching may be necessary. The use of corticosteroids has been shown to improve the likelihood of complete recovery. Due to the association of viruses with Bell palsy, the use of antiviral medications such as acyclovir or valacyclovir is recommended. Studies regarding the use of these medications have shown inconsistent results, but two recent studies show benefit when these drugs are combined with corticosteroids.[47] Surgical decompression of the nerve has not been shown to confer great benefit.[47]

KEY POINTS

- Bell palsy, or neuropathy of the facial nerve, results in paralysis of the muscles on one side of the face. Often a self-limiting condition with unknown cause, Bell palsy may last only a few days or weeks.
- Treatment is supportive, and spontaneous recovery usually occurs.

SUMMARY

A traumatic event, such as a spinal cord injury, or a chronic neurologic disease, such as dementia, can transform an individual from a relatively healthy state to one of almost complete dependence. At best, some of the neurologic states described in this chapter may resolve spontaneously or require only minor lifestyle adjustment, but more commonly, chronic neurologic conditions require lifetime rehabilitation.

The process of life care planning includes taking stock of current health status, future health care concerns, appropriate resources, and associated costs to address lifelong disability and illness management.

In general, the goal of rehabilitation is to increase self-care and promote a meaningful lifestyle that incorporates the neurologic disability. The primary goal of such tertiary prevention is to help the affected individual maintain the highest possible level of wellness.

REFERENCES

1. Centers for Disease Control and Prevention: Epilepsy. Available at: http://www.cdc.gov/Epilepsy/.
2. McPhee SJ, Papadakis MA , editors: *Current medical diagnosis and treatment,* ed 46, New York, 2007, McGraw Hill.
3. Walker MC: Treatment of nonconvulsive status epilepticus, *Int Rev Neurobiol* 81:287-297, 2007.
4. Adams SM, Knowles PD: Evaluation of a first seizure, *Am Fam Physician* 75(9):1342-1348, 2007.
5. Adelman AM, Daly MP: Initial evaluation of the patient with suspected dementia, *Am Fam Physician* 71(9):1745-1750, 2005.
6. Alzheimer's Association: Alzheimer News, March 20, 2007. Available at: http://www.alz.org/news_and_events_rise.asp.
7. Forero DA, Casadesus G: Synaptic dysfunction and oxidative stress in Alzheimer's disease: emerging mechanisms, *J Cell Mol Med* 10(3):796-805, 2006.
8. Beatty GE: Shedding light on Alzheimer's, *Nurse Pract* 31(9):32-43, 2006.
9. Moreira PI, Zhu X: Compensatory responses induced by oxidative stress in Alzheimer disease, *Biol Res* 39(1):7-13, 2006.
10. Noseworthy JH, editor: *Neurological therapeutics: principles and practice,* ed 2, Boca Raton, Fla, 2006, Informa Healthcare.
11. Bonner LT, Peskind ER: Pharmacologic treatments of dementia, *Med Clin North Am* 86:657-674, 2002.
12. Delagarza VW: Pharmacologic treatment of Alzheimer's disease: An Update, *Am Fam Physician* 68(7):1365-1372, 2003.
13. Grossman H, Bergmann C: Dementia: a brief review, *Mt Sinai J Med* 73(7):985-992, 2006.
14. Langa KM, Foster NL: Mixed dementia: emerging concepts and therapeutic implications, *J Am Med Assoc* 292(23):2901-2909, 2004.
15. Zhu X, Smith MA et al: Vascular oxidative stress in Alzheimer disease, *J Neurol Sci* 257(1-2):240-246, 2007.
16. Tsuang DW, Bird TD: Genetics of dementia, *Med Clin North Am* 86:591-614, 2002.
17. Alzheimer's Disease, *Prescriber's Letter* 13(10):57, 2006.
18. Rayner AV, O'Brien JG: Behavior disorders of dementia: recognition and treatment, *Am Fam Physician* 73(4):647-652, 2006.
19. National Parkinson Foundation: About Parkinson Disease. Available at: http://www.parkinson.org/NETCOMMUNITY/Page.aspx.
20. Savitt JM, Dawson VL: Diagnosis and treatment of Parkinson disease: molecules to medicine, *J Clin Invest* 116(7):1744-1754, 2006.
21. Hermanowicz N, Haske-Palomino M: Parkinson disease: Essentials of diagnosis, *Consultant* 46(12):1313-1317, 2006.
22. Brown TP, Rumsby PC: Pesticides and Parkinson's disease: is there a link? *Environ Health Perspect* 114(2):156-164, 2006.
23. Rao SS, Hofman LA: Parkinson's disease: diagnosis and treatment, *Am Fam Physician* 74(12):2046-2056, 2006.
24. Hermanowicz N, Haske-Palomino M: Parkinson disease: New insights, new treatment options, *Consultant* 46(12):1333-1340, 2006.
25. Krigger KW: Cerebral Palsy: an overview, *Am Fam Physician* 73(1):91-100, 2006.
26. Merck Manual: Cerebral Palsy (CP) Syndromes. Available at: http://www.merck.com/mmpe/sec19/ch283/ch283.html.
27. United Cerebral Palsy: Cerebral Palsy—facts & figures. Available at: http://www.ucp.org/ucp_generaldoc.cfm.
28. Bjornson K, Hays R: Botulinum toxin for spasticity in children with cerebral palsy: A comprehensive evaluation, *Pediatrics* 120(1):49-58, 2007.
29. Verrees M, Selman W: Management of normal pressure hydrocephalus, *Am Fam Physician* 70(6):1070-1086, 2004.
30. Hydrocephalus Association: About endoscopic third ventriculostomy. Available at: http://www.hydroassoc.org/newsletter/etv.html.
31. National MS Society: Epidemiology. Available at: http://www.nationalmssociety.org
32. Lunemann JD, Kamradt T: Epstein-Barr virus: environmental trigger of multiple sclerosis, *J Virol* 81(13):6777-6784, 2007.
33. Inglese M: Multiple sclerosis: New insights and trends, *Am J Neuroradiol* 27:954-957, 2006.
34. Calabresi PA: Diagnosis and management of multiple sclerosis, *Am Fam Physician* 70(10):1935-1944, 2004.
35. National MS Society: Living with MS, Treatments, Medications Used in MS. Available at: http://www.nationalmssociety.org/site/PageServer?pagename=HOM_LIVE_meds-natalizumab.html.
36. Behrman RE, Kliegman RM , editors: *Nelson textbook of pediatrics,* ed 17, Philadelphia, 2004, Saunders.
37. Amyotrophic Lateral Sclerosis Association: About ALS. Available at: http://www.alsa.org
38. Amyotrophic Lateral Sclerosis Association: ALS in the Military: Unexpected consequence of military service, May 16, 2007. Available at: http://www.alsa.org/files/pdf/ALS_Military_Paper.pdf.
39. Shoesmith CL, Strong MJ: Amyotrophic lateral sclerosis: update for family physicians, *Can Fam Physician* 52:1563-1569, 2006.
40. Mayo Clinic: Spinal cord injury. Available at: http://www.mayoclinic.com/health/spinal-cord-injury/DS00460/DSECTION=3.
41. Fleming JC, Norenberg MD: The cellular inflammatory response in human spinal cords after injury, *Brain* 129:3249-3269, 2006.
42. Qiao F, Atkinson C: Complement plays an important role in spinal cord injury and represents a therapeutic target for improving recovery following trauma, *Am J Pathol* 169(3):1039-1047, 2006.
43. Blackmer J: Rehabilitation medicine: 1. Autonomic dysreflexia, *Can Med Assoc J* 169(9):931-935, 2003.
44. Bailes JE, Petschauer M: Management of cervical spine injuries in athletes, *J Athl Train* 42(1):126-134, 2007.
45. National Institute of Neurological Disorders and Stroke: Guillain-Barré Syndrome Fact Sheet. Available at: http://www.ninds.nih.gov/disorders/gbs/detail_gbs.htm.
46. Hughes RA, Wijdicks EF: Supportive care for patients with Guillain-Barré Syndrome, *Arch Neurol* 62:1194-1198, 2005.
47. Tiemstra JD, Khatkhate N: Bell's palsy: diagnosis and management, *Am Fam Physician* 76(7):997-1004, 2007.

chapter 46

Alterations in Special Sensory Function

Joni D. Nelsen-Marsh

MEDIA RESOURCES

Additional Material for Study, Review, and Further Exploration

 CD Companion ■ Review Questions and Answers ■ Glossary (with audio pronunciations for selected terms) ■ Disease Profiles ■ Animations

evolve **Website** at http://evolve.elsevier.com/Copstead/
■ Case Studies ■ Disease Profiles ■ WebLinks ■ Key Points Review

 Online Course (Module 18)

KEY QUESTIONS

■ What are the general manifestations of hearing impairment?
■ How do conductive and sensorineural mechanisms of hearing loss differ in etiology and treatment?
■ What are the predisposing factors, clinical manifestations, and management of otitis media?

■ What are the general manifestations of visual impairment?
■ What are the causes, clinical manifestations, and management of common visual disorders, including errors of refraction, strabismus, cataract, and retinopathies?
■ How do open-angle and closed-angle glaucoma differ?
■ How do the two forms of macular degeneration differ?

CHAPTER OUTLINE

The human body has countless sense organs that fall into two main categories: general sense organs and special sense organs. By far the most numerous are the general sense organs or receptors. The receptors function to produce the general or somatic senses. Examples of these senses are touch, temperature, and pain, and the receptors that initiate various reflexes necessary for maintaining homeostasis (see Chapter 43). The largest general sense organ in the body is the skin.

Special sense organs, by comparison, function to produce the unique sensations of hearing, balance, vision, smell, and taste. These senses allow humans to interact with their environment in a meaningful way.

Alterations in sensory function may be acute/short-term, chronic/long-term, or progressive in nature. They may result from such factors as genetics, disease, infection, trauma, and normal aging. Alterations in special sensory function require prompt assessment, evaluation, and treatment from appropriate health professionals. Equally important is an assessment of how the sensory impairment affects the individual's activities of daily living. This chapter discusses special sensory function with regard to physiologic processes, sensory impairment, and the diagnosis and management of these impairments.

Hearing and Balance

STRUCTURE AND FUNCTION OF THE EAR

External Ear

Hearing results from normal functioning of several complex structures both external and internal to the body. Sound consists of waves of vibrations in the air, produced in the environment. These vibrations travel much like ripples in a pool of water. Externally, these vibrations are caught and funneled into the ear canal by the auricles (Figure 46-1). Even though the auricles are in a fixed position and lie close to the head, their shape serves to concentrate sound waves, especially high-frequency waves. The auricles also have an important role in sound localization.

The ear canal has a somewhat "S" shape from its opening to its termination at the tympanic membrane. This configuration affords both protection from airborne foreign objects and access to sound. The outer portion of the ear canal contains hair to filter out unwanted substances. Along the ear canal are also glands that secrete cerumen. This brown, wax-like substance coats the hairs in the canal to help prevent the entrance of foreign bodies into the ear canal. After entering the ear canal, sound waves strike the tympanic membrane (eardrum) and

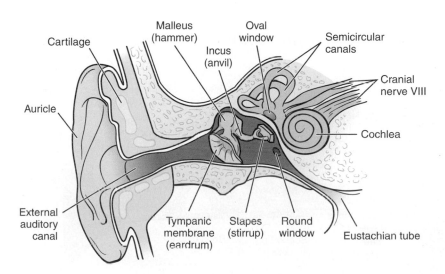

FIGURE 46-1 Anatomic structures of the ear.

cause it to vibrate. The tympanic membrane is a thin, elastic membrane that is very sensitive to changes in pressure.

Middle Ear

The middle ear is a bony, air containing space that functions primarily as a structure by which sound energy is transmitted from the air to the fluids of the inner ear. The tympanic membrane is connected to the first of the **ossicles,** the malleus (hammer), followed by the incus (anvil) and stapes (stirrup). The ossicles further amplify the sound waves and then transfer airborne sound waves to the fluid-filled inner ear at the oval window.

The eustachian tube is also part of the middle ear, and although it does not contribute directly to the transmission of sound through the ear, absence of proper function can greatly affect hearing. This tube has a mucosal lining and extends from the middle ear cavity to the nasopharynx. It makes equalization of pressure against the inner and outer surfaces of the tympanic membrane possible, thus improving mobility of the membrane for sound transduction. A patent eustachian tube prevents membrane rupture and discomfort that marked pressure differences can produce.

Inner Ear

The inner ear is composed of the oval window, the cochlea, and the semicircular canals. Within the cochlea are three parallel tubes: the scala vestibuli, the scala media, and the scala tympani. Movement of the perilymph, a fluid much like cerebrospinal fluid, in the scala vestibuli and the scala tympani is eventually dissipated by movement of the round window (Figure 46-2). The scala tympani and the scala vestibuli are continuous with one another at the apex of the cochlea through an opening called the *helicotrema*.

Transmission of the sound stimulus from the scala vestibuli to the vestibular membrane results in displacement of the endolymph, the fluid contained in the membranous labyrinth of the scala media and the basilar membrane. The organ of Corti, which contains the receptors for hearing, lies on the basilar membrane. Perilymph and endolymph transmit the mechanical vibrations from the footplate of the stapes to the organ of Corti. Endolymph also transports nutrients to the organ of Corti. No direct communication between endolymph and perilymph is normally present.

The organ of Corti consists of a series of sensory hair cells and supporting cells. These cells are innervated by the sensory fibers from the vestibulocochlear nerve (cranial nerve VIII). Overhanging the organ of Corti is a flexible flap of tissue called the *tectorial membrane* (Figure 46-3). Hairs of the sensory cells of the organs of Corti are in contact with the tectorial membrane. The wave of perilymph induces movement of the basilar membrane, which causes a pull or shearing force on the hair cells in contact with the tectorial membrane. This action transforms the mechanical energy of sound into electrical

FIGURE 46-2 Movement of fluid in the cochlea after forward thrust of the stapes.

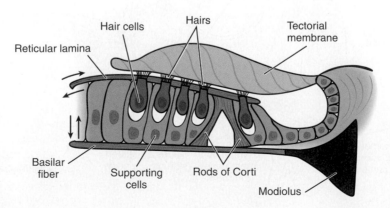

FIGURE 46-3 Stimulation of hair cells by the back-and-forth movement of the hair cells in the tectorial membrane.

impulses stimulating the vestibulocochlear nerve. Impulses are relayed through nuclei in the medulla, pons, midbrain, and thalamus before reaching the auditory area of the temporal lobe.

Balance

The ear has dual sensory functions. In addition to its role in hearing, it also functions as the sense organ of **equilibrium.** The stimulation or "trigger" responsible for balance involves activation of receptor hair cells contained in the semicircular canals. Movement of the head causes movement of the endolymph contained in the semicircular canals. The receptor hair cells in turn create a nerve impulse in the vestibular portion of the vestibulocochlear nerve (cranial nerve VIII), where the stimulus is transmitted to the brain. Not only are signals from the inner ear involved in keeping individuals upright; they are also involved in controlling the eye muscles so that the eyes can remain fixed on the same point despite changes in the position of the head.

Vertigo. Vertigo is a common symptom of vestibular disorders rather than a well-defined disease. It is either a sensation of motion without any actual motion or an exaggerated sense of motion; it is not simply a sensation of "spinning." Accompanying symptoms may include nausea, vomiting, pallor, and sweating. **Nystagmus** often is also noted. It is not associated with a loss of consciousness or a feeling of impending loss of consciousness more common to syncope. Vertigo can have a peripheral vestibular cause or central causes. In the case of Meniere disease (discussed later in this chapter), a disorder in which vertigo is common, the cause is unknown.

Disorders of the brainstem or cerebellum that may also cause vertigo include tissue ischemia secondary to atherosclerosis, tumors, or conditions such as psychiatric disorders, migraine headaches, or multiple sclerosis. However, in these cases, additional neurologic signs and symptoms are typically present. Drugs may also cause vertigo (alcohol, anticonvulsants, sedatives).[1] Management of vertigo is usually aimed at the cause if known. Medications such as antihistamines and anticholinergics can be helpful.[2]

GENERAL MANIFESTATIONS OF HEARING IMPAIRMENT

Hearing impairment is a very common disorder and a leading chronic health problem in the United States along with arthritis and hypertension.[3] One in three adults older than 65 and one half of those older than 75 have some level of hearing loss.[4]

Hearing may be impaired in many ways, and impairments can occur across the age spectrum. Disorders may affect the outer ear, such as impacted cerumen and foreign bodies in the ear canal. The middle ear may be affected by fluid **effusion,** infection (otitis media), tumors, or diseases such as otosclerosis. Hearing loss may also be caused by repeated exposure to loud sounds or **ototoxic** medications such as aminoglycoside antibiotics, chemotherapeutic agents, and high-dose loop diuretics. Some of these medications can cause hearing loss

even when administered at therapeutic doses.[3,5] Other causes of hearing loss, especially in children, include infection (measles, meningitis), environmental teratogens (radiation), intrauterine infections (cytomegalovirus, herpes simplex virus, human immunodeficiency virus, and *Toxoplasma*), maternal metabolic disorders (diabetes, hypothyroidism), and exposure to industrial chemicals (solvents or pesticides).[6-8] By whatever mechanism hearing impairment occurs, the signs and symptoms are similar.

Symptoms of hearing impairment may be manifested in behavior such as inattentiveness, speaking out of turn in conversations, withdrawal from social situations, increased volume of voice when speaking, increased volume of radio or television, confusion, loss of reaction to loud sounds, and emotional outbursts. Children with hearing impairment may demonstrate inattentiveness and difficulty with articulation and the development of speech. Alterations in hearing function can generally be classified into two categories, conductive and sensorineural, depending on the cause of the impairment. Some hearing impairments have a component of both. The following alterations in hearing function are categorized according to the primary cause of dysfunction.

HEARING IMPAIRMENT DISORDERS

Conductive Hearing Impairment

Conductive hearing loss occurs when sound cannot reach the cochlea. Individuals with conductive hearing impairment have a decreased sensitivity to sound. This type of hearing impairment is caused by dysfunction in the external or middle ear. Four mechanisms, each resulting in impairment of the passage of sound vibrations to the inner ear, lead to conductive hearing impairment: (1) obstruction (cerumen impaction), (2) mass loading (middle ear effusion), (3) stiffness effect (otosclerosis), and (4) discontinuity (ossicular disruption). Conductive hearing loss is generally correctable with medical or surgical therapy—or in some cases both.[5]

Loss Caused by Cerumen Impaction and Foreign Body Occlusion

Etiology. Cerumen impaction is a common and frequently overlooked cause of conductive hearing loss, especially in the elderly. In most cases, cerumen impaction is self-induced through attempts at cleaning the ear with objects such as cotton swabs. Foreign bodies in the ear canal occur most frequently in children. Objects such as small stones, pieces of wood, peas, beans, and paper are fairly common.

Clinical Manifestations and Treatment. Sometimes no symptoms are present and the foreign body is discovered on routine examination. If the foreign body is an insect, beating of its wings and movement may cause distress. When symptomatic, however, foreign bodies can cause pain or drainage of pus from the ear. The external ear canal is very sensitive to touch and bleeds easily, which increases the risk for subepithelial hematomas from minor trauma. Therefore, removal of solid foreign bodies carries a risk of additional trauma to the ear canal, as well as tympanic membrane rupture, if the individual is not completely cooperative or removal is difficult. Light anesthesia may be necessary. Firm materials may be removed from the canal with loop or hook instruments, taking care not to push the object further into the canal. Irrigation should not be performed on organic foreign bodies (beans, peas) because water may cause them to swell. Living insects may be immobilized with lidocaine before removal.[5] Excess cerumen may be removed with gentle irrigation.

Otosclerosis

Etiology. Otosclerosis is a progressive conductive sensorineural or mixed hearing impairment caused most often by stapedial fixation. Resorption of bone is followed by the formation of new spongelike bony lesions usually occurring on and around the ossicles of the middle ear. Lesions involving the footplate of the stapes cause decreased transmission of sound waves to the oval window. However, when otosclerotic lesions impinge on the cochlea, permanent sensorineural hearing loss can occur. The basic initiating factors are unknown, but up to 50% of individuals with clinical otosclerosis have a history of the disease in the family.[9] The disease is most common in Caucasian middle-aged women. Pregnancy may accelerate the otosclerotic process.[9] Viral infections are also thought to be a possible cause. The age of onset is variable due to the insidious progression of the disorder, but the most common ages are between 15 and 45. There may be periods of symptom worsening, followed by times of little apparent change.[10]

Diagnosis and Treatment. The diagnosis of otosclerosis is made through careful history taking and radiologic studies, along with audiometric studies. Generally hearing loss begins in one ear, but 80% to 90% of affected individuals will develop bilateral impairment.[10] Although hearing loss may be severe, speech discrimination is preserved except in the instance of cochlear involvement. The individual may report being able to hear better in a noisy environment than in a quiet one.[10] **Tinnitus** is often present. Hearing tests reveal a conductive loss of varying severity.

Management of otosclerosis at this point is generally surgical, in an effort to prevent the conductive hearing loss. The limitation on treatment options for otosclerosis is related largely to the lack of exact knowledge regarding the cause and pathogenesis of the disease. The universally accepted operation for otosclerosis is stapedectomy, or removal of the focus of the disease by removing the stapes and inserting a prosthesis. In the case of otosclerosis involving the cochlea, treatment with oral sodium fluoride, and calcium supplements is associated with some decrease in development of the sensorineural hearing loss.[5,9,10] Amplification with hearing aids is another approach.[10]

Sensorineural Hearing Impairment

In sensorineural hearing impairment, the hearing mechanism is disturbed in the inner ear in the cochlea or the vestibulocochlear nerve to the brain. Long-term exposure to loud sounds, ototoxic medication, trauma, metabolic causes, aging, and certain disease states cause sensorineural hearing impairment. Sensorineural hearing loss is usually irreversible.[5]

Loss Caused by Ototoxic Medications.
Drug toxicity is an increasingly important cause of sensorineural hearing loss. The drugs most well known for this effect are the aminoglycoside antibiotics, salicylates, quinine and related antimalarials, and cytotoxic antineoplastic drugs. Most ototoxic drugs affect the hair cells of the cochlea. Unfortunately, these ototoxic effects may not become apparent during drug administration but may occur days to weeks after the therapy has been terminated. Ototoxicity may also be unilateral. Aspirin can produce a temporary hearing loss and tinnitus in individuals receiving high doses. In most cases, however, both disappear after aspirin use is terminated.

Loss Caused by Trauma

Etiology. Acquired sensorineural hearing loss caused by chronic, repeated exposure to loud sounds is common in the U.S. population. Ten million Americans have suffered irreversible noise-induced hearing loss. Approximately 30 million workers are exposed to hazardous noise on the job.[4] Noise-induced hearing loss can be associated with the use of firearms, personal stereo systems, and power tools and with occupations such as firefighting, construction, agriculture, mining, manufacturing, transportation, and the military.

The loudness of sound/noise is measured in the logarithmic units of decibels (dB). A normal whisper is measured at approximately 30 dB, a conversation at 3 feet at 50 to 60 dB. In contrast, ambulance sirens have been measured at 120 dB, lawnmowers and motorcycles at 90 dB.[11] Sounds exceeding 85 dB are considered potentially injurious, and chronic noise exposure is the most damaging.[5] If exposure is severe enough, most structures of the inner ear can be damaged, including the organ of Corti. Sensory hair cells and supporting cells are lost because of overexposure. Noise-induced hearing loss typically is bilateral and affects higher (speech) frequencies first.

Noise exposure has two phases: the first is a temporary *threshold* shift. When the ear is exposed to a loud sound, it will show a loss of sensitivity (a rise in the threshold for sound). If the hearing returns to normal after the sound has been removed, the shift was temporary and no permanent damage has occurred. If hearing does not return to normal, damage has occurred and the hearing impairment is permanent. Such a permanent threshold shift is the second phase of the damage.[12] The ears of some individuals are more easily affected by noise, and considerable damage may occur before individuals are aware of the hearing loss.

Clinical Manifestations. Individuals with hearing loss caused by noise trauma report that they are unable to discriminate words, particularly in noisy environments. Complaints about tinnitus are expressed more often than complaints about hearing loss. A diagnosis of noise-induced hearing loss is made through careful history and audiometric testing. Because noise-induced hearing loss is irreversible, no medical therapy can help once the problem has been established. Prevention is presently the only treatment for this type of hearing impairment.

Sensorineural hearing impairment can also occur with head trauma and subsequent damage to the structures of the inner ear. If blood is coming from the ear or the temporal bone is fractured, damage should be suspected. As a rule, hearing loss from trauma or head injury is permanent if the cochlea is damaged.

Presbycusis. Presbycusis is a sensorineural hearing loss and the most common form of hearing loss in older adults. Approximately 25% of people age 65 to 75 and 50% of those older than 75 suffer from age-related hearing loss.[5] Typically, the hearing impairment is of gradual onset, is bilateral, and results in difficulty hearing high-pitched tones and conversational speech. Presbycusis can progress to involve the middle and lower tones. Frequently, individuals complain that people are mumbling to them but deny any other type of hearing loss.

Etiology. Four categories of presbycusis have been theorized: (1) sensory, characterized by atrophy and degeneration of the sensory and supporting cells; (2) neural, typified by loss of neurons in the cochlea and central nervous system; (3) metabolic, characterized by atrophy of the wall of the cochlea affecting central auditory processing; and (4) mechanical, in which the middle ear undergoes changes in properties with a resulting conductive hearing loss.[13,14] Some of these age-related changes are shown in Geriatric Considerations: Changes in Hearing. An endless list of genetic, environmental, and disease states can also cause hearing loss in an older adult, many of which may occur concurrently. Thus uncertainty remains regarding the exact cause of presbycusis.

Diagnosis. Assessment of an individual with suspected presbycusis should begin with exclusion of all other causes of hearing impairment. Diseases such as diabetes, stroke, and heart disease may produce effects similar to those seen with hearing loss and must be ruled out. The diagnosis is made with a careful history and audiometric studies. Individuals with presbycusis respond well to hearing aids that amplify sound. Many simple lifestyle adjustments that will be mentioned at the end of this section can dramatically improve the quality of life for an individual experiencing presbycusis. It is important in these patients to avoid excessive noise exposure and ototoxic drugs, which may further their hearing loss.[15]

Meniere Disease

Etiology and Pathogenesis. Meniere disease is an excessive accumulation of endolymph in the membranous labyrinth. The volume of endolymph increases with distention of the scala media until the membrane ruptures. Consequently, the neural end organs of the cochlea degenerate. Many conditions including allergies, viral and bacterial infections (such as syphilis), head trauma, metabolic derangements, and chronic stress have been suggested as causative agents, but the precise cause cannot be established in most cases.[5,10] Men and women are equally affected by this disorder, and the onset of symptoms typically occurs between the ages of 20 and 50.[16]

Clinical Manifestations. Clinical manifestations of Meniere disease include tinnitus, fluctuating sensorineural hearing loss, vertigo, and sensations of ear fullness. In the early stages, hearing loss fluctuates, with return to normal after the rupture heals. Remissions and exacerbations are typical. The hearing loss is usually in the low tones. As the disease progresses, hearing loss becomes permanent. Symptoms initially usually are unilateral, however up to 40% of patients develop bilateral symptoms within 20 years.[17]

GERIATRIC CONSIDERATIONS

Changes in Hearing

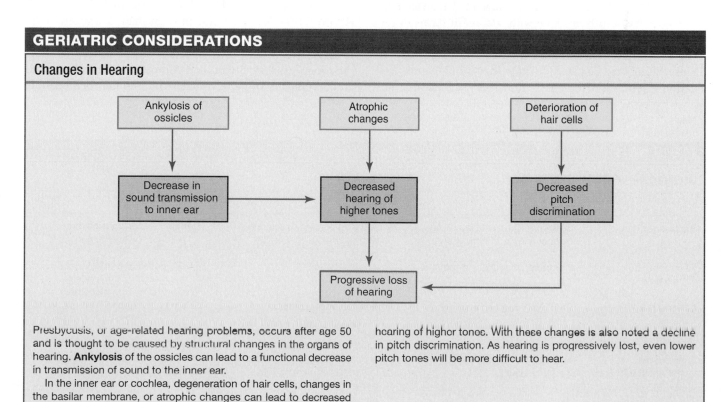

Presbycusis, or age-related hearing problems, occurs after age 50 and is thought to be caused by structural changes in the organs of hearing. **Ankylosis** of the ossicles can lead to a functional decrease in transmission of sound to the inner ear.

In the inner ear or cochlea, degeneration of hair cells, changes in the basilar membrane, or atrophic changes can lead to decreased hearing of higher tones. With these changes is also noted a decline in pitch discrimination. As hearing is progressively lost, even lower pitch tones will be more difficult to hear.

Episodes of vertigo may be immediately preceded by the sensation of pressure in the ear, increased hearing loss, increased tinnitus, or an alteration in the quality of these symptoms. The onset of vertigo is usually sudden, reaches maximal intensity within a few minutes, usually lasts for an hour or more, and either subsides completely or continues as a sensation of unsteadiness for several hours or days. The tinnitus is typically a low buzzing or blowing sound and is frequently louder before the attack of vertigo. The attacks are not precipitated by positional changes and may be several weeks or months apart. In the initial stages of the disease they may be years apart. If not treated, the episodes may become more frequent and severe. Nystagmus, which occurs only during acute attacks, may be directed to the side opposite the involved ear. **Diagnosis and Treatment.** Physical examination, including neurologic and otolaryngologic examination, is generally normal in those with Meniere disease. Radiologic studies are often used to rule out other causes of the symptoms of Meniere disease such as acoustic neuroma. Electrophysiologic studies, such as auditory brainstem response testing and electrocochleography and audiometric tests, can lead to a diagnosis of Meniere disease.[16] Caloric testing (irrigating the ears with warm and cool water) commonly reveals loss or impairment of thermally induced nystagmus on the involved side.[5]

Treatment for Meniere disease consists of giving symptomatic relief during acute episodes with antiemetics and anticholinergics such as meclizine. Between acute attacks, a low-sodium diet and diuretics may help reduce the volume of endolymph. Cessation of smoking, stress management, and elimination of caffeine from the diet are also suggested. Vasodilators have also been used with mixed success.[16] Aggressive management of allergies has also been done with success in terms of decreasing the symptoms of this disorder.[10]

Several surgical interventions are used to manage Meniere disease. Shunts can be placed to drain excess endolymph, and ablation of portions of the eighth cranial nerve and destruction of the labyrinth are options. These interventions have different indications, risks, and benefits associated with them. Almost all patients who choose surgical intervention have failed to respond to medical treatment.[5,10,16]

OTITIS MEDIA

Otitis media is an inflammation of the middle ear. It is almost always due to poor functioning of the eustachian tube and is often diagnosed by the presence of **effusion.** It is the most common reason for a child to require medical attention.[6]

Otitis media is more common in the winter months when viral and bacterial infections are most prevalent. Upper respiratory tract infections can cause eustachian tubes to become blocked and predispose individuals to middle ear inflammation. Children are especially susceptible because of shorter, more flexible and horizontally positioned eustachian tubes. The dysfunction of the eustachian tube prevents middle ear secretions from draining and creates negative pressure in the middle ear space. Negative pressure leads to the introduction of infected nasopharyngeal secretions into the middle ear. Risk factors for otitis media include use of pacifiers, secondhand cigarette smoke exposure, gastroesophageal reflux, poor socioeconomic conditions, daycare attendance, and propped bottles. Males, Native Americans, Eskimo children, children with craniofacial abnormalities such as cleft palate, and individuals with Down syndrome have a higher incidence of otitis media.[6,18,19]

Much confusion surrounds the use of terminology in categorizing otitis media. This confusion relates to the presence of effusion and the length of illness (Table 46-1). *Acute Otitis Media.* Acute otitis media is characterized by the sudden onset of ear pain in association with symptoms of upper respiratory tract infection and is usually of short duration (less than 3 weeks).[18] Although older children and adults complain of pain, younger children may demonstrate

TABLE 46-1

Comparison of Otitis Media Types

Type	Onset/Duration	Symptoms	Treatment Options
Acute otitis media	Sudden onset, associated with upper respiratory infections	Reddened tympanic membrane with poor mobility, may be bulging or ruptured, ear pain	Antibiotics, analgesics, antipyretics, or "watch and wait"
Recurrent acute otitis media	3 or more episodes in 6 months	Same as above	Daily doses of prophylactic antibiotics in some cases, ventilation tube placement
Chronic otitis media	Duration of more than 12 wk, may develop as consequence of acute otitis media	Thick immobile tympanic membrane, purulent drainage from ear, may have conductive hearing loss, pain is rare	Removal of debris from middle ear, ventilation tube placement
Otitis media with effusion	May precede or follow any type of otitis media	Ear popping, feeling of pressure in middle ear, hearing loss, retraction of tympanic membrane, fluid line or bubbles	Treat acute otitis media, "watch and wait"

irritability as well as difficulty eating and sleeping, or tugging at the affected ear as well as fever. Physical examination reveals a reddened tympanic membrane that has poor mobility. Bulging or rupture of the tympanic membrane may also be present.

Management of acute otitis media generally includes a 10- to 14-day course of antibiotics effective against *Streptococcus pneumoniae* and *Haemophilus influenzae* (the bacteria commonly involved).[5] Most individuals receiving antibiotic therapy should have significant improvement in symptoms within 48 hours. Additional therapy such as analgesics and antipyretics will assist with symptom management. Follow-up examination is extremely important to determine that appropriate antibiotic selection and resolution have occurred. However, recent concern relating to antibiotic-resistant strains of bacteria has stimulated controversy regarding the use of antibiotics to manage acute otitis media. Evidenced-based guidelines suggest a "watch and wait" approach for those in whom the diagnosis is uncertain or whom illness is mild. Management of pain is necessary regardless of the decision to treat with antibiotics.[20] This approach does not appear to have long-term drawbacks, but may help decrease antibiotic resistance.[21,22] Re-evaluation is also important for these patients. Recurrent acute otitis media, defined as three or more episodes of acute otitis media in 6 months, may be managed with daily doses of prophylactic antibiotics, however this is another area of controversy.[6] Surgical placement of ventilation tubes in the tympanic membrane is also done in cases of recurrent otitis media. Complications of unresolved otitis media include hearing loss, mastoiditis, meningitis, osteomyelitis of the skull bones, and facial paralysis.

Chronic Otitis Media. Chronic otitis media is inflammation in the middle ear lasting longer than 12 weeks. Irreversible damage has occurred to structures in the middle ear. This damage comes in many forms, including atrophy or perforation of the tympanic membrane or adhesions in the middle ear causing tympanic membrane retraction. Calcification of the ossicles may occur, as may the formation of cholesteatomas (benign, slowly growing collections of skin tissue) within the middle ear space. The hallmark clinical sign of chronic otitis media is purulent drainage from the ear. Pain is an uncommon finding, and conductive hearing loss may occur. Chronic otitis media generally develops as a consequence of acute otitis media, but it may follow other diseases or trauma. Management of chronic otitis media generally includes surgical removal of debris in the middle ear, placement of ventilation tubes in the tympanic membrane, and adenoidectomy to assist with eustachian tube function.

INTERVENTIONS FOR INDIVIDUALS WITH HEARING IMPAIRMENT

In general, interventions for individuals with hearing loss are aimed at maximizing whatever hearing ability the individuals possess and allowing for compensation with other senses. To improve communication, adequate visual contact should be made. Lighting and positioning should be such that the individual can see the speaker's lips. Reductions should be made in background noise. Speech should be at a normal rate and rhythm and at normal volume. Shouting can distort sounds and actually make them more difficult to hear. The speaker should use shorter sentences and gestures such as pointing when appropriate.

Devices that amplify sound or transform sounds into tactile or visual signals may be helpful. Amplifiers for the telephone, television, or radio; closed-captioned television; and teletypewriters are examples of these devices. Others include doorbells and telephones that light up as well as ring, and flashing smoke detectors and alarm clocks.

Implanted hearing devices such as cochlear implants may be helpful for patients over the age of 2 years with profound hearing loss. Surgically implanted cochlear electrodes work together with an external processor that converts sound waves to electrical signals that can be recognized by the brain. These devices can improve communication and provide psychosocial benefits.

KEY POINTS

- Perception of sound requires that sound waves be transmitted through the outer ear canal, across the tympanic membrane, and through the ossicles to the oval window. Movement of the oval window initiates movement of perilymph, which causes movement of endolymph through the vestibular membrane. This fluid's motion stimulates the neurosensory organs of hearing, the hair cells. Bending of the hair cells induces action potentials in the cochlear nerve, which projects to the brainstem. Neural projections to the auditory area in the temporal lobe result in sound perception.
- Balance is controlled by hair cells contained in the semicircular canals. Stimulation of these cells by head movement causes nerve impulses to be transmitted to the brain to keep individuals upright and control eye movement.
- Vertigo, the sensation of motion or aggravation of motion, is a cardinal symptom of disorders of the vestibular system. Vertigo is often associated with nystagmus and nausea.
- Hearing loss may result from interruptions in any part of the sound transmission pathway. Disorders of the outer and middle ear are generally termed *conductive* because sound waves are not reliably conducted to sensory organs of hearing. Accumulation of wax in the outer ear, ossification of bones, and middle ear infections and edema may result in conductive hearing loss. Conductive hearing loss is amenable to treatment.
- Sensorineural hearing loss is due to dysfunction of the hair cells or neural pathways to the brain. Chronic exposure to loud noise, ototoxic drugs, head trauma, and aging changes may lead to sensorineural hearing loss. Sensorineural hearing loss is not as amenable to treatment as conductive loss.

- Otosclerosis is a disorder characterized by resorption of healthy bone and deposition of weak, spongelike bone in the ossicles of the middle ear, most frequently the stapes. These bony lesions lead to progressive conductive hearing loss.
- Presbycusis is a gradual sensorineural hearing loss common in older adults. Its cause is unclear and difficult to distinguish from other types of hearing loss, especially noise trauma.
- Meniere disease is a chronic inner ear disease of unknown cause characterized by vertigo and progressive unilateral sensorineural hearing loss.
- Otitis media, or inflammation of the middle ear, is most frequently seen in children and commonly results from eustachian tube dysfunction after upper respiratory infections. Otitis media can be both acute and chronic.

Vision

Healthy vision requires three basic processes to function appropriately: formation of an image on the retina, stimulation of rods and cones, and conduction of nerve impulses to the brain. Malfunction of any of these processes can disrupt normal vision.

STRUCTURE OF THE EYE

The eye is a spherical structure contained in the bony cavity of the eye socket, composed of three basic layers: the sclera, the choroid, and the retina (Figure 46-4). The sclera is white and opaque, and is made up of dense connective tissue. It aids in protecting the inner structures of the eye, and helps maintain the shape of the eye. The sclera merges with the coverings of the optic nerve on the posterior of the eye. The clear front portion of the sclera is the cornea. The cornea is also composed of dense connective tissue and has a greater curvature than the sclera that causes it to protrude from the sclera. No blood vessels are located in the cornea. Deep within the anterior portion of the sclera, at its conjunction with the cornea, lies a ring-shaped venous sinus, the canal of Schlemm. Affixed to the sclera are the **extraocular** muscles that control eye movement.

The choroid layer of the eye is highly vascularized and darkly pigmented. Attached to this layer is the iris. The iris is a muscular diaphragm whose pigments are responsible for eye color. The iris controls the size of the pupil, the opening through which light stimuli enter the posterior portion of the eye. Behind the pupil is a clear lens. The lens is a transparent, avascular elastic membrane. This elasticity assists in focusing light stimuli on the retina.

The eye is composed of anterior and posterior chambers separated by the lens and iris. The anterior chamber is filled with aqueous humor, the transparent protein-free liquid that is formed in the ciliary body and drained through the canal of Schlemm (Figure 46-5). Aqueous humor provides oxygen and nutrients to the lens and cornea and is continually being formed and reabsorbed. The balance between formation and reabsorption of aqueous humor regulates the total volume and pressure of the **intraocular fluid**. The posterior chamber is the portion of the eye behind the lens that contains a thicker fluid, vitreous humor.

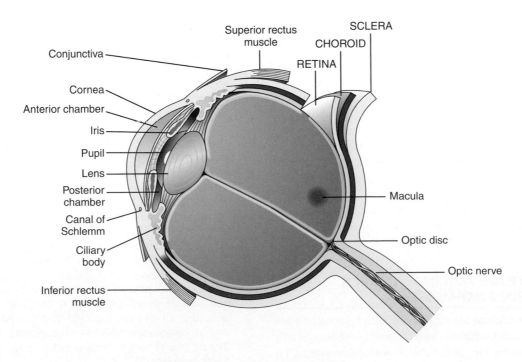

FIGURE 46-4 Anatomic structures of the eye.

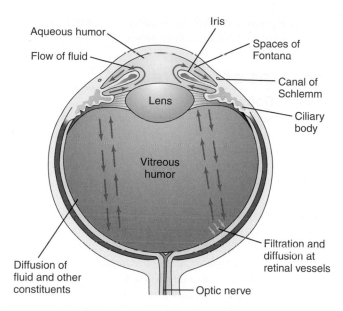

FIGURE 46-5 Circulation of the aqueous and vitreous humor of the eye.

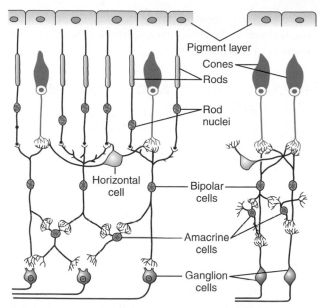

FIGURE 46-6 Three-neuron organization of the retina. (Redrawn from Guyton AC, Hall JE: *Textbook of medical physiology*, ed 11, Philadelphia, 2006, Saunders, p 635.)

VISUAL PATHWAYS

The innermost layer of the eye is the retinal layer. It is here that light waves are transformed into nerve impulses. Three layers of neurons make up the major portion of the retina (Figure 46-6). The outermost layer is composed of **photoreceptor** neurons, the rods and cones. Cones are responsible for daylight vision, color vision, and visual acuity. The greatest concentration of cones occurs in the macula. This area is devoid of retinal vessels and is responsible for the most detailed vision. Rods are important for nighttime and peripheral vision and outnumber cones by nearly 20 to 1. The pigmented layer of the retina or the retinal pigment epithelium is one cell thick. It functions to protect and nourish the retina. The retinal pigment epithelium also removes metabolic cellular debris from the photoreceptor cells, prevents new blood vessel growth into the retina, and absorbs light to diminish scattering and thereby enhance vision.

Action potentials from the rods and cones are communicated throughout the other layers of the retina. All axons of the ganglion neuron extend back to a small circular area in the posterior of the eye, the optic disk, where the optic nerve passes through the sclera. When an image is focused on the retina, it is projected upside down and reversed left to right. An object in the upper temporal visual field of the right eye reflects its image on the lower nasal area of the retina. The optic disk is a blind spot because it does not contain any rods or cones. The optic nerve maintains the spatial arrangement of upside-down and reversed images, and at the optic chiasm just anterior to the pituitary gland half of the nerve fibers cross over to the other side of the brain (Figure 46-7). The left optic tract contains fibers from the left half of each retina, and the right optic tract contains fibers from the right half of each

FIGURE 46-7 Visual pathways. (From Jarvis C: *Physical examination and health assessment*, ed 5, Philadelphia, 2008, Saunders, p 303.)

retina. The nerve impulse travels through the optic nerves to connections in the thalamus and finally connects with the neurons of the occipital cortex.

GENERAL MANIFESTATIONS OF VISUAL IMPAIRMENT

Visual impairment may occur or become evident at any time during the life span. If these impairments occur during infancy or early childhood and are not immediately detected and managed, vision may not develop normally. In older children, academic performance may suffer. In adults and elderly individuals, poor eyesight affects activities of daily living and can limit an individual's ability to function normally and meaningfully in the environment. The various effects of aging on the eye can be seen in Geriatric Considerations: Changes in the Eyes.

Clues that may indicate a visual impairment include squinting, closing one eye, tilting the head, redness of the eye, excessive tearing, and eye rubbing. These signs are especially helpful in identifying children who may be unable to verbalize visual difficulties. In older children and adults, complaints of blurred vision, halos, "floaters" in the visual fields, headaches, and eye pain may indicate a visual impairment. A thorough health history and physical examination along with *visual acuity testing* and *ophthalmoscopic examination* will provide health care providers with the necessary information to appropriately treat or refer individuals with visual impairment.

DISORDERS OF THE EYE

Errors of Refraction

Focusing a clear image on the retina is essential for good vision. In a normal eye, light rays enter the eye and are focused into a clear, upside-down image on the retina. The brain can easily "right" the upside-down image in conscious perception but cannot correct an image that is not sharply focused (Figure 46-8).

Myopia, Hyperopia, Presbyopia, and Astigmatism. If the eye is elongated, the image focuses in front of the retina rather than on it. The retina receives only a fuzzy image. This condition, called *myopia* or nearsightedness, can be corrected with concave contact lenses or glasses. Frequently seen in late childhood or early adolescence, individuals with myopia are unable to see distant objects clearly.

If the eye is shorter than normal, the image focuses behind the retina, also producing a fuzzy image. This condition, called *hyperopia* or farsightedness, can be corrected with convex lenses. *Presbyopia* is the loss of **accommodative capacity.** This inability to see near objects clearly occurs most commonly in middle age and is frequently corrected with reading glasses. An irregularity in curvature of the cornea or lens, termed

---

GERIATRIC CONSIDERATIONS

Changes in the Eyes

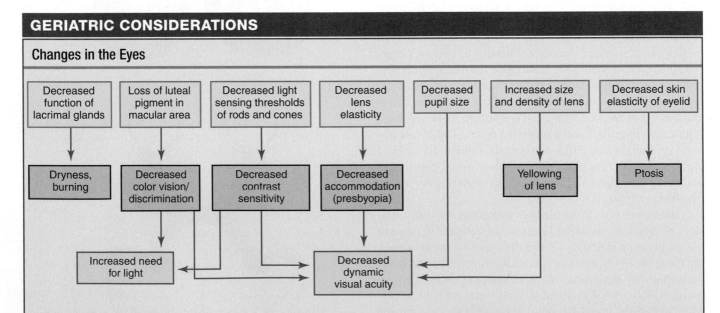

Aging affects all parts of the eye. Minor changes include decreased skin elasticity, changes in lacrimal gland function, and shrinking of the vitreous body. The changes in the lens and retina of the eye are more significant. These changes cause a decrease in color vision and discrimination, reduced contrast sensitivity, and diminished accommodation. As a result, the elderly need brighter light to see and do not differentiate color well. The elderly also have less dynamic visual acuity.

The retina is affected by a loss of the luteal pigment in the macular areas, as well as reduced light-sensing thresholds of the rods and cones. These changes lead directly to a slowing of dark adaptation and a decrease in the ability to discern brightness and colors, particularly shorter light wavelengths such as blues and greens.

A primary change in the aging eye is the development of presbyopia. Presbyopia is caused by a decrease in the elasticity of the lens and decrease in the effectiveness of the ciliary muscle, which lead to an inability to focus on near objects.

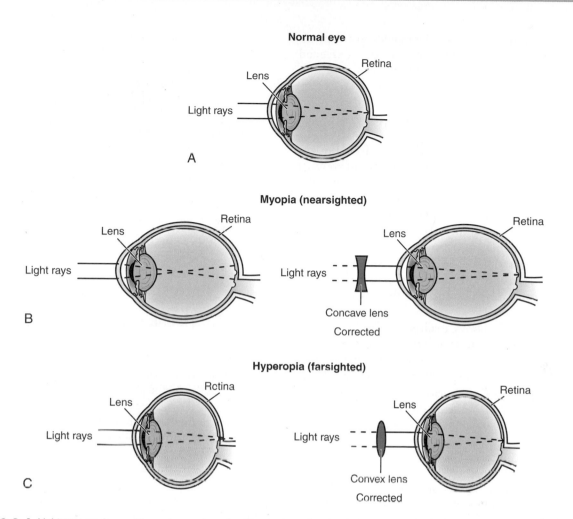

FIGURE 46-8 A, Light rays are focused to produce a clear visual image (emmetropia). **B,** In myopia, light rays are focused in front of the retina. A concave lens moves the focus back onto the retina and results in a clear image. **C,** In hyperopia, light rays are focused behind the retina. A convex lens moves the focus forward so that the light rays fall directly on the retina.

astigmatism, produces a distorted image, and is corrected with glasses or contact lenses that are formed with the opposite curvature.

Age-Related Disorders

Strabismus. To make visual perceptions meaningful, the visual images in the two eyes normally fuse with each other on corresponding points of the two retinas. Strabismus, also called *squint* or *cross-eyedness,* is a condition of ocular misalignment. The eyes appear misaligned on examination. Symptoms include squinting and frowning when reading, closing one eye to see, having trouble picking up objects, dizziness, and headache. Strabismus is often caused by an abnormal "set" of the fusion mechanism of the visual system and is most commonly found in children. Strabismus affects approximately 4% of children younger than 6 years of age.[6]

In the early efforts of the child to fixate the two eyes on the same object, one of the eyes fixates satisfactorily but the other fails to fixate, or both eyes fixate satisfactorily but never simultaneously. Soon the patterns of conjugate movements of the eyes become abnormally set so that the eyes never fuse.

Treatment of strabismus includes occlusion therapy, or patching of the good eye to force use of the weak eye, corrective lenses, surgery on the eye muscles, use of prisms, and eye exercises. If management of strabismus is begun before 24 months of age, amblyopia may be prevented.

Amblyopia. Amblyopia is poor vision, even with the proper optical correction, in one or both eyes. It is the most common cause of decreased vision in the pediatric population, affecting 2 to 3 out of every 100 children.[23] It results from altered visual development despite normal-appearing retinal and optic nerve pathways. Amblyopia occurs when the normal course of visual development is interrupted, such as when visual images do not fuse as in the case of untreated strabismus, or when severe refractive errors are present. Conditions such as congenital cataracts may also interfere with visual development.[24]

The diagnosis of amblyopia is confirmed when a complete ophthalmologic examination reveals a decrease in visual acuity that cannot be explained by organic causes. Although screening for it is much easier in older children, treatment is more difficult at this point. Therefore, screening must take place at an early age. Successful management of amblyopia depends on several factors. The most important is the age of onset and the length of time between onset and the commencement of treatment. Management of amblyopia includes the use of atropine to blur vision or patching of the "stronger" eye. This forces the brain and weaker eye to work together to stimulate vision.[23,24]

Cataracts. Cataracts are a clouding or opacity of the lens that leads to gradual, painless blurring of vision and eventual loss of sight. More than half of all Americans age 80 and older have a cataract, or have had cataract surgery.[25] Cataracts result from the process of aging (senile), trauma (causing lens rupture and swelling), congenital factors (Down syndrome, intrauterine rubella infection), metabolic disease (diabetes mellitus, hypoparathyroidism), and certain medications (systemic corticosteroids). Cigarette smoking and heavy alcohol consumption may also increase the risk of cataract formation.[5,26]

Oxidative stress and exposure to ultraviolet light are factors contributing to the development of cataracts.[26] Both eyes may be affected, but at different rates. Patients with cataracts may experience increased glare at night, blurred vision, and altered color perception. Persons with opacity in the central portion of the lens can generally see better in dim light when the pupil is dilated. The degree of visual loss corresponds to the density of the cataract.

A diagnosis of cataracts can be made through examination of the eye with an ophthalmoscope or slit lamp. As the cataract worsens or "matures," visualization of the retina becomes increasingly difficult until finally the pupil appears white and the retina cannot be visualized at all. Treatment for cataracts involves surgical removal and replacement of the lens. This procedure is completed on an outpatient basis, with individuals returning home immediately after surgery.

Retinopathy

Retinopathy is any disorder of the retina. Damage to the retina impairs vision because even a well-focused image cannot be perceived if some or all of the light receptors do not function properly. Retinopathies can result from a variety of causes, the most common being trauma and vascular disease, especially in individuals with diabetes mellitus and hypertension.

Retinal Detachment. Detachment of the retina is usually spontaneous but may be secondary to trauma such as sudden blows to the head. Spontaneous detachment occurs most frequently in individuals older than 50 years.[5] Eye tumors, myopia, and cataract extraction are other common predisposing factors. Retinal detachments are classified into three categories. Exudative (or serous) detachments result from accumulation of serous or hemorrhagic fluid in the subretinal space, generally due to hydrostatic factors (e.g., severe, sudden hypertension), inflammation (sarcoidosis), or neoplastic effusions. The second type, tractional retinal detachment, occurs when mechanical forces on the retina caused by fibrosis and scarring pull it away from the underlying epithelium (injury or surgery to the eye). The third type of retinal detachment

FIGURE 46-9 Retinal detachment.

is spontaneous or rhegmatogenous. As individuals age, the vitreous humor shrinks and traction develops causing separation.[27]

Tearing of the retina allows vitreous fluid to flow behind the retina and cause traction and progressive detachment (Figure 46-9). The area of detachment increases rapidly, and visual loss is progressive. Common manifestations of retinal detachment include the sudden appearance of floating spots that may decrease over a period of weeks and odd flashes of light that appear when the eye moves. Others include blurring of vision in a single eye that appears as though "a curtain is being pulled down over the eye." If untreated, the retina may detach entirely and result in total blindness in the affected eye. However, if diagnosed and treated early, permanent vision loss can be prevented.[28] Retinal detachments may also cause vitreous hemorrhage.

Retinal detachments are diagnosed through ophthalmoscopic examination. The retina appears to hang in the vitreous humor like a gray cloud. One or more retinal tears, generally crescent-shaped, are usually present. Management of retinal detachment is aimed at closing tears in the retina and positioning the fragments of the retina so that reattachment can occur. Surgical intervention is common, and 80% of rhegmatogenous cases of retinal detachment can be cured with one operation.[5,28]

Diabetic Retinopathy

Etiology and Pathogenesis. Diabetic retinopathy is the leading cause of new cases of blindness in the United States. Nearly all individuals with type 1 diabetes and greater than 60% of patients with type 2 diabetes will have evidence of retinopathy within 20 years after onset of the disease.[29] Diabetic retinopathy is a disease of the vasculature of the retina. In diabetes, the retinal capillary becomes diseased; it loses the ability to transport red blood cells and thus oxygen and nourishment to the retina, with consequent tissue hypoxia and ischemia. Diabetic retinopathy can be divided into two categories: nonproliferative and proliferative.

In nonproliferative diabetic retinopathy, retinal veins become dilated and microaneurysms develop. This effect is a result of damaged vascular epithelium. Small retinal hemorrhages and cotton-wool spots (infarctions in the nerve fibers) occur. Early in the process, visual changes may be minimal or resolve after a few days. As the disease progresses, retinal edema occurs. If the edema involves the macular area, visual acuity is noticeably affected.

Proliferative diabetic retinopathy is characterized by the development of new but abnormal blood vessels (neovascularization) caused by the loss of retinal blood flow and ischemia. These new vessels affect vision in two ways: first, because they are abnormal, they are prone to leakage of blood into the vitreous cavity and may thus result in vitreous hemorrhage. Second, the vessels firmly attach themselves to the retina and grow out into the vitreous humor. The subsequent traction on the retina increases the risk for retinal detachment.[5]

Clinical Manifestations. Diabetic retinopathy is associated with complaints of blurred, darkened, and distorted vision. Visual changes may fluctuate in severity. Some individuals complain of being unable to read or have vague changes in vision.

Diagnosis and Treatment. The diagnosis of diabetic retinopathy is made through careful history taking, visual acuity testing, ophthalmologic examination, and retinal angiography. The most important factor in the management of diabetic retinopathy is prevention. Intensive blood sugar control and blood pressure management have been shown to slow the progression or reduce the risk of developing diabetic retinopathy.[29] Laser treatments are also used to prevent further vision loss. Because the retina is nervous system tissue, it does not regenerate efficiently. Therefore, treatment may prevent any further injury to eye tissue, but it cannot restore vision.

Management of proliferative diabetic retinopathy must be instituted as soon as possible to prevent blindness. Surgical intervention and laser procedures are used in conjunction with the measures used for nonproliferative retinopathy. Because of the risk of diabetic retinopathy, it is recommended that individuals with diabetes mellitus have annual ophthalmologic examinations.

Age-Related Macular Degeneration

Etiology and Pathogenesis. Age-related macular degeneration (AMD) is the leading cause of permanent visual loss in the elderly.[5] Approximately 2% of people in their 50s and 30% of individuals older than 75 are affected.[30] The cause of macular degeneration is unknown, but the outcome is bilateral progressive macular deterioration with central vision loss. Risk factors for developing AMD include female gender, smoking, family history of AMD, increased serum cholesterol, cardiovascular disease, hypertension, obesity, and significant cumulative sunlight exposure.[30,31] There is also a strong relationship between AMD and nutrition.[30,31] Dietary supplements have been shown to delay progression from intermediate to advanced disease; however, some studies suggest they do not prevent the disease.[32] AMD includes a wide spectrum of findings that can be divided into two subgroups. Manifestations, diagnosis, and management of each subgroup differ.

"Dry" or atrophic AMD is the most common form, affecting approximately 80% of patients with AMD.[30] Atrophic AMD causes visual loss due to degeneration of the outer retina, the pigmented layer, and the choroidal layer. There are subretinal accumulations of cellular debris known as *drusen*, along with metabolic dysfunction of the retina. Hard drusen may be seen during ophthalmologic examination and appear as discrete yellow deposits on the retina. Atrophic AMD often affects just one eye initially but later develops in the unaffected eye.

In "wet" or exudative AMD, visual loss is usually more rapid in onset and causes more severe visual disruption. Impairment of barrier function allows for subretinal fluid collections, which may cause retinal detachments and/or neovascularizations. These fluid buildups may be visualized on retinal examination.

Clinical Manifestations. AMD is generally painless. In the atrophic form, the initial symptom is slightly blurred vision and decreased ability to see fine detail. Often patients need more light for completing fine tasks such as reading and needlework. As the disorder progresses, the area of central vision loss becomes larger and darker.

Exudative AMD may also be manifested by a progressive blurring of vision. A hallmark of this form of AMD is the wavy appearance of straight lines. This occurs due to distortion of the retina from fluid accumulations behind it. Vision may be lost rapidly or occur suddenly in previously undiagnosed patients due to retinal detachment or hemorrhage.

Diagnosis and Treatment. AMD is diagnosed with thorough history and physical examination to rule out other causes of visual loss, visual acuity testing, dilated retinal examination, and use of the Amsler grid (Figure 46-10). If AMD is suspected, fluorescein angiography may be completed by the ophthalmologist. In this examination, fluorescein dye is injected into the patient. Photos of the retina show characteristic changes of the choroidal vascular layer.

Management of AMD depends on the type and severity of the disease. Antioxidant/zinc vitamin supplementation has been shown to slow/delay the progression of AMD.[29,30] Other treatment modalities are aimed at correcting the vascular changes and include laser photocoagulation and photodynamic therapy. As with all progressive diseases, patients with AMD should have regular comprehensive eye examinations and daily self-evaluation using the Amsler grid.

Glaucoma

Glaucoma is characterized by increased intraocular pressure and progressive loss of vision. As fluid pressure inside the eye and against the retina increases, blood flow through the retina slows. Reduced blood flow causes degeneration of the retina and thus loss of vision. Glaucoma can be categorized into two main types: open angle and closed (narrow) angle (Figure 46-11).

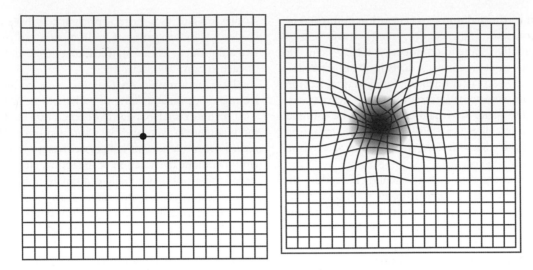

FIGURE 46-10 *Left,* What an Amsler grid looks like to an individual with normal vision. *Right,* What an Amsler grid might look like to an individual with macular degeneration. (From Macular Degeneration Network. Available at: http://www.macular-degeneration.org/WetDry/WetamslerMain.html.)

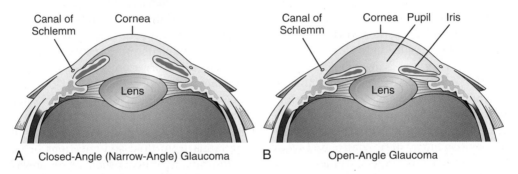

FIGURE 46-11 Closed-angle (narrow-angle) glaucoma compared with open-angle glaucoma. **A,** In closed-angle glaucoma, the outflow of aqueous humor is obstructed by the iris root of the dilated pupil. **B,** In open-angle glaucoma, the obstruction to outflow of aqueous humor is in the drainage canals.

Glaucoma is more common in the elderly, African Americans, those with a family history, those with myopia, and individuals with diabetes. There is also a weak association between systemic hypertension, migraine with vasospasm, and the development of glaucoma.[26]

Open-Angle Glaucoma

Etiology and Pathogenesis. The cause of open-angle glaucoma is not clear. The drainage channels for aqueous humor appear normal. The disease is often bilateral and has a genetic component. Open-angle glaucoma accounts for 90% of all cases of glaucoma.[5]

Open-angle glaucoma has an insidious onset with no symptoms in the early stages. However, the intraocular pressure is consistently elevated, and, over a period of months or years, symptoms including gradual loss of vision in the periphery resulting in tunnel vision appear. Affected individuals may have complaints of vague but persistent dull eye pain or an inability to distinguish colors. Halos may appear around lights if the intraocular pressure is markedly elevated.

Diagnosis and Treatment. The diagnosis of open-angle glaucoma is made through intraocular pressure measurement, ophthalmoscopic examination of the optic disk, and central visual field testing. Because of the insidious nature of the disorder, it is recommended that all individuals older than 40 years have an intraocular pressure measurement and ophthalmoscopic examination every 3 to 5 years. If a family history of glaucoma is present, more frequent examination is recommended.

Management of open-angle glaucoma is aimed at increasing drainage of aqueous humor and decreasing intraocular pressure. β-Adrenergic blocking eye drops, such as timolol, are used to help decrease intraocular pressure by decreasing aqueous humor production. Miotics such as pilocarpine are also useful in that they constrict the pupil and thereby stimulate the ciliary muscles to pull on the trabecular meshwork surrounding the canal of Schlemm to increase the flow of aqueous humor. If the intraocular pressure elevation persists or the optic nerve damage progresses despite treatment, laser surgery aimed at the trabecular meshwork may be done to lower intraocular pressure.[26]

Closed-Angle (Narrow-Angle) Glaucoma

Etiology and Pathogenesis. Closed-angle (narrow-angle) glaucoma is caused by abnormality of the angle between the pupil and lateral cornea. This angle is narrow and blocks outflow of aqueous humor when the pupil is dilated. Closed-angle glaucoma is much less common than open-angle glaucoma but is more prevalent in the elderly, hyperopes, and Asian populations.[5,28] This form of glaucoma has a rapid onset and is treated as an emergency. Closed-angle glaucoma is associated with pupillary dilation and thus might occur when an individual is sitting in a darkened room or during times of stress. Forward displacement of the iris toward the cornea with dilation narrows or closes the chamber angle, obstructing the outflow of aqueous humor (see Figure 46-11).[20]

Manifestations of closed-angle glaucoma include severe eye pain, nausea and vomiting, blurred vision with halos around lights, redness of the eye, a steamy cornea, and a dilated pupil that is nonreactive to light. Closed-angle glaucoma is an emergency situation because permanent blindness can occur within 2 to 5 days after onset of symptoms.[28]

Diagnosis and Treatment. Diagnosis of closed-angle glaucoma involves the same tests as used for diagnosis of open-angle glaucoma. Treatment again in this case is aimed at decreasing intraocular pressure. Acutely, carbonic anhydrase inhibitors such as acetazolamide and miotics may be used to decrease aqueous humor production and blockage. Laser iridectomy usually results in a permanent cure.

Visual Field Deficits
Visual Field Loss

Etiology and Pathogenesis. Visual field loss can be caused by changes in the eye itself, as is the case in cataracts, or result from tumors, vascular lesions, and demyelinating lesions near or in the neural pathways of the retina, optic nerve, or the visual cortex of the brain.

Damage to the visual pathway does not always result in a total loss of vision. Depending on where the damage occurs, only part of the visual field may be affected (Figure 46-12). Monocular field loss indicates disease of the retina or optic nerve. For example, a certain form of neuritis often associated with multiple sclerosis can cause loss of only the center of the visual field, called a *scotoma*.

Damage or lesions may also cause bilateral visual field losses or loss of half of the visual field, called **hemianopsia.** Lesions of the optic chiasm, usually caused by pituitary tumors, characteristically produce a bitemporal hemianopsia. Lesions occurring behind the optic chiasm cause a homonymous hemianopsia, which is a visual field loss involving the same side in both eyes. The more posterior the lesion in the visual pathway, the more congruous (similar size, shape, location) are the defects in the two eyes. Cerebrovascular accidents (strokes) and tumors are responsible for most of these lesions.

Diagnosis and Treatment. Visual field deficits are easily and rapidly assessed through confrontation (i.e., comparison of a person's vision to the examiner's own). Visual field deficits should be suspected if patients demonstrate one-sided neglect of their environment or eye deviation toward the side of the lesion. Treatment for visual field loss includes managing the underlying cause (tumor removal), adapting the patient's environment and teaching compensatory techniques.

INTERVENTIONS FOR INDIVIDUALS WITH VISION IMPAIRMENT

Once the visual impairment of an individual has been thoroughly investigated, specific interventions may be prescribed. Interventions may be thought of in three general categories: assistive devices, environment, and behavior. Proper care and cleaning of contact lenses and eyeglasses directly influences the effectiveness of the prosthesis. Tinted lenses are generally available and may be effective in reducing glare for some individuals. Pocket magnifiers are frequently useful for persons with an acuity impairment. Large print is now available on many household items (e.g., watches, playing cards, telephones, books), and various textures are used in further modifications for the visually impaired.

An unchanging, structured environment where items are kept in fixed locations familiar to the visually impaired person promotes safety and independence. Attempts to structure temporary environments, such as by introducing personal items into a hospital room, might yield positive results if consistently considered by the staff. Attention to adequate lighting, glare reduction, and appropriate use of contrasting colors enhances safety and independent function of those with visual impairment.

Behavioral techniques for the health care professional and visually impaired individuals can promote client comfort, safety, and independence. Such techniques for the professional include announcing oneself at all interactions and explaining sensory occurrences. Encouraging independence and social interaction often benefits individuals inasmuch as they may experience anger, frustration, or changes in self-concept as a result of their visual deficit.

Visually impaired individuals may be taught to wait several minutes for changes in dark-light adaptation and avoid abrupt changes in lighting. Individuals should be discouraged from looking directly into bright lights to reduce glare. Assessment of the visually impaired patient's ability to summon help in the health care and home settings is advised.

KEY POINTS

- Visual acuity depends on the formation of discrete patterns of light on the retina. Errors of refraction such as myopia and hyperopia cause light to focus in front of or behind the retina. Irregular curvature of the cornea results in astigmatism. These disorders are correctable with lenses to refract the light to the appropriate retinal location.
- Strabismus occurs when both eyes do not focus together to form a single image. If this is not corrected, the brain may ignore the image from one eye in an attempt to avoid double imaging; eventually, amblyopia can result.
- Cataracts are due to opacification of the lens that blocks and scatters light. Cataracts may be congenital, traumatic, or associated with aging.

1. Retinal damage
   • Macula—central blind area (e.g., diabetes):

   • Localized damage—blind spot (scotoma) corresponding to particular area:

   • Increasing intraocular pressure—decrease in peripheral vision (e.g., glaucoma). Starts with paracentral scotoma in early stage:

   • Retinal detachment. Person has shadow or diminished vision in one quadrant or one half of visual field:

2. Lesion in globe or optic nerve. Injury here yields one blind eye, or unilateral blindness:

3. Lesion at optic chiasm (e.g., pituitary tumor)—injury to crossing fibers only yields a loss of the nasal part of each retina and a loss of both temporal visual fields. Bitemporal (heteronymous) hemianopsia:

4. Lesion of outer uncrossed fibers at optic chiasm (e.g., aneurysm of left internal carotid artery exerts pressure on uncrossed fibers). Injury yields left nasal hemianopsia:

5. Lesion of right optic tract or right optic radiation. Visual field loss in right nasal and left temporal fields. Loss of same half of visual field in both eyes is homonymous hemianopsia:

FIGURE 46-12 Visual field losses. (From Jarvis C: *Physical examination and health assessment,* ed 5, Philadelphia, 2008, Saunders, p 337.)

- Retinopathy is any disorder affecting the retina. Trauma and systemic disorders such as diabetes mellitus, hypertension, and vascular disease are the most common causes of retinopathy.
- Retinal detachment is characterized by tearing of the retina away from the choroid layer of the eye, with seepage of vitreous humor behind the retina causing further detachment.
- Diabetic retinopathy is a disorder of the retinal vessels characterized by the formation of microaneurysms and hemorrhage (nonproliferative) or neovascularization and subsequent leakage and retinal detachment (proliferative)
- Macular degeneration is an age-related, progressive loss of central vision due to atrophic or exudative changes to the macula of the retina.
- Glaucoma occurs when intraocular pressure is increased by a decrease in the outflow of aqueous humor from the anterior chamber of the eye. Open-angle glaucoma has an unclear cause because no clear obstruction impedes the outflow of aqueous humor. Closed-angle (narrow-angle) glaucoma occurs when the angle between the pupil and lateral aspect of the cornea is narrow and blocks outflow when the pupil is dilated.
- Visual field losses are caused by lesions anywhere along the visual pathways. The location of the lesion determines monocular or binocular involvement and the portion of vision lost.

Smell and Taste

The senses of smell and taste allow separation of noxious or even lethal agents from those that are desirable. The sense of smell has a protective function in signaling danger: animals use smell to recognize the proximity of other animals, and humans use smell to sense harmful substances, such as smoke or spoiled food items, in the environment. The sense of taste allows a person to select food in accordance with desire and perhaps also in accordance with tissue needs. Both senses are strongly tied to primitive emotional and behavioral functions of the nervous system. These chemical senses are interrelated and will be discussed together.

Nerve fibers of the **olfactory** system have their cell bodies in the mucous membrane of the upper and posterior parts of the nasal cavity. The sense of smell begins with chemical stimulation of these cells. Axons of these receptor cells pass through the cribriform plate and travel to the olfactory area of the cortex through the first cranial nerve. These nerves lie under the frontal lobes of the brain. Olfactory impulses reach the cerebral cortex without relay through the thalamus; in this respect, olfaction is unique among the sensory systems.[12]

Like stimuli for smell, stimuli for taste are chemical. Food particles dissolved in fluid stimulate sensory receptors (taste buds) located on the surface of the tongue and in lesser density on the palate, pharynx, and larynx.[12] Stimulation from the sensory receptors is conducted through the cranial nerves of

taste (VII, IX, X) to connections in the brainstem and thalamus with eventual termination in the **gustatory** cortex in the parietal lobe. The gustatory sensory receptors have a heightened sensitivity for one of the primary taste sensations (sweet, salty, sour, or bitter); however, they can respond to a variety of stimuli. The number of sensory receptors for taste diminishes with age, often affecting nutritional status.

Disorders of Smell and Taste

Etiology and Pathogenesis. Olfactory disorders range from loss or reduction in the sense of smell to distortions and olfactory hallucinations. Commonly the sense of smell is diminished because of smoking and conditions involving congestion and swelling of the nasal mucosa, such as allergies and sinusitis. Head trauma often results in the loss of smell because of actual shearing of the neuronal fibers as they traverse the cribriform plate. Tumors and large cerebral aneurysms of the anterior cerebral and anterior communicating arteries are lesions capable of diminishing olfactory sense. Epilepsy and psychiatric disorders may be associated with olfactory hallucinations.[12]

A decreased gustatory sense can also result from heavy smoking, as well as extreme dryness of the tongue and mucous membranes. A variety of medications are known to alter the sense of taste, including certain antidepressant, antithyroid, antirheumatic, and anticancer medications. In addition, influenza-like illnesses and lesions on the thalamus and parietal lobe may impair taste sensation.

Clinical Manifestations. Individuals with smell dysfunction frequently complain of a diminished ability to taste. They may experience a decreased appetite and use excessive amounts of salt, sugar, or other seasonings on their foods. These individuals may stop reacting to strong smells and not notice their own body odor. Smell dysfunction increases the risk of accidents in that these individuals may not detect signs of imminent danger such as gas or smoke. In addition, spoiled food may be ingested, and excessive use of salt is associated with health risks.

Diagnosis and Treatment. Assessment of the sense of smell is done by asking the individual to smell different known odors while keeping the eyes closed. Irritating substances such as ammonia should be avoided because they stimulate the trigeminal nerve. Assessment of gustatory sense should include the primary taste sensations in appropriate areas of the tongue, with the surface of the tongue wiped clean between substances. Questions regarding weight loss and appetite add valuable information to the assessment data.

Interventions for those with smell and taste dysfunction focus on augmenting the stimulus, teaching the individual to rely on other senses, and changing the environment. Because their senses of smell and taste are unreliable in identifying spoiled foods, people with these dysfunctions are encouraged to adhere to a strict schedule for discarding leftovers and be aware of expiration dates on food products. Because significant nutritional problems may occur, it is important to educate and monitor the individual's diet. The creative use of seasonings and spices along with variations in the texture and presentation of food may enhance appetite. Individuals with taste impairments are encouraged to avoid blended foods and to practice frequent oral hygiene. Smoke detectors should be installed in all rooms where smell-impaired individuals sleep, and fire safety should be emphasized.

KEY POINTS

- The senses of smell and taste result from chemical stimulation of specialized nerve fibers located in the nose and the tongue and are closely related to each other. Nerve impulses travel through the cranial nerves to separate areas of the brain.

- Changes in smell and taste most commonly result from smoking and inflammation caused by colds, sinusitis, or allergies. A change in smell or taste sensation in the absence of an obvious cause may indicate a brain tumor and should prompt a thorough neurologic evaluation.

SUMMARY

Humans interact with their environment by means of the special senses of hearing, vision, smell, and taste. Through a variety of stimuli, including chemicals, light, and sound, individuals are able to enjoy everything from a symphony performance to a hot fudge sundae. The special senses also protect individuals from harm by allowing the perception of smoke or alarms. Only when these special senses are impaired does their importance become apparent.

Loss of these senses may result from congenital conditions, trauma, tumors, illness, or unknown causes. Loss may also be a consequence of aging. The mechanism of impairment may be a disruption of the mechanical aspect of the special sense, as in the obstruction of sound waves from cerumen impaction in the ears, or may be a neurologic event, as in the occurrence of homonymous hemianopsia after a stroke.

Regardless of the cause of loss of the sense of hearing, vision, smell, or taste, prompt intervention and treatment can make tremendous differences in outcome. The loss may be totally corrected, or its progression may be slowed. Treatment may be aimed at the underlying cause of the sensory impairment or at altering the individual's behavior or environment to maximize the remaining function. In working with individuals who have alterations in special sensory function, health care professionals have the opportunity to make a great difference in that person's quality of life.

REFERENCES

1. Labuguen RH: Initial evaluation of vertigo, *Am Fam Physician* 73(2):244-251, 2006.
2. Swartz R, Longwell P: Treatment of vertigo, *Am Fam Physician* 71(6):1115-1122, 2005.
3. The Cleveland Clinic Health and Information Center: Hearing loss. Available at: http://www.clevelandclinic.org/health/health-info/docs/2700/2733.asp?index=10059.
4. National Institute on Deafness and other Communication Disorders: Statistics about hearing disorders, ear infection and deafness. Available at: http://www.nidcd.nih.gov/health/statistics/hearing.asp.
5. McPhee SJ, Papadakis MA, Tierney LM, editors: *Current medical diagnosis and treatment,* ed 46, New York, 2007, McGraw-Hill.
6. Behrman RE, Kliegman RA, Jenson, HB, editors: *Nelson textbook of pediatrics,* ed 17, Philadelphia, 2004, Saunders.
7. Centers for Disease Control and Prevention: Noise and Hearing Loss Prevention. Available at: http://www.cdc.gov/niosh/topics/noise/.
8. Kutz JW, Simon LM, Chennupati SK et al: Clinical predictors for hearing loss in children with bacterial meningitis, *Arch Otolaryngol Head Neck Surg* 132:941-945, 2006.
9. Holt JJ: Cholesteatoma and otosclerosis: Two slowly progressive causes of hearing loss treatable through corrective surgery, *Clin Med Res* 1(2):151-154, 2003.
10. Miller MH, Schein JD: Selected complex auditory disorders, *J Rehabil Res Dev* 42(4 Suppl 2):1-8, 2005.
11. The Mayo Clinic: Senior Health, hearing loss. Available at: http://www.mayoclinic.com/health/hearing-loss/DS00172/DSECTION=4.
12. Snow JB, Ballenger JJ, editors: *Ballenger's otorhinolaryngology: Head and neck surgery,* ed 16, Hamilton ONT, Canada, 2003, BC Becker.
13. Martin JS, Jerger JF: Some effects of aging on central auditory processing, *J Rehabil Res Dev* 42(4 Suppl 2):25-44, 2005.
14. Merck Manual On-line: Ear, Nose and Throat and Dental Disorders, Hearing loss. Available at: http://www.merck.com/mmpe/print/sec 08/ch085/ch085a.html.
15. Bogardus ST, Yueh B, Shekelle PG: Screening and management of adult hearing loss in primary care: Clinical applications, *JAMA* 289(15):1986-1990, 2003.
16. American Academy of Otolaryngology—Head and Neck Surgery: Meniere's disease. Available at: http://www.entnet.org/healthinfo/balance/menier.cfm.
17. Havia M, Kentala E: Progression of symptoms of dizziness in Meniere's disease, *Arch Otolaryngol Head Neck Surg* 130(4):431-435, 2004.
18. Donaldson JD: Middle ear, acute otitis media, medical treatment. Available at: http://www.emedicine.com/ent/topic212.htm.
19. Lubianco Neto JF, Hemb L, Silva DB: Systematic literature review of modifiable risk factors for recurrent acute otitis media in childhood, *J Pediatr* (Rio J) 82(2):87-96, 2006.
20. Neff MJ: American Academy of Pediatrics; American Academy of Family Physicians: AAP, AAFP release guideline on diagnosis and management of acute otitis media, *Am Fam Physician* 69(11):2713-2715, 2004.
21. Spiro DM, Tay KY, Arnold DH et al: Wait-and-see prescription for the treatment of acute otitis media: a randomized controlled trial, *JAMA* 296(10):1235-1241, 2006.
22. Little P, Moore M, Warner G et al: Longer term outcomes from a randomised trial of prescribing strategies in otitis media, *Br J Gen Pract* 56(524):176-182, 2006.
23. National Eye Institute: Amblyopia. Available at http://www.nei.nih.gov/health/amblyopia.
24. Doshi NR, Rodriguez ML: Amblyopia, *Am Fam Physician* 75(3):361-367, 2007.
25. National Eye Institute: Cataract. Available at: http://www.nei.nih.gov/health/cataract_facts.asp.
26. Silverston B et al, editors: *Lighthouse handbook on vision impairment and vision rehabilitation,* vol 1, New York, 2000, Oxford University Press.
27. Gariano RF, Kim CH: Evaluation and management of suspected retinal detachment, *Am Fam Physician* 69(7):1691-1698, 2004.
28. Pokhrel PK, Loftus SA: Ocular emergencies, *Am Fam Physician* 76(6):829-836, 2007.
29. Fong DS, Aiello L, Gardner TW et al: Diabetic retinopathy, *Diabetes Care* 26(Suppl 1):S99-S102, 2003.
30. National Eye Institute: Age-related macular degeneration. Available at: http://www.nei.nih.gov/health/maculardegen/armd_facts.asp.
31. Clemons TE, Milton RC, Klein R et al: Risk factors for the incidence of advanced age-related macular degeneration in the age-related eye disease study (AREDS) AREDS report No. 19. *Ophthalmology* 112(4):533-539, 2005.
32. Chong EW, Wong TY, Kreis AJ et al: Dietary antioxidants and primary prevention of age related macular degeneration: systematic review and meta-analysis, *BMJ* 355(7623) Epub 2007.

Pain

Joni D. Nelsen-Marsh • Jacquelyn L. Banasik

MEDIA RESOURCES

Additional Material for Study, Review, and Further Exploration

CD Companion ▪ Review Questions and Answers
- Glossary (with audio pronunciations for selected terms)
- Disease Profiles ▪ Animations

evolve **Website** at http://evolve.elsevier.com/Copstead/
- Case Studies ▪ Disease Profiles ▪ WebLinks ▪ Key Points Review

Online Course (Module 18)

KEY QUESTIONS

- How do the processes of transduction, transmission, perception, and modulation relate to the phenomenon of nociception?
- How is neurotransmission of pain signals modulated at the receptor, spinal cord, and brain?
- How do acute pain and chronic pain differ with regard to cause and clinical manifestations?
- Why are some painful sensations perceived at a distance from the site of injury (referred)?
- Why is it important to adequately manage pain?

CHAPTER OUTLINE

Pain is a complex physiologic and perceptual phenomenon. Because pain is very much a subjective experience, defining and assessing it are difficult. Merskey defined pain as "an unpleasant sensory and emotional experience associated with actual or potential tissue damage or described in terms of such damage."[1] McCaffery offered a clinically useful definition: "Pain is whatever the experiencing person says it is, existing whenever the experiencing person says it does."[2] Accurate assessment and optimal management of pain are extremely important not only because relief of pain and suffering is ethically desirable but also because unrelieved pain is physiologically harmful. Studies have documented the benefits of adequate pain control on the rate of recovery, health care costs, and postoperative morbidity. In fact, the Joint Commission on Accreditation of Healthcare Organizations (JCAHO) has developed standards of care regarding the assessment and management of pain that must be followed by all accredited agencies. Pain has been referred to as the fifth vital sign.

PHYSIOLOGY OF PAIN

The physiologic mechanisms involved in the pain phenomenon are termed **nociception.** Nociception can be divided into four stages: transduction, transmission, perception, and modulation. Transduction is the process of converting painful stimuli to neuronal action potentials at the sensory receptor.

Transmission refers to the movement of action potentials along neurons that make their way from the peripheral receptor to the spinal cord and then centrally to the brain. Perception occurs when the brain receives pain signals and interprets them as painful. The complex mechanism whereby synaptic transmission of pain signals is altered is called modulation. It is clinically useful to conceptualize pain physiology according to these four processes because each stage provides an opportunity for intervention in the pain experience (Figure 47-1).

Transduction

Most pain begins in the periphery when free nerve endings called **nociceptors** are stimulated. Nociceptors transduce noxious stimuli into neuronal action potentials that progress centrally to the spinal cord and then the brain. Nociceptors are found in skin; muscle; connective tissue; the circulatory system; and the abdominal, pelvic, and thoracic viscera. Stimulation can be the result of direct damage to nerve endings, or it can result from release of chemicals at the site of injury.

Numerous substances participate in the initiation of nociceptive impulses. Some of these substances are released as a direct result of tissue injury, whereas others may be produced as part of the inflammatory response to the injury. Important chemical mediators of pain include K^+, H^+, lactate, histamine, serotonin, bradykinins, and prostaglandins.[3] These chemicals alter the membrane potential of the pain receptor, and if depolarization is sufficient, action potentials are generated. When these impulses are conducted centrally, the second step, transmission, is initiated.

Prostaglandin involvement in the process of nociceptor stimulation is of particular interest because prostaglandin inhibitors such as aspirin and other nonsteroidal antiinflammatory drugs (NSAIDs) are commonly used to manage pain. Prostaglandins are formed when cells are damaged and an enzyme, phospholipase A, breaks down phospholipids in the cell membrane and converts them to arachidonic acid[4] (Figure 47-2). Arachidonic acid undergoes further breakdown by

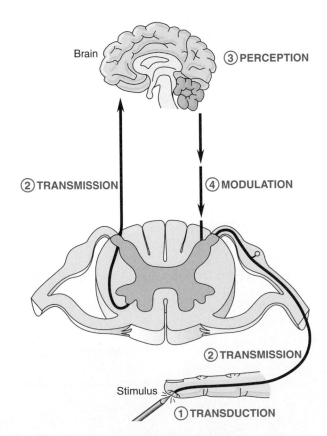

FIGURE 47-1 The four processes of pain signaling: transduction, transmission, perception, and modulation.

FIGURE 47-2 Tissue injury results in the release of prostaglandins from the breakdown of phospholipids in cell membranes. Nonsteroidal antiinflammatory agents *(NSAIDs)* inhibit the cyclooxygenase enzyme and block the production of prostaglandins.

the enzyme cyclooxygenase to form prostaglandins. Sensitization by prostaglandins lowers the threshold of nociceptive fibers so that stimuli that would not cause pain under normal circumstances are now pain producing. NSAIDs prevent prostaglandin production by inhibiting the action of cyclooxygenase.

Transmission

Stimulated nociceptors transmit impulses to the central nervous system (CNS) by means of specialized sensory fibers. The primary sensory fibers involved in the transmission of nociceptive impulses are the Aδ and C fibers.[4] The characteristics and functions of these fibers are summarized in Table 47-1. In general, the larger, myelinated Aδ fibers transmit the nociceptive impulses very quickly as an initial response to tissue injury. The nature of the pain carried by the fast-traveling Aδ fibers is characterized as sharp, stinging, and highly localized. In contrast, unmyelinated C fibers transmit pain more slowly. Pain transmitted by C fibers is poorly localized and has a dull or aching quality that lingers long after the initial sharp pain

abates. The majority of pain sensations travel via C fibers and project to areas of the brain that evoke emotional responses such as displeasure and anxiety.

Most sensory afferent pain fibers enter the spinal cord by way of the posterior nerve roots (Figure 47-3). The cell bodies of pain neurons are located in the dorsal root ganglion. As the afferent neurons enter the dorsal horn, collateral branches spread up and down the spinal cord for two to three segments by way of the tract of Lissauer. These spinal connections are important for reflex postural adjustments when a painful body part is suddenly withdrawn from the painful stimulus.

Sensory afferent neurons synapse with interneurons, anterior motor neurons, and sympathetic preganglionic neurons in specific regions of the spinal cord (see Figure 47-3). Aδ fibers and C fibers carry excitatory impulses from cutaneous pain receptors in small, localized areas of the skin to interneurons in lamina I. Many of the neurons originating in lamina I cross the spinal cord to activate neurons in the anterolateral tract.

Laminae II and III represent a key anatomic region of the cord involved in pain transmission known as the **substantia gelatinosa.** The substantia gelatinosa is characterized by multiple synaptic connections among primary sensory afferent neurons, interneurons, and anterolateral ascending fibers. There is much opportunity at this point for pain signal transmission to be modulated by other sensory input or from CNS activity. Pain signals can be either enhanced or blocked at these synapses.

Another key synaptic area involved in nociception is lamina V. Numerous Aδ and C fibers deliver somatic input from mechanical, thermal, and chemical receptors in the periphery to lamina V. Sensory afferent neurons from visceral receptors also terminate in lamina V. The convergence of both somatic and visceral fibers in lamina V may help explain the phenomenon of referred pain, in which pain from a visceral organ is perceived at the body surface.[4,5] The remaining, deeper

TABLE 47-1		
Afferent Sensory Pain Fibers		
Feature	Aδ Fibers	C Fibers
Structure	Myelinated	Unmyelinated
Amount	10%	90%
Source	Thermal, mechanical stimuli	Polymodal stimuli (mechanical, thermal, chemical)
Speed	Fast traveling, 5-10 m/sec	Slower traveling, 0.6-2 m/sec
Sensory quality of pain mediated	Sharp, stinging, cutting, pinching	Dull, burning, aching

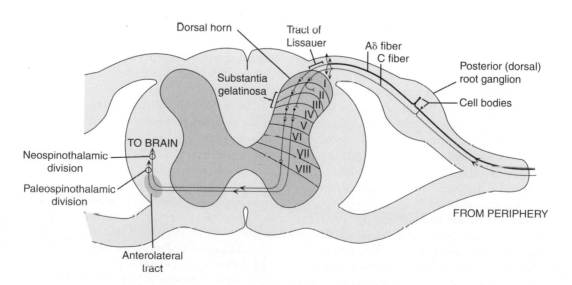

FIGURE 47-3 A spinal cord segment showing primary afferent pain fibers, Aδ and C fibers, entering the dorsal horn, synapsing on interneurons, crossing to the opposite side, and traveling to the brain in the anterolateral tract.

laminae VI to VIII receive sensory input from muscles, joints, and visceral afferent fibers.

A number of neurotransmitters and neuropeptides are involved in synaptic transmission in the spinal cord. Substance P is a well-known example. Others include excitatory amino acids (glutamate), GABA, cholecystokinin, and calcitonin gene–related peptide. These neurotransmitters bind to the next neurons in the pathway and thereby initiate action potentials. The pain signal is propelled along its pathway toward the brain. Interruption of these synaptic processes can inhibit pain transmission. The synapses in the spinal cord are extremely important points of pain modulation by both endogenous and exogenous means.

The excitatory neurotransmitter glutamate is involved in carrying the nociceptive message from primary afferent fibers to secondary neurons. Glutamate binding to its *N*-methyl-D-aspartate (NMDA) receptors on the postsynaptic neuron is thought to induce a kind of synaptic memory in the pain pathway. Excessive or repeated stimulation of C fibers sensitizes the spinal cord neurons so that even mild stimulation may be perceived as painful.[6] This phenomenon has been termed "wind-up" and may be an important mechanism in the development of chronic pain syndromes. Drugs that inhibit glutamate production may impede the wind-up response, thereby controlling pain before synaptic memory of the pain develops in the pain pathways.

Pain signals transmitted by the spinal interneurons are then conducted to the brain by ascending spinal pathways (Figure 47-4). The major pathway for pain signal transmission up the spinal cord is the anterolateral tract, so named because it travels in the anterolateral portion of the white matter of the spinal column. This tract is also called the *spinothalamic tract* in some texts and has two divisions: the neospinothalamic tract and the paleospinothalamic tract. Both divisions cross at the spinal segment and carry pain signals up the contralateral (opposite) side of the cord. Thus nociceptor input from the right side of the body travels in the anterolateral tracts on the left side of the cord, whereas signals from the left side of the body travel on the right side of the cord.

The neospinothalamic division has fewer synapses in the cord and projects first to the thalamus and then to the primary somatosensory cortex. Aδ fiber signals are transmitted in this tract and reach the brain quickly to provide specific information about pain location with little emotional connotation. C fiber impulses travel mainly in the paleospinothalamic division, which makes a greater number of synapses and reaches the brain more slowly. The paleospinothalamic tract projects to widespread brain areas and stirs aversive emotional responses. The paleospinothalamic tract travels with the neospinothalamic tract in the anterolateral portion of the spinal cord to the level of the medulla and then sends diffuse projections to the reticular formation, the mesencephalon, and, finally, the thalamus. From the thalamus, further projections to the cerebral cortex, limbic system, and basal ganglia occur. The pain sensation from C fibers is poorly localized, longer lasting, and more distressing than Aδ fiber pain. Pain

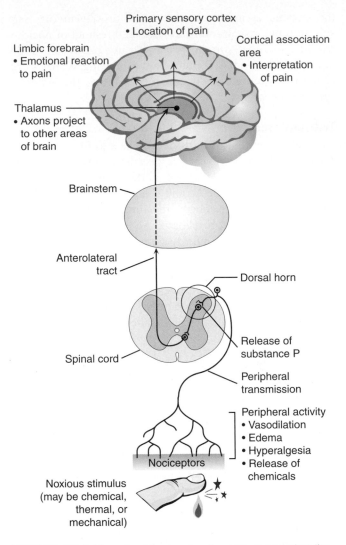

FIGURE 47-4 The anterolateral nociceptive pathways travel up the spinal cord and project to the thalamus, somatosensory cortex, cortical association areas, and limbic structures.

impulses entering the brainstem reticular activating formation, thalamus, and other lower brain centers cause conscious perception of pain, but the cortex is important in interpreting pain quality.[4]

The brain can localize a pain sensation to a particular part of the body because nociceptor pathways are kept in specific anatomic order in the cord and somatosensory cortex. Each spinal nerve contains the nociceptor fibers for a particular area of the body surface, called a *sensory dermatome* (Figure 47-5). Dermatomal maps are useful for locating a source of neurologic pain. Pain that follows a dermatomal distribution is due to spinal nerve compression or trauma and is called a *radiculopathy*. Vertebral disk disease is a common cause of radiculopathy. Peripheral neuropathies, in contrast, do not follow a dermatomal pattern. Examples of peripheral neuropathies are carpal tunnel syndrome (median nerve) and diabetic neuropathy, which often affects both legs in a stocking-like pattern.

FIGURE 47-5 Sensory dermatomes. Pain located in the pattern of a dermatome occurs with spinal nerve injury and is referred to as *radiculopathy*.

Perception

Perception is the result of neural processing of pain sensations in the brain. Perception includes an awareness and interpretation of the meaning of the sensation. Pain perception is influenced by attention, distraction, anxiety, fear, fatigue, and previous experience and expectations. Pain perception is not localized to a specific brain area.[4] In fact, patients who have had a complete hemispherectomy have near normal pain sensation.[5] Numerous neuronal networks are necessary to localize, process, and interpret painful sensations. The primary somatosensory cortex, association cortex, frontal lobe, and limbic structures all participate in this processing.

Pain perception can be described in terms of pain threshold and pain tolerance. Pain threshold is the level of painful stimulation required to be perceived and is remarkably similar from one individual to another. Pain tolerance is the degree of pain that one is willing to bear before seeking relief. Pain tolerance varies widely among individuals and within the same individual under differing conditions. Age, culture, family upbringing, gender, and previous pain experience influence tolerance to pain. Environmental factors, including noise, bright light, and interrupted sleep, may affect pain tolerance.

Pain expression is the way in which the pain experience is communicated to others. Pacing, writhing, jaw clenching, facial grimacing, muscle guarding, crying, moaning, groaning, and verbal descriptions may be used to express pain. Thus the highly variable nature of pain expression among individuals makes accurate pain assessment difficult.

Modulation

Modulation of pain signals occurs at multiple sites along the pain pathway. A fair amount is known about pain modulation at the spinal cord, where neurons from nociceptors, somatosensory receptors, and descending neurons from the CNS all converge and interact. Modulation also occurs at the peripheral nociceptor ending and within the brain; however, these mechanisms are less well understood.

Attempts to decrease the perception of painful stimuli may be initiated spontaneously by the person experiencing pain. Rubbing, pressing, or shaking the painful area may reduce the intensity of pain. In 1965, Melzack and Wall proposed the gate control theory to explain how stimulation of large "touch" neurons could inhibit the transmission of nociceptor impulses.[7] This theory was very useful in focusing efforts to understand pain signal processing at the spinal cord level.

Central to the gate control theory is the capacity for interneurons in the spinal cord to modify the transmission of nociceptor impulses. The original gate control theory suggested that impulses carried by large myelinated cutaneous fibers (Aβ) could "close the gate" on nociceptor impulses so that pain signals would be blocked in the spinal cord and not allowed to progress centrally to the brain. The physiologic process underlying the closing-the-gate mechanisms has been the subject of much study. Numerous interneurons, neurotransmitters, and neuropeptides have been implicated in this complex gating mechanism.

Descending pathways from the brain to the dorsal horn region of the spinal cord are important modulators of the pain response (Figure 47-6). These descending pathways originate in a brainstem nucleus called the *raphe magnus* and project to the dorsal horn regions of laminae I, II, and IV.[5] Neurotransmitters released by these neurons can inhibit synaptic transmission of pain signals. One way to inhibit synaptic transmission is through presynaptic inhibition of substance P release from nociceptor neurons (Figure 47-7). **Opioids** such as **endorphins** are thought to be the mediators of presynaptic inhibition. A similar inhibitory effect can be achieved by administering opioid drugs, such as morphine, that bind to opioid receptors and mimic the effect of endorphins.

The raphe magnus receives input from two other brain areas important in the pain response: the periaqueductal gray (PAG) area in the midbrain and the rostral pons in the brainstem. The PAG area has a high concentration of endogenous opioids (endorphins and enkephalins) that are known to produce analgesic effects similar to narcotic drugs. Stimulation of the PAG area causes release of these endogenous opioids and also sends nerve impulses to the raphe magnus. Serotonin (5-hydroxytryptamine, 5HT) is the neurotransmitter that conveys analgesic signals from the PAG area to the raphe magnus. This finding helps explain the pain-relieving action of drugs

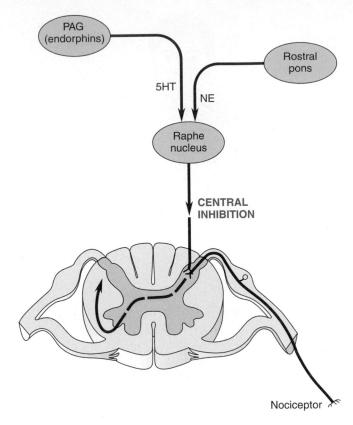

FIGURE 47-6 Descending pathways from the brain are thought to regulate pain impulse transmission in the dorsal horn. These regulatory neurons originate in the brainstem raphe magnus, which receives input from the periaqueductal gray *(PAG)* and the rostral pons. Stimulation of these brain areas induces analgesia. *5HT,* Serotonin; *NE,* norepinephrine.

that enhance serotonin activity in the brain, such as tricyclic antidepressants.

The neurons projecting to the raphe magnus from the rostral pons secrete norepinephrine as the neurotransmitter. Stimulation of these neurons also produces an analgesic effect. Clonidine, a drug that mimics the effect of norepinephrine in the brain, has been shown to have pain-relieving properties.

The descending pathways from the brain provide an important means for gating the flow of pain impulses from the periphery to the brain. The PAG area is well apprised of the flow of pain signals because it receives input by way of the thalamus and limbic structures.

Pain modulation occurs not only at the cord level but also in the brain itself. Opioids produced in the brain are thought to be important modulators of pain perception. Specific opioid receptors were identified within the brain in the early 1970s.[8] Also discovered around this time were the naturally occurring morphine-like substances termed *endorphins.* The word *endorphin* is a combination of two words, *endogenous* (coming from within the body) and *morphine* (from the Latin word *morpheus,* meaning "sleep inducing"). The term endorphin actually refers to two groups of naturally occurring peptides: enkephalins (which are pentapeptides) and three

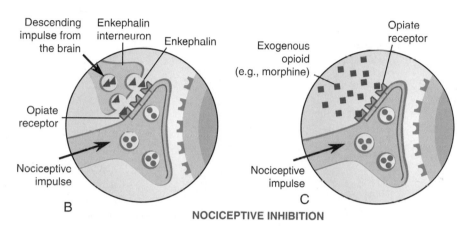

FIGURE 47-7 Pain transmission and inhibition at the molecular level. **A,** Nociceptive transmission to higher levels of the central nervous system. **B,** Nociception inhibited through binding of endogenous opioids (e.g., enkephalin). The release of substance P is prevented. **C,** Nociception inhibited through binding of exogenous opioid (e.g., morphine). Release of substance P is prevented.

types of endorphin polypeptides (α-, β-, and γ-endorphin). Of these, most is known about β-endorphin.

During times of stress, pain, or emotion, the brain apparently creates its own analgesia through the secretion of endogenous opioids—a process known as *stress-induced analgesia*. Stress-induced analgesia is reversed by naloxone, a drug that blocks opioid receptors, thus supporting the role of endogenous opioids in the process.[5] As previously described, the PAG area produces large quantities of endogenous opioids that are thought to inhibit pain signal perception within the brain. High concentrations of β-endorphin are also found in the pituitary gland, and it is likely that release of pituitary stress hormones (adrenocorticotropic hormone) is accompanied by the release of endorphins. The adrenal glands also produce endogenous opioids as a sympathetic response to stress. Endorphins released into the bloodstream by the pituitary gland and adrenal gland have their effects in the periphery because they cannot effectively cross the blood-brain barrier.

Opioids have different effects depending on the types of receptors they activate. Four types of opioid receptors have been identified: mu (μ), kappa (κ), sigma (σ), and delta (δ) (Table 47-2). The distribution of the specific opioid receptors varies throughout the body. The μ and κ receptors have analgesic activities. The μ receptors are found in high concentration in the brain, where they are thought to modulate pain perception.

TABLE 47-2	
Opioid Receptor Activity	
Opioid Receptor	**Activity**
Mu (μ)	Analgesia
	Sedation
	Respiratory depression
	Pupil constriction
	Nausea and vomiting
	Constipation
	Urine retention
	Pruritus
Kappa (κ)	Analgesia
	Sedation
	Respiratory depression
	Pupil constriction
	Diuresis
Sigma (σ)	No analgesia
	Vasomotor stimulation
	Tachypnea
	Pupil dilation
	Psychotomimetic effects (hallucinations, paranoia, delirium)
Delta (δ)	No analgesia
	Respiratory depression
	Nausea and vomiting
	Pruritus

TABLE 47-3

Receptor Affinity of Commonly Used Opioids

Drug	Receptor Affinity	Agonist		Antagonist	
		Pure	Partial	Pure	Partial
Morphine, meperidine, hydromorphone, methadone, fentanyl	Mu (μ)	X			
	Kappa (κ) *(morphine only)*	X			
	delta (δ)	X			
Buprenorphine	Mu (μ)	X			
	Kappa (κ)	X		X	
Butorphanol	mu (μ)				X
	Kappa (κ)	X		X	
	Sigma (σ)	X		X	
Nalbuphine	mu (μ)			X	
	Kappa (κ)	X			
	Sigma (σ)		X		
Pentazocine	mu (μ)	X		X	
	Kappa (κ)	X			
	Sigma (σ)				
Naloxone	mu (μ)			X	
	Kappa (κ)			X	
	Sigma (σ)				
	delta (δ)				
Naltrexone	mu (μ)			X	
	Kappa (κ)			X	

The κ receptors are concentrated primarily in the spinal cord, where they contribute to pain modulation by CNS descending pathways. Each opioid receptor subtype is associated with a number of undesirable side effects. Depending on the affinity for certain receptors, different drugs may have differing analgesic potency and side effect profiles (Table 47-3).

KEY POINTS

- Nociception can be conceptualized as four interdependent processes: stimulus transduction, signal transmission, pain perception, and pain modulation.
- Nociceptor activity is transmitted to the spinal cord by two types of neurons: large, myelinated Aδ fibers, which transmit sharp, localized sensations; and small, unmyelinated C fibers, which transmit dull, aching, poorly localized sensations.
- Pain signals are transmitted by afferent fibers that enter the spinal cord through the dorsal horn, synapse on interneurons, and then cross the cord and project centrally in the anterolateral tract.
- The anterolateral tract has two divisions: the neospinothalamic tract, which carries Aδ fiber input and projects to the thalamus and then the sensory cortex; and the paleospinothalamic tract, which carries C fiber input and projects diffusely to the reticular formation, mesencephalon, and thalamus.

- Perception of painful stimuli involves several brain structures, including the primary somatosensory cortex, association areas, and limbic structures. Pain perception is influenced by culture, environment, and physical status and varies widely among individuals.
- Afferent pain signals can be modulated at several levels. Descending pathways project from the PAG area and rostral pons by way of the raphe magnus to inhibit pain neurons in the dorsal aspect of the spinal cord. Pain is also modulated within the brain/spinal cord by endogenous opioids (enkephalins, endorphins).

Types of Pain

Pain can be categorized into two major subtypes: physiologic pain and pathologic pain. Physiologic pain occurs when tissue injury has occurred, and aides in prevention of further injury or in some cases survival. This is the pain felt when a person for example has touched a hot stove. This injury will likely heal, and the memory of the experience will hopefully prevent future similar injuries. Pain of an acute appendicitis also may be considered physiologic pain as it alerts a person to a serious problem. In contrast, pathologic pain occurs after tissue injury, but long-term changes occur both within the peripheral and central nervous systems. These changes occur along somatosensory pathways from the periphery to the cortex. The pain sensation can be significantly enhanced (**hyperalgesia**), or non-noxious stimuli may cause pain (**allodynia**). These changes in pain perception and modulation serve no beneficial purpose to learning or survival. These underlying changes are theorized to be the cause of neuropathic pain, fibromyalgia, and other chronic pain syndromes.[9]

Pain most commonly is classified according to duration (acute, chronic), source (cancer, neuropathic, ischemic), or location and referral pattern. Pain is a symptom of an underlying problem rather than a primary disorder; attempts to alleviate pain should be accompanied by efforts to locate and manage the underlying etiology. The character, location, and duration of pain can provide helpful clues to aid the diagnostic process.

ACUTE PAIN

Pain is categorized as being acute or chronic, depending on the duration of symptoms. Acute pain results from tissue injury and resolves when the injury heals, usually in less than 3 months. Acute pain is typically accompanied by clinical signs and symptoms of pain that result from stimulation of the sympathetic nervous system. These signs and symptoms include an elevated heart rate, respiratory rate, and blood pressure, as well as pallor, sweating, and nausea (Table 47-4). Persons experiencing acute pain may express pain behavior such as pacing, grimacing, crying, or moaning. Short-term therapy with nonopioid and opioid agents is often helpful. The risk of becoming dependent on pain medications is small in persons experiencing acute pain. Adequate management of pain during an acute episode may help prevent the development of some types of chronic pain syndromes.

Headache

Etiology and Pathogenesis. Headache is one of the most common causes of acute pain, accounting for approximately 13 million visits each year in the Unites States to physician's offices, urgent care clinics, and emergency departments.[10] Headaches are classified according to etiologic categories (e.g., tension, migraine, sinus). However, it is very common for headache type to be misdiagnosed, migraines frequently being labeled as tension or sinus headache. In the Unites States over 45 million people experience chronic recurring headaches, 28 million of these suffering from migraines.[11] Previous theories of migraine included simply a vascular causation. It was thought that cerebral vessels spasmed, and then vasodilation caused the throbbing pain typical of migraine. Current theories involve stimulation of the trigeminal nerve in combination with changes in neurotransmitter levels in the CNS and blood vessel tone.

Migraines probably result from dysfunction of the brainstem areas involved with modulation of craniovascular afferent fibers. There is a release of inflammatory chemicals including local release of calcitonin gene related peptide, which causes vasodilation. The inflammatory cascade that results in migraine can be initiated by many "migraine triggers." There is a genetic predisposition for sensitivity to these headache triggers. The brainstem becomes activated, causing stimulation

TABLE 47-4

Physiologic Responses to Acute Pain

Criteria	Response
Signs and symptoms	↑ Heart rate
	↑ Blood pressure
	↑ Respiratory rate
	Dilated pupils
	Pallor and perspiration
	Nausea and vomiting
	Urine retention
Physiologic response	Blood shifts from superficial vessels to striated muscle, heart, lungs, and brain
	Bronchioles dilate to ↑ oxygenation
	↑ Gastric secretions
	↑ Gastrointestinal motility
	↑ Circulating blood sugar
	Hypomotility of the bladder and ureters

Adapted from Merck Manual: Pain. Available at: http://www.merck.com/mmpe/print/sec16/ch209/ch209a.html; Boswell MV, Cole, BE editors: *Weiner's Pain Management: a practical guide for clinicians,* ed 7, Boca Raton, FL, 2006, Taylor and Francis.

of the trigeminal nucleus caudalis. This activation causes pain signals to be sent to the thalamus and cerebral cortex where pain is perceived and is responsible for many signs/symptoms of migraine. Any of the branches of the trigeminal nerve can refer pain signals along this pathway. If left untreated, continuous activation of the trigeminal nucleus caudalis may result in central sensitization and more refractory pain.

Clinical Manifestations. Typical signs of a migraine headache include severe unilateral pounding or throbbing pain that may be accompanied by nausea, vomiting, photophobia, phonophobia, and lacrimation. The pain is increased by routine physical activity. Some migraines may be preceded by an aura such as flashing lights or other visual disturbances, and unilateral paresthesias. Other symptoms may include sinus/nasal congestion, neck muscle stiffness and pain, vertigo, and changes in bowel pattern.

Diagnosis and Treatment. Headaches are diagnosed through careful history and physical examination. Brain tumors, infection, hydrocephalus, and increased intracranial pressure must be ruled out. Physical assessment should include ears, nose and throat, sinuses, temporomandibular joint, neck musculature, cranial nerves, and retinal examination. General cognitive, neurologic, and motor function should also be examined. Headaches caused by trauma, following a worsening pattern, accompanied by other neurologic symptoms, or those of sudden onset that are the worst experienced by an individual require neuroimaging. The International Headache Society has established criteria for a migraine diagnosis, and this has been adopted by many health care providers (Box 47-1). However, many whose migraines do not meet the criteria have been diagnosed with sinus headache (a relatively rare cause of

BOX 47-1

International Headache Society Diagnostic Criteria for Migraine

Migraine without aura	Migraine with aura
Recurrent headache attacks lasting 4-72 hours and having at least 2 of the following: ■ unilateral location ■ pulsating quality ■ moderate or severe intensity ■ aggravation by routine physical activity At least one of the following characteristics is present: ■ Nausea and/or vomiting ■ Photophobia and phonophobia Can evolve to a very frequent (chronic) migraine condition with or without acute or analgesic medication overuse.	Recurrent disorder manifesting in attacks of reversible focal neurological symptoms that usually develop gradually over 5-20 minutes and last for less than 60 minutes. Typical aura consists of visual and/or sensory and/or speech symptoms. Headache with the same features as migraine without aura usually follows the aura symptoms. Less commonly, headache lacks migrainous features or is completely absent.

Data from Headache Classification Subcommittee of the International Headache Society: The International Classification of Headache Disorders, 2nd edition. *Cephalgia* 24(supp 1): 23-135, 2004.

headaches, according to ear-nose-throat experts) or tension-type headache. Out of 28 million individuals with migraines, 14.6 million will be misdiagnosed.[11] As a result, patients may experience inadequate control of their headache pain, creating disability for the patients and an economic burden resulting from sick days and lost work productivity.

Headaches are managed with a wide variety of therapies and medications, each aimed at a different piece of the pathophysiologic puzzle. Depending on the type and frequency of the headache, prophylactic medications may also be used. One mainstay of nonpharmacologic migraine therapy is the avoidance of headache triggers. Patients are encouraged to eliminate vasoactive substances from their diets including cheese, chocolate, foods containing nitrates and nitrites, and monosodium glutamate. Regular sleep-wake schedules are helpful as are the use of stress management techniques in preventing the occurrence of migraines. Other nonpharmacologic therapies for headache include resting in a quiet, darkened room or applying cold packs to the head and back of the neck. There are numerous medications used to control migraines and other types of headaches. A key to successful treatment is the prompt use of these agents at the onset of pain. Prophylactic therapy with antidepressants (selective serotonin reuptake inhibitors, tricyclic antidepressants), β-blockers (propranolol), α-blockers (clonidine), and calcium channel blockers (verapamil) may be necessary. Refer to Table 47-5 for a comparison of pharmacologic therapies for the acute management of migraine headache.

CHRONIC PAIN

Pain is considered chronic when it lasts more than several months beyond the expected healing time (usually more than 6 months). When chronic pain is not due to a malignancy, its cause is often difficult to ascertain. Chronic pain is generally not associated with signs and symptoms of sympathetic activity. As the body becomes accustomed to pain, the nervous system desensitizes itself to the noxious input; therefore, symptoms are more often psychological. Lack of sleep because of pain causes fatigue and irritability. Loss of a job or loss of body image because of pain causes personal and family difficulties. Treatment failures may create a sense of hopelessness or distrust of caregivers.

Depression is a common finding in individuals experiencing chronic pain. In many cases the cause of the chronic pain cannot be determined, and therefore treatment is difficult. The use of narcotic pain relievers is discouraged because of the necessity of long-term therapy and therefore has a risk of dependency. Satisfactory treatment may require numerous coordinated approaches, and the patient may benefit from the services of a pain clinic that specializes in multimodal therapies.

Fibromyalgia Syndrome

Etiology and Pathogenesis. Fibromyalgia syndrome (FMS) is a chronic pain syndrome affecting an estimated 11 million people in the United States. Women are affected more frequently than men, with a ratio of 9:1.[12] FMS is a collection of symptoms without a clear physiologic cause. It is neither degenerative nor progressive. Patients have a history of chronic widespread pain affecting all four extremities. FMS is a controversial diagnosis once classified at a psychosomatic illness. It can now be objectively identified using criteria set forth by the American College of Rheumatology.

The cause of FMS is unknown. However, etiologic studies have identified several risk factors for the development of the syndrome. Individuals with a medical history of excessive stress, trauma (both physical and emotional), sexual abuse, viral infections (parvovirus, hepatitis C, Epstein-Barr), and endocrine disorders (hypothyroidism) are more commonly affected. Disordered pain mechanisms in the CNS are a suspected factor in FMS. Patients with FMS have a lower threshold for pain than those without the disorder. Pain maintenance and modulation mechanisms in the brain and spinal cord are also suspect. Studies have demonstrated a higher level of substance P in the cerebrospinal fluid of FMS patients. Lower levels of pain-inhibitory

TABLE 47-5

Acute Migraine Therapies

Drug	Route of Administration	Comments
Serotonin Receptor Agonists (Triptans)		
Sumatriptan (Imitrex)	PO, nasal spray, SC injection, dissolvable tablet	Increases serotonin; cannot be given with monoamine oxidase inhibitors, contraindicated in renal/hepatic failure, risk of serotonin syndrome if given with selective serotonin reuptake inhibitors
Zolmitriptan (Zomig)		
Rizatriptan (Maxalt)		
Naratriptan (Amerge)		
Eletriptan (Relpax)		
Ergot Alkaloids		
Ergotamine with caffeine (Wigraine, Ercaf, Cafergot)	IV, IM, SC, PO, rectal suppository, inhaler	Rarely used due to development of newer agents with less side effects. Increases serotonin; intracerebral vasoconstriction; best if given early after onset; contraindicated in patients with cardiovascular disease and pregnancy, may cause nausea/vomiting
Dihydroergotamine mesylate (DHE, Migranal)		Used rarely now
Nonsteroidal Antiinflammatories and Nonopiates		
Acetaminophen (Tylenol)	PO, IV, IM	May cause gastrointestinal upset/bleeding; frequent use may cause "rebound" headache
Ketorolac (Toradol)		
Naproxen Sodium (Naprosyn, Aleve)		
Ibuprofen (Motrin, Advil)		
Aspirin		
Barbiturate-Hypnotic Combinations		
Butalbital with aspirin and caffeine (Fioricet, Fioricet with codeine)	PO	High abuse/addictive potential; may cause sedation; rebound headache with frequent use, withdrawal potential
Opiates/Combinations		
Acetaminophen with codeine, oxycodone, or hydrocodone (Tylenol no. 3/4, Percocet, Lorcet)	PO, nasal spray (Stadol only)	High abuse/addictive potential; may cause sedation, considered "rescue medications"
Butorphanol (Stadol)		

Adapted from McPhee SJ, Papadakis MA, editors: *Current medical diagnosis and treatment*, ed 46, New York, 2007, McGraw-Hill.

neurochemicals are also found.[13] Other theories include growth hormone deficiency, abnormalities in the hypothalamic-pituitary-adrenal axis, and abnormal activation of the sympathetic stress response.[14]

Clinical Manifestations. Patients complain of pain that waxes and wanes, and does not follow a dermatomal pattern. The pain tends to be exacerbated by physical exertion. Hyperalgesia and allodynia are common. Musculoskeletal examinations are generally normal. Other symptoms commonly seen associated with FMS include sleep disturbance/insomnia with non-restorative sleep and irritable bowel syndrome. Fatigue is a hallmark of the syndrome. Depression and anxiety are also common along with cognitive difficulties such as problems with attention and short-term memory.

Diagnosis and Treatment. FMS is a diagnosis of exclusion. Thyroid disorders, myopathies, rheumatoid arthritis, and chronic viral infections (e.g., human immunodeficiency virus) must be ruled out. In FMS there is a lack of objective or laboratory findings. However, the American College of Rheumatology has established criteria to assist in the diagnosis

of FMS. An individual must complain of widespread pain in all four extremities that has been present for 3 months or more and have pain in 11 of 18 "trigger" or "tender" points when pressure is applied to these areas (Figure 47-8).

Management of FMS begins with patient education. Although sometimes disabling, FMS is not a fatal illness and does not affect life span. Treatment includes a variety of medications including antidepressants, such as the selective serotonin reuptake inhibitors and the tricyclic antidepressants. Restoration of sleep patterns seems to be a key factor of successful treatment. NSAIDs and muscle-relaxing agents are also helpful. Opioid medications and corticosteroids are generally avoided as these are not effective long-term therapies.[14] There is currently only one FDA approved therapy for the pain of FMS. Pregabalin (Lyrica) is an analogue of the neurotransmitter GABA (gamma-amino butyric acid). Originally developed as an anticonvulsant, it decreases release of the chemicals glutamate and substance P.[13] Nonpharmacologic therapies include regular physical exercise, good nutrition, and psychological counseling.

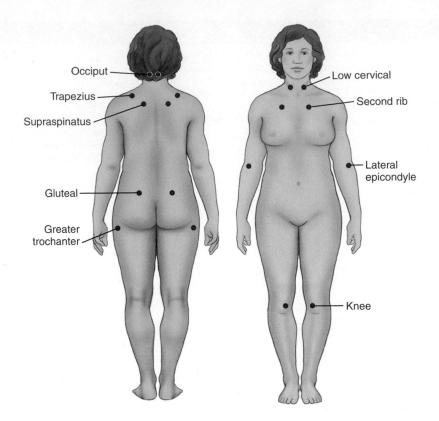

FIGURE 47-8 Posterior and anterior trigger points. (Adapted from the American College of Rheumatology: Fibromyalgia. Available at: http://www.rheumatology.org/public/factsheets/fibromya_new.asp.)

CANCER-RELATED PAIN

Cancer pain is a subcategory of chronic pain, although it may be associated with acute pain episodes. Malignant pain differs from nonmalignant chronic pain in that it often has an identifiable cause. Pain associated with cancer may result from infiltration of organs or compression of structures by an expanding tumor, or it may occur as a result of treatments that damage tissue such as radiation therapy or chemotherapy. In patients with cancer pain, clinical signs and symptoms are often a mixture of sympathetic nervous system activation and behavioral changes. Unremitting cancer pain requires a multifaceted approach and use of potent medications. Often the quality of life is a larger consideration than the length of life, and adequate pain control is a major factor affecting the quality of life.

NEUROPATHIC PAIN

Neuropathic pain is a complex, often disabling chronic pain that results from tissue injury in which the nerves themselves become damaged or dysfunctional. This may occur in the peripheral or central nerves. The pain results from the actual damage or dysfunction of the nerves rather than stimulation of the pain receptors.[5] Nerve injury from surgery, tumor growth, metastasis, radiation therapy, chemotherapy, elevated blood glucose, viral infection, or trauma often causes neuropathic

pain. It is characterized by constant aching sensations that may be interrupted by bursts of burning or shock-like pain in the affected area. Allodynia is common. Neuropathic pain may not occur immediately after an injury. Days, weeks, or even months after the tissue-damaging source of pain has resolved, the onset of neuropathic pain can initiate a new and complex pain state. Pain often seems to be out of proportion to the area of tissue damage.

Neuropathic pain is thought to result from altered central processing of nociceptive input. Nerve injury may initiate excitotoxic and apoptic cell death of neurons within the spinal cord dorsal horn. GABAergic interneurons are significantly depleted. GABA is an inhibitory neurotransmitter in the spinal cord, and a reduction in GABA-secreting neurons may be the cause of the hyperalgesia and allodynia. In some cases, excessive responsiveness to ongoing stimulation of afferent pain fibers appears to be important; however, central perception of pain may occur in the absence of any nociceptor input.[5,6] Examples of neuropathic pain include postherpetic neuralgia, diabetic neuropathy, trigeminal neuralgia, epidural spinal cord compression, cauda equina compression, plexus injuries, and phantom limb pain. Sympathetically maintained pain is a unique type of neuropathic pain that may occur in the absence of nerve injury. Sympathetically maintained pain is attributed to hyperactivity of the sympathetic nervous system. Release of norepinephrine from sympathetic nerve endings sensitizes nociceptors such that they respond to a lower level of nociceptor stimuli.[5,15] Not all sufferers of this type of pain exhibit the same symptoms, but most prevalent are allodynia, hyperalgesia, atrophy of the affected extremity, coldness in the affected area, and dystrophic changes, most often manifested as hair loss and a shiny appearance of the skin. Neuropathic pain is difficult to manage. It is frequently unresponsive to opioid or other pharmacologic therapy.

Trigeminal Neuralgia

Etiology and Pathogenesis. Trigeminal neuralgia is a form of neuropathic pain that can be quite disabling for patients. It is sudden, momentary, but excruciating pains along the second and third divisions of the trigeminal nerve. Trigeminal neuralgia is more common in women than in men, and occurs more frequently in middle-aged or older individuals.[16] If trigeminal neuralgia occurs at an earlier age, multiple sclerosis should be ruled out.[10] Other causes of trigeminal neuralgia include lesions or tumors of the brainstem. Chronic compression of the trigeminal nerve by a vessel is suspected in most cases. This causes demyelination of the trigeminal nerve and interruption and alteration in nerve signaling. Herpes simplex virus infections have also been implicated.[16]

Clinical Manifestations. The pain of trigeminal neuralgia is often described as sharp or shooting; some have compared it to the pain of an electrical shock. Patients may be pain free between episodes or complain of a dull ache in the affected area. Sometimes patients may only have a few episodes of pain followed by a long remission period. However, others may unfortunately experience an increase in frequency and duration of the pain. Anxiety is common, as patients worry about when their next attack may occur.

Diagnosis and Treatment. Diagnosis of neuralgia is most frequently based on the clinical history. The result of neurologic evaluation is normal if there is no underlying lesion. Management of trigeminal neuralgia includes antiseizure medications such as carbamazepine (Tegretol), phenytoin (Dilantin), or gabapentin (Neurontin). Surgical nerve decompression has been used successfully for trigeminal neuralgia in patients who do not respond to or cannot tolerate the medications. Gamma radiosurgery is the newest treatment for this condition, and early results appear promising.[10,16]

Diabetic Neuropathy

Etiology and Pathogenesis. One of the most common complications of diabetes, diabetic neuropathy affects approximately 50% of all individuals with diabetes, both type 1 and type 2.[10] Diabetic neuropathy is caused by damage to the peripheral nerves. The exact pathogenetic mechanism is unknown, but this damage is thought to be mediated by occult inflammation and demyelination of the larger peripheral nerves, leaving an excess of smaller myelinated fibers. This causes a loss of inhibitory input from the spinal cord with unopposed nociceptive afferent bombardment. Ischemic damage to nerves is also a contributing factor. Some also hypothesize that hyperglycemia and related biochemical changes in the nerve microenvironment cause nerve malfunction and injury. The newest research examining diabetic neuropathy has found that the nerve damage associated with each type of diabetes is slightly different. In type 1 diabetes, the neuropathy progresses more rapidly and shows a more marked decline in nerve conduction velocity. This is attributed to reduced blood flow to the neuron, malfunction of the neuron ion channels causing axonal swelling and disruption of axonal junctions. This finding is rare in type 2 diabetes. Moreover, abnormalities in the nociceptive C fibers are more severe in type 1 diabetes. These findings are regardless of blood sugar control. A proposed mechanism is the proinsulin C-peptide deficiency that occurs in type 1 diabetes, but that is not found in type 2 disease.[17] The role of C-peptide in this process is still unknown, but this provides a novel target of treatment of diabetic neuropathy in type 1 diabetics.

Clinical Manifestations. Although pain is the most common feature, patients also complain of numbness and tingling, mild weakness, and loss of vibratory sense and proprioception. Fine touch and vibratory sensation are decreased. Patients complain of burning pain in the distal bilateral lower extremities, often with a symmetric distribution. Pain is frequently worse at night.

Diagnosis and Treatment. Diabetic neuropathy is confirmed through careful physical examination. Diabetic patients are encouraged to keep tight control of their blood glucose to prevent neuropathy. Management of this disorder includes the use of a wide variety of topical and systemic pain medications. Systemic therapeutic agents include tricyclic antidepressants, serotonin/norepinephrine reuptake inhibitors, and anticonvulsants.[10] Although opioids can help with pain relief of diabetic neuropathy, their use has been limited due to tolerance and dependence issues. Side effects of all of these medications can limit their usefulness, especially in elderly patients or those with other comorbid conditions. Many patients use a combination of topical and systemic therapies. An important nonpharmacologic treatment for diabetic neuropathy is the prevention of further complications. Diabetic patients are strongly encouraged to perform daily foot examinations, taking precautions against the development of foot sores and ingrown toenails. The combination of numbness and impaired circulation make diabetic patients at high risk for undetected injuries that do not heal and become easily infected. Amputation is a common outcome.[18]

Postherpetic Neuralgia

Etiology and Pathogenesis. A common but disabling complication of the varicella virus is herpes zoster. Years after an individual has recovered from the chickenpox virus, herpes zoster (shingles) may occur. This is a reactivation of the latent virus that has lain dormant along the nerve roots.

Postherpetic neuropathy is persistent pain that lasts for more than 8 weeks after the onset of skin lesions. Approximately 10% to 15% of patients with herpes zoster develop postherpetic neuralgia.[10] Risk factors for the development of this neuralgia are advanced age and history of immune compromise.

Clinical Manifestations. Herpes zoster is characterized by a burning pain that follows along a dermatomal pathway and is accompanied by a blistering rash. It occurs in individuals who have a history of varicella infection (chickenpox). Frequently the pain is present prior to the eruption of the blisters.

Diagnosis and Treatment. The diagnosis is most often made clinically; however, cultures can be used to determine the presence of the virus. The early use (within 72 hours of eruption of rash) of antiviral medications such as acyclovir (Zovirax) can decrease the risk of developing postherpetic neuralgia.[10]

Management of the neuralgia includes both topical and systemic therapies. Transdermal lidocaine and capsaicin cream may be helpful in mild cases. Anticonvulsants and tricyclic antidepressants are also useful. NSAIDs and opioids may be mildly helpful as well.[10] There is also a vaccine that adults may receive that will prevent or lessen the severity of a varicella zoster outbreak, and decrease the risk of post herpetic neuralgia.

ISCHEMIC PAIN

Pain resulting from a sudden or profound loss of blood flow to the tissues in a particular part of the body may result in ischemic pain. Decreased perfusion leads to tissue hypoxia and injury, with release of inflammatory and pain-producing chemicals. Ischemic pain is described as aching, burning, or prickling (paresthesia). The symptoms of ischemic pain depend on the origin of the ischemia. For example, pain of cardiac origin is visceral and radiates to the arm or jaw. This pain is perceived as being deep, aching, diffuse, and pressing. Ischemia resulting from acute deep venous occlusion is also aching and has a deep quality and gradual onset. Acute arterial occlusion may be felt as either burning or aching but has a sudden onset.

Chronic ischemic pain can occur in atherosclerotic syndromes. Arteriosclerosis obliterans occurs gradually as plaque develops in the intima of the arteries, most often arteries of the lower extremities. In the early stages, the pain, called *intermittent claudication,* is associated with physical activity and alleviated with rest and has a cramping quality. In severe cases, ischemic neuropathy may ensue and cause a more consistent burning, shooting pain in the leg or foot.

Management of ischemic pain is directed at improving blood flow and reducing tissue hypoxia. Acute ischemia is usually associated with a thrombus or embolus and can be managed with drugs to dissolve the clot or surgery to remove it. Chronic ischemia is most often associated with atherosclerosis and may be improved through lifestyle changes, including smoking cessation, weight loss, lipid lowering, and regular exercise. Surgical bypass procedures or placement of intravascular stents are also utilized.

REFERRED PAIN

Referred pain is perceived in an area other than the site of the injury. It is often felt at some distance from the point of nociceptor activation. A familiar example is the pain of myocardial infarction that is felt in the jaw or left arm. Other examples of referred pain include shoulder pain after pelvic procedures, diaphragmatic irritation from peritonitis, and cutaneous abdominal pain experienced with visceral irritation or tension. Common patterns of referral are shown in Figure 47-9. Pain is generally referred to other structures in the same sensory dermatome. Convergence of nociceptors from internal organs with somatic afferents from the body surface occurs in the dorsal horn of the spinal cord.[6] The brain cannot differentiate

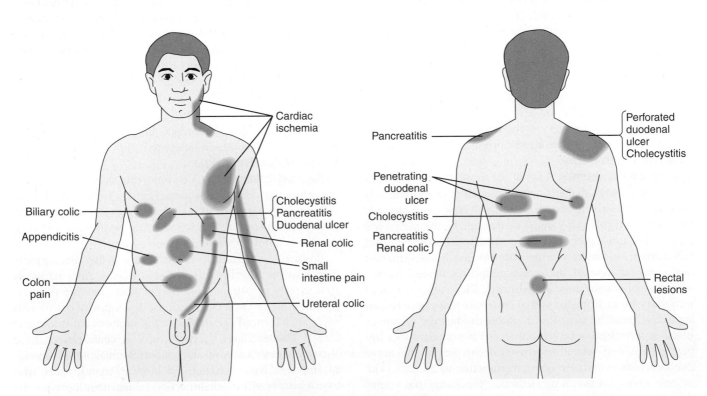

FIGURE 47-9 Areas of referred pain.

the two sources of pain signals and tends to attribute the visceral pain to a body surface location. Patterns of referred pain are fairly uniform and can be used to help locate a source of visceral pathologic process.[5]

PHYSIOLOGIC RESPONSES TO PAIN

The autonomic nervous system, which is responsible for much of the physiologic response to pain, includes both the sympathetic and parasympathetic divisions. Activation of the sympathetic nervous system results in a predictable cluster of physical signs and symptoms, including an elevated heart rate, blood pressure, and respiratory rate, as well as dilated pupils, perspiration, and pallor[4] (see Table 47-4). Sympathetic stimulation results in constriction of superficial vessels to divert blood to striated muscle, heart, and lungs; bronchodilation; increased cardiac contractility; and increased circulating blood glucose. In addition, although gastrointestinal motility and secretion decrease, sphincter tone increases. Nausea, vomiting, and even paralytic ileus may develop. Hypomotility of the bladder and ureters can also result from sympathetic activation and lead to urine retention. Pain stimulates the release of numerous stress hormones, including antidiuretic hormone, aldosterone, and cortisol. These hormones help the kidneys conserve fluid and stimulate the release of glucose from the liver.

The sympathetic responses to pain may be physiologically helpful in the short term but become deleterious if excessive or prolonged. The body cannot sustain this level of activation for long periods. Eventually, physiologic adaptation occurs and the observed sympathetic response to pain abates. Thus the heart rate, blood pressure, and respiratory rate return toward normal or baseline. Signs and symptoms of sympathetic nervous system activation may be an important clue in pain assessment when present, but their absence does not guarantee the absence of pain sensations.

PAIN IN THE YOUNG AND THE ELDERLY

Many myths and misconceptions surround the issue of pain, especially in the very young and the elderly. As a result, often the young and the old receive inadequate treatment of their pain. It was previously thought that neonates were unable to perceive pain. Because their CNS had not yet fully developed and they were unable to remember painful events, neonates often did not receive pain medication or anesthesia for surgery. It has since been found that infants do indeed have pain perception and that inadequate pain control may lead to hemodynamic instability, catabolism, and poor surgical outcomes, especially for premature infants.[19]

In the elderly, it has also been theorized that pain perception is decreased. Research in this area has been inconclusive. Social expectations interfere with the adequacy of pain control in the elderly, as pain is often an expected part of aging. Cognitive factors also hinder pain treatment, especially in patients with dementia who are unable to communicate their need for pain medication. However, it has been found that

pain has a significant effect on an elderly individual's quality of life. No matter what the age of the patient, adequate pain control is important to his or her care.

KEY POINTS

- Acute pain results from tissue injury and generally resolves when the injury resolves. The clinical manifestations result from activation of the sympathetic nervous system (elevated heart rate, blood pressure, and respiratory rate; dilated pupils; perspiration; and pallor).
- Headaches are a common but disabling cause of acute pain. Migraine headaches are caused by an interaction between neurotransmitters and cerebrovascular mechanisms and may be triggered by factors such as stress, foods, and sleep deprivation. There are a variety of treatments for headaches, but all must be initiated early in the course of the headache.
- Chronic pain lasts several months beyond the expected healing time and is often not associated with sympathetic manifestations of pain owing to physiologic adaptation. Instead, changes in personality or lifestyle may occur. Individuals may experience acute and chronic pain simultaneously, as commonly occurs in advanced cancer.
- Fibromyalgia syndrome (FMS) is a poorly understood cause of chronic pain. It is more common in women and has many associated signs and symptoms. FMS is best treated with multiple approaches, both pharmacologic and nonpharmacologic.
- Neuropathic pain results from injury to peripheral or central nerves as a consequence of surgery, tumor, trauma, or drugs and has a constant, achy, or shock-like quality. The sympathetic nervous system may maintain neuropathic pain by releasing norepinephrine onto nociceptors.
- Ischemic pain occurs when inadequate blood flow to tissues results in cellular injury and release of chemicals that stimulate and/or damage nociceptors.
- Referred pain is a painful sensation perceived at some distance from an injury but generally within the same dermatome. Referred pain is thought to occur because of the convergence of visceral nociceptor activity with primary somatic afferents in the posterior horn of the cord.

Treatment Modalities

PHARMACOLOGIC AND NONPHARMACOLOGIC PAIN MANAGEMENT

Many pain management strategies are available. By understanding the basic mechanisms of pain transmission, one can readily identify potential sites where various types of treatment modalities could interrupt pain transmission and perception. Pain management interventions can be directed at three points: (1) interrupting peripheral transmission of nociception; (2) modulating pain transmission at the spinal cord level; and (3) altering the perception and integration of nociceptive impulses in the brain. Recently, the terms *balanced analgesia* and *pre-emptive analgesia* have been used to describe approaches to pain management aimed at multiple sites and applied before stimulation of pain receptors when possible. These approaches are based on the observation that pain memory and hyperalgesia are not prevented by drugs that affect only perception in the brain.[5]

Interrupting Peripheral Transmission of Pain

Modalities that interrupt the peripheral transmission of nociceptive impulses are often the first step in controlling pain. The basic action of splinting an injured limb or area of the body alters the peripheral transmission of pain by minimizing or reducing tissue injury. Applying heat or cold to an injured area also helps reduce peripheral nociception by altering blood flow to the area or by reducing swelling.

Pharmacologic treatments such as NSAIDs or local anesthetic agents also exert their analgesic effects by interrupting peripheral transmission at an early stage. NSAIDs and local anesthetic agents are used as a primary intervention for pain management.[4,5,10] Inhibition of prostaglandin production by NSAIDs reduces the number of pain chemicals available to stimulate nociceptors in the peripheral tissues. NSAIDs include indomethacin, ibuprofen, naproxen, sulindac, piroxicam, ketorolac, and many others. Blocking the production and action of prostaglandins is not without side effects. For example, prostaglandins are responsible for maintenance of the gastric mucosa, and blocking their actions can result in gastrointestinal bleeding. Prostaglandin inhibition can also lead to decreased platelet aggregation and renal insufficiency. Knowledge of the risks and prescribing guidelines is essential for safe patient care, especially for prolonged periods. Many of these agents are available over the counter, and patient teaching regarding benefits and precautions may be needed.

Local anesthetic agents can be applied either to nerve endings at the site of injury or to the nerve plexus supplying the area. By providing localized or regional blockade, peripheral pain transmission is interrupted. Local anesthetic agents diminish or block conduction of the nociceptive impulses by blocking sodium influx during phase 0 of the action potential. The degree of blockade achieved with local agents depends on the amount of drug applied and hence the extent of sodium channel blockade. Local infiltration of a wound or surgical site with local anesthetic agents such as bupivacaine or lidocaine is common practice, even when the patient is also receiving a general anesthetic.

Modulating Pain Transmission at the Spinal Cord

Numerous procedures and agents are used to modulate pain transmission at the level of the spinal cord. Nonpharmacologic techniques that inhibit pain transmission include several types of cutaneous stimulation. Cutaneous stimulation activates and recruits large sensory fibers that can block the central progression of nociceptive transmission at the interneurons. Examples of cutaneous stimulation include transcutaneous electrical nerve stimulation (TENS), massage, acupuncture, application of heat or cold, and therapeutic touch.

Pharmacologic measures that act at the level of the spinal cord include epidural and intrathecal analgesia. Spinal analgesia can be achieved with opioids, local anesthetics, and α-adrenergic blocking agents. Intraspinal opioids work by binding with opioid receptors in the posterior horn of the spinal cord, thereby decreasing the release of neurotransmitters such as substance P. Intraspinal local anesthetic agents block nerve conduction at the posterior nerve root. Epidural administration of an α-adrenergic blocking agent such as clonidine is thought to achieve analgesic effects by blocking sympathetically mediated pain transmission.

Dorsal column stimulators, sometimes used in chronic pain management, also work at the level of the spinal cord to "close the pain gate" by modulating descending input from the brain to the spinal cord.

Altering the Perception and Integration of Pain

The traditional modality for managing moderate to severe pain is the administration of systemic opioids. This pharmacologic intervention has stood the test of time. Opioids work at specific receptor sites that are located throughout the body but are highly concentrated in the brain. Opioid analgesic agents such as morphine and other derivatives alter the perception of pain by the brain. Opioid analgesics have similar mechanisms of action but vary widely in potency. This difference in potency has led to the development of equianalgesic tables to help clinicians prescribe these drugs appropriately (Table 47-6).

Systemic opioids work best for suppressing pain at rest and are less effective during function (moving, coughing).[4] Opioid administration is associated with numerous side effects that

TABLE 47-6

Equianalgesic Table for Common Opioid Analgesics

Drug	Approximate Equianalgesic Dose	
	Oral	Parenteral
Morphine	30 mg q3-4h	10 mg q3-4h
Codeine	30-60 mg	—
Controlled-release morphine (MS Contin)	90-120 mg q12h	—
Hydrocodone	5 mg q4-6h	—
Hydromorphone (Dilaudid)	7.5 mg q3-4h	1.5 mg q3-4h
Meperidine (Demerol)	300 mg q2-3h	100 mg q3h
Methadone	20 mg q6-8h	10 mg q6-8h

Data from McPhee SJ, Papadakis MA, editors: *Current medical diagnosis and treatment,* ed 46, New York, 2007, McGraw-Hill.

may limit effectiveness (nausea, vomiting, respiratory depression, constipation). Long-term use of opioids leads to physical dependence and tolerance.[4] Although the incidence of opioid addiction in persons experiencing acute pain is very low, fears about addiction contribute to inadequate pain therapy. Physical dependence is characterized by withdrawal symptoms if treatment is stopped abruptly. Tolerance to opioids is characterized by the need for increasing dosages to achieve the same analgesic effect. Dependence and tolerance are expected responses to long-term opioid therapy. Drug addiction is a behavioral pattern characterized by craving and preoccupation with obtaining the drug.

Nonpharmacologic techniques of pain management include such activities and procedures as distraction, imagery, relaxation, biofeedback, and hypnosis. With distraction, the number of generalized stimuli reaching the brain increases. Because the brain has a limited capacity to sort and attend to multiple and varied stimuli, it is less able to integrate the pain experience when other competition is present. Imagery may alter the perception of painful stimuli in the higher centers of the brain and produce relaxation as well as analgesia. Biofeedback is a conditioned response that can be learned as a pain-control strategy. Biofeedback is thought to control pain by increasing blood flow (usually as a consequence of relaxation) to targeted body areas. The increased blood flow decreases the concentration of pain-inducing chemicals in the area. Biofeedback may also increase the amount of endorphins produced and released.

A combination of nonpharmacologic and pharmacologic strategies may help reduce the need for high doses of medications. The choice of drug therapy should correspond to the severity of the pain. It has been recommended that mild pain be managed with nonopioid analgesics such as NSAIDs or acetaminophen, whereas moderate pain may require low-potency opioids such as codeine.[4] Severe pain requires larger and more potent doses of opioids like morphine and fentanyl. Recently, the value of combination therapy in blocking pain transmission at multiple sites has been recognized.

SUMMARY

The human experience of pain, although unpleasant, is a normal and expected phenomenon in response to injury. Pain sensations alert the individual to a physiologic problem and help ensure that timely treatment is sought. However, prolonged severe pain serves no good purpose and can be physiologically and psychologically harmful. Appropriate efforts to alleviate pain may enhance recovery from illness and prevent the development of some types of chronic pain syndromes. As understanding of pain physiologic mechanisms grows, treatment strategies can more effectively combine the best of pharmacologic and nonpharmacologic therapies.

REFERENCES

1. Pain terms: a list with definitions and notes on usage. Recommended by the IASP Subcommittee on Taxonomy, *Pain* 6(3):249, 1979.
2. McCaffery M: *Nursing practice theories related to cognition, bodily pain and man-environment interactions,* Los Angeles, 1968, University of California, Los Angeles (master's thesis).
3. Merck: Pain. Available at: http://www.merck.com/mmpe/print/sec16/ch209/ch209a.html.
4. Boswell MV, Cole BE, editors: *Weiner's pain management: a practical guide for clinicians,* ed 7, Boca Raton, Fla, 2006, Taylor and Francis.
5. Hudspith MJ, Siddall PJ: Physiology of pain. Available at: http://intl.elsevierhealth.com/e-books/pdf/1198.pdf.
6. Staud R: Biology and therapy of fibromyalgia: Pain in fibromyalgia syndrome, *Arthritis Res Ther* 8(3):208, 2006.
7. Melzack R, Wall PD: Pain mechanisms: a new theory, *Science* 150(699):971-979, 1965.
8. Melzack R, Wall PD, editors: *The challenge of pain,* ed 2, Harmondworth, UK, 1988, Penguin.
9. Zhuo M: Neuronal mechanism for neuropathic pain, *Mol Pain* 3:14, 2007.
10. McPhee SJ, Papadakis MA, editors: *Current medical diagnosis and treatment,* ed 46, New York, 2007, McGraw-Hill.
11. Lipton RB, Diamond S, Reed M et al: Migraine diagnosis and treatment: results from the American migraine study II, *Headache* 41(7):638-645, 2001.
12. Jones KD, Adams DG: Fibromyalgia: Rational management in primary care, *Clinician Reviews* 16(5):42-48, 2006.
13. Arnold LM: Biology and therapy of fibromyalgia: New therapies in fibromyalgia, *Arthritis Res Ther* 8(4):212, 2006.
14. Peterson EL: Fibromyalgia—management of a misunderstood disorder, *J Am Acad Nurse Pract* 19(7):341-348, 2007.
15. Merck: Neuropathic pain: Available at: http://www.merck.com/mmpe/sec16/ch209/ch209c.html.
16. Bagheri SC, Farhidvash F, Perciaccante VJ: Diagnosis and treatment of patients with trigeminal neuralgia, *J Am Dent Assoc* 135(12):1713-1717, 2004.
17. Ekberg K, Brismar T: C-Peptide replacement therapy and sensory nerve function in Type 1 diabetic neuropathy, *Diabetes Care* 30(1):71-76, 2007.
18. Aring AM, Jones DE: Evaluation and prevention of diabetic neuropathy, *Am Fam Physician* 71(11):2123-2128, 2005.
19. Gupta A, Giordano J: On the nature, assessment, and treatment of fetal pain: Neurobiological bases, pragmatic issues, and ethical concerns, *Pain Physician* 10(4):525-532, 2007.

KEY POINTS

- Treatment is aimed at moderating pain transmission at specific points along the pain pathways. Potential sites of pain moderation are at the peripheral nociceptor, spinal cord, and brain.
- Nociceptor activation can be altered by prostaglandin inhibitors (NSAIDs), heat and cold, and local anesthetics that block sodium influx through fast channels.
- Spinal cord transmission can be altered by cutaneous stimulation (gate control theory), intraspinal analgesics (opioids, local anesthetics, α-adrenergic blockers), and dorsal column stimulators.
- The perception of pain can be altered within the brain by systemic opioids and by nonpharmacologic means such as hypnosis, distraction, and biofeedback.

Biological Markers of Depression and Schizophrenia

Sheila K. Smith • David W. Metzler • Michael J. Kirkhorn

Depression occurs at some time in the lives of most individuals. It can be described as a temporary sadness, the blues, loneliness, or part of normal life, or it can result in a very deep sadness called *major depression*. Major depression is a syndrome resulting in lack of sleep, lack of desire to do things, depressed mood, poor appetite, anxious feelings, and suicidal thoughts. It may end in a completed suicide, devastating a person's family and ending a once-promising life.

Researchers have identified categories of individuals who are most likely to develop depression. The number and variety of these categories suggest that depression is a common problem. As many as 8% of Americans may suffer serious depression at any one time.

Recent epidemiologic studies have demonstrated that young women are more than twice as likely to suffer depression as young men. Depression among the elderly is common, especially if they suffer other illnesses, as many elderly individuals do. However, health care professionals who have infrequent contact with individual patients may overlook it, or if they do diagnose depression, they are likely to undertreat it, resulting in significant morbidity.

People with chronic illnesses may also have chronic depression. Depression has been found increasingly among persons with multiple sclerosis, in which depression is studied both as a possible symptom and as a precipitating factor in the disease. Depression is also commonly found in individuals suffering from dementia of the Alzheimer type, which is characterized by memory loss and intellectual disabilities. Other chronic illnesses frequently accompanied by depression include cancer, heart disease, and advanced lung disease.

Researchers have noted differences in the emotional outlook of individuals who have suffered a single ischemic stroke to the right hemisphere as compared to the left hemisphere. Those with right hemisphere damage were found to have less anxiety than those with left hemisphere stroke, leading researchers to speculate that this decreased anxiety in patients with right hemisphere damage was misunderstood and described in clinical notes as indifference and failure to recover as expected. Research also indicates a relationship between depression and immunity. One study argues that immunocompetence is lower among persons with depression.

The use of biological markers in depression may one day prove to be important, but to this point they are not

PET scan of glucose use in a depressed subject showing frontal hypometabolism on left side (top). *Improvement after treatment with antidepressant medication. Note increased glucose metabolism in frontal lobe* (bottom). *(From Stuart GW, Laraia MT:* Principles and practice of psychiatric nursing, *ed 7, St Louis, 2001, Mosby, p 109.)*

Neuropsychological Function

helpful in the diagnosis and treatment of depression. A family tendency for depression may have a genetic component or more likely multiple genetic causes, but these will likely remain elusive for the foreseeable future. Greater availability of newer antidepressant agents has noticeably influenced mental health care. The use of these agents and other psychotropic medications has increased dramatically during the past decade.

Like depression, schizophrenia can be a severely disabling disease characterized by serious brain chemistry dysfunction in many areas of the brain. Schizophrenia is a chronic disease that typically affects the young. More than three fourths of sufferers become ill before the age of 25, are unlikely to return to normal function without treatment, and may suffer continued decline after repeated episodes. More than 2 million Americans have been diagnosed with schizophrenia, and 200,000 new cases are diagnosed every year.

Over nearly two generations, researchers have followed a hypothesis suggesting that schizophrenia patients suffer from functional changes in the central dopaminergic systems of their brains. This hypothesis is being refined, given the evolution of new antipsychotic medications that affect both the dopamine and the serotonin systems.

Although researchers agree that schizophrenia produces brain dysfunctions, there is still no clear agreement on exactly how and where the brain harbors the disease. For many decades, scientists suspected that they might find a genetic explanation for schizophrenia. Researchers at the National Institute of Mental Health believe that genetic susceptibility accounts for about 60% of the probability of developing the disease. Genotyping is now underway among families with an ill family member to identify characteristics of the disease shared among families. Up to 10 different genetic variations have been linked to schizophrenia. One researcher theorizes that the more of these genetic variations a person has acquired, the more likely their risk of developing the disease. Environmental factors linked to development of schizophrenia include viral, respiratory, and CNS infections; prenatal bereavement or deprivation; obstetric complications such as low birth weight, CNS damage, hypoxia, or pre-eclampsia; and adolescent street drug use, or significant mental health stressors. Some research suggests that in families with a history of mental illness, schizophrenia prevention might be possible by avoiding exposure to environmental stressors and maintaining the healthiest possible social and emotional environments.

Neurobiology of Psychotic Illnesses

Lee-Ellen C. Copstead • Patricia A. Garber

◼ MEDIA RESOURCES

Additional Material for Study, Review, and Further Exploration

CD Companion ◼ Review Questions and Answers
◼ Glossary (with audio pronunciations for selected terms)
◼ Disease Profiles ◼ Animations

evolve Website at http://evolve.elsevier.com/Copstead/
◼ Case Studies ◼ Disease Profiles ◼ WebLinks ◼ Key Points Review

Online Course (Module 19)

◼ KEY QUESTIONS

- What genetic, gestational, and neurologic risk factors are related to schizophrenia?
- What are the "positive" and "negative" symptoms of schizophrenia?
- How are dopamine D_1 and D_2 receptors related to positive and negative symptoms of schizophrenia?

- How is schizophrenia managed?
- What is the neurobiology of major depression?
- What are the hallmark symptoms of major depression?
- What are the subtypes of bipolar disorder?
- How are major depression and bipolar disorder managed?

◼ CHAPTER OUTLINE

Psychosis is a term used to describe a serious and debilitating mental state. The hallmark symptoms of psychosis are delusions, hallucinations, cognitive disorganization, and altered reality. These symptoms characterize a small number of specific mental disorders; however, a wide range of different physical and mental conditions can produce psychotic symptoms. The neurobiological basis of psychosis can be summarized as acute or chronic alterations in neuron anatomy and physiology and cellular biochemical processes. Thought disorders and mood disorders are only two categories of mental disorders with symptom profiles that may include psychosis. Symptoms of psychosis may also occur with substance disorders, delirium, dementia, and acute stress disorder.

Groundbreaking research in brain imaging techniques and psychopharmacology now allow highly precise definitions of the various biochemical pathways associated with psychosis. This chapter addresses four disorders: schizophrenia, delusional disorder, major depression, and bipolar disorder.

Schizophrenia. Disturbance and deterioration of cognitive, social, and emotional functioning characterize **schizophrenia.** Schizophrenia appears to be more a syndrome with unique symptoms then a single disease. Reports of persons described as suffering from these unique symptoms have been recorded for thousands of years in all cultures. The global incidence rate of schizophrenia has consistently been estimated to be about 1% of the world population.[1] The term *schizophrenia* literally is defined as "split mind." Once believed to be a disorder that caused the personality to split into multiple subtypes that communicated with each other, thanks to Eugene Bleuler, who first coined the term, schizophrenia now is correctly understood as a split or separation among normally well-synchronized brain functions. This loss of synchronized brain functioning leads to thoughts, behaviors, and feelings that are disordered, disorganized, and disconnected from reality—a condition generally referred to as *psychosis*.

Etiology and Neurobiology. Most persons first diagnosed with schizophrenia are 15 to 54 years old. The most common age of symptom onset and clinical diagnosis is between 25 and 35 years for women and 15 and 25 years for men. Psychiatrists once disagreed over the likelihood that schizophrenia could first emerge after the age of 45. Most experts now place far less emphasis on first age of symptom onset and focus instead on the presenting symptoms regardless of age.

Antipsychotic medications, first discovered in the 1950s, were the first interventions to truly relieve many of the common symptoms of schizophrenia. Although far from being universally effective and often causing profound side effects, the first generation of antipsychotic medications, also known as neuroleptics, eased suffering, made discharge possible for long-term and seriously ill patients, and radically shifted the focus of treatment from inpatient to outpatient care. The effectiveness of the first generation of antipsychotic medications primarily was attributed to their effectiveness in blocking specific dopamine receptor activity in the brain. This observation was confirmation that schizophrenia was a neurophysiologic illness with complex biopsychosocial symptoms that could be managed pharmacologically. This advance made it possible to more accurately describe the illness, but the exact cause of schizophrenia remains unclear and may, in fact, be a result of many contributing factors.[2]

Dopamine Effects. Because dopamine antagonists (competitive) reduce symptoms of schizophrenia and dopamine agonists (complementary) produce them, abnormalities in dopaminergic pathways in specific regions of the brain were hypothesized as the etiologic key to schizophrenia. Dopamine-specific neurons in the brain primarily are located in the ventral tegmentum of the mesencephalon, medial and superior to the substantia nigra. These regions, as a whole, are referred to as the *mesolimbic dopaminergic system*. The long nerve fibers leaving this system mainly project into the medial and anterior portions of the limbic system. The limbic system contains three powerful centers of behavior control: the nucleus accumbens, the amygdala, and the anterior caudate nucleus (Figure 48-1).

Generally speaking, decreased neurotransmission and connectivity appear to be the neurobiological basis of schizophrenia. This conclusion, reported in findings from an international conference on synaptic dysfunction and schizophrenia,[3] represents the core biochemical process of schizophrenia. As summarized by these experts, the two core neurochemical processes involved are an excess of subcortical dopaminergic transmission at dopamine D_2 receptors and a deficit of glutamate transmission at N-methyl-D-aspartate (NMDA)

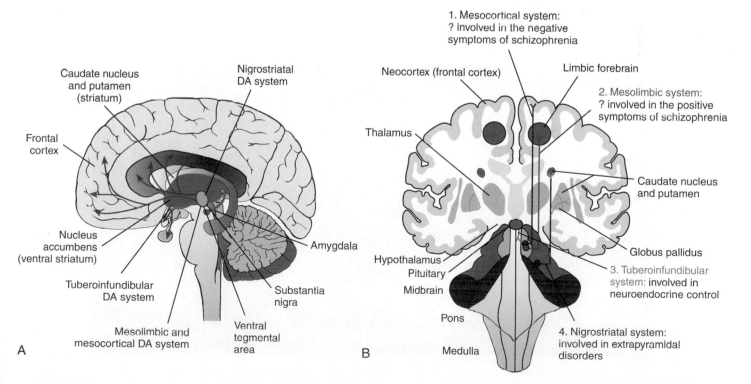

FIGURE 48-1 A, A midsagittal section shows the approximate anatomic routes of the four dopamine (DA) tracts. **B,** A coronal section shows the sites of origin and the targets of all four tracts. (Modified from Kandel E, Schwartz J, Jessell T: *Principles of neural science,* ed 3, New York, 1991, Elsevier. In Stuart GW, Laraia MT: *Principles and practice of psychiatric nursing,* ed 8, St Louis, 2005, Mosby, p 398.)

receptors. The dopamine pathogenesis of schizophrenia can be thought of as disordered synaptic organization. In the brain, normal synaptic organization implies the provision for normal brain cell–to–brain cell communication.

That said, dopamine receptor activity and synaptic transmission are subject to a variety of mediators such as brain-derived neurotrophic factor (BDNF), a neurotrophin that increases synaptic activity and neurotransmitter output.[4] Dopamine synaptic activity also has been closely linked with stress-related cortisol activity and drugs of abuse (cocaine, amphetamine, morphine, nicotine, and ethanol).[5] Although dopamine dysregulation clearly is the driving force[6] behind the neurochemical processes of psychosis, other experts caution against this purely biological model of illness. If schizophrenia were merely a biochemical process, the correct biochemical intervention would be expected to reverse the process instantly. Since this is not the case, critics note that the affected person's cognitive, psychodynamic, and cultural contexts shape the expression of biochemical dysregulation.[6]

Positron emission tomography (PET) brain images have enabled researchers to further examine the overall role of dopamine activity in psychosis and schizophrenia. PET studies have demonstrated low glucose metabolism rates in the frontal cortex and dopamine regions[7] of the brains of persons with schizophrenia (Figure 48-2). Of the many different types of dopamine brain cell receptors identified, dopamine D_2 receptors once again were found to be strongly associated with symptoms of schizophrenia. Similar research has shown that dopamine D_2 receptors are particularly responsive to antipsychotic drugs.

Thus, the **dopamine hypothesis,** which postulates that schizophrenia symptoms result from presynaptic dysregulation of dopamine transmission, continues to be the focus of neurobiological studies. The specific neuropathologic mechanism of schizophrenia appears to be a functional excess of postsynaptic dopamine receptor activity and dopamine receptor hypersensitivity, either alone or in combination.

Genetic Effects. For individuals who are genetically predisposed to schizophrenia, symptoms are largely determined by the biopsychosocial characteristics.[8] Researchers continue to study the actual versus potential genetic risks of schizophrenia. For example, it was once thought that individual genetic predisposition to schizophrenia was triggered by severe stress. For example, severe physical or sexual abuse during vulnerable periods of growth and development might trigger symptoms in persons who are genetically vulnerable. In other words, what factors appear to be most reliably associated with symptom onset? Absent any other condition, having a family history of schizophrenia does not alone lead to schizophrenia. Schizophrenia can and often does develop in persons with no family history of psychopathology. Nevertheless, significant genetic factors have been identified.

Initial interest in identifying possible genetic contributions to schizophrenia was based on early research on monozygotic (identical) and dizygotic twins. In identical twins born to parents with schizophrenia but reared apart from their parents, the percentage of offspring who do and who do not develop schizophrenia is about equal.[9] Children of two parents with schizophrenia have a 40% to 68% risk of developing the illness, whereas children with one parent with schizophrenia have

Controls

Schizophrenics

FIGURE 48-2 Individual variation in positron emission tomography (PET) scans. Four normal individuals *(top row)* and four schizophrenics *(bottom row)* show range of hypofrontality and diminished basal ganglia metabolism. (From Buchsbaum MS, Haier RJ: Functional and anatomical brain imaging: impact on schizophrenia research, *Schizophr Bull* 13(1):115-132, 1987. Reproduced by permission of Monte S. Buchsbaum, MD.)

a 9% to 16% risk.[9] At 8% to 14%, the risk in a non-twin sibling of a brother or sister with schizophrenia is slightly less. The obvious limitation of these findings is that they do not explain why an at-risk offspring does not develop schizophrenia.

Several additional conditions are thought to be involved in the transformation from genetic risk to actual illness. Factors such as prenatal infections, malnutrition, birth complications, and brain injury have been associated with the development of schizophrenia in persons who have increased genetic risk.[10] Moreover, different gene locations appear to also be relevant to the illness onset. Experts question whether inherited genetic risk for schizophrenia could explain observed differences in incidence and prevalence rates based on gender and race. Lastly, genetic models of schizophrenia typically do not address risk in terms of the subtype of schizophrenia, such as symptoms with versus symptoms without paranoia. Given the high standards of proof required for gene typing, a purely genetic explanation of an illness as complex as schizophrenia

seems unlikely. Increased genetic risk of schizophrenia appears to be a critical part of a puzzle composed of many pieces.

Gestational Effects. Early findings noted that in persons with schizophrenia, pyramidal cells in the hippocampus were not lined up like a "picket fence," as they were in control subjects (Figure 48-3). Instead, the cells appeared to be rotated at 70° to 90° angles.[11] Pyramidal cells migrate during the second trimester of gestation and later become fastened by neuronal cell adhesion molecules (N-CAMs). Researchers focused on the possibility of pyramidal cell misalignment and lost N-CAM adhesive effects as links between gestation and schizophrenia. Researchers noted that in pregnant women living in Scandinavia and England who were exposed to the 1957 flu epidemic during their second trimester, 300% more of their children were diagnosed with schizophrenia than those of women who experienced flu during the first or third trimester.

These findings were considered significant for two reasons: (1) neuronal migration peaks during the second trimester,

FIGURE 48-3 Photographic comparison of hippocampal tissue at CA 2/3 interface in a control *(top)* and in a person with chronic schizophrenia *(bottom).* (Original magnification of the Nissl-stained tissue, ×100.) (From Kovelman JA, Scheibel AB: A neurohistological correlate of schizophrenia, *Biol Psychiatry* 19:1601-1621, 1984.)

and (2) the influenza virus is one of a very few viruses that produce capsular neuraminidase, an enzyme that can change the adhesive properties of N-CAMs.[12] Hippocampus, para-hippocampal gyrus, and amygdala neurons process information and emotional expression. Researchers speculated that the symptoms of schizophrenia might be due to failed neuronal connections and distorted interpretation of incoming messages to the brain that reduce the brain's ability to filter out extraneous stimuli. Other researchers have suggested that delivery complications could be an additional factor, playing a mediating role between prenatal influenza exposure and later development of schizophrenia.[13]

In an effort to explain why gestational exposure to influenza might manifest years later in young adults, a 29-year longitudinal study, conducted by the University of Southern California and Danish researchers,[14] followed 207 Danish children born to mothers with severe schizophrenia. The teams examined reports of elementary school behavior in an attempt to identify children with early behavioral dysfunctions. The study revealed that children who later developed negative symptoms of schizophrenia as young adults had been described by their elementary teachers as withdrawn, isolated, and passive. The children who later developed more positive symptoms of schizophrenia, including hallucinations, delusions, and inappropriate behavior, had been described as high-strung and aggressive with behavior problems. These findings indicate that although the full onset of the illness may not occur at early stages of growth and development, related alterations can be observed.

More recent studies of gestational abnormalities focused on specific brain regions and stages of prenatal neurodevelopment.[15] This research is exemplified in a well-controlled Canadian study that examined the association of hippocampus formation abnormalities and first adult episode of schizophrenia. The main functions of the hippocampus are learning and new-memory formation. Both abilities may be lost when hippocampal functioning is impaired. Macroscopic cell abnormalities, such as fewer synapse connections and diminished synapse activity, result in reduced hippocampal volume. Reduced hippocampal volume has been associated with severe stress, mood disorders, and schizophrenia.[16] The Canadian researchers hypothesized that schizophrenia was associated with incomplete formation of the hippocampus during the second trimester of development. They used magnetic resonance images to compare the brains of newly diagnosed patients with healthy matched controls. Although the number of participants in the study was too small to allow for generalizations to be drawn, the magnetic resonance images of the newly diagnosed patients clearly showed enlarged hippocampal fissures or disrupted hippocampal formation. Interestingly, obstetric complications during pregnancy were not significant factors.

Neurologic Effects. Observed neuroanatomic differences in persons with schizophrenia led researchers to study anatomic and functional abnormalities in the limbic and frontal brain. Structural abnormalities in these brain regions would suggest that abnormal functioning might contribute to the disrupted cognitive processes or symptoms of schizophrenia. Beginning in 1976, computed tomography (CT) studies revealed enlarged brain ventricles in persons with schizophrenia. A ground-breaking 1980 study showed that the neurochemical basis of schizophrenia might involve two processes: dopamine neurotransmission dysregulation and abnormal cerebral structure.[17]

Magnetic resonance imaging (MRI) studies of persons with chronic schizophrenia indicated larger-than-normal lateral and third ventricles and reduced temporal lobe gray matter[18] (Figure 48-4). MRI findings also showed reduced frontal lobe

Unaffected   Affected

FIGURE 48-4 Loss of brain volume associated with schizophrenia is clearly shown by magnetic resonance images comparing the size of ventricles (butterfly-shaped, fluid-filled spaces in the midbrain) of 44-year-old male identical twins, one of whom has schizophrenia *(right)*. The ventricles of the person with schizophrenia are larger, suggesting structural brain changes associated with the illness. Note that such magnetic resonance images cannot be used to diagnose schizophrenia in the general population because of normal genetic variation in ventricle size; many unaffected people have large ventricles. (From Fortinash KM, Worret PA: *Psychiatric mental health nursing,* ed 3, St Louis, 2004, Mosby, p 240. Courtesy Daniel Weinberger, MD, Clinical Brain Disorders Branch, Division of Intramural Research Program, NIMH, 1990. Updated December 11, 2000.)

Active in
frontal cortex

Less active in
frontal lobe and
cingulate gyrus

Normal
control

Schizophrenia
patient

FIGURE 48-5 Positron emission tomography (PET) scan with ^{18}F-deoxygluose shows metabolic activity in a horizontal section of the brain in a control subject *(left)* and in an unmedicated client with schizophrenia *(right)*. Red and yellow indicate lower activity in the white matter areas of the brain. The frontal lobe is magnified to show reduced frontal activity in the prefrontal cortex of the client with schizophrenia. (From Fortinash KM, Worret PA: *Psychiatric mental health nursing,* ed 3, St Louis, 2004, Mosby, p 259. Courtesy Monte S. Buchsbaum, MD, Mt. Sinai School of Medicine, New York.)

National Institute of Mental Health Clinical Neuropsychiatry
rCBF Percent Change Activation

Normal
patients
(n=25)

Schizophrenic
patients
(n=24)

Left   Right

FIGURE 48-6 Regional cerebral blood flow *(rCBF)* maps showing lateral views of cerebral cortex with frontal pole at *left*, occipital pole at *right*. Lateral view of percent change in rCBF in left and right hemisphere during the Wisconsin Card Sorting (WCS)/number matching tasks. Data are for 25 normal subjects *(top)* and 24 patients with schizophrenia treated with neuroleptic agents *(bottom)*. Note that the normal subjects show striking rCBF increases during WCS/number matching tasks. (Redrawn from Berman KF, Zec RF, Weinberger DR: Physiologic dysfunction of dorsolateral prefrontal cortex in schizophrenia II. Role of neuroleptic treatment, attention, and mental effort., *Arch Gen Psychiatry* 43(2):126-135, 1986.)

blood flow and relative decreases in frontal lobe metabolic activity. Prefrontal cortex structure and functioning deficits were consistently observed when the subject was simultaneously placed under stress (Figure 48-5). The stress used in the study was primarily psychological, such as contingency planning exercises or divergent thinking during performance of a cognitive task that utilized specific regions of the prefrontal cortex[19] (Figure 48-6).

Subsequent studies of brain structure with persons with severe schizophrenia replicated the earlier findings of abnormal limbic-cortical structures and smaller, misarranged hippocampal pyramidal cells. This includes replication of MRI findings of reduced bilateral temporal lobe volume, decreased hippocampal volume, and reduced volume in the parahippocampal gyrus region of the brain. Studies of brain regions other than the limbic system revealed frontal lobe structural alterations in the dorsolateral area of the prefrontal cortex and in the cingulate and motor cortices. The finding of decreased frontal lobe glucose metabolism associated with schizophrenia also has been replicated.[20]

Postmortem brain tissue studies of deceased patients indicated fewer nicotinic receptors present in the hippocampus. Tobacco dependence is a common secondary disorder with schizophrenia. The finding of fewer nicotinic receptors was of particular interest to researchers in that previous studies had shown that smoking could temporarily normalize auditory sensory gating that typically becomes impaired with schizophrenia.[21] Since then, researchers found that a neurophysiologic deficit at chromosome 15, at the OC7-nicotinic receptor gene, may partially explain the inheritance of this neurophysiologic symptom.[22] Although the development of schizophrenia is associated with any number of specific abnormalities, early neurodevelopmental alterations that result in dysfunction of the limbic and prefrontal regions of the brain appear to be critical.

Clinical Manifestations. **Positive symptoms**[23] of schizophrenia are thought to result from excessive dopamine D_2 receptor activity in the brain. Positive symptoms are more apparent to the casual observer than negative symptoms. Common symptoms include disorganized thinking (inability to logically connect thoughts), unusual speech (e.g., invented words, tangential ideas), odd behavior, delusions (systematic fixed false beliefs), and hallucinations (sensory perceptions with no apparent stimulus). Delusions often are persecutory, grandiose, or religious in nature. Auditory hallucinations are most common, but hallucinations may affect vision, smell, taste, and touch. Antipsychotic medications that effectively decrease brain dopamine activity tend to be effective in relieving and managing positive symptoms of schizophrenia.

Negative symptoms[23] of schizophrenia are thought to be associated with dopamine D_1 receptor activity in the brain. Negative symptoms represent deficits in functioning and thus can be more difficult to recognize than positive symptoms. Common examples of negative symptoms include social withdrawal and isolation, dull or blunted emotional affect, poverty of speech (limited verbal communication), posturing or remaining in one position for prolonged periods, and autism. Antipsychotic medications that effectively block dopamine D_1 receptors tend to be effective in relieving and managing negative symptoms of schizophrenia.

Disorganization, in comparison with previous functioning, is generally accepted as a behavioral hallmark of schizophrenia. This includes some degree of impairment in work or academic performance, interpersonal relating, and self-care. Disorganization and disturbance in language and communication may be the most common observation made of persons with schizophrenia. The person finds it difficult if not impossible to conform to accepted rules governing behavior, appearance, and speech, and these discrepancies cannot be attributed to intelligence, education, or cultural background.

Speech manifestations of schizophrenia include tangential ideas, words with private or approximate rather than generally accepted meanings, and neologisms. Neologisms are invented words with invented, special, or private meanings. Loose associations are seemingly unrelated ideas presented as though they are related. Speech symptoms are a serious source of frustration for persons with schizophrenia. Loss of ability to communicate with others is isolating, and the inability to understand others can become alarming. Box 48-1 summarizes problems of cognitive functioning in schizophrenia, including those related to speech.

Delusions are systematic false beliefs that persist despite evidence to the contrary. The beliefs or ideas have meaning and are true to the individual rather than to reality and are not merely reflections of cultural values or ideals. Delusional content varies from person to person. Common delusional systems are grandiose, persecutory, or religious in nature. A person with delusions of persecution might believe he or she is being poisoned, watched, harassed, cheated, or otherwise plotted against by a powerful group or individual. Fearful convictions that one's thoughts, feelings, or actions are under the control of others can occur. Thought broadcasting is the belief that one's thoughts are being broadcasted and made audible to others. Inversely, thought insertion is the belief that others are able to place thoughts into one's mind. Believing that one can control the thoughts, feelings, and actions of others also occurs. Delusions generally have themes of control and passivity and have been referred to as *first-rank symptoms.*

Hallucinations indicate the breakdown of perceptual selectivity. The ability to sort and process sensory information is lost. Perceptions (vision, hearing, taste, smell, touch) occur without objectively discernible stimuli. Hallucinations usually are auditory, but any or all of the five senses can be affected. Clear conscious awareness of hearing one's own thoughts or hearing voices, known or unknown, argue, comment, comfort, threaten, or appraise is not uncommon. Command hallucinations are the least predictable form of auditory hallucinations with the tremendous potential for tragic effects. Command hallucinations are experienced as impulses that the person has no choice but to carry out.

Affect, or emotional tone, may become blunted, shallow, flat, inappropriate, or silly. Loss of emotional tone is characterized by an unchanging, inexpressive facial expression, lack of eye contact, few gestures, and little to no tone or inflection in speech.

Anhedonia, or the absence of pleasure or interest, is observed with many disorders, including schizophrenia. The

---

BOX 48-1

Problems in Cognitive Functioning

Memory
Difficulty retrieving and using stored memory
Impaired short-term/long-term memory

Attention
Difficulty maintaining attention
Poor concentration
Distractibility
Inability to use selective attention

Form and Organization of Speech (Formal Thought Disorder)
Loose associations
Tangentiality
Incoherence/word salad/neologism
Illogicality
Circumstantiality
Pressured/distractible speech
Poverty of speech

Decision Making
Failure to abstract
Indecisiveness
Lack of insight (anosognosia)
Impaired concept formation
Impaired judgment
Illogical or concrete thinking
Lack of planning and problem-solving skills
Difficulty initiating tasks

Thought Content
Delusions
Paranoid
Grandiose
Religious
Somatic
Nihilistic
Thought broadcasting
Thought insertion
Thought control

From Stuart GW, Laraia MT: *Principles and practice of psychiatric nursing,* ed 8, St Louis, 2005, Mosby, p 389.

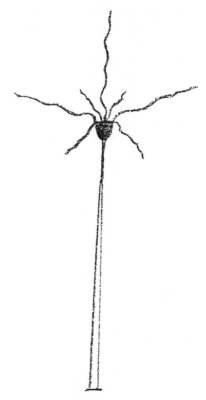

FIGURE 48-7 A person actively experiencing psychosis was asked to draw a tree. Black was chosen from a selection of colors. The slender, tapered tree trunk may represent the instability of the Ego. The branching structure is reminiscent of religious symbolism and poverty of hope. (Courtesy Chris Rost, RNC, MN, Spokane, Wash.)

affected individual may feel little pleasure from pleasurable experiences or may no longer engage in pleasurable experiences.

Self-identity disturbances with schizophrenia can be profound. Generally, having a sense of oneself means being able to differentiate one's physical self from the physical environment (Figure 48-7). This can take the form of a cosmic feeling of being one with the universe or being limitless. The disturbance is related to impaired perceptual and cognitive recognition of boundaries (Figure 48-8). Self-identity disturbances also are psychological. Identity requires discernment of self as distinct from others. Without this, people can feel exposed and defenseless.

Autism is a term used to indicate profound detachment. In autism, the external world becomes inaccessible, leaving the person alone in a separate world. Behavior, communication, and mood may reflect this separate world and thus, to casual observers, appear inappropriate.

Motor behavior is affected by schizophrenia. Posturing, mannerisms, pacing, bizarre rituals, clumsiness, grimacing, and aimless activity are examples of impaired psychomotor behavior (Figure 48-9). These behavioral symptoms of schizophrenia can be confused with extrapyramidal side effects of antipsychotic medications.

Sleep disturbance with acute schizophrenia generally takes the form of being unable to sleep. Tension, anxiety, psychomotor hyperactivity, active delusions, and hallucinations literally keep people awake. Those who are able to find sleep may spend close to the normal amount of time sleeping but

FIGURE 48-8 This drawing was created by a person with a thought disorder and demonstrates absence of boundaries between sky and sea. The isolation and powerlessness are underscored by the island and body position of the person. Negation of vital life is represented by the decaying tree. The fish and birds and squirrel maintain a menacing quality. Although a full color range of markers was available, the person used only black. (Courtesy Chris Rost, RNC, MN, Spokane, Wash.)

their sleep is not restful, including less deep sleep or rapid eye movement (REM) sleep, frequent awakenings, nightmares, and early-morning awakening. As a result, the normal wake-up time tends to shift from morning to early afternoon.

Pharmacologic Treatment. Newer antipsychotic medications are intended to generally manage psychosis as well as both the positive and negative schizophrenia symptoms. Older antipsychotic medications were less effective in managing negative schizophrenia symptoms. They mainly acted as dopamine antagonists, blocking the dopamine receptors (D_2). This action diminishes the amount of dopamine received by the receptor sites (Figure 48-10). Specific schizophrenia symptoms have been associated with neurotransmission dysregulation that diminished or elevated dopamine activity. Hyperdopaminergic states have primarily been associated with positive symptoms of schizophrenia such as hallucinations, delusions, and psychosis. Hypodopaminergic states have primarily been associated with negative symptoms of schizophrenia such as cognitive difficulties, lack of energy and motivation, and depression.[24] Dopamine D_2 receptors have been associated with positive symptoms and psychosis, whereas dopamine D_1 receptors have been associated with negative symptoms. Effective antipsychotic medications have significant dopamine effects; however, schizophrenia symptoms are highly complex and likely to involve other neurotransmitters, particularly serotonin and norepinephrine (Table 48-1).

When effective, antipsychotic medications[25] can be expected to diminish or remit hallucinations or reduce their impact on functioning. The ability to reason should improve; ambivalence, delusions, and suspiciousness should be greatly reduced; agitation and confusion should be relieved; and social behavior should improve. Antipsychotic medications are designed to have specific effects on targeted neurotransmitters. Dopamine and serotonin have been the most important neurotransmitters associated with the symptoms of schizophrenia. Antipsychotic medications employ different biochemical methods to achieve similar objectives, the primary objective being the reduction of dopamine activity in the limbic system and the frontal cortex.

Newer antipsychotic medications are equally effective in this regard but they vary in their side effect profiles and their potential for interacting with other medications. First-generation antipsychotic medications (e.g., chlorpromazine) had relatively nonspecific neurotransmitter effects and

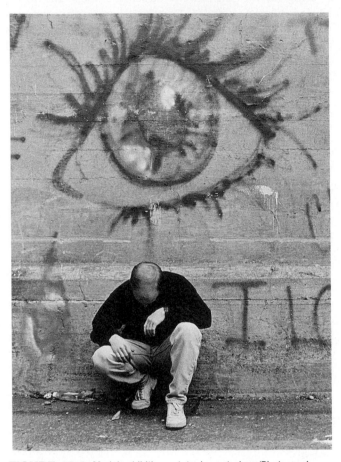

FIGURE 48-9 Model exhibiting catatonic posturing. (Photographer: Kathleen Kelly, Spokane, Wash.)

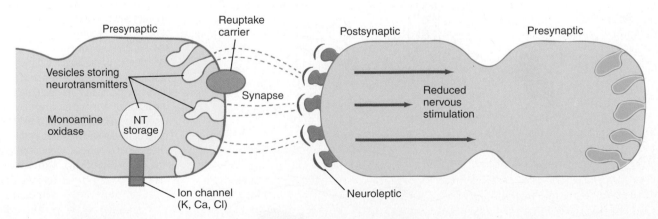

FIGURE 48-10 Neuroleptic (antipsychotic) action. Neurotransmitter *(NT)* action at the synapse is modified by neuroleptics, which block postsynaptic receptor sites to reduce nervous stimulation (reducing symptoms of schizophrenia). (From Fortinash KM, Worret PA: *Psychiatric mental health nursing,* ed 4, St Louis, 2008, Mosby, p 254.)

TABLE 48-1

Neurotransmitters in Schizophrenia: Type and Function

Neurotransmitter	Type	Function
Dopamine	Catecholamine	Regulates motor behavior in extrapyramidal nerve tracts and also transmits in the cortex. Increases vigilance and may increase aggression. Too much may produce psychosis; too little may cause movement disorders (EPS).
Serotonin	Indolamine	Brainstem transmitter; modulates mood; lowers aggressive tendencies. A deficiency may be responsible for some forms of schizophrenia.
Acetylcholine	Cholinergic	Transmits at nerve-muscle connections (central nervous system and autonomic nervous system). A deficiency may increase confusion and acting out behavior. Controls EPS.
Norepinephrine	Catecholamine	Transmits in the sympathetic nervous system. Induces the "flight or fight" syndrome (hypervigilance). May be insufficient in clients with schizophrenia who display anhedonia (loss of pleasure).
Cholecystokinin	Peptide	Excites the limbic neurons. A deficiency is related to avolition (lack of motivation) and a flat affect.
Glutamate	Amino acid	Excitatory neurotransmitter. Impairment in the N-methyl-D-aspartate affects glutamate metabolism, which can lead to problems with cognition, delusions, and possibly some negative symptoms of schizophrenia.
γ-Aminobutyric acid (GABA)	Amino acid	Inhibitory neurotransmitter; predominantly a brain transmitter. Promotes a balance between dopamine and glutamate and thus inhibits impulsive behaviors.

From Fortinash KM, Worret PA: *Psychiatric mental health nursing,* ed 3, St Louis, 2004, Mosby, p 241.
EPS, Extrapyramidal symptoms.

numerous side effects. Haloperidol was the first high-potency antipsychotic medication that had significantly less anticholinergic and hypotensive side effects. By 1990, atypical antipsychotics became widely available. The first atypical antipsychotic, clozapine, was quickly followed by a generation of new atypical antipsychotics (risperidone, olanzapine, and quetiapine), each promising still fewer side effects, better relief of both positive and negative schizophrenia symptoms, and minimal risk of tardive dyskinesia (the one antipsychotic medication side effect that can become irreversible).

Dopamine D_2 remains the lead neurotransmitter target of the atypical antipsychotics.[25] Researchers found that the most common side effects of antipsychotic medication could be reduced if the drug's impact on dopamine D_2 receptors was not excessive. Lower receptor occupancy, less receptor affinity, and faster release[26] of the receptor were methods shown to be associated with fewer side effects. More recently, the aim for effective antipsychotic medication is to stabilize rather than reduce dopamine activity. These medications, such as aripiprazole and ziprasidone, show greater affinity for serotonin receptors (negative symptoms) and moderate affinity for dopamine and norepinephrine receptors (positive symptoms).[26]

Pharmacologic Side Effects. Metabolic side effects of the new atypical antipsychotic medications can be significant. Some worrisome side effects are clinically significant weight gain, glucose dysregulation, and dyslipidemia.[27,28] Experts have speculated that hyperglycemia may have to do with dopamine receptor involvement in the regulation of insulin secretion. Numerous explanations for weight gain as a major side effect of antipsychotic medication continue to be developed and tested. The glutamate neurobiological model[29] of psychosis

and schizophrenia, an alternative to the dopamine model, may be the basis for the next new generation of antipsychotic medications.

The *glutamate deficit*[29] model attempts to focus attention on the cause of excessive dopamine receptor activity rather than the excessive activity itself. γ-Aminobutyric acid (GABA) is the most important inhibitory brain neurotransmitter. GABA synthesis depends on and is controlled by the enzyme glutamic acid decarboxylase (GAD). GAD activity is modulated by the glutamate receptor NMDA. GAD dysregulation is thought to lead to insufficient GABA activity and, consequently, excessive dopamine activity. Reduced GAD activity has been observed in the dorsolateral prefrontal cortex and hippocampus of patients with schizophrenia. The interesting observation for pharmacological researchers is that a broad range of different drugs has been shown to be capable of affecting GAD activity. Although the glutamate deficit model is not new, the model might yet lead to a class of antipsychotic medications unlike any generation before.

KEY POINTS

- Schizophrenia is characterized by altered perceptions of reality and disordered thinking. Genetic predisposition and environmental factors are thought to interact to produce biological changes in the brain, particularly in the hippocampus, temporal lobes, and dopaminergic pathways that project to the limbic system. Exposure to influenza virus during the fifth to sixth months of gestation appears to predispose to schizophrenia. The age

- at onset is 15 to 25 years for men and 25 to 35 years for women. There is a higher incidence in industrialized societies. Stress and childhood experiences may affect the expression of schizophrenia. Lack of safety, security, order, and predictability and low self-worth are probable contributing factors in relation to increased stress.
- Neurologic abnormalities found in those with schizophrenia and children who later develop schizophrenia include abnormal blinking and blink reflex, abnormal pupil reflex and facial movements, enlarged lateral and third ventricles, reduced temporal gray matter, decreased blood flow, and decreased glucose metabolism in frontal lobes.
- The positive symptoms of schizophrenia are thought to be due to excessive dopamine D_2 receptor activation in the brain. Disorganized thinking (inability to connect thoughts logically), disorganized speech (rambling, tangentiality), delusions (fixed system of false beliefs), and hallucinations (sensory perceptions when no apparent stimulus exists) are typical positive symptoms. Delusions are often persecutory, grandiose, or controlling. Hallucinations are most often auditory but may also be visual, olfactory, or tactile. Positive symptoms respond to drugs that decrease dopamine activity in the brain (e.g., olanzapine, quetiapine).
- Negative symptoms are thought to be mediated by dopamine D_1 receptors in the brain. Drugs that block D_1 receptors (e.g., clozapine) may alleviate some of the negative symptoms, which include social withdrawal, flat affect, poverty of speech, ritualistic posturing, and autism.

Delusional Disorder. **Delusional disorder** does not present a clear clinical picture. The disorder is characterized by behaviors that are dominated by systematic false beliefs that persist despite objective contradictory evidence. Unlike the delusions typically associated with schizophrenia, the delusions are highly systematic with very limited themes. The actual content and process of the delusions remain constant. Usually other symptoms of disordered thinking are absent or are rare. Systematic delusions are persistent and pervasive and may impact several aspects of daily life. Delusional disorder is similar to schizophrenia in that acute psychosis can occur.

Etiology and Neurobiology. Delusional disorder may eventually prove to be a form of schizophrenia or schizophrenia spectrum disorder.[30] Presently most experts consider delusional disorder a separate disorder with neurophysiological properties that overlap with those of schizophrenia. Unlike schizophrenia, delusional disorder can dramatically reshape personality and character traits. Also, learned suspiciousness resulting from overwhelming interpersonal stress and negative life experiences is not uncommon with delusional disorder. In fact, the onset of delusional symptoms can coincide with stressful life events that the affected person perceives as overwhelming and inexplicable. Although actual misfortune, suffering, disadvantagement, and disappointment may have been experienced, actual events do not become the basis for systematic false beliefs. The beliefs are better understood as cognitive symptoms in reaction to actual events, which does not imply that the onset of delusional disorder is triggered by the experience of disturbing life events. The etiologic progression of delusional disorder continues to be studied.

A key characteristic of delusional disorder is the readiness and ease with which new, neutral, and coincidental life experiences become incorporated into the system of delusional beliefs. Once a delusional system has been developed, actual life experiences are likely to be viewed through the lens of the delusional system. In this way, life seems always to confirm rather than challenge the delusions. Life experiences thought to be associated with the onset of delusional disorder tend to be profound experiences that generate intense feelings of failure or personal inadequacy. In effect, the delusions appear to function as a massive psychological defense against further injury or damage to self-esteem. Given its low incidence, believed to be 3 to 4 cases per 100,000, and low prevalence, believed to be less than 0.10%, delusional disorder is a relatively rare condition. That said, low incidence and prevalence rates also could be explained by the observation that few persons with delusional disorder are likely to recognize their condition and seek mental health care.

Clinical Manifestations. Delusions[31] are the hallmark or defining symptom of delusional disorder. With this disorder, delusions typically take the form of false beliefs that are systematic without being bizarre. The core feature of these false beliefs is that the beliefs in theory could be true but are nevertheless highly unlikely. Mental and cognitive functions that are not directly involved in the delusions remain intact. Two common delusional systems are the belief that one is having a secret relationship with a famous person and the belief that one is being pursued by a powerful government agency intent on destroying the individual. Grandiose delusions also are extremely common. In this case the person believes she or he possesses great attributes or is in some way extraordinary. Jealousy delusions often have to do with a sexual partner who is perceived as unfaithful or untrustworthy. Less obvious delusions involve litigation and persistent legal actions to seek redress for perceived wrongs or slights. Retaliation or the unpredictable use of aggression or violence is a constant concern with any person who is delusional and feels unfairly wronged or slighted.

Reality testing[31] or the ability to evaluate and appreciate the difference between internal experiences and external experiences is, by definition, impaired by delusions. Delusional beliefs are unaffected by the lack of objective evidence. Normal reality testing implies that, in the face of compelling evidence to the contrary, the belief no longer is accepted as valid. With delusional disorder, impaired reality testing maintains the delusions. In other words, impaired reality testing indicates that the person is unable, rather than unwilling, to perceive reality.

KEY POINTS

- Delusional disorder is a psychotic illness dominated by a tenacious system of false beliefs. It is a slowly developing disorder that may begin with a "grain of truth" and then escalate to delusional proportions as the person assigns false meaning to life experiences. Delusional beliefs often have themes of jealousy, secret love, grandiosity, persecution, and legal retaliation for perceived wrongs (litigiousness).
- The biochemical and structural basis of delusional disorder is unknown. Some commonality with schizophrenia is suspected.

TABLE 48-2

Risk Factors for Major Depressive and Bipolar Disorders

Risk Factor	Major Depression	Bipolar Disorder
Lifetime prevalence (%)	F: 5-9	0.6-0.9
M/F ratio	1:2	1:1.2
Age at onset (yr)	Mid to late 30s	Late teens to early 20s
Social class	No relationship	Slight increase in upper classes
Race	No relationship	No relationship
Family history		
Major depression in relatives (%)	17	15
Bipolar depression in relatives (%)	2-3	8

From Hirschfeld RMA, Goodwin PR: Mood disorders. In Talbott JA, Hales RE, Yudofsky SC, editors: *The American Psychiatric Press textbook of psychiatry,* Washington, DC, 1988, American Psychiatric Press, p 410.

Major Depression. Once referred to as endogenous depression, or depression that arises from characteristics of the person, major depression now is understood to be a complex illness involving inherited genetic susceptibility and symptoms associated with specific alterations in brain structures and functioning. According to the *Diagnostic and Statistical Manual of Mental Disorders,*[31] the American Psychiatric Association reference guide that is updated about every 10 years, a diagnosis of major depression requires the presence of multiple symptoms that are intense enough to cause distress and to persistently impair psychosocial functioning. Depression with one or two symptoms that last 2 years or more is commonly referred to as minor depression or **dysthymia.**

Major depression is a leading cause of suicide. This illness frequently occurs as a comorbid disorder with serious physical illness as well as other mental disorders. Major depression also can develop as a serious secondary illness or illness complication. For example, as early as 1937, researchers were able to show that cardiac patients with severe depression had higher cardiac death rates than their counterparts. More recent studies of depression and mortality during the first year following myocardial infarction showed significantly greater risk for 1-year mortality in patients who were depressed.[32]

Evidence of a possible genetic susceptibility to major depression partially explains why female rates consistently are twice the rates observed in males, but significant rates of major depression are observed in all age, race, education, and income groups.[33] The complexity of managing severe depression in adolescents[34] and older adults[35] has made these population groups particularly concerning. As a result of the potentially serious disability, morbidity, and mortality risks directly associated with the illness, the World Health Organization (WHO) ranks major depression among the top five global health problems.[36]

Etiology and Neurobiology. Improved neurobiological research techniques have made possible the accomplishment of basic scientific advances in determining the neurobiological mechanisms of major depression. Nevertheless, the specific cause of major depression remains unknown. Table 48-2 summarizes mood disorder risk factors.

Cognitive-behavioral[33] models of depression, particularly learned helplessness,[34] have been shown to correlate with the basic neurobiology of depression. Avoidant persons, when faced with a highly stressful situation, anxiously withdraw from or avoid confronting the situation, despite opportunities to do so. Persistent avoidance eventually conditions the person to automatically respond to stressful situations with strong feelings of helplessness. Helpless response to a stressful situation exposes the person to the full negative impact of the stress, which in turn promotes more withdrawal, more avoidance, more helplessness, and, most importantly, higher levels of stress.

Neurobiological changes associated with major depression are thought to involve neurotransmission dysregulation,[35] altered hippocampal and prefrontal cortex cell structure and functioning,[37] and hypothalamic-pituitary-adrenal (HPA) system activation[38] (Table 48-3). Based on observations of low central nervous system levels of serotonin (Figure 48-11) in persons with severe symptoms of depression, the basic neurobiology of depression has been hypothesized to be reduced brain serotonin neurotransmission activity either through excessive presynaptic uptake or through stress-related downregulation of postsynaptic receptors (Figure 48-12). Chronic or persistent vulnerability to depression is thought to be related to decreased hippocampal volume or capacity[39] and suppressed hippocampal neurogenesis.[40]

Research focused on the biological model supports a biological basis for mood disorders. Some of the biological factors associated with depression are illustrated in Figure 48-13.

HPA axis dysfunction has been associated with depression. Genetic susceptibility to depression appears to mediate the link between stress and depression.[41] Comparison studies of stress-induced cortisol levels in depressed persons and healthy control subjects showed significant links between stress hormones and depression, but far more information is needed before the precise nature of the link can be understood.[42]

TABLE 48-3

Prefrontal Cortex and Serotonin Interconnections: Implications in Depression

Interconnected Brain Structures	Hypothesized Role of These Interconnections in Depression
Prefrontal cortex	Covering the frontal lobes, it is unique within the central nervous system for its strong interconnections with all other areas of the brain; it receives information that has already been processed by other sensory areas and then merges this information with other emotional, historical, or relevant information, thus attending to both feelings and intellect.
Limbic system structures	The prefrontal cortex modulates limbic system activities (emotional and instinctive) by way of these three structures: Hippocampus — Major importance in cognitive function, including memory. Amygdala — Major importance in modulating feelings such as aggression, anger, love, and shyness. Cingulate gyrus — Involved in motivation and interest.
Brainstem	Responsible for regulating the general state of arousal and tone of brain function; also the location of structures that manufacture various neurotransmitters, such as serotonin (5-HT), norepinephrine (NE) and dopamine (DA).
Raphe nuclei	Located in the brainstem, they manufacture 5-HT; they also modulate excessive stimuli, and the organization and coordination of appropriate responses to these stimuli.
Hypothalamus	This interconnection allows for direct prefrontal input into neuroendocrine function via the hypothalamic-pituitary axes.
Suprachiasmatic nucleus	Located in the hypothalamus, it regulates circadian (24-hr) rhythms and circannual rhythms; thus it is also implicated in seasonal affective disorder.

From Stuart GW, Laraia MT: *Principles and practice of psychiatric nursing,* ed 8, St Louis, 2005, Mosby, p 341.

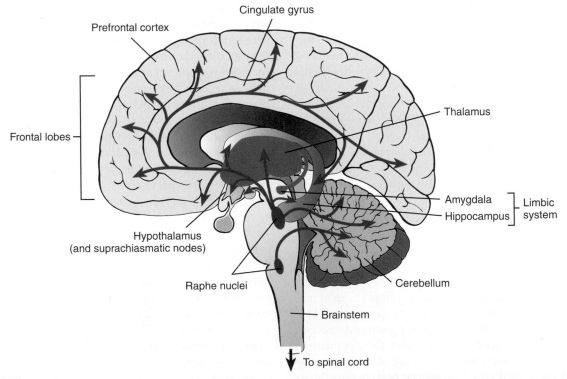

FIGURE 48-11 The serotonin neurotransmitter system implicated in depression. (From Stuart GW, Laraia MT: *Principles and practice of psychiatric nursing,* ed 8, St Louis, 2005, Mosby, p 340.)

One of a number of stress and depression theories proposes that increased stress hormone levels can lead to significant decreases in the expression of brain-derived neurotrophic factor (BDNF). Reduced BDNF has been shown to lead to hippocampal cell atrophy and, consequently, reduced neurotransmission activity in this area of the brain.[43] According to the researchers, effective antidepressant medications seemed to improve BDNF activity and thereby promote the growth and survival of serotonin neurons in this vital brain region. Significant reduction in BDNF activity, as a result of severe stress, has also been demonstrated in research animals. The HPA model of depression supports the development of novel

FIGURE 48-12 Levels of postsynaptic serotonin (5-HT) receptors. More receptors are present when there is too little 5-HT (up-regulation) and fewer receptors when there is too much 5-HT (down-regulation). (From Stuart GW, Laraia MT: *Principles and practice of psychiatric nursing,* ed 8, St Louis, 2005, Mosby, p 372.)

FIGURE 48-14 A, Normal sleep architecture. **B,** Depressed sleep architecture. Green areas indicate rapid eye movement *(REM)* sleep. (From Stuart GW, Laraia MT: *Principles and practice of psychiatric nursing,* ed 8, St Louis, 2005, Mosby, p 342.)

FIGURE 48-13 Biological factors related to depression. *EEGs,* Electroencephalograms, *TRH,* thyroid-releasing hormone, *DST,* dexamethasone suppression test. (From Stuart GW, Laraia MT: *Principles and practice of psychiatric nursing,* ed 8, St Louis, 2005, Mosby, p 342.)

treatments that can target cortisol activity (e.g., mifepristone) rather than serotonin activity (e.g., selective serotonin reuptake inhibitors, SSRIs).[44]

Sleep studies of depression have shown significantly reduced slow-wave (delta) sleep (stages 3 and 4) and increased light sleep (stage 1). The periods of REM sleep latency with depression are shortened, but the total number of REM periods does not decrease (Figure 48-14). Sleep is restorative for brain cells. Among the numerous restoration activities that occur, mood-related hormone activity during sleep appears to decrease although severe reductions in serotonin activity have been associated with less restful sleep. Because of the link between fluctuations in mood-related hormones and sleep, disturbed sleep is a hallmark symptom of depression. The classic sleep disturbances include difficulty falling asleep, early-morning waking, and decreased total sleep time.[45]

Circadian rhythms (synchronizing cycles) are closely associated with symptoms of major depression. The pineal gland in the brain produces the hormone melatonin. Brain melatonin levels can fluctuate significantly, with annual and daily increases and decreases in light and dark periods. Melatonin helps regulate circadian rhythms; in turn, these cycles govern body temperature changes and the urge to sleep. Depressed persons have been shown to suffer from low melatonin levels when their symptoms include disturbed sleep. Depression symptoms that predictably occur when the daily hours of daylight decrease in the winter then remit when the hours of natural light increase in the spring is known as **seasonal affective disorder**. In theory, natural light acts as a *zeitgeber*, or a biological clock synchronizer that is based on the 24-hour day-night cycle. It has been hypothesized that persons with seasonal affective disorder who are exposed to additional natural light will experience improvement in their sleep-wake cycle and, consequently, improved mental health.

Clinical Manifestations. Depressed mood and the loss of interest or pleasure (anhedonia) are hallmark symptoms of major depression. This change in mood is relatively constant and is recognized both by the depressed person and by others. Depressed mood associated with major depression is qualitatively different from the normal sadness or grief associated with loss. Depressed mood typically is experienced as painful, numbing, and bottomless. Loss of interest or pleasure can be more difficult to recognize. Others may notice this change before the depressed person does but the loss may be absolute, meaning that if the person engages in such activities, interest and pleasure are not experienced. In effect, the capacity for interest and pleasure appears to be lost.

Fatigue or loss of energy is a common yet somewhat alarming symptom of depression. Depressed people may associate their severe or sudden fatigue with serious physical illness such as cancer, diabetes, or cardiovascular disease. The fatigue associated with depression can make ordinary daily activities, once performed automatically, nearly impossible. The fatigue of depression is not relieved by rest or sleep and, when severe, can become immobilizing.

Restless, irritable agitation associated with depression can range from mild hyperactivity and sarcasm to hostility and aggression. Compulsive yet meaningless physical activities such as pacing are not uncommon. Often the person attempts to engage the restlessness with activities such as "organizing" papers.

Impaired concentration is experienced as a highly disturbing symptom of depression. Decreased ability to concentrate, attend, and think is common with severe depression. Thoughts slow down and the process of thinking literally becomes difficult. Thought content typically is dominated by highly depressive themes. Impaired decision making is one of many consequences of thinking that is slowed and narrowed. Minor choices and simple preferences become difficult, but more importantly, the decision to seek or accept treatment for depression can be affected.

Low self-esteem is the psychological hallmark of depression. Negative self-appraisals range from pointless guilt to self-hate. In some cases, the guilt reaches delusional proportions or is markedly disproportionate to actual misdeeds or perceived failings. Loss of self-esteem with depression differs from the ordinary day-to-day waxing and waning of self-esteem. People generally find ways to protect their self-esteem from the normal assaults of daily life. With severe depression, self-esteem can be absent and only rarely is the loss related to actual life events.

Negative thinking, expressed as negative views of self, life, and the future, is a symptom of severe depression that is common but often misunderstood. Severe depression is an empty experience that makes life itself seem futile. Expressions of negative thinking essentially reflect this deep psychological experience. Negative thinking associated with depression can be mistaken as willful or so unpleasant that others avoid contact with the depressed person.

Vegetative states associated with depression manifest as slowed or reduced physical activity. Normal daily activities, particularly bathing and dressing, may not be performed. Vegetative symptoms typically are described as feeling as though one is sleep walking, living in slow motion, or has become a robot.

Sleep disturbances of depression follow the neurobiological and cognitive-behavioral symptoms of depression. Insomnia is most common, but some people may sleep more or shift their sleep hours from nighttime to daytime. Sleep symptoms include difficulty falling asleep, early-morning awakening, frequent awakenings, and waking tired. The cognitive activity generated by obsessive negative thinking disturbs sleep essentially by preventing it or by literally waking the person.

Appetite disturbance associated with depression ranges from increased to decreased appetite to marked change in food preferences. Severely depressed persons can become unaware of their hunger or thirst. Diminished salivary and gastric activity can dampen appetite. Weight loss of 10 to 20 pounds over relatively short periods is not uncommon. Overeating also occurs, but this disturbance appears to be related more to restlessness than to appetite. People who normally use food for emotional comfort may, when depressed, increase their consumption of high-fat, high-sugar, high-salt foods.

Psychosis associated with major depression is thought to result from extreme symptom severity, prolonged symptom duration, or comorbid illness complications. Hallucinations, delusions, and disorganization may become prominent and require treatment with antipsychotic medications. Severely depressed older adults are at increased risk of depression-associated psychosis.

Pharmacologic Treatment. Most antidepressants currently available act by improving brain norepinephrine and serotonin activity. Earlier generations of antidepressants had less specific effects on these neurotransmitters and significantly more side effects. Monoamine oxidase inhibitors (MAOIs) blocked the destruction of norepinephrine and serotonin once it was released into the synaptic cleft. Tricyclic antidepressants (TCAs) blocked the reuptake of norepinephrine and serotonin, thereby allowing more neurotransmitter activity. SSRIs became widely available in the 1990s and were the first antidepressants with selective serotonin effects. SSRIs such as fluoxetine, paroxetine, and sertraline have been shown to relieve depression symptoms three times faster than earlier medications with far fewer side effects.

SSRIs quickly became the primary class of antidepressants; some have multiple treatment indications for additional disorders. Although the side-effect profile of SSRIs represents real improvement over earlier antidepressants, SSRIs are not side effect free.[46] Serotonin syndrome[47] is a serious side effect that results from excessive serotonin activity. This side effect can be caused by drug-drug interactions or individual sensitivity to serotonergic drugs. Symptoms of serotonin syndrome include altered mental status, restless agitation, myoclonus, hyperreflexia, sweating, shivering, tremor, gastrointestinal upset, ataxia, and headache.

Sexual dysfunction also is thought to result from SSRI-induced excessive serotonin activity. Onset can be immediate or gradual, with effects ranging from loss of interest, to impaired arousal, to anorgasmia. Less severe but equally troublesome side effects include gastrointestinal upset, headache, allergy, dry mouth, constipation, urination difficulties, sweating, and significant weight gain.

SSRI cellular and neurochemical mechanisms continue to be the subject of a great deal of basic and clinical research. It would appear that the SSRIs share the basic action of boosting neurotransmission activity of mood-related monoamines. More recent research findings suggest that SSRIs may also alter the genetics-based expression of BDNF and cell neurogenesis in the hippocampus.[48]

Bipolar Disorder

Etiology and Neurobiology. Bipolar disorder is a highly complex mood disorder characterized by recurring symptoms of depression and elation that can become severe enough to produce psychosis. Decades of clinical and genetic research findings indicate that the increased risk of developing the illness is both inherited and acquired (Figure 48-15). Symptom onset leading to the initial diagnosis of bipolar disorder typically does not occur before late adolescence or early young adulthood. However, childhood onset and older age onset also can occur. The most recognizable course of illness with bipolar disorder is the sudden onset of severe mania lasting from weeks to months. Mania is the hallmark symptom of bipolar disorder; however, when the initial symptoms of mania are severe enough to produce psychosis, bipolar disorder can be mistaken for schizophrenia. Accurate diagnosis of bipolar disorder when the initial symptom profile is depression can be quite difficult or long delayed.

Efforts to identify the neurobiological factors that characterize bipolar disorder have yielded mixed results. First, the similarities between psychosis associated with mania, psychosis associated with depression, and psychosis associated with schizophrenia are a major hurdle. Second, the depression associated with bipolar disorder differs very little from the depression that characterizes major depression. Third, when bipolar symptom onset is gradual, changes in behavior can be mistaken for personality disorder or substance use disorder.

Thus far there is little evidence of a stable genetic or biochemical distinction between bipolar disorder, schizophrenia, and major depression. However, as with schizophrenia and major depression, the significant inherited risks of bipolar disorder have been documented. The findings of twin studies and parent-child studies show significant inherited risk of bipolar disorder.[31] The risk in monozygotic twins of a parent with bipolar disorder is 75%. The risk in a person with two parents with bipolar disorder is 60%. The risk in first-degree relatives is 20%, and the risk in the general population is 1%.

The neurotransmission model of bipolar disorder follows the basic *catecholamine hypothesis* for major depression and schizophrenia. Neurotransmission activity deficits are thought to promote depression symptoms associated with bipolar disorder, whereas excessive activity is thought to promote symptoms of mania and psychosis. The assumption is that the depression and mania of bipolar disorder are the result of two different neurobiological processes. The alternative hypothesis is that bipolar disorder is the result of a specific form of neurotransmission dysregulation that results in the loss of mood stabilization. Given the fact that with bipolar disorder a mixed mood state that includes symptoms of both mania and depression is not uncommon, the mood destabilization hypothesis is of great interest. Both models focus on serotonin, norepinephrine, and dopamine as the neurotransmitters involved.[49]

Neuroimaging studies of brain structural changes associated with bipolar disorder indicate findings potentially similar to those of major depression. For example, ventricular enlargement, increased numbers of T2 signal hyperintensities, and tissue loss in the basal ganglia, lateral and mesial temporal structures, and cortical regions have been observed. At the same time, other researchers have reported no significant tissue changes associated with bipolar disorder. Experts suggest that tissue changes probably are linked with greater mania symptom severity and duration. For example, symptom onset in older age has been related to greater tissue changes.[49] Neurobiological studies of the evidence of tissue changes associated with bipolar disorder thus far have not linked specific changes with depression, elation, or mania. Nevertheless, impaired functioning has consistently been associated with tissue changes. Findings such as these lend important support to the hypothesis of impaired emotion processing and impaired regulation of emotional behavior as the probable neurobiological mechanism of bipolar disorder.[49]

Clinical Manifestations. The two basic forms of bipolar disorder are bipolar I and bipolar II. A diagnosis of bipolar I disorder requires at least one episode of mania as well as major depression. A diagnosis of bipolar II disorder requires no episodes of mania and at least one episode of hypomania and major depression.

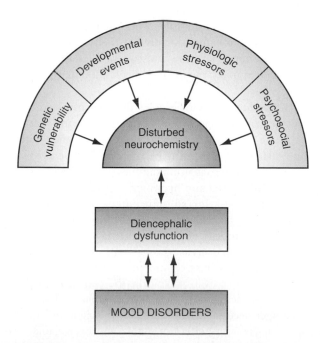

FIGURE 48-15 Unified model of mood disorders. (Redrawn from Stuart GW, Sundeen SJ: Disturbances of mood. In Stuart GW, Sundeen SJ, editors: *Principles and practice of psychiatric nursing,* ed 4, St Louis, 1991, Mosby, p 429.)

Three additional types have been proposed (types II1/2, III, and IV) which go beyond the previous two types and better represent the clinical complexity of bipolar symptoms.[50] This suggests the concept of a bipolar spectrum and allows for earlier and more accurate diagnosis and treatment of persons who clearly suffer from mood dysregulation but who do not meet the narrow symptom criteria for bipolar I or bipolar II disorder.

Mania or full mania is characterized by apparent symptoms and marked impairment. Overwhelming increase in energy and drive manifest as nonstop activity, grandiose thinking, impulsivity, euphoria, impaired judgment, acting-out behaviors, and hypersexuality. Changes in thinking, appearance, speech, personality, and emotions can be dramatic and last weeks to months with or without evidence of psychosis. Anger, belligerence, and aggression can develop quickly when others attempt to set limits or interfere. The person sleeps very little if at all and may believe that he or she either is too busy to eat or no longer requires food. Highly inappropriate phone calls, attempts to contact public officials or famous persons, excessive spending, and "schemes" can result in very serious financial and legal consequences.

Hypomania or partial mania can include any symptoms of mania but without the loss of reality testing, without psychosis (e.g., hallucinations, delusions), and without impaired functioning. The individual experiencing hypomania may insist that the sudden onset of increased energy, expanded self-esteem, and decreased anxiety has improved his or her productivity or that it is an acceptable *natural high.* Unlike mania, it is possible for an episode of hypomania to run its course without being recognized as hypomania.

Depression or dysphoria can have a sudden onset and include symptoms similar in number and intensity to those of major depression (see the Major Depression section).

Euphoria or expanded mood is a hallmark symptom of both mania and hypomania. Extreme cheerfulness, enthusiasm, and optimism are present, but the joyful, buoyant mood is disproportionate to events and surroundings.

Racing thoughts, also referred to as "flights of ideas," grossly impair cognitive ability and speech. People who experience racing thoughts typically describe having thoughts "flying through my mind" at such a volume and speed that they cannot talk fast enough or move fast enough to keep up.

Irritable mood occurs with both mania and hypomania, particularly after prolonged symptom duration. Sarcasm, hurtful criticism, fault finding, and general unpleasantness predominate. Attempts to limit the activities of a person who is hypomanic or fully manic can quickly be met with dramatic displays of aggressive irritability.

Grandiosity or wildly inflated self-esteem is expressed through self-appraised importance, claims of limitless expertise, and insulting put-downs. When grandiose, the person with bipolar disorder has little or no tolerance for being criticized, questioned, or contradicted. This perceived self-importance can reach delusional proportions resulting in the person's attempting to act on his or her importance, genius, and infallibility. Serious negative consequences of grandiose actions as well as financial and criminal schemes are not uncommon.

Energy level with mania and hypomania can appear to be limitless. At lower levels, increased energy can be productive. But more often, increased energy produces aimless hyperactivity with constantly shifting interests and distractions. Signs of physical fatigue become obvious, but the hyperactivity continues. Dangerously low sensitivity to fatigue as well as increased risk of injury and self-harm can occur. At extremely high levels of energy, the person becomes disorganized if not psychotic. Compulsive collecting and hoarding of meaningless objects is common.

Speech disturbance with bipolar disorder can become dramatic. The most common disturbance with mania is loud, rapid, constant, pressured, or explosive speech that may not be interpretable. At early stages, pressured speech may seem an adroit and humorous play with words. Entertaining jokes, rhymes, and puns are common. At later stages, clang associations, runaway thoughts, and invented words make communication extremely difficult. Untreated, eventually speech becomes incoherent.

Hallucinations and **delusions** can occur with the psychosis that typically develops with severe, prolonged mania. Unlike the hallucinations and delusions associated with schizophrenia, the alterations in perceptions and thinking that occur with mania generally are mood congruent. In other words, grandiose mood is likely to be mirrored by grandiose delusions and hallucinations.

Impulsive action is a hallmark symptom of mania and hypomania. This mood state typically is characterized by behavior with little to no consideration of effects or consequences. People who become impulsive when manic or hypomanic are truly unable to explain or predict their actions and may be unable to appreciate the consequences of their actions. Impulsivity can make the affected person a potential danger to self or others.

Impaired judgment with bipolar disorder can lead to significant deviancy. Socialized behavior is behavior that conforms to the social rules defining right and wrong. Without this internal switch governing behavior, primitive drives can take over. The more common examples of impaired judgment associated with mania and hypomania have to do with inappropriate sexual behavior, substance abuse, inappropriate and excessive spending, thrill seeking, and rule breaking.

Appetite is indirectly affected by mania and hypomania in that food intake can decrease dramatically, resulting in significant weight loss and loss of appetite. No single explanation holds true for all cases, but typically the person either is too busy with other activities to stop or insists that food and water are no longer necessary. In effect, loss of weight and appetite occurs as a secondary effect of mania and hypomania. True loss of appetite, as with major depression, is rare, meaning that the person may be hungry but is too distracted or busy to eat.

Sleep disturbance with mania and, in some cases, with hypomania takes the form of little or no sleep. Sleeping can become difficult and, as with food, the person may insist that sleep is unnecessary. Days without sleep may force the person to take brief naps but, without treatment, restorative sleep can become unattainable.

Hypersexuality associated with mania and hypomania creates high-risk situations and potentially serious consequences. Combined with impulsivity and impaired judgment, a sudden increase in the drive for sex can lead to highly uncharacteristic and unpredictable behavior. This includes serious risk of the patient being victimized or exploited by others as well as carrying out harmful behaviors toward others. Marriages and long-term relationships can suffer greatly from indiscriminate sexual behavior that the person cannot explain. The risk of atypical sexual behaviors or activity involving persons with whom the patient might normally not have contact is a serious source of concern.

Pharmacologic Treatment. Medications presently indicated for use as mood stabilizers include lithium, anticonvulsants, and atypical antipsychotics. Appropriate pharmacologic treatment for bipolar disorder requires accurate diagnosis. Before bipolar disorder diagnosis and treatment are considered, the possibility of a primary medical condition or drug reaction as the cause of depression, elation, mania, or psychosis must be considered (Table 48-4). Because of the many overlapping symptoms, it is not uncommon for persons with bipolar disorder to be misdiagnosed as depressed or schizophrenic.[51]

Lithium is the standard mood stabilization medication used to manage bipolar disorder. Recent, well-controlled clinical treatment studies confirm lithium's effectiveness in the management of bipolar I and bipolar II disorders.[52] That said, many individuals with severe bipolar disorder symptoms nonetheless require additional antidepressant and antipsychotic medications to achieve optimal symptom management. Antipsychotic medications have been found to be effective in remitting symptoms of psychosis as well as in preventing their recurrence. Managing the depression symptoms of bipolar disorder can prove more complicated. In some cases antidepressant medications can trigger mood switching or destabilize mood.

Growing numbers of anticonvulsants now are being considered for use as mood stabilizers. These include various reformulations of carbamazepine, divalproex, and lamotrigine. Many of the pharmacodynamic and pharmacokinetic properties of the commonly used mood-stabilizing medications have been well defined.[53] A variety of potential mechanisms have been proposed for lithium. The neurotransmission effects of lithium have been attributed to calcium-dependent cell wall depolarization. Through this process, dopamine and norepinephrine are released, and major secondary messenger neurotransmitter signals are released.

Lithium is absorbed in the gastrointestinal tract but is not metabolized; more than 90% is excreted by the renal system. Any interference with the excretion of lithium (e.g., fluid volume depletion, angiotensin-converting enzyme inhibitors, diuretics) can lead to rapidly increasing plasma lithium levels and toxicity. Continuous patient education and routine plasma lithium level checks help to reduce the risk of toxicity.

Early symptoms of lithium toxicity include confusion, nausea, and fatigue. Prelithium assessment of liver, renal, and thyroid functioning is required. In some cases, lithium leads to hypothyroidism that requires treatment. Lastly, lithium treatment for bipolar disorder requires multiple daily doses, generally twice a day or more often. Multiple daily doses can exacerbate patient ambivalence about taking lithium. Euphoria, mania, and long symptom-free periods typically are misperceived as signs that lithium no longer is needed.

Divalproex often is the next best choice when lithium cannot be taken. This anticonvulsant has been found to have neuroprotective effects similar to those of lithium.[53] Unlike lithium, divalproex is highly bioavailable, is metabolized by the liver, produces an active metabolite, has a long half-life, and can be used to manage acute mania. Persons with impaired liver functioning or liver disease cannot take divalproex, and the routine evaluation of plasma levels is required to reduce the risk of toxicity.

Several atypical antipsychotic medications show promise as potentially effective mood-stabilizing medications. Of these, olanzapine, risperidone, quetiapine, and ziprasidone have received considerable attention. These medications exhibit a range of dopaminergic, serotonergic, and norepinephrinergic effects that improve many bipolar symptoms, particularly when the symptoms include full mania rather than hypomania. Once-daily dosing is an important advantage.

KEY POINTS

- Affective disorders are due to disordered emotions or affect. Included in this category of psychoses are bipolar disorder (periods of mania and depression) and unipolar depression. The average age at onset is 30 years for bipolar disorder and 40 years for unipolar depression. Depression affects women twice as often as men.

- A biochemical basis for **bipolar disorder** is supported by observations that brain monoamines (norepinephrine, serotonin) are below normal or the ratio of norepinephrine to serotonin is altered. Depression is thought to occur when serotonin and norepinephrine activity in the brain is low. Mania may be due to a relative excess of norepinephrine in the context of low serotonin or acetylcholine activity. Plasma membrane transport of small molecules such as lithium also is different. Bipolar disorder has a familial pattern of expression, suggesting a genetic cause.

- Psychosocial factors that may affect the development and expression of mood disorders include loss (real, anticipated, or perceived) and low self-esteem. Sleep disorders accompany both extremes of mood. Depression is associated with altered REM sleep and decreased slow-wave sleep. Mania is associated with short sleep and reduced fatigue.

- **Depression** is manifested by low energy, inability to experience joy, difficulty initiating tasks, reduced decision-making ability, difficulty sleeping, poor appetite, weight loss, and decreased libido. Thoughts may focus

TABLE 48-4

Selected Physical Illnesses and Drug Reactions Associated with Psychiatric Conditions

Cause	Psychiatric Symptoms Associated with Specific Disorders			
	Depression	Mania	Paranoia	Anxiety
Infectious processes	Influenza; viral hepatitis infectious mononucleosis; general paresis (tertiary syphilis); tuberculosis	Influenza; St. Louis encephalitis; Q fever; general paresis (tertiary syphilis)		
Endocrine disorders	Myxedema; Cushing disease; Addison disease	Hyperthyroidism	Addison disease; Cushing disease; hypothyroidism; hypoparathyroidism; hyperparathyroidism	Hyperadrenalism (Cushing disease); hypothyroidism; hyperthyroidism
Neoplastic disorders	Occult abdominal malignancies (e.g., carcinoma of head of pancreas)			Secreting tumors (carcinoid, insulinoma, pheochromocytoma)
Collagen disorders	Systemic lupus erythematosus	Systemic lupus erythematosus; rheumatic chorea	Systemic lupus erythematosus	Systemic lupus erythematosus
Neurologic disorders	Multiple sclerosis; cerebral tumors; sleep apnea; dementia; Parkinson disease; non-dominant temporal lobe lesions	Multiple sclerosis; diencephalic and third ventricular tumors	Brain tumors; temporal lobe epilepsy; Alzheimer disease; Pick disease; Huntington disease; Parkinson disease; multiple sclerosis; cerebral atherosclerosis; hypertensive encephalopathy; multi-infarct dementia	Encephalopathies (infectious, sleep apnea; metabolic, toxic); essential tremor; intracranial mass lesions; postconcussional syndrome; complex partial seizures; vertigo
Nutritional states	Pellagra; pernicious anemia		Vitamin B$_{12}$ deficiency	Caffeine; monosodium glutamate; vitamin deficiency diseases; anemias
Reactions to drugs	Steroidal contraceptives, reserpine; methyldopa; physostigmine; alcohol; sedative-hypnotics; amphetamine withdrawal	Steroids; levodopa; amphetamines; methylphenidate; cocaine; monoamine oxidase inhibitors; tricyclic antidepressants; thyroid hormones	Amphetamines; cocaine; hallucinogens (LSD, PCP); marijuana; mescaline; withdrawal syndromes (alcohol, sedative-hypnotics, barbiturates, benzodiazepines)	Akathisia (secondary to antipsychotic drugs); anticholinergic toxicity; digitalis toxicity; hallucinogens; hypotensive agents; stimulants (cocaine, amphetamines, related drugs); withdrawal syndromes (alcohol, sedative-hypnotics); bronchodilators (theophylline)
Metabolic disorders			Hypoglycemia; liver failure; uremia	Hyperthermia; hyponatremia; hyperkalemia; hypocalcemia; hypoglycemia; menopause; porphyria (acute intermittent)
Cardiovascular disorders				Angina arrhythmias; congestive heart failure; hypertensive; hypovolemia; myocardial infarction; syncope (of multiple causes); valvular disease; vascular collapse (shock)
Respiratory disorders				Asthma; chronic obstructive pulmonary disease; pneumonia; pneumothorax; pulmonary edema; pulmonary embolism

Data from Whybrow P, Akiskal H, McKinney W: *Mood disorders: toward a new psychology*, New York, 1984, Plenum Press; Hyman SE, Jenike MA: *Manual of clinical problems in psychiatry*, Boston, 1990, Little, Brown; Rosenbaum JF: The drug treatment of anxiety, *N Engl J Med* 306:401–404, 1982.

on guilt, futility, emptiness, hopelessness, helplessness, and suicide. The management of unipolar depression is aimed at increasing norepinephrine and serotonin activity in the brain. MAOIs reduce the rate of neurotransmitter destruction; TCAs inhibit reuptake; newer agents (fluoxetine) selectively prevent serotonin reuptake.

- **Mania** is manifested by high energy; inflated self-esteem; hyperactivity; inability to focus or concentrate; low sensitivity to fatigue, injury, or pain; rapid or incoherent speech; hallucinations; delusions; increased appetite and libido; decreased sleep; poor judgment; and poor impulse control. Mania is managed with lithium, a compound that inhibits the action of norepinephrine and serotonin in the brain.

GERIATRIC CONSIDERATIONS

- Schizophrenia and delusional disorder may continue into old age or may appear later in life. Late-onset schizophrenia, which emerges after age 45 years, occurs more often in women than in men.
- Psychiatric admissions of older individuals are characterized by significantly more major depression and less dysthymia than that seen in younger adults. The incidence of bipolar disorder in the geriatric age group should approach that of lifetime risk. It is extremely rare for bipolar disorder to emerge after age 60 years, and all bipolar disorder patients who survive to old age continue to be vulnerable to that illness.
- Mood disorders in the elderly are likely to be associated with concomitant illnesses or their treatments.
- Management of late-appearing psychoses is complicated by a number of factors. Older patients are more sensitive to medication than younger patients, and their response varies more than that of younger patients; they may suffer cognitive impairment; they may have visual or auditory impairment; they may be taking drugs for other chronic disorders; and they may forget to take their medications or take wrong doses. In addition, older patients may suffer side effects such as tardive dyskinesia, a disorder related to antipsychotic drug dosage and duration and characterized by involuntary chewing motions and darting of the tongue.

SUMMARY

The clinical symptoms, causes, and neurobiological mechanisms of schizophrenia, major depression, and bipolar disorder have been presented. Significant risk of psychosis is a common characteristic shared among these seemingly unrelated disorders. Brief overviews of the neurobiological basis of medications used to manage the symptoms of these disorders reflect the tremendous neurobiological advances that have been accomplished. Nevertheless, these three illnesses are potentially disabling conditions that all too often rob the affected person of academic goals, meaningful work, close relationships, self-actualization, and, in some circumstances, survival. Psychosis is associated with a wide range of illnesses and disorders; this chapter has covered three of the most common mental disorders.

REFERENCES

1. Thaker GK, Carpenter WT Jr: Advances in schizophrenia, *Nat Med* 7(6):667-671, 2001.
2. Manish S, Phansalkar S, Kablinger AS: Biological markers and the future of early diagnosis and treatment in schizophrenia, *Psychiatric Times* 24(2):19-21, 2007.
3. Frankle WG, Lerma J, Laruelle M: The synaptic hypothesis of schizophrenia, *Neuron* 39(2):205-216, 2003.
4. Goggi J, Pullar IA, Carney SL et al: Signaling pathways involved in the short-term potentiation of dopamine release by BDNF, *Brain Res* 968(1):156-161, 2003.
5. Saal D, Dong Y, Bonci A et al: Drugs of abuse and stress trigger a common synaptic adaptation in dopamine neurons, *Neuron* 37(4):577-582, 2003.
6. Kapur S: Psychosis as a state of aberrant salience: a framework linking biology, phenomenology, and pharmacology in schizophrenia, *Am J Psychiatry* 160(1):13-23, 2003.
7. Portin P, Alanen YO: A critical review of genetic studies of schizophrenia: II. Molecular genetic studies, *Acta Psychiatr Scand* 95(2):73-80, 1997.
8. Harrop C, Thrower P: *Why does schizophrenia develop at late adolescence? A cognitive-developmental approach to psychosis,* West Sussex, England, 2003, Wiley.
9. Rinomhota AS, Marshall P: *Biological aspects of mental health nursing,* Edinburgh, 2000, Churchill Livingstone.
10. Javitt DC, Coyle JT: Decoding schizophrenia, *Sci Am* 290(1):48-55, 2004.
11. Weinberger DR: Implications of normal brain development for the pathogenesis of schizophrenia, *Arch Gen Psychiatry* 44(7):660-669, 1987.
12. Susser E, Lin SP, Brown AS et al: No relation between risk of schizophrenia and prenatal exposure to influenza in Holland, *Am J Psychiatry* 151(6):922-924, 1994.
13. Venables PH et al: Prenatal influenza exposure and delivery complications: implications for the development of schizophrenia, *Fam Community Health* 30(2):151-159, 2007.
14. Baxter RD, Liddle PF: Neuropsychological deficits associated with schizophrenic syndromes, *Schizophr Res* 30(3):239-249, 1998.
15. Nasralla HA, Smeltzer DJ: *Contemporary diagnosis and management of the patient with schizophrenia,* Newtown, Pa, 2002, Handbooks in Health Care.
16. Smith GN, Lang DJ, Kopala LC et al: Developmental abnormalities of the hippocampus in first-episode schizophrenia, *Biol Psychiatry* 53(7):555-561, 2003.
17. Jampala VC, Taylor MA, Abrams R: The diagnostic implications of formal thought disorder in mania and schizophrenia: a reassessment, *Am J Psychiatry* 146(4):459-463, 1989.
18. Milev P, Ho BC, Arndt S et al: Initial magnetic resonance imaging volumetric brain measurements and outcome in schizophrenia: a prospective longitudinal study with 5-year follow-up, *Biol Psychiatry* 54(6):608-615, 2003.
19. Jessen F, Scheef L, Germeshausen L et al: Reduced hippocampal activation during encoding and recognition of words in schizophrenia patients, *Am J Psychiatry* 160(7):1305-1312, 2003.
20. Holden C: Neuroscience: deconstructing schizophrenia, *Science* 299(5605):333-335, 2003.
21. Schmitz Y et al: Presynaptic regulation of dopaminergic neurotransmission, *J Neurochem* 87(2):273-289, 2003.
22. Evans JD, Heaton RK, Paulsen JS et al: The relationship of neuropsychological abilities to specific domains of functional capacity in older schizophrenia patients, *Biol Psychiatry* 53(5):422-430, 2003.
23. Fadem B: *High-yield behavioral science,* ed 2, Philadelphia, 2001, Lippincott Williams & Wilkins.
24. Keltner NL: Neuroreceptor function and psychopharmacologic response, *Issues Ment Health Nurs* 21(1):31-50, 2000.
25. Kapur S, Seeman P: Does fast dissociation from the dopamine d(2) receptor explain the action of atypical antipsychotics? A new hypothesis, *Am J Psychiatry* 158(3):360-369, 2001.
26. Keltner NL, Folks DG: *Psychotropic drugs,* ed 4, St Louis, 2005, Elsevier.

27. Nasrallah HA: Atypical antipsychotic-induced metabolic side effects: insights from receptor-binding profiles, *Mol Psychiatry* 13(1):27-35, 2007.

28. Aquila R: Management of weight gain in patients with schizophrenia, *J Clin Psychiatry* 63(Suppl 4):33-36, 2002.

29. Kalkman HO, Loetscher E: GAD(67): the link between the GABA-deficit hypothesis and the dopaminergic and glutamatergic theories of psychosis, *J Neural Transm* 110(7):803-812, 2003.

30. Winokur G, Clayton P, editors: *The medical basis of psychiatry,* ed 2, Philadelphia, 1994, Saunders.

31. American Psychiatric Association: *Diagnostic and statistical manual of mental disorders,* ed 4, text revision, Washington, DC, 2000, The Association.

32. Frasure-Smith N, Lespérance F, Gravel G et al: Social support, depression, and mortality during the first year after myocardial infarction, *Circulation* 101(16):1919-1924, 2000.

33. Zubenko GS, Hughes 3rd HB, Stiffler JS et al: D2S2944 identifies a likely susceptibility locus for recurrent, early-onset, major depression in women, *Mol Psychiatry* 7(5):460-467, 2002.

34. Brent DA, Birmaher B: Clinical practice: adolescent depression, *N Engl J Med* 347(9):667-671, 2002.

35. Insel TR, Charney DS: Research on major depression: strategies and priorities, *JAMA* 289(23):3167-3168, 2003.

35a. "Major Depression Fact Sheet," National Association for the Mentally Ill. www.nami.org. Arlington, VA. Accessed 2008.

36. Racagni G, Brunell N: Physiology to functionality: the brain and neurotransmitter activity, *Int Clin Psychopharmacol* 14(Suppl 1):S3-S7, 1999.

37. Stockmeir CA, Shi X, Konick L et al: Neurokinin-1 receptors are decreased in major depressive disorder, *Neuroreport* 13(9):1223-1227, 2002.

38. Young E, Korszun A: Psychoneuroendocrinology of depression. Hypothalamic-pituitary-gonadal axis, *Psychiatr Clin North Am* 21(2):309-323, 1998.

39. Jacobs BL, van Praag H, Gage FH: Depression and the birth and death of brain cells, *Am Sci Online* 88(4):340-347, 2000.

40. Caspi A, Sugden K, Moffitt TE et al: Influence of life stress on depression: moderation by a polymorphism in the 5-HTT gene, *Science* 301(5631):386-389, 2003.

41. Posener JA, DeBattista C, Williams GH et al: 24-hour monitoring of cortisol and corticotropin secretion in psychotic and non-psychotic major depression, *Arch Gen Psychiatry* 57(8):755-760, 2000.

42. Shimizu E, Hashimoto K, Okamura N et al: Alterations of serum levels of brain derived neurotrophic factor (BDNF) in depressed patients with or without antidepressants, *Biol Psychiatry* 54(1):70-75, 2002.

43. Manji HK et al: Enhancing neuronal plasticity and cellular resilience to develop novel improved therapeutics for difficult-to-treat depression, *Biol Psychiatry* 53(8):707-742, 2003.

44. Phillips ML, Drevets WC, Rauch SL et al: Neurobiology of emotion perception II: implications for major psychiatric disorders, *Soc Biol Psychiatry* 54(5):515-528, 2003.

45. Nierenberg AA, Ostacher MJ, Huffman JC et al: A brief review of antidepressant efficacy, effectiveness, indications, and usage for major depressive disorder, *J Occup Environ Med* 50(4):428-436, 2008.

46. Pearson G: Psychopharmacology. In Mohr WK: *Psychiatric-mental health nursing,* ed 6, Philadelphia, 2006, Lippincott Williams & Wilkins.

47. Sheline YI: Neuroimaging studies of mood disorder effects on the brain, *Biol Psychiatry* 54(3):338-352, 2003.

48. "Major Depression Fact Sheet." National Association for the Mentally Ill. www.nami.org. Arlington, VA. Accessed 2008.

49. Stahl SM: *Essential psychopharmacology: neuroscientific basis and practical applications,* ed 2, Cambridge, UK, 2000, Cambridge University Press.

50. Akiskal HS: The bipolar spectrum in psychiatric and general medical practice, *Primary Psychiatry* 11(9):30-35, 2004.

51. Tugrul K: The nurse's role in the assessment and treatment of bipolar disorder, *J Am Psychiatr Nurs Assoc* 9(6):180-186, 2003.

52. Suppes T, Dennehy EB: Evidence-based long-term treatment of bipolar I disorder, *J Clin Psychiatry* 63(Suppl 10):29-33, 2002.

53. Keck PE, McElroy SL: Clinical pharmacodynamics and pharmacokinetics of antimanic and mood-stabilizing medications, *J Clin Psychiatry* 63(Suppl 4):3-11, 2002.

Neurobiology of Nonpsychotic Illnesses

Lee-Ellen C. Copstead • Patricia A. Garber

MEDIA RESOURCES

Additional Material for Study, Review, and Further Exploration

CD Companion ■ Review Questions and Answers
■ Glossary (with audio pronunciations for selected terms)
■ Disease Profiles ■ Animations

ⓔvolve **Website** at http://evolve.elsevler.com/Copstead/
■ Case Studies ■ Disease Profiles ■ WebLinks ■ Key Points Review

 Online Course (Module 19)

KEY QUESTIONS

■ What neurobiological alterations have been associated with anxiety symptoms?
■ What neurobiological alterations have been associated with personality disorders?
■ What neurobiological alterations have been associated with anorexia?

CHAPTER OUTLINE

The neurobiological mechanisms of mental disorders that do not cause psychosis may prove to be more similar than different from those of mental disorders associated with psychosis. These conditions already show similarity in that altered neuronal structures and functioning, genetic risk factors, and neurotransmission dysregulation characterize them. A major difference between psychotic and nonpsychotic illnesses is that individual variations in nonpsychotic conditions can be extensive. Greater individual variations increase the difficulty of defining the hallmark symptomatology and neurobiological basis of the condition. In addition, much has been learned about the neurobiological impact of stress response systems in psychotic illnesses, whereas the impact of stress response systems in nonpsychotic illnesses is less well understood. In the past, simple comparisons, such as comparing schizophrenia with eating disorders, invited the false assumption that one disorder may be more or less serious than another. For the affected person, such comparisons are unhelpful. Any mental disorder has the potential of causing profound suffering and disability.

The purpose of this chapter is to briefly demonstrate the complexity of nonpsychotic illnesses. Three representative illnesses—anxiety disorders, personality disorders, and eating disorders— are described. **Anxiety disorders** are characterized by highly distressing physical and emotional symptoms that are difficult to control. The three anxiety disorders reviewed are panic disorder, generalized anxiety disorder, and obsessive-compulsive disorder. **Personality disorders** are characterized by rigid patterns of thinking and behaving that are highly maladaptive, negatively impact all aspects of daily life, and expose the affected person to increased risk for comorbid substance disorders. The two disorders reviewed are borderline personality disorder and antisocial personality disorder. **Eating disorders** are characterized by food and weight obsessions and compulsions, and gravely distorted body image.

ANXIETY DISORDERS

This section presents three anxiety disorders: panic disorder, generalized anxiety disorder (GAD), and obsessive-compulsive disorder (OCD). Anxiety disorders are characterized by similar physical symptoms, but they differ greatly in terms of symptom onset triggers, symptom duration, and symptom management. Because anxiety disorders primarily are characterized by physical symptoms, physical illnesses (e.g., hyperthyroidism) and medication reactions (e.g., antidepressants, steroids, anticholinergic medications) must be ruled out before a diagnosis of anxiety disorder can be made.

Panic Disorder. Panic disorder is characterized by acute episodes of anxiety symptoms that are unexpected, sudden, recurrent, and generate intense feelings of fear. Sudden symptom onset can cause affected persons to seek emergency health care for what they believe is a cardiac arrest, respiratory arrest, or "nervous breakdown."

Depending on subtype, panic anxiety or panic disorder is diagnosed two to three times more often in women than in men.[1] Rates of 1% to 2% are most commonly reported. Initial illness onset usually is in late adolescence or young adulthood, with a mean age of onset of 26.6 years. Initial symptom onset in older age adults is less typical. Persons diagnosed with panic disorder typically report that their first panic episode occurred relatively early in life. Panic disorder is characterized by two important psychological symptoms: anticipatory anxiety and avoidance anxiety.

Anticipatory anxiety refers to fearful expectation of panic anxiety onset. With panic disorder, no single experience consistently triggers symptom onset. People with the disorder tend to develop a morbid dread of events or experiences that they come to believe *might* trigger panic anxiety. In short, they try to anticipate their anxiety.

Avoidance refers to personal strategies used to increase feelings of control and thereby decrease the risk of panic anxiety. True panic disorder without avoidance anxiety is unlikely. Persons with panic disorder strive to avoid situations and circumstances they associate with their symptoms. For example, panic disorder and agoraphobia (the phobic avoidance of public spaces beyond personal control, e.g., airports and shopping malls) often coexist.

Etiology and Neurobiology. The risk of anxiety disorder symptom onset has been associated with significant genetic, psychological, and biological system alterations.[2] Family,

twin, and adoptive family studies have consistently shown a strong genetic liability for these disorders. However, experts now speculate that the etiology question no longer is nature versus nurture. Current models seek to explain the *interactions* of nature and nurture that can create susceptibility to anxiety. Brain regions that underpin the experiences of fear, anxiety, and stress are thought of as circuits that can be shaped and altered by a wide range of forces. Neurobiological conditioning is one force shown to impact such circuits and thus is of particular importance to understanding the development of anxiety disorders.

Brain serotonin activity has been shown to interact with both genes and environment, and these interactions contribute to what has come to be referred to as *synaptic plasticity*.[2] In this way, genes are linked with brain cell neurochemistry and psychological characteristics such as temperament. More specifically, evidence of genetic variability in negative emotions, such as anxiety, has been found in studies of serotonin transporter cells. In this research, gene variability is in gene allele length. For example, family studies have shown that siblings with serotonin transporter cells with the short-form gene allele had higher neuroticism scores than their siblings with the long-form gene allele. Research aimed at gene typing mental disorders clearly is in its infancy and findings such as these are inconclusive, but they demonstrate the possibility of genetics-based neurobiological models of anxiety.

Susceptible persons who breathe air with high levels of carbon dioxide will experience an acute onset of panic anxiety symptoms.[3] A small study of persons with panic anxiety disorder, using an infusion of doxapram (respiratory stimulant) to cause profound hyperventilation, examined the effectiveness of cognitive interventions to reduce respiratory anxiety symptoms.[4] Cognitive interventions were designed to minimize misinterpretation of drug-induced hyperventilation as a sign of danger and thereby reduce the odds of the respiratory stimulant triggering panic anxiety. Breath-by-breath analyses of the patients and healthy controls were performed. The researchers[4] hypothesized that if the respiration anxiety symptoms were the result of dysregulation within the brain respiratory control center, cognitive interventions would not be particularly effective. They found that less fearful thinking did reduce panic, but some respiratory anxiety symptoms persisted despite less fearful thinking. In other words, respiratory anxiety symptoms appeared to result both from anticipatory anxiety and from dysregulation within the brain respiratory center.

Surges of physiologic activation and physiologic instability are thought to be the hallmark neurobiological processes underlying panic anxiety disorder.[5] Multiple organ systems, including the cardiovascular and respiratory systems, are thought to be involved. Observations such as these help to explain why, for example, caffeine triggers panic anxiety symptoms in susceptible individuals. All anxiety disorders are thought to share key symptom characteristics, but physiologic instability appears to be unique to panic. Physiologic instability may prove to be the key to identifying a genetics-based marker for susceptibility to panic. However, the biopsychological marker for the disorder is likely to be the overinterpretation of physical anxiety symptoms (e.g., sudden increase in heart rate) as life threatening. This thinking, referred to as *learned panic,* is thought to result from inordinately high levels of life stress in early childhood.

Overwhelming life stress can increase the level of circulating glucocorticoids (stress hormones) and stimulate the release of glutamate (which inhibits neurogenesis).[6] Early-childhood life stress, specifically abuse and neglect, have been studied as possibly predictors of various adult-onset anxiety disorders. These models are based on altered serotonin, norepinephrine, and dopamine neurotransmission; glutamate release; and physiologic instability. Repeated and prolonged childhood exposure to overwhelming stress is thought to create adult susceptibility to anxiety disorders. The leading theory is that early life stress leads to *overspecialized* or excessive stress response.

Early life stress is thought to produce adult susceptibility to anxiety by altering critical neuron structures and functioning during this critical stage of human growth and development. Brain regions most vulnerable to alteration as a result of early life stress include the hippocampus (glucocorticoid receptors), amygdala (γ-aminobutyric acid [GABA] and benzodiazepine receptors), corpus callosum (glial cells critical to myelination), cerebellar vermis (glucocorticoid receptors), and the prefrontal cortex (glucocorticoid receptors, dopamine projections, and inhibition of hypothalamic-pituitary-adrenal axis [HPA] activation).[6,7] When the developing brain of a young child is exposed to overwhelming life stress, the stress response system appears to adapt by overbuilding or building additional brain stress-response pathways. Later, under less stressful adult circumstances, this overbuilt stress response system becomes maladaptive. Like a very large overpowered car on a small, winding road, the overbuilt stress response system could become the source of physiologic instability that has come to be associated with panic anxiety.[8]

Clinical Manifestations. Physical symptoms include respiratory distress, heart palpitations, tachycardia, pounding heart, chest pain, smothering or choking sensation, dizziness, light-headedness, faintness, sweating, trembling, shaking, hot flushes, chills, numbness, tingling, nausea, abdominal distress, and urinary frequency.[9]

Psychological and *cognitive* symptoms include expressed fears of dying, fear of cardiac arrest, fear of losing control, fear of nervous breakdown, derealization, depersonalization, and perceptual distortions.

Behavioral symptoms include hyperkinesis, pressured speech, and exaggerated startle response.

Pharmacologic Treatment. Panic anxiety disorder can be effectively managed with cognitive-behavioral therapy aimed at reducing fearful thinking and desensitization of cognitive and physical stress responses. When panic symptoms are disabling, medication for symptom management is recommended. Long-acting benzodiazepines, such as clonazepam, are the sedatives of choice when short term calming and symptom

relief are mandatory. Tolerance to benzodiazepines develops with continuous use regardless of dosage. Misuse of benzodiazepines represents a serious health hazard. Many atypical psychiatric medications that can target serotonin, dopamine, or norepinephrine receptors have been clinically tested and shown to be effective treatment for anxiety symptoms. Examples of such medications found to be helpful include paroxetine, sertraline, citalopram, and fluoxetine. Unless contraindicated, β-blocker medications that dampen physical anxiety symptoms may also be helpful.

Generalized Anxiety Disorder. Generalized anxiety disorder is characterized by worry that is chronic and persistent, as well as physical anxiety symptoms. Persistent worry that is difficult to control typically leads to multiple anxiety symptoms including restlessness, fatigue, impaired concentration, irritability, muscle tension, muscle pain, and disturbed sleep. Lacking clear symptom onset patterns, GAD is easily overlooked or misdiagnosed.

Etiology and Neurobiology. Generalized anxiety disorder[10] differs from other anxiety disorders in that the cognitive, psychological, and behavioral symptoms of GAD are relatively constant. Psychoanalysts developed most of the original etiology theories concerning persistent worry. What now is referred to as persistent worry was then described as anxious expectation. Even at that early stage of discovery, it was apparent that generalized anxiety rarely occurred without comorbid conditions such as depression. This *psychodynamic* view of generalized anxiety prevailed until the late 1980s and early 1990s. At that time, the disorder still was so poorly understood that the diagnosis was used to refer to what was then thought to be leftover or residual anxiety symptoms from other disorders. Technologically advanced research methods have now made it possible to precisely define GAD symptoms in terms of their actual qualities, intensity, and duration, but physical GAD symptoms continue to be viewed as *somatic* expressions of psychological problems.[10]

Unlike other anxiety disorders, GAD onset typically is gradual with symptom duration measured in years. As has been observed with other anxiety disorders, vulnerability to GAD likely is inherited. Twin and family study findings indicate a 30% increase in risk of GAD among the relatives of persons with the disorder. Efforts to describe the neurobiological basis of GAD will no doubt be greatly advanced by theoretical models of inherited vulnerability as well as improved understanding of GAD symptoms, but critical questions remain unanswered. The most important unanswered question likely will have to do with the fact that the alterations in brain structure and functioning shown to be associated with GAD also are consistent with alterations observed with other disorders.

Preliminary positron emission tomography (PET) studies measuring brain glucose metabolism rates in GAD have shown higher than normal rates in patients at rest.[11] With GAD, apparently some brain regions undergo both increases and decreases in glucose metabolism rates. This mixed response is most apparent in the frontal and cingulate areas of the cortex, the brain region associated with worry and hypervigilance.

Findings such as these lend support to the basic GAD explanatory hypothesis of anxiety symptoms as manifestations of hyperactive brain circuits. Just the opposite condition (hypoactive brain circuits) is thought to be the fundamental basis of depressive disorders.[11]

Neurotransmitter findings with GAD, as with other disorders that produce mood, thinking, and behavior symptoms, point to alterations in GABA receptors, benzodiazepine receptors, norepinephrine systems, serotonin systems, HPA axis activation, and plasma cortisol. Thus far, no specific alterations that can consistently explain GAD symptoms have been identified.[11] Nevertheless, one interesting observation shows considerable promise. At rest, no obvious alterations in neurotransmission are noted in GAD patients. Only when subjected to laboratory activities designed to induce stress responses is significant neurotransmitter overactivity observed. Evidence of norepinephrine receptor down-regulation lends additional support to this stress response model. Attempting to modulate overactive responses, receptor down-regulation is thought to occur automatically when subjected to prolonged, recurrent, excessive, or hyperactive neurotransmitter activity.

Whereas norepinephrine activity is thought to be associated with physical symptoms of GAD, anticipatory and avoidance symptoms are thought to be associated with activity along a key serotonin pathway linking the amygdala and frontal cortex. As might be expected, insufficient serotonin activity in specific brain regions is thought to be associated with GAD. Given the obvious symptom overlap between stress and anxiety, hyperactivity within the HPA axis and high plasma cortisol levels continue to be leading models in GAD research. Much of the difficulty in defining the neurobiological basis of GAD has to do with significant individual variations in GAD symptomatology. Uncontrollable worry (frontal cortex) is the only symptom likely to show meaningful consistency over time and from individual to individual. A second major research difficulty has to do with the frequency with which GAD symptoms co-occur with depression symptoms—so much so that some experts now view mixed depression-anxiety as a specific disorder.

Clinical Manifestations. *Physical* symptoms vary too greatly to allow for a meaningful listing, but common GAD symptoms include muscle tension, lightheadedness, sweating, palpitations, dizziness, and stomach distress.

Psychological symptoms also vary over time and from individual to individual, but a few symptoms are essential for a diagnosis of GAD. These are uncontrollable worry with no areas of life excluded, fearfulness, and foreboding. Worry is not limited to any single area of concern (e.g., children). Concentration typically is severely impaired, and irritability is common. Diffuse anticipatory anxiety, avoidance anxiety, and dysphoria are common.

Behavioral symptoms include severe sleep disturbance and fatigue. Although much of the behavior associated with GAD is likely to be the result of maladaptive methods of coping with physical and psychological GAD symptoms, impaired social and academic/employment functioning are common.

Pharmacologic Treatment. Effective psychological and drug treatments for GAD can be relatively complex. Comorbid conditions such as alcohol abuse are not uncommon and, when present, may extend the duration of needed treatment. Duration of treatment also is likely to be prolonged when GAD symptoms are long-standing and highly disabling. Lastly, neurobiological research findings indicate that effective drug treatment is likely to require one or more medications that are reliable modulators of multiple neurotransmission systems across multiple brain regions. Medications shown to relieve and in some cases remit GAD symptoms include long-acting benzodiazepines (e.g., clonazepam), partial serotonin (5-HT_{1A}) agonists (e.g., buspirone), tricyclic antidepressants (e.g., imipramine), selective serotonin reuptake inhibitors (e.g., sertraline), serotonin-norepinephrine reuptake inhibitors (e.g., venlafaxine), and long-acting β-blockers (e.g., propranolol).[12]

Obsessive-Compulsive Disorder.
Obsessive-compulsive disorder is one of the most severe anxiety disorders. Even modest OCD symptomatology can become disabling. The disorder is characterized by persistent involuntary thoughts that then provoke anxiety and involuntary anxiety management rituals. Unlike the acute onset and short duration of panic anxiety symptoms or the chronic symptoms of GAD, the obsessions and compulsions that characterize OCD are localized but nevertheless impact all areas of functioning.

People with OCD strive to avoid disclosing their symptoms to relatives, friends, and health professionals, so that accurate incidence and prevalence statistics are nearly impossible to determine. The lifetime OCD prevalence rate for the general population is 2.2%, whereas the risk in first-degree relatives is 9.2%. Some experts consider this general-population estimate to be an underestimate, but disabling OCD is not thought to be common. The median age of symptom onset is about 23 years, with 15 to 39 being the peak-onset age range.

Etiology and Neurobiology. True OCD symptoms cause a great deal of emotional distress, are very time consuming, and significantly interfere with normal functioning. Neurobiological research findings indicate strong genetic or inherited risks of OCD. Family studies show that when an adult family member is diagnosed with the disorder, child relatives also may be diagnosed. Depression, anorexia, and Tourette syndrome are common OCD comorbid disorders. Close links between OCD and the hereditary neurologic disorder Tourette syndrome have been reported, but it is not clear whether this link represents an increased risk of OCD or if Tourette syndrome and OCD are related in some other way.

OCD studies using PET brain scans have shown significant increases in glucose metabolism rates in the frontal lobes, caudate nucleus, and cingulate gyrus regions of the brain (Figure 49-1). These brain regions are directly associated with response to strong emotions. However, several OCD models of altered brain functioning have been hypothesized. One model proposes that a causal pathway for OCD exists between the frontal cortex region and basal ganglia region of the brain. This model draws on the observation that similar illnesses

FIGURE 49-1 Hyperactivity of the orbitofrontal cortex has been a consistent finding in more than a decade of brain-imaging research on patients with obsessive-compulsive disorder *(OCD)*. These positron emission tomographic images are from the initial report of this finding by a UCLA group. This excessive metabolic activity could generate spurious "error detection" signals that result in patients with obsessive-compulsive disorder experiencing repetitive adventitious feelings that "something is wrong." (Originally adapted from Baxter LR Jr et al: Local cerebral glucose metabolic rates in obsessive-compulsive disorder. A comparison with rates in unipolar depression and in normal controls, *Arch Gen Psychiatry* 44(3):211-218, 1987. As published in Schwartz JM: Obsessive-compulsive disorder, *Sci Med* 4:16, 1997.)

with well-defined etiologic factors have been shown to involve both cognitive and motor brain regions. Predictably, serotonin activity dysregulation and dysfunction also represent possible OCD models.

As shown in Figure 49-1, PET scans of the brain of a person with OCD reveal significant increases in glucose metabolism activity in the prefrontal cortex brain region. Magnetic resonance imaging (MRI) findings have suggested widely distributed cellular abnormalities such as significantly lower amounts of total white matter (connection fibers) and greater cortex cell volume. More recent models of OCD focus on the possibility of deficient serotonin inhibitory action in the basal ganglia region of the brain, which then permits excessive release of dopamine, a stimulating neurotransmitter.

PET, functional MRI (fMRI), and single-photon emission computed tomography (SPECT) studies of persons with OCD have confirmed the correlation between OCD symptoms and abnormal brain circuit activity in the orbitofrontal cortex, caudate nucleus, anterior cingulate cortex, and thalamus.[13] An fMRI study of medicated OCD patients and comparison subjects explored the possibility of meaningful links between anterior cingulate cortex activity and the severity of OCD symptoms by observing this activity under laboratory stress designed to trigger symptom onset. Patients attempted to successfully perform the computer-based tasks quickly without error, but the program had been designed to increase their error rate and generate doubt. Comparison subjects were faster than OCD patients; otherwise few group behavior differences were noted. Hyperactivity was observed only in one brain region (anterior cingulate cortex) and was significantly related to error making and expressed doubt. That study showed the possibility of developing a neurobiological model of disabling self-correction urges associated with OCD.[13]

Clinical Manifestations. Obsessions are strong, persistent, intrusive, uncontrollable thoughts. Obsessive thoughts manifest as ideas, images, and urges that dominate normal thinking and functioning. Affected persons recognize that their obsessions are products of their own mind and may judge them as senseless. Nevertheless, they are unable to stop, govern, or resist their obsessions.

Compulsions are repetitive, ritualistic actions performed with urgency. Compulsions typically are content related to obsessions. Performance of compulsions neutralizes or prevents the anxiety triggered by obsessions. True compulsions absorb inordinate amounts of time daily and are performed despite negative consequences. Realization that a compulsion is unreasonable, senseless, and excessive has little impact on the urge to perform the action. Examples of common compulsions are counting, symmetry, touching, checking, cleaning, and picking. Hoarding (inability to dispossess meaningless, worthless objects) is one example of more complex compulsions.[14] A case study of 20 individuals noted the onset of severe anxiety associated with the thought of discarding hoarded objects. In that study, the items most commonly hoarded were newspapers/magazines, junk mail, old clothing, receipts, lists, food, and gifts for others. The magnitude of hoarding ranged from clutter in all closets and one or two rooms to all closets filled, garage filled, and more than one room filled. These hoarding compulsions were in addition to primary OCD compulsions (e.g., symmetry, checking, cleaning). Ninety percent of the study patients had one or more relatives with OCD symptoms.[14] Clinically significant hoarding behaviors, such as described in this study, occur in about 25% to 30% of individuals with OCD.[15]

Pharmacologic Treatment. Cognitive-behavioral therapy with effective medication treatment can effectively diminish OCD obsessions and compulsions. Nevertheless, the disorder itself makes entering treatment extremely difficult if not impossible. To be successful, cognitive-behavioral therapy must target the person's obsessions and compulsions. This would require full disclosure, and disclosure is very difficult. Higher doses of anti-anxiety and antidepressant medications (fluvoxamine, paroxetine, sertraline, venlafaxine, fluoxetine) have generally proved effective in reducing OCD symptoms. Atypical antipsychotics, such as risperidone, in combination with antidepressants and β-blockers may be considered when OCD symptoms are disabling. Effective OCD symptom relief has been reported with the tricyclic antidepressant clomipramine, and some experts recommend the seizure medication gabapentin.[16]

KEY POINTS

- Anxiety disorders are characterized by irrational and debilitating fears. The three major categories of anxiety disorders are panic disorder, generalized anxiety disorder, and obsessive-compulsive disorder. These disorders show some evidence of heritability, and biochemical correlates are suspected. Defects in serotonin pathways have been proposed as etiologic factors.
- Panic disorder is characterized by acute episodes of severe anxiety accompanied by dyspnea, chest pain, and a sense of impending doom. Palpitations, hyperventilation, dizziness, paresthesias, and diaphoresis may occur during an attack, which may last 5 to 30 minutes. Anticipatory anxiety and phobic avoidance may develop in individuals with panic disorder. Efforts to avoid future episodes may result in agoraphobia.
- Generalized anxiety disorder is characterized by a continuous but moderate degree of anxiety without discrete periods of acute attacks. Agoraphobia rarely develops, but chronic headaches, muscle tension, abdominal discomfort, and sleep disturbances are common.
- Obsessive-compulsive disorder is characterized by obsessive thoughts and compulsive behavior. Obsessions (persistent, intrusive, compelling thoughts) commonly have themes of committing violent acts, being a victim of violence, or fear of contamination. In contrast to schizophrenia, such persons realize that the obsessive thoughts are from their own minds but are helpless to control them. Compulsions (repetitive, ritualistic behavior) include such actions as excessive washing and grooming, repeated checking to ensure safety, and elaborate measures to avoid contact with dirt or bodily wastes. If the individual is prevented from performing compulsive rituals, a high state of anxiety ensues.
- Benzodiazepines and antidepressants may be used to manage anxiety disorders.

PERSONALITY DISORDERS

Personality disorder refers to pervasive and persistent disturbance of emotions and behavior. The disturbance is stable and sufficiently predictable that emotions and behaviors appear to be rigid. Given that personality dramatically influences how individuals interact with others, personality disorder symptoms significantly impact all areas of interpersonal functioning. It is not unusual for affected persons to fully deny any link between their emotions and behaviors and problems in their life. More often, they believe their disturbed emotions and behaviors are acceptable.[16]

Persons with personality disorder maintain global views of self, others, and the world that can be extremely maladaptive. Evidence of maladaptive life views, if not actual disturbances in emotions and behavior, may be recognized in early childhood but rarely is the formal diagnosis of personality disorder made before late adolescence or young adulthood. Hallmark symptoms make it possible to group specific personality disorders into general groups. Cluster A disorders are characterized by unusual behavior (schizotypal, schizoid, paranoid). Cluster B disorders are characterized by instability (antisocial, borderline, histrionic, narcissistic). Cluster C disorders are characterized by anxiety (avoidant, dependent, obsessive compulsive).[17] Additional diagnoses, such as depressive personality disorder[18] and further subtyping, such as treatment seeker and treatment rejector[19] continue to be explored. Comparative studies of monozygotic versus dizygotic twins confirm the common observation that personality disorder attributes, rather than personality disorder per se, show significant genetic inheritability.

Borderline Personality Disorder. The term **borderline** originally was intended to suggest a condition that bordered both psychosis and neurosis. Now the term refers to instability as the hallmark characteristic of the disorder. With borderline personality disorder, dramatic lack of stability is evident in mood, behavior, interpersonal relationships, and self-esteem. Behavior can become highly unpredictable and impulsive. Mood states, whether positive or negative, tend to be extreme and labile, but the disorder actually is characterized by persistent feelings of alienation and emotional emptiness. These characteristics result in a basic lifestyle that is dominated by crisis.[20]

Etiology and Neurobiology. Biological models of borderline personality disorder are used to determine the underlying basis of extreme symptoms such as impulsive aggression. Both self-directed and other-directed impulsive aggression has been shown to be associated with serotonin activity in brain regions that process emotions.[21] Findings such as these support apparent links between trauma, as the most consistent antecedent to diagnosis, and borderline personality disorder. Sexual and physical abuse are among the most commonly observed forms of trauma. One theory holds that undergoing trauma of this magnitude contributes to the overdevelopment of brain stress response systems that lead to altered serotonin activity. Yet brief increases in dopamine activity also have been observed and linked with impulsive aggression that, in extreme cases, can produce psychotic-like symptoms. Family studies have yielded mixed results, leading researchers to speculate that specific traits may be inherited and that in susceptible individuals these traits may lead to the development of borderline personality disorder.[21] In other words, borderline personality disorder may reflect selective interaction of high-risk genetic, family, and environmental characteristics.

Possible models of neurotransmission dysregulation that might explain the instability and impulsive aggressive behavior of borderline personality disorder have focused on hyperresponsive HPA axis activity as a biological linkage between the stress and trauma of childhood abuse and adult illness onset.[21] Comparisons of abused and nonabused individuals with borderline personality disorder and healthy controls showed hyperresponsiveness of corticotropin and cortisol activity in women with a history of sustained childhood abuse. However, these links did not appear to be exclusive to borderline personality disorder. For example, as might be expected, links also were observed between childhood abuse and adult posttraumatic stress disorder.

Other neurobiological models focus on alterations in brain structure and functioning using advanced electrophysiologic tools such as electroencephalograms. A review of that line of research[22] showed inconclusive findings. In some studies, electroencephalographic abnormalities such as slowing and spikes were observed but no consistent abnormalities were noted. The lack of clear findings might have to do with the high rate of comorbid conditions found with borderline personality disorder. Nevertheless, electroencephalographic findings are promising enough to represent a third line of research in addition to fMRI and PET studies. The implication here is that the development of a useful biological model of borderline personality disorder will likely require the combined application of these technologies.[22]

Although somewhat more difficult to interpret, models that address specific borderline personality disorder traits also show promise. For example, one of the many interpersonal instability characteristics of borderline personality disorder has come to be referred to as *abandonment issues.* A study of women diagnosed with borderline personality disorder who had a history of childhood sexual or physical abuse asked the women to prepare narratives of personal experiences of abandonment.[23] Brain scans were performed as each woman's narrative was read back to her and during the reading of neutral experiences. Compared with healthy controls, the women with borderline personality disorder showed increased blood flow in the right dorsolateral prefrontal cortex region of the brain and decreased blood flow in the anterior cingulate and in the hippocampus-amygdala regions as they listened to the abandonment narratives. These three brain regions process strong emotions. Similar alterations in volume measures have been reported for the same brain regions. Volume refers to brain structures rather than the neurobiological functions of the brain structure. Significant reduction in hippocampus and amygdala volumes have been observed in women with borderline personality disorder.[24] Findings such as these help demonstrate the complex structural and functional neurobiological alterations thought to underlie the defining characteristics of the disorder.

Clinical Manifestations. *Interpersonal instability* is evident in relationships and interactions with others.

Splitting refers to a predictable pattern of alternately devaluing and idealizing others. Devaluation appears to be unpredictably triggered by sudden angry responses to perceived or actual interpersonal loss.

Manipulation refers to the relating to others as objects for the purpose of achieving unstated goals. Manipulation may be covert or overt, but the aim almost always is to obtain caretaking responses from others.

Self-harm and *suicidal ideation* refer to impulsive harmful behaviors toward self that vary widely in severity. Self-harm sometimes is intended to elicit a rescue response from others but also may be used to relieve severe feelings of emptiness, numbness, frustration, anger, or interpersonal tension. Common self-harm behaviors include cutting and burning, hitting objects, and drug overdose. Suicidal thoughts and attempted suicide in response to perceived or actual trauma or crisis characterize severe forms of the disorder.

Anger and **dysphoria** are commonly experienced or chronic negative mood states. Displays of negative emotions can vary greatly but can reach levels of intensity that simply overwhelm the affected person. Negative emotions also include loneliness and boredom. Complaints of never experiencing good or happy emotions may not be an overstatement.

Derealization refers to transient experiences in which nothing seems real. When derealization also includes depersonalization, the affected person does not feel *real* and instead feels like a disembodied observer. Although short lived, the experience is highly disturbing to the affected person. Bizarre activities intended to regain a sense of realness are not uncommon.

Impulsive aggression is common. This propensity may manifest as alarming episodes of substance abuse, promiscuity, fighting, and self-harm. Flight or escape in response to impulsive aggression can be anticipated.

Pharmacologic Treatment. Medications used to manage symptoms of borderline personality disorder are determined by the person's immediate treatment needs. Persons with this disorder are at increased risk for depression, anxiety, stress, panic, and substance abuse. In some cases of borderline personality disorder, long-term use of antidepressants may prove helpful. Severe impulsive aggression may require short-term treatment with an atypical antipsychotic medication (e.g., risperidone, olanzapine) that produces multiple neurotransmitter effects. Mood stabilization medications (e.g., gabapentin) might improve severe mood instability. Given the somewhat unpredictable mixture of clinical symptoms that can be associated with a diagnosis of borderline personality disorder, psychotherapy treatment must be emphasized. The primary psychotherapeutic goals for borderline personality disorder include crisis prevention and management and stabilization of object relations. In effect, therapy provides opportunities for the patient to explore and experience success and stability and to learn how to safely manage overwhelming emotions. Treatment effectiveness is associated with treatment duration, but both long-term psychodynamic and cognitive-behavioral therapy have been shown to be effective.[25,26]

Antisocial Personality Disorder. *Psychopath* and *sociopath* are early terms once used to describe the condition now referred to as *antisocial personality disorder*. The term literally refers to patterns of mood, thinking, and behaviors that consistently show absolute disregard for others. In effect, persons with antisocial personality disorder are against and separate from the people, norms, rules, and laws that define society.

Etiology and Neurobiology. No single psychological, social, or neurobiological factor explains the onset of antisocial personality disorder. That said, a great deal of useful information has been generated. Males with antisocial personality disorder typically are the sons of antisocial fathers. This parental link is less apparent in females with antisocial personality disorder. Horrific experiences found to be associated with the onset of this disorder include childhood traumatic loss; physically or emotionally absent parents; childhood abuse and neglect; rigid, punishing childrearing practices; overwhelming childhood stress; and emotional trauma. Absent such experiences, childhood identification with an antisocial adult also significantly increases the risk of developing this highly disturbing disorder.

Persons with antisocial personality disorder can appear dangerous but are far more likely to be charismatic and charming. The many damaging effects of antisocial personality disorder include the ability to design and *wear* a public face that bears no relationship to the person's actual antisocial thoughts, feelings, and actions. Many characteristics of the disorder actually are personality characteristics that are absent. Antisocial personality disorder is not associated with feelings of anxiety, depression, remorse, concern, or empathy. Delusions or evidence of thought disorder are highly uncommon. Evidence of apparent intelligence and calculated cleverness are common. Dishonesty and deceit are hallmark characteristics of antisocial personality disorder. Antisocial personality disorder is distinct from sadistic personality disorder, a proposed diagnosis under consideration; however, persons with antisocial personality disorder can behave in a highly sadistic manner.

It should be noted that considerable disagreement exists among experts who study antisocial personality disorder. For example, traditionally the disorder has been viewed as a specific diagnosis, but many experts note that the presence of many overlapping characteristics of the cluster B disorders argues against this framework. They propose that rather than being a diagnostic category, antisocial personality disorder should be viewed in terms of behavior on a continuum that ranges from histrionic, narcissistic, and borderline to antisocial and sadistic.[27] The continuum model emphasizes specific characteristics, such as intelligence, that might better predict antisocial behavior. For example, extremely low intelligence has been shown to be associated with more frequent impulsive aggression.[28]

The debate regarding the proper classification of various antisocial behaviors speaks volumes in terms of the confounding nature of this inexplicable disorder. Others argue that difficulty comprehending antisocial behavior is a hallmark characteristic of the disorder. That said, researchers interested in developing causal models of antisocial personality disorder have attempted to apply various continuum models. For example, researchers have noted that substance dependence, antisocial behaviors, and disinhibition typically co-occurred. *Externalization* was identified as a key factor predicting advancement along the continuum of increasingly dangerous behaviors.[28] Progressive externalization appeared to be inherited. If this turns out to be a generalizable finding, externalization might reliably predict antisocial behavior.

Biosocial models of violent antisocial personality disorder have strived to understand the interactions of genetics, biological, environmental, and social risk factors.[29] Relying both on family studies and on PET and fMRI findings, and attempting to account for potentially protective biological and environmental factors, researchers have identified biological and environmental interactions that may prove more predictive of antisocial behavior than any single risk factor. Nevertheless, models that attempt to explain antisocial personality disorder based on the interactions of multiple factors, such as birth complications and negative home environments, are likely to be exceedingly complex. National programs designed to reduce the risk of prenatal and negative home environment as lifelong risk factors have long been in operation.

Strictly neurobiological models of antisocial personality disorder attempt to rely solely on brain scan findings to more fully characterize the disorder rather than to predict behavior. For example, in an fMRI study that compared prison inmates with and without an antisocial diagnosis,[30] researchers hypothesized that antisocial inmates would show less brain activation than healthy controls or criminals not diagnosed with an antisocial disorder. Inmates were asked to respond to emotionally neutral and emotionally negative words. No group differences were observed with neutral words, but antisocial inmates showed significantly less emotional limbic and frontal cortex activation.[30] Less activation suggested that the antisocial inmates used different, nonemotional ways of processing negative emotional experiences. In other words, their emotions did not influence their thinking. This finding is consistent with the "cold" lack of emotion associated with antisocial personality disorder.

Clinical Manifestations. *Disregard for others* is a hallmark symptom of antisocial personality disorder. Although persons with this disorder are likely to be described as predators, indifference to others is more accurate.

Charm ironically is a common characteristic among persons with antisocial personality disorder. Possibly as a result of their indifference to others, they are able to project charm and may even be charismatic. These normally positive attributes tend to be little more than masks used to disarm or to create opportunities to manipulate and exploit others.

Blaming is a hallmark symptom of antisocial personality disorder. Others consistently are blamed for the person's actions and consequences of their actions. Often rather than a calculated ploy, blaming reflects the lack of self-awareness. When confronted with their actions they automatically look to explanations outside of themselves.

Impulsivity is observed with all cluster B personality disorders; however, with antisocial personality disorder, impulsivity frequently takes the form of thoughtless, harmful, or dangerous actions toward others.

Rule breaking refers to the ease with which norms, rules, and laws are disregarded. Calm contempt for others practically ensures recurrent antisocial behavior despite society's efforts to discourage such behavior. Few persons with this disorder are without a history of criminal activity. However, criminal activity should be distinguished from a criminal record of arrest, conviction, and incarceration. Large portions of prison inmate populations are persons with antisocial personality disorder. But antisocial personality disorder also can be observed among people of wealth, power, and standing who have the resources to avoid the legal system or successfully defend themselves in a legal action.

Deceitfulness and *deceptiveness* are hallmark symptoms of antisocial personality disorder.

Aggression and *assault* with antisocial personality disorder can occur on impulse or may reflect coldly calculated planning. This behavior is viewed as natural, appropriate, or "just the way it is." A matter-of-fact manner is typical.

Irresponsibility with antisocial personality disorder is evidenced by disregard for the expectations of others. Family members, employers, and others are likely to expect responsible actions, but from the perspective of the person with antisocial personality disorder, the expectations of others are not his or her concern.

Pharmacologic Treatment. As with other personality disorders, treatment for antisocial personality disorder typically is determined by the presenting symptomatology. Substance disorders are common comorbid disorders; however, when these disorders are present all too often they dominate treatment with too little emphasis given to the antisocial personality disorder diagnosis. When specific antisocial personality disorder symptoms are the focus of treatment, the symptoms commonly include impulsivity, anger, and aggression. Serotonin-activating medications, including antidepressants (e.g., paroxetine) and atypical antipsychotics (e.g., quetiapine) may be helpful in reducing chronic negative mood states. In some cases, atypical antipsychotic medications such as olanzapine may reduce agitation and impulsivity. Symptom-focused treatment may improve behavior management, but long-term adaptive improvements can require extensive care. Psychotherapy using cognitive-behavioral methods and behavior contracts can be useful when development of insight and behavior alternative training are needed. However, much of the promised effectiveness of these therapies is based on involuntary inmate populations. Until reliable neurobiological findings can be used to inform medication treatment for antisocial personality disorder, limited symptom remission methods are a reasonable treatment alternative.

KEY POINTS

- Personality disorders are characterized by behavior deemed "inappropriate" or deviant within the cultural context. Behavioral patterns are recognizable by adolescence and include paranoid, schizophrenia-like, narcissistic, self-absorbed, antisocial, compulsive, passive-aggressive, and dependent.
- Borderline personality disorder is characterized by unstable and dependent interpersonal relationships. Exclusive possession of another person is desired. To this end the individual may exhibit clinging, manipulation (complaints of illness, threatened suicide), self-destruction, and lying. Fear of abandonment may be ever present. Impulsiveness, substance abuse, loneliness, and lack of life goals are common. Psychosocial and biochemical factors are thought to be contributory; poor early mother-child relationships, child abuse, separation, or abandonment are significant contributing factors. Biological deficits in mood regulation could contribute to poor child-parent bonding.
- Antisocial personality disorder is characterized by failure to internalize moral and ethical values consistent with societal norms. Lack of anxiety and guilt, cold-bloodedness, and careless indifference or contempt for others are hallmarks of the disorder. The diagnosis of antisocial personality disorder is based on repeated antisocial behavior before age 15, along with failure to establish an occupational history after age 18. Psychosocial and biological factors are thought to be contributory and include lack of adequate parental role models, child abuse, inconsistent parenting, emotional deprivation, and having an alcoholic parent. A genetic component has been proposed.

EATING DISORDERS

Eating disorders can be subtyped as conditions characterized either by undereating (anorexia), overeating (bulimia), or compulsive eating (binge eating). Although extremely common, eating disorders are profoundly complex conditions manifested by dysregulation of psychological, behavioral, metabolic, and neurobiological systems. The exemplar disorder presented in this section is anorexia nervosa (AN). Once primarily observed in well-educated, very young women from middle- and high-income households, anorexia increasingly is observed in all age, income, educational, and ethnic groups.

Dieting has long been assumed to be a possible trigger of eating disorder onset, but this assumption may not be supported by research. Ordinary weight loss dieting has not been shown to be related to eating disorder onset unless the eating disorder preceded dieting; reliable evidence of a relationship between "yo-yo" weight loss and eating disorder onset has not been found; and the risk of negative psychological outcomes related to dieting is unknown.[31] Whatever the relationship between dieting and eating disorder onset, adolescents appear to be highly vulnerable.

The incidence of eating disorders in a sample of high school girls up to age 18 was found to be 2.8%; for ages 19 to 24 the incidence was 1.3%.[32] However, the incidence of psychological disorders, particularly depression, was 89.5%, and evidence of impaired functioning and increased risk of adult-onset mental disorders well exceeded expectations.[32] The age of onset for anorexia tends to be much younger than the age of onset for bulimia. But a finding of unique interest is that, in addition to low incidence rates, in young girls, these eating disorders may be transient and short-lived.

Nevertheless, the high incidence of depression demands that experts continue to strive to determine what, if any, relationship exists between depression and anorexia. Are young depressed women more likely to explore disordered eating? Or are young eating-disordered women significantly more likely to become seriously depressed? Longitudinal studies of eating disorder risk transference from childhood to adolescence to adulthood suggest that the greatest risk is from adolescence to young adulthood.[33] Findings such as these would suggest that, although severe eating disorders in young females are less common than depression, early age onset might predict adult disordered eating.

Genetic studies of anorexia and major depression have shown a 58% concordance rate of anorexia in female twins.[34] Findings such as these indicate substantial heritability for anorexia. PET studies have shown a connection between emotionality and dopamine activity in areas of the brain associated with appetite and the risk of anorexia, but completely different neurobiological factors appear to underlie eating for survival and eating for emotional reward.[35] Neurobiological alterations affecting survival eating may be more closely related to anorexia. However, PET studies showing significant brain glucose hypometabolism in the parietal cortex of underweight patients with anorexia further complicate the model.[36] As yet, it is unclear whether less brain glucose metabolism and altered survival appetite drive characterize anorexia or are the result of excessive weight loss. Clear discernment of the direction of such findings is likely to remain difficult. Currently, cause-and-effect associations are absolutely clear only in studies such as the measurement of anorexia effects on bone reabsorption rates (serum osteocalcin levels) in severely underweight patients.[37]

Anorexia Nervosa. Anorexia nervosa is characterized by severe restriction of total calorie intake, refusal to maintain a healthy body weight, fear of weight gain, and fear of obesity.[38] Calorie restriction methods can include compulsive rituals that are dangerous, peculiar, or irrational. Normal dieting and successful weight loss may precede the onset of anorexia. Obsessive body dysmorphic thoughts and severe body image disturbance are hallmark symptoms of the disorder. This obsessive thinking in dangerously underweight persons can maintain the drive for calorie restriction and weight loss without consideration for actual hunger or body weight. That said, anorexia starts out as volitional behavior, but severe undereating can become compulsive. Loss of voluntary control of calorie intake can make it difficult for even dangerously emaciated persons to stop restricting their calorie intake.

Etiology and Neurobiology. Phobic avoidance anxiety associated with weight; neurotransmitters (serotonin, norepinephrine, dopamine, dysregulation); altered hunger-satiety signals; and psychological, physiologic, and autoimmune mechanisms have been studied as possible models of AN. Early AN models focused on the loss of secondary sex characteristics that accompanied extreme weight loss. Those models generally attributed anorexia to psychological fears of impregnation. Later models focused on intense struggles for power and control between very young women with anorexia and their parents. These psychodynamic models seemed only to explain a very small portion of the illness experience. More recent psychodynamic models focus on attributes such as obsessive-compulsive perfectionism.[39]

Researchers now are exploring neurobiological models of anorexia that involve hypothalamic dysfunction; metabolic dysfunction; comorbid psychological disorders; stress response dysregulation; and altered norepinephrine, serotonin, and dopamine neurotransmission systems. The findings of long-term survival studies make plain the need for more sophisticated biological models of anorexia. A 30-year study found that 93% of 208 individuals survived anorexia.[40] In addition to malnutrition, the causes of death were liver failure, cardiac arrest, pneumonia, suicide, convulsion, and acute alcohol toxicity. Of these causes, the incidence of alcohol-related deaths far exceeded expectations. Similar findings were observed in a 21-year study.[41]

The search for strong causal models of anorexia has been underway for decades, yet the most convincing findings continue to describe survival analysis and comorbid illnesses. In other words, although currently understood to be an eating disorder that can persist, the disorder may be far more complicated. For example, early stages appear to be far less complex than later stages, and anorexia with depression or alcohol abuse appears to be more dangerous than anorexia alone. Neurobiological findings for these comorbid disorders would suggest that alterations in brain structures and functioning associated with anorexia are likely to be related to age of illness onset and symptom duration.

Clinical Manifestations. *Calorie restriction* is the hallmark symptom of AN. These restrictions can take the form of elaborate rituals and rules that govern all calorie intake. Weight loss is viewed as evidence of successful calorie restriction.

Appetite suppression may go unnoticed, but AN does not produce true loss of appetite until dangerously low body weight is reached. Persons with AN must battle against their hunger, a battle that of course is not always successful. Any lapse is likely to be met with redoubled efforts.

Bingeing and *purging* can occur with AN when the disorder essentially includes both anorexia and bulimia.

Physical symptoms of AN in younger adolescent girls and boys include delayed psychosexual development, hypothermia, dependent edema, bradycardia, hypotension, and languor. Amenorrhea is predictable when young girls maintain a body weight insufficient for reproductive health. Severe, potentially life-threatening physical symptoms include hypokalemia and QRS rhythm changes. Cardiac arrhythmias typically are the actual cause of death in severe cases of AN. These physical symptoms are reversed by adequate calorie intake and normal weight. However, remission of physical symptoms of AN does not necessarily lead to remission of the psychological symptoms that may have triggered the disorder.

Pharmacologic Treatment. Recovery from AN is considered to be a long and costly process, with fewer than 50% of patients achieving recovery in less than 6 years.[42] Severity is clearly a factor. The more severe the weight loss at the outset, the more difficult and more prolonged recovery will be. Individuals with anorexia may have a host of treatment needs and remain vulnerable to serious health crisis for years. Treatment is further complicated by the existence of profound comorbid disorders such as alcoholism, depression, anxiety, bipolar disorder, and personality disorder. For profoundly low-weight persons, the process of *refeeding* for weight gain is in itself slow and difficult, and other treatment goals may have to be secondary. With these concerns in mind, recent treatment guidelines for anorexia recommend a comprehensive care plan that includes medication treatments, psychosocial interventions, and nutritional interventions.[43] Selective serotonin reuptake inhibitors are the medications of choice when depression is a comorbid disorder. In some cases, antidepressant medications may exert central effects on appetite that may prove helpful. Severely underweight patients must be closely monitored for medication side effects such as dizziness.

KEY POINTS

- Anorexia nervosa is an eating disorder characterized by excessive dietary restriction, significant weight loss (>15%), irrational fears of gaining weight, and disturbed body image. The disorder appears to have a genetic predisposition and affects females almost exclusively. The average age at onset is 13 to 15 years. Afflicted individuals tend to be secretive about their food restrictions. Self-induced vomiting and laxative abuse may also occur. Manifestations of AN include amenorrhea, hypothermia, edema, hypotension, and fluid and electrolyte imbalance. Potassium imbalance may lead to the serious consequence of cardiac dysrhythmias.

SUMMARY

Hypotheses regarding the cause and pathogenesis, clinical manifestations, and implications for management of representative subsets of three large categories of illnesses have been presented. It is important to recognize that these illnesses represent mixtures of biological, psychological, social, and environmental factors. Researchers have yet to unlock the mysteries surrounding the neurobiological mechanisms of nonpsychotic illnesses.

REFERENCES

1. American Psychiatric Association: *Diagnostic and statistical manual of mental disorders*, ed 4, text revision, Washington, DC, 2000, The Association.
2. Lesch KP: Molecular foundation of anxiety disorders, *J Neural Transm* 108(6):717-746, 2001.
3. Gorman JM, Kent J, Martinez J et al: Physiological changes during carbon dioxide inhalation in patients with panic disorder, major depression, and premenstrual dysphoric disorder: evidence for a central fear mechanism, *Arch Gen Psychiatry* 58(2):125-131, 2001.
4. Abelson JL, Weg JG, Nesse RM et al: Persistent respiratory irregularity in patients with panic disorder, *Biol Psychiatry* 49(7):588-595, 2001.
5. Wilhelm FH, Trabert W, Roth WT: Physiologic instability in panic disorder and generalized anxiety disorder, *Biol Psychiatry* 49(7):596-605, 2002.
6. Mathew SJ, Coplan JD, Gorman JM: Neurobiological mechanisms of social anxiety disorder, *Am J Psychiatry* 158(10):1558-1567, 2001.
7. Heim C, Newport DJ, Bonsall R et al: Altered pituitary-adrenal axis responses to provocative challenge tests in adult survivors of childhood abuse, *Am J Psychiatry* 158(4):575-581, 2001.
8. Teicher MH, Andersen SL, Polcari A et al: The neurobiological consequences of early stress and childhood maltreatment, *Neurosci Biobehav Rev* 27(1-2):33-44, 2003.
9. Sheikh JI: Anxiety in older adults. Assessment and management of three common presentations, *Geriatrics* 58(5):44-45, 2003.
10. Rickels K, Rynn MA: What is generalized anxiety disorder? *J Clin Psychiatry* 62(Suppl 11):4-12, 2001.
11. Nutt DJ: Neurobiological mechanisms in generalized anxiety disorder, *J Clin Psychiatry* 62(Suppl 11):22-27, 2001.
12. Davidson JR: Pharmacotherapy of generalized anxiety disorder, *J Clin Psychiatry* 62(Suppl 11):46-50, 2001.
13. Ursu S, Stenger VA, Shear MK et al: Overactive action monitoring in obsessive-compulsive disorder: evidence from functional magnetic resonance imaging, *Am Psychol Soc* 14(4):347-353, 2003.
14. Winsber ME, Cassic KS, Koran LM: Hoarding in obsessive-compulsive disorder: a report of 20 cases, *J Clin Psychiatry* 60(9):591-597, 1999.
15. Brown WA: Hoarding, *Psych Times* 24(13):50-52, 2007.
16. Endler NS, Kocovski NL: Personality disorders at the crossroads, *J Personal Disord* 16(6):487-502, 2002.
17. McDermut W, Zimmerman M, Chelminski I: The construct validity of depressive personality disorder, *J Abnorm Psychol* 112(1):49-60, 2003.
18. Tyrer P, Mitchard S, Methuen C et al: Treatment rejecting and treatment seeking personality disorders: type R and type S, *J Personal Disord* 17(3):263-268, 2003.
19. Coolidge FL, Thede LL, Jang KL: Heritability of personality disorders in childhood: a preliminary investigation, *J Personal Disord* 15(1):33-40, 2001.
20. Skodol AE et al: The borderline diagnosis II: biology, genetics, and clinical course, *Biol Psychiatry* 51(12):951-963, 2002.
21. Rinne T, de Kloet ER, Wouters L et al: Hyperresponsiveness of hypothalamic-pituitary-adrenal axis to combined dexamethasone/corticotropin-releasing hormone challenge in female borderline personality disorder subjects with a history of sustained childhood abuse, *Soc Biol Psychiatry* 52(11):1102-1112, 2002.
22. Boutros NN, Torello M, McGlashan TH: Electrophysiological aberrations in borderline personality disorder: state of the evidence, *J Neuropsychiatry Clin Neurosci* 15(2):145-154, 2003.
23. Schmahl CG, Elzinga BM, Vermetten E et al: Neural correlates of memories of abandonment in women with and without borderline personality disorder, *Soc Bio Psychiatry* 54(2):142-151, 2003.
24. Tebartz van Elst L, Hesslinger B, Thiel T et al: Frontolimbic brain abnormalities in patients with borderline personality disorder: a volumetric magnetic resonance imaging study, *Soc Biol Psychiatry* 54(2):163-171, 2003.
25. Gabbard GO: Psychotherapy of personality disorders, *J Psychother Pract Res* 9(1):1-6, 2000.

26. Leichsenring F, Leibing E: The effectiveness of psychodynamic therapy and cognitive behavior therapy in the treatment of personality disorders: a meta analysis, *Am J Psychiatry* 160(7):1223-1232, 2003.

27. Murphy C, Vess J: Subtypes of psychopathy: proposed differences between narcissistic, borderline, sadistic, and antisocial psychopaths, *Psychiatr Q* 74(1):11-29, 2003.

28. Krueger RF, Hicks BM, Patrick CJ et al: Etiologic connections among substance dependence, antisocial behavior, and personality: modeling the externalizing spectrum, *J Abnorm Psychol* 111(3):411-424, 2002.

29. Raine A: Biosocial studies of antisocial and violent behavior in children and adults: a review, *J Abnorm Child Psychol* 30(4):311-326, 2002.

30. Kiehl KA, Smith AM, Hare RD et al: Limbic abnormalities in affective processing by criminal psychopaths as revealed by functional magnetic resonance imaging, *Soc Biol Psychiatry* 50(9):677-684, 2001.

31. National Task Force on the Prevention and Treatment of Obesity: Dieting and the development of eating disorders in overweight and obese adults, *Arch Intern Med* 160(17):2581-2589, 2000.

32. Lewinsohn PM, Striegel-Moore RH, Seeley JR: Epidemiology and natural course of eating disorders in young women from adolescence to young adulthood, *J Am Acad Child Adolesc Psychiatry* 39(10):1284-1292, 2000.

33. Kotler LA, Cohen P, Davies M et al: Longitudinal relationships between childhood, adolescent, and adult eating disorders, *J Am Acad Child Adolesc Psychiatry* 40(12):1434-1440, 2001.

34. Wade TD, Bulik CM, Neale M et al: Anorexia nervosa and major depression: shared genetic and environmental risk factors, *Am J Psychiatry* 157(3):469-471, 2000.

35. Volkow ND et al: Brain dopamine is associated with eating behaviors in humans, *Int J Eat Disord* 33:136-142, 2003.

36. Delvenne V, Goldman S, De Maertelaer V et al: Brain glucose metabolism in eating disorders assessed by positron emission tomography, *Int J Eat Disord* 25(1):29-37, 1999.

37. Hotta M, Fukuda I, Sato K et al: The relationship between bone turnover and body weight, serum insulin-like growth factor (IGF) I, and serum IGF-binding protein levels in patients with anorexia nervosa, *J Clin Endocrinol Metab* 85(1):200-206, 2000.

38. Mehler PS: Diagnosis and care of patients with anorexia nervosa in primary care settings, *Ann Intern Med* 134(11):1048-1059, 2001.

39. Halmi KA, Sunday SR, Strober M et al: Perfectionism in anorexia nervosa: variation by clinical subtype, obsessionality, and pathological eating behavior, *Am J Psychiatry* 157(11):1799-1805, 2000.

40. Korndörfer SR, Lucas AR, Suman VJ et al: Long-term survival of patients with anorexia nervosa: a population-based study in Rochester, Minn, *Mayo Clin Proc* 78(3):278-284, 2003.

41. Zipfel S, Löwe B, Reas DL et al: Long-term prognosis in anorexia nervosa: lessons from a 21-year follow-up study, *Lancet* 355(9205):721-722, 2000.

42. Finfgeld DL: Anorexia nervosa: analysis of long-term outcomes and clinical implications, *Arch Psychiatr Nurs* 16(4):176-186, 2002.

43. American Psychiatric Association Work Group on Eating Disorders: Practice guidelines for the treatment of patients with eating disorders (revision), *Am J Psychiatry* 157(1 Suppl):1-39, 2000.

chapter

50

Structure and Function of the Musculoskeletal System

Carol L. Danning

MEDIA RESOURCES

Additional Material for Study, Review, and Further Exploration

 CD Companion ■ Review Questions and Answers
■ Glossary (with audio pronunciations for selected terms)
■ Disease Profiles ■ Animations

evolve **Website** at http://evolve.elsevier.com/Copstead/
■ Case Studies ■ Disease Profiles ■ WebLinks ■ Key Points Review

 Online Course (Module 20)

KEY QUESTIONS

■ What are the functions of osteoblasts and osteoclasts in bone remodeling?
■ What is the relationship between joint structure and joint mobility?
■ Why is articular cartilage particularly susceptible to degenerative changes?

■ What factors determine tendon strength and compliance?
■ How does the striated structure of skeletal muscle relate to its contractile function?
■ How does an action potential in the α-motor neuron lead to a contraction in the muscle cells of the motor unit?

CHAPTER OUTLINE

Movement is one of the most characteristic and visible aspects of human life. Ease of movement adds to self-worth and well-being because the ability to move is closely connected to independence. A working knowledge of the system responsible for body movement is imperative to the health care provider. This chapter examines the basic characteristics of the firm support of bone and joint structures that make motion possible and the properties of skeletal muscles that are responsible for actually moving the body's framework.

STRUCTURE AND FUNCTION OF BONE

The primary purposes of the skeletal system are to protect internal organs, provide bony attachments for muscles and ligaments, present rigid levers to allow functional movement of the body and its separate parts, and store mineral and marrow elements for forming new blood cells. Bone is highly vascular and is metabolically active from birth to death.

Composition

The organic component of bone is 90% to 95% collagen fibers, which extend along lines of tension and give bone its great tensile strength.[1] Bone can remodel itself throughout life in response to external forces (or loads) such as the pull of tendons and body weight during activities. Bone is the hardest connective tissue in the body, having a high content of inorganic material (mineral salts) combined with an organic matrix. This combination provides for a hard, rigid structure that is both flexible and resilient.

Similar to other connective tissue, bone consists of a cellular component, ground substance, and fibrous component. The cellular component consists of fibroblasts, fibrocytes, osteoblasts, osteocytes, osteoclasts, and osteoprogenitor cells. **Fibroblasts** and **fibrocytes** are needed for collagen production. **Osteoblasts,** which lay down bone, are formed from **osteoprogenitor** cells, which are bone stem cells lining bone surfaces. **Osteocytes** are mature bone cells. **Osteoclasts** are responsible for bone resorption. **Ground substance** is a homogeneous gelatinous substance composed of extracellular fluid and proteoglycans, chondroitin sulfate, and hyaluronic acid, which help control the deposition of calcium salts.[2]

The mineral portions of bone, mainly calcium and phosphate, account for 65% to 75% of the dry weight of bone and give bone its solid structure. Bone is also a source of essential minerals, especially calcium. Bone mineral is embedded in fibers of protein collagen, the fibrous aspect of the extracellular matrix. Collagen fibers are tough, pliable, and resistant to stretching. Collagen composes approximately 95% of the extracellular matrix and accounts for 25% to 35% of the dry weight of bone. Collagen is the chief fibrous component of the musculoskeletal system.

A ground substance surrounds collagen fibers in bone. Ground substance consists of protein polysaccharides, or **glycosaminoglycans,** mainly in a molecule called **proteoglycan.** Glycosaminoglycans serve as cement between layers of collagen fibers.

Water accounts for approximately 25% of the weight of live bone. Most of the water is located in the organic matrix surrounding collagen fibers and ground substance. Another 15% of the water is located in canals that carry nutrition to bone tissue.

Microscopically, the basic unit of bone is the **osteon** or the **haversian system** (Figure 50-1). The haversian canal lies at the center of each osteon and contains blood vessels and nerve fibers. A concentric series of lamellae of mineralized matrix surrounds the central canal. Bordering the lamellae are small cavities (lacunae) that contain a bone cell, the **osteocyte.** Many small channels, the canaliculi, connect adjacent lamellae with each other and eventually with the main haversian canal. This canal system allows nutrients from blood vessels in the haversian canal to reach osteocytes. Collagen fibers connect one lamella to another within the osteon and increase the mechanical strength of bone.

At the tissue level, bones are classified as two types: **cancellous** or **trabecular** bone and **compact** or **cortical** bone (Figure 50-2). **Cancellous bone** is formed in thin plates called **trabeculae.** Trabeculae are laid down in response to stress and shape to accommodate loads placed on the bone. Cancellous bone is covered by compact bone. **Compact bone** is quite resistant to compression and is dense in structure. Compact bone is laid down in concentric layers. A tough fibrous membrane called the *periosteum* covers all bones. The periosteum is highly vascularized and provides nutrition for bone via Volkmann canals (see Figure 50-1). An inner layer of the periosteum contains **osteoblasts,** which are responsible for bone growth and repair. The periosteum covers the entire bone except for the ends, which are covered by hyaline cartilage.

In longer bones, a central cavity (**medullary cavity**) is present (see Figure 50-2). A thin membrane called the **endosteum** covers this cavity. The central cavity is filled with fatty marrow. Osteogenic cells are located in the endosteum.[3]

FIGURE 50-1 Microscopic anatomy of bone. The section has been enlarged to show the periosteum, osteoblasts, the haversian system, lacunae, and osteoclasts.

Blood vessels are distributed through the haversian canals. Living cells in bone communicate with each other and the haversian system via threadlike processes.

Functional Properties

Growth and Ossification

The process of longitudinal bone growth involves endochondral ossification. In this type of growth, cartilage is replaced by bone as in embryonic development, fracture healing, and some bone tumor growth. In children, fracture through the shaft of a long bone stimulates bone growth, possibly because of increased nutrition to growth cartilage from the hyperemia associated with fracture healing. Particular attention to bone alignment or overlapping of fracture ends must be paid when managing a fracture in a child between 2 and 10 years of age since predictable bone overgrowth can lead to limb length discrepancies.[4]

Circumferential bone growth occurs via intramembranous ossification. In this case, connective tissue is transformed into bone. Interstitial growth is not possible in bone. Bone can grow in length only by a process of growth within cartilage, followed by endochondral ossification (Figure 50-3). Two sites of cartilage growth are available in a long bone: articular cartilage and epiphyseal plate cartilage. In longer

bones, the epiphysis provides the only growth plate for the entire bone.

Continuous Growth

The **epiphyseal plate** (see Figure 50-3) allows for lengthening of the metaphysis and diaphysis of a long bone and is the site of continuous growth. Growth and thickening of cartilage cells of the plate move the epiphysis away from the metaphysis. Calcification and replacement of cartilage occur on the metaphyseal surface (endochondral ossification). Injuries to this growth plate in children may lead to limb length discrepancies. In addition, inflammatory arthritis in children (particularly of the knee) can lead to increased blood flow to the epiphyseal plate, which also may accelerate growth or lead to premature plate closure. This also can lead to leg length abnormalities.

The function of the epiphyseal plate in the growth process may be illustrated by examining the specific zones of the plate (Figure 50-4) and how they contribute to the growth process. The **zone of resting cartilage** maintains adherence of the plate to the epiphysis. Immature chondrocytes and vessels penetrate this first zone from the epiphysis and nourish the plate. The **zone of young proliferating cartilage** demonstrates the most active cartilage cell growth. The **zone of maturing**

Epiphysis — Articular cartilage
— Epiphyseal line
— Spongy bone/cancellous (trabecular) bone
— Compact bone
— Medullary cavity

Diaphysis

— Nutrient foramen
— **Endosteum**
— Periosteum

Epiphysis
— Articular cartilage

FIGURE 50-2 Structure and composition of a typical long bone. (From Applegate E: *The anatomy and physiology learning system*, 2nd ed, Philadelphia, 2000, Saunders, p 93.)

cartilage contains the enlarged and mature cartilage cells as they migrate toward the metaphysis. The final zone is the **zone of calcifying cartilage,** which is a very thin line of chondrocytes and the weakest segment of the epiphyseal plate. These chondrocytes are no longer living because of calcification of the matrix.

Bone is also deposited quite actively on the metaphyseal side of the plate. With the addition of new bone, the metaphysis becomes longer.

Osteoblasts in the inner layer of the periosteum are responsible for growth in the width of bones. This process is called **intermembranous ossification.** Resorption of bone, through a process of osteoclastic resorption, causes the medullary cavity to enlarge, causing additional widening of bone.

Hormones influence bone growth. Too little secretion of thyroxine by the thyroid gland or too little growth hormone from the pituitary gland results in dwarfism. Oversecretion of growth hormone results in giantism. Sex hormones, such as estradiol, are produced in higher amounts during and after puberty and can cause more rapid maturation and fusion of the epiphyseal plates. These hormones may limit the growth spurts of puberty, and early sexual maturity, especially in girls, can lead to shorter stature.[3]

Response to Injury, Stress, and Aging

The ability of bone to remodel after injury is important. Although remodeling of bone continues throughout life, death of the osteon or removal of calcium from bone requires that new bone be deposited to retain strength and function.

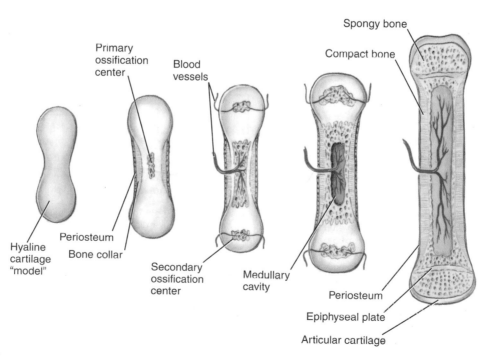

FIGURE 50-3 Events in endochondral ossification. (From Applegate E: *The anatomy and physiology learning system,* 2nd ed, Philadelphia, 2000, Saunders, p 95.)

Primary ossification center
Blood vessels
Spongy bone
Compact bone

Hyaline cartilage "model"
Periosteum
Bone collar
Secondary ossification center
Medullary cavity
Periosteum
Epiphyseal plate
Articular cartilage

Mechanical Principles

The amount of tension that a muscle can generate is dictated by a number of mechanical concepts or principles of relationship. These principles include the length-tension relationship, load-velocity relationship, force-time relationship, and effects of muscle temperature and muscle fatigue. Muscle tension, fatigue, and prestretching are other important factors in muscle force production. A brief review follows.

Length-Tension Relationship

Maximal tension is produced when muscle is at its usual resting length because this position allows actin and myosin filaments to overlap and provide the maximal number of cross-bridges between filaments. At a short resting length, little tension or muscle shortening is possible inasmuch as myosin filaments abut the Z line. If muscle fiber is held at lengths beyond the resting length, tension decreases because actin and myosin do not overlap and therefore no active tension is present.

Load-Velocity Relationship

The velocity of the shortening of a muscle contracting concentrically is inversely related to the load applied. The lower the weight, the higher the velocity is. The greater the weight, the slower the contraction of the muscle is. An isometric contraction occurs when the load equals the amount of force that the muscle exerts. If the load exceeds the force generated by the muscle, an eccentric contraction occurs. Greater load leads to faster eccentric lengthening.

Force-Time Relationship

The longer the time of contraction, the greater the force that the muscle can generate until the muscle reaches its point of maximal tension. An increase in the duration of force allows higher levels of tension to be produced by the contractile structures.

Effects of Temperature Change

Conduction velocity across the sarcolemma increases with a rise in muscle temperature. Temperature elevation increases the enzymatic activity of muscle metabolism and the elasticity of collagen in elastic components. Muscle temperature increases when athletes warm up as a result of the increased blood flow and heat generated by metabolism. Both changes increase the amount of force that a muscle can produce.

Effects of Fatigue

The availability of ATP determines muscles' ability to contract and relax. Prolonged activity of muscles can be sustained only when the muscle has an adequate supply of nutrients and oxygen to synthesize ATP. If the activity is of sufficient intensity to deplete ATP faster than it can be replaced, muscle tension will gradually weaken and at some point drop to zero. When muscle returns to its original state, creatine phosphate, a major storage form of energy in muscle, must be re-synthesized and glycogen stores replaced. This revitalization process requires energy, so the muscle will continue to consume oxygen at high rates even after termination of activity. Heavy, rapid breathing continues after a period of strenuous exercise to provide adequate oxygen for ATP synthesis. This oxygen is also essential for removing lactic acid from muscle. Resting muscle uses oxygen to re-form glucose and glycogen from lactic acid and to oxidize the lactic acid to carbon dioxide and water.[1]

Response to Movement and Exercise

Early mobilization may prevent muscle atrophy after surgery or injury. With early motion, muscle fibers position themselves in a more parallel alignment as opposed to the fibers in an immobilized individual. With movement, capillarization occurs more rapidly and tensile strength improves more quickly. With immobilization, the cross-sectional area of muscles decreases and oxidative enzyme activity is reduced. Early mobility prevents atrophy. Afferent impulses from the muscle spindles are increased, thus improving the stimulation of some muscle fibers.

Physical training and conditioning increase the cross-sectional area of muscle fibers. An increase in area coincides with an increase in muscle bulk and strength. In addition, stretching exercises are effective in preventing injury and improving performance, as well as increasing muscle flexibility, maintaining and improving joint motion, and enhancing the elasticity and length of the musculoskeletal unit.

KEY POINTS

- The fundamental unit of muscle contraction is the sarcomere.
- A sarcomere extends from one Z line to the next and consists of interdigitating thick and thin filaments.
- Muscle contraction occurs when myosin head regions bind to sites on the actin filament to form cross-bridges.
  - After binding, myosin tugs on the actin filament, which causes thick and thin filaments to overlap more.
  - Myosin then releases and proceeds to bind at another point farther along the actin filament. Each cross-bridge cycle requires one molecule of ATP.
- For contraction to occur, the cytoplasm must have sufficient calcium ions.
  - In the absence of calcium, tropomyosin covers binding sites on the actin filament and prevents cross-bridge formation.
  - Another regulatory protein, troponin, controls the position of tropomyosin.
  - When calcium is bound to troponin, tropomyosin is moved to expose binding sites on actin, and cross-bridge formation ensues.
- Calcium ions are stored in the sarcoplasmic reticulum and released into the cytoplasm when the muscle cell depolarizes during an action potential.
- A group of skeletal muscle cells innervated by a single motor neuron is called a *motor unit*. All of the cells in the unit contract simultaneously when the motor neuron depolarizes.
  - An action potential in the α-motor neuron releases acetylcholine at the motor end-plate. Acetylcholine binds to receptors on the muscle cell membrane and

triggers an action potential in the cell. To generate more force in the muscle, a greater number of motor units can be activated, a process termed *recruitment*.

■ Activation of a motor unit by a single action potential results in a brief twitch contraction.

■ A train of action potentials in the motor neuron results in a sustained contraction, in which calcium is released into the cytoplasm faster than it is removed.

■ Sustained contraction in response to repetitive stimulation is termed *summation*.

■ Muscle contraction does not always result in muscle shortening.

  ■ Isometric contraction refers to contraction with no change in muscle length.

  ■ Eccentric contraction occurs when the muscle lengthens while contracting (because of a high load).

  ■ Muscle shortening with contraction is termed *concentric*.

  ■ Isometric contraction generates greater tension than concentric contraction does; eccentric contraction may generate the highest tension.

■ The behavior of contracting muscle is governed by several mechanical principles:

  ■ Length-tension relationship: Up to a point, a greater resting length of the muscle generates a greater force of contraction. Optimal actin-myosin overlap occurs at about the usual resting muscle length.

  ■ Load-velocity relationship: The velocity of muscle shortening is inversely related to the applied load.

  ■ Force-time relationship: A longer contraction is associated with a greater force of contraction.

■ Creatine phosphate is a storage form of energy that is quickly converted to ATP when cellular ATP levels fall.

■ Fatigue results when energy and nutrient supply are insufficient.

■ A higher rate of muscle oxygen consumption occurs during and for a period after muscle activity.

■ Lack of muscle use (disuse) leads to a reduction in muscle mass and slowing of oxidative enzyme activity.

■ Early activity after injury is associated with quicker recovery of tensile strength, less atrophy, and better circulation.

GERIATRIC CONSIDERATIONS

Changes in the Muscular System

With aging, the size and number of muscle cells decrease. The remaining muscle cells undergo atrophy, decreased muscle fiber diameter, and reduced elastic tissue. These changes result in reduced muscle mass. Within muscle cells, extracellular sodium, chloride, water, and lipofuscin pigment increase, with diminished intracellular potassium. The loss of muscle protein may not be obvious because of increased collagen and fat replacement.

Because fewer capillaries are available to supply the muscles, removal of metabolites is decreased. Hormonal stimulation of muscle by testosterone, somatotropin, and thyrotropin is decreased, in addition to reduced muscle uptake of glucose during exercise.

Muscle response to nervous system stimulation is decreased with decreased muscle norepinephrine. Muscles are also less responsive to neurotransmitters, including acetylcholine at the myoneural junction, and cholinesterase activity is decreased as well.

The muscle, neural, and hormonal changes of aging that affect the muscular system lead to a functional decrease in muscle strength of 30% to 50%, reduced muscle endurance, diminished muscle tone, and increased fatigability. Muscular decline rises with increasing age and usually occurs earlier in men; however, the extent of muscular system decline varies. An elderly individual with good nutritional balance and protein intake combined with adequate active exercise maintains muscle function and strength.

SUMMARY

The musculoskeletal system provides movement for the body. Alterations in function of the musculoskeletal system that decrease the efficiency of movement can often magnify the stress placed on uninvolved structures and increase the potential for degeneration, joint laxity, and pain.

A sound knowledge base of the anatomy, physiology, and mechanics of movement makes the diagnosis of aberrant movement and function easier and thus aids in planning the necessary care and education of patients. Too often, in attempts to provide relief for patients with musculoskeletal dysfunction, the tissue involved or the mechanism of activity causing the injury is not properly identified. Short-lived relief of pain may be provided through the use of analgesics. However, return to activity exacerbates pain and the restriction of movement present before medical care.

Familiarity with the musculoskeletal system also allows health care providers to identify basic tissues involved in injury or disease. Such awareness empowers the clinician to provide relief of pain as well as address quality-of-life issues. Determination of the type of activity that creates the problem and identification of segments of the musculoskeletal system affected provide the basis to achieve positive long-lasting improvement. Weakness, instability, or decreased motion of structures involved in the dysfunction must be identified. Analysis of physical limitations can lead to patient education and referral to sources that can reduce the impact of physical limitations. In addition, the use of tested exercise, modification of living and working environments, and education of family members will help affected individuals achieve optimal motor function and prevent further injury. The effects of aging on the muscular system are described in Geriatric Considerations: Changes in the Muscular System.

REFERENCES

1. Guyton AC, Hall JE: *Human physiology and mechanisms of disease*, ed 10, Philadelphia, 2000, Saunders.
2. Ruddy S, Harris ED, Sledge CB, editors: *Kelley's textbook of rheumatology*, ed 6, Philadelphia, 2001, Saunders.
3. Favus MJ, editor: *Primer on the metabolic bone diseases and disorders of mineral metabolism*, ed 4, Philadelphia, 1999, Lippincott-Raven.
4. Chapman MW et al, editors: *Chapman's orthopaedic surgery*, ed 3, Philadelphia, 2001, Lippincott Williams & Wilkins.
5. Wolff J: *Des Gesetz der Transformation der Knochen*, Berlin, 1892, Hirschwold.
6. Giangregorio L, Blimkie CJ: Skeletal adaptations to alterations in weight-bearing activity: a comparison of models of disuse osteoporosis, *Sports Med* 32(7):459-476, 2002.
7. Koopman WJ, editor: *Arthritis and allied conditions*, ed 14, Philadelphia, 2001, Lippincott Williams & Wilkins.
8. Klippel JH, editor: *Primer on the rheumatic diseases*, ed 12, Atlanta, 2001, Arthritis Foundation.
9. Beers MH, Berkow R, editors: *The Merck manual of geriatrics*, Rahway, NJ, 2000, Merck.

Alterations in Musculoskeletal Function: Trauma, Infection, and Disease

Carol L. Danning

MEDIA RESOURCES

Additional Material for Study, Review, and Further Exploration

CD Companion ■ Review Questions and Answers
■ Glossary (with audio pronunciations for selected terms)
■ Disease Profiles ■ Animations

 Website at http://evolve.elsevier.com/Copstead/
■ Case Studies ■ Disease Profiles ■ WebLinks ■ Key Points Review

Online Course (Module 20)

KEY QUESTIONS

- What is the process and duration of normal bone healing after a fracture?
- How are osteoporosis and osteomalacia or rickets similar, and how do they differ?
- What are the clinical findings and management of bone infections?
- What terminology is used to describe primary bone tumors?

- How can clinical manifestations of soft-tissue injuries be used to differentiate non-contractile and contractile injuries?
- What are the manifestations and management of compartment syndrome?
- What are the cause and pathogenesis of muscular dystrophy and myasthenia gravis?

CHAPTER OUTLINE

A smoothly functioning musculoskeletal system facilitates a complete range of human actions, including walking, talking, running, breathing, and a myriad of voluntary physical activities. Any abnormality in the musculoskeletal system decreases the efficiency of movement and increases mechanical stress. Ballistic requirements of many sports and occupations, such as skiing and driving an automobile, have increased the potential for trauma. Diseases also disrupt the integrity of the musculoskeletal system. Infectious processes, genetic abnormalities, immune-mediated inflammatory disorders, and nutritional deficiencies may all affect movement.

Clinicians who work with patients experiencing dysfunctions of the musculoskeletal system must have a solid background in evaluation and management of such disorders. Without this preparation, interventions will not be sufficient to promote maximal functional return. This chapter discusses disorders particular to the musculoskeletal system as they affect the skeletal frame, soft tissue, and muscles.

BONE AND JOINT TRAUMA

The skeletal system is subject to alterations in function from mechanical stress and infection. The purposes of the skeletal system are to protect internal organs, contribute to mineral homeostasis, produce blood cells, and provide muscle attachment sites and thus facilitate body movement. Bone is one of the body's hardest structures, as well as one of its most dynamic and metabolically active tissues. Bone is vascular with a capacity for repair. It adapts to mechanical demands placed on it and alters its configuration in response to those mechanical stresses.

Types of Bone

Two basic forms of bone are present in the human body: cortical bone and cancellous bone. **Cortical bone** forms the cortex, or outer shell, of the bone. Cortical bone is designed to tolerate compression and shearing forces, but tension forces may exceed the tolerance of cortical bone. Most fractures are due to tension failures in which bone is pulled apart. With bending, twisting, or straight tension, stress may exceed the bone's tolerance, and a fracture occurs on the convex side of the bend. **Cancellous bone,** which has a spongy or lattice-like appearance, is found in the interior of bones. Unlike cortical bone, cancellous bone does not tolerate compression stress. Cancellous bone provides structural support to cortical bone and increases a bone's potential to withstand stress.

Fracture

A **fracture** is a break in continuity of a bone, an epiphyseal plate, or a cartilaginous joint surface. Trauma generating enough energy to fracture a bone also produces force sufficient to traumatize adjacent soft tissue. With that concept in mind, the remainder of this section will address injury to the bony component of the musculoskeletal system.

Types of Fracture

Fracture type reflects the type of tension stress placed on bone (Figure 51-1). A **transverse** fracture occurs in a straight line at approximately a 90-degree angle to the longitudinal axis of the bone. **Spiral** fractures are the result of rotational forces and cause bone to separate in the form of an *S* around the bone. **Longitudinal** fractures split bone along its length. **Oblique** fractures result from a rotational force, but unlike spiral fractures, the break is along an oblique course (45-degree angle) and does not rotate around the entire bone. **Comminuted** fractures consist of more than one fracture line and more than two bone fragments. These fragments may be shattered or crushed. Comminuted fractures often present considerable treatment problems because of associated soft-tissue damage and multiple bone fragments. An **impacted** fracture is caused by excessive force that telescopes or drives one fragment into another. A **greenstick** fracture is an incomplete break in the bone with the intact side of the cortex flexed. It is usually seen in children. A **stress** fracture is a failure of one cortical surface of the bone, often caused by repetitive activity such as running. Without proper treatment, a stress fracture can become a complete fracture with two distinct fragments. An **avulsion** fracture is separation of a small fragment of bone at the site of attachment of a ligament or tendon.

Of special concern are fractures at or near a joint line in children. This location of a fracture may suggest an epiphyseal growth plate fracture (Figure 51-2). With epiphyseal injuries, the potential for disruption of growth of the long bones is present. Proper reduction and fixation are necessary to avoid growth disturbance in fractures through the growth plate. Crush injury to the epiphyseal plate commonly leads to premature growth cessation. Cancellous bone does not tolerate compression stress; it buckles and then cracks. Therefore, **crush** or **compression** fractures (Figure 51-3) are consistent with cancellous bone trauma. In children, a compression injury to cancellous bone of the metaphysis of a long bone is identified as a **buckle** fracture, where bone buckles and eventually cracks. In adults, compression fractures are often found

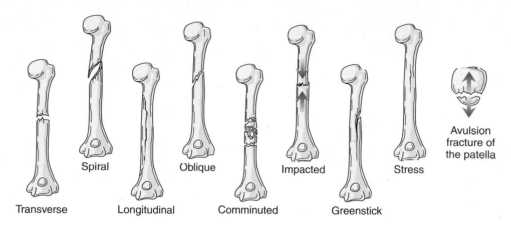

FIGURE 51-1 Types of fractures.

FIGURE 51-2 Epiphyseal injury.

FIGURE 51-3 Compression fracture.

in a vertebral body of the spine, especially in older individuals with osteoporosis.

Extent of Fracture

Fractures can be classified according to extent and depth. A **displaced** fracture is one in which the ends of fracture fragments are separated. In a **nondisplaced** fracture, the fracture fragments remain in alignment and position. With a **depressed** fracture, the fragment is displaced below the level of the surface of the bone, usually in the skull. A **complete** fracture is one in which the fracture line disrupts bone continuity through the whole thickness of the bone, including the cortex (Figure 51-4). In an **incomplete** fracture, the cortex of the bone buckles or cracks; however, bone continuity is not disrupted. Incomplete fractures tend to occur in the more

flexible, growing bones of children. Fractures can also be classified as **open** (compound) or **closed** (simple) (Figure 51-5). An open fracture occurs when bone is broken and an external wound leads to the fracture site. These fractures present an increased risk of infection and are therefore difficult to manage. A closed fracture is a fracture in which the fragments do not extend through mucous membrane or skin and skin is not broken.

In cases of open fractures, a wound classification system may be used that ranges from type I to type IIIC in increasing degree of severity. Type I is a wound smaller than 1 cm, moderately clean with minimal contamination. The fracture is simple transverse or an oblique fracture with a bone spike piercing the skin. Soft-tissue damage is minimal. Type II wounds are larger than 1 cm with moderate contamination. The fracture might be a moderate comminution or crush injury with moderate soft-tissue damage. Type III wounds have a high degree of contamination. The fracture is severely

Complete
fracture

Incomplete
fracture

FIGURE 51-4 Comparison of complete and incomplete fractures.

Open (compound)

Closed (simple)

FIGURE 51-5 Comparison of open and closed fractures.

comminuted and unstable. It is accompanied by much soft-tissue damage involving muscle, skin, and neurovascular structures. Traumatic amputations would be classified here. With type IIIA wounds, soft-tissue coverage of the fracture is sufficient. Segmental or severely comminuted fractures occur with these wounds. Type IIIB wounds with open fractures include extensive injury or loss of soft tissue, as well as periosteal stripping and bone exposure. Fractures are severely comminuted. Massive contamination is found with such wounds. Type IIIC wounds include any open fracture associated with arterial injury requiring repair regardless of the extent of soft-tissue injury.[1]

Healing Process

When a fracture occurs, the continuity of both cortical and cancellous bone is usually compromised. The five stages of fracture healing are described in Chapter 50.

Healing in a Cortical Bone. At the time of fracture in a cortical bone, blood vessels in the haversian systems are torn. After a period of bleeding, clotting occurs at the fracture site and for a short distance on both sides of the fracture. Because of lack of circulation, a small section of bone distal to the fracture site undergoes necrosis (Figure 51-6). The avascular bone eventually is replaced by living bone through resorption and bone deposition. The majority of bleeding occurs from arteries in the periosteal sleeve.

The hematoma that forms becomes the medium for early stages of healing. Osteogenic cells, which develop from the periosteum, form the external and internal callus. If the periosteum is severely torn, healing cells must proliferate from the mesenchymal cells of surrounding soft tissue. During the early stages of repair, the amount of osteogenic tissue is extensive.

Within the first few weeks, the thick mass of osteogenic tissue has formed a fracture callus.

During the initial stages of **callus formation,** no bone cells are present within the matrix. The callus is quite soft but becomes progressively firmer. With consolidation of the fracture callus, new bone formation begins. Initially, new bone forms at the edges of the periosteum, where the blood supply is more substantial. Where blood supply is sufficient, osteogenic cells differentiate into osteoblasts and primary woven bone. Near the fracture site, where the blood supply is less adequate, osteogenic cells initially differentiate into chondroblasts (cartilage).

As both the external callus (which unites cortical bone) and the internal callus (which unites cancellous bone) harden from the cartilage stage through ossification, the fracture site becomes firm and stable. No movement is detected by the medical evaluator or patient. At this point the fracture is clinically united. Although stable, cartilage and primary woven bone may be found intermixed at the site of healing.

With time, the primary callus is replaced by mature bone, and any excess callus is reabsorbed. This phase is the remodeling (last) stage of bone healing. When all immature bone cells have been replaced by mature lamellar bone, the fracture is said to be consolidated (radiographic union).

Healing in a Cancellous Bone. Cancellous fracture healing occurs mainly through development of an internal callus. The rich blood supply present in cancellous bone prevents necrosis of bone at the fracture site. If the fracture is nondisplaced, the healing process is much more rapid than that of cortical bone. Osteogenic cells in the trabeculae form the primary woven bone in the internal fracture hematoma (Figure 51-7). The internal callus fills the open space of cancellous bone and crosses

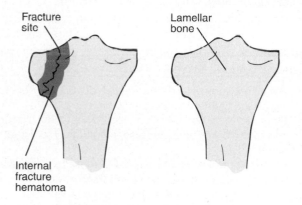

FIGURE 51-6 A, Stages of healing of cortical bone. **B,** Bone healing (schematic representation). *1,* Bleeding at broken ends of the bone with subsequent hematoma formation. *2,* Organization of hematoma into fibrous network. *3,* Invasion of osteoblasts, lengthening of collagen strands, and deposition of calcium. *4,* Callus formation: new bone is built up as osteoclasts destroy dead bone. *5,* Remodeling is accomplished as excess callus is reabsorbed and trabecular bone is laid down. **(B,** From Lewis SM, Heitkemper MM, Dirksen SR: *Medical-surgical nursing,* ed 6, St Louis, 2004, Mosby, p 1658.)

FIGURE 51-7 Healing of cancellous bone.

the fracture site. Woven bone develops and is eventually replaced by lamellar bone. As noted earlier, cancellous bone is susceptible to compression forces, and the majority of injuries incurred are compression-type fractures. With a compression fracture, fragments of bone are impacted together, which provides a more suitable environment for healing of cancellous bone. Rapid union occurs because fracture fragments move in unison.

Treatment. Medical treatment for a fracture consists of stabilization of the fracture site until healing is sufficient to allow stress to be placed on the structure. Rehabilitation of a patient with a fracture really begins at the time of release from treatment, when the fracture has had time to heal.

Complications in Bone Healing

Delayed Healing. Fracture healing may not always progress smoothly without complications. Delayed union, malunion, and nonunion of the fracture are all complications that might occur. Delayed union is usually identified anywhere from 3 months to 1 year after the fracture, when bone pain and tenderness are continuously increasing beyond the expected healing period for the wound type. Healing is slowed. The cause of delayed union might be either distraction of fracture fragments or systemic causes such as infection. Bone healing can be delayed by additional factors such as smoking, malnutrition, use of corticosteroids, and poor vascular circulation to the area.[1]

Malunion results when unequal stresses of muscle pull and gravity lead to improper alignment of fracture fragments. It often happens in the case of fractures managed with cast immobilization after skeletal traction. Malunion may also happen if an ambulatory device is applied before the fracture is firm or if the extremity is subjected to weight bearing too early in the healing process. Primary features of malunion are external deformity and radiographic evidence of internal derangement. Prevention is adequate reduction and immobilization of the fracture and adherence to specific activity and positioning restrictions.[1]

Nonunion occurs when a fracture has not healed by 4 to 6 months after a fracture. Failure to heal is due to poor blood supply and repetitive stress on the fracture site, and can be the result of interposition of muscle, tendon, or soft tissue between fracture pieces; prolonged or excessive traction; poor immobilization that allows motion at the fracture site; poor internal fixation; or wound infection after internal fixation.

Treatment. Treatment includes bone grafting, internal/external fixation, electrical bone stimulation, or any combination of these methods.[1] Bone grafts bridge gaps in bone. In normal bone healing, when bone is compressed, it becomes electronegative, thus stimulating bone formation. Negative current applied through the use of a bone stimulator is believed to induce bone formation similar to that stimulated by bone compression.[1]

Soft-Tissue Complications in Bone Healing. Soft tissue as well as bone is subjected to insult when the stress is of sufficient magnitude to cause a fracture. Soft tissue is also stressed with the immobilization requirements of a healing fracture. Rehabilitation of a fracture site is, in reality, rehabilitation of soft tissue surrounding the site. Although soft-tissue injuries are discussed in more depth later in this chapter, compartment syndrome and neurovascular injuries are discussed here.

Although bone may heal without complication, surrounding tissues may have complications. Compartment syndrome and neurovascular injuries are two examples. A compartment is an area in the body where muscles, nerves, and blood vessels are enclosed within tissue such as fasciae. **Compartment syndrome** is a result of high pressure in a muscle compartment in the closed fascial space. Capillary pressure is reduced below what is essential for tissue viability. Compartment syndrome may be classified as acute, chronic, or crush. In the case of a fracture, the acute classification is of concern because it is the most severe form and often requires surgery urgently.

Compartment syndrome can be triggered by injury to the tissues surrounding bone with soft tissue inflammation, swelling, and, in some cases, hemorrhage into the area. Decreased blood flow from arterial damage can also occur, which leads to hypoxia of the cells of capillary walls. Capillary integrity is diminished, and colloid proteins and fluid escape into the extravascular tissues causing further swelling. Intracompartment pressures increase because the fasciae enclosing the compartment are restrictive. If the tissue pressure exceeds the intravascular pressure, blood vessels will collapse impeding blood flow and leading to further hypoxia and worsening edema. Intracompartment pressures of 30 to 40 mm Hg can compromise microcirculation in muscle. The excessive compartment pressures lead to hypoxia, damage, and eventual necrosis of the soft tissue, especially muscles and nerves. Emergent decompression is needed to preserve limb viability. Compartment syndrome can also occur due to extrinsic compression, such as that of a cast on an injured, swollen limb.[1] Symptoms of compartment syndrome are pain out of proportion to the injury, paralysis, paresthesia, pallor, and pulselessness.

Neurovascular injury after a fracture may be due to either the fracture or the treatment for the fracture. Neurovascular damage occurring at the time of fracture may be the result of either the force causing the fracture, fracture fragments, hemorrhage, joint dislocation, or the body position assumed after trauma. Neurovascular damage related to treatment may be due to moving or splinting the fracture, manipulation at the time of reduction of the fracture, application of stabilizing devices such as a cast or splint, or hemorrhage or edema.

Dislocations and Subluxations

Two additional mechanical alterations in the musculoskeletal system are dislocations and subluxations. A **dislocation** is displacement of a bone from its normal position to the extent that articulating surfaces completely lose contact.[1] A **subluxation** is displacement of a bone from its normal joint position to the extent that articulating surfaces partially lose contact.[1] A dislocation or subluxation can occur when forces cause one aspect of the joint complex to move beyond its normal anatomic limit. A considerable amount of tissue damage occurs in dislocation and subluxation, including possible ligament tear or rupture. With any dislocation, especially first-time dislocation, evaluation for a fracture is necessary. Although almost any joint may dislocate, some joints are more prone to dislocation than others. Joints most commonly dislocated are small joints of the fingers, the patella, and the shoulder. Symptoms of dislocation are pain, alteration in the normal contour of the joint, change in extremity length, and loss of normal mobility. Treatment must include consideration of local soft-tissue trauma and healing.

KEY POINTS

- Bones are subject to different types of fracture, depending on the type of tension stress imposed.
- Fractures can be classified according to the orientation of the break as transverse, longitudinal, oblique, or spiral.
- A comminuted fracture consists of more than one fracture line and more than two bone fragments.
- A greenstick fracture is an incomplete break.
- Fractures are classified as open or compound when the skin is penetrated and as closed or simple when the skin is not broken.
- Healing of fractured cancellous bone occurs more quickly than healing of cortical bone.
- Trauma causes hematoma formation, followed by callus formation.
- The callus is initially soft and cartilaginous; then it progressively ossifies to become firm and stable.
- The fracture is clinically stable when no movement at the break is detectable.
- Radiographically apparent union occurs when the callus has been completely replaced by mature bone.
- Healing of fractured bone is contingent on stabilization and time.
- Complete separation of joint articulating surfaces is termed *dislocation*. Subluxation refers to partial separation. Soft-tissue damage is the primary problem.

ALTERATIONS IN BONE MASS AND STRUCTURE

Scoliosis

Etiology and Pathogenesis. **Scoliosis** is a lateral curvature of the spine resulting in an S- or a C-shaped spinal column with vertebral rotation. Scoliosis can be a consequence of numerous congenital, connective tissue, and neuromuscular disorders. Seventy-five percent to 85% of all cases of scoliosis are classified as idiopathic.[1] Scoliosis occurs in approximately 5% of children screened for scoliosis. About half of the children, in whom scoliosis is diagnosed, require treatment, with the majority being female.

Clinical Manifestations. Scoliosis may be described as either structural or nonstructural. Nonstructural scoliosis resolves when the patient bends to the affected side. No vertebral rotation or bony deformity of the vertebrae is present, and the condition is not progressive. When the patient bends laterally, the spine usually appears symmetric. The scoliotic curve will disappear on forward flexion. Nonstructural scoliosis may be related to postural problems, hysteria, nerve root irritation, inflammation, or compensation caused by leg length discrepancy or contracture (in the cervical spine).[1]

Structural scoliosis is a lateral curve of the spine that fails to correct itself on forced bending against the curvature and has vertebral rotation. This type of scoliosis is more serious and involves deformity of the vertebrae and asymmetric changes in hip, shoulder, and rib cage positions. The patient lacks normal flexibility, and side bending becomes asymmetric. This type of scoliosis is progressive, and the curve does not disappear on forward flexion. Severe structural scoliosis may require intensive therapy or surgical intervention to halt progression and correct deformities.

Scoliosis is detected by typical asymmetric changes (Figure 51-8), including: (1) uneven shoulders or hips, (2) shoulder or scapular prominence, (3) rib or chest hump when bending over, and (4) a C- or S-shaped spine. A scoliometer can be used to assess the angle of trunk rotation when the patient is bent in a forward flexion position. Scoliosis is usually diagnosed after puberty because of a tendency for the curve to be accentuated during periods of rapid skeletal growth. The diagnosis is confirmed by radiographic examination of the spine. The degree of curvature is determined from radiographs and is classified as right or left, depending on the direction of convexity. Mild degrees of curvature may be managed conservatively with exercise and frequent reevaluation to assess progression to more significant deformity. Surgery is indicated for curvatures of 40 to 50 degrees or greater, or in cases of significant progression of scoliosis in spite of bracing and other conservative therapies.

In addition to body image disturbances, scoliosis predisposes a patient to a number of physiologic problems. Respiratory difficulties from restricted expansion of the lungs may occur. Severe forms may be associated with significant pain. Gastrointestinal dysfunction can result from compression of abdominal organs. If uncorrected, scoliosis may progressively worsen with age owing to increased upper body weight and gravitational forces exacerbating the vertebral deformity. Over time, significant degenerative changes to the intervertebral disks can occur.

Treatment. Treatment for structural scoliosis is aimed at correcting spinal malalignment. Nonsurgical measures include primarily braces and exercises. Bracing applies constant pressure to the spinal convexity to straighten the curve. Braces must be worn for prolonged periods each day to be effective. Compliance is a major difficulty because the braces are stiff and uncomfortable. Spinal muscle strengthening should accompany brace therapy because trunk musculature loses tone after prolonged bracing.[1] Surgical intervention includes spinal realignment, fusion, and bracing with internal appliances, and most surgical procedures require prolonged body immobilization postoperatively.

Conditioning exercises to strengthen muscles and correct posture are used to treat nonstructural, or postural, scoliosis.

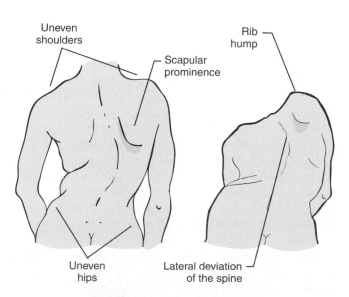

Uneven shoulders

Scapular prominence

Rib hump

Uneven hips

Lateral deviation of the spine

FIGURE 51-8 Structural scoliosis.

KEY POINTS

- Scoliosis is a lateral deformity of the spinal column that is detected from asymmetry of the shoulders, hips, and chest wall.
- Scoliosis may be described as structural or nonstructural.
- Severe scoliosis can compromise lung expansion and lead to a restrictive respiratory disorder.

Osteoporosis

Etiology and Pathogenesis. **Osteoporosis,** the most common metabolic bone disease, affects approximately one in two women and one in five men older than 60 years. It occurs when the rate of bone resorption is greater than that of bone formation. The normal osteoblastic and osteoclastic balance is disrupted, and mineral and protein matrix components are decreased. Trabeculae are decreased in amount, and width and bone mass is decreased. This process leads to fragile bone and thus fractures. Cancellous bone is lost faster than cortical bone, with fractures happening sooner in cancellous bone (vertebrae) than in cortical bone (femoral neck). A current definition of osteoporosis is based on gradations of low bone mass. The World Health Organization defines osteoporosis as bone mineral density (BMD) greater than or equal to 2.5 standard deviations below the mean peak BMD of young normal women.[2]

The specific cause of osteoporosis is not known. However, the rate of bone loss is influenced greatly by age, genetics, estrogen, and risk factors. A family history of osteoporosis is a major risk factor. The normal bone loss that occurs with aging is accelerated during menopause, with the most rapid phase of loss occurring in the first 5 years due to the sudden decrease in estrogen. The exact mechanisms of estrogen action are unclear, but estrogen derivatives may influence osteoblast activity and the production of local cytokines and growth factors that modulate the balance of bone resorption and formation. Estrogen deficiency increases the risk of osteoporosis by stimulating bone resorption over formation.[3] Other risk factors include small frame, Caucasian or Asian race, early surgically induced menopause, high doses of thyroid hormone supplementation, use of corticosteroid drugs (such as prednisone), a diet low in sources of calcium and vitamin D, physical inactivity, and smoking or increased alcohol intake. Patients with chronic renal disease often have abnormal parathyroid function, as well as altered calcium and vitamin D metabolism, which can lead to a decline in bone mass. Furthermore, chronic inflammatory diseases, such as rheumatoid arthritis or systemic lupus erythematosus, can be associated with increased risk of osteoporosis, even independent of corticosteroid use.[3]

Clinical Manifestations. On physical examination the patient may have a Colles fracture, femoral or hip fractures, or vertebral compression fractures. Obvious kyphosis of the thoracic spine (dowager's hump) may be present. The patient often has shortened stature, muscle wasting or spasms of back muscles, and difficulty bending over. The patient may complain of impaired breathing (because of deformities of the spine and rib cage) and poor dentition. Screening bone density measurement is generally accomplished using dual energy x-ray absorptiometry (DXA). Laboratory tests may show normal urinary and serum calcium, phosphorus, and alkaline phosphatase but elevated serum osteocalcin levels. Radiographic and computed tomographic findings may show diffuse radiolucency of bones, sparse transverse trabeculae, normal vertical trabeculae, indistinct articular cortices, wedge-shaped thoracic vertebrae, biconcave lumbar vertebral bodies, and possibly old or new compression fractures.

Treatment. Treatment varies depending on the cause. Adequate dietary intake of calcium and vitamin D is important,

and moderate, regular exercise such as walking or riding a stationary bicycle is valuable. Physical therapy exercises for individuals who are immobilized or paralyzed are helpful as well. Estrogen replacement therapy may be indicated for postmenopausal osteoporosis, though recommendations must take into account risk factors for vascular thrombosis, endometrial cancer, and breast cancer. For women not wishing to use estrogen replacement therapy, a selective estrogen receptor modulator (raloxifene) can be prescribed. Bisphosphonates can suppress osteoclast-mediated bone resorption. Several agents in this class of drugs are available such as alendronate, etidronate, ibandronate, or risedronate. Other treatment options include calcitonin and the newest agent, a recombinant human parathyroid hormone (rhPTH 1-34). For symptomatic relief of pain and muscle spasms, analgesics and muscle relaxants may be necessary.

Other Causes of Osteoporosis. **Disuse osteoporosis** may occur with prolonged bed rest, which leads to an increase in osteoclastic activity and resorption of bone greater than osteoblastic buildup. Stress placed on bone as a result of weight bearing is necessary for osteoblast function. The stress of exercise stimulates new bone growth as a result of changes in electrical charges on the bone surface.

The loss of bone density following a period of reduced weight bearing may be restored upon return to normal activity, although recovery may not be complete.[4] Osteoporosis may also occur when collagen formation is impaired in such conditions as scurvy, protein deficiency, or Cushing syndrome.

Rickets and Osteomalacia

Clinical Manifestations. **Rickets** and **osteomalacia** are characterized by deficits in mineralization of newly formed bone matrix in the growing skeleton (rickets) or of the mature skeleton (osteomalacia) with resulting soft osteopenic bone. Vitamin D deficiency prevents maintenance of normal levels of calcium and phosphorus. Children may have either vitamin D–resistant rickets or congenital hypophosphatasia. In rickets, cartilage that occurs in the growing epiphyses fails to calcify. Cartilage is not replaced by bone and continues to enlarge. Bone is poorly calcified and less rigid. Kyphosis, genu valgum ("knock knee"), and genu varum ("bowleg") are common deformities.

Osteomalacia is the adult counterpart of rickets. Osteomalacia is always due to an inadequate concentration of vitamin D, calcium, and/or phosphorus in the body as a result of either decreased intestinal absorption of vitamin D and calcium due to poor intake or malabsorption, poor vitamin D metabolism due to decreased sun exposure, renal disease (especially renal tubular acidosis), or a combination of these conditions.[2] In the case of vitamin D deficiency, calcification fails to occur and the bone is soft. All bones are affected, but weight-bearing structures may collapse and cause compression-type fractures.

Treatment. Treatment involves correction of the underlying deficiency with adequate intake of vitamin D supplementation (calcidiol, calcitriol, or ergocalciferol). Adequate intake of calcium and phosphate is also indicated by dietary adjustments

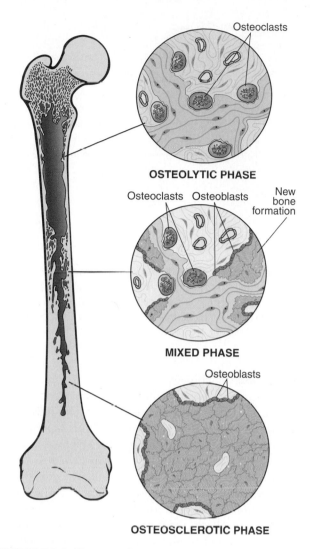

FIGURE 51-9 Diagrammatic representation of Paget disease of bone demonstrating the three phases in the evolution of the disease. (From Kumar V et al: *Robbins basic pathology,* ed 7, Philadelphia, 2003, Saunders, p 764.)

or supplements. Exposure to sunlight increases vitamin D metabolism and absorption, especially for elderly individuals.

Paget Disease. **Paget disease of bone** (osteitis deformans) is a slowly progressive metabolic bone disease characterized by an initial phase of excessive bone resorption, mediated by osteoclasts, followed by excessive bone formation (Figure 51-9). The end product is a disorganized mosaic of bone matrix made up of woven and lamellar bone at affected sites of the skeleton. This new bone is less compact, more vascular, and more fragile, which accounts for the deformities and fractures of Paget disease.[3]

Etiology and Pathogenesis. The specific cause of Paget disease is unknown, but the disease has a familial tendency suggesting a genetic component. It has also been theorized that a viral infection may affect osteoclastic function leading to aberrant bone remodeling. Changes in certain cytokines produced in the local bone marrow environment may also influence the

bone formation/resorption balance.[3] In the United States, about 3% of individuals older than 50 years have Paget disease, with males being affected slightly more than females. It also tends to be more prevalent in individuals of northern European descent.

Clinical Manifestations. In the early stages the disease may not cause any symptoms; however, when pain develops, it is severe and persistent. In the initial stages of Paget disease, affected bones soften and tend to bend. As the disease progresses, irregular subperiosteal bone formation occurs and causes bone to become thick and hard. Thickening of cranial bones may cause compression of cranial nerves and result in vertigo, blindness, deafness (with or without tinnitus), headaches, and facial paralysis. Other complications may include hypertension, arthritis, calcific periarthritis, and pain.

Treatment. During active stages of the disease, treatment focuses on preventing deformity and fracture, often with the use of calcitonin or bisphosphonates (such as etidronate, alendronate, or pamidronate, among others). These medications have been shown to decrease bone resorption, stabilize the fragile bone lesions, and reduce pain and the risk of fractures.[3]

KEY POINTS

- Bone density is a product of the rate of bone resorption and bone deposition.
- Osteoporosis occurs when the rate of bone resorption is greater than that of bone formation. A reduction in bone mass predisposes to fractures.
- Hormone deficiencies (estrogen, androgen), poor calcium intake, and lack of use are common factors in the rate of bone loss.
- Vitamin D deficiency is associated with rickets and osteomalacia, disorders characterized by soft, weak bones.
- Paget disease may be genetic. It has also been theorized that a viral infection may affect osteoclastic function leading to aberrant bone remodeling. Painful deformities or bone fractures may result.

INFECTIONS OF THE BONE

Osteomyelitis. **Osteomyelitis** is a severe pyogenic infection of bone and local tissue that requires immediate treatment. Organisms may reach bone by one of three routes: (1) via the bloodstream (hematogenous osteomyelitis), (2) from adjacent soft tissue (contiguous focus), and (3) by direct introduction of the organism into the bone.[1]

Etiology and Pathogenesis. *Hematogenous osteomyelitis,* in which the infectious agent may be introduced by blood from infection elsewhere in the body, is the most common type of osteomyelitis. It occurs most often in children younger than 16 years (mean age of 6 years old) and adults older than

Sinuses

Reactive bone (involucrum)

Trapped necrotic bone (sequestrum)

Periosteum

FIGURE 51-10 Osteomyelitis. The bacteria reach the metaphysis through the nutrient artery. Bacterial growth results in bone destruction and formation of an abscess. From the abscess cavity, the pus spreads between the trabeculae into the medulla, through the cartilage into the joint, through the haversian canals of the compact bones to the outside. These sinuses traversing the bone persist for a long time and heal slowly. The pus destroys the bone and sequesters parts of it in the abscess cavity. Reactive new bone is formed around the focus of inflammation. (From Damjanov I: *Pathology for the health-related professions,* ed 3, Philadelphia, 2006, Saunders, p 437.)

50 years.[1] It involves bone rich in red marrow. In children as well as infants, these are long bones and the infection usually begins acutely in the metaphyseal region of the bone. Blood-borne bacteria reach the marrow space via the nutrient artery, or after blunt trauma a hematoma develops; thus a pathway for the organism to reach the bone is present (Figure 51-10).

Clinical Manifestations. In children, acute hematogenous osteomyelitis manifests as a high fever and pain at the site of bone involvement. The infection may remain localized if it becomes walled off by fibrotic tissue reaction, a condition referred to as a *Brodie abscess.* Muscle spasms, redness, and swelling are common, and the child may refuse to move the limb. In adults, hematogenous osteomyelitis is more difficult to detect. Symptoms are vague and may include fever, malaise, anorexia, night sweats, and weight loss. Pain at rest is common. The diagnosis may be supported by radiographic signs of bone destruction. The most common causative organism is *Staphylococcus aureus,* with gram-negative bacillary infections increasing in frequency. In children between 2 months and 3 years of age, *Haemophilus influenzae* can also be a cause.[1]

Osteomyelitis secondary to an introduced or contiguous focus of infection can occur after burns, sinus disease, trauma, malignant tumor necrosis, periodontal infection, or an infected pressure ulcer. Again, *S. aureus* is the most common pathogen; however, some infections are polymicrobial and include gram-negative and anaerobic agents.[1]

Direct invasion of the organism into bone can occur as a result of open fractures, penetrating wounds; surgical contamination; or insertion of prostheses, metal plates, or screws. The latter three can act as a focus for bacterial reproduction.

During the acute stage of osteomyelitis, bacteria remain in bone and proliferate where the circulation is not optimal. Before puberty the bacteria grow in the metaphyseal sinusoidal vein, which leads to infection of the metaphysis near the growth

plate. The loose attachment of overlying periosteum permits exudate to accumulate in the subperiosteal area. Uncontrolled infection can disrupt the cortex and lead to joint infection or septic arthritis, which can lead to osteoarthritis later in life. In infants, medullary infection can reach the epiphysis and joint surfaces via capillaries crossing the growth plate, and stunted growth and angular deformities can result. The growth plate in children is avascular, so infection is limited. The inflammatory reaction leads to pus formation, edema, and vascular congestion. Pus collects and is confined within bone, thus increasing pressure and adding to vascular occlusion, ischemia, and, finally, necrosis of bone. Volkmann and haversian canals allow a route for release of pus and thus spread of bacteria. Blood and therefore antibiotics cannot reach bone tissue when vascular system pressure equals arteriolar pressure. As a result, the course and virulence of the osteomyelitis are affected. Even after meticulous treatment, the organism can reappear years later in a context of trauma or immunosuppression.

Healing Complications. If osteomyelitis is not managed or if the treatment is not sufficient, the resulting necrotic bone can separate from healthy bone into dead segments called *sequestra.* A sequestrum is then a medium for the continued bacterial proliferation described as chronic osteomyelitis. Sequestra can enlarge and extrude through bone into soft tissue, where it is possible that it might revascularize and resolve as a result of the body's defense mechanisms.

Osteoblasts may try to heal infected bone by isolating the dead tissue and forming an involucrum (a layer of new bone around old bone). Involucrum formation prevents successful effects of antibiotics and phagocytosis and leads to chronic infection.[1]

Any type of osteomyelitis may become chronic, especially if the treatment was inadequate during the acute phase. It may be manifested months or years after assumed cure, especially after acute hematogenous disease. Drainage via a sinus tract to the skin can occur.

Treatment. Treatment usually includes 4 to 6 weeks of parenteral antibiotic therapy for acute osteomyelitis. A shorter period of parenteral therapy followed by oral antibiotics can be effective if the infection is under control and a therapeutic blood level of the antibiotic can be maintained. Antibiotic choice is based on culture and sensitivity results.

If acute osteomyelitis is complicated by an abscess or extensive necrosis, the involved area is debrided and antibiotic therapy is instituted. If a prosthesis is involved, it is usually removed. After debridement, dead space is usually filled with packing, bone grafts, muscle pedicles, or skin grafts. In osteomyelitis associated with peripheral vascular disease, amputation is performed if antibiotic therapy is unsuccessful.[1]

Tuberculosis

Etiology and Pathogenesis. Bone and joint tuberculosis (TB) is an extrapulmonary form of TB that occurs after lymphohematogenous spread from a primary lung lesion. As the incidence of TB increases in the United States, one can expect to see more cases of skeletal TB. Persons with skeletal TB may have a history of pulmonary TB, drug abuse, crowded and poor living conditions, diseases that depress the immune system, and immigration to the United States after 1991. Musculoskeletal TB is not communicable to others unless an open wound exists. *Mycobacterium tuberculosis,* the organism responsible for the destruction of bone and joint, is transmitted via the airborne route. Initially, infectious droplets are inhaled and infect lungs; then *M. tuberculosis* spreads hematogenously from lungs or lymphatic drainage to bone. The bacterium may lie dormant for a long while before it is detected.

Clinical Manifestations. When involving the bone or joint, *M. tuberculosis* likely first infects bone where the blood supply is richest after which the infection spreads into the bone and possibly joint spaces (tuberculous arthritis). The most common site of skeletal TB is the vertebral column, particularly the lower thoracic and lumbar vertebrae (often called *Potts disease*). Vertebral infection results in destruction of the bone, anterior wedging, and collapse. On x-ray, the appearance is of a lytic lesion in the bone without local sclerotic (new bone formation) reaction. When the infection spreads to adjacent disks, paraspinal fluid may accumulate as a "cold abscess."[5] Symptoms may include local pain, low-grade fever, and possible neurologic symptoms due to impingement.

Other common sites of skeletal TB or tuberculous arthritis include weight-bearing joints such as hips, knees, and ankles, although any joint or bone could be involved.[5]

Risk Factors. Persons most at risk for TB are those at extremes of age or individuals who are immunosuppressed or undernourished. Children are at higher risk for skeletal TB because of extreme vascularity. In acquired immunodeficiency syndrome, knowledge of the patient's human immunodeficiency virus status is critical to optimize the therapeutic plan for the patient.[5]

Treatment. Treatment for skeletal TB requires long-term combination antibiotic therapy. Agents such as isoniazid,

rifampin, pyrazinamide, ethambutol, and others are used in combinations for 9 to 12 months. Therapeutic response can be complicated by development of drug resistance. Surgical intervention may be indicated in cases of spinal TB when severe deformities or neurologic deficits are seen.

> ### KEY POINTS
>
> - Bone infections may be from blood-borne organisms or direct traumatic infection.
> - Osteomyelitis—organisms reach the bone by one of three routes: bloodstream (hematogenous osteomyelitis), adjacent soft tissue (contiguous focus), and direct introduction of the organism into the bone.
> - TB of the bone—infection is spread via lung or lymphohematogenous drainage.
> - Antibiotic therapy can help to reduce the progression of bone infection and is the main treatment; however, abscess formation and chronic infection may occur.

BONE TUMORS

Neoplasms occurring in the musculoskeletal system can be benign or malignant. Benign tumors often go undiagnosed because they cause no pain. The most common benign bone tumor is a fibrous cortical defect often referred to as a *developmental anomaly.* An osteochondroma (exostosis) can occur in multiple locations such as the femur, pelvis, and shoulder. The tumor grows with skeletal growth. Malignant neoplasms are referred to as *sarcomas.* More common than sarcomas are metastatic lesions, which have spread to bone from primary carcinomas. These metastatic tumors usually occur when patients are in their 60s or 70s. Primary carcinomas that most commonly metastasize to bone are breast, prostate, lung, and kidney carcinomas. Other malignancies that can metastasize to bone include thyroid, bladder, uterine, colorectal, and vaginal cancer. Common sites of bone metastases are the vertebral bodies, pelvis, proximal ends of the femur and humerus, and ribs. Metastases occur via direct spread within a body cavity or by hematogenous or lymphatic spread.

Thus although the majority of bone tumors are metastatic, a number of primary tumors of bone can be identified. Some bone tumors are benign (Figure 51-11).

Osteochondroma

Etiology, Pathogenesis, and Clinical Manifestations. Osteochondroma, the most common bone tumor, is a cartilage-forming benign tumor that accounts for 35% to 50% of all benign bone tumors and 10% to 15% of all primary bone tumors.[1] Osteochondroma is hereditary and usually occurs in individuals 30 years or younger.

Bony projections on the external surface of the bone are capped with cartilage. Exostoses are usually asymptomatic and found by chance. Pressure on surrounding soft tissue

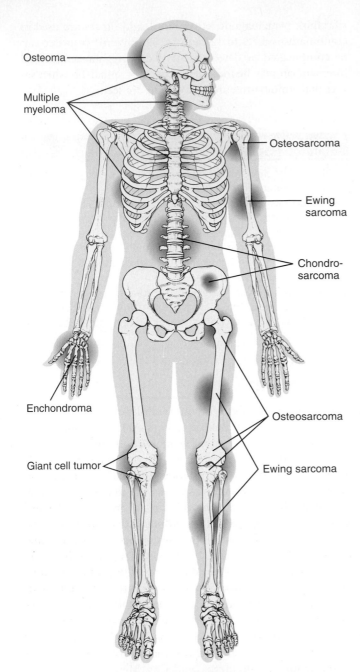

Osteoma

Multiple myeloma

Osteosarcoma

Ewing sarcoma

Chondro-sarcoma

Enchondroma

Osteosarcoma

Giant cell tumor

Ewing sarcoma

FIGURE 51-11 Schematic presentation of the most common sites of origin of bone tumors. Most often, osteosarcomas originate in the metaphyses of long bones, chondrosarcomas arise in the axial skeleton, Ewing sarcomas develop in the diaphyses of long bones, and giant cell tumors originate in the epiphyses of long bones. Osteomas occur most often in the skull and enchondromas in the small bones of the hand. Multiple myelomas involve the calvaria, vertebrae, and ribs, but also other bones that contain hematopoietic bone marrow. (From Damjanov I: *Pathology for the health-related professions,* ed 3, Philadelphia, 2006, Saunders, p 445.)

may cause pain. These tumors are usually located on the metaphyses of long bones such as the proximal end of the tibia and distal part of the femur, the shoulder, and the pelvis (see Figure 51-11).

Chondroma. **Chondroma** or enchondroma is a cartilage-forming tumor in bone that can be located in the medullary cavity or in the subperiosteal layers of bone.[1] It is believed to arise from remnants of epiphyseal cartilage. Chondromas arise most often in the small bones of the hands and feet but can develop in other areas. Tumor growth may erode the cortex of bone and expand the contour. Chondroma usually occurs in persons 30 to 40 years of age.

Osteoid Osteoma. **Osteoid osteoma** is a painful but benign bone-forming tumor that accounts for approximately 10% to 13% of symptomatic benign tumors.[1] Sharp or dull pain can be felt, often worse at night and alleviated by aspirin or other nonsteroidal anti-inflammatory drugs. This small lesion is often found in the cortex of the tibia and femur, but any bone may be involved. Radiographs show the lesion enclosed in a sclerotic shell. This tumor usually occurs in persons 10 to 20 years old.

Giant Cell Tumor. A **giant cell tumor,** or osteoclastoma, is benign but aggressive with richly vascularized tissue consisting of plump spindle-shaped cells and numerous giant cells. These lesions account for about 4% to 5% of all primary bone tumors.[1] In some cases, giant cell tumors undergo transformation to sarcomas. The cells can metastasize without malignant transformation. Giant cell tumors commonly occur between the ages of 20 and 40 years and do not have any gender predilection. The area of development includes the distal end of the femur, proximal part of the tibia, distal part of the radius, and proximal end of the humerus (see Figure 51-11). Pain is the initial complaint.

Osteosarcoma

Etiology and Pathogenesis. Osteosarcoma, an extremely malignant bone-forming tumor, is the most common primary malignant bone tumor that develops in the metaphyseal region of long bones. It is characterized by the formation of bone or osteoid by tumor cells. The majority of victims are children, adolescents, and young adults 10 to 30 years of age, although a second peak in incidence can be seen in adults 60 to 70 years old.[6] The most active epiphyseal growth areas—the distal end of the femur, proximal end of the tibia, fibula, and proximal end of the humerus—are common sites of involvement (see Figure 51-11). Lesions can also be seen in flat bones of the pelvis, skull, scapula, ribs, or spine.[6]

Clinical Manifestations. Osteosarcoma grows rapidly and is quite destructive; destruction of the cortex of the metaphyseal region predisposes it to pathologic fracture. Metastasis to lungs is noted early in disease development. Pain is consistent and progressively more intense. Joint function may be compromised as a result of the proximity of the metaphysis.

Treatment. Although amputation may be necessary, conservative surgery and chemotherapy have provided positive results, with studies showing 5-year disease-free survival between 41% and 87%.[6]

Chondrosarcoma

Pathogenesis. A **chondrosarcoma** is a malignant cartilage-forming tumor. These tumors usually develop slowly, so pain is not a prominent clinical symptom. Even with a slow rate of development, the tumor will eventually metastasize, typically to the lung. Chondrosarcomas tend to develop in the pelvic and shoulder girdles and the proximal ends of long bones (see Figure 51-11).

Secondary chondrosarcoma is a benign lesion, like osteochondroma or multiple enchondromatosis, which undergoes malignant transformation. It occurs in the pelvis and proximal ends of the femur and humerus in individuals between 20 and 40 years of age. Evidence of malignant transformation may include pain, an irregular border, or an increase in cap size after patient growth is complete.[6]

Clinical Manifestations. Primary chondrosarcoma is characterized by the formation of cartilage by tumor cells. This tumor has a higher cellularity and greater pleomorphism than a chondroma. It usually occurs in the femur, pelvis, ribs, and scapula in individuals between 30 and 60 years of age.

Ewing Sarcoma

Pathogenesis. Ewing sarcoma is the third most common primary sarcoma of bone and is characterized as a rapidly growing malignant round cell tumor. This tumor most often develops in the long bones of children between the ages of 10 and 15 years. Ewing tumor is composed of densely packed small cells with round nuclei. It arises in the medullary canal of bone and perforates the cortex of the shaft producing a painful soft-tissue mass overlying the involved bone. The tumor favors long tubular bones, such as the femur, tibia, proximal fibula, or humerus (see Figure 51-11); however, it can arise in the pelvis and flat bones where it may be more difficult to diagnose.[6]

Clinical Manifestations and Treatment. Ewing sarcoma metastasizes quite early in its development to the lungs and other bones. Because of the rapid rate of growth, pain is a dominant symptom that increases in severity. Ewing sarcoma is often confused with osteomyelitis because patients often appear systemically ill and may develop fever, anemia, leukocytosis, and an increased sedimentation rate.[6] Treatment includes radiotherapy and possible adjunct surgical therapy.

Multiple Myeloma

Etiology and Pathogenesis. Multiple myeloma is a slowly growing bone marrow malignancy with neoplastic proliferation of a single clone of plasma cells. The annual incidence is approximately 4 per 100,000 and represents about 1% of all malignant cancers.[6]

Clinical Manifestations and Treatment. Although multiple myeloma is not a sarcoma, its symptoms and radiographic findings are similar. On radiographs, evidence of bone destruction by a lytic, or bone-destroying, process and bone marrow involvement can be seen. Homogeneous immunoglobulin is also present in urine or serum. Because multiple myeloma is a slow-growing lesion, it takes a long time to become symptomatic. Bone pain is the most common symptom, particularly of the chest and back, and is related to excessive accumulation of abnormal plasma cells in the bone marrow (Chapter 11). Although it can affect any bone, multiple myeloma most commonly occurs in the thoracic and lumbar vertebrae. Patients experience hypercalcemia and pathologic fractures where bone has been destroyed. This disease can also cause kidney dysfunction, lung or pleural involvement, and neurologic symptoms due to nerve compression.[6] Treatment often requires aggressive combination chemotherapy, although at times local radiation may be useful for refractory bone pain.

KEY POINTS

- Most bone tumors are secondary to metastasis from other sites. Osteochondroma, chondroma, osteoid osteoma, and giant cell tumors are benign, primary bone tumors.
- Malignant bone tumors include osteosarcoma, chondrosarcoma, and Ewing sarcoma.
- Multiple myeloma is a slow-growing bone marrow malignancy in which plasma cells proliferate. This disease affects the kidneys and the immune and circulatory systems.

Soft-Tissue Injuries

In addition to injuries of the bony skeleton, soft tissue may also be traumatized. At times it is difficult to differentiate among the types of soft tissue. In an attempt to differentiate the exact site of a lesion, Cyriax[7] described two types of soft tissue: contractile and inert. **Contractile** tissue is composed of structures involved in the contraction of muscle and includes not only the muscle belly but also the tendon and bony insertion. Although not involved in a pure contraction, as is the muscle belly, the tendon and its insertion into bone are mechanically linked to tension generated by the muscle. According to Cyriax, pain may be elicited by active contraction and by passive stretching in the opposite direction.[7] Pain with resisted contraction may also occur at a fracture site near a muscular insertion, lymphatic gland, or bursa, or an abscess situated under a muscle.

INERT SOFT-TISSUE INJURIES

Inert, or **noncontractile,** tissue possesses no ability to contract or relax. Inert soft tissues include joint capsules, ligaments, bursae, fasciae, dura mater, and nerve roots. Passive stretching provokes pain from inert tissue. Evaluation of inert tissue lesions requires identification of all structures involved: the capsule of a joint, a section of a ligament or a nerve, or mechanical displacement of the meniscus.

Ligament Injuries

A **ligament** is a dense connective tissue with parallel-fibered collagenous tissues designed to connect bone to bone. Ligaments contribute to mechanical stability of the joint,

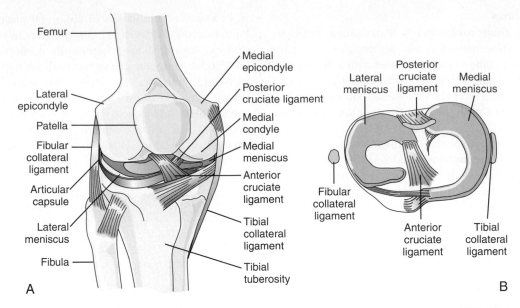

FIGURE 51-12 The principal structures of the interior of the knee joint. **A,** From the front. **B,** From above with the femur removed.

guide motion, and prevent excessive motion. Injuries to ligaments occur when loading exceeds the physiologic range of motion. Microfailure precedes total failure of the ligament. With total failure of a ligament, damage to surrounding soft tissue occurs. Ligament injuries are classified by the extent of tear and may be described as mild, moderate, or severe. With a mild injury, a few ligament fibers are damaged, but ligament strength is not lost.

Clinical Manifestations. A common site of ligament injury, particularly among athletes, is the knee with the anterior cruciate ligament (Figure 51-12). Symptoms may include a sudden "tearing" sensation or "popping" in the knee followed by pain with weight bearing and often acute swelling of the knee. Another common site for ligament injury is the anterior ankle (talofibular ligament).[8]

Treatment. Treatment is geared primarily toward relief of symptoms, and recovery is usually complete. A moderate ligament injury is a definite tear in some component of the ligament with loss of strength. The fibers are not widely separated. Treatment is primarily protection of the ligament. With a severe ligament injury, the ligament is completely torn and no longer functions. Potentially the fragments are widely separated. Treatment may require surgical restoration of ligament continuity, when possible.

Joint Capsule Injuries

Another inert structure that is intimately involved in stabilization of a synovial joint is the **joint capsule** (Figure 51-13). The joint capsule is composed of an inner and outer layer. The inner layer is highly vascularized but has minimal innervation. It synthesizes the hyaluronic acid component of synovial fluid, produces matrix collagen, and is essential for joint nutrition.[9] The outer layer of the capsule is attached to the periosteum of the bones through Sharpey fibers. The capsule is reinforced by

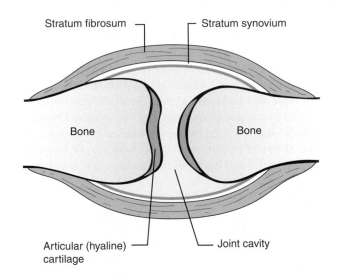

FIGURE 51-13 Joint capsule.

ligaments and musculotendinous structures. The outer layer of the capsule is poorly vascularized but richly innervated by joint receptors. Joint receptors are able to detect the rate and direction of motion, proprioception, compression and tension, vibration, and pain.[9]

After injury to the joint capsule, the ensuing increase in vascularity and development of fibrous tissue lead to a thick capsule. Any effusion into the joint cavity may lead to stretching of the capsule and its associated ligaments. The joint capsule, like ligaments, provides joint stability. The capsule, however, has an interesting mechanical adaptation: capsular redundancy. An example of the importance of the redundancy has been identified by Hettinga[10]: "The inferior medial portion of the shoulder joint capsule is a loose, redundant sac that becomes tense only when the shoulder is fully abducted or flexed. The posterior capsule of the knee is loose in flexion but so tight in extension that it becomes an important stabilizer."

Capsular redundancy provides for a stable joint at the end ranges of movement. Any injury or edema in the joint that causes scarring in the lax section of the capsule prevents full range of motion. Prolonged immobilization of a joint causes loss of mobility and extensibility of the capsule, with subsequent loss of motion. Immobilization of a joint causes an alteration in the flow of synovial fluid and contracture of the joint capsule and periarticular muscle. The altered flow of synovial fluid prevents fluid diffusion into and out of cartilage and causes compression and distention of cartilage. Nutrition of the joint components stagnates, leading to degenerative changes in the joint that become permanent. Contracture of the joint capsule and periarticular muscle results when fatty tissue proliferates in the joint space. This increase in connective tissue leads to adhesions that limit joint motion. The increase in connective tissue is due to failure to keep the latticework of tissue stretched open, which is usually kept open by normal flexion and extension of muscle. The muscles bridging the immobilized joint also shorten.

Frozen Shoulder. An example of such a restriction is loss of function in the shoulder after even a minor injury leading to a "frozen shoulder," also called adhesive capsulitis. With an injury to any component of the shoulder complex, inflammation occurs in the joint along with swelling and distention of the joint capsule. With prolonged immobilization, thickening of the capsule may ensue possibly due to proliferation of fibroblasts and capsular contraction. Capsular tightness leads to a loss of movement and an increase in pain especially at night. Excessive joint motion may cause a tearing of the capsule, similar to a ligamentous tear, and render the joint unstable. Conservative treatment of the frozen shoulder is usually recommended with intra-articular corticosteroid injections, gentle stretching and physical therapy, and anti-inflammatory medication. Prevention of adhesive capsulitis involves avoiding prolonged or excessive immobilization of the shoulder after minor injuries and early gentle stretching.[9]

Internal Joint Derangement

Internal joint derangement may be caused by injury to inert soft-tissue structures. Meniscal tears at the knee, labrum tears at the glenohumeral joint, and disk tears in the temporomandibular joint all cause restrictions of the joint and may lead to soft-tissue dysfunction in the form of weakness, loss of motion, or pain. Tears of the medial and lateral menisci in the knee are common causes of knee pain, with the medial meniscus being torn more often. A meniscal tear is usually the result of a twisting motion.

The anterior and posterior cruciate ligaments prevent anterior and posterior displacement of the tibia relative to the femur, respectively (see Figure 51-12). These ligaments can be torn in varying degrees of severity. Injury to either ligament leads to some degree of instability in the knee joint.

Injuries to Fasciae and Bursae

Fasciae and **bursae** may also be causes of pain and restriction of movement of the musculoskeletal system.

Fasciae. When connective tissues of the body are arranged in sheaths that envelop muscles, they are designated **fasciae.** Individual muscles are surrounded by a thin fascia called the **perimysium.** Trauma to fascia, as with any soft tissue, may cause edema and scarring. Restrictions in fascia movement cause a restriction in joint function.

Bursae. In many locations between muscles or between muscle or tendon and bone, connective tissue forms a pocket lined with synovium that contains fluid. These pockets are identified as **bursae.** Bursae are located in areas of high friction and are designed to dissipate some of the stress. With faulty mechanics of the joint, repetitive movement, or direct trauma, the bursal sac may become inflamed (bursitis) and extremely painful. Bursitis, because of its strategic position at stress points of muscle function, causes major disruption of movement. An inflamed bursa may restrict any movement of the joint and lead to restriction in capsular function or muscle dysfunction as a result of edema. Some of the more common sites of bursitis include the trochanteric bursa (lateral hip), subacromial bursa (shoulder), pes anserine bursa (medial knee), and olecranon bursa (elbow).

Injuries to Nerves, Nerve Roots, or Dura Mater

Trauma to any soft tissue may lead to adhesive constriction of the nerve, nerve root, or dura mater. Irritation or entrapment of a nerve causes pain that radiates along the structures innervated by that nerve. Pain, altered sensation (numbness and tingling), motor weakness, and diminished reflexes may result from trauma to these essential soft-tissue components of the musculoskeletal system.[2]

An example is trauma to vertebrae in the lumbosacral area with nerve root impingement. Components of the intervertebral disk can herniate and cause pressure on nerve roots (Figure 51-14). The intervertebral disk is a shock absorber located between vertebrae. The center is a gelatinous-like material, the nucleus pulposus, which has a high water content. The nucleus pulposus is surrounded by the fibrous annulus fibrosus. Trauma to the back can cause unequal pressure on the disk leading to herniation. Common sites of disk problems are at L3 to L4, which affects the L4 nerve root; L4 to L5, which affects the L5 nerve root; and L5 to S1, which affects the S1 nerve root.

CONTRACTILE SOFT-TISSUE INJURIES

Injury to Tendons

Injury to tendons occurs along a continuum from minor strain, in which a few fibers of the tendon are torn, to a complete tear or rupture. The sheath in which a tendon slides may also be traumatized. Inflammation of the tendon within the sheath is called **tendinitis.** This inflammation may be due to infection, direct injury, or injury from repetitive motion. Tendons are injured when the stress placed on them is greater than the fibers can tolerate. Muscle tendons that are subjected to high tensile stress or compression are more prone to injury. Frequently

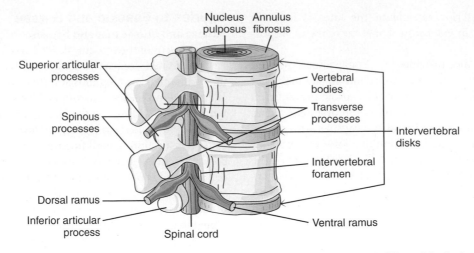

FIGURE 51-14 Lateral view (somewhat superior) of a segment of the lumbar part of the vertebral column.

injured tendons include the following: extensor pollicis brevis and abductor pollicis longus of the thumb (de Quervain syndrome), rotator cuff of the shoulder, biceps brachii tendon, tendons of the patellar complex, quadriceps tendon, hamstring tendon, Achilles tendon, and posterior tibialis tendon.

Muscle and Tendon Strains

Muscle trauma compromises the contractile unit. As in the case of injury to a tendon, tears in a muscle may range from a minor tear to complete rupture. Most injuries to muscle are due to abnormal muscle contraction. Muscle and tendon strains are often categorized by the severity of injury[11]:

Grade I: Minute tear of connective tissue and muscle fiber.

Grade II: Tear of a large portion of the contractile unit, with a segment still intact.

Grade III: Total rupture or loss of continuity of the contractile structure.

Blunt Trauma

A soft-tissue contusion or crush injury also compromises the contractile structure. Any blunt trauma that causes bleeding into the muscle belly may lead to an inability to contract the muscle. Hemorrhage in a muscle belly has the potential to coagulate and calcify. This abnormal calcification in a muscle results in a painful condition called **myositis ossificans.** Calcification prevents a normal and strong contraction of the muscle involved.

Compartment Syndrome

Compartment syndrome is due to trauma to soft tissue caused by the unyielding structure of inert tissue. Causes of compartment syndrome may be divided into three categories: decreased compartment size, increased compartment content, or externally applied pressure. With an injury, edema causes an increase in pressure within the compartment. Because volume is expanding in a confined area, pressure reduces capillary flow. Muscle and nerves become ischemic, with a resultant excruciating pain. Besides pain, the skin looks pale, the pulse may be absent, and sensation is diminished. Compartment

syndrome is a medical emergency requiring immediate decompression. Nerves can survive only 2 to 4 hours of ischemia and muscles approximately 6 to 8 hours. However, muscles do not have the ability to regenerate, and if the muscle becomes necrotic, it will be replaced by fibrous connective tissue and fat. Compartment syndromes are noted most often in the leg (anterior, deep posterior, superficial posterior, and lateral), forearm (dorsal and volar), upper arm (deltoid and biceps), hand (interosseous), buttock (gluteal), and thigh (quadriceps). For additional discussion of compartment syndrome, see the Complications in Bone Healing section earlier in this chapter.

Evaluation of Contractile Injuries

Cyriax[7] has provided a functional guide to the evaluation of contractile injuries. The patterns of function deal with pain and strength rather than excessive motion noted during evaluation of ligamentous injury.

Strong and pain free: Indicates that the contractile structure being tested does not have a lesion, regardless of how tender the muscle is on palpation. The muscle functions painlessly and is not the source of the patient's pain.

Strong and painful: Indicates a local lesion of the muscle or tendon, previously listed as a grade I or II muscle strain. No limitation of passive movement is noted unless secondary joint restriction from disuse is present. Stiffness in the joint would then take precedence in treatment.

Weak and painful: Indicates a severe lesion around the joint, such as a fracture. Weakness is usually due to reflex inhibition of the muscles around the joint.

Weak and pain free: Indicates rupture of a muscle or involvement of the nerve supplying the muscle.

If all movements are painful, pain may be due to fatigue, emotional hypersensitivity, or emotional problems.

Soft-Tissue Healing After Trauma

Trauma to soft tissue results in disruption of the circulatory and lymphatic systems. Hemorrhage, fluid loss, and cell death result. Blood vessels at the site of trauma constrict, which

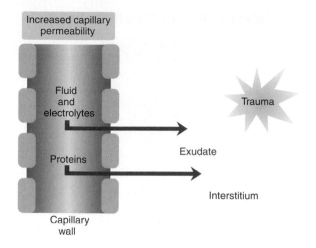

FIGURE 51-15 Edema formation. With trauma, increased capillary permeability and dilation cause leaking into tissue space. Initially clear, the exudate in the tissue space becomes more viscous with an increase in plasma protein.

limits blood loss from the affected area. Norepinephrine mediates this initial constriction response, which may last a few minutes. Serotonin (from mast cells of connective tissue) and platelets prolong vasoconstriction. It may also contribute to vasodilation in inflamed tissue.

Platelets adhere to collagen fibers and release serotonin and adenosine diphosphate, which causes platelets to adhere to the traumatized endothelial wall and form a platelet plug that temporarily decreases bleeding. Trauma to the endothelial surface triggers release of an enzyme that initiates clotting by converting prothrombin to thrombin, which converts fibrinogen to fibrin. The endothelial surfaces of small vessels are also compressed, thereby ensuring that vessels remain closed after vasoconstriction has ceased. In the early stages of inflammation, the endothelial margins of the venules may be covered with neutrophilic leukocytes, a process called neutrophilic margination. At this point the release of histamine from mast cells, basophils, and platelets causes vasodilation and increased permeability of venules. With the increase in permeability, serous fluid containing cells and plasma proteins accumulates as edema in tissue spaces (Figure 51-15). This edema fluid contains fibrinogen, which forms fibrin through an interaction with thrombin. Fibrin seals damaged lymphatics and confines the inflammatory reaction to an area immediately surrounding the injury.

Wound Repair

The inflammatory response prepares injured tissue to progress to the healing process of repair and reorganization. Figures 51-16 and 51-17 provide a summary of the phases of wound repair. The acute response lasts about 2 weeks, and the subacute phase lasts another 2 weeks. When the wound is clear of foreign substances, an infiltrate of macrophages and fibroblasts is noted. A matrix of collagen, hyaluronic acid, and fibronectin develops. Lymphatics form in the matrix, prevent additional edema, and assist in preventing infection. This granulation tissue develops in the wound space. Macrophages have an important role in wound repair.

Next in the process of wound repair is reepithelialization of the wound surface. Epidermal cells migrate over established epidermal cells until the defect is closed. The formation of basement membrane follows. This membrane is first laid down at the wound periphery and then progresses to the center of the wound. A strong bond forms between epidermal cells and the newly formed basement membrane to complete reepithelialization (granulation tissue formation).

Wound tensile strength is a result of the deposition of collagen. Collagen production begins approximately 5 days after myofibroblast migration into the wound space. Hyaluronic acid, found in the extracellular matrix, assists glycosaminoglycans to stimulate fibroplasia. Myofibroblasts secrete an extracellular matrix, which induces cell migration and proliferation, and synthesize proteoglycans, which stimulate collagen formation and increase tissue resilience and tensile strength. By the end of the first month, tensile strength begins to increase, but several months are required to achieve the maximal level. Collagen reaches its maximal strength approximately 3 months after injury. Maximal tensile strength is only 70% to 80% of preinjury levels.

Revascularization (angiogenesis or growth of new blood vessels) must take place to ensure survival of the new tissue. Vascularization occurs through the development of new circulatory networks in the wound and reattachment of existing vessels. Extracellular matrix, endothelial cell development, lactic acid, and heparin are a few of the factors that stimulate revascularization.

Wound closure or contraction is the final phase of healing in soft-tissue injuries. Contraction begins soon after injury and is completed in approximately 2 weeks. Myofibrils assist in wound closure. Interaction between extracellular matrix and granulation tissue results in a contractile unit called a *fibronexus*. Cytoplasmic actin binds to the fibronexus and draws tissue together to ensure a stable wound. As tension increases across the wound, collagen fibers are reoriented and collagen phagocytosis increases. Complete organization and concentration of collagen may require more than 40 weeks. In the case of rupture of soft-tissue structures, surgical intervention may be necessary to ensure that the traumatized tissue is in close enough proximity to allow healing.

KEY POINTS

- Soft-tissue injury refers to injuries of noncontractile elements (joint capsule, ligament, bursa, fascia, dura mater, and nerve root) and contractile elements (muscle and tendons).
- Passive stretching causes pain in noncontractile tissue injury, whereas active contraction is painful in contractile injury.

HEALING BY FIRST INTENTION

HEALING BY SECOND INTENTION

24 hours

— Scab

— Neutrophils

— Clot

3 to 7 days

— Mitoses

— Granulation tissue

— Macrophage

— Fibroblast

— New capillary

Weeks

— Fibrous union

Wound contraction

FIGURE 51-16 Steps in wound healing by first intention and second intention. In the latter, the resultant scar is much smaller than the original wound because of wound contraction. (From Kumar V et al: *Robbins basic pathology,* ed 8, Philadelphia, 2007, Saunders, p 75.)

- Noncontractile tissue injuries generally cause altered range of motion around a joint as a result of pain, edema, adhesion, or fibrosis.
- Contractile tissue injuries are characterized by decreased muscle strength.
- Compartment syndrome is a dangerous complication of soft-tissue injury that results from swelling of injured tissue within a restrictive fascia. Unless pressure is quickly reduced, compressed tissue may become ischemic and necrotic.

- Manifestations of compartment syndrome include severe pain, pallor, pulselessness, paralysis, and paresthesia.
- Soft-tissue injury results in local inflammation and initiates the process of wound healing. Strength of the injured tissue is improved by the deposition of collagen. Normalization of collagen may require more than 40 weeks.

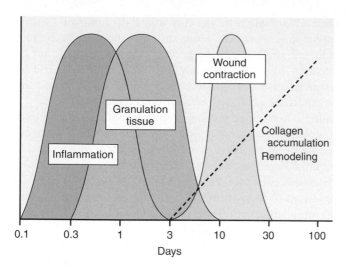

FIGURE 51-17 Orderly phases of wound healing. (Modified from Clark RA: In Goldsmith LA, editor: *Physiology, biochemistry and molecular biology of the skin,* ed 2, vol 1, New York, 1991, Oxford University Press, p 577. In Kumar V et al: *Robbins basic pathology,* ed 8, Philadelphia, 2007, Saunders, p 74.)

Diseases of Skeletal Muscle

Skeletal muscle, the most abundant tissue in the human body, accounts for approximately 40% of total body weight.[9] Skeletal muscle performs dynamic work (locomotion) and static work (posture). As with other tissue of the musculoskeletal system, muscle atrophies in response to disuse and immobilization, and hypertrophies when subjected to increased stress.

MUSCULAR DYSTROPHY

Muscular dystrophy comprises a group of genetically determined myopathies characterized by progressive muscle weakness and degeneration as muscle tissue is replaced by fat and fibrous connective tissue. The dystrophies are classified by their pattern of inheritance, age of onset, and distribution of muscular weakness.

Duchenne Muscular Dystrophy

Etiology and Pathogenesis. Duchenne muscular dystrophy, the most common and most severe form of muscular dystrophy, is inherited as an X-linked trait and therefore afflicts only males. The incidence is 1 in 3500 male births. Due to a genetic mutation, muscle cells are deficient in the protein dystrophin, a deficiency that weakens the cell membrane and allows extracellular fluid to leak into the cell. Proteases and inflammatory processes are activated leading to muscle fiber necrosis and muscle degeneration.[12]

The disease begins at birth and is usually apparent by the age of 3 years, with initial involvement of the pelvic girdle and progression to the shoulder girdle.

Clinical Manifestations. The calf muscles of an individual with Duchenne muscular dystrophy are noticeably enlarged because of the infiltration of fat cells and degeneration of muscle fibers. Distal muscle involvement leads to frequent falling by the age of 5 or 6 years, and by age 12 to 14 years most children are confined to a wheelchair. Some muscles, such as those in the hands, face, jaw, pharynx, larynx, and eyes, are spared to the end. Survival to age 20 is rare. Cardiac failure or pulmonary infection is the usual cause of death.[12]

Treatment. Treatment in muscular dystrophy is focused on appropriate education for the patient and family, preservation of physical function as long as possible, and prevention of contractures. In some cases, corticosteroid therapy may be useful to delay loss of muscle strength and prolong independent ambulation, but eventual steroid-induced osteoporosis is a risk. Immunosuppressive therapies have also been tried but with limited success.

Becker Muscular Dystrophy

Etiology, Pathogenesis, and Clinical Manifestations. Becker muscular dystrophy is a milder form of inherited muscle degeneration, somewhat less common than the Duchenne type with an annual incidence of 5 per 100,000. The genetic mutation leads to production of a reduced amount of an abnormal dystrophin protein and a slower muscular degeneration. Calf hypertrophy is still prominent and often painful with progressive loss of strength and ability to ambulate. The mean age of symptom onset is somewhat later (5 to 15 years) with patients requiring a wheelchair by the age of 30 years.[12]

Facioscapulohumeral Muscular Dystrophy

Etiology and Pathogenesis. Facioscapulohumeral muscular dystrophy is an inherited autosomal dominant trait that affects the muscles of the shoulder girdle and the face. It is rare with an annual incidence of 1 in 20,000. The onset of disease can occur at any age, but it usually begins in the second decade. Facial muscles are involved early, with later involvement of scapular and upper arm musculature. It progresses slowly with periods of arrest and can ultimately involve more distal muscles of the upper and lower extremities. Both males and females are affected, and most live to a normal age, although approximately 20% of these patients require a wheelchair eventually.[12]

Other Disorders of Muscle

Myasthenia Gravis. Myasthenia gravis is a chronic autoimmune disease affecting the neuromuscular function of voluntary muscles and characterized by profound muscle weakness and fatigability. Its peak onset in females occurs at 20 to 30 years of age. Men may experience it after 40 years of age. Women are affected more often than men. Characteristically, weakness begins with ocular and cranial muscles, and then limb muscles can also be involved. During times of emotional stress, respiratory muscles may be included.

In myasthenia gravis, acetylcholine receptor antibodies are produced that destroy or block acetylcholine receptors of the muscle end-plate of the neuromuscular junction. These antibodies impair the transmission of acetylcholine across the junction. The result is the muscle weakness and fatigability so prevalent in this disease.[12]

Treatment. Anticholinesterase inhibitors (e.g., pyridostigmine bromide, neostigmine) may be used to inhibit breakdown of acetylcholine in the neuromuscular synapse. Increased synaptic acetylcholine enhances the activation of postsynaptic receptors and improves skeletal muscle contraction force. Because myasthenia gravis is an autoimmune disorder, corticosteroids, intravenous immune globulin, plasmapheresis, and immunosuppressive agents may be used to regulate the immune system. In severe cases, respiratory muscle fatigue may necessitate mechanical ventilation. Thymectomy for hyperplasia, which is often apparent in 85% of patients, is often recommended. If done within the first 2 years of the disease, thymectomy induces remission of symptoms in about 40% of patients. Women seem to achieve greatest benefit from thymectomy.[12]

Myasthenia crisis can be due to insufficient medication, emotional stress, trauma, infection, or surgery. A sudden increase in blood pressure and pulse is noted. Other symptoms include cyanosis from hypoxia, absent cough and gag reflexes, restlessness, increased secretions and lacrimation, diaphoresis, decreased urine output, bowel and bladder incontinence, dysarthria, and respiratory distress.

Cholinergic crisis is usually due to excessive medication. Patients experiencing such a crisis will have fasciculations, especially around the mouth; difficulty chewing, swallowing, and speaking; advancing muscle weakness approximately 1 hour after anticholinesterase medication; nausea and vomiting; cramps and diarrhea; increased secretions (salivary, perspiration, lacrimal, bronchial); headache; confusion; irritability and anxiety; syncope; and respiratory distress leading to respiratory arrest.

CHRONIC MUSCLE PAIN

Fibromyalgia Syndrome

Etiology and Pathogenesis. The cause of **fibromyalgia syndrome** (FMS) is unknown. No laboratory abnormalities have been found, muscle biopsy findings are nonspecific, and patients are usually normal on psychological testing. The condition is not an inflammatory process but rather a "pain syndrome," with recent studies suggesting that changes in the central nervous system may lead to amplification of pain fiber impulses, a theory called *central sensitization*. This generalized increase in pain sensitivity may involve both ascending and descending neural pathways and a variety of neurotransmitters and neuropeptides.[13]

FMS is characterized by chronic pain in muscles and surrounding structures often of months or years duration. Additional symptoms include fatigue, sleep dysfunction, headache, numbness and tingling, joint pain, memory and concentration difficulties, irritable bowel syndrome, depression, edema of the hands, and sensitivity to cold.[8] Patients may either have no other musculoskeletal disease or may have rheumatoid arthritis, osteoarthritis, Lyme disease, or sleep apnea. FMS is characterized by a strong female preponderance (more than 75% in most epidemiology studies), with a peak incidence between 20 and 60 years of age.

Clinical Manifestations. Patients with FMS complain of widespread musculoskeletal pain, stiffness, and fatigability. Joint pain and swelling may be perceived by the patient, but the swelling, if present, is usually soft-tissue "puffiness" and not a true inflammatory process. Complaints of muscle pain and weakness are expressed without objective demonstration. In addition to pain and fatigue, sleep disturbances are a common complaint. The examination of a patient with FMS is characterized by an excessive number of reported symptoms with minimal objective findings other than muscular tenderness. Proposed criteria for the diagnosis of FMS established by the American College of Rheumatology include widespread pain in combination with tenderness of at least 11 of 18 (9 bilateral sites) specific tender point sites:[8]

1 Occiput—bilaterally at suboccipital muscle insertions
2 Low cervical—bilaterally at anterior aspects of the intertransverse spaces at C5 to C7
3 Trapezius—bilaterally at the midpoint of the upper border
4 Supraspinatus—bilaterally at the origins above the scapular spine near the medial border
5 Second rib—bilaterally at the second costochondral junctions, just lateral to junctions on the upper surfaces
6 Lateral epicondyle—bilaterally, 2 cm distal to the epicondyles
7 Gluteal—bilaterally in the upper outer quadrants of the buttocks in the anterior fold of the muscle
8 Greater trochanter—bilaterally, posterior to the trochanteric prominence
9 Knee—bilaterally at the medial fat pad proximal to the joint line

Although these tender points are the most common and are included in the criteria for fibromyalgia, in actuality, nearly any muscle in the human body could contain a tender point.

Treatment. FMS is neither a psychiatric condition nor life threatening. Because the cause of FMS is unknown, treatment focuses on maintaining functionality and reducing symptoms. Patient education is important and may be associated with improved outcomes and better prognosis. An exercise regimen is essential and should include regular stretching; improvement in physical conditioning via low-impact aerobic exercise (biking, swimming, walking); and measures of pacing, muscle protection, and relaxation. Because pain and fatigue may be aggravated by stress and other psychological factors, counseling may be helpful.[14]

Blinded, randomized, placebo-controlled studies of amitriptyline, cyclobenzaprine, zolpidem, and alprazolam administered at bedtime have indicated that all are effective FMS therapy. Treatment begins at the lowest possible doses and increases as tolerated, with the goal being to improve quality of sleep without drug side effects, such as daytime somnolence or excessive dry mouth. Other medications under investigation in FMS are meant to lower pain sensitivity. The selective serotonin reuptake inhibitors that have been studied in FMS include fluoxetine, sertraline, and citalopram. Although their efficacy as monotherapy is modest at best, they may prove beneficial in combination with other agents. Most recently, pregabalin (an anticonvulsant agent) has been shown to be effective in reducing pain and is the first FDA-approved drug for the treatment of FMS.[8] Additional medications that may have a role include venlafaxine and duloxetine (both serotonin-norepinephrine reuptake inhibitors), and tramadol (an opioid-like analgesic) among many other agents being investigated.[8,13]

KEY POINTS

■ Muscular dystrophy comprises a group of genetic disorders characterized by degeneration of skeletal muscle.

■ Duchenne muscular dystrophy is inherited as an X-linked disorder and affects only males.

■ Facioscapulohumeral muscular dystrophy is an autosomal dominant disorder in which degenerating muscle fibers are replaced by connective tissue such that muscles may gain in bulk even though muscle strength is lost.

■ Myasthenia gravis is an autoimmune disorder characterized by progressive weakness as the muscles are used. Antibodies against acetylcholine receptors in the motor end-plate interrupt neuromuscular transmission.

■ FMS is a poorly characterized chronic disorder associated with generalized pain, stiffness, sleep dysfunction, and fatigability.

SUMMARY

A solid working knowledge of the anatomy, physiology, and biomechanics of movement is extremely important when dealing with any type of alteration in the musculoskeletal system. With a grasp of the mechanics involved in function, the clinician is able to approach each aberration with an awareness of the time requirements for healing, stress tolerances, and expected management outcomes.

The injuries and diseases discussed in this chapter are a small representation of the many dysfunctions that may afflict the musculoskeletal system. An ability to determine the specific type of tissue involved (contractile or inert) allows the clinician to be cognizant of activities that would aggravate trauma, types of injury that require supportive devices, and injuries that respond to medical intervention.

An awareness of the tissue response to healing enhances the clinician's evaluative skills and provides a signal regarding when intervention has achieved the expected results within an appropriate time frame. It is the responsibility of the practitioner to become knowledgeable about the variety of dysfunctions that occur. This knowledge base must continue to expand as technological advancements provide increasingly complex levels of information and new diagnostic tools become available.

REFERENCES

1. Chapman MW et al, editors: *Chapman's orthopaedic surgery*, ed 3, Philadelphia, 2001, Lippincott Williams & Wilkins.
2. Hochberg MC et al, editors: *Rheumatology*, ed 4, Philadelphia, 2008, Elsevier Limited.
3. Favus MJ, editor: *Primer on the metabolic bone diseases and disorders of mineral metabolism*, ed 4, Philadelphia, 1999, Lippincott-Raven.
4. Giangregorio L, Blimkie CJ: Skeletal adaptations to alterations in weight-bearing activity: a comparison of models of disuse osteoporosis, *Sports Med* 32(7):459-476, 2002.
5. Iseman MD: *A clinician's guide to tuberculosis*, Philadelphia, 2000, Lippincott Williams & Wilkins, pp 162-167.
6. Abeloff MD et al, editors: *Clinical oncology*, ed 2, New York, 2000, Churchill Livingstone.
7. Cyriax J: *Textbook of orthopedic medicine: diagnosis of soft tissue lesions*, ed 8, London, 1982, Bailliere Tindall.
8. Klippel JH et al, editors: *Primer on the rheumatic diseases*, ed 13, New York, 2008, Arthritis Foundation.
9. Ruddy S, Harris ED, Sledge CB: *Kelley's textbook of rheumatology*, ed 6, Philadelphia, 2001, Saunders.
10. Hettinga DL: Inflammatory response of synovial joint structures. In Gould J, editor: *Orthopedic and sports physical therapy*, ed 2, St Louis, 1990, Mosby, p 100.
11. Richardson JK, Iglarsh ZA: *Clinical orthopedic physical therapy*, Philadelphia, 1993, Saunders.
12. Oldman L, Bennett JC, editors: *Cecil textbook of medicine*, ed 21, Philadelphia, 2000, Saunders.
13. Rao SG: The neuropharmacology of centrally-acting analgesic medications in fibromyalgia, *Rheum Dis Clin North Am* 28(2):235-259, 2002.
14. Bennett RM: The rational management of fibromyalgia patients, *Rheum Dis Clin North Am* 28(2):181-199, 2002.

chapter

52

Alterations in Musculoskeletal Function: Rheumatic Disorders

Carol L. Danning

MEDIA RESOURCES

Additional Material for Study, Review, and Further Exploration

 CD Companion ▪ Review Questions and Answers
▪ Glossary (with audio pronunciations for selected terms)
▪ Disease Profiles ▪ Animations

evolve **Website** at http://evolve.elsevier.com/Copstead/
▪ Case Studies ▪ Disease Profiles ▪ WebLinks ▪ Key Points Review

 Online Course (Module 20)

KEY QUESTIONS

▪ How are osteoarthritis and rheumatoid arthritis differentiated on the basis of cause, clinical findings, and treatment?
▪ What are the similarities and differences among rheumatoid arthritis, systemic lupus erythematosus, and scleroderma?

▪ What are the infective organisms associated with joint inflammation and Lyme disease?
▪ What is the pathogenesis of gouty arthritis?
▪ How do the three subtypes of juvenile rheumatoid arthritis differ?

CHAPTER OUTLINE

Arthritis is the most common disabling musculoskeletal condition in the United States. The National Arthritis Foundation estimates that approximately 46 million people have arthritis with the numbers increasing yearly as the population ages. More than 150 defined rheumatologic diseases have been identified. This chapter discusses the more common rheumatologic diseases.[1]

LOCAL DISORDERS OF JOINT FUNCTION

Osteoarthritis. Osteoarthritis (degenerative joint disease) is the most common arthritis worldwide. It is a progressive, noninflammatory disease of diarthrodial joints, especially those that bear weight. It is characterized by a progressive loss of articular cartilage and by formation of thick subchondral bone and new bone at the joint margins. Osteoarthritis (OA) becomes more prevalent with increasing age. Individuals older than 70 years have the highest incidence. In postmenopausal women, the knees and hands are most frequently affected by OA.[1] It is difficult to estimate the exact prevalence of OA due to difficulties associated with diagnosis, lack of longitudinal data, and difficulty defining disease onset.

Etiology and Pathogenesis. The etiologic progression of OA varies widely. Development of OA may be related to factors that increase the likelihood of abnormal "wear and tear" on joints such as obesity, joint trauma, and congenital disorders (i.e., hip dysplasia, joint laxity, leg length discrepancy). Other predisposing conditions include lifestyle factors and occupation (stress to joints), genetic predisposition, and hormonal status (postmenopausal).[1]

Biomechanical, biochemical, inflammatory, and immunologic factors may all be involved in the development of OA (Figure 52-1). An initial injury causes release of proteolytic and collagenolytic enzymes from chondrocytes. A breakdown of the matrix of proteoglycan and collagen occurs. The decreased hydration of cartilage that occurs with aging can increase the likelihood of wear and damage. Collagen fatigue and microfracture occur with the stress of weight bearing. The ability of the structure to absorb shock is decreased due to subcortical bone and cartilage microfractures. Breakdown of joint integrity overloads the capacity for repair, with resultant degenerative changes.

Structural breakdown of the cartilage involves fissuring, pitting, and erosion. Erosion can become so extensive that the articular surface denudes the full thickness of the cartilage. Osteophyte spur formation, sclerosis of subchondral bone, and cyst formation are also examples of structural changes present in OA. Cartilage fragments may break off into joints and form "loose bodies" (Figure 52-2). Joint effusions are common in advanced cases. Synovium becomes inflamed and secretes an increased amount of synovial fluid, which causes the joint to distend.

Clinical Manifestations. Bony enlargement of joints, crepitus with movement, morning stiffness lasting less than 30 minutes (that improves with joint mobility), and pain with function are typical clinical manifestations of OA. These signs and

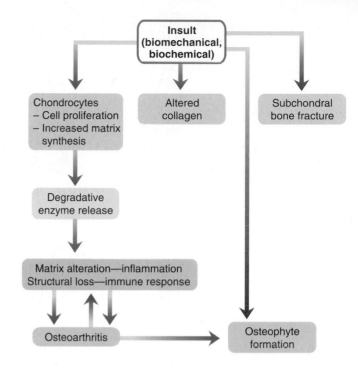

FIGURE 52-1 Pathogenesis of osteoarthritis.

symptoms are usually local. Although any joint may be affected, weight-bearing joints such as the hips and knees, cervical and lumbosacral joints, and interphalangeal joints are most frequently involved. Degenerative arthritis or OA may occur in an isolated joint, or multiple joints can be involved, especially in hands. Mechanical dysfunction, anatomic anomalies, or trauma may cause breakdown of joint surface. It is imperative to establish a differential diagnosis and to rule out a systemic or medical problem. While OA is localized, rheumatoid arthritis (RA) is a systemic autoimmune disorder that causes a highly inflammatory, symmetric, peripheral arthritis.

Radiologic abnormalities are normally consistent with clinical symptoms. Classic findings include bony proliferation at the joint margins (i.e., osteophytes or bone spurs), asymmetric narrowing of the joint space, and subchondral bone sclerosis. Later, malalignment of the joints and cyst formation in subchondral bone can also be seen. When significant synovial fluid accumulates in the joint, it is usually translucent noninflammatory fluid containing less than 2000 white blood cells per cubic millimeter.[1]

The most common deformity of the hands occurs in the distal interphalangeal (DIP) joints (Figure 52-3). Enlargement is caused by bone spurs *(Heberden nodes)* that form on the dorsolateral and medial aspects of the joint. Similar enlargements in the proximal interphalangeal (PIP) joints are called *Bouchard nodes.* The knees and hips are also common locations for OA. Local pain over joint margins, tenderness, crepitus, and muscle atrophy are common findings. Loss of cartilage in medial or lateral compartments of the knee may lead to such structural changes as genu valgus or varus (Figure 52-4).

FIGURE 52-2 Schematic presentation of the pathologic changes in osteoarthritis. Fragmentation and loss of cartilage denude the subchondral bone, which undergoes sclerosis and cystic change. Osteophytes form on the lateral side and protrude into the adjacent soft tissues, causing irritation, inflammation, and fibrosis. (From Damjanov I: *Pathology for the health-related professions,* ed 3, Philadelphia, 2006, Saunders, p 448.)

Pain is relieved by rest during initial stages, though stiffness can be a complaint after prolonged sitting. Because cartilage does not contain nociceptors (pain receptors), pain originates from intraarticular and periarticular structures. Although an acute inflammatory response is often the result of a specific traumatic incident and may cause synovitis in the joint capsule, acute inflammation is not commonly associated with OA. As breakdown in structure progresses, even light activity elicits discomfort, and pain at night is common.

Treatment. Initial treatment is designed to decrease stress on the joint and protect it from additional trauma. Acetaminophen is often the initial analgesic agent recommended for management of mild OA symptoms. Nonsteroidal antiinflammatory drug (NSAID) therapy decreases swelling and pain. Most NSAIDs are nonselective, but anti-inflammatory agents that target the cyclooxygenase-2 (COX-2) enzyme have clinical benefit equal to traditional NSAIDs and may have potentially fewer gastrointestinal side effects. The only COX-2 inhibitor presently available in the United States is celecoxib (Celebrex). All NSAIDs (selective or nonselective) have the potential for renal toxicity and possibly even cardiovascular side effects. Visco-supplementation, the intraarticular injection of hyaluronan or its derivatives, may increase joint lubrication, reduce inflammation, and alleviate pain. These agents are currently only available for use in knee OA. Intraarticular corticosteroid injections can provide temporary pain relief, but too frequent usage (i.e., more than 3 injections per year in the same joint) may accelerate cartilage deterioration.

Physical therapy to improve range of motion, muscle strength, and joint conditioning as well as weight reduction can improve symptoms and prevent loss of function. Assistive devices, such as a cane or walker, afford mechanical relief of weight-bearing stress as can supportive shoe wear. Surgical intervention may be necessary if the joint surface loses enough integrity to prevent joint function. OA is the most common cause for total hip and total knee replacement.

Infectious Arthritis. Infectious or septic arthritis may be defined as an invasion of the synovial membrane by bacteria or another pathogen, leading to a closed-space infection. The pathogen can invade the joint space via hematogenous route, extension of adjacent infection, or direct inoculation following trauma or invasive procedure. Infection causes both synovium and cartilage to deteriorate.

Etiology and Pathogenesis. The basic cause of bone and cartilage destruction is the interaction of antigenic bacterial cell wall components, the toxic effects of bacteria, the destruction caused by the purulent inflammatory exudate, and the local immune-mediated synovial or cartilage response.

FIGURE 52-4 Genu varus and genu valgus.

FIGURE 52-3 Comparison of Heberden nodes (seen in patients with osteoarthritis) with Bouchard nodes (seen in patients with osteoarthritis).

If the bacterial infection is not managed, cartilage can be destroyed, and this can lead to ankylosis of the joint.

Clinical Manifestations. A warm, very swollen joint is symptomatic of any type of infectious arthritis. Usually only a single joint is involved, but polyarticular joint infections can occur in 10 to 20% of cases, most often in debilitated or immunosuppressed individuals. Synovial fluid analysis reveals a very high white cell count (often ≥100,000 cells/mm³), and diagnosis is established by recovery of bacteria from synovial fluid. Blood cultures are also used to provide a medical diagnosis.

The patient with septic arthritis presents with joint pain, fever, chills, and leukocytosis. Fever may range from mild to high fever with shaking chills. In neonates, children older than 4 years, and adults, *Staphylococcus aureus* is the most common causative organism. In children 6 months to 5 years of age, *Haemophilus influenzae* type B is most common. *Neisseria gonorrhoeae* is a causative organism in some adults younger than 30 years of age.[2]

Treatment. Treatment of a septic joint should include appropriate antibiotic therapy (often initially intravenous and then oral) with the average duration required being 4 to 6 weeks.

This therapy is most effective when the bacteria can be isolated and identified from the synovial fluid and antibiotic sensitivities can be used to determine the most effective antibiotic to be used. In addition, the infected joint usually requires repetitive drainage to facilitate bacterial clearance, decrease pain, and prevent loss of function. This can be done either through repeated joint aspiration or arthroscopy with tidal lavage or open surgical drainage.

Joint Prosthesis Infection

Bacterial arthritis (aerobic or anaerobic organisms) may be found in patients after total joint replacement. *Staphylococcus epidermidis* can be a common agent in the prosthetic joint infection but is rarely seen in a native septic joint. Generally, a prosthetic joint infection requires removal of the prosthesis followed by a rigorous course of intravenous antibiotic therapy, often for 6 weeks or longer. Antibiotic beads may also be placed in the wound. The prosthesis is replaced when cultures from the wound show no growth.[2]

KEY POINTS

- Osteoarthritis is a local degenerative joint disorder associated with aging and wear and tear from repetitive stress.
- OA is characterized by loss of articular cartilage, wear of underlying bone, and the formation of bone spurs. The process is noninflammatory. Weight-bearing joints are often affected.
- Signs and symptoms of OA are localized (not systemic) and include joint pain and crepitus with movement.
- Joint infection may be due to a variety of infectious agents, but bacteria are the most problematic. The route of infection is usually by way of the bloodstream. Signs and symptoms are due to localized infection and the systemic manifestation of inflammation.

SYSTEMIC DISORDERS OF JOINT FUNCTION

Immune-Mediated Disorders

Rheumatoid Arthritis. **Rheumatoid arthritis** is a systemic autoimmune inflammatory disease. In the United States, approximately 1% to 2% of the population is affected.[1] Women are two to three times more likely to develop RA than men, with a peak incidence in the fourth and fifth decades. Gender difference disappears in older age. RA affects all races, and its prevalence is not affected by climate. Eighty percent of RA patients test rheumatoid factor (RF) positive. RA occurs two to three times more often in women with a familial history of RA.[3]

Etiology and Pathogenesis. The specific cause of RA is unknown. An infectious agent has long been sought as a cause, but reproducible evidence of a particular bacteria or virus has not been found. A more likely theory is that RA is caused by an abnormal autoimmune response (possibly triggered by a bacterial or viral antigen) occurring in individuals who have a genetic predisposition to the disease.

Current research suggests that susceptibility to RA is determined by gene products of the major histocompatibility system. β-Lymphocyte alloantigen human leukocyte antigen DR4 (HLA-DR4) has been noted in 60% to 70% of adult Caucasian patients with RA, although it is likely that several genes are involved.[3] These genes possibly control humoral and cell-mediated immune mechanisms believed to contribute to the pathogenesis of RA. A particular amino acid sequence of the third hypervariable region of DR beta chains (called the "shared epitope") is seen more commonly in RA patients. The cause and type of stimulus of immunologic abnormalities are not known, but they might be due to an infectious agent, environmental influences, or other lifestyle factors (such as tobacco use.) Trauma to the joint is also a possible cause. An increase in physical and/or psychological stress has also been associated with precipitating acute exacerbation of the disease.

Initially, pathologic changes in RA occur when the immune response localizes in synovial tissue. Here lymphocytes (T and B cells) and macrophages are activated by an unknown antigen trigger. B cells produce RF antibodies against immunoglobulin G (IgG) to form immune complexes. Although immunoglobulins are natural human antibodies, the body produces an antibody (RF) against its own antibody (IgG). Activated lymphocytes, macrophages, and antigen-antibody complexes activate the complement system, stimulate recruitment of other immune cells into the synovium, and produce an extensive array of inflammatory cytokines, metalloproteinases, and other mediators. These products of macrophages and lymphocytes are believed to be critical in RA pathogenesis because they stimulate and perpetuate the inflammation in the joint. Key proinflammatory cytokines demonstrated in the synovium include tumor necrosis factor α (TNF-α), and interleukins-1β (IL-1β), 8, 15, and 18, although many more are also being studied. Newer biological therapies are designed to target these cytokines as well as activated inflammatory cells and cell co-stimulatory markers.

The escalating inflammatory response in the rheumatoid joint leads to accumulation of dense aggregates of immune cells and infiltration of the synovium. The cells produce more cytokines and growth factors, which also stimulate edema, neovascularization, and proliferation of the synovium (which expands in a tumorlike manner.) This hypertrophied synovium invades such surrounding tissue as cartilage, ligaments, joint capsule, and tendons. Granulation tissue forms, covering articular cartilage and leading to pannus formation. Pannus is vascularized tissue made up of lymphocytes, macrophages, histiocytes, fibroblasts, and mast cells. Pannus can erode and destroy articular cartilage, resulting in bone erosion, bone cysts, and fissures (Figure 52-5). The expansion and destruction of joint structures can lead to inflammation, shortening, and even rupture of tendons as well as ligament laxity, joint subluxations, contractures, and deformities.[1]

Clinical Manifestations. RA has a number of clinical features. In 1987, the American Rheumatism Association revised the then 30-year-old criteria for classification of RA. There are seven criteria, and RA is defined by the presence of four or more criteria. Criteria 1 to 4 must present for a minimum of 6 weeks. The criteria are as follows:

1. Morning stiffness in and around joints lasting at least 1 hour before maximal improvement.
2. Soft-tissue swelling (arthritis) of three or more joint areas (including the right and left proximal PIP, metacarpophalangeal [MCP], wrist, elbow, knee, ankle, and metatarsophalangeal [MTP] joints).
3. Swelling of at least one wrist, MCP, or PIP joint.
4. Simultaneous symmetric swelling in joints listed in criterion 2.
5. Subcutaneous rheumatoid nodules.
6. Presence of rheumatoid factor.
7. Radiographic erosions and/or periarticular osteopenia in hand and/or wrist joints.[4]

Malaise, fatigue, and diffuse musculoskeletal pain are common manifestations during acute flare-ups of the disease. It is interesting to note that symmetric patterns involving the joints of the hands, wrists, elbows, and shoulders are evident. DIP joints are usually spared. This symmetry and the noninvolvement of the DIP joint assist in making the diagnosis of RA.

The hands, wrists, knees, and feet are most commonly involved. In the spine, the upper cervical area is most often affected. However, any diarthrodial joint is potentially at risk. The development of pannus followed by inflammatory destruction of the soft tissue leads to laxity of the ligaments and tendons and results in biomechanical dysfunction. This mechanical stress causes the typical deformities of RA.

Swelling in the hands is a typical sign of MCP and PIP joint involvement. Pain is elicited on palpation of the joints. Gradually, progressive synovial damage leads to characteristic ulnar deviation in the MCP joint (Figure 52-6). In advanced situations, a swan-neck deformity develops in the fingers. Swan-neck deformity is a hyperextension of the PIP joint with flexion of the MCP and DIP joints due to contractures

TNF-α (etanerc…
available for par…
effective at slow…
symptoms. Othe…
phocytes (rituxir…
(abatacept) are a…

Systemic L…

erythematosus

autoimmune dis…
erbations and re…
affected at differe…

Etiology and Patl…

demonstrated in…
occurs in all races…
among African Ar…
mon in Africa.[6] Ei…
mal burns, and ot…
development of S…
peak incidence bet…
hormonal factors i…

SLE is the resu…
body against its o…
body has a decrea…
mechanisms is B-ly…
autoantibody prod…
of antibodies direc…
gens located in cel…
tibodies, those dire…
antibodies, or AN…
patients.[6] Antigen-a…
ment membranes c…
brain, and joints. Ii…
ment and trigger th…
sponsible for tissue…

Clinical Manifestatio…

systems such as th…
joints, lungs, and ga…
fected simultaneousl…
of exacerbation and…
years.

Arthralgias and sy…
most patients noting…
of the disease. In lup…
movement, and mor…
the capsule, ligamen…
ing reducible deform…
arthropathy). Defor…
fingers, to hyperexter…
thumb, to subluxatio…
steroid therapy, tendc…

Skin lesions may b…
ous lupus erythemato…
terfly (malar) rash, th…
can be present in 80%…
acerbated during syste…
noted, and sunlight o…

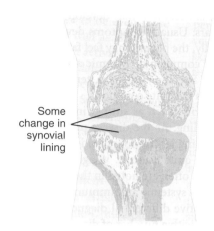
Some change in synovial lining

INITIATION PHASE

Influx of immune cells: B cells, T cells, macrophages, Ag–Ab complexes

IMMUNE RESPONSE PHASE
Hyperplasia of synovium

INFLAMMATORY PHASE
Oxygen radicals, arachidonic acid radicals, and lysosomes destroy synovial tissue

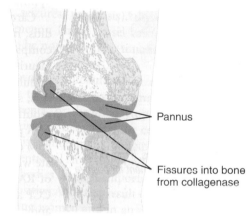
Pannus

Fissures into bone from collagenase

DESTRUCTION PHASE

FIGURE 52-5 Schematic presentation of the pathologic changes in rheumatoid arthritis. The inflammation (synovitis) leads to pannus formation, obliteration of the articular space, and finally, ankylosis. The periarticular bone shows disuse atrophy in the form of osteoporosis. (From Black JM et al: *Medical-surgical nursing, clinical management for positive outcomes,* ed 6, Philadelphia, 2001, Saunders.)

Ulnar drift

FIGURE 52-6 Typical deformity of the hand seen in patients with rheumatoid arthritis. Note ulnar deviation. (From Black JM, Hawks JH: *Medical-surgical nursing, clinical management for positive outcomes,* ed 8, Philadelphia, 2009, Saunders, p 2058.)

of intrinsic muscles and tendons.[5] A boutonnière deformity, consisting of flexion of the PIP joints and hyperextension of the DIP joints, is also a common dysfunctional position due to rupture or excess laxity of extensor tendons over the fingers (Figure 52-7). Loss of strength and the ability to achieve a strong pinch is frequently noted in the hand affected by RA. A rupture of tendons and loss of the ability to extend the fingers are common findings in later stages of the disease.

The wrist is commonly involved. The synovium around the wrist becomes boggy and affects the tendon sheaths. Limitation of movement, especially dorsiflexion of the wrist, is often noted. Proliferation of the synovium on the volar or palmar aspect of the wrist may cause compression of the median nerve and development of carpal tunnel syndrome. Flexion contractures and swelling of the elbow are other common manifestations; in later stages of the disease, shoulder involvement may occur. Typical signs of shoulder involvement

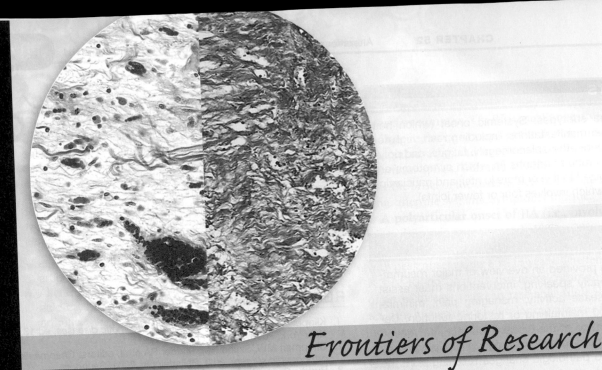

Frontiers of Research

Wounds and Wound Healing

Sheila K. Smith

Through accidents, surgery, war, violence, infections, and debilitation, millions are inflicted with wounds each year. Many of these wounds become chronic, often due to underlying vascular or metabolic pathology. Even with modern treatment, chronic wounds may not heal quickly and may leave a scarred reminder of severe trauma or underlying disease. In the United States, chronic wounds are usually the afflictions of cancer patients, individuals with diabetes, patients with vascular disease, patients confined to bed for long periods, the elderly, individuals with nerve system damage, or those whose immune systems and metabolic processes have been compromised. Chronic wounds are painful and dangerous. They are prone to infection, which can then lead to sepsis, sometimes with antibiotic-resistant organisms. The debilitated, chronically ill patient undergoing major surgery is particularly susceptible to slow-healing wounds. Open heart surgery in the setting of poorly controlled diabetes has been found to be particularly susceptible to infection and lack of healing at the wound site.

After a wound occurs, almost immediately the specialized cells that contribute to healing rush to the site, attracted by chemical signals. Growth factors are released, unusually rapid cell proliferation begins, and the process of healing starts. For some time, researchers have known that endogenous growth factors

released at the location of a wound are conducive to wound healing. Multiple molecules involved in local intercellular communication and/or chemoattraction have been identified and intensively studied. It appears that some growth factors are active at every stage of wound healing. The process of wound healing is incredibly complex, and it has been difficult to affect it favorably by simple manipulations of individual factors. However, in some pathologic states individual growth factors have shown success in clinical trials. For example, topical platelet-derived growth factor has shown significant benefit in certain cases of diabetic foot ulcers. In addition, it is now understood that deep wound debridement activates endogenous growth factors necessary to starting reparative tissue development.

The first response to a bleeding injury or a surgical wound is the formation of a fibrin clot by a protein called *fibrinogen,* which circulates in the bloodstream and seals damaged blood vessels. Platelets also adhere to the damaged blood vessels. Next, inflammatory changes occur as release of local chemical mediators attracts leukocytes to the damaged area. Polymorphonuclear leukocytes and activated macrophages digest damaged tissue components, modify the extracellular matrix, and kill bacteria. They also release growth factors and other soluble products that

Granulation tissue showing numerous blood vessels, edema, and a loose extracellular matrix containing occasional inflammatory cells (left); *minimal mature collagen* (blue) *can be seen at this point. Mature scar, showing dense collagen, with only scattered vascular channels* (right). (*From Kumar V et al: Robbins and Cotran pathologic basis of disease, ed 8, Philadelphia, 2007, Saunders, p 71.*)

FIGURE 52-7 S
JM, Hawks JH: *Medi
outcomes,* ed 8, Phila

are limitations of
of the coracoid p
of the joint capsul

Involvement of
mon finding. Dest
tebrae (such as th
for subluxation of
cord. Laxity in the
of the vertebral art
Limitation of moti
and headache in th

Abnormalities
signs noted when
sular involvement
comes extensive, se
involvement in the
ceps atrophy, contr
nous bursa (Baker
articular surface, b
instability. One col
foot is retrocalcane
ment include swelli
to subluxation of th
deviation of the firs

Integumentary System

magnify and extend the healing process. Soon a migratory and proliferative process occurs. On the surface of the wound, locally produced growth factors encourage epidermal migration with re-epithelialization. Beneath this, vascular endothelial budding and migrating fibroblasts form the new vessels and collagen of granulation tissue.

Under normal postoperative circumstances, by the fifth day the processes of re-epithelialization, neovascularization, and fibroblast migration have formed a wound that can maintain its integrity to minor tension. Over the ensuing months, the extracellular matrix consisting of proteins and mucopolysaccharides is extensively remodeled to further strengthen the wound. The final product is a relatively acellular scar (made up primarily of strong collagen bundles) that affords about 70% of the strength of normal skin.

Wound healing is strongly affected by the age, nutritional status, immunocompetence, cardiopulmonary condition, and habits of the patient seeking care. Age is a major consideration in wound healing. Older patients heal more slowly than younger patients, but the outcome is likely to be the same if the requirements of age are taken into account. Aged skin is more fragile, and the elderly are less able to defend themselves against infection. They may be poorly nourished, and decreased perfusion may slow down the healing process. Chronic disease, medications, motivation, and social habits are other factors that need to be taken into account. Oxygenation, nutritional supplementation, ambulation, monitoring for infection, and maintenance of good metabolic control all help with wound healing and recovery in the debilitated patient.

Because it decreases capillary and arteriolar flow to the skin, decreases oxygenation, and damages connective tissues, cigarette smoking retards wound healing. Health care professionals find that cigarette smoke, which contains nicotine, carbon monoxide, and hydrogen cyanide, reduces healing. Nicotine reduces blood flow to the skin and may also directly inhibit fibroblast function; carbon monoxide reduces oxygen transport and metabolism; and hydrogen cyanide inhibits metabolism and oxygenation after a variety of surgeries.

However miraculous the processes of wound healing and tissue regeneration may be, extensively damaged or lost tissues frequently cannot be restored without extensive and skilled surgical reconstruction. Such therapies, while of great benefit, are costly, time-consuming, painful, and still largely out of reach of many individuals who've suffered disfiguring injuries. The body and its tissues are not endlessly reparable, a basic fact that is essential to remember in providing the best possible health care for the prevention, management, and healing of wounds.

Alterations in the Integumentary System

Lee-Ellen C. Copstead • Ruth E. Diestelmeier • Michael R. Diestelmeier

MEDIA RESOURCES

Additional Material for Study, Review, and Further Exploration

CD Companion ■ Review Questions and Answers
■ Glossary (with audio pronunciations for selected terms)
■ Disease Profiles ■ Animations

evolve **Website** at http://evolve.elsevier.com/Copstead/
■ Case Studies ■ Disease Profiles ■ WebLinks ■ Key Points Review

Online Course (Module 20)

KEY QUESTIONS

■ How does the aging process affect the integumentary system?
■ Why is it important to differentiate primary from secondary skin lesions?
■ What lesion characteristics are assessed to aid in determination of the lesion's cause?
■ How do systemic disorders affect nail and hair growth?
■ Which skin disorders are more likely to occur more commonly in certain age groups, including infants, children, adolescents, and the elderly?

■ How does ultraviolet radiation affect the skin?
■ How do superficial and deep pressure ulcers differ in clinical and etiologic features?
■ How can malignant melanoma be differentiated from other skin lesions?

CHAPTER OUTLINE

This chapter focuses on altered structure and function of the integumentary system. The etiologic factors, pathogenesis, and clinical manifestations of selected skin disorders, as well as general considerations regarding treatment modalities and their therapeutic application are described.

AGE-RELATED CHANGES

The skin undergoes dramatic changes from birth through the mature years. Healthy infants and young children have relatively smooth and unwrinkled skin characterized by elasticity and flexibility. Because skin tissues are in an active phase of new growth, healing of skin injuries is often rapid and efficient. Young children and elderly individuals have fewer sweat glands than adults do, so their bodies rely more on increased blood flow to maintain a normal body temperature.

As adulthood begins at puberty, hormones stimulate the development and activation of sebaceous glands and sweat glands. After the sebaceous glands become active, especially during the initial years, they may overproduce sebum and thus give the skin an unusually oily appearance. Sebaceous ducts may become clogged or infected and form acne pimples or other blemishes on the skin. Activation of apocrine sweat glands during puberty causes increased sweat production, an ability needed to maintain an adult body properly, and also the possibility of increased "body odor." Body odor is caused by wastes produced by bacteria that feed on the organic compounds found in apocrine sweat and on the surface of the skin.

INFECTIOUS PROCESSES

Viral Infections

Verrucae

Etiology and Pathogenesis. Verrucae, or warts (Figure 53-4), are common benign papillomas caused by DNA-containing papillomaviruses. Although warts vary in appearance depending on their location, the histologic characteristics of all lesions are similar. A wart is actually an exaggeration of normal skin composition, with the stratum corneum being irregularly thickened. The human papillomaviruses, the subgroup of papovaviruses that causes human warts, are not found in other animals and invade only the skin and mucous membranes of humans.

Warts may resolve spontaneously if immunity to the virus develops, but the immune response can be delayed for years and is not reliably activated in every case. In 95% of cases, untreated warts will resolve within 5 years,[2] but they may multiply into hundreds of lesions and can involve any body site. Current surgical treatment may be directed at removal of the wart by laser. Liquid nitrogen or acid chemicals, cryotherapy, and salicylic acid paint or plasters have also been effective medical treatments. Topical blistering agents, immunomodulators, and intralesional injections of various agents may also be effective.

Herpes Simplex Virus

Etiology and Pathogenesis. Herpes simplex virus (HSV) infections of the skin and mucous membranes are common (Figure 53-5). Two types of herpesviruses infect humans: type 1 and type 2. Most HSV-1 infections occur above the waist.[3] HSV-1 may result when external infection is spread to the other parts of the body through the occupational hazards that exist in professions such as dentistry and medicine and some athletics. HSV-2 is responsible for most infections in the genital region.[3]

Herpesvirus lesions usually begin with a burning or tingling sensation. Vesicles and erythema follow and progress to pustules, ulcers, and crusts before healing. The lesion is most common on the lips, face, and mouth. Pain is common, and

FIGURE 53-4 Plantar warts. (From Callen JP et al: *Color atlas of dermatology,* ed 2, Philadelphia, 2000, Saunders, p 92.)

healing takes place in 10 to 14 days.[4] After the initial infection, the herpesvirus persists in latent form in the trigeminal and other ganglia. Recurrent lesions are common and may be precipitated by stress, sunlight exposure, menses, or injury.[5,6] The vast majority of patients have at least one episode of herpesvirus reactivation, and some individuals may have 10 or more outbreaks per year. Recently, concern has arisen over the identification of infectious viral shedding in the absence of symptomatic lesions.[5]

Treatment. No cure for herpes simplex is known, and most treatment measures are palliative. Lidocaine (Xylocaine) or diphenhydramine (Benadryl) application and aspirin help relieve pain. Cold compresses help in the acute stages. Acyclovir, famciclovir, or valacyclovir are recommended to shorten the duration of active disease outbreaks; in certain situations, these drugs may be used for daily prophylaxis.

Herpes Zoster

Etiology and Pathogenesis. Herpes zoster (shingles) is an acute localized inflammatory disease of a dermatomal segment of the skin (Figure 53-6). It is caused by the same herpesvirus that causes chickenpox (varicella-zoster). It is believed to be the result of reactivation of a latent varicella-zoster virus that has been present in the sensory dorsal ganglia since childhood infection. During an attack of shingles, the reactivated virus travels from the ganglia to the skin of the corresponding dermatome.

Clinical Manifestations and Treatment. The clinical manifestations of shingles include the eruption of vesicles with erythematous bases that are restricted to skin areas supplied by sensory neurons of a single or associated group of dorsal root ganglia. Eruptions generally follow a unilateral dermatomal distribution and most often occur on the thorax, trunk, and face. In immunosuppressed persons, the lesions may extend beyond the dermatome. New crops of vesicles erupt for 3 to 5 days along the nerve pathway.[3] Lesions are deeper and more confluent than those of chickenpox. The vesicles dry, form crusts, and eventually fall off. Lesions usually clear in 2 to 3 weeks.[3] Severe pain and paresthesias are common. In the elderly, herpes-zoster is a particularly serious condition that may be long lasting. Pain reports from elderly individuals indicate an increased severity and lengthy episodes of up to 1 year.[3] Systemic treatment with acyclovir, famciclovir, or valacyclovir should be initiated as soon as possible, preferably within the first 48 to 72 hours.

Postherpetic neuralgia is the most important complication occurring in people older than 50 years.[3] Eye involvement can result in permanent blindness.

Treatment. Management of shingles includes oral antiviral drugs of which acyclovir (Zovirax) is one example. Topical agents such as Burrow compresses or aqueous alcohol shake lotions may also be used. Pain medication may be indicated in severe cases. Systemic corticosteroids have also been effective in healthy persons older than 50 years with severe pain, but their use remains controversial. High doses of interferon, an antiviral glycoprotein, have been used in persons with cancer when the herpetic lesions are limited to the dermatome.[7]

FIGURE 53-5 Herpes simplex virus (HSV), types 1 and 2. **A,** Herpes simplex labialis—recurrent lesions. **B,** Herpetic whitlow: herpes simplex infection of the finger. **C,** Vaginal primary herpes simplex virus. **D,** Penile lesions of recurrent herpes simplex infection. **E,** Recurrent blistering on the elbow of this patient was treated as recurring impetigo before being correctly diagnosed as HSV infection. **F,** The histopathologic appearance of HSV reveals an intraepidermal bulla with bizarre multinucleated balloon cells. **G,** A positive Tzanck smear from a herpes simplex blister. (**A-E,** From Callen JP et al: *Color atlas of dermatology,* ed 2, Philadelphia, 2000, Saunders, p 92. **F** and **G,** From Callen JP et al: *Color atlas of dermatology,* Philadelphia, 1993, Saunders, p 168.)

FIGURE 53-6 Herpes zoster. **A,** Recurrent infection with the varicella-zoster virus. The eruption is usually dermatomal but can become generalized. **B,** Disseminated herpes zoster. **C,** Herpes zoster ophthalmicus. (From Callen JP et al: *Color atlas of dermatology,* ed 2, Philadelphia, 2000, Saunders, p 92.)

Additionally, vaccination is becoming an important tool in preventing Herpes zoster.

Fungal Infections

Superficial Fungal Infections. Three genera of **fungi** (**dermatophytes**) commonly infect human skin: *Microsporum, Trichophyton,* and *Epidermophyton.* These organisms can cause an infection termed **tinea** in any cutaneous area, including the hair and nails. Infections in different locations are named after the location: tinea capitis (scalp) (Figure 53-7), tinea barbae (beard), tinea faciei (face) (Figure 53-8), tinea

corporis (trunk) (Figure 53-9), tinea manus (hand), tinea cruris (groin), and tinea pedis (foot).

Clinical Manifestations. The clinical signs of superficial fungal infection vary depending on the physical location and the host's response to the invading organism. Often fungal infections are manifested as erythematous macules or plaques with peripheral scaling and some central clearing. Vesicular lesions often accompany the dry scaling on the feet. Because of the variability of signs and symptoms, superficial dermatophytosis must be considered when evaluating even a weeping, crusted area more suggestive of eczema or impetigo. Dermatophyte

FIGURE 53-7 Tinea capitis, localized patch. (From Callen JP et al: *Color atlas of dermatology,* Philadelphia, 1993, Saunders, p 106.)

FIGURE 53-9 Tinea corporis. Annular scaly plaques in superficial basal cell epithelioma. (From Callen JP et al: *Color atlas of dermatology,* Philadelphia, 1993, Saunders, p 106.)

FIGURE 53-8 Tinea faciei. (From Callen JP et al: *Color atlas of dermatology,* ed 2, Philadelphia, 2000, Saunders, p 89.)

FIGURE 53-10 Dermatophyte infection of the nails resulting in onycholysis. (From Callen JP et al: *Color atlas of dermatology,* Philadelphia, 1993, Saunders, p 347.)

infection of the nails, or onychomycosis, is usually seen as a white or yellow opaque discoloration that often progresses to a thickened, crumbed, or deformed nail (Figure 53-10).
Treatment. Topical management of localized superficial dermatophyte infections is very effective. Among the topical antifungal preparations available in cream and solution form are miconazole nitrate, clotrimazole, econazole nitrate, ciclopirox olamine, and terbinafine. A 4-week course of twice-daily applications will usually clear the symptoms. For more extensive infections involving the hair, nails, or resistant organisms, systemic therapy (e.g., griseofulvin or intraconazole and terbinafine) is required. Treatment duration ranges from 3 to 4 weeks (tinea corporis) to 12 months (onychomycosis).

Yeast Infections. The yeast *Candida albicans* is another common source of superficial infection (Figure 53-11). It is manifested in newborns as the white lesions of **thrush,** in infants and bedridden patients as **intertrigo,** and in immuno-impaired individuals as the systemic disorder **mucocutaneous candidiasis.** Mucocutaneous candidiasis may actually be the presenting sign in an individual with a previously undiagnosed immunodeficiency disorder.

Localized yeast infections such as oral candidiasis (thrush) may be managed with nystatin mouth rinse or clotrimazole troches (throat lozenges). The topical antifungal medications mentioned earlier may also be used in the management of localized yeast infections. Widespread or systemic infections respond well to oral ketoconazole or fluconazole (Diflucan).

Bacterial Infections
Impetigo
Etiology and Clinical Manifestations. Impetigo is an acute, contagious skin disease characterized by the formation of

FIGURE 53-11 Candida albicans infection of the tongue in chronic mucocutaneous candidiasis. (From Berger TG et al: *Andrews' diseases of the skin: clinical dermatology*, ed 9, Philadelphia, 2000, Saunders, p 385.)

FIGURE 53-12 Impetigo. (From Swartz MH: *Physical diagnosis, history and examination,* ed 4, Philadelphia, 2002, Saunders, p 713.)

vesicles, pustules, and yellowish crusts (Figure 53-12). The most common cause of infection of the skin, impetigo is caused by staphylococci or streptococci. Approximately 5% of the population each year sustains *Staphylococcus* infections of a severity sufficient to require medical attention.[8] Approximately 20% of adults are chronic carriers of the bacterium *Staphylococcus aureus,* and another 60% are intermittent carriers.[8] The bacterium is carried in the nasal area and may pass onto the skin and produce disease. Staphylococcal infections are a special problem for hospitalized patients, who may become infected from the infected hospital staff.

Treatment. Treatment for impetigo includes topical application of 2% mupirocin ointment (Bactroban) or 1% retapamulin (Altabax) ointment. If a large area of skin is involved or if the person is febrile, impetigo may be managed systemically with oral dicloxacillin, cephalexin, or erythromycin.

Syphilis

Etiology and Clinical Manifestations. A variety of sexually transmitted diseases caused by bacteria can infect the genitalia. The most serious is **syphilis,** which is caused by *Treponema pallidum.* If the person remains untreated, three stages can occur. In primary syphilis, a chancre (ulcer) generally occurs as a single lesion on the genitalia; the spirochetal microorganism that causes syphilis can be seen in a scraping of the chancre. Secondary syphilis is characterized by a disseminated rash that cannot be clearly distinguished from other rashes. Both the primary and secondary stages of syphilis are contagious.

Treatment. Studies to detect serum antibodies against syphilis (such as the Venereal Disease Research Laboratory, VDRL) and examination of the pustules for the spirochete are required to achieve a diagnosis. Penicillin is very effective in eradicating syphilis in the primary and secondary stages, but unfortunately damage caused by tertiary syphilis to the cardiovascular and central nervous systems is permanent.

Leprosy. **Leprosy** is a chronic infectious disease of the skin caused by the intracellular bacillus *Mycobacterium leprae.* Approximately 11 million people worldwide have leprosy.[8] The diagnosis is made with a skin biopsy. Leprosy has a low rate of infectivity and is usually responsive to sulfone drugs like dapsone. For chronic deformities, corrective orthopedic surgery may be required.

INFLAMMATORY CONDITIONS

Lupus Erythematosus. Lupus erythematosus (LE) is an inflammatory disease that has cutaneous manifestations. Systemic LE and chronic discoid LE are clinically dissimilar but basically related diseases. The two diseases differ with regard to characteristic skin lesions, subjective complaints, other organ involvement, LE cell test findings, response to treatment, and eventual prognosis. Discoid lupus presents with scaly red plaques with scarring that involve sun-exposed skin. Classically, systemic lupus presents with a butterfly-shaped erythema involving the cheeks and nose; discoid lesions may be seen as well. A comparison of the two conditions is found in Table 53-4. Figure 53-13 illustrates characteristic skin lesions of both conditions.

Seborrheic Dermatitis

Clinical Manifestations and Treatment. Seborrheic dermatitis (Figure 53-14) is a papulosquamous skin disease manifested by various degrees of scaling and erythema in areas of high oil gland concentration such as the scalp, eyebrows, glabellae, eyelids, nasolabial folds, pinna and posterior sulcus of the ears, sternum, axillae, umbilicus, and anogenital area. Common manifestations of this disease are cradle cap in newborns and dandruff in adolescents and adults.

Although seborrheic dermatitis is not curable, it may be controlled with topical medication. The regular use of tar,

TABLE 53-4

Comparison of Chronic Discoid with Systemic Lupus Erythematosus

Parameter	Chronic Discoid LE	Systemic LE
Primary lesions	Red, scaly, thickened, well-circumscribed patches with enlarged follicles and elevated border	Red, mildly scaly, diffuse, puffy lesions. Purpura also seen
Secondary lesions	Atrophy, scarring, and pigmentary changes	No scarring; mild hyperpigmentation
Distribution	Face, mainly in the "butterfly" area, but also on the scalp, ears, arms, and chest. May not be symmetric	Face in the "butterfly" area, arms, fingers, and legs; usually symmetric
Course	Very chronic with gradual progression; slow healing under therapy; no effect on life	Acute onset with fever, rash, malaise, and joint pains. Most cases respond rather rapidly to steroid and supportive therapy, but the prognosis for life is poor
Season	Aggravated by intense sun exposure or radiation therapy	Same
Sex incidence	Almost twice as common in females	Same
Systemic pathology	None obvious	Nephritis, arthritis, epilepsy, pan-carditis, hepatitis, etc.
Laboratory findings	Biopsy characteristic in classic case LE cell test negative, as are other laboratory tests	Biopsy less useful

From Sauer GC: *Manual of skin diseases,* ed 6, Philadelphia, 1991, Lippincott, p 253.
LE, Lupus erythematosus.

FIGURE 53-13 A and **B,** Discoid lupus erythematosus. Round or oval cutaneous lesions occurring in patients with lupus erythematosus. **C,** Subacute cutaneous lupus erythematosus. (From Callen JP et al: *Color atlas of dermatology,* ed 2, Philadelphia, 2000, Saunders, pp 15, 16.)

FIGURE 53-14 Annular seborrheic dermatitis of the ear. (From Callen JP et al: *Color atlas of dermatology,* ed 2, Philadelphia, 2000, Saunders, p 246.)

FIGURE 53-15 Psoriasis vulgaris. (From Callen JP et al: *Color atlas of dermatology,* ed 2, Philadelphia, 2000, Saunders, p 280.)

zinc, selenium sulfide, or salicylic acid shampoos often clears the symptoms and signs of seborrheic dermatitis in the scalp; mild topical corticosteroids (e.g., 1% hydrocortisone) clear lesions on the face and ears.

Psoriasis

Etiology and Clinical Manifestations. **Psoriasis** is a common chronic skin disease characterized by papules and plaques with an overlying silvery scale. The specific cause of psoriasis is unknown, but it appears to be a multifactorial inherited condition in which minor aberrations of the immune system promote inflammation and hyperproliferation within the skin. The disease may affect, with varying degrees of severity, people of all ages. Lesions can appear on any area of the body; however, they seem to have a predilection for the knees, elbows, lower part of the back, scalp, and nails (Figure 53-15). Disease progression is unpredictable, and the patient may periodically experience spontaneous exacerbations or remission.

Treatment. No cure for psoriasis is known. Treatments, both topical and systemic, are directed at clearing and controlling the lesions. Therapies include topical corticosteroids (most commonly used), a vitamin D derivative (calcipotriene ointment [Dovonex]), ultraviolet light exposure, topical tar preparations, and combinations of ultraviolet light with topical tar or systemic psoralen. Systemic therapies with methotrexate and hydroxyurea are also effective in clearing psoriasis but carry considerable risk of toxicity. Newer, highly effective biological agents are now available for use by injection but are very expensive and also carry risks of significant side effects.

Lichen Planus

Etiology and Pathogenesis. **Lichen planus** is a relatively common, chronic, pruritic disease involving inflammation and papular eruption of the skin and mucous membranes. Idiopathic lichen planus is of unknown cause but can be stimulated by a variety of drugs and chemicals in susceptible persons. The characteristic lesion is a shiny, white-topped, purplish, polygonal papule. Lesions appear on the wrists, ankles, and trunk (Figure 53-16). Mucous membrane lesions are

FIGURE 53-16 Linear lichen planus as a result of Koebner phenomenon. (From Callen JP et al: *Color atlas of dermatology,* ed 2, Philadelphia, 2000, Saunders, p 249.)

white and lacy and may become bullous. Pruritus is severe, and new lesions develop as a result of scratching (Koebner phenomenon). Nails are affected in approximately 10% of people with lichen planus.[9]

Treatment. In the majority of people, lichen planus is a self-limiting disease. Treatment measures include discontinuing all medications, followed by the administration of topical corticosteroids and occlusive dressings. Systemic corticosteroids may be indicated in severe cases, and antipruritic agents are helpful in reducing the itch.

Pityriasis Rosea

Etiology, Pathogenesis, and Treatment. Pityriasis rosea is a rash of unknown origin that primarily affects young adults. The incidence is highest in spring and fall. It has been speculated to be viral in origin, but to date no virus has been isolated. The characteristic lesion is a macule or papule with surrounding erythema. The lesion spreads with central clearing, much like tinea corporis. This initial lesion is a solitary lesion, called

FIGURE 53-17 **A** and **B,** Acne vulgaris with papules and pustules. (From Callen JP et al: *Color atlas of dermatology,* ed 2, Philadelphia, 2000, Saunders, p 151.)

the herald patch, and is usually located on the trunk or neck. As the lesion enlarges and begins to fade away (2 to 10 days), successive crops of lesions appear on the trunk and neck.[10] The extremities, face, and scalp may be involved, and mild to severe pruritis may occur. The disease is self-limiting and usually disappears within 2 to 10 weeks.[10] Treatment is palliative and includes topical steroids, antihistamines, and colloid baths. Systemic corticosteroids may be indicated in severe cases. Systemic antibiotics, especially erythromycin, may also shorten the course.

Acne Vulgaris

Etiology and Pathogenesis. Acne, an extremely common disease of the pilosebaceous unit, affects up to 90% of all individuals and produces unsightly lesions and sometimes permanent scarring and disfigurement[11] (Figure 53-17). Etiologically, acne involves multiple factors such as sex hormones, heredity, bacterial flora of the skin, stress, mechanical occlusion, and cosmetics use. Acne arises when sludging of sebaceous oils and deposition of loose epithelial cells cause an obstruction of the follicular canal. Continued oil production and bacterial growth in this obstructed follicle may cause rupture of the wall or sebaceous gland and result in an inflamed lesion.

Treatment. No cure for acne is known. Treatment modalities are directed to clearing the lesions and maintaining a clear complexion. Topical therapy works for most patients. Such

medications are designed to cause increased peeling of the stratum corneum and loosening of the follicular plugs.

Many products are available to achieve this goal. Soaps, lotions, and gels containing sulfur, resorcinol, salicylic acid, or benzoyl peroxide all enhance drying and peeling. Astringents, which are liquids primarily composed of alcohol with acetone, are used as solvents to remove the surface lipid and loose skin cells, as well as to enhance drying. Topical retinoids, of which there are several, are a mainstay of treatment. Retinoic acid, a derivative of vitamin A, is one example of this class of drugs.[4] A peeling agent, it is very useful in dealing with open comedones and papules. Topical antibiotics are also available, the most effective being liquid preparations of erythromycin and clindamycin (Cleocin T) with an alcohol base.

For cases characterized by inflammatory lesions, pustules, or nodules, systemic therapy can be useful. Antibiotics, especially tetracycline and erythromycin, have long been used in such treatments. In cases that are resistant, minocycline, sulfamethoxazole-trimethoprim, and sulfones are occasionally used. Isotretinoin, a vitamin A derivative, is effective in the management of nodular and cystic acne.[12] Birth control pills, especially the estrogen-dominant type, can be of value in managing severe recalcitrant acne in females. However, androgen-dominant contraceptives can aggravate or precipitate acne.

As with any medication regimen, both systemic and topical acne treatments can produce unwanted side effects in sensitive patients. Systemic tetracycline may cause gastrointestinal upset, nausea, diarrhea, and vaginal *Monilia* overgrowth. Tetracycline should not be used in children because their uncrupted teeth may be severely and permanently discolored. Topical antibiotics can cause irritant or allergic contact dermatitis.

Other useful acne treatments include corticosteroid injection into cysts and nodules and surgery, which involves extraction of the comedones and drainage of fluctuant cystic lesions.[6]

Pemphigus. A group of related disorders (**pemphigus group** of vulgaris, vegetans, foliaceus, and erythematosus) is characterized by bullous eruptions (blisters). These disorders are thought to be caused by autoimmune reactions. Patients show antibodies against keratinocytes and basement membranes. The autoantibodies perhaps cause the keratinocytes to separate from one another to form blisters. Of the group of related diseases, **pemphigus vulgaris** has the worst prognosis (Figure 53-18). Bullae can erupt on the skin and mucous membranes (e.g., esophagus), and toxemia and infection can cause death if proper treatment (cortisone) is not administered.

ALLERGIC SKIN RESPONSES

Atopic Dermatitis

Etiology and Clinical Manifestations. Atopy, or **allergy,** is indicated by a personal and sometimes family history of asthma, allergic rhinitis, or the most commonly seen manifestation, eczematous dermatitis (Figures 53-19 to 53-21). The highest incidence of atopic dermatitis occurs in children, with most

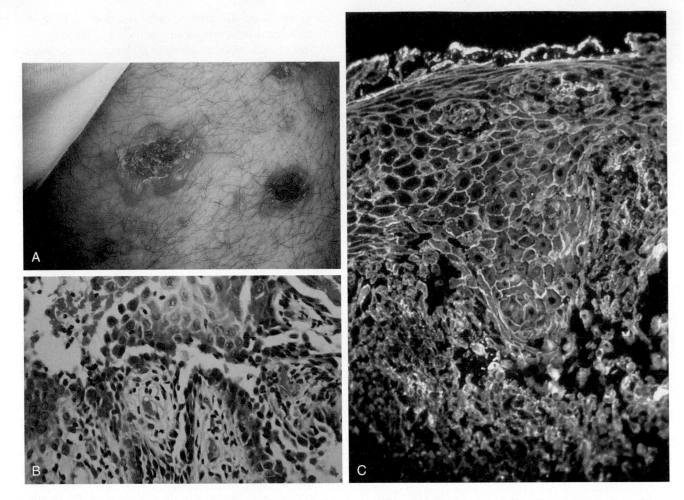

FIGURE 53-18 Pemphigus vulgaris. **A,** Bullae are transient in this disorder; erosion is more characteristic. **B,** The blister is suprabasilar within the epidermis. Individual cells are unattached within the bulla (acantholytic cells). **C,** Deposition of IgG in the intercellular areas of the epidermis is characteristic of pemphigus. (From Callen JP et al: *Color atlas of dermatology,* Philadelphia, 1993, Saunders, p 163.)

cases developing in those younger than 5 years.[13] The characteristic features depend on the age at onset, but pruritus is always present. In infants, the disease characteristically appears on the face, scalp, or extensor surfaces of the extremities; the predominant lesion is an oozing, crusting, coalescent papule. The disease in children is most often seen as erythema, papules, and lichenification of the flexor surfaces of the extremities, especially the antecubital and popliteal areas, the wrists, and the nape of the neck. Older children and young adults have thickening of the skin, or lichenification, along with fine, dry scaling and some papules. These changes are again seen on the flexor surfaces of the extremities and the scalp, face, and upper chest. Retrospective studies show that in nearly half of all patients with childhood atopic dermatitis, the disease improves or clears with age.[14]

Treatment. Treatment of atopic dermatitis is usually carried out on an outpatient basis. The most important considerations are moisturization of the skin and prevention of continued drying and water loss. The drying and scaling that are characteristic features of atopic dermatitis impair the skin's ability not only to retain moisture but also to repel such external invaders as chemical irritants and surface bacteria. Milder cases of atopic eczema can be managed conservatively by decreasing the frequency of bathing, using tepid water in baths, eliminating alkaline soaps, and using moisturizing creams (especially after baths and washing). In more severe cases that involve an inflammatory response to skin breakdown, topical steroids are an important part of therapy. Short courses of systemic antibiotics such as erythromycin have also been helpful in controlling the severity of atopic eczema by reducing the concentration of cutaneous bacterial flora. Even after all these measures have been executed, some patients with severe atopic dermatitis are hospitalized for continuous wet dressings and topical steroids.

An important feature of all atopic dermatitis that must be dealt with is pruritus. The topical treatments mentioned previously are helpful in reducing itch. If additional measures are needed, systemic antihistamines (e.g., hydroxyzine and diphenhydramine) are effective.

Contact Dermatitis

Etiologies and Clinical Manifestations. Contact dermatitis is a cutaneous reaction to topical irritation or allergy. Irritant contact dermatitis develops in any person exposed to a sufficiently

FIGURE 53-19 Atopic dermatitis. An extremely pruritic condition. **A,** Multiple excoriations, vesiculation, and marked lichenification are seen in this patient. **B,** Minute excoriations with marked lichenification in the antecubital fossa. (From Callen JP et al: *Color atlas of dermatology,* Philadelphia, 1993, Saunders, p 192.)

FIGURE 53-20 Papular eczema. (From Callen JP et al: *Color atlas of dermatology,* Philadelphia, 1993, Saunders, p 192.)

FIGURE 53-21 Chronic eczema of the feet. (From Callen JP et al: *Color atlas of dermatology,* Philadelphia, 1993, Saunders, p 192.)

high concentration of the irritating agent. Some of the more active irritants are acids, alkalis, and hydrocarbons.

Allergic contact dermatitis indicates delayed acquired hypersensitivity to a specific allergen. Dermatologic problems may appear after years of asymptomatic exposure to the precipitating agent. Chromates, nickel, ethylenediamine, paraphenylenediamine, neomycin, formaldehyde, and lanolin components may cause allergic contact dermatitis.

Aside from reactions to various industrial chemicals, the most common type of allergic contact dermatitis reaction is to plants. **Rhus dermatitis** encompasses allergy to poison ivy, poison oak, and poison sumac. Clinically, rhus dermatitis begins within 48 hours of contact. The first symptom is pruritus, followed by erythema and vesicle formation, sometimes in linear fashion (Figure 53-22). As long as the allergen remains on the surface of the skin, it can be spread to nonexposed areas. Therefore, thorough washing can help prevent spread by hand contact. Exposure to blister fluid does not spread poison ivy lesions.

Treatment. Contact dermatitis from exposure to poison ivy can range from mild to severe. For the mildest cases, application of topical steroids or cooling shake lotions of camphor and menthol may effectively decrease discomfort. Severe cases may require hospitalization for cooling baths and wet dressings, which dry the lesions and decrease the tense, pruritic blisters. Discomfort and generalized edema often respond to systemic steroids administered over a 10- to 14-day period.

Drug Eruptions

Etiology and Clinical Manifestations. Adverse or undesirable reactions to medically administered drugs are common, yet cutaneous reactions are uncommon (0.1%) within the overall prescription-taking population.[15] Cutaneous reactions to medication usually begin within a week of drug exposure,

FIGURE 53-22 Rhus dermatitis with the characteristic linear groups of vesicles. (From Berger TG et al: *Andrews' diseases of the skin: clinical dermatology,* ed 9, Philadelphia, 2000, Saunders, p 101.)

FIGURE 53-23 Fixed-drug eruption. An early lesion may be manifested as an urticarial plaque. This lesion frequently resolves with macular hyperpigmentation. (From Callen JP et al: *Color atlas of dermatology,* ed 2, Philadelphia, 2000, Saunders, p 217.)

although reactions to penicillins may occur later. Women experience more cutaneous drug eruptions than men do. The drugs that most frequently result in adverse cutaneous eruptions are ampicillin, penicillin, cephalosporins, and barbiturates. Blood transfusions also occasionally produce cutaneous reactions identical to a drug eruption.

The most common type of adverse cutaneous drug eruption is an erythematous maculopapular exanthem (rash). These often pruritic lesions are usually widely dispersed, and clearing is gradual and continues for several weeks after the drug has been discontinued. Other common drug reactions include urticaria, erythema multiforme (including Stevens-Johnson syndrome), exfoliative dermatitis, photosensitivity, vasculitis, and fixed-drug eruption.

Exanthem-type eruptions can be caused by such medications as barbiturates, griseofulvin, penicillin, thiazides, and sulfonamides. Urticarial eruptions may result from the use of barbiturates, penicillin, chloramphenicol, phenolphthalein, salicylates, sulfonamides, or tetracycline. Erythema multiforme is seen with erythromycin, penicillin, phenolphthalein, salicylate, diphenylhydantoin, and thiazides. Exfoliative dermatitis can be caused by barbiturates, gold, penicillin, phenothiazides, and sulfonamides, and photosensitivity is seen with chlordiazepoxide, fluoroquinolones, griseofulvin, phenothiazines, sulfonamides, tetracycline, and thiazides. Cutaneous vasculitis may be triggered by iodines, erythromycin, penicillin, quinidine, sulfonamides, and thiazides. Fixed-drug eruption (Figure 53-23) is a round to oval, violaceous macule or slightly palpable plaque that is often recurrent, especially in previously affected sites, on re-exposure to the irritating medication. This effect can be caused by barbiturates, gold, phenolphthalein, sulfonamides, and tetracycline. These drug lists are not inclusive, and several substances are known to cause multiple adverse cutaneous reactions.[16]

Treatment. Management of drug eruptions includes discontinuation of the offending drug and administration of oral antihistamines and antipruritic lotions of hydrocortisone, menthol, camphor, or other proven substances for relief of pruritus. For more severe eruptions, a 2- to 3-week course of systemic corticosteroids should be considered. In addition, the patient should be counseled regarding use of the offending medication and an appropriate notation placed in the patient's medical record.

Vasculitis

Etiology. When antigen and antibody react in blood vessels in the skin, severe **necrotizing inflammation (vasculitis)** can appear. This condition can be caused by drug allergies; disorders such as SLE, rheumatoid arthritis, and glomerulonephritis; and certain infectious diseases such as hepatitis B. **Polyarteritis nodosa** is a form of systemic vasculitis that can cause inflamed arteries in visceral organs, brain, and skin.

Treatment. Immunofluorescent studies reveal antigens and serum immunoglobulins trapped in the wall of the blood vessel that is inflamed by neutrophils. Acute vasculitis can cause damage not only to skin but also to the brain and visceral organs. When the vasculitis is severe, systemic corticosteroids may be administered in high doses.

PARASITIC INFESTATIONS

Scabies. *Sarcoptes scabiei* is a mite, and infestation with this mite in humans is called **scabies.** Scabies begins with eggs laid in the stratum corneum. These eggs hatch into larvae within 3 to 4 days and grow to adulthood within 2 months. Scabies is usually contracted after close personal contact with an infested individual.

Clinically, scabies lesions are small (1 to 4 mm) erythematous papules, some with an overlying dry scale or crust (Figure 53-24). In some cases, linear burrows are seen. Scabies mites have a predilection for the finger webs, wrists, umbilicus, and groin area. The history related by most patients is an intensely pruritic eruption that spreads over a period of weeks from a single area of the body to other areas.

Scabies treatment consists of topical permethrin cream (Elimite), γ-benzene hexachloride (Lindane), or crotamiton (Eurax). For infants, 5% to 6% precipitated sulfur in petrolatum applied twice daily for a week is usually adequate.

Fleas. Three types of flea commonly bite and cause cutaneous reactions in humans: the human flea *(Pulex irritans)*, the cat flea *(Ctenocephalides felis)*, and the dog flea *(Ctenocephalides canis)*. Flea bites may appear as small erythematous macules, erythematous papules, wheals, or a vesicle (Figure 53-25).

Diethyltoluamide or pyrethrin insect repellents are effective in preventing flea infestation. Indoor carpeting, an ideal environment for fleas, should be treated with an appropriate insecticide.

The milder papular form of flea bites can be managed with soothing shake lotions of menthol and camphor or with topical steroids. More severe reactions (e.g., vesicles or bullae) may require a course of systemic steroids.

Lice. *Phthirus pubis* (crab lice), *Pediculus humanus* var. *capitis* (head lice), and *Pediculus humanus* var. *corporis* (body lice) are the types of lice most often found on humans. They are surface dwelling, unlike the burrowing scabies mite, and they usually can be seen without magnification. Control and

FIGURE 53-24 A, Scabies. **B,** An extremely pruritic infestation. **C,** Crusted (Norwegian) scabies. **(A,** From Callen JP et al: *Color atlas of dermatology,* ed 2, Philadelphia, 2000, Saunders, pp 170, 283.)

FIGURE 53-25 Insect bites (fleas) led this patient to scratch. (From Swartz MH: *Physical diagnosis, history and examination,* ed 4, Philadelphia, 2002, Saunders, p 163.)

eradication are possible with one of the following: permethrin cream rinse or pyrethrin and piperonyl butoxide liquid, gel, or shampoo.

Chiggers. Chiggers are mites that reside in grass and bushes. They are common in the southern United States but can be found as far north as Canada. Puncture of the skin by the mite to obtain nourishment produces pruritic papules commonly seen wherever it encounters resistance, such as the top of socks, at the belt line, or around the neckband area (Figure 53-26). Secondary lesions are excoriations from scratching that have become infected by bacteria. Treatment is palliative, and the use of insect repellent is encouraged for prevention.

Bedbugs. The common bedbug, *Cimex lectularius,* is a reddish brown insect 3 to 6 mm long that turns purple after feeding. Like most parasites, bedbugs feed on human blood. Importantly, they can also alternate between human and animal hosts, and they live up to and sometimes beyond 1 year.[8] When not feeding, bedbugs stay hidden in the cracks and crevices of furniture, mattresses, wallpaper, picture frames, baseboards, flooring, door locks, or any darkened area. Unless their source is eliminated, recurrence is inevitable. Professional extermination is advised because of their many hiding places. Bedbugs have been known to feed on animal populations when forced from their living quarters. On rehabitation in the same quarters, the bedbug can easily return to human hosts.

They are nocturnal feeders, and, when crushed, they emit a foul odor. The bedbug bite is painless and produces a pruritic oval or oblong wheal with a small hemorrhagic punctum at the center. Bullous lesions are not uncommon. Usually, lesions are multiple and arranged in rows or clusters on the face, neck, hands, and arms. No area is exempt. The wheal is probably a type 1 sensitivity reaction to the anticoagulant saliva of the bedbug. Secondary excoriation and bacterial infections may occur.

The diagnosis depends on the time of the day when the lesions appear. Because of the painless bite, it is not uncommon

FIGURE 53-26 Chigger bites. (From Berger HL et al: *Andrews' diseases of the skin: clinical dermatology,* ed 9, Philadelphia, 2000, Saunders, p 569.)

for the victim to awake with one or several pruritic papules. Topical antipruritics are used as treatment.

Mosquitoes. Most people have experienced mosquitoes and are familiar with their bites. The typical lesion is a raised wheal on an erythematous base, accompanied by pruritus within 45 minutes of the bite. A second type of reaction is the delayed response. Eight to 12 hours after the bite, the lesion becomes raised, erythematous, and indurated, with extensive pruritus or pain. This reaction peaks 24 hours to 72 hours after the bite.[9] The saliva of the mosquito is believed to be the source of the skin reaction. Although severe skin reactions are possible, they are rare. Insect repellents are recommended for prevention; local antipruritics are used for treatment.

Blood Flukes. Bathers in the freshwater lakes of Wisconsin, Michigan, and Minnesota are prone to periodic attacks of inflammatory, papular, urticarial, and vesicular eruptions on the uncovered areas of the body, mainly the legs. This pruritic eruption, commonly called "swimmer's itch," usually subsides within a week and is caused by invasion of the skin by cercariae (larvae) of the schistosomes (worms) of ducks and mammals. The life cycle of these various species of schistosomes includes the snail as an intermediate host. On invasion of the abnormal definitive host, the human skin, the cercariae die, and the resulting skin eruption is the skin's reaction in ridding itself of the foreign bodies. Repeated attacks are met with stronger resistance, and the dermatitis becomes increasingly severe. Secondary infection, edema, and lymphangitis can occur.

Swimmer's itch is best prevented by destruction of the snails through careful addition of a combination of copper sulfate and hydrated lime to the lake water. Rapid drying of the swimmer with a towel apparently prevents penetration of the cercariae. Active therapy is directed to relief of the itching and prevention of secondary infection.

Ticks. Ticks are insects that live in woods and underbrush. They attach to human and animal hosts and burrow in the epidermis, where they feed on blood. The tick bite itself is not problematic, but the infectious bacteria or viruses that ticks carry to human hosts create problems. Many tick-borne illnesses are known, including Central European encephalitis, Q fever, babesiasis, relapsing fever, Rocky Mountain spotted fever (RMSF), and Lyme disease. Both RMSF and Lyme disease are relatively common in the United States.

Rocky Mountain Spotted Fever

Etiology, Pathogenesis, Clinical Manifestations. **Rocky Mountain spotted fever** is caused by a tick that carries *Rickettsia rickettsii*. In the past RMSF was localized to the Rocky Mountain area, but by 1982 most states had reported a case of RMSF.[8]

The initial tick bite appears as a papule or macule, with or without a central punctate area. The tick burrows in and enlarges as it feeds. The tick must be attached to the human host for 4 to 6 hours before the rickettsiae are activated by the blood.[8] Rickettsiae are found in the tick feces and body parts. The rickettsiae then enter the bloodstream and multiply in body tissues. Within 4 to 8 days the patient experiences fever, headache, muscle aches, nausea, and vomiting.[8] A rash then appears on the wrist or ankle. The characteristic rash is a macular or maculopapular one that spreads to the rest of the body. Other symptoms include generalized edema, conjunctivitis, petechial lesions, photophobia, lethargy, confusion, and cranial nerve deficits.

Treatment. Treatment for RMSF requires hospitalization and antibiotic therapy. The most important measure is to prevent tick bites by using insect repellents while engaged in activities in the woods. Once a tick has attached itself, it is important to remove all the body parts to limit the possibility of infection. One can remove ticks by dousing them with mineral oil or alcohol before slowly pulling them out with tweezers. The practice of applying a hot match to the end of the tick is not an effective method for removal because the tick may regurgitate into the open wound.[8]

Lyme Disease

Etiology. Lyme disease is caused by the bite of a tick that carries the spirochete *Borrelia burgdorferi*. White-tailed deer and white-footed mice are the main reservoirs of this disease-causing spirochete. Lyme disease causes multiple symptoms affecting the skin, nervous system, heart, and musculoskeletal system.

Pathogenesis, Clinical Manifestations, and Treatment. The disease has three clinical stages. Stage I usually occurs in the summer and early fall with single or multiple erythematous papules that may itch, sting, or burn. The thighs, groin, and axillae are particularly common sites of involvement. This disease is often accompanied by flulike symptoms (fatigue,

headache, chills, fever, sore throat, stiff neck, nausea, myalgias, and arthralgias). If the patient remains untreated, stage II Lyme disease appears weeks to months later. This stage is characterized by meningitis, cranial nerve palsies, and peripheral neuropathy; occasionally, cardiac involvement is noted. In stage III, oligoarticular arthritis occurs. In early Lyme disease, treatment includes antibiotic therapy such as doxycycline, amoxicillin, or erythromycin for 10 to 21 days. Neurologic disease, arthritis, or cardiac disease is managed with doxycycline or amoxicillin for 1 month or with intravenous penicillin for 10 to 14 days.

OTHER DISORDERS OF THE DERMIS

Scleroderma. **Scleroderma** is characterized by massive collagen deposition with fibrosis accompanied by inflammatory reactions and vascular changes in the capillary network. The process by which these changes occur is not known but may represent an autoimmune mechanism or primary vasculopathy.

The two forms of scleroderma, localized and diffuse, are clinically dissimilar except for some common skin histopathologic features. Localized scleroderma (morphea) is a benign disease; diffuse scleroderma (progressive systemic sclerosis) is serious, progressive, and fatal.

Localized Scleroderma. Localized scleroderma has an unknown etiology, no systemic involvement, and no known treatment. Disability is confined to the area involved. Lesions tend to involute (shrivel) slowly and spontaneously. Relapses are rare. Primary skin lesions are single or multiple, violet colored, firm, inelastic macules and plaques that enlarge slowly. The progressing border retains a violet hue while the center becomes whitish and slightly depressed beneath the skin surface. Bizarre lesions occur, such as long linear bands on extremities, "saber cut" lesions in scalp, or lesions involving one side of the face or the body. Secondary lesions include mild or severe scarring after healing, permanent hair loss from the scalp lesions, and, rarely, ulceration. The trunk, extremities, and head are most frequently involved (Figure 53-27).

Diffuse Scleroderma. Diffuse scleroderma is a rare systemic collagen disease of unknown cause characterized by a long course of progressive disability resulting from lack of mobility of the areas and the organs affected. The skin becomes hardened like hide, the esophagus and the gastrointestinal tract semirigid, the lungs and the heart fibrosed, the bones resorbed, and the overlying tissue calcified. Figure 53-28 illustrates the "hidelike" skin on the face of a woman with diffuse scleroderma.

Another rare collagen disorder, **dermatomyositis**, is characterized by the acute or insidious onset of muscle pain, weakness, fever, arthralgia, and, in some cases, a puffy erythematous eruption that is usually confined to the face and the eyelids. Progression of the disease results in muscle atrophy and contractures, skin telangiectasias (vascular lesions formed by blood vessel dilation) and atrophy, and generalized organ involvement. Death occurs in 50% of cases.[12,17]

Sunburn and Photosensitivity

Effects of Sunlight

Sunlight is an extremely harmful environmental agent because it produces the short ultraviolet wavelength that is responsible for sunburn, thickening of the stratum corneum, suntan, and increased melanin production. Sunlight produces direct local effects on the skin in the form of elastotic

FIGURE 53-27 Extensive morphea (localized scleroderma). (From Berger TG et al: *Andrews' diseases of the skin: clinical dermatology,* ed 9, Philadelphia, 2000, Saunders, p 195.)

syndromes, keratoacanthomas, premalignant diseases, basal cell epitheliomas, and squamous cell epitheliomas. Both indirect and direct effects can produce malignant melanomas.[18]

Sunburn is initially manifested as erythema, pain, heat, and occasionally blistering, edema, and tenderness. In severe sunburn, these symptoms may also be accompanied by the constitutional symptoms of chills, fever, nausea, and generalized discomfort.

The most effective treatment is to avoid or limit exposure to sunlight. Wearing protective clothing is effective; sunscreens are also quite useful in preventing sunburn and the chronic solar changes of the skin. Para-aminobenzoic acid is the most widely used sunscreen. People sensitive to para-aminobenzoic acid may use cinnamates and benzophenones as substitutes. Opaque screens such as zinc oxide and titanium dioxide also work well. However, these white preparations are not cosmetically elegant. Recently, titanium dioxide has been incorporated into foundation makeup for women.

Sunburn can be managed symptomatically with cold water baths or compresses; topical steroids are often effective in relieving the discomfort of localized severe burns. For widespread sunburn, a 10- to 14-day course of systemic steroids may suppress the symptoms.

Ulcers

An unfortunate problem for a bedridden person may be the development of **pressure sores,** or **decubitus ulcers.** Because thinning epithelial cells and blood vessels have a slower rate of repair, the incidence of decubitus ulcers is higher and the ulcer more severe in the elderly, and healing of damaged skin is slower.

Pressure sores are localized areas of cellular necrosis resulting from prolonged pressure between any bony prominence and an external object such as a bed or wheelchair. The tissues are deprived of blood supply and eventually die. Areas frequently affected in older persons include the heels, greater trochanter, sacrum, dorsal (especially in thin kyphotic persons) and scapular regions of the spine, and elbows.

FIGURE 53-28 Hidelike skin on the face of a woman with diffuse scleroderma (progressive systemic sclerosis). (From Berger TG et al: *Andrews' diseases of the skin: clinical dermatology,* ed 9, Philadelphia, 2000, Saunders, p 197.)

TABLE 53-5

Clinical Description of Pressure Sores

Grade/Stage	Description
1	Acute inflammatory response primarily in the epidermis with minimal soft-tissue swelling and warmth; erythema of intact skin; it is erythematous and, unless abraded, the erythema will blanch; blanchable erythema (reactive hyperemia) can be expected to be present for 30 to 45 minutes following exposure to pressure; it is usually very discretely bordered; reversible with intervention
2	Pressure sore representing an inflammatory and fibroblastic response extending through the epidermis into the dermis; there is partial thickness or superficial skin loss involving the epidermis and/or the dermis; it may present as blistering with erythema and/or induration; the ulcer may also present as an abrasion or shallow crater; the wound base is moist and pink; the wound is painful but free of necrotic tissue
3	Pressure sore clearly penetrating the subcutaneous layers; often there is exposed muscle, fat, and tendons; the full-thickness tissue loss extends through the dermis to involve the subcutaneous tissue; damage or necrosis of dermis may extend down to, but not through, underlying fascia; the ulcer presents clinically as a deep crater with or without undermining of adjacent tissue; this stage may also include sinus tract formation, exudates, and/or infection; the wound base is usually painful
4	Pressure sore extending beyond the deep fascia, almost always to the bone; deep-tissue destruction occurs, extending through the subcutaneous tissue and fascia; there is full-thickness skin loss with extensive tissue necrosis and damage to muscle, bone, and supporting structures (tendons and joint capsules); undermining sinus infection may be present; the wound base is usually not painful

Long-term pressure increases vulnerability to decubitus ulcer development. High pressure maintained for a short time is less dangerous than low pressure continued for a long time. Predisposing factors include poor nutrition, aging, immobility, superficial sensory loss, and disturbed autonomic function (loss of bowel and bladder control).[19] Older people with dementia are particularly prone to the development of pressure sores because of arteriosclerotic changes in the vessels, loss of subcutaneous tissue and tissue elasticity, and clouding of the sensorium.[19]

Pressure sores can be evaluated clinically using the staging system described in Table 53-5. Pressure sores are superficial (benign) or deep (malignant). Superficial sores are reddened areas involving only the outer skin layers. They are less dangerous than deep sores and are caused by friction, shearing stresses, trauma, infection, and saturation with urine or other wet agents. The lesions are frequently painful but are easily treated and prevented. Treatment consists of keeping the area clean, dry, and free from infection or further pressure; a covering with a nonstick dressing also promotes healing. Measures such as frequent turning (every 2 hours), getting the person out of bed and into a chair, keeping the vulnerable areas clean and dry, and keeping the weight of the bed coverings off the feet are most effective in warding off superficial pressure sores.

Deep sores develop quickly as a result of thrombosis of the vessels in deep tissue overlying bony prominences. Muscle and fat layers are more vulnerable than the dermis, and involvement of these layers causes deep, large ulcers. The sore begins as a reddening of the skin with unobservable necrosis in the deep underlying tissue. In 1 to 2 days, the lesion bursts through the skin like an abscess to reveal a deep cavity full of black or infected slough, which may go through to the bone.[19]

BOX 53-1

Prevention of Deep Pressure Sores

Change position every 2 hours.
Do not oversedate or undersedate.
Avoid or correct malnutrition.
Avoid dehydration; maintain blood pressure and cardiac output.
Use an alternating-pressure airbed or waterbed.

Data from Rosen T et al, editors: *Nurse's atlas of dermatology,* Boston, 1981, Little, Brown.

Skin loss from such a large area results in extensive scarring. The appearance of deep pressure sores with an illness can delay recovery and may even be fatal.

Prevention is more difficult with deep pressure sores, especially in the elderly. The risk of these lesions developing is greatest during the 10 days after the onset of illness or admission to the hospital, which coincides with the period of greatest immobility.[19] A deep sore that develops early and penetrates deeply is most dangerous to an older person. Early signs of deterioration include apathy, loss of appetite, and incontinence. Some measures that can help prevent deep pressure sores are described in Box 53-1.

Treatment consists primarily of reinforcing preventive measures, including maintenance of fluid and protein stores that are lost through serous and purulent discharge, repair of tissues by giving vitamin supplements, avoidance of general infections such as pneumonia or cystitis, and remediation of anemia. The lesions should be cleaned and dressed, with care taken to manage local infection. To promote granulation and healing, the wound should be irrigated with warm saline every day. Irrigation washes out the debris, reduces the growth of anaerobes, promotes separation of the slough, and decreases the pocketing of infection in deeper tissues. Infection must be eradicated and the slough must separate before healing can take place.

Altered Cell Growth
Epidermal Proliferation

Keratinocytes produce keratin. Rare, inherited defects in keratinocytes can occur, and the inherited disease **congenital ichthyosis** is characterized by an excessive growth of keratinocytes and keratin, which gives the skin a fish scale appearance (Figure 53-29).

Corns and **calluses** result from **hyperkeratosis.** Stimulation of the epidermis by intermittent pressure elicits hyperkeratosis (corn and callus formation). By contrast, *atrophy* of the epidermis can arise from a decreased blood supply.

Benign or malignant **neoplasms** commonly arise from keratinocytes. **Warts** (verrucae), for instance, are caused by a virus that provokes a benign proliferation of keratinocytes. **Squamous cell carcinomas** (arising from keratinocytes) often occur in areas of skin excessively exposed to sunlight.

Tumors. Each cell type of the skin can give rise to either benign or malignant tumors. Benign tumors, including squamous papillomas, arise from keratinocytes, common moles (**nevi**) arise from melanocytes, lipomas from adipose cells, vascular tumors (hemangiomas) from blood vessels, dermatofibromas from fibroblasts, and neuromas from nerves.

Kaposi sarcoma arises from reticulocytes and is multifocal, metastasizing, and malignant. Kaposi sarcoma is classified as an opportunistic neoplasm because it occurs in persons with pre-existing immunodeficiency: for example, individuals with primary immunodeficiency, those who undergo therapeutic immunosuppression, and persons with human immunodeficiency virus (HIV) infection. Figures 53-30 and 53-31 show some of the cutaneous diseases associated with HIV infection.

Cancer. Cancer of the skin is common. Most skin cancers are slowly progressive, but certain types can be rapidly lethal. Excessive exposure to sunlight by a person with fair skin often leads to skin cancer. In addition to sunlight, exposure to irritating chemicals, recurrent trauma, and irradiation are associated with a high risk of skin cancer.

Basal cell carcinomas are the most common skin tumors and the most benign[20] (Figure 53-32). Squamous cell carcinomas are the next most common malignancy[20] (Figure 53-33). They can occasionally metastasize. By contrast, melanoma is rare but can be highly malignant (Figure 53-34). Melanoma is notoriously unpredictable; however, the prognosis is based on size, depth of invasion of the tumor, and the presence of metastasis.[21] Lumps that increase rapidly in size, change color, ulcerate, or bleed should undergo biopsy and be examined microscopically to rule out malignancy. Complete surgical excision is the treatment of choice for skin cancers.

Pigmentation Alterations

Vitiligo. **Vitiligo** (**leukoderma**) is a condition in which pigment disappears from a patch of skin. The onset is sudden and may be associated with pernicious anemia, hyperthyroidism, and diabetes mellitus.

Vitiligo is a concern to darkly pigmented individuals of all races. It also affects light-skinned individuals, but not as often. The lesion is a depigmented patch with definite borders on the face, axillae, neck, or extremities (Figure 53-35). The borders are smooth. Size varies from small to large macules involving large areas of the skin surface. The large macular type is much more common. Depigmented areas, which burn in sunlight, appear bone colored or grayish blue.

Vitiligo appears at any age, in men and women alike, and usually occurs before the age of 21.[22] Its incidence has been increasing in India, Pakistan, and Far Eastern countries.[22] Although the cause is unknown, inheritance and autoimmune factors have been implicated. Affected areas spread over time.

Treatment may consist of various topical immunomodulating agents as well as the use of various types of ultraviolet light. Cosmetics such as Derma Blend may be used to camouflage the areas of depigmentation.

Albinism

Etiology and Pathogenesis. Melanocytes produce melanin. A partial or total absence of melanin arises as an inborn error in metabolism in individuals with **albinism.** Albinism, also

FIGURE 53-29 Ichthyosis. (From Callen JP et al: *Color atlas of dermatology,* ed 2, Philadelphia, 2000, Saunders, p 14. Courtesy Donald Hazelrigg, MD, Evansville, Ind.)

FIGURE 53-30 Cryptococcosis associated with HIV infection. (From Callen JP et al: *Color atlas of dermatology,* Philadelphia, 1993, Saunders, p 229.)

FIGURE 53-31 Seborrheic dermatitis associated with HIV infection. (From Callen JP et al: *Color atlas of dermatology,* Philadelphia, 1993, Saunders, p 372.)

FIGURE 53-32 Basal cell carcinoma. Notice the rolled, well-defined margin. (From Swartz MH: *Physical diagnosis, history and examination,* ed 4, Philadelphia, 2002, Saunders, p 144.)

termed *oculocutaneous albinism,* is characterized by a generalized lack of pigmentation of the skin and the hair. In addition, the eyes may show nystagmus and a lack of pigmentation of the fundi and translucent irises. The condition is recessively inherited. Biochemically, albinism occurs because of impaired or absent melanin synthesis. The long-term consequences of

albinism may include solar keratoses and basal and squamous cell cancers.

Education regarding the use of sunscreens and clothing for protection against ultraviolet light–induced damage is indicated. Sunglasses and magnifiers are beneficial for the ocular symptoms.

FIGURE 53-33 **A** and **B,** Squamous cell carcinomas. (From Callen JP et al: *Color atlas of dermatology,* ed 2, Philadelphia, 2000, Saunders, p 367.)

FIGURE 53-34 **A** and **C,** Superficial spreading malignant melanoma. **B,** Cross-section through a melanoma. Note the nests of melanoma cells in the dermis. (From Swartz MH: *Physical diagnosis, history and examination,* ed 4, Philadelphia, 2002, Saunders, p 145.)

FIGURE 53-35 Vitiligo. (From Callen JP et al: *Color atlas of dermatology,* ed 2, Philadelphia, 2000, Saunders, p 282.)

inflammation rather than cure. Antibiotics may be used to prevent or manage lesion superinfections.

- Skin allergies are associated with substances that cause erythema and itching. Atopic dermatitis (eczema), commonly seen in young children, may be aggravated by substances to which the individual is allergic. Contact dermatitis occurs in anyone coming in contact with a certain substance. Drug reactions are allergic responses manifested as widely dispersed, often pruritic rashes. Antigen-antibody reactions within cutaneous blood vessels can result in severe necrotizing vasculitis.
- The skin is subject to invasion by a number of different bugs, ticks, and parasites. Lesions tend to be singular or grouped and in areas exposed to the particular pest. Scabies commonly occurs on the hands and wrists and may appear as linear burrows. Bites from fleas, mites, bedbugs, and mosquitoes often induce pruritic macules or papules. Tick bites are usually painless but may be problematic because ticks may carry diseases such as RMSF and Lyme disease.
- Scleroderma is a collagen disease of unknown cause. It may be localized to the skin or produce systemic involvement. The skin is discolored, thick, and hardened.
- Ultraviolet rays in sunlight are associated with acute damage to the skin (sunburn) and also increase the long-term risk of skin cancer.
- Pressure ulcer is a significant problem of immobility caused by prolonged pressure on bony prominences. Superficial sores are reddened areas involving the outer skin layers. Deep sores are due to thrombosis of vessels deep in tissue. Deep sores may be unnoticed initially and then burst through the skin like an abscess.
- Abnormalities of skin cell growth may result in such benign processes as corns and calluses or the more serious consequence of cancer. Basal cell and squamous cell carcinomas are slowly progressive and generally amenable to surgical excision. Malignant melanoma is more prone to metastasis and carries a poorer prognosis.
- Abnormal pigmentation may occur in response to skin injury, infection, or inflammation or may be genetically determined. Albinism is due to lack of melanin production. Vitiligo is a depigmented patch of skin that is most noticeable in dark-skinned individuals. The cause of vitiligo is unknown.

KEY POINTS

- Skin infections may be caused by viral, fungal, or bacterial organisms.
- Viruses are associated with warts (human papillomavirus), cold sores (herpes simplex), and shingles (herpes zoster). Warts are painless. They may be surgically removed but often resolve spontaneously. Herpes simplex lesions are painful, may be managed symptomatically, and often recur in times of stress. Herpes zoster inhabits sensory dorsal ganglia neurons and causes pain along a dermatome.
- Superficial fungal infections (tinea, ringworm) are often characterized by central clearing and peripheral scaling. They may be effectively managed with topical antifungals. Yeast infections tend to occur in moist areas such as mucous membranes and are managed with systemic or topical drugs.
- Impetigo is caused by staphylococcal or streptococcal infection and is characterized by yellowish pustules and crusts. It responds to antibiotic therapy.
- The cause of noninfectious inflammatory diseases is usually unknown. Lupus erythematosus, seborrheic dermatitis, psoriasis, lichen planus, pityriasis rosea, and acne are in this category. Treatment is aimed at reducing

SPECIAL CHARACTERISTICS OF DARK SKIN

A number of disorders of the skin exclusively affect people with dark skin. Pigmentary disturbances from many causes, both hypopigmentation and hyperpigmentation, are common. Postinflammatory hyperpigmentation, for example, may occur in African-American individuals when melanocytes are stimulated by inflammation. Hyperpigmentation in any person with dark skin can occur after traumatic injury, skin infection, or inflammatory skin disease. Patchy areas of

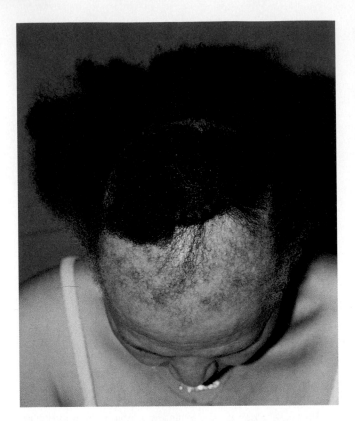

FIGURE 53-36 Traction alopecia from tight braiding and use of a hot comb. (From Callen JP et al: *Color atlas of dermatology,* Philadelphia, 1993, Saunders, p 363.)

FIGURE 53-37 Hot comb damage resulting in scarring alopecia. (From Callen JP et al: *Color atlas of dermatology,* Philadelphia, 1993, Saunders, p 366.)

depigmentation (vitiligo), described earlier, are more noticeable in persons with dark skin because of the color contrast. Some lesions, such as those causing erythema, may show no visible color change in darkly pigmented individuals. For example, petechiae, which cause pinpoint purplish red lesions, are usually observable only on the oral mucosa or conjunctiva.

Disorders such as seborrheic dermatitis and keloids are seen with greater frequency in African Americans.[23] The custom of tightly plaiting the hair or using hot oil and tension on the scalp leads to gradual damage to hair follicles, hair thinning, and, eventually, hair loss. Known as **traumatic alopecia,** this condition is also seen with greater frequency in African Americans (Figures 53-36 and 53-37).

Conversely, many skin disorders that affect light-skinned people, such as squamous cell or basal cell carcinoma, senile keratoses, and psoriasis, only rarely affect darker-skinned persons.

Psoriasis is rare among the African-American population. If present, it may be difficult to detect. The typical bright red color is not present. The plaques assume a blue or violet hue because of stimulation of melanocytes. The characteristic silvery scale is often absent.

Literature related specifically to abnormalities of dark skin is also rare. Normal variants such as the Mongolian spot in infants, Futcher or Voigt lines, and linear nail pigmentation are frequently mistaken for disorders. Box 53-2 presents tips for assessing dark skin.

KEY POINTS

- Certain skin disorders are manifested differently or appear in greater or lesser frequency in individuals with dark skin. Normal variants such as the Mongolian spot in infants, Futcher or Voigt lines, and linear nail pigmentation are frequently mistaken for disorders.
- Disorders such as seborrheic dermatitis and keloids are seen more often in African Americans.
- Traumatic alopecia occurs more often in African Americans because of tight plaiting of the hair or the use of hot oil and tension on the scalp.
- Squamous cell or basal cell carcinoma, senile keratoses, and psoriasis only rarely affect darker-skinned persons.

BOX 53-2

Tips for Assessing Dark Skin

Skin color should be observed in the sclerae, conjunctivae, buccal mucosa, tongue, lips, nail beds, palms, and soles.

Inspection should be accompanied by palpation, especially if inflammation or edema is suspected.

Findings should always be correlated with the patient's history to arrive at a diagnosis.

Pallor in brown-skinned patients may appear as a yellowish brown tinge to the skin. In a black-skinned patient the skin will appear ash gray. Pallor can be difficult to determine. In dark-skinned individuals it is characterized by absence of the underlying red tones in the skin.

Jaundice may be observed in the sclera but should not be confused with the normal yellow-pigmented sclera of a dark-skinned black patient. The best place to inspect is in the portion of the sclera that is observable when the eye is open. If jaundice is suspected, the posterior portion of the hard palate should also be observed for a yellowish cast, which is most effective when done in bright daylight.

The *oral mucosa* of dark-skinned individuals may have a normal freckling of pigmentation that may also be evident on the gums, the borders of the tongue, and the lining of the cheeks. The gingiva may normally have a dark blue color that may appear blotchy or be evenly distributed.

Petechiae are best observed over areas of lighter pigmentation — the abdomen, gluteal areas, and volar aspect of the forearm. They may also be seen in the palpebral conjunctiva and buccal mucosa.

To differentiate petechiae and ecchymosis from erythema, remember that pressure over the area will cause erythema to blanch but will not affect either petechiae or ecchymosis.

Erythema is usually associated with increased skin temperature, so palpation should also be used if an inflammatory condition is suspected.

Edema may reduce the intensity of the color of an area of skin because of the increased distance between the external epithelium and the pigmented layers. Therefore, darker skin would appear lighter. On palpation the skin may feel "tight."

Cyanosis can be difficult to determine in dark-skinned individuals. Familiarity with the precyanotic color is often helpful. However, if it is not possible to determine cyanosis from the skin, close inspection of the nail beds, lips, palpebral conjunctiva, palms, and soles should show evidence of cyanosis.

Rashes may be assessed by palpating for changes in skin texture.

Integumentary Manifestations of Systemic Disease

The skin reflects the status of many organ systems. For example, the endocrine, cardiovascular, renal, respiratory, and hepatic systems all have possible dermal manifestations. Metabolic disorders and internal malignancies also cause cutaneous alterations. Certainly, skin manifestations of internal malignancy can be obvious. The late-appearing features of **cachexia** (wasting), pallor, and cutaneous metastases are obvious signs of malignancy. Abnormalities in endocrine function also produce a myriad of cutaneous changes. In general, systemic disease states are expressed through altered color, sensation, texture, and temperature of the skin; altered growth, texture, color, and lubrication of the hair; and changes in nail shape, color, and texture.

Skin

Color

Color changes in the skin can signal the presence of systemic disease. The entire color spectrum (red, orange, yellow, green, blue, indigo, and violet) is represented through possible coloration changes in the skin.

Redness (**erythema**) may be generalized, as with carbon monoxide poisoning, or localized, as with rashes or on the palms. Although erythema is often visible in lighter-skinned individuals, it may be less apparent in those whose skin is dark; however, the affected part may become an even deeper shade of brown. Redness may accompany inflammation.

When inflammation is suspected in a dark-skinned person, other parameters can be assessed by palpation, among them increased skin temperature, tight skin suggestive of edema, induration of deep tissue or blood vessels, and tenderness. Because the dorsal skin surface of the fingers is more sensitive to subtle skin temperature differences than the palmar surface is, the examiner should use the dorsal portion of the fingers to move from one skin area to another for comparison. The patient's family and friends are also helpful in validating color change, particularly when it has occurred gradually.

Orange discoloration can occur from the deposition of carotene. Protein-calorie malnutrition can cause hypopigmentation in African-American children, with the hair and skin appearing orange.

Yellow discoloration can occur locally when lipids are deposited in skin secondary to a metabolic defect in blood lipids. More commonly, a generalized yellow (jaundiced) appearance arises because of liver disease. Bilirubin accumulates in blood and saturates the tissues. **Jaundice** is observed in the usual sites (e.g., mucous membranes, nail beds). Because many factors can alter these findings, one single positive finding should not be held as conclusive. Other parameters, such as environmental temperature, drugs, smoking, amount of hemoglobin, and the color of urine or stool, can support a description of cyanosis or jaundice. In both dark-skinned and light-skinned individuals, yellow sclerae may indicate jaundice, but other factors can cause yellow scleral pigmentation; fatty deposits that contain carotene are a common finding in dark-skinned individuals. To determine whether the yellow sclerae signify jaundice, observe the hard palate in bright daylight. Jaundice can be detected there quite early (i.e., when serum bilirubin is 2 to 4 mg/100 ml) if the palate does not have heavy melanin pigmentation.[24] If the hard palate does not show jaundice when the sclerae are yellow, the pigmentation may be due to some other factor, such as carotene accumulation. All these factors support the importance of repeated observation and accurate description of what is seen. As often as possible, the same individual should perform the entire examination and confirm specific findings in one area with additional data from other areas.

When jaundice is severe, **biliverdin** also accumulates. A person with obstructed bile ducts can become green-yellow because of biliverdin.

Blueness of the skin (**cyanosis**) often occurs on the tips of the fingers, toes, nose, and lips in individuals with cardiac or respiratory problems that prevent oxygenation of blood. Localized blueness with pain of the fingers on exposure to cold is termed *Raynaud disease.* It frequently arises from cryoglobulins, which solidify in the cold, and is also associated with disorders of the immune system, such as lymphoma and acquired immunodeficiency syndrome.[25]

Indigo discoloration occurs locally, as in gangrene of the toes from severe generalized arteriosclerosis. The skin can darken from increased melanin synthesis, as in chronic adrenal insufficiency. Also, silver poisoning can make the skin dusky. Violet-colored palms (palmar erythema) can be seen in some individuals with liver disease and occasionally in pregnant women as a response to hyperestrogenism.

Shades of violet occur on the legs as a result of vascular insufficiency or when cardiopulmonary function is compromised.

The primary sites for assessing skin **pallor** are the nail beds, lips, and conjunctivae. When observing the lower eyelid (inferior palpebral conjunctiva) for pallor, the examiner should lower the lid sufficiently to see the conjunctiva near not only the outer canthus but also the inner canthus because the former is often darker. Greater perception is necessary when assessing a darkly pigmented individual for pallor because the changes are subtle. Red tones may be absent; a brown-skinned person may appear more yellowish brown, and a black-skinned person may appear ash gray. This variability supports the need for accurate baseline data for comparison.

Sensation

Sensory innervation is generally responsible for the itching (**pruritis**) and **pain** that accompany most skin diseases. *Itching* is often the initial symptom in such conditions as atopic eczema, allergic contact dermatitis, scabies, dermatophytosis, psoriasis, and varicella. It can also be associated with systemic disorders, including carcinoma, diabetes, thyroid disease, uremia, and obstructive biliary disease. Other dermatologic conditions, such as herpes simplex, aphthous stomatitis, herpes zoster, furuncles, and cellulitis, produce considerable *pain.*

Texture

Normal aging produces an alteration in the texture of skin. Loose and wrinkled skin that lacks tone may also indicate **dehydration** (an abnormal finding). Dehydration may also be

apparent through inspection of the oral cavity. On inspection, a dry, leathery appearance of the tongue is *not* a reliable indicator of dehydration inasmuch as mouth breathing frequently makes the tongue look dry even when the individual is well hydrated. A more reliable method of assessing hydration of the oral cavity is to palpate the mucous membranes along the area of the gum and cheek where the membranes approximate. If the membranes are dry and the finger does not slide easily, dehydration is evident.

To evaluate **fluid excess,** palpate the skin over the hands, feet, ankles, and sacrum. If the skin is firm and indents easily (pitting edema) on moderate pressure from the fingertips, fluid excess is present.

Feeling the deeper portions of the skin may reveal areas of **induration** (hardness) such as those resulting from multiple intramuscular or subcutaneous injections of medication. **Lipodystrophies** consist of smooth, large depressions in the skin that indicate atrophy of the subcutaneous fat layer, which has a spongy consistency. Both induration and lipodystrophy are often seen at sites of repeated insulin injections.

Temperature

If the skin feels warm and dry in a person who is febrile (feverish), the blood temperature is probably rising, an indication that the thermoregulatory mechanism of sweating may not be functioning. Likewise, if the skin is warm and wet, the temperature can be expected to fall owing to the cooling mechanism of sweating.

Sweating can also occur when the blood glucose concentration falls rapidly with a resultant rise in the blood epinephrine level. Hypoglycemic sweating can usually be distinguished from other causes of sweating because of the additional symptoms of weakness, tachycardia, hunger, headache, and "inward nervousness" manifested as mental irritability and confusion.

Because skin temperature depends on the amount of blood circulating through the dermis, decreased localized blood flow (resulting in coolness), often to the feet, may indicate a peripheral vascular dysfunction. Generalized skin coolness may indicate decreased metabolism such as that occurring after general anesthesia. If the temperature is very low, signs of shock may be evident.

On the other hand, an increase in skin temperature may indicate a **hypermetabolic state,** such as that occurring in hyperthyroidism and after sun exposure or sunburn.

Hair

Disturbances in body function are often reflected in changes in growth pattern, amount, texture, color, and lubrication of the hair.

Growth

The high speed of growth of the scalp hair makes it more susceptible to damage from systemic disease, toxic drugs, radiation, and stress. The rate of growth varies with general health and age, and hair growth is dependent on circulating hormonal factors (primarily testicular or adrenal androgens). Thus hormonal imbalances or shifts (e.g., those accompanying childbirth) may also result in disturbances in the hair growth cycle. Nutritional factors, although often promoted in the nonmedical literature, have little effect on hair growth except in cases of severe malnutrition.

Amount

Alterations in the amount of body hair can be extremely anxiety provoking for both males and females. In females with hypertrichosis, or **hirsutism,** hair growth is intensified on the upper lip, chin, cheeks, and chest, around the nipples, and from the pubic crest to the umbilicus (along the linea alba); the downy hair on the arms, legs, and back becomes coarse. The pubic hair often takes on the upright triangular distribution typical of the male as opposed to the female's usual inverted triangle. An endocrine malfunction such as excess androgen production may sometimes be associated with hirsutism, but the ethnic background (Mediterranean groups predominantly) may also be responsible for the excessive hair growth. This propensity is especially true of the hair on the arms, legs, back, and face. Other ethnic group members such as full-blooded African-American females and male Native Americans rarely have facial hair. Distribution of the hair in family members and ethnic background are thus important considerations in ascertaining hair growth.

Hypertrichosis lanuginosa is typically a congenital, autosomal dominant disorder in which excessive hair is distributed over the entire body throughout life. The condition is usually associated with other congenital anomalies such as spina bifida.[26] In some cases, such as with certain internal carcinomas, hypertrichosis lanuginosa is an acquired disorder; the degree of hairiness is variable and usually involves the face.

Color

Perhaps the most common color change in the hair is the generalized graying that accompanies the aging process.

Texture

Normal aging also produces a decrease in hair thickness.

Disturbances of the thickness of scalp hair are common. Baldness (**alopecia**) or thinning of the hair that is generalized or creates a receding hairline is often genetically determined (Figure 53-38). Some rare genetic defects in the hair shaft itself may produce breaking of the hairs and be erroneously diagnosed as alopecia. Generalized and localized baldness may result from treatment modalities such as radiation therapy or chemotherapy. In addition, various types of scalp diseases (e.g., fungal, lupus) and telogen effluvium (transient hair loss occurring 2 to 3 months after general anesthesia, febrile illness, or giving birth) can cause hair loss. Other traumatic types of hair loss may result from pulling of the hair because of a nervous habit, hair styles such as tight braids or ponytails, or wearing of constrictive apparel such as a hat.

FIGURE 53-38 Male pattern baldness (androgenetic alopecia) in a woman. (From Callen JP et al: *Color atlas of dermatology,* Philadelphia, 1993, Saunders, p 365.)

Lubrication

Hyperfunction of the sebaceous glands is associated with androgen stimulation such as occurs with the excessive scalp oiliness and facial acne in adolescence. Dry, brittle hair is commonly the result of excessive washing or the application of chemical agents (coloring, bleach, or detergent shampoos) to the hair.

In addition to direct observation of the scalp and face, correlation of the findings with data from the patient history helps determine dysfunctional states of health.

Nails

Because nails are derived from a highly active tissue, they may be affected by any serious systemic illness. Moreover, any local skin disease that affects the epidermis may also affect the nail matrix (epidermal cells that give rise to the nail plate) and lead to an abnormal (**dystrophic**) nail. By measuring the distance between abnormalities (pits, grooves, and lines) and the proximal nail border, one may estimate the time of initial illness.

Shape

Transverse furrows (**Beau lines**) in the nail indicate that nail growth has been disturbed (Figure 53-39). These furrows can result from infection, systemic disease, or injury. Nails with a concave curve are known as spoon nails, or **koilonychia.** This may signal a form of iron-deficiency anemia and is also associated with other disorders such as coronary disease, syphilis, or the use of strong soaps. Destruction of the nails (**onycholysis**) may accompany a great variety of unrelated conditions ranging from the application of false nails to hyperthyroidism, fungal nail infection, or psoriasis (Figures 53-40 to 53-42). Certain medications may also cause onycholysis (Figure 53-43). **Splinter hemorrhages** may be linked to bacterial endocarditis and trichinosis. These red or brown splinters or streaks run parallel to the finger in the nail bed (Figure 53-44). **Clubbing** of the fingers is characterized by a flattening of the angle of the base of the nail. It may occur in association with

FIGURE 53-39 Beau lines. This patient had major surgery 5 months previously. (From Callen JP et al: *Color atlas of dermatology,* ed 2, Philadelphia, 2000, Saunders, p 334.)

FIGURE 53-40 *Candida albicans* infection resulting in onycholysis. (From Callen JP et al: *Color atlas of dermatology,* ed 2, Philadelphia, 2000, Saunders, p 333.)

FIGURE 53-41 Psoriasis resulting in onycholysis. (From Callen JP et al: *Color atlas of dermatology,* Philadelphia, 1993, Saunders, p 347.)

FIGURE 53-42 Onycholysis secondary to false "sculptured" nails. (From Callen JP et al: *Color atlas of dermatology,* ed 2, Philadelphia, 2000, Saunders, p 367.)

FIGURE 53-43 Drug-induced onycholysis. (From Callen JP et al: *Color atlas of dermatology,* ed 2, Philadelphia, 2000, Saunders, p 334.)

FIGURE 53-44 Splinter hemorrhages in a patient with leukocytoclastic vasculitis. (From Callen JP et al: *Color atlas of dermatology,* ed 2, Philadelphia, 2000, Saunders, p 337.)

cardiovascular disease, subacute bacterial endocarditis, and pulmonary disease.

Color

Nail color indicates the amount of blood oxygenation. Bluish or purplish discoloration of the nail beds occurs with **cyanosis,** whereas **pallor** often indicates anemia. To compare color of the nail beds, apply slight pressure on the free edge of the second or third fingernail. The blanching that results is then compared with the normal color of the nail. The rate of color return also indicates the quality of peripheral vasomotor function.

Texture

Thickening of the nail may result from nutritional disturbances, repeated trauma, inflammation, and local infection. Along with thickening, toenails may become discolored and grooved, and debris may accumulate under the nail. This condition may be exacerbated as the distal portion of the nail works free from the underlying nail bed and more debris is accumulated; fungal infections may also follow. Treatment usually consists of periodic debridement of the nail plate; however, a return to normal nail structure rarely occurs after thickening.

KEY POINTS

- Many systemic diseases are associated with alterations in skin, hair, and nails. Skin reflects systemic inflammation and fever as erythema. A rising fever is manifested as warm, dry skin, whereas warm, moist skin indicates a fever beginning to decline. Poor oxygenation and circulation may be manifested by cyanosis, pallor, or coolness. Jaundice indicates altered bilirubin metabolism, usually caused by liver or biliary disease. Fluid balance may be manifested in the skin as decreased turgor or edema. Sympathetic activation may be indicated by cool, pale, diaphoretic skin.
- Hair growth, strength, texture, and color are affected by systemic diseases such as endocrine abnormalities, extreme malnutrition, and drugs. Excessive androgen may result in hirsutism. Alopecia may result from chemotherapeutic drugs or radiation therapy.
- Abnormalities of nail growth (pits, grooves, lines) occur as a result of nearly any serious systemic illness. Certain nail defects are characteristic of particular diseases: spoon nails may indicate iron-deficiency anemia; clubbing is associated with cardiopulmonary disease. Nail color is commonly assessed to determine the adequacy of oxygenation and perfusion.

Treatment Implications

A distinct advantage in treating the skin is the ease of direct observation of the pathologic process and the effects of treatment. Culture, macroscopic examination of skin scrapings,

and biopsy also facilitate diagnosis. A correct diagnosis can help prevent complications from improper therapy but does not lessen the importance of choosing an appropriate delivery system.

Topical Treatment

Wet Dressings

Wet dressings, the application of a liquid in compress form, are a very important part of the dermatologic therapy delivery system. The applied liquid can be plain water or water with additives (e.g., sodium, magnesium, or aluminum salts).

Wet dressings are a versatile, even paradoxical therapeutic approach in that they can dry or hydrate as necessary. Intermittently applied, they serve as an effective astringent for the weeping, oozing lesions that accompany stasis and decubitus ulcers and impetigo. Vesicular lesions, including those seen in dyshidrotic eczema, herpes zoster, and pemphigus, also respond nicely to treatment with intermittent wet dressings. By drying disease-related lesions, intermittent dressings help speed recovery.

Continuous wet dressings, on the other hand, are effective in rapidly hydrating the skin. This technique, used most often in severe cases of atopic eczema, normally requires hospitalization. Wet dressings of gauze soaked in tap water are applied directly to the skin and covered with an insulating agent such as towels, large thick gauze pads, or even long underwear to prevent evaporation. It is very important that the dressings remain moist. Therefore, they must be resoaked and changed every 3 hours around the clock throughout the course of treatment. Once the desired state of hydration has been achieved, the dressings can be discontinued and emollient creams used to prevent redrying of the treated area.

Lotions

Shake lotions are mixtures of small suspended particles in a liquid vehicle such as water or alcohol. These are especially useful for application directly to moist or exudative processes such as rhus dermatitis. As the liquid phase dissipates, the evaporative effect cools and dries the skin.[27]

Emollient lotions are a mixture of oil in water and have a slightly greasy consistency. These preparations are useful when skin moisturization is needed such as in xerotic conditions. Lotions are often used as a vehicle for other medications such as topical steroids that must be applied over large areas of skin.[27]

Gels

Most gels are clear, colorless, volatile substances. They generally penetrate better than creams. Gels are very convenient to use on wet lesions because of their astringent tendencies. Because they do not leave the white or oily residue of creams and ointments, they are appropriate for use on scalp lesions.

Creams

Creams are the most widely used dermatologic delivery system. Many different bases are used in creams, but the "vanishing" type is most common and allows application with no surface residue. Creams penetrate well and have some moisturizing capability. They are used most frequently in the management of dry to slightly moist dermatoses.

Ointments

The medication in most ointments is carried in a petrolatum-type base, which facilitates penetration into the upper skin layers. Ointments are frequently used on skin lesions that have overlying dry scaling and crusting, but they are also very effective on severe dermatoses requiring an increased medication dosage. Ointments are semiocclusive and often not appropriate for use on lesions that are oozing and discharging a transudate or exudate.

Aerosols and Foams

Aerosols, fine particle sprays of medication usually delivered by gas under pressure, are a cosmetically elegant way of treating dermatoses, especially on hairy areas of the body. Many topical medications are now available as foams that can be used in a similar fashion.

Intralesional Injection

Intralesional injection, or the deposition of medication directly into the lesion, can be done with a conventional needle and syringe or with an instrument (Dermajet) that injects fine particles of medication through the skin with air pressure. This delivery form is especially useful in delivering higher concentrations of corticosteroids to lesions (usually with deep dermal components) that do not respond to topical medication.

Selection of a Delivery System

Delivery system selection depends on the disease being treated, the type of lesions clinically present, and the practitioner's preferred medication routine. For instance, weeping exudative lesions require drying (wet dressings) and perhaps corticosteroids. Initial delivery as a gel would increase the drying tendency; as the lesion dries, a cream may be used to prevent overdrying and fissure formation.

In a disease state such as chronic atopic eczema with lichenoid or thickened skin, the prescriber may choose an ointment to enhance penetration of the medication into the lesion. The ointment's occlusive nature reduces moisture loss from the skin.

Seborrhea and psoriasis in the scalp may be treated with aerosols, which are quick and easy to use and are associated with a high degree of patient compliance. Patients often find them cosmetically superior to the identical medication in cream form. Keloids, which require highly concentrated medication to be delivered to a small area, are ideal candidates for intralesional injection of corticosteroids.

Corticosteroids

Corticosteroids are a very important tool in the practice of dermatology. Dermatologists administer steroids systemically and topically. Steroids may be characterized as short acting

(cortisone or hydrocortisone), intermediate acting (prednisone, prednisolone, methylprednisolone, or triamcinolone), or long acting (dexamethasone or betamethasone).

Systemic Steroids

Administration of systemic steroids in dermatologic disease is usually oral. Intermediate-acting steroids (prednisone, prednisolone, methylprednisolone) are used most often. The greatest benefit of oral administration is the ability to adjust dosage schedules quickly if required. Once-daily doses, divided daily dosage, or alternate-day regimens are all effective.

Intramuscular administration of corticosteroids is also common. Preparations such as triamcinolone acetonide are used most often. These drugs, which may reduce inflammation for more than 4 weeks, ensure that an unreliable patient will receive appropriate doses of medication.

Systemic corticosteroids are generally used for relatively short periods. Therefore, the complications commonly associated with corticosteroid use are not usually seen in dermatologic treatment. However, the long-term use of corticosteroids in diseases such as pemphigus and SLE often results in cushingoid features such as a round, puffy face and a "buffalo hump." Additional adverse effects include fatiguing, weakness, and acne.

Topical Steroids

Corticosteroids can also be applied topically to suppress inflammation. Although this approach does not cure the disease, the reduction in erythema, edema, and pruritis promotes healing. Topical steroids are available in a variety of forms. Based on their capacity to cause cutaneous vasoconstriction, topical steroids are divided into seven groups, with group 1 being the most potent (augmented betamethasone dipropionate [Diprolene AF] and clobetasol dipropionate [Temovate]) and group 7 being the least potent (1% hydrocortisone).

KEY POINTS

- Selection of topical treatment depends largely on whether the goal is to moisturize or dry the affected area. Continuous wet dressings, lotions, creams, and ointments tend to be moisturizing. Intermittent wet dressings and gels tend to be astringents for weeping, oozing lesions.
- Corticosteroids are commonly administered to reduce inflammation. They may be given topically, intralesionally, or systemically.

Developmental Considerations

The skin and the skin problems of special groups warrant consideration. Certain skin problems are seen only in infants and children (e.g., cradle cap and diaper rash) (Figure 53-45). Other dermatoses are seen in both children and adults, but

CONGENITAL DERMATOSES   IRRITATIVE AND INFLAMMATORY DERMATOSES

FIGURE 53-45 Sites of common dermatoses in infants and small children.

in children these dermatoses may appear different from the adult counterpart. Still other dermatoses affect primarily older individuals.

INFANCY

Infancy connotes soft, flawless skin. In general, this is a true image. Several congenital skin lesions, such as Mongolian spots, hemangiomas, and nevi (moles), are nevertheless associated with the early neonatal period.

Mongolian spots are caused by selective pigmentation. They usually occur on the buttocks or sacral area and are commonly seen in Asian Americans or African Americans.

Hemangiomas are vascular disorders of the skin. Two types of hemangiomas are commonly seen in infants and small children: bright red, raised *strawberry hemangiomas* and flat, reddish purple *port-wine stain hemangiomas.* Strawberry hemangiomas begin as small red lesions shortly after birth. They may remain as small superficial lesions or extend to involve subcutaneous tissue. Strawberry hemangiomas usually disappear before the child reaches 5 to 7 years of age without leaving an appreciable scar.[28] Port-wine stain hemangiomas are rare, usually occur on the face and neck, and can be quite disfiguring. They do not disappear with age and no satisfactory medical

treatment is available, although laser surgery may be effective in some cases. Coverage using cosmetic makeup such as Derma Blend may sufficiently conceal their disfiguring effects.

Nevi may vary in shape or size, and they may be present at birth or develop later in life.

Infant skin is also exquisitely sensitive to irritation, injury, and extremes of temperature. Prolonged exposure to a warm humid environment can lead to **prickly heat,** and too frequent bathing can cause excessive dryness. Soiled diapers, left unchanged, can lead to **contact dermatitis** and bacterial infections. **Cradle cap** is a harmless and usually self-limited scaly condition of the scalp. Figure 53-45 illustrates common skin problems of infants and small children.

The primary factor in preventing infant skin disorders is careful and meticulous skin care. Baby lotions are helpful in maintaining skin moisture, whereas baby powder acts as a drying agent. Both are helpful aids when used selectively and according to the nature of the skin problem (excessive moisture or dryness).

Baby powders containing talc can cause serious respiratory problems if inhaled; therefore, containers should be kept out of the reach of small children. Corn starch is preferable to talc, and baby powders containing corn starch are readily available. Unnecessary bathing should be avoided, and

SUMMARY

In systemic diseases, the color, texture, and composition of the skin mirror and participate in widespread pathophysiologic events. For example, internal disease states such as acquired immunodeficiency syndrome; collagen diseases such as scleroderma and dermatomyositis; diabetes; gout; malignancies; neurologic diseases; liver disease; muscle weakness; and vascular, inflammatory, and metabolic disorders all exhibit cutaneous manifestations. Because the skin mirrors the interior condition of the body, it is important in the diagnosis of disease. Cutaneous manifestations may be caused by bodily changes such as pregnancy or obesity. They may also be caused by external factors such as climate, industrial contamination, indoor heating systems, clothing, plant life, and toxic or allergic reactions to drugs and cosmetics.

A distinct advantage in treating individuals with skin disease is the ability to observe the pathology and the effects of treatment. In addition to a careful history, a culture, skin scraping, or biopsy provides good diagnostic information. A correct diagnosis can help prevent complications from improper therapy, but it does not lessen the importance of choosing an appropriate delivery system.

REFERENCES

1. Gupta AK, Jain HC, Lynde CW et al: Prevalence and epidemiology of onychomycosis in patients visiting physicians' offices: a multicenter Canadian survey of 15,000 patients, *J Am Acad Dermatol* 43(2 Pt 1):244-248, 2000.
2. Spanos NP, Williams V, Gwynn MI: Effects of hypnotic, placebo, and salicylic acid treatments on wart regression, *Psychosom Med* 52(1):109-114, 1990.
3. Gulick R: Herpes virus infections. In Arndt KA et al, editors: *Cutaneous medicine and surgery: an integrated program in dermatology*, vol 1, Philadelphia, 1996, Saunders, pp 1074-1092.
4. Dicken CH: Retinoids: a review, *J Am Acad Dermatol* 11(4):541-552, 1984.
5. Yeung-Yue KA, Brentjens MH, Lee PC et al: Herpes simplex viruses 1 and 2, *Dermatol Clin* 20(2):249-266, 2002.
6. Epstein JH: Phototherapy and photochemotherapy, *N Engl J Med* 322(16):1149-1151, 1990.
7. Groopman JE: Neoplasms in the acquired immune deficiency syndrome: the multidisciplinary approach to treatment, *Semin Oncol* 14(2 suppl 3):S1-S6, 1987.
8. Benenson AS, editor: *Control of communicable diseases manual*, ed 16, Washington, DC, 1995, American Public Health Association.
9. Ackerman AB, Cockerell CJ: Papules, *Cutis* 37(4):242-245, 1986.
10. Gonzalez E: Pityriasis rosea. In Arndt KA et al, editors: *Cutaneous medicine and surgery: an integrated program in dermatology*, vol 1, Philadelphia, 1996, Saunders, 218-220.
11. Strauss JS: Biology of the sebaceous gland and the pathophysiology of acne vulgaris. In Soter NA, Baden HP, editors: *Pathophysiology of dermatologic diseases*, New York, 1991, McGraw-Hill, pp 195-210.
12. Callen JP: The value of malignancy evaluation in patients with dermatomyositis, *J Am Acad Dermatol* 6(2):253-259, 1982.
13. Kristal L, Clark RAF: Atopic dermatitis. In Arndt KA et al, editors: *Cutaneous medicine and surgery: an integrated program in dermatology*, vol 1, Philadelphia, 1996, Saunders, 195-202.
14. Roth HL, Kierland RR: The natural history of atopic dermatitis. A 20-year follow-up study, *Arch Dermatol* 89:209-214, 1964.
15. Shear B, Stern RS: Cutaneous reactions to drugs and biologic response modifiers. In Arndt KA et al, editors: *Cutaneous medicine and surgery: an integrated program in dermatology*, vol 1, Philadelphia, 1996, Saunders, 412-425.
16. Sober AJ, Fitzpatrick TB: Adverse drug reactions. In Sober AJ, Fitzpatrick TB, editors: *Year book of dermatology*, St Louis, 1990, Mosby, pp 109-120.
17. Rockerbie NR, Woo TY, Callen JP et al: Cutaneous changes of dermatomyositis precede muscle weakness, *J Am Acad Dermatol* 20(4):629-632, 1989.
18. Gilchrest BA, Yaar M: Ageing and photoageing of the skin: observations at the cellular and molecular level, *Br J Dermatol* 127 (Suppl 41):25-30, 1992.
19. Pieper B: Mechanical forces, pressure, shear, and friction. In Bryant RA, Nix DP, editors: *Acute and chronic wounds,* ed 3, St Louis, 2007, Mosby, pp 205-234.
20. Friedman RJ et al: Skin cancer: basal cell and squamous cell carcinoma. In Holleb AI, Fink DJ, Murphy GP, editors: *Clinical oncology,* ed 7, New York, 1991, American Cancer Society, pp 290-303.
21. Sherman CD et al: Malignant melanomas. In Rubin P, editors: *Clinical oncology: a multidisciplinary approach for physicians and students,* ed 7, Philadelphia, 1993, Saunders, pp 667-675.
22. Boissy RE, Nordlund JJ: Vitiligo. In Arndt KA et al, editors: *Cutaneous medicine and surgery: an integrated program in dermatology,* vol 1, Philadelphia, 1996, Saunders, 1210-1218.
23. Berardesca E, Maibach HI: Sensitive and ethnic skin: a need for special skin-care agents? *Dermatol Clin* 9(1):89-92, 1991.
24. Martin S: Variants of normal skin in blacks. In Rosen T, Martin S, editors: *Atlas of black dermatology,* Boston, 1981, Little, Brown, pp 1-16.
25. Ackerman AB, Cockerell CJ: Cutaneous lesions: correlations from microscopic to gross morphologic features, *Cutis* 37(2):137-138, 1986.
26. Berger TG, Odom RB, James WD: Diseases of the skin appendages. In Berger TG, Odom RB, James WD, editors: *Andrew's diseases of the skin: clinical dermatology,* ed 9, Philadelphia, 2000, Saunders, pp 943-990.
27. Leyden JJ, Rawlings AV: *Skin moisturization*, New York, 2002, Marcel Dekker.
28. Cohen S: Programmed instruction: skin rashes in infants and children, *Am J Nurs* 78(6 Suppl):S1-S32, 1978.
29. Johnson ML: *Skin diseases.* In Wyngaarden JB, Smith LH Jr, Bennett CJ, editors: *Cecil textbook of medicine,* ed 19, vol. 2, Philadelphia, 1992, Saunders, pp 2280-2330.
30. Dunkle LM, Arvin AM, Whitley RJ et al: A controlled trial of acyclovir for chickenpox in normal children, *N Engl J Med* 325(22):1539-1544, 1991.
31. Arvin AM: Varicella-zoster virus, *Clin Microbiol Rev* 9(3):361-381, 1996.
32. Gilchrest BA: Dermatologic disorders in the elderly. In Rossman I, editor: *Clinical geriatrics,* ed 3, Philadelphia, 1986, Lippincott, pp 375-387.
33. Goldman R: Decline in organ function with aging. In Rossman I, editor: *Clinical geriatrics,* ed 2, Philadelphia, 1979, Lippincott, pp 23-52.
34. Smith L: Histopathologic characteristics and ultrastructure of aging skin, *Cutis* 43(5):414-424, 1989.
35. Cerimele D, Celleno L, Serri F: Physiological changes in ageing skin, *Br J Dermatol* 122(suppl 35):S13-S20, 1990.

Burn Injuries

Julio Bird • K. John Hartman • Nirav Patel

MEDIA RESOURCES

Additional Material for Study, Review, and Further Exploration

CD Companion ▪ Review Questions and Answers ▪ Glossary (with audio pronunciations for selected terms) ▪ Disease Profiles ▪ Animations

evolve **Website** at http://evolve.elsevier.com/Copstead/
▪ Case Studies ▪ Disease Profiles ▪ WebLinks ▪ Key Points Review

Online Course (Module 20)

KEY QUESTIONS

- What are the most common causes of burn injuries?
- How are burn degree and severity determined?
- What are the principles that guide the management of burn injuries?

- What are the potential complications associated with burn injuries?
- What are the outcomes following burn injuries?

CHAPTER OUTLINE

urns are injuries to tissues caused by contact with dry heat (flame or hot surfaces), moist heat (steam or hot liquids), electricity (current or lightning), chemicals (corrosive substances), friction, or radiant and electromagnetic energy. Approximately 500,000 individuals seek medical attention for burn injuries annually in the United States, of which approximately 40,000 necessitate acute hospitalization.[1] In recent decades, burn mortality rates have decreased significantly, with most patients achieving excellent functional and cosmetic outcomes. Improved outcomes have clearly been related to an improved understanding of the pathophysiologic mechanism of burns, advances in burn care management, and the development of a comprehensive, treatment-oriented approach to care.[1,2,3] The American Burn Association in conjunction with the American College of Surgeons Committee on Trauma has been instrumental in promoting the development of burn centers, of which there are now 125 in the United States.[4] Advanced burn life support prehospital and provider courses have also been developed to provide emergency care personnel the skills and information to facilitate rapid assessment, stabilization, and transport of burn victims to appropriate emergency facilities, and providing hospital caregivers guidelines in the assessment and treatment of burn patients during the first 24 hours after injury.[5] The priorities for assessment and treatment of burn victims are no different from that of other trauma patients. However, depending on the cause, burn injuries influence a variety of systemic, circulatory, and metabolic changes. As a result, in order to make appropriate treatment decisions and recognize potential complications such as inhalation injuries, cardiac arrhythmias, compartment syndrome, and rhabdomyolysis, a clear understanding of the pathophysiologic processes associated with the burn injury is necessary.

THERMAL INJURY

Etiology

Thermal injuries are burns caused by contact with or exposure to extremes of temperature. Thermal injuries from dry heat result most commonly from exposure to flames or hot surfaces and often occur in the absence of any clear external stigmata such as with inhalation injuries. This also applies to injuries resulting from contact with or exposure to moist heat on one end of the spectrum, and hypothermia and frostbite on the other.

Incidence and Mortality

According to the American Burn Association's 2007 fact sheet, more than 500,000 thermal burn injuries occur in the United States each year.[6] This incidence has declined significantly from the 2 million annual injuries estimated in the first report of the National Health Interview Survey (NIHS), drawn from 1957 to 1961 data. As of the early 1990s, the rate of reportable burn injuries in the United States had declined from about 10 per 10,000 to 4.2 per 10,000.[5] Thermal injuries result in approximately 40,000 hospitalizations per year, of which

approximately half are to specialized burn treatment centers, and the other half to the nation's approximately 5000 other hospitals.[5] According to the U.S. Centers for Disease Control and Prevention (CDC), in 2006 there were 2580 deaths, not including fire fighters, as a result of fire/burn injuries in the United States.[5] Eighty-five percent of all fire deaths occurred in residential fires, with most of the victims succumbing to smoke inhalation. Although cooking remains the leading cause of residential fires, smoking-related fires remain the leading cause of mortality.[7-9] A dramatic decline in mortality rates has been observed with thermal injuries as a result of advances in our understanding of the pathophysiologic mechanisms, a multidisciplinary team-oriented approach, improved fluid resuscitation strategies, infection control, early surgical excision, skin-grafting techniques, advances in skin substitute development, and rehabilitation techniques.[10-14]

The fire loss record in the United States is the worst in the industrialized world, with the fire-related mortality double that of most countries on a per capita basis. In 2005, residential fires in the United States caused nearly $7 billion in property damage.[7] Ignition of upholstered furniture and mattresses by cigarettes was the single leading cause of fire-related mortality. In addition, approximately 200 deaths per year were associated with fires resulting from the use of cigarette lighters, with 125 of these victims being younger than 5 years of age.[9]

A half century ago, burns over 50% total body surface area (TBSA) resulted in a greater than 50% mortality in pediatric patients.[15] Currently, most children survive burns of this size, and more than half survive burns of more than 90% of their TBSA.[16] Early mortality generally occurred as a result of inadequate initial resuscitation. As vigorous resuscitation protocols were developed, a significant reduction in mortality occurred. Unfortunately, the reduction in mortality was replaced by an increased number of survivors with wound sepsis. The advent of topical and systemic antimicrobials, recognition of the importance of maintaining nutrition, early wound excision, and grafting has resulted in a significant reduction in mortality. As a result of these advances, acute mortality in patients with thermal injuries remains relatively low. The primary cause of death in this population now occurs in the subacute setting as a result of pulmonary sepsis, often occurring secondary to inhalation injury. More than 80% of patients sustaining burns have involvement of less than 20% of their TBSA and are treated on an outpatient basis. Despite burn degree, the associated physical and emotional sequelae are often extensive and prolonged. As a result, this unique population requires vigilant follow-up.

Risk Factors

The CDC has identified the following groups as being at high risk for fire-related injuries and deaths: children younger than 4 years; adults 65 years and older; Native Americans and African Americans; economically challenged individuals; people living in rural areas; and those residing in manufactured homes or substandard housing. Children younger than 15 years old account for one third of all admissions to burn units

FIGURE 54-1 All burns in children must be carefully evaluated with a consideration for nonaccidental or intentional injury. This 2-year-old boy was immersed by his father in a bathtub of hot water and sustained burns over 55% of his total body surface area. One feature that characterizes abuse burns is a clear demarcation between burned and unburned skin and the absence of drip, spill, or splatter marks. (Courtesy Michael Peck, MD, University of North Carolina Burn Center, Chapel Hill.)

and one third of all deaths from burns and burn-related injuries.[7] Each year, 116,600 children sustain burns severe enough to warrant medical attention, with 528 deaths due to these injuries.[8] Scald injuries are the most common in this population and account for up to 60% of all burn injuries. In 2002, nearly 22,600 children were treated for scald injuries.[6] Most of these injuries are due to accidental spills; however, 20% or more involve an element of abuse or neglect (Figure 54-1).[3,17] Other causes of pediatric burns include flame injuries (30%), contact with hot surfaces (10%), and chemical and electrical burns (2%) (Table 54-1).[15,17]

Approximately 3000 seniors are injured in home fires annually. The population over 65 years of age accounts for approximately 25% of all burn/fire-related deaths in the United States. Burns in the elderly carry a high mortality rate as a result of preinjury disability, age-related immunosuppression, and impaired healing responses (see Table 54-1).[7]

Environmental and lifestyle factors influence the frequency and magnitude of thermal burn injuries. Alcohol and drug abuse contributes to approximately 40% of all residential fire-related deaths. Neurologic and psychiatric disorders have also been found to increase the risk of accidental burn injury, with one study finding 3% of patients admitted to the burn unit had thermal injuries associated with neurologic disorders.

Integument Effects

The skin is the largest organ of the body and constitutes approximately 20% of the total body weight. It consists of two layers, the epidermis and dermis, which rest on the hypodermis (or subcutaneous layer). The epidermis contains two main cell types, melanocytes and keratinocytes, as well as multiple appendages such as hair, nails, and glands (sweat and sebaceous). The appendages, although originating from the

epidermal layer, are anatomically located in both the epidermis and the dermis. Keratinocytes constitute 95% of the epidural binary cell system and synthesize keratin. The melanocytes are scattered throughout the basal layer (stratum germinativum) and produce melanin, a pigment that shields deeper structures of the skin from sunlight. Two types of sweat glands are found in the skin. Apocrine glands, the large sweat glands, are rudimentary structures with no known useful purpose. They respond to autonomic nerve stimulation rather than thermal stimulation to produce an odorless, viscous, milk-like droplet from the hair shaft. Apocrine glands are more numerous in women and are located in the axilla, areola of nipples, groin, perineum, and perianal and periumbilical regions. Eccrine glands are small sweat glands distributed over the body that act as true secretory glands and produce the sweat responsible for heat regulation. At environmental temperatures above 31° C or 32° C (90° F), sweating occurs over the entire body; at lower temperatures, microscopically visible droplets are secreted periodically as part of the total insensible water loss from the body. Sweat normally provides skin with an acid mantle (average pH, 5.7 to 6.4) that retards growth of the many bacteria that reside in the keratin layer, glands, and hair follicles. The function of sweat glands is severely altered in areas of thermal injury after healing, and they become hypersecretory (Box 54-1).

Sebaceous glands secrete sebum, a complex mixture of lipids that is emptied into the hair shaft. The rate of production of sebum and its location depend on androgens, which initiate and continue production. During the hypermetabolic state that follows major thermal injury, production of sebum is decreased, leading to the dry skin conditions commonly found after recovery.

Thermal injury to the integument occurs in two phases. The first is immediate and is a result of direct cellular injury. The second is delayed and occurs as a result of the associated progressive dermal ischemia.

The degree of tissue destruction is related to the duration of exposure and the temperature, or the amount of energy, to which the skin is exposed. The cellular damage is the product of protein denaturation. There are three zones of injury described in the burn wound. The first is the zone of necrosis and is the area in the burn wound where coagulation necrosis has occurred. This area is surrounded by the zone of stasis, a region with decreased blood flow, which can be returned to normal with appropriate resuscitation or converted to necrosis in the case of dehydration, infection, or decreased perfusion. The zone of hyperemia surrounds the zone of stasis and is comprised of minimally injured tissue that usually recovers normal function within 1 week.[18]

In response to thermal injury, keratinocytes develop from cells in the basal layer of the epidermis and progress upward from the stratum germinativum to the stratum corneum over a 14-day period. Over this time the wound develops a light pink or reddish coloration, with normal skin color restored in a delayed fashion by the melanocytes. Regeneration of hair and nails is dependent on viability of

TABLE 54-1

Physiologic Changes Associated with Age

Body System	Pediatric	Elderly
Cardiovascular	**Symptoms of shock:** Increased heart rate Decreased blood pressure Decreased urine output Cardiac output dependent on heart rate Decreased myocardial compliance Stroke volume plateaus at lower filling pressures **Peripheral cyanosis:** Neonates: a normal finding Children: decreased cardiac output	Increased chronic disease processes Decreased vascular elasticity results in increased systolic blood pressure Decreased cardiac output Decreased β-adrenergic responsiveness Decreased cardiac stress response Decreased intrinsic heart rate Decreased blood flow Decreased vascular permeability Increased myocardial irritability Decreased myocardial perfusion Increased dysrhythmias Conduction system changes
Pulmonary	Small trachea is easily obstructed Neck hyperextension leads to epiglottal or tracheal obstruction At <8 yr, cricoid cartilage is narrowest airway point At <8 yr, no cuff is needed on endotracheal tube Hypoxemia leads to decreased heart rate in neonates Hypoxemia leads to decreased heart rate in children Diaphragmatic breathing Lower airways are easily obstructed Decreased O_2 reserve	Increased need for ventilatory support Increased incidence of inhalation injury Increased pneumonia Decreased lung elasticity Decreased chest wall muscle Decreased oxygen saturation Decreased tidal volume Decreased vital capacity Decreased pulmonary capillary circulation
Thermoregulation and metabolism	Increased resting metabolic rate Increased resting O_2 consumption Increased BSA in relation to body weight Increased hypothermia Increased heat loss from evaporation and convection At <6 mo, inability to shiver to increase body heat Stress leads to hypoglycemia Glycosuria is a sign of infection At <2 yr, buffering capacity is decreased Increased metabolic demands of growth	Increased burn wound infection Increased sepsis Poor or delayed wound healing Increased preexisting malnutrition Decreased febrile response Increased hypothermia
Gastrointestinal and renal	Decreased endogenous calorie stores Increased diarrhea with fluid and calorie deficits At <2 yr, gastric emptying is delayed At <2 yr, increased gastric distention At <30% TBSA burn, can take sufficient caloric supplementation At >30% TBSA burn, requires caloric supplementation At <12 mo, poor renal filtration and absorption	Increased volume sensitivity Decreased nutritional status Increased likelihood of hypotensive or hypertensive renal damage Increased incidence of type 2 diabetes mellitus Decreased creatinine clearance
Neurocognitive	Increased incidence of cerebral edema with fluid resuscitation Increased irritability Increased regressive behavior Increased risk taking behavior Immature judgment	Decreased brain mass Decreased cerebral nerve cells Decreased brain cortex layer Decreased cerebellar cortical cells Decreased nerve conduction velocity Decreased memory Decreased electroencephalographic activity Slower reaction time Decreased taste Decreased smell Decreased vision Decreased hearing Increased pain threshold Decreased judgment and cognitive abilities
Immune	Immature immune system Decreased immunocompetence	Decreased number of leukocytes Decreased immunocompetence Decreased T-cell response

From Carrougher GJ, editor: *Burn care and therapy*, St Louis, 1998, Mosby, p 100.

BSA, Body surface area; *TBSA,* total body surface area.

BOX 54-1

Normal Physiologic Functions of the Skin Altered or Lost After Thermal Injury

Protection
Barrier between the internal organs and the external environment
Continuous with the mucous membrane at the external openings of organs of the digestive, respiratory, and urogenital systems
Acidic skin (pH 4.2 to 5.6) and perspiration protect against bacterial invasion
Thickened skin of palms and soles provides padding

Percutaneous Absorption
Epidermis is relatively impermeable to most chemical substances; some may be absorbed through the epidermis or the orifices of hair follicles

Sensory Processing
Receptor skin nerve endings allow constant monitoring of the environment by sensing warm and cold temperature, pain, touch, and pressure

Production
Endogenous production of vitamin D_3, which is necessary for synthesis of vitamin D

Barrier
Skin prevents water and electrolyte loss, maintains moist subcutaneous tissues, and prevents water absorption during immersion

Thermoregulation
The body continuously produces heat as a by-product of cellular metabolism; heat is dissipated through skin
Internal body temperature is regulated by radiation, conduction, or convection
Rate of heat loss depends primarily on the surface temperature of skin, which is a function of skin blood flow

Immunologic
The major site of immune complexes is the dermal-epidermal junction and the dermal vessels of skin
Monocyte/macrophage system is mobilized by local tissue mediators

Circulatory
Skin temperature depends on the rate of blood flow through the skin
Circulatory system distributes pharmacologic agents to local tissues

Aesthetic
Provides the individual identity of a person

---

the hair follicle and nail matrix. With intact follicles, hair generally grows back at approximately 1 cm per month. New nail formation is often irregular and of abnormal thickness as regrowth occurs.

Major burns produce a chain of pathophysiologic changes characterized by the onset of shock and related hypoperfusion, acid-base imbalance, erosion of tissues, bacterial infection, and organ dysfunction or failure. The body responds to serious burns with increases in energy expenditure, enhanced catabolism, and accelerated loss of lean body mass. Patients with severe burns are susceptible to systemic inflammatory response syndrome, adult respiratory distress syndrome, and multiple organ dysfunction syndromes.[19]

Burn injury activates the immune system. The body responds to burn injury by producing inflammation, which might be seen as a summoning of the forces that are needed to repair damaged tissue. After the injury occurs, blood vessels constrict to reduce blood loss, clots form, and healing cells migrate to the wound. Edema, a potentially dangerous condition, may begin to emerge almost immediately and continue for several days. The inflammatory period lasts about 2 weeks.[19]

As the inflammatory period progresses, cells called *fibroblasts* contribute to wound repair by producing the structural protein collagen, which strengthens the damaged dermis. Fibroblasts also produce elastin, a protein that adds elasticity to the wound, but its contribution is considerably less significant than that of collagen. As these proteins and other elements begin the healing process, macrophages respond to the inflammation by attacking bacteria and other foreign substances.

New vascular networks begin to form during the inflammatory period and continue their development in the subsequent proliferative stage. New epithelial cells move inward from the edges of the injury and wound contraction begins, although deeper burns require wound excision and skin grafting to facilitate healing.

Depth Classification

Depth of burn injury is divided into four classifications: first-degree (superficial), second-degree (superficial and deep partial-thickness), third-degree (full-thickness), and fourth-degree (full-thickness with bone or muscle involvement), based on criteria established by the American Burn Association (Table 54-2).[20]

First-Degree Burns

Superficial Burns. First-degree burns involve only superficial tissue destruction in the outermost layers of the epidermis, with no associated compromise of the function of the skin (see Table 54-2). These burns are often associated with local discomfort, erythema, and mild systemic responses such as headache, chills, nausea, and vomiting. Erythema, a thermovascular response that occurs in first-degree burns in the absence of direct trauma to the dermis, is probably related to the release of tissue contents in the superficial circulation. First-degree burns are generally self-limiting, require no fluid resuscitation, and are therefore not included in estimates of the percentage of TBSA burned. However, in infants and elderly, first-degree burns may lead to systemic dehydration,

TABLE 54-2

Burn Wound Classification

Degree of Burn	Cause of Injury	Depth of Injury	Wound Characteristics	Treatment Course
First-degree burn	Prolonged ultraviolet light exposure, brief exposure to hot liquids	Limited damage to epithelium, skin intact	Erythematous, hypersensitive, no blister formation	Complete healing within 3-5 days without scarring
Superficial partial-thickness burn: second degree	Brief exposure to flash, flame, or hot liquids	Epidermis destroyed, minimal damage to superficial layers of dermis, epidermal appendages remain intact	Moist and weepy, pink or red, blisters, blanching, hypersensitive	Complete healing within 21 days with minimal or no scarring
Deep partial-thickness burn: second degree	Intense radiant energy; scalding liquids or hot semiliquids (e.g., tar) or solids; flame	Epidermis destroyed, underlying dermis damaged, some epidermal appendages remain intact	Pale, decreased moistness, blanching absent or prolonged; intact sensation to deep pressure but not to pin-prick	Prolonged healing (often longer than 21 days), may require skin grafting to achieve complete healing with better functional outcome
Full-thickness burn: third degree	Prolonged contact with flame, scalding liquids, steam; hot objects; chemicals; electrical current	Epidermis, dermis, and epidermal appendages destroyed; injury through dermis	Dry, leatherlike; pale, mottled brown, or red; thrombosed vessels visible; insensate	Requires skin grafting
Full-thickness burn: fourth degree	Electrical current, prolonged contact with flame (e.g., unconscious victim)	Epidermis, dermis, and epidermal appendages destroyed; injury involves connective tissue, muscle, and possibly bone	Dry; charred, mottled brown, white, or red; no sensation; limited or no movement of involved extremities or digits	Requires skin grafting, amputation of involved extremities or digits likely

From Carrougher GJ, editor: *Burn care therapy,* St Louis, 1998, Mosby, p 138.

necessitating intravenous resuscitation. Therapy generally includes simple analgesia. These injuries typically heal in 3 to 6 days without scarring or pigmentation changes.

Second-Degree Burns

Superficial Partial-Thickness Burns. Superficial partial-thickness burns involve the epidermis to the level of the dermis and appear red to pale ivory. Moist, thin-walled blisters often form within minutes of the injury (Figure 54-2). Pain is a major clinical feature of this depth of injury as tactile and pain sensors remain intact (see Table 54-2). Injuries typically heal in 7 to 21 days in the absence of wound infection. The amount of scarring that follows is a genetically determined trait, with some groups of people tending to scar excessively (African Americans and Caucasians with red hair) or minimally (Native American and Asian groups). Hair follicles remain intact and will regrow hair in the area of injury. Hair usually reappears 7 to 10 days after injury.

Deep Partial-Thickness Burns. Deep partial-thickness burns may involve the entire dermis and leave only the epidermal skin appendages located in the hair follicles. The area of injury has a mottled appearance, with large areas of waxy-white tissue surrounded by light pink or red tissue. The surface is generally dry, and blisters tend to resemble flat, dry tissue paper rather than the fluid-filled raised areas seen with superficial partial-thickness injury. Tactile and pain sensors are either absent or greatly diminished in the area of deepest tissue destruction, but this area is usually surrounded by margins of lesser depth of injury in which pain and tactile sensors remain intact. Deep partial-thickness injury is visually and clinically indistinguishable from full-thickness injury at the time of injury. These wounds heal spontaneously in previously healthy individuals in about 4 weeks in the absence of secondary infection. The longer the time to healing, the more significant the scarring and depigmentation is observed. As a result, these burns are often excised early and subsequently treated with a skin graft in an effort to diminish scarring and achieve early wound closure.

Third-Degree Burns

Full-Thickness Burns. Third-degree burns may also involve the entire epidermis, the dermis, and the underlying subcutaneous tissue. Immediately following injury, these areas appear white, cherry red, or black. Deep blisters may be present under a dry layer of dehydrated skin. Superficial blood vessels coagulated by the heat of injury may be visible through the skin as thrombosed veins. One of the physiologic characteristics of the skin that is lost (see Box 54-1) is the elasticity of the dermis, resulting in a wound with a dry, hard, leathery texture. The massive edema that accompanies major burn injury combined with the loss of elasticity may result in a tourniquet-like effect when the injury occurs circumferentially around a limb or torso. This often necessitates escharotomies or, rarely, fasciotomies to restore distal circulation.

FIGURE 54-2 This young child sustained a hot water scald burn on the heel of the right foot that resulted in a superficial second-degree burn. A superficial second-degree (partial-thickness) burn will re-epithelialize within 3 weeks. These burns are characterized by loss of epidermis (blistering) and by a shiny, sensate, vascularized dermis. (Courtesy Michael Peck, MD, University of North Carolina Burn Center, Chapel Hill.)

These burns are painless to touch, as all superficial nerve endings in the skin have been destroyed. However, as with partial-thickness injuries, rarely are burn injuries totally uniform, and an area of lesser injury in which pain and tactile sensors are intact is usually located on the periphery. Areas of full-thickness injury require skin grafting with the patient's own skin as all dermal elements have been destroyed, leaving no residual tissue for regeneration. However, small injuries often heal by secondary intention as a result of ingrowth of dermal elements from the margins of the wound.

Fourth-Degree Burns

Full-thickness injuries that extend beyond the dermis to involve muscle, bone, or both are often classified as fourth-degree. These injuries often occur in victims of high-voltage electrical injury or those who have had prolonged exposure to intense heat, such as unconscious fire victims.

Extent of Injury

Extent of injury refers to the percentage of TBSA burned. Estimates can be calculated with the rule of nines (Figure 54-3) or the Lund and Browder chart (Figure 54-4). The rule of nines is commonly used in prehospital settings and emergency departments, and provides a rough estimate of TBSA involved. The Lund and Browder chart, or a variation of it, is generally used in burn centers and is more precise particularly in assessing TBSA in children under the age of 10 years (see Figure 54-4).

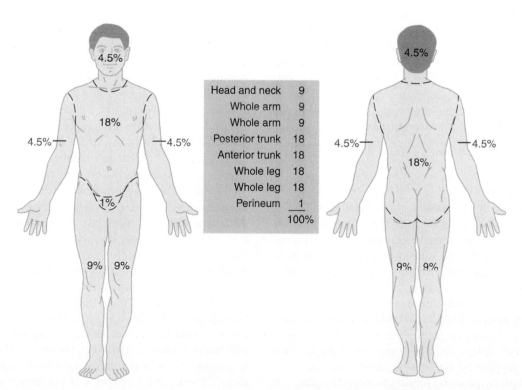

Head and neck	9
Whole arm	9
Whole arm	9
Posterior trunk	18
Anterior trunk	18
Whole leg	18
Whole leg	18
Perineum	1
	100%

FIGURE 54-3 The rule of nines is a commonly used assessment tool that permits a timely and useful estimate of the percentage of total body surface area burned.

Head	7.0
Neck	2.0
Anterior trunk	13.0
Posterior trunk	13.0
Right buttock	2.5
Left buttock	2.5
Genitalia	1.0
Right upper arm	4.0
Left upper arm	4.0
Right lower arm	3.0
Left lower arm	3.0
Right hand	2.5
Left hand	2.5
Right thigh	9.5
Left thigh	9.5
Right leg	7.0
Left leg	7.0
Right foot	3.5
Left foot	3.5
	100%

FIGURE 54-4 The Lund and Browder chart. The areas of the body are presented in sections, which permits a more accurate estimation of burn size.

Severity Classification

The severity of a burn injury is determined by the extent to which the physiologic functions of the skin are disrupted beyond the body's normal ability to respond with compensatory mechanisms. The American Burn Association[20] classifies burn injury as minor, moderate, and major (Table 54-3). The severity of the burn injury and the eventual morbidity and mortality associated with it are related to a combination of factors: the patient's medical history, the extent and depth of the burn, the body area involved, the presence of concomitant trauma sustained at the time of the burn, and the patient's age.

Acute Management

The first priority in burn management is the elimination of the source of burn. People whose clothing has caught fire tend to run, thereby increasing exposure time and extent of the injury. This is compounded by inhalation injury due to their burning garments. A national campaign to educate the public, the "stop, drop, and roll" campaign, has had a significant impact in decreasing the severity and extent of flame burns associated with clothing fires. The physical rolling helps extinguish flames from the mechanical standpoint, whereas the supine position also serves to keep the flames away from the face and airway. People familiar with the "stop, drop, and roll" concept may instinctively run, and hearing somebody repeat this phrase will often initiate the action. If the appropriate action is not seen, despite reinforcing the concept, attempts should

be made to assist the individual in accomplishing it. However, extreme caution must be exercised to ensure that the rescuer does not become a victim. If available, water should be used to put out the fire, as it not only eliminates the source of the heat but also enables cooling of the underlying skin. The water need not be sterile or even clean, as the primary objective is elimination of the fire. In the absence of any available water, flames may be smothered with a blanket, coat, or any other nonflammable covering that will aid in deprivation of oxygen required for combustion. Once the flames are eliminated, the cover should be promptly removed to enable escape of the underlying heat, thereby minimizing injury depth. Scald injuries are best treated initially with cool water, which allows cooling of the scalding liquid as well as the underlying skin. Contact burns from chemicals are managed by removing the clothing; dusting off any powdered chemicals; and subsequent dilution of the chemicals by copious flushing with water.[21] No attempts, however, should be made to neutralize chemicals on the skin, as neutralization is a heat-producing chemical reaction resulting in a compounding thermal injury component. Burns from tar, asphalt, or melted plastics are also initially treated with water. If no water is available, the material is allowed to cool to room temperature, which generally occurs within 2 to 3 minutes. However, the increased exposure duration often results in significant increase in burn extent. Once cooled, the material acts as a sterile dressing; therefore no attempt should be made to remove it unless it is causing a life-threatening airway compromise.

TABLE 54-3

American Burn Association Burn Severity Classification Schedule

Classification	Assessment Criteria
Minor burn injury	<15% TBSA burn in adults <40 yr old <10% TBSA burn in adults >40 yr old <10% TBSA burn in children <10 yr old *and* <2% TBSA full-thickness burn without risk of cosmetic or functional impairment or disability
Moderate burn injury	12%-25% TBSA burn in adults <40 yr old 10%-20% TBSA burn in adults >40 yr old 10%-20% TBSA burn in children <10 yr old *and* 10% TBSA full-thickness burn without cosmetic or functional risk to burned area involving the face, eyes, ears, hands, feet, or perineum
Major burn injury	>25% TBSA burn in adults <40 yr old >20% TBSA burn in adults >40 yr old >20% TBSA burn in children <10 yr old *or* >10% TBSA full-thickness burn (any age) *or* Injuries involving the face, eyes, ears, hands, feet, or perineum likely to result in functional or cosmetic disability *or* High-voltage electrical burn injury *or* All burn injuries with concomitant inhalation injury or major trauma

Modified from American Burn Association guidelines. In Carrougher GJ, editor: *Burn care and therapy*, St Louis, 1998, Mosby, p 94.

TBSA, Total body surface area.

BOX 54-2

Burn Unit Referral Criteria

Partial-thickness burns greater than 10% TBSA
Burns that involve the face, hands, feet, genitalia, perineum, or major joints
Third-degree burns in any age group
Electrical burns, including lightning injury
Chemical burns
Inhalation injury
Burn injury in patients with pre-existing medical disorders that could complicate management, prolong recovery, or affect mortality
Any patients with burns and concomitant trauma (such as fractures) in which the burn injury poses the greatest risk of morbidity or mortality; in such cases, if the trauma poses the greater immediate risk, the patient may be initially stabilized in a trauma center before being transferred to a burn unit; physician judgment will be necessary in such situations and should be in concert with the regional medical control plan and triage protocols
Burned children in hospitals without qualified personnel or equipment for the care of children
Burn injury in patients who will require special social, emotional, or long-term rehabilitative intervention

From American College of Surgeons Committee on Trauma. *Resources for optimal care of the injured patient*, Chicago, 1999, The College, p 55.

TBSA, Total body surface area.

Assessment

Patients with thermal burn injuries are trauma patients, and initial management should focus on stabilizing the ABCs (airway-breathing-circulation).[3] Common signs of inhalation injury include cough, stridor, hoarseness, singed nasal hair, carbonaceous sputum, oropharyngeal edema, and blisters. These injuries generally evolve over time often progressing to complete airway obstruction secondary to edema. Unfortunately, no clinical variables accurately predict which patients will progress to airway compromise, therefore consideration should be given early to bronchoscopy and endotracheal intubation.[22] Compromise of breathing in burn patients is often attributed to underlying inhalation injury or circumferential full-thickness burns resulting in impaired chest excursion. Although such injuries do occur, burn patients, like other trauma patients, are also at risk for pneumothorax or hemothorax, as well as chest wall instability from multiple segmental fractures (flail chest). These conditions should be investigated and, if identified, appropriately treated. Vascular access is preferentially obtained peripherally through unburned tissue if possible. If no such sites are available, access may be established through burned skin. The patient is then evaluated by a complete head-to-toe examination for any other associated traumatic injuries, which are identified and managed as required. TBSA is then determined using a standardized chart such as the Lund and Browder (see Figure 54-4). Fluid resuscitation requirements are subsequently determined and initiated while the patient is placed on clean sheets and the burned areas are wrapped in sterile dressings. The wounds, however, should not be treated with any topical agent such as Silvadene in the acute setting. Burns should not be covered with cool wet sheets as these quickly become cold wet sheets, and with the loss of the burned skin's ability to regulate body temperature, hypothermia can quickly ensue. A Foley catheter is also placed to monitor urine output during resuscitation, and in patients with burns greater than 20% TBSA, if possible, a nasogastric tube should be placed to allow for gastric decompression and to minimize the risk of abdominal bloating and aspiration. Transfer of patients to burn units or other facilities with appropriate resources is initiated during the course of the initial assessment. The American College of Surgeons Committee on Trauma has developed a set of burn unit referral criteria to assist initial evaluators in triage (Box 54-2).

Burn Shock and Acute Resuscitation

Two different but simultaneous mechanisms occur in cases of major burns: local wound pathophysiologic processes related to the loss of skin integrity and systemic pathophysiologic

CAPILLARY DURING BURN SHOCK   CAPILLARY AFTER BURN SHOCK

FIGURE 54-5 Direction of fluid and electrolyte shifts associated with burn shock. During burn shock, K^+ is moving out of the cell, and Na^+ and H_2O are moving in. After burn shock, K^+ moves in, and Na^+ and H_2O move out.

processes related to sequelae of the burn injury. The most immediate systemic change identified is burn shock and includes pathophysiologic changes in the cardiovascular system that are profound, systemic, and lethal without timely and appropriate medical intervention to support the patient's failing cardiovascular system.

Within minutes of a burn injury, the cardiovascular system, which is normally a closed, semipermeable system, becomes an open system through which the patient's circulating volume leaves the circulatory system. This phenomenon, known as "capillary leak," occurs within a few minutes of injury and persists for 24 hours. Burn shock is not confined to the burn area but, rather, is a systemic process. As the capillary system throughout the body becomes leaky, fluid lost in the area of the burn leaks through the burn into the environment in an evaporative fashion, whereas fluid loss internally collects in the nearby soft tissues, producing extensive interstitial edema (Figure 54-5).

Restoration of the patient's circulating volume is an essential part of acute burn management. The rate and volume of fluids lost are related directly to the severity of burn. Therefore, the extent and depth of the burn injury must be ascertained during the initial clinical assessment.

The most widely used formula to guide fluid resuscitation within the first 24 hours of burn injury is the Parkland formula (Box 54-3). The formula utilizes lactated Ringer solution as the resuscitation fluid, as it most closely approximates the fluid it is replacing and thereby minimizes the profound electrolyte imbalances often seen with large-volume resuscitation. Colloid is rarely used in the acute phase of fluid resuscitation (Box 54-4). The standardized formulas provide an excellent guideline for initiating fluid resuscitation but do not ensure adequacy of resuscitation. Depending on the underlying pathophysiologic state and degree of burn, few patients will require less than the predicted 4 ml/kg/% TBSA. Patients with

---

BOX 54-3

Parkland Formula for Fluid Resuscitation in Burn Shock

During the first 24 hours after a burn, administer intravenous LRS at the following rate:

4 ml LRS/% TBSA burn/kg body weight,

where
- Time is calculated from the time of burn injury
- TBSA is total body surface area
- Half of the total fluid is administered in the first 8 hours after burn
- One fourth of the total is administered in the second 8 hours
- One fourth of the total is administered in the third 8 hours or in quantities to maintain adult urine output at 30 ml/hr or child urine output at 1 ml/kg/hr

Example of formula calculation in a 70-kg patient with a 50% TBSA burn:

4 ml × 70 kg × 50% TBSA burn = 14,000 ml (14 L) LRS in 24 hr

- Administer 7000 ml in the first 8 hours at 875 ml/hr
- Administer 3500 ml in the second 8 hours at 437 ml/hr
- Administer 3500 ml in the third 8 hours at 437 ml/hr

Data from Baxter CR: Guidelines for fluid resuscitation, *J Burn Care Rehabil* 2:279-286, 1981.

LRS, Lactated Ringer solution; *TBSA,* total body surface area.

accompanying inhalation injury, burns extending into muscle, and those in whom fluid resuscitation is delayed often require more fluid volume. In Cartotto's series, 30 patients with mean TBSA of burns of 27% received 6.7 ± 2.8 ml/kg/% TBSA burn in the first 24 hours to ensure adequate resuscitation.[23] Adequacy of resuscitation is determined by the global response of the patient to the fluid administration and not by

BOX 54-4

Plasma Requirements and Evaporative Water Loss After Burn Injury

Colloid Replacement
Twenty percent of blood volume given as fresh-frozen plasma or plasma expander
Adult males: 20% = 5 ml/kg body weight
Adult females and children: 20% = 8 ml/kg

Maintenance Fluids Until Wound Closure Is Achieved
Basal fluid requirements:
 1500 ml fluid/m^2 TBSA = 24-hour requirement
Evaporative water loss from burn wound until healed:
 Adults: (25 + % TBSA burn) × m^2 BSA = ml/hr requirement
 Children: (35 + % TBSA burn) × m^2 BSA = ml/hr requirement
Maintenance fluids equal basal fluid requirements plus evaporative water loss and may be administered intravenously, orally, or by nasogastric or jejunal tube, according to patient need.

BSA, Body surface area; *TBSA,* total body surface area burned.

one single variable.[24] Markers commonly used to reflect adequacy of resuscitation include normalization of mental status, blood pressure, pulse, capillary refill, arterial pH, base deficit, and maintenance of urine output at 0.5 to1 ml/kg per hour for adults and 1 to 1.5 ml/kg per hour for children. In addition to the fluid volumes calculated by the standardized formulas, the patient should also receive appropriate maintenance fluid over the first 24-hour period.

Approximately 24 hours following the acute burn injury, the capillary leak syndrome begins to resolve as cardiovascular integrity is restored. At this time, a colloid solution such as albumin may be administered according to a formula, which differs by gender and age (see Box 54-4), in an effort to replace the protein lost during the acute burn shock phase.

One of the major functions of intact skin is to serve as a barrier to water evaporation. With major burn injury, this ability of the skin to regulate evaporative loss is disrupted. In a classic study done in 1962, Moncrief and Mason[25] attempted to determine the magnitude of such a loss and found that daily evaporative loss was in the range of 20 times normal during the early phase of burn injury, with gradual decreases as wound closure was achieved. Further studies revealed that the insensible water loss through burned skin is not caused by evaporation of water from sweat glands but rather by water vapor formed within the body and lost through the skin.[26,27] As the patient progresses to the subacute phase of resuscitation, it is imperative that attention be paid to these unaccountable losses.

Children and older patients require special care. Older patients are more likely to have cardiopulmonary disease, chronic illnesses, and weakened immune systems, all of which complicate fluid resuscitation. Children are also sensitive to resuscitation volumes that are insufficient or exceed requirements. Table 54-1 summarizes the physiologic changes associated with age that increase the vulnerability of children and elderly persons.[28-30]

Organ Dysfunction
Cardiovascular Dysfunction

Burn shock is often accompanied by a precipitous drop in cardiac output that does not parallel the gradual reduction in blood volume and is refractory to restoration of the circulating volume. This finding of low cardiac output in the presence of vigorous intravenous fluid resuscitation and massive catecholamine release has led to the suggestion of a specific myocardial depressant factor.[31-36] The pathophysiologic mechanism behind this myocardial dysfunction is poorly understood. There appears to be no simple, specific myocardial depressant factor but rather a cascade of events involving metabolic and immunologic factors (Figure 54-6).[17]

Respiratory Dysfunction

Respiratory dysfunction following burn injury generally is the result of obstruction, interstitial alterations, and metabolic changes. Obstruction may occur as a result of edema of the upper airway secondary to direct injury, or more often due to the generalized edema that occurs following fluid resuscitation in the face of an ongoing capillary leak syndrome that accompanies burn injuries. On occasion, burns of the oral cavity and upper airway occur as superheated air is inhaled or scalding water enters the mouth. The pulmonary system is extremely efficient at dissipating heat and prevents the inhalation of superheated air beyond the bronchi, but steam may permeate further into the lung parenchyma (see Figure 54-6).[18,22]

Airway obstruction secondary to edema generally has its onset within the first few hours following burn injury but tends to manifest clinically 2 to 4 hours later as resuscitation is undertaken. Endotracheal intubation is recommended prophylactically when impending airway obstruction is identified. The endotracheal tube is preferably secured with cotton twill tape that enables readjustment to allow for the increase in head and face circumference related to increasing facial and soft-tissue edema.[37]

Smoke or fume inhalation often leads to acute hypoxia that is refractory to oxygen administration. Inhalation injury directly results in the chemical denaturing of pulmonary tissue, and the subsequent edema results in increased distances over which oxygen must diffuse to the capillaries. This may progress to acute respiratory distress (ARDS) syndrome and is usually seen within six days of admission, although it can be seen up to one month later. Whether or not the actual inhalation injury causes susceptibility towards ARDS is debatable. However, it is clear that many factors play a role in this condition due to the intense inflammatory response to the burn in addition to contributions from sepsis, shock, pneumonia, multiple organ failure, and increasing duration of mechanical support. However, the treatment of ARDS mandates ventilator support. With newer guidelines toward ventilator management in ARDS, which consists of low tidal volumes and increased frequency of breaths, there is a much lower incidence of associated mortality that is comparable to similar individuals who have not developed ARDS.[34,38] The efficiency of ventilator management is monitored by the patients end

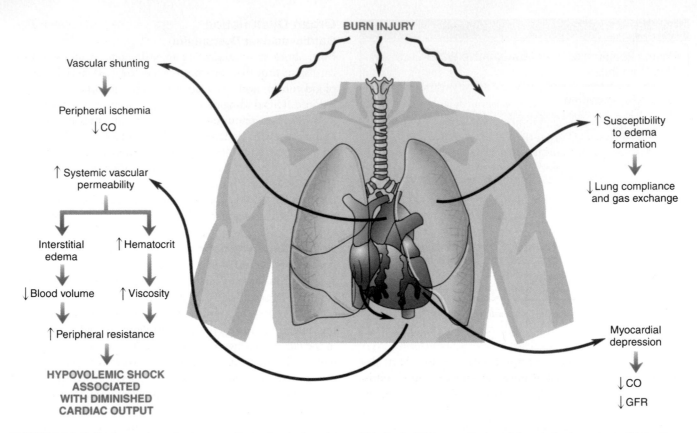

FIGURE 54-6 Cardiovascular and pulmonary effects of major burn injury within the first 24 hours after burn injury, during burn shock. *CO,* Cardiac output; *GFR,* glomerular filtration rate.

tidal carbon dioxide levels, arterial blood gases, and oxygen saturation on pulse oximetry.

Smoke inhalation is also responsible for the majority of cases of inadvertent carbon monoxide poisoning. Carbon monoxide is in direct competition with oxygen and has much greater affinity for the oxygen binding sites on hemoglobin. Once bound, carbon monoxide causes a change in hemoglobin (carboxyhemoglobin), which decreases its ability to off-load oxygen to peripheral tissues. It is also responsible for inactivation of cytochrome oxidase, which is an enzyme that aides in utilization of oxygen. Therefore carbon monoxide poisoning diminishes both delivery and utilization of oxygen in peripheral tissue. The vast range of clinical symptoms can include vague constitutional symptoms such as headache, nausea, and fatigue, or may be much more severe leading to lactic acidosis, seizures, and coma. The degree of carboxyhemoglobin is largely dependent on amounts of carbon monoxide and oxygen in the native environment, duration of exposures, and the patient's minute ventilation.

Carbon monoxide poisoning is diagnosed with a compatible history and physical in conjunction with the presence of elevated carboxyhemoglobin levels. Carboxyhemoglobin can be directly measured on arterial blood gas samples, although these levels may not correlate with the development of neurological sequelae. In addition, pulse oximetry plays no role in monitoring patients with carbon monoxide poisoning as it cannot differentiate between oxyhemoglobin and carboxyhemoglobin.

Treatment of carbon monoxide poisoning involves removal of carbon monoxide from hemoglobin via its direct competition with oxygen. Normal half life of carbon monoxide in a patient breathing room air is 300 minutes. If high-flow oxygen is delivered by a face mask, the half life can be decreased to 90 minutes. Therefore treatment involves removal of the patient from the source of inhalation and immediate institution of high-flow 100% oxygen via non-rebreather face mask. In cases of severe poisoning manifested by a carboxyhemoglobin level greater than 25 percent, loss of consciousness, severe metabolic acidosis, or evidence of ischemic change in any organ system, the treatment should involve institution of hyperbaric oxygen. This will reduce the half life of carbon monoxide even further to approximately 30 minutes, and it also increases the amount of oxygen dissolved in the blood (unbound to hemoglobin) from 0.3 to 6 milliliters per deciliter. In addition to assisting with elimination of carbon monoxide, the addition of hyperbaric oxygen improves delivery of oxygen to peripheral tissues, even in the presence of elevated carboxyhemoglobin levels.[39,40]

Renal Dysfunction

Acute renal failure (ARF) after burn injury can be classified as early or late. Early renal failure occurs during the first five days postburn. It is caused by low intravascular volumes and the presence of myoglobin in the bloodstream, which is filtered by the kidneys. Myoglobin is a product of muscle injury as a result of the burn. The process causing release of myoglobin into the bloodstream due to muscle injury is termed rhabdomyolysis. The etiology of kidney failure in rhabdomyolysis is twofold. Dead muscle tissue causes fluid to shift into muscle from the intravascular space resulting in lower blood volume and less flow to the kidneys. Also, the by-products of myoglobin can be toxic to the kidneys causing damage by precipitation in the renal tubules. Prevention of this complication is focused on adequate fluid resuscitation as well as fasciotomy to relieve high intra-compartmental pressures that may be causing additional muscle breakdown. Late ARF, defined as occurring greater than five days postburn, is less of a result of the initial burn and may generally be caused by several factors including onset of sepsis or the use of medications with nephrotoxic effects. Most patients will require either intermittent hemodialysis or continuous renal replacement therapy in this acute setting. Continuous venovenous hemofiltration (CVVH) has been used with success in treating ARF in burns and is associated with less vascular complications than arteriovenous hemodialysis.[47] Prognosis is generally poor for the burn patient who develops ARF. Mortality rates from 50% to 100% have been described.[48] Survival is dismal for patients with early-onset ARF associated with rhabdomyolysis. However, even in the face of severe ARF, renal function will generally recover over time in those patients who survive.[49]

Metabolic Changes

Acute burn injury results in changes in the body's metabolism related to the massive release of catecholamines into the general circulation as part of the "fight-or-flight" response to major trauma. The metabolic reaction to the stress of a major burn injury involves the sympathetic nervous system and other homeostatic regulators. Hypermetabolism is manifest as a sustained heart rate in the 120 to 140 beats/min range, and oxygen consumption increases to about 150% of normal. The hypermetabolism of burn injury generally persists until the burn wound is reduced to less than 20% of TBSA. This burn-related hypermetabolism poses a major challenge in the treatment of these patients. Many modalities for ameliorating hypermetabolism have been attempted, including reduction of metabolic rate using propranolol, administration of counterregulatory hormones such as insulin and insulin-like growth factor, and stimulation of anabolism using growth hormones and steroids (natural or synthetic). A study from Shriner's Burns Institute in Galveston, Texas, randomized 56 children with major burns to receive supplemental growth hormone, propranolol, or both. Propranolol markedly reduced resting heart rate and energy expenditure measured by indirect calorimetry and improved net muscle protein synthesis. Interestingly, the addition of growth hormone did not enhance these effects.[29] Muscle protein wasting appears to be caused primarily by accelerated protein breakdown. Although protein synthesis is also increased, it fails to keep pace with proteolysis and amino acid mobilization. Thomas

and colleagues evaluated the effect of continuous infusions of insulin (to maintain blood glucose levels between 100 and 140 mg/dl) on preservation of muscle mass in a randomized controlled clinical trial in 18 children with major burns. Evaluation of each patient when the burn wounds were 95% healed showed that insulin-treated patients had improved lean body mass, less muscle wasting, and reduced length of hospital stay in comparison with controls.[39]

Gianotti and colleagues studied temporal fluctuations in insulin-like growth factor type I and its binding protein in a group of burn patients, and demonstrated that both decline for the first 14 days after the burn, paralleling decreases in prealbumin and transferrin.[41] However, plasma levels of growth hormone remained unchanged. In a small study of burned children, administration of insulin-like growth factor type I and insulin growth factor binding protein appeared to exert widespread effects in ameliorating acute inflammation by reducing the synthesis of type 1 and 2 acute phase proteins and interleukin 6 (IL-6) while increasing synthesis of constituted protein such as prealbumin and transferrin. Anabolic steroids, including testosterone and its analogs, such as oxandrolone, are widely used to ameliorate muscle wasting in patients with cancer and acquired immunodeficiency syndrome. However, studies have suggested limited benefits associated with their use in burn patients.

Cellular Changes

Major burn injury affects the entire body, but survival ultimately depends on its effects at the cellular level. The cellular response to burn injury occurs as a metabolic and an immunologic pathophysiologic process. The basic pathologic condition, named the "sick cell syndrome" by Welt[42] in 1967, is a cell membrane transport defect related to an alteration in the steady-state composition, characterized by high intracellular concentrations of sodium. Entry of sodium into the intracellular space occurs simultaneously with entry of water, which leads to cellular edema and, possibly, rupture of the cell wall. Trunkey and coworkers[43] found a marked decrease in primate muscle extracellular water and an increase in intracellular sodium and water during burn shock. An associated decrease in resting membrane potential occurs as the transmembrane potential is disrupted and results in a decrease in amplitude of the action potential and prolongation of the repolarization and depolarization time.[44,45] As sodium and water enter the cell, the sodium-potassium pump is disrupted and potassium moves out, thus further exacerbating the electrolyte imbalance intracellularly.[46] Calcium channel transport is disrupted, along with a loss of intracellular magnesium and phosphate[47] and an increase in serum lactate dehydrogenase levels.[48] The cascade of events that occurs at the level of the cell membrane suggests impairments of basic cellular function as the underlying cause of the diminished membrane potentials. Although the pathophysiologic mechanism has not been completely described, data suggest a decrease in the efficiency of the sodium-potassium pump, a change that can be reversed over time with adequate fluid resuscitation.

Evidence suggests that the burn wound itself at least partially mediates the physiologic response to burn injury at both the local and systemic level. Burn tissue inflammation can lead to vasodilation, increased capillary permeability, and edema, which are normal conditions that promote wound healing. Massive injury results in increased metabolic demands and consumption of inflammatory mediators by the wound, when the priority for survival should be transport of these mediators to healthy tissue.

The extensive evaporative water loss that accompanies burn injury is a heat-consuming process, with the energy need met in part by increased visceral heat production. This hypermetabolic state persists during rest, sleep, and external cooling. The increased oxygen consumption cannot be accounted for on the basis of elevated body temperature alone; thus, an increased basal metabolic rate, not a thermoregulatory drive, is responsible for the increased heat production.

Immune Response

The immune system normally protects the body from disease by recognizing foreign material and mobilizing the body's defenses to maintain homeostasis. When the body is burned, the effects on normal immune response are immediate and extensive. Burn, which upsets homeostasis more than any other injury, can profoundly suppress the immune system and thereby increase the risk of infection. The result in individuals surviving burn shock is immunosuppression with increased susceptibility to potentially fatal system burn wounds, pulmonary sepsis, or both.

Local and systemic physiologic changes are caused by the release of cytokines from burn wounds.[50] Cytokines act directly on the burn wound and also activate other agents, including those that release oxidants, arachidonic acid metabolites, and proteases, thereby contributing to further local and systemic inflammation and, potentially, multisystem organ dysfunction. Recent studies have shown a relationship between decreased cellular cytotoxicity in burned patients and increased production of the cytokines IL-4 and IL-10. Research also shows that the administration of immunopotentiators such as IL-12 improves mortality rates and resistance to bacterial infection.[51]

A host of chemicals found in altered concentrations in burn plasma may also play a role in burn shock. These substances include vasoactive amines (histamine, serotonin), products of complement activation (C3a, C5a), prostaglandins, kinins, endotoxin, and metabolic hormones (catecholamines, glucocorticoids). A decrease in the complement components C3a and C5a in the circulation after burn injury suggests nonspecific activation of the complement system. Activation of the complement system in injured tissue results in an inflammatory response caused by the release of histamine and serotonin by C3a and C5a. Because both histamine and serotonin alter capillary permeability, some investigators propose this mechanism as a cause for burn shock as these vasoactive amines initiate the inflammatory response along with kinin polypeptides and other chemical mediators. As a result of these

vascular changes, fluid and fibrinogen leave the dilated, permeable vessels.

Elements of Burn Injury Survival

The emergent phase of burn care refers to the time between the end of burn shock and closure of the burn wound to less than 20% TBSA. Three elements are essential for survival after a major burn injury: meticulous wound management, adequate nutritional support to establish positive nitrogen balance, and early surgical excision and grafting of full-thickness wounds. The goal of burn management is wound closure in a manner to promote survival.

Management of Wounds

Meticulous wound management consists of measures to limit bacterial proliferation on the wound and adjacent tissue as a result of the loss of the first line of defense—the skin. Burn wounds are sterile initially as a result of thermal decontamination. However, bacterial flora soon re-establish colonies on the burned skin, or eschar. This medium is favorable for pathogenic growth because of the necrotic tissue and warm environment that exist within the burn wound dressing. Benign microorganisms normally found on skin, in the gastrointestinal tract, and in the pulmonary system become lethal as they colonize the burn wound, often resulting in burn progression, invasive sepsis, and death.

The most common source of burn wound bacteria is the patient's own hair follicles, sweat glands, pulmonary tract, and gastrointestinal system, although poor hand-washing technique by staff members can contribute to infection through cross-contamination from other patients.

The goals of wound care are to cleanse and debride the wound of necrotic tissue and debris that promote bacterial growth, minimize further destruction of viable tissue, prevent cross-contamination, preserve body heat and energy, and promote patient comfort. Initial care of the burn wound involves debridement with soap and water. The excision of blisters is controversial and varies from institution to institution. Some argue that the blister provides a moist and protective environment for healing, while others state that large tense blisters put pressure on the underlying wound bed (which impedes healing) and the contained fluid may serve as a nidus for infection. The decision to debride a blister should take into consideration the size and type of the blister. Blisters less than six millimeters in size are unlikely to rupture or put pressure on underlying tissue and should not be debrided. Thick walled blisters due to thick skin particularly on the hands and feet should be left intact as they are not likely to become infected and debridement often leads to limited mobility of the affected extremity. Large tense blisters or those with thin walls that are likely to rupture and become infected can impede wound healing, and debridement of these lesions should be considered.[52] This debridement may also allow for further evaluation of the depth of injury in the underlying wound bed. Additional wound care requires daily observation and management, which includes bathing the patient at least once each day with mild soap and water. Burn wounds are washed to remove accumulated bacteria and previously applied ointments and to debride necrotic tissue. Cleansing of wounds is the most stressful and painful experience that burn patients endure. Pain medication diminishes the pain only marginally because the most effective analgesics work best on visceral or deep pain rather than pain at superficial skin nerve endings. Benzodiazepines are often added to decrease anxiety and provide a degree of amnesia.

After the wound is clean, topical antibacterial agents are applied and covered with a light dressing (Table 54-4). Systemic antibiotics are not helpful in controlling burn wound flora because the burn eschar has no blood supply, limiting local antibiotic bioavailability. Topical burn agents penetrate the eschar, thereby inhibiting bacterial invasion of the wound. Systemic antibiotics are administered when the patient demonstrates signs of systemic infection and are used prophylactically at times of surgical procedures. Appropriate antibiotic selection

TABLE 54-4

Topical Antibiotic Therapy for Thermal Injury Wounds

Drug	Indications for Use	Advantages	Disadvantages	Method of Use
Bacitracin	Bland ointment with minimal antibiotic properties used to promote comfort in patients with minor injury (<25% TBSA)	Prevents drying of wounds, keeps eschar soft and pliable, economical, works well on facial burns to promote healing and patient comfort without facial dressings, painless upon application	No major antibiotic properties; oil based, so it is difficult to wash away	1. Apply to cleansed wound twice daily, cover with Adaptic and Kerlix 2. Apply to facial burns twice daily 3. Apply to recently grafted or healed areas twice daily, wrap with Adaptic and Kerlix
Silver sulfadiazine (Silvadene)	Partial- and/or full-thickness thermal injury (>25% TBSA); small wounds that require topical antibiotic therapy such as frostbite	Wide-spectrum bacteriostatic action and painless on application; organisms resistant to silver nitrate are usually sensitive to silver sulfadiazine; eschar remains soft and pliable; water-miscible base promotes ease of removal	Not effective against fungal organisms, can cause leukopenia, expensive; sulfa component can produce allergic reactions in sensitive patients; resistance can emerge with prolonged use	Apply to cleansed wound 1-3 times daily; may leave wound open or cover with light dressing
Silver nitrate	Partial- and/or full-thickness burns (>25% TBSA), fungal infections, patients with sulfa allergy	Wide-spectrum bacteriostatic action, effective against fungal infections, comfortable, economical, no sensitivity reported, painless on application, no resistant organisms	Can cause severe electrolyte imbalances (hyponatremia and hypochloremia), which are corrected with oral and intravenous NaCl; poor penetration into wound; requires bulky dressing, thereby severely limiting motion; messy and time consuming to use	0.5% solution in distilled water applied to wet dressing every 2 hr; dressing changes twice daily
Mafenide acetate (Sulfamylon)	Electrical injury, ear burns, wounds colonized with organisms resistant to other topical agents because it penetrates eschar more deeply	Wide-spectrum bacteriostatic action; active penetration allows delayed therapy to be effective; requires no dressing, thereby promoting motion; resistant organisms do not develop with prolonged use; drug of choice for all	Causes severe metabolic alterations within 72 hr when used on >20% TBSA wounds; carbonic anhydrase inhibition with HCO_3^- excretion and chloride retention; compensation is by hyperventilation with subsequent CO_2 decreased or depletion	Apply to cleansed wound acetate 1-2 times daily; leave open because wrapping produces maceration

From Kravitz M: Thermal injuries. In Cardona VD et al, editors: *Trauma nursing: from resuscitation through rehabilitation*, Philadelphia, 1988, Saunders, p 723.

TBSA, Total body surface area.

is based on laboratory cultures of the patient's wound tissue to identify and deliver antibiotics to which the bacteria are sensitive.

Healing of burn wounds begins when white blood cells have surrounded the burn wound and phagocytosis begins. Necrotic tissue begins to slough. Fibroblasts begin to lay down matrices of the collagen precursors that eventually form granulation tissue. Kept free from infection, a partial-thickness burn will heal from the edges and from below in a process that occurs over a 14- to 21-day period. Full-thickness burns require autografting to achieve wound closure because no dermal elements are available to form new skin.

Burn Surgery

The third element essential to survival after major burn injury is surgical excision of dead skin, or burn eschar, followed by skin grafting with the patient's own skin (autograft). Areas of full-thickness burn are excised. In some cases, it is difficult to assess the depth of the burn. In these cases, it may be appropriate to wait 7 to 10 days to allow the area to declare its depth. This is especially true in young children with scald burns. In burns involving the face, scalp, and ears, it may be appropriate to wait as long as 3 weeks for the area to declare itself. These sites are particularly dense areas of dermal appendages and may heal without grafting if given time. Current surgical management of burn wounds involves early removal of the necrotic tissue followed by split-thickness autografts. This therapy has changed the management of burn care in the past 20 years from one of daily bathing and mechanical debridement of necrotic tissue for months after burn injury to one of early surgical removal of the burn wound and a dramatic reduction in hospitalization time. In the past, patients with major burns had low rates of survival because healing and wound coverage took so long that death from infection usually occurred before healing. Now, mortality and morbidity are greatly decreased as a result of early surgical intervention.

Excision and Grafting. The two types of surgical excision are tangential excision and full-thickness excision. Both tangential and full-thickness excision procedures involve massive blood loss often requiring red blood cell transfusion. Traditionally, to avoid this bleeding, the wound would be treated locally until the eschar separated and then covered with a graft. This process resulted in long hospital stays of approximately 3 to 5 weeks with increased bacterial colonization of wounds leading to higher incidences of sepsis and multiple organ failure. It is now accepted practice to perform early excision and grafting of wounds 2 to 7 days after injury. Although blood loss is a concern with early excision, improvements in intensive care management of these patients have made this issue more manageable. The benefits of early excision of burns are seen as a decrease in wound infections, decreased lengths of hospital stay, and improved survival.[56]

In tangential excision, eschar is removed in thin layers with an instrument called a *dermatome* until viable tissue is visible. Full-thickness excision using a surgical scalpel removes eschar to the level of fascia. Full-thickness excision often leaves an uneven contour postexcision, which is difficult to graft, with resultant poor cosmetic effects. After bleeding has been controlled in the area of excision, application of an autograft, skin substitute, or dressing follows. In some cases, the area may need to be covered with wet dressings soaked in antibiotic solutions for 24 hours with delayed autografting. Some studies have shown a benefit for usage of a vacuum-assisted closure device to promote blood circulation in the wound bed allowing for earlier placement of an epidermal graft.[60]

Skin Substitutes. Several temporary biological dressings are available for patients with extensive burns that do not permit initial autografting. Products available for temporary coverage include homograft (skin harvested from cadavers), xenograft (skin harvested from pigs), synthetic skin (a variety of products for temporary coverage), and amnion (amniotic lining of human placenta harvested from afterbirth following human delivery). Temporary skin substitutes can be used in superficial burns and functions mainly to decrease pain and augment healing. It is important to make sure that all nonviable tissue is removed, as dead tissue under a graft causes a marked increase in muscle wasting and impaired immune defenses. Bioactive dermal components added to the graft help to stimulate healing and include elastin, fibronectin, growth factors, glycosaminoglycans and hyaluronic acid. In deep burns or large burns in which not enough skin is present to completely close the wound, it may be necessary to utilize a permanent skin substitute. These grafts often provide a good functional and cosmetic result and have rapid and excellent adherence properties. Grafts may consist of a bilayer membrane that provides a dermal matrix of bovine collagen and an epidermal or silicone layer to prevent desiccation (drying), or the dermal and epidermal components may be replaced separately.[54] The composition of a permanent skin substitute often includes the patient's own cells in either the dermal or epidermal layer. The dermal matrix allows ingrowth of capillaries and fibroblasts. This matrix is slowly degraded as a neodermis develops. The silicone layer acting as the epidermal barrier is then removed and autograft is applied over the neodermis.[53]

These dressings promote patient comfort while partially restoring the water vapor barrier and some antibacterial properties to the wound until an autograft is available. The unburned area of the patient from which skin is harvested in a paper-thin sheet is referred to as the *donor site*. Donor sites heal in about 5 to 7 days in the presence of adequate nutritional support and the absence of infection and can be reharvested at that time. Donor sites can be repeatedly harvested depending on graft thickness, enabling increased wound coverage, which thereby permits survival in some patients with TBSA injury as large as 90%. To expand the surface area that a sheet of autograft will cover, harvested skin is cut in a manner that resembles a net or mesh by using an instrument called a *skin mesher*. The skin may then be expanded, depending on the size of the mesh, to cover two, three, four, or more times its original size. This combination of repeated harvesting and meshing allows autografting of massive burn injuries over a period of a few weeks. After grafting, the areas must be protected from infection, pressure, shearing, and trauma that produce bruising or bleeding under the graft. Major causes of graft loss include infection, blisters, or hematoma underneath the graft that interferes with revascularization. Negative pressure dressings or vacuum-assisted closure devices (VAC) placed over a graft improves the contact surface of the graft as well as prevents underlying accumulation of serum or blood. Use of these devices when compared to standard bulky dressings have demonstrated a decrease in loss of graft, decreased need for secondary grafting procedures on the same wound, and a resulting decrease in hospital stay for these procedures.[58]

The greatest risk of infection is after postoperative day 3, as the bacteria begin to recolonize the area. Grafts are usually stable by postoperative day 4, at which time physical and occupational therapy can begin.[9,57]

Surgical wound management of elderly burn patients is determined by the philosophy of the burn center. Elderly patients do not generally tolerate any surgical procedure as well as younger patients; this knowledge has been applied to the management of burn wounds in some patients, and conservative, nonsurgical wound management for weeks after injury has produced acceptable survival rates in elderly patients.[59] Others report that early excision of eschar and early wound closure are associated with increased survival and decreased length of stay for older patients with burns.[61] Children younger than 2 years have a high mortality rate with major burn injury, but older children recover at a high rate with proper medical management.[12,14,29] Table 54-5 summarizes physiologic changes related to the aging process that can affect surgical outcome.

Nutritional Support for Positive Nitrogen Balance

Healing occurs only in a state of positive nitrogen balance. Hypermetabolism characterizes the metabolic response to thermal injury; with the magnitude of the physiologic alteration related to the extent of the burn injury. One of the most significant advances in recent burn management is

TABLE 54-5

Physiologic Changes Related to the Aging Process That Can Affect Surgery

Physiologic Changes	Effects	Potential Postoperative Complication
Cardiovascular ↓ Elasticity of blood vessels ↓ Cardiac output ↓ Peripheral circulation	↓ Circulation to vital organs Slower blood flow	Shock (hypotension), thrombosis with pulmonary emboli, delayed wound healing, postoperative confusion, hypervolemia, decreased response to stress
Respiratory ↓ Elasticity of lungs and chest wall ↑ Residual lung volume ↓ Forced expiratory volume ↓ Ciliary action Fewer alveolar capillaries	↓ Vital capacity ↓ Alveolar volume ↓ Gas exchange ↓ Cough reflex	Atelectasis, pneumonia, postoperative confusion
Urinary ↓ Glomerular filtration rate ↓ Bladder muscle tone Weakened perineal muscles	↓ Kidney function Stasis of urine in bladder Loss of urinary control	Prolonged response to anesthesia and drugs, overhydration with intravenous fluids, hyperkalemia, urinary tract infection, urinary retention
Musculoskeletal ↓ Muscle strength Limitation of motion	↓ Activity	Atelectasis, pneumonia, thrombophlebitis, constipation or fecal impaction
Gastrointestinal ↓ Intestinal motility Metabolic	Retention of feces	Constipation or fecal impaction
↓ γ-Globulin level ↓ Plasma proteins	↓ Inflammatory response	Delayed wound healing, wound dehiscence or evisceration
Immune System Fewer killer T cells ↓ Response to foreign antigens	↓ Ability to protect against invasion by pathogenic microorganisms	Wound infection, wound dehiscence, pneumonia, urinary tract infection

From Keeling AW, Muro GA, Long BC: Preoperative nursing. In Phipps WJ et al, editors: *Medical-surgical nursing: concepts and clinical practice*, ed 5, St Louis, 1995, Mosby.

recognition of the critical importance of early nutrition to the wound-healing process. The magnitude of nutritional support required by burn patients depends on two factors: the patient's preburn nutritional status and the extent of the TBSA burn. Patients with minor burns require no nutritional support beyond a regular diet, whereas those with moderate and large burns require additional carbohydrate and protein supplementation. Patients with poor preburn nutritional status are classified as having a critical injury regardless of the burn size due to the associated immune deficiencies and limited metabolic reserves. The most easily recognized and documented finding in the absence of adequate nutritional support after burn injury is massive loss of body weight. Maintenance of body protein appears to be critical for survival. Loss of one fourth to one third of the protein mass from the body is predictably fatal; this degree of negative nitrogen balance in humans is associated with a 40% to 50% body weight loss.

Patients with greater than a 40% TBSA burn demonstrate the maximal stress response within predictable ranges of body mass. In these hypermetabolic patients, providing early protein and caloric support of at least the predicted energy requirement is necessary for optimal outcome and may be essential for survival. Providing early nutrition in enteral form may also help by blunting the hypermetabolic response to thermal injury.[69] Weight loss after thermal injury is not an obligatory component of the response to trauma but rather a reflection of the difference between the total energy requirements and the ability to supply them in the form of adequate caloric intake.[16] Kao and colleagues demonstrated that enteral feeding should begin within 18 hours of admission with a Dobhoff feeding tube.[62] These feedings should be continuous and should not be stopped when the patient goes to the operating room. With vigorous nutritional support, erosion of total body mass and subsequent starvation leading to immunologic alteration are not inevitable in a massively burned patient.[46,63,64]

General formulas are used to estimate the caloric requirements of burn patients, all of which are based on either preburn body weight and % TBSA burn or square meters of body surface area and % TBSA burn. The two most widely used formulas are the Curreri formula for adults and the Polk formula for children. Curreri and colleagues[65] demonstrated that caloric requirements in adult burn patients could be expressed by the following formula:

$$(25) \times (\text{body weight in kg}) + (40) \times (\%\text{TBSA burn}) =$$
$$\text{Ideal 24-hour caloric needs}$$

The requirements in children[67] are predicted as follows:

$$(60) \times (\text{body weight in kg}) + (36) \times (\%\text{TBSA burn}) =$$
$$\text{Ideal 24-hour caloric needs}$$

If the ideal daily caloric intake can be maintained, then the amount of weight loss post burn could be minimized. It is important to emphasize that these formulas represent more than just total caloric intake; they are used to predict positive nitrogen balance for each patient. Thus if the patient is losing tremendous amounts of nitrogen or is not absorbing glucose,

the net caloric utilization will be much less than the intake, even though the adult patient may be receiving as much as 5000 kcal/day. Monitoring of daily nitrogen balance by indirect calorimetry is essential throughout the course of burn treatment to ensure a positive nitrogen balance (nonprotein kilocalorie to nitrogen ratio of 100:1 and at least 2 g of protein per kilogram per day). The serum prealbumin concentration is a useful indicator of nutritional progress.

The routes for initiating caloric support after major burn injury are either enteral or parenteral. Any patient with a functioning gastrointestinal tract should receive enteral nutrition orally, by tube feeding, or by a combination of both. Early enteral nutrition has shown to preserve gastrin secretion, promote motility of the gastrointestinal tract, and maintain mucosa barrier function, which serves to decrease bacterial translocation, lower incidence of intestinal ischemia, and decrease inflammatory mediators.[66] In some burn patients, enteral feeding may not be possible, and total parenteral nutrition may become the only method available for providing nutritional support. The possibility of infection is increased when parenteral nutrition is used.

Hart and colleagues demonstrated that the catabolic response may continue for 4 to 6 months in adults and as long as 9 months in children.[68] Given this information, the nutritional status and dietary habits of burn patients should be continually evaluated for many months after their discharge from the burn unit.

Rehabilitation Phase

The rehabilitation phase begins when the burn size is reduced to less than 20% TBSA and the patient is capable of assuming some self-care. This phase may occur as early as 2 weeks or as long as 2 to 3 months after the burn and, in the case of a major debilitating or disfiguring injury, may last many years. Goals for this period are to assist the patient in resuming a functional role in society and to accomplish functional and cosmetic reconstruction.[9,11,13]

Wound Healing

During the rehabilitation phase, the pathophysiologic mechanism of hypermetabolism and the impaired immune function have begun to normalize, although some changes will persist beyond discharge from the hospital. The major pathophysiologic process of this phase is related to the dysfunctional results of wounds healing in a manner that causes flexor contractures, excessive scarring, and keloid formation. The burn wounds have healed either by primary intention or by autografting. Layers of epithelialization begin building back the tissue structure destroyed by the burn injury. Collagen fibers present in the new scar tissue help healing and add strength to weakened areas. After healing, the new skin appears flat and pink, even in dark-skinned people.

In approximately 4 to 6 weeks the area becomes raised and hyperemic. If adequate range-of-motion exercises are not instituted early in the hospital course, the new tissue will shorten and a contracture will result (Figure 54-7).[9,11] Mature healing

FIGURE 54-7 Physical and occupational therapy is necessary from the time of injury. This 8-year-old girl was burned 4 years previously in a house fire. Inadequate follow-up because of parental neglect led to severe scar contractures and hand disability. (Courtesy Michael Peck, MD, University of North Carolina Burn Center, Chapel Hill.)

FIGURE 54-8 The custom-fitted antiscar support garment modeled here effectively provides pressure therapy over wounds, which helps to minimize the development of hypertrophic scarring. (From Black JM, Matassarin-Jacobs E, editors: *Medical-surgical nursing: clinical management for continuity of care,* ed 6, Philadelphia, 2001, Saunders, p 1356. Courtesy Medical Z, San Antonio, Texas.)

is reached in 6 to 12 months, when suppleness has returned and the pink or red color has faded to a slightly lighter hue than the surrounding unburned tissue. It takes longer for darker skin to regain its color because many of the melanocytes were destroyed, and often the skin never returns to its original color. The mesh pattern in meshed autograft fades with time, but in larger expansions such as 4:1 or greater the pattern may persist.

Scarring has two components: discoloration and contour. The discoloration of scars fades with time and can be covered with makeup on visible body surface areas. However, scar tissue tends to develop altered contours; that is, the skin is no longer flat but becomes raised above the contour of the surrounding area (also known as hypertrophic scarring). Areas of the face tend to scar in an even plane—a process that distorts the natural contours around the nose, chin, and mouth and thus greatly alters a patient's appearance. Scarring on the cheeks can contract and pull the lower eyelid down sufficiently to prevent closure and protection of the eye normally afforded by the eyelid—a condition called ectropion. Burns on the eyelid can also result in ectropion and must be corrected by reconstructive surgery. Pressure can help keep a scar flat if the pressure is slightly greater than capillary pressure and is continuous during the healing process. This knowledge led to the development of burn garments, which are custom made for each patient to contour with pressure over the area of burn for about 12 to 18 months after burn injury. Except for bath times, the garments must be worn continuously; patient compliance often becomes an issue (Figure 54-8).

Excessive and sometimes debilitating discomfort from itching occurs in the healing burn wound and persists for many months. The exact pathophysiologic process is not known but is related to the absence of sebaceous glands in the area and to the hyperactivity of sweat glands. Topical lotions and orally administered antihistamines give partial relief of symptoms, but tolerance to the drugs develops and patients often require a series of different medications over time. The newly formed skin is extremely sensitive to trauma, and blisters form after very slight pressure or friction. The newly healed areas may be hypersensitive or hyposensitive to cold, heat, or touch. Ward and colleagues[70] studied loss of cutaneous sensibility after grafting in 60 patients and found that 97% demonstrated markedly diminished or absent responses to sharp/dull, hot/cold, and light touch stimuli over the grafted areas. Grafted areas are more likely to be hyposensitive until peripheral nerve regeneration occurs, although donor sites harvested several times will show all the same healing pathologic process as healed burn wounds.

Scarring is a genetically inherited trait. Some people will have minimal scarring, whereas others, especially African Americans and Caucasians with red hair, tend to have significant scarring and keloid formation in which the scar tissue actually outgrows the boundary of the original wound. Healed burn wounds must be protected from direct sunlight for 1 year to prevent hyperpigmentation.

The most common complications during the rehabilitation phase are related to the formation of skin and joint contractures. Because of pain associated with movement, the patient will want to assume the position of comfort, which is with all extremities flexed, but this position predisposes to contracture formation. To minimize contracture formation, positioning in extension, splinting in the position of function, and active range-of-motion exercises are initiated on admission and continue throughout the course of treatment. The areas most subject to contracture formation include the anterior and lateral neck areas, axillae, antecubital fossae, fingers, groin areas, popliteal fossae, and ankles. Not only do contractures develop in the skin, but the underlying tissues such as ligaments and tendons also have a tendency to shorten during the healing process. Therapy is aimed at extension of body parts to ensure that the flexors are longer than the extensors.[9]

KEY POINTS

- The emergent phase is the time between the end of burn shock and closure of the wound to less than 20% TBSA. Wound management, nutritional support, and surgical grafting of full-thickness wounds are the priorities of treatment during the emergent phase.
- Wound management is necessary to prevent bacterial colonization of the wound and subsequent septicemia. Early surgical wound management is essential. Topical antibiotics are used because systemic antibiotics cannot reach the wound because of a lack of blood supply.
- Nutritional requirements after burn injury are high. A high-calorie, high-protein diet is needed. Persons with major burns usually cannot ingest sufficient nutrients and require parenteral and enteral supplementation. A positive nitrogen balance is essential for healing.
- Early surgical excision and skin grafting are the treatment of choice for deep burns. Excision procedures result in significant blood loss requiring blood transfusions. Skin grafts are taken from a healthy portion of the patient's skin. Temporary grafts (e.g., cadaver skin, synthetics, pig skin) may be used to cover the wound until an autograft can be obtained.
- The rehabilitation phase begins when the burn is reduced to less than 20% TBSA. Problems during this phase include skin contracture and excessive scarring. Healing is complete at 6 to 12 months. Positioning in extension and range-of-motion exercises are important to prevent contracture.

Factors That Increase Risk of Burn Injury

Environmental and lifestyle factors influence the frequency and magnitude of burn injury. Conditions that impair judgment or hinder the ability to obtain a safe distance from a fire will increase the risk of injury. Certain factors that increase the risk of accidental burn injury include alcohol or drug abuse, neurologic or psychiatric disorders, and immobilizing physical disabilities. Alcohol use contributes to an estimated 40% of residential fire deaths. One study found that 3.25% of patients admitted to a burn unit had both thermal injury and neurologic disorders. The occurrence of burns during pregnancy is rare but often results in fetal death, even with relatively small maternal TBSA burns. In cases of electrical burns, the fetal mortality rate is 15% to 73%, and in the case of lightning strike it is 50%. The high fetal death rate is caused

by adaptive mechanisms that identify the gravid uterus and fetal-placental circulation as low priority in the presence of diminished circulating blood volume such as occurs with burn injury.[71]

ELECTRICAL INJURY

Incidence and Mortality

Electrical injury accounts for fewer than 2% of admissions to burn facilities, but injury from electricity has been increasing in the United States.[74] Electrical injuries are classified as high-voltage (1000 volts or greater) or low-voltage. Household currents of 120 and 220 volts typically cause low-voltage electrical injury. High-voltage injuries are frequently due to high-tension sources, which commonly carry from 7200 to 19,000 volts (Figure 54-9) but may involve 100,000 to 1 million volts.[75]

Burn facilities serving rural areas report a higher percentage of electrical injury admissions than do facilities serving urban areas.[74] Few of these injuries are the result of household accidents, although toddlers are occasionally injured when they insert metal objects into electrical outlets. Teething infants may sustain electrical burns to the mouth by chewing on electrical cords,[76-78] but electrical current rarely passes through the body.

Lightning injuries kill between 150 and 300 people per year in the United States.[78] Lightning carries a direct current of 100 million or more volts and up to 200,000 amperes, and it can injure either by a direct strike or by a side flash as a result of the flow of current between the victim's body and a nearby object struck by lightning.[78]

FIGURE 54-9 High-voltage electrical injuries produce devastating injuries, such as the damage to the right hand of this electrician who inadvertently contacted a 17,000-V line. The underlying muscle damage is often greater than the thermal skin burn. Myoglobinuria, if inadequately managed, can lead to acute tubular necrosis. Early fasciotomies are mandatory, and amputation may be necessary to control rhabdomyolysis. (Courtesy Michael Peck, MD, University of North Carolina Burn Center, Chapel Hill.)

Pathophysiology

The pathophysiologic mechanism of electrical injury is related to the subsequent tissue damage as electrical energy is converted to heat. Workplace electrocutions account for 5% of all worker deaths.[79] In children, electrical burns account for 2% to 3% of all burns, and 60% to 70% of these result from biting extension cords.

Arcing electricity produces surface heat, which may ignite clothing and destroy superficial tissue, but internal damage is absent; this injury is actually a flame or thermal injury and not electrical. These injuries are properly classified as heat injuries, for which the treatment plan is identical to that for other heat injuries.[74] True electrical injury occurs as electrical current enters the body, traverses a portion of the body, and exits at another body site. Electrical injuries are usually deeper than full-thickness skin injury and are often classified as fourth-degree injury.

Voltage, type of current (direct or alternating), and length of contact all influence the extent of damage. Alternating current (AC) produces prolonged tetanic muscle contraction. At low voltages it can cause ventricular fibrillation, tetanic contraction of the respiratory muscles, superficial burns, and rhabdomyolysis. At lower voltage, AC is associated with low mortality. High-voltage AC or direct current (DC) causes ventricular fibrillation, a single sustained contraction, rhabdomyolysis, and higher overall mortality.[80]

Each true electrical injury produces an entrance wound and at least one exit wound, with the most extensive damage commonly occurring at the exit point. Electrical current follows the path of least resistance: in humans, this path is through blood vessels, nerves, tendons, and bone. Skin has high resistance; thus the current enters through the skin but goes deeper to travel the path of least resistance until it exits the body. The current rarely produces direct visceral damage, but severe injuries to the extremities are common. The amputation rate after severe electrical injury exceeds 90%. The pathophysiologic process, in addition to direct tissue destruction, involves heat coagulation of blood vessels, which leaves distal areas without blood supply. Electrical injuries produce both systemic and local alterations. The systemic changes produce three common complications during the acute period: arrhythmias or cardiac arrest, metabolic acidosis, and myoglobinuria. Electrical injury may also cause direct myocardial necrosis. Arrhythmias are exacerbated by any given voltage of AC. Higher voltage may also cause asystole. Locally, electrical injury produces direct cellular denaturation; areas of healthy tissue are devascularized as a result of heat coagulation of arteries and veins. These events are followed 48 to 72 hours after injury by gross tissue necrosis and subsequent gangrene resulting from lack of blood flow. Amputation is required early in electrical injury to prevent the development of deep soft-tissue infections and sepsis leading to death.

Management and Complications

Once the patient is admitted, airway management is the primary focus; patients with major electrical injury often require endotracheal intubation to ensure a patent airway. A condition similar to burn shock develops within a few minutes of major electrical injury and requires similar fluid resuscitation measures. No formula exists to predict fluid requirements for patients with electrical injury shock because often the only apparent damage is the entrance and exit wounds and no assessment of internal damage is possible. An adult patient is given a 1-L bolus of Ringer lactate solution intravenously within the first 15 minutes after intravenous line placement; children are given a smaller, size-appropriate amount. Thereafter, fluid is infused at a rate to produce a urine volume of 100 ml/hr in adults and 1 to 2 ml/kg per hour in children. Adult patients frequently require 1 to 2 L of fluid per hour to support the cardiovascular system.

Patients have traditionally been on cardiac monitoring for the first 24 hours after injury. Bailey and colleagues determined that this is unnecessary if the initial electrocardiogram (ECG) is normal, there was no loss of consciousness at the scene, and the patient is an adult. Twenty-four-hour monitoring is indicated in adult patients with an abnormal initial ECG, a history of cardiac disease, positive loss of consciousness at the scene, and/or voltage greater than 240 volts.[80] Measurement of cardiac enzymes initially reveals elevated values, also suggesting acute myocardial damage, but in such patients these findings are not indicative of a cardiac pathologic process.

Electrical injury also produces a profound, potentially lethal metabolic acidosis. These patients often have initial serum pH values of 6.8 to 7.2 on admission. Treatment consists of intravenous administration of sodium bicarbonate in amounts to correct the values toward normal. Metabolic acidosis is a recurring problem requiring ongoing treatment until the problem resolves 24 to 48 hours after injury. The pathophysiologic mechanism is related to the release of intracellular contents into the general circulation from areas of tissue damage and to the lactic acidosis that accompanies hypotensive shock states.

Myoglobinuria follows electrical injury as myoglobin, a component of muscle tissue, is released from muscles damaged by electrical current and enters the systemic circulation.[81] Myoglobin is a large protein that precipitates in the renal tubules and leads to cast formation. Subsequently the tubules become obstructed and renal tubular acidosis develops. This accumulation is prevented by maintaining urine output at 100 to 200 ml/hr in adults and 2 ml/kg per hour in children until the urine clears. Mannitol, an osmotic diuretic, is administered along with large volumes of intravenous fluids to prevent the development of acute tubular necrosis, a totally preventable sequela of electrical injury with proper management. Sodium bicarbonate is often administered to alkalinize the urine, thereby increasing the solubility of myoglobin.

Local effects of electrical injury are related to alterations in tissue perfusion. Surgical decompression of areas of electrical burn by fasciotomy is performed for the purpose of releasing any increased compartment pressures that may be compromising blood flow. Amputation may be required during the initial surgery for devascularized areas. Because of the continued presence of necrotic tissue, areas of surgical decompression or initial amputation are not closed surgically.[82]

Central nervous system alterations can be noted in patients with major electrical injury. Memory deficits can occur for several weeks. This condition improves gradually and usually resolves within 4 to 6 weeks after injury. Other central nervous system deficits after electrical injury include ataxia and gait alterations accompanied by sensory deficits. These alterations may or may not improve over time.

Electrically injured patients experience all the challenges of rehabilitation plus possible adjustments to amputation and gait instability related to central nervous system impairment. Skin grafting in areas adjacent to amputation presents challenging prosthetic problems that may delay independent ambulation and restoration of self-care abilities.[83] In general, patients with major electrical injury experience longer rehabilitation periods than do thermally injured patients.

A unique complication of electrical injury is the formation of corneal cataracts,[84] the cause of which is unknown. The cataracts may be detected on ophthalmic examination as early as 1 month or as late as 12 months after injury and may occur in one or both eyes. The electrical injury does not have to be on or near the head for the condition to develop. Progression is rapid, with the cornea becoming completely opaque within months. Ophthalmic examinations should be performed monthly for the first year and then every 3 months during the second year after injury to identify this pathologic process early. The patient will usually complain of blurring vision, but young children may not mention blurring because they do not recognize the concept. Treatment consists of corneal transplantation.[84]

SUMMARY

In recent decades, burn mortality rates have decreased significantly, with most patients achieving excellent functional and cosmetic outcomes. Improved outcomes have clearly been related to an improved understanding of the pathophysiologic mechanism of burns, advances in burn care management, and the development of a comprehensive, treatment-oriented approach to care.

The priorities for assessment and treatment of burn victims are no different from that of other trauma patients. However, depending on the cause, burn injuries influence a variety of systemic, circulatory, and metabolic changes. As a result, in order to make appropriate treatment decisions and recognize potential complications, a clear understanding of the pathophysiologic processes associated with the burn injury is necessary.

REFERENCES

1. Arturson G: Pathophysiology of the burn wound and pharmacological treatment, *Burns* 22(4):255-274, 1996.
2. Nguyen TT et al: Current treatment of severely burned patients, *Ann Surg* 223(1):14-25, 1996.
3. Sheridan RL: Burns, *Crit Care Med* 30(11 Suppl):S500-S514, 2002.
4. American College of Surgeons Committee on Trauma: *Resources for optimal care of the injured patient*, Chicago, 1999, The College, p 55.
5. National Center for Injury Prevention and Control. Fire Deaths and Injuries: [cited 27 February 2008]. Available at: http://www.cdc.gov/ncipc/factsheets/fire.htm.
6. National SAFE KIDS Campaign (NSKC): *Burn Injury Fact Sheet*, Washington (DC), 2007, NSKC.
7. Istre GR et al: Residential fire related deaths and injuries among children: fireplay, smoke alarms, and prevention, *Inj Prev* 8(2):128-132, 2002.
8. Safe Kids Worldwide (SKW): *Burn and Scalds Safety*, Washington DC, 2007, SKW.
9. Richard R: OT/PT forum, *J Burn Care Rehabil* 23(3):220, 2002.
10. Ho WS, Ying SY, Burd A: Outcome analysis of 286 severely burned patients: retrospective study, *Hong Kong Med J* 8(4):235-239, 2002.
11. Young A: Rehabilitation of burn injuries (review), *Phys Med Rehabil Clin North Am* 13(1):85-108, 2002.
12. Stoddard FJ et al: Treatment of pain in acutely burned children, *J Burn Care Rehabil* 23(2):135-156, 2002.
13. Partridge J: Psychosocial rehabilitation after burn injuries, *Nurs Times* 97(48):47, 2001.
14. Sheridan RL et al: Long-term outcome of children surviving massive burns, *JAMA* 283(1):69-73, 2000.
15. Muller MJ, Pegg SP, Rule MR: Determinants of death following burn injury, *Br J Surg* 88(4):583-587, 2001.
16. Gore DC et al: Hyperglycemia exacerbates muscle protein catabolism in burn-injured patients, *Crit Care Med* 30(11):2438-2442, 2002.
17. Gibran NS, Heimbach DM: Current status of burn wound pathophysiology, *Clin Plast Surg* 27(1):11-22, 2000.
18. Arturson G: Forty years in burns research—the postburn inflammatory response, *Burns* 26(7):599-604, 2000.
19. Nebraska Burn Institute: *Advanced burn life support provider's manual*, Lincoln, Nebraska, 1994, Burn Institute.
20. American Burn Association [cited 27 February 2008]. Available at: http://www.ameriburn.org.
21. Berkowitz Z et al: Hazardous substances emergency events in the agriculture industry and related services in four mid-western states, *J Occup Environ Med* 44(8):714-723, 2002.
22. Holm C et al: The relationship between oxygen delivery and oxygen consumption during fluid resuscitation of burn-related shock, *J Burn Care Rehabil* 21(2):147-154, 2000.
23. Cartotto RC et al: How well does the Parkland formula estimate actual fluid resuscitation volumes? *J Burn Care Rehabil* 23(4):258-265, 2002.
24. Tompkins RG: ABA 2002 presidential address: The American Burn Association in the new millennium, *J Burn Care Rehabil* 22:369-374, 2001.
25. Moncrief JA, Mason AD Jr: Water vapor loss in the burned patient, *Surg Forum* 13:38-41, 1962.
26. Moncrief JA: Burns. In Schwartz SI et al, editors: *Principles of surgery*, ed 2, New York, 1974, McGraw-Hill, pp 253-274.
27. Roe CF, Kinney JM: Water and heat exchange in third-degree burns, *Surgery* 56:212-220, 1964.
28. White DJ et al: Cardiomyocyte intracellular calcium and cardiac dysfunction after burn trauma, *Crit Care Med* 30(1):14-22, 2002.
29. Sheridan RL, Schnitzer JJ: Management of the high-risk pediatric burn patient, *J Pediatr Surg* 36(8):1308-1312, 2001.
30. Wibbenmeyer LA et al: Predicting survival in an elderly burn patient population, *Burns* 27(6):583-590, 2001.
31. Baxter CR, Cook WA, Shires GT: Serum myocardial depressant factor of burn shock, *Surg Forum* 17:1-2, 1966.
32. Lefer AM, Martin J: Origin of myocardial depressant factor in shock, *Am J Physiol* 218(5):1423-1427, 1970.
33. Ribeiro CA et al: Association between early detection of soluble TNF-receptors and mortality in burn patients, *Intensive Care Med* 28(4):472-478, 2002.
34. No authors listed: Ventilation with lower tidal volumes as compared with traditional tidal volumes for acute lung injury and the acute respiratory distress syndrome. The Acute Respiratory Distress Syndrome Network, *N Engl J Med* 342(18):1301-1308, 2000.

35. Sukuki M et al: Correlation between QT dispersion and burn severity, *Burns* 28(5):481-485, 2002.

36. Steinvall I et al: Acute respiratory distress syndrome is as important as inhalation injury for the development of respiratory dysfunction in major burns, *Burns* 34(4):441-451, 2008 [Epub ahead of print].

37. Turnage RH et al: Mechanisms of pulmonary microvascular dysfunction during severe burn injury (review), *World J Surg* 26(7):848-853, 2002.

38. Liffner G et al: Inhalation injury assessed by score does not contribute to the development of acute respiratory distress syndrome in burn victims, *Burns* 31(3):263-268, 2005.

39. Thomas JA et al: IRAK contributes to burn-triggered myocardial contractile dysfunction, *Am J Physiol Heart Circ Physiol* 283(2):H829-H836, 2002.

40. Clardy PF, Manaker S: Carbon monoxide poisoning, *UpToDate Online* 15.3, January 18, 2007.

41. Gianotti L et al: Activity of GH/IGF-1 axis in burn patients: comparison with normal subjects and patients with GH deficiency, *J Endocrinol Invest* 25(2):116-124, 2002.

42. Welt LG: Membrane transport defect: the sick cell, *Trans Assoc Am Physicians* 80:217-226, 1967.

43. Trunkey DD et al: The effect of hemorrhagic shock on intracellular muscle action potentials in the primates, *Surgery* 74(2):241-250, 1973.

44. Cunningham JN Jr, Shires GT, Wagner Y: Changes in intracellular sodium and potassium content of red blood cells in trauma and shock, *Am J Surg* 122(5):650-654, 1971.

45. Rosenthal SM, Tabor H: Electrolyte changes and chemotherapy in experimental burn and traumatic shock and hemorrhage, *Arch Surg* 51:244-252, 1945.

46. Turinsky J, Gonnerman WA, Loose LD: Impaired mineral metabolism in post-burn muscle, *J Trauma* 21(6):417-423, 1981.

47. Sun IF et al: Continuous arteriovenous hemodialysis and continuous venovenous hemofiltration in burn patients with acute renal failure, *Kaohsiung J Med Sci* 23(7):344-351, 2007.

48. Deets DK, Glaviano VV: Plasma and cardiac lactic dehydrogenase activity in burn shock, *Proc Soc Exp Biol Med* 142(2):412-416, 1973.

49. Mustonen KM, Vuola J: Acute renal failure in intensive care burn patients (ARF in burn patients), *J Burn Care & Research* 29(1):227-237, 2008.

50. Ogura H et al: Long-term enhanced expression of heat shock proteins and decelerated apoptosis in polymorphonuclear leukocytes from major burn patients, *J Burn Care Rehabil* 23(2):103-109, 2002.

51. Rose JK, Herndon DN: Advances in the treatment of burn patients, *Burns* 23(Suppl 1):S19-S26, 1997.

52. Sargent RL: Management of blisters in the partial-thickness burn: an integrative research review, *J Burn Care & Research* 27(1):66-81, 2006.

53. Boyce ST et al: The 1999 clinical research award: cultured skin substitutes combined with Integra Artificial Skin to replace native skin autograft and allograft for the closure of excised full-thickness burns, *J Burn Care Rehabil* 20(6):453-461, 1999.

54. Demling R et al: Use of skin substitutes, Burnsurgery.org [Cited March 26, 2008.]

55. Mann R et al: Prospective trial of thick vs. standard split-thickness skin grafts in burns of the hand, *J Burn Care Rehabil* 22(6):390-392, 2001.

56. Ong Y et al: Meta-analysis of early excision of burns, *Burns* 32(2):145-150, 2006.

57. Latenser BA, Kowal-Vern A: Pediatric burn rehabilitation (review), *Pediatr Rehabil* 5(1):3-10, 2002.

58. Llanos S et al: Effectiveness of negative pressure closure in the integration of split thickness skin grafts, *Ann Surg* 244(5):700-705, 2006.

59. Housinger T et al: Conservative approach to the elderly patient with burns, *Am J Surg* 148(6):817-820, 1984.

60. Adamkova M et al: First experience with the use of vacuum assisted closure in the treatment of skin defects at the burn center, *Acta Chir Plast* 47(1):24-27, 2005.

61. Slater AL, Slater H, Goldfarb IW: Effect of aggressive surgical treatment in older patients with burns, *J Burn Care Rehabil* 10(6):527-530, 1989.

62. Kao CC, Garner WL: Acute burns, *Plast Reconstr Surg* 105(7):2482-2492, 2000.

63. Deveci M et al: Comparison of lymphocyte populations in cutaneous and electrical burn patients: a clinical study, *Burns* 26(3):229-232, 2000.

64. Pratt VC et al: Alterations in lymphocyte function and relation to phospholipid composition after burn injury in humans, *Crit Care Med* 30(8):1753-1761, 2002.

65. Curreri PW et al: Dietary requirements of patient with major burns, *J Am Diet Assoc* 65(4):415-417, 1974.

66. Chen Z et al: A comparison study between early enteral nutrition and parenteral nutrition in severe burn patients, *Burns* 33(6):708-712, 2007.

67. Haynes BW Jr: The management of burns in children, *J Trauma* 5:267-277, 1965.

68. Hart DW et al: Persistence of muscle catabolism after severe burn, *Surgery* 128(2):312-319, 2000.

69. Wasiak J et al: Early versus delayed enteral nutrition support for burn injuries, *Cochrane Database of Syst Rev* 3 (CD005489), 2006.

70. Ward RS et al: Sensory loss over grafted areas in patients with burns, *J Burn Care Rehabil* 10(6):536-538, 1989.

71. Deitch EA, Rightmire DA, Clothier J et al: Management of burns in pregnant women, *Surg Gynecol Obstet* 161(1):1-4, 1985.

72. Biddle EA, Hartley D: Fire and flame related events with multiple occupational injury fatalities in the United States, 1980-1995, *Inj Control Saf Promot* 9(1):9-18, 2002.

73. Quinney B et al: Thermal burn fatalities in the workplace, United States, 1992 to 1999, *J Burn Care Rehabil* 23(5):305-310, 2002.

74. Artz CP: Electrical injury. In Artz CP, Moncrief JA, Pruitt BA Jr, editors: *Burns: a team approach,* Philadelphia, 1979, Saunders, pp 351-362.

75. Luce EA, Gottlieb SE: "True" high-tension electrical injuries, *Ann Plast Surg* 12(4):321-326, 1984.

76. Leake JE, Curtin JW: Electrical burns of the mouth in children, *Clin Plast Surg* 11(4):669-683, 1984.

77. Port RM, Cooley RO: Treatment of electrical burns of the oral and perioral tissues in children, *J Am Dent Assoc* 112(3):352-354, 1986.

78. Jain S, Bandi V: Electrical and lightning injuries, *Crit Care Clin* 15(2):319-331, 1999.

79. American Burn Association: *American Burn Association Committee on Specific Optimal Criteria for Hospital Resources for Care of Patients with Burn Injury,* San Antonio, 1976, The Association.

80. Bailey B, Gaudreault P, Thivierge RL: Experience with guidelines for cardiac monitoring after electrical injury in children, *Am J Emerg Med* 18(6):671-675, 2000.

81. David WS: Myoglobinuria, *Neurol Clin* 18(1):215-243, 2000.

82. Holliman CJ, Saffle JR, Kravitz M et al: Early surgical decompression in the management of electrical injuries, *Am J Surg* 144(6):733-739, 1982.

83. Ward RS et al: Prosthetic use in patients with burns and associated limb amputations, *J Burn Care Rehabil* 11(4):361-364, 1990.

84. Saffle JR, Crandall A, Warden GD: Cataracts: a long-term complication of electrical injury, *J Trauma* 25(1):17-21, 1985.

Appendix
Clinical and Laboratory Values

TABLE A-1

Blood, Plasma, and Serum Values

Test	Normal Values*	Significance of a Change
Acid phosphatase	*Women:* 0.01-0.56 sigma U/ml *Men:* 0.13-0.63 sigma U/ml	↑ in kidney disease ↑ in prostate cancer ↑ after trauma and in fever
Alanine aminotransferase (ALT, SGPT)	7-56 U/L	↑ in liver damage
Albumin	3.5-5.0 g/dl	↓ in liver disease ↓ in malnutrition
Alkaline phosphatase	*Adult:* 38-110 IU/L *Child:* up to 104 IU/L	↑ in bone disorders ↑ in liver disease ↑ during pregnancy ↑ in hypothyroidism
Amylase	20-110 U/L	↑ in pancreatitis
α_1-Antitrypsin	110-270 mg/dl	↓ in genetic emphysema
Aspartate aminotransferase (AST, SGOT)	0-35 U/L	↑ in liver damage
Bicarbonate (arterial)	22-26 mEq/L	↑ in metabolic alkalosis ↓ in respiratory alkalosis ↓ in metabolic acidosis ↑ in respiratory acidosis
Blood urea nitrogen (BUN)	5-25 mg/dl	↑ with increased protein intake ↑ in kidney failure
Blood volume	*Women:* 65 ml/kg body weight *Men:* 69 ml/kg body weight	↓ during hemorrhage
Calcium Total Ionized	8.4-10.5 mg/dl (2.1-2.6 mmol/L) 4.6-5.3 mg/dl	↑ in hypervitaminosis D ↑ in hyperparathyroidism ↑ in bone cancer and other bone diseases ↓ in hypoparathyroidism ↓ in avitaminosis D (rickets and osteomalacia)
Carbon dioxide content (venous bicarbonate)	24-32 mEq/L	↑ in severe vomiting ↑ in hypoventilation disorders ↑ in obstruction of intestines ↓ in metabolic acidosis ↓ in severe diarrhea ↓ in kidney disease

TABLE A-1

Blood, Plasma, and Serum Values—cont'd

Test	Normal Values*	Significance of a Change
Chloride	98-110 mEq/L	↑ in hyperventilation ↑ in kidney disease ↑ in Cushing syndrome ↓ in severe diarrhea ↓ in severe burns ↓ in Addison disease
Cholesterol		
Total	<200 mg/dl	↑ in chronic hepatitis ↑ in hyperthyroidism ↑ in atherosclerosis ↓ in acute hepatitis ↓ in hypothyroidism
High-density lipoprotein (HDL)	>40 mg/dl	↑ with regular exercise
Low-density lipoprotein (LDL)	<130 mg/dl	↑ with high-fat diet ↑ in diabetes mellitus ↓ in chronic obstructive pulmonary disease
Triglycerides	<165 mg/dl	↑ in cardiovascular disease ↑ in diabetes mellitus ↓ in hyperthyroidism ↓ with exercise
Clotting time (bleeding time)	5-10 min	↓ in hemophilia ↓ in platelet deficiency or defects
Copper	100-200 µg/dl	↑ in some liver disorders
Cortisol (at 8 AM)	5-20 µg/dl	↑ in Cushing disease ↓ in Addison disease
Creatine phosphokinase (CPK)	32-260 U/L	↑ in Duchenne muscular dystrophy ↑ during myocardial infarction ↑ in muscle trauma
Creatinine	0.6-1.5 mg/dl	↑ in some kidney disorders
Ferritin	*Women:* 4-161 ng/ml *Men:* 16-300 ng/ml	↑ in hemochromatosis ↑ in iron deficiency
α-Fetoprotein	0-15 ng/ml	↓ in neural tube defects
Fibrinogen	175-433 mg/dl	↑ may increase risk of thrombus ↓ in disseminated intravascular coagulation
Folic acid (RBC)	165-760 ng/dl	↓ in macrocytic anemia
Glucose	60-100 mg/dl (fasting)	↑ in diabetes mellitus ↑ in liver disease ↑ during pregnancy ↑ in hyperthyroidism ↓ in hypothyroidism ↓ in Addison disease ↓ in hyperinsulinism
Glycolated hemoglobin (HbA$_{1c}$)	3.9%-6.9%	↑ in hyperglycemia
Hematocrit (packed cell volume)	*Women:* 38%-47% *Men:* 40%-54%	↑ in polycythemia ↑ in severe dehydration ↓ in anemia ↓ in leukemia ↓ in hyperthyroidism ↓ in cirrhosis of liver

(continued)

TABLE A-1

Blood, Plasma, and Serum Values—cont'd

Test	Normal Values*	Significance of a Change
Hemoglobin	*Women:* 12-16 g/dl *Men:* 13-18 g/dl *Newborn:* 14-20 g/dl	↑ in polycythemia ↑ in chronic obstructive pulmonary disease ↑ in congestive heart failure ↓ in anemia ↓ in hyperthyroidism ↓ in cirrhosis of liver
Iron	50-150 μg/dl (can be higher in men)	↑ in liver disease ↓ in iron-deficiency anemia
Iron-binding capacity (TIBC)	250-460 μg/dl	↑ in iron deficiency
Lactic dehydrogenase (LDH)	88-230 U/L	↑ during myocardial infarction ↑ in anemia (several forms) ↑ in liver disease ↑ in acute leukemia and other cancers
Lipase	0-160 U/L	↑ in pancreatitis
Magnesium	1.8-3.0 mg/dl	↑ in excessive intake ↓ in alcoholism, renal disease
Mean corpuscular hemoglobin concentration	31%-36%	↓ iron-deficiency anemia
Mean corpuscular volume (RBC)	82-98 fl	↑ or ↓ in various forms of anemia
Osmolality	285-295 mOsm/L	↑ or ↓ in fluid and electrolyte imbalances
Paco₂	35-43 mm Hg	↑ in severe vomiting ↑ in hypoventilation disorders ↑ in obstruction of intestines ↓ in metabolic acidosis ↓ in severe diarrhea ↓ in kidney disease
Pao₂	75-100 mm Hg (breathing standard air)	↓ in cyanotic heart defects ↓ in chronic obstructive pulmonary disease
Partial thromboplastin time (activated PTT)	25-35 sec	↑ in intrinsic pathway defects
pH	7.35-7.45	↑ during hyperventilation ↑ in Cushing syndrome ↓ during hypoventilation ↓ in acidosis ↓ in Addison disease
Phosphorus	2.5-4.5 mg/dl	↑ in hypervitaminosis D ↑ in kidney disease ↑ in hypoparathyroidism ↑ in acromegaly ↓ hyperparathyroidism ↓ in hypovitaminosis D (rickets and osteomalacia)
Plasma volume	*Women:* 40 ml/kg body weight *Men:* 39 ml/kg body weight	↑ or ↓ in fluid and electrolyte imbalances ↓ during hemorrhage
Platelet count	150,000-400,000/μl	↑ in heart disease ↑ in some forms of cancer ↑ in cirrhosis of liver ↑ after trauma ↓ in anemia (some forms) ↓ during chemotherapy ↓ in some allergies
Potassium	3.5-5.1 mEq/L	↑ in hypoaldosteronism ↑ in acute kidney failure ↓ in vomiting or diarrhea ↓ in starvation

Paco₂ and Pao₂ use subscripts: Pa_{CO_2} 35-43 mm Hg; Pa_{O_2} 75-100 mm Hg.

TABLE A-1

Blood, Plasma, and Serum Values—cont'd

Test	Normal Values*	Significance of a Change
Prostate-specific antigen	0-4 ng/ml	↑ in prostate cancer
Protein		
Total	6-8.4 g/dl	↑ (total) in severe dehydration
Albumin	3.5-5 g/dl	↓ (total) during hemorrhage
Globulin	2.3-3.5 g/dl	↓ (total) in starvation
Prothrombin time (PT)	11-15 sec	↑ in extrinsic pathway defects
Red blood cell count	*Women:* 4.2-5.4 million/μl *Men:* 4.5-6.2 million/μl	↑ in polycythemia ↑ in dehydration ↓ in anemia (several forms) ↓ in systemic lupus erythematosus
Reticulocyte count	33,000-135,000/μl (0.5%-1.5% of RBC count)	↑ in hemolytic anemia ↑ in leukemia and metastatic carcinoma ↓ in pernicious anemia ↓ in iron-deficiency anemia ↓ during radiation therapy
Sodium	135-145 mEq/L	↑ in dehydration ↑ in trauma or disease of the central nervous system ↑ or ↓ in kidney disorders ↓ in excessive sweating, vomiting, diarrhea ↓ in burns (sodium shift into cells)
Specific gravity	1.058	↑ or ↓ in fluid imbalances
Thyroid-stimulating hormone (TSH)	0.4-6 μU/ml	↑ in hypothyroidism (primary) ↓ in hyperthyroidism (primary)
Thyroxin (T_4)—total	5-11 μg/dl	↑ in hyperthyroidism ↓ in hypothyroidism
Transferrin	190-375 mg/dl	↓ in certain anemias
Troponin I	<0.05 ng/ml	↑ in myocardial infarction
Uric acid	*Women:* 1.5-6.0 mg/dl *Men:* 3-9 mg/dl	↑ in gout ↑ in toxemia of pregnancy ↑ during trauma
Viscosity	1.4-1.8 times the viscosity of water	↑ in polycythemia ↑ in dehydration
Vitamin B_{12}	140-820 pg/ml	↓ in pernicious anemia
White blood cell count		
Total	4500-11,000/μl	↑ in acute infections ↑ in trauma ↑ in some cancers ↓ in anemia (some forms) ↓ during chemotherapy
Basophils	0.5%-1% of total	↓ in severe allergies
Eosinophils	2%-4% of total	↑ in allergies
Lymphocytes	20%-25% of total	↑ during antibody reactions
Monocytes	3%-8% of total	↑ in chronic infections
Neutrophils	60%-70% of total	↑ in acute infection

Adapted from Thibodeau GA, Patton KT: *Anatomy & physiology,* ed 5, St Louis, 2003, Mosby, pp 1023-1026.

*Values vary with the analysis method used.

TABLE A-2

Characteristics of Urine

Test	Normal Values*	Significance of a Change
Routine Urinalysis		
Acetone and acetoacetate	0	↑ during fasting ↑ in diabetic acidosis
Albumin	0-trace	↑ in hypertension ↑ in kidney disease ↑ after strenuous exercise (temporary)
Ammonia	20-70 mEq/L	↑ in liver disease ↑ in diabetes mellitus
Bile and bilirubin	—	↑ during obstruction of the bile ducts
Calcium	<150 mg/day	↑ in hyperparathyroidism ↓ in hypoparathyroidism
Color	Transparent yellow, straw-colored, or amber	Abnormal color or cloudiness may indicate blood in urine, bile, bacteria, drugs, food pigments, or high solute concentration
Odor	Characteristic slight odor	Acetone odor in diabetes mellitus (diabetic ketosis)
Osmolality	500-800 mOsm/L	↑ in dehydration ↑ in heart failure ↓ in diabetes insipidus ↓ in aldosteronism
pH	4.6-8.0	↑ in alkalosis ↑ during urinary infections ↓ in acidosis ↓ in dehydration ↓ in emphysema
Potassium	25-100 mEq/L	↑ in dehydration ↑ in chronic kidney failure ↓ in diarrhea or vomiting ↓ in adrenal insufficiency
Sodium	75-200 mg/day	↑ in starvation ↑ in dehydration ↓ in acute kidney failure ↓ in Cushing syndrome
Creatinine	1-2 g/day	↑ in infections ↓ in some kidney diseases ↓ in anemia (some forms)
Creatinine clearance	100-140 ml/min	↑ in kidney disease
Glucose	0	↑ in diabetes mellitus ↑ in hyperthyroidism ↑ in hypersecretion of adrenal cortex
Urea	25-35 g/day	↑ in some liver diseases ↑ in hemolytic anemia ↓ during obstruction of bile ducts ↓ in severe diarrhea
Urea clearance	>40 ml blood cleared per min	↑ in some kidney diseases
Uric acid	0.6-1.0 g/day	↑ in gout ↓ in some kidney diseases

(continued)

TABLE A-2

Characteristics of Urine—cont'd

Test	Normal Values*	Significance of a Change
Microscopic Examination		
Bacteria	<10,000/ml	↑ during urinary infections
Blood cells (RBC)	0-trace	↑ in pyelonephritis ↑ from damage by calculi ↑ in infection ↑ in cancer
Blood cells (WBC)	0-trace	↑ in infection
Blood cell casts (RBC)	0	↑ in pyelonephritis
Blood cell casts (WBC)	0	↑ in infection
Crystals	0-trace	↑ in urinary retention Very large crystalline masses are calculi
Epithelial casts	0-trace	↑ in some kidney disorders ↑ in heavy metal toxicity
Granular casts	0-trace	↑ in some kidney disorders
Hyaline casts	0-trace	↑ in some kidney disorders ↑ in fever

Adapted from Thibodeau GA, Patton KT: *Anatomy & physiology,* ed 6, St Louis, 2007, Mosby, p 1054.

*Values vary with the analysis method used.

Glossary

A

A band A dark band corresponding to an area where actin and myosin filaments overlap in skeletal or cardiac muscle.

Abruptio placentae Premature separation of the placenta prior to delivery; the separation may be partial or complete and may result in overt or concealed hemorrhage.

Absolute anemia Anemia involving a decrease in the number of red blood cells (as opposed to a decrease in the percent of cells).

Acalculous cholecystitis An important subgroup of acute cholecystitis. It tends to occur in the setting of major surgery, critical illness, trauma, or burn-related injury and does not occur in association with gallstones.

Accelerated (malignant) high blood pressure Rapidly progressing, potentially fatal form of hypertension in which diastolic blood pressure exceeds 120 mm Hg.

Acclimatization A normal adaptive response to environmental changes, such as changes in altitude. For example, the red blood cell count increases when an individual moves to a high altitude.

Accommodative capacity Ability of the eye to adjust to see objects at changing distances. This is a function of the ciliary muscle's ability to flatten or thicken the lens, thereby focusing the image on the retina.

Achalasia A disorder of esophageal smooth muscle function resulting in difficulty in swallowing both liquids and solids.

Acid A substance that releases hydrogen ions in solution and from which hydrogen may be displaced by a metal to form a salt. An increase in acid concentration produces a decrease in pH.

Acidemia The state in which the blood is overly acidic; usually defined as a pH <7.35.

Acidosis Presence of a condition that tends to make body fluids overly acidic.

Acne vulgaris A disease of the skin common where sebaceous glands are numerous (face, upper back, and chest). Characteristic lesions include open (blackhead) and closed (whitehead) comedones, inflammatory papules, pustules, nodules, and cysts.

Acquired immunodeficiency syndrome (AIDS) A syndrome caused by the human immunodeficiency virus (HIV) in which the CD4 lymphocyte count is <200/μl or an AIDS-indicator condition is present.

Acquired or secondary immunodeficiency An immunodeficiency that develops after birth and is the result of an illness rather than a genetic defect. Examples include impaired immune function secondary to poor nutrition or medication. This type of immunodeficiency may be reversible.

Acromegaly A chronic metabolic condition characterized by excessive growth of bone, soft tissues, and organs in adults due to abnormally high levels of growth hormone.

Acrosome Covering on the head of the sperm that contains large quantities of hydrolytic (water-splitting) enzymes that are released during capacitation.

Actin A cytoskeletal protein that makes up the thin filament of the muscle sarcomere in skeletal and cardiac muscle. It is also present in nonmuscle cells and is an important component of cell movement.

Actinic keratosis A horny premalignancy of skin epithelium caused by excessive exposure to sunlight.

Acute Relatively severe but running a short course.

Acute HAV infection A viral hepatitis infection caused by the hepatitis A virus characterized by jaundice and fatigue.

Acute renal failure An abrupt reduction of renal function that is potentially reversible.

Acute rheumatic fever An inflammatory disease following a β-hemolytic group A streptococcal pharyngeal infection.

Acute viral hepatitis Inflammatory liver disease usually caused by hepatitis A virus, hepatitis B virus, and hepatitis C virus.

Adaptation An alteration in structure or function in response to a changed environment, which enhances or promotes survival.

Adapting Making an adjustment to a change in internal or external conditions or circumstances.

Addison disease Primary adrenocortical insufficiency thought to be autoimmune in etiology.

Adenosine triphosphate (ATP) A nucleoside with three phosphate groups and an adenine base, which functions as the principal source of energy in cells.

Affect The outward expression of emotion associated with a mental state or in response to a stimulus.

Afferent neuron A neuron that transmits impulses from the periphery (sensory receptors) to the central nervous system.

Affinity The "tightness" of a ligand-receptor bond; the tendency of ligand and receptor to remain bound at low ligand concentration.

Afterload The impedance or resistance that must be overcome in order to eject blood from a cardiac chamber. Systemic vascular resistance is the primary determinant of left ventricular afterload.

Colored terms have audio pronunciation available on the CD-ROM included with this book.

Agoraphobia Irrational fear of open spaces. In panic disorder, agoraphobia is a fear of any place or situation in which assistance would be unavailable in case of an unexpected panic attack; also called *phobic avoidance*.

Airway resistance Relationship between pressure and flow of gas, as determined by the radius of the airway.

Alagille syndrome An autosomal dominant condition associated with typical bony and vascular malformations and paucity of intrahepatic bile ducts; also called *arteriohepatic dysplasia*.

Alarm The initial response to stress. The major features of the alarm reaction are attributable to activation of the sympathetic nervous system.

Albinism Partial or total absence of pigment in skin, hair, and eyes.

Alcohol abuse Overingestion of alcohol to the point of an individual's being dependent on the substance.

Alcoholic fatty liver An accumulation of fat in the liver cells resulting from chronic alcohol consumption; also called *steatosis*.

Alcoholic hepatitis An active inflammation, especially of the centrilobular region of the liver, resulting from acute or chronic alcohol consumption.

Alcoholic liver disease Manifested by fatty liver, hepatitis, and cirrhosis. One or more of these manifestations may be found in alcoholic patients.

Aldosterone A mineralocorticoid synthesized by the adrenal cortex in response to angiotensin II that conserves sodium, producing increased water retention and consequently increased blood volume.

Alkalemia The state in which the blood is overly alkaline; usually defined as a pH >7.45.

Alkalosis Presence of a condition in which body fluids are overly alkaline.

Allele One of two or more alternative forms of a gene located at the same site on homologous chromosomes.

Allergic contact dermatitis Indicates delayed acquired hypersensitivity to a specific allergen on the skin. Chromates, nickel, ethylenediamine, paraphenylenediamine, neomycin, formaldehyde, and lanolin components may cause allergic contact dermatitis.

Allergy Type I hypersensitivity of the immune system to environmental agents. Antigens that trigger an allergic response are often called *allergens*.

Allodynia Perception of pain in response to normally nonpainful sensory stimuli.

Allogeneic Referring to transplanted tissue that was obtained from a closely matched donor, usually a sibling, parent, or child.

All-or-none response In a skeletal muscle, all of the muscle fibers innervated by a motor unit will respond as one to its maximum or they will not contract at all. In a nerve, a depolarization will result in either a full amplitude action potential or none at all.

Alopecia Loss of hair, usually referring to the scalp.

α₁-Antitrypsin A plasma protein produced primarily in the liver; it is an acute phase reactant that inhibits the activity of elastase, cathepsin G, trypsin, and other proteolytic enzymes.

Alveolar period The last stage in fetal lung development when alveolar ducts form from terminal sacs and alveoli mature by increasing in size and in number.

Amenorrhea Absence or suppression of menstrual bleeding, usually due to an altered pattern of hormonal functioning that interrupts the normal sequence of endometrial proliferation and sloughing.

Amniocentesis A procedure in which fluid is obtained from the amniotic cavity by an ultrasound-guided needle. The fluid contains fetal cells that can be used to screen for chromosomal and other defects.

Amniotic cavity The space between the amniotic sac and the developing embryo. It is filled with a clear amniotic fluid that keeps the embryo moist and provides a measure of protection against mechanical injury.

Amphipathic Having different characteristics. For example, membrane lipids are partly hydrophobic and partly hydrophilic, and hence are amphipathic.

Ampulla A flasklike cavity or dilatation of a tubular structure.

Amyloid plaque A microscopic lesion in the cerebral cortex composed of fragmented axon terminals and dendrites surrounding a core of β-amyloid as found in Alzheimer disease.

Amyloid precursor protein A member of a large family of proteins that is associated with cell membranes, and a precursor to β-amyloid, a component of brain plaques in Alzheimer disease.

Amyotrophic lateral sclerosis A progressive degenerative disease affecting both the upper and lower motor neurons characterized by muscle wasting and atrophy of the hands, arms, and legs; also called *Lou Gehrig disease*.

Anabolism The energy-requiring phase of metabolism through which molecules, cells, and tissues are created.

Anagen The growing phase of the hair cycle.

Anaplasia A lack of differentiated features in a tumor cell as evidenced by variations in cell size and shape and presence of abnormal nuclei.

Androgenic Producing masculine characteristics such as the androgenic hormone testosterone.

Anemia A decrease in the quantity of hemoglobin, hematocrit, and/or red blood cells.

Anergy Diminished immune responsiveness to antigens.

Aneuploidy An abnormal number of chromosomes—either too few (hypoploidy) or too many (hyperploidy, polyploidy).

Aneurysm Local dilation of arterial wall or muscular chamber (e.g., cardiac ventricle).

Angina pectoris A paroxysmal chest pain most often due to cardiac ischemia associated with atherosclerotic coronary artery disease.

Anhedonia Loss of interest in and withdrawal from all regular and pleasurable activities, often associated with depression.

Ankylosing spondylitis An arthritis of the axial skeleton including the sacroiliac joints, spine, hips, and shoulders. Marked limitation of motion develops, and a flexed spinal posture with flexed hips and knees may predominate.

Anorexia Loss of appetite.

Anorexia nervosa A refusal to eat or an aberration in eating patterns to the point of danger. The clinical syndrome may be due to an intense fear of becoming obese or to emotional states such as anxiety, irritation, or anger. Affected individuals become obsessed with the desire to become thin, and food intake is restricted even as weight falls well below minimal normal value for age and height. Periods of fasting may alternate with periods of bingeing.

Anosognosia Lack of insight or denial of a neurologic defect, or illness in general (especially paralysis), on one side of the body.

Anthropometric Pertaining to measurements of the body or body parts such as height and weight for the purposes of understanding human physical variation.

Antibody Protein produced by B cells that destroys or inactivates a specific antigen.

Anticipatory anxiety Anxious anticipation of an anxiety-provoking event.

Anticodon Sequence of three nucleotides in a transfer RNA molecule that is complementary to the messenger RNA codon.

Antigen Macromolecule that provokes an immune system response.

Antimicrobial A chemical or agent that inhibits microbial growth, as in "antimicrobial resistance"; this is conferred to microorganisms that have developed mechanisms to evade antimicrobial actions.

Antisocial personality disorder A mental disorder characterized by failure to acquire the conditioned responses that are necessary for the learning of avoidance behaviors, conventional morality, and socialized positive responses to others; also called *antisocial reaction.*

Anuria Severe decrease or lack of urine output of less than 100 ml per day.

Anxiety disorders General group that comprises three major diagnoses: panic disorder, generalized anxiety disorder, and obsessive-compulsive disorder. Anxiety disorders are characterized by irrational fears and have great potential to cause disability in affected individuals.

Aortic valve The cardiac valve that lies between the left ventricle and the aorta. It is open during ventricular systole and closed during ventricular diastole. Aortic valve closure contributes to heart sound S_2.

Aphasia A global disorder of language involving impaired speech (expressive aphasia) and impaired ability to understand the spoken word (receptive aphasia).

Apocrine sweat gland A sweat gland that becomes functional only after puberty and discharges its products onto the skin through the hair follicle (hair pore).

Apoprotein A polypeptide chain not yet complexed to its specific prosthetic group.

Apoptosis Programmed cell death, characterized by DNA degradation and cell dissolution, but without necrosis.

Appendicitis Inflammation of the vermiform appendix due to an obstruction. This inflammation may lead to necrosis of the appendix, with subsequent abscess formation and peritonitis.

Apraxia An inability to execute previously learned skills, usually following a stroke.

Arachnoidal villi Fingerlike projections in the delicate membrane between the dura mater and the pia mater of the brain.

Arnold-Chiari II malformation A congenital anomaly associated with meningomyelocele and hydrocephalus in which the cerebellum and medulla oblongata protrude into the cervical spinal canal through the foramen magnum.

Arterial pulse pressure The difference between systolic and diastolic blood pressure.

Arteriosclerosis Generalized term for pathologic conditions resulting in decreased distensibility of arteries; also called *hardening of the arteries.*

Arteriovenous fistula Abnormal communication between an artery and a vein.

Arteriovenous malformation (AVM) A congenital disorder of the connections between veins and arteries in the vascular system.

Arteritis Inflammation of an artery. May be associated with an autoimmune reaction.

Articular (hyaline) cartilage Connective tissue that forms a smooth, resilient, low-friction surface for articulation of two bones. It is without nerves, is avascular in adults, and derives nourishment from synovial fluid. It tolerates extreme compression stress.

Articulation A point of contact between bones; also called *joint.*

Ascites Abnormal accumulation of fluid in the peritoneal cavity. Causes include liver disease, heart failure, constrictive pericarditis, infection, malnutrition, pancreatitis, lymphatic obstruction or leakage, renal disease, hypothyroidism, collagen vascular diseases, and malignancy.

Aspiration Inadvertent entry of food substances, liquids, or gastric content into the respiratory system. This potentially life-threatening occurrence is normally prevented by the coordinated set of actions performed by the muscles in the pharynx during swallowing.

Asthenia The lack or loss of strength or energy; weakness.

Asthma A respiratory condition characterized by increased responsiveness of the trachea and bronchi to various stimuli and manifested by widespread narrowing of the airways and inflammation.

Ataxia Failure of muscular coordination, resulting in incoordination and disturbances in posture and gait.

Atelectasis Full or partial collapse of the lung alveoli.

Atherosclerosis A type of arteriosclerosis characterized by proliferation of smooth muscle cells and lipid collection within the walls of arteries, resulting in narrowed lumina and impaired ability to dilate.

Atopic 1. Displaced or ectopic. 2. Pertaining to atopy.

Atopy A genetic predisposition to allergies.

Atresia Congenital failure to develop (absence) or abnormal closure of a normally open passage.

Atrial fibrillation A completely disorganized and irregular atrial rhythm accompanied by an irregular ventricular rhythm of variable rate.

Atrophy A reduction in size and function of a cell or tissue; wasting.

Aura A peculiar sensation preceding the appearance of more definite symptoms, as in migraine and seizure.

Auscultatory gap The time during cuff deflation after systolic blood pressure when the Korotkoff sounds disappear.

Autism A mental disorder primarily characterized by abnormal development of social interaction and communicative skills. Affected individuals may manifest an inability to perceive or understand others' feelings or to express their own feelings, and may adhere to rigid, nonfunctional behaviors or rituals.

Autocrine Relating to hormone-like chemicals in which the target cell is the same cell that secretes the chemical.

Autocrine signaling The secretion of factors that feed back onto the cell that secreted them. Usually used in reference to growth factors.

Autografting Surgical procedure to move skin from one area of the body to an area of injury. The purpose is to provide permanent skin coverage to the injured area.

Autoimmune liver disease Hepatic injury from self-reactive antibodies produced by errant B lymphocytes.

Autoimmunity An inappropriate and excessive response of the immune system to self antigens causing disease. Disorders that result from an autoimmune response are called *autoimmune diseases.*

Autonomic dysreflexia Hyperreflexia; an uninhibited and exaggerated reflex of the autonomic nervous system in response to stimulation in spinal cord patients.

Autoregulation The intrinsic tendency of an organ or tissue to maintain adequate blood flow despite changes in metabolism or blood pressure.

Autosomal dominant polycystic kidney disease Hereditary disorder associated with defects on chromosome 16 (95% of cases) or chromosome 4 (5% of cases), resulting in dilation of all collecting ducts and impaired renal function.

Autosomal recessive polycystic kidney disease Congenital disorder linked to a defect on chromosome 6, which results in dilations of the renal collecting ducts and hepatic fibrosis.

Autosome Any ordinary paired chromosome, as distinguished from a sex chromosome.

Avoidance Refers to conscious or subconscious defensive reactions used to increase feelings of control and decrease the risk of anxiety.

Avulsion fracture A separation of a small fragment of bone at the site of attachment of a ligament or tendon.

Axoneme 1. Central core of a cilium or flagellum, consisting of two central fibrils surrounded by nine peripheral fibrils. 2. Motor apparatus of the sperm's tail.

Azotemia Increased levels of nitrogenous waste products, especially urea nitrogen, in the blood indicative of impaired renal clearance.

B

B cell A type of lymphocyte that can produce antibodies that attack pathogens or directs other cells to attack them. B cells that are actively producing antibodies are called *plasma cells*.

Bacillus A genus of aerobic, Gram-positive, or facultatively anaerobic, spore-bearing, rod-shaped bacterium that may or may not be motile.

Bacterial enzyme An enzyme that aids in a microorganism's ability to spread or invade tissues, such as fibrinolysin, coagulase, and hyaluronidase.

Ball-and-socket joint Formed by a ball-like surface fitting into a concave socket. Ball-and-socket joints permit flexion-extension, adduction-abduction, and rotational movements, such as those of the hip and shoulder.

Barrett esophagus A complication of chronic gastroesophageal reflux disease that represents replacement of the normal squamous epithelium of the distal esophagus by columnar tissue. Considered to be a preneoplastic condition.

Basal energy expenditure A term used to describe the calculated caloric expenditure at rest also called the basal metabolic rate.

Basal ganglia Groups of cell bodies (nuclei) located deep within the cerebral hemispheres that help plan and execute motor activities, including the caudate, putamen, globus pallidus, substantia nigra, and subthalamus.

Basal metabolic rate The amount of energy required for an individual to maintain vital processes at rest, such as respiration, digestion, and circulation.

Base 1. The nonacid part of a salt. 2. A substance that accepts hydrogen ions in solution to form salts and increases pH.

Basophil/basophilic granulocyte A leukocyte that is functionally and chemically related to the mast cell and has a kidney-shaped nucleus and large deep basophilic granules, which contain vasoactive amine and heparin and are important in IgE binding.

Beau line Transverse furrow in the nail that indicates a disturbance in nail growth.

Becker dystrophy A milder form of inherited muscle degeneration than the Duchenne type and somewhat less common, with an annual incidence of 5 per 100,000. The genetic mutation leads to production of a reduced amount of an abnormal dystrophin protein and slower muscular degeneration.

Bell palsy An acute idiopathic unilateral paresis or paralysis of the facial nerve involving an inflammatory reaction at or near the stylomastoid foramen or in the bony facial canal.

Bence Jones proteins Proteins found in the urine of patients with plasma cell (multiple) myeloma. They are derived from overproduction of light chain fragments of antibodies by malignant plasma cells. Bence Jones proteins are nephrotoxic and may contribute to development of kidney disease.

Benign breast disorders A group of lesions affecting the breast, which are usually divided into two categories: fibrocystic breast disease and benign neoplasms of the breast.

Benign prostatic hyperplasia/hypertrophy (BPH) A noncancerous enlargement of the prostate gland.

Benign tumor A type of tumor that is strictly local, usually well differentiated, and does not metastasize.

β-Amyloid A protein fragment snipped from a larger molecule (called *amyloid precursor protein*) during metabolism. Abnormal β-amyloid is a component of neuritic plaques found in Alzheimer disease.

Biaxial joint A joint that has two axes of movement and permits movement in two planes.

Bile A substance produced by hepatocytes in the liver and stored in the gallbladder. It is composed primarily of water, electrolytes, bile salts, cholesterol, and phospholipids. The major functions of bile are to aid in the digestion of dietary lipids through emulsification and to transport waste products, particularly bilirubin, into the intestine for disposal or reabsorption.

Biliary atresia A congenital or acquired disorder of the bile ducts. The acquired type occurs in the setting of certain autoimmune illnesses and is one of the principal forms of chronic rejection of a transplanted liver allograft. It is a common birth defect, occurring in 1 in 10,000 to 1 in 15,000 live births; also called *extrahepatic ductopenia* or *progressive obliterative cholangiopathy*.

Biliary cirrhosis Inflammation and scarring of the liver as a result of bile duct obstruction with obliteration of the bile ductules.

Biliary colic Persistent epigastric pain related to intermittent obstruction of the cystic duct, usually by a gallstone. A typical episode lasts several hours.

Bilirubin A substance formed from the degradation of hemoglobin from erythrocytes by the reticuloendothelial cells.

Biliverdin A greenish bile pigment formed in the breakdown of hemoglobin and converted to bilirubin.

Bipennate Pertaining to a muscle with a central tendon toward which the fibers converge on either side like the barbs of a feather.

Bipolar disorder A mood disorder characterized by alternating periods of mania and depression.

Bladder calculus A solid mass (stone) formed from debris within the bladder.

Blast An immature precursor of a lymphoid or myeloid white blood cell. Blasts are not normally found in the peripheral blood because they are retained in the marrow until mature. Blasts in the peripheral blood indicate leukemia.

Blood urea nitrogen (BUN) Urea is an end product of amino acid metabolism, measured in the blood as BUN and excreted primarily by the kidney.

Blunted affect A severe reduction in the intensity of externalized feelings.

Body fluid The water contained in the body plus the substances dissolved in it.

Body mass index (BMI) A weight reference standard. The formula for BMI is weight (kg) divided by height squared (m^2).

Body water All of the water contained in the body.

Bolus 1. A round mass of food that has been softened and formed into an appropriate size for swallowing by the action of chewing. 2. A concentrated mass of pharmaceutical preparation.

Bone and joint tuberculosis An extrapulmonary form of tuberculosis that occurs after lymphohematogenous spread from a primary lung lesion.

Borderline personality disorder Personality disorder that represents a pervasive and persistent disturbance in ways of handling events and situations. Personalities influenced by this disorder are unstable, unpredictable, impulsive, and often moody and self-deprecating. Some overlap with depression is suggested.

Brainstem Portion of the brain made up of the midbrain, pons, and medulla oblongata and the mesencephalon.

Branched-chain amino acids A group of amino acids that includes valine, leucine, and isoleucine, which are mainly metabolized in the muscle for energy.

Bronchiectasis A disorder characterized by destruction of the elastic and muscular structures leading to dilation of the bronchi.

Bronchiolitis Inflammation of small bronchi.

Bronchitis Widespread inflammation of bronchi and bronchioles due to infectious agents or allergic reactions.

Bronchospasm Narrowing of the bronchi and bronchioles because of an abnormal contraction of the smooth muscles of the bronchial walls.

Bruit Sound generated by turbulent blood flow auscultated over a blood vessel.

Brush border Covering of the microvilli projecting from the intestinal villi. This fuzzy coating contains many digestive enzymes.

Buck fascia or fascia of Buck Thick fibrous envelope surrounding the tunica albuginea, which encloses each of the erectile bodies of the penis.

Buckle fracture A fracture in children whereby the bone buckles and eventually cracks as a result of a compression injury to cancellous bone of the metaphysis of a long bone.

Buffer A chemical that releases hydrogen ions when a fluid is too alkaline and takes up hydrogen ions when a fluid is too acidic.

Bulbourethral glands Two glands that produce viscous fluid, which is secreted into the urethra near the base of the penis; also called *Cowper glands*.

Bulbous urethra The proximal portion of the penile urethra. The bulbous urethra is surrounded by the bulb of the urethra and bulbospongiosus muscle.

Bulimia nervosa Recurrent episodes of binge eating followed by self-induced vomiting or diarrhea, excessive exercise, strict dieting or fasting, and an exaggerated concern about body shape and weight.

Bulla Large, thin-walled cyst. Commonly used in reference to lung or skin.

Bursa Pocket of connective tissue lined with liquid-containing synovium, located between muscles or between muscle or tendon and bone.

Byler syndrome A rare autosomal recessive disorder involving severe jaundice, pruritus, and malabsorption caused by an error in bile salt metabolism; also called *progressive intrahepatic cholestasis* and *progressive familial intrahepatic cholestasis*.

C

Cachexia A combination of symptoms, including anorexia, weight loss, muscle wasting, and weakness, which is associated with the severe malnutrition of chronic diseases such as cancer.

Calcitonin A hormone produced by thyroid parafollicular cells; it influences the processing of calcium by bone cells.

Calculus A mass of solid mineral or metabolic substance. A stone.

Callus (bone) The bony deposit formed between and around the broken ends of a fractured bone during healing; also called *keratoma*.

Calluses (skin) Common, usually painless thickenings of the stratum corneum at locations of external pressure or friction.

Cancellous bone Bone with a spongy or lattice-like appearance, found in the interior of bones. Cancellous bone does not tolerate compression stress.

Cancer cachexia The severe nutritional effects of cancer. See *cachexia*.

Capacitation The multiple changes that activate sperm and enhance their ability to participate in the final process of fertilization.

Capillary hydrostatic pressure The outward push of the vascular fluid against the capillary walls from blood pressure.

Capillary osmotic pressure The inward pull of particles in the vascular fluid from dissolved proteins in the blood.

Carbohydrates The main energy source for the body consisting of simple or complex sugars. They must be supplied in a fairly constant manner to meet the energy requirements for normal body functioning. Provides 4 kcal/g.

Carbonic anhydrase The enzyme that catalyzes the reversible conversion of carbon dioxide and water to carbonic acid.

Carcinogen A substance that initiates or promotes the development of cancers. Most carcinogens cause cancer by damaging DNA to produce mutations.

Cardiac asthma Results from bronchospasm precipitated by congestive heart failure.

Cardiac cycle A cardiac cycle includes one diastolic and one systolic phase.

Cardiac index A measure of the heart's pumping ability taking into account body surface area. The cardiac index is calculated by dividing cardiac output by body surface area. A cardiac index less than 2.0 L/min/m^2 is considered to be insufficient for adequate peripheral perfusion.

Cardiac output A measure of the amount of blood pumped by the heart in 1 minute, usually expressed in liters per minute.

Cardiac tamponade Abnormal external pressure on the heart resulting in poor cardiac filling and decreased cardiac output.

Cardiomyopathy Diseases that primarily affect myocardial cells, often of unknown cause. Three common types of cardiomyopathy are dilated, hypertrophic, and restrictive.

Carina A ridgelike structure at the base of the trachea that projects from the area that separates the left and right bronchi.

Carpal joint A synovial joint between the carpal bones.

Carrier A person who harbors a recessive gene for a particular trait. A recessive heterozygote.

Carrier proteins Proteins located in lipid bilayers that transport ions and small molecules through the membrane by first binding on one side and then moving to the other side by changing conformation.

Cartilaginous joint A joint that connects bony segments by fibrocartilage or hyaline growth cartilage.

Casts White or red blood cells that collect in a protein meshwork in a nephron tubule and conform to the shape of the tubule; their presence indicates infection or inflammation of the kidney.

Catabolism The process of converting large molecules of carbohydrate, protein, and fat to smaller molecules to be utilized for energy.

Catecholamine A hormone (e.g., epinephrine and norepinephrine) that stimulates glycogenolysis and gluconeogenesis. An amine neurotransmitter (e.g., norepinephrine, dopamine).

Catecholamine hypothesis A hypothesis that abnormally low catecholaminergic neurotransmission leads to depression and abnormally high catecholaminergic neurotransmission leads to mania.

Caudal Signifying a position toward the distal end of the body, or an inferior position.

Caudate nuclei Portion of each cerebral hemisphere that, together with the lentiform nuclei, forms the corpus striatum of the basal ganglia.

Celiac disease A disease that is characterized by intolerance of gluten, a protein in wheat and wheat products that causes abdominal distention and malabsorption.

Cell cycle The phases through which a cell progresses during cellular reproduction, including gap 1, synthesis, gap 2, and mitosis.

Centromere Constricted region that holds two sister chromatids together. The centromere is the site of attachment to the microtubules, which pull the chromatids apart during mitosis.

Centrosome A centrally located organelle that organizes microtubules in the cell. It acts as the spindle pole during mitosis.

Cerebellum Portion of the brain, attached to the brainstem, which has an essential role in maintaining muscle tone, posture, and coordinating normal movements.

Cerebral dysrhythmia An abnormality in an otherwise normal rhythmic pattern, as seen on electroencephalography.

Cerebral palsy Refers to a diverse group of crippling syndromes that appear during childhood and involves permanent, nonprogressive encephalopathic damage to the developing brain.

Cerebrospinal fluid Fluid found in the cavities and canals of the brain and spinal cord.

Cerebrotendinous xanthomatosis A steroid hydroxylase deficiency that leads to premature atherosclerosis and encephalopathy; also called *van Bogaert disease*.

Cerebrum Portion of the brain that controls consciousness, memory, sensations, emotions, and voluntary movements. The largest part of the brain, it consists of two hemispheres.

Ceruminous gland A special variety or modification of apocrine sweat gland. The mixed secretions of sebaceous and ceruminous glands form a brown waxy substance called *cerumen*, which protects the ear canal from dehydration.

Chagas disease Caused by *Trypanosoma cruzii* and transmitted to humans by bloodsucking insects. It is a common cause of acquired myocarditis and megacolon in Central and South America but is rarely seen in the United States.

Chancre Painless, ulcerative lesion arising at the original port of entry of the spirochete that causes syphilis.

Chancroid An ulcerative, infectious disease of the genital tract caused by the sexually transmitted bacillus *Haemophilus ducreyi*. Unlike the chancre in syphilis, the lesion in chancroid is painful, tender, and often multiple.

Channel proteins Proteins located in lipid bilayers, which form porelike structures that allow ions to pass through by diffusion when appropriately stimulated.

Chemodissolution Use of chemical substances, such as bile acids or organic solvents, to dissolve gallstones. Used as a nonoperative method to treat gallstones.

Chemotaxis The movement of cells according to chemical gradients (chemotaxins) that attract them.

Chest physiotherapy Use of percussion and postural drainage to mobilize secretions from specific segments of the lungs.

Chickenpox A common communicable childhood disease that is caused by the *Varicella zoster* virus, which is also the causative agent in shingles. The characteristic skin lesion occurs in three stages: macule, vesicle, and granular scab; also called *varicella*.

Chlamydia Genus of a microorganism that lives as an intracellular bacterium. *Chlamydia trachomatis* inhabits the epithelium of the urethra and cervix and is responsible for the highly contagious systemic infection lymphogranuloma venereum.

Chloride shift An exchange of chloride ions for HCO_3^- in red blood cells in peripheral tissues in response to changes in P_{CO_2} of blood.

Cholecalciferol Precursor substance of active vitamin D.

Cholecystectomy Surgical removal of the gallbladder.

Cholecystitis Inflammation of the gallbladder wall; may be acute or chronic and usually is associated with cholelithiasis.

Cholecystokinin Hormone secreted from the small intestinal mucosa; two of its chief functions are stimulation of the release of pancreatic enzymes during a meal and contraction of the gallbladder.

Cholelithiasis Formation of stones in the gallbladder.

Cholinergic-noradrenergic imbalance hypothesis A hypothesis that suggests that a relative increase in the ratio of acetylcholine activity to norepinephrine activity produces depression and that mania is the result of a relative increase in the ratio of norepinephrine activity to acetylcholine activity.

Chondroma A cartilage-forming tumor located within bone that accounts for about 15% of benign bone tumors; also called *enchondroma*.

Chondrosarcoma A malignant cartilage-forming tumor; chondrosarcomas tend to develop in the pelvic and shoulder girdles and the proximal ends of long bones.

Chordae tendineae Bands of fibrous connective tissue that anchor the atrioventricular valves to the papillary muscles of the ventricular chambers.

Chorionic villus sampling A procedure in which tissue is obtained from the placenta by ultrasound-guided biopsy. Chorionic villus sampling can be performed earlier in pregnancy (10 to 12 weeks) than amniocentesis (16 weeks).

Chromatid One copy of a chromosome formed by DNA replication that may be joined to the other copy (sister chromatid) at the centromere.

Chromosome A linear thread of nuclear DNA that becomes visible under the microscope during cell mitosis.

Chronic Refers to a condition that lasts for a long time (months to years).

Chronic active hepatitis A progressive, destructive inflammatory disease that extends beyond the portal triad to the hepatic lobule (piecemeal necrosis).

Chronic bronchitis A condition characterized by excessive secretion of bronchial mucus and manifested by productive cough for 3 or more months in at least 2 consecutive years in the absence of any other disease process that may cause this symptom.

Chronic hepatitis Ongoing inflammation of the liver, usually of more than 6 months duration, following viral hepatitis or due to autoimmune disease.

Chronic persistent hepatitis A benign disease in which the inflammation is confined to the portal triads without destruction of normal liver functions despite elevated serum transaminase levels; also called *triaditis* or *transaminitis*.

Chronic renal failure Gradual loss of renal function that is progressive and irreversible.

Chronic venous insufficiency Varicosity of the deep veins that prevents effective return of blood from the periphery. Usually manifests as edema.

Chylothorax An accumulation of chylous fluid attributable to leakage of chyle (lymph fluid) from the thoracic duct or to rheumatoid pleural effusion or tuberculous pleuritic; also called *chylous pleural effusion.*

Chyme Viscous, semifluid contents of the stomach following the mixture of ingested nutrients with gastric secretions. Chyme then passes through the pylorus into the duodenum, where further digestion occurs.

Cilia Motile hairlike processes on the surface of some cells.

Circadian rhythm The regular recurrence of certain biological phenomena in approximately 24-hour cycles, regardless of constant darkness or other conditions of illumination.

Circumferential burn A burn injury that wraps completely around an extremity or the trunk. Loss of elasticity of skin results in a tourniquet effect, compromising circulation to distal tissues or respiratory expansion of chest. Escharotomy or fasciotomy is necessary.

Cirrhosis A diffuse, irreversible scarring of the liver resulting in abnormal nodules of liver cells surrounded by fibrosis.

Clang association Association of words similar in sound but not in meaning, or words having no logical connection; may include rhyming and punning.

Clinical dehydration The combination of extracellular fluid volume deficit and hypernatremia.

Clinical manifestations The functional consequences of the structural and associated alterations in cells or tissues that are either characteristic of the disease or diagnostic of the process.

Clonic Characterized by alternating periods of involuntary muscular contraction and relaxation in rapid succession.

Closed fracture A type of fracture that occurs when fragments of a fracture do not extend through mucous membranes or skin and skin is not broken.

Closing volume Lung volume at which airways in the lower lung zones collapse and ventilation ceases.

Clubbing A process characterized by flattening of the angle of the base of the nail. It may occur in association with cardiovascular disease, subacute bacterial endocarditis, and pulmonary disease.

CO$_2$ Carbon dioxide; this gas is produced by cells during metabolism and is excreted by the lungs.

Coagulation The process of blood clot formation.

Coagulopathy An abnormality in blood clot formation.

Cocci Round nonmotile bacteria.

Codon Sequence of three nucleotides in DNA or messenger RNA that represents the instruction for a particular amino acid in a polypeptide chain.

Collagen Most abundant protein in the body. The major protein of the white fibers of connective tissue. Has tensile strength similar to that of steel and is responsible for functional integrity of connective tissue.

Colloid osmotic pressure Pressure produced by passage of fluid from an area of less concentration to an area of higher concentration of colloids (large charged molecules such as proteins); also called oncotic pressure.

Colonization Harmless inhabitation of the skin or mucous membranes by microorganisms.

Colostomy Establishment of an artificial opening of the colon on the abdominal wall; usually performed following removal of a diseased or injured bowel segment.

Comminuted fracture A fracture consisting of more than one fracture line and more than two bone fragments.

Compact bone Hard, dense bone that is usually found at the periphery of skeletal structures.

Compartment syndrome A syndrome resulting from trauma to soft tissue caused by swelling within the unyielding structure of a nonelastic tissue or device (e.g., a cast).

Compensation The counterbalancing of any defect of structure or function. For example, a process that tends to restore pH to normal by making other blood chemistry values abnormal.

Complement A group of proteins that participate in a cascade of reactions resulting in inflammation and cell lysis. Complement activation can occur by the classical or the alternative pathways.

Complete fracture A fracture whose line disrupts bone continuity through the whole thickness of the bone, including the cortex.

Compliance A measure of the ease of elastic distensibility of a hollow organ.

Complication A new or separate process that may arise secondarily because of some change produced by the original entity. For example, bacterial pneumonia may be a complication of viral infection of the respiratory tract.

Compression fracture Consistent with cancellous bone trauma; also called *crush fracture.*

Compulsion Repetitive ritualistic behavior that has a driven quality.

Concentric contraction A type of isotonic muscle contraction. During isotonic contraction, the muscle maintains a constant tension as it moves. Isotonic contractions can be eccentric (lengthening) or concentric (shortening). Concentric contraction of a musle occurs when the muscle force generates sufficient tension to overcome the resistance of the limb. One example is lifting a cup of water to one's mouth.

Condyloid joint A joint that permits flexion and extension at one axis and adduction and abduction around another axis, like the metacarpophalangeal joint of the hand.

Condylomata acuminatum; condylomata acuminata Genital wart(s) caused by papillomavirus forms.

Conformational change A movement or alteration in the three-dimensional formation of a protein without any change in amino acid structure.

Congenital adrenal hyperplasia Overproduction of adrenal androgens due to a lack of an enzyme needed for cortisol production. Symptoms include virilization of the female infant's genitalia.

Congenital ichthyosis An inherited disease characterized by an excessive growth of keratinocytes and keratin, which gives the skin a fish-scale appearance.

Congenital immunodeficiency Rare condition that results from improper development of immune system components before birth.

Congenital malformation A general term meaning a defect in form or function that is present at birth.

Congestive heart failure Dysfunctional cardiac pumping that results in congestion of blood behind the dysfunctional cardiac pump. Right-sided heart failure is associated with systemic venous congestion. Left-sided heart failure is associated with pulmonary congestion.

Consanguinity Mating of blood-related individuals.

Consolidation The process of tissues becoming firm and solid, as when the lung alveoli become firm as air spaces are filled with exudate in pneumonia.

Constipation A condition of having small, infrequent, and difficult bowel movements. Authorities have established a norm of fewer than three stools per week as a guideline for defining constipation.

Contact dermatitis A cutaneous reaction to topical irritation or allergy. Irritant contact dermatitis can develop in any person exposed to a sufficiently high concentration of the irritating agent. Some of the more active irritants are acids, alkalis, and hydrocarbons.

Contractile tissue Tissues involved in the contraction of muscle, including not only the muscle belly but also the tendon and bony insertion.

Contractility The force and velocity of cardiac muscle shortening in response to stimuli that increase cytoplasmic free calcium ion levels.

Contraction time The time from initial tension development to peak tension.

Contralateral Referring to the opposite side of the body.

Convalescence The stage of recovery after a disease, injury, or surgical operation.

Coombs antiglobulin test The direct test is an assay for antibody that is attached to red cells; the indirect test is an assay for antibody circulating in serum.

Coping A measure of an individual's resourcefulness and ability to deal with stress and stressors.

Corns Horny masses of condensed epithelial cells overlying bony prominences. Corns result from chronic friction and pressure.

Cor pulmonale Right ventricular hypertrophy secondary to pulmonary diseases that increase right ventricular afterload.

Corpora cavernosa Two paired erectile bodies that lie dorsally in the penis.

Corpus luteum Anatomic structure on the surface of the ovary that grows in the ruptured ovarian follicle following ovulation and acts as a temporary endocrine organ that secretes progesterone.

Corpus spongiosum Erectile body in the penis containing the urethra.

Correction A process whereby normal values are restored when the underlying cause is addressed. An example would be restoring pH to normal by addressing the underlying cause of an acid-base imbalance.

Cortical bone The dense cortex or outer shell of bone, designed to tolerate compression and shearing forces.

Corticosteroid A hormone produced by the adrenal gland that stimulates gluconeogenesis and contributes to insulin resistance (e.g., cortisol) or a drug that has similar effects.

Cortisol A glucocorticoid (steroid hormone) released by the adrenal gland that causes an increase in blood glucose level by promoting liver gluconeogenesis.

Coryza A head cold with profuse nasal drainage.

Costovertebral angle Area lateral to the sacrospinalis muscle and beneath the 12th rib used as an external landmark for the kidneys.

Cowper glands Two glands that produce viscous fluid, which is secreted into the urethra near the base of the penis; also called *bulbourethral glands*.

Crackles Rales; discontinuous fine crackling sounds, usually heard on inspiration, that are indicative of air moving through fluid.

Cradle cap A seborrheic condition in infants characterized by scaling of the scalp. Occurs as a result of infrequent or inadequate washing of the scalp.

Creatine kinase An enzyme that catalyzes the transfer of a phosphate group between adenosine triphosphate and creatine. The isoenzyme found in cardiac muscle is called *CK-MB* (the MB fraction of creatine kinase).

Creatinine End product of muscle metabolism that is filtered freely through the glomeruli and excreted by the kidney only. Creatinine clearance is used as a measure of glomerular filtration rate.

Cretinism Extreme hypothyroidism during infancy and childhood that causes mental and physical abnormalities.

Cricothyroidotomy Incision through the site below the thyroid cartilage for emergency opening of the tracheal passageway.

Crigler-Najjar syndrome A rare autosomal recessive disorder marked by severe unconjugated hyperbilirubinemia seen shortly after birth.

Crohn disease An inflammation of the gastrointestinal tract that extends through all layers of the intestinal wall, most commonly affecting the terminal ileum. It may affect multiple portions of the intestine, leaving intervening normal areas in between the affected regions. The manifestations of Crohn disease differ in some respects from those of *ulcerative colitis*, although some overlap may occur. In Crohn disease, abdominal pain is the predominant symptom.

Cross-bridge The interaction between thick and thin filaments of the contractile apparatus when myosin heads bind to actin.

Cross-bridge theory This theory of muscle contraction is suggested by the anatomic configuration of the sarcomere. Muscle shortening is accomplished by increasing the amount of overlap of actin and myosin filaments; also called *sliding filament theory*.

Crush fracture A fracture that is consistent with cancellous bone trauma; also called *compression fracture*.

Cryptogenic cirrhosis Advanced liver disease in patients with neither a suggestive history nor any detectable markers that would place them in any of the four main groups of cirrhosis.

Cryptorchidism Undescended testes.

Culture An integrated pattern of customs, attitudes, values, and shared beliefs that bind people together to form a society.

Cushing disease Hyperfunctioning of the adrenal cortex with increased glucocorticoid (cortisol) secretion because of excessive secretion of adrenocorticotropic hormone (ACTH) from the anterior pituitary gland.

Cushing syndrome The clinical features of hypercortisolism, regardless of cause.

Cutaneous membrane Thin, flat organ, also known as *skin*. It is composed of two main layers: an outer thinner layer called the *epidermis*, and an inner thicker layer called the *dermis*.

Cyanosis A blue coloration of the skin as a result of poor saturation of hemoglobin with oxygen. Cyanosis is usually not evident until saturation falls below 75%.

Cystic fibrosis An autosomal recessive condition with abnormal chloride channel function, producing lung and pancreatic disease in children.

Cystitis Inflammation of the urothelium (lining of the bladder) resulting from infection, irritation, presence of a foreign body, or trauma.

Cystocele Protrusion of a portion of the urinary bladder into the anterior vagina at a weakened part of the vaginal musculature. Predisposing factors include obesity, aging, inherent weakness, history of heavy-object lifting, or injury during childbirth or surgery.

Cytokine A peptide factor released by cells to influence the behavior of target cells. Cytokines have signaling, inflammatory, growth, and inhibitory functions.

Cytopathic Pertaining to significant cellular injury or death.

Cytoskeleton System of protein filaments in the cytoplasm of a cell that give the cell its shape and the capacity for purposeful movement.

D

Decubitus ulcer Localized area of cellular necrosis resulting from prolonged pressure between a bony prominence and an external object such as a bed or wheelchair. The tissues are deprived of blood supply and eventually die; also called *pressure sore.*

Deep partial-thickness burn A burn characterized by destruction of the entire dermis, leaving only epidermal skin appendages. All physiologic functions of skin are absent; also called *second-degree burn.*

Degranulate The release of granules by mast cells and basophils; the granules contain proinflammatory chemicals.

Degranulation Exocytosis of stored molecules contained in cytoplasmic vesicles.

Delusion A fixed, false belief that is held despite considerable contradictory evidence.

Delusional disorder A behavioral constellation dominated by a system of fixed, false beliefs that are tenacious and typically refractory to contrary evidence.

Dementia Syndrome characterized by a general loss of intellectual abilities caused by either reversible or progressive disorders, most typically Alzheimer disease or multi-infarct dementia.

Demyelination Destruction, removal, or loss of the myelin sheath of a nerve or nerve fibers.

Deoxyribonucleic acid (DNA) The biomolecule that carries genetic information in the cell. DNA is composed of covalently linked nucleotides that form long polymers.

Depressed fracture A fracture in which the fragment is displaced below the level of the surface of the bone, usually in the skull.

Depressed mood A hallmark symptom of major depression. This change in mood is relatively constant and is recognized both by the depressed individual and by others.

Depression can have a sudden onset and may include symptoms similar in number and intensity to those of major depression.

Dermatitis Inflammation of the skin.

Dermatome An area of skin that is innervated by a specific spinal cord segment.

Dermatomyositis A rare collagen disorder characterized by the acute or insidious onset of muscle pain, weakness, fever, arthralgia, and, in some cases, a puffy erythematous eruption that is usually confined to the face and the eyelids.

Dermatophyte A fungus that causes infection of the skin. The most common dermatophytes are *Microsporum, Trichophyton,* and *Epidermophyton.*

Dermatosis Any disorder of the skin, especially those not associated with inflammation.

Dermis Inner, thicker layer of the cutaneous membrane.

Dermoepidermal junction The specialized area where the cells of the epidermis meet the connective tissue cells of the dermis.

Desensitization The process of manipulating or "training" the hypothalamus to react less forcefully to a perceived threat or stressor. This technique works by changing the predominant brain waves of the individual from beta waves to alpha waves that are slower and more normal.

Desquamation The shedding of epithelial elements from the skin surface.

Detrusor muscle Smooth muscle of the bladder body.

Diabetes insipidus An endocrine deficiency of antidiuretic hormone manifesting as excretion of large quantities of very dilute urine and excessive thirst.

Diabetes mellitus An endocrine disorder characterized by impaired glucose entry into insulin-sensitive cells due to an absolute or relative deficiency of insulin.

Dialysate fluid Prepared solution with varying concentrations of glucose and electrolytes used to aid dialysis.

Dialysis An artificial process that replaces the renal functions of diffusion and filtration necessary to maintain homeostasis.

Diaper rash A skin irritation resulting from feces or the ammonia and alkali by-products of urine breakdown.

Diarrhea An increase in the frequency and fluidity of bowel movements. It is usually a primary sign of gastrointestinal tract disorders.

Diarthrosis A freely movable joint in which a contiguous bony surface is covered by articular cartilage and connected by a fibrous connective tissue capsule lined with a synovial membrane; also called *synovial joint.*

Diastole A phase of the cardiac cycle in which the ventricles are relaxing and filling with blood.

Diastolic blood pressure The lowest measured pressure in the arteries just prior to the next ventricular ejection.

Diencephalon "Between" brain; part of the brain between cerebral hemispheres and the midbrain.

Diffusion Movement of a gas from an area of high concentration to low concentration, or the process by which solutes move across a semipermeable membrane from an area of greater concentration to one of lesser concentration.

Diffusion coefficient A constant that depends on the properties of the tissue and the solute; the rate of movement of a solute is proportional to the diffusion coefficient.

Diploid Containing two sets of homologous chromosomes and, therefore, two copies of each gene, one from each parent.

Disconjugate An abnormal positioning of the eyes such that they deviate from one another in the direction of gaze.

Disease Sum of the deviations from normal structure or function of any part, organ, or system (or combination thereof) of the body manifested by a characteristic set of symptoms and/or signs and whose cause, pathogenesis, and prognosis may be known or unknown.

Dislocation Displacement of a bone from its normal position in a joint to the degree that the articulating surfaces lose contact.

Displaced fracture A fracture in which the ends of fragments are separated.

Disuse atrophy The tendency of cells and tissues to reduce size and function in response to lack of trophic stimuli.

Disuse osteoporosis Reduction in quantity of bone or atrophy of skeletal tissue in response to lack of weight-bearing activity. May occur with prolonged bed rest.

Diuresis Excretion of large amounts of urine, sometimes as a result of the actions of a diuretic.

Diurnal variation The regular (24-hour) recurrence of certain biological phenomena under conditions of illumination; recurring during the daytime, or period of light.

Diverticulitis Inflammation of one or more diverticula, or outpouchings, in the intestinal wall.

Diverticulosis The presence of diverticula, or outpouchings, in the wall of the colon.

Diverticulum Outpouching of one or more layers of the wall of a structure in the gastrointestinal tract, especially in the colon or esophagus.

DNA polymerase An enzyme complex that binds to DNA, using it as a template for synthesis of a complementary DNA strand.

Dominant Referring to the gene allele that is overtly expressed in the cell's phenotype. Opposite of recessive.

Dopamine hypothesis A hypothesis that postulates that schizophrenia is the result of neuronal overactivity dependent on dopamine.

Down-regulation A decrease in the number or functionality of cell receptors for a specific hormone usually resulting from the cell's prolonged exposure to high concentrations of the hormone. Down-regulation results in a decrease in the target cell response to a hormone.

Drug-induced asthma Asthma related to an ingested drug. An attack may occur within minutes of ingestion or may be delayed up to 12 hours. Nonsteroidal antiinflammatory drugs including indomethacin (Indocin) and ibuprofen (Motrin, Advil) are common causes.

Duchenne muscular dystrophy The most common and most severe form of muscular dystrophy, inherited as an X-linked trait and therefore afflicting only males.

Ductus deferens Thick, muscular tube that is continuous with the epididymis. The ductus deferens travels along the pelvic wall and joins with the seminal vesicle duct at the prostate to form the ejaculatory duct; also called *vas deferens*.

Dumping syndrome The rapid emptying or "dumping" of stomach contents into the proximal small intestine due to loss of pyloric regulation of gastric emptying. This loss of function may occur following a gastrectomy.

Dysconjugate See *disconjugate*.

Dysfunctional uterine bleeding Abnormal endometrial bleeding not associated with tumor, inflammation, pregnancy, or trauma. It is most common around the time of menarche and menopause.

Dysmenorrhea Pain associated with menstruation, usually classified as primary (unrelated to an identifiable disease) or secondary (related to the presence of an underlying disease).

Dysphagia Difficulty in swallowing as perceived by the individual. It may include the inability to initiate swallowing and/or the sensation of ingested substances sticking in the esophagus.

Dysphoria The constant experience of unpleasant emotions.

Dysplasia An alteration in cellular growth in which cell morphologic characteristics are variable and disorderly. Dysplastic cells may become cancerous and therefore are often termed *preneoplastic*.

Dyspnea Breathlessness or difficulty breathing.

Dysrhythmia An abnormality of heart rhythm, including altered rates or sites of impulse initiation and abnormal conduction pathways; also called arrhythmia.

Dysthymia A state of chronic depression.

Dystrophic Abnormal tissue growth that impairs function. May result from disordered growth (trophic) signals.

E

Eating disorder Anorexia nervosa or bulimia nervosa. See *anorexia nervosa* and *bulimia nervosa*.

Eccentric contraction A lengthening contraction that occurs when the load is greater than the amount of tension that the muscle is able to generate, such as walking down stairs (eccentric contraction of the quadriceps muscles).

Ecchymosis Bluish discoloration of the skin (bruise) caused by escape of blood into the tissues.

Eccrine sweat gland A sweat gland that opens directly onto the skin surface.

Ectasia Dilation of a tubular structure, as in mammary duct ectasia (in which the collecting ducts beneath the nipple and areola become dilated, thinned, and filled with secretions).

Ectopic In an abnormal location.

Ectopic ureter A single ureter that implants during fetal growth in any position other than normal, or an additional ureter.

Ectopy (cardiac) A cardiac impulse initiated at a site other than the sinoatrial node.

Edema An excess of fluid in the interstitial compartment.

Efferent neuron A neuron that carries information away from the central nervous system to the muscle cells, glands, or postganglionic neurons.

Effusion Presence of fluid in a contained space, causing pressure on structures within the space.

Ejaculation Expulsion of the ejaculate from the posterior urethra through the urethral meatus.

Ejection fraction Stroke volume divided by end-diastolic volume; indicates pumping efficiency of the ventricle.

Elastin A protein found in tendons and ligaments that imparts elasticity or extensibility.

Elastosis Skin wrinkling due to changes in collagen with fibers becoming cross-linked and rearranged in thicker bundles.

Electrochemical gradient A difference in concentration of charged particles across a membrane. Driving force that moves charged particles across a membrane due to the combined influences of concentration gradient and electrical charge gradient.

Electroencephalogram Graphic tracing of brain's action potentials; used to evaluate nervous tissue function.

Electrolyte Substance that releases charged particles (ions) when dissolved.

Electromyography A technique for evaluating muscle contraction; using electromyography, aspects of the contractile process such as time relationships between the beginning of electrical activity and the actual contraction of the muscle can be studied.

Electron transport chain A series of proteins on the inner mitochondrial membrane that move an electron from a higher to a lower energy level and create a proton gradient.

Embolus A collection of material (thrombus, air, fat, tumor cells, bacteria, amniotic fluid) propelled by blood flow to another site, where it lodges and causes obstruction of flow.

Embryoscopy A procedure in which a scope is passed through the mother's abdominal wall and into the uterus to visualize and sample embryonic tissues.

Emission One of the two phases of ejaculation. During emission, secretions from the periurethral glands, seminal vesicles, and prostate are deposited with sperm into the prostatic urethra.

Emphysema A chronic obstructive respiratory condition characterized by abnormal, permanent enlargement of air spaces distal to the terminal bronchiole with destruction of their walls and without obvious fibrosis.

Empyema Accumulation of pus in a body cavity, especially the pleural space.

Encapsulation Physiologic process of enclosure in a sheath composed of a substance not normal to the part. Prevents opsonization (recognition and binding) by antibodies and thus prevents the microorganism from being phagocytized.

Encopresis Fecal holding with constipation and fecal soiling.

Endocardium A layer of endothelial cells that lines the chambers of the heart. The layer of heart muscle just under the endocardium is called the subendocardium.

Endocrine organ Any organ that manufactures and secretes hormones into the bloodstream.

Endocrine system The cells and organs that produce and secrete hormones into the bloodstream.

Endocytosis Cellular ingestion of extracellular molecules.

Endogenous depression Major depression arising from characteristics within the individual as opposed to depression resulting from identifiable external events.

Endometrioma A mass of endometrial tissue that grows outside the lining of the uterine cavity in the condition known as endometriosis.

Endometriosis Growth of endometrial tissue outside the lining of the uterine cavity; an abnormal condition with potentially destructive effects on the pelvic organs.

Endometrium The innermost lining of the uterus, consisting of two layers: a thin deep layer, called the basilar layer, and a thick superficial layer, referred to as the functional layer. During a woman's reproductive years, the endometrium displays a constant cyclic activity of alternate proliferation and sloughing of the functional layer in response to hormonal secretion.

Endomysium The connective tissue that surrounds the sarcolemma of an individual muscle fiber.

Endorphin One of a group of potent endogenous opioid peptides derived from cells in the hypothalamus, also found in the periaqueductal gray matter of the brain. β-Endorphin has been found to have analgesic properties.

Endoscopic retrograde cholangiopancreatography (ERCP) A procedure whereby an optical scope is passed through the mouth, esophagus, stomach, and duodenum, and then guided in a retrograde fashion into the pancreaticobiliary system. Using this technique, physicians can perform a number of therapeutic procedures without performing a laparotomy.

Endoscopic sclerosis A procedure of the esophageal varices that is accomplished by passing a flexible needle through the gastroscope and injecting various sclerosant solutions into and around the bleeding varix.

Endosteum The thin membrane that covers the medullary cavity in longer bones.

Endotoxin A heat-stable lipopolysaccharide derived from the cell wall of Gram-negative bacteria that induces the release of pyrogens and inflammatory mediators from immune cells.

Energy The capacity to operate or work, measured in kilocalories (kcal); 1 kcal represents the amount of energy required to raise the temperature of 1 kg of water from 15° C to 16° C.

Enteropathic arthritis Refers to joint manifestations of inflammatory bowel diseases such as ulcerative colitis and Crohn disease.

Enuresis Involuntary voiding; the term is generally used when referring to inappropriate wetting in children.

Eosinophil A leukocyte that is the same size as a neutrophil but contains a two-lobed nucleus and large, coarse, eosinophilic granules that fill the cell; these participate in allergic and inflammatory responses.

Epicardium A layer of epithelial cells that covers the outer surface of the heart and forms the inner (visceral) layer of the pericardial sac.

Epidemic An outbreak of a disease that occurs suddenly and affects numbers of individuals clearly in excess of normal expectancy.

Epidemiology The study of patterns of disease among human populations for the purpose of establishing programs to prevent and control their spread.

Epidermal proliferating unit Group of active basal cells, together with vertical columns of migrating keratinocytes, which are undergoing mitosis.

Epidermis Outer, thinner layer of the cutaneous membrane.

Epididymis Tightly coiled tube in which sperm mature and develop the ability to swim; lies along the top of and behind the testes.

Epididymitis Inflammation of the epididymis.

Epileptogenic focus Cellular focus in the brain with the capacity to induce epilepsy.

Epimysium The connective tissue surrounding a muscle.

Epinephrine A catecholamine neurotransmitter that produces some of the same effects as norepinephrine but has a greater influence on cardiac action. Epinephrine enhances myocardial contractility, increases heart rate, and increases venous return to the heart, thus increasing cardiac output and blood pressure.

Epiphyseal plate A segment of a long bone between metaphysis and epiphysis developed from a center of ossification and distinct from the shaft. An area of growth in a bone.

Epispadias A congenital anomaly in which the urethra opens on the dorsal aspect of the penis at a point proximal to the glans.

Epistaxis Hemorrhage from the nose; nosebleed.

Epitope A site on the surface of an antigen that is specifically recognized by an immune cell, thus stimulating an immune response.

Equilibrium Sense of balance.

Erection A complicated interaction of vascular, neurologic, and hormonal factors that enables the penis to increase in length and diameter and become stiffened.

Erythema Diffuse redness of the skin.

Erythroblastosis Presence of erythroblasts in the blood due to premature release from the bone marrow.

Erythromelalgia Painful erythema (redness of the skin) of the palms and soles due to congestion of the capillaries.

Erythron The blood as a single body system.

Erythropoiesis The process of red blood cell production.

Erythropoietin Hormone produced primarily by the kidney that stimulates bone marrow to produce erythrocytes.

Eschar Burn tissue.

Escharotomy A surgical incision through eschar of a circumferential extremity burn for the purpose of restoring distal blood flow, or through eschar of the chest to restore respiratory expansion.

Esophageal atresia Congenital anomaly in which the esophagus is closed off in a blind pouch at some point. It occurs in about 1 in every 4000 live births and requires immediate surgical correction.

Esophageal varix (pleural; varices) Abnormally dilated blood vessel lying just below the mucous membrane of the esophagus that connects the hypertensive portal system with the systemic circulation. Esophageal varices may rupture, causing massive hemorrhage.

Esophagitis Inflammation or infection of the esophagus.

Essential amino acids Amino acids that must be supplied in the diet because the body cannot manufacture them.

Estrogen One of a group of ovarian hormones that promote the development of female secondary sex characteristics. During the menstrual cycle, estrogen renders the female reproductive tract suitable for fertilization of the ovum, implantation of the zygote, and nutrition of the early embryo.

Etiology Study of the assignment of causes or reasons for phenomena.

Euchromatin Chromatin that is less densely packed and potentially open to transcription, as opposed to heterochromatin, which is condensed and not open to transcription.

Eukaryote A cell that has a true nucleus bounded by a nuclear membrane.

Euphoria A hallmark symptom of both mania and hypomania. Extreme cheerfulness, enthusiasm, and optimism are present, but the joyful, buoyant mood is disproportionate to events and surroundings; also called *expanded mood*.

Ewing sarcoma A malignant round cell tumor (marrow tumor) that is relatively uncommon but rapidly growing.

Exacerbation A relatively sudden increase in the severity of a disease or any of its signs and symptoms.

Exercise-induced asthma Asthma that manifests 5 to 10 minutes after the exercise period begins. The increased rate and depth of respiration during exercise, especially in cold air, leads to cooling and dehydration of the lower airways.

Exhaustion A stage in the stress response that occurs when the stressor is too great or prolonged, resulting in depletion of energy reserves.

Exocytosis The process of cellular secretion.

Exon The portion of an RNA transcript that remains after unwanted sections (introns) have been removed from the primary transcript. A linear section of DNA that serves as a template for synthesis of a particular RNA sequence.

Exophthalmos Protrusion of the eyeball.

Exotoxin Toxins, such as enzymes or pore-forming proteins, produced by bacteria that cause physiologic dysfunction in the host.

Extracellular fluid Body fluid that is not inside the cells; includes vascular, interstitial, and transcellular fluids.

Extraocular Outside the globe of the eyeball.

Extrapyramidal system or tracts Part of the brain that includes the corpus striatum, subthalamic nucleus, substantia nigra, and red nucleus, and the interconnections with the reticular formation, cerebellum, and cerebrum. As distinct from the corticospinal tract (pyramidal motor tract) which traverses the medullary pyramids in the brainstem.

Extrapyramidal tract A functional rather than anatomical unit comprising the nuclei and fibers, excluding those of the pyramidal tract of the brain; comprises the nuclei and fibers involved in motor activities that control and coordinate postural, static, support, and locomotor mechanisms.

Extrinsic Originating from sources outside of the individual.

Extrinsic asthma An asthma condition that commonly affects children and young adults. Attacks are related to specific antigens and are immunoglobulin E mediated; also called *allergic asthma*.

Extrinsic pathway of clotting The mechanism that produces fibrin following tissue injury, beginning with formation of an activated complex between tissue factor and activated factor VII and leading to activation of factor X, which induces the reactions of the common pathway of coagulation

Exudate Fluid of high protein content that moves into tissues or cavities as part of a reaction to inflammation or injury.

F

Fascia A sheath of connective tissue that envelops muscles or other parts of the body.

Fasciculus Bundle of muscle fibers that compose individual muscles.

Fascioscapulohumeral muscular dystrophy A rare inherited autosomal dominant trait that affects the muscles of the shoulder girdle and the face and upper arms.

Fast twitch (type II, white) A muscle fiber that can develop high tension rapidly. It is usually innervated by a single α motor neuron and has low fatigue resistance, low capillary density, low levels of aerobic enzymes, and low oxygen availability.

Fat The most concentrated dietary source of energy, derived from either animals or vegetables. Provides 9 kcal/g.

Fatigue A lack of physical or emotional energy or power.

Fatty acid An organic acid with a long, straight hydrocarbon chain that is a fundamental component of lipids. Some fatty acids are manufactured by the body; others are essential and must be supplied in the diet.

Fetotoxic Referring to a substance that is damaging to a developing fetus.

Fibrillation Cardiac dysrhythmia characterized by rapid, random myocardial contractions and discoordinated pumping action.

Fibrinolysis Dissolution or breakup of a fibrin clot.

Fibroblast A cell that produces components of collagen fibers, which compose the bulk of the dermis.

Fibrocystic breast disease A condition in which palpable breast masses (cysts) correspond to fluctuations in the menstrual cycle; the masses may be associated with pain and tenderness.

Fibromyalgia syndrome A painful, noninflammatory musculoskeletal disorder associated with fatigue, and multiple somatic complaints.

Fibrosis Condition of decreased elasticity because of excessive deposition of fibrin and collagen in the tissue (e.g., restrictive process characterized by thickening of the alveolar interstitium).

Filtration Movement of fluid across capillary walls, as a net result of opposing hydrostatic and oncotic forces.

First-degree burn Superficial tissue destruction in the outermost layers of the epidermis. All physiologic functions of the skin remain intact.

Fistula An abnormal tubelike passage between two organs or between an internal organ and the body surface.

Flagellum Motile (whiplike) appendage that allows a cell to move or swim.

Flat affect Lack of appropriate emotional expression.

Fomite An inanimate object that transmits a pathogen to a new host.

Foreskin Penile skin that overlies the glans and is removed in circumcision; also called *prepuce*.

Fossa navicularis Area of widening near the end of the penile urethra.

Fournier gangrene A rare condition involving a gangrenous necrosis of the scrotum, penis, or perineum.

Fourth-degree burn A full-thickness burn that penetrates the dermis to reach muscle or bone.

Fracture A break or disruption in continuity of a bone, an epiphyseal plate, or cartilage.

Frank-Starling law of the heart Describes the relationship between diastolic stretch and subsequent increased strength of contraction; also called *length-tension relationship*.

Free-living bacteria Bacteria that can live outside the host cell.

Free radical An extremely reactive compound that avidly makes molecular bonds with other compounds.

Full-thickness burn A burn characterized by destruction of epidermis, dermis, and underlying tissue. All physiologic functions of the skin are absent. This burn will not heal and requires autografting; also called *third-degree burn*.

Full-thickness excision Removal by surgical knife of complete eschar to fascia. Full-thickness excision often leaves an uneven contour, which presents difficulty with grafting, resulting in poor cosmesis.

Functional disorder of the endocrine system An endocrine disorder caused by a nonendocrine disease (e.g., chronic renal failure, liver disease, or heart failure).

Functional incontinence Loss of urine or feces as a result of factors external to the urinary or digestive tract, such as physical or cognitive impairment.

Functional syncytium A multinucleate mass of protoplasm that results from the merging of cells. It is characteristic of the gastrointestinal tract and heart, meaning that its separate cells have the ability to function in concert with one another in a unified manner.

Fungal infection Any inflammatory condition caused by a fungus.

Fungus A nonphotosynthetic, eukaryotic protist that is disseminated throughout the environment.

G

Gallbladder A distensible sac of about 30 to 50 ml capacity that stores bile and connects the common hepatic duct to the common bile duct via the cystic duct.

Ganglion A group of neuronal cell bodies located outside of the central nervous system.

Gangrene Cellular death involving a large area of tissue; may be characterized as wet, dry, or gaseous.

Gap junction A cell-to-cell communication pore that allows small biomolecules to flow from the cytoplasm of one cell to the cytoplasm of an adjacent cell.

Gastrectomy Surgical removal of all or, more commonly, part of the stomach. This procedure may be used to remove a chronic peptic ulcer, to stop hemorrhage in a perforating ulcer, or to remove a malignancy.

Gastrin An intestinal hormone that is released in response to certain types of food. Gastrin increases acid secretion by stomach parietal cells.

Gastritis Inflammation of the stomach lining. It may occur following the ingestion of irritating substances or in the presence of viral, bacterial, or chemical toxins.

Gastroenteritis Inflammation of the stomach and intestines, which may occur on an acute or chronic basis and is commonly caused by viruses.

Gastroesophageal reflux disease (GERD) Backflow of gastric contents into the esophagus through the lower esophageal sphincter. GERD may or may not produce symptoms. The most common manifestations of GERD are heartburn, regurgitation, chest pain, and dysphagia.

Gay bowel syndrome Transmission of and subsequent infection with enteric pathogens through sexual contact. These disorders are not limited to the homosexual community and may be transmitted among any individuals who engage in direct or indirect fecal-oral contact.

Gene A unit of heredity made up of a segment of DNA nucleotides that encodes a messenger RNA capable of being translated into a protein.

General adaptation syndrome The total organism's nonspecific response to stress. The term was coined by Hans Selye.

Generalized anxiety disorder (GAD) A disorder characterized by the continual presence of a moderate degree of anxiety without discrete periods of acute attacks. GAD symptoms include chronic anxiety and tension accompanied by headaches, abdominal problems, or sleep disturbances. Agoraphobia is rarely seen in GAD.

Generalized seizure A seizure that involves the whole brain surface and impairs consciousness.

Genome The entire complement of genes located on chromosomes in the nucleus of a cell.

Genotype The genetic constitution of an individual, often described by listing the allele types at a certain gene locus.

Gestational diabetes mellitus A disorder of glucose tolerance first diagnosed in the mother during pregnancy. Usually disappears after delivery of the infant.

Ghon tubercle A nodule or swelling containing *Mycobacterium tuberculosis*.

Giant cell tumor A benign but aggressive tumor with richly vascularized tissue consisting of plump spindle-shaped cells and numerous giant cells; also called *osteoclastoma*.

Gilbert syndrome A common, benign autosomal dominant condition that results in mild unconjugated (indirect) hyperbilirubinemia.

Ginglymus A type of joint that permits flexion and extension like the interphalangeal joint of the finger, the elbow, or the knee; also called *hinge joint*.

Glasgow Coma Scale Scale developed by G. Teasdale and B. Jennett for the purpose of objectively assessing coma and impaired consciousness.

Glomerular filtration rate The rate of fluid filtration through the glomeruli into Bowman capsule per minute; normally 125 ml/min.

Glomerulonephritis Inflammation of the glomerular capillary walls causing impaired filtration and renal function.

Glucagon Hormone produced by the α cells of the pancreas, which stimulates glycogenolysis and gluconeogenesis in the liver.

Glucocorticoid resistance model This model proposes a specific link between stress, immunity, and disease. Rather than viewing disease as a result of increased vulnerability due to stress, this model proposes that overwhelming stress reduces the sensitivity of the immune system to cortisol.

Glucocorticoids A class of steroid hormones secreted by the adrenal cortex, necessary for use of sugars, fats, and proteins and for the body's normal response to stress.

Gluconeogenesis The production of glucose from amino acids and other substrates in the liver.

Glycogen A carbohydrate consisting of branched chains of glucose produced by the muscle and liver as a storage form of glucose.

Glycogenesis Production of glycogen from glucose in hepatic and muscle tissue.

Glycogenolysis Production of glucose from the breakdown of glycogen in hepatic and muscle tissue.

Glycolysis The anaerobic process of breaking down sugars into simpler molecules, with the net production of two adenosine triphosphate and two pyruvate molecules per glucose molecule.

Glycosaminoglycan A protein polysaccharide contained in ground substances surrounded by collagen fibers in bone.

Glycosylated hemoglobin An index of glycemic control; the quantity of glucose attached to hemoglobin molecules, reflecting mean blood glucose values for a period of 120 days.

Goiter Enlargement of the thyroid gland.

Golgi apparatus A membrane-bound organelle in which the proteins and lipids that are synthesized in the endoplasmic reticulum are modified and sorted in preparation for transport to the lysosomes or plasma membrane.

Gomphosis joint An articulation created by the insertion of a conical process into a socket, such as the insertion of a root of a tooth into an alveolus of the mandible or the maxilla. Gomphosis is not a connection between true bones but is considered a type of fibrous joint.

Gonad An organ that produces sex cells. Derived from the urogenital ridge, the undifferentiated and primitive gonads become the testes in males and the ovaries in females.

Gonorrhea Common sexually transmitted disease involving the inflammation of epithelial tissue by the organism *Neisseria gonorrhoeae*. Characteristic symptoms include urethritis, dysuria, purulent urethral discharge, and redness and swelling at the site of the infection.

Gout A condition caused by lack of the enzyme uricase and the inability to oxidize uric acid into a soluble compound; characterized by recurrent attacks of articular and periarticular inflammation, accumulation of tophi (crystalline deposits) in bony and connective tissue, renal impairment, and uric acid calculi.

Grading Assignment of degree of differentiation of tumor cells by histologic examination. The degree of anaplasia usually correlates with the degree of malignancy.

Gram stain A process that determines whether a type of bacteria can retain a basic dye after iodine fixation; used to differentiate species into two groups, based on the properties of the bacteria's cell wall. This ability is the basis for classifying bacteria into Gram-negative and Gram-positive organisms.

Granulocyte A leukocyte with polymorphic nuclei and cytoplasmic granules. Neutrophils, basophils, and eosinophils are types of granulocytes.

Granulocytopenia An abnormal decrease in the total number of granulocytes in the blood.

Granuloma Tissue that forms into a nodular mass as a result of inflammation, infection, or injury.

Granuloma inguinale An ulcerative disease of the genital tract caused by the bacterium *Calymmatobacterium granulomatis*. The communicability of the disease is relatively low, and it is generally believed that repeated exposure is necessary for infection.

Granulomatous Relating to granulomas, chronic inflammatory lesions characterized by an accumulation of macrophages; epithelioid macrophages, with or without lymphocytes; and giant cells into a discrete granule.

Graves disease Hyperthyroid state characterized by exophthalmos and goiter from autoimmune stimulation of the thyroid.

Greenstick fracture An incomplete break in the bone with the intact side of the cortex flexed; it is usually seen in children.

Ground substance A material composed of a hydrated network of proteins, mainly glycoproteins and proteoglycans; serves as the "cement" between layers of collagen fibers; also called *matrix*.

Growing pain A common soft tissue syndrome in children. The most common symptom is nocturnal pain that usually occurs in the calves, shins, and thighs; also called *nonarticular rheumatism*.

Growth hormone A hormone secreted by the anterior pituitary gland with wide-ranging action, including effects on energy metabolism and increasing lean body mass.

Guillain-Barré syndrome An inflammatory demyelinating disease of the peripheral nervous system; also called *acute idiopathic polyneuropathy* or *polyradiculoneuropathy*.

Gustatory Pertaining to the sense of taste.

Gyrus A raised ridge or convolution on the surface of a structure (e.g., cerebral cortex).

H

H$^+$ Hydrogen ion; released by acids; determines pH; also called *proton*.

HCO$_3^-$ Bicarbonate ion; a base that binds and buffers H$^+$.

H$_2$CO$_3$ Carbonic acid; this acid is removed from the body in the form of carbon dioxide and water during exhalation.

H zone Corresponds to a region occupied solely by myosin filaments with no actin filament overlap in cardiac and skeletal muscle.

Hair Keratinized, threadlike outgrowth of the skin that covers most of the body.

Hair follicle Slender, cylindrical tube of epidermal cells in which hair grows.

Hallucination A perception for which there are no real sensory data.

Haploid Containing only one set of chromosomes (as distinct from diploid), as in a sperm cell or egg cell.

Hapten Incomplete, lipid-soluble particle that is incapable of being an antigen by itself, but that becomes an antigen inside the body when it binds with a host protein called a carrier. When a hapten penetrates the epidermis and binds to a carrier, it can cause contact hypersensitivity.

Haustral churning The mixing movement of the haustra (the outpouchings in the colon wall) when material is in the proximal end of the colon.

Haversian system The basic unit of bone; also called *osteon*.

HBV infection Hepatitis B virus infection. Vertical transmission from an HBsAg-positive mother to the infant is a common mechanism of spread. Features suggesting immune complex disease such as arthritis, fever, papular acrodermatitis (a rash not seen in adults), renal disease, and hematologic complications are more common in children.

HCV infection Hepatitis C virus infection. A type of hepatitis transmitted most commonly by blood transfusion or percutaneous inoculation.

HDV infection Hepatitis D virus infection. A form of hepatitis that occurs only in patients coinfected with hepatitis B. HDV relies on HBV replication and cannot replicate independently. The disease usually progresses to a chronic state.

Heimlich maneuver An emergency procedure for dislodging an obstruction from the trachea. It consists of grasping the choking person from behind and placing the hands around the victim's waist just below the sternum, in a fist, thumb side in, and pulling inward and upward with force to dislodge the obstruction.

Helicobacter pylori An infectious gastrointestinal tract bacterium first identified in 1982. Since then, *H. pylori* has generated worldwide attention for its role in the promotion of chronic gastritis, peptic ulcer disease, and gastric carcinoma. The mode of transmission of *H. pylori* is still unclear, although person-to-person, fecal-oral spread is suspected because of the tendency of *H. pylori* infections to cluster in families.

Hemarthrosis Blood in a joint cavity.

Hematemesis Blood in vomitus.

Hematochezia Feces containing bright red blood.

Hematoma A mass caused by extravasation of blood into a tissue or cavity.

Hematopoiesis Production of cells in the bone marrow, including red cells, white cells, and platelets.

Hematuria Blood in the urine.

Hemianopsia Partial loss of vision in both eyes.

Hemiparesis Motor weakness affecting one side of the body, usually occurring with lateral cerebral injuries.

Hemiplegia Paralysis of one side of the body.

Hemochromatosis A disorder (usually genetic) of iron metabolism characterized by excess absorption of iron and deposition in organs such as the liver.

Hemodynamics Principles of blood flow.

Hemoglobin Oxygen-carrying protein in red blood cells.

Hemolysis Separation of hemoglobin from red blood cells and its appearance in the fluid in which the corpuscles are suspended; red blood cell lysis.

Hemoptysis Spitting up of blood, the origin of which is the lungs or bronchial tubes.

Hemostasis Arrest of bleeding; prevention of blood loss.

Hemothorax Accumulation of blood and fluid in the pleural space.

Hepatitis An inflammatory condition of the liver. Potential causes include viral, bacterial, fungal, and protozoal infections; drugs and toxins; autoimmune disorders; and metabolic disorders.

Hepatocellular carcinoma A common form of primary hepatic malignancy. Signs and symptoms include hepatomegaly, abdominal pain, weight loss, nausea, and, in advanced cases, jaundice and ascites; also called *hepatoma*.

Hepatocellular failure Acute or chronic loss of essential liver function resulting in portal systemic encephalopathy and a variety of other problems, including coagulopathy, renal failure, bleeding, infection, hypoglycemia, respiratory failure, and death.

Hepatoma A primary liver cancer arising from cells normally found in the liver, not to be confused with cancer metastatic to the liver from a distant site.

Hereditary hemochromatosis An autosomal recessive disorder caused by the activity of a mutant gene called *HFE*, which allows excessive and uncontrolled iron absorption by the GI tract.

Herpesviruses Important group of viral agents producing infections in humans. Two types of herpes simplex viruses, referred to as types 1 and 2, may be sexually transmitted.

Herpes zoster (shingles) An acute localized inflammatory disease of a dermatomal segment of the skin caused by the same herpesvirus that causes chickenpox.

Heterochromatin A type of chromatin (DNA) that is tightly compacted and genetically inactive.

Heterozygous Having two different alleles for a specific gene product.

HEV infection Hepatitis E virus infection. A self-limited type of hepatitis acquired by ingestion of fecally contaminated water or food.

Hiatal hernia A defect in the diaphragm that allows a portion of the stomach to protrude through the diaphragmatic opening into the thorax.

High blood pressure A consistent elevation of blood pressure above 140 mm Hg systolic and/or 90 mm Hg diastolic (in adults).

Hilum Concave portion of the kidney that faces the vertebral column through which the nerves, blood vessels, and ureter enter and exit the kidney.

Hinge joint A joint that permits flexion and extension like the interphalangeal joint of the finger, the elbow, or the knee; also called *ginglymus joint*.

Hirschsprung disease A congenital disorder of the large intestine in which the autonomic nerve ganglia in the smooth muscle are absent or markedly reduced in number, which causes poor or absent peristalsis.

Hirsutism Excessive growth of the hair or presence of hair in unusual places.

Histiocyte A type of cell normally present in small numbers around blood vessels, but in pathologic conditions it can migrate in the dermis as a tissue monocyte. It can also form abundant reticulum fibers. When it phagocytizes bacteria and particulate matter, it is referred to as a *macrophage*.

Histone A protein around which linear DNA is wrapped.

Histrionic Theatrical, dramatic.

Hodgkin disease A progressive malignancy of the lymph node characterized by the presence of Reed-Sternberg cells and slow, predictable spread through the lymphatic vessels.

Homeostasis A dynamic steady state, representing the net effect of all the turnover reactions.

Homologous Corresponding in structure. For example, the labia majora are *homologous* with the scrotum of the male.

Homologous chromosomes A pair of chromosomes in a diploid cell that contain similar gene loci, each being derived from a different parent.

Homozygous Having two identical alleles for a specific gene product.

Hormone A blood-borne chemical messenger that affects target cells anatomically distant from the secreting cells.

Hormone agonist A chemical that binds to a hormone receptor and initiates intracellular activities identical to those caused by hormones. Some medications exert their therapeutic effects through this process.

Hormone antagonist A chemical that competes with hormones for cell receptors. Antagonists bind to cell receptors and prevent the occurrence of intracellular activities associated with hormone-receptor binding. Some medications produce their therapeutic effects through this process.

Hormone receptor A protein on or within a target cell that binds to circulating hormones and allows the cellular response to a specific hormone. Hormone-receptor binding is the first step in the cellular response to a particular hormone.

Host-parasite relationship The interaction between the host and the microorganisms that reside on or in it.

Human immunodeficiency virus (HIV) A retrovirus that affects the immune system, causing a defect in cell-mediated immunity and failure of the immune system to function properly.

Human leukocyte antigen (HLA) complex The major histocompatibility complex (MHC) in human leukocytes.

Hyaline membranes Membranes in alveolar tissue that look like glass. The alveoli are filled with proteinaceous fluid and epithelial cells.

Hydrocele Accumulation of fluid in the tunica vaginalis testis; one of the most common causes of scrotal swelling.

Hydrocephalus Increase in the amount of cerebrospinal fluid due to blocked circulation or absorption and the consequent enlargement of the ventricles.

Hydrophilic Soluble in water but insoluble in lipid.

Hydrophobic Insoluble in water but soluble in lipid.

Hydropic swelling An increase in intracellular fluid volume and changes in intracellular organelles in association with cell injury; also called *oncosis*.

Hydrostatic pressure Pressure exerted by a liquid.

Hydroureter Distention of a ureter with urine, usually resulting from an obstruction process.

Hyperacusis Exceptionally acute hearing, the hearing threshold being unusually low. It may or may not be accompanied by pain.

Hyperalgesia An increased sensitivity to painful stimuli characterized by a lower than normal pain threshold.

Hypercalcemia Serum calcium concentration above normal.

Hypercapnia An abnormally high amount of carbon dioxide in the blood.

Hypercortisolism Elevated serum level of cortisol.

Hyperemesis gravidarum A Latin term meaning "excess vomiting in pregnant women." Unlike the transient nausea and vomiting that occurs in about half of women in the first trimester of pregnancy, hyperemesis gravidarum continues throughout the entire pregnancy. It is often severe and can have life threatening consequences.

Hyperemia Localized redness produced by increased blood flow.

Hyperkalemia Serum potassium concentration above normal.

Hyperkeratosis Horny overgrowth of epidermis, such as callus formation.

Hypermagnesemia Serum magnesium concentration above normal.

Hypermetabolic state A condition of abnormally high basal metabolic rate. May be indicated by an increase in skin temperature, such as that occurring in hyperthyroidism and after sun exposure or sunburn.

Hypernatremia Serum sodium concentration above normal; results from gain of salt relative to water or loss of water relative to salt; water deficit.

Hyperphosphatemia Serum phosphate concentration above normal.

Hyperplasia Abnormal multiplication or increase in the number of normal cells in normal arrangement in a tissue.

Hypersensitivity An abnormal excessive response to a sensitizing antigen.

Hypertension A consistent elevation of blood pressure above 140 mm Hg systolic and/or 90 mm Hg diastolic (in adults).

Hyperthyroidism Overactivity of the thyroid gland.

Hypertonic fluid Fluid that has a higher particle concentration (osmolality) than normal body fluid; causes a net flow of water across cell membranes out of cells.

Hypertrichosis lanuginosa Excessive hair growth over the entire body.

Hypertrophy An increase in cell or tissue size and function.

Hypocalcemia Serum calcium concentration below normal.

Hypochromia An abnormal decrease in the hemoglobin content of the erythrocytes.

Hypodermis Loose subcutaneous layer rich in fat and areolar tissue lying beneath the dermis; also called *superficial fascia*.

Hypoglycemic sweating Sweating caused by low blood glucose. Usually distinguishable from other causes of sweating due to the additional symptoms of weakness, tachycardia, hunger, headache, and "inward nervousness" manifested as mental irritability and confusion.

Hypokalemia Serum potassium concentration below normal.

Hypomagnesemia Serum magnesium concentration below normal.

Hypomania A disorder that may include any symptoms of mania, but without the loss of reality testing, without psychosis (e.g., hallucinations, delusions), and without impaired functioning; also called *partial mania*.

Hypomenorrhea A deficient amount of menstrual flow, usually the result of an endocrine or systemic disorder that interferes with hormonal function. It may also result from partial obstruction of the menstrual flow by the hymen or a narrowing of the cervical os.

Hyponatremia Serum sodium concentration below normal; results from gain of water relative to salt or loss of salt relative to water; water intoxication.

Hypophosphatemia Serum phosphate concentration below normal.

Hypophysis The pituitary gland, which consists of anterior and posterior lobes.

Hyposensitization Reduction in sensitivity to an allergen, accomplished by administering low doses of the allergen, which binds with immunoglobulin G.

Hypospadias A congenital anomaly in which the urethral meatus is located on the undersurface of the penis or on the perineum.

Hypothalamic-pituitary-adrenal (HPA) axis Refers to a hierarchy of control mechanisms whereby the hypothalamus regulates the anterior pituitary gland and the pituitary gland regulates the secretion of hormones from the adrenal cortex.

Hypothalamus A group of nuclei at the base of the brain concerned with regulation of body processes: temperature, thirst, hunger, satiety, and adaptive sexual behaviors.

Hypothyroidism Underactivity of the thyroid gland.

Hypotonic fluid Fluid that has a lower particle concentration (osmolality) than normal body fluid; causes a net flow of water across cell membranes into cells.

Hypoventilation Decreased exchange of air in the alveoli in relation to oxygen consumption, influenced by a decreased rate and depth of respiration.

Hypoxemia An abnormally low amount of oxygen in the blood.

Hypoxia A reduction in oxygen at the tissue level that may lead to failure of aerobic production of adenosine triphosphate.

I

I bands "I" is for "isotropic"; these bands are light in color and correspond to the position of thin actin filaments extending in both directions from the Z line in striated muscle.

Iatrogenic Resulting from the activity of a medical intervention.

Icterus A yellow discoloration of the skin, mucous membranes, and sclerae of the eyes, caused by greater than normal amounts of bilirubin in the blood; also called *jaundice*.

Idiopathic Without known cause.

Idiopathic hypertension High blood pressure of unknown cause; also called *primary hypertension*.

Ileocecal valve Sphincter between the small and large intestines that is normally closed, so that the contents of the large intestine cannot move in a retrograde fashion back into the small intestine. It opens in response to a peristaltic contraction, bringing intestinal contents toward it.

Illusion The misperception of a real sensory stimulus.

Immobilization A mechanical action of limiting or preventing movement at a joint. Prolonged immobilization may cause a shortening of connective tissue, a breakdown of cartilage, a weakening of ligaments, and a decrease in the muscles' ability to contract, as well as increased bone resorption.

Immunity A state of active resistance to a particular pathogen, which requires functional T- and B-cell memory cells.

Immunization Exposure of a susceptible host to an altered pathogen that does not cause disease but causes the host to create antibodies to that pathogen.

Immunodeficiency Failure of immune system mechanisms to defend against pathogens. There are two broad categories of immunodeficiencies, based on the mechanism of lymphocyte dysfunction: primary and acquired.

Immunogen Foreign substance, cell, toxin, or protein that causes the components of the immune system to react and respond, inducing the formation of antibodies; also called *antigen*.

Immunogenicity The ability to stimulate an immune response.

Immunosuppression The inability to produce an immune response to an antigen, resulting in reduced resistance to infection.

Impacted fracture A fracture caused by excessive force that telescopes or drives one fragment into another.

Impaired fasting glucose A disorder of glucose tolerance, not diagnostic of diabetes, which is characterized by a fasting blood glucose value between 100 and 125 mg/dl.

Impaired glucose tolerance A disorder of glucose tolerance, not diagnostic of diabetes, which is characterized by a 2-hour postprandial blood glucose value of between 140 and 200 mg/dl.

Impetigo An acute, contagious skin disease characterized by the formation of vesicles, pustules, and yellowish crusts.

Impotence Failure to achieve and maintain an erection of the penis; also called erectile dysfunction.

Impulsivity Spontaneous acting out of impulses accompanied by failure to plan ahead, predict consequences, or consider other possibilities.

Incomplete fracture A fracture in which the cortex of the bone buckles or cracks without disrupting bone continuity.

Induration Hardness, such as that resulting from multiple intramuscular or subcutaneous injections of medication.

Inert tissue Soft tissue that possesses no ability to contract or relax; this includes the joint capsule, ligament, bursa, fascia, dura mater, and nerve root.

Infectious disease A pathologic process caused by a microorganism that is transmissible from one host to another.

Infiltrate Fluid or material that has moved into tissues.

Inflammation The body's protective response at the site of injury or tissue destruction. Although infectious agents can produce inflammation, infection is not synonymous with inflammation.

Inflammatory bowel disease A general term for inflammatory diseases of the bowel of uncertain cause, such as ulcerative colitis and Crohn disease.

Inhalation injury Cellular injury to lung tissue as a result of inhalation of a toxic substance such as smoke. Smoke inhalation significantly increases the morbidity and mortality from burn injury.

Innate immune response Part of the host defense system that is composed of mechanical and biochemical barriers, phagocytes, and chemical mediators.

Inotropy The force or energy of cardiac contraction; similar to contractility.

Insulin Hormone produced by the β cells of the pancreas; has wide-ranging effects on energy metabolism and protein synthesis.

Insulin resistance The condition of requiring an increased amount of insulin for the same level of tissue glucose influx.

Integrins A large family of transmembrane proteins that mediate adhesion of cells to the extracellular matrix.

Integument Covering; refers to the skin.

Integumentary system The skin and its appendages, including the hair and nails.

Intercurrent Occurring during the course of an already existing disease.

Intermembranous ossification The process in which osteoblasts in the inner layer of the periosteum are responsible for the increase in the width of bones.

Interstitial fluid Fluid that lies between the cells; a component of extracellular fluid.

Interstitial space The space between cells.

Intertrigo An erythematous irritation of opposing skin surfaces caused by friction.

Intestinal villi Fingerlike projections, numbering in the millions, that line the small intestine and serve to increase the surface area of the intestine for digestion and absorption of nutrients.

Intra- Within. For example, in intra-aortic balloon counterpulsation, a catheter with a balloon at the distal segment is inserted through the femoral artery and positioned in the aorta just distal to the left subclavian artery.

Intracellular fluid Fluid that is inside the cells.

Intracellular obligate parasites Bacteria that must live inside a living cell.

Intraocular Inside the globe of the eyeball.

Intravenous pyelography A diagnostic procedure in which an iodine-based contrast material is injected into the vascular system to allow visualization of the kidneys and urinary tract.

Intrinsic Originating from within the individual.

Intrinsic asthma Asthma caused by pathophysiologic disturbances that do not involve IgE-mediated mechanisms. This type of asthma frequently develops in middle age. Psychological stress factors, pulmonary irritants, and exercise may precipitate an asthma attack.

Intrinsic nervous system Neural structures belonging entirely to the gastrointestinal (GI) system that control most GI functions and are responsible for many reflexes occurring locally in the GI tract. It is composed of two layers: the myenteric plexus and the submucosal plexus.

Intrinsic pathway of coagulation A sequence of reactions leading to fibrin formation, beginning with the contact activation of factor XII, followed by the sequential activation of factors XI and IX, and resulting in the activation of factor X, which in activated form initiates the common pathway of coagulation.

Intron The portion of a primary RNA transcript that is removed prior to translation of the RNA message.

Intussusception A telescoping of a portion of the bowel into an adjacent distal portion. It is most common in infants and occurs three times more often in males than in females.

Ipsilateral Referring to the same side of the body.

Irritable bowel syndrome The presence of alternating diarrhea and constipation accompanied by abdominal cramping in the absence of any identifiable pathologic process in the gastrointestinal tract.

Ischemia Inadequate flow through the arterial system, producing tissue hypoxia.

Ischemic A lack of blood or oxygen supply to tissue.

Isoimmunity The condition occurring when an individual's immune system reacts against antigens on tissues from other members of the same species, such as a blood transfusion reaction in which an individual with type A blood reacts against a transfusion with type B blood.

Isolated systolic hypertension An elevation in systolic blood pressure above 140 mm Hg without an increase in diastolic blood pressure. It most commonly occurs in the elderly.

Isolated urinary tract infection A first infection or an infection that occurs more than 6 months after a previous infection.

Isometric contraction A contraction in which no movement takes place and the muscle maintains its specific length. For example, holding a weight in the hand with elbow flexed produces an isometric contraction.

Isotonic fluid Fluid that has the same particle concentration (osmolality) as normal body fluid.

J

Jaundice Yellowness of skin.

Joint A point of contact between bones; also called *articulation*.

Joint capsule A dense layer of connective tissue surrounding a synovial joint. The capsule is solidly attached to the periosteum of the adjacent bony components. The joint capsule provides strength to the joint and, through its neural receptors, detects motion, compression, tension, vibration, and pain.

Juxtaglomerular apparatus The collection of macula densa cells in the distal convoluted tubule, afferent and efferent arterioles, and the juxtaglomerular cells located around the arterioles, which work together to control glomerular filtration rate.

Juxtamedullary nephron A nephron with long loops of Henle that extend deep into the medulla and create a concentrated interstitium via the countercurrent mechanism.

K

Keratin Tough, water-repellent protein produced by keratinocytes and found in hair, nails, and horny tissue.

Keratinocyte One of several types of epithelial cells. Keratinocytes are able to produce keratin.

Keratosis Any skin lesion in which there is overgrowth and thickening of the cornified epithelium.

Kernicterus An abnormal toxic accumulation of bilirubin in central nervous system tissues caused by hyperbilirubinemia.

Ketone bodies The result of fatty acids in the liver that are transformed to acetyl coenzyme A, which is then processed into one of three compounds known as ketone bodies.

Kilocalorie The unit of measure for energy value of foods.

Kinin A vasoactive peptide produced during inflammation and injury.

Koilonychia Dystrophy of the fingernails, in which the nails are concave; also called *spoon nail*.

Korotkoff sounds Sounds heard during auscultation of arterial blood pressure. As the pressure in the blood pressure cuff is released, blood begins to flow turbulently through the artery, producing Korotkoff sounds.

L

Lactation Formation and secretion of milk from the breasts for the nourishment of the infant.

Lactic acidosis An increase in the anaerobic production of lactate, which, when released into the bloodstream, creates a condition of metabolic acidosis.

Laminar flow Flow of air or fluid in which there is no turbulence and the direction of flow is linear and parabolic.

Langerhans cell One of several types of epithelial cell. Langerhans cells are thought to have a role in immunologic reactions that affect the skin and may serve as a defense mechanism for the body.

Laparoscopic cholecystectomy Surgical removal of the gallbladder using an optical scope and instruments inserted through small abdominal incisions.

Laparoscopy Examination of the abdominal cavity via a small incision to permit the insertion of a variety of optical scopes for diagnosis or therapy.

Latency period A period of time when there is no apparent change in status. The time required for elastic structures to tighten to prepare for the development of tension.

Leiomyoma Benign neoplasm of the smooth muscle of the uterus that is characteristically firm, well circumscribed, and round. Uterine leiomyomas usually appear and exhibit growth activity during the reproductive years.

Leprosy A chronic infectious disease of the skin caused by the intracellular bacillus *Mycobacterium leprae*.

Leptomeninges The combined structures of the pia mater and arachnoid mater.

Lesion A demonstrable structural change produced in the course of a disease. Lesions may be evident at a gross or microscopic level.

Leukemia A malignant disease of bone marrow stem cells, with accumulation of immature blasts in the marrow and peripheral blood.

Leukocyte A cell that mediates immune function. Leukocytes protect the body by phagocytosis of microorganisms and production of antibodies and memory cells; also called *white blood cell*.

Leukoderma Patch of depigmentation; also called *vitiligo*.

Leukopenia A deficiency of white blood cells in the peripheral circulation, which is usually indicative of bone marrow failure.

Leydig cell An interstitial cell in the testes that produces and secretes testosterone.

Libido Sexual drive; feeling of sexual desire.

Lichen planus A relatively common, chronic, pruritic disease involving inflammation and papular eruption of the skin and mucous membranes.

Ligament A dense connective tissue with parallel-fibered collagenous tissues designed to connect bone to bone.

Limbic system A group of structures surrounding the corpus callosum that produce various emotional feelings.

Lipid bilayer A double layer of lipid molecules that forms cellular membranes, including the plasma membrane, organelle membranes, and vesicles.

Lipodystrophy A group of conditions due to defective metabolism of fat, resulting in atrophy of subcutaneous fat.

Lipolysis Production of free fatty acids resulting from the breakdown of fat in adipose tissue.

Lipoproteins A group of biomolecules composed of differing amounts of cholesterol, triglyceride, and protein, such as high-density lipoprotein (HDLs) and low-density lipoprotein (LDLs).

Lithotripsy Mechanical or chemical fragmentation of a calculus.

Liver transplantation Surgical transfer of an appropriately matched donor liver into a host who has inadequate liver function to sustain life.

Longitudinal fracture Fracture in which a bone is split along its length.

Loose association Flow of thought in which ideas shift from one subject to another in a completely unrelated or noncohesive way. When severe, speech may be unintelligible.

Lower esophageal sphincter The circular band of muscular tissue at the lower end of the esophagus. It serves to prevent the highly acidic gastric contents from moving in a retrograde motion back into the esophagus.

Lumpectomy Surgical removal of only the malignant tumor or "lump" from an affected breast.

Lunula "Little moon"; the crescent-shaped white area nearest the root of the nail body.

Lusitropy Relaxation of cardiac muscle and chambers.

Lyme disease An infectious, immune-mediated multisystem disease caused by a tick-borne spirochete. It is characterized by an erythema migrans rash in which the area of redness begins at the site of the tick bite. The site is generally flat, warm, and indurated, but not painful. Headache, neck stiffness, fever, chills, myalgia, arthralgia, malaise, and fatigue accompany skin involvement, and arthritis of the large joints may develop.

Lymphadenopathy A pathologic lymph node enlargement, which is usually painless and may be associated with malignancy, especially lymphoma. Lymphadenopathy must be distinguished from normal reactive lymph node enlargement in response to infection. Reactive nodes are usually tender and are situated "downstream" from a site of infection.

Lymphedema Swelling produced by an obstruction of lymphatic flow.

Lymphocyte A white blood cell derived from the lymphoid stem cell that is not affected by diseases of the myeloid stem cell. Lymphocytes are of three basic types: T, B, and natural killer cells.

Lymphogranuloma venereum Highly contagious systemic infection caused by a number of strains of *Chlamydia*. It has progressive stages of development in which an initial lesion forms, and systemic disease occurs following dissemination via the lymphatic system.

Lymphoid group Dermal cells consisting of lymphocytes commonly found in inflammatory lesions of the skin.

Lymphopoiesis Formation of lymphocytes.

Lysosome An organelle containing hydrolytic enzymes that function to digest intracellular materials.

Lysozyme An enzyme secreted by macrophages and neutrophils to control foreign particle activity.

M

M line Marks the center of the A band and the midpoint of myosin filaments in striated muscle.

Macrocyte An abnormally large erythrocyte.

Macrophage A mature monocyte that migrates from the blood vessels to sites in the lymphoid tissues. Macrophages are powerful phagocytes and secrete a number of cytokines that stimulate inflammation.

Major histocompatibility complex (MHC) The gene regions on chromosome 6 that contain the genes for MHC proteins. Class I proteins are present on virtually all nucleated cells. Class II proteins are found mainly on antigen-presenting cells: B cells, macrophages, and dendritic cells.

Malabsorption Failure of the gastrointestinal tract to absorb or normally digest one or more dietary constituents.

Maladaptation Ineffective, inadequate, or inappropriate change in response to new or altered circumstances.

Malignant tumor A type of tumor that has a tendency to invade local tissues and spread to distant sites (metastasis). Malignant tumors are generally poorly differentiated and are associated with a poor prognosis if not promptly managed.

Mallory-Weiss syndrome Mild to massive bleeding due to a tear in the mucosa or submucosa of the cardia or lower esophagus. The tear is usually longitudinal and is caused by forceful or prolonged vomiting during which the upper esophageal sphincter fails to relax.

Mania A condition characterized by an overwhelming increase in energy and drive; manifests as nonstop activity, grandiose thinking, impulsivity, euphoria, impaired judgment, acting-out behaviors, and hypersexuality; also called *full mania*.

Mass lesion Any lesion in the cranium that behaves like a space-occupying mass. Mass lesions tend to progress and cause signs and symptoms of increased intracranial pressure.

Mast cell Mast cells have intracytoplasmic basophilic metachromatic granules containing heparin and histamine. The normal skin contains relatively few mast cells, but their number is increased in many different skin conditions, particularly the itching dermatoses; also called *histiocytic cell*.

Mastectomy Surgical removal of a breast. See *modified radical mastectomy* and *radical mastectomy*.

McBurney point The point located in the lower right quadrant of the abdomen situated in the normal area of the appendix midway between the umbilicus and the anterior iliac crest.

Mean arterial pressure The average pressure in the arterial system through the cardiac cycle. It is calculated by adding the systolic pressure to two times the diastolic reading and dividing the sum by 3.

Measles Known as *hard measles*, *7-day measles*, or *rubeola*. This is a communicable viral disease caused by paramyxovirus of the genus *Morbillivirus* with a characteristic macular and blotchy rash; sometimes the macules become confluent.

Mediastinum The area of the chest between the sternum and vertebral column and between the lungs. Mediastinal structures include the trachea, esophagus, aorta, heart, and lymph nodes.

Medullary cavity Central cavity in longer bones.

Megakaryocyte A large bone marrow cell that sheds platelets in the bone marrow from its cytoplasm.

Megaloblastic dysplasia Abnormal development of large red cells and nonlymphocytic bone marrow cells.

Megaloblasts Large abnormal hematopoietic bone marrow cells.

Meiosis A type of cell division that results in daughter cells with one half the normal number of chromosomes. Meiosis occurs in gonadal germ cells.

Melanin Dark pigment found in melanocytes that gives color to hair and skin.

Melanocyte One of several types of epithelial cells. Melanocytes contribute color to the skin and serve to filter ultraviolet light.

Melena Tarry, black feces due to the action of gastrointestinal secretions on blood in the intestine.

Membranous urethra The urethral segment that passes through the muscular layers of the urogenital diaphragm.

Menarche The first menstrual period at the time of puberty, usually occurring around age 12 years in North America.

Meninges Membranes surrounding the brain and spinal cord, which include the dura mater, arachnoid, and pia mater.

Meningocele Hernial protrusion of meninges through a neural tube defect in the skull or vertebral column.

Meniscus Curved, fibrous cartilage located in the knee and other joints. Menisci facilitate rotation at the knee by allowing better contact of the tibial surfaces with the femoral condyles.

Menopause A process by which the supply of ovarian follicles and estrogen hormones declines, usually beginning between the ages of 45 and 55 years.

Menorrhagia An increase in the amount or duration of menstrual bleeding, usually resulting from a lesion of the female reproductive organs.

Menstrual cycle The rhythmic pattern of changes in hormonal secretions and in sexual organs occurring approximately every 28 days during a female's reproductive years. The cycle culminates in the production of an ovum and the preparation of the uterus for implantation of a fertilized ovum.

Merkel cells One of several types of epithelial cells. Merkel cells consist of free nerve endings attached to modified epidermal cells. It is generally agreed that Merkel cells function as touch receptors.

Mesoblastic nephroma Benign congenital renal tumor.

Mesonephros One of three distinct stages in the development of the renal system. Mesonephros, which is the middle stage, corresponds to the mature excretory organ of some amphibians. In humans, it begins developing at about the fourth to fifth week of gestation.

Metabolic acidosis Any of the types of acidosis resulting from accumulation in the blood of noncarbonic, nonvolatile acids; characterized by a low HCO_3^- concentration.

Metabolic alkalosis A disturbance in which the acid-base balance shifts to the alkaline because of uncompensated loss of acids, ingestion or retention of excess base, or potassium depletion.

Metabolism Synthesis and breakdown of molecules in a living organism. Metabolism involves both the use and the release of energy.

Metanephros The final stage of development of the renal system. The metanephros begins in the fourth week when the ureteral bud grows out of the mesonephric duct.

Metaplasia Transformation of one kind of tissue to another fully differentiated tissue.

Metastasis Dissemination of cancer cells from the location of origin to other distant areas in the body.

Methemoglobin A transformation product of oxyhemoglobin, formed when the iron of the hemoglobin molecule is oxidized to the ferric state (Fe^{3+}).

Metrorrhagia Bleeding between menstrual periods, usually the result of slight physiologic bleeding from the endometrium during ovulation. It may also result from other causes such as uterine malignancy, cervical erosions, endometrial polyps, or estrogen therapy.

Microbial adherence The ability of the microorganism to latch onto and gain entrance into the host.

Microcytic Referring to an abnormally small erythrocyte.

Micropenis A small, normally formed penis with a stretched length more than 2 standard deviations below the mean, or a stretched length less than 2.5 cm.

Mineralocorticoids A class of steroid hormones, secreted by the adrenal cortex, that regulate the mineral salts (electrolytes) and water balance in the body.

Mitochondrion A membrane-bounded organelle that carries out oxidative phosphorylation to synthesize most of the adenosine triphosphate in a eukaryotic cell.

Mitosis A type of cell division that results in daughter cells with chromosomes that are identical to the parent cell. Mitosis occurs in somatic cells.

Mitral valve The cardiac valve that lies between the left atrium and left ventricle. The valve is normally closed during ventricular systole and open during ventricular diastole. Mitral valve closure contributes to heart sound S_1; also called *bicuspid atrioventricular valve.*

Mixed acid-base imbalance A combined disturbance of acid-base balance in which a primary respiratory disorder and primary metabolic disorder coexist.

Mixed incontinence Loss of bladder control with symptoms of both stress incontinence and urge incontinence.

Modified radical mastectomy Surgical removal of the breast accompanied by dissection of a portion of the axillary lymphatic system.

Molluscum contagiosum A viral skin disease with two forms. One form affects children and is spread through indirect contact; the other is sexually transmitted and occurs in young adults. It is characterized by pink and white lesions on the genitalia with an exudative core.

Mongolian spots Caused by selective pigmentation. They usually occur on the buttocks or sacral area and are commonly seen in Asian Americans and African Americans.

Monocyte An immature circulating macrophage.

Monosaccharide A simple sugar (e.g., glucose, fructose).

Monosomy Having only one member of a homologous chromosome pair, as in monosomy X; also called *Turner syndrome.*

Monounsaturated fatty acid A fatty acid with one double bond.

Mood Sustained expression of an emotion that affects one's outlook.

Mood disorder A disturbance of mood that may be caused by either organic damage to the brain or chemical alterations in neurotransmission. Mood disorders may also have no known biological basis.

Mood swings Oscillation between periods of euphoria (elevated mood) and depression or anxiety.

Morphogen A substance that triggers growth, proliferation, and differentiation of cells in a concentration-dependent manner.

Morphogenesis Arrangement of cells in a particular order during the development of complex organisms.

Morphologic changes Structural and associated functional alterations in cells or tissues that are either characteristic of the disease or diagnostic of the etiologic process.

Motor end-plate The points of contact between an α motor neuron and the skeletal muscle cells it innervates.

Mucocutaneous candidiasis Candidal infection of the mucous membrane and the skin.

Mucosal edema Swelling of mucous membranes.

Müllerian ducts A pair of embryonic ducts that become the fallopian tubes, uterus, and vagina in females; also called *paramesonephric ducts* because they develop alongside the mesonephric ducts.

Multipennate muscle A muscle with several central tendons toward which the muscle fibers converge like the barbs of feathers.

Multiple myeloma (plasma cell myeloma) A malignant disorder of antibody-secreting plasma cells that produce large quantities of monoclonal antibodies and have a predilection to settle in the skeleton, where osteoclastic bone lesions are produced.

Multiple sclerosis A chronic demyelinating disease of the central nervous system that causes significant disability in young adults. It is thought to be an autoimmune disorder that results in inflammation and scarring (sclerosis) of the myelin sheaths covering nerves.

Muscular dystrophy Term referring to a group of genetically determined myopathies characterized by progressive degeneration of muscle fibers.

Mutagen A physical or chemical agent capable of causing alterations in an organism's DNA by inducing mutations.

Mutation A heritable change in the nucleotide sequence of a chromosome, which is passed on to daughter cells when the cell divides.

Myasthenia gravis A chronic autoimmune disease affecting the neuromuscular function of voluntary muscles and characterized by profound muscle weakness and fatigability.

Mycosis Infection caused by a fungus.

Myeloid group Cells of the dermis consisting of polymorphonuclear leukocytes and eosinophilic leukocytes. These cells occur commonly with allergic dermatoses.

Myelomeningocele or meningomyelocele Hernial protrusion of meninges, spinal fluid, and a portion of the spinal cord with its nerves through a defect in the skull and vertebral column.

Myocardial infarction Localized area of cardiac necrosis most often associated with coronary heart disease.

Myocardium The middle layer of the heart, composed of cardiac muscle tissue.

Myosin A cytoskeletal protein that makes up the thick filament of the muscle sarcomere in skeletal and cardiac muscle. It is also present as a contractile filament in other types of cells. Myosin binds with actin during muscular contraction.

Myositis ossificans An abnormal calcification within a muscle.

Myxedema Nonpitting edema caused by advanced hypothyroidism in adulthood.

N

Narcissism Self-absorption; excessive self-love.

Necrosis Death and degradation of body cells or tissues in response to injurious events.

Necrotizing enterocolitis A disorder occurring most often in premature infants (less than 34 weeks gestation) and infants with low birth weight (less than 5 lb or 2.25 kg). This disorder is characterized by diffuse or patchy intestinal necrosis accompanied by sepsis.

Necrotizing inflammation This response can occur when antigen and antibody react in blood vessels in the skin. Necrotizing inflammation can be caused by drug allergies; disorders such as systemic lupus erythematosus, rheumatoid arthritis, and glomerulonephritis; and certain infectious diseases such as hepatitis B; also called *vasculitis*.

Negative feedback A term used to explain homeostatic mechanisms. Negative feedback causes the controller to respond in a manner that opposes or negates deviation from normal level (set point). Most body systems operate on the principle of negative feedback.

Negative nitrogen balance The condition of protein breakdown exceeding daily protein intake and synthesis.

Negative symptoms (schizophrenia) Symptoms of schizophrenia that are thought to be mediated by dopamine D_1 receptors in the brain. Drugs that block D_1 receptors may alleviate some of the negative symptoms, which include social withdrawal, flat affect, poverty of speech, ritualistic posturing, and autism.

Neologism 1. A new word that is often created by combining syllables of other words. 2. A word given special or private significance.

Neoplasia New growth. The term implies an *abnormality* of cellular growth and may be used interchangeably with the term *tumor.*

Neoplasm A new and abnormal proliferation of cells. If malignant, the growth infiltrates tissue, metastasizes, and often recurs, even after attempts at surgical removal.

Nephralgia Renal pain.

Nephroblastoma (Wilms tumor) The most common childhood malignant kidney tumor, resulting from a defect on chromosome 13.

Nephrolithiasis The presence of a stone or calculus anywhere in the urinary tract.

Nephron Functional unit of the kidney composed of epithelial cells forming the glomerulus, proximal convoluted tubule, loop of Henle, distal convoluted tubule, and collecting duct.

Nephropathy A pathologic process in the kidney, including inflammatory, degenerative, and sclerotic conditions. Many disorders can lead to nephropathy, as in diabetic nephropathy, toxic nephropathy, ischemic nephropathy, and obstructive nephropathy.

Nephrotic syndrome A common set of symptoms caused by damage to the glomeruli, in which proteins cross the glomerulus and are lost in the urine at a rate of >3.5 g/day.

Nephrotoxic Poisonous to the kidney.

Neural thread protein Microscopic protein thread that binds and helps stabilize microtubules (the cell's internal support structure or skeleton). In Alzheimer disease, the threads become chemically altered and twist into paired helical filaments, known as *neurofibrillary tangles.* See *tau protein.*

Neurofibrillary tangle An abnormal bundle of twisted threads inside a nerve cell that is the collapsed remains of the neuron's microtubules, which normally provide structural support.

Neurogenic bladder Bladder dysfunction caused by a lesion at any level in the nervous system.

Neurogenic shock Often called "fainting," neurogenic shock may be caused by severe pain, fear, an unpleasant sight, or other strong stimuli that overwhelm the usual regulatory capacity of the nervous system.

Neuroglia, glia A group of cell types (including astrocytes, microglia, ependymal cells, and oligodendrocytes) that support nerve cells and do not conduct action potentials.

Neuropathic osteoarthropathy A neurologic disease that leads to bone abnormalities and joint involvement. The mechanics of disease development are probably a combination of neurovascular and neurotraumatic processes.

Neurovascular injury An injury that affects the nerves that control the caliber of blood vessels.

Neutropenia A type of leukopenia in which the absolute neutrophil count is below 500 cells/µl. Neutropenia is associated with a high risk of bacterial sepsis.

Neutrophilia A high blood neutrophil count.

Neutrophil/neutrophilic granulocyte A cell that contains small lysosomal granules and a segmented nucleus with 2 to 5 lobes. These cells compose 57% to 67% of leukocytes.

Nevus A congenital discoloration of a circumscribed area of the skin; also called *mole* or *birthmark.*

Nociception Activation of nociceptors by potentially tissue-damaging stimuli, resulting in the perception of pain by the central nervous system. Nociception includes the processes of receptor transduction, signal transmission, perception, and signal modulation.

Nociceptor Pain receptor.

Nonarticular rheumatism A common soft tissue syndrome in children. The most common symptom is nocturnal pain that usually occurs in the calves, shins, and thighs; also called *growing pain.*

Noncontractile tissue Soft tissue that possesses no ability to contract or relax; this includes the joint capsule, ligament, bursa, fascia, dura mater, and nerve root; also called *inert tissue.*

Nondisjunction The failure of homologous chromosomes to separate normally during meiosis or mitosis, resulting in unequal distribution of chromosomes to daughter cells.

Nondisplaced fracture A fracture in which the fragments remain in alignment and position.

Non-Hodgkin lymphoma A varied group of malignant disorders of lymph node cells involving B cells, T cells, and natural killer cells. In comparison with Hodgkin disease, these lymphomas tend to spread unpredictably and metastasize early, and thus carry an overall worse prognosis.

Non–Q-wave infarct A subendocardial infarct affecting only the inner third to half of the ventricular wall and generally associated with less severe symptoms.

Nonspecific immune response Referring to a series of mechanical, biochemical, and phagocytic barriers to infection; also called *innate immune system.*

Norepinephrine A major catecholamine neurotransmitter involved in the etiologic development of mood disorders. See *serotonin.*

Nuclei A cluster of neuronal cell bodies located in the central nervous system.

Nucleocapsid The core of the human immunodeficiency virus (HIV), which contains two strands or chains of RNA, protein, and enzymes.

Nucleotide A biomolecule composed of a purine or pyrimidine base linked to a ribose or deoxyribose sugar, with one or more phosphate groups attached to the sugar. DNA and RNA are polymers of nucleotides.

Nucleus A cellular organelle that contains chromosomal DNA.

Nutritional screening A method for quickly determining the nutritional status of an individual from a selected group of anthropometric and biochemical tests.

Nutritional status The state of an individual's nutrition, resulting from the consumption and utilization of nutrients to meet metabolic needs.

Nystagmus Involuntary, rapid, rhythmic movements of the eyeball; these occur commonly in a horizontal direction, but can also occur in a vertical or a rotational direction.

O

Oblique fracture Fracture resulting from a rotational force; however, unlike a spiral fracture, the break is along an oblique course (45-degree angle) and does not rotate around the entire bone.

Obsession A powerful, persistent, intrusive thought, impulse, or image that dominates the mental life of the individual to the extent of seriously interfering with normal living.

Obstruction An anomaly that compromises or prevents flow because of abnormal narrowings. Stenosis or atresia (failure to develop) of valves, and coarctation of the aorta are the most common cardiac obstructive defects.

Occupational asthma Resembles allergic asthma and may be accompanied by positive skin test reactions to protein allergens in the work environment.

Odynophagia A severe sensation of burning squeezing pain with swallowing; may accompany *dysphagia,* or difficulty with swallowing.

Ogilvie syndrome The idiopathic syndrome of intestinal pseudo-obstruction; may result in megacolon.

Olfactory Pertaining to the sense of smell.

Oligomenorrhea Infrequent menstruation, usually the result of failure to ovulate due to inappropriate hormonal function.

Oligosaccharide A compound consisting of 2 to 10 joined monosaccharide units.

Oliguria Urine output of less than 500 ml/day.

Omphalocele Congenital anomaly in which a herniation of viscera at the base of the umbilical cord is present; requires surgical correction.

Oncocytoma Benign renal tumor consisting of large eosinophilic cells that have granular cytoplasm and round, uniform nuclei.

Oncogene A gene associated with the initiation of cancerous behavior in a cell.

Onycholysis Separation of the nail from its bed.

Oogonia The cells present in the female ovaries during prenatal development that ultimately develop into ova. The entire lifetime supply of ova is established prenatally; no new oogonia arise after birth.

Open fracture Fracture occurring when bone is broken and an external wound leads to the fracture site.

Ophthalmia neonatorum Purulent gonococcal conjunctivitis and keratitis in the newborn resulting from exposure of the infant's eyes to infected maternal secretions during the passage through the vagina at birth.

Ophthalmoscopic examination Examination of the extraocular and intraocular structures of the eye using an ophthalmoscope.

Opioid Any of a group of drugs with an affinity for opioid receptors in the central nervous system. Morphine is the standard opioid with which others are compared for characteristics and potency.

Opportunistic infection An infection caused by organisms that are usually nonpathogenic but that become pathogenic because of decreased function of the immune system.

Opsonization The process of proteins, usually antibodies or complement fragments, binding to an antigen in order to make the antigen easier for phagocytic cells to locate. Phagocytic cells have receptors for opsonins.

Organelles The membrane-bound structures in the cell cytoplasm, including nucleus, mitochondria, endoplasmic reticulum, and Golgi apparatus.

Orthopnea Difficulty with breathing that is brought on or exacerbated by lying horizontal.

Orthostatic (postural) hypotension A form of low blood pressure that occurs after positional change from supine to standing. Diagnosed by an increase in heart rate of more than 15% or a decrease in either systolic blood pressure by more than 15 mm Hg, or diastolic blood pressure by more than 10 mm Hg.

Osmolality A measure of degree of concentration; number of particles per kilogram of solvent.

Osmosis Movement of water across a semipermeable membrane to equalize the particle concentration of the fluid on both sides of the membrane.

Ossicle One of several small bones in the middle ear responsible for transmitting sound waves to the inner ear.

Osteoarthritis A common degenerative joint disease characterized by progressive loss of articular cartilage and by formation of new bone from subchondral bone at joint margins.

Osteoblast A bone-forming cell that is derived from the embryonic mesenchyme and, during the early development of the skeleton, differentiates from a fibroblast to function in the formation of bone tissue.

Osteochondroma A benign bone tumor consisting of bone and cartilage.

Osteoclast A cell responsible for bone resorption.

Osteocyte A mature bone cell.

Osteoid osteoma A painful but benign bone-forming tumor that is often found in the cortex of the tibia and femur.

Osteomalacia An abnormal condition of lamellar bone, characterized by a loss of calcification of the matrix and consequent softening of the bone. The condition is the result of an inadequate amount of phosphorus and calcium available in the blood for mineralization of the bones.

Osteomyelitis A severe pyogenic infection of bone and local tissue that requires immediate management.

Osteon The basic unit of bone; also called *Haversian system*.

Osteoporosis A common metabolic bone disease in which reduction in bone mass results from bone resorption proceeding at a rate faster than that of new bone formation.

Osteoprogenitor A type of bone stem cell that lines bone surfaces.

Osteosarcoma A malignant bone-forming tumor and the most common primary malignant bone tumor that develops in the metaphyseal region of long bones.

Ototoxic Damaging to the structures of the inner ear.

Ovarian cyst A sac on an ovary that contains fluid or semisolid material. It may develop at any time between puberty and menopause; the cause is presently unknown.

Overflow incontinence Loss of bladder control associated with urinary retention and bladder distention due to obstruction, detrusor underactivity or inactivity, or sphincteric malfunction.

Oviduct Another term for *fallopian tube*. Each oviduct runs laterally from the uterus to the uterine end of the ovary. The free end of the oviduct adjacent to the ovary is called the *infundibulum*.

Oxygen consumption The amount of oxygen used by the tissues in 1 minute, usually expressed as VO_2.

Oxygen delivery The amount of oxygen delivered to the tissues each minute. Oxygen delivery (DO_2) is calculated by multiplying cardiac output and arterial oxygen content.

Oxytocin Hormone secreted by the posterior pituitary gland. It causes uterine contraction and is thought to have a major role in promoting increased uterine contractility during parturition. After birth, it is secreted in response to suckling by the infant and stimulates the release of milk, called the *milk ejection reflex*.

P

Paco₂ Partial pressure of carbon dioxide in arterial blood; an indicator of the effectiveness of respiratory excretion of carbonic acid.

Paget disease A slowly progressive metabolic bone disease characterized by an initial phase of excessive bone resorption followed by a reactive phase of abnormal excessive bone formation; also called *osteitis deformans*.

Pain An unpleasant sensation caused by noxious stimulation of the sensory nerve endings, or perceived as such.

Pallor Paleness of skin; primarily assessed by skin pallor of the nail beds, lips, and conjunctivae. A possible symptom of anemia.

Pancreas Gland located in the abdomen; has both endocrine and exocrine functions. The endocrine pancreas produces insulin, glucagon, amylin, and somatostatin.

Pancreatitis Inflammation of the pancreas; may be acute or chronic.

Pancytopenia Decreased production of red blood cells, white blood cells, and platelets.

Pandemic An epidemic that affects large geographic regions, possibly spreading worldwide.

Panhypopituitarism A condition of deficiency in all pituitary hormones.

Panic disorder Psychiatric disorder characterized by recurrent, unexpected episodes of acute anxiety, fear, and panic, often accompanied by the subject's belief that he or she may be having a heart attack, is unable to breathe, is losing control, or that death is imminent.

Panmyelosis Overproduction of normal red blood cells, white blood cells, and platelets.

Papillary layer One of two layers of the dermis. The papillary layer consists of bumps (papillae) that project into the epidermis.

Papillary muscles Muscles within the ventricles that connect the chordae tendineae to the ventricular wall. Papillary muscles contract during ventricular systole to place tension on the valves and prevent backflow through them.

Paracrine Referring to hormone-like chemicals, the target cell of which is located next to the cell secreting the chemical.

Parametritis An infection of the connective tissue between the broad ligaments underlying the female reproductive organs.

Paraneoplastic syndrome A cluster of systemic conditions associated with cancer, such as hypercalcemia, hyponatremia, or Cushing syndrome.

Paraphimosis Painful constriction of the glans penis by foreskin, which has been retracted behind the corona.

Parasite One of a variety of protozoa (single-celled animals), nemathelminths (roundworms), platyhelminths (flatworms), and arthropods (invertebrate animals with jointed appendages). Parasites depend on another organism for survival.

Parkinsonism Parkinson disease symptoms. A neurologic disorder caused by various lesions in the extrapyramidal motor system. It is characterized by rest tremor; muscle rigidity; hypokinesia; slow shuffling gait; and difficulty in chewing, swallowing, and speaking.

Paroxysm A sudden outburst or change from the norm, as in a sudden burst of electrical activity seen on electroencephalography, as occurs with seizure activity.

Paroxysmal nocturnal dyspnea A sudden severe feeling of suffocation, which usually occurs at night and wakes the individual from sleep.

Partial seizure A seizure in which part of the brain surface is involved.

Parturition The process by which an infant is born.

Pathogen An agent that causes disease.

Pathogenesis Development or evolution of disease. A description of the pathogenesis includes everything that happens in the body from the initial stimulus to the ultimate expression of manifestations of the disease.

Pathology Study of the causes, characteristics, and effects of disease.

Pathophysiology The study of the etiology, pathogenesis and clinical manifestations of disease.

Pauciarticular onset Affecting four or fewer joints; used in association with juvenile rheumatoid arthritis.

Pedigree Genetic lineage or family history of traits, used to trace the pattern of inheritance.

Pelvic inflammatory disease Any acute or subacute recurrent or chronic infection of the oviducts and ovaries with involvement of the adjacent reproductive organs.

Pemphigus A group of disorders including vulgaris, vegetans, foliaceus, and erythematosus. The pemphigus group disorders are characterized by bullous eruptions (blisters) thought to be caused by autoimmune reactions.

Pemphigus vulgaris Included in the pemphigus group of disorders, pemphigus vulgaris has the worst prognosis. Bullae can erupt on the skin and mucous membranes (e.g., esophagus), and toxemia and infection can cause death if proper treatment (cortisone) is not administered.

Penile urethra The longest segment of the male urethra, extending about 15 cm in length from the membranous urethra to the external meatus.

Penis Male organ of copulation and urinary excretion.

Penumbra The margin or fringe surrounding a central part. In the case of stroke, a penumbra of viable tissue surrounds the necrotic core that can survive if optimal conditions exist and if it is not subject to further insults.

Peptic ulcer disease Disorder of the upper gastrointestinal tract caused by the action of acid and pepsin. This disorder may include injury to the mucosa of the esophagus, stomach, or duodenum, and may range from a slight mucosal injury to severe ulceration.

Percutaneous Referring to a procedural approach that traverses the skin and is less traumatic than open surgical methods.

Pericardium A protective covering of the heart that is made of two layers separated by a fluid-filled space. The inner (visceral) layer is attached to the heart itself, whereas the outer (parietal) layer forms a sac around the heart.

Perimysium The connective tissue surrounding the fasciculi.

Peripheral vascular dysfunction Decreased localized blood flow resulting in coolness, often to the feet, because skin temperature depends on the amount of blood circulating through the dermis.

Peristalsis The basic propulsive movement of the gastrointestinal (GI) tract. During normal functioning, this coordinated, rhythmic, serial contraction of smooth muscle propels the contents of the GI tract in a downward direction.

Permissive hypothesis A hypothesis positing that poor dampening by serotonin of other neurotransmitter systems (e.g., norepinephrine and dopamine) allows wide variations in mood.

Permissiveness The process in which one hormone increases the number of cellular receptors for a second hormone, thus increasing the cellular response to the second hormone.

Peroxisome (microbody) Small membrane-bound organelle that uses molecular oxygen to degrade organic molecules.

Perseveration Persisting response to a previous stimulus after a new stimulus has been presented.

Personality disorder A disorder that represents immature, inflexible, and persistently maladaptive ways of dealing with the intrapersonal and interpersonal aspects of life.

Petechiae Nonblanching, pinpoint red or purple spots caused by capillary hemorrhages.

Peyronie disease Formation of palpable, fibrous plaques on the surface of the corpora cavernosa.

pH The negative logarithm of the hydrogen ion concentration; a measure of the acidity of a solution.

Phagocytosis Ingestion and destruction of pathogens by leukocytes.

Phagosome A cellular lysosome containing substances obtained by phagocytosis.

Phenotype The physical, biochemical, and biological makeup of an individual, expressed as recognizable traits.

Pheochromocytoma Tumor of the adrenal gland that secretes catecholamines, resulting in elevated blood pressure. An example of a condition that causes secondary high blood pressure.

Phimosis A condition in which the penile foreskin fits so tightly over the glans that it cannot be retracted.

Phlebitis Inflammation of a vein.

Photoreceptor A receptor found in the eye that responds to light.

Physiologic jaundice of the newborn A harmless, short-term condition caused by immature bilirubin conjugation and transport mechanisms, characterized by yellowish staining of the skin and sclera.

Physiology The study of the specific characteristics and functions of a living organism and its parts.

Pigmentary disturbance Interruption of any organic coloring material produced in the body, such as melanin.

Pinocytosis A process of ingesting fluids and small particles that is common to most cell types; also called *cellular drinking*.

Pituitary gland A gland located at the base of the hypothalamus. It consists of anterior and posterior lobes; also called *hypophysis*.

Pityriasis rosea A rash of unknown origin that primarily affects young adults. The characteristic lesion of a macule or papule with surrounding erythema is thought to be viral in origin, but no virus has been isolated to date.

Pivot joint A synovial joint that allows rotation as its single axis movement. Examples include the superior radioulnar joint of the elbow and the union between the first and second vertebrae; also called *trochoid joint*.

Placenta A highly vascularized organ through which the fetus receives nutrients and by which wastes are removed. It also is an endocrine organ, producing several hormones, most notably human chorionic gonadotropin.

Placenta previa Condition of pregnancy in which the placenta is implanted abnormally over the internal cervical os. It occurs in varying degrees of severity and may result in sudden massive hemorrhage following dilatation of the internal os.

Plasma A complex, aqueous liquid in blood and lymph containing a number of organic and inorganic substances.

Plasma cell 1. An antibody-secreting B lymphocyte. 2. A dermal cell rarely seen in normal skin secretions, occurring in small numbers in most chronic inflammatory diseases of the skin and in larger numbers in granulomas.

Plasma membrane The membrane that surrounds a living cell.

Plasmapheresis Removal of plasma from withdrawn blood, with retransfusion of the formed elements into the donor.

Platelet A circulating cytoplasmic fragment of megakaryocytes that is essential in the formation of blood clots and in the control of bleeding.

Pleural effusion A collection of fluid in the pleural cavity resulting from a disease process.

Pleurodesis Instillation of a chemically irritating drug (e.g., tetracycline, sterile talc, bleomycin, doxycycline) into the pleural space to stimulate inflammation and adhesion.

Pneumonia An acute inflammation of lung tissue caused by an infectious agent or by aspiration of chemically irritating fluid.

Pneumothorax Accumulation of air in the pleural space.

Polyarteritis nodosa A form of systemic vasculitis that can cause inflamed arteries in visceral organs, brain, and skin.

Polyarticular onset (oligoarticular) Affecting five or more joints; used in association with juvenile rheumatoid arthritis.

Polycystic kidney disease A progressive disease characterized by multiple dilations of the collecting ducts of the kidneys, which appear as if they are fluid-filled cysts, as a result of renal pathologic processes.

Polycythemia An excess of circulating red blood cells.

Polydipsia Excessive thirst.

Polygenic Referring to a trait determined by multiple genes at different loci, all having additive effects.

Polymenorrhea An increased frequency of menstruation, which may be associated with ovulation due to endocrine or systemic factors.

Polymorphism Inherited structural differences in proteins as a result of many alleles for a particular gene locus.

Polymorphonuclear neutrophil (PMN) A cell that contains small lysosomal granules and a segmented nucleus with two to five lobes. PMNs compose 57% to 67% of leukocytes.

Polymyositis Inflammation of many muscles, usually accompanied by deformity, edema, insomnia, pain, sweating, and tension.

Polyp A general descriptive term used for any mass of protruding tissue. Polyps may be either benign or malignant, although the term usually refers to the benign form.

Polyploidy Having more than two sets of homologous chromosomes.

Polysaccharide A saccharide containing 10 to 10,000 monosaccharide units.

Polysomy Having greater than the usual number of autosomal chromosomes.

Polyunsaturated fatty acid A fatty acid with several double bonds.

Polyuria Excretion of large amounts of urine.

Portal hypertension Abnormally high blood pressure in the blood vessels draining the intra-abdominal alimentary tract, pancreas, gallbladder, and spleen. It may be due to increased resistance to blood flow, as in cirrhosis, or, rarely, to abnormally increased blood flow, as in arteriovenous communications.

Portal systemic encephalopathy A neuropsychiatric syndrome caused by liver dysfunction and resulting in mental status changes ranging from mild cerebral dysfunction to deep coma (hepatic coma) and death.

Positive end-expiratory pressure A method in which a ventilator is used to maintain positive airway pressure at the end of expiration, resulting in increased functional residual capacity and decreased shunt.

Positive feedback A term used to explain homeostatic mechanisms. Positive feedback increases deviation from the set point. Although most systems of the body operate on the principle of negative feedback, sneezing and childbirth are two examples of positive feedback.

Positive nitrogen balance The condition of dietary intake of proteins exceeding output.

Positive symptoms (schizophrenia) Symptoms of schizophrenia that are thought to be due to excessive dopamine D_2 receptor activation in the brain. Disorganized thinking (inability to connect thoughts logically), disorganized speech (rambling, tangentiality), delusions (fixed system of false beliefs), and hallucinations (sensory perception when no apparent stimulus exists) are typical positive symptoms.

Positron emission tomography (PET) A technique of brain imaging. PET studies measure changes in tissue utilization of glucose.

Postictal phase The phase following a seizure during which the person is sleepy and confused.

Postobstructive diuresis Increased urinary output after resolution of partial or total obstruction of the urinary tract.

Potter syndrome Congenital condition often associated with renal agenesis, but always manifesting with the following anomalies: wide-spaced eyes with epicanthal folds, low-set ears, broad and flat nose, hypoplastic lungs, and limb deformities.

Poverty of speech Speech that gives little information owing to vagueness, empty repetitions, or obscure phrases.

Preeclampsia-eclampsia Elevated blood pressure during pregnancy associated with edema and proteinuria. Blood pressure returns to normal after delivery. Eclampsia is present when preeclampsia progresses to seizures; also called *pregnancy-induced hypertension*.

Pregnancy-induced hypertension The rapid rise of arterial blood pressure associated with a loss of large amounts of protein in the urine occurring during pregnancy. Women at risk for pregnancy-induced hypertension include teenagers and women in their late 30s and early 40s; also called *toxemia of pregnancy* and *preeclampsia-eclampsia*.

Preload The volume of blood in the cardiac chamber just prior to systole (end-diastolic volume).

Prepuce Penile skin that overlies the glans and is removed with circumcision; also called *foreskin*.

Presbyesophagus Presence of slow or disorganized esophageal motility in the older adult.

Pressure sores Localized areas of cellular necrosis resulting from prolonged pressure between any bony prominence and an external object such as a bed or wheelchair. The tissues are deprived of blood supply and eventually die; also called *decubitus ulcers*.

Priapism Painful, persistent erection.

Prickly heat A rash caused by midepidermal obstruction and rupture of the sweat glands from prolonged exposure to a warm and humid environment.

Primary biliary cirrhosis A slowly progressive disease that destroys small to medium-sized bile ducts and results in cirrhosis and liver failure.

Primary dysthymia A long-term state of chronic depression not associated with any other disorder. It is neither a prelude to major depression nor a state existing between episodes of a cyclic form of mood disorder.

Primary endocrine disorder Direct malfunction of a hormone-producing gland not induced by the pituitary gland.

Primary glomerulopathy Disease states resulting from alterations in the structure and function of the glomerular capillary circulation, in which the kidney is the only or primary organ involved.

Primary (essential, idiopathic) hypertension High blood pressure of unidentified cause. Accounts for 90% of cases of high blood pressure.

Primary lesion Injury that originates in the skin and has not been altered by scratching or by treatment.

Primary prevention The first level of health promotion, designed to prevent disease.

Prodromal period The period preceding the onset of a disorder. Symptoms indicate an impending seizure, migraine, or other problem.

Progesterone A hormone produced by the corpus luteum and adrenal cortex during the luteal phase of the menstrual cycle that promotes uterine changes essential for the implantation and growth of the fertilized ovum.

Prognosis A forecast about the probable outcome of a disease; the prospect of recovery from a disease indicated by the nature, signs, and/or symptoms of the case.

Progressive familial intrahepatic cholestasis A rare autosomal recessive disorder comprising severe jaundice, pruritus, and malabsorption due to a defect in bile salt excretion.

Proinsulin Precursor to insulin produced by the β cells of the pancreas.

Prokaryote A cell that does not have a membrane-bound nucleus or other membrane-bound organelles (e.g., bacteria).

Prolactin Hormone secreted by the anterior pituitary gland. Following birth of an infant, prolactin stimulates milk production.

Pronephros One of three distinct phases in the development of the renal system. The pronephros is the earliest state in humans, corresponding to the mature structure in primitive vertebrates.

Prostate Gland located below the bladder; its secretions help activate sperm and maintain their motility.

Prostatic urethra The widest and most distensible part of the male urethra.

Prostatitis Inflammation of the prostate.

Prostatodynia Pain in the prostate.

Protein A molecule composed of nitrogen, carbon, hydrogen, oxygen, and occasionally sulfur; when hydrolyzed, proteins yield amino acids.

Proteoglycan Any of a group of polysaccharide-protein conjugates occurring primarily in the matrix of connective tissue and cartilage, composed mainly of polysaccharide chains, particularly glycosaminoglycans, as well as minor protein components.

Proto-oncogene A normal cellular gene that is growth promoting and usually inhibited in nonproliferating cells. When erroneously activated, it becomes an oncogene and promotes cancer.

Provirus The viral DNA that is spliced into the host cell's DNA.

Pruritus Itching of the skin.

Pseudocyst A collection of fluid within or adjacent to the pancreas that often has a direct communication to the pancreatic duct. It is the most common localized complication of acute pancreatitis.

Pseudoglandular period The first stage in fetal lung development when the bronchial divisions are differentiated and the major elements of lung tissue are present except for those involved in gas exchange: the respiratory bronchioles and alveoli.

Pseudomembranous enterocolitis An acute inflammation and necrosis of the small and large intestines caused by *Clostridium difficile,* usually affecting the mucosa but sometimes extending to other layers.

Psoriasis A common chronic skin disease characterized by papules and plaques with an overlying silvery scale. Lesions can appear on any area of the body but especially the knees, elbows, lower part of the back, scalp, and nails.

Psoriatic arthritis An inflammatory arthritis associated with psoriasis occurring in approximately 0.1% of the population in the United States. Peak age of onset is 30 to 55 years of age, and the arthritis can occur in patients who have had psoriasis for many years.

Psychogenic Produced or caused by emotional or psychological factors rather than organic factors.

Psychosis The most serious and debilitating of mental disorders. The hallmarks of psychosis are delusions and hallucinations, thought disorders, and inappropriate emotional responses or social behavior.

Psychosomatic medicine The discipline involving the physiologic impact of psychic stress on the emergence of disease.

Pulmonic valve The cardiac valve that lies between the right ventricle and the pulmonary artery. It is open during ventricular systole and closed during ventricular diastole. Pulmonic valve closure contributes to heart sound S_2.

Pulse pressure The difference between the systolic and diastolic blood pressures.

Purpura Hemorrhagic lesions 2 to 4 mm in diameter; petechiae that occur in groups or patches, caused by a vascular or bleeding disorder.

Putamen nuclei The larger, darker, and more lateral part of the lentiform nucleus.

Pyelonephritis An infection of the kidney medulla or cortex.

Pylorus Muscular sphincter between the stomach and the duodenum that controls gastric emptying and limits the reflux of bile from the small intestine.

Pyogenic Producing or produced by fever.

Pyrosis A substernal burning sensation that may radiate to the neck or throat. It is caused by the reflux of gastric contents into the esophagus; also called *heartburn.*

R

Radical mastectomy Surgical removal of the entire breast, lymphatic drainage, and underlying pectoral muscles.

Radiolysis Lysis or splitting of water molecules into H^+ and OH^- by action of radioactive particles.

Rapidly progressing glomerulonephritis A syndrome that combines abrupt hematuria and proteinuria followed by a swift decline in renal function.

Rarefaction Decrease in density and weight of bone, but not in volume.

Raynaud phenomenon Blanching or cyanosis of fingers or hands on exposure to cold or emotional stress. The phenomenon is attributed to vasospasm and structural disease of blood vessels. Puffiness and swelling of the hands and fingers are noted clinically.

Reality testing The act of evaluating and considering the differences between internal experiences and external events.

Receptor activation Binding of a ligand to a cellular receptor, resulting in a change in intracellular cell signaling or function.

Receptor specificity The principle of allowing intracellular processes to be activated only by certain hormones. If a cell does not have the specific receptors for a hormone, it will not respond to the hormone.

Recessive Referring to a gene allele that fails to be expressed in the phenotype when a dominant allele is present. The trait carried in a recessive allele is apparent only when two identical copies are present.

Recruitment The process of calling in additional motor units in response to an increase in stimulation of motor nerves.

Rectocele Protrusion of the anterior rectal wall into the posterior vagina at a weakened part of the vaginal musculature. It usually results from an injury during childbirth or surgery; it may also be the result of the aging process or an inherent weakness in the vaginal wall.

Recurrent urinary tract infection Repeated infections within a short period of time following verified resolution of an earlier infection.

Red blood cell (erythrocyte) Cell responsible for transporting oxygen to the tissues, removing carbon dioxide from the tissues, and buffering blood pH.

Reed-Sternberg cell A malignant cell type found in affected lymph nodes of patients with Hodgkin disease. The presence of Reed-Sternberg cells differentiates Hodgkin disease from all other forms of malignant lymphoma.

Re-entry The proposed mechanism for many dysrhythmias, including premature complexes and fibrillation. Re-entry occurs when an impulse is able to activate the cardiac muscle more than once due to abnormalities in conduction through a portion of the heart.

Reflex incontinence Urine loss that occurs without sensory warning or awareness.

Reflux Retrograde flow of urine from the bladder to the kidney.

Refractory period The time during which a nerve or muscle membrane is unable to respond to a stimulus by generating an action potential.

Regurgitation (valvular) Retrograde blood flow through a cardiac valve when the valve is supposed to be closed.

Reiter syndrome Seronegative arthritis that appears 2 to 6 weeks after onset of an infection, characterized clinically by diffuse swelling of fingers and toes, swelling in the Achilles tendon or plantar fascia, and low back pain.

Relative anemia Anemia characterized by normal total red blood cell mass with disturbances in the regulation of plasma fluid volume resulting in low hematocrit.

Relative polycythemia Polycythemia characterized by normal total red blood cell mass with disturbances in the regulation of plasma volume resulting in elevated hematocrit.

Relaxation time The period between peak tension and zero tension in a muscle.

Releasing hormone A hormone secreted by the hypothalamus that stimulates the anterior pituitary gland to secrete other hormones.

Remission Disappearance of clinical manifestations of disease. In leukemia, complete remission is determined by the absence of leukemic blasts in the bone marrow aspirate and peripheral blood. Malignant stem cells still may be present, and remission does not imply cure.

Renal adenoma A tumor smaller than 3 cm with a cellular makeup similar to that of renal cell carcinoma.

Renal agenesis Failure of one or both kidneys to develop.

Renal angiomyolipoma (hamartoma) Benign renal tumor composed of abdominal blood vessels, clusters of fat cells, and sheets of smooth muscle.

Renal calculus Concretion of crystals of material (e.g., uric acid, calcium phosphate, struvite) that initially form in the calices or pelvis of the kidney. Calculi may migrate down the urinary tract and cause pain, obstruction, and infection.

Renal cell carcinoma Most common malignant tumor of the kidney.

Renal or ureteral colic Intermittent flank or abdominal pain caused by spasms in the kidneys and/or ureters.

Renin An enzyme stored and released by the juxtaglomerular cells; converts angiotensinogen to angiotensin I.

Resident flora Microorganisms that usually reside in a certain environment on the host without causing disease.

Resistance In the stress response, resistance occurs when sympathetic activity declines while secretion of adrenocortical hormones is high.

Respiratory acidosis A pulmonary hypoventilation condition that tends to cause an excess of carbonic acid and that may result in acid-base imbalance.

Respiratory alkalosis A pulmonary hyperventilation condition that tends to cause a deficit of carbonic acid and that may result in acid-base imbalance.

Respiratory quotient The ratio of the volume of carbon dioxide exhaled to the volume of oxygen absorbed in the alveoli.

Respiratory syncytial virus A member of a subgroup of myxoviruses that in tissue culture cause formation of giant cells or syncytia.

Reticular formation Fibers in the brainstem that arouse the cerebrum.

Reticular layer One of two layers of the dermis; consists of a denser reticulum (network) of fibers than the papillary layer above it. The reticular layer is made of collagen and elastin and contains skeletal (voluntary) and smooth (involuntary) muscle fibers.

Reticulocytosis Increase in the number of circulating reticulocytes (immature red blood cells).

Reticulohisticytic group Cells of the dermis consisting of fibroblasts, histiocytes, and mast cells. Immature cells of the reticulohisticytic group are called *reticulum cells.*

Retrodisplacement Posterior displacement (such as an alteration in the position of the uterus) in which the body of the uterus is displaced from its normal location overlying the bladder to a position in the posterior pelvis.

Retroperitoneal Referring to the anatomic space in the abdomen behind the peritoneal cavity, where the kidneys reside.

Retrovirus An RNA virus capable of transcribing its own RNA into DNA, which can be integrated into the host genome through the actions of a viral polymerase; also called *reverse transcriptase.*

Reverse transcriptase An enzyme that allows certain viruses to convert RNA to DNA and incorporate their genome into the DNA of the host cell.

Reye syndrome Primarily a children's disease, it is characterized by fatty infiltration of the liver with severe hepatic dysfunction.

Rheumatoid arthritis A systemic, inflammatory, connective tissue disease of unknown cause. Enzymes are released into the joint fluid, causing inflammation, proliferation of synovium, and tissue damage. The hands, wrists, knees, and feet are most commonly involved. Joint involvement is symmetric. Other systems affected include integumentary, ocular, otolaryngologic, pulmonary, cardiac, gastrointestinal, renal, neurologic, and hematologic.

Rhinorrhea Drainage of a watery fluid from the nasal mucosa.

Rhonchus Coarse, bubbling sound usually heard on expiration, but which also can be heard on inspiration due to secretions in the airways.

Rhus dermatitis An inflammatory reaction to poison ivy, poison oak, and poison sumac. Clinically, rhus dermatitis begins within 48 hours of contact. The first symptom is pruritus, followed by erythema and vesicle formation, sometimes in linear fashion.

Rhythmicity The ability to beat regularly without external stimuli; also called *automaticity.*

Ribonucleic acid (RNA) A nucleic acid, found in both the nucleus and cytoplasm of cells, which has several roles in the translation of the genetic code and the assembly of proteins.

Ribosome A cellular structure containing ribosomal RNA and proteins that bind to mRNA and perform the task of translating the RNA message into a protein.

Rickets A condition caused by the deficiency of vitamin D, seen primarily in infancy and childhood and characterized by abnormal bone formation.

Rigor mortis The stiffening of muscles throughout the body after death due to formation of permanent actin-myosin cross-bridges.

Risk factor Characteristic related to the probability of a certain outcome; a risk factor may be shown to cause an outcome or may be correlated with an outcome.

RNA polymerase An enzyme complex that binds to a gene segment of DNA, using it as a template for the synthesis of an RNA strand.

Rocky Mountain spotted fever An infection caused by a tick that carries *Rickettsia rickettsii*. The characteristic rash is a macular or maculopapular one that spreads to the rest of the body. Other symptoms include generalized edema, conjunctivitis, petechial lesions, photophobia, lethargy, confusion, and cranial nerve deficits.

Roseola infantum A contagious viral disease that generally affects children younger than 4 years and usually those about 1 year of age. It produces a characteristic maculopapular rash covering the trunk and spreading to the appendages.

Rostral A positional term referring to the head end.

Rough endoplasmic reticulum A portion of the endoplasmic reticulum that is studded by ribosomes. Ribosomes attached to the endoplasmic reticulum synthesize proteins that are destined for the plasma membrane or lysosomes.

Rubella A childhood disease caused by the Rubella virus. It is characterized by a diffuse, punctate, macular rash that begins on the trunk and spreads to the arms and legs; also called *3-day measles* or *German measles*.

Rugae Folds in the lining of the body of a hollow organ, for example in the bladder that allow the bladder muscle to distend to accommodate urine or in the stomach to accommodate a meal.

S

Saddle joint A joint in which the surfaces are convex in one plane and concave in the other, permitting both flexion extension and adduction-abduction movements; the surfaces of a saddle joint fit together as a saddle fits a horse. The carpometacarpal joint of the thumb is a saddle joint; also called *sellar joint*.

Saline deficit Extracellular fluid volume deficit.

Saline excess Extracellular fluid volume excess.

Saline imbalances Extracellular fluid volume imbalances.

Salivary amylase Digestive enzyme contained in saliva, which initiates carbohydrate digestion in the mouth; also called *ptyalin*.

Sarcolemma The membrane that encloses a muscle cell.

Sarcomere The unit of muscle contraction in striated muscle. A sarcomere extends from one Z disk to another and consists of overlapping actin and myosin filaments.

Sarcoplasm The cytoplasm of the muscle fiber.

Sarcoplasmic reticulum A calcium-storing structure in muscle cells analogous to the endoplasmic reticulum; it fills the space between myofibrils and forms sacs.

Saturated fatty acid Having the maximal number of hydrogen atoms present so that only single bonds exist in the carbon chain, as in saturated fatty acids.

Saturation The condition of being saturated. The degree of hydrogen saturation refers to the number of double bonds between the carbon atoms in the hydrocarbon chain.

Scabies Infestation with the mite *Sarcoptes scabiei* in humans. Scabies begins with eggs laid in the stratum corneum. These eggs hatch into larvae within 3 to 4 days and reach adulthood within 2 months.

Scarlet fever A systemic reaction to the toxins produced by group A β-hemolytic streptococci. It occurs when the individual is sensitized to the toxin-producing variation of streptococci. Scarlet fever frequently occurs in association with streptococcal sore throat (strep throat), but it may also be associated with a wound, skin infection, or puerperal infection.

Schizoid Indifferent to social interaction and possessing a limited range of emotional experience and expression.

Schizophrenia A syndrome or combination of mental disorders characterized by deterioration of mental function and disturbance of psychological processes.

Scleroderma A disorder characterized by massive collagen deposition with fibrosis accompanied by inflammatory reactions and vascular changes in the capillary network.

Scoliosis A lateral deviation of the spine resulting in an S- or C-shaped spinal column. The disorder, most common in adolescent girls, can be a consequence of congenital, connective tissue, or neuromuscular disorders.

Scrotum Pouchlike sac containing the testes, epididymis, and spermatic cord.

Seasonal affective disorder A condition in which lethargy results from seasonal changes of decreased periods of daylight and longer nights.

Sebaceous gland Oil- or sebum-producing gland that anoints hair and skin.

Seborrheic keratosis Benign skin tumor common in the elderly, composed of immature epithelial cells.

Second messenger An intracellular signal that is produced in response to an extracellular signal.

Secondary dysthymia A long-term state of chronic depression that is associated with some other non-mood disorder, which may be a classic mental disorder (e.g., anorexia nervosa) or a physical illness.

Secondary endocrine disorder A malfunction of the hypothalamus/pituitary cells that control the hormone-producing gland.

Secondary glomerulopathy Alterations in the structure and function of the glomerular capillary circulation resulting from drug exposure, infections, or glomerular injury in the setting of multisystem or vascular abnormalities.

Secondary hypertension High blood pressure in which the cause can be identified.

Secondary lesion Injury modified by normal progress over time or by such external agents as scratching.

Secondary prevention The second level of health promotion, based on early detection and screening.

Second-degree burn See *superficial partial-thickness burn* and *deep partial-thickness burn*.

Secretin A digestive hormone that is produced by the S cells lining the duodenum and jejunum when protein of partially digested food enters the intestine from the stomach; it stimulates the pancreas.

Segmentation contractions A set of movements that occur in the small intestine. The primary effect of these contractions is progressive mixing of solid chyme particles with secretions of the small intestine.

Seizure A transient neurologic event of paroxysmal abnormal or excessive cortical electrical discharges that is manifested by disturbances of skeletal motor function, sensation, autonomic visceral function, behavior, or consciousness.

Self-identity disturbance In schizophrenic patients, self-identity disturbances can be profound, both in terms of the ability to differentiate one's physical self from the physical environment and the psychological discernment of self as distinct from others.

Semen Male reproductive fluid that contains spermatozoa; released with ejaculation.

Seminal vesicles Two glands that contribute rich nutrients to the seminal fluid.

Sequela, sequelae A condition or conditions caused by and following a disease.

Serotonin A major monoamine neurotransmitter that is an etiologic factor in mood disorder; *also called 5-hydroxytryptamine (5-HT).*

Sertoli cell An elongated cell that supports and provides nutrition to attached spermatids until they mature into spermatozoa.

Sex chromosome A chromosome that confers gender to the individual. In humans, females are designated as 46XX, whereas males are 46XY. The Y chromosome confers male gender.

Sexually transmitted disease One of many diseases that can be transmitted by sexual contact, regardless of whether the disease has manifestations in the genital organs (previously referred to as *venereal disease*).

Sharpey fibers Fibers that attach tendons to bones; they are continuous with the perimysium.

Shock A condition of severe hemodynamic and metabolic disturbance resulting in an imbalance between oxygen supply and oxygen demand at the cellular level. The common types of shock are cardiogenic, hypovolemic, obstructive, and distributive.

Short-bowel syndrome Severe diarrhea and significant malabsorption that develop following the surgical removal of large portions of the small intestine. The severity of the manifestations depends on the amount and location of the bowel resected.

Shunt (right-to-left) An abnormal route of blood flow through the heart or lungs that allows movement of blood into the arterial system without passing through areas of the lung.

Sickle cell A red blood cell containing abnormal hemoglobins that cause the cell to assume a sickle shape under decreased oxygen tension.

Sign Objectively identifiable aberration of the disease. Fever, reddening of the skin, and a palpable mass are *signs* of disease.

Skeletal muscle Striated muscle that is attached to bone. Constituting 40% of total body weight, skeletal muscle enables bones to move at the joint and provides strength and protection to the skeleton by distributing and absorbing shock.

Skeletal system Rigid system of bony structures designed to protect internal organs and provide bony attachments for muscles and ligaments; presents rigid levers to allow for functional movement of the body and its separate parts.

Skin A relatively flat membrane composed of an outer, thinner layer (epidermis) and an inner, thicker layer (dermis).

Skin cancer A cutaneous neoplasm caused by ionizing radiation, certain genetic defects, or chemical carcinogens (including arsenics, petroleum, tar products, and fumes from some molten metals), or by overexposure to the sun or other sources of ultraviolet light.

Sleep study Recording of electroencephalogram (EEG) motor activity and respiration during sleep to determine duration and type of sleep and number of awakenings.

Sliding filament theory This theory of muscle contraction is suggested by the anatomic configuration of the sarcomere. Muscle shortening is accomplished by increasing the amount of overlap of actin and myosin filaments; also called *cross-bridge theory.*

Slow twitch (type I, red) A muscle fiber that develops tension more slowly than a fast-twitch fiber. This fiber is usually fatigue resistant and relies on oxidative phosphorylation for energy.

Slow-wave electrical activity One of the basic types of electrical activity in the gut. Slow waves represent an ongoing basic oscillation in membrane potential occurring in the smooth muscle of the gastrointestinal tract between 3 and 12 times per minute.

Smooth endoplasmic reticulum A portion of the endoplasmic reticulum that has no ribosomes. Smooth endoplasmic reticulum is a site of lipid synthesis.

Soft tissue injury Any trauma to soft tissue with disruption of circulatory and lymphatic systems.

Solar elastosis Wrinkled, weather-beaten appearance of skin caused by overexposure to sunlight.

Somatosensory receptors Specialized nerve endings located in the dermis of all skin areas. Receptors permit the skin to serve as a sense organ, transmitting sensations of pain, pressure, touch, and temperature.

Somatotopic Referring to the sequential arrangement of neurons related to sensory or motor function in specific anatomic regions.

Specific immune response Creation of specific antibodies by the host against a specific pathogen that leads to the destruction of the pathogen.

Spermatid An immature sperm cell.

Spermatocele A painless, cystic mass containing sperm.

Spermatogenesis Production of sperm cells.

Spermatozoon A mature sperm cell.

Spherocyte An abnormal spherical erythrocyte that is less biconvex than a normal erythrocyte.

Spike potential Sudden increase in membrane potential in the smooth muscle of the gastrointestinal tract that appears on the peaks of slow waves in response to certain conditions, including stimulation by stretching or the effects of acetylcholine or parasympathetic excitation.

Spina bifida A developmental anomaly characterized by defective closure of the bony encasement of the spinal cord (neural tube) through which the spinal cord and meninges may or may not protrude.

Spinal shock A temporary physiologic suspension of spinal cord function and reflexes below the level of cord injury.

Spiral [bacteria] Referring to any bacterium of the genus *Spirochaeta* that is motile and spiral-shaped with flexible filaments. See *spirochete.*

Spiral fracture A fracture resulting from rotational forces and causing bone to separate in the form of an *S* around the bone.

Spirochete Spiral-shaped bacterium.

Splinter hemorrhage A linear hemorrhage, appearing as a red or brown streak, running parallel to the finger in the nail bed; may be linked to bacterial endocarditis and trichinosis.

Spontaneous abortion Expulsion of the products of conception from the uterus before the period of fetal viability. It is usually called "miscarriage" by laypersons, and is differentiated from an elective abortion.

Squamous cell carcinoma A type of cancer that often occurs in areas of skin excessively exposed to sunlight and arising from keratinocytes.

Staging The process of determining the extent and location of cancer in an individual.

Stasis A "staying" of a substance in an anatomic location. A *stasis* of bile in the gallbladder promotes an increase in gallstone formation.

Status asthmaticus Severe asthma attack that does not respond to routine therapy.

Status epilepticus Rapid succession of seizures without intervals of consciousness. Brain damage may result.

Steatorrhea Passage of high fat content in the feces; seen in malabsorption diseases where there is lack of pancreatic enzymes.

Stenosis (valvular) Obstruction to blood flow through cardiac valves that open incompletely.

Steroid A hormone synthesized from cholesterol; includes glucocorticoids, mineralocorticoids, estrogens and androgens.

Still disease Systemic-onset juvenile rheumatoid arthritis.

Stomatitis An inflammation of the tongue and oral mucosa that may extend to the buccal mucosa, lips, and palate.

Stratum Layer.

Stratum corneum Outermost layer of the epidermis, composed of flat, compact cells that have lost their nuclei.

Stratum germinativum The final (fifth) layer of the epidermis is a line of cuboidal cells that marks the lowest boundary of the epidermis and divides it from the dermis; also called *basal cell layer*.

Stratum granulosum Third layer of the epidermis, comprising flatter cells that contain protein granules, called *keratohyalin granules*.

Stratum lucidum Second layer of the epidermis, appearing as a translucent line of flat cells. This layer of the skin is present only on the palms and the soles.

Stratum spinosum Fourth layer of the epidermis, composed of upwardly migrating and maturing keratinocytes. This layer forms the bulk of the epidermis over most of the body.

Strawberry hemangioma A soft vascular nevus, usually present on the face or neck, occurring at birth or shortly afterward.

Strawberry tongue Bright red papillated tongue, characteristic of scarlet fever.

Stress The sum of biological reactions produced when an organism's homeostasis is disrupted.

Stress fracture A fracture of one cortical surface of the bone, often caused by repetitive activity such as running.

Stress incontinence Loss of bladder control caused by increased intra-abdominal pressure combined with pelvic muscle laxity.

Stressor An agent or condition capable of producing stress. The term denotes both physical (gravity, mechanical force, pathogen, injury) and psychological (fear, anxiety, crisis, joy) forces that an individual may experience.

Striation The typical pattern of banding apparent upon microscopic inspection of a skeletal muscle cell.

Stricture A narrowing or constriction of the lumen of a tube, duct, or hollow organ, such as the ureter or urethra.

Stroke volume The volume of blood ejected from the ventricle in one contraction (end-diastolic volume minus end-systolic volume).

Structural scoliosis A lateral curve of the spine that fails to correct itself on forced bending against the curvature and has vertebral rotation.

Subarachnoid space The space between the arachnoid and the pia mater.

Subendocardium The part of the myocardium lying in proximity to the endocardial surface.

Subluxation Displacement of a bone from its normal position (articulating surface) in a joint; less severe than dislocation.

Substantia gelatinosa Another term for areas in laminae II and III that are important in the transmission of pain signals in the spinal cord.

Substantia nigra The layer of gray matter separating the tegmentum of the midbrain from the crus cerebri part of the basal ganglia.

Sudden cardiac death Death due to cardiac causes within 1 hour of symptom onset; also called sudden cardiac arrest.

Sulcus A deep furrow or groove on the surface of a structure (e.g., cerebral cortex).

Summation The additive response to repetitive stimuli.

Superficial fascia Loose subcutaneous layer rich in fat and areolar tissue, which lies beneath the dermis; also called *hypodermis*.

Superficial partial-thickness burn A burn characterized by destruction of the epidermis and dermis. The water vapor barrier is absent, but all tactile and pain sensors are intact; also called *second-degree burn*.

Suppurative disease A disease that produces purulent material (pus).

Surface film Thin film of emulsified material spread over the surface of skin.

Surfactant A surface tension–reducing agent produced by type II pneumocytes in the lung.

Suture joints A joint that unites bone with a thin but dense layer of fibrous tissue. Found only in the skull.

Sweat gland Most numerous of the skin glands. Sweat glands are of two types: apocrine and eccrine.

Symphysis joint A joint that connects bony segments by a fibrocartilaginous plate or disk.

Symptom Subjective feeling of discomfort that an affected individual can report to an observer. Nausea, malaise, and pain are *symptoms* of disease.

Symptomatically Defined by symptoms.

Synarthrosis A fibrous or cartilaginous (nonsynovial) joint.

Synchondrosis A joint connecting cartilage to a bony component; allows bone growth while providing stability.

Syncytium A complex of fused cells that act in concert.

Syndesmosis A fibrous joint in which opposing surfaces that are relatively far apart are connected by ligaments.

Syndrome A collection of signs and symptoms that occur together.

Syndrome of inappropriate antidiuretic hormone secretion (SIADH) Excessive antidiuretic hormone secretion either from the posterior pituitary gland or from other tissues; results in retention of water, hemodilution, and hyponatremia.

Synostosis The bony union that results from the fusion of a suture joint.

Synovial fluid A clear, pale yellow, viscous fluid similar to blood plasma but containing hyaluronic acid and a glycoprotein called lubricin. Synovial fluid reduces friction between the capsule and joint surfaces, lubricates the surface of the cartilage, resists shear forces, and provides nourishment for cartilage. Viscosity of the fluid is inversely related to joint velocity or rate of shear. High temperature decreases viscosity, and low temperature increases viscosity.

Synovial joint Freely movable joint in which a contiguous bony surface is covered by articular cartilage and connected by a fibrous connective tissue capsule lined with a synovial membrane.

Synovial sheath A dense layer of connective tissue surrounding synovial joints. The capsule is solidly attached to the periosteum of the adjacent bony components. The synovial sheath provides strength to the joint and, through its neural receptors, detects motion, compression, tension, vibration, and pain; also called *joint capsule*.

Syphilis Sexually transmitted disease caused by the spirochete *Treponema pallidum* and characterized by distinct stages of effects over a period of years.

Systemic lupus erythematosus A chronic inflammatory disease resulting from an immunoregulatory disturbance. It is a multisystem relapsing disease that can affect skin, mucosa, lung, heart, kidneys, central and peripheral nervous systems, and blood components. Arthralgias and synovitis are common features. Skin lesions are often present as a butterfly rash. Renal failure is the leading cause of death with this disease.

Systemic vascular resistance The impedance to blood flow exerted by the arterioles; determined primarily by vascular diameter.

Systole A phase of the cardiac cycle in which the ventricles are contracting to develop force and eject blood.

Systolic blood pressure The maximal pressure in the aorta and major arteries during ventricular ejection of blood.

T

T cell Lymphocyte that provides cellular immunity, has regulatory functions, and attacks antigen in association with other cells. T cells mature in the thymus.

Tangential excision Excision to remove eschar in thin layers until viable tissue is visible; also called *full-thickness excision.*

Target cell or target organ The cell or organ that is stimulated by the effects of a hormone.

Tau protein Neuronal protein that organizes microtubules. It becomes chemically altered in Alzheimer disease and twists into abnormal bundles called *neurofibrillary tangles;* also called *neural thread protein.*

Telangiectasia A lesion created by dilated blood vessels.

Telogen The resting phase of hair growth.

Telomerase An enzyme that permits addition of nucleotides to the tips of the chromosomes to prevent progressive shortening of the telomeres during cell division. Telomerase is produced by cancer cells, enabling them to become immortal.

Telomere The end cap of the chromosome; this section shortens with each cell division in certain cell types.

Tendinitis Inflammation of the tendon within the sheath.

Teratogen An agent or factor that causes damage or physical defects in a developing embryo.

Terminal hair Long, coarse, thick, visible strands of tightly fused keratinized epidermal cells.

Terminal sac period The third stage in fetal lung development when terminal sacs become thinner, preparing the lung tissue for gas exchange. Proliferation of pulmonary capillaries is also prominent during this period.

Tertiary prevention The third phase of health promotion, based on supporting independent function and preventing further disease-related deterioration.

Testis The male gonad or reproductive gland that produces spermatozoa and houses the Leydig cells.

Testosterone Male sex hormone produced by interstitial cells in the testes.

Thalamus Portion of diencephalon; mass of gray matter involved in relay of sensory information, emotion, arousal, and complex reflexes.

Thoracentesis Surgical perforation of the chest wall and pleural space with a needle to aspirate fluid for diagnostic or therapeutic purposes or to remove a specimen for biopsy.

Thoracotomy Surgical opening of the chest wall.

Threshold The lowest level at which a stimulus can produce a response.

Thrill Vibration palpated over a blood vessel or cardiac chamber reflecting turbulent blood flow.

Thrombocyte Circulating cytoplasmic fragment of a megakaryocyte that is essential in the formation of blood clots and in the control of bleeding; also called *platelet.*

Thrombocytopenia A deficiency of platelets (thrombocytes) in the peripheral blood. Any reduction in platelet count below normal is called *thrombocytopenia,* but significant risk of bleeding does not occur until the count drops below about 20,000/μl.

Thromboembolus An embolus that originated as a thrombus, most commonly in the venous system of the lower extremities.

Thrombophlebitis Inflammation of a vein accompanied by the formation of a clot.

Thrombus Stationary blood clot formed within a vessel.

Thrush Candidiasis of the tissues of the mouth. The condition is characterized by the appearance of creamy white patches of exudates on an inflamed tongue or buccal mucosa.

Thyroid storm Extreme thyrotoxicosis. Massively elevated levels of thyroid hormones cause an increased basal metabolic rate, tachycardia, hypertension, and fever, eventually leading to cardiovascular collapse.

Thyroxine (T₄) A hormone secreted by the thyroid gland which contains 4 iodides.

Tight junction Cell-to-cell junction that seals adjacent epithelial cells together and prevents the passage of most substances through the epithelial sheet.

Tinea The infection caused by fungal infections of the skin in any cutaneous area, including the hair and nails.

Tinnitus Ringing, buzzing, or roaring in the ears, commonly associated with exposure to loud noise or disorders, such as Ménière disease.

Tonic Referring to continuous stimulation or muscular contraction.

TORCH complex An acronym used to describe the usual offending infectious agents that commonly cause congenital anomalies: *t*oxoplasmosis, *o*thers, *r*ubella, *c*ytomegalovirus, *h*erpesvirus.

Torsion Act of twisting or condition of being twisted. Applies to the state of the testes when abnormally rotated.

Trabecular bone Cancellous bone cells arranged in response to mechanical stress placed on the bone. Configuration of bone cells increases strength of bone.

Tracheoesophageal fistula Congenital anomaly in which an abnormal opening between the trachea and esophagus exists. It requires immediate diagnosis and surgical correction.

Transcellular fluid Body fluid contained in special compartments, such as the synovial or cerebrospinal compartments; a component of extracellular fluid.

Transcription The process by which a segment of DNA is used as a template to produce a complementary sequence of messenger RNA.

Transient flora Microorganisms that temporarily reside in a certain environment on the host.

Transitional flow Airflow occurring in the larger airways, especially at bifurcations; also called *mixed pattern of airflow.*

Translation Formation of a polypeptide chain in a sequence dictated by messenger RNA.

Translocation Shifting of a segment of one chromosome into another chromosome.

Transmission of infection The process by which a pathogenic organism is transferred from one host to another.

Transmural Denoting the entire thickness of a wall (e.g., the myocardial wall). A transmural myocardial infarction extends throughout the entire cardiac muscle layer.

Transudate Fluid of low protein content that passes through membranes because of a difference in hydrostatic pressure.

Transverse fracture Occurs in a straight line at approximately a 90-degree angle to the longitudinal axis of the bone.

Traumatic alopecia Hair loss as a result of tight plaiting of hair or use of hot oil and tension on the scalp. Gradual damage to hair follicles occurs, leading to hair thinning and loss.

Triad asthma A subcategory of drug-induced asthma representing a combination of intrinsic asthma, aspirin sensitivity, and nasal polyposis.

Triaxial joint A joint that permits movement around three axes so that motion can occur in three planes. Permits gliding movement between two bones as exemplified by the carpal joints of the hand.

Tricuspid valve The cardiac valve that lies between the right atrium and right ventricle. The valve is normally closed during ventricular systole and open during ventricular diastole. Tricuspid valve closure contributes to heart sound S_1.

Triglyceride A simple fat compound consisting of three molecules of fatty acid and glycerol.

Trigone Triangular area usually referring to the bladder muscle.

Tri-iodothyronine (T$_3$) A hormone secreted by the thyroid gland which contains 3 iodides.

Trisomy Having three homologous chromosomes instead of the usual pair, as in trisomy 21; also called *Down syndrome*.

Tropic/trophic hormone A hormone released by the anterior pituitary gland that stimulates the release of other hormones, which then act on target organs.

Tropical sprue Inflammation of the mucosa of the small intestine secondary to infection.

Tropomyosin A structural protein involved in regulation of actin-myosin cross-bridge formation. Associated with the thin filament of the sarcomere in skeletal and cardiac muscle, where it blocks cross-bridge formation when intracellular calcium levels are low.

Troponin A regulatory protein involved in regulation of actin-myosin cross-bridge formation. Associated with tropomyosin and actin in the thin filament of the sarcomere. Troponin binds calcium ion in the cell and regulates the position of tropomyosin, allowing muscle contraction when intracellular calcium levels rise.

Tumor marker Biochemical substance, such as a specific enzyme, receptor, or surface protein, that helps identify the tumor cell.

Tumor suppressor gene A gene that regulates a group of growth-promoting genes and suppresses tumor formation. Mutation and underexpression of tumor suppressor genes are associated with the development of cancer.

Tunica albuginea Fascial layer covering the testes and erectile bodies of the penis.

Turbulent airflow The friction and increased resistance caused by air movement from the nasal cavity through the large bronchi.

Turnover and regeneration time Time required for a population of cells to mature and reproduce. As the surface cells of the stratum corneum are lost, replacement of keratinocytes by mitosis must occur.

Twitch The mechanical response to a single stimulus of a motor unit.

Type 1 diabetes mellitus Insulin-dependent diabetes mellitus, characterized by an absolute deficiency of insulin.

Type 2 diabetes mellitus Non–insulin-dependent diabetes mellitus; characterized by tissue insulin resistance and impaired insulin production by the pancreas.

U

Ulcerative colitis An inflammatory disease of the mucosa of the rectum and colon. Most commonly it affects the most distal portions of the colon, but eventually it may affect the entire colon. It is typically characterized by exacerbations and remissions. The clinical manifestations of ulcerative colitis are abdominal pain, diarrhea, and rectal bleeding.

Ultrafiltration Filtration through a filter capable of removing colloidal particles from a dispersion medium, as in the filtration of plasma at the capillary membrane.

Ultrasound An imaging modality that uses sound waves to assess the size, structure, and function of internal organs, tissue, or the fetus.

Uniaxial joint A joint that allows motion around a single axis.

Unipennate A muscle with a lateral tendon to which the fibers are attached obliquely, like one half of a feather.

Unipolar depression Depression without periods of mania.

Unresolved urinary tract infection A urinary tract infection (UTI) in which bacteriuria remains after initial antibiotic treatment.

Unsaturated (fatty acid) Referring to an organic compound in which one or more pairs of carbon atoms are united by double or triple bonds, as in unsaturated fatty acids.

Up-regulation An increase in the number of cell receptors or activity for a specific hormone usually resulting from chronically low concentrations of the hormone. Up-regulation helps maintain the target cell response to a hormone, even when circulating hormone levels are low.

Urea Substance produced in the liver from the breakdown of protein and excreted in the urine.

Uremia A clinical syndrome related to the deleterious effects of azotemia on other body systems.

Ureter One of a pair of fibromuscular, mucosa-lined narrow tubes that connect the kidneys to the bladder.

Ureterocele Congenital cystic dilatation of the distal ureter.

Ureteropelvic junction obstruction Disruption of urinary flow from the kidney(s) into one or both ureters.

Urethral stricture A fibrotic narrowing of the urethra, usually composed of scar tissue.

Urethral valve The most common cause of urinary obstruction in male newborns and infants. Posterior in location, occurring in the distal prostatic urethra, urethral valves are mucosal folds that resemble thin membranes and cause obstruction when the child attempts to void.

Urethrorectal fistula A rare congenital anomaly almost always associated with an imperforate anus. The fistula results from failure of the urorectal septum to develop completely, leading to a persistent communication between the rectum posteriorly and the urogenital tract anteriorly.

Urge incontinence A strong and immediate urge to void brought about by involuntary detrusor overactivity.

Urinary bladder Muscular sac located in the anterior inferior pelvic cavity that holds urine until it is excreted through the urethra.

Urothelial tumor A malignant tumor of the lining of the renal pelvis, calyces, ureter, and bladder.

Urothelium Epithelial lining of the urinary tract from the renal pelvis to the bladder.

Urticaria A pruritic skin eruption characterized by transient wheals of varying shapes and sizes with well-defined erythematous margins and pale centers.

Uterine prolapse A sinking of the uterus from its normal position. It usually occurs when supporting structures, such as the uterosacral ligaments and cardinal ligaments, relax, altering the relationship of the uterus to the vaginal axis.

V

Varicose veins Incompetency of the superficial veins of the extremities, producing engorgement.

Vas deferens Thick, muscular tube that is continuous with the epididymis. It travels along the pelvic wall and joins with the seminal vesicle duct at the prostate to form the ejaculatory duct; also called *ductus deferens*.

Vascular fluid Fluid that is in blood vessels; a component of extracellular fluid.

Vasculitis Inflammation of the lining (intima) of a blood vessel.

Vasospasm Sudden, involuntary constriction of a blood vessel, producing obstruction of flow.

Vellus Tiny hair strands that are almost unnoticeable. Vellus covers the whole body, except the palms and soles.

Ventilation The process of moving air into the lungs and distributing air within the lungs to gas exchange units (alveoli) for maintenance of oxygenation and removal of CO_2.

Ventricle A fluid-filled compartment as in brain or heart.

Ventriculoperitoneal shunt A shunt that extends all the way from the ventricular system of the brain to the peritoneal cavity of the body.

Verrucae Circumscribed elevations of the epidermis; commonly called *warts*.

Verumontanum A small elevation that is marked by a midline opening from the prostatic utricle, a remnant of the Müllerian duct system.

Vesicle A portion of the cell membrane that surrounds extracellular material and pinches off to be internalized. This is part of the process of endocytosis.

Vesicoureteral reflux Retrograde movement of urine from the bladder to the kidney as a result of a disruption in the normal valvular mechanism at the ureter-bladder junction.

Vibrissae Large hairs of the nasal cavity.

Virion A virus particle.

Virulence The capacity of a microorganism to successfully evade host defenses and cause disease.

Virulent Referring to a microorganism's ability to evade host defenses and cause disease.

Viruses Tiny genetic parasites that are totally dependent on the host cell for survival. They utilize the host cell "machinery" for energy and replication.

Visual acuity The ability of the eyes to focus clearly on an image at a known distance; it is assessed with a Snellen chart and often expressed as the ability of an individual to accurately discern characters of various sizes at a distance of 20 feet.

Vitamin An organic substance that is essential in the diet and is required for the body's utilization of energy-containing nutrients.

Vitiligo Patch of depigmentation; also called *leukoderma*.

Voiding dysfunction A failure in the normal process of bladder emptying that results in urinary retention and/or incontinence.

Volvulus A twisting of the bowel on itself, which results in blood vessel compression.

W

Wallerian degeneration Complete disintegration of the distal portion of an axon that has been severed from the cell body. The axon, myelin sheath, and terminal arborization all disintegrate.

Wart An epidermal tumor caused by a virus that provokes a benign proliferation of keratinocytes; also called *verruca*.

Water imbalance Imbalance of body fluid concentration; osmolality imbalance; hypernatremia and hyponatremia.

White blood cell A cell that mediates immune function. White blood cells protect the body from foreign material and microorganisms; also called *leukocyte*.

White-coat phenomenon Elevated blood pressure readings when measured in a clinical setting by a nurse or physician.

Wilson disease A rare autosomal recessive disorder in which excessive amounts of copper accumulate in the liver or other organs; also called *hepatolenticular degeneration*.

Wolffian ducts Mesonephric ducts that develop as nephric ducts but go on to form male genital ducts.

Wolff's law States that the bone is laid down where it is needed and resorbed where it is not needed.

X

Xerostomia Dryness of the mouth caused by cessation of normal salivary secretion.

Z

Z line A dark band that defines a sarcomere; Z lines are perpendicular to actin and myosin filaments. A sarcomere extends from one Z line to the next.

Zeitgeber A synchronizer of the biological clock.

Zona pellucida The thick covering of the ovum.

Zone of calcifying cartilage A very thin line of chondrocytes and the weakest segment of the epiphyseal plate.

Zone of maturing cartilage Contains the enlarged and mature cartilage cells as they migrate toward the metaphysis.

Zone of resting cartilage Maintains adherence of the plate to the epiphysis.

Zone of young proliferating cartilage Demonstrates the most active cartilage cell growth.

Zygote The developing ovum, from the time it is fertilized until it is implanted in the uterus.

Page numbers followed by f indicate figures; t, tables; b, boxes. Bold entries designate diseases or syndromes

Prefixes and Suffixes Commonly Used in Medical Terminology

Prefix	Meaning	Suffix	Meaning
a-	Without, not	-al, -ac	Pertaining to
af-	Toward	-algia	Pain
an-	Without, not	-aps, -apt	Fit; fasten
ante-	Before	-arche	Beginning; origin
anti-	Against; resisting	-ase	Signifies an enzyme
auto-	Self	-blast	Sprout; make
bi-	Two; double	-centesis	A piercing
circum-	Around	-cide	To kill
co-, con-	With; together	-clast	Break; destroy
contra-	Against	-crine	Release; secrete
de-	Down from, undoing	-ectomy	A cutting out
dia-	Across; through	-emesis	Vomiting
dipl-	Twofold, double	-emia	Refers to blood condition
dys-	Bad; disordered; difficult	-flux	Flow
ectop-	Displaced	-gen	Creates; forms
ef-	Away from	-genesis	Creation, production
em-, en-	In, into	-gram	Something written
endo-	Within	-graph(y)	To write, draw
epi-	Upon	-hydrate	Containing H2O (water)
eu-	Good	-ia, -sia	Condition; process
ex-, exo-	Out of, out from	-iasis	Abnormal condition
extra-	Outside of	-ic, -ac	Pertaining to
hapl-	Single	-in	Signifies a protein
hem-, hemat-	Blood	-ism	Signifies "condition of"
hemi-	Half	-itis	Signifies "inflammation of"
hom(e)o-	Same; equal	-lemma	Rind; peel
hyper-	Over; above	-lepsy	Seizure
hypo-	Under; below	-lith	Stone; rock
infra-	Below, beneath	-logy	Study of
inter-	Between	-lunar	Moon; moonlike
intra-	Within	-malacia	Softening
iso-	Same, equal	-megaly	Enlargement
macro-	Large	-metric, -metry	Measurement, length
mega-	Large; million(th)	-oid	Like; in the shape of
mes-	Middle	-oma	Tumor
meta-	Beyond, after	-opia	Vision, vision condition
micro-	Small; millionth	-oscopy	Viewing
milli-	Thousandth	-ose	Signifies a carbohydrate (especially sugar)
mono-	One (single)	-osis	Condition, process
neo-	New	-ostomy	Formation of an opening
non-	Not	-otomy	Cut
oligo-	Few, scanty	-penia	Lack
ortho-	Straight; correct, normal	-philic	Loving
para-	By the side of; near	-phobic	Fearing
per-	Through	-phragm	Partition
peri-	Around; surrounding	-plasia	Growth, formation
poly-	Many	-plasm	Substance, matter
post-	After	-plasty	Shape; make
pre-	Before	-plegia	Paralysis
pro-	First; promoting	-pnea	Breath, breathing
quadr-	Four	-(r)rhage, -(r)rhagia	Breaking out, discharge
re-	Back again	-(r)rhaphy	Sew, suture
retro-	Behind	-(r)rhea	Flow
semi-	Half	-some	Body
sub-	Under	-tensin, -tension	Pressure
super-, supra-	Over, above, excessive	-tonic	Pressure, tension
trans-	Across; through	-tripsy	Crushing
tri-	Three; triple	-ule	Small, little
		-uria	Refers to urine condition

From Thibodeau GA, Patton KT: Anatomy & physiology, ed 5, St Louis, 2003, Mosby.